International Textbook of Diabetes Mellitus

SECOND EDITION

International Textbook of
Diabetes Mellitus

SECOND EDITION

Edited by

K.G.M.M. Alberti

The Medical School, Newcastle upon Tyne, UK

P. Zimmet

International Diabetes Institute, Caulfield, Australia

R.A. DeFronzo

University of Texas Health Science Center, San Antonio, USA

Honorary Editor

H. Keen

United Medical and Dental Schools, Guy's Hospital, London, UK

VOLUME 1

Zimmer

JOHN WILEY & SONS
Chichester • New York • Weinheim • Brisbane • Singapore • Toronto

Other Wiley Editorial Offices

John Wiley & Sons, Inc., 605 Third Avenue,
New York, NY 10158-0012, USA

VCH Verlagsgesellschaft mbH, Pappelallee 3,
D-69469 Weinheim, Germany

Jacaranda Wiley Ltd, 33 Park Road, Milton,
Queensland 4064, Australia

John Wiley & Sons (SEA) Pte Ltd, 2 Clementi Loop #02-01,
Jin Xing Distripark, Singapore 129809

John Wiley & Sons (Canada) Ltd, 22 Worcester Road,
Rexdale, Ontario M9W 1L1, Canada

British Library Cataloguing in Publication Data

A catalogue record for this book is available from the British Library

ISBN 0 471 93930 7

Typeset in 10/12pt Times by Laser Words, Madras, India
Printed and bound in Great Britain by Bookcraft (Bath) Ltd
This book is printed on acid-free paper responsibly manufactured from sustainable forestation,
for which at least two trees are planted for each one used for paper production.

About the Editors

Professor K.G.M.M. Alberti is Dean and Professor of Medicine and Head of the Human Diabetes and Metabolism Research Centre at the University of Newcastle upon Tyne, as well as Head of the WHO Collaborating Centre for Research and Development in Laboratory Techniques in Diabetes. He is a former editor of *Diabetologia*, President of the EASD and Vice President of the IDF and currently Vice Chairman of the British Diabetic Association.

Professor P. Zimmet is Foundation Chief Executive Officer, International Diabetes Institute, and Professor of Diabetes, Monash University, Melbourne, as well as Head of the WHO Collaborating Centre for the Epidemiology of Diabetes Mellitus and Health Promotion for Non-communicable Disease Control. His major research interests are the health effects of life-style change in newly industrialized nations in the Pacific and Indian Ocean region and the socio-economic and public health aspects of diabetes in these populations, as well as studies of the aetiology and pre-diagnosis of insulin dependent diabetes, particularly in adults. In 1991 he received the ADA's Kelly West Award for outstanding contributions to research in the field of epidemiology of diabetes. In 1994 he was awarded the Lilly Lectureship of the IDF.

Professor R.A. DeFronzo is Professor of Medicine, Chief of the Diabetes Division and member of the Nephrology Division, at the University of Texas Health Sciences Center and the South Texas Veterans Health Care System—Audie L. Murphy Division, San Antonio, Texas. He also is the Deputy Director of the Texas Diabetes Institute and the Director of the Diabetes Research Unit of the Clinical Research Center. He has served on the Board of Directors of the American Diabetes Association, and as Chairman of the ADA's Research Policy Committee and its Medical and Scientific Committee. He is the Editor of *Diabetes Reviews*, an official journal of the ADA, and was the recipient of the ADA's most prestigious Lilly Award in 1988.

Contents

Biochemistry and Pathophysiology of Diabetes

Contents

Management of Diabetes

VOLUME 2

Contributors

Lloyd M. Aiello   Joslin Diabetes Center, One Joslin Place, Boston, MA 02215, USA

K.G.M.M. Alberti   Department of Medicine, The Medical School, Framlington Place, Newcastle upon Tyne, NE2 4HH, UK

James H. Anderson Jr   Department of Medicine, Regenstrief Health Center, Indiana University Medical Center, 1001 West 10th Street, Indianapolis, IN 46202, USA

Morsi Arab   40 Safia Zagloul Street, Alexandria, Egypt

J.-P. Assal   Diabetes Treatment and Teaching Unit, Hôpital Cantonal Universitaire, 1211 Geneva 4, Switzerland

Shigeaki Baba   International Institute for Diabetes Education and Study (IIDES), Sankyo Seiko Daiichi Sky Building #103, 101 Edomachi, Chuo-ku, Kobe, Hyogo 650, Japan

Clifford J. Bailey   Department of Pharmaceutical and Biological Sciences, Aston University, Aston Triangle, Birmingham, B4 7ET, UK

Stephen C. Bain   Department of Medicine, University of Birmingham, Birmingham Heartlands Hospital, Bordesley Green East, Birmingham, B9 5SS, UK

Anthony H. Barnett   Department of Medicine, University of Birmingham, Birmingham Heartlands Hospital, Bordesley Green East, Birmingham, B9 5SS, UK

Peter H. Bennett   Phoenix Epidemiology and Clinical Research Branch, National Institute of Diabetes and Digestive and Kidney Diseases, Phoenix, Arizona, USA

Michael Berger   Klinik für Stoffwechselkrankheiten und Ernährung, Heinrich Heine Universität Düsseldorf, Moorenstrasse 5, 40001 Düsseldorf, Germany

Rudy W. Bilous   Diabetes Care Centre, Middlesbrough General Hospital, Middlesbrough, TS5 5AZ, UK

Per Björntorp   Department of Heart and Lung Diseases, University of Göteborg, Sahlgren's Hospital, S-413 45 Göteborg, Sweden

Lorenz M. Boehlen   Medizinische Universitäts-Poliklinik, Inselspital, Freiburgstrasse 6, CH-3010 Bern, Switzerland

Riccardo C. Bonadonna   Division of Metabolic Diseases, University of Verona School of Medicine, Verona, Italy

Knut Borch-Johnsen   Medical Department C, Glostrup University Hospital, DK-2600 Glostrup, Denmark

Peter Bressler	Diabetes Division, University of Texas Health Science Center, 7703 Floyd Curl Drive, San Antonio, TX 78284-7886, USA
Michael Brownlee	Albert Einstein College of Medicine, 1300 Morris Park Avenue F-531, Bronx, NY 10461, USA
G. Calabrese	Istituto di Medicina Interna e Scienze Endocrine e Metaboliche, Via E dal Pozzo, 06126 Perugia, Italy
Rob Carter	NHMRC National Centre for Health Program Evaluation, Yarra House, Fairfield Hospital, Yarra Bend Road, Fairfield, Australia 3078
Jerry D. Cavallerano	Joslin Diabetes Center, One Joslin Place, Boston, MA 02215, USA
David A. Cavan	Department of Medicine, St Thomas's Hospital, Lambeth Palace Road, London, SE1 7EH, UK
Antonio Ceriello	Chair of Internal Medicine, University of Udine, P.le S. Maria della Misericordia, 33100 Udine, Italy
A. Cesarini	Pretura Circondariale, Perugia, Italy
Stella S.J. Chale	Muhimbili Medical Centre, PO Box 65243, Dar es Salaam, Tanzania
Erik Christiansen	Steno Diabetes Center, Niels Stensensvej 2, 2820 Gentofte, Denmark
Anne Clark	Diabetes Research Laboratories, Radcliffe Infirmary, Woodstock Road, Oxford, OX2 6HE, UK
P.M.S. Clark	Department of Clinical Biochemistry, Addenbrooke's Hospital, Hills Road, Cambridge, CB2 2QR, UK
Matthew Cohen	International Diabetes Institute, 260 Kooyong Road, Caulfield, Victoria 3162, Australia
John A. Colwell	Medical University of South Carolina, Division of Endocrinology-Metabolism-Nutrition, 171 Ashley Avenue, Charleston, SC 29425-2222, USA
Philip E. Cryer	Division of Endocrinology, Diabetes and Metabolism, Washington University School of Medicine, St Louis, MO 63110, USA
Mayer B. Davidson	Diabetes Clinical Programs, UCLA School of Medicine, City of Hope National Medical Center, Los Angeles, CA, USA
Matthew D. Davis	Department of Ophthalmology, University of Wisconsin-Madison, WARF Building, 610 N Walnut Street, Madison, WI 53705, USA
J.L. Day	Ipswich Diabetes Centre, Ipswich Hospital, Heath Road, Ipswich, IP4 5PD, UK
Torsten Deckert	Steno Memorial Hospital, Niels Steensenvej 2, DK-2820 Gentofte, Denmark
Maximilian de Courten	International Diabetes Institute, 260 Kooyong Road, Caulfield, Victoria 3162, Australia

Ralph A. DeFronzo   Diabetes Division, University of Texas Health Science Center,
                                    7703 Floyd Curl Drive, San Antonio, TX 78284-7886, USA

Eelco J.P. de Koning   Diabetes Research Laboratories, Radcliffe Infirmary, Woodstock Road,
                                    Oxford, OX2 6HE, UK

Stefano Del Prato   Cattedra di Malattie del Metabolismo, Via Giustiniani 2, 35128 Padova, Italy

Richard M. Denton   Department of Biochemistry, School of Medical Sciences, University Walk,
                                    Bristol, BS8 1TD, UK

Steve F. DePaul   Division of Diabetes Translation, Centers for Disease Control and Prevention,
                                    1600 Clifton Road (NE), Atlanta, GA 30333, USA

M.A. Desai   Evans Medical Ltd, Gaskill Road, Speke, Liverpool, L24 9GR, UK

Francesco Dotta   Department of Endocrinology, University of Rome 'La Sapienza', Rome, Italy

Gary Dowse   Midwest Public Health Unit, PO Box 68, Geraldton, WA 6531, Australia

Pilar Durruty   Diabetes Unit, Medicine Service, Hospital San Juan de Dios, Santiago, Chile

M.E. Edmonds   Diabetic Department, King's College Hospital, Denmark Hill,
                                    London, SE5 9RS, UK

George S. Eisenbarth   Barbara Davis Center for Childhood Diabetes, University of Colorado Health
                                    Sciences Center, 4200 East 9th Avenue, Denver, CO 80262, USA

Johan Eriksson   Diabetes and Genetic Epidemiology Unit, Department of Epidemiology and
                                    Health Promotion, National Public Health Institute, Mannerheimintie 166,
                                    FIN-00300 Helsinki, Finland

Ole K. Faber   Øresund Hospital, Denmark

Eleuterio Ferrannini   Metabolism Unit, CNR Institute of Clinical Physiology, Via Savi 8,
                                    56126 Pisa, Italy

S. Edwin Fineberg   Department of Medicine, Regenstrief Health Center, Indiana University
                                    Medical Center, 1001 West 10th Street, Indianapolis, IN 46202, USA

Brian M. Frier   Department of Diabetes, Royal Infirmary of Edinburgh, 1 Lauriston Place,
                                    Edinburgh, EH3 9YW, UK

Jan Frystyk   Institute of Experimental Clinical Research, Aarhus Kommune Hospital,
                                    Norrebrogade 44, 8000 Aarhus C, Denmark

Greg R. Fulcher   Department of Endocrinology, Royal North Shore Hospital, Pacific Highway,
                                    St Leonards, NSW 2065, Australia

Manuel García de los Ríos   Avda Vitacura 5566 Depto 152, Santiago, Chile

Andrea Giaccari   Diabetes Division, Department of Medicine, University of Texas
                                    Health Science Center, San Antonio, TX 78284, USA

Gary W. Gibbons   Division of Vascular Surgery, New England Deaconess Hospital,
                                    110 Francis Street, Boston, MA 02215, USA

Geoffrey V. Gill	The Diabetes Centre, Walton Hospital, Rice Lane, Liverpool, L9 1AE, UK
Dario Giugliano	Faculty of Medicine, University of Naples, Piazza Miraglia, 80131 Naples, Italy
Barry J. Goldstein	Department of Medicine, Jefferson Medical College of Thomas Jefferson University, Philadelphia, PA 19107, USA
Daryl K. Granner	Department of Molecular Physiology and Biophysics, 707 Light Hall, Vanderbilt University Medical School, Nashville, TN 37232-0615, USA
Derek W.R. Gray	Nuffield Department of Surgery, Oxford Radcliffe Hospital, The John Radcliffe, Headington, Oxford, OX3 9DU, UK
Rosaire P. Gray	165 Ferme Park Road, Crouch End, London, N8 9BP, UK
Carl G. Groth	Department of Transplantation Surgery, Huddinge Hospital, S-141 86 Huddinge, Sweden
Uwe Gudat	Klinik für Stoffwechselkrankheiten und Ernährung, Heinrich Heine Universität Düsseldorf, Moorenstrasse 5, 40001 Düsseldorf, Germany
Sarah T. Gwangwa'a	Centre for Nutrition, Institute of Medical Research and Study of Medicinal Plants, Ministry of Scientific and Technical Research, Yaounde, Cameroon
C.N. Hales	Department of Clinical Biochemistry, Addenbrooke's Hospital, Hills Road, Cambridge, CB2 2QR, UK
Richard F. Hamman	Department of Preventive Medicine and Biometrics, University of Colorado School of Medicine, 4200 East Ninth Avenue, Denver, CO 80262, USA
U. Hanson	Departments of Obstetrics and Gynaecology, Karolinska Hospital, Stockholm, Sweden
Maureen I. Harris	National Diabetes Data Group, NIDDK/NIH, Westwood Building, Bethesda, MD 20892, USA
Svend G. Hartling	Department of Endocrinology, University of Copenhagen, Herlev Hospital, Denmark
Leif Sparre Hermann	Meda AB, Box 138, S-40122 Göteborg, Sweden
S.P.J. Higson	Department of Chemistry, Manchester Metropolitan University, All Saints, Manchester, M15 6BA, UK
William Hollingworth	Health Services Research Group, Institute of Public Health, University of Cambridge, Robinson Way, Cambridge, CB2 2SR, UK
Philip D. Home	Department of Medicine, The Medical School, Framlington Place, Newcastle upon Tyne, NE2 4HH, UK
David Hopkins	Diabetes and Endocrinology Research Group, Department of Medicine, University of Liverpool, Liverpool, L69 3BX, UK
Barbara V. Howard	Medlantic Research Institute, 108 Irving Street NW, Washington DC 20010, USA

P.A. In't Veld Department of Clinical Genetics, Erasmus University and Academic Hospital, Rotterdam, The Netherlands

Alan M. Jacobson Mental Health Unit, Joslin Diabetes Center, One Joslin Place, Boston, MA 02215, USA

Rudolf Jokl Medical University of South Carolina, Division of Endocrinology-Metabolism-Nutrition, 171 Ashley Avenue, Charleston, SC 29425-2222, USA

C. Ronald Kahn Elliott P. Joslin Research Laboratory, Joslin Diabetes Center, One Joslin Place, Boston, MA 02215, USA

Steven E. Kahn Division of Endocrinology and Metabolism, VA Medical Center, 1660 South Columbian Way, Seattle, WA 98108, USA

Harry Keen Unit for Metabolic Medicine, UMDS, Guy's Hospital, London, SE1 9RT, UK

Friedrich W. Kemmer Klinik für Stoffwechselkrankenheiten und Ernährung, Heinrich Heine Universität Düsseldorf, Moorenstrasse 5, 40001 Düsseldorf, Germany

Timothy S. Kern Department of Ophthalmology, University of Wisconsin-Madison, WARF Building, 610 N Walnut Street, Madison, WI 53705, USA

Miller H. Kerr Division of Diabetes Translation, Centers for Disease Control and Prevention, 1600 Clifton Road (NE), Atlanta, GA 30333, USA

B.A.K. Khalid Faculty of Medicine, Universiti Kebangsaan Malaysia, Jalan Raja Muda Abdul Aziz, 50300 Kuala Lumpur, Malaysia

Ronald Klein Department of Ophthalmology and Visual Sciences, University of Wisconsin Medical School, 600 Highland Avenue, Madison, WI 53792-3220, USA

Günter Klöppel Department of Pathology, University of Kiel, Michaelisstrasse 11, 24105 Kiel, Germany

William C. Knowler National Institute of Diabetes and Digestive and Kidney Diseases, Phoenix, AZ, USA

Jerzy W. Kolaczynski Department of Medicine, Jefferson Medical College of Thomas Jefferson University, Philadelphia, PA 19107, USA

Markku Laakso Department of Medicine, Kuopio University Hospital, FIN-70210 Kuopio, Finland

M.F. Laker Department of Clinical Biochemistry and Metabolic Medicine, The Medical School, Framlington Place, Newcastle upon Tyne, NE2 4HH, UK

R.E. LaPorte Department of Epidemiology, Graduate School of Public Health, University of Pittsburgh, Pittsburgh, PA 15025, USA

H.E. Lebovitz Department of Medicine, Kings County Hospital, Brooklyn, NY, USA

Pierre J. Lefèbvre Department of Medicine, Division of Diabetes, Nutrition and Metabolic Disorders, CHU Sart Tilman, B-4000 Liège 1, Belgium

R.D.G. Leslie	Department of Diabetes and Metabolism, St Bartholomew's Hospital, London, EC1A 7BE, UK
N.J. Lewis-Barned	Department of Human Nutrition, University of Otago, Dunedin, New Zealand
Frank W. LoGerfo	Division of Vascular Surgery, New England Deaconess Hospital, 110 Francis Street, Boston, MA 02215, USA
Maria F. Lopes-Virella	Division of Endocrinology-Diabetes-Medical Genetics, Medical University of South Carolina, 171 Ashley Avenue, Charleston, SC 29425, USA
N.-O. Lunell	Departments of Obstetrics and Gynaecology, Huddinge Hospital, Stockholm, Sweden
Sten Madsbad	Department of Endocrinology, Hvidovre Hospital, 2650 Hvidovre, Denmark
W.J. Malaisse	Laboratory of Experimental Medicine, Université Libre de Bruxelles, Route de Lennik 808, B-1070 Brussels, Belgium
J.I. Mann	Department of Human Nutrition, University of Otago, Dunedin, New Zealand
S.M. Marshall	Department of Medicine, The Medical School, Framlington Place, Newcastle upon Tyne, NE2 4HH, UK
M. Massi Benedetti	Istituto di Medicina Interna e Scienze Endocrine e Metaboliche, Via E dal Pozzo, 06126 Perugia, Italy
Jean-Claude Mbanya	Diabetes and Endocrine Unit, Department of Internal Medicine, Faculty of Medicine and Biomedical Sciences, University of Yaounde I, BP 8046, Yaounde, Cameroon
David K. McCulloch	Virginia Mason Medical Center, Seattle, WA, USA
Marg McGill	The Diabetes Centre, QE II Building, Royal Prince Alfred Hospital, 59 Missenden Road, Camperdown, NSW 2050, Australia
D.G. McLarty (deceased)	Muhimbili Medical Centre, Dar es Salaam, Tanzania
Arne Melander	Department of Clinical Pharmacology, Malmö General Hospital, S-214 01 Malmö, Sweden
V. Mohan	MV Diabetes Specialities Centre (P) Ltd, 44 Royapetta High Road, Royapetta, Madras 600 014, India
Peter J. Morris	Nuffield Department of Surgery, Oxford Radcliffe Hospital, The John Radcliffe, Headington, Oxford, OX3 9DU, UK
Scot E. Moss	Department of Ophthalmology and Visual Sciences, University of Wisconsin Medical School, 600 Highland Avenue, Madison, WI 53792-3220, USA
P.J. Nestel	Division of Human Nutrition, CSIRO, Adelaide 5000, Australia
Richard M. O'Brien	Department of Molecular Physiology and Biophysics, 707 Light Hall, Vanderbilt University Medical School, Nashville, TN 37232-0615, USA

Hans Ørskov Institute of Experimental Clinical Research, Aarhus Kommune Hospital, Norrebrogade 44, 8000 Aarhus C, Denmark

Pan Xiao-Ren Department of Endocrinology, China-Japan Friendship Hospital, Yinghua East Road, Hepingli, Beijing 100029, China

Michelle A. Penny Division of Virology, MRC National Institute for Medical Research, The Ridgeway, Mill Hill, London, NW7 1AA, UK

Bengt Persson St Göran's Children's Hospital, S-11281 Stockholm, Sweden

Anne L. Peters Clinical Diabetes Program, UCLA School of Medicine, 200 UCLA Medical Plaza, Los Angeles, CA 90095-1693, USA

Daniel Porte Jr Division of Endocrinology and Metabolism, VA Medical Center, 1660 South Columbian Way, Seattle, WA 98108, USA

P. Pozzilli Department of Diabetes and Metabolism, St Bartholomew's Hospital, London, EC1A 7BE, UK

D.A. Pyke 17 College Road, Dulwich Village, London, SE21 7BG, UK

Kalevi Pyörälä Department of Medicine, Kuopio University Hospital, FIN-70210 Kuopio, Finland

Leslie J. Raffel Division of Medical Genetics, Departments of Medicine and Pediatrics, Cedars-Sinai Medical Center, 8700 Beverly Boulevard, Los Angeles, CA 90048, USA

A. Ramachandran Diabetes Research Centre and MV Hospital for Diabetes, 5 Main Road, Royapuram, Madras 600 013, India

Lawrence I. Rand 164 Bigelow Road, West Newton, MA 02165, USA

Philip Raskin University of Texas Southwestern Medical Center, Department of Internal Medicine, 5323 Harry Hines Boulevard, Dallas, TX 75235-8858, USA

Daiva Rastenytė Department of Epidemiology and Health Promotion, National Public Health Institute, Mannerheimintie 166, FIN-00300 Helsinki, Finland

Gérard Reach INSERM U341, Diabetes Department, Hôtel-Dieu, 1 Place du Parvis Notre Dame, 75004 Paris, France

G.P. Rigby Department of Medicine, Clinical Biochemistry Section, University of Manchester, Hope Hospital, Salford, M6 8HD, UK

Arlan L. Rosenbloom University of Florida, College of Medicine, Health Science Center, Department of Pediatrics, Gainesville, FL 32610-0296, USA

Luciano Rossetti Department of Medicine, Albert Einstein College of Medicine, Bronx, NY 10461, USA

Jerome I. Rotter Division of Medical Genetics, Departments of Medicine and Pediatrics, Cedars-Sinai Medical Center, 8700 Beverly Boulevard, Los Angeles, CA 90048, USA

Julio V. Santiago   St. Louis Children's Hospital, One Children's Place, St. Louis, MO 63110, USA

Christopher D. Saudek   Osler Building, Johns Hopkins Hospital, Baltimore, MD 21287-5576, USA

Maren T. Scheuner   Division of Medical Genetics, Departments of Medicine and Pediatrics, Cedars-Sinai Medical Center, 8700 Beverly Boulevard, Los Angeles, CA 90048, USA

Colin J. Schwartz   Department of Pathology, University of Texas Health Science Center, 7703 Floyd Curl Drive, San Antonio, TX 78284-7750, USA

Leonie Segal   NHMRC National Centre for Health Program Evaluation, Yarra House, Fairfield Hospital, Yarra Bend Road, Fairfield, Australia 3078

A. Sekikawa   Department of Epidemiology, Graduate School of Public Health, University of Pittsburgh, Pittsburgh, PA 15025, USA

A. Signore   Cattedra di Endocrinologia (I), Clinica Medica II, University of Rome 'La Sapienza', Rome, Italy

Donald C. Simonson   Department of Medicine, Brigham and Women's Hospital, 221 Longwood Avenue, Boston, MA 02115, USA

Jay S. Skyler   Diabetes/Endocrinology Unit, University of Miami Hospitals and Clinics, 1475 NW 12th Avenue, Miami, FL 33136, USA

Thomas J. Songer   Department of Epidemiology, Graduate School of Public Health, University of Pittsburgh, Pittsburgh, PA 15261, USA

Peter Sönksen   Department of Endocrinology and Chemical Pathology, St. Thomas's Hospital, Lambeth Palace Road, London, SE1 7EH, UK

Michael P. Stern   Division of Clinical Epidemiology, Department of Medicine, University of Texas Health Science Center, 7703 Floyd Curl Drive, San Antonio, TX 78231-7873, USA

M.W. Stewart   Department of Medicine, The Medical School, Framlington Place, Newcastle upon Tyne; NE2 4HH, UK

William S. Stirewalt   Departments of Obstetrics and Gynecology, and Molecular Physiology and Biophysics, University of Vermont, Burlington, Vermont, USA

Suzanne M. Strowig   University of Texas Southwestern Medical Center, Department of Internal Medicine, 5323 Harry Hines Boulevard, Dallas, TX 75235-8858, USA

Calum Sutherland   Department of Molecular Physiology and Biophysics, 707 Light Hall, Vanderbilt University Medical School, Nashville, TN 37232-0615, USA

M.R. Taskinen   Third Department of Medicine, University Central Hospital, 00290 Helsinki, Finland

Jeremy M. Tavaré   Department of Biochemistry, School of Medical Sciences, University Walk, Bristol, BS8 1TD, UK

P.K. Thomas   Department of Neurological Science, Royal Free Hospital School of Medicine, Rowland Hill Street, London, NW3 2PF, UK

Annika Tibell   Department of Transplantation Surgery, Huddinge Hospital, S-141 86 Huddinge, Sweden

Antonio Tiengo   Istituto di Medicina Clinica dell'Università di Padova, Via Giustiniani 2, 35128 Padova, Italy

John E. Tooke   Department of Vascular Medicine, Postgraduate Medical School, University of Exeter, Barrack Road, Exeter, EX2 5DW, UK

Elaine Y.L. Tsui   Mount Sinai Hospital, 600 University Avenue, Toronto, Ontario, M5G 1X5, Canada

Jaakko Tuomilehto   Diabetes and Genetic Epidemiology Unit, Department of Epidemiology and Health Promotion, National Public Health Institute, Mannerheimintic 166, FIN-00300 Helsinki, Finland

Eva Tuomilehto-Wolf   Diabetes and Genetic Epidemiology Unit, Department of Epidemiology and Health Promotion, National Public Health Institute, Mannerheimintie 166, FIN-00300 Helsinki, Finland

Matti Uusitupa   Department of Clinical Nutrition, University of Kuopio, FIN-70211 Kuopio, Finland

P.M. Vadgama   Department of Medicine, Clinical Biochemistry Section, University of Manchester, Hope Hospital, Salford, M6 8HD, UK

Anthony J. Valente   Department of Pathology, University of Texas Health Science Center, 7703 Floyd Curl Drive, San Antonio, TX 78284-7750, USA

Timo Valle   Diabetes and Genetic Epidemiology Unit, Department of Epidemiology and Health Promotion, National Public Health Institute, Mannerheimintie 166, FIN-00300 Helsinki, Finland

Frank Vinicor   Division of Diabetes Translation, Centers for Disease Control and Prevention, 1600 Clifton Road (NE), Atlanta, GA 30333, USA

M. Viswanathan   Diabetes Research Centre and MV Hospital for Diabetes, 5 Main Road, Royapuram, Madras 600 013, India

Mark Walker   Department of Medicine, The Medical School, Framlington Place, Newcastle upon Tyne, NE2 4HH, UK

J.D. Ward   Department of Diabetes, Royal Hallamshire Hospital, Glossop Road, Sheffield, S10 2JF, UK

P.J. Watkins   Diabetic Department, King's College Hospital, Denmark Hill, London, SE5 9RS, UK

Peter Weidmann   Medizinische Universitäts-Poliklinik, Inselspital, Freiburgstrasse 6, CH-3010 Bern, Switzerland

Neil H. White   St. Louis Children's Hospital, One Children's Place, St. Louis, MO 63110, USA

Charles Williams   William Harvey Hospital, Ashford, Kent, TN24 0LZ, UK

D.R.R. Williams	Division of Epidemiology and Public Health, Nuffield Institute for Health, University of Leeds, Fairbairn House, 71-75 Clarendon Road, Leeds, LS2 9PL, UK
Gareth Williams	Diabetes and Endocrinology Research Group, Department of Medicine, University of Liverpool, Liverpool, L69 3BX, UK
John S. Yudkin	UCL Medical School, Academic Division of Medicine, Whittington Hospital, Archway Road, London, N19 3UA, UK
D.K. Yue	The Diabetes Centre, QE II Building, Royal Prince Alfred Hospital, 59 Missenden Road, Camperdown, NSW 2050, Australia
Paul Zimmet	International Diabetes Institute, 260 Kooyong Road, Caulfield, Victoria 3162, Australia
Bernard Zinman	Mount Sinai Hospital, 600 University Avenue, Toronto, Ontario, M5G 1X5, Canada

Foreword to the Second Edition

The Editors were at work commissioning the Second Edition of ITDM before the ink was dry on the First. Such is the editorial responsiveness to readers' comments and to the pace of scientific advance that this Edition contains 31 new subject headings and over 80 new authors. The disappearance of familiar names from the contents pages should not be misconstrued. Some have gone off in hot pursuit of knowledge elsewhere; some, laudably, to spend more time with their patients. Some will 'sit this one out', hopefully to reappear in some future edition with renewed verbal vigour. New material has pushed itself forward, sometimes at the expense of the old; the whole oeuvre has been revised and rewritten.

Diabetes is advancing on a broad front, from molecular biology on one flank to the health economics and sociology of diabetes on another. The recent celebration of the 75th anniversary of Banting and Best's epic success with the isolation of pancreatic insulin highlights the spectacular speed of subsequent advance, defining its composition, its configurations, its complex synthesis and processing, the information on its surfaces and its intermolecular interactions. The black box of the cell is progressively becoming a goldfish bowl; we are now close to the full blueprint of interlocking molecular mechanisms by which insulin regulates the cellular machinery. There are even claims to have improved on the insulin molecule itself—at any rate for the treatment of diabetes. Genetic re-engineering of the C-terminal end of the B chain has created a monomeric form which is more rapidly absorbed from the injection site and so more briskly enters the circulation. Molecular modifications to slow absorption are emerging. Promising though these developments may be for improved metabolic correction, we must maintain high levels of vigilance for undesirable effects of novel molecules.

Clinically, the grail of normoglycaemia has been even more sanctified by the results of the landmark Diabetes Control and Complications Trial (DCCT). It must be the best-conducted, most compelling (and perhaps most expensive) clinical trial in history. We all suspected how it would come out but that was no alternative to really knowing. In an era of evidence-based medicine it is the rock-solid argument we need to persuade the ever-reluctant disbursers of finance and resource. Professional enthusiasm, though, should not blind us to the patient's-eye-view. Here is another mountain to climb, with some tricky traverses and frightening hypoglycaemic chasms to negotiate. Health professionals can shout instructions and encouragement from the safety of the base camp; the patient has to do the climbing. The easier and safer it can all be made, the better. Quality of life ranks at least equally with quality of glycaemic control. In this regard, the implantable closed-loop device and the transplantable islet organ still elude us in any meaningful clinical sense. It can surely only be a matter of time before they are on stream—but how long?

In the interim, much more is now known to lighten the burden of diabetes, particularly of its complications. Glycation, polyol production, glycosaminoglycan synthesis, rheological dysfunction notwithstanding, we are little closer to understanding the sequence which links the molecular disorder of the diabetic state to the structural disorganization of the complications. Besides glycaemic rectitude, a number of 'non-glycaemic' interventions are now firmly established to influence the pathogenetic processes of the complications and protect and preserve vulnerable organ function. They work.

Now the challenge is to put the complex pattern of evaluation and care together and deliver it, appropriately customized, to all who need it. By identifying susceptible individuals and applying the right interventions promptly and effectively, vision can be preserved, limbs saved, renal function protected, heart attacks and strokes prevented, life prolonged. To realize this heartening potential, what is wanted is the will and the wherewithal. Modern diabetes care delivery recognizes that the person with diabetes is not so much a consumer as a co-producer of care, an essential member of the therapeutic partnership. All this is good news for patients and professionals; it must also be so powerfully proclaimed as to convince even the most short-termist of care-purchasers that the investment in good services pays enormous dividends.

As this Second Edition goes to press, the World Health Organization, the International Diabetes Federation, and regional and national diabetes associations are once again reviewing diabetes criteria, remodelling terminology and remaking classifications. It is too facile to dismiss this as just another exercise in intellectual bureaucracy. It is that, but much more beside. Our perception of the (man-made) concept of diabetes mellitus and how we tackle its elucidation and correction can be expressed only in names and numbers. As perceptions enlarge and change, the names and the numbers we use must follow suit. We do useful things with today's names and numbers; the only justification for changing them can be that the new ones are even more useful. Some day, perhaps, the notion of diabetes will dissolve altogether, but not yet.

Harry Keen

Introduction

It is 4 years since the first edition of 'ITDM' appeared. At that time we attempted to give a broader sweep to our coverage of diabetes than was customary in the available 'Northern' textbooks. This was due in part to the pandemic of diabetes that was, and still is, sweeping the globe, and in part to the lack of texts dealing with diabetes in non-Europids. We felt that much could be learned by considering diabetes in relation to different ethnic groups, cultures and geographical settings. We also attempted to cover the whole of diabetes, from the gene and cell biology to the social and economic aspects. Further background to the rationale of ITDM is given in the original introduction which is reprinted below.

We have been encouraged by the response to the first edition: hence the present volumes. This second edition does not, however, just represent a reworking of the previous volumes. Several new chapters have been added, others replaced, and many new authors introduced. We hope that we have been able to enhance the previous edition and also remain current and relevant.

K.G.M.M. Alberti
P.Z. Zimmet
R.A. DeFronzo

INTRODUCTION TO FIRST EDITION

A modern textbook of diabetes should be international in scope. Not only does it draw on the knowledge and expertise of people from all over the world, but it also reminds us that no race of mankind is immune from the diabetic state. Ethnic susceptibility to diabetes varies tremendously, a variation in liability which must depend both upon the widely differing conditions in which the human species exists and upon the diversity of the genetic endowment. It is important to our understanding of the nature of diabetes mellitus and our attempts to prevent and treat it that we view the diabetic state as the outcome of the interplay of a multiplicity of causal factors, potentially varying in both the genetic and the environmental components of the mix. Although the diabetic state can itself be clearly defined—We, after all, are responsible for creating the definition—it is, nevertheless, heterogeneous in its causation and in its consequences. In investigating its mechanisms we should be prepared to find differences between, and even within, populations in the nature of the underlying susceptibility and in the factors that provoke its emergence and its pathological sequelae.

Before attempting to explain the diabetic state, we should agree upon its definition. Those who coined the term *diabetes mellitus* had little doubt: originally, it described a grave sickness characterized by dramatic symptoms—intense thirst, profuse urination, rapid wasting, inexorably proceeding through the stages of vomiting and drowsiness to coma and death. The term *diabetes* was no more than a description of these characteristic symptoms; *mellitus* was added when the sweetness of the urine indicated its high sugar content and distinguished it from the insipid, sugar-free variety.

Identification of the urinary sugar as glucose can be said to have ushered in the era of clinical chemistry. However, it was not until laboratory methods were sufficiently refined that the central importance of hyperglycaemia in the diabetic state and its primacy in diabetes diagnosis were recognized. This transition from clinical to chemical diagnosis had a profound effect on the diagnostic concept of diabetes: it resulted in the addition to the same diagnostic rubric of ever-larger numbers of cases with ever-lessening degrees of symptomatology. This conceptual inflation reached its limits with the application of pre-emptive screening tests for diabetes to large sections of the general population. Now, the diagnosis was called upon to accommodate cases without symptoms or signs, sometimes even without glucose in the urine. The existence of a state of 'pathological hyperglycaemia' had become the main justification for including in the same diagnostic category a spectrum of abnormality which ranged from a totally asymptomatic transgression of an arbitrary blood glucose norm at the one extreme, to a potentially lethal metabolic catastrophe at the other. A further justification for retaining the single diagnostic term was the common liability to the ultimate development of a characteristic set of organ and tissue abnormalities—the complications of diabetes.

Population surveys for diabetes, with the new diagnostic perspectives that they generated, stemmed from the recognition of the high prevalence of unsuspected diabetes and the hope that early detection and treatment might avert its complications. Large population samples were tested, many being submitted to measurements of blood glucose concentration in response to a glucose challenge. It was difficulty with interpretation of the results of such surveys that brought the diagnostic definition of diabetes to critical review. Unexpectedly large numbers of apparently healthy people had blood glucose levels at the suspiciously high end of the range, their frequency increasing with age. At no age could a 'natural' dividing line be found separating normal from diabetic glycaemic responses. Depending on which set of diagnostic criteria were adopted, the estimates of diabetes frequency in a given population could vary as much as tenfold. As a consequence, an individual diagnosed as unquestionably diabetic by one doctor could be equally emphatically reassured of normality by another. Add to this the substantial variation introduced by differences in the methods of diagnostic testing, and the reasons for the moves towards national and international standardization of the 1970s and early 1980s become clear. A measure of order was introduced in consensus meetings of a number of national diabetes organizations, principally the US National Diabetes Data Group, and soon after by the World Health Organization. They agreed upon a set of glycaemic criteria for diabetes diagnosis and interposed a new category of 'impaired glucose tolerance' (IGT) between clearly normal and clearly diabetic glycaemic responses. Although these proposals are by no means above criticism, they have been increasingly widely applied in both clinical practice and epidemiological investigation, and provide a degree of comparability and uniformity that was previously lacking.

The international perspective is also appropriate to the classification of the diabetic state, which also has been the subject of concern and revision over the past decade. The two major types of diabetes mellitus, insulin dependent (IDDM or type 1) and non-insulin dependent (NIDDM or type 2), are essentially defined by their clinical characteristics, although these largely correspond (in people of European origin) to underlying aetiological mechanisms and, perhaps, to genetic liabilities. The frequency of IDDM or type 1 diabetes—the severe disease of classic description—is notably higher in peoples of European origin, although it has been reported almost universally in others. NIDDM also has rather different characteristics in Europeans, compared with most other ethnic groups: its prevalence is lower, it appears later in life and it

is, perhaps, less liable to lead to renal failure, possibly because of its later appearance. Malnutrition related diabetes mellitus (MRDM) appeared in the most recent WHO classification as an independent type. Its existence as a tropical variant of diabetes, secondary to pancreatic damage and aetiologically related to dietary protein deficiency or to toxic food contaminants, has been the subject of debate and investigation in recent years. More systematic investigation is needed before the size and nature of this problem can be confidently documented.

NIDDM is by far the largest problem numerically on a global scale. In the most susceptible populations, up to one person in two may expect to develop the disease. The Pima tribe of American Indians, currently topping the league tables for diabetes prevalence, have shown what appears to be an explosive increase in incidence over the course of this century. The tribe was visited in the early 1930s by Dr E. P. Joslin, the doyen of diabetes in the USA, who was interested in the reputed rarity of diabetes among its members. This dramatic transformation must have been the response to some widespread environmental change affecting a relatively inbred population carrying some underlying genetic susceptibility to the disease: a steeply rising prevalence of obesity is widely held to have been the environmental determinant; the genetic susceptibility factor has as yet eluded definition. At the present pace of genetic research and discovery, its detection can only be a matter of time. When it is found, however, will it prove to be the same as that determining susceptibility to NIDDM in other populations? On the face of it, it seems unlikely that NIDDM is a single homogeneous entity *within* populations, let alone *between* them. Its associations with age, adiposity and clinical progression appear so diverse that a multiplicity of underlying mechanisms appears probable.

In recent years some part of this broad spectrum of NIDDM and IGT have been linked with a number of other common disorders and conditions, such as hypertension, hyperlipidaemia and hyperinsulinaemia. From this has emerged the view that this form of glucose intolerance may only be part—and not an obligatory part at that—of some much more general disturbance of adaptation to the conditions of modern life. Characterized by diminished tissue sensitivity to the effects of insulin and associated with a centripetal distribution of body fat and increased liability to atherosclerosis, this so-called syndrome X currently attracts the attention of many investigators. In a continuum of interacting mechanisms which may contribute to a number of important human disorders, glucose intolerance or diabetes may have a small or even non-existent role. Other broad classes of NIDDM may be described, without obesity, with early age of onset and with evidence of islet autoimmunity, which highlight its probable heterogeneity.

It is the so-called complications of diabetes that today constitute the main burden for patients, their families and the societies in which they live. Blindness due to retinopathy, such a dreaded hazard a generation ago, is now in large part a preventable disaster provided that facilities for eye screening and timely photocoagulation are available. The long period of ill-health as diabetic renal disease neared its termination in end-stage renal failure can now be reversed with modern renal substitution methods of dialysis and transplantation; there is reason to suppose that the stage of renal failure may be postponed and the number of patients entering renal failure greatly diminished, again depending upon facilities for the early recognition of those at risk and their appropriately monitored treatment. There is some evidence that people with the increased arterial disease risk of diabetes are sharing in the general diminution in coronary heart disease morbidity and mortality documented in some societies over the past 20 years. This strongly suggests that much of the aggravated risk of atherosclerotic disease in diabetes could be reduced. Even the morbid effects of that most intransigent of diabetic complications—neuropathy—can be ameliorated by the application of quite simple preventative measures. The scope of diabetes care has expanded dramatically in recent years, with the promise of longer and healthier years of life for many and (that prize so beloved of health politicians) a reduction in the enormous costs of health-care provision for diabetic complications. The remarkable advances of knowledge have firmly placed on the agenda even the prevention of diabetes itself.

It is our hope that we have been able, in this book, to cover most of this broad panorama of diabetes, from the molecular structures responsible for susceptibility, through the hormonal and biochemical mechanisms responsible for the clinical manifestations and complications of the disease, to the therapeutic agencies and their availability to ameliorate, arrest, reverse, or even prevent its damaging impact. Much remains to be discovered; we are still far short of a full understanding of the disease. Much that is known remains to be applied; it is important to translate what we know into what we do. We hope that this book will enhance the understanding of diabetes mellitus and help in applying that understanding to the better care of people with diabetes.

Harry Keen
George Alberti
Ralph DeFronzo
Paul Zimmet

Preamble: the History of Diabetes

D.A. Pyke

Diabetic Department, King's College Hospital, London, UK

The discovery of insulin in 1921 was one of the most dramatic events in the history of medicine; it overshadows everything else in the story of diabetes. But it is not the beginning of our story; diabetes had been described more than 2000 years earlier.

The first description is usually credited to Arataeus of Cappadocia in Asia Minor in the first century AD, who gave the disease its name. This was because diabetes was thought to be like water passing through a siphon. However, Celsus also described the disorder a few years earlier. Both had noticed one of the essential clinical features, an excessive volume of urine. This observation is all the more creditable as the disease seems to have been uncommon in those days, or at least not commonly diagnosed. Galen said he had seen only two cases.

The sweet taste of the urine in diabetes is usually said to have been noticed first in the seventeenth century by the Oxford physician, Thomas Willis (who also described the arteries at the base of the brain). It was an original observation by him but Willis was not the first to make it. Avicenna, an Arab physician of the eleventh century, described many of the clinical features. It was also observed by the ancient Indians, who referred to diabetes as Madhumeha, in the fourth century BC (some writers have described this observation as being in the fourth century AD, an error equivalent to the time from Magna Carta to the present day!). The ancient Indians are said to have noticed ants congregating around the urine of diabetics, so perhaps the ants deserve the credit for discovering the sweetness of diabetic urine. Similar observations were also made in China in the seventh century AD by Chen Chhuan, who gave a good description of the main features, including the sweet urine. An excellent account of the history of diabetes is included in Medvei (1993) [1].

The distinction between the sweet tasting urine of the common type of diabetes, called mellitus for this reason, and the non-sweet taste in diabetes insipidus was made by Willis. This has always seemed to me to be a remarkable achievement in view of the great rarity of diabetes insipidus, but perhaps one case was enough for him to make the distinction. Willis suspected that the fault in diabetes derived from the blood and not, as others had thought, from a weakness of the kidneys.

That the sweet taste of diabetic urine was due to sugar was proved by Matthew Dobson a century after Willis, and he also made the crucial observation of the excess of sugar in the blood. Dobson referred to alimentary matter being drawn off by the kidneys before it is perfectly assimilated, showing an understanding that diabetes is a generalized disease. Forty years later the sweetness of urine was proved by Michel Chevreul to be due to sugar.

Attempts at treatment began when no more was known of diabetes than the polyuria. John Rollo, Surgeon-General to the Royal Artillery, treated Captain Meredith in 1796 by dietary restriction, with considerable success for the patient survived for at least a year. Rollo's next patient was a general; he was less obedient, did not follow the diet and came to grief. Rollo also noticed the smell of acetone on the breath of diabetics, presumably those in the advanced stage of type 1 diabetes, and he observed cataracts in diabetics.

Another observation at the same time was by Thomas Cawley, that the pancreas of a patient who had died of diabetes showed stones and tissue damage, but the significance of this vital clue of 1788 was appreciated only 101 years later, when Minkowski removed the pancreas from a dog and unexpectedly produced diabetes.

International Textbook of Diabetes Mellitus, Second Edition. Edited by K.G.M.M. Alberti, P. Zimmet, R.A. DeFronzo, and H. Keen (Honorary)
© 1997 John Wiley & Sons Ltd

CLAUDE BERNARD

The greatest figure in the history of diabetes in the first half of the nineteenth century was Claude Bernard. He was an extraordinary man. He trained as a pharmacist but fancied himself as a literary man. He wrote a romantic play and took it to St Marc Girardin, a professor at the Sorbonne, who read the play, then said to Claude Bernard, 'You have done some pharmacy, why not take up medicine?'. That must be the best advice ever given. Claude Bernard became a professor of the Collège de France and a dominant figure in physiology and medicine in France and indeed in Europe. When he died in 1878 he was given a state funeral, the only scientist to be so honoured. For all his scientific greatness, he was a sad figure. He was deserted by his wife and two daughters who hated his experiments on live animals, in particular dogs with stomach fistulas who wandered about the house. Claude Bernard's writings are still very well worth reading. The only one published in English is his *Study of Experimental Medicine*. For diabetologists his *Leçons de Physiologie* and *Leçons sur le Diabète* are of absorbing interest, especially the first.

Bernard's important discoveries were first, that the liver stored glycogen and secreted a sugary substance into the blood. He assumed that it was an excess of this secretion which caused diabetes. As it was known that the nervous system controlled secretory organs he assumed that this function too was under nervous control. This reasoning led to his second, though less important, discovery, that pricking the brain stem in the conscious animal resulted in a temporary diabetes. He thought that this resulted from stimulation of the origin of the vagus nerve but proved himself wrong by finding that cutting the vagus did not prevent the diabetes. He concluded that the effect was mediated by the sympathetic system, in which he was correct. He made other observations which, like 'piqûre' diabetes, are still of uncertain significance, for example that curare and morphine led to hyperglycaemia.

Claude Bernard was such a dominating figure that his view that diabetes was due to an oversecretion of glucose by the liver held universal sway. But not for long.

DIABETES AND THE PANCREAS

In 1879 came one of those extraordinary strokes of chance that instantaneously change men's minds, the discovery that removing the pancreas caused diabetes. Von Mering, a German physician in Strasburg, was interested in digestion. He wanted to know what role the pancreas played. He wanted to try the effect of removing it but thought that this was impossible. His colleague Oscar Minkowski said, 'Bah, I can take out the pancreas'. He could and he did. Then the unexpected happened. The next day the laboratory technician complained that the dog was urinating all over the cage, in spite of having been house-trained. Minkowski realised at once what this might mean, tested the urine and found glucose. He had produced diabetes by removing the pancreas, therefore the pancreas contained an antidiabetic substance. Von Mering was only mildly interested; the rest of the story is Minkowski's. He was working in the laboratory of Bernard Naunyn, who was interested in diabetes, and he needed no help in realising the importance of his discovery. Minkowski, who was also the first person to associate the pituitary with acromegaly, lived to see the introduction of insulin in 1922. He once memorably rebuked Zuelzer, who at a meeting in Berlin claimed that he was the true discoverer of insulin, 'I, too, wish I had discovered insulin'.

The discovery was more difficult to develop than Minkowski or anyone else expected. Try as they did they could not extract the antidiabetic substance from the pancreas. They knew that the main function of the pancreas was to produce digestive enzymes and that these might be interfering with the extraction of the antidiabetic substance, but they could not find a way around this difficulty. Neither could the many other workers in Europe and North America. There was no lack of appreciation of what was at stake.

The idea that the antidiabetic substance might come from the islets of Langerhans was widely held. The islets, named after a German medical student who observed the little islands of tissue quite different in appearance from the rest of the gland, presumably had a different function from the rest of the pancreas. They were not connected to any ducts, so it was reasonable to suppose that their secretion, whatever it was, went straight into the circulation.

Several people got very near to solving the problem but none did so. Nicolas Paulesco of Bucharest came as near as any but he was dogged by 'toxic' effects, i.e. hypoglycaemia, whose meaning he did not understand. Canadian and American investigators also got very close, but none found a complete and convincing answer to the problem of producing an effective, stable extract of pancreas which would predictably and consistently produce a fall of blood glucose in diabetic animals.

THE DISCOVERY OF INSULIN

The final triumph came from a surprising quarter. In 1921, in Canada, Frederick Banting was an unsuccessful orthopaedic surgeon (in itself something of a rarity) who, on reading of the association of the destruction of the pancreas with diabetes, became convinced that he could find the antidiabetic substance. He was so ignorant that he did not know how many other people had tried in the 40 years since Minkowski. That was his strength; he did not realise how difficult the problem was. Nothing would stop him. He persuaded J.J.R. Macleod, the Professor of Physiology at Toronto who did understand the problem and its difficulties, to let him try. Macleod assigned a young medical student, Charles Best, to work with him and later (when the process of extraction and stability of the pancreas secretion was proving difficult) he put a visiting professor J.B. Collip, a biochemist, on to the problem with dramatic results.

Banting's original idea had been that it was the external secretions of the pancreas which destroyed the 'insulin'. So he tied off the pancreatic duct, waited some weeks for the glandular part of the pancreas to atrophy, then made an extract of the remaining gland. In the end this logical process proved not to be effective and insulin was obtained by standard chemical methods of extraction. Finally, an extract was made which could be tried on patients. It had a dramatic effect. For the first time levels of blood glucose were lowered. Young patients who had been slowly dying of their diabetes lost their consuming thirst, recovered their strength and regained their lost weight. It was a miraculous transformation. A universally fatal disease had been cured—no, not cured but controlled; so long as they took their daily insulin injections the patients could be restored to normal life.

We can easily forget today, when insulin treatment is universally available and successful, what type 1 diabetes meant before this discovery. Death was a slow one. Some of those youngsters who were the first to be treated with insulin had been wasting away for years, losing ground all the time but kept alive by ferocious dieting. 'Dieting' meant starvation. Those early diabetologists—Elliott Joslin in Boston and Frederick Allen in New York—were puritans and had to be. They had nothing else to offer but starvation. If the patient got an infection and the diabetes got worse the answer was even stricter starvation. It was a miserable situation for diabetics and heart-rending for their parents.

Then came insulin and the great revival it brought. Nowhere is this more vividly expressed than by a nurse at Frederick Allen's 'physiatric' hospital in New York, who wrote 10 years later:

> ... the mere illusion of new hope cajoled patient after patient into new life. Diabetics who had not been out of bed for weeks began to trail weakly about, clinging to walls and furniture. Big stomachs, skin-and-bone necks, skull-like faces, feeble movements, all ages, both sexes—they looked like an old Flemish painter's depiction of a resurrection after famine. It was a resurrection, a crawling stirring, as of some vague springtime.

The patients heard that Dr Allen had come back from Toronto:

> Bed immediately after dinner was the rule for our patients. But not that evening. My office opened on the big center hallways. I could see them drifting in, silent as the bloated ghosts they looked like. Even to look at one another would have painfully betrayed some of the intolerable hope that had brought them. So they just sat and waited, eyes on the ground.
>
> It was growing dark outside. Nobody had yet seen Doctor Allen. His first appearance would be at his dinner, which followed the patients' dinner hour. We all heard his step coming along the covered walk, past the entrance to the main hallways. His wife was with him, her quick tapping pace making a queer rhythm with his. The patients' silence concentrated on that sound. When he appeared through the open doorway, he caught the full beseeching of a hundred pairs of eyes. It stopped him dead. Even now I am sure it was minutes before he spoke to them, his voice curiously mingling concern for his patients with an excitement that he tried his best not to betray. 'I think,' he said, 'I think we have something for you.' [2]

News spread all over the medical world. Within weeks leaders came to Toronto to verify the rumours, then to learn from the Toronto workers how to produce the insulin, and from the pharmaceutical company Eli Lilly of Indianapolis, whose fortunes were revived by the discovery. August Krogh of Denmark, a Nobel Prize winner for his research on capillaries, was in the USA at the time to talk about his work but found that everyone he met talked of nothing but insulin, so he went to Toronto. When he returned to Denmark with H.C. Hagedorn he laid the foundation of the great Danish insulin manufacturing industry. They set up the Nordisk Insulin Company, a non-profit-making concern which, together with the Novo Company, was responsible for making Denmark the main insulin-producing country outside the USA, where Eli Lilly held the near-monopoly.

Britain was slower to respond. Sir Henry Dale of the Medical Research Council came to Toronto, realised the significance of the discovery, and saw also the need for a properly controlled trial to assess the effect, applicability and risks of insulin. But the British pharmaceutical industry did not respond as the Danes did and they were never a major force outside the British Isles.

The discovery of insulin transformed the work of physicians looking after diabetic patients. For some it also transformed their lives. Robin Lawrence, a young British doctor who was training as a surgeon, developed diabetes and was likely to die. He went out to Florence to spend his last few years practising among the English community there. He was summoned back to London by a laconic telegram from G.A. Harrison, a biochemist at King's College Hospital in London; 'I have got insulin. It works. Come back immediately'. He did, it did and he lived for another 45 years. He became the leading British diabetologist and created the Diabetic Department at King's College Hospital. He taught hundreds of doctors and thousands of diabetic patients about the diabetic life. When he died in 1968 at the age of 76 he had no complications of diabetes.

The first type of insulin was quick- and short-acting ('soluble' or 'regular' insulin). It had to be injected twice daily. There was an obvious clinical need for a longer-acting preparation and in 1936 protamine zinc insulin was introduced, in 1954 the lente insulins. The number of new preparations has steadily increased since then and new types continue to be produced. But even with the best modern insulins we are a long way from imitating nature, in that we still cannot achieve continuous precision control of blood glucose.

The earlier insulin preparations were crude and impure. The first patients had to endure injections of 5–10 ml intramuscularly. Pain and abscesses were common. As this was going to be a life-long treatment, injections had to be made acceptable. Purity greatly improved and the volume of injections—even with the dilute preparations of 40 units/ml then in use—could be reduced to 1 ml or less in most cases, but there were still local reactions in some patients, especially in the early weeks.

INSULINS

Impurities in insulin preparations were in most cases due to other pancreatic peptides which were present in tiny concentrations. The Danes produced a purer type of insulin, 'monocomponent' insulin, and other 'highly purified insulins' were made. When the Danes tried to capitalize on these improved products by introducing them to the American market the Americans reacted by producing 'human' insulin, i.e. genetically engineered insulin, which now dominates the scene. Previously insulin had come from animal sources, mainly cattle in the USA and the UK, pigs in Denmark. Although human, pig and cattle insulin differ from each other in one to three of their amino acids, they are equally effective.

Insulin was crystallized in 1926 by J.J. Abel. Its composition, two chains of 51 amino acids linked by disulphide bridges, was discovered by very highly skilled and patient chemistry by Frederick Sanger of Cambridge. For this work he got a Nobel Prize in 1955. For later work he got another. He is one of only two men to win two Nobel Prizes in science (John Bardeen, physicist, of the USA was the other; Linus Pauling's second Nobel Prize was for peace, which does not count in my reckoning!).

The three-dimensional structure of the insulin molecule was discovered 14 years later at Oxford, by the crystallographer Dorothy Hodgkin. A few years

later she did the same for Vitamin B_{12}. She got only one Nobel Prize.

The scientific investigation of diabetes, and hence our understanding of its causes, were greatly improved by the discovery of the technique of immunoassay by Solomon Berson and Rosalind Yalow in 1957. Minute concentrations of insulin, and later of other hormones, could be exactly and consistently measured, a huge improvement on the previous methods of bioassay. In diabetes these methods had been pioneered by Joe Bornstein of Melbourne, working with R.D. Lawrence at King's College Hospital, London. Solomon Berson died prematurely and Rosalind Yalow survived to get the Nobel Prize that Berson would certainly have shared. Their discovery transformed all endocrinology.

A discovery of much theoretical, but still little practical, interest was that in 1967 of the natural insulin precursor proinsulin by the Chicago biochemist, Donald Steiner. Proinsulin consists of insulin, connecting peptide and linking amino acids and is the inactive storage form of insulin.

IMPACT OF THE DISCOVERY OF INSULIN

With the discovery of insulin it was obvious that Claude Bernard's ideas needed revising or, in some people's view, overthrowing. Thus Joslin said that '...the spell of Claude Bernard... hung over the disease and confusion regarding its aetiology reigned'. That was true for insulin dependent diabetes, which was due to lack of insulin, not oversecretion of glucose by the liver. But it is too sweeping a condemnation to apply to all diabetes. We know that the commoner type 2 diabetes is produced by an entirely different mechanism from type 1. We do not know what the mechanism is but it is certainly not an immune-mediated destruction of pancreatic B cells. We still do not know what role, if any, is played by glucose over-secretion or nervous control in type 2 diabetes. If the ill effect of Claude Bernard's work was to concentrate minds on the breakdown of liver glycogen as the cause of diabetes, perhaps one could say that the ill effect of the discovery of insulin was to concentrate minds exclusively on islet B cell deficiency.

Thus, the seeming capacity of insulin deficiency to explain all diabetes obscures some other discoveries which may or may not be relevant to the cause of type 2 diabetes, but which are certainly of physiological importance. Bernardo Houssay, one of Argentina's two Nobel Prize winners, observed in 1924 that hypophysectomy produced extreme sensitivity to insulin and improved experimental diabetes. Frank Young, Professor of Biochemistry in London and later in Cambridge, noted in 1937 that pituitary growth hormone when given to a growing animal produced excessive growth but when given to a mature animal produced diabetes.

With these observations and our own inability to explain the role of obesity, insulin resistance and genetic factors, we are forced into a wider approach. We now appreciate, perhaps more than ever before, how right Claude Bernard was when he said that, 'we know less about diabetes than we thought we knew'. In our understanding of the causes of diabetes we have come a long way—and, in doing so, have discovered how far there is still to go. The distinction between the two main types of diabetes—insulin dependent and non-insulin dependent—was an important advance. All previous work was distorted by the need to find *a* cause for a single disease, diabetes. Thus the findings (a) from twin studies, that the genetic influences were, contrary to expectations, apparently stronger in type 2 than type 1 diabetes because concordance rates in identical twins were only about 35% in type 1 but 80–100% in type 2, and (b) that type 1 diabetes was tightly linked to certain HLA types, were important clues to understanding. The second of these findings encouraged, even if it did not account for, the highly important evidence of how an immune process worked in destroying islet B cells.

The *clinical* distinction between the two types of diabetes had long been appreciated by physicians, but they could not know that they expressed two pathogenetic mechanisms. Important biochemical differences had been shown by Harold Himsworth, who in 1936 demonstrated insulin *sensitivity* in type 1 and insulin *resistance* in type 2 diabetes.

TREATMENT BY MOUTH

The hope of being able to treat diabetes by mouth is an old one. Insulin cannot be given by mouth because, being a peptide, it is broken down in the gut by digestive enzymes. It still cannot, in spite of a prediction I remember Charles Best making in the 1950s that insulin would be given by mouth within 10 years.

Some forms of oral treatment for non-insulin-dependent diabetes had been in existence since the 1930s; aspirin had been used, also 'synthalin', a mild hepatotoxic agent, but none was really effective. That was true before an unexpected and happy chance befell a scientist who was not interested in diabetes—just as Minkowski's great discovery came when he was looking elsewhere.

Montpellier is a beautiful university town in the South of France. In 1942, halfway through the Second World War, the Germans, having previously occupied half of France, seized the rest of it including Montpellier. University life and research were difficult. Professor M.J. Janbon, Professor of Pharmacology, was working on a therapy for typhoid, still a fairly common disease, especially in war time. He was testing a substance on animals, a sulphonylurea, and found that it sometimes produced a bizarre toxic effect. He quickly suspected the cause, hypoglycaemia. He asked the Professor of Medicine, August Loubatières, to try it on diabetic patients. It worked, producing undoubted fall of blood glucose. The research workers had a potential treatment for diabetes. They explored the mechanism of action and found that it was ineffective in animals after removal of the pancreas. The inference was that sulphonylureas stimulated the secretion of insulin but could not substitute for it. It was useless in insulin-deficient diabetes.

Their work was published in France in 1944. The war was still on, people had other things to think about and the discovery attracted little attention—until 10 years later, when Franke and Fuchs in Berlin rediscovered the sulphonylureas, applied them clinically and published their results widely and in English.

That started a great effort to discover the clinical use of the sulphonylureas and their mode of action. It was soon confirmed that they did stimulate insulin secretion by the pancreas, although this did not entirely explain their actions. By an odd chance, the first sulphonylurea given serious clinical trial, carbutamide, was toxic to the bone marrow. Many sulphonylureas have been developed since then; none has any serious toxicity. The modern treatment of non-insulin dependent diabetes still relies heavily on these drugs.

An altogether different type of drug, the biguanides was introduced by G. Unger. As with the sulphonylureas, the first—phenethylbiguanide (dibotin)—had a toxic effect, rare but serious, lactic acidosis. By the time this had been discovered another biguanide, dimethylbiguanide (metformin), had been introduced which rarely, if ever, produced lactic acidosis.

COMPLICATIONS OF DIABETES

At first insulin was regarded as almost a cure for diabetes; I say 'almost' because, of course, insulin treatment had to be continued indefinitely, but 'cure' because it seemed to have restored the patient's health. It gradually emerged that it did not. Complications of diabetes affecting the eyes, diabetic retinopathy, had been described before the discovery of insulin. It was thought to be a rarity—it was a rarity because few patients lived long enough to develop retinopathy. With insulin they did. They also lived long enough to develop glomerulosclerosis, which gradually progressed to renal failure and death. The condition was named the Kimmelstiel–Wilson syndrome after its

American and British co-discoverers in 1936. Also, with longer survival of diabetic patients, complications affecting the peripheral, and later the autonomic, nervous system were described.

Before the discovery of insulin, successful pregnancy in a diabetic woman was a rarity. Now it became possible. Whereas many diabetic women used to die in pregnancy, with insulin they hardly ever did so. Nevertheless there was still a heavy fetal loss, about 40%. With improved and concentrated care of the mother's diabetes, needing two or three daily injections of insulin, frequent hospital visits, prompt treatment of any relapse, early admission to hospital, close fetal monitoring (such as it was in those days) and early delivery, usually by caesarian section, Lawrence, Oakley and Peel at King's College Hospital, and Priscilla White at the Joslin Clinic in Boston, were able to produce a progressive reduction in fetal loss rate. This was achieved not by any dramatic discovery, apart from insulin, but by good medical care. Diabetic pregnancy is one of the most successful chapters in the story of diabetes care.

ORGANIZATIONS CONCERNED WITH DIABETES

The British Diabetic Association was founded in 1938 by R.D. Lawrence and the writer H.G. Wells, himself a diabetic, in conjunction with others, to look after the interests of diabetics. Although many doctors joined the BDA it was essentially an organization of patients. It was concerned with their education and all other aspects of their care. It did valiant work in the Second World War to ensure that diabetics obtained a fair ration and the money to pay for it. A medical and scientific section of the BDA was formed in 1960 with F.G. Young as chairman. It has held highly successful meetings of doctors, scientists and others who are professionally interested in diabetes, twice yearly. As with all medical and scientific meetings, the number of those attending increases continuously.

The American Diabetes Association founded in 1942 is rather different. It is an organization of doctors and others who care for diabetic patients, not of diabetic patients themselves. It holds large and important annual

meetings and publishes a monthly journal, *Diabetes*. Many other national diabetes associations were set up, resulting in improvement in knowledge of diabetes and in its care.

The European Association for the Study of Diabetes (EASD) was founded in 1965. It was largely created by Albert Renold, a leading biochemist from Switzerland who had spent many years in Boston at the Joslin Clinic. When he returned to Geneva he noticed a relative lack of organization of European compared to American doctors and scientists, so with the support of J.F. Hoet, the Belgian pioneer of diabetes research and care, he organized the EASD. It holds an annual scientific meeting and publishes the journal *Diabetologia*. The world organization concerned with diabetes, the International Diabetes Federation, was founded in 1952. It holds 3-yearly meetings, the first at Leyden; since then meetings have been held in all continents.

The World Health Organization has a wide remit and is only peripherally concerned with diabetes, but with the decline of most infectious diseases (abolition in the case of smallpox) it has been able to give more attention to the chronic diseases. It has published a number of reports on diabetes and has been helpful in producing diagnostic standards of blood glucose levels and providing useful information on the worldwide epidemiology of diabetes.

CONCLUSION

This has been a gallop through the history of diabetes to 1974. For the more recent history and the future of the subject you will have to read the rest of this book.

REFERENCES

1. Medvei C. The history of endocrinology, 2nd edn. New York: Parthenon, 1993.
2. Bliss M. The discovery of insulin. Edinburgh: Paul Harris Publishing, 1983. (A superb account, all the better for being written not by a doctor but by a professor of history. Anyone interested in diabetes would enjoy reading it.)

Diagnosis, Epidemiology and Aetiology of Diabetes

1

Classification of Diabetes Mellitus and Other Categories of Glucose Intolerance

Maureen I. Harris* and Paul Zimmet†

* National Institutes of Health, Bethesda, Maryland, USA, and
†International Diabetes Institute, Melbourne, Victoria, Australia

INTRODUCTION

A major requirement for orderly epidemiologic and clinical research on, and indeed for management of, diabetes mellitus is an appropriate classification. Furthermore, a hallmark in the process of understanding the etiology of a disease and studying its natural history is the ability to identify and differentiate its various forms and place them into a rational etiopathologic framework. While there have been a number of sets of nomenclature and diagnostic criteria proposed for diabetes, no systematic categorization existed until just over a decade ago. Now diabetes mellitus is recognized as being a syndrome, a collection of disorders that have hyperglycemia and glucose intolerance as their hallmark, due either to insulin deficiency or to impaired effectiveness of insulin's action, or to a combination of these.

The contemporary classification of diabetes and other categories of glucose intolerance (Table 1), based on research on this heterogeneous syndrome, was developed in 1979 by an international workgroup sponsored by the National Diabetes Data Group (NDDG) of the National Institutes of Health, USA [1, 2]. The World Health Organization (WHO) Expert Committee on Diabetes in 1980 and later the WHO Study Group on Diabetes Mellitus endorsed the substantive recommendations of the NDDG [3, 4]. These groups recognized two major forms of diabetes in Western countries, insulin dependent diabetes mellitus (IDDM, type 1 diabetes) and non-insulin dependent diabetes mellitus (NIDDM, type 2 diabetes).

Credit for the initial recognition that diabetes is not a single disorder rests with two Indian physicians, Chakrata and Susruta (600 BC), who differentiated two forms of the disease, although most of the descriptions in the classic literature probably relate to what we know today as IDDM. During the eighteenth and nineteenth centuries, a less clinically symptomatic variety of the disorder, identified by marked glycosuria, often detected in later life and commonly associated with overweight rather than wasting, was noted which today is recognized as NIDDM. In the twentieth century, when screening programs for diabetes commenced, it became apparent that there were many people who could be classified as having diabetes but who were generally 'asymptomatic'. It has become apparent subsequently that the term diabetes mellitus covers a wide spectrum of disease, from the acute and sometimes explosive onset of IDDM to asymptomatic individuals whose NIDDM is discovered by accident.

In the mid-1930s, Himsworth [6] proposed that there were at least two clinical types of diabetes, insulin-sensitive and insulin-insensitive, the former being due to insulin deficiency. Confirmation of his clinical observations came with Bornstein's development of a bioassay for insulin [7], and when radioimmunoassay for

International Textbook of Diabetes Mellitus, Second Edition. Edited by K.G.M.M. Alberti, P. Zimmet, R.A. DeFronzo, and H. Keen (Honorary)
© 1997 John Wiley & Sons Ltd

Table 1 Classification of diabetes mellitus and other categories of glucose intolerance

Class.	Former terminology	Associated factors	Characteristics
Insulin dependent diabetes mellitus (IDDM, type 1)	Juvenile diabetes, juvenile-onset diabetes, juvenile-onset type diabetes, JOD, ketosis-prone diabetes, brittle diabetes	Evidence regarding etiology suggests genetic and environmental or acquired factors, association with certain HLA types, and abnormal immune responses, including autoimmune reactions	Persons in this subclass are dependent on injected insulin to prevent ketosis and to preserve life, although there may be preketotic, non-insulin-dependent phases in the natural history of the disease. In the preponderance of cases, onset is in youth, but IDDM may occur at any age. Characterized by insulinopenia. Islet cell and GAD antibodies are frequently present at diagnosis in this type
Non-insulin dependent diabetes mellitus (NIDDM, type 2) (a) Non-obese (b) Obese	Adult-onset diabetes, maturity-onset diabetes, maturity-onset type diabetes, MOD, ketosis-resistant diabetes, stable diabetes	There are probably multiple etiologies for this class, the common outcome being derangement of carbohydrate metabolism. Evidence on familial aggregation of diabetes implies genetic factors, and this class includes diabetes presenting in children and adults in which autosomal dominant inheritance has been clearly established (formerly termed the MODY type, maturity-onset diabetes in the young). Environmental factors superimposed on genetic susceptibility are probably involved in the onset of the NIDDM types. Obesity is suspected as an etiologic factor and is recommended as a criterion for dividing NIDDM into two subclasses, according to the presence or absence of obesity	Persons in this subclass are not insulin-dependent or ketosis-prone, although they may use insulin for correction of symptomatic or persistent hyperglycemia and they can develop ketosis under special circumstances, such as episodes of infection or stress. Serum insulin levels may be normal, elevated, or depressed. In the preponderance of cases, onset is after age 40, but NIDDM is known to occur at all ages. About 60–90% of NIDDM subjects are obese and constitute a subtype of NIDDM; in these patients, glucose tolerance is often improved by weight loss. Hyperinsulinemia and insulin resistance characterize most patients in this subtype
Malnutrition-related diabetes mellitus (MRDM) (a) Fibrocalculous pancreatic diabetes (b) Protein-deficient pancreatic diabetes	Tropical diabetes, pancreatic diabetes, ketosis-resistant diabetes of the young	Occurs in tropical developing countries, in which young diabetics often present with a history of nutritional deficiency and a constellation of symptoms, signs and metabolic characteristics which fail to meet the criteria used to classify IDDM and NIDDM. Distinctive clinical features and coarse, uncertain etiology and pathophysiology	Characterized by stone formation in the main pancreatic duct and its branches, together with extensive fibrosis of the pancreas Characterized by ketosis resistance, insulin resistance, extreme degrees of wasting and emaciation, onset of symptoms before age 35; pancreatic calcification and fibrosis are absent

Gestational diabetes (GDM)	Gestational diabetes	Glucose tolerance with onset during pregnancy is thought to be due to complex metabolic and hormonal changes which are incompletely understood. Insulin resistance may be responsible in part for gestational diabetes	Glucose intolerance that has its onset or recognition during pregnancy. Thus, diabetics who become pregnant are not included in this class. Associated with increased perinatal complications and with increased risk for progression to diabetes within 5–10 years after parturition. Requires reclassification after pregnancy terminates into PrevAGT, DM or IGT
Other types of diabetes, including diabetes associated with certain conditions and syndromes: (a) Pancreatic disease (b) Hormonal (c) Drug or chemical induced (d) Insulin receptor abnormalities (e) Certain genetic syndromes	Secondary diabetes	This subclass contains a variety of types of diabetes, in some of which the etiologic relationship is known (e.g. diabetes secondary to pancreatic disease, endocrine disease or administration of certain drugs). In others, an etiologic relationship is suspected because of a higher frequency of association of diabetes with a syndrome or condition (e.g. a number of the genetic syndromes). See Table 2 for a list of these conditions and syndromes	In addition to the presence of the specific condition or syndrome, diabetes mellitus is also present
Impaired glucose tolerance (IGT) (a) Non-obese IGT (b) Obese IGT (c) IGT associated with pancreatic disease, hormonal conditions; drug- or chemical-induced, insulin receptor abnormalities, certain genetic syndromes	Asymptomatic diabetes, chemical diabetes, subclinical diabetes, borderline diabetes, latent diabetes	Mild glucose intolerance in subjects in this class may be attributable to normal variation of glucose tolerance within a population. In some subjects, IGT may represent a stage in the development of NIDDM or IDDM although the majority of persons with IGT remain in this class for many years or return to normal glucose tolerance	Non-diabetic fasting glucose levels and glucose intolerance of a degree between normal and diabetic. Some studies have shown increased prevalence of arterial disease symptoms and electrocardiographic abnormalities and increased susceptibility to atherosclerotic disease associated with known risk factors including hypertension, hyperlipidemia, adiposity and age. Clinically significant renal and retinal complications of diabetes are absent

(continued overleaf)

Table 1 (*continued*)

Class	Former terminology	Associated factors/Characteristics
Previous abnormality of glucose tolerance (PrevAGT)	Latent diabetes, prediabetes	This class is restricted to those persons who now have normal glucose tolerance but who have previously demonstrated diabetic hyperglycemia or impaired glucose tolerance, either spontaneously or in response to an identifiable stimulus. Individuals who have been gestational diabetics and returned to normal glucose tolerance after parturition form an obvious subclass of PrevAGT. Another small but important group of individuals in this class are former obese diabetics whose glucose tolerance has returned to normal after losing weight. Clinical studies have shown that many patients under acute metabolic stress due to trauma or injury experience transient hyperglycemia. Apart from studies of former gestational diabetics, there has been little systematic investigation of the later liability of persons who have exhibited glucose intolerance to develop diabetes. However, it is likely that this is increased and that there is utility in including all those with a history of glucose intolerance, now normal, in this PrevAGT class
Potential abnormality of glucose tolerance (PotAGT)	Prediabetes, potential diabetes	This class includes persons who have never exhibited abnormal glucose tolerance but who are at substantially increased risk for the development of diabetes. Individuals who are at increased risk for IDDM include (in decreasing order of risk): persons with islet cell antibodies; monozygotic twin of an IDDM diabetic; sib of an IDDM diabetic, especially one with identical HLA haplotypes; offspring of an IDDM diabetic. Individuals who are at increased risk for NIDDM include (in decreasing order of risk): monozygotic twin of a NIDDM diabetic; first-degree relative of a NIDDM diabetic (sib, parent or offspring); mother of a neonate weighing more than 4 kg; obese individuals; members of racial or ethnic groups with a high prevalence of diabetes, e.g. a number of American Indian tribes. The degree of risk for many of these circumstances is not well established as yet

insulin became available a decade later [8], Bornstein's observations were confirmed. The widespread acceptance of the terms 'juvenile-onset' and 'maturity-onset' diabetes at this time was affirmation of the concept that there were at least two major forms of the disease.

The NDDG/WHO classification system incorporated data from research conducted during the previous several decades, which clearly established that diabetes mellitus is an etiologically and clinically heterogeneous group of disorders that share glucose intolerance in common. The evidence in favor of this heterogeneity is overwhelming and includes the following: (a) there are many distinct disorders, most of which are individually rare, in which glucose intolerance is a feature; (b) there are large differences in prevalence of the major forms of diabetes among various racial or ethnic groups worldwide; (c) glucose intolerance presents with variable clinical features, for example the differences between thin, ketosis-prone, insulin-dependent diabetes and obese, non-ketotic, insulin-resistant diabetes; (d) genetic, immunologic and clinical studies show that, in Western countries, the forms of diabetes with their onset primarily in youth or in adulthood are distinct entities; and (e) a type of non-insulin-requiring diabetes in young people, which is inherited in an autosomal dominant fashion, is clearly different from the classic acute-onset diabetes of juveniles; (f) in tropical countries, several clinical presentations occur, including fibrocalcific pancreatitis and malnutrition-related diabetes. These and other collective evidence have been used in Table 1 to divide diabetes mellitus into four distinct types, in each of which subtypes have been identified.

Table 1 presents certain salient features associated with each class and highlights the different clinical presentations and genetic and environmental etiologic factors that permit discrimination among the types of diabetes. The classification includes four types of diabetes mellitus, all of which are characterized by either fasting, hyperglycemia or levels of plasma glucose during an oral glucose tolerance test (OGTT) above defined limits (see Chapter 2 for diagnostic criteria). In addition, it includes the category 'impaired glucose tolerance' (IGT), in which plasma glucose levels during an OGTT lie above normal but below those defined as diabetes. Finally, the classification includes high risk classes that may be part of the natural history of diabetes but in which there currently are no abnormalities of glucose tolerance, namely, 'previous abnormality of glucose tolerance' and 'potential abnormality of glucose tolerance'.

The classification highlights the marked heterogeneity of the diabetic syndrome. Such heterogeneity has important implications not only for clinical management of diabetes but also for biomedical research. Thus,

it indicates that the distinct disorders grouped together under the rubric 'diabetes' differ markedly in pathogenesis, natural history and responses to therapy and preventive measures. In addition, it demonstrates that different genetic and environmental etiologic factors can result in similar diabetic phenotypes.

The scheme in Table 1 serves as a useful model for categorizing patients and determining appropriate treatment modalities for individuals who have been diagnosed as having diabetes. In addition, the classification is being used as a uniform framework for conducting clinical and epidemiologic research, so that more meaningful and comparable data can be obtained internationally on the scope and impact of the various forms of diabetes and other categories of glucose intolerance.

The classification is based on current knowledge of diabetes and also represents some compromises of different points of view. It is a mixture of clinical manifestations (e.g. insulin-dependent, non-insulin-dependent) and etiopathogenesis (e.g. malnutrition-related, gestational). Despite such anomalies, it works reasonably well in practice but, as knowledge of diabetes continues to develop with future research advances, it is likely that the classification will be revised. For example, a definitive etiology is not well established for any of the diabetes subclasses. However, it is anticipated that genetic markers for diabetes will be discovered which will provide a sounder basis for classifying patients into the various types of diabetes and for establishing the occurrence of a prediabetic or diabetes-susceptible state in a subject. It is also anticipated that further heterogeneity in both etiology and pathogenesis that can be ascribed to specific factors will be demonstrated. These research advances may allow separation of diabetes and glucose intolerance and their predecessor stages into even more types than those shown in Table 1. They will also permit more refined definitions of specific subtypes of diabetes based on etiopathologic grounds.

The final word with respect to the classification of diabetes is still to come, and neither the NDDG nor the WHO expert groups discounted this possibility. Research into diabetes is continuing and dynamic, and epidemiological and clinical studies are emerging which will permit revision and refinement of the classification system.

INSULIN DEPENDENT DIABETES MELLITUS

This subclass of diabetes, insulin dependent diabetes mellitus (IDDM) or type 1 diabetes, is generally characterized by abrupt onset of severe symptoms, dependence on exogenous insulin to sustain life, and proneness to ketosis even in the basal state, all of which are caused by absolute insulin deficiency (insulinopenia). IDDM is the most prevalent type of diabetes among children and young adults in developed countries, and it was formerly termed 'juvenile diabetes'. However, classification based on age at onset has been discontinued, since clinical onset can occur at any age. Onset of IDDM in adult subjects is not uncommon. In Minnesota, USA, 32% of subjects with IDDM had been diagnosed after the age of 30 years [10]. In Finland, 15% of IDDM subjects were in this older-onset group [11]. In New Zealand, as many as 14.4% of adults with diabetes were insulin treated and most of these (83%) had commenced insulin as permanent treatment within 12 months of diagnosis [5].

All of the characteristics of IDDM mentioned above can be attributed to the diminution of insulin-secretory capacity associated with destruction of pancreatic B cells as a result of autoimmunity. IDDM should not be confused with malnutrition-related diabetes in which the etiology may be ascribed to specific environmental, nutritional and toxic factors that act directly on the pancreas. The etiology of IDDM is still unclear, but the disease appears to be a heterogeneous category in that it is associated with various genetic and environmental factors [12], and as evidenced by the wide variability of its occurrence. The incidence of IDDM is highest in Scandinavia, with more than 30 cases/year/100 000 persons, of medium incidence in Europe and the USA (approximately 10–15 cases/year/100 000), and lowest in Oriental groups (0.5 cases/year/100 000) and populations living in the tropics [13]. It appears to be virtually absent in some populations, e.g. North American Indians and Pacific Islanders. Genetic determinants are important risk factors for IDDM, in particular certain histocompatibility antigens (HLA) located on chromosome 6. Recently, several other genes have been implicated, although with a much smaller contribution to risk than the HLA antigens [41]. In Europe and North America, about 95% of young IDDM patients have either HLA DR3, or DR4, or both, compared to only about 20% of the general population [14, 15]. The strongest associations have been described with the DQB region [42]. However, concordance rates for identical twins are about 35–50%, well below the rate required if genetic factors were the only determinants of the disease, although rates reach 70% for twin pairs who have both DR3 and DR4 [16]. Some evidence indicates that IDDM might be distinguished by the type of HLA present. Thus, HLA DR3 appears to be associated with a more slowly progressive form of the disease [17] and some evidence suggests that onset of IDDM in HLA DR3-positive cases is not seasonal [18]. Abnormal immune responses and autoimmunity play an etiologic role, and multiple immunologic abnormalities have been found in patients with IDDM [19]. In particular, islet cell antibodies are frequently present at diagnosis in this type of diabetes. Often as many as 70% of newly diagnosed patients have islet-cell antibodies, compared with only 3% of age- and sex-matched controls [20, 21]. Insulin autoantibodies have also been found in increased frequency in newly diagnosed IDDM patients before the institution of insulin therapy [22]. Antibodies to glutamic acid decarboxylase (GAD) have been detected up to 8 years before diagnosis [66] and are present in 75% of newly diagnosed IDDM subjects [67]. IDDM has a seasonal incidence, with a diagnosis peak occurring in the winter months in many studies. However, no such peak was found in patients living in an urban area in the USA, in contrast to the seasonality found in rural cases of IDDM [23]. Partly because of seasonality, viral infections have been implicated as possible initiators of the autoimmune process in the etiology of IDDM. However, many of the circumstances surrounding onset of IDDM may simply reflect the end stage in a long pathogenetic process, since islet cell antibodies, insulin antibodies, and antibodies to GAD can be present months or even years before onset in persons who develop IDDM. A further characteristic, which is a consequence of deficient insulin synthesis, is the relative absence of C-peptide, a by-product of the production of insulin from proinsulin. All of these characteristics may be used to place an individual in the IDDM class, namely: insulin deficiency; low levels of C-peptide; presence of islet cell, insulin and GAD antibodies; presence of HLA DQB; and association with an infectious process. In the absence of these measurements, allocation to the IDDM class depends on clinical judgement supported by evidence of ketosis, absence of obesity, and consistent insulin use since onset of diabetes.

At times, classification may need to be made after onset of IDDM by reference to the clinical record. If the record shows clear evidence of ketosis and/or the patient has required insulin consistently since diagnosis apart from relatively short breaks, assignment to the IDDM class may be made. Problems in classification may arise when a newly-diagnosed patient goes into temporary remission and may cease using insulin for weeks to months (the 'honeymoon period'). This remission is often part of the natural history of IDDM, but the clinical situation inevitably progresses to relapse with absolute requirement for insulin. A confusing situation is the patient who appears to have NIDDM but fails to respond adequately to diet and/or oral antidiabetic therapy and is placed on insulin to achieve adequate metabolic control. When that patient is obese, is not ketonuric and may have stopped insulin for periods without experiencing ketosis, the condition is unlikely to represent IDDM. However, for less obese patients who are treated with insulin for control of symptoms or hyperglycemia, the proper classification may be less clear, and there may be a small group of unassignable patients in whom insulin dependency is uncertain. This category has been variously labeled as 'type $1\frac{1}{2}$' diabetes [9] and 'latent autoimmune diabetes in adults' [68] and is discussed in more detail below.

NON-INSULIN DEPENDENT DIABETES MELLITUS

This subclass of diabetes, non-insulin dependent diabetes mellitus (NIDDM) or type 2 diabetes, greatly outnumbers all other forms of diabetes. In Western countries it constitutes approximately 90% of all cases of diabetes and, in certain groups such as North American Indians and populations in the South Pacific, it is virtually the only form of diabetes [69]. In contrast to IDDM, patients with NIDDM are not dependent on exogenous insulin for prevention of ketonuria and are not prone to ketosis. However, they may require insulin for correction of fasting hyperglycemia if this cannot be achieved with the use of diet or oral agents, and they may develop ketosis under special circumstances such as severe stress precipitated by infections or trauma. In the basal state there may be normal levels of insulin, mild insulinopenia, or above normal levels of insulin associated with insulin resistance. In response to a glucose or meal challenge, a range of insulin levels from low to supranormal has been found in the group of diabetics in this subclass.

Although diagnosis in most patients with NIDDM is made in adult years, the disease also occurs in young persons who do not require insulin and are not ketotic, and hence could not be considered to have IDDM. In addition, the age at diagnosis of NIDDM now tends to occur much earlier in high prevalence groups such as North American Indians and Pacific Islanders [70]. Consequently, age at onset is not recommended as a criterion by which to determine whether a patient should be classified as NIDDM, and the previously used terms 'adult-onset' and 'maturity-onset' diabetes have been abandoned. Although some NIDDM patients may be treated with insulin, this alone does not indicate that they should be classified as having developed IDDM. Complete insulin deficiency, characteristic of persons with IDDM, is thought to develop in only about 3% of patients with NIDDM [24]. However, two studies suggest that as many as 20% of subjects who present initially with NIDDM may have slowly-progressive IDDM [68, 71].

Although the etiology of NIDDM is unclear, the disease has a strong genetic basis, as evidenced by the frequent familial pattern of occurrence, its high prevalence in certain ethnic groups, and genetic admixture studies. Identical twins have been particularly important in establishing the influence of genetic factors in the etiology of NIDDM. About half of co-twins of persons with NIDDM develop NIDDM themselves, and the discordance indicates that environmental factors are also involved in the etiology of NIDDM [16, 25]. Included in NIDDM are persons with maturity onset diabetes of youth (MODY), which occurs in families in which NIDDM is inherited in an autosomal dominant fashion, even in children and young adults [27]. While NIDDM is strongly associated with genetic factors, it is undoubtedly heterogeneous in its etiology, since a variety of lifestyle and environmental factors have been identified as being risk factors for the condition. Nevertheless, except for specific mutations to key enzymes in rare syndromes of familial diabetes, the rare mitochondrial DNA point mutations [72], and the link between some MODY families and mutations to the glucokinase gene in liver and islet B cells [73], the gene(s) causing most cases of NIDDM remain obscure.

In all probability the causes of NIDDM lie in environmental and lifestyle factors superimposed on genetic susceptibility. Prominent among these factors is obesity, and about 50–90% of all NIDDM patients are obese. However, a portion remain non-obese, and because of this disparity the NIDDM subclass has been divided according to whether or not obesity is present. The definition of obesity is complex and no satisfactory index of obesity has been devised. However, it has been shown that, of measures employing height and weight, the body mass index [BMI, weight (kg) divided by height^2 (m^2)] has the highest correlation with both skinfold thickness and body density. In addition, BMI is linearly related to the index of percentage desirable weight (PDW). The latter has been endorsed by several international conferences on obesity [28] as the recommended standard for weight in relation to height. A PDW of 120% corresponds to a BMI of 27 for men and 25 for women, and values equal to or greater than these have been recommended as the criteria for obesity. A strong association between upper body obesity (central obesity) and NIDDM prevalence and incidence [74] has been demonstrated. Some studies have determined that intra-abdominal (rather than central subcutaneous) fat is the important site conveying enhanced risk for NIDDM [75]. Many international groups are now attempting to define the levels of risk associated with various levels of waist:hip ratio and other indices of abdominal obesity.

HETEROGENEITY IN THE CLINICAL COURSE OF IDDM AND NIDDM

A situation sometimes encountered is the individual who presents clinically with NIDDM, yet within a year or so is insulin-dependent. Conversely, individuals who appeared at first to have IDDM may lose their insulin dependence. How do such individuals fit into the current classification? In short, they do not, and there appears to be a 'gray zone' between IDDM and NIDDM.

The former situation has been labeled provisionally as 'type $1\frac{1}{2}$' diabetes. It is clear that IDDM can occur after a prolonged period of what is clinically suggestive of and accepted as NIDDM [29, 30]. Presenting with typical clinical NIDDM features, these individuals can be treated with diet alone, or with diet and oral hypoglycemic agents, for up to several years before progressing to insulin dependency. This subgroup has distinctive immunologic and metabolic features which distinguish its members from NIDDM subjects [29, 76]. Thus, among a group of adults with non-ketotic diabetes who were treated with diet or oral hypoglycemic agents for at least 1 year after diagnosis, 14% had islet cell antibodies (ICA) and lower C-peptide levels which showed little increase after glucagon stimulation [31]. During 2 years of follow-up, islet B-cell function deteriorated significantly in 41% of the ICA-positive patients and a larger proportion required insulin. These patients were suggested to have 'latent' IDDM, characterized by persistent ICA, progressive loss of B cells, and a high frequency of thyrogastric autoimmunity. Furthermore, there was an excess frequency of HLA DR3 and DR4 in these subjects, confirming an earlier report [32]. Measurement of antibodies to GAD has provided further strength to the hypothesis that this group belongs to the IDDM category [68]. Patients who had initially been non-ketotic and non-insulin-dependent for ≥ 6 months were classified according to glucagon-stimulated C-peptide levels into an insulin-deficient group and a non-insulin-deficient group. Anti-GAD occurred in 76% of the insulin-deficient group compared with 12% of the non-insulin-deficient group. Thus, in a proportion of adults who present with NIDDM, a slowly evolving autoimmune insulitis can be revealed by testing for anti-GAD. This could have important implications not only for the correct classification of diabetes but also for early intervention. These patients clearly cannot be defined by the current NDDG and WHO classifications but will need to be recognized if further studies confirm these findings. The name 'latent autoimmune diabetes in adults' (LADA) has been suggested [68].

In regard to the clinical presentation of IDDM progressing to NIDDM, an atypical form of diabetes in young Afro-Americans which presents as IDDM has been described [33]. Insulin dependence was transient, and the subsequent clinical course was typical of NIDDM. Clinical, familial, immunologic, genetic and metabolic features distinguish this group from classically defined IDDM, and it is more akin to maturity onset diabetes of youth (MODY) [27]. This is supported by the autosomal dominant inheritance demonstrated in family studies and, on the basis of available evidence, these subjects could be categorized within the NIDDM subclass. A similar form of diabetes has been reported in young Indians in India [34] and another group of Afro-Americans in New York [77]. Again, the clinical features are the same as MODY and are distinct from those of malnutrition-related diabetes mellitus which is frequent in Indian diabetics, and these subjects could be classified as NIDDM. By contrast, young ketosis-prone insulin-dependent diabetic subjects have been described in East Africa in whom virtually none have autoimmune markers [78]. Clearly, attention will need to be given to this area when an expert group next considers classification of diabetes.

It has been suggested that basal serum C-peptide and/or stimulated C-peptide (post-glucose or post-glucagon) can be used to discriminate between IDDM and NIDDM and thus aid in classification of diabetes. Fasting C-peptide level was used to confirm the classification of patients into IDDM and NIDDM in 94.5% of diabetic subjects [35]. In the remaining subjects, 73% were receiving insulin therapy, and they may represent the group who can be categorized as 'type $1\frac{1}{2}$' diabetes. A study of Europid IDDM subjects and Pima Indians with NIDDM support these findings [36]. Similarly, fasting and post-glucagon C-peptide concentration are both able to distinguish IDDM and NIDDM subjects [37]. It is likely that a combination of C-peptide and antibodies to GAD will provide even better discrimination. These findings highlight the need for a review of the classification of diabetes within the next few years.

MALNUTRITION-RELATED DIABETES MELLITUS (MRDM)

The 1985 WHO Study Group on Diabetes [3] elevated the heterogeneous syndrome generally known as tropical diabetes from the 'other types' category to an independent entity with the name malnutrition-related diabetes mellitus (MRDM). This has not been without debate and the comment has been made that 'the latest WHO Study Group on Diabetes report has raised these variants from "other types" to a single entity, "malnutrition related diabetes" which automatically legitimizes what may yet prove to be a child or children of indeterminate origin' [38]. There are a number of comprehensive reviews on this form of diabetes [38, 39, 40, 79, 80, 81] as well as a chapter in this volume (Chapter 9, Diabetes in the Tropics).

The term MRDM covers the variety of types known previously as tropical diabetes, pancreatogenic diabetes, endocrine pancreatic syndrome and ketosis-resistant diabetes of the young [3]. There are at least two subclasses—fibrocalculous pancreatic diabetes and protein-deficient pancreatic diabetes [39]. In both subclasses, the subjects are inhabitants of relatively poor tropical countries, are characteristically underweight or emaciated, and have clinical signs of present or past malnutrition and other dietary deficiency states. A history of cassava ingestion is often present. Three major features appear to distinguish the fibrocalculous form:

(a) Recurrent attacks of abdominal pain often extending back to childhood.

(b) Pancreatic fibrosis and calcification.

(c) Clinical evidence of pancreatic endocrine and exocrine malfunction.

Several comprehensive reviews highlight the apparent magnitude of the problem [39, 79, 80]. There is a strong case for more detailed epidemiologic studies on the prevalence, incidence and global distribution of this syndrome in order to assess its true magnitude [3], particularly to confirm whether the syndrome's importance justifies its newly elevated status.

MRDM remains a controversial area [79]. A new set of diagnostic criteria have been proposed by the combined Kobe/Suribaya team [81]. They recommend exocrine pancreatic deficiency, rather than malnutrition, as the pathognomonic feature of this form of diabetes. Familial aggregation has been described and a genetic basis has thus been attributed, but in this situation it is difficult to exclude environmental factors shared by family members.

OTHER TYPES OF DIABETES

This subclass, which is discussed in detail in Chapters 10 and 11, is numerically small and etiologically very heterogeneous, since diabetes can be associated with a variety of other conditions and syndromes. In certain instances, abnormal glucose tolerance is secondary to the condition (e.g. specific endocrine diseases), whereas in others the relationship is apparently causal but not yet explained (e.g. certain genetic syndromes). On this basis, the subclass is defined according to the known or presumed etiologic relationship or the strong association with other conditions. These conditions are listed in Table 2, which shows that diabetes may be secondary to (a) pancreatic disease

or removal of pancreatic tissue, (b) endocrine diseases such as acromegaly, Cushing's syndrome, pheochromocytoma, glucagonoma, somatostatinoma and primary aldosteronism, or (c) the administration of certain hormones, drugs (e.g. thiazide diuretics, corticosteroids) and chemicals that cause hyperglycemia. Diabetes may also be associated with rare amino acid substitutions in the insulin molecule and with defects of insulin action caused by abnormalities in number or affinity of insulin receptors, or by antibodies to receptors with or without associated immune disorders. Diabetes (or glucose intolerance) is found in increased frequency with a large number of genetic syndromes (see Chapter 3, Genetics of Diabetes). The heterogeneity of the diabetic syndrome is clearly illustrated by the variety of conditions listed in Table 2 with which glucose intolerance is associated.

Gestational Diabetes (GDM)

This class is restricted to pregnant women in whom the onset or recognition of diabetes or IGT first occurs during pregnancy. Thus, diabetic women who become pregnant are not included in this class. After parturition, a woman who had GDM must be reclassified, either into diabetes mellitus or IGT, if postpartum plasma glucose levels meet the criteria for those classes, or into previous abnormality of glucose tolerance (PrevAGT). In the majority of gestational diabetics, glucose tolerance becomes more normal postpartum [43] and the subject can be reclassified as PrevAGT. However, lifetime risk for impaired glucose tolerance and NIDDM is substantially increased in women who have had GDM [44, 82].

GDM is found in about 3–5% of unselected pregnancies in Western countries. Age is the single most reliable correlate of abnormal OGTT in pregnancy, and the incidence of GDM appears to be no higher in patients selected on the basis of several potential risk factors, including prior macrosomic infant or prior pregnancy loss, once age is considered [83, 84]. Clinical recognition of GDM is important because, when the hyperglycemia is not effectively treated, offspring are at increased risk of macrosomia and perinatal mortality, although congenital anomalies appear to be no more frequent than in pregnancies of women with normal glucose tolerance [45, 85, 86].

Serious questions about the association of glucose intolerance with pregnancy, and whether GDM should even be considered a separate entity, have been raised by a number of reports. Several studies found that abnormalities of glucose tolerance and insulin secretion exist in patients for months or even years after pregnancy [46, 47]. The proportion of young, non-pregnant women who meet criteria for GDM is similar to the proportion of pregnant women meeting these

Table 2   Conditions and syndromes associated with diabetes mellitus and impaired glucose tolerance*

1. *Pancreatic Disease*
   (a) Neonatal
       Congenital absence of the pancreatic islets
       Transient diabetes of the newborn
       Functional immaturity of insulin secretion
       Converse of infants of diabetic mothers
   (b) Postinfancy
       Acquired—traumatic, infectious, toxic,
           neoplastic
       Inherited—cystic fibrosis, hereditary relapsing
           pancreatitis, hemochromatosis

2. *Hormonal*
   (a) Hypoinsulinemic
       Endocrine overactivity
           Catecholamines, e.g. pheochromocytoma
           Somatostatinoma
           Mineralocorticoids, e.g. aldosteronoma
       Underactivity
           Hypoparathyroidism—hypocalcemia
           Type-1 isolated growth hormone deficiency
           Multitropic pituitary deficiency
           Laron dwarfism
           Hypothalamic lesions—'piqûre' diabetes (of
               Claude Bernard)
   (b) Hyperinsulinemic—states of insulin resistance
       Overactivity
           Glucocorticoids
           Progestins and estrogens
           Growth hormone—acromegaly
           Glucagon
       Underactivity
           Type-2 isolated growth hormone deficiency

3. *Drugs and Chemical Agents†*
   (a) Diuretics and antihypertensive agents
       Chlorthalidone (Hygroton, Combipres,
           Regroton)
       Clonidine (Catapres, Combipres)
       Diazoxide (Hyperstat, Proglycem)
       Furosemide (Lasix)
       Metalazone
       Thiazides (several forms, many trade names)
       ‡   Bumetamide
       ‡   Clopamide
       ‡   Clorexolone
       ‡   Ethacrynic acid (Edecrin)
           (Note: hyperglycemic response to diuretics may
           be independent of K^+ fluctuations)
   (b) Hormonally active agents
       Adrenocorticotropin (Acthar)
       ‡   Tetracosactrin
       Glucagon
       Glucocorticoids (natural and synthetic)
       Oral contraceptives
       Somatotropin
       Thyroid hormones (thyrotoxic doses)
           Dextrothyroxine (Choloxin)
       ‡   Calcitonin (Calcimar)
       ‡   Medroxyprogesterone (AMEN, Depo-Provera,
           Provera)
       ‡   Prolactin

Drugs and Chemical Agents (continued).
   (c) Psychoactive agents
       Chlorprothixene (Teractan)
       Haloperidol (Haldol)
       Lithium carbonate (Eskalith, Lithane, others)
       Phenothiazines
           Chlorpromazine (Thorazine)
           Perphenazine (Trilafon, Etrafon, Triavil)
       ‡   Clopenthixol
       Tricyclic Antidepressants
           Amitriptyline (Elavil, Endep, Etrafon,
               Triavil)
           Desipramine (Norpramin, Pertofran)
           Doxepin (Adapin, Sinequan)
           Imipramine (Presamine, Tofranil, Imavate)
           Nortriptyline (Aventyl)
       ‡   Marijuana
   (d) Catecholamines and other neurologically active
       agents
       Diphenylhydantoin (Dilantin)
       Epinephrine (Adrenalin Chloride, Asthma-
           Meter, Sus-Phrine)
       Isoproterenol (Isuprel)
       Levodopa (Bendopa, Dopar, Larodopa,
           Sinemet)
       Norepinephrine (levarterenol, Levophed)
       ‡   Buphenine (Nylidrin)
       ‡   Fenoterol
       ‡   Propranolol (Inderal)
   (e) Analgesic, antipyretic, and anti-inflammatory
       agents
       Indomethacin (Indocin)
       ‡   Acetaminophen (overdose amounts) (Tylenol,
           Nebs, others)
       ‡   Aspirin (overdose amounts)
       ‡   Morphine
   (f) Antineoplastic agents
       Alloxan
       L-asparaginase
       Streptozotocin
       ‡   Cyclophosphamide (Cytoxan)
       ‡   Megestrol Acetate (Megace)
   (g) Miscellaneous
       Isoniazid (INAH, Nydrazid, others)
       Nicotinic acid (Cerebro-Nicin, Nicobid, others)
       ‡   Carbon disulfide
       ‡   Cimetidine
       ‡   Edetic acid (EDTA)
       ‡   Ethanol
       ‡   Heparin
       ‡   Mannoheptulose
       ‡   Nalidixic acid (NegGram)
       ‡   Nickel chloride
       ‡   Niridazole
       ‡   Pentamidine (Lomidine)
       ‡   Phenolphthalein (Ex-Lax)
       ‡   Rodenticide (Vacor)
       ‡   Thiabendazole
4. *Insulin Receptor Abnormalities*
   (a) Defect in insulin receptor
       Congenital lipodystrophy
       Associated with virilization, acanthosis
           nigricans

Table 2 (*continued*)

(b) Antibody to insulin receptor-associated immune disorders	Friedreich's ataxia
5. *Genetic Syndromes*	Alstrom's syndrome
(a) Inborn errors of metabolism	Laurence–Moon–Biedl syndrome
Glycogen-storage disease type 1	Retinopathy, hypogonadism, mental retardation, nerve deafness
Acute intermittent porphyria	Pseudo-Refsum's syndrome
Hyperlipidemia	(d) Progeroid syndrome
Hyperglycerolemia	Cockayne's syndrome
(b) Insulin-resistant syndromes	Werner syndrome
Ataxia telangiectasia	(e) Syndromes with glucose intolerance secondary to obesity
Myotonic dystrophy	Prader–Willi syndrome
Mendenhall's syndrome	Achondroplasia
Lipoatrophic syndromes	(f) Miscellaneous
(c) Hereditary neuromuscular disorders	Steroid-induced ocular hypertension
Optic atrophy, diabetes mellitus, diabetes insipidus, nerve deafness	Epiphyseal dysplasia and infantile onset diabetes
Muscular dystrophies	(g) Cytogenetic disorders
Late-onset proximal myopathy	Down's syndrome
Huntington's chorea	Turner's syndrome
Machado's disease	Klinefelter's syndrome
Herrman syndrome	

*It is acknowledged that this list is not all-inclusive, and it is anticipated that it will change with future research advances.

†For many of these agents, it cannot be determined now whether the hyperglycemic response represents solely a pharmacologic action or is an interaction between a predisposition for abnormal glucose tolerance and the pharmacologic effects of the agent. Drugs exacerbating pre-existing diabetes have been excluded from this list. A number of agents shown to cause hyperglycemia in animals but with no reported effect in humans also are not listed.

‡Association not clearly established for one of the following reasons: (1) confounded by the simultaneous administration of other drugs; (2) limited to a single case report; (3) conflicting or contradictory evidence; (4) drug has been reported to cause interference with laboratory test for serum glucose.

criteria (3–5%), indicating that GDM may not be etiologically related to pregnancy but simply represents pre-existing glucose intolerance that is detected during the metabolic testing that normally accompanies prenatal care [48]. This area clearly deserves further research and close scrutiny when the diabetes classification system undergoes future review.

DIFFICULTIES IN ASSIGNMENT OF A PATIENT TO A SUBCLASS OF DIABETES

Each of the subtypes of diabetes described above has characteristics that distinguish it from the others. A thorough investigation of each patient should precede assignment of that individual to a particular subclass of diabetes. This process goes hand-in-hand with determining the most appropriate therapy for the particular type of diabetes. However, when presented with a patient who has previously been diagnosed as having diabetes, it may be difficult to assign that individual to one subclass because inadequate information has been obtained on the clinical characteristics of the patient. Thus, distinguishing between an IDDM patient and a thin NIDDM patient who has been prescribed insulin may require stopping insulin therapy and monitoring the course of their disease, which may not be feasible. On the other hand, antibodies to GAD may discriminate this group in about 75% of cases and, unlike islet cell autoantibodies (ICA) and anti-insulin antibodies (IAA), the GAD antibodies may persist for over 20 years after diagnosis of diabetes [67]. The tests and measurements used to determine whether a patient has diabetes secondary to some other condition may not have been done, and without this information some patients may be incorrectly classified as IDDM or NIDDM when they have diabetes secondary to another condition. Further, there are stages in the natural history of each type of diabetes that mimic features of the other types, e.g. the remission phase of IDDM or the ketonuria a NIDDM patient develops under metabolic stress. If these discrete stages are considered alone rather than in the context of the historical progression of the diseases, misclassifications may result. In addition, there will on occasion be patients whose plasma glucose levels in the fasting state or after an oral glucose challenge have been improperly measured or are equivocal, such that they do not meet the required criteria for diabetes (see Chapter 2). In each of these situations, classification should be held in abeyance until adequate clinical and diagnostic information is obtained.

IMPAIRED GLUCOSE TOLERANCE (IGT)

Several longitudinal research studies have provided the scientific basis for defining the condition termed impaired glucose tolerance (IGT), in which plasma glucose levels are intermediate between those considered normal and those considered to be diabetic. To designate persons as having IGT, their fasting plasma glucose concentration must be less than that required for a diagnosis of diabetes (i.e. < 140 mg/dl,

< 7.8 mmol/l) and their plasma glucose response during the OGTT must be intermediate between normal and diabetic (140–199 mg/dl, 7.8–11.0 mmol/l). Thus, the IGT class is defined not by clinical manifestations but by plasma glucose criteria, and an OGTT is necessary to place a subject in this class. The diagnostic criteria are discussed in Chapter 2. In analogy to the subclasses within diabetes mellitus, it is suggested that clinicians and researchers might find it advantageous to characterize IGT individuals with regard to the presence of conditions or syndromes suspected of inducing glucose intolerance and whether or not obesity is present (Tables 1 and 2).

Individuals in this class are not diabetic, and the clinically significant microangiopathic renal and retinal complications characteristic of diabetes are virtually absent in subjects with IGT [49–51]. However, individuals with IGT have an increased prevalence of arterial disease and electrocardiographic abnormalities and increased susceptibility to atherosclerotic disease associated with known risk factors including hypertension, hyperlipidemia, and adiposity [52–54]. Thus, particularly in otherwise healthy and ambulatory individuals, IGT may have prognostic implications and should not be ignored or taken lightly. However, since these individuals do not have diabetes, they are appropriately designated as having IGT to avoid the social, psychologic and socio-economic stigma of the term diabetes. The older terms 'chemical', 'borderline', 'subclinical', 'asymptomatic' and 'latent' diabetes, which had been applied to persons in this class, have been abandoned.

IGT may represent a stage in the natural history of diabetes, since persons with IGT are at higher risk than the general population for the development of NIDDM. When retested 5–10 years after being initially ascertained as IGT, about one-third have OGTTs that would qualify as diabetic. However, a similar proportion have normal glucose tolerance and a proportion remain in the IGT class for many years. Evidence from the long-term prospective study in Bedford, UK, gave no indication that treatment with tolbutamide reduced the proportion who developed clinical diabetes. Improvement in glucose tolerance can be effected over the short term by caloric restriction or weight loss [55, 56], although the long-term impact on development of clinical diabetes in persons with IGT is not known. The clinical significance of IGT and its prognostic significance for the development of complications remain to be fully investigated.

PREVIOUS ABNORMALITY OF GLUCOSE TOLERANCE (PrevAGT)

This class includes persons who now have normal glucose tolerance but who have previously demonstrated diabetic hyperglycemia or IGT, either spontaneously or in response to an identifiable stimulus. It is believed that these persons will again develop hyperglycemia if subjected to such stresses, but few data exist to substantiate this assertion. Apart from studies of former gestational diabetics, there has been little systematic investigation of the later liability of persons who have exhibited transient glucose intolerance to develop IGT or diabetes. However, it is likely that this risk is increased and hence there is utility in including all those with a history of glucose intolerance, now normal, in the separate class PrevAGT. The terms 'latent diabetes' and 'prediabetes' have been used in the past to describe persons in this class. However, these terms have been abandoned because PrevAGT individuals are not diabetic and because of the psychosocial and economic sanctions that would erroneously be placed on these individuals by use of the term diabetes.

Individuals who had abnormal glucose tolerance detected during pregnancy (GDM), and returned to normal glucose tolerance after parturition, form a subclass of PrevAGT discussed above. Another small but important group of individuals in the class PrevAGT are former obese diabetics whose glucose tolerance has returned to normal since they lost weight.

Clinical studies have demonstrated that a large proportion of patients in the acute phase of myocardial infarction have hyperglycemia or impaired glucose tolerance [57, 87]. Hyperglycemia is also a common feature in patients with acute stroke [26, 88]. Elevated blood glucose is observed in patients with other traumatic events, including burns, accidents resulting in bone injury, war wounds, abdominal surgery and infections [58–62]. Often these individuals return to normal glucose tolerance as time elapses after termination of the metabolic stress and should be reclassified as PrevAGT. Since interpretation of the OGTT applies only to otherwise healthy and ambulatory individuals under carefully standardized conditions and not individuals with acute or chronic illnesses, the initial interpretation of abnormal or impaired glucose tolerance in the states described above has to be questioned.

POTENTIAL ABNORMALITY OF GLUCOSE TOLERANCE (PotAGT)

This is a statistical risk class that includes persons who have never exhibited glucose intolerance, but who are at increased risk over that of the general population for development of diabetes for a variety of reasons. Like PrevAGT, PotAGT should never be applied as a diagnosis to a patient, although knowledge of factors that increase risk for diabetes may be of value in counseling non-diabetic subjects. The purpose of PotAGT in this classification lies primarily in identifying groups of individuals who could be used in prospective research studies.

Individuals who are at increased risk for NIDDM include: the monozygotic twin of a NIDDM patient; a first-degree relative of a NIDDM patient, i.e. a sibling, parent or offspring; obese individuals; and members of racial or ethnic groups that have a high prevalence of diabetes, such as certain North American Indian tribes and South Pacific populations and, to a lesser extent, Hispanic and Black Americans, and Maltese. Individuals who are at increased risk for IDDM include: persons with islet cell antibodies; the monozygotic twin of an IDDM patient; the sibling of an IDDM patient—HLA identical, haploidentical and HLA non-identical; and offspring of an IDDM patient. The degree of risk for any of these circumstances is not well established as yet, and further studies on groups of persons with these characteristics are needed.

In addition to its ketosis-prone stage, IDDM can also be recognized in a preketosis-prone stage before the development of overt disease. Prospective testing in siblings of insulin-dependent diabetics has disclosed patients with normal fasting plasma glucose levels but with abnormal glucose tolerance who progress rapidly to the ketotic form, usually within 2 years after recognition, but occasionally after longer periods of time [63]. Persons with islet cell antibodies, even though they have normal glucose tolerance, are also at increased risk for development of IDDM [64]. This has been shown not only in children but also in adults [31, 65].

The terms 'prediabetes' and 'potential diabetes' have been used to describe persons in this class. However, glucose tolerance is normal in these individuals and these terms are not recommended, since these convey the meaning that a clinical form of diabetes exists in these persons, which invokes unjustified social, psychological and economic sanctions. 'Prediabetes' should be used in a retrospective fashion, exclusively referring to the period of life before diagnosis of diabetes.

REFERENCES

1. National Diabetes Data Group. Classification and diagnosis of diabetes mellitus and other categories of glucose intolerance. Diabetes 1979; 28: 1039–57.
2. Harris MI, Hadden WC, Knowler WC, Bennett PH. International criteria for the diagnosis of diabetes and impaired glucose tolerance. Diabetes Care 1985; 8: 562–7.
3. World Health Organization. Second report of the WHO expert committee on diabetes mellitus. Technical Report Series 646. Geneva: WHO, 1980.
4. World Health Organization. Diabetes mellitus, report of a WHO study group. Technical Report Series 727. Geneva: WHO, 1985.
5. Scott RS, Brown LJ. Prevalence and incidence of insulin-treated diabetes mellitus in adults in Canterbury, New Zealand. Diabet Med 1991; 8: 443–7.
6. Himsworth HP. Diabetes mellitus: its differentiation into insulin-sensitive and insulin-insensitive types. Lancet 1936; i: 117–19.
7. Bornstein J, Lawrence RD. Plasma insulin in human diabetes mellitus. Br Med J 1951; 2: 1541–4.
8. Berson SA, Yalow RS. Antigens in insulin determinants of specificity of porcine insulin in man. Science 1963; 139: 844–5.
9. Editorial. Insulin dependent? Lancet 1985; ii: 89.
10. Melton LJ, Palumbo PJ, Chu C-P. Incidence of diabetes mellitus by clinical type. Diabetes Care 1983; 6: 75–81.
11. Laakso M, Pyorala K. Age at onset and type of diabetes. Diabetes Care 1985; 8: 114–17.
12. Rossini AA, Greiner DL, Friedman HP, Mordes JP. Immunopathogenesis of diabetes mellitus. Diabetes Rev 1993; 1: 43–75.
13. Diabetes Epidemiology Research International Group. Secular trends in incidence of childhood IDDM in 10 countries. Diabetes 1990; 39: 858–64.
14. Nerup J. HLA autoimmunity and insulin-dependent diabetes mellitus. In Creutzfeldt W, Kobberling J, Neel JV (eds) The genetics of diabetes mellitus. Berlin: Springer, 1976: pp 348–54.
15. Cudworth AG, Woodrow JC. Genetic susceptibility in diabetes mellitus: analysis of the HLA association. Br Med J 1976; 2: 846–9.
16. Kaprio J, Tuomilehto J, Koskenvuo M, Romanov K, Reunanen A, Eriksson J, Stengard J, Kesaniemi YA. Concordance for type 1 (insulin-dependent) and type 2 (non-insulin-dependent) diabetes mellitus in a population-based cohort of twins in Finland. Diabetologia 1992; 35: 1060–7.
17. Ludvigsson J, Samuelsson U, Beauforts C et al. HLA-DR3 is associated with a more slowly progressive form of Type 1 (insulin-dependent) diabetes. Diabetologia 1986; 29: 207–10.
18. Weinberg CR, Dornan TL, Hansen JA et al. HLA-related heterogeneity in seasonal patterns of diagnosis in Type 1 (insulin-dependent) diabetes. Diabetologia 1984; 26: 199–202.
19. Drell DW, Notkins AL. Multiple immunological abnormalities in patients with Type 1 (insulin-dependent) diabetes mellitus. Diabetologia 1987; 30: 132–43.
20. Kolb H, Dannehl K, Gruneklee D et al. Prospective analysis of islet cell antibodies in children with Type 1 (insulin-dependent) diabetes. Diabetologia 1988; 31: 189–94.
21. Bingley PJ, Bonifacio E, Shattock M et al. Can islet cell antibodies predict IDDM in the general population? Diabetes Care 1993; 16: 45–51.
22. Atkinson MA, Maclaren NK, Riley WJ et al. Are insulin autoantibodies markers for insulin-dependent diabetes mellitus? Diabetes 1986; 35: 894–932.
23. Allen C, Palta M, D'Alessio DJ. Incidence and differences in urban–rural seasonal variation of Type 1 (insulin-dependent) diabetes in Wisconsin. Diabetologia 1986; 29: 629–33.
24. Laakso M, Sarlund H, Pyorala K. Prevalence of insulin deficiency among initially non-insulin-dependent middle-aged diabetic individuals. Diabetes Care 1986; 9: 228–31.
25. Newman B, Selby JV, King MC et al. Concordance for Type 2 (non-insulin-dependent) diabetes mellitus in male twins. Diabetologia 1987; 30: 763–8.
26. Woo J, Lam CW, Kay R, Wong AH. The influence of hyperglycemia and diabetes mellitus on immediate and

3-month morbidity and mortality after acute stroke. Arch Neurol 1990; 47: 1174-7.

27. Tattersall RB, Fajans SS. A difference between the inheritance of classical juvenile-onset and maturity-onset type diabetes of young people. Diabetes 1974; 24: 44-53.

28. Foster WR, Burton BT (eds). Health implications of obesity; National Institutes of Health consensus development conference. Ann Intern Med 1985; 102: 981-1077.

29. Zimmet P, King H. Classification and diagnosis of diabetes mellitus. In Alberti KGGM, Krall L (eds) Diabetes annual 3. Amsterdam: Elsevier, 1987: pp 1-22.

30. Lyons IJ, Kennedy L, Atkinson AB et al. Predicting the need for insulin therapy in late onset (40-60 years) diabetes mellitus. Diabet Med 1984; 1: 105-8.

31. Groop LC, Bottazzo GF, Doniach D. Islet cell antibodies identify latent Type 1 diabetes in patients aged 35-75 years at diagnosis. Diabetes 1986; 35: 237-41.

32. Di Mario, Irvine WJ, Borsey DO et al. Immune abnormalities in diabetic patients not requiring insulin at diagnosis. Diabetologia 1983; 25: 392-6.

33. Winter WE, Maclaren NK, Riley WJ et al. Maturity-onset diabetes of youth in Black Americans. New Engl J Med 1987; 316: 285-7.

34. Mohan V, Ramachandran A, Snehalatha C et al. High prevalence of maturity-onset diabetes of the young (MODY) amongst Indians. Diabetes Care 1985; 8: 371-4.

35. Welborn TA, Garcia-Webb P, Bonser AM. Basal C-peptide in the discrimination of Type I from Type II diabetes. Diabetes Care 1981; 4: 616-20.

36. Katzeff HL, Savage PJ, Barclay-White B et al. C-peptide measurement in the differentiation of Type I (insulin-dependent) diabetes mellitus. Diabetologia 1985; 28: 264-8.

37. Laakso M, Sarlund H, Pyorala K. Clinical characteristics in the discrimination between patients with low or high C-peptide level among middle-aged insulin-treated diabetics. Diabetes Res 1987; 4: 95-9.

38. Abu-Bakare A, Gill GV, Taylor R et al. Tropical or malnutrition-related diabetes: a real syndrome? Lancet 1986; i: 1136-7.

39. Bajaj JS. Malnutrition-related fibrocalculous pancreatic diabetes. In Serrano-Rios M, Lefèbvre PJ (eds) Diabetes 1985. Amsterdam: Excerpta Medica, 1986: pp 1055-68.

40. Mohan V, Ramachandran A, Viswanathan M. Tropical diabetes. In Alberti KGGM, Krall LP (eds) Diabetes annual 2. Amsterdam: Elsevier, 1986: pp 30-45.

41. Davies JL, Kawaguchi Y, Bennett ST, Copeman JB, Cordell HJ, Pritchard LE et al. A genome-wide search for human type 1 diabetes susceptibility genes. Nature 1994; 371:130-6.

42. Bonifacio E, Bottazzo GF. Immunology of IDDM (type 1 diabetes)—entering the '90s. In Alberti KGMM, Krall LP (eds) Diabetes annual 6. Amsterdam: Elsevier, 1991: pp 20-47.

43. Kjos SL, Buchanan TA, Greenspoon JS, Montoro M, Bernstein GS, Mestman JH. Gestational diabetes mellitus: the prevalence of glucose intolerance and diabetes mellitus in the first two months postpartum. Am J Obstet Gynecol 1990; 163: 93-8.

44. Coustan DR, Carpenter MW, O'Sullivan PS, Carr SR. Gestational diabetes mellitus: predictors of subsequent disordered glucose metabolism. Am J Obstet Gynecol 1993; 168: 1139-45.

45. O'Sullivan JB, Mahan CD, Charles D et al. Gestational diabetes and perinatal mortality rate. J Obstet Gynecol 1973; 116: 7-14.

46. Damm P, Kuhl C, Hornnes P, Molsted-Pedersen L. A longitudinal study of plasma insulin and glucagon in women with previous gestational diabetes. Diabetes Care 1995; 18: 654-65.

47. Metzger BE, Bybee DE, Freinkel N et al. Gestational diabetes mellitus: correlations between the phenotypic and genotypic characteristics of the mother and abnormal glucose tolerance during the first year postpartum. Diabetes 1985; 34 (suppl 2): 111-15.

48. Harris MI. Gestational diabetes may represent the discovery of pre-existing glucose intolerance. Diabetes Care 1988; 11: 402-11.

49. Klein R, Barrett-Connor EL, Blunt BA, Wingard DL. Visual impairment and retinopathy in people with normal glucose tolerance, impaired glucose tolerance, and newly diagnosed NIDDM. Diabetes Care 1991; 14: 914-18.

50. Pettitt DJ, Knowler WC, Lisse JR et al. Development of retinopathy and proteinuria in relation to plasma glucose concentration. Lancet 1980; ii: 1050-2.

51. McCartney P, Keen H, Jarrett RJ. The Bedford survey: observations on retina and lens of subjects with impaired glucose tolerance and in controls with normal glucose tolerance. Diabète Métab 1983; 9: 303-5.

52. Harris MI. Impaired glucose tolerance in the U.S. population. Diabetes Care 1989; 12: 464-74.

53. Fuller JH, Shipley MJ, Rose G, Jarrett RJ, Keen H. Coronary heart disease risk and impaired glucose tolerance. The Whitehall Study. Lancet 1980; 1: 1373-6.

54. Fujimoto WY, Leonetti DL, Kinyoun JL, Shuman WP, Stolov WC, Wahl PW. Prevalence of complications among second-generation Japanese-American men with diabetes, impaired glucose tolerance, or normal glucose tolerance. Diabetes 1987; 36: 730-9.

55. Sartor G, Schersten B, Carlstrom S et al. Ten-year follow-up of subjects with impaired glucose tolerance. Diabetes 1980; 29: 41-9.

56. Long SD, O'Brien K, MacDonald KG et al. Weight loss in severely obese subjects prevents the progression of impaired glucose tolerance to Type II diabetes. Diabetes Care 1994; 17: 372-5.

57. Datey KK, Nanda NC. Hyperglycemia after acute myocardial infarction. New Engl J Med 1967; 276: 262-5.

58. Allison SP. Intravenous glucose insulin, and free fatty acids levels in burned patients. Lancet 1968; ii: 1113-15.

59. Pearson D. Intravenous glucose tolerance in myocardial infarction. Postgrad Med J 1971; 47: 648-52.

60. Howard JMH. Studies of the absorption and metabolism of glucose following injury. Ann Surg 1955; 141: 321-4.

61. Ross H. Effects of abdominal operations on glucose tolerance. Lancet 1966; ii: 563-6.

62. Chupin M. Glucose intolerance in viral hepatitis. Diabetes 1978; 27: 661-5.

63. Fajans SS, Cloutier MC, Crowther RL. Clinical and etiologic heterogeneity of idiopathic diabetes mellitus. Diabetes 1978; 27: 1112-20.

64. Srikanta S, Ganda OP, Jackson RA et al. Pre-Type 1 (insulin-dependent) diabetes: common endocrinological

course despite immunological and immunogenetic heterogeneity. Diabetologia 1984; 27: 146-8.

65. Gleichmann H, Zorcher B, Greulich B et al. Correlation of islet cell antibodies and HLA-DR phenotypes with diabetes mellitus in adults. Diabetologia 1984; 27: 90-2.

66. Palmer JP, McCulloch DK. Prediction and prevention of IDDM—1991. Diabetes 1991; 40: 943-7.

67. Rowley MJ, Mackay IR, Chen Q-Y, Knowles WJ, Zimmet PZ. Antibodies to glutamic acid decarboxylase discriminate major type of diabetes mellitus. Diabetes 1992; 41: 548-51.

68. Tuomi T, Groop LC, Zimmet PZ, Rowley MJ, Knowles W, Mackay IR. Antibodies to glutamic acid decarboxylase reveal latent autoimmune diabetes mellitus in adults with a non-insulin-dependent onset of disease. Diabetes 1993; 42: 359-62.

69. Zimmet P, Dowse G, Serjeantson S, Finch C, King H. The epidemiology and natural history of NIDDM—lessons from the South Pacific. Diabet Metab Rev 1990; 6: 91-124.

70. Zimmet PZ, Collins VR, Dowse GK, Knight LT. Hyperinsulinaemia in youth is a predictor of type 2 (non-insulin-dependent) diabetes mellitus. Diabetologia 1992; 35: 534-41.

71. Hagopian WA, Karlsen AE, Gottsater A, Landin-Olsson M, Grubin CE, Sundkvist G et al. Quantitative assay using recombinant human islet glutamic acid decarboxylase (GAD65) shows that 64K autoantibody positivity at onset predicts diabetes type. J Clin Invest 1993; 91: 368-74.

72. van der Ouweland JMW, Lemkes HHPJ, Trembath RC, Ross R, Velho G, Cohen D, Froguel P, Maassen JA. Maternally inherited diabetes and deafness is a distinct subtype of diabetes and associates with a single point mutation in the mitochondrial tRNA-Leu (UUR) gene. Diabetes 1994; 43: 746-51.

73. Vionnet N, Stoffel M, Takeda J, Yasuda K, Bill GI, Zouali H et al. Nonsense mutation in the glucokinase gene causes early-onset non-insulin-dependent diabetes mellitus. Nature 1992; 356: 721-2.

74. Hamman RF. Genetic and environmental determinants of non-insulin-dependent diabetes mellitus (NIDDM). Diabet Metab Rev 1993; 8: 287-338.

75. Bergstrom RW, Newell-Morris LL, Leonetti DL, Shuman WP, Wahl PW, Fujimoto WY. Association of elevated fasting C-peptide level and increased intraabdominal fat distribution with development of NIDDM in Japanese-American men. Diabetes 1990; 39:104-11.

76. Gottsäter A, Landin-Olsson M, Fernlund P, Lernmark Å, Sundkvist G. β-Cell function in relation to islet cell antibodies during the first 3 years after clinical diagnosis of diabetes in type II diabetic patients. Diabetes Care 1993; 16: 902-8.

77. Banerji MA, Chaiken R, Huey H, Tuomi T, Norin AJ, Mackay IR, Rowley MJ, Zimmet PZ, Lebovitz HE. GAD antibody negative NIDDM in adult black subjects with DKA and increased frequency of HLA DR3 and DR4. Diabetes 1994; 43: 741-5.

78. McLarty DG, Athaide I, Bottazzo GF, Swai ABM, Alberti KGMM. Islet cell antibodies are not specifically associated with insulin-dependent diabetes in rural Tanzanian Africans. Diabetes Res Clin Pract 1990; 9: 219-24.

79. Yajnik CS. Diabetes in tropical developing countries. In Alberti KGMM, Krall LP (eds) Diabetes Annual 6. Amsterdam: Elsevier, 1991; pp 62-81.

80. McMillan DE. The role of cyanide indigestion in tropical malnutrition and the diabetes associated with it. In Rifken H, Caldwell JA, Taylor SI (eds) Diabetes 1991. Amsterdam: Elsevier Science Publishers, 1991; pp 955-9.

81. Zimmet P. Malnutrition-related diabetes mellitus or tropical diabetes? An overview. In Baba S, Tjokropawiro A, Kaneko T, Iwaj S (eds) Malnutrition-related diabetes mellitus (MRDM) 1989. Kobe: International Center for Medical Research, 1989; pp 82-90.

82. Henry OA, Beischer NA. Long-term implications of gestational diabetes for the mother. Baillière's Clinical Obstetrics and Gynecology 1991; 5: 461-83.

83. Marquette GP, Klein VR, Niebyl JR. Efficacy of screening for gestational diabetes. Am J Perinatol 1985; 2: 7-9.

84. Coustan DR, Nelson C, Carpenter MW, Carr SR, Rotondo L, Widness JA. Maternal age and screening for gestational diabetes: a population-based study. Obstet Gynecol 1989; 73: 557-61.

85. Pettit DJ, Knowler WC, Baird HR, Bennett PH. Gestational diabetes: infant and maternal complications of pregnancy in relation to third-trimester glucose tolerance in Pima Indians. Diabetes Care 1980; 3: 458-64.

86. Berkus MD, Langer O. Glucose tolerance test: degree of glucose abnormality correlates with neonatal outcome. Obstet Gynecol 1993; 81: 344-8.

87. O'Sullivan JJ, Conroy RM, Robinson K, Hickey N, Mulcahy R. In-hospital prognosis of patients with fasting hyperglycemia after first myocardial infarction. Diabetes Care 1991; 14: 758-60.

88. Matchar DB, Divine GW, Heyman A, Feussner JR. The influence of hyperglycemia on outcome of cerebral infarction. Ann Intern Med 1992; 117: 449-56.

2

Diabetes Diagnosis

Harry Keen* and K.G.M.M. Alberti†

*United Medical and Dental Schools, Guy's Hospital, London, and †Medical School, University of Newcastle upon Tyne, UK

IN THE BEGINNING

In its historical origins, the term 'diabetes mellitus' was purely descriptive. It was derived from a readily recognizable and characteristic set of symptoms which usually then followed a predictable and catastrophic course. With the growth of medical understanding and in particular the science of biochemistry, the diagnostic term acquired a more precise chemical identity with excessive urinary and (later) blood glucose as its central feature. As the diagnostic concept of diabetes expanded to include the chemically defined disorder, greatly increased numbers of people were identified qualifying for the diagnosis. In the 1940s, 1950s and 1960s these numbers became so large and the qualifying glycaemic criteria so variable that the whole diagnostic process came under national and international scrutiny. From this emerged the current, more rigorous definition of diabetes mellitus and, short of this, but still 'at risk', the state of impaired glucose tolerance, both described and discussed below. Over the past decade, there has been increasing acceptance and adoption of this set of internationally recommended standardized criteria. They define the minimum glycaemic requirements for a diagnosis of the glucose intolerant states; for the classical clinical syndrome, recognition and diagnostic confirmation have changed little this century.

The state of diabetes mellitus, as it is now defined, therefore spans a very broad clinical spectrum. At one extreme lie the (more numerous) oligosymptomatic or asymptomatic individuals, qualifying solely on the basis of meeting minimal glycaemic criteria; at the other are severely ill patients, *in extremis* with diabetic ketoacidosis. The single defining feature that unifies this variegated clinical array under the rubric of 'diabetes mellitus' is the diagnostic demonstration of hyperglycaemia. In the broadest terms, the severity of the characteristic clinical symptoms and signs of the diabetes parallels the degree of hyperglycaemia. The symptoms and signs are intensified and modified by its accompanying biochemical disturbances.

Definition—the Role of Hyperglycaemia

The diabetic state is constituted by the sustained elevation of the blood glucose above specified concentrations (see Table 1). In practice, glucose concentrations in diabetes often exceed the normal upper limits by a large margin. This hyperglycaemia may be associated with disturbances—sometimes major—in the concentrations of other metabolic products, notably ketone bodies [1], but these play no part in the diagnostic definition. In non-diabetic people under normal conditions of life, blood glucose concentration is regulated at values between about 3 mmol/l (54 mg/dl) and 6 mmol/l (108 mg/dl); it rises a little after meals, rarely and transiently to values as high as 8–10 mmol/l (144–180 mg/dl) after the ingestion of large quantities of rapidly absorbed carbohydrate [2–4]. In people with diabetes, both glycaemic setting levels and homeostatic corrective mechanisms are deranged in varying, sometimes gross, degree. Blood glucose values in untreated diabetes are often found to be in the

International Textbook of Diabetes Mellitus, Second Edition. Edited by K.G.M.M. Alberti, P. Zimmet, R.A. DeFronzo, and H. Keen (Honorary)
© 1997 John Wiley & Sons Ltd

Table 1 Oral glucose tolerance test: diagnostic glycaemic criteria for adults (data from reference 52)*

	Glucose concentration in mmol/l (mg/dl)			
	Plasma		Whole blood	
	Venous	Capillary	Venous	Capillary
Diabetes mellitus				
Fasting value	≥7.8 (140)	≥7.8 (140)	≥6.7 (120)	≥6.7 (120)
or				
2-hour value	≥11.1 (200)	≥12.2 (220)	≥10.0 (180)	≥11.1 (200)
Impaired glucose tolerance				
Fasting value	<7.8 (140)	<7.8 (140)	<6.7 (120)	<6.7 (120)
and				
2-hour value	7.8–11.1 (140–200)	8.9–12.2 (160–220)	6.7–10.0 (120–180)	7.8–11.1 (140–200)

*For children, WHO [50, 52] has recommended that the test load of glucose should be 1.75 g per kg body weight up to a total of 75 g. In general, glycaemic criteria are as for adults but the interpretation and management of glucose intolerance short of DM remain the subject of research.

In pregnancy, if abnormal glucose tolerance is found for the first time, WHO recommends the criteria above for diagnosis of gestational DM and IGT (GDM and GIGT) and that the management of GIGT should be the same as for GDM. This differs from the procedure and interpretation of GDM recommended by NDDG [49, 53] (see text and Table 2).

range of 15–25 mmol/l (270–450 mg/dl) and may rise considerably higher. Not only may basal blood glucose concentration be raised (sometimes massively so) but the swings of glycaemia, in response to food, physical and emotional stimuli, trauma and infection are also greatly increased with delayed return to lower values.

RECOGNITION OF THE DIABETIC STATE

The state of diabetes mellitus (DM) as it is now defined has been enormously expanded from its classical origins. Historically, it was first recognized by its combination of striking symptoms and signs, partial descriptions of which can be found in the earliest written records [5]. A morbid sequence of events, comprising unassuageable thirst, profuse urination and rapidly progressive body wasting, terminating in stupor, coma and death, was described in ancient writings [6, 7]. The first use of the term 'diabetes' (describing the drinking and polyuria—'flowing as through a siphon') is attributed to Demetrios of Apamaia (second century BC). To Aretaeus (Aretaios) of Cappadocia (AD 81–3) must go credit for the first, graphic clinical description which has been little bettered—'a wonderful but not very frequent affection among men, being a melting down of the flesh and limbs into urine … life is short, offensive and distressing, thirst unquenchable, death inevitable'. The sweetness of the urine was referred to in the Indian Sanskrit Susruta (third century BC) which also recorded its attractiveness to insects. The more modern history of diabetes began with Thomas Willis's account in 1674 of the 'pissing evil' [8]. He clearly documented the sweet taste of the urine (although he ascribed it to an excess of sulphur and salts) and firmly established the disease on the English scene. It was not until a century later that Matthew Dobson [9], a

highly observant Liverpool physician, showed that the sweet, white residue left after evaporation of diabetic urine consisted largely of a yeast-fermentable sugar. He made the further observations that the blood plasma of the diabetic patient also tasted sweet and that it was milky in appearance. To him therefore must be credited the first documentation of diabetic glycosuria, hyperglycaemia and lipaemia. It was 1835 before Bouchardat [10] identified the sugar in the urine, and some years later that in the blood, as glucose.

Glycaemia

It was not until the middle of the nineteenth century and the seminal work of Claude Bernard [11] that the importance of hyperglycaemia as the source of the urinary glucose was appreciated. The classical view of Galen (AD 124–99) that diabetes was a disorder of the kidney was widely accepted before that. Thomas Sydenham assigned it an alimentary origin; others ascribed the condition to disease of the liver and even the lung. The late recognition of raised blood glucose concentration was due to the technical difficulty of estimating the small quantities in the circulation. Because of this, Claude Bernard long denied the suggestion that glucose was present at all in normal systemic blood, regarding its appearance in diabetes as due to centrally initiated and neurologically mediated pathological release from liver glycogen. Francis Pavy, a little recognized physician of Guy's Hospital, London, was among the first to expound the firm link between hyperglycaemia and glycosuria. Thus emerged the notion of normal blood glucose homeostasis and its grave disturbance which is the foundation for today's perception of the nature of the diabetic state.

Glycosuria and Hyperglycaemia

Despite the recognition of the essential role of hyperglycaemia in the diabetic state, the detection of glucose in the urine was originally (and often still is) the first indicator of the diagnosis. Glycosuria is a valuable but inadequate pointer to the diagnosis of diabetes [12]. Heavy glycosuria may coexist with normal blood glucose concentrations in the condition of renal glycosuria (sometimes misnamed renal diabetes) when the glucose load filtered at the renal glomeruli exceeds the tubular reabsorptive capacity. Positive tests may also result from transient elevation of blood glucose above the renal threshold [12] or from the presence of other sugars or reducing substances unless glucose-specific urine tests are used. Even when heavy glycosuria is accompanied by ketonuria in a person with diabetic symptoms, the diagnosis must still be confirmed by demonstrating abnormally raised blood glucose.

Just as the presence of glycosuria does not establish a diagnosis of diabetes, so its absence does not absolutely exclude it. The renal threshold for glucose, low enough in youth to permit occasional alimentary glycosuria, rises with age [13]. In population surveys with an initial urine screening for glucose, subsequent tests of glucose tolerance on aglycosuric subjects reveal, especially in older people, degrees of glucose intolerance ranging up to the unequivocally diabetic [13]. Individuals with lesser degrees of glucose intolerance (impaired glucose tolerance—see below) are characteristically aglycosuric most of the time. The specificity of a positive test is relatively high although sensitivity is low. Sensitivity can be increased by testing postprandially.

With these caveats, a positive urine test for glucose remains the single most commonly encountered pointer to underlying diabetes. The urine test retains an important place in the routine clinical examination of the patient. A positive result should never be ignored and, in the absence of diabetic symptoms, calls for a blood glucose screening test. If symptoms such as thirst, polyuria and weight loss are present, a single on-the-spot measurement may be so high as to establish the diagnosis, obviating the need for formal tests of glucose tolerance. Methods for urine testing and blood glucose estimation are dealt with in detail in Chapters 50 and 51.

Other Diagnostic Prompts

It is probably in a minority of those in whom diabetes is diagnosed that the characteristic symptoms of thirst, polyuria and weight loss are responsible for bringing the diagnosis to light. Other circumstances must also prompt diagnostic suspicion. As mentioned earlier these include the chance finding of glycosuria, or its discovery in routine employment or insurance examinations. The chance of finding diabetes is also increased where there is a first-degree relative with diabetes, in the presence of overweight and obesity [14, 15] particularly if the fat is central [16, 17], and on achieving the sixth decade of life [18–20]—or earlier in life in some specially susceptible ethnic groups [21, 22]. More compelling is the complaint of unexplained weight loss without reduction of appetite, genital itching, impairment of visual acuity, repeated skin sepsis and unaccountable pains and paraesthesia in the limbs. The long-term use of some common therapeutic agents, especially thiazide diuretics and corticosteroids, may unmask or even provoke glucose intolerance. The evaluation of glucose homeostasis during pregnancy is of particular interest [23] (see Tables 1 and 2, and also Chapter 57). A high level of diagnostic suspicion is indicated in women with a history of glucose intolerance in a previous pregnancy, in those who have borne an unusually heavy baby (e.g. over 4.5 kg), or when there is a history of pregnancies with toxaemia

Table 2 National Diabetes Data Group [49, 53] recommendations for diagnosis of gestational diabetes mellitus*

Initial screening procedure

- Positive if venous plasma glucose 1 hour after 50-g oral glucose load is 7.8 mmol/l (140 mg/dl) or more

Establishing diagnosis in positives

100-g oral glucose challenge in morning after 8–14 hour overnight fast preceded by 3 days unrestricted carbohydrate intake and physical activity

Venous plasma glucose measured fasting and 1, 2 and 3 hours after load. Enzymatic method preferable. Subject seated and smoking prohibited for test

- Positive if two or more of following values are met or exceeded in venous plasma glucose concentration

Gestational diabetes mellitus

Fasting value	≥5.8 mmol/l	(105 mg/dl)
1-hour value	≥10.6 mmol/l	(190 mg/dl)
2-hour value	≥9.2 mmol/l	(165 mg/dl)
3-hour value	≥8.1 mmol/l	(145 mg/dl)

*Modified to meet recommendations of Third International Workshop Conference on Gestational Diabetes Mellitus (Chicago, Illinois, November 1990).

or ending in miscarriage or stillbirth. Many recommend that glucose tolerance should be routinely tested in all pregnancies [23] using specially modified methods and interpretative criteria [24] (Table 2), although that view is not universally held [25, 26]. It is worth emphasizing that more and more countries outside North America are using the WHO criteria [52] (Table 1) rather than those of NDDG (Table 2). Apart from greater simplicity, a recent report has shown greater sensitivity using WHO criteria [90].

Even using these prompts to diagnosis it is likely that many people with asymptomatic or oligosymptomatic diabetes will escape diagnosis. Diabetes is still often diagnosed virtually by chance and sometimes not until the advent of its complications brings it to attention, e.g. visual impairment due to diabetic retinopathy or cataract, or presentation with chronic foot ulceration or incipient gangrene. This raises once more the still debatable issue of widespread, diagnostic population screening for diabetes (to be clearly distinguished from scientifically based epidemiological surveys). Although expert opinion on this receded from the uncritical enthusiasm for the unselective 'diabetes detection drives' of the middle decades of this century [27] to the more reserved view of the 1970s and 1980s [28], the emergence of the new diagnostic criteria and the broader perception of the implications of glucose intolerance now make the question ripe for comprehensive review.

Diabetes Sequelae

Though not strictly part of the diagnostic definition of diabetes mellitus, the syndrome is inadequately portrayed without consideration of the high risk of the eventual development of the somewhat stereotyped and specific pattern of damage to particular organs and tissues, collectively known as the complications of diabetes. These complications include disease of the retina, the renal glomeruli and damage to peripheral nerves, with the consequent correspondingly high risk of visual impairment, renal failure and severe sensorimotor and autonomic abnormalities as a result (see Chapters 65–77). They have a particular importance in that risk of these 'complications' determines the glycaemic criteria for diagnosis of diabetes. Aggravated atherosclerotic disease is also characteristic both of diabetes and of the lesser degrees of glucose intolerance, with increased liability to ischaemic disease of heart, leg and brain. These complications are so closely identified with the diabetic state as to have come to be regarded as an integral part of it. Indeed there was a view, no longer widely current, that these were not complications of the diabetic state so much as an independent morphological expression of it.

THE GLUCOSE TOLERANCE TEST

Since the 1920s the glucose tolerance test has been used diagnostically to evaluate the glycaemic response to an exogenous glucose load, administered by mouth—the oral glucose tolerance test (OGTT)—or intravenously—the intravenous glucose tolerance test (IVGTT). The intravenous test remains almost exclusively a research procedure and is not considered in this section. The oral test has had innumerable methodological variants and its results a diversity of interpretations. Its early history, development and multiple versions were comprehensively reviewed by Kelly M. West [29]. The size and the nature of the glucose load have varied, the former twofold to threefold. Blood has been drawn at a variety of times after the glucose challenge and submitted to many different analytical methods giving substantially different results. The curve of rise and fall of the blood glucose has been interpreted in many ways, with much disputation particularly as to what constituted the demarcation between the normal and the diabetic response. So great was the diversity that the rate of abnormality in a collection of responses from a given population sample could vary as much as tenfold depending upon the criteria adopted [30]. West [31] graphically described what this could mean to the individual. On the basis of written opinions he collected from 20 recognized expert physicians in diabetes, he showed that a given glycaemic response to an oral glucose load could be unequivocally diagnosed as diabetic by several of the experts and equally firmly dismissed as normal by others. Siperstein [32] was so disaffected by the shortcomings of the OGTT that he advocated its abandonment. Standardization of test procedures and interpretation of results was clearly highly desirable and has now been achieved (see below). However, the test is grossly overused in the clinical setting when quicker and less resource-consuming measurements would be entirely satisfactory in establishing diagnosis. This has been emphasized repeatedly [91].

New Criteria

It was the era of mass screening and population surveys for diabetes that brought the unsatisfactory diagnostic situation to a head. When large, unselected populations were submitted to OGTT, a wide spectrum of response was found. Frequency distributions of glucose tolerance and intolerance showed no natural break between normal and diabetic responses [33–34], so diagnostic cut-off values were relatively arbitrarily imposed upon a continuum of results. Application of the then prevailing British Diabetic Association diagnostic criteria for diabetes [35] would have classified 14% of the population of the small British town of Bedford as diabetic [12]. Similar findings in other studies also cast doubt on the validity of applying the stigmatizing diagnostic label of diabetes to large numbers of people with no more than trivial deviations from arbitrary blood glucose norms. Particularly called into question was the widely accepted assumption that lesser degrees of glucose intolerance represented 'early diabetes' which was almost inevitably destined to worsen [36]. Follow-up studies showed that many such individuals reverted apparently spontaneously to normal glucose tolerance; some remained in the equivocal zone, while a relatively small proportion showed progressive deterioration of glucose tolerance (Figures 1 and 2) [37–43]. The development of the specific microvascular complications of diabetes was not observed in people with these lesser degrees of glucose intolerance over periods of up to 10 years of follow-up. For these reasons it was deemed inappropriate to apply the term 'diabetes', however qualified, to individuals with 'borderline' OGTT responses. However, because these subjects had a greater likelihood of progressing to diabetes and, in some studies, of developing arterial disease [44–48], they could not be dismissed as normal and so were assigned to a new 'risk class' of impaired glucose tolerance (IGT). A number of authoritative and representative bodies [49–51] therefore set out to seek agreement on new diagnostic criteria based so far as possible on sound scientific data and at the same time sufficiently acceptable to the clinical community to make their recommendations very broadly applicable.

The National Diabetes Data Group and World Health Organization Expert Committee

In 1979, the US National Diabetes Data Group (NDDG) [49] published a set of methodological and diagnostic recommendations and proposed a new classification for diabetes mellitus and allied metabolic disorders. This was shortly followed by the second report of the World Health Organization (WHO) Expert Committee on Diabetes Mellitus [50]. Based upon a consideration of the epidemiological evidence and the progression over substantial periods of time of individuals characterized by standard OGTT at baseline, they proposed revised glycaemic criteria for the diagnosis of diabetes mellitus and defined the new class of impaired glucose tolerance (see Table 1). There were very broad areas of agreement between the NDDG and WHO. Differences in detail remained, most of which have subsequently been resolved [52, 53].

The revised values of fasting and postload glycaemia that define the minimum criteria for the diagnosis of DM represent a degree of glucose intolerance that

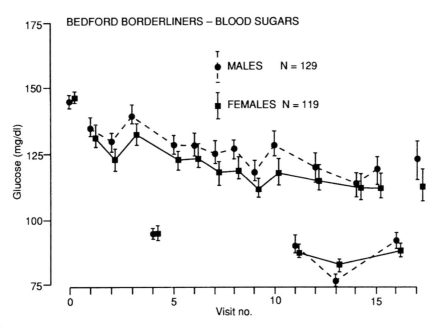

Figure 1 Mean capillary blood glucose in 129 men and 119 women first ascertained in the Bedford population survey (1962) (visit 0 on abscissa) as having impaired glucose tolerance ('borderline diabetes') defined as 2 h post 50-g glucose capillary blood glucose (ferricyanide reduction method) ≥120 mg/dl (6.7 mmol/l) <200 mg/dl (11.1 mmol/l). Visit 4 blood was collected fasting, visits 11, 13 and 16 without any special preparation (i.e. 2–4 h after midday meal). Early (visits 0–1, 1–2) fall probably largely due to 'regression to mean' statistical phenomenon. Individuals 'worsening to diabetes' (i.e. 2 consecutive or 3 non-consecutive 2 h BG ≤200 mg/dl) contribute to mean values up to and including the visit where that definition is met. Female post-load values slightly but consistently lower than male. Steady falling trend due in part to selective loss of those worsening to diabetes from groups

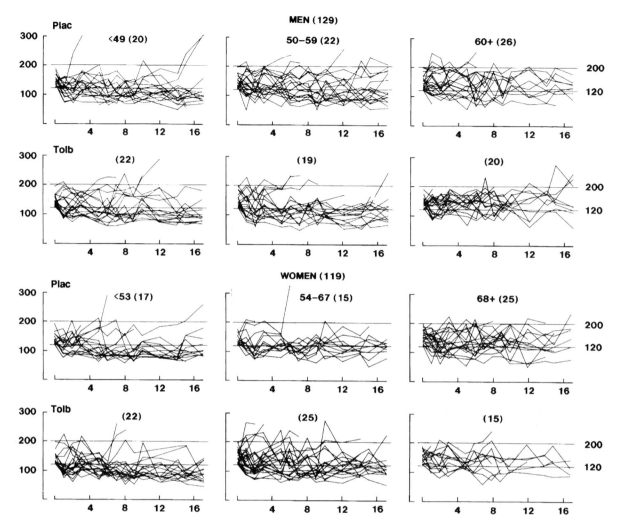

Figure 2 'Spaghettogram' demonstrating the variable behaviour over 10 years of follow-up (1962–1972) of 2 h post load blood glucose in individuals originally ascertained in the Bedford population survey (1962) with impaired glucose tolerance (visits 0 (ascertainment) to 17 on abscissa). Subjects found at 0 with 2 h capillary blood glucose 120–199 mg/dl (6.7–11.1 mmol/l) (ordinate) separated into age groups (vertically) and different treatment groups (horizontally, Plac = placebo, Tolb = tolbutamide 1 g/day). Capillary blood glucose measured 2 h after 50 g glucose by mouth. Values for visit 4 (fasting) and visits 11, 13 and 16 (no preparation—random) omitted from individual records (see Figure 1)

all clinical authorities accept as being unquestionably diagnostic. They have been shown to be associated cross-sectionally and longitudinally with the risk of developing specific diabetic microangiopathy. The diagnostic cut-off values selected for DM also correspond approximately to the intersection of the upper and lower subdistributions of OGTT responses in those populations where the responses are bimodally distributed [54–56] and in which follow-up studies have demonstrated restriction of specific diabetic complications to those in the upper subdistribution.

The class of IGT accommodates the intermediate range of glucose intolerance within which informed opinions were in disagreement, some regarding them as 'high normal', others as 'mild diabetes'. This pragmatic solution to the general problem of creating categories

within a continuum and the specific defining values selected have inevitably provoked much debate over the past decade [22, 57–62]. The WHO/NDDG diagnostic recommendations have nevertheless been applied in non-pregnant adults, apparently without major difficulty, to both the requirements of individual patient diagnosis and to epidemiological enquiry into the prevalence and incidence of DM and IGT in a number of populations [63–72].

Glycaemic Criteria for Diabetes Diagnosis

When the symptoms characteristic of the diabetic state are evident, a single measurement of the blood glucose concentration usually reveals such a high value as to make further diagnostic investigation unnecessary

Table 3 Diagnostic indication from unstandardized (casual, random) blood glucose values [50, 52]

	Glucose values in mmol/l (mg/dl)				
	Plasma			Whole blood	
Diabetes mellitus	Venous	Capillary		Venous	Capillary
Likely	≥11.1 (200)	≥12.2 (200)		≥10.0 (180)	≥11.1 (200)
Uncertain	Values intermediate between those above and below				
Unlikely	<5.5 (100)	<5.5 (100)		<4.4 (80)	<4.4 (80)

A single, unstandardized blood glucose value may suffice to indicate diagnosis, especially when diabetic symptoms are present. OGTT may be considered for those with values in uncertain range, if indicated, abbreviated to the 2-hour value in some cases. 'The clinician must always feel confident that the diagnosis of diabetes is fully established since the consequences for the patient are considerable and lifelong' (WHO, 1985) [52].

(Table 3). Except under the highly stressed conditions following myocardial infarction, major surgery, trauma or overwhelming infection, a casual or random reading in excess of 11.1 mmol/l in venous plasma or 10.0 mmol/l in capillary whole blood is very unlikely to be met with in the absence of diabetes. In the symptomatic individual, glucose concentrations are often found to be between 15 mmol/l (270 mg/dl) and 25 mmol/l (450 mg/dl), leaving little room for diagnostic doubt. In such cases, urine tests for ketones and clinical evaluation for acidosis and dehydration become part of the evaluatory process and may be the prelude to prompt therapeutic intervention. In the absence of supporting clinical or biochemical data, or when associated with a highly stressful event, a high value of blood glucose must have further confirmatory measurements before the diagnosis of diabetes can be considered established. Even the best laboratories make mistakes.

WHO/NDDG Standard Oral Glucose Tolerance Test

Methods of preparation for the OGTT and its performance were agreed between the WHO and NDDG [49, 50, 52]. While closely resembling methods already generally in use, a major difference was the recommendation of an oral glucose load of 75 g or its anhydrous equivalent as partial starch hydrolysates (or 1.75 g/kg body weight up to 75 g for children).

The OGTT should be administered in the morning after at least 3 days of unrestricted diet (more than 150 g carbohydrate daily) and normal physical activity. The test should be preceded by 10–16 hours of fasting, during which drinking plain water is permitted. It is carried out in the seated subject; smoking is not allowed on the morning of the test. Factors that could influence the test's interpretation (e.g. medications, infection, recent trauma, departure from recommended test methods, etc.) must be recorded.

Following collection of the fasting blood sample, the glucose load dissolved in 250–300 ml of water is drunk over the course of about 5 minutes. A diagnostic blood sample must also be collected 2 hours after the test load. Mid-test samples, usually taken at 1 hour

but sometimes more frequently, may be collected for special purposes. The NDDG originally required the 1-hour sample for interpretation of the OGTT [49] but it has subsequently endorsed [53] the simpler WHO procedure which requires only fasting and 2-hour samples. For epidemiological or screening purposes the 2-hour sample alone may be adequate.

If the glucose concentration cannot be determined immediately, the blood sample should be preserved in a container with sodium fluoride (6 mg/ml whole blood) and centrifuged immediately to separate the plasma if necessary. Plasma should be frozen until the glucose is estimated. It is generally not appreciated that even in fluoride blood glucose levels can fall by up to 15% in 2 hours if the sample is kept at room temperature.

Test results are interpreted according to the values shown in Table 1.

Abbreviated Screening Test

A single measurement of blood glucose 2 hours after a 75 g oral glucose load [73] is a useful test for individuals in whom casual blood glucose measurements have given equivocal values (see Table 3) or when a simple test is required to screen for diabetic status. If standardized conditions are required (e.g. in epidemiological studies) the test should be conducted in the morning after an overnight fast. As an initial individual screening measurement, the test may be carried out without special dietary preparation at any time of day. Values should be interpreted against the 2-hour blood glucose criteria in Table 1. Those falling in the DM range will require further confirmation before diagnosis can be considered established. Those in the range of IGT call for fuller evaluation with the standard OGTT. Values in the normal range exclude glucose intolerance, but obviously relate only to the time of the test.

Diagnostic Variability

After allowing for the effects of time of day, drastic changes in carbohydrate or total food energy consumption, trauma, sepsis and certain medications on the glycaemic response to oral glucose, there remains substantial unexplained individual variability in the OGTT response, little of which is attributable to variation in absorption of the glucose load. The substantial diagnostic implications of spontaneous variation were recognized in the early studies of MacDonald et al [74], who showed that despite remarkable reproducibility of the population distributions of glucose tolerance over six retests, the position of individuals within those distributions could vary enormously. Individual variability has been repeatedly demonstrated to the present day [75, 76] and is of particular importance to the final diagnosis in those found to have glucose intolerance in screening surveys or as a chance finding. In such individuals the statistical phenomenon of regression to the mean on retest will also operate. Although this latter effect will cause higher values to fall on average, the more extreme the abnormality in the initial test, the less likely is a change of diagnostic category on retest. Equally, the chance of categorical change on retest rises as the initial response approaches the limiting values. Bounded by both upper and lower limiting values, individuals falling into the category of IGT are particularly liable to change on retest, with many 'improving' to normal tolerance and others 'worsening' to diabetes. In the study of Eriksson and Lindegärde [77], fewer than one-third of those initially classified as IGT and one-half of those classified as DM remained in their original category on retest after 1 month. In a study in Tanzania nearly 80% of those found to be IGT on the first test had reverted to normal when retested 1–3 days later [92]. Overall repeatability, as well as the significance of, IGT has been reviewed recently [42, 93].

In practical terms in a clinical setting, this variability emphasizes the need for confirmatory diagnostic measurements, especially when the test has been performed in the absence of symptoms of (or other diagnostic prompts for) diabetes, or when the result falls near the diagnostic cut-off values. If the confirmatory test disagrees categorically with the initial result the individual concerned should still be considered at risk for the higher category of abnormality. A series of tests, perhaps of the abbreviated 2-hour type, may be necessary before a confident judgement can be made of the true diagnostic status.

GLYCATION PRODUCTS IN DIABETES DIAGNOSIS

Glucose reacts non-enzymatically with proteins to form ultimately stable ketoamine adducts. Their abundance is closely related to the ambient concentration of glucose and the duration of exposure of the protein to it [78] (see Chapter 52). In the circulation this results in the formation, *inter alia*, of glycated haemoglobin derivatives (HbA_{1a}, HbA_{1b} and HbA_{1c}) and glycated

plasma proteins (known collectively as fructosamine) [79]. Present in the circulation of non-diabetic individuals [80], these glycated proteins are increased in people with sustained hyperglycaemia. The proportion of protein glycated correlates well with the average blood glucose concentration of people with diabetes, over the previous 8–10 weeks in the case of haemoglobin and 10–20 days in the case of fructosamine. Both estimations have found an important place in the regular monitoring of glycaemic control in those with established diabetes.

Since certain of these adducts are relatively insensitive to short-term fluctuations in blood glucose concentration and the completed glycation reaction is irreversible, no special dietary preparation or timing is necessary before the test sample is taken. This would seem to offer an attractive prospect for application in the diagnostic setting and many investigators have turned their attention to this [81–89]. In general, their conclusions have been disappointing. Both glycated haemoglobin and fructosamine lack sensitivity and specificity in detecting individuals with lesser degrees of IGT or even those with asymptomatic diabetes, fulfilling the WHO diagnostic OGTT criteria. It is only with symptomatic (so-called overt) diabetic patients that glycated haemoglobin and fructosamine values separate reasonably clearly from the normal range. In such patients, a single on-the-spot measurement of blood glucose level is very likely to be unequivocally and diagnostically elevated (Table 3). The screening and diagnostic values of this technically demanding and relatively expensive estimation of glycated haemoglobin and of the simpler, cheaper but even less sensitive fructosamine are thus limited, and their use for primary diagnostic purposes cannot at present be recommended. Nonetheless, a recent careful study has suggested that HbA_{1c} is very nearly as specific and sensitive as the 2-h post glucose load plasma glucose value in predicting outcome [94]. However, due to the expense and lack of standardization, HbA_{1c} is unlikely to replace measurement of blood glucose as a diagnostic test in the near future.

NEW DEVELOPMENTS

Recently, there has been an increasing view that the diagnostic criteria for the diagnosis of diabetes should be re-examined. There is now more than 10 years' experience with the NDDG and WHO criteria and many studies have been carried out using these. There is also a considerable body of data available concerning the outcome of IGT [93], which should allow better assessment of the cut-off points between IGT and diabetes, and also definition of non-diabetic fasting glucose values. As a result both the American Diabetes

Association and WHO have convened groups to re-examine the criteria and should be reporting in 1997. The main discussion points are: (a) whether the OGTT should be retained; (b) whether the cut-off points for fasting and 2-hour glycaemic levels should be altered; and (c) whether blood glucose measurement should be replaced by measurement of another variable.

The arguments against retaining the oral glucose tolerance test are, first and foremost, its variability (see above) and poor reproducibility. Mooy et al [95] showed an intra-individual coefficient of variation for the 2-hour value of 16.7% compared with 6.4% for fasting plasma glucose. Secondly, the OGTT is cumbersome, more expensive than a single measurement and not particularly pleasant for the recipient. On the other hand, the 75 g OGTT is now well standardized, there is a wealth of comparative data using it, it is not indeed necessary clinically for many cases (except gestational diabetes), and the diagnosis of IGT, an important high risk category, can only be made using it. There are proponents for using fasting plasma glucose alone but there are fewer comparative data available and there is always slight uncertainty as to whether subjects have indeed been fasting. It is also worth noting that McCance et al in their Pima Indian study [94] found the fasting plasma glucose to have slightly lower specificity and sensitivity than the 2-hour level.

One major problem has been the lack of equivalence of current fasting and 2-hour post glucose load criteria. Nearly all those with a fasting plasma glucose level of 7.8 mmol/l (140 mg/dl) or higher in the NHANES survey had a diagnostic 2-hour value, but only 25% of those with a 2-hour value above 11.1 mmol/l (200 mg/dl) had a raised fasting level [96]. Several groups have now re-assessed the fasting glucose value for diagnosis. Using contingency tables we found that a plasma glucose value of 7.0 mmol/l (126 mg/dl) best equated to the 2-hour value of 11.1 mmol/l (200 mg/dl) [97] in a range of Pacific populations, whilst Harris et al [96] found a value of 5.6 mmol/l (117 mg/dl) in NHANES II and McCance et al reported 6.8 mmol/l (123 mg/dl) in Pima Indians based on their prospective data.

There may also be a case for adjusting the 2-hour value, as 11.1 mmol/l is below the nadir values found in those populations with a bimodal distribution, but most would suggest that the arguments are not strong and that it is probably not as necessary to change the 2-hour level as the fasting level.

Finally, arguments still continue as to the usefulness of glycated haemoglobin measurement as the primary diagnostic test. For the reasons cited above, this seems premature. Only one study has shown reasonable sensitivity as well as specificity and there are problems of standardization. It is likely, therefore, that the new fasting glucose level and the 2-hour post glucose value will be the dominant diagnostic criteria for the next decade.

REFERENCES

1. Alberti KGMM, Press CM. The biochemistry of the complications of diabetes. In Keen H, Jarrett J (eds) Complications of diabetes, 2nd edn. London: Edward Arnold, 1982: 231–70.
2. Kopf A, Tchobroutsky G, Eschwege E. Serial postprandial blood glucose levels in 309 subjects with and without diabetes. Diabetes 1973; 22: 834–46.
3. Lefebvre PJ, Luyckx AS. The breakfast tolerance test: a return to physiology. Diabète Métab 1976; 2: 15–19.
4. Tchobroutsky G. Blood glucose levels in diabetic and non-diabetic subjects. Diabetologia 1991; 34: 67–73.
5. von Engelhardt D (ed.). Diabetes: its medical and cultural history. Berlin: Springer; 1989.
6. Frank LL. Diabetes mellitus in the text of old Hindu medicine. Am J Gastroenterol 1957; 27: 76–81.
7. Papaspyros NS. The history of diabetes mellitus, 2nd edn. Stuttgart: 1964. Originally published by Robert Stockwell Ltd, London: 1952.
8. Willis T. Therapeutice Rationalis (London) 1674; 4: 113.
9. Dobson M. Experiments and observations on the urine in a diabetic. Medical Observations and Inquiries by a Society of Physicians in London 1776; 5: 298–316.
10. Bouchardat A. Du diabète sucré ou glycosurie; son traitement hygiénique. Paris: 1851.
11. Young FG. Claude Bernard and the discovery of glycogen. A century of retrospect. Br Med J 1957; 2: 1431–7.
12. Keen H. The Bedford survey: a critique of methods and findings. Proc Roy Soc Med 1964; 51: 196–202.
13. Butterfield WJH, Keen H, Wichelow M. Renal glucose threshold variations with age. Br Med J 1967; 4: 505–7.
14. West KM. Epidemiology of diabetes and its vascular lesions. New York: Elsevier North-Holland, 1978: pp 231–48.
15. Felber JP, Golay A, Jéquier E, Curchod B, Temier E, DeFronzo RA, Ferrannini E. The metabolic consequences of long term human obesity. Int J Obesity 1988; 12: 377–89.
16. Vague J. The degree of masculine differentiation of obesities. A factor determining predisposition to diabetes, atherosclerosis, gout and uric-calculous disease. Am J Clin Nutr 1956; 4: 20–34.
17. Kissebah AH, Vydelingum N, Murray R. Relation of body fat distribution to metabolic complications of obesity. J Clin Endocrinol Metab 1982; 54: 254–60.
18. Harris MI, Hadden WC, Knowler WC, Bennett PH. Prevalence of diabetes and impaired glucose tolerance and plasma glucose levels in US population aged 20–74 yr. Diabetes 1987; 36: 523–34.
19. Shurakata H, Muller DC, Fleg JL, Soskin J, Ziemba AW, Andres R. Age as an independent determinant of glucose tolerance. Diabetes 1991; 40: 44–51.
20. Davidson MB. The effect of aging on carbohydrate metabolism: a review of the English literature and a practical approach to the diagnosis of diabetes mellitus in the elderly. Metabolism 1979; 28: 688–705.

21. Mather HM, Keen H. The Southall Diabetes Survey, prevalence of known diabetes in Asians and Europeans. Br Med J 1985; 291: 1081–4.

22. Ramaiya KL, Swai ABM, McLarty DG, Bhopal RS, Alberti KGMM. Prevalences of diabetes and cardiovascular risk factors in Hindu Indian subcommunities in Tanzania. Br Med J 1991; 303: 271–6.

23. Summary and recommendations of the Third International Workshop-Conference on Gestational Diabetes 1991; 40 (suppl 2).

24. O'Sullivan JM, Mahan CM. Criteria for the oral glucose tolerance test in pregnancy. Diabetes 1964; 13: 278–85.

25. Jarrett RJ. Diabetes mellitus and gestational diabetes. In Wald N (ed.) Antenatal and neonatal screening. Oxford University Press, 1984: pp 382–95.

26. Ales KL, Santini DL. Should all pregnant women be screened for gestational glucose intolerance? Lancet 1989; i: 1187–91.

27. West KM. Epidemiology of diabetes and its vascular lesions. New York: Elsevier North-Holland, 1978: pp 41–67.

28. Herron CA. Screening in diabetes mellitus: report of the Atlanta Workshop. Diabetes Care 1979; 2: 357–62.

29. West KM. Epidemiology of diabetes and its vascular lesions. New York: Elsevier North-Holland, 1978: pp 74–126.

30. Kobberling J, Creutzfeldt W. Comparison of different methods for evaluation of the oral glucose tolerance test. Diabetes 1970; 19: 870–4.

31. West KM. Substantial differences in the diagnostic criteria used by diabetes experts. Diabetes 1975; 24: 641–4.

32. Siperstein MD. The glucose tolerance test: a pitfall in the diagnosis of diabetes mellitus. Adv Int Med 1975; 20: 297–323.

33. Keen H. Diabetes epidemiology, a frontiersman's tool. In Alberti KGMM, Mazze RS (eds) Frontiers of diabetes research: Current trends in non-insulin-dependent diabetes mellitus. Amsterdam: Excerpta Medica, 1989.

34. Gordon T. Glucose tolerance of adults. Washington, DC: National Centre for Health Statistics, US Public Health Service Series 11, no. 2, 1964.

35. Fitzgerald MG, Keen H. Diagnostic classification of diabetes. Br Med J 1964; 1: 1568–9.

36. Jarrett RJ, Keen H. Hyperglycaemia and diabetes mellitus. Lancet 1976; ii: 1009–12.

37. O'Sullivan JB, Mahan CM. Prospective study of 352 young patients with chemical diabetes. New Engl J Med 1968; 278: 1038–41.

38. Jarrett RJ, Keen H, Fuller JH, McCartney M. Worsening to diabetes in men with impaired glucose tolerance ('borderline diabetes'). Diabetologia 1979; 16: 25–30.

39. Keen H, Jarrett RJ, McCartney P. The ten-year follow-up of the Bedford Survey (1962–1972): glucose tolerance and diabetes. Diabetologia 1982; 22: 73–8.

40. Sartor G, Schersten B, Carlstrom S, Melander A, Norden A, Persson G. Ten year follow-up of subjects with impaired glucose tolerance: prevention of diabetes by tolbutamide and diet regulation. Diabetes 1980; 29: 41–9.

41. King H, Zimmet P, Raper LR, Balkau B. The natural history of impaired glucose tolerance in the Micronesian population of Nauru: a six-year follow-up study. Diabetologia 1984; 26: 39–43.

42. Yudkin JS, Alberti KGMM, McLarty DG, Swai ABM. Impaired glucose tolerance. Is it a risk factor for diabetes or a diagnostic ragbag? Br Med J 1990; 301: 397–401.

43. Saad MF, Knowler WC, Pettit DJ, Nelson RG, Mott DM. The natural history of impaired glucose tolerance in the Pima Indians. New Engl J Med 1988; 319: 1500–6.

44. Fuller JH, Shipley MJ, Rose G, Jarrett RJ, Keen H. Coronary heart disease risk and impaired glucose tolerance: the Whitehall study. Lancet 1980; i: 1373–6.

45. Fuller JH, Shipley MJ, Rose G, Jarrett RJ, Keen H. Mortality from coronary heart disease and stroke in relation to degree of glycaemia: the Whitehall Study. Br Med J 1983; 287: 867–70.

46. Keen H, Rose G, Pyke DA, Boyns D, Chlouverakis C, Mistry S. Blood sugar and arterial disease. Lancet 1965; ii: 505–8.

47. Grabauskas VJ. Glucose intolerance as a contributor to non communicable disease morbidity and mortality. WHO Integrated Programme for Community Health in Noncommunicable Disease. Diabetes Care 1988; 11: 253–7.

48. Wingard DL, Barrett-Connor E. Family history of diabetes and cardiovascular disease risk factors and mortality among euglycemic borderline hyperglycemic and diabetic adults. Am J Epidemiol 1987; 125: 948–58.

49. National Diabetes Data Group. Classification and diagnosis of diabetes mellitus and other categories of glucose intolerance. Diabetes 1979; 28: 1039–57.

50. World Health Organisation Expert Committee. Second report on diabetes mellitus. Technical Report Series 646. Geneva: WHO, 1980.

51. Keen H, Jarrett RJ, Alberti KGMM. Diabetes mellitus: a new look at diagnostic criteria. Diabetologia 1979; 16: 283–5.

52. WHO. Diabetes mellitus: report of a WHO Study Group. Technical Report Series 727. Geneva: WHO, 1985.

53. Harris MI, Hadden WC, Knowler WC, Bennett PH. International criteria for the diagnosis of diabetes and impaired glucose tolerance. Diabetes Care 1985; 8: 562–7.

54. Bennett PH, Rushforth NB, Miller M, Lecompte P. Epidemiologic studies in diabetes in the Pima Indians. Rec Prog Horm Res 1976; 32: 333–76.

55. Zimmet P, Whitehouse S. Bimodality of fasting and two-hour glucose tolerance distributions in a Micronesian population. Diabetes 1978; 27: 793–800.

56. Rosenthal M, McMahan CA, Stern MP, Eiffler CW, Haffner SM, Hazuda HP, Franco LJ. Evidence of bimodality of two hour plasma glucose concentrations in Mexican Americans: results from the San Antonio heart study. J Chron Dis 1985; 38: 5–16.

57. Stern MP. Type II diabetes. Interface between clinical and epidemiological investigation. Diabetes 1988; 11: 119–26.

58. Massari V, Eschwege E, Valleron AJ. Imprecision of new criteria for the oral glucose tolerance test. Diabetologia 1983; 24: 100–6.

59. Jarrett RJ. Do we need IGT? Diabet Med 1987; 4: 544–5.

60. Sasaki A. Assessment of the new criteria for diabetes mellitus according to 10-year relative survival rates. Diabetologia 1981; 20: 195–8.

61. Stern MP, Rosenthal M, Haffner S. A new concept of impaired glucose tolerance. Relation to cardiovascular risk. Arteriosclerosis 1985; 5: 311–14.

62. Modan M, Harris MI, Halkin H. Evaluation of WHO and NDDG criteria for impaired glucose tolerance: results from two national samples. Diabetes 1989; 38: 1630–5.

63. King H, Zimmet P. Trends in the prevalence and incidence of diabetes: non insulin dependent diabetes mellitus. Wld Hlth Statist Quart 1988; 41: 190–6.

64. Schranz AG. Abnormal glucose tolerance in Malta. A population-based longitudinal study of the natural history of NIDDM and IGT in Malta. Diabetes Res Clin Pract 1989; 7: 7–16.

65. Harlan LC, Harlan WR, Landes JR, Goldstein NG. Factors associated with glucose tolerance in adults in the United States. Am J Epidemiol 1987; 126: 674–84.

66. Stengård JM, Tuomilehto J, Salomaa V, Korhonen M. The prevalence of impaired glucose tolerance and diabetes does not vary between east and west Finland. Diabetes 1991; 40 (suppl 1): 375A.

67. King H, Rewers M. Geographic patterns of diabetes mellitus (DM) and impaired glucose tolerance (IGT) in adults. Diabetes 1991; 40 (suppl 1): 304A.

68. Dowse GK, Hassain G, Zimmet P et al. High prevalence of NIDDM and impaired glucose tolerance in Indian, Creole and Chinese Mauritians. Diabetes 1990; 39: 390–6.

69. Glatthar C, Welborn TA, Stenhouse NS, Garcia-Webb P. Diabetes and impaired glucose tolerance; a prevalence estimate based on the Busselton 1981 survey. Med J Austr 1985; 143: 436–40.

70. French LR, Boey JR, Martinez AM, Rushhouse SA, Sprafky JM, Goetz FC. Population based study of impaired glucose tolerance and Type II diabetes in Wadena, Minnesota. Diabetes 1990; 39: 1131–7.

71. Harris MI. Impaired glucose tolerance in the US population. Diabetes Care 1988; 11: 23–9.

72. Forrest RD, Jackson CA, Yudkin JS. Glucose intolerance and hypertension in North London. The Islington diabetes survey. Diabet Med 1986; 3: 338–42.

73. Forrest RD, Jackson CA, Yudkin JS. The abbreviated glucose tolerance test in screening for diabetes: the Islington diabetes survey. Diabet Med 1988; 5: 557–61.

74. MacDonald GW, Fisher GF, Burnham C. Reproducibility of the oral glucose tolerance test. Diabetes 1965; 14: 473–8.

75. Harding PE, Oakley NW, Wynn V. Reproducibility of oral glucose tolerance data in normal and mildly diabetic subjects. Clin Endocrinol 1973; 2: 387–93.

76. Balkau B, Eschwege E. Repeatability of the oral glucose tolerance test for the diagnosis of impaired glucose and diabetes mellitus. Diabetologia 1991; 34: 201–2.

77. Eriksson KF, Lindegärde F. Impaired glucose tolerance in a middle-aged male urban population: a new approach for identifying high-risk cases. Diabetologia 1990; 33: 526–31.

78. Duncan BB, Heiss G. Reviews and commentary: non enzymatic glycosylation of proteins: new loci for assessment of cumulative hyperglycemia in epidemiologic studies, past and future. Am J Epidemiol 1984; 120: 169–89.

79. Baker JR, O'Connor JP, Metcalf PA, Lawson MR, Johnson RN. The clinical usefulness of serum fructosamine estimation as a screening test for diabetes mellitus. Br Med J 1983; 287: 683–7.

80. Simon D, Senan C, Garner P, Saint-Paul M, Papoz L. Epidemiological features of glycated haemoglobin A_{1c} distribution in a healthy population. The Telecom Study. Diabetologia 1989; 32: 864–9.

81. Ferrell RE, Harris CL, Aguilar L et al. Glycosylated hemoglobin determination from capillary blood samples: utility in an epidemiologic survey of diabetes. Am J Epidemiol 1984; 199: 159–66.

82. Hall PM, Cook JGH, Sheldon J et al. Glycosylated hemoglobins and glycosylated plasma proteins in the diagnosis of diabetes mellitus and impaired glucose tolerance. Diabetes Care 1984; 7: 147–50.

83. Modan M, Halkin H, Karasik A, Lusky A. Effectiveness of glycosylated hemoglobin, fasting plasma glucose and a single post-load plasma glucose level in population screening for glucose intolerance: the Israel study of glucose intolerance, obesity and hypertension. Am J Epidemiol 1984; 199: 431–44.

84. Albutt EC, Nattrass M, Northam BE. Glucose tolerance test and glycosylated haemoglobin measurement for diagnosis of diabetes mellitus; an assessment of the criteria of the WHO Expert Committee on Diabetes Mellitus. Ann Clin Biochem 1985; 22: 67–73.

85. Forrest RD, Jackson CA, Gould BJ, Casburn-Budd M, Taylor JE, Yudkin JS. Four assays of glycated haemoglobin compared as screening tests for diabetes mellitus: the Islington diabetes survey. Clin Chem 1988; 34: 145–8.

86. Guillausseau PJ, Charles M-A, Paolaggi F et al. Comparison of HbA_1 and fructosamine in diagnosis of glucose tolerance abnormalities. Diabetes Care 1983; 13: 898–900.

87. Verillo A, de Teresa A, Golia R, Nunziata V. The relationship between glycosylated haemoglobin levels and various degrees of glucose intolerance. Diabetologia 1983; 24: 391–3.

88. Swai ABM, Harrison K, Chuwal M, Makene W, McLarty D, Alberti KGMM. Screening for diabetes: does measurement of serum fructosamine help? Diabet Med 1988; 5: 648–52.

89. Shima K, Abe F, Chikakiyo H, Ito N. The relative value of glycated albumin, haemoglobin A_{1c} and fructosamine when screening for diabetes mellitus. Diabetes Res Clin Pract 1989; 7: 243–50.

90. Deerochanawong C, Putiyanun C, Wongsuryrat M, Serirat S, Jinayon P. Comparison of National Diabetes Data Group and World Health Organization criteria for detecting gestational diabetes mellitus. Diabetologia 1996; 39: 1070–3.

91. Stolk RP, Grobee DE, Orchard TE. Why use the oral glucose tolerance test? Diabetes Care 1995; 18: 1045–9.

92. Swai ABM, McLarty DG, Kitange HM et al. Study in Tanzania of impaired glucose tolerance—methodological myth? Diabetes 1991; 40: 516–20.

93. Alberti KGMM. The clinical implications of impaired glucose intolerance. Diabet Med 1996; 13: 927–37.

94. McCance DR, Hanson RL, Charles MA et al. Comparison of tests for glycated haemoglobin and fasting and two-hour plasma glucose concentrations as diagnostic methods for diabetes. Br Med J 1994; 308: 1323–8.

95. Mooy JM, Grootenhuis PA, de Vries H et al. Intra-individual variation of glucose, specific insulin and proinsulin concentrations measured by two-hour oral glucose tolerance tests in a general Caucasian population: the Hoorn Study. Diabetologia 1996; 39: 298–305.

96. Harris MI, Hadden WC, Knowler WC, Bennett PH. Prevalence of diabetes and impaired glucose tolerance and plasma glucose levels in the US population aged 20-74 years. Diabetes 1987; 36: 523-34.

97. Finch CF, Zimmet PZ, Alberti KGMM. Determining diabetes prevalence; a rational basis for the use of fasting plasma concentrations. Diabet Med 1990; 7: 603-10.

3

Genetics of Diabetes

Maren T. Scheuner, Leslie J. Raffel and Jerome I. Rotter

Division of Medical Genetics, Departments of Medicine and Pediatrics, Cedars-Sinai Medical Center and UCLA School of Medicine, Los Angeles, California, USA

INTRODUCTION

It is clearly established that diabetes mellitus is not a single disease but a genetically heterogeneous group of disorders with glucose intolerance as a common feature [5–12]. The concept of genetic heterogeneity, i.e. that different genetic and/or environmental etiologic factors can result in similar phenotypes, has significantly altered the genetic analysis of this common disorder. It is now apparent that diabetes and glucose intolerance are not diagnostic terms but, like anemia, simply describe symptoms and/or laboratory abnormalities which can have a number of distinct etiologies.

DIFFICULTIES IN GENETIC STUDIES OF DIABETES

The geneticist is confronted with a number of obstacles in his/her attempts to unravel the genetics of diabetes. These include differences in the definition of affected individuals, modification of the expression of the diabetic genotype by environmental factors, and variability in the age of onset of the disease. One of the major sources of confusion in the study of diabetes mellitus has been the definition of an 'affected' individual. Some investigators have labeled an individual as diabetic only if he has clinical symptoms of the disease, while others have accepted a mildly abnormal glucose tolerance test.

Another problem in the definition of affected individuals is the marked clinical variability of diabetes. The phenotypic expression of the diabetes genotype (or genotypes) appears to be modified by a variety of environmental factors, including diet, obesity, infection and physical activity, as well as sex and parity. Obese non-insulin dependent diabetic individuals may lose all signs of the disorder, clinical as well as chemical, if their weight returns to normal. Because of the marked variability in the age of onset of the disease, at any given time only a fraction of those individuals possessing the diabetic genotype may be recognized. Thus, longitudinal studies are required to detect those genetically affected family members who will eventually manifest clinical disease.

The high prevalence of diabetes in the population presents additional difficulties for the geneticist. Is a relative affected because he has the same genotype, because she shares the same environment, or because he/she has a chance occurrence of a common disorder? Furthermore, the diabetic syndromes are sufficiently common that two genetically different forms of them may occasionally occur in the same family.

The most important impediment to genetic analysis has been a lack of knowledge concerning the basic defect(s) in each of the disorders leading to diabetes. Because of this, there is no certain method for detecting all individuals with disease-predisposing genotypes prior to their clinical manifestations: that is, individuals who possess the diabetic genotypes but have no signs of abnormal carbohydrate metabolism.

Despite all these obstacles, considerable progress has been made through increasing recognition of the genetic heterogeneity of diabetes and its delineation by a variety of lines of evidence, as discussed below.

International Textbook of Diabetes Mellitus, Second Edition. Edited by K.G.M.M. Alberti, P. Zimmet, R.A. DeFronzo, and H. Keen (Honorary)
© 1997 John Wiley & Sons Ltd

DIABETES IN FAMILIES AND TWINS

Familial Aggregation of Diabetes

It is widely recognized that diabetic individuals have an 'increased family history' of the disease [15]. In most reports the frequency of diabetic individuals with positive family histories of the disease ranges from 25% to 50%. Since the frequency of a positive family history of diabetes in non-diabetic individuals has usually been found to be below 15%, this family history information has been used to support the hypothesis that diabetes mellitus is a hereditary disorder. However, these types of data are not very powerful. A more accurate method of assessing familial aggregation is to compare diabetes prevalence in specific relatives of affected individuals with that found among similar relatives of non-diabetic controls. Pincus and White [16] were the first to use this method, when they established statistically the increased prevalence of diabetes among relatives of patients with the disease, since confirmed by many other investigators [12]. Using more sensitive markers of the diabetic genotype, such as oral, intravenous and cortisone-induced glucose tolerance tests, the prevalence of affected individuals among the relatives of diabetic patients is even higher (usually between 10% and 30% of the parents, sibs or close relatives, as compared to 1–6% of the similar relatives of non-diabetic individuals).

Early Twin Studies

Familial aggregation of a trait may be caused by either genetic or environmental factors. Twin studies represent one approach to resolving this question. The frequency of concordance (both members of the twin pair affected) of monozygotic (identical) twins is compared with that of dizygotic (fraternal) twins. Monozygotic twins share all genes, and thus should theoretically be concordant for those disorders with pure genetic etiology. Dizygotic twins share only half their genes and thus are no more alike genetically than any pair of siblings.

Twin studies have confirmed the importance of genetic factors in the etiology of diabetes. Using clinical diabetes as the criterion, most investigators have reported a concordance rate for monozygotic twins between 45% and 96%, and for dizygotic twins between 3% and 37%. When NIDDM is considered separately and glucose tolerance tests are performed in the 'non-diabetic' monozygotic co-twins, the concordance rate is usually above 70%. The available data suggest that dizygotic twin risk appears to be approximately equivalent to that of siblings, arguing that whatever environmental factors contribute, these are present in the majority of a given population, and suggesting that there is not a large contribution from

unique family environments. As will be discussed, the monozygotic concordance rates are very different for IDDM and NIDDM.

GENETIC HETEROGENEITY IN DIABETES

Although studies of familial aggregation and twins leave no doubt as to the importance of genetic factors in the etiology of diabetes, for many years there was little agreement as to the nature of these factors. This confusion can largely be explained by the genetic heterogeneity which is now known to exist in diabetes. The hypothesis of genetic heterogeneity proposed in 1966 was based on several lines of evidence. Indirect evidence included: (a) the existence of distinct, mostly rare genetic disorders (now numbering over 70) [12], that have glucose intolerance as one of their features (Table 1); (b) genetic heterogeneity in diabetic animal models; (c) ethnic variability in prevalence and clinical features; (d) clinical variability between the thin, ketosis-prone, insulin dependent, juvenile onset diabetic vs. the obese, non-ketotic, insulin resistant, adult onset diabetic patient; and (e) physiologic variability, i.e. the demonstration of decreased plasma insulin in younger vs. the relative hyperinsulinism of older diabetic patients. In addition, some direct evidence for heterogeneity came from clinical genetic studies which suggested that insulin-dependent and non-insulin dependent patients differed genetically within families [9, 14].

Heterogeneity between Type 1 Diabetes (IDDM) and Type 2 Diabetes (NIDDM)

A number of lines of clinical and genetic evidence led to the eventual separation of type 1 (IDDM) and type 2 diabetes (NIDDM) as clearly distinct groups of disorders (Table 2). Clinical differences which tended to run true in families provided some of the first evidence [17–29]. In addition, the extensive monozygotic twin studies by Pyke et al in the UK strongly supported the separation of IDDM and NIDDM patients [30]. Among 200 pairs of monozygotic (identical) twins, concordance for diabetes was shown to be less than 50% for IDDM twins, but close to 100% for NIDDM, suggesting a greater role of non-genetic factors in NIDDM.

Physiologic studies further supported the separation of IDDM and NIDDM, and immunologic studies pinpointed the importance of immune mechanisms in the etiology of IDDM, but not NIDDM. Direct evidence for an autoimmune role in the pathogenesis of IDDM (see Chapter 5) came from the discovery of organ-specific cell-mediated immunity to pancreatic islets, and the demonstration of antibodies to the islet cells of the pancreas [31–33]. While these antibodies were first detected only in IDDM subjects with coexistent

Table 1 Genetic syndromes associated with glucose intolerance and diabetes mellitus

Syndromes	Types of DM	Associated clinical findings	Pattern of inheritance	*McKusick
Syndromes associated with pancreatic degeneration				
Congenital absence of the pancreas	IDDM (congenital)	IUGR, poor adipose and muscle development, malabsorption, dehydration	AD,?AR	260 370
Congenital absence of the islets of Langerhans	IDDM (congenital)	IUGR, dehydration, ± fatal secretory diarrhea	?AR or XR	304 790
Congenital pancreatic hypoplasia	IDDM (infancy)	IUGR, pancreatic exocrine deficiency	?AR	260 370
Renal–hepatic–pancreatic dysplasia	IDDM	Renal cystic dysplasia, biliary dysgenesis, pancreatic fibrosis and cysts, ± polysplenia	AD	263 200
Hereditary relapsing pancreatitis	IGT → IDDM	Abdominal pain, chronic pancreatitis	AD	167 800
Cystic fibrosis	IGT → IDDM	Malabsorption, chronic respiratory disease	AR	219 700
Polyendocrine deficiency disease (Schmidt's syndrome)	IDDM	Autoimmune endocrine disease, hypothyroidism, hypoadrenalism	?AR,AD	269 200
IgA deficiency, malabsorption and diabetes	IDDM	IgA deficiency, malabsorption	?AD	137 100
Hemochromatosis	NIDDM	Hepatic, pancreatic, skin, cardiac and endocrine complications of iron storage	AR	235 200
Thalassemia	IGT → NIDDM	Anemia, iron overload	AR	141 900
Alpha-1-antitrypsin deficiency	IGT	Emphysema, cirrhosis	AR	107 400
Hereditary endocrine disorders with glucose intolerance				
Isolated growth hormone deficiency	NIDDM	Proportionate dwarfism	AD AR	173 100 262 400
Hereditary panhypopituitary dwarfism	NIDDM	Proportionate dwarfism, hypogonadism ± TSH & ACTH deficiency	AR XR	262 600 312 000
Johanson–Blizzard syndrome	IDDM	Hypoplastic nasal alae, deafness, hypothyroidism, growth retardation, mental retardation, malabsorption	AR	243 800
Laron dwarfism	NIDDM	Proportionate dwarfism	AR	262 100
Nesidioblastosis	NIDDM	Hyperinsulinism, hypoglycemia in infancy can evolve into late glucose intolerance	AR	256 450

continued overleaf

Table 1   (*continued*)

Syndromes	Types of DM	Associated clinical findings	Pattern of inheritance	*McKusick
Pheochromocytoma	IGT	Hypertension, tremor, paroxysmal sweating	AD	171 300
Multiple endocrine adenomatosis	IGT	Pituitary (acromegaly), parathyroid (renal stones) and pancreatic adenomas (peptic ulcer)	AD	131 100

Inborn errors of metabolism with glucose intolerance

Alaninuria (Stimmler's syndrome)	IDDM (infancy)	Mental retardation, microcephaly, IUGR, dwarfism, enamel hypoplasia, high blood pyruvate, lactate and alanine	?AR	202 900
Glycogen storage disease type 1 (von Gierke's disease)	IGT	Hepatomegaly, early hypoglycemia	AR	232 200
Acute intermittent porphyria	IGT	Paroxysmal abdominal pain, hypertension	AD	176 000
Hyperlipidemias	NIDDM	Hyperlipidemia, coronary artery disease	AD	144 250
Fanconi's syndrome— hypophosphatemia	NIDDM	Renal tubular dysfunction, metabolic bone disease	AR	227 700
Thiamine responsive megaloblastic anemia	IGT, IDDM	Megaloblastic anemia, deafness	AR	249 270

Syndromes with non-ketotic insulin resistant early onset diabetes mellitus

Ataxia telangiectasia	Insulin resistant	Ataxia, telangiectasia, IgA deficiency	AR	208 900
Myotonic dystrophy	Insulin resistant	Myotonia, cataracts, balding, testicular atrophy	AD	160 900
Lipoatrophic diabetes:				
Seip–Berardinelli syndrome	Insulin resistant	Hepatomegaly, acanthosis nigricans, elevated BMR, polycystic ovaries, clitoral hypertrophy	AR	269 700
Brunzell syndrome	Insulin resistant	Same as Seip–Berardinelli, with cystic angiomatosis of soft tissue and bone (?same syndrome)	AR	272 500

Syndromes	Types of DM	Associated clinical findings	Pattern of inheritance	*McKusick
Familial partial lipodystrophy (Kobberling–Dunnigan syndrome) Type A: confined to limbs, sparing face and trunk Type B: trunk also affected, with exception of vulva	Insulin resistant	Hyperlipidemia, xanthomata, acanthosis nigricans	?AD,XD	151 660
Partial lipodystrophy with Rieger anomaly	IGT → NIDDM	Rieger anomaly, midface hypoplasia, short stature, hypotrichosis	AD	151 680
Aredlyd syndrome (acrorenal and ectodermal dysplasia)	Insulin resistant	IUGR and growth retardation, lipoatrophy, hepatosplenomegaly, unusual facies, hypotrichosis, dental abnormalities, scoliosis, hyperostosis of cranial vault, hand malformations, hypoplasia of breasts, genital abnormalities, ectodermal dysplasia	AR	207 780
Alstrom's syndrome	Insulin resistant	Retinal degeneration, nerve deafness, obesity	AR	203 800
Bloom syndrome	Insulin resistant	IUGR, sun-sensitive telangiectatic rash	AR	210 900
Edwards' syndrome	Insulin resistant	Mental retardation, deafness, retinitis pigmentosa, obesity, hypogonadism, ± acanthosis nigricans	AR	268 020
Hoepffner syndrome (combined deficiency of action of insulin, IGF-I and EGF)	Insulin resistant	Lipodystrophy, scleroderma-like skin joint contractures, bird-like facies	AR	233 805
Leprechaunism (point mutations in insulin receptor gene)	Insulin resistant	IUGR and growth retardation, large hands, feet and genitals, acanthosis nigricans, decreased subcutaneous fat, hirsutism	AR	246 200
Seemanova syndrome	Insulin resistant	Obesity, mental retardation, delayed puberty, macroorchidism, acanthosis nigricans, curly hair	AD	100 600

continued overleaf

Table 1 (*continued*)

Syndromes	Types of DM	Associated clinical findings	Pattern of inheritance	*McKusick
SHORT syndrome	Insulin resistant	Short, hyperextensibility, ocular depression, Rieger anomaly, delayed teething, lipodystrophy	AR	269 880
Rabson–Mendenhall syndrome	Insulin resistant	Unusual facies, enlarged genitals, precocious puberty, acanthosis nigricans, hirsutism, pineal hyperplasia	AR	262 190
Acanthosis nigricans insulin resistant diabetes syndromes				
Type A	Insulin resistant, decreased receptors	Acanthosis nigricans, ovarian hirsutism, accelerated growth	AD	147 670
Type A with acral hypertrophy and cramps	Insulin resistant (post-receptor defect)	Large hands, acanthosis nigricans, muscle cramps, enlarged kidneys, polycystic ovaries	?AR	
Type A with brachydactyly and dental anomalies	Insulin resistant	Acanthosis nigricans, bitemporal narrowing, acral hypertrophy, decreased body fat, brachydactyly, dental anomalies	?AR	
Type A with muscle cramps and coarse facies	Insulin resistant (post-receptor defect)	Coarse facies, muscular women, acanthosis nigricans, headaches, muscle cramps, hyperprolactinemia, no ovarian dysfunction	AD	
Type B	Insulin resistant (circulating inhibitor)	Acanthosis nigricans, immunological disease	?	
Hereditary neuromuscular disorders associated with glucose intolerance				
Anosmia–hypogonadism syndrome (Kallmann's syndrome)	IGT or IDDM	Anosmia, hypogonadotrophic hypogonadism, hearing loss ± cleft lip and palate	XR ?AR ?AD	308 700 244 200 147 950
Fryn's syndrome	IDDM	Mental retardation, craniofacial dysmorphism, hypogonadism, seizures	AR	229 850
Muscular dystrophies	IGT → NIDDM	Muscular dystrophy	AD AR XR	158 900 253 600 310 200
Late onset proximal myopathy	IGT → NIDDM	Myopathy, cataracts	?AR	600 109
Huntington's disease	IGT → NIDDM	Chorea, dementia	AD	143 100
Machado disease	NIDDM	Ataxia	AD	109 150

Syndromes	Types of DM	Associated clinical findings	Pattern of inheritance	*McKusick
Herrmann syndrome	NIDDM	Photomyoclonus, deafness, nephropathy, dementia	AD	172 500
Diabetes mellitus–optic atrophy–diabetes insipidus–deafness syndrome (Wolfram, DIDMOAD syndrome)	IDDM	Optic atrophy, diabetes insipidus, deafness, neurologic symptoms	AR	222 300
Friedreich's ataxia	IDDM or NIDDM	Spinocerebellar degeneration	AR	229 300
Ramon syndrome	IDDM	Gingival fibromatosis, cherubism, mental retardation, epilepsy, JRA, vascular skin lesions	AR	266 270
Pseudo-Refsum syndrome	NIDDM	Muscle atrophy, ataxia, retinitis pigmentosa	AD	158 500
Stiff man syndrome	IDDM	Fluctuating muscle rigidity with painful spasm, characteristic EMG, autoimmune disease of nervous and endocrine system	?AD (most sporadic)	184 850
Roussy–Levy syndrome	NIDDM	Ataxia, areflexia with amyotrophy	AD	180 800
Progeroid syndromes associated with glucose intolerance				
Cockayne's syndrome	IGT	Dwarfism, progeria, mental retardation, deafness, blindness	AR	216 400
Metageria	NIDDM	Early atherosclerosis, tall and thin, bird-like facies and aged appearance, normal sexual development, atrophic mottled skin, telangiectasia, little subcutaneous fat	?AR	201 200
Werner syndrome	NIDDM	Premature aging, cataracts, arteriosclerosis	AR	277 700
Mitochondrial syndromes				
Ballanger–Wallace syndrome	IDDM/NIDDM	Deafness, cardiomyopathy, retinopathy		520 000
MELAS syndrome	IDDM/NIDDM	Myopathy, encephalopathy, lactic acidosis, stroke-like episodes		540 000
Rotig syndrome	IDDM/NIDDM	Proximal tubulopathy, cerebellar ataxia, myopathy, skin abnormalities		560 000

continued overleaf

Table 1 (*continued*)

Syndromes	Types of DM	Associated clinical findings	Pattern of inheritance	*McKusick
Syndromes with glucose intolerance secondary to obesity				
Achondroplasia	IGT	Disproportionate dwarfism, relative obesity	AD	100 800
Bardet–Biedl syndrome	IGT → NIDDM	Mental retardation, retinal degeneration, polydactyly, hypogonadism and obesity	AR	209 900
Prader–Willi syndrome	NIDDM	Obesity, short stature, acromicria, mental retardation, disproportionate dwarfism	15q abnormal	176 270
Miscellaneous syndromes associated with glucose intolerance				
Christian syndrome	IGT → NIDDM	Short stature, ridged metopic suture, mental retardation, fusion of cervical vertebrae, thoracic hemivertebrae, scoliosis, sacral hypoplasia, abducens palsy, carrier females may have NIDDM or IGT	XR	309 620
Steroid-induced ocular hypertension	IGT	Steroid-induced ocular hypertension	AD	137 760
Epiphyseal dysplasia and infantile onset diabetes mellitus (Wolcoff–Rallison syndrome)	IDDM (congenital)	Epiphyseal dysplasia, tooth and skin defects	AR	226 980
Progressive cone dystrophy, degenerative liver disease, endocrine dysfunction, and hearing defect	MODY	Color blindness, liver disease, deafness, hypogonadism	AR	268 315
Symmetric lipomatosis	IGT → NIDDM	Diffuse symmetric lipomas of neck and trunk, stiff skin, muscle cramps, decreased sensation, hearing loss, urolithiasis, hypertension, peptic ulcers	AD	151 800
Woodhouse–Sakati syndrome	NIDDM	Unusual facies, hypogonadism, absent breast tissue, sparse hair, mental retardation, sensineural deafness and ECG abnormalities	AR	241 080

Syndromes	Types of DM	Associated clinical findings	Pattern of inheritance	*McKusick
Cytogenetic disorders associated with glucose intolerance				
Down's syndrome	IGT	Mental retardation, short stature, typical facies	Trisomy 21	
Klinefelter's syndrome	IGT → NIDDM	Hypogonadism, tall stature, mental retardation	47,XXY	
Turner's syndrome	IGT → NIDDM	Short stature, gonadal dysgenesis, web neck	45,XO	

Abbreviations: AD, autosomal dominant; AR, autosomal recessive; BMR, basal metabolic rate; IDDM, insulin dependent diabetes mellitus (type 1); IGT, impaired glucose tolerance; IUGR, intrauterine growth retardation; JRA, juvenile rheumatoid arthritis; MODY, maturity onset type diabetes of the young; NIDDM, non-insulin dependent diabetes mellitus (type 2); XR, X-linked recessive, XD, X-linked dominant. *McKusick refers to the catalog of single gene conditions [443]. (Table modified from reference 444, with permission.)

Table 2 Separation of IDDM from NIDDM

Distinguishing characteristics	IDDM (type 1) (juvenile onset type)*	NIDDM (type 2) (maturity onset type)*
Clinical	Thin: ketosis prone; insulin required for survival; onset predominantly in childhood and early adulthood	Obese; ketosis resistant; often treatable by diet or drugs; onset predominantly after age 40 years
Family studies	Increased prevalence of juvenile or type 1	Increased prevalence of maturity or type 2
Twin studies	<50% concordance in monozygotic twins	Close to 100% concordance in monozygotic twins
Insulin response to a glucose load	Flat	Variable
Associated with other autoimmune endocrine diseases and antibodies	Yes	No
Islet cell antibodies and pancreatic cell-mediated immunity	Yes	No
HLA associations and linkage	Yes	No

*Older nomenclature.

autoimmune endocrine disease, it soon became apparent that they were common (60–80%) in newly diagnosed IDDM subjects. Islet cell antibody studies supported the differentiation of insulin dependent from non-insulin dependent diabetes, as autoantibodies were present in 30–40% of the former group (even after onset), as opposed to 5–8% of the latter. Of interest, many (possibly the majority) of the non-insulin dependent, yet antibody-positive, patients appear to become insulin dependent with time. They have flat insulin responses to a glucose load, and they also have the HLA-associated DR3 and DR4 antigens [34]. This has suggested that etiologically these cases belong in the insulin dependent category; i.e., they are in a transitional state on the way to eventual insulin dependence and share the same underlying pathogenetic mechanisms as IDDM [34–38]. Thus, immunologic studies have served both to separate disorders (IDDM vs. NIDDM) and combine others (insulin dependent and non-insulin dependent yet antibody positive).

Finally, the clear and consistent association of IDDM, but not NIDDM, with specific HLA antigens became a major argument for etiologic differences between these two disorders; approximately 95% of IDDM patients have DR3 or DR4 or both [10, 19, 32, 39, 40–43].

A few cautions are in order. Just because we are able to separate the bulk of patients and families into IDDM and NIDDM forms does not mean this phenotypic distinction is absolute. There is at least some evidence that families of either type have more of the other type of diabetes than do families in the general population [44, 45]. Part of this overlap may be attributed to the insulin independent phase of the insulin dependent type (the frequency of which is still being defined) [35–38, 46]. This observation may also be the result of even further etiologic heterogeneity (see below). Finally, while the distinction between insulin dependence and independence provides the primary basis for dividing the two main subtypes of diabetes, age of onset and other clinical differences should not be dismissed summarily. For example, delineation of a distinct form of non-insulin dependent diabetes which has been termed 'maturity onset diabetes of the young' (MODY) [47, 48] clearly demonstrated that age of onset is a useful clinical criterion for classification purposes. Similarly, there is evidence that age of onset may still be helpful as an additional classification criterion in IDDM, in that those individuals with DR3/DR4 have the youngest age of onset.

INSULIN DEPENDENT DIABETES MELLITUS (IDDM, TYPE 1)

The molecular genetics of type 1 diabetes is covered in detail in Chapter 6, so this chapter will concentrate on the following aspects: difficulties in genetic analysis; differences between HLA-DR3- and DR4-associated type 1 diabetes; environmental factors; and genetic counseling.

Difficulties in Genetic Analysis

With the discovery of HLA associations with IDDM, the genetic region that provides the major (but not sole) genetic susceptibilities to IDDM was located. The genetics of IDDM remains an area of some confusion, however, with no complete consensus as to which gene or combination of genes in the major histocompatibility complex is responsible for the HLA-related susceptibility, or how many other genes outside of the HLA region (in most cases on other chromosomes) are involved. Several major difficulties continue to confound attempts to analyze the genetics of IDDM. These include the reduced penetrance of the disorder, the confounding of linkage and association, and the heterogeneity within the disorder.

When the mode of inheritance is unknown, the only estimate we have for penetrance of the IDDM genotype comes from identical twin concordance data. The largest twin data set (the UK diabetic twin study) reported concordance for IDDM of some 50% [30, 52]. However, it is clear that this sample is an unrepresentative one, with only a fraction of the twins in the UK identified, and thus a presumed bias toward concordant pairs [53]. Reports from less biased, but much smaller, samples report concordances of approximately 20% [44, 54]. Finally, a prospective study of twins from the UK group yielded a concordance estimate of about 36%, which is probably the best estimate available [55]. This reduced penetrance indicates that what is inherited in IDDM is disease susceptibility; other factors, presumably environmental, are required to convert genetic susceptibility into clinical disease. This view is supported both by the observations that the onset of

IDDM clusters in families and twin pairs [55, 56] and by the epidemiologic, experimental animal and clinical evidence for viral infections as a supervening factor in at least some cases [57, 58] (see below). However, it is not the only explanation, as the somatic recombination that occurs within the immune system is also a potential explanation for the reduced penetrance (see below).

A second problem in the genetics of IDDM is that relationships between genes in the HLA region and IDDM have been found in studies of families and of the population at large. The former observation connotes linkage, the latter connotes association. Linkage and association were classically characterized as being entirely distinct phenomena, although it is now appreciated that the two can occur together (see below). Linkage is a reflection of the relative proximity of gene loci on the chromosome map. If two genes are linked (that is, located close to one another on the same chromosome), they tend to accompany one another through meiosis and therefore travel together vertically down a pedigree, even though the two genes may have totally unrelated functions. Thus, once it has been demonstrated that a disease and a marker locus cosegregate, a gene or locus which is polymorphic (such as a variable number tandem repeat sequence [VNTR]) can be used as a marker locus to infer who within a given family has inherited predisposition to a disease. However, because of crossing-over or recombination, specific alleles at the linked loci will not be associated with the disease throughout a population. In contrast, disease association studies examine the prevalence of a well defined genetic trait, such as blood groups, serum enzyme polymorphisms or DNA polymorphisms of a candidate gene, among individuals with and without the disease of interest. If the disease occurs more commonly with a particular allele of a well defined genetic locus (e.g. a positive association such as the increased frequency of blood group O among individuals with duodenal ulcer) then the genetically determined trait is usually considered to be important in the pathogenesis of the disorder [59, 60]. Association usually implies that there is some etiologic relationship between the gene marker allele and disease. Classically, this was considered to be quite distinct from the concept of linkage. For example, the association between blood group O and duodenal ulcer does not imply any linkage between the ABO locus and a duodenal ulcer gene. Thus, linkage is usually a phenomenon within families and not across populations, whereas association is a phenomenon across a population, and not necessarily within families. For many years, most mathematical techniques for linkage detection included the assumption that there was no population association between the disease (phenotype) under study and the genetic marker alleles.

However, the genetics of the HLA region (discussed in detail in Chapter 6) violate the cardinal rule of separation between linkage and association. Certain pairs of HLA antigens, which are linked because they are close to one another on the chromosome, also occur together in the population in greater frequency than would be expected by chance (estimated by multiplying their individual frequencies), i.e. they are associated. Such pairs of HLA antigens are said to be in 'linkage disequilibrium'. The most popular explanation for linkage disequilibrium is that selective forces exist that tend to select for and thus retain certain advantageous combinations of antigens. One of the major speculations regarding the etiology of various autoimmune diseases is that we are seeing today the residual effects of the selective advantage of these antigenic associations against the infectious diseases that our species was exposed to in the past [61, 62]. In some situations, however, linkage disequilibrium may occur simply because of the close physical proximity of two loci to each other. If a given mutation associated with disease susceptibility has occurred relatively recently in human evolution, there may not have been enough time for multiple recombination events to have occurred between the disease gene and other genetic regions close by. Linkage disequilibrium, which reflects the haplotype of the ancestral chromosome region on which the disease-causing mutation occurred, may therefore be observed. This latter type of linkage disequilibrium occurs with much greater frequency than was previously appreciated. Whereas it was initially seen as a complication for genetic studies, confounding our ability to identify the disease-causing gene within a chromosomal segment, this type of linkage disequilibrium is now actually being exploited to aid in identifying genes. Use of linkage disequilibrium for positional cloning was involved in identifying the gene for cystic fibrosis and exclusively in locating the gene for diastrophic dysplasia, a rare form of dwarfism [63].

The HLA Region and IDDM

HLA associations with IDDM and possible mechanisms are described in Chapter 6.

The IDDM association is unusual among HLA disease associations, because it involves two antigens, HLA-DR3 and DR4. In addition, the relative risk for IDDM in individuals who have both DR3 and DR4 (compound heterozygotes) is greater than in those homozygous for either DR3 or DR4 [41–43]. This finding of the increased risk of the DR3/DR4 heterozygote was the first suggestion that more than one gene may predispose to IDDM, and thus was the first evidence for heterogeneity within IDDM using HLA data [62, 68].

Further evidence for at least two forms of IDDM susceptibility comes from the observation that familial aggregation of IDDM suggests that DR3 susceptibility acts in a recessive fashion, with most DR3-carrying IDDM patients also having a second high-risk HLA haplotype (containing either DR3 or DR4). DR4-related IDDM susceptibility, on the other hand, appears to act in a dominant fashion, as demonstrated by the observation of many DR4-carrying IDDM patients who do not carry a second high-risk haplotype [73, 93–95].

Phenotypic heterogeneity is also apparent between HLA-DR3 and DR4-associated IDDM, and further supports the concept that there is more than one form of genetic susceptibility encoded within the HLA region (Table 3) [38, 96–100]. The DR3 form of the disease (autoimmune form) is characterized by a greater persistence of pancreatic islet cell antibodies and antipancreatic cell-mediated immunity, but a relative lack of antibody response to exogenous insulin. This form apparently has onset throughout life and probably accounts for a significant fraction of older-onset IDDM. In the older age groups, this form of IDDM may be treatable without insulin for a significant period of time, but the presence of islet cell antibodies predicts eventual insulin dependence [35, 37, 38]. The second form of IDDM is associated with DR4. While not as strongly associated with autoimmune disease or islet cell antibodies, this form is accompanied by an increased antibody response to exogenous insulin [99, 101]. Thus, in this type of IDDM, some individuals with the highest insulin antibody titers may have been treated with insulin for less than 5 years, thus indicating that prolonged duration of treatment is not the only explanation for an exaggerated immune response to insulin [75]. The relation between HLA-DR4 and insulin immunogenicity can also be seen before the initiation of exogenous insulin therapy, with the occurrence of insulin antibodies prior to disease onset [102, 103]. DR4-associated IDDM also appears to have an earlier age of onset, exhibits seasonality, and may be related to viral infections.

Given the variety of linkage, association and phenotypic data described above, it is clear that the mechanism of IDDM susceptibility produced by gene(s) within the HLA region is complex. As it remains unsure which gene(s) in the HLA region are responsible for IDDM susceptibility (see Chapter 6), there is likely to be even more genetic heterogeneity than is apparent from DR3 and DR4 alone. This view is supported by the growing evidence that the DQ and DP loci are also involved in IDDM. A more complete understanding of the modes of inheritance of IDDM susceptibility must await further clarification of both the number and identity of the HLA-linked genes which account for IDDM risk.

Non-HLA Region Genes and IDDM

Estimates of the proportion of genetic susceptibility to IDDM accounted for by the HLA region vary, but

Table 3 Heterogeneity within IDDM

Evidence	DR3	DR4	Combined form (DR3/DR4)
Linkage disequilibrium	A1, B8	B15, DQB1*0302	↑ penetrance in monozygotic twins, risk to siblings
Insulin antibodies	Non-responder (low antibody titers)	High responder (high antibody titers)	↑ occurrence in familial cases
Islet cell antibodies	Persistent	Transient	
Insulin autoantibodies	Less frequent	Increased frequency	Highest titers
Antipancreatic cell-mediated immunity	Increased	Not increased	
Thyroid autoimmunity in IDDM	Yes	Less frequent	
Associated with other autoimmune endocrine diseases	Yes	No	
IgA deficiency in IDDM	Increased	Not increased	
Age of onset	Any age	Younger age	Youngest
Ketoacidosis at clinical onset	Lesser frequency	Greater frequency	
Levels of C peptide	Preserved longer	Absent after shorter duration	Lowest

even the highest estimates are in the range of 60–70% [445], clearly indicating that other, non-HLA loci must also exist which play a role in IDDM. Over the past 20 years, a number of non-HLA candidate genes have been studied, and as many as ten loci have now been identified by mapping (Table 4). Several of these are discussed in detail in Chapter 6.

Table 4 Human IDDM loci

Locus	Chromosome no.
*IDDM*1 (HLA)	6p
*IDDM*2 (5′ Insulin Gene VNTR)	11p
*IDDM*3	15q
*IDDM*4	11q
*IDDM*5	6q
*IDDM*7	2q
Other potential loci	3q,4q,6q,13q

It will only be after the genes are cloned that the interactions among the various loci will be understood. It may well be that in any given individual, only a portion of the IDDM genes will be involved in disease causation. Whether the loci will all be additive in their effects, as appears to be the case for HLA and the insulin gene region, or whether there will be synergistic interactions among some loci, remains to be seen.

Support for the importance of non-HLA region genes in susceptibility to IDDM also comes from animal models of diabetes as discussed in Chapter 6. As many as 15 loci have been mapped which are involved in the development of insulitis and IDDM in the NOD mouse [138–140] (Table 5). These loci are scattered throughout the genome, although the mapping data suggest the presence of more than one IDDM locus on some chromosomes, as in the case of mouse chromosomes 1 and 3 [138, 141–143].

Initially there was the hope that mouse IDDM loci identification would aid in the localization of human IDDM genes. Unfortunately, with the exception of the MHC in the mouse and HLA in humans, no clear evidence exists that the same genes are responsible for IDDM susceptibility in mouse and man. Although the existence of homologous susceptibility loci has not been excluded, it now appears that extension of the human mapping studies will be necessary to identify human IDDM loci.

Given the growing data from both human and animal models that multiple genes participate in IDDM susceptibility, the potential for genetic complexity is great. Not only can several loci provide susceptibility and/or protection, but there may be epistatic interactions among the various loci as well [147]. Data collected thus far suggest that some

Table 5 Candidate IDDM loci in the NOD mouse

Murine locus	Murine chromosome no.	Human syntenic region, chromosome no.	Reference
Idd-2	9	11q (Thy-1/Alp-1 region)	[133]
Idd-3	3, proximal	1 or 4	[143]
Idd-4	11	17	[143]
Idd-5	1, proximal	2q	[141]
'Peri-insulitis'	1, distal	1, 2 or 18	[142]
Idd-6	6	12p12	[144]
Idd-7	7	19q13	[138]
Idd-8	14	10q24 or 3p	[138]
Idd-9	4	1p	[145]
Idd-10	3, distal	1p13	[138]
Idd-11	4		[140]
Idd-12	14		[146]
Idd-13	2		[140]
Idd-14	13		[140]
Idd-15	5		[140]

loci will act independently, while others will display epistasis. Thus, for example, although one study has suggested that the 5′ insulin gene region provides risk preferentially to HLA-DR4-positive individuals [123], most studies of the IDDM risk afforded by this region suggest that it acts independently of HLA [122, 148]. By contrast, there does appear to be interaction between the HLA region and the Gm locus; Field et al [107] reported that the immunoglobulin heavy chain allotype G1m(2) was associated with increased IDDM risk in HLA-DR3 individuals, while G3m(5) resulted in increased risk in HLA-DR4 individuals. The interactions among loci may be even more complex; specific Gm allotypes have been reported to interact with an RFLP of the T cell receptor beta chain in IDDM [149] and interactions between HLA-DR and Gm have been reported to occur as a function of sex [116, 150].

Pathophysiology of IDDM

It is now apparent that IDDM is a chronic autoimmune disorder that gradually develops over many years. A variety of abnormalities in immune function and insulin release precede the abrupt development of the diabetic syndrome in patients genetically predisposed to diabetes [70, 151–155] and these are discussed in Chapter 5.

Non-obese diabetes (NOD) mice and Biobreeding (BB) rats appear to be excellent models of the autoimmune form of IDDM [152, 156]. It has been suggested that major histocompatibility complex (MHC) Class II genes and T lymphocytes are both important in the pathogenesis of islet B-cell destruction [157, 158]. Indeed, activated T lymphocytes from acute-diabetic BB rats and NOD mice can transfer diabetes to other animals [159].

Similar evidence for the interaction of the MHC region and T lymphocytes in human diabetes comes from the studies of pancreatic transplantation between identical twins [160, 161]. When a pancreas is transplanted from a non-diabetic twin to a diabetic monozygotic co-twin without immunosuppression, islet cell destruction with massive T-cell infiltration and relapse of the diabetes occurs within weeks. Thus, the basic defect in IDDM appears to be extrinsic to the pancreas and related to the activation of T lymphocytes, which then mediate the destruction of the islets.

T-cell activation through gene rearrangement may well be the proximate step in the development of IDDM in an individual who is genetically predisposed to the disease. The various environmental agents discussed below may well operate in triggering or selecting the appropriate T-cell receptor rearrangement, and the specific HLA type may be necessary for the interaction of these activated T cells and islet B cell-directed antibodies with the pancreas. In support of this concept are the tentative data for T-cell receptor associations [112–114, 120].

The Role of Environmental Factors in IDDM

The monozygotic twin data, which show an IDDM concordance of approximately 20–40%, raise the possibility that there are important environmental components to the etiologies of IDDM. Immunologic gene rearrangements could also provide an explanation for such a reduced penetrance [162, 163]. Yet the possibility of environmental factors having a significant role must be thoroughly investigated, especially with regard to the implications for preventive strategies. Environmental agents could play one of several roles [56, 164, 165]. They might function as initiating factors, i.e. factors which begin or continue the etiologic processes which eventually terminate in IDDM. If environmental factors function in this role, then more than one agent (for example, several different viruses, or viruses and chemical agents) might be involved in the etiology (or etiologies). Alternatively, environmental factors could act mainly as precipitating factors—that is, factors which convert pre-clinical diabetes into clinical disease. In either role (or both), what is clear is that environmental factors must act on genetically susceptible individuals for IDDM to occur. Several classes of environmental agents (infectious, chemical and dietary) have been implicated in the etiology of IDDM.

Infectious Agents

A viral etiology for diabetes has been suggested for many years, with case reports of diabetes following an episode of an infectious disease dating back to the 1800s [57, 166–168]. The current evidence for a role of viral agents comes from several sources, including case reports, epidemiologic studies, clinical studies and evidence from animal and human models.

Anecdotally, a 'viral-like' illness is known to precede the onset of many cases of IDDM [57, 165]. Epidemiologic evidence is also consistent with an infectious etiology. Thus, it has been noted that trends in age at onset of diabetes are consistent with a viral etiology [165]. These data are most consistent with infectious agents playing a precipitating role in IDDM, and the total number of infections during the preceding year has been shown to correlate with IDDM risk [169]. One study suggests that sibling pairs are more likely to have their onset of diabetes within a year of one another than would be expected by chance [165] and the period of discordance for IDDM in monozygotic twins has been reported to be less than 3 years in 60% of those twin pairs where both ultimately develop IDDM [170].

There is also limited evidence for an infectious agent's role (e.g. mumps, Coxsackie) from studies comparing viral and bacterial antibody titers in IDDM patients and non-diabetic controls [171–176]. Others have found no evidence of increased titers to Coxsackie B viruses in new onset cases [177, 178], while still others have suggested that Coxsackie B3 and B4 titers are actually decreased in IDDM [179]. More recent studies have utilized molecular techniques to determine the prevalence of viral DNA. Human cytomegalovirus (CMV) genes were detected (by molecular hybridization with a human CMV-specific probe) in 22% of IDDM patients as compared to 2.6% of controls [180]. There was a strong correlation between the CMV gene and islet cell antibodies in the diabetic patients, suggesting that persistent CMV infection may be relevant to

pathogenesis in some cases of IDDM. A study of the incidence of IDDM in relationship to the introduction of the measles–mumps–rubella vaccination and the subsequent disappearance of mumps in Finland suggested that elimination of natural mumps infection has decreased the incidence of IDDM [181]. Measles vaccination itself was also correlated with a lower risk of IDDM [169].

Evidence from clinical studies also suggests a role for infectious agents in IDDM. The insulitis which has been noted in early IDDM could be consistent with viral infection of the pancreas, and autopsy studies have clearly documented pancreatic islet B-cell damage in children dying from overwhelming viral infections [182]. Coxsackie B-specific antigens have specifically been found in the islets and the B4 virus itself has been isolated from the pancreas of a child dying of acute onset IDDM [183]. Several types of viruses are known to be capable of infecting human pancreatic islet B cells *in vitro*, and there are data to suggest that Coxsackie B virus, rubella virus and possibly cytomegalovirus are capable of producing pathologic islet B-cell changes *in vivo*.

There is a region of sequence homology between glutamic acid decarboxylase (GAD) and the P2-C protein of Coxsackie B virus, raising the possibility that Coxsackie virus infection can trigger an anti-islet B cell autoimmune response by molecular mimicry [184]. Antibodies to GAD species and to the P2-C protein have been shown to cross-react in some but not all studies, further supporting the idea that molecular mimicry may be a mechanism by which viral infection can affect the development of IDDM [185–187].

Evidence from animal studies is strongly suggestive of a viral component to the etiology of IDDM. Thus the M strain of the encephalomyocarditis (EMC) virus infects islet B cells, and produces a diabetes-like disease in some strains of mice [188, 189]. This model has been widely studied, and it is now clear that the EMC-D variant (but not the EMC-B variant of the M strain) causes direct viral destruction of the islet B cells in certain genetically susceptible (SJL/JH; C3H/HeJ) mouse lines [190–199]. In addition, in other mouse strains (for example, Balb/cBy), EMC M strains appear to initiate an immunologically mediated form of diabetes, suggesting that the same virus can have multiple effects, depending on the genetic predisposition of the host [200, 201]. Diabetes in SJL/J mice can be prevented by vaccinating animals with live-attenuated EMC vaccine [202, 203]. In BB/WOR diabetes-resistant rats, Kilham's rat virus (KRV) has been found to reproducibly induce IDDM [204]. KRV does not produce diabetes in non-BB rats, however, clearly indicating that genetic factors are also necessary in order for IDDM to develop. Several other promising animal models of infectious agents and diabetes have been, or are currently being, developed.

That only some strains of mice are susceptible to virally-induced diabetes strongly suggests a genetic component to disease susceptibility. The fact that only certain strains of virus are capable of inducing diabetes in specific animal models indicates that genetic factors in the agent are also important. The genetic/strain specificity of the agent may be particularly important in viruses which change their genetic characteristics rapidly in the population. This specificity may explain several puzzling aspects of IDDM epidemiology; specifically, the possible changing incidence of IDDM over time, as well as the interesting observation that the proportion of complicated mumps cases who were ICA+ decreased rapidly from the late 1970s to the mid-1980s [205].

The animal models suggest that infectious agents can cause diabetes or diabetes-like syndromes by at least four different mechanisms: (a) by acute infection of the islet B cell, leading to necrosis (EMC and reovirus models); (b) through autoimmune mechanisms (rubella and KRV models); (c) through persistent infection, leading to decreased growth and life-span of the islet B cell (lymphocytic choriomeningitis model); and (d) through biochemical alterations in the cell or cell membrane which lead to decreased insulin synthesis/release (Venezuelan encephalitis model) [188, 206]. While our knowledge of infectious agents in human diabetes is less advanced, it is possible that all four mechanisms also occur in human diabetes.

The animal models have also raised the hope that vaccination against promoting or initiating viral agents may protect genetically susceptible individuals against IDDM. Vaccination against EMC virus in SJL/J mice, and against pertussis (whole cell vaccine) in CD-1 mice with streptozotocin-induced diabetes, suggests that islet B-cell destruction can either be prevented or halted in at least some mouse models [202, 207].

The best human models of infectious agents in IDDM come from studies of individuals with the congenital rubella syndrome and from serial studies of children with viral infections who subsequently develop IDDM. The incidence of IDDM and other autoimmune diseases among children and young adults with the congenital rubella syndrome is markedly increased over that in the general population, and may be as high as 15-40%. Those cases of congenital rubella with IDDM have an increased frequency of HLA-DR3 and DR4 and a decreased frequency of HLA-DR2, much as in non-rubella IDDM cases [210]. A significant proportion of patients with congenital rubella syndrome have T-cell subset abnormalities, and a variety of autoimmune antibodies, including anti-thyroid microsomal, antithyroglobulin and anti-islet cell and islet cell surface antibodies, suggesting an autoimmune etiology for their IDDM [210, 211]. Rubella virus has been isolated from the pancreas of several cases with congenital rubella syndrome [212], and at least one case is known of insulitis and B-cell destruction in an infant with congenital rubella infection who died of acute diabetes [213]. This evidence suggests that rubella can indeed infect and damage the B cell, that the diabetes seen in congenital rubella syndrome could be due either to initiation of an immune process by the rubella virus, or be directly due to persistent pancreatic rubella infection.

Dietary Agents and Molecular Mimicry

An area of recent interest as an environmental trigger for IDDM has been dietary exposure. Several studies [216-223] reported an association of the introduction of cows' milk and cessation of breast feeding with IDDM risk. Elevated antibodies to several cows' milk proteins have also been reported in children with IDDM [224-226]. When it was reported that one epitope of bovine serum albumin, a 17 amino acid peptide (ABBOS), cross-reacts with p69, an islet B-cell surface protein, it was suggested that early introduction of cows' milk into the infant diet could result in initiation of autoimmune injury to the B-cell via this molecular mimicry [227, 228]. Some studies of infant nutrition have not supported the association of autoimmunity to cows' milk and IDDM risk; in fact very preliminary findings of the DAISY study actually suggest a protective effect of early cows' milk feeding [229-232]. Therefore, the importance of cows' milk in IDDM remains unresolved at present, but the possible role of early infant and childhood diet requires further investigation [233].

Genetic Counseling in Insulin Dependent Diabetes

Because the mode of inheritance in IDDM is not straightforward, most genetic counseling for IDDM is based upon empiric risk estimates which have been developed from both population-based and family-based epidemiologic studies (Table 6). These recurrence risks are frequently reassuring to families, as the risks are often less than the family has feared, particularly for siblings of the IDDM patient. The empiric risk of recurrence for IDDM is dependent upon the relationship of the individual in question to the affected family member. For siblings the empiric risk is approximately 5-10%. If the father is affected, the risk to his offspring is 4-6%, as compared to 2-3% if the mother is affected [234, 235]. For further refinement

Table 6 Empiric recurrence risks for insulin dependent diabetes

Reference	Proband	Risk to sibs (%)	Risk to offspring (%)	Comments
Harris (1950) [22]	<30	4.1		Interview
Working Party, College of General Practitioners (1965) [29]	<30	4.8	1.4	Predicted by age 40 Interview
Simpson (1962) [27]	<20	5.7	0.9	Interview
Simpson (1968) [28]	<20	2.4	1.8	Mailed questionnaire
Kobberling (1969) [24]	<25	10.9 ± 3.9		Predicted by age 25
Darlow and Smith (1973) [65]	<25	4.7–7.6		Predicted by age 25
Tattersall and Fajans (1975) [48]	<25	11		Interview and GTT
Nerup et al (1976) [66]	Juvenile	9.7		HLA typed
Degnbol and Green (1978) [20]	<20	6.2 ± 1.3	5.4 ± 2.9*	Questionnaire interview—predicted by age 35
West et al (1979) [67]	<17	4.1		Medical record review
Gottlieb (1980) [45]	<20	4.5	3.1	Mailed questionnaire of proband and relatives
Gamble (1980) [56]	<16	5.6		Observed by age 16—mailed questionnaire of families
Kobberling and Bruggeboes (1980) [13]	Insulin treated since diagnosis		2.4	Medical questionnaire—includes both parents affected
			1.5	Only mother affected
Wagener et al (1982) [438]	<17	3.3–6 10.5+		+ If parent also affected
Chern et al (1982) [248]	Insulin treated since diagnosis	4.6 ± 0.8++ 8.5 ± 2.0**		++ If proband diagnosed >10 years of age ** If proband diagnosed ≤ 10 years of age
Tillil and Kobberling (1987) [69]	Insulin within $1\frac{1}{2}$ years of diagnosis	6.6 ± 1.1	4.9 ± 4.9	Lifetime risk
Warram et al (1988) [235]	<20; insulin dependent		2.1 ± 0.5	Offspring of diabetic mothers—cumulative risk to age 20
			6.1 ± 1.8	Offspring of diabetic fathers—cumulative risk to age 20

*Actual observed recurrence 2.8%.

of sibling risks, HLA testing can be used to determine haplotype sharing with the diabetic sib [236, 237]. If two haplotypes are shared, the risk increases to 16–17%, and is 20–25% if the haplotypes contain both DR3 and DR4 [12]. Siblings who share one haplotype have a risk in the range of 5–7%, while the risk is approximately 1–2% if no haplotypes are shared [12].

It is important to realize that the sibling of an individual with IDDM still has a risk for IDDM that is increased above that of the general population, even when the sib shares no HLA haplotypes in common with the diabetic in the family. Based on our understanding of the genetics of IDDM, there are at least three possible explanations for this persistent risk. Since the IDDM gene or genes within the HLA region have not yet been absolutely identified, it is possible for siblings to have inherited the HLA-related IDDM susceptibility genes but, due to recombination, to have inherited different HLA types. Also, because the high-risk HLA haplotypes (i.e. those containing DR3 or DR4) occur fairly commonly in the general population, it is possible that one or both parents of a child with IDDM may actually carry two high-risk haplotypes. Thus, a child may inherit diabetes susceptibility genes, even though he/she shares no HLA haplotypes with the diabetic sibling. Lastly, it is possible that the increased risk is due to one or more of the non-HLA region susceptibility genes.

There is some concern regarding the benefit of performing HLA typing for the siblings of an individual with IDDM when this information would not lead to any alteration in management (see also Chapter 89). Particular attention must be paid to the potential negative effects of stigmatization and the risks of the child being treated as though he is ill; it must be stressed that HLA testing at best identifies someone to be more susceptible to developing IDDM but does not guarantee that he will develop diabetes. The potential for other negative effects, such as possibly being ruled ineligible for health, life and/or disability insurance due to the presence of a 'pre-existing' condition, must also be discussed with every family contemplating more refined testing.

What *is* clear is that HLA testing is not appropriate as a screening tool for the general population. Approximately 50% of the non-diabetic population have the same HLA-DR types as patients with IDDM. Thus, at least 98% of the people with DR3 or DR4 will never develop IDDM. For every 1000 persons with HLA-DR3 or DR4 in the population, only 2–4 will develop IDDM (Table 7). Thus, population screening using HLA-DR serological typing will result in more 'false' positive results than 'true' positives in terms of genetic risk. Even molecular testing of the class II genes, using for example DQ-α and DQ-β molecular probes, will result in many more false positives than true positives and will be fraught with the difficulties of different allelic associations depending upon the ethnic and racial background of the individuals being tested. Islet cell or GAD antibody testing is also not yet specific enough to be effective for screening in the general population (see also Chapters 5 and 89).

Screening for Other Autoimmune Disorders

Diabetes is not the only autoimmune disorder for which relatives of an individual with IDDM are at risk. Family members, as well as the patient, are at increased risk for autoimmune thyroid disease (Hashimoto thyroiditis, Graves' disease), pernicious anemia secondary to autoimmune gastritis, autoimmune adrenal disease (Addison's disease), myasthenia gravis, vitiligo, and coeliac disease [12, 238–240] (see also Chapter 5). One study found that 21% of individuals with IDDM and 22% of their first-degree relatives had evidence of autoimmune disease [241]. Of patients with persistent islet cell antibodies (ICA), 57% had other autoimmune conditions, as compared to 15% of those not found to have persistent ICAs [241]. Seventy-five percent of the autoimmune disease in relatives occurred in families in which there was a proband with autoimmune disease [241], indicating that there may be increased genetic susceptibility to other autoimmune disorders in certain IDDM families.

The most common form of autoimmune disease in families with IDDM is thyroid disease [241, 242]. Although the proportion of IDDM patients with clinical or subclinical thyroid disease has been reported to be as high as 35%, the actual proportion is thought to be closer to 15–20% [241, 243]. By contrast, the prevalence of autoimmune thyroid disease in non-diabetic Europids is about 4.5% [244]. The prevalence of clinical or subclinical autoimmune thyroid disease in first-degree relatives of individuals with IDDM is estimated to be 15–25% [241, 243]. As is true with autoimmune thyroid disease in the general population, female family members have higher rates of thyroid and gastric autoimmunity than do males [242].

Other autoimmune disorders are also seen with increased frequency in IDDM individuals and their

Table 7 Risks for IDDM

Population risks	Overall	1/500
	HLA-DR related:	
	No high risk allele	1/5000
	1 high risk allele, i.e. DR3/x or DR4/x	1/400
	HLA-DR4 subset defined by molecular techniques	1/300
	HLA-DR3/3 or DR4/4	1/150
	HLA-DR3/4	1/40
Risks in relatives:		
Siblings	Overall	1/14
	HLA haplotypes shared with diabetic siblings:	
	0 haplotypes shared	1/100
	1 haplotype shared	1/20
	2 haplotypes shared	1/6
	2 haplotypes shared and DR3/4	1/5 to 1/4
Offspring	Overall	1/25
	Offspring of affected female	1/50 to 1/40
	Offspring of affected male	1/20
Monozygotic twin of diabetic		1/3

relatives. Autoimmune gastritis is seen in 5–12% of individuals with IDDM and 2.5–6% of their first-degree relatives [241, 243, 244]. The prevalence of adrenal autoantibodies is 1–3% in individuals with IDDM, compared to less than 0.6% in non-diabetic individuals [241, 245].

Interestingly, one autoimmune disease may actually be protective for IDDM. Alopecia areata is associated with autoimmune disease such as thyroid disease and probably pernicious anemia as well. Relatives of alopecia areata patients have an increased frequency of IDDM, yet the alopecia patients themselves do not [246].

It is particularly important for the relatives of patients with IDDM to be made aware of this increased risk for autoimmune disease. Although most physicians know of the association of IDDM with other autoimmune disease, the fact that close relatives are also at risk is not as well appreciated, even though approximately 40% of all families which include an individual with IDDM will have at least one other family member with latent or clinical autoimmune disease [241]. Since many of these autoimmune disorders can have relatively insidious onsets, with fairly non-specific symptoms, earlier diagnosis may be possible if relatives and their physicians are made aware of the increased risk.

Given this increased risk, periodic screening of individuals with IDDM and all their first-degree relatives is warranted, particularly for thyroid dysfunction and vitamin B_{12} deficiency. In the future, it may also be possible to screen for atrophic gastritis directly by measuring the pepsinogen I/pepsinogen II ratio [250].

Pregnancy and IDDM

It is well known that women with IDDM have a higher rate of pregnancy complications than do non-diabetic women (see also Chapter 57). It should be emphasized that although the risks can be lowered by achieving optimal glycemic control of the diabetes prior to pregnancy, all diabetic pregnancies must be considered high-risk and will benefit from a multispecialty management approach.

From the genetic counseling perspective, the most important issue related to pregnancy and IDDM is the markedly increased risk of fetal anomalies in the offspring [252, 253]. In the general population, the risk of having a child with a birth defect is 2–3%. For women with IDDM, the risk is increased threefold, to 6–10% [253–255]. The malformations seen in infants born to diabetic women tend to be more severe than those seen in infants of non-diabetic women and include abnormalities of the skeletal, renal, cardiac and central nervous systems [252, 254, 256–258]. Virtually all anomalies occur with increased frequency in infants

of diabetic mothers, but those which have the highest relative risk are caudal regression, renal agenesis, transposition of the great vessels, ventricular septal defects, atrial septal defects, situs inversus, and neural tube defects (anencephaly and meningomyelocele). For example, the relative risk for caudal regression in the offspring of a diabetic woman has been estimated to be as high as 200 [257]. The relative risks for the other defects are not as high, due in large part to their higher incidence in the general population [252].

The disruption of embryogenesis leading to fetal abnormalities occurs prior to the eighth week of pregnancy, i.e. often before a woman realizes that she is pregnant [259]. There is evidence to suggest that elevated glycated hemoglobin (HbA_{1c}) levels are associated with a high risk for malformations, and vigorous control of blood glucose levels prior to conception appears to reduce significantly the incidence of congenital malformations [259–262]. Although it is beneficial to optimize diabetes control even in women who present when they are already pregnant, postconceptional intervention is less likely to reduce the malformation risk.

Because of the increased risk for major structural malformations, prenatal diagnostic tests should be recommended for all pregnant women who have IDDM. These should be performed during the second trimester (usually between 16–20 weeks' gestation), providing women with abnormal results with the opportunity to obtain genetic counseling regarding the anomaly (i.e. prognosis, treatment options) and to make informed decisions regarding pregnancy options. For women who have normal results, the information obtained via prenatal diagnosis can be very reassuring and help alleviate anxiety for the remainder of the pregnancy. Ultrasonography can be used to evaluate fetal growth and to rule out major fetal structural anomalies such as renal agenesis, neural tube defects and caudal regression. Fetal echocardiography, performed at 18–22 weeks following the first day of the last menstrual period, enables prenatal diagnosis of major structural cardiac malformations. Elevations of maternal serum α-fetoprotein (MSAFP) have been associated with open neural tube defects such as anencephaly and meningomyelocele [263, 264]; thus, MSAFP screening is recommended for all pregnant diabetics. Because MSAFP levels are altered in pregnant diabetic (as compared to non-diabetic) women, tables specific for diabetic women should be used when calculating their MSAFP values and it is therefore important that the laboratory performing the assay be made aware that the patient has diabetes [265–267]. There is evidence that, in the general population, folic acid supplementation begun prior to conception is helpful in decreasing the risk for neural tube defects [268]. Although studies looking specifically at infants of diabetic mothers have not been reported, folic acid supplementation prior to conception should be strongly considered, as the potential benefits outweigh any known risks.

NON-INSULIN DEPENDENT DIABETES (NIDDM)

Evidence of a Genetic Contribution to NIDDM

Several lines of evidence suggest the importance of genetic susceptibilities underlying the development of NIDDM. Genetic epidemiologic studies provide convincing descriptive data including population and ethnic differences, studies of familial aggregation, familial transmission patterns and comparisons of twin concordance rates. Animal models of NIDDM and studies of specific genetic syndromes that feature glucose intolerance provide further data supporting the etiologic role of genetic factors in the pathogenesis of NIDDM. Finally, the genetic etiologies for NIDDM have been more convincingly determined using genetic markers in population association and family studies.

Evidence from Animal Models

Relevant animal models provide the opportunity to study genes and pathophysiologic mechanisms which may have application to human diabetes. However, finding animal models that have pathophysiologic mechanisms similar to those found in human disease is problematic. The advantages of animal studies are numerous, and include a large resource of genetically characterized animals which are homozygous at many loci. This allows extensive study of the genetic aspects of phenotypic traits through breeding studies. The environment can also be modified, to allow investigation of the interaction of genes and the environment. Further, since the genetics of mice and rats are known so well, linkage studies can be conducted to try to pinpoint the actual genes of interest.

Variability in blood glucose levels does indeed occur between different strains of inbred mice and rats [269]. Among the more intensively studied mouse models of NIDDM are the ob/ob (obesity and hyperglycemia) and db/db (diabetic obese) syndromes [270–272]. The diabetes and obesity seen in conjunction with these two mutations are modified by the genetic background of the strain of mouse in which they occur [273, 274]. For example, on the C57BL/KsJ (BL/Ks) background, diabetes is severe and life-shortening, while on the C57BL/6J background, the diabetes is transient and well compensated. These studies suggest that, at least

in mice, diabetes can be modified by genes other than those directly responsible for obesity and/or diabetes.

Recently the *ob* gene was cloned in the mouse, followed rapidly by isolation of the rat and human homologues [275]. In the ob/ob mouse, the obesity and diabetes phenotype results from a non-sense mutation, which generates a stop codon. Further proof that the inability to produce leptin, the *ob* gene product, is responsible for the diabetes and obesity has come from the demonstration by several researchers that infusion of leptin results in dramatic weight loss in ob/ob mice [276–278], with concomitant reductions in plasma glucose [276, 277]. Although there is a high degree of homology among the mouse, rat and human *ob* genes, studies in obese humans have failed to identify any mutations in this gene [279, 280] and it appears unlikely that this gene is responsible for many, if any, cases of obesity and/or diabetes in humans.

The *db* gene, which maps to mouse chromosome 4 and rat chromosome 5 (the homologous fatty [*fa*] locus), has not yet been cloned [281, 282]. Based on early parabiosis experiments [270], the db/db mouse model has long been thought to be due to resistance to the *ob* gene product. This hypothesis now appears to have been proven; thus (a) db/db mice have elevated circulating and adipose tissue levels of the *ob* protein as compared to lean control animals [277]; and (b) infusion of *ob* protein fails to result in any reduction in weight [277, 278], even though diet-induced obese mice and, to a lesser extent, lean control animals show decreased body weight and food intake in response to ob infusion [277, 278].

Some researchers have suggested that the db/db and ob/ob mutants are not good models for human NIDDM [269], and several other models have been proposed as being more relevant. These include the C57BL/6J mouse strain subjected to dietary stress (without the ob/ob or db/db mutation) [283, 284], the DBA/2J and C57BL/6J mouse strains [269], and the SHR/N-cp rat [285, 286]. The C57BL/6J model appears to be a diet-sensitive form of diabetes which is characterized by impaired glucose-stimulated insulin secretion [269, 283]. Multiple genes may be involved in the metabolic disturbances seen in this model [269, 284] and it appears that the insulin resistance and hyperglycemia may be due to different genetic loci [284]. The SHR/N-cp rat is normoglycemic when lean, but has an increased insulin response to low levels of glucose, and a markedly impaired insulin response to high levels of glucose after being fed a high sucrose diet [286]. Further studies are required to determine the utility and applicability of these models to the study of human NIDDM genetics.

Evidence from Population Studies

Population-based studies of the distribution of a phenotypic trait can be helpful as a first step in evaluating whether the trait is likely to be controlled by a' major gene' or by multiple factors (either genetic or environmental). Several studies suggest that in populations with a high prevalence of NIDDM, the distribution of glucose tolerance may be bimodal; that is, fasting glucose levels appear to be distributed around two distinct mean values (see Chapter 8). Thus, in the Pima Indians, the Oklahoma Seminoles and several South Pacific populations, the distribution of glucose tolerance values in adults is consistent with an underlying bimodal distribution. This is usually interpreted as suggesting that there is a major gene which influences glucose tolerance [287–290]. However, in most populations, blood glucose values in the population appear to be distributed unimodally. This is probably due to the heterogeneous nature of most other populations under study.

Evidence from Twin Studies and Family Studies

Studies in twins and families have long suggested a 'genetic', or at least a strong familial component to the susceptibility to NIDDM. Twin studies demonstrate almost complete concordance for NIDDM in monozygotic twins [30, 52], yet the familial aggregation of clinical disease or glucose levels is not consistent with a single, simple mode of inheritance [10]. Genetic heterogeneity would seem the most likely explanation. In addition, environmental factors are known to be important as well. The close to 100% concordance in monozygotic twins suggests that, in the urbanized Western world, the environment is sufficiently constant (and diabetogenic) that genetic susceptibility is the primary determinant for development of NIDDM. In studying a specific phenotype related to NIDDM development, Tremblay and co-workers found tentative evidence for genetic factors influencing insulin sensitivity in response to short-term exercise training in male monozygotic twin pairs [291].

Difficulties in Studying the Genetics of NIDDM

NIDDM and other common chronic diseases present a number of difficult analytic challenges to the geneticist. The late and variable age of onset of NIDDM, probably resulting from interactions of genetic and environmental factors, can result in an underestimation of the number of individuals who are genetically susceptible to NIDDM. This is a particularly vexing problem for family studies, in which linkage of NIDDM with genetic markers is often the goal. While there is typically no confusion about the status of an affected living member of the family, unaffected individuals who carry the requisite gene(s), but who have not yet lived long enough to express diabetes, will not be recognizable. In addition, at the time a family is studied, many affected members in the older generations will be deceased and may have had their diabetes diagnosed (or not diagnosed) years ago, using perhaps less-than-optimal diagnostic criteria. The late age of onset also means that some individuals who are genetically 'affected' will die of other causes prior to developing diabetes.

Another difficulty in studying the genetics of NIDDM is the strong environmental component involved in many forms of diabetes. In industrialized or 'Westernized' countries, high monozygotic twin concordance rates suggest that the environment is sufficiently uniform (and 'diabetogenic') that most individuals with the genetic predisposition will develop diabetes. On the other hand, in non-Westernized countries, studies of the genetics of NIDDM are far more difficult to carry out. Many people with the requisite genes will never manifest clinical disease under existing environmental conditions.

Studies in populations which have had a rapid change in diet and/or exercise levels give some indication of the strength of the environmental component in the etiology of NIDDM. For example, among the Nauruans of the South Pacific, documented prevalence of diabetes has increased from low rates to more than 50% of the adult population in a time period of about 30 years [292, 293]. Similar increases in prevalence with Westernization have been noted in other populations as diverse as the natives of Australia, African and Near Eastern immigrants to Israel, Japanese immigrants to the USA, and certain Native American populations [294–298].

Another element of complexity in studying the genetics of NIDDM is the high disease frequency of NIDDM in many populations. This probably means that the genes for at least some of the more common forms of NIDDM occur with a relatively high gene frequency in some populations. Once again, this presents particular problems in family studies, as it can be unclear whether two affected individuals in a pedigree actually share the same disease genes, or whether several types of diabetes are occurring by chance in the same family.

In all probability, at least some forms of NIDDM require the presence of more than one gene defect to cause clinical diabetes. There is increasing evidence that a large proportion of the adult population has peripheral insulin resistance, yet most of these individuals have neither clinical diabetes nor impaired glucose tolerance. The most parsimonious explanation for this is that other defects, either genetically or environmentally determined, are required for the development of

NIDDM. As was discussed above regarding the genetics of IDDM, the requirement of multiple genetic loci for disease occurrence adds considerably to the difficulties in understanding the genetic predispositions to a disease or group of diseases.

Perhaps the most problematic aspect of studying the genetics of NIDDM is the probably extensive etiologic heterogeneity which underlies this disease. Genetic defects could influence any of the many steps involved in glucose metabolism. Each of these defects, either alone or in concert with other defects, could result in NIDDM. While such etiologic complexity by no means precludes genetic investigations, extensive etiologic heterogeneity implies that to understand particular pathogenetic mechanisms, one must be able to measure physiologic 'defects' at a more specific level than the gross phenotype of glucose intolerance.

Evidence Supporting Heterogeneity in NIDDM

Family Physiologic Studies

The study of physiologic traits associated with NIDDM within families can be useful on several levels, including dissection of disease heterogeneity. First, it may allow characterization of early stages of, and variability in, the natural history of the disease (see also Chapter 31). It also allows for comparison between families, which may be helpful in separating etiologic sub-types. Finally, it can lead to better studies of mode of inheritance and linkage to genetic markers, as more of the genetically 'affected' individuals in the pedigree will be identified.

The first physiologic studies in families with NIDDM were conducted using glucose tolerance as the phenotype. Even with this relatively crude measure of glucose metabolism, there was evidence that in normal healthy subjects glucose and insulin responses have an appreciable genetic component [299]. In their studies of large pedigrees with NIDDM, Beaty and Fajans [300] also assessed the role of genetic determinants of fasting blood glucose levels. Their data were consistent with a role for additive genetic factors, although a large proportion of the intrafamilial variability could not be explained by genetic factors. Familial studies of liability for hyperglycemia in Pacific Nauruans have also been interpreted as consistent with the effect of a major gene [301]. However, in studies of Japanese-Americans, Williams et al [302] concluded that heritability of fasting blood glucose within families was low, and they could find no evidence for a major gene. Similar results were reported from a study of families in Jerusalem [303].

Studies in the Mexican-American population, a high-risk population with a high prevalence of NIDDM, have demonstrated a genetic 'dosage effect' on fasting insulin levels [304]. An increase in fasting insulin levels was a function of whether an individual had 0, 1 or 2 diabetic parents, suggesting that insulin resistance is familial. In an elegant study in Pima Indians (another high-risk group), Lillioja et al [305] demonstrated that *in vivo* insulin action has a familial component. Glucose uptake at maximally stimulating insulin concentrations showed a high degree of familiality which was independent of age, sex or degree of obesity. To control for familial correlations in dietary intake, subjects were placed on a standard diet for at least 7 days. Thus, the 'familial' component, which was estimated to explain 38% of the variance in insulin action, appeared to be due to genetic rather than environmental similarities.

Genetic/environmental influences on the insulin response to glucose have been studied for many years at the Karolinska Hospital in Sweden [306–308]. In studying insulin release after a glucose infusion in family members, as well as fasting and stimulated glucose and insulin levels, it was first concluded that their data showed considerable intrafamilial correlation, and was consistent with a major recessive gene common in the Swedish population (with a gene frequency perhaps as high as 20%) [307]. More recent studies of insulin release and sensitivity in these families still suggest that these variables are genetically regulated, although the evidence for a major gene is no longer as convincing [308].

Other studies have also looked at physiologic abnormalities of insulin secretion in relatives of people with diabetes [309]. O'Rahilly et al [310] studied the pulsatile release of insulin in first-degree relatives of NIDDM subjects. Compared to controls, the first-degree relatives lacked the normal oscillations in insulin secretion following an intravenous glucose challenge. Since these relatives had only mild glucose intolerance and high-normal fasting glucose levels, this lack of pulsatile insulin release may be the first expression of NIDDM in these high-risk relatives [311].

Population Studies

Comparisons of phenotypic characteristics between populations can be useful in separating etiologic sub-types within heterogeneous disorders such as NIDDM. When surveys of glucose tolerance have been performed in populations of European ancestry, the number of individuals found to have asymptomatic undiagnosed diabetes has been approximately equal to that with known diabetes. Among the Eskimo, however, clinical diabetes is extremely rare, but abnormal glucose tolerance tests have been found to be very common [312]. Thus, abnormal glucose tolerance in the Eskimo appears to be a chemical trait that rarely leads to clinical diabetes. The maximum plasma insulin response to an oral glucose challenge in normal Navajo and Pima Indians was over three times as great as that observed in Western Europeans [313, 314]. In addition, the insulin output of NIDDM patients was also clearly different in the American Indians than in the Europeans. Finally, physiologic studies of Asian Indians with NIDDM suggest that they are more insulin resistant than are Europid NIDDM subjects, even when the degree of obesity is comparable [315]. These findings suggest that there may be distinct sub-types of NIDDM in different populations or ethnic groups, and it is possible that these differences are genetically determined.

Clinical Heterogeneity in NIDDM

Even early clinical genetic studies suggested heterogeneity within NIDDM. When Kobberling [316] divided his adult-onset probands into low, moderate and markedly overweight categories, he found a significantly higher frequency of affected siblings in the light-proband category (38%) and a significantly lower frequency in the heavy-proband category (10%). Irvine et al [23] observed a different clinical range of diabetes in the relatives of the non-obese and obese insulin dependent propositi.

Fajans [317] and co-workers demonstrated metabolic heterogeneity in non-obese latent diabetes. These investigators were able to divide their latent diabetic patients into two broad groups: those with an insulinopenic form of glucose intolerance, and those with high levels of plasma immunoreactive insulin. The high responders and low responders remained consistent and distinct over many years of follow-up, suggesting that they represented different metabolic disorders.

There is remarkable variability in the physiologic abnormalities seen in patients with NIDDM, ranging from structural and numeric abnormalities of pancreatic A and B cells, to abnormalities in pancreatic insulin secretion and decreased insulin sensitivity in the liver and peripheral tissues. As discussed by Fajans [318], there is now considerable evidence for even further physiologic heterogeneity in NIDDM. Among patients with mild NIDDM or impaired glucose tolerance are individuals with early insulin responses that range from supernormal to subnormal. Similar variability has been documented for the late insulin response in such patients [318]. Fajans has proposed six possible pathophysiologic 'sub-types' of NIDDM as a working hypothesis [318]. The basic defects responsible for diabetes in these sub-types include: decreased islet B cell insulin reserves (group 1); delayed insulin response (groups 2 and 3); decreased insulin sensitivity and/or biologic activity of insulin (groups 4 and 5); and peripheral insulin resistance (group 6). That so much

variability is seen in individuals with presumably early stages of diabetes strongly suggests that NIDDM is not caused by a single defect. Genetic studies, as discussed below, support this notion.

Genetic Approaches in NIDDM

Two major strategies can be used for teasing out the heterogeneous etiologies of NIDDM [59, 319, 320]: one starts with a specific physiologic trait or defect and then works backwards to determine the genetic defect (working from the phenotype down); the other starts with a gene or allele proposed to be related to diabetes, establishes a genetic relationship, and works forward (working from the genotype up) to determine the physiologic trait associated with this gene or gene defect. Either strategy can be applied to studies of physiologic variability in animal or human populations, and may include comparisons of affected and unaffected individuals within a population or family.

Genetic studies can use a systematic 'marker gene' approach (studying a number of genetic markers spaced throughout the genome) or a 'candidate gene' approach (studying specific genes which might play a role in the susceptibility to diabetes). The former approach has only recently been used in type 2 diabetes and has not yet yielded many results. Investigators have used the candidate gene approach with mixed success, as described below (and summarized in Table 8).

Maturity Onset Diabetes of the Young (MODY)

The greatest success in determining the genetic basis of a form of NIDDM has been with maturity onset diabetes of the young (MODY).

MODY was originally described in 1964 [321] and was clearly identified as an autosomal dominant sub-type of NIDDM in the 1970s [47]. In addition to the criteria for the diagnosis of diabetes, the following criteria must be met for diagnosis of MODY: (a) age of onset for at least one family member under 25 years; (b) correction of fasting hyperglycemia for at least 2 years without insulin; and (c) non-ketotic diabetes [323]. Using these criteria, many families with clearly dominant inheritance have been identified. However, there is considerable clinical heterogeneity among MODY, and this is now appreciated to be due in large measure to genetic heterogeneity. In the French population, using rather stringent criteria, it is estimated that MODY may account for as much as 10–15% of familial diabetes cases, but less of general or later-onset NIDDM [324].

Although MODY is a relatively rare disorder, accounting for at most a few percent of all NIDDM cases, it has taken on great importance in the

Table 8 Candidate gene studies in NIDDM

Gene	Population associations	Family/linkage studies	Mutation studies	References
Insulin	+/− NIDDM associations in Europids, Japanese, Indians	No evidence for linkage	Mis-sense mutations found in less than 0.5% of NIDDM subjects	[105, 343–367]
Insulin receptor	+ NIDDM associations in Europids and Hispanics + Gestational diabetes associations in Europids and African-Americans	No evidence for linkage	Mutations inherited in an autosomal recessive fashion cause severe insulin resistance (leprechaunism, Rabson–Mendenhall syndrome, lipoatrophic diabetes, type A extreme insulin resistance). May play a role in a small percentage of NIDDM	[362, 370–383]
Insulin receptor substrate-1	+ NIDDM associations in Danish	No evidence for linkage	None identified	[385, 386]
Glucagon-like peptide-1 receptor	No association in African-Americans	No evidence for linkage	None identified	[387]
Prohormone convertase 2	+ NIDDM association in Japanese	NT	$G \rightarrow T$ transition in exon 1, ? if it has functional consequences	[388]
Gc phenotype	+ association with fasting insulin levels in Dogrib Indians	NT	None identified	[389]
Glut1	+ NIDDM association in English, Italians, US Europids, Chinese- and African-Americans; conflicting results in other similar populations, however	NT	None identified	[393–398]
Glut2	None found	Possible linkage with acute insulin response but not with NIDDM in Pimas. No linkage in US Europids	No mutations with phenotypic effects	[395, 397, 400, 401, 403, 446]
Glut4	None found	NT	No mutations with phenotypic effects	[395, 401, 405–407, 447]
Glucokinase	+ NIDDM association in Mauritian Creoles, African-Americans, Japanese and Finns	Linkage with glucose response to oral glucose challenge in Chinese	Mutations in GCK are responsible for the majority of MODY families but are rarely seen in non-MODY NIDDM	[324, 330, 332–335, 409–424]
Adenosine deaminase	No association in Chinese	No evidence for linkage	None identified	[325, 404, 418]
HLA region	Associations with different class 1 and class 2 genes and varying alleles reported in Pimas, Nigerians, Indians, Chinese, African-Americans, and Northern European Europids	Possible linkage between DR4 and diabetes in families with both NIDDM and IDDM	None identified	[425–437, 439]

(continued overleaf)

Table 8 (*continued*)

Gene	Population associations	Family/linkage studies	Mutation studies	References
Apolipoprotein A1/C3/A4 gene cluster	+ NIDDM association in obese Chinese-Americans and Poles	NT	None identified	[374, 442]
Apolipoprotein B	+ NIDDM association in lean Chinese-Americans	NT	None identified	[374]
Apolipoprotein E	? + NIDDM association in Europids (study may have included mostly IDDM)	NT	None identified	[71, 72, 74, 76]
Lipoprotein lipase	+ associations with fasting insulin, triglyceride and HDL levels in non-diabetics, and + association with fasting insulin in diabetic Hispanics and Europids	NT	None identified	[77–81]
Fatty acid binding protein 2	+ weak NIDDM association in Finns, English and Welsh	Linkage with maximal insulin action in Pimas and Mexican-Americans	None identified	[82, 83, 251]
Glycogen synthase	+ NIDDM associations in Finns, French and Japanese. In the Finnish study, + association also seen with hypertension and insulin-stimulated glucose storage	No evidence for linkage	None identified	[89, 91, 92, 406]
Beta 3 adrenergic receptor	+ association with earlier NIDDM onset in Pimas and Finns + association with decreased resting metabolic rate in Pimas + association with capacity to gain weight in the French	NT	Mis-sense mutation in the first intracellular loop affects several diabetes and obesity-related phenotypes	[106, 108, 109]
Mitochondrial DNA	− NIDDM association in Pimas. Excess maternal transmission of diabetes has been reported in US Europids, French, Mexican-Americans and Taiwanese and in German MODY pedigrees. This could potentially be due to mitochondrial alterations	Maternal transmission of mitochondrial mutations has been documented	Mutation in nucleotide 3243 can cause isolated diabetes, diabetes with deafness, or MELAS. A 10.4 kb deletion in this region of the mitochondrial genome also causes diabetes and deafness. These mitochondrial mutations impair insulin secretion	[119, 121, 124–130]

NT, not tested.

past decade because of the lessons it has taught about the loci involved in NIDDM and genetic heterogeneity. The first MODY locus was identified by Bell et al [325] with the demonstration of linkage of MODY with the adenosine deaminase (ADA) locus on the long arm of chromosome 20 in one large MODY family (the RW pedigree). Interestingly, clear delineation of linkage was only possible after exclusion of certain branches of the RW pedigree from analysis, following appreciation of the fact that non-MODY NIDDM was occurring in these branches. Subsequent to the report of linkage in the RW pedigree, only a few other pedigrees have been shown to be linked to chromosome 20, suggesting that this locus (MODY1) accounts for a minority of MODY subjects. MODY1 has not yet been cloned, although the candidate gene region has been narrowed to 5–8 million base pairs contained within a YAC contig [326].

Not long after linkage to chromosome 20 was reported for the RW pedigree, linkage with the glucokinase gene (GCK) on chromosome 7p was reported in other MODY families [327, 328]. Unlike the ADA locus on chromosome 20, which was tested simply as a polymorphic marker in a systematic mapping approach, GCK was tested as a candidate gene because of its role in glucose sensing by the islet B cell and in the deposition of glucose in the liver [324, 329, 330]. Most MODY patients have a decreased insulin response to glucose, suggesting a primary pancreatic B-cell defect [331], so the glucokinase gene was an excellent candidate for genetic investigations. Following the demonstration of linkage, actual mutations within the coding region were identified [332–334]. Mutations in glucokinase account for a major portion of MODY pedigrees; 60% of French MODY families have GCK mutations [335].

A significant number of MODY pedigrees are not linked to either chromosome 20 or glucokinase. A third MODY locus was mapped to 12q [336], but the responsible gene has yet to be identified. MODY3 accounts for approximately 25% of French MODY families [337]. Thus, although GCK and MODY3 together explain the majority of MODY families, there must be at least one more MODY locus still to be found.

With the identification of genetically separate groups of MODY families, it has become possible to distinguish clinical differences among MODY families due to different loci. GCK mutations cause a relatively mild form of diabetes, or only impaired glucose tolerance, in most affected individuals. Frank diabetes (as opposed to impaired glucose tolerance) is found in 46% [338]. They rarely require insulin and usually do not develop vascular complications [339]. Members of the RW pedigree linked to chromosome 20, however, demonstrate a wider spectrum of diabetes severity.

Approximately 30% require insulin treatment and vascular complications are fairly common [339]. MODY3 on chromosome 12q also causes a more severe form of diabetes, with the prevalence of diabetes rather than impaired glucose tolerance reported to be 97% [338]. Mutations in GCK are thought to alter the set point of the islet B cell so that a higher circulating glucose level is necessary to trigger insulin secretion [340]. Studies of the RW pedigree suggest that this form of MODY results from abnormalities in insulin secretion as well. Herman et al [341] found that there was a difference in the response to prolonged intravenous glucose infusion in non-diabetic family members who carry the linked marker on chromosome 20, as compared to those who do not. Individuals with the marker demonstrated both decreased mean plasma C-peptide levels and a decrease in the amplitude of insulin secretory oscillations during glucose infusion. Similar abnormalities were present in the diabetic family members as well, suggesting that these secretory changes may be the earliest manifestations of MODY in this family. MODY3 is probably also an insulin secretory defect, but the mechanism is not as clear [338].

The discovery that at least four genetically distinct forms of MODY exist suggests that there is likely to be even greater genetic heterogeneity within 'classical' NIDDM. Just as different MODY defects appear to cause varying degrees of diabetes severity and complications, the clinical and physiologic differences among NIDDM patients may well result from genetically separate forms of diabetes.

Candidate Genes and NIDDM

Insulin Gene

Several studies have suggested that impaired insulin secretion is an early defect in the development of NIDDM [306, 309, 311, 342]. It has also been shown that insulin release is genetically regulated [308]. These pathophysiologic traits could conceivably be due to variations near or within the insulin gene—variations which may affect the production and/or secretion of insulin.

Mutation studies. A number of patients have now been described with discrete point mutations in the insulin gene, which result in the production of abnormal insulins of greatly reduced biologic activity [343]. Patients with these mutations present with hyperglycemia, hyperinsulinemia, normal C-peptide levels, and a normal responsiveness to exogenous insulin. The mutant insulin trait is transmitted in an autosomal dominant pattern and carriers of a mutant insulin gene usually are not diabetic until adulthood. Additional mutations in the insulin gene lead to hyperproinsulinemia. The clinical presentation of the latter is similar to the hyperinsulinemic mutant insulins, and autosomal dominant transmission is seen within pedigrees [343].

Three well-characterized mis-sense mutations leading to mutant insulins and hyperinsulinemia have been discovered: insulin Chicago (amino acid substitution B25 phenylalanine to leucine); insulin Los Angeles (B24 phenylalanine to serine); and insulin Waykayama (A3 valine to leucine). Several families have been described with point mutations at the cleavage site of the C-peptide, resulting in hyperproinsulinemia [344, 345], and it is likely that additional mutations will be found which alter the structure or processing of the insulin molecule. These mutant insulins can be detected in serum by means of variant migration on high performance liquid chromatography (HPLC) and in DNA by alterations in restriction enzyme cleavage sites [346–350].

In a population of NIDDM subjects screened for mutant insulins, however, fewer than 0.5% were found to have such mutations [351]. In a study of 100 African-American NIDDM subjects, single strand confirmation polymorphism (SSCP) and direct sequencing of the coding and promoter regions of the insulin gene were employed to search for variations in the insulin gene [352]. Not a single mutation was found in the coding portions of the gene. Eight allelic variants were described, with only one in the coding region. The authors suggest that two of these polymorphisms may have biologic consequences. The deletion of a cytosine nucleotide at the −90 position in the proximal promoter might alter transcription of the gene, and a four-nucleotide insertion at position 46 alters the consensus sequence of the 5′-splice donor site of the first intron, which might alter proinsulin mRNA processing. In a similar study of a small number of diabetic Pima Indians ($n = 6$) and Nauruans ($n = 2$), using direct sequencing techniques, the nucleotide sequences of the coding and adjacent regions of the insulin gene were identical to previously published insulin gene sequences of non-diabetic subjects [353].

The 5′ Insulin Gene Polymorphism

Population studies. In the 5′ flanking region of the insulin gene (located on chromosome 11) there is a hypervariable DNA region. Initial studies of this region in NIDDM suggested an association of the large class 3 alleles with NIDDM [354]. Subsequent studies in Europid populations have for the most part been negative [105, 355–357], although a study of healthy Italian subjects did suggest an association between the class 3 allele and a reduced ability to secrete insulin following glucose infusion [358]. Studies in other ethnic groups

have had mixed results. In Japanese-Asian and southern Indian NIDDM subjects an association with the class 3 allele has been noted [359–361], particularly in those subjects who also had a positive family history of diabetes. However, in a study of Punjabi Sikhs (northern Indians), no differences in the frequencies of the hypervariable region alleles were found between diabetic and control subjects, even when the diabetic subjects were subdivided for a positive family history of diabetes [362].

A *Pst*I restriction site polymorphism, due to a point mutation in the 3′ untranslated region at position 1628, has also been identified [363]. Elbein et al [364] found this marker to be non-polymorphic in Europids, Pima Indians and African-Americans, and therefore concluded that the β allele represented an isolated mutation. However, a study of this allele in Punjabi Sikhs has shown that the presence of this allele depends upon the frequency of the class 3 hypervariable region allele, and that the two alleles are in linkage disequilibrium [365]. Unfortunately, this marker did not appear to be better at predicting diabetes than the class 3 allele in this population. In a German and Polish diabetic patient population characterized by a positive family history and fasting hyperinsulinemia with normal C-peptide levels, the β allele of the *Pst*I restriction digest was more often associated with the diabetic patients than the controls ($p = 0.05$) [366]. The authors of this study suggest that this mutation may have an effect on the stability or persistence of the transcribed mRNA product, thus influencing the insulin levels.

Family studies. Results of family studies suggest that mutations in the insulin gene and its surrounding area are unlikely to play a major role in most idiopathic forms of NIDDM. For example, in the 23 Utah pedigrees analyzed by Elbein and colleagues, most families either showed no evidence for linkage to this locus, or were uninformative [367]. Similarly, in two Punjabi Sikh families studied by Hitman et al [362], no linkage could be established with the hypervariable region of the insulin gene and diabetes in one family, while the other family was uninformative.

In conclusion, the current data suggest that the insulin gene plays a minor role in predisposing to NIDDM. While in a few families NIDDM is directly the result of mutations in the insulin gene, these mutations account for only a very small proportion of NIDDM. It remains possible that in some populations the insulin gene or genes nearby may contribute some degree of NIDDM susceptibility.

Insulin Receptor Gene

Since NIDDM patients often have peripheral insulin resistance, and in some populations this appears to be a primary defect contributing to the development of NIDDM, there has been interest in genes coding for and/or regulating the insulin receptor. The insulin receptor gene consists of 22 exons spanning about 150 000 base pairs on chromosome 19p (19p13.2–p13.3) [368]. The insulin receptor is a transmembrane protein consisting of two α and two β chains. The α chain is extracellular and binds insulin. The β chain spans the membrane, and the molecule's tyrosine kinase domain is found in the cytoplasmic region [369] (see Chapter 21).

Population studies. A number of restriction fragment length polymorphisms (RFLPs) in or around the insulin receptor gene have been described. *Bgl*II and *Bam*HI polymorphisms were evaluated in Punjabi Sikh and British Europid diabetic and control subjects, with negative results [362].

An *Sst*I RFLP of the insulin receptor gene was investigated in American-Europid and Hispanic NIDDM patients and control subjects [370]. A significant association with a 5.8 kb fragment was observed, occurring in 7.7% of the normal control subjects and 23.5% of the diabetic subjects ($p < 0.05$). Interestingly, non-diabetic subjects carrying this allele were found to be hyperinsulinemic and/or to have elevated glucose levels. This 5.8 kb polymorphism had been described previously, however, and not found to be associated with NIDDM in a Europid population [371]. An association study in a large population of African-American subjects demonstrated a significant negative correlation with NIDDM [372]. These conflicting results are difficult to assess. It may be that a relationship exists between the insulin receptor and NIDDM, but through different mechanisms in different populations [370].

Raboudi et al [373] investigated an *Rsa*I RFLP of the insulin receptor gene in Mexican-American and non-Hispanic White diabetic and control subjects. Alleles of 6.7 kb (allele A), 6.2 kb (allele B), and 3.4 kb (allele C) were identified. The C allele was observed in Mexican-American subjects only. Diabetic Mexican-Americans were twice as likely to be homozygous for the C allele than control subjects, with an age-adjusted 4.7-fold increase in risk of diabetes among Mexican-Americans with the CC genotype compared with Mexican-Americans without this genotype. Additionally, there was a trend toward a younger age of diabetes onset in CC homozygote cases than in heterozygotes or non-C allele homozygotes. The high-risk C allele was also found in high frequency (34%) among the Pima Indians [371]. Thus, it will be interesting to determine whether this marker is simply a marker of 'Native American genes', or truly plays a role in the development of NIDDM in these high-risk populations.

In a Chinese-American population, frequencies of RFLPs and haplotypes of the insulin receptor gene in diabetic and non-diabetic subjects were compared [374]. Seven polymorphic restriction sites were identified (*Pst*I, *Xba*I(A), *Rsa*I, *Sst*I, *Xba*I(B), *Kpn*I, *Bgl*II). There were no significant differences in the allelic frequencies between the diabetic and control subjects. However, haplotype differences between these groups were seen, with the haplotypes *Xba*I(A) allele 2, *Rsa*I allele 2, and *Kpn* allele 2 haplotype, and the *Xba*I(A) allele 1, *Rsa*I allele 3, *Kpn*I allele 2 haplotype found significantly more frequently among control subjects than in the diabetic group. These findings suggest a protective effect of these insulin receptor gene haplotypes, which would imply that genes in this region may indeed be important in the development of NIDDM.

In a study of Europid-American, African-American and Hispanic-American women, the *Kpn*I restriction polymorphism was compared in women with gestational diabetes and in a group of control subjects [375]. Among Black and Europid subjects, the 15.5 kb *Kpn*I band was associated with NIDDM. In addition, this allele also significantly interacted with body mass index (BMI) and history of diabetes in the subject's mother. In the Europid group, a significant interaction between this *Kpn*I 15.5 kb allele and an insulin-like growth factor II allele (*Bam*HI 1.2 kb band) was also observed. No allelic frequency differences were observed in a Hispanic group of women, however, suggesting genetic differences among these groups.

Family studies. Linkage studies in Punjabi Sikh families [362] and Europid families [376, 377] have failed to find linkage of NIDDM and a variety of insulin receptor gene RFLPs. In addition, scanning of the β chain exons 13–21 of the insulin receptor locus (mutations here presumed to be involved in post-receptor defects) by SSCP, with subsequent DNA sequencing, identified only silent mutations not likely to result in defective insulin receptor function [378]. In further direct sequence analysis of exon 17, which binds ATP and appears essential to tyrosine kinase activity, a valine-to-methionine substitution was found at codon 985 in three diabetic members within three generations of one pedigree. Carriers of this mutation were found to have higher 1 h and 2 h post-glucose load glucose levels than non-carriers, suggesting that this valine-to-methionine substitution may be predisposing to insulin resistance in this pedigree.

Mutation studies. Mutations in the insulin receptor gene are involved in a number of syndromes associated with severe insulin resistance, including leprechaunism, the Rabson–Mendenhall syndrome (extreme insulin resistance, acanthosis nigricans, abnormalities of teeth and nails, and pineal hyperplasia), lipoatrophic diabetes, and type A extreme insulin resistance (triad of insulin resistance, acanthosis nigricans and hyperandrogenism). Homozygous mutations in the insulin receptor gene are responsible for most cases, although many of the patients with type A insulin resistance have mutations in only one allele [379]. Five classes of disease-causing mutations have been described [379]: class 1 mutations, which decrease the level of insulin receptor mRNA; class 2 mutations, which impair the transport of receptors through the endoplasmic reticulum and Golgi apparatus to the plasma membrane; class 3 mutations, which decrease the affinity to bind insulin; class 4 mutations, which impair receptor tyrosine kinase activity; and class 5 mutations, which accelerate the degradation of insulin receptors.

Many of the heterozygous parents of patients with these genetic syndromes are insulin resistant [380, 381]. Indeed, many have levels of insulin resistance similar to common forms of NIDDM, consistent with the hypothesis that mutations in the insulin receptor gene may contribute to the insulin resistance seen in a subgroup of patients with NIDDM. Theoretical calculations suggest that about 0.1–1.0% of the general population are heterozygous for a mutation in the insulin receptor gene, and it may be that these individuals constitute a subpopulation of NIDDM [379].

In a UK population of 30 diabetic and 13 control subjects, O'Rahilly et al [382] investigated exons 17–21 (β chain locus tyrosine kinase domain) and found five silent mutations in exon 17, as well as the met985 mutation described above in the family study by Elbein and Sorensen [378]. The met985 mutation was found in only one diabetic subject and in one of the normoglycemic control subjects (fasting glucose < 5.7 mmol/l (103 mg/dl), $HbA_{1c} < 6.1\%$, and no family history of diabetes). An additional mis-sense mutation in exon 18, a lysine-to-glutamic acid substitution at codon 1068, was described in one of the diabetic subjects. This mutation results in the replacement of a basic residue by a highly acidic one, an alteration that is unlikely to be biologically silent. Both the Val985 and Lys1068 residues are located within the highly conserved tyrosine kinase domain of the receptor, and both are conserved in the insulin receptor of other mammalian species, marking their relative importance and providing further support for the significance of these findings.

In a Japanese population of 35 individuals (28 diabetic and seven control subjects), studied using SSCP, a mutation in exon 20 substituting leucine for proline at codon 1178 of the insulin receptor gene was found in a diabetic patient with moderate insulin resistance associated with morbid obesity, acanthosis nigricans and polycystic ovary syndrome [383]. Proline 1178 is a part of a characteristic sequence motif common to many protein kinases, located near the autophosphorylation sites of the insulin receptor's tyrosine kinase domain. Thus, the substitution of leucine for proline at codon 1178 may be a functionally relevant mutation.

In conclusion, the insulin receptor locus does not appear to play a major role in diabetes susceptibility in the population at large. The population association studies provide conflicting results regarding the possible association of the insulin receptor locus and NIDDM. The available family studies suggest that the insulin receptor gene locus is unlikely to act as a major locus in the susceptibility to NIDDM, while investigations which have used SSCP and direct sequencing of the insulin receptor cDNA have provided limited evidence for a contribution of the insulin receptor gene to NIDDM in a small subset of cases

Insulin Receptor Substrate-1 Gene

The protein designated as insulin receptor substrate-1 (IRS-1) is a major substrate for the insulin receptor tyrosine kinase. It is phosphorylated by the insulin receptor kinase when the latter is activated by insulin. The gene encoding this protein maps to chromosome 2, bands q35–q36.1 [384]. This protein is ubiquitous in insulin-sensitive and insulin-like growth factor I (IGF-I) sensitive tissues, including those that determine glucose production and utilization and those with regulatory effects on pancreatic B-cell function. IRS-1 has a central role as an adaptor molecule that links the insulin receptor and IGF-I receptor kinases with enzymes that regulate cellular metabolism and growth; thus it is an excellent candidate gene for NIDDM.

Population studies. In a population of Danish Europids, SSCP and direct sequencing techniques were employed to investigate associations of this genetic locus with diabetes [385]. Two amino acid polymorphisms were identified, one at codon 972 (arginine to glycine) and one at codon 513 (alanine to proline). The frequency of these IRS-1 polymorphisms was about three times higher in patients with NIDDM than in control subjects ($p = 0.02$). Ten of the diabetic subjects and only three of the control subjects were heterozygous for the codon 972 polymorphism and six of the diabetic subjects and two of the control subjects were heterozygous for the codon 513 polymorphism. None of the polymorphism carriers had both amino acid variants. Both amino acid substitutions are located close to tyrosine phosphorylation motifs that are putative recognition sites for insulin and IGF-I signal transmission proteins. Subjects with NIDDM who had IRS-1 variants did not differ in their degree of insulin resistance from subjects without known IRS-1 polymorphisms. However, heterozygotes for the codon 972 polymorphism had significantly lower fasting plasma insulin and C-peptide, suggesting that this genetic locus may play an etiologic role in NIDDM.

Family studies. The only reported linkage study investigating the IRS-1 gene was carried out in 31 Mexican-American families ascertained through a proband with NIDDM [386]. No evidence for linkage was found, but additional studies in other ethnic groups are necessary to exclude a role for this candidate gene in NIDDM.

Glucagon-like Peptide-1 Receptor Gene

Glucagon-like peptide-1 (GLP-1) is a fragment of proglucagon secreted by intestinal L-cells. It has potent glucose-dependent insulin secretory effects and also suppresses gastric acid secretion in the stomach. The actions of GLP-1 are mediated by the GLP-1 receptor. Because of this important regulatory role in insulin secretion, the GLP-1 receptor is a candidate gene for NIDDM. The GLP-1 receptor gene is localized to chromosome 6, band p21.1, about 20 centimorgans (cM) from the HLA region [387].

Population studies. Two highly polymorphic simple sequence repeat regions (SSRs) have been identified in association with the GLP-1 receptor. Several polymorphic alleles for both sequences have been defined in African-Americans and Europid-Americans. In a large population of African-Americans the allele frequencies of the two SSRs did not differ between diabetic and control subjects [387].

Family studies. The GLP-1 receptor gene SSRs were used for linkage analysis in 16 Utah Mormon pedigrees with NIDDM, and linkage was rejected under both dominant and recessive models [387]. Examination of individual families did not suggest heterogeneity at this locus, and all individual LOD scores were 1 or less. However, under the models of intermediate or low penetrance the GLP-1 locus could not be excluded (LOD score < -2). Thus, although unlikely to be a major susceptibility gene, the GLP-1 receptor gene locus may still be a contributor to the development of NIDDM and further studies are warranted.

Prohormone Convertase 2 Gene

Proinsulin is converted to insulin by two proteases, prohormone convertase 2 and prohormone convertase 3. Prohormone convertase 2 cleaves the proinsulin molecule where the C-peptide and the A-chain domains are joined. The gene has been cloned and it is localized to chromosome 20, band p11.2. A simple tandem repeat exists in intron 2. Because NIDDM is associated with increased proinsulin and proinsulin-like molecules, the

prohormone convertase 2 gene is a candidate gene for NIDDM.

Population studies. In a population of Japanese diabetic and control subjects matched for age and BMI, the A1 allele of the intron 2 tandem repeat, consisting of 21 CA repeats, was significantly associated with NIDDM [388]. The 12 exons of the gene were screened for mutations in 60 diabetic subjects. In one subject a G-to-T substitution was identified in exon 1, two base pairs before the translational start site. This created an in-frame methionine codon, generating a protein with two methionines at its NH2 terminus, the functional consequences of which are not known.

Given the positive association, additional population and family studies are warranted to investigate this candidate gene further.

Gc Genotype

Serum group-specific component (Gc) binds vitamin D, a metabolically active form which is known to be involved in the regulation of insulin. In studies in the Dogrib Indian population of Canada, the homozygous Gc phenotype 1F-1F was found to be associated with the lowest levels of fasting insulin [389]. In addition, the Gc genotype was found to be the only significant predictor of fasting insulin level in multivariate analysis, after correcting for adiposity. This would suggest that the Gc gene (or genes nearby it) may play a role in insulin regulation in this population.

Glut1

The Glut1 gene is approximately 35 kb in size and is located on chromosome 1p (1p31.3–35) [390]. It codes for a 492-residue glucose transport protein that can be translocated from an intracellular position to a membrane compartment in 3T3-L1 adipocytes on stimulation with insulin [391]. This gene product is the major glucose transporter gene of brain, erythrocytes and placenta, and it is expressed to a variable extent in heart, skeletal muscle, adipose tissue, intestine, kidney and liver [392].

Population studies. Population association studies with a variety of RFLPs have produced conflicting results. The most extensively studied is an *Xba*I RFLP in intron 2 of the gene which has alleles X1 (size 6.2 kb) and X2 (5.9 kb).

Li et al [393] investigated this RFLP in three populations; English-Europids, Italian-Europids, and Japanese. The *Xba*I RFLP marker demonstrated significant associations between the genotypes X1X1, X1X2, and X2X2 in NIDDM patients and controls in all three populations, with the X1 allele having a greater frequency in the diabetic subjects vs. the control subjects. Cox et al [394] studied the same *Xba*I polymorphism in Europid-Americans, Chinese-Americans and African-Americans living in the San Francisco area. In comparing the allele frequencies, they found an increase of the X1 allele in diabetic subjects vs. controls in the three different ethnic groups, but this increase was not statistically significant. Oelbaum et al [395], studying the *Xba*I marker as well as a *Stu*I RFLP (alleles 3.2 and 2.6) in an English-Europid population, found no significant differences between the allelic or genotypic frequencies at either marker between diabetic patients, non-diabetic controls or a subgroup of diabetic patients with a positive family history of diabetes. Haplotype frequencies of the *Xba*I/*Stu*I markers, which can be more specific than the study of individual markers, also failed to show any statistically significant difference between the diabetic subjects and controls. The *Xba*I RFLP was also examined in an African-American population [396]. Although an association was found, it was not statistically significant upon correction for multiple comparisons. A number of other RFLPs (*Bgl*II, *Taq*I, *Pst*I) have been examined, with no allele, genotype or haplotype associations with NIDDM observed [394, 396].

In conclusion, there are conflicting results regarding the association of the Glut1 gene with NIDDM. The X1 allele of the *Xba*I marker within intron 2 of the Glut1 gene appears to have the strongest relationship with diabetes, but the preponderance of the data does not support a significant association between the Glut1 gene and NIDDM.

Family studies. Linkage studies have not provided any further evidence for an association between the Glut1 gene and NIDDM. Elbein et al [397] tested the relationship between two markers (*Xba*I and *Stu*I) and NIDDM in 18 large Europid pedigrees from Utah. Using an alternative linkage analysis approach, the affected sib-pair method, similar negative results were obtained [398]. Both the *Msp*I RFLP marker located adjacent to the Glut1 gene at an estimated 0.2 recombination frequency, and the *Xba*I marker occurring within intron 2 of the gene, failed to demonstrate any significant evidence for linkage between NIDDM and the Glut1 gene. This conclusion held true when both alleles were evaluated separately and when combined as haplotypes.

Glut2

Glut2 is the facilitative glucose transporter expressed in pancreatic B cells and hepatocytes. This protein is a high capacity, low affinity glucose transporter that allows uptake of glucose at concentrations in the physiological range. In the B cell, Glut2 may act as a glucose sensor. In the hepatocyte, Glut2 mediates the uptake of glucose after a meal and its release in the postabsorptive state. Therefore mutations in this gene may cause NIDDM by increasing the threshold for glucose-stimulated insulin secretion in B cells and by reducing uptake and promoting release of glucose by the liver, as well as by having effects on glucose absorption in the small intestine and reabsorption from urine in the kidney [399].

The gene for Glut2 maps to chromosome 3 and has 11 exons, spanning about 30 kb. Markers which have been used in genetic studies include multiple RFLPs and, more recently, three highly polymorphic tandem repeat sequences in introns 1 and 4a, and a 168 base pair insertion/deletion polymorphism in intron 3 [399].

Population studies. In a British-Europid population, no significant differences in the frequencies of several diallelic RFLPs (*Eco*RI, *Taq*I, *Bcl*I) and their haplotypes were found between diabetic and control subjects [400]. In a similar population (British-Europid), using the restriction enzymes *Bgl*I, *Hind*III, *Taq*I, and *Kpn*I, all of which yielded two allele polymorphisms, there were no significant differences in allelic, genotypic or haplotype frequencies in control subjects, diabetic subjects, or diabetic subjects with a positive family history of diabetes [395]. Matsutani et al [401] found similar negative results in an African-American population using (*Eco*RI and *Taq*I) RFLPs.

The Glut2 *Taq*I RFLP was also studied in diabetic patients with a family history of NIDDM (at least one sibling with NIDDM) [446]. The allele frequencies of diabetic patients with a family history of NIDDM were significantly different from those in a matched control group who did not have a personal or family history of NIDDM. Yet, when diabetic subjects who had an unknown or indeterminate family history of diabetes were compared with the control population, the allele frequencies were no longer significantly different, although a similar trend was seen.

Family studies. A study of 18 large, Europid pedigrees from Utah tested linkage of the Glut2 diallelic *Eco*RI RFLP and a highly polymorphic (six-allele) dinucleotide repeat with NIDDM [397]. The LOD scores for the Glut2 locus were < -4.0 under all models tested, thus excluding linkage.

Janssen et al [403] investigated the association of the Glut2 locus with NIDDM and with the acute insulin response (AIR), a measure of pancreatic B cell function, in Pima Indian volunteers. It was shown that the AIR aggregated in families both before and after adjusting for sex and percentage body fat ($p < 0.0002$), with large differences between families and small mean variation within families. Analysis of 117 sib-pairs from 38 families provided borderline evidence for linkage between dinucleotide repeat polymorphisms of the Glut2 locus and a measure of AIR ($\log_{10}$ of mean plasma insulin concentration from 3, 4 and 5 minutes after an IVGTT), but no linkage was observed between Glut2 and NIDDM. To investigate this association further, SSCP followed by direct DNA sequencing was used and a mis-sense mutation in exon 3 was identified (ACT110–ATT110) which changed the amino acid threonine to isoleucine in the second membrane-spanning domain of the Glut2 protein. However, no significant phenotypic associations (NIDDM, AIR) could be demonstrated in individuals with or without this mutation.

In summary, the preponderance of genetic evidence does not link the Glut2 locus with NIDDM in the populations which have been studied thus far, including Northern European Europids, American-Europids, African-Americans and Pima Indians.

Glut4

Abnormal or reduced insulin-mediated glucose disposal is a major feature of NIDDM and may be partially genetically determined [305]. Therefore Glut4, the insulin-sensitive muscle/adipose glucose transporter, was considered a strong candidate gene for NIDDM.

Population studies. Genetic association and linkage studies have been limited because of the paucity of informative polymorphic markers. The *Kpn*I diallelic polymorphism is the only RFLP marker that has been described, and its association with NIDDM has been investigated in a British-Europid population [395], an Italian population [447] and an African-American population [401]. In each study there were no significant differences in allelic or genotypic frequencies between diabetic subjects and controls.

The development of SSCP, allele specific oligonucleotide (ASO) hybridization and direct DNA sequencing have facilitated the study of the promoter and coding regions of the Glut4 gene. A common silent polymorphism at codon 130 of Glut4 was studied in a randomly selected subgroup of Welsh diabetic patients and control subjects. There were no significant differences in the allelic or genotypic frequencies between the diabetic and control subjects [405]. Bjørbaek et al [406] scanned the entire coding region of the Glut4 gene in seven Danish-Europid diabetic subjects by SSCP, using cDNA generated from total RNA isolated from muscle biopsies, and the polymorphism at codon 130 was also seen. The promoter region of the gene was also investigated by SSCP of genomic DNA in 30 diabetic subjects. Direct sequencing identified three different variations, all single nucleotide substitutions at positions −580, 1 and 30. None of these

variants were identified to have any major impact on Glut4 expression in skeletal muscle of individuals heterozygous for one or all of the promoter sequence variations. Because a reduced Glut4 mRNA content has been observed in adipose tissue, but not in muscle tissue from NIDDM patients, it is not known if any of the three identified variants may have an impact on Glut4 expression in adipose tissue.

Family studies. A study of the expression of Glut4 mRNA and its protein product in muscle biopsies taken from 14 insulin-resistant patients with NIDDM, 10 of their first-degree relatives and in 12 insulin-sensitive control subjects failed to demonstrate an inherited tendency for Glut4 abnormalities [407]. The levels of Glut4 mRNA were significantly higher in the diabetic patients than the control subjects. However, the Glut4 mRNA levels in the relatives were not significantly different from those observed in the control subjects, and the Glut4 protein levels did not significantly differ between control subjects, diabetic patients and relatives.

In conclusion, although the glucose transporter genes initially appeared to be good NIDDM candidate genes, the studies performed to date do not support a significant role for Glut1, Glut2 or Glut4 in NIDDM.

Glucokinase

As discussed above, mutations in the glucokinase (GCK) gene are a cause of approximately one-third of MODY pedigrees [330, 409]. The gene has also been investigated as a candidate gene in non-MODY NIDDM.

Population studies. Microsatellite (CA)n repeats near the 3′ and 5′ end of the glucokinase gene have been identified and used as genetic markers (GCK1 and GCK2 respectively) in both population and family studies [324]. The GCK1 alleles have been most informative. The most common number of 3′ repeats is known as allele Z; the other alleles differ from the Z allele by the number of nucleotides (Z + 2, Z + 4, Z + 10, etc.). Five alleles have been identified in American Blacks, four in Mauritian Creoles, four in the Japanese, six in Whites, and four in Pimas [324, 410–412]. The GCK2 alleles have been less instructive in identifying an association with diabetes. The most common allele is called the O allele and, similarly, the other alleles differ from the O allele by the number of nucleotides (O-2, O-4, etc.)

A significant association between the GCK1 marker and diabetes was described in the Mauritian Creoles [410]. The frequency of the Z + 2 allele was greater in the NIDDM subjects than in controls (23.8% vs. 8.9%, $p = 0.008$) and the frequency of the common

Z allele was lower in the NIDDM subjects than in controls (60% vs. 75.6%, $p = 0.03$). By contrast, no association between GCK1 and NIDDM was observed in the Mauritian-Indian population.

The frequency of the Z + 4 GCK1 allele was significantly associated with diabetes in American Blacks, occurring in 20% of diabetic subjects vs. 12% of non-diabetic subjects, and the common Z allele was significantly negatively associated with diabetes, occurring in 60% of diabetic vs. 50% of non-diabetic subjects. After adjusting for age, sex and BMI, the Z + 4 allele still had a significant positive association with NIDDM, and the Z allele had a significant negative association with diabetes [411].

A similar population association study was performed in Japanese subjects using the GCK1 marker and the GCK2 marker [412]. The Z + 4 allele was found to occur more frequently in the diabetic subjects than in the control subjects. There were no phenotypic differences associated with the different allele types in the diabetic subjects. There were no significant differences in the frequencies of GCK2 alleles between the diabetic and non-diabetic subjects. Additionally, when the GCK1 and GCK2 alleles were used in combination to define a haplotype, there were no significant frequency differences between the diabetic and non-diabetic subjects.

Population association studies using the GCK1 and GCK2 alleles in Europid populations have been inconsistent. In a study of Welsh-Europids the frequencies of both the GCK1 and GCK2 alleles did not differ between diabetic and non-diabetic subjects, nor did the frequencies of haplotypes derived from the two alleles. There was also no observed difference between plasma glucose or insulin responses to meal glucose tolerance tests with the GCK haplotypes or alleles [413]. Conversely, a significant association between the GCK1 locus Z + 2 allele and glucose intolerance (as defined by WHO criteria) has been described in an elderly Finnish population, with a frequency of 0% in control subjects, 6.5% in subjects with impaired glucose tolerance, and 12.2% in diabetic subjects. Individuals with this allele had 2-h glucose levels which were significantly higher than those seen in individuals without the allele [414]. Similarly to the previously mentioned studies, the GCK2 allele and haplotypes derived from the two markers in the Finnish men showed no statistically significant associations with glucose tolerance.

Family studies. In linkage analyses of Europid pedigrees from Utah ($n = 18$), France ($n = 79$), and Oxford, UK ($n = 12$), there was no evidence that the glucokinase gene plays a major role in late-onset non-insulin dependent diabetes or glucose intolerance [415–417]. A mis-sense mutation in exon 7 was found in one of the French families in all diabetic members. However, this family was probably a MODY family, as four younger members carrying this mutation were found to be hyperglycemic [417]. In a Taiwanese-Chinese population of 94 nuclear families, using sib-pair linkage analysis, significant linkage was established between glucose response to an oral glucose challenge and the GCK locus (haplotypes based on two tightly linked GCK markers) [418]. By contrast, measures of insulin response to the oral glucose challenge did not show any evidence for linkage. These physiologic results would be analogous to the physiology in GCK MODY families.

Mutation analyses. Despite the above-described significant GCK1 association findings in the American Black population, the Mauritian Creoles, the Japanese, and the Finnish, mutations in the coding sequence of the glucokinase gene are rare in non-MODY NIDDM, and it appears that primary structural changes in the glucokinase enzyme do not play a significant role in the common form of NIDDM. The glucokinase mutations which have been identified in the UK and French MODY pedigrees were not identified in a sampling of unrelated NIDDM subjects in either the UK and French populations [332, 333] or in the American Black population. The sequence variants that have been described do not affect the amino acid sequence of the gene product [419]. Thus, either the above association findings are spurious, or they may be attributable to mutations in adjacent regulatory regions of the gene that have yet to be identified. Similarly, mutations within the coding sequence of the glucokinase gene do not appear to be prevalent in the Japanese population [420–422], although a few Japanese families have been found to have a mutation which co-segregates with glucose intolerance or late-onset diabetes in family members [423, 424]. In both cases the mutation was located in exon 5 [at positions 186 and 188] and all individuals with this mutation demonstrated impaired insulin secretion in response to a glucose challenge. There are no frequency differences in the variations in the glucokinase gene promoter region in Japanese diabetic subjects and control subjects [422], suggesting that mutations in the glucokinase promoter region in NIDDM are rare and are likely to have a limited role in the pathogenesis of NIDDM in this group.

In summary, the population association data suggest that the glucokinase gene may be an important etiologic contributor to non-insulin dependent diabetes. Unfortunately, the sequencing data described for the glucokinase structural gene in the American Black, Japanese and Europid populations have been unsuccessful in identifying any common mutations. An explanation for this discrepancy may be that regulatory regions near the structural locus are responsible for the population associations, although an initial investigation in the Japanese population has failed to support this hypothesis.

The Adenosine Deaminase (ADA) Locus on Chromosome 20q

Even though the region of chromosome 20q near the ADA locus has been linked to one large MODY pedigree, the ADA locus does not appear to be a major diabetes susceptibility gene in NIDDM. An affected sib-pair study of the ADA locus in UK and Italian pedigrees did not identify any statistically significant linkage [404]; neither was any evidence for linkage observed in a Chinese population [418].

The HLA Region on Chromosome 6

Population studies. While most forms of NIDDM do not appear to be immunologically mediated, there has been some interest in looking at HLA markers in NIDDM patients from populations with high rates of NIDDM. In several populations, associations have been reported with various HLA-A and -B antigens, including A2 (Pima Indians), A10 and Aw32 (Nigerian Blacks), B22/Bw56 (Nauruans), Bw61 (Indians from northern India), and Bw54 (Chinese) [425–431]. The significance of these associations is not entirely clear; they could reflect either real differences in disease susceptibility or biases inherent in the population samples. They are probably an example of genetic background or polygenic contribution, analogous to many differences in diabetes seen with different genetic backgrounds in the various rodent models (reviewed above).

Several population studies examining traits of insulin sensitivity and autoimmunity have shed some light on these HLA associations. In an elderly Finnish population composed of diabetic and non-diabetic subjects, significant HLA associations were found [432]. High-risk IDDM haplotypes were investigated among the elderly Finnish men, and found to be present in 94% of diabetic subjects, 79% of subjects with impaired glucose tolerance, and in only 13% of non-diabetic subjects. In this population, the sensitivity, specificity and predictive values of these high-risk HLA haplotypes were very high (90%, 87% and 97% respectively). Mean fasting blood glucose determinations did not differ significantly between men with or without the high-risk haplotypes, although blood glucose values 2 h after a glucose load were significantly higher in men with the high-risk haplotypes. These findings provide evidence for an etiologic role for the HLA region in subjects who appear phenotypically to have NIDDM.

In African-Americans, Banerji and Lebovitz [433] have reported that NIDDM exists in two forms: one with a primary defect in insulin action (insulin-resistant variant), the other with normal insulin action and a primary defect in insulin secretion (insulin-sensitive) as determined by the euglycemic insulin clamp and C-peptide response to oral glucose. In a population of diabetic and control African-American subjects, Banerji et al [434] have shown that the frequency of the HLA-DQW7 allele in the insulin-resistant diabetic population (76%) was significantly greater than in the insulin-sensitive diabetic population (32%) or the normal control population (21%). The frequency of the HLA-DQW6 allele was also significantly increased in the insulin-sensitive diabetic subjects (76%) as compared with the normal control subjects (33%). Banerji et al interpret these associations with the two variant forms of NIDDM in the African-American population as supporting the hypothesis that these variants are genetically distinct and are probably not related to environmental factors, such as differing degrees of obesity or hyperglycemia.

In a population of American Blacks who presented with diabetic ketoacidosis, yet whose clinical course was consistent with NIDDM, the frequencies of HLA class II alleles DR3 and DR4 were higher than in non-diabetic control subjects (65% vs. 30%, $p < 0.012$) [435]. All but one subject was insulin-resistant, as measured using the euglycemic insulin clamp. Antibodies to glutamic acid decarboxylase (GAD) and islet cell cytoplasmic proteins (ICP) were absent, however, and thus B-cell destruction may not be a factor in the development of diabetes in these subjects. Therefore, the increased frequencies of the HLA-DR3 and -DR4 alleles in these predominantly insulin-resistant diabetic subjects are probably not related to an autoimmune insulitis occurring in the subgroup of NIDDM patients described by Tuomi et al [435].

Further support for the HLA loci in NIDDM susceptibility comes from a report of a significantly increased frequency of HLA-A33, -DR2, -DR9 and -BF-S in African-American women with gestational diabetes who required insulin therapy during pregnancy, as compared to control subjects [436]. Furthermore, the gestational diabetic women who went on to develop NIDDM had a significantly higher frequency of -B41, -DR2, and -BF-S and a lower frequency of -DR1 and -DR6 than control subjects. Even after controlling for age and BMI, -B41 and -DR2 were independent predictors of developing insulin-requiring gestational diabetes and NIDDM in gestational diabetic subjects. In a population of Europids of Northern European ancestry, the HLA-DR4 antigen was found to be associated with non-insulin dependent diabetes and glucose intolerance, defined by an oral glucose tolerance test [437].

Family studies. Further evidence for the role of HLA genes in NIDDM was found in family studies of IDDM probands. Epidemiologic data suggest that a parental history of NIDDM increases the risk of IDDM in siblings of an IDDM proband, consistent with a shared genetic susceptibility between IDDM and NIDDM [438]. In a study by Rich et al [439], the frequency of the HLA-DR4 antigen was higher in IDDM diabetic subjects with a NIDDM parent than in IDDM subjects whose parents did not have diabetes. Additionally, a -DR4 haplotype was transmitted from the NIDDM parent to the IDDM offspring more often than expected. These data, as suggested by the authors, are consistent with the hypothesis that families with a NIDDM parent and an IDDM child, heavily determined by HLA-DR4 linked factors, may represent a homogeneous subset of diabetes susceptibility.

In summary, several population association studies in insulin-resistant diabetic subjects and in gestational diabetic women provide evidence for an HLA-related genetic susceptibility to NIDDM. The family studies also suggest that the HLA locus is a contributor to NIDDM, possibly within a subset of diabetes that can present phenotypically as either NIDDM or IDDM in different family members.

Genes Involved in Lipid Metabolism/Insulin Resistance

Because of the relationship between diabetes, insulin resistance and atherosclerosis in the syndrome X phenotype (see Chapter 12), a number of studies have examined genes involved in lipid metabolism as candidate genes in NIDDM as well.

Apolipoproteins—population studies. Lipid metabolism is often abnormal in diabetic patients, and therefore, the genes encoding for enzymes and protein products involved in lipid metabolism are candidate genes for NIDDM. An association with Lp(a), an LDL particle with an associated atherogenic apo(a) apolipoprotein, has been described by Dahlen and Berg. As early as 1976 they reported that individuals who were positive for the Lp(a) antigen had lower mean insulin levels than Lp(a)-negative individuals [440, 441].

An association of the apolipoprotein A1 gene (*apo*-A1) with NIDDM has been described in a Polish population of 100 diabetic patients and 100 controls [442]. Upon *Eco*RI digestion of genomic DNA, a 2.5 kb allele was found in 13 of the diabetic patients and in 2 of the controls, both of whom had a family history of diabetes. Thus, the *apo*A1 gene appears to be associated with NIDDM in this population. In a study of Chinese Americans, Xiang et al [374] reported evidence that genetic variations in the apolipoprotein A1/C3/A4 gene cluster and the *apo*-B gene contribute to the risk for NIDDM. Their studies suggest that the *apo*-A1/C3/A4 locus and the *apo*-B locus are associated with the development of NIDDM in obese subjects

and lean subjects, respectively, supporting the notion that NIDDM in lean and obese individuals may have distinct genetic etiologies. This study, similar to others, also found associations of the *apo*-A1/C3/A4 and *apo*-B loci with atherosclerosis, suggesting a common mechanism underlying both disease processes.

The association of diabetes and the three common apolipoprotein E alleles (E-2, E-3, E-4) has been investigated in several populations with conflicting results. No differences in the *apo*-E allele frequencies were found between diabetic and control subjects in two Japanese studies [71, 72]. In a study of Europid insulin-treated diabetic subjects (the majority of whom may have had IDDM) there was an 8-fold increase in the prevalence of E2/E2 individuals and a 3-fold decrease in the observed number of E2/E3-typed individuals over the frequency expected, assuming Hardy–Weinberg equilibrium [74]. In a diabetic Mexican-American population the *apo*-E allele frequencies were in Hardy–Weinberg equilibrium and they did not differ from a random sample from the same population [76]. In this study, differences among the *apo*-E alleles were found for LDL cholesterol and β-lipoprotein cholesterol values but not for hypertriglyceridemia, which was a finding common in the Japanese diabetics possessing the E2 allele [71, 72].

Lipoprotein lipase—population studies. The lipoprotein lipase (LPL) gene has also been investigated as a candidate gene contributing to the insulin resistance syndrome (syndrome X). LPL catalyzes the hydrolysis of the core triglycerides of chylomicrons and very low density lipoproteins. Two common RFLPs using the enzymes *Pvu*II and *Hind*III have been investigated in population association studies.

In a population of non-diabetic Hispanics, the presence of the *Hind*III restriction site was found to be associated with elevated fasting insulin and triglycerides, and decreased HDL levels [77]. Similar findings among non-diabetic subjects were seen in a Mediterranean population [78] and in non-Hispanic Whites [79]. Among diabetic subjects, the *Hind*III polymorphism was significantly associated with fasting insulin levels, while the *Pvu*II polymorphism showed no association with any trait [79]. Absence of the *Pvu*II restriction site has, however, been found to be associated with elevated fasting insulin levels in non-diabetic Hispanic men [80] and hypertriglyceridemia in Europids [81].

These population association studies suggest that the LPL locus, or genes nearby, may play a role in the development of insulin resistance—a metabolic derangement which may contribute to the development of NIDDM. Additional population and family studies may provide further insight into the importance of this locus in NIDDM susceptibility.

Fatty acid binding protein 2. This genetic locus was the first to be identified in a systematic search for linkage with a NIDDM-related phenotype. Using the sib-pair linkage analysis method in a population of Pima Indians, linkage of the trait of maximal insulin action was established with a region on chromosome 4q26 [82]. The intestinal fatty acid-binding protein gene (FABP2) and the annexin V gene were candidate genes in this region which could conceivably affect insulin action. Support for the role of the FABP2 locus was found in a family study of Mexican-Americans from San Antonio. Using the sib-pair method, evidence was found for linkage of BMI, fasting insulin, 2-h insulin, and fasting C-peptide with the FABP2 gene located at 4q28–q31 region [251]. In a population association study of a trinucleotide repeat near the FABP2 gene in Finnish, UK Europid, and Welsh individuals, there were no significant associations between allele frequencies and glucose intolerance in any of the populations [83]. However, the A3 allele was approximately twice as common in the NIDDM subjects as in the control subjects in the Finnish and UK populations, and log-linear analysis across all three populations indicated that this was of borderline significance. These results may indicate that the FABP2 locus is a determinant of insulin resistance in the Native American Indian and Mexican-American population (who probably derive their diabetogenic genes from the admixture of Native American genes), but that this locus does not appear to be of great importance in predominantly European Europid populations. Further investigations of this locus are warranted.

Glycogen Synthase

Glycogen synthase is a key enzyme in glucose metabolism, accounting for more than 90% of the non-oxidative glucose metabolism in skeletal muscle [84]. Impaired stimulation of non-oxidative glucose metabolism by insulin is characteristic of insulin resistance in patients with NIDDM and their first-degree relatives [85, 86]. In diabetic individuals and their relatives, the rate of insulin-stimulated glucose storage is decreased compared to normal control subjects, and there is a significant correlation with impaired muscle glycogen synthase activity, $p < 0.001$ [87]. Given these biochemical and genetic epidemiologic data, the glycogen synthase gene is an excellent candidate for predisposition to NIDDM.

Population studies. The glycogen synthase gene has been localized to chromosome 19, band q13.3 [88]. An *Xba*I RFLP has been identified and two alleles are described, A1 and A2 [89]. In a Finnish population the frequency of the A2 allele was significantly increased in diabetic subjects vs. controls lacking a family history

(30% vs. 8%). In addition, the diabetic subjects with the A2 allele were characterized by a stronger family history of NIDDM, a higher prevalence of hypertension, and a greater defect in insulin-stimulated glucose storage than diabetic subjects with the A1 allele [89]. In a French population the frequency of the A1 allele was significantly higher (96% vs. 88%) and the A2 allele significantly lower (4% vs. 12%) among the patients with diabetes than among the normal subjects, and the diabetic subjects with the A1 allele were more likely than the control group to have a personal and family history of both diabetes and hypertension, $p = 0.023$ [322].

The *Xba*I polymorphism was also studied in a Japanese population of non-obese NIDDM and control subjects, but the A2 allele was not found. A simple tandem repeat polymorphism (TG)n in the human glycogen synthase gene was recently identified [90] and was used as an alternative genetic marker in this Japanese study population [91]. Nine alleles were identified and the overall frequency distribution varied significantly between the diabetic and control subjects. The 2G allele was found more frequently in diabetic than in non-diabetic subjects (17.7% vs. 8.7%). The 2G allele was not associated with any particular subgroup of diabetic subjects, although there was a tendency towards a higher prevalence of positive family history of diabetes in the diabetic patients with the 2G allele.

Linkage and mutation analyses. Linkage analysis using another simple tandem repeat polymorphism located approximately 15 kb from the 3′ end of the glycogen synthase gene was performed in 346 members of 16 Utah Europid families [92], and linkage of this marker with NIDDM was rejected under multiple models, with LOD scores of -1.36 to -5.22. In these Utah pedigrees the *Xba*I-A2 allele was rare and was not shared by any two diabetic siblings, suggesting that the *Xba*I RFLP is not a useful marker in this population.

Genetic variants in the coding region and the promoter region of the glycogen synthase gene have also been investigated in 52 Europid-Danish NIDDM subjects and 25 age-matched healthy volunteers [406]. Using SSCP analysis and DNA sequencing, five nucleotide substitutions were discovered in the promoter region. The three most common variants could be excluded from having a major impact on glycogen synthase mRNA expression in muscle. Scanning of the coding sequence of the glycogen synthase gene revealed only one silent common polymorphism at codon 342. Thus none of the variants discovered in either region appear to make a major contribution to the predisposition to NIDDM in these Europid subjects. The significance of the population associations thus remains in question; the findings may be spurious, there may be mutations in genetic regions near the glycogen synthase gene not yet studied, or the glycogen synthase gene may be an important genetic contributor to NIDDM in some but not all populations.

β3-Adrenergic Receptor Gene

The $\beta3$-adrenergic receptor is expressed in visceral adipose tissue and it is thought to contribute to the regulation of the resting metabolic rate and lipolysis, making it a candidate gene for NIDDM and obesity. This locus has recently been investigated in the Pima Indians, the French and the Finns. In Pima Indians, SSCP and sequence analysis identified a mis-sense mutation [106] in which a C-to-T substitution results in the replacement of tryptophan by arginine at position 64 in the first intracellular loop of the receptor. The allelic frequency of this mutation in Pimas was 0.31, in Mexican-Americans 0.13, in African-Americans 0.12 and in Europid-Americans 0.08. In Pima subjects who were homozygous for this mutation, the age of NIDDM onset was significantly lower than in heterozygotes, and subjects with the mutation tended to have lower resting metabolic rates. In the Finnish population, diabetic subjects with the mutation also had an earlier age of NIDDM onset than those without the mutation [108]. Among non-diabetic subjects, those with the mutation had a significantly higher waist–hip ratio, a greater increase in serum insulin response after an oral glucose challenge, a higher diastolic blood pressure, and a lower rate of glucose disposal during a hyperinsulinemic–euglycemic clamp study than those non-diabetic subjects without the mutation. In a population of morbidly obese (BMI >40) French subjects, individuals with the arginine-to-tryptophan mutation had an increased capacity to gain weight within a 25-year time interval than those without the mutation [109]. Thus, these data support a role for the $\beta3$-adrenergic receptor in the etiology of insulin resistance and the associated diagnoses of NIDDM, hypertension and obesity.

Mitochondrial Mutations and Maternal Transmission

In early studies of NIDDM and MODY-like families, Dorner and colleagues [110, 111] reported evidence that diabetes occurred more frequently on the maternal than on the paternal side of families ascertained through a diabetic proband. In addition, significantly more mothers (18.2%) than fathers (9.1%) of the MODY individuals were themselves diabetic [111]. Among a large population of Europid NIDDM patients, Alcolado and Alcolado [402] found a similar significant excess of diabetic mothers vs. fathers of cases. Further support for this finding was described in a study of French-Europid NIDDM patients who had a significant excess of diabetic mothers and maternal relatives (aunts and uncles) compared to fathers and paternal relatives [408]. Pettitt and co-workers, studying the inheritance of diabetes in Pima Indian NIDDM families, also have evidence which supports the importance of maternal diabetes in determining the risk for diabetes in the offspring [115]. In these studies, 45% of the offspring of women diabetic prior to pregnancy were themselves diabetic by age 20–24 years, compared to 1.4% and 8.6% of the offspring of non-diabetic and 'prediabetic' women (women who became diabetic later), respectively. The paternal diabetic status appeared to contribute little additional risk to the offspring, after correcting for maternal diabetes and other risk factors [115]. Significant excess maternal transmission of diabetes and an insulin-resistant phenotype characterized by heart disease, stroke and hypertension, was also described in a Mexican-American population of NIDDM subjects [117], although these findings were not confirmed in a similar population [448]. Finally, Lin et al [118] have described a maternal excess of diabetes inheritance in a Taiwanese population, with an odds ratio for reporting maternal diabetes of 2.64 (95% CI 1.12–5.71) in diabetic patients as compared to non-diabetic subjects.

Mitochondrial mutations could explain this excess of maternal transmission, and indeed, mitochondrial inheritance of a genetic mutation leading to defects in glucose tolerance has been identified by several investigators. The human mitochondrial genome consists of a double-stranded, circular DNA molecule approximately 16 000 base pairs in length. It is maternally inherited and uses its own genetic code, coding for 13 subunits of the respiratory chain complexes, 22 transfer RNAs (tRNA) and two ribosomal RNAs. Several investigators have identified a mutation at nucleotide pair 3243 in diabetes with maternal transmission history and associated hearing loss, a conserved position in the mitochondrial gene for tRNA Leu(UUR). This mutation alters the dihydrouridine loop in this tRNA, leading to impairment of mitochondrial transcription termination. This may cause defects in mitochondrial translation and protein synthesis. This is also the mutation responsible for the more dramatic MELAS syndrome (mitochondrial myopathy, encephalopathy, lactic acidosis, and stroke-like episodes) [119]. Individuals with this mutation have been characterized as having insulin secretory defects along with an increased prevalence of sensorineural deafness, or maternal inherited diabetes and deafness (MIDD) [121, 124–127]. Additionally, some of these individuals with the nucleotide pair 3243 mutation have been characterized as islet cell antibody-positive NIDDM patients who go on to require exogenous insulin therapy, due to islet B-cell destruction and/or failure [128]. Ballinger et al [129] have also described a 10.4 kb deletion in the mitochondrial genome which was associated with maternal transmission of diabetes and deafness. These mitochondrial mutations are likely to account for only a small amount of NIDDM. Thus, for example, a screen of Pima Indians failed to detect any individuals with this specific mutation [130]. However, mitochondrial mutations may be candidates for individuals or families who have defects in insulin secretion, especially at an early age, such as some of the MODY pedigrees.

Several other hypotheses have been generated to explain this excess maternal transmission. These include: (a) a metabolic (teratogenic) effect of a diabetic or subclinical diabetic ('pre-diabetic') environment during pregnancy; (b) an imprinted gene that is only expressed when it is passed through a female meiosis; and (c) reporting bias. Reporting bias seems an unlikely explanation, as this phenomenon has also been observed in rats. Results from crosses between Goto-Kakizaki rats (which exhibit spontaneous NIDDM) and outbred non-diabetic Wistar rats have demonstrated an effect of maternal inheritance on diabetes in offspring of the first generation [131]. These hypotheses are not exclusive and one or more may be interacting to cause excess maternal transmission of disease.

Several reports have identified low birth-weight as a risk factor for NIDDM and insulin resistance, suggesting a mechanism which may support a maternal transmission [132, 134–136]. Decreased numbers of islet B cells and impaired B-cell function have been associated with low birth-weight. However, a lack of correlation between low birth-weight and the subsequent development of diabetes was noted, suggesting that additional genetic or environmental factors are necessary for the development of NIDDM [137]. Furthermore, there were no differences in the birth-weights of individuals with NIDDM, IGT or normoglycemic subjects when the offspring of hyperglycemic and normoglycemic mothers were considered separately [137]. Thus, these data do not provide conclusive evidence for a fuel-mediated teratogenic mechanism, since diabetic mothers were no more likely than non-diabetic mothers to have babies of low birth-weight.

Further research examining mitochondrial and sex-influenced autosomal loci and further studies to evaluate maternal environmental factors are warranted.

Genetic Counseling for NIDDM

For the most part, genetic counseling must depend on empiric recurrence risks (Table 9). For relatives of an individual with NIDDM, the empiric recurrence risk to first-degree relatives is of the order of 10–15% for

clinical diabetes and 20–30% for IGT. This increased risk appears to be only for NIDDM, not for IDDM, although (as discussed above) in some studies there is a somewhat increased risk for both forms of diabetes [438]. For MODY, an autosomal dominant disorder, the risk to siblings and offspring is 50%.

Table 9 Risks for NIDDM and IGT in relatives of individuals with NIDDM

	NIDDM	IGT
Population risk	1/20	1/20
Risk in relatives		
Siblings	1/10–1/7	1/5–1/3
Offspring	1/10–1/7	1/5–1/3
Monozygotic twin	3/4–∼ 1	∼ 1

Screening and Prevention of NIDDM
(see Chapter 89)

Screening of first-degree relatives of NIDDM diabetic subjects can be accomplished by periodic glucose tolerance testing. Those relatives with IGT should be advised to attain ideal body weight through diet and exercise, as this will improve glucose tolerance. This is strongly to be encouraged, with the goals being to delay or prevent progression to frank diabetes and minimize the cardiovascular risks associated with IGT. Screening and intervention for other risk factors for cardiovascular disease, e.g. hypertension and hyperlipidemias, is strongly encouraged.

Further refinement of genetic risk can only currently be done in MODY families and in those rare forms of NIDDM due to mutant insulins, insulin receptor variants, or mitochondrial mutations. In such families, individuals at risk can potentially be identified at any age at which DNA can be obtained, e.g. even in childhood or prenatally. The issues which must be considered before going to DNA studies are complex, however. Particularly with forms of diabetes which have a later (e.g. adult) onset, it is not clear what the benefit of childhood carrier detection will be, and there is the risk of stigmatization as well as the risk of adversely impacting insurability. Therefore the pros and cons of DNA analysis should be discussed carefully prior to any testing.

NIDDM and Pregnancy

Although attention is usually focused on the pregnant patient with IDDM (see above), women with NIDDM are also at increased risk for complications during pregnancy. In general, the more severe the hyperglycemia, the poorer the pregnancy outcome. Women with NIDDM have a significantly increased risk of delivering a child with fetal malformations [208, 252, 253], but the risk is less than that for women with

IDDM. Becerra et al [208] reported that the relative risk for major malformations for women with IDDM was 7.9 (95% CI 1.9–33.5) as compared to non-diabetic women, while the relative risk for women with NIDDM who required insulin treatment during pregnancy was 3.4 (95% CI 1.0–11.7). The excess risk in insulin-treated NIDDM women was due primarily to an increased risk of cardiovascular malformations.

In the USA, the trend toward delaying pregnancy into the 30s and 40s, coupled with the increasing proportion of the population which is of Hispanic ethnic background, suggests that NIDDM in pregnancy will be seen with increasing prevalence and may, without appropriate intervention, become an increasingly important cause of fetal malformations [209]. Although the risk of malformations appears to be somewhat less in pregnancies complicated by NIDDM as compared to IDDM, careful monitoring of the pregnant woman with NIDDM is of great importance. Women with NIDDM should be counseled about the risks associated with diabetes in pregnancy and encouraged to optimize diabetes control prior to conception and during pregnancy, even though studies assessing the efficacy of such optimization have for the most part been performed in women with IDDM.

The prenatal diagnostic tests discussed above for IDDM pregnancies should also be recommended for all pregnant women who have NIDDM.

OTHER FORMS OF DIABETES MELLITUS

The separation of idiopathic diabetes into IDDM and NIDDM by no means exhausts the potential heterogeneity within the diabetic phenotype. There could well be genetically distinct forms of diabetes whose phenotypic presentation could include either IDDM or NIDDM. The atypical form of diabetes among American Blacks reported by Winter et al [214] may be an example. There is ample precedent for this phenomenon in other common diseases: examples include combined gastric and duodenal ulcer, which appears to be a separate disorder from either solitary duodenal ulcer or solitary gastric ulcer [215], and familial combined hyperlipidemia, where a given individual in a family can present with either an elevated cholesterol, an elevated triglyceride, or both [247]. Evidence for 'overlap' phenotypes in diabetes includes suggestions of too high a frequency of either type in family members of the other type compared to the general population, and reports that NIDDM in parents of IDDM patients increased the risk to other siblings for IDDM [44, 248, 438]. Some of this may be due to the occurrence of a NIDDM-like phase in IDDM patients with a more protracted natural history, but it possibly reflects further heterogeneity. In addition, it has been reported that in some non-Europid (South African, Indian, and Black) populations, regardless of the type of diabetes in the index case, there was an increase in NIDDM in first-degree relatives [249]. In addition, low order of magnitude HLA associations have been reported with HLA antigen Bw61 in diabetes of Indian subcontinent origin [428], and with HLA antigen A2 in Pima Indian diabetes [431]. The genetic–etiologic relationship of these HLA associations with diabetes in these non-Europid populations would seem fundamentally different from that of HLA and IDDM in Europid populations. Since there is no evidence for the role of immunologic factors in these NIDDM types of diabetes, these HLA associations may have a polygenic background role more analogous to that of the mouse H2 locus and the effect of strain differences. Essentially, there are whole groups or classes of diabetes for which our knowledge of nosology, etiology and genetics is minimal. This includes not only most forms of diabetes in the developing world (discussed in Chapter 9), but also gestational diabetes (see Chapter 57).

FINAL CONSIDERATIONS AND SPECULATIONS

Evolutionary Aspects

Heterogeneity within both the insulin dependent and non-insulin dependent types appears extensive. An important question arises from the population genetic viewpoint. These diabetic disorders, whose susceptibility appears to be primarily genetically determined, are deleterious, and thus reproductive fitness should be impaired. As regards NIDDM, a possible explanation is the concept of a 'thrifty' genotype, as first proposed by Neel [1]. He proposed that the diabetic genotype allowed more efficient utilization of foodstuffs by the body in periods of famine, to which primitive man was often exposed. Such a 'thrifty' gene would therefore have a selective survival advantage and would tend to increase in frequency. However, in the modern Western world, with its continuous abundance of calories, such a gene would lead to diabetes and obesity. Neel's hypothesis has received support from observations in both man and animals. The extremely high frequency of diabetes and obesity in populations such as the Pima Indians [2] and Pacific islanders [4], and its apparent increase with modernization and urbanization, are entirely consistent with the thrifty genotype hypothesis. Direct support comes from studies which have shown that heterozygotes for rodent diabetes–obesity genes exhibit a much better ability to survive fasting than normal rodents [3].

What might be the selective advantage of the genes that predispose to IDDM? Since IDDM is a disorder in which autoimmunity and immune response genes seem implicated, a possible role in the resistance to infectious agents has been proposed. However, the problem of the selective advantage of IDDM is much greater than for NIDDM. Before the onset of insulin therapy, IDDM was usually a lethal disorder, at least in genetic terms (i.e. failure to reproduce). This is both because of its severity and because its onset is earlier. Since the susceptibility seems to be provided even by single HLA-linked susceptibility genes, negative selection is much greater than that for recessive genetic disorders such as sickle cell anemia, where negative selection operates only on homozygotes. Thus, one would suppose that the positive selective advantage would of necessity be dramatic, and that it should have continued into modern human history. Otherwise the incidence of the disorder would have been decreasing dramatically prior to the advent of insulin therapy. Yet no such positive selective advantage has been discerned, at least postnatally.

Evidence has now accumulated that suggests a potential selective advantage mechanism for IDDM, and at the same time provides a partial explanation of the recent recognition that the risk for IDDM appears to be higher for offspring of males with IDDM than for offspring of females with IDDM (at least in the first 20 years of life) [13, 20, 234]. What has been observed is preferential transmission of diabetogenic HLA haplotypes, not only to affected offspring, but to unaffected offspring as well [49, 50]. In addition, while this occurs for both high-risk (DR3- and DR4-associated) diabetic alleles/haplotypes in fathers, it has been reported to occur for only the DR3-associated haplotypes in mothers, providing an explanation for the increased paternal risk. Furthermore, the available evidence suggests that this occurs via *in utero* selection [49, 51]. These data thus provide an explanation for the maintenance of the high population frequency for this previously genetically lethal disease. In addition, it has been suggested that this prenatal selection could occur via immunologically mediated events, raising the theoretical possibility that an additional consequence of these events, in fetuses that survive, might be immune changes that presage the eventual development of IDDM [64].

REFERENCES

1. Neel JV. Diabetes mellitus: a 'thrifty' genotype rendered detrimental by 'progress?' Am J Hum Genet 1962; 14: 353–62.
2. Knowler WC, Pettitt DJ, Savage PJ, Bennett PH. Diabetes incidence in Pima Indians: contributions of obesity and parental diabetes. Am J Epidemiol 1981; 113: 144–56.
3. Coleman DL. Obesity genes: beneficial effects in heterozygous mice. Science 1979; 203: 663–5.
4. Zimmet P. Epidemiology of diabetes and its macrovascular manifestations in Pacific population—the medical effects of social progress. Diabetes Care 1979; 2: 144–53.
5. Creutzfeldt W, Kobberling J, Neel JV (eds). The genetics of diabetes mellitus. Berlin: Springer-Verlag, 1976.
6. Fajans SS, Cloutier MC, Crowther RL. Clinical and etiologic heterogeneity of idiopathic diabetes mellitus. Diabetes 1978; 27: 1112–25.
7. Friedman JM, Fialkow PJ. The genetics of diabetes mellitus. In Steinberg AG, Bearn Ag, Motulsky AG, Childs B (eds) Progress in medical genetics, vol IV. Philadelphia: WB Saunders, 1980; 199–232.
8. Kobberling J, Tattersall R. The genetics of diabetes mellitus. London: Academic Press, 1982.
9. Rotter JI, Rimoin DL, Samloff IM. Genetic heterogeneity in diabetes mellitus and peptic ulcer. In Morton NE, Chung CS (eds) Genetic epidemiology. New York: Academic Press, 1978; 381–414.
10. Rotter JI, Rimoin DL. Etiology: genetics. In Brownlee M (ed.) Handbook of diabetes mellitus, vol 1. New York: Garland STPM Press, 1981; 13–93.
11. Rotter JI, Rimoin DL. The genetics of the glucose intolerance disorders. Am J Med 1981; 70: 116–26.
12. Rotter JI, Vadheim CM, Rimoin DL. Diabetes mellitus. In King RA, Rotter JI, Motulsky AG (eds) The genetic basis of common disease. New York: Oxford University Press, 1992; 413–81.
13. Kobberling J, Bruggeboes B. Prevalence of diabetes among children of insulin-dependent diabetic mothers. Diabetologia 1980; 18: 459–62.
14. Simpson NE. A review of family data. In Creutzfeldt W, Kobberling J, Neel JV (eds) The genetics of diabetes mellitus. Berlin: Springer-Verlag, 1976; 12–20.
15. Rimoin DL, Schimke RN. Endocrine pancreas. In Genetic disorders of the endocrine glands. St Louis: CV Mosby, 1971; 150–216.
16. Pincus G, White P. On the inheritance of diabetes mellitus. I. An analysis of 675 family histories. Am J Med Sci 1933; 186: 1–14.
17. Cammidge PJ. Diabetes mellitus and heredity. Br Med J 1928; ii: 738–41.
18. Cammidge PJ. Heredity as a factor in the etiology of diabetes mellitus. Lancet 1934; i: 393–5.
19. Cudworth AG. Type 1 diabetes mellitus. Diabetologia 1978; 14: 281–91.
20. Degnbol B, Green A. Diabetes mellitus among first- and second-degree relatives of early onset diabetics. Ann Hum Genet 1978; 42: 25–34.
21. Harris H. The incidence of parental consanguinity in diabetes mellitus. Ann Eugenics 1949; 14: 293–300.
22. Harris H. The familial distribution of diabetes mellitus: a study of the relatives of 1241 diabetic propositi. Ann Eugenics 1950; 15: 95–110.
23. Irvine WJ, Toft AD, Holton DE, Prescott RJ, Clarke BF, Duncan LJP. Familial studies of type I and type II idiopathic diabetes mellitus. Lancet 1977; ii: 325–8.
24. Kobberling J. Untersuchungen zur Genetik des Diabetes Mellitus. Eine geeignete Methode zur Durchfuhrung von Alterskorrekturen. Diabetologia 1969; 5: 392–6.
25. Lestradet H, Battistelli J, Ledoux M. L'hérédité dans le diabète infantile. Le diabète 1972; 2: 17–21.

26. MacDonald MJ. Equal incidence of adult-onset diabetes among ancestors of juvenile diabetics and non-diabetics. Diabetologia 1974; 10: 767–73.

27. Simpson NE. The genetics of diabetes: a study of 233 families of juvenile diabetics. Ann Hum Genet 1962; 26: 1–12.

28. Simpson NE. Diabetes in the families of diabetics. Can Med Assoc J 1968; 98: 427–32.

29. Working Party, College of General Practitioners. Family history of diabetes. Br Med J 1965; i: 960–62.

30. Pyke DA. The genetic connections. Diabetologia 1979; 17: 333–43.

31. Bottazzo GF, Florin-Christensen A, Doniach D. Islet-cell antibodies in diabetes mellitus with autoimmune polyendocrine deficiencies. Lancet 1974; ii: 1279–82.

32. Cahill GF Jr, McDevitt HO. Insulin-dependent diabetes mellitus: the initial lesion. New Engl J Med 1981; 304: 1454–64.

33. MacCuish AC, Barnes EEW, Irvine WJ, Duncan LJP. Antibodies to pancreatic islet cells in insulin-dependent diabetics with coexistent autoimmune disease. Lancet 1974; ii: 1529–31.

34. Groop L, Miettinen A, Groop PH, Meri S, Koskimies S, Bottazzo GF. Organ-specific autoimmunity and HLA-DR antigens as markers for beta-cell destruction in patients with type II diabetes. Diabetes 1988; 37: 99–103.

35. Groop LC, Bottazzo GF, Doniach D. Islet cell antibodies identify latent type I diabetes in patients aged 35–75 years at diagnosis. Diabetes 1986; 35: 237–41.

36. Irvine WJ, Gray RS, McCallum CJ, Duncan LJP. Clinical and pathogenic significance of pancreatic islet cell antibodies in diabetics treated with oral hypoglycemic agents. Lancet 1977; i: 1025–7.

37. Kilvert A, Fitzgerald MG, Wright AD, Nattrass M. Clinical characteristics and etiological classification of insulin-dependent diabetes in the elderly. Q J Med 1986; 60: 865–72.

38. Wilson RM, van Der Minne P, Deverill I, Heller SR, Gelsthorpe K, Reeves WG, Tattersall R. Insulin dependence: probems with the classification of 100 consecutive patients. Diabet Med 1985; 2: 167–72.

39. Nerup J, Cathelineau C, Seignalet J, Thomsen M. HLA and endocrine diseases. In Dausset J and Svejgaard A (eds) HLA and disease. Copenhagen: Munksgaard, 1977; 149–61.

40. Maclaren N, Riley W, Skordis N, Spillar R, Silverstein J, Klein R, Vadheim C, Rotter J. Inherited susceptibility to insulin-dependent diabetes is associated with HLA-DR1 (and DR3 and DR4) while DR5 (and DR2) are protective. Autoimmunity 1988; 1: 197–205.

41. Platz P, Jakobsen BD, Morling N, Ryder LP, Svejgaard A, Thomsen M et al. HLA-D and DR antigens in genetic analysis of insulin-dependent diabetes mellitus. Diabetologia 1981; 21: 108–15.

42. Rotter JI, Anderson CE, Rubin R, Congleton JE, Terasaki PI, Rimoin DL. HLA genotype study of insulin-dependent diabetes, the excess of DR3/DR4 heterozygotes allows rejection of the recessive hypothesis. Diabetes 1983; 32: 169–74.

43. Wolf E, Spencer KM, Cudworth AG. The genetic susceptibility to type 1 (insulin-dependent) diabetes: analysis of the HLA-DR association. Diabetologia 1983; 24: 224–30.

44. Cahill GF Jr. Current concepts of diabetic complications with emphasis on hereditary factors: a brief review. In Sing CF, Skolnick MH (eds) Genetic analysis of common diseases: applications to predictive factors in coronary heart disease. New York: Alan R. Liss, 1979; 113–29.

45. Gottlieb MS. Diabetes in offspring and siblings of juvenile and maturity-onset type diabetes. J Chronic Dis 1980; 33: 331–9.

46. Irvine WJ, Sawen JSA, Prescott RJ, Duncan LJP. The value of islet cell antibody in predicting secondary failure of oral hypoglycemic agent therapy in diabetes mellitus. J Clin Lab Immunol 1979; 2: 23–6.

47. Tattersall RB. Mild familial diabetes with dominant inheritance. Q J Med 1975; 43: 339–57.

48. Tattersall RB, Fajans SS. A difference between the inheritance of classical juvenile onset and maturity onset type diabetes of young people. Diabetes 1975; 24: 44–5.

49. Vadheim CM, Rotter JI, Maclaren NK, Riley WJ, Anderson CE. Preferential transmission of diabetic alleles within the HLA gene complex. New Engl J Med 1986; 315: 1314–18.

50. Thivolent CH, Beaufrere B, Betuel H, Gebuhrer, Chatelain P, Durand A et al. Islet cell and insulin autoantibodies in subjects at high risk for development of type 1 (insulin-dependent) diabetes mellitus: the Lyon family study. Diabetologia 1988; 31: 741–6.

51. Vadheim CM, Rotter JI, Riley WJ, Akkina JE, Anderson CE. Prenatal selection for diabetes HLA genes and the onset of IDDM. Diabetes 1985; 34: 21A.

52. Barnett AH, Eff C, Leslie RDG, Pyke DA. Diabetes in identical twins: a study of 200 pairs. Diabetologia 1981; 20: 87–93.

53. Pyke DA. Twin studies in diabetes. In Nance WE, Allen G, Parisi P (eds) Twin research, Part C, Clinical studies. New York: Alan R. Liss, 1978; 1–12.

54. Gottlieb MS, Root HF. Diabetes mellitus in twins. Diabetes 1968; 17: 693–704.

55. Olmos P, Hern RA, Heaton DA, Millward BA, Risley D, Pyke DA, Leslie RDG. The significance of the concordance rate for type 1 (insulin-dependent) diabetes in identical twins. Diabetologia 1988; 31: 747–50.

56. Gamble DR. An epidemiological study of childhood diabetes affecting two or more siblings. Diabetologia 1980; 19: 341–4.

57. Craighead JE. Viral diabetes mellitus in man and experimental animals. Am J Med 1981; 70: 127–33.

58. Rayfield EJ, Seto Y. Etiology: viruses. In Brownlee M (ed.) Handbook of diabetes mellitus, vol. 1. New York: Garland STPM Press, 1981; 95–120.

59. Rotter JI, Rimoin DL. Diabetes mellitus: the search for genetic markers. Diabetes Care 1979; 2: 215–26.

60. Rotter JI, Rimoin DL. The genetics of insulin-dependent diabetes. In Martin JM, Ehrlich RM, Holland FJ (eds) Etiology and pathogenesis of insulin-dependent diabetes mellitus. New York: Raven Press, 1981; 37–59.

61. McMichael A, McDevitt H. The association between the HLA system and disease. In Steinberg AG, Bearn AG, Motulsky AG, Child B (eds) Progress in medical genetics, vol 11. Philadelphia: WB Saunders, 1977; 39–100.

62. Svejgaard A, Platz P, Ryder LP, Staub-Nielsen L, Thomsen M. HLA and disease association —a survey. Transplant Rev 1975; 22: 3–34.

63. Hastbäcka J, de la Chapelle A, Mahtani MM, Clines G, Reeve-Daly MP, Daly M et al. The diastrophic dysplasia gene encodes a novel sulfate transporter: positional cloning by fine-structure linkage disequilibrium mapping. Cell 1994; 78: 1073-87.

64. Vadheim CM, Rotter JI, Riley WJ, Maclaren NK, Petersen GM, Cantor RM. An interaction of genetic susceptibility and birth order in type I diabetes. Clin Res 1987; 35: 186A.

65. Darlow JM, Smith C. A statistical and genetical study of diabetes III. Empiric risks to relatives. Ann Hum Genet 1973; 37: 157-74.

66. Nerup J, Platz P, Ortved-Anderson O, Christy M, Egeberg J, Lyngsoe JE et al. HLA, autoimmunity, and insulin dependent diabetes. In Creutzfeldt W, Kobberling J, Neel JV (eds) The genetics of diabetes mellitus. Berlin: Springer-Verlag, 1976; 106-14.

67. West R, Belmonte MM, Colle E, Crepeau P, Wilkins P, Poirier R. Epidemiologic survey of juvenile-onset diabetes in Montreal. Diabetes 1979; 28: 690-3.

68. Rotter JI, Rimoin DL. Heterogeneity in diabetes mellitus—update 1978: evidence for further genetic heterogeneity within juvenile onset insulin-dependent diabetes mellitus. Diabetes 1978; 27: 599-608.

69. Tillil H, Kobberling J. Age-corrected empirical genetic risk estimates for first-degree relatives of IDDM patients. Diabetes 1987; 36: 93-9.

70. Maclaren NK. How, when and why to predict IDDM. Diabetes 1988; 37: 1591-4.

71. Eto M, Watanabe K, Iwashima Y, Morikawa A, Oshima E, Sekiguchi M, Ishii K. Apolipoprotein E polymorphism and hyperlipemia in type II diabetics. Diabetes 1986; 35: 1374-82.

72. Imari Y, Koga S, Ibayashi H. Phenotype of apolipoprotein E and abnormalities in lipid metabolism in patients with non-insulin dependent diabetes mellitus. Metabolism 1988; 37: 1134-8.

73. Thomson G, Robinson WP, Kuhner MK, Joe S, MacDonald JS, Gottschall JL et al. Genetic heterogeneity, modes of inheritance and risk estimates for a joint study of Caucasians with insulin dependent diabetes mellitus. Am J Hum Genet 1988; 43: 799-816.

74. Winocour PH, Tetlow L, Durrington PN, Ishola M, Hillier V, Anderson VD. Apolipoprotein E polymorphism in insulin treated diabetes mellitus. Atherosclerosis 1989; 75: 167-73.

75. Anderson CE, Hodge SE, Rubin R, Rotter JL, Terasaki PI, Irvine WJ, Rimoin DL. A search for heterogeneity in insulin-dependent diabetes mellitus (IDDM): HLA and autoimmune studies in simplex, multiplex and multigenerational families. Metabolism 1983; 32: 471-7.

76. Shriver MD, Boerwinkle E, Hewett-Emmett D, Hanis CL. Frequency and effects of apolipoprotein E polymorphism in Mexican-American NIDDM subjects. Diabetes 1991; 40: 334-7.

77. Ahn YI, Ferrell RE, Hamman RF, Kamboh MI. Association of lipoprotein lipase gene variation with the physiological components of the insulin-resistance syndrome in the population of the San Luis Valley, Colorado. Diabetes Care 1993; 16: 1502-6.

78. Mitchell RJ, Earl L, Bray P, Fripp YJ, Williams J. DNA polymorphisms at the lipoprotein lipase gene and their association with quantitative variation in plasma high-density lipoproteins and triacylglycerides. Human Biology 1994; 66: 383-97.

79. Ahn YI, Kamboh MI, Hamman RF, Cole SA, Ferrell RE. Two DNA polymorphisms in the lipoprotein lipase gene and their associations with factors related to cardiovascular disease. J Lipid Res 1993; 34: 421-8.

80. Cole SA, Aston CE, Hamman RF, Ferrell RE. Association of a PvuII RFLP at the lipoprotein lipase locus with fasting insulin levels in Hispanic men. Genet Epidemiol 1993; 10: 177-88.

81. Chamberlain JC, Thorn JA, Oka K, Galton DJ, Stocks J. DNA polymorphisms at the lipoprotein lipase gene: associations in normal and hypertriglyceridaemic subjects. Atherosclerosis 1989; 79: 85-91.

82. Prochazka M, Lillioja S, Tait JF, Knowler WC, Mott DM, Spraul M et al. Linkage of chromosomal markers on 4q with a putative gene determining maximal insulin action in Pima Indians. Diabetes 1993; 42: 514-9.

83. Humphreys P, McCarthy M, Tuomilehto J, Tuomilehto-Wolf E, Stratton I, Morgan R et al. Chromosome 4q locus associated with insulin resistance in Pima Indians. Studies in three European NIDDM populations. Diabetes 1994; 43: 800-4.

84. Shulman GI, Rothman DL, Jue T, Stein P, DeFronzo RA, Shulman RG. Quantitation of muscle glycogen synthesis in normal subjects and subjects with non-insulin-dependent diabetes by ^{13}C nuclear magnetic resonance spectroscopy. New Engl J Med 1990; 322: 223-8.

85. Eriksson J, Franssila-Kallunki A, Ekstrand A, Saloranta C, Widen E, Schalin C, Groop L. Early metabolic defects in persons at increased risk for non-insulin-dependent diabetes mellitus. New Engl J Med 1989; 321: 337-43.

86. Gulli G, Ferrannini E, Stern M, Haffner S, DeFronzo RA. The metabolic profile of NIDDM is fully established in glucose-tolerant offspring of two Mexican-American NIDDM parents. Diabetes 1992; 41: 1575-86.

87. Schalin-Jäntti C, Härkonen M, Groop LC. Impaired activation of glycogen synthase in people at increased risk for developing NIDDM. Diabetes 1992; 41: 598-604.

88. Lehto M, Stoffel M, Groop L, Espinosa R 3d, Le Beau MM, Bell GI. Assignment of the gene encoding glycogen synthase (GYS) to human chromosome 19, band q13.3. Genomics 1993; 15: 460-1.

89. Groop LC, Kankuri M, Schalin-Jäntti C, Ekstrand A, Nikula-Ijäs P, Widén E et al. Association between polymorphism of the glycogen synthase gene and non-insulin-dependent diabetes mellitus. New Engl J Med 1993; 328: 10-14.

90. Vionnet N, Bell GI. Identification of a simple tandem repeat DNA polymorphism in the human glycogen synthase gene and linkage to five markers on chromosome 19q. Diabetes 1993; 42: 930-2.

91. Kuroyama H, Sanke T, Ohagi S, Furuta M, Furuta H, Nanjo K. Simple tandem repeat DNA polymorphism in the human glycogen synthase gene is associated with NIDDM in Japanese subjects. Diabetologia 1994; 37: 536-9.

92. Elbein SC, Hoffman M, Ridinger D, Otterud B, Leppert M. Description of a second microsatellite marker and linkage analysis of the muscle glycogen synthase locus in familial NIDDM. Diabetes, 1994; 43: 1061-5.

93. MacDonald MJ, Gottschall J, Hunter JB, Winter KL. HLA-DR4 in insulin-dependent diabetic parents and their diabetic offspring: a clue to dominant inheritance. Proc Natl Acad Sci USA 1986; 83: 7049–53.

94. Louis EJ, Thomson G. Three-allele synergistic mixed model for insulin-dependent diabetes mellitus. Diabetes 1986; 35: 958–63.

95. Thomson G, Robinson WP, Kuhner MK, Joe S, Klitz W. HLA and insulin gene associations with IDDM. Genet Epidemiol 1989; 6: 155–60.

96. Knip M, Ilonen J, Mustonen A, Akerblom HK. Evidence of an accelerated B-cell destruction in HLA-Dw3.Dw4 heterozygous children with type 1 (insulin-dependent) diabetes. Diabetologia 1986; 29: 347–51.

97. Ludvigsson J, Lindblom B. Human lymphocyte antigen DR types in relation to early clinical manifestations in diabetic children. Pediatr Res 1984; 18: 1239–41.

98. Ludvigsson J, Samuelsson U, Beauforts C. HLA-DR3 is associated with a more slowly progressive form of type 1 (insulin-dependent) diabetes. Diabetologia 1986; 29: 207–10.

99. Rotter JI. The modes of inheritance of insulin-dependent diabetes. Am J Hum Genet 1981; 33: 835–51.

100. Schernthaner G. The relation between clinical, immunological and genetic factors in insulin-dependent diabetes mellitus. In Kobberling J, Tattersall RB (eds) The genetics of diabetes mellitus. London: Academic Press, 1982; 99–114.

101. Sklenar I, Nerit M, Berger W. Association of specific immune responses to pork and beef insulin with certain HLA-DR antigens in type I diabetes. Br Med J 1982; 285: 1451–3.

102. Karjalainen J, Knip M, Mustonen A, Ilonen J, Akerblom HK. Relation between insulin antibody and complement-fixing islet cell antibody at clinical diagnosis of IDDM. Diabetes 1986; 35: 620–2.

103. Srikanta S, Ricker AT, McCulloch DR, Soeldner JS, Eisenbarth GS, Palmer JP. Autoimmunity to insulin, beta cell dysfunction and development of insulin-dependent diabetes mellitus. Diabetes 1986; 35: 139–42.

104. Barbosa J, Rich SS, Dunsworth T, Swanson J. Linkage disequilibrium between insulin-dependent diabetes and the Kidd blood group Jkb allele. J Clin Endocrinol Metab 1982; 55: 193–5.

105. Bell GI, Horita S, Karam JH. A polymorphic locus near the human insulin gene is associated with insulin-dependent diabetes mellitus. Diabetes 1984; 33: 176–83.

106. Walston J, Silver K, Bogardus C, Knowler WC, Celi FS, Austin S et al. Time of onset of non-insulin-dependent diabetes mellitus and genetic variation in the β(3)-adrenergic receptor gene. New Engl J Med 1995; 333: 343–7.

107. Field LL, Anderson CE, Neiswanger K, Hodge SE, Spence MA, Rotter JI. Interaction of HLA and immunoglobulin antigens in type 1 (insulin-dependent) diabetes. Diabetologia 1984; 27: 504–8.

108. Widen E, Lehto M, Kanninen T, Walston J, Shuldiner AR, Groop LC. Association of a polymorphism in the β(3)-adrenergic-receptor gene with features of the insulin resistance syndrome in Finns. New Engl J Med 1995; 333: 348–51.

109. Clement K, Vaisse C, Manning BSJ, Basdevant A, Guy-Grand B, Ruiz J et al. Genetic variation in the β(3)-adrenergic receptor and an increased capacity to gain weight in patients with morbid obesity. New Engl J Med 1995; 333: 352–4.

110. Dorner GA, Mohnike E, Steindel. On possible genetic and epigenetic modes of diabetes transmission. Endokrinologie 1975; 66: 225–7.

111. Dorner GA, Mohnike A. Further evidence for a predominantly maternal transmission of maturity-onset type diabetes. Endokrinologie 1976; 68: 121–4.

112. Hoover ML, Capra JD. HLA and T-cell receptor genes in insulin-dependent diabetes mellitus. Diabetes Metab Rev 1987; 3: 835–56.

113. Ito M, Tanimoto M, Kamura H, Yoneda M, Morishima Y, Takatsuki K, Itatsu T, Saito H. Association of HLA-DR phenotypes and T-lymphocyte-receptor beta-chain-region RFLP with IDDM in Japanese. Diabetes 1988; 37: 1633–6.

114. Millward BA, Welsh KI, Leslie RDG, Pyke DA, Demaine AG. T cell receptor beta chain polymorphisms are associated with insulin-dependent diabetes. Clin Exp Immunol 1987; 70: 152–7.

115. Pettitt DJ. The long-range impact of diabetes during pregnancy: the Pima Indian experience. IDF Bulletin 1986; 31: 70–1.

116. Rich SS, Weitkamp LR, Guttormsen S, Barbosa J. Gm, Km, and HLA in insulin-dependent type 1 diabetes mellitus: a log-linear analysis of association. Diabetes 1986; 35: 927–32.

117. Scheuner MT, Wang SJ, Raffel LJ, Vadheim CM, Ipp E, Rotter JI. Maternal transmission of the insulin resistance syndrome (IRS) in familial Hispanic non-insulin dependent diabetes (NIDDM). Am J Hum Genet 1993; 53: A502.

118. Lin RS, Lee WC, Lee Y-T, Chou P, Fu C-C. Maternal role in type 2 diabetes mellitus: indirect evidence for a mitochondrial inheritance. Int J Epidemiol 1994; 23: 886–90.

119. Goto Y-I, Nonaka I, Horai S. A mutation in the tRNA$^{\text{Leu(UUR)}}$ gene associated with the MELAS subgroup of mitochondrial encephalomyopathies. Nature 1990; 348: 651–3.

120. Hibberd ML, Millward BA, Wong FS, Demaine AG. T-cell receptor constant beta chain polymorphisms and susceptibility to type 1 diabetes. Diabet Med 1992; 9: 929–33.

121. Reardon W, Ross RJM, Sweeney MG, Luxon LM, Pembrey ME, Harding AE, Trembath RC. Diabetes mellitus associated with a pathogenic point mutation in mitochondrial DNA. Lancet 1992; 340: 1376–9.

122. Raffel LJ, Vadheim CM, Klein R, Moss S, Riley WJ, Maclaren NK, Rotter JI. HLA-DR and the 5′ insulin gene polymorphism in insulin dependent diabetes. Metabolism 1991; 40: 1244–8.

123. Julier C, Hyer RN, Davies J, Merlin F, Soularue P, Briant L et al. The insulin-IGF2 region on chromosome 11p encodes a gene implicated in HLA-DR4-dependent diabetes susceptibility. Nature 1991; 354: 155–9.

124. Kadowaki T, Kadowaki H, Mori Y, Tobe K, Sakuta R, Suzuki Y et al. A subtype of diabetes mellitus associated with a mutation of mitochondrial DNA. New Engl J Med 1994; 330: 962–8.

125. van den Ouweland JMW, Lemkes HHPJ, Ruitenbeek W, Sandkuijl LA, de Vijlder MF, Struyvenberg PAA et al. Mutation in mitochondrial tRNA$^{\text{Leu(UUR)}}$ gene in a large pedigree with maternally transmitted

type II diabetes mellitus and deafness. Nature Genetics 1992; 1: 368–71.

126. van den Ouweland JMW, Lemkes HHPJ, Trembath RC, Ross R, Velho G, Cohen D et al. Maternally inherited diabetes and deafness is a distinct subtype of diabetes and associates with a single point mutation in the mitochondrial tRNA$^{Leu(UUR)}$ gene. Diabetes 1994; 43: 746–51.

127. Katagiri H, Yamanouchi T, Oka Y. Mitochondrial diabetes: clinical characterization of patients with mitochondrial tRNA$^{Leu(UUR)}$ gene mutation. Diabetes 1993; 42: 109A.

128. Oka Y, Katagiri H, Yazaki Y, Murase T, Kobayashi T. Mitochondrial gene mutation in islet-cell-antibody-positive patients who were initially non-insulin-dependent diabetics. Lancet 1993; 342: 527–8.

129. Ballinger SW, Shoffner JM, Hedaya EV, Trounce I, Polak MA, Koontz DA, Wallace DC. Maternally transmitted diabetes and deafness associated with a 10.4 kb mitochondrial DNA deletion. Nature Genet 1992; 1: 11–15.

130. Sepehrnia B, Prezant TR, Rotter JI, Pettitt DJ, Knowler WC, Fischel-Ghodsian N. Screening for MtDNA diabetes mutations in Pima Indians with NIDDM. Am J Med Genet 1995; 56: 198–202.

131. Gauguier D, Nelson I, Bernard C, Parent V, Marsac C, Cohen D, Froguel P. Higher maternal than paternal inheritance of diabetes in GK rats. Diabetes 1994; 43: 220–4.

132. Phipps K, Barker DJP, Hales CN, Fall CHD, Osmond C, Clark PMS. Fetal growth and impaired glucose tolerance in men and women. Diabetologia 1993; 36: 225–8.

133. Prochazka M, Leiter EH, Serreze DV, Coleman DL. Three recessive loci required for insulin-dependent diabetes in non-obese diabetic mice. Science 1987; 237: 286–9.

134. Robinson S, Walton RJ, Clark PM, Barker DJP, Hales CN, Osmond C. The relation of fetal growth to plasma glucose in young men. Diabetologia 1992; 35: 444–6.

135. Barker DJP, Hales CN, Fall CHD, Osmond C, Phipps K, Clark PMS. Type 2 (non-insulin-dependent) diabetes mellitus, hypertension and hyperlipidaemia (syndrome X): relation to reduced fetal growth. Diabetologia 1993; 36: 62–7.

136. Valdez R, Athens MA, Thompson GH, Bradshaw BS, Stern MP. Birthweight and adult health outcomes in a biethnic population in the USA. Diabetologia 1994; 37: 624–31.

137. Cook JTE, Levy JC, Page RCL, Shaw JAG, Hattersley AT, Turner RC. Association of low birth weight with β cell function in the adult first degree relatives of non-insulin dependent diabetic subjects. Br Med J 1993; 306: 302–6.

138. Ghosh S, Palmer SM, Rodrigues NR, Cordell JH, Hearne CM, Cornall RJ et al. Polygenic control of autoimmune diabetes in non-obese diabetic mice. Nature Genet 1993; 4: 404–9.

139. Miyazaki J, Ishii M, Tashiro F. [Current studies on the identification of susceptibility genes for IDDM in NOD mice]. Nippon Rinsho [Japanese Journal of Clinical Medicine] 1994; 52: 2772–7.

140. Mouse Genome Database (MGD), Mouse Genome Informatics Project, The Jackson Laboratory, Bar Harbor, Maine. World Wide Web (URL: http//www.informatics.jax.org). July, 1995.

141. Cornall RJ, Prins JB, Todd JA, Pressey A, DeLarato NH, Wicker LS, Peterson LB. Type 1 diabetes in mice is linked to the interleukin-1 receptor and *Lsh/Ity/Bcg* genes on chromosome 1. Nature 1991; 353: 262–5.

142. Garchon HJ, Bedossa P, Eloy L, Bach JF. Identification and mapping to chromosome 1 of a susceptibility locus for periinsulitis in non-obese diabetic mice. Nature 1991; 353: 260–2.

143. Todd JA, Aitman TJ, Cornall RJ, Ghosh S, Hall JRS, Hearne CM et al. Genetic analysis of autoimmune type 1 diabetes mellitus in mice. Nature 1991; 351: 542–7.

144. International Committee for Standardized Genetic Nomenclature, The Seventh International Mouse Genome Conference, Hamamatsu, Japan, November, 1993.

145. Rodrigues NR, Cornall RJ, Chandler P, Simpson E, Wicker LS, Peterson LB, Todd JA. Mapping of an insulin-dependent diabetes locus, Idd9, in NOD mice to chromosome 4. Mammalian Genome 1994; 5: 167–70.

146. Serreze DV, Prochazka M, Reifsnyder PC, Bridgett MM, Leiter EH. Use of recombinant congenic and congenic strains of NOD mice to identify a new insulin-dependent diabetes resistance gene. J Exp Med 1994; 180: 1553–8.

147. Risch N, Ghosh S, Todd JA. Statistical evaluation of multiple-locus linkage data in experimental species and its relevance to human studies: application to non-obese diabetic (NOD) mouse and human insulin-dependent diabetes mellitus (IDDM). Am J Hum Genet 1993; 53: 702–14.

148. Bain SC, Prins JB, Hearne CM, Rodrigues NR, Rowe BR, Pritchard LE et al. Insulin gene region-encoded susceptibility to type 1 diabetes is not restricted to HLA-DR4 positive individuals. Nature Genet 1992; 2: 212–5.

149. Field LL, Stephure DK, McArthur RG. Interaction between T cell receptor beta chain and immunoglobulin heavy chain region genes in susceptibility to insulin-dependent diabetes mellitus. Am J Hum Genet 1991; 49: 627–34.

150. Propert DN, Tait BD, Harrison LC. Interaction of immunoglobulin allotypes (Gm and Km), HLA, and sex in insulin-dependent (type 1) diabetes. Disease Markers 1991; 9: 43–5.

151. Atkinson MA, Maclaren NK, Riley WJ, Winter WE, Fisk DD, Spillar RP. Are insulin autoantibodies markers for insulin-dependent diabetes mellitus? Diabetes 1986; 35: 894–8.

152. Eisenbarth G. Type I diabetes mellitus: a chronic autoimmune disease. New Engl J Med 1986; 314: 1360–8.

153. Gorsuch AN, Spencer KM, Lister J. Evidence for a long pre-diabetic period in type I (insulin-dependent) diabetes mellitus. Lancet 1981; ii: 1363–5.

154. Tarn AC, Smith CP, Spencer KM, Bottazzo GF, Gale EAM. Type 1 (insulin dependent) diabetes: a disease of slow clinical onset? Br Med J 1987; 294: 342–5.

155. Tarn AC, Thomas JM, Dean BM, Ingram D, Schwarz G, Bottazzo GF, Gale EAM. Predicting insulin-dependent diabetes. Lancet 1988; i: 845–50.

156. Jackson R. Animal models of diabetes. In Farid NR (ed.) Immunogenetics of endocrine disorders. New York: Alan R. Liss, 1988; 89–110.

157. Mordes JP, Desemone J, Rossini AA. The BB rat. Diabetes Metab Rev 1987; 3: 725–50.

158. Rossini AA, Slavin S, Woda BA, Geisberg M, Like AA, Mordes JP. Total lymphoid irradiation prevents diabetes mellitus in the biobreeding/Worcester (BB/W) rat. Diabetes 1984; 33: 543–7.

159. Koevary SB, Williams DE, Williams RM, Chick WL. Passive transfer of diabetes from BB/W to Wistar–Furth rats. J Clin Invest 75; 1985: 1904–7.

160. Sutherland DER, Goetz FC, Sibley RK. Recurrence of disease in pancreas transplants. Diabetes 1989; 38 (suppl 1): 85–7.

161. Sutherland DER, Sibley RK, Za XZ, Michael A, Srikanta S, Taub F et al. Twin to twin pancreas transplantation reversal and re-enactment of the pathogenesis of type I diabetes. Trans Assoc Am Phys 1984; 97: 80–7.

162. Eisenbarth GS. Genes, generator of diversity, glyco-conjugates, and auto-immune B cell insufficiency in type I diabetes. Diabetes 1987; 36: 355–64.

163. Rimoin DL, Rotter JI. Progress in understanding the genetics of diabetes mellitus in genetic disorders. In Berg K (ed.) Medical genetics: past, present and future. New York: Alan R. Liss, 1985; 393–412.

164. Bosi E, Todd I, Pujol-Borrell R, Bottazzo GF. Mechanisms of autoimmunity: relevance to the pathogenesis of type 1 (insulin-dependent) diabetes mellitus. Diabetes Metab Rev 1987; 3: 893–924.

165. Gamble DR. The epidemiology of insulin-dependent diabetes, with particular reference to the relationship of viral infections to its etiology. Epidemiol Rev 1980; 2: 49–70.

166. Gunderson E. Is diabetes of infectious origin? J Infect Dis 1927; 41: 197–202.

167. McCrae WM. Diabetes mellitus following mumps. Lancet 1963; i: 1300–1.

168. Peig M, Ercilla G, Milian M, Gomis R. Post-mumps diabetes mellitus. Lancet 1981; i: 1007.

169. Blom L, Nystrom L, Dahlquist G. The Swedish childhood diabetes study. Vaccinations and infections as risk determinants for diabetes in childhood. Diabetologia 1991; 34: 176–81.

170. Kumar D, Gemayel S, Deapen D, Kapadia D, Yamashita PH, Lee M et al. North American twins with IDDM: genetic, etiological and clinical significance of disease concordance according to age, zygosity and the interval after diagnosis in first twin. Diabetes 1993; 42: 1351–63.

171. Banatvala JE, Bryant J, Schernthaner G, Borkenstein M, Schodber E, Brown D et al. Coxsackie B, mumps, rubella and cytomegalovirus-specific IgM responses in patients with juvenile-onset, insulin-dependent diabetes mellitus in Britain, Austria and Australia. Lancet 1985; i: 1409–12.

172. Champsaur HF, Bottazzo GF, Bertrams J, Assan R, Bach C. Virologic, immunologic, and genetic factors in insulin-dependent diabetes mellitus. J Pediatr 1982; 100: 15–20.

173. Gamble DR, Kinsley ML, Fitzgerald MG, Bolton R, Taylor KW. Viral antibodies in diabetes mellitus. Br Med J 1969; iii: 627–30.

174. King ML, Bidwell D, Voller A, Bryant J, Banatvala JE. Coxsackie B viruses in insulin-dependent diabetes mellitus. Lancet 1983; ii: 915–16.

175. King ML, Shaikh A, Bidwell D, Voller A, Banatvala JE. Coxsackie B virus-specific IgM responses in children with insulin-dependent (juvenile-onset; type I) diabetes mellitus. Lancet 1983; i: 1397–9.

176. Schernthaner G, Banatvala JE, Scherbaum W, Bryant J, Borkenstein M, Schober E, Mayer WR. Coxsackie B virus-specific IgM responses, complement-fixing islet cell antibodies, HLA-DR antigens and C-peptide secretion in insulin-dependent diabetes mellitus. Lancet 1985; ii: 630–2.

177. Orchard TJ, Atchison RW, Becker D, Rabin B, Eberhardt M, Kuller LH et al. Coxsackie infection and diabetes. Lancet 1983; ii: 631.

178. Frisk G, Friman G, Tuvemo T, Fohlman J, Diderhom H. Coxsackie B virus IgM in children at onset of type 1 (insulin-dependent) diabetes mellitus: evidence for IgM induction by a recent or current infection. Diabetologia 1992; 35: 249–53.

179. Palmer JP, Cooney MK, Ward RH, Hansen JA, Brodsky JB, Ray CG et al. Reduced Coxsackie antibody titres in type 1 (insulin-dependent) diabetic patients presenting during an outbreak of Coxsackie B3 and B4 infection. Diabetologia 1982; 22: 426–9.

180. Pak CY, Eun HM, McArthur RG, Yoon JW. Association of cytomegalovirus infection with autoimmune type 1 diabetes. Lancet 1988; ii: 1–4.

181. Hyöty H, Hiltunen M, Reunanen A, Leinikki P, Vesikari T, Lounamaa R et al. Decline of mumps antibodies in type 1 (insulin-dependent) diabetic children and a plateau in the rising incidence of type 1 diabetes after introduction of the mumps–measles–rubella vaccine in Finland. Childhood Diabetes in Finland Study Group. Diabetologia 1993; 36: 1303–8.

182. Jenson AB, Rosenberg HS, Notkins AL. Pancreatic islet cell damage in children with fatal virus infections. Lancet 1980; ii: 354–8.

183. Yoon JW, Austin M, Onodera T, Notkins AL. Virus-induced diabetes mellitus: isolation of a virus from the pancreas of a child with diabetic ketoacidosis. New Engl J Med 1979; 300: 1173–9.

184. Kaufman DL, Erlander MG, Clare-Salzer M, Atkinson MA, Maclaren NK, Tobin AJ. Autoimmunity to two forms of glutamate decarboxylase in insulin-dependent diabetes mellitus. J Clin Invest 1992; 89: 283–92.

185. Hou J, Said C, Franchi D, Dockstader P, Chatterjee NK. Antibodies to glutamic acid decarboxylase and P2-C peptides in sera from Coxsackie virus B4-infected mice and IDDM patients. Diabetes 1994; 43: 1260–6.

186. Atkinson MA, Bowman MA, Campbell L, Darrow BL, Kaufman DL, Maclaren NK. Cellular immunity to a determinant common to glutamate decarboxylase and Coxsackie virus in insulin-dependent diabetes. J Clin Invest 1994; 94: 2125–9.

187. Richter W, Mertens T, Schoel B, Muir P, Ritzkowsky A, Scherbaum WA, Boehm BO. Sequence homology of the diabetes-associated autoantigen glutamate decarboxylase with Coxsackie B4-2C protein and heat shock protein 60 mediates no molecular mimicry of autoantibodies. J Exp Med 1994; 180: 721–6.

188. Rayfield EJ, Ishimura K. Environmental factors and insulin-dependent diabetes mellitus. Diabetes Metab Rev 1987; 3: 925–57.

189. Yoon JW, Notkins AL. Virus-induced diabetes mellitus. VI. Genetically determined host differences in the replication of encephalomyocarditis virus in pancreatic beta cells. J Exp Med 1976; 143: 1170–85.

190. Boucher DW, Notkins AL Virus-induced diabetes mellitus. I. Hyperglycemia and hypoinsulinemia in mice infected with encephalomyocarditis virus. J Exp Med 1973; 137: 1226–39.

191. Craighead JE, Higgins DA. Genetic influences affecting the occurrence of a diabetes mellitus-like disease in mice infected with the encephalomyocarditis virus. J Exp Med 1974; 139: 414–26.

192. Gould CL, Trombley ML, Bigley NJ, McMannama KG, Giron DJ. Replication of diabetogenic and non-diabetogenic variants of encephalomyocarditis (EMC) virus in ICR Swiss mice. Proc Soc Exp Biol Med 1984; 175: 449–53.

193. Gould CL, McMannama KG, Bigley NJK, Giron DJ. Virus-induced murine diabetes: enhancement by immunosuppression. Diabetes 1985; 34: 1217–21.

194. Hayashi K, Boucher DW, Notkins AL. Virus-induced diabetes mellitus. II. Relationship between beta cell damage and hyperglycemia in mice infected with encephalomyocarditis virus. Am J Pathol 1974; 75: 91–102.

195. Iwo K, Bellomo SC, Mukai N, Craighead JE. Encephalomyocarditis virus-induced diabetes mellitus in mice: long-term changes in the structure and function of islets of Langerhans. Diabetologia 1983; 25: 39–44.

196. Onodera T, Yoon J, Brown K, Notkins AL. Evidence for a single locus controlling susceptibility to virus-induced diabetes mellitus. Nature 1978; 276: 693–6.

197. Yoon JW, McClintock PR, Onodera T, Notkins AL. Virus-induced diabetes mellitus. XVIII. Inhibition by a non-diabetogenic variant of encephalomyocarditis virus. J Exp Med 1980; 152: 878–82.

198. Yoon JW, Rodriques MM, Currier C, Notkins AL. Long-term complications of virus-induced diabetes mellitus in mice. Nature 1982; 296: 566–9.

199. Yoon JW, Cha CY, Jordan GW. The role of interferon in virus-induced diabetes. J Infect Dis 1983; 147: 155–9.

200. Huber SA, Babu G, Craighead JE. Genetic influences on the immunologic pathogenesis of encephalomyocarditis (EMC) virus-induced diabetes mellitus. Diabetes 1985; 34: 1186–90.

201. Jordan GW, Cohen SH. Encephalomyocarditis virus-induced diabetes mellitus in mice: model of viral pathogenesis. Rev Infect Dis 1987; 9: 917–24.

202. Yoon JW, Notkins AL. Virus-induced diabetes in mice. Metabolism 1983; 32: 37–40.

203. Yoon JW, Ray UR. Perspectives on the role of viruses in insulin-dependent diabetes. Diabetes 1985; 8: 39–44.

204. Guberski KL, Thomas VA, Shek WR, Like AA, Handler ES, Rossini AA et al. Induction of type I diabetes by Kilham's rat virus in diabetes-resistant BB/Wor rats. Science 1991; 254: 1010–13.

205. Helmke K, Otten A, Willems WR, Brockhaus R, Mueller-Eckhardt G, Stief T et al. Islet cell antibodies and the development of diabetes mellitus in relation to mumps infection and mumps vaccination. Diabetologia 1986; 29: 30–3.

206. Yoon JW. Induction and prevention of type 1 diabetes mellitus by viruses. Diabète Métab 1992; 18: 378–86.

207. Huang SW, Taylor G, Basid A. The effect of pertussis vaccine on the insulin-dependent diabetes induced by streptozotocin in mice. Pediatr Res 1984; 18: 221–6.

208. Becerra JE, Khoury 0MJ, Cordero JF, Erickson JD. Diabetes mellitus during pregnancy and the risks for specific birth defects: a population-based case-control study. Pediatrics 1990; 85: 1–9.

209. Contreras-Soto J, Forsbach G, Vazquez-Rosales J, Alvarez-Garcia C, Garcia G. Non-insulin dependent diabetes mellitus and pregnancy in Mexico. Int J Gynaecol Obstet 1991; 34: 205–10.

210. Rubinstein P, Walker ME, Fedun B, Witt ME, Cooper LZ, Ginsberg-Fellner F. The HLA system in congenital rubella patients with and without diabetes. Diabetes 1982; 31: 1088–91.

211. Rabinowe SL, George KL, Loughlin R, Soeldner JS, Eisenbarth GS. Congenital rubella: monoclonal antibody-defined T-cell abnormalities in young adults. Am J Med 1986; 81: 779–82.

212. De Prins F, Van Assche FA, Desmyter J, De Groote G, Gepts W. Congenital rubella and diabetes mellitus. Lancet 1978; i: 439–40.

213. Patterson K, Chandra RS, Jenson AB. Congenital rubella, insulitis and diabetes mellitus in an infant (letter). Lancet 1981; i: 1048–9.

214. Winter WE, MacLaren NK, Riley WJ, Clarke DW, Kappy MS, Spillar RP. Maturity-onset diabetes of youth in Black Americans. New Engl J Med 1987; 316: 285–91.

215. Rotter JI. Gastric and duodenal ulcer are each different diseases. Dig Dis Sci 1981; 26: 154–60.

216. Borch-Johnsen K, Joner G, Mandrup-Poulsen T, Christy M, Zachan-Christiansen B, Kastrup B, Nerup J. Relation between breast-feeding and incidence of insulin-dependent diabetes mellitus. Lancet 1984; ii: 1083–6.

217. Blom L, Dahlquist G, Nystome L, Sandstrom A, Wall S. The Swedish Childhood Diabetes Study: social and perinatal determinants for diabetes in childhood. Diabetologia 1989; 32: 7–13.

218. Dahlquist G, Blom L, Lonnberg G. The Swedish childhood diabetes study—a multivariate analysis of risk determinants for diabetes in different age groups. Diabetologia 1991; 34: 757–62.

219. Kostraba JN, Dorman JS, LaPorte RE, Scott FW, Steenkiste AR, Gloninger M, Drash AL. Early infant diet and risk of IDDM in blacks and whites. A matched case-control study. Diabetes Care 1992; 15: 626–31.

220. Kostraba JN, Cruickshanks KJ, Lawler-Heavner J, Jobim LF, Rewers MJ, Gay EC et al. Early exposure to cow's milk and solid foods in infancy, genetic predisposition, and risk of IDDM. Diabetes 1993; 42: 288–95.

221. Virtanen SM, Rasanen L, Ylonen K, Aro A, Clayton D, Langholz B et al. Childhood Diabetes in Finland Study Group: early introduction of dairy products associated with increased risk of IDDM in Finnish children. Diabetes 1993; 42: 1786–90.

222. Gerstein HC. Cow's milk exposure and type 1 diabetes mellitus: a critical overview of the clinical literature. Diabetes Care 1994; 17: 13–19.

223. Verge CF, Howard NJ, Irwig L, Simpson JM, Mackerras D, Silink M. Environmental factors in childhood IDDM. A population-based, case-control study. Diabetes Care 1994; 17: 1381–9.

224. Karjalainen J, Saukkonen T, Savilahti E, Dosch H-M. Disease-associated anti-bovine serum albumin antibodies in type 1 (insulin-dependent) diabetes mellitus are detected by particle concentration fluoroimmunoassay, and not by enzyme-linked immunoassay. Diabetologia 1992; 35: 985–90.

225. Dahlquist G, Savilahti E, Landin-Olsson M. An increased level of antibodies to β-lactoglobulin is a risk determinant for early-onset type 1 (insulin-dependent) diabetes mellitus independent of islet cell antibodies and early introduction of cow's milk. Diabetologia 1992; 35: 980–4.

226. Virtanen SM, Saukkonen T, Savilahti E, Ylonen K, Rasanen L, Aro A et al. Diet, cow's milk protein antibodies and the risk of IDDM in Finnish children. Childhood Diabetes in Finland Study Group. Diabetologia 1994; 37: 381–7.

227. Robinson BH, Dosch H-M, Martin JM, Akerblom HK, Savilahti E, Knip M, Ilonen J. A model for the involvement of MHC class II proteins in the development of type 1 (insulin-dependent) diabetes mellitus in response to bovine serum albumin peptides. Diabetologia 1993; 36: 364–8.

228. Karjalainen J, Martin JM, Knip M, Ilonen J, Robinson BH, Savilahti E et al. A bovine albumin peptide as a possible trigger of insulin-dependent diabetes mellitus. New Engl J Med 1992; 327: 302–7.

229. Atkinson MA, Bowman MA, Kao KJ, Cambell L, Dush PJ, Shah SC et al. Lack of immune responsiveness to bovine serum albumin in insulin-dependent diabetes. New Engl J Med 1993; 329: 1853–8.

230. Bodington MJ, McNally PG, Burden AC. Cow's milk and type 1 childhood diabetes: no increase in risk. Diabet Med 1994; 11: 663–5.

231. Fava D, Leslie RD, Pozzilli P. Relationship between dairy product consumption and incidence of IDDM in childhood in Italy. Diabetes Care 1994; 17: 1488–90.

232. Norris JM, Beaty B, Eisenbarth GS, Hamman RF, Rewers M. Lack of association between infant diet and prediabetic autoimmunity in high genetic risk children. The Diabetes Autoimmunity Study in the Young (DAISY). Diabetes 1995; 44 (suppl 1): 6A.

233. Kostraba JN. What can epidemiology tell us about the role of infant diet in the etiology of IDDM? Diabetes Care 1994; 17: 87–91.

234. Warram JH, Krolewski AS, Gottlieb MS, Kahn RC. Differences in risk of insulin-dependent diabetes in offspring of diabetic mothers and fathers. New Engl J Med 1984; 311: 149–52.

235. Warram JH, Krolewski AS, Kahn RC. Determinants of IDDM and perinatal mortality in children of diabetic mothers. Diabetes 1988; 37: 1328–34.

236. Gorsuch AN, Spencer KM, Lister J, Wolf E, Bottazzo GF, Cudworth AG. Can future type I diabetes be predicted? A study in families of affected children. Diabetes 1982; 31: 862–6.

237. Rotter JI, Vadheim CM, Petersen GM, Cantor RM, Riley WJ, Maclaren NK. HLA haplotypes sharing and proband genotype in IDDM. Genetic Epidemiology 1986; 3(suppl 1): 347–52.

238. Eisenbarth S, Wilson P, Ward F, Lebovitz HE. HLA type and occurrence of disease in familial polyglandular failure. New Engl J Med 1978; 298: 92–4.

239. Riley WJ, Maclaren NK, Lezotte DC, Spillar RP, Rosenbloom AL. Thyroid autoimmunity in insulin-dependent diabetes mellitus: the case for routine screening. J Pediatr 1981; 98: 350–4.

240. Bottazzo GF, Mann JI, Thorogood M, Baum JD, Doniach D. Autoimmunity in juvenile diabetics and their families. Br Med J 1978; ii: 165–8.

241. Betterle C, Zanette F, Pedini B, Presotto F, Rapp LB, Monsciotti CM, Rigon F. Clinical and subclinical organ-specific autoimmune manifestations in type 1 (insulin-dependent) diabetic patients and their first degree relatives. Diabetologia 1984; 26: 431–6.

242. Gorsuch AN, Dean BM, Bottazzo GF, Lister J, Cudworth AG. Evidence that type 1 diabetes and thyrogastric autoimmunity have different genetic determinants. Br Med J 1980; i: 145–7.

243. Fialkow PJ, Zavala C, Nielson K. Thyroid autoimmunity: increased frequency in relatives of insulin dependent diabetes patients. Ann Intern Med 1975; 83: 170–6.

244. Riley WJ, Toskes PP, Maclaren NK, Silverstein JH. Predictive value of gastric parietal cell autoantibodies as a marker for gastric and hematologic abnormalities associated with insulin dependent diabetes. Diabetes 1982; 31: 1051–5.

245. Riley WJ, Maclaren NK, Neufeld M. Adrenal autoantibodies and Addison's disease in insulin-dependent diabetes mellitus. J Pediatr 1980; 97: 191–5.

246. Wang SJ, Shohat T, Vadheim CM, Shellow W, Edwards J, Rotter JI. Increased risk for type 1 (insulin dependent) diabetes in relatives of patients with alopecia areata. Am J Med Genet 1994; 51: 234–9.

247. Motulsky AG. The genetic hyperlipidemias. New Engl J Med 1976; 294: 823–7.

248. Chern MM, Anderson VE, Barbosa J. Empirical risk for insulin-dependent diabetes (IDD) in sibs. Further definition of genetic heterogeneity. Diabetes 1982; 31: 1115–/8.

249. Omar MAK, Asmal AC. Family histories of diabetes mellitus in young African and Indian diabetics. Br Med J 1983; 286: 1786.

250. Samloff IM, Varis K, Ihamaki T, Siurala M, Rotter JI. Relationships among serum pepsinogen I, serum pepsinogen II, and gastric mucosal histology. A study in relatives of patients with pernicious anemia. Gastroenterology 1982; 83: 204–9.

251. Mitchell B D, Kammerer C M, O'Connell P, Harrison CR, Manire M, Shipman P et al. Evidence for linkage of postchallenge insulin levels with intestinal fatty acid-binding protein (FABP2) in Mexican-Americans. Diabetes 1995; 44: 1046–53.

252. Mills JL. Malformation in infants of diabetic mothers. Teratology 1982; 25: 385–94.

253. Kitzmiller JL, Cloherty JP, Younger MD. Diabetic pregnancy and perinatal morbidity. Am J Obstet Gynecol 1978; 131: 560–80.

254. Gabbe SG. Congenital malformations in infants of diabetic mothers. Obstet Gynecol 1977; 32: 125–32.

255. Cousins L. Congenital anomalies among infants of diabetic mothers. Etiology, prevention, prenatal diagnosis. Am J Obstet Gynecol 1983; 147: 333–8.

256. Neave C. Congenital malformations in offspring of diabetics. Perspect Pediatr Pathol 1984; 8: 213–22.

257. Kucera J. Rate and type of congenital anomalies among offspring of diabetic women. J Reprod Med 1971; 7: 73–82.

258. Soler NG, Walsh CH, Malins JM. Congenital malformations in infants of diabetic mothers. Q J Med 1976; 45: 303–13.

259. Mills JL, Baker L, Goldman AS. Malformations in infants of diabetic mothers occur before the seventh gestational week. Diabetes 1979; 28: 292–3.

260. Miller E, Hare JW, Cloherty JP, Dunn PJ, Gleason RE, Soeldner JS, Kitzmiller JL. Elevated maternal hemoglobin A1c in early pregnancy and major

congenital anomalies in infants of diabetic mothers. New Engl J Med 1981; 304: 1331–4.

261. Hanson U, Persson B, Thunell S. Relationship between hemoglobin A1c in early type 1 (insulin-dependent) diabetic pregnancy and the occurrence of spontaneous abortion and fetal malformations in Sweden. Diabetologia 1990; 33: 100–4.

262. Kitzmiller JL, Gavin, LA, Gin GD, Jovanovic-Peterson L, Main EK, Zigrang WD. Preconception care of diabetes: glycemic control prevents congenital anomalies. JAMA 1991; 265: 731–6.

263. Brock DJH, Sutcliffe RG. Alpha-fetoprotein in the antenatal diagnosis of anencephaly and spina bifida. Lancet 1972; ii: 197–9.

264. Wald NJ, Cuckle H. Maternal serum alpha-fetoprotein measurement in antenatal screening for anencephaly and spina bifida in early pregnancy. United Kingdom Collaborative Study. Lancet 1977; i: 1323–32.

265. Milunsky A, Alpert E, Kitzmiller JL, Younger MD, Neff RK. Prenatal diagnosis of neural tube defects VIII. The importance of serum alpha-fetoprotein screening in diabetic pregnant women. Am J Obstet Gynecol 1982; 142: 1030–2.

266. Reece AE, Davis N, Mahoney MJ, Baumgarten A. Maternal serum alpha-fetoprotein in diabetic pregnancy: correlation with blood glucose control. Lancet 1987; ii: 275.

267. Baumgarten A, Robinson J. Prospective study of an inverse relationship between maternal glycosylated hemoglobin and serum alpha-fetoprotein concentrations in pregnant women with diabetes. Am J Obstet Gynecol 1988; 159: 77–81.

268. Czeizel AE, Dudas I. Prevention of the first occurrence of neural tube defects by periconceptional vitamin supplementation. New Engl J Med 1992; 327: 1832–5.

269. Kaku K, Fiedorek FT, Province M, Permutt MA. Genetic analysis of glucose tolerance in inbred mouse strains. Diabetes 1988; 37: 707–13.

270. Coleman DL. Obese and diabetes, two mutant genes causing diabetes–obesity syndromes in mice. Diabetologia 1978; 14: 141–8.

271. Coleman DL. Diabetes–obesity syndromes in mice. Diabetes 1982; 31: 1–6.

272. Curry DL, Stern JS. Dynamics of insulin hypersecretion by obese Zucker rats. Metabolism 1985; 34: 791–6.

273. Coleman DL, Hummel KP. The influence of genetic background on the expression of the obese (*ob*) gene in the mouse. Diabetologia 1973; 9: 287–93.

274. Hummel KP, Coleman DL, Lane PW. The influence of genetic background on expression of mutations at the diabetes locus in the mouse, I C57BL/KsJ and C57BL/6J strains. Biochem Genet 1972; 7: 1–13.

275. Zhang Y, Proenca R, Maffei M, Barone M, Leopold L, Friedman JM. Positional cloning of the mouse obese gene and its human homologue. Nature 1994; 372: 425–32.

276. Pelleymounter MA, Cullen MJ, Baker MB, Hecht R, Winters D, Boone T, Collins F. Effects of the obese gene product on body weight regulation in *ob/ob* mice. Science 1995; 269: 540–3.

277. Halaas JL, Gajiwala KS, Maffei M, Cohen S, Chait BT, Rabinowitz D et al. Weight-reducing effects of the plasma protein encoded by the obese gene. Science 1995; 269: 543–6.

278. Campfield LA, Smith FJ, Guisez Y, Devos R, Burn P. Recombinant mouse Ob protein: evidence for a peripheral signal linking adiposity and central neural networks. Science 1995; 269: 546–50.

279. Masuzaki H, Ogawa Y, Isse N, Satoh N, Okazaki T, Shigemoto M et al. Human obese gene expression. Adipocyte-specific expression and regional differences in the adipose tissue. Diabetes 1995; 44: 855–8.

280. Considine RV, Considine EL, Williams CJ, Nyce MR, Magosin SA, Bauer TL et al. Evidence against either a premature stop codon or the absence of obese gene mRNA in human obesity. J Clin Invest 1995; 95: 2986–8.

281. Bahary N, Leibel RL, Joseph L, Friedman JM. Molecular mapping of the mouse db mutation. Proc Natl Acad Sci USA 1990; 87: 8642–6.

282. Truett GE, Bahary N, Friedman JM, Leibel RL. Rat obesity gene fatty (*fa*) maps to chromosome 5: evidence for homology with the mouse gene diabetes (*db*). Proc Natl Acad Sci USA 1991; 88: 7806–9.

283. Surwit RS, Kuhn CM, Cochrane C, McCubbin JA, Feinglos MN. Diet-induced type II diabetes in C57BL/6J mice. Diabetes 1988; 37: 1163–7.

284. Surwit RS, Seldin MF, Kuhn CM, Cochrane C, Feinglos MN. Control of expression of insulin resistance and hyperglycemia by different genetic factors in diabetic C57BL/6J mice. Diabetes 1991; 40: 82–7.

285. Michaelis OE, Patrick DJ, Hansen CT, Canary JJ, Werner RN, Carswell N. Animal models of human disease insulin dependent diabetes mellitus (type II) spontaneous hypertensive/NIH-corpulent rat. Am J Pathol 1986; 123: 398–400.

286. Voyles NR, Powell AM, Timmers KI, Wilkins SD, Bhathena SJ, Hansen C et al. Reversible impairment of glucose-induced insulin secretion in SHR/N-cp rats. Diabetes 1988; 37: 398–404.

287. Elston RC, Namboodiri KK, Nino HV, Pollitzer WS. Studies on blood and urine glucose in Seminole Indians: indications for segregation of a major gene. Am J Hum Genet 1974; 26: 13–34.

288. Raper LR, Taylor R, Zimmet P, Milne B, Balkau B. Bimodality in glucose tolerance distributions in the urban Polynesian population of Western Samoa. Diabetes Res 1984; 1: 19–26.

289. Rushforth NB, Bennett PH, Sternberg AG, Burch TA, Miller M. Diabetes in the Pima Indians, evidence of bimodality in glucose tolerance distributions. Diabetes 1971; 20: 756–65.

290. Zimmet P, Whitehouse S. Bimodality of fasting and two-hour glucose tolerance distributions in a Micronesian population. Diabetes 1978; 27: 793–800.

291. Tremblay A, Poehlman E, Nadeau A, Perusse L, Bouchard C. Is the response of plasma glucose and insulin to short-term exercise-training genetically determined? Horm Metab Res 1987; 19: 65–7.

292. Zimmet P. Type 2 (non-insulin-dependent) diabetes—an epidemiologic overview. Diabetologia 1982; 22: 399–411.

293. Zimmet P, Kirk R, Serjeantson S, Whitehouse S, Taylor R. Diabetes in Pacific populations—genetic and environmental interactions. In Melish JS, Hamma J, Baba S (eds) Genetic environmental interactions in diabetes mellitus. Amsterdam: Excerpta Medica, 1982; 9–17.

294. Cohen AM, Fidel J, Cohen B, Furst A, Eisenberg S. Diabetes, blood lipids, lipoproteins, and change

of environment: restudy of the 'new immigrant Yemenites' in Israel. Metabolism 1979; 28: 716–28.

295. Modan M, Karasik A, Halkin H, Fuchs Z, Lusky A, Shitrit A, Modan B. Effect of past and current body mass index on prevalence of glucose intolerance and type 2 (non-insulin dependent) diabetes and on insulin response. Diabetologia 1986; 29: 82–9.

296. O'Dea K, Spargo RM, Nestel PJ. Impact of Westernization on carbohydrate and lipid metabolism in Australian Aborigines. Diabetologia 1982; 22: 148–53.

297. Schraer C, Lanier A. Diabetes mellitus in Alaska natives. Centers for Disease Control Arctic Investigation Laboratory 1987; Program Notes No. 6.

298. Sievers ML, Fisher JR. Diabetes in North American Indians. In National Diabetes Data Group. Diabetes in America; diabetic data compiled 1984. U.S. Dept. of Health and Human Services NIH publication, #85-1468, 1985; XI 1–20.

299. Lindsten J, Cerasi E, Luft R, Morton N, Ryman N. Significance of genetic factors for plasma insulin response to glucose in healthy subjects. Clin Genet 1976; 10: 125–34.

300. Beaty TH, Fajans SS. Estimating genetic and nongenetic components of variance for fasting glucose levels in pedigrees ascertained through noninsulin dependent diabetes. Ann Hum Genet 1982; 46: 355–62.

301. Serjeantson SW, Zimmet P. Diabetes in the Pacific: evidence for a major gene. In Baba S, Gould M, Zimmet P (eds) Diabetes mellitus: recent knowledge on aetiology, complications and treatment. Sydney: Academic Press, 1984; 23–30.

302. Williams WR, Morton NE, Rao DC, Gulbrandsen CL, Rhoads GG, Kagan A. Family resemblance for fasting blood glucose in a population of Japanese Americans. Clin Genet 1983; 23: 287–93.

303. Friedlander Y, Kark JD, Bar-On H. Family resemblance for fasting blood glucose: the Jerusalem Lipid Research Clinic. Clin Genet 1987; 32: 222–34.

304. Haffner SM, Stern MP, Hazuda HP, Mitchell BD, Patterson JK. Increased insulin concentrations in nondiabetic offspring of diabetic parents. New Engl J Med 1988; 319: 1297–1301.

305. Lillioja S, Mott DM, Zawadzki JK, Young AA, Abbott WGH, Knowler WC et al. *In vivo* insulin action is familial characteristic in non-diabetic Pima Indians. Diabetes 1987; 36: 1329–35.

306. Cerasi E, Luft R. 'What is inherited—what is added', hypothesis for the pathogenesis of diabetes mellitus. Diabetes 1967; 16: 615–27.

307. Iselius L, Lindsten J, Morton NE, Efendic S, Cerasi E, Haegermark A, Luft R. Evidence for an autosomal recessive gene regulating the persistence of insulin response to glucose in man. Clin Genet 1982; 22: 180–94.

308. Iselius L, Lindsten J, Morton NE, Efendic S, Cerasi E, Haegermark A, Luft R. Genetic regulation of the kinetics of glucose-induced insulin release in man. Clin Genet 1985; 28: 8–15.

309. O'Rahilly SP, Rudenski AS, Burnett MA, Nugent Z, Hosker JP, Darling P. Beta-cell dysfunction, rather than insulin insensitivity, is the primary defect in familial type 2 diabetes. Lancet 1986; ii: 360–64.

310. O'Rahilly SP, Turner RC, Matthews DR. Impaired pulsatile secretion of insulin in relatives of patients with non-insulin-dependent diabetes. New Engl J Med 1988; 318: 1225–30.

311. Polonsky KS, Giben BD, Hirsch LJ, Tillil H, Shapiro ET, Beebe C et al. Abnormal patterns of insulin secretion in non-insulin-dependent diabetes mellitus. New Engl J Med 1988; 318: 1231–9.

312. Schaefer O. Carbohydrate metabolism in Eskimos. Arch Environ Health 1969; 18: 143–7.

313. Arnoff SL, Bennett PH, Gorden P, Rushforth N, Miller M. Unexplained hyperinsulinemia in normal and 'prediabetic' Pima Indians compared with normal Caucasians. Diabetes 1977; 26: 827–40.

314. Rimoin DL. Ethnic variability in glucose tolerance and insulin secretion. Arch Intern Med 1969; 124: 695–700.

315. Sharp PS, Mohan V, Levy JC, Mather HM, Kohner EM. Insulin resistance in patients of Asian Indian and European origin with non-insulin dependent diabetes. Horm Metab Res 1987; 19: 84–5.

316. Kobberling J. Studies on the genetic heterogeneity of diabetes mellitus. Diabetologia 1971; 7: 46–9.

317. Fajans SS. The natural history of idiopathic diabetes mellitus. Heterogeneity in insulin responses in latent diabetes. In Creutzfeldt W, Kobberling J, Neel JV (eds). The genetics of diabetes mellitus. Berlin: Springer-Verlag, 1976; 64–78.

318. Fajans SS. Heterogeneity of insulin secretion in type II diabetes. Diabetes Metab Rev 1986; 2: 347–61.

319. O'Rahilly S, Wainscoat JS, Turner RC. Type 2 (non-insulin-dependent) diabetes mellitus. New genetics for old nightmares. Diabetologia 1988; 31: 407–14.

320. Rotter JI. Genetic predispositions to common adult disease. In Kaback MM, Shapiro LJ. Frontiers in genetic medicine (Proceedings of the 92nd Ross Conference on Pediatric Research). Columbus, OH: Ross Laboratories, 1987; 35–43.

321. Fajans SS, Conn JW. Prediabetes, subclinical diabetes, and latent clinical diabetes: interpretation, diagnosis and treatment. In Leibel DS, Wrenshall GS (eds) On the nature and treatment of diabetes. International Congress Series, vol. 84. Amsterdam: Excerpta Medica, 1965; 641–56.

322. Zouali H, Velho G, Froguel P. Polymorphism of the glycogen synthase gene and non-insulin-dependent diabetes mellitus New Engl J Med 1993; 328: 1568.

323. Tattersall RB. The present status of maturity-onset type of diabetes mellitus. In Kobberling J, Tattersall RB (eds) Genetics of diabetes mellitus. New York: Academic Press, 1982; 261–70.

324. Permutt MA, Chiu KC, Tanizawa Y. Glucokinase and NIDDM: a candidate gene that paid off. Diabetes 1992; 41: 1367–72.

325. Bell GI, Xiang K-S, Newman MV, Wu S-H, Wright LG, Fajans SS et al. Gene for non-insulin-dependent diabetes mellitus (maturity-onset diabetes of the young subtype) is linked to DNA polymorphism on human chromosome 20q. Proc Natl Acad Sci USA 1991; 88: 1484–8.

326. Bell GI. Polygenic complexity of human and animal NIDDM. Presentation to the Genetics of Diabetes Symposium, American Diabetes Association Annual Meeting, Atlanta, GA, June, 1995.

327. Froguel Ph, Vaxillaire M, Velho G, Zouali H, Butel MO, Lesage S et al. Close linkage of glucokinase locus on chromosome 7p to early-onset non-insulin-dependent diabetes mellitus. Nature 1992; 356: 162–4.

328. Hattersley AT, Turner RC, Permutt MA, Patel P, Tanizawa Y, Chiu KC et al. Linkage of type 2 diabetes to the glucokinase gene. Lancet 1992; 339: 1307–10.

329. Magnuson MA. Glucokinase gene structure: functional implications of molecular genetic studies. Diabetes 1990; 39: 523–7.

330. Nishi S, Stoffel M, Xiang K, Shows TB, Bell GI, Takeda J. Human pancreatic beta-cell glucokinase: cDNA sequence and localization of the polymorphic gene to chromosome 7, band p13. Diabetologia 1992; 35: 743–7.

331. Fajans SS. Scope and heterogeneous nature of MODY. Diabetes Care 1990; 13: 49–64.

332. Vionnet N, Stoffel M, Takeda J, Yasuda K, Bell GI, Zouali H et al. Non-sense mutation in the glucokinase gene causes early-onset non-insulin-dependent diabetes mellitus. Nature 1992; 56: 721–2.

333. Stoffel M, Patel P, Lo Y-MD, Hattersley AT, Lucassen AM, Page R et al. Mis-sense glucokinase mutation in maturity-onset diabetes of the young and mutation screening in late-onset diabetes. Nature Genet 1992; 2: 153–6.

334. Blanche H, Hager J, Sun F, Dausset J, Cohen D, Froguel P, Cohen N. Non-radioactive screening of glucokinase mutations in maturity onset diabetes of the young. Biotechniques 1994; 16: 866–8, 870, 873–6.

335. Froguel P, Velho G. Maturity-onset diabetes of the young. Curr Opin Pediatr 1994; 6: 482–5.

336. Vaxillaire M, Boccio V, Phillipi A, Vigouroux C, Terwilliger J, Passa P et al. A gene for maturity onset diabetes of the young (MODY) maps to chromosome 12q. Nature Genet 1995; 9: 418–23.

337. Vaxillaire M, Boccio V, Philippi A, Velho G, Lathrop MG, Froguel P. A third gene for maturity-onset diabetes of the young maps to chromosome 12q. Diabetes 1995; 44 (suppl 1): 41A.

338. Velho G, Clement K, Pueyo ME, Vaxillaire M, Passa P, Robert J-J, Froguel P. MODY linked to chromosome 12q markers: clinical and metabolic profiles. Diabetes 1995; 44 (suppl 1): 233A.

339. Fajans SS, Bell GI, Bowden DW, Halter JB, Polonsky KS. Maturity-onset diabetes of the young. Life Sci 1994; 55: 413–22.

340. Velho G, Froguel P, Clement K, Pueyo ME, Rakotoambinina B, Zouali H et al. Primary pancreatic beta-cell secretory defect caused by mutations in glucokinase gene in kindreds of maturity onset diabetes of the young. Lancet 1992; 340: 444–8.

341. Herman WH, Fajans SS, Ortiz FJ, Smith MJ, Sturis J, Bell G et al. Abnormal insulin secretion, not insulin resistance, is the genetic or primary defect of MODY in the RW pedigree. Diabetes 1994; 43: 40–6.

342. Mitrakou A, Kelley D, Mokan M, Veneman T, Pangburn T, Reilly J, Gerich J. Role of reduced suppression of glucose production and diminished early insulin release in impaired glucose tolerance. New Engl J Med 1992; 326: 22–9.

343. Sanz N, Karam JH, Horita S, Bell GI. Prevalence of insulin-gene mutations in non-insulin-dependent diabetes mellitus. New Engl J Med 1986; 314: 1322–3.

344. Elbein SC, Gruppuso P, Schwartz R, Skolnick M, Permutt MA. Hyperproinsulinemia in a family with proposed defect in conversion is linked to the insulin gene. Diabetes 1985; 34: 821–4.

345. Gruppuso PA, Gorden P, Kahn CR, Cornblath M, Zeller WP, Schwartz R. Familial hyperproinsulinemia due to a proposed defect in conversion of proinsulin to insulin. New Engl J Med 1984; 11; 629–34.

346. Given BD, Mako ME, Tager HS, Baldwin D, Markese J, Rubenstein AH et al. Diabetes due to secretion of an abnormal insulin. New Engl J Med 1980; 302: 129–35.

347. Haneda M, Polonsky KS, Bergenstil RM, Jaspan JB, Shoelson SE, Blix PM et al. Familial hyperinsulinemia due to a structural abnormal insulin, definition of an emerging new clinical syndrome. New Engl J Med 1984; 310: 1288–94.

348. Seino S, Funakoshi A, Fu ZZ, Vinik A. Identification of insulin variants in patients with hyperinsulinemia by reversed-phase, high-performance liquid chromatography. Diabetes 1985; 34: 1–7.

349. Shoelson S, Haneda M, Blix P, Nanjo A, Sanke T, Inouye K et al. Three mutant insulins in man. Nature 1983; 302: 540–3.

350. Tager HS. Abnormal products of the human insulin gene. Diabetes 1984; 33: 693–9.

351. Sanz N, Karam JH, Horita S, Bell GI. Prevalence of insulin-gene mutations in non-insulin dependent diabetes mellitus. New Engl J Med 1986; 314: 1322.

352. Olansky L, Janssen R, Welling C, Permutt MA. Variability of the insulin gene in American Blacks with NIDDM. Analysis by single-strand conformational polymorphisms. Diabetes 1992; 41: 742–9.

353. Raben N, Barbetti F, Cama A, Lesniak MA, Lillioja S, Zimmet P et al. Normal coding sequences of insulin gene in Pima Indians and Nauruans, two groups with highest prevalence of type II diabetes. Diabetes 1991; 40: 118–22.

354. Owerbach D, Nerup J. Restriction fragment length polymorphism of the insulin gene in diabetes mellitus. Diabetes 1982; 31: 275–7.

355. Rotwein PS, Chirgwin J, Province M, Knowler WC, Pettitt DJ, Cordell B et al. Polymorphism in the 5′ flanking region of the human insulin gene: a genetic marker for non-insulin-dependent diabetes mellitus. New Engl J Med 1983; 308: 65–71.

356. Hitman GA, Jowett NI, Willians LG, Humphries S, Winter RM, Galton DJ. Polymorphisms in the 5′ flanking region of the insulin gene and non-insulin-dependent diabetes. Clin Sci 1984; 66: 383–8.

357. Mandrup-Poulsen T, Owerbach D, Nerup J, Johansen K, Ingerslev J, Tybjærg Hansen A. Insulin-gene flanking sequences, diabetes mellitus and atherosclerosis: a review. Diabetologia 1985; 28: 556–64.

358. Cocozza S, Riccardi G, Monticelle A, Capaldo B, Genovese S, Krogh V et al. Polymorphism of the 5′ end flanking region of the insulin gene is associated with reduced insulin secretion in healthy individuals. Eur J Clin Invest 1988; 18: 582–6.

359. Nomura M, Iwama N, Mukai M, Saito Y, Kawamori R, Shichiri M, Kamada T. High frequency of class 3 allele in the human insulin gene in Japanese type 2 (non-insulin-dependent) diabetic patients with a family history of diabetes. Diabetologia 1986; 29: 402–4.

360. Awata T, Shibasaki Y, Hirai H, Okabe T, Kanazawa Y, Takaku F. Restriction fragment length polymorphism of the insulin gene region in Japanese diabetic and non-diabetic subjects. Diabetologia 1985; 28: 911–13.

361. Kambo PK, Hitman GA, Mohan V, Ramachandran A, Snehalatha C, Suresh S et al. The genetic predisposition to fibrocalculous pancreatic diabetes. Diabetologia 1989; 32: 45–51.

362. Hitman GA, Karir PK, Mohan V, Rao PV, Kohner EM, Levy JC, Mather H. A genetic analysis of type 2 (non-insulin-dependent) diabetes mellitus in Punjabi

Sikhs and British Caucasoid patients. Diabetic Med 1987; 4: 526–30.

363. Bell GI, Picket RL, Rutter WJ, Cordell B, Tischer E, Goodman HM. Sequence of the human insulin gene. Nature 1980; 284: 26–32.

364. Elbein SC, Corsetti L, Permutt MA. New polymorphisms at the insulin locus increase its usefulness as a genetic marker. Diabetes 1985; 34: 1139–44.

365. Hitman GA, Kambo PK, Viswanathan M, Mohan V. An analysis of amplified insulin gene products in diabetics of Indian origin. J Med Genet 1991; 28: 97–100.

366. Horst-Sikorska W, Zoll B, Kwiatkowska J, Willms B, Kraszewski A, Horst A, Slomski R. Prevalence of beta allele of the insulin gene in type II diabetes mellitus. Hum Genet 1994; 93: 325–8.

367. Elbein SC, Corsetti L, Goldgar D, Skolnick M, Permutt MA. Insulin gene in familial NIDDM. Lack of linkage in Utah Mormon pedigrees. Diabetes 1988; 37: 569–76.

368. Seino S, Seino M, Nishi S, Bell GI. Structure of the human insulin receptor gene and characterization of its promoter. Proc Natl Acad Sci USA 1989; 86: 114–18.

369. Kasuga M, Zick Y, Blith DL, Karlsson FA, Karing HU, Kahn CR. Insulin stimulation of phosphorylation of the beta-subunit of the insulin receptor. J Biol Chem 1982; 257: 9891–4.

370. McClain RA, Henry RR, Ullrich A, Olefsky JM. Restriction-fragment-length polymorphism in insulin-receptor gene and insulin resistance in NIDDM. Diabetes 1988; 37: 1071–5.

371. Elbein SC, Corsetti L, Ullrich A, Permutt MA. Multiple restriction fragment length polymorphisms at the insulin receptor locus. Proc Natl Acad Sci USA 1986; 83: 5223–7.

372. McGill J, Corsetti L, Elbein SC. Restriction fragment length polymorphisms at the insulin receptor in a population of diabetic and nondiabetic blacks (abstr). Diabetes 1987; 36 (suppl 1): 21A.

373. Raboudi SH, Mitchell BD, Stern MP, Eifler CW, Haffner SM, Hazuda HP, Frazier ML. Type II diabetes mellitus and polymorphism of insulin-receptor gene in Mexican Americans. Diabetes 1989; 38: 975–80.

374. Xiang K-S, Cox NJ, Sanz N, Huang P, Karam JH, Bell GI. Insulin-receptor and apolipoprotein genes contribute to development of NIDDM in Chinese Americans. Diabetes 1989; 38: 17–23.

375. Ober C, Xiang K-S, Thisted RA, Indovina KA, Wason CJ, Dooley S. Increased risk for gestational diabetes mellitus associated with insulin receptor and insulin-like growth factor II restriction fragment length polymorphisms. Genet Epidemiol 1989; 6: 559–69.

376. Elbein SC, Sorensen LK, Taylor M. Linkage analysis of insulin-receptor gene in familial NIDDM. Diabetes 1992; 41: 648–56.

377. Karir PK, Niven MJ, Mohan V, Levy JC, Rao PV, Mather H et al. An association exists of insulin receptor gene polymorphisms in Caucasoid non-insulin dependent diabetes but not Asian diabetics. Diabet Med 1986; 3: 566A.

378. Elbein SC, Sorensen LK. Genetic variation in insulin receptor beta-chain exons among members of familial type 2 (non-insulin-dependent) diabetic pedigrees. Diabetologia 1991; 34: 742–9.

379. Taylor SI. Lilly lecture: molecular mechanisms of insulin resistance. Lessons from patients with mutations in the insulin-receptor gene. Diabetes 1992; 41: 1473–90.

380. Kadowaki T, Bevins CL, Cama A, Ojamaa K, Marcus-Samuels B, Kadowaki H et al. Two mutant alleles of the insulin receptor gene in a patient with extreme insulin resistance. Science 1988; 240: 787–90.

381. Lekanne-Deprez RH, Potter van Loon BJ, van der Zon GC, Moller W, Lindhout D, Klinkhamer MP et al. Individuals with only one allele for a functional insulin receptor have a tendency to hyperinsulinemia but not to hyperglycemia. Diabetologia 1989; 32: 740–4.

382. O'Rahilly S, Choi WH, Patel P, Turner RC, Flier JS, Moller DE. Detection of mutations in insulin-receptor gene in NIDDM patients by analysis of single-stranded conformation polymorphisms. Diabetes 1991; 40: 777–82.

383. Kim H, Kadowaki H, Sakura H, Odawara M, Momomura K, Takahashi Y et al. Detection of mutations in the insulin receptor gene in patients with insulin resistance by analysis of single-stranded conformational polymorphsims. Diabetologia 1992; 35: 261–6.

384. Stoffel M, Espinosa R, Keller SR, Lienhard GE, LeBeau MM, Bell GI. Human insulin receptor substrate-1 gene (IRS1): chromosomal localization to 2q35-q36.1 and identification of a simple tandem repeat DNA polymorphism. Diabetologia 1993; 36: 335–7.

385. Almind K, Bjorbaek C, Vestergaard H, Hansen T, Echwald S, Pedersen O. Amino acid polymorphisms of insulin receptor substrate-1 in non-insulin-dependent diabetes mellitus. Lancet 1993; 342: 828–32.

386. Shipman P, Kammerer C, O'Connell P, Stern M. Insulin receptor substrate-1 is not linked to type II diabetes in Mexican Americans. Diabetes 1994; 43 (suppl 1): 168A.

387. Tanizawa Y, Riggs AC, Elbein SC, Whelan A, Donis-Keller H, Permutt MA. Human glucagon-like peptide-1 receptor gene in NIDDM. Identification and use of simple sequence repeat polymorphisms in genetic analysis. Diabetes 1994; 43: 752–7.

388. Yoshida H, Ohagi S, Sanke T, Furuta H, Furuta M, Nanjo K. Association of the prohormone convertase 2 gene (PCSK2) on chromosome 20 with NIDDM in Japanese subjects. Diabetes 1995; 44: 389–93.

389. Szathmary EJE. The effect of Gc genotype on fasting insulin levels of Dogrib Indians. Hum Genet 1987; 75: 368–72.

390. Shows TB, Eddy RL, Byers MG, Fukushima Y, DeHaven CR, Murray JC, Bell GI. Polymorphic human glucose transporter gene (GLUT) is on chromosome 1p31.3–p35. Diabetes 1987; 36: 546–9.

391. Gould GW, Derechin V, James DE, Tordjman K, Ahern S, Gibbs EM et al. Insulin-stimulated translocation of the HepG2/erythrocyte-type glucose transporter expressed in 3T3-L1 adipocytes. J Biol Chem 1989; 264: 2180–4.

392. Fukumoto H, Seino S, Imura H, Seino Y, Bell GI. Characterization and expression of human HepG2/erythrocyte glucose-transporter gene. Diabetes 1988; 37: 657–61.

393. Li SR, Baroni MG, Oelbaum RS, Stocks J, Galton DJ. Association of genetic variant of the glucose transporter with non-insulin-dependent diabetes mellitus. Lancet 1988; ii: 368–70.

394. Cox NJ, Xiang K-S, Bell GI, Karam JH. Glucose transporter gene and non-insulin-dependent diabetes (letter). Lancet 1988; ii: 793-4.

395. Oelbaum RS. Analysis of three glucose transporter genes in a Caucasian population: no associations with non-insulin-dependent diabetes and obesity. Clin Genet 1992; 42: 260-6.

396. Kaku K, Matsutani A, Mueckler M, Permutt MA. Polymorphisms of HepG2/erythrocyte glucose transporter gene. Diabetes 1990; 39: 49-56.

397. Elbein SC, Hoffman MD, Matsutani A, Permutt MA. Linkage analysis of GLUT1 (HepG2) and GLUT2 (liver/islet) genes in familial NIDDM. Diabetes 1992; 41: 1660-7.

398. Baroni MC, Alcolado JC, Gragnoli C, Franciosi AM, Cavallo MG, Fiore V et al. Affected sib-pair analysis of the GLUT1 glucose transporter gene locus in non-insulin-dependent diabetes mellitus (NIDDM): evidence for no linkage. Hum Genet 1994; 93: 675-80.

399. Takeda J, Toshiaki K, Fukomoto H, Bell GI. Organization of the human GLUT2 (pancreatic beta-cell and hepatocyte) glucose transporter gene. Diabetes 1993; 42: 773-7.

400. Patel P, Bell GI, Cook JTE, Turner RC, Wainscoat JS. Multiple restriction fragment length polymorphisms at the GLUT2 locus: GLUT2 haplotypes for genetic analysis of type 2 (non-insulin-dependent) diabetes mellitus. Diabetologia 1991; 34: 817-21.

401. Matsutani A, Koranyi L, Cox N, Permutt MA. Polymorphisms of GLUT2 and GLUT4 genes. Use in evaluation of genetic susceptibility to NIDDM in Blacks. Diabetes 1990; 39: 1534-42.

402. Alcolado JC, Alcolado R. Importance of maternal history of non-insulin dependent diabetic patients. Br Med J 1991; 302: 1178-80.

403. Janssen RC, Bogardus C, Takeda J, Knowler WC, Thompson DB. Linkage analysis of acute insulin secretion with GLUT2 and glucokinase in Pima Indians and the identification of a mis-sense mutation in GLUT2. Diabetes 1994; 43: 558-63.

404. Baroni MG, Alcolado JC, Needham EWA, Pozzilli P, Stocks J, Galton DJ. Sib-pair analysis of adenosine deaminase locus in NIDDM. Diabetes 1992; 41: 1640-3.

405. O'Rahilly S, Krook A, Morgan R, Rees A, Flier JS, Moller DE. Insulin-responsive glucose transporter (GLUT4) mutations and polymorphisms in a Welsh type 2 (non-insulin-dependent) diabetic population. Diabetologia 1992; 35: 486-9.

406. Bjørbaek C, Echwald SM, Hubricht P, Vestergaard H, Hansen T, Zierath J, Pedersen O. Genetic variants in promoters and coding regions of the muscle glycogen synthase and the insulin-responsive GLUT4 genes in NIDDM. Diabetes 1994; 43: 976-83.

407. Eriksson J, Koranyi L, Bourey R, Schalin-Jäntti C, Widén E, Mueckler M et al. Insulin resistance in type 2 (non-insulin-dependent) diabetic patients and their relatives is not associated with a defect in the expression of the insulin-responsive glucose transporter (GLUT-4) gene in human skeletal muscle [published erratum appears in Diabetologia 1992(Jun); 35: 594]. Diabetologia 1992; 35: 143-7.

408. Thomas F, Balkau B, Vauzelle-Kervroedan F, Papoz L; CODIAB-INSERM-ZENECA Study Group. Maternal effect and familial aggregation in NIDDM. Diabetes 1994; 43: 63-7.

409. Koranyi LI, Tanizawa Y, Welling CM, Rabin DU, Permutt MA. Human islet glucokinase gene. Isolation and sequence analysis of full-length cDNA. Diabetes 1992; 41: 807-11.

410. Chiu KC, Province MA, Dowse GK, Zimmet PZ, Wagner G, Serjeantson S, Permutt MA. A genetic marker at the glucokinase gene locus for type 2 (non-insulin-dependent) diabetes mellitus in Mauritian Creoles. Diabetologia 1992; 35: 632-8.

411. Chiu KC, Province MA, Permutt MA. Glucokinase gene is genetic marker for NIDDM in American blacks. Diabetes 1992; 41: 843-9.

412. Noda K, Matsutani A, Tanizawa Y, Neuman R, Kaneko T, Permutt MA, Kaku K. Polymorphic microsatellite repeat markers at the glucokinase gene locus are positively associated with NIDDM in Japanese. Diabetes 1993; 42: 1147-52.

413. Tanizawa Y, Chiu KC, Province MA, Morgan R, Owens DR, Rees A, Permutt MA. Two microsatellite repeat polymorphisms flanking opposite ends of the human glucokinase gene: use in haplotype analysis of Welsh Caucasians with type 2 (non-insulin-dependent) diabetes mellitus. Diabetologia 1993; 36: 409-13.

414. McCarthy MI, Hitman GA, Hitchins M, Riikonen A, Stengård J, Nissinen A et al. Glucokinase gene polymorphisms: a genetic marker for glucose intolerance in a cohort of elderly Finnish men. Diabet Med 1994; 11: 198-204.

415. Elbein SC, Hoffman M, Chiu K, Tanizawa Y, Permutt MA. Linkage analysis of the glucokinase locus in familial type 2 (non-insulin-dependent) diabetic pedigrees. Diabetologia 1993; 36: 141-5.

416. Cook JT, Hattersley AT, Christopher P, Bown E, Barrow B, Patel P et al. Linkage analysis of glucokinase gene with NIDDM in Caucasian pedigrees. Diabetes 1992; 41: 1496-500.

417. Zouali H, Vaxillaire M, Lesage S, Sun F, Velho G, Vionnet N et al. Linkage analysis and molecular scanning of glucokinase gene in NIDDM families. Diabetes 1993; 42: 1238-45.

418. Wu DA, Bu X, Shen D, Fuh M, Warden CH, Reaven GM et al. The glucokinase locus is an important contributor to glucose variation in the Chinese population at high risk for type II diabetes. Am J Hum Genet 1994; 55: A208.

419. Chiu KC, Tanizawa Y, Permutt MA. Glucokinase gene variants in the common form of NIDDM. Diabetes 1993; 42: 579-82.

420. Nishi S, Hinata S, Matsukage T, Takeda J, Ichiyama A, Bell GI, Yoshimi T. Mutations in the glucokinase gene are not a major cause of late-onset type 2 (non-insulin-dependent) diabetes mellitus in Japanese subjects. Diabet Med 1994; 11: 193-7.

421. Eto K, Sakura H, Shimokawa K, Kadowaki H, Hagura R, Akanuma Y et al. Sequence variations of the glucokinase gene in Japanese subjects with NIDDM. Diabetes 1993; 42: 1133-7.

422. Shimokawa K, Sakura H, Otabe S, Eto K, Kadowaki H, Hagura P et al. Analysis of the glucokinase gene promoter in Japanese subjects with non-insulin-dependent diabetes mellitus. J Clin Endocrinol Metab 1994; 79: 883-6.

423. Katagiri H, Asano T, Ishihara H, Inukai K, Anai M, Miyazaki J et al. Non-sense mutation of glucokinase gene in late-onset non-insulin-dependent diabetes mellitus. Lancet 1992; 340: 1316-17.

424. Shimada F, Makino H, Hashimoto N, Taira M, Seino S, Bell GI et al. Type 2 (non-insulin-dependent) diabetes mellitus associated with a mutation of the glucokinase gene in a Japanese family. Diabetologia 1993; 36: 433–7.

425. Bennett PH, Knowler WC, Pettitt DJ, Carraher MJ, Vasquesz B. Longitudinal studies of the development of diabetes in the Pima Indians. In Escheg E (ed.) Diabetes Epidemiol INSERM Symposium No. 22. New York: Elsevier 1982; 65–74.

426. Lee TD, Zhao T, Chi Z, Wong H, Shen M, Rodey G. HLA-A, B, and HLA-DR phenotypes in mainland Chinese patients with diabetes mellitus. Tissue Antigens 1983; 22: 92–5.

427. Omar MAK, Hammond MG, Motala AA, Seedat MA. HLA Class I and II antigens in South African Indians with NIDDM. Diabetes 1988; 37: 796–9.

428. Serjeantson SW, Ryan DP, Zimmet P. HLA and non-insulin dependent diabetes in Fiji Indians. Med J Australia 1981; 1: 462–4.

429. Serjeantson SW, Ryan DP, Zimmet P, Taylor R, Cross R, Charpin M, Gonidec G. HLA antigens in four Pacific populations with non-insulin dependent diabetes mellitus. Ann Hum Biol 1982; 9: 69–84.

430. Serjeantson SW, Owerbach D, Zimmet P, Nerup J, Thoma K. Genetics of diabetes in Nauru: effects of foreign admixture, HLA antigens, and insulin-gene linked polymorphism. Diabetologia 1983; 25: 13–5.

431. Williams RC, Knowler WC, Butler WJ, Pettitt DJ, Lisse JR, Bennett PH et al. HLA-A2 and type 2 (insulin-independent) diabetes mellitus in Pima Indians: an association of allele frequency with age. Diabetologia 1981; 21: 460–3.

432. Tuomilehto-Wolf E, Tuomilehto J, Hitman GA, Nissinen A, Stengard J, Pekkanen J et al. Genetic susceptibility to non-insulin dependent diabetes mellitus and glucose intolerance are located in HLA region. Br Med J 1993; 307: 155–9.

433. Banerji MA, Lebovitz HE. Insulin-sensitive and insulin-resistant variants in NIDDM. Diabetes 1989; 38: 784–92.

434. Banerji MA, Chaiken RL, Norin AJ, Lebovitz HE. HLA-DQ associations distinguish insulin-resistant and insulin-sensitive variants of NIDDM in black Americans. Diabetes Care 1993; 16: 429–33.

435. Tuomi T, Groop LC, Zimmet PZ, Rowley MJ, Knowles W, Mackay IR. Antibodies to glutamic acid decarboxylase reveal latent autoimmune diabetes mellitus in adults with a non-insulin-dependent onset of disease. Diabetes 1993; 42: 359–62.

436. Acton RT, Roseman JM, Bell DS, Goldenberg RL, Tseng ML, Vanichanan C et al. Genes within the major histocompatibility complex predict NIDDM in African-American women in Alabama. Diabetes Care 1994; 17: 1491–4.

437. Rich SS, French LR, Sprafka JM, Clements JP, Goetz FC. HLA-associated susceptibility to type 2 (non-insulin-dependent) diabetes mellitus: the Wadena city health study. Diabetologia 1993; 36: 234–8.

438. Wagener DK, Sacks JM, LaPorte RE, Macgregor JM. The Pittsburg study of insulin-dependent diabetes mellitus. Risk for diabetes among relatives of IDDM. Diabetes 1982; 31: 1115–18.

439. Rich SS, Panter SS, Goetz FC, Hedlund B, Barbosa J. Shared genetic susceptibility of type 1 (insulin-dependent) and type 2 (non-insulin-dependent) diabetes mellitus: contributions of HLA and haptoglobin. Diabetologia 1991; 34: 350–5.

440. Dahlen G, Berg K. Pre-beta 1-lipoprotein and Lp(a) antigen in relation to triglyceride levels and insulin release following an oral glucose load in middle-aged males. Acta Med Scand 1976; 199: 413–19.

441. Dahlen G, Berg K. Confirmation of an influence of the inherited Lp(a) variation on serum insulin and glucose levels. Clin Genet 1979; 16: 418–27.

442. Buraczynska M, Hanzlik J, Grzywa M. Apolipoprotein A-I gene polymorphism and susceptibility of non-insulin-dependent diabetes mellitus. Am J Hum Genet 1985; 37: 1129–37.

443. McKusick VA. Mendelian inheritance in man, 11th edn. Baltimore: Johns Hopkins University Press, 1994.

444. Raffel LJ, Scheuner MT, Rimoin DL, Rotter JI. Diabetes mellitus. In Rimoin DL, Connor JM, Pyeritz RE, Emery AEH (eds) Principles and practice of medical genetics, 3rd edn. London: Churchill Livingstone, 1996.

445. Rotter JI, Landaw EM. Measuring the genetic contribution of a single locus to a multilocus disease. Clin Genet 1984; 24: 529–42.

446. Alcolado JC, Baroni MG, Li SR. Association between a restriction fragment length polymorphism at the liver/islet cell (GluT2) glucose transporter and familial Type 2 (non-insulin-dependent) diabetes mellitus. Diabetologia 1991; 34: 734–6.

447. Baroni MG, Oelbaum RS, Pozzilli P, Stocks J, Li SR, Fiore V et al. Polymorphisms at the GLUT1 (hepG2) and GLUT4 (muscle/adipocyte) glucose transporter genes and non-insulin-dependent diabetes mellitus (NIDDM). Hum Genet 1992; 88: 557–61.

448. Mitchell BD, Reinhart L. No evidence for excess maternal transmission of NIDDM in Mexican Americans. Diabetes 1994; 43 (suppl 1): 26A.

4

Epidemiology of Insulin Dependent Diabetes Mellitus

A. Sekikawa and R.E. LaPorte

Department of Epidemiology, University of Pittsburgh, Pennsylvania, USA

More is now known about the epidemiology of IDDM than about the epidemiology of almost any other chronic disease. The disease is being accurately monitored in more countries than any other chronic disease, and we know more about the temporal trends in incidence for this disorder than for almost any other disease. Ten years ago, almost nothing was known, so it is worth documenting the changes which have transformed this subject in the intervening period.

HISTORICAL BACKGROUND

In the early 1980s little was known concerning the epidemiology worldwide of IDDM, particularly in childhood. It was clear that this was an important and costly disorder, yet we did not even know how frequently it occurred. In the USA, for example, there were few data, and the data which were available were not standardized, and thus not directly comparable [1, 2]. This was also the case in other countries, with almost no data available [3, 4].

The turning-point came when the Juvenile Diabetes Foundation sponsored a meeting in Philadelphia to review what was known concerning the epidemiology of childhood diabetes in 1983. Results presented at the meeting hinted at remarkable global variation in incidence of the disease, and suggested that the disease could easily be studied cross-culturally.

It was recognized at that meeting how important registries would be for the investigation of the epidemiology of IDDM. A simple set of criteria was developed for the registries: cases were to be under the age of 15 years at onset, diagnosed as having diabetes, on insulin at the time of diagnosis, and a resident of a defined community [5]. This definition of childhood diabetes has proved to be remarkably easy to implement, and robust even in the poorest country. The disease lends itself to the development of registries: children who develop the disease are easily recognized; the symptoms are easily identifiable; and the disease can easily be confirmed with a simple blood or urine test. In addition, the disease is severe, so that children will come to medical attention (because their mothers are afraid) but it is not so severe that cases typically die immediately at onset, before receiving medical attention. This may, however, occur in some developing countries or where access to medical care is difficult. Also, it is a 'countable' disease, as it is frequent but not too frequent. Thus, a dedicated person—even working alone—can develop a registry.

The findings that stimulated interest at the meeting in 1983 are presented again here. The enormous international variation of the disease was recognized: a child in Finland was almost 40 times more likely to develop the disease than a child in Japan [5]. Investigators soon wanted to know where their country would fit onto the graph, and registries started to proliferate.

The second big event occurred when the WHO Multinational Project for Childhood Diabetes (*Diabète Mondiale*, DiaMond) was approved in Geneva [6]. The WHO DiaMond project reduced the potential political

International Textbook of Diabetes Mellitus, Second Edition. Edited by K.G.M.M. Alberti, P. Zimmet, R.A. DeFronzo, and H. Keen (Honorary)
© 1997 John Wiley & Sons Ltd

problems of the global program. Also, the image of the research effort was raised, and this permitted more people to join, and to raise local resources to develop the registration systems. Registration has grown enormously over the 20-year life of IDDM epidemiology, and the 6-year life of the WHO DiaMond project. Currently there are over 150 centers in over 70 countries [7]. The registries range in size from those monitoring the incidence of IDDM in less than 50 000 children to an enormous registry in China monitoring IDDM incidence in over 23 million children (representing 25% of the children in China).

GEOGRAPHIC VARIATION IN IDDM

The finding of variation around the world was exciting. The first area of development has been that of mapping out the geographic variation of the disease. Figure 1 presents the latest information available concerning geographic variations of the incidence and mortality of chronic diseases [8–11]. Some of these diseases show remarkable variation, over 300-fold for liver cancer. IDDM is one of the few chronic diseases where a 300-fold difference in risk has been confirmed [8, 9]. The place where a child lives is one of the most potent determinants of risk of the disease. If we knew why

there was such a variation, we might understand why people develop the disease.

We can look at the geographic variation by region, as presented in Figure 2. In every region there is remarkable variation, even in Asia where the incidence is low.

Marked variation has also been found within racial groups (except for Japanese). For Europids, the variation is fivefold [5]; for blacks, threefold [5, 12–14]. Variations in Chinese are also high [9]. It thus appears that across almost all racial and ethnic groups there is geographic variation in the incidence of the disease.

ETIOLOGY OF IDDM: GENES AND ENVIRONMENT

With childhood diabetes, as with all other chronic diseases, there is continuing interest in the relative contributions of genes and the environment in producing disease. Analyses have not been specifically targeted towards the identification of the type of factor responsible for the development of IDDM, but rather the degree to which two distinct groups of factors, genetic and environmental, contribute to the development of the disease.

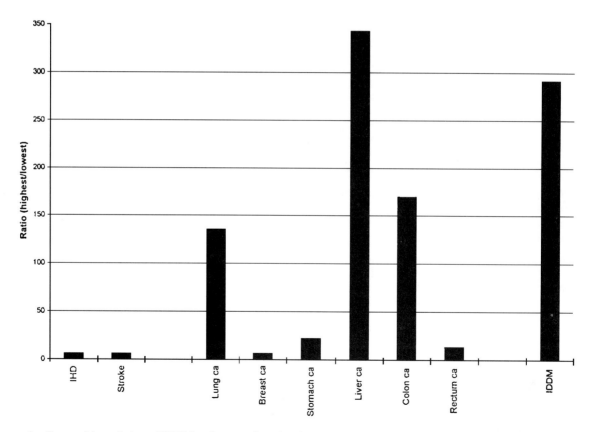

Figure 1 Geographic variation of IDDM and some other chronic diseases. Highest incidence over lowest incidence shown for IDDM and cancer (data from references 8, 9, 11). Highest mortality over lowest mortality shown for ischemic heart disease (IHD) and stroke (data from reference 10)

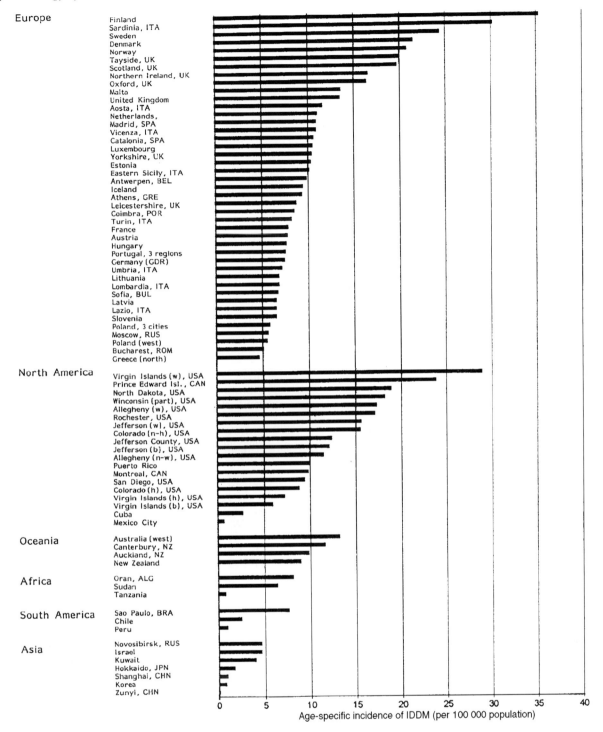

Figure 2 Geographic variation of IDDM by region. Abbreviations: w, white; n-w, non-white; n-h, non-hispanic; b, black (data from references 8 and 9)

Twin Studies

One method has been to evaluate twin studies. The latest twin studies from Finland [15] and Denmark [16] from the twin registries present a somewhat different set of findings. In Finland, the concordance rate of identical twins was greater than that for fraternal twins (23% vs. 5%). In Denmark, the concordance rate for identical twins was also greater than that for non-identical twins (53% vs. 11%). The frequency differed across the two studies, perhaps as a result of small numbers, but the results are consistent with a major

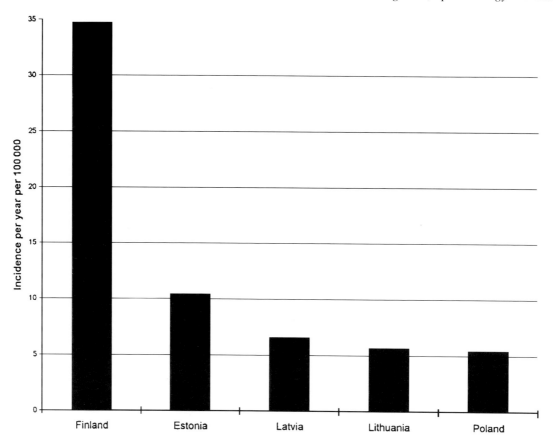

Figure 3   Incidence of IDDM in five Baltic countries (from reference 17, with permission)

contribution of the environment to the development of diabetes.

Geographic Variation Among Similar Ethnic Groups

The IDDM registries also present graphic evidence for the role of the environment in the etiology of IDDM. As presented in Figure 3, the incidence of disease in the Baltic Countries varies dramatically [17]. The Estonians are genetically very similar to the Finns, whereas the Latvians and Lithuanians are more similar to middle Europe. When the incidence rates were determined, it was clear that the incidence of disease amongst the Estonians was considerably lower than that of the Finnish. However, this does not rule out the important contribution of genetics, as the incidence of IDDM among native Estonians was greater than for Russian children who lived in Estonia [18], as well as being greater than the incidence of the disease in Latvia and Lithuania.

Migration

Further evidence for environmental factors comes from data on incidence of IDDM within migrant populations,

as compared with incidence in their native country (Figure 4). Such migrant studies demonstrate a powerful effect of migration, that varies by racial and ethnic group [18–21]. In some cases, as with Jewish children in Canada, there is an almost fourfold greater incidence in the migrant population. In other comparisons the effect is smaller, but still very evident. A fourfold increase with migration would represent one of the most powerful migratory effects for any disease, and would imply a powerful environmental agent.

Temporal Trends

Evidence for the contribution of environmental agents also comes from studies of temporal trends. There is little question that IDDM exhibits strong temporal trends. This does not fit with a purely genetic disease. The pattern of change has typically been a steadily increasing incidence. A second pattern would be an increase punctuated by sharp epidemics. Most North European countries have exhibited the former pattern, with a steady rise in incidence [8, 22]. The annual change in Sweden [23] and Norway [24] is 3.3%, in Finland 2.4% [25]. Outside Europe we see epidemics of the disease [8, 14, 26, 27]. Figure 5 presents evidence for one such epidemic [14]. What is striking about the

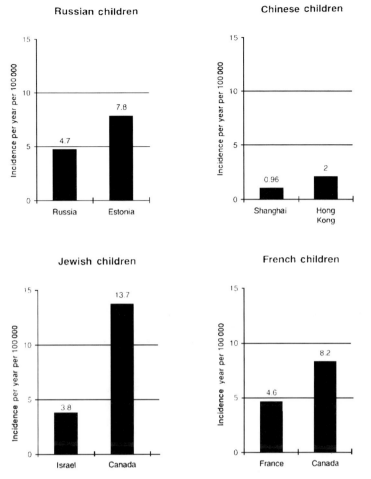

Figure 4   Incidence of IDDM in native and adopted countries (data from references 18–21)

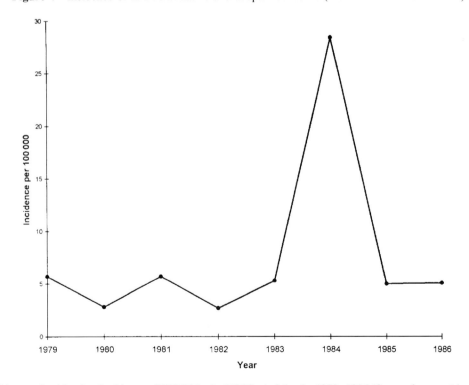

Figure 5   Evidence of epidemics. Incidence of IDDM in the US Virgin Islands, 1979–1986 (from reference 14, with permission)

epidemics is that for most chronic diseases epidemics do not appear, yet for IDDM there can be a doubling of the incidence in only a year or two, something unheard of for most chronic conditions.

We thus know much about the descriptive epidemiology of childhood diabetes. Disappointingly, despite having much data on the geographic and temporal trends of the disease, we still know little about what is driving the patterns. Some clues have been provided, but not enough.

We have argued that it is in the epidemics that we will find the answer to the environmental factors causing the disease. Epidemics exist, and they are frequent. However, by the time they are identified, 1–5 years afterwards, the environmental agents causing the disease are long since past. We thus need widespread and timely monitoring of IDDM [26]. Perhaps registries need to be supplemented by alternative means to obtain wider coverage, more accurately.

It would appear that the development of local to national IDDM monitoring systems is the means for early identification of IDDM epidemics. There are few national systems: they exist only in Norway, Sweden, Finland, Austria, Cuba, Chile, plus a few more countries. However, the registration approach will not work in larger countries where the incidence is high, such as the USA. Therefore a new approach to disease monitoring using capture–recapture may be the best means by which rapid disease monitoring can take place [28, 29].

Seasonal Variation

In addition to the temporal trends in disease, there is a fascinating seasonal pattern [8, 30, 31] as presented in Figure 6. In practically all registries there is a decline in the incidence of the disease during the warm summer months. The seasonal pattern is quite consistent, with about a 10–15% dip during the summer time. The reason for this dip has never been explained, although infectious agents, nutrition or hormonal cycles have been suggested.

Age at Onset

The age-at-onset pattern also appears universal for IDDM, with one notable exception. In general, during childhood there is an increase in the incidence with increasing age. Some countries exhibit an increase at about age 4–5 years, whereas others do not. Almost all show an increase to the age of puberty, followed by a steep decline. The exception is that of Finland. The pattern in Finland in the early years of the registry was as presented above. However, now that the

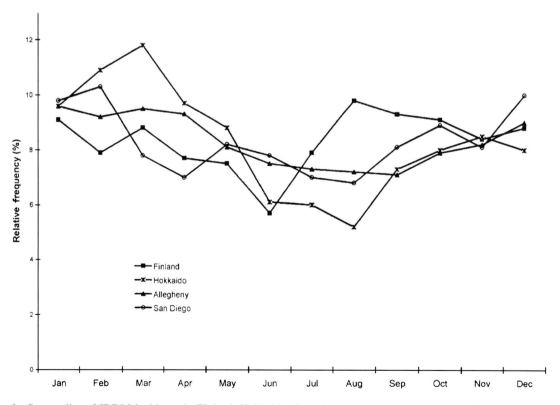

Figure 6 Seasonality of IDDM incidence in Finland, Hokkaido (Japan), Allegheny (USA) and San Diego (USA) (data from references 8, 30, 31)

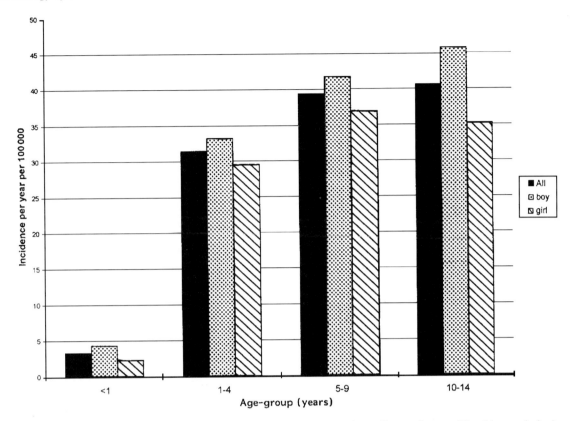

Figure 7   Incidence of IDDM in Finland by age-group (years) and sex (from reference 25, with permission)

age-specific incidence has risen to over 35 per 100 000, the age-at-onset pattern of the disease has changed, with even very young children having an incidence not much different from children at puberty [25]. Whatever is increasing the incidence of IDDM in Finland is also flattening out the age-at-onset curve (Figure 7).

THE FUTURE OF IDDM EPIDEMIOLOGY

At the end of this century we will have the results of the WHO Multinational Project for Childhood Diabetes, with the incidence monitored for a decade in over 70 different countries. It is then that we will have the largest study ever completed on a non-communicable disease. We will know how the incidence of disease has changed this decade, and should be able to extrapolate into the future.

It is to be hoped that by then we will have been able to 'catch' several epidemics and identify the causative agents producing the disease.

These registries are also proving to be rich material for molecular epidemiologic studies as developed by Dorman [32], and for studies of the epidemiology of the complications of diabetes, as developed by Orchard. They will be especially important for prevention trials, as the incidence will have been defined.

REFERENCES

1. Sultz HA, Schlesinger ER, Mosher WE, Feldman JG. Long-term childhood illness. Pittsburgh: University of Pittsburgh Press, 1972; 223–48.
2. Palumbo PJ, Elveback LR, Chu CP, Connolly DC, Kurland LT. Diabetes mellitus: incidence, prevalence, survivorship and causes of death in Rochester, Minnesota, 1945–1970. Diabetes 1976; 25: 566–73.
3. Reunanen A, Akerblom HK, Kaar ML. Prevalence and ten-year (1970–1979) incidence of insulin-dependent diabetes mellitus in children and adolescents in Finland. Acta Paediatr Scand 1982; 71: 893–9.
4. Ustvedt HJ, Olsen E. Incidence of diabetes mellitus in Oslo, Norway 1956–65. Br J Prev Soc Med 1977; 31: 251–7.
5. LaPorte RE, Tajima N, Akerblom HK, Berlin N, Brosseau J, Christy M et al. Geographic differences in the risk of insulin-dependent diabetes mellitus: the importance of registries. Diabetes Care 1985; 8 (suppl. 1): 101–7.
6. WHO Diamond Project Group. WHO multinational project for childhood diabetes. Diabetes Care 1990; 13: 1062–8.
7. LaPorte RE, Matsushima M, Chang Y. Prevalence and incidence of insulin-dependent diabetes. In Harris MI, Cowie CC, Stern MP, Boyko E, Reiber GE, Bennett PH (eds) Diabetes in America. Bethesda: National Diabetes Data Group, NIH publ. no. 95-1468, 1995: 37–46.
8. Karvonen M, Tuomilehto J, Libman I, LaPorte R for the World Health Organization DiaMond Project Group. A review of the recent epidemiological data on

the worldwide incidence of type 1 (insulin-dependent) diabetes mellitus. Diabetologia 1993; 36: 883–92.

9. Sino–US Diabetes Epidemiology Research Group. Ascertainment corrected IDDM incidence rates (95% CI) in 21 areas in China in WHO DiaMond project in China. (Personal communication).

10. Anthony PP. Cardiovascular disease. In Racial and ethnic differences in disease. Oxford: Oxford University Press, 1989: 125–67.

11. Anthony PP. Cancers. In Racial and ethnic differences in disease. Oxford: Oxford University Press, 1989; 168–224.

12. Rewers M, LaPorte RE, King H, Tuomilehto J. Trends in the prevalence and incidence of diabetes: insulin-dependent diabetes mellitus in childhood. Wld Health Statist Q 1988; 41: 179–89.

13. Lipman TH. The epidemiology of type 1 diabetes in children 0–14 years of age in Philadelphia. Diabetes Care 1993; 16: 922–5.

14. Tull ES, Roseman JM, Christian CLE. Epidemiology of childhood IDDM in U.S. Virgin Islands from 1979 to 1988. Diabetes Care 1991; 14: 558–64.

15. Kaprio J, Tuomilehto J, Koskenvuo M, Romanov K, Reunanen A, Eriksson J et al. Concordance for type 1 (insulin-dependent) and type 2 (non-insulin-dependent) diabetes mellitus in a population-based cohort of twins in Finland. Diabetologia 1992; 35: 1060–7.

16. Kyvik KO, Green A, Beck-Nielsen H. Concordance rates of insulin dependent diabetes mellitus: a population based study of young Danish twins. Br Med J 1995; 311: 913–17.

17. Tuomilehto J, Podar T, Brigis G, Urbonaite B, Rewers M, Adojaan B, et al. Comparison of the incidence of insulin-dependent diabetes mellitus in childhood among five Baltic populations during 1983–1988. Int J Epidemiol 1992; 21: 518–27.

18. Podar T, LaPorte RE, Tuomilehto J, Shubnikov E. Risk of childhood type 1 diabetes for Russians in Estonia and Siberia. Int J Epidemiol 1993; 22: 262–7.

19. Diabetes Epidemiology Research Institute. Preventing insulin dependent diabetes mellitus: the environmental challenge. Br Med J 1987; 295: 479–81.

20. Gary WKW, Sophei SFL, Stephen JO. Epidemiology of IDDM in Southern Chinese children in Hong Kong. Diabetes Care 1993; 16: 926–8.

21. Hua F, Shui-xian S, Zhao-wen C, Jia-jun W, Ting-ting Y, LaPorte RE, Tajima N. Shanghai, China, has the lowest confirmed incidence of childhood diabetes in the world. Diabetes Care 1994; 17: 1206–8.

22. Diabetes Epidemiology Research International Group. Secular trends in incidence of childhood IDDM in 10 countries. Diabetes 1990; 39: 858–64.

23. Dahlquist G, Blom L, Holmgren G, Hagglof B, Larsson Y, Sterky G, Wall S. The epidemiology of diabetes in Swedish children 0–14 years—a six-year prospective study. Diabetologia 1985; 28: 802–8.

24. Joner G, Sovik O. Incidence, age at onset and seasonal variation of diabetes mellitus in Norwegian children. Acta Paediatr Scand 1981; 70: 329–35.

25. Tuomilehto J, Lounamaa R, Tuomilehto-Wolf E, Reunanen A, Virtala E, Kaprio A, Akerblom HK and the Childhood Diabetes in Finland (DiMe) Study Group. Epidemiology of childhood diabetes mellitus in Finland—background of a nationwide study of type 1 (insulin-dependent) diabetes mellitus. Diabetologia 1992; 35: 70–6.

26. WHO DiaMond Project Group on Epidemics. Childhood diabetes, epidemics and epidemiology: an approach for controlling diabetes. Am J Epidemiol 1992; 135: 803–16.

27. Dokheel TM for the Pittsburgh Diabetes Epidemiology Research Group. An epidemic of childhood diabetes in the United States? Evidence from Allegheny County, PA. Diabetes Care 1993; 16: 1606–11.

28. Fienberg SE. The multiple recapture census for closed populations and incomplete 2k contingency tables. Biometrics 1972; 59: 591–603.

29. Green A, Gale EAM, Patterson CC for the EURODIAB ACE study. Incidence of childhood-onset insulin-dependent diabetes mellitus: the EURODIAB ACE study. Lancet 1992; 339: 905–9.

30. Karvonen M, Tuomilehto J, Virtala E, Pitkaniemi J, Reunanen A, Tuomilehto-Wolf E, Akerblom KA for the Childhood Diabetes in Finland (DiMe) Study Group. Seasonality in the clinical onset of insulin-dependent diabetes mellitus in Finnish children. Am J Epidemiol 1996; 143: 167–76.

31. Tajima N, LaPorte RE. Incidence of IDDM outside Europe. In Levy-Marchal C, Czernichow P (eds) Epidemiology and etiology of insulin-dependent diabetes in the young. Basel: Karger, 1992: 31–41.

32. Dorman JS. Genetic epidemiology of insulin-dependent diabetes mellitus: international comparisons using molecular genetics. Ann Med 1992; 24: 393–9.

5

Immunopathogenesis of Type 1 Diabetes in Western Society

Francesco Dotta* and George S. Eisenbarth†

*University of Rome, La Sapienza, Rome, Italy, and †University of Colorado Health Sciences Center, Denver, Colorado, USA

Type 1 diabetes mellitus or insulin dependent diabetes is becoming one of the most intensively studied autoimmune disorders. The intensity of study probably reflects the existence of (a) many individuals with the disease (e.g. 0.3% of the US population), and (b) two excellent animal models (the BB rat and NOD mouse). The disease is characterized by the selective destruction of the pancreatic islet insulin-producing cells. This destruction results in a series of complex metabolic aberrations associated with long-term sequelae with significant morbidity and mortality. Once considered a disease of acute onset, there is now compelling evidence that type 1 diabetes is a genetically determined chronic autoimmune disorder with a long subclinical prodromal phase [1]. The prodromal phase, which begins in genetically susceptible individuals, can last for years and is associated with a series of immunologic and metabolic abnormalities. Some of these abnormalities can be used to detect those individuals at high risk of developing type 1 diabetes. Over the past 5 years there has been a dramatic increase in the biochemical identification of islet autoantigens and in the definition of alleles associated with diabetes susceptibility. With increasing ability to predict the disorder, trials for the prevention of type 1 diabetes have begun.

STAGES IN THE DEVELOPMENT OF THE DISEASE.

Progression to overt type 1 diabetes can be divided into distinct stages starting with genetic susceptibility. In genetically susceptible subjects, a precipitating event (either mutational or environmental) presumably triggers the autoimmune attack against the pancreatic B cells. The presence at this stage of antibodies directed against islet-related antigens, including islet cell antibodies (ICA) [2], anti-insulin autoantibodies (IAA) [3], anti-64 kDa protein antibodies [4], anti-ICA69 [5] and anti-ICA512 [39], can be used for the detection of individuals at high risk of developing the disease. With the progression of the islet destructive process, besides the immune abnormalities, individuals show a progressive loss of first-phase insulin release (as shown by intravenous glucose tolerance testing). During the early phases of loss of insulin secretion individuals are still euglycemic [6]. Impaired insulin secretion is one of the first metabolic aberrations to occur during the 'preclinical' phase of the disease. In the 18 months preceding the clinical onset of the disease, a subclinical rise of blood glucose levels is frequently detected [6]. The loss of first-phase insulin release is followed by hyperglycemia and the clinical onset of the disease. C-peptide secretion can still be

International Textbook of Diabetes Mellitus, Second Edition. Edited by K.G.M.M. Alberti, P. Zimmet, R.A. DeFronzo, and H. Keen (Honorary)
© 1997 John Wiley & Sons Ltd

present for a period following the onset of diabetes, but ends once the autoimmune process destroys the remaining islet B cells.

GENETIC FACTORS

The autoimmune destruction of pancreatic B cells has been documented in three different species: man, non-obese diabetic (NOD) mouse and Bio-Breeding (BB) rat. In all three species at least one diabetogenic gene within the major histocompatibility complex (MHC) is necessary for the development of the disease [7, 8, 9, 10]. Among type 1 diabetic patients, 95% are HLA-DR3 and/or -DR4 positive compared to the 40% of the general population [10]. Conversely, the haplo-type DR2 is negatively associated with the occurrence of the disease, since HLA-DR2-positive type 1 diabetics are rare [11]. It is also noteworthy that type 1 diabetic patients expressing the DR2 haplotype have unusual DQβ gene sequences that are positively correlated with type 1 diabetes susceptibility. (On the island of Sardinia a haplotype associated with type 1 diabetes consists of DR2, DQA1*0102, DQB1*0502. We have reported the HLA typing for three brothers in a single family with type 1 diabetes and DR2, DQA1*0101, DQB1*0402.) Consequently, nearly all individuals developing this disease express a diabetes-associated class II gene. Most type 1 diabetic subjects express both DR3 and DR4. DR4-associated haplotypes can be subdivided by DQB typing, with DQB1*0302 a high risk allele and DQB1*0301 of moderate risk. The DR4 haplotype is more common in younger diabetic individuals and it is associated with the presence of anti-insulin autoantibodies. DR3 is primarily associated with type 1 diabetes in Europids and in American Blacks.

Recently, it has been proposed that HLA-DQ might be even closer to the HLA-linked susceptibility gene than HLA-DR. With nucleotide sequences now available each polymorphic allele is assigned a number for its DQA and DQB chain. Polymorphism of the HLA-DQβ chain at position 57 might play a role in determining susceptibility or resistance to the development of type 1 diabetes [12]. In Europids, alanine, valine and serine at residue 57 are present in DQβ alleles positively associated with type 1 diabetes. Conversely, an aspartic acid at this position has negative or neutral association with the disease. Interestingly, the I-Aβ gene (the murine equivalent to the human DQ) of the NOD mouse has a serine at position 57. Most other mouse strains have an aspartic acid at position 57. However, the presence in Oriental populations of a diabetogenic HLA-DQβ allele that has an aspartic acid at residue 57 suggests that the negative association between the occurrence of type 1 diabetes and the presence of this amino acid at residue 57 is not absolute. Although the protective allele DQB1*0602 has aspartic acid at position 57, its protective effect (dominantly expressed) greatly exceeds that of other Asp57 alleles (e.g. DQB1*0301). Sheehy et al have presented evidence that alleles at both DQ and DR are essential for diabetes susceptibility [13].

Genes outside the MHC complex are necessary for the development of the disease. Within families, the risk of developing type 1 diabetes is not equal among siblings and depends also on the number of HLA haplotypes shared with the proband. Among sibling pairs with type 1 diabetes, approximately 60% share both HLA haplotypes, 37% share one haplotype and fewer than 5% share none. The risk for developing type 1 diabetes in the second of identical twins varies between 30 and 50%. Approximately 40% of the offspring of two type 1 diabetics develop diabetes, but only 17% of siblings HLA-identical to a sibling with type 1 diabetes become diabetic. These data suggest the presence of a diabetogenic gene outside the major histocompatibility complex (MHC).

Several studies clearly indicate that polymorphisms of the insulin gene on chromosome 11 are associated with diabetes risk [14]. These polymorphisms are outside the coding region of the gene. The specific polymorphism determining diabetes risk is most likely a region 5' to the insulin gene consisting of repetitive DNA sequences [40, 41]. Polymorphisms of the insulin gene are non-randomly associated with each other (linkage disequilibrium) and thus haplotypes increased in patients with type 1 diabetes can be defined. Researchers identify a standard polymorphism of the insulin gene by PCR (polymerase chain reaction) amplification of sequences 3' of the insulin gene, followed by digestion of the DNA with the FOK restriction enzyme. By such FOK typing, individuals have either an A or B FOK allele. Approximately 90% of patients with type 1 diabetes are A/A homozygous compared with 60% of control populations. There are conflicting reports about whether there is imprinting of the insulin gene (i.e. differential influence of maternal vs. paternal inheritance). Studies from France and the USA [14, 15] (but not the UK) give strong evidence for maternal imprinting of the insulin gene. The B allele only 'protects' from type 1 diabetes when inherited from one's father and not one's mother. We speculate that this genetic effect of the insulin gene may relate to expression of insulin in the thymus. Expression of insulin within the thymus of individuals with B haplotypes would be imprinted (suppressed) by maternal inheritance.

It is likely that additional genetic loci will influence diabetes susceptibility. The biochemical and computational tools are now available to search for such additional genes. National repositories with DNA from multiplex families are now available to interested investigators. Non-MHC genes may not only determine diabetes susceptibility in an autosomal dominant pattern, but also influence the age of onset of the disease, and a series of potential loci are being identified [42, 43]. Besides classical type 1 diabetes, pancreatic B cell dysfunction takes place in several genetic disorders including trisomy 21 (Down's syndrome) and Wolfram's syndrome. Down's syndrome shows a very high incidence of type 1 diabetes and of other autoimmune disorders [16]. The gene(s) responsible for the autoimmune phenomena in these patients have not yet been identified, but the long arm of chromosome 21 contains genes determining levels of interferon receptors. Wolfram's syndrome or DIDMOAD syndrome (diabetes insipidus, diabetes mellitus, optic atrophy, deafness) is characterized by juvenile onset insulin dependent diabetes mellitus, optic atrophy, diabetes insipidus and neural deafness [17, 44]. Diabetes mellitus appears in virtually all patients, being usually also the first manifestation. Little is known about the specific cellular abnormalities associated with this syndrome. Pancreatic islets from Wolfram's syndrome patients show almost no insulin-containing cells, whereas cells producing glucagon, somatostatin and pancreatic polypeptide (PP) are regularly present, suggesting a selective loss of B cells. These histological findings, together with the lack of markers of an autoimmune process, suggest that this syndrome is caused by genetically programmed selective B-cell and neuronal death. To date we have observed only one patient with type 1 diabetes and the protective HLA alleles DQA1*0102/DQB1*0602. This individual has the autoimmune polyendocrine syndrome (APS) type 1 (mucocutaneous candidiasis, hypoparathyroidism, Addison's disease). Type 1 diabetic patients with DQB1*0602 are at increased risk of having one of the above rare genetic syndromes.

How diabetogenic gene products predispose to the development of the disease is so far unknown. These genes might impair the immune response (T cell deficiency, lack of tolerance to specific islet antigens) or induce the expression of polymorphic antigens on pancreatic B cells. Bottazzo et al suggested that in type 1 diabetes target cells (pancreatic B cells) express class II MHC molecules. However, in the animal models of type 1 diabetes (NOD mouse and BB rat), class II expression cannot be demonstrated in the early phases of the disease. In humans, class II-bearing islet cells have only been studied after the clinical onset of the disease, when the vast majority of B cells have already been destroyed. In addition, within the pancreas, class II expression can also be detected in the ductal cells, which clearly are not targets of autoimmunity.

AUTOIMMUNE POLYENDOCRINE SYNDROMES

Insulin dependent diabetes has been associated with over 20 different genetic disorders. The autoimmune polyendocrine syndromes (APS) [18] represent a group of endocrine and non-endocrine autoimmune diseases, often clustered in the same individual or in members of the same family. The study of these syndromes is important. There are similarities in the genetics and in the etiology of the different diseases, and treatment used for one disease might thus be applicable to the treatment of others.

Type 1 and 2 APS are the best characterized among these syndromes (Table 1). Only the type 2 APS is HLA-associated (DR3 and DR4) [19]; inheritance of type 1 APS is independent of HLA [45]. Type 1 APS occurs mainly in children. The syndrome is characterized by the presence of Addison's disease, idiopathic hypoparathyroidism and mucocutaneous candidiasis. Type 1 diabetes (4% of patients), chronic active hepatitis (13%), pernicious anemia (13%) and vitiligo (8%) can also be present in this syndrome. Type 1 diabetes, Addison's disease, autoimmune thyroid disease and myasthenia gravis are the most characteristic disorders in type 2 APS.

Table 1 Autoimmune disorders associated with type 1 and type 2 autoimmune polyendocrine syndrome

Type 1	Type 2
Addison's (67%)	Addison's (100%)*
Hypoparathyroidism (82%)	Hyperthyroidism (69%)
Mucocutaneous candidiasis (73%)	Hypothyroidism (69%)
Type 1 diabetes (5%)	Type 1 diabetes (52%)
Hypogonadism (17%)	Hypogonadism (3.5%)
Pernicious anemia (13%)	Pernicious anemia (?)
Vitiligo (8%)	Vitiligo (4.5%)
Chronic active hepatitis (13%)	

*By one definition of APS type 2.

Several organ-specific autoantibodies are associated with these two syndromes and assays for their determination vary in clinical utility. Antigastric, antimicrosomal and antithyroglobulin antibodies are not highly predictive of future disease, whereas a subset of islet cell antibodies (ICA), adrenal cortical antibodies, anti-endomysial antibodies (celiac disease) and steroidal cell antibodies are markers of subsequent disease. Islet cell antibodies usually disappear soon after disease onset in type 1 diabetics, whereas they persist for years in patients with type 2 APS. Type 1 diabetic patients have an increased risk of developing any of the other APS 2 diseases and have other circulating organ-specific autoantibodies, particularly antiparietal cell and antithyroid autoantibodies. Patients with the type 2 APS frequently express a form of cytoplasmic islet cell autoantibodies that are not highly predictive of future diabetes [20, 21]. This type of ICA has been termed 'restricted' (reacting with rat and human but not mouse islets), or 'selective' (reacting selectively with B cells within islets), and consists of high titers of autoantibodies reacting with the intracytoplasmic enzyme glutamic acid decarboxylase (GAD, formerly the 64K autoantigen). Such anti-GAD autoantibodies are similar to the antibodies found in patients with stiff man syndrome.

In addition to type 1 and 2 APS, other genetic disorders involving multiple endocrine organs include: (a) trisomy 21 with thyroiditis and diabetes; (b) Turner's syndrome with gonadal dysgenesis; and (c) POEMS syndrome—polyneuropathy, organomegaly, endocrinopathy (diabetes, hypogonadism), immunoglobulin-M spike—a disease where local irradiation of a plasmocytoma may lead to amelioration of the diabetes.

TRIGGERING EVENTS

Concordance for the development of type 1 diabetes of only 50% in identical twins has been proposed as evidence for the presence of environmental factors involved in initiating the autoimmune process. Congenital rubella infection is the only 'environmental' factor clearly linked with the development of type 1 diabetes. Such infection is also associated with other autoimmune endocrine disorders and with abnormalities in resting T-cell subsets [22]. The incidence of congenital rubella is very low and a clear epidemiologic association between type 1 diabetes and other viruses (mumps, Coxsackie B3 and B4, reovirus type 3, herpes viruses) has never been proven. Mechanisms of viral action might be direct B-cell destruction, or a cross-reactivity of viral and islet B-cell antigens resulting in B-cell destruction. Karounis et al have described a 52 kDa islet autoantigen, which reacts with a monoclonal antirubella virus antibody. Studies of the NOD mouse indicate that viral infections can also inhibit the development of diabetes.

Current knowledge of human genetics suggests that environmental factors are not obligatory for the development of type 1 diabetes. The enormous diversity of immunoglobulin and T-cell receptor genes is due to a stochastic process that combines genes to form complete antibody or T-cell receptor genes. This mechanism [generator of diversity, or GOD] explains why, as far as the differentiation of T and B lymphocytes is concerned, identical twins are no longer identical for key immunologic genes. The autoimmune B-cell destruction process might also be activated by a somatic mutation similar to that reported as the mechanism determining differential penetrance observed in selected hereditary cancers [23]. Hereditary retinoblastoma is due to an autosomal dominant gene on chromosome 13, but the disease affects only 85% and not the expected 100% of individuals carrying such a gene. Disease apparently only occurs if a somatic mutation inactivates the one normal gene in a single retinal cell that then results in a malignant clone of cells.

Environmental factors may influence the development of autoimmunity. In the last 40 years the global incidence of diabetes appears to have increased at a rate exceeding potential changes in the genetic pool leading to diabetes susceptibility. Currently, responsible environmental factors have not been identified but there is epidemiologic evidence that the introduction of bovine albumin into diets of young infants increases the risk of diabetes. It is hypothesized that the limited amino acid homologies between bovine albumin and the ICA69 islet autoantigen may contribute to the development of type 1 diabetes [24].

TARGET ANTIGENS

The presence of autoantibodies directed against islet antigens represents the hallmark of the humoral immune abnormalities associated with type 1 diabetes. Antibodies against a variety of islet-related antigens can be observed in the circulation well before the clinical onset of the disease (Figure 1), but only high-titer cytoplasmic ICA (>40 JDF units, see below), anti-insulin autoantibodies detected by radiobinding fluid phase assay, anti-GAD autoantibodies (formerly termed anti-64K antibodies), and antibodies to 37 kDa, 40 kDa autoantigen (ICA512/IA-2 and IA-2β) have shown enough diabetes-specificity to be used as markers of increased diabetes risk in first-degree relatives (Table 2).

Cytoplasmic Islet Cell Autoantibodies (ICA)

High-titer cytoplasmic ICA are present in 60–80% of new onset type 1 diabetics, in approximately 3% of first-degree relatives of patients with type 1 diabetes, and in 0.2% of the general population. They can be present in circulation years before the clinical onset of the disease. Cytoplasmic ICA are IgG antibodies which can react on frozen sections of human, rat or mouse pancreas (Figure 2). Cytoplasmic ICA which react with human and rat, but not mouse pancreas are usually high titer anti-GAD autoantibodies [20,

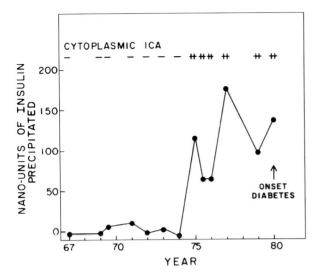

Figure 1 The appearance of insulin autoantibodies and of cytoplasmic islet cell antibodies in the monozygotic twin of a diabetic patient, 5 years before the onset of type 1 diabetes mellitus. In 1975 this patient also started to express anti-64 kDa protein antibodies (from Soeldner et al, reprinted by permission of the New England Journal of Medicine 1985; 313: 893)

Table 2 Diabetes-specific antibodies to molecularly characterized autoantigens

	Prediabetic (%)	Control (%)	ICA-negative relatives (%)
Anti-insulin (RIA)	76	1	4.6
Anti-GAD (64K) (recombinant RIA)	91	1	9.0
Anti-ICA512 (recombinant RIA)	40	1	1.5
Anti-GM2-1 (TLC Staining)	≃80	≃5	NT*
A + B + C**			
At least 1	98	3	12.3
At least 2	80	0	2.6
All 3	31	0	0

*NT = not tested
**Combinations of insulin autoantibodies (IAA), GAD autoantibodies utilizing recombinant human GAD (GAA) and ICA512.

21]. Non-GAD autoantibodies reacting with human islets but not rat or mouse islets also exist. Although ICA have been studied since 1974, their target antigen has not yet been fully characterized. For antibodies which react with all three species (human, rat and mouse), the target antigen is resistant to fixation with acetone that removes neutral lipids, is resistant to pronase digestion (arguing against protein involvement) and is removed by methanol (suggesting a glycolipid antigen). In addition, ICA binding could be ablated by neuraminidase treatment, which selectively cleaves sialic acid residues. It was also sensitive to mild periodate oxidation, and after periodate treatment antigenicity was restored by borohydride reduction, confirming the involvement of sialic acid. These data strongly suggest that the target antigen is a sialic acid-containing glycolipid (by definition a ganglioside) [25]. Pre-incubation of ICA-positive sera with pancreatic glycolipid extracts blocks subsequent staining. These glycolipid extracts can similarly block the binding of monoclonals directed against islet gangliosides, but not of monoclonals reacting with islet cell proteins. It has also been shown that, within the pancreatic glycolipid extract, the blocking activity resides in the monosialoganglioside fraction. Employing high-performance liquid chromatography, we have demonstrated that human islets express monosialogangliosides that are minimally, if at all, detectable in whole human pancreas. One such monosialoganglioside has now been sequenced and is termed GM2-1.

Several workshops have been held in order to standardize ICA assays by comparing reproducibility, sensitivity and specificity of the assays performed in different laboratories. Standard ICA-positive sera were identified by the majority of the assays, but several laboratories identified as ICA-positive some of the control blood donor sera. The detection limit for the assays varied considerably, with some assays detecting as little as 5 JDF units (JDF or Juvenile Diabetes Foundation unit is an arbitrary unit based on a single standard positive serum defined as having 80 JDF units), and others with a detection limit of 40 or 80 JDF units. Assays with a higher detection limit, like those employing protein A as detecting reagent or detecting complement-fixing ICA, appear to have a higher positive predictive value (since they are specific to individuals at high risk for subsequent disease onset) and a lower negative predictive value. Using protein A or complement-fixing assays, the prevalence of ICA in normal controls is 0.25% compared with 1.7% using standard ICA assays, and is 2.5% in first-degree relatives vs. 4.9%. Individuals identified as positive employing protein A or complement-fixing assays become diabetic five times more often than those identified as positive using only standard ICA assays. Low-titer ICA (<40 JDF units) have a low positive predictive value (<5%) for diabetes development and it is not yet certain whether the islet antigen detected with such weakly positive sera is identical to the antigen reacting with high-titer sera.

Anti-insulin Autoantibodies (IAA)

Like ICA, competitive anti-insulin autoantibodies (IAA) can be detected in the circulation well before the clinical onset of type 1 diabetes, representing another

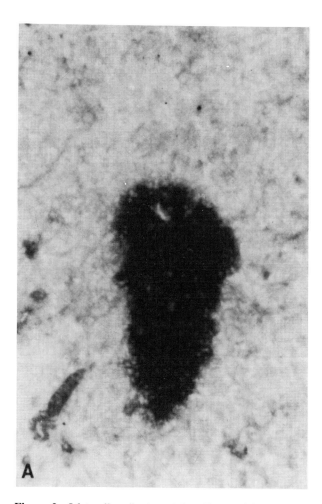 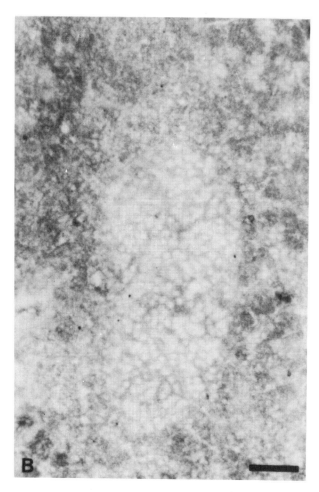

Figure 2   Islet cell antibody staining (A = positive, B = negative) on a frozen section of rat pancreas. Peroxidase-conjugated protein A has been used as detecting reagent (from Colman et al, Diabetes Care 1988; 11: 367, with permission)

immunological marker for the detection of individuals at risk of developing the disease. IAA are present in about 60% of new onset type 1 diabetics prior to insulin therapy and show a marked inverse age correlation. By employing a sensitive competitive radiobinding assay [26], anti-insulin antibodies have been detected in one study in 100% (18/18) of new onset diabetic children under the age of 5 years, but in fewer than 20% of individuals developing type 1 diabetes after the age of 15 years. IAA concentration appears to be closely linked to the rate of the autoimmune B-cell destructive process and therefore represents an important tool for predicting the duration of the 'prediabetic' phase. In our studies IAA are present in 60% of ICA-positive and 2.7% of ICA-negative first-degree relatives. Anti-insulin autoantibodies of prediabetic individuals are of high affinity and low capacity and recognize a conformational epitope of the insulin molecule. The epitope recognized is critically dependent upon the A13 leucine which is at the base of a pocket in the three-dimensional structure of insulin.

The autoantibody-binding epitope is not within the receptor binding region of the insulin molecule [3].

Two general types of assays have been used to measure these antibodies: either fluid phase radioassays with ^{125}I-labelled insulin in which antibody-bound insulin is precipitated with polyethylene glycol, or ELISA assays in which insulin is adsorbed to plastic wells and insulin-binding antibodies are detected with anti-immunoglobulin reagents. Data obtained from screening new onset diabetics, first-degree relatives and a non-diabetic control population suggest that radioimmunoassay (RIA) methods and ELISA methods give different results. Laboratories employing RIAs found IAA in 3.4% of ICA-negative first-degree relatives and in 40% to 80% of prediabetic relatives, while those employing ELISA methods found IAA in 20% of ICA-negative first-degree relatives and in 44% of new onset diabetics. Considering that only approximately 3% of all first-degree relatives subsequently develop diabetes, it is likely that the majority of the ELISA-positive patients will remain free of the disease. Recent workshop comparisons of identical sera assayed for IAA by RIA and ELISA indicate that the two assay formats may actually measure qualitatively different antibodies and the ELISA assays utilized in the workshops do not detect antibodies associated with risk of type 1 diabetes [27].

Anti-GAD and Anti-64K Autoantibodies

The discovery that a major subset of anti-64K autoantibodies react with the enzyme glutamic acid decarboxylase (which converts glutamate to the neurotransmitter GABA) has led to the development of a series of biochemical assays for anti-GAD autoantibodies [4, 46]. It has also led to the realization that GAD (and thus the 64K autoantigen) is not B-cell specific in human islets (being expressed by A- and D-cells as well) and that it is an intracytoplasmic molecule associated with synapse-like microvesicles. The assays using recombinant GAD have a higher positive predictive value for disease. Nevertheless, relatives with the highest levels of anti-GAD autoantibodies (who frequently express restricted ICA [21]) rarely progress to type 1 diabetes. Harrison et al have hypothesized that such relatives produce antibodies but not a T-cell response to GAD [28].

A 37 kDa islet molecule reported to be a trypsin fragment of a non-GAD 64K autoantigen is also the target of autoantibodies [29]. Autoantibodies reacting with this molecule are more predictive of eventual diabetes development than anti-GAD autoantibodies amongst ICA-positive relatives of patients with type 1 diabetes. The higher association with diabetes risk may, however, result from the observation that autoantibodies of patients with restricted ICA are anti-GAD antibodies. The 37 kDa molecule is not yet characterized but a potentially related molecule, termed ICA512, has been cloned and sequenced. Antibodies to ICA512 measured with a radioassay format are highly specific for type 1 diabetes [39].

Anti-ICA69 Autoantibodies

Dosch et al have reported that the great majority of individuals with new onset type 1 diabetes have antibodies reacting with bovine albumin [24]. The disease specificity and reproducibility of assays for anti-albumin antibodies associated with type 1 diabetes is questionable, but a novel islet molecule with three short regions of homology to bovine albumin has recently been cloned by Dosch et al and by Pietropaolo et al [5]. ICA69 is a hydrophilic 55 kDa antigen which aberrantly migrates at 69 kDa on polyacrylamide gel electrophoresis. The majority of individuals developing type 1 diabetes express autoantibodies reacting with ICA69 and thus this molecule will contribute to the panel of biochemically characterized autoantibodies available to screen for diabetes risk.

Combinatorial Autoantibody Screening

The great majority of individuals developing type 1 diabetes express autoantibodies reacting with more than one autoantigen. Relatives expressing a single autoantibody (e.g. anti-GAD with restricted ICA or anti-insulin amongst ICA-negative relatives) show a lower rate of and slower progression to overt diabetes or develop additional autoantibodies. One novel study of several individuals who died while expressing 'restricted' ICA found no islet lesions upon examination of the pancreas. The variety of autoantibodies detected with ICA testing, coupled with the difficulties of standardizing this test which utilizes human pancreas, leads to the obvious need to replace this test with biochemical autoantibody assays. A combination of screening for anti-insulin, anti-GAD, and anti-ICA512 antibodies with a combinatorial algorithm has a higher sensitivity and specificity (if at least two of these autoantibodies are included) for prediction of type 1 diabetes than ICA testing (Table 2).

PRODROMAL METABOLIC ABNORMALITIES

The appearance of ICA and of other diabetes-associated antibodies can precede the onset of the disease by a decade or more. In order to study B-cell function, glucose-stimulated first-phase insulin secretion has been studied in detail, because it has been shown that a series of islet injuries results in a selective loss of B-cell response to glucose compared with other secretagogues.

Abnormalities of first-phase insulin secretion in response to intravenous glucose can precede the onset of type 1 diabetes in both ICA-positive and ICA-negative relatives [6, 30–34]. The Joslin family study performed intravenous glucose tolerance testing (IVGTT) on 43 non-diabetic ICA-positive first-degree relatives with a mean follow-up period of more than 3 years. The sum of the 1 and 3 minute insulin values after a rapid intravenous infusion (3 minutes) of glucose (0.5 mg/kg body weight) was used as an index of first-phase insulin response. The results are expressed as a percentile of the response in 225 healthy non-obese individuals with no family history of diabetes.

Nineteen of the 43 ICA-positive relatives who underwent an IVGTT developed type 1 diabetes. Eighteen of the 43 ICA-positive relatives had an IVGTT result below the first percentile; to date, 15 of these 18 (83%) have progressed to overt diabetes compared with only four (16%) of the 25 individuals with a normal insulin response to an IVGTT. Among the four individuals who developed type 1 diabetes with no documented IVGTT below the first percentile, one was last tested 3 years prior to overt diabetes and the other three were children. In ICA-positive children, progression may be more rapid than in adults; therefore in young individuals it may be necessary to repeat the IVGTT as frequently as 3-monthly, in order to document loss of first-phase insulin release. In addition, in some ICA-positive first-degree relatives followed over a period of up to 4 years prior to diabetes, although remaining within the normal range, the fasting blood glucose level exhibited a striking linear rise over time, as did the blood glucose level at 60 minutes on IVGTT. This increase began approximately 1.5 years prior to the onset of diabetes and all individuals whose fasting blood glucose exceeded 108 mg/dl (6 mmol/l) developed overt diabetes within 1.5 years [6]. Consequently, the development of type 1 diabetes in ICA-positive relatives seems to be a chronic metabolic process with progressive rise of glucose levels in the majority of patients in the last 1.5 years.

A topic of debate relates to whether B-cell destruction in prediabetic relatives is a progressive, linear process with more B cells destroyed over time. We favor this hypothesis, with the rate of destruction varying dramatically between individuals. In addition, many autoantibody-positive relatives (e.g. those expressing restricted ICA) show no evidence of B-cell destruction. The IVGTT insulin response has a coefficient of variation of almost 30% so until insulin release is very low a large amount of random variation is evident. Children under the age of 8 years, particularly on initial testing, can have low insulin secretion which improves on subsequent testing.

PREDICTION OF TYPE 1 DIABETES

The identification of asymptomatic individuals at risk of developing type 1 diabetes is of crucial importance, since an intervention during the prodromal phase is the most likely to prevent subsequent morbidity and mortality. The identification of individuals developing this disease can be important:

(a) To prevent morbidity at onset, since epidemiologic studies have shown that 1 in 200 children die at the onset of type 1 diabetes.

(b) To aid in career and family decisions (e.g. the advisability of training to be an airline pilot or for a military career).

(c) To avoid circumstances in which the development of type 1 diabetes would be an unacceptable risk (e.g. renal donor).

(d) In research, for example to help in the discovery of successful preventive therapies.

Psychological stress represents the major disadvantage of identifying individuals at risk of future diabetes, but we believe that the advantages of the knowledge gained (see above) outweigh the disadvantages. However, clinical screening extended to the general population will not, in our opinion, become clinical practice until current assays are standardized and a reliable preventive therapy becomes available.

The usefulness of screening relatives for 'prediabetes' relies on the accuracy of the available tests for disease susceptibility. The prevalence of the disease, together with the sensitivity and specificity of the assays, determines the clinical utility of a screening program. Among the general population, 3 per 1000 individuals will develop type 1 diabetes. Screening 100 000 individuals without a family history of diabetes, using an assay with 98% specificity and 90% sensitivity, will detect 270 of the 300 prediabetics. Unfortunately, among the 99 700 who will not develop diabetes, this assay would identify 1994 as antibody-positive and potential diabetics, giving a positive predictive value of only 12%—270/(1994 + 270). Applying the same assay to a population of 100 000 first-degree relatives, of whom 3000 will develop diabetes, 2700 will be appropriately identified as prediabetics, but 1940 individuals who will not develop the disease will also be identified as positive, giving a positive predictive value of 58%, still far from reaching a value of clinical utility. However, it is possible to increase the positive predictive value of an assay by increasing specificity and 'sacrificing' sensitivity, defining positivity at a higher 'cut-off' point. For instance, screening 100 000 relatives using an assay with 99.75% specificity and 60% sensitivity (such as current protein A and complement-fixing cytoplasmic islet cell antibody assays), one would identify 1800 of the 3000 who will develop diabetes, while 242 relatives would be incorrectly identified as at risk. The positive predictive value would be 88%, approaching clinical utility. It is likely that in order to identify individuals at risk of developing type 1 diabetes, a combination of highly specific assays will have to be employed, such as a combination of biochemically defined autoantibodies and insulin secretion following IV glucose. At present a combination of ICA and IV glucose tolerance testing can identify a subgroup of relatives with a risk of type 1 diabetes exceeding 90% within 4 years. This has allowed the development of preventive trials.

THE PREVENTION OF TYPE 1 DIABETES

The immediate goal of clinical research in the prediction of type 1 diabetes is obviously its prevention. Immunotherapeutic trials using immunosuppressive drugs such as cyclosporin A or azathioprine have been performed only after diabetes onset, giving modest results from the metabolic point of view, presumably because by diabetes onset most of the pancreatic islets have already been destroyed, with the consequent impossibility of restoring truly normal insulin production [35]. In the trials to date, by 3 years almost all patients lose their non-insulin requiring remission. It is noteworthy that Biostator treatment for 2 weeks at the onset of type 1 diabetes, followed by subcutaneous insulin therapy in a randomized trial has been reported to preserve C-peptide secretion as long as 1 year later [36]. In animal models (NOD mouse and BB rat), 'resting' B cells with insulin therapy prevents diabetes, insulitis and B-cell destruction [37].

In the light of the failure to maintain remission with immunotherapy after diabetes diagnosis, it would seem more logical to evaluate immunotherapy prior to overt diabetes. The combination of highly specific immunological tests with the measurement of first-phase insulin release during an IVGTT can be used to detect individuals at risk of developing diabetes within 3 years. In such a population, treatment protocols could be tested to halt further B-cell destruction; and with an improved predictive ability, it now becomes possible to evaluate fairly rapidly whether a new treatment is effective or not. A pilot trial of intravenous insulin therapy followed by low dose subcutaneous insulin has been carried out in relatives expressing high titer cytoplasmic ICA, insulin autoantibodies and low first-phase insulin secretion [38] (Figure 3). Such therapy appears to have resulted in a marked inhibition or delay in the development of diabetes, and a large National Institutes of Health national trial for the prevention of type 1 diabetes is about to begin. To date, in this pilot trial all seven non-treated relatives developed diabetes within 2 years, while two of five treated relatives have become diabetic (one after 1 year and the other after 4 years of therapy). Nevertheless, the two relatives to progress to diabetes had the lowest first-phase insulin secretion of the treated relatives. This suggests that earlier identification may be essential, or that more effective therapy may be required for this subgroup.

In NOD mice and BB rats, several therapies can prevent the onset of diabetes; these include administration of cyclosporin A, anti-T cell antibodies or nicotinamide, bone marrow transplantation, insulin therapy, injection of an expanding series of peptides and proteins (e.g. GAD, insulin B chain, Freund's adjuvant)

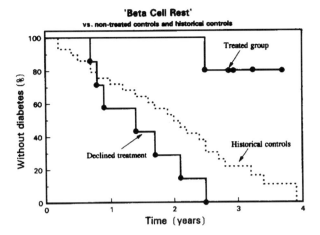

Figure 3 Pilot trial of insulin therapy for prevention of type 1 diabetes (from Keller et al, Lancet 1993; 341: 928, with permission)

and even oral insulin (presumably inducing oral tolerance to insulin). Whether one or more of these treatments would be safe and effective in man is currently unknown, but with the present understanding of the autoimmune process leading to diabetes and with the development of better immunomodulatory protocols, the prevention of diabetes may soon become a clinical reality.

REFERENCES

1. Eisenbarth GS. Type 1 diabetes mellitus: a chronic autoimmune disease. New Engl J Med 1986; 314: 1360–8.
2. Bottazzo GF, Gorsuch AN, Dean BM, Cudworth AG, Doniach D. Complement fixing islet cell antibodies in type 1 diabetes: possible monitors of active beta cell damage. Lancet 1980; 1: 668–72.
3. Castano L, Ziegler A, Ziegler R, Shoelson S, Eisenbarth GS. Characterization of insulin autoantibodies in relatives of patients with insulin dependent diabetes mellitus. Diabetes 1993; 42: 1202–9.
4. Baekkeskov S, Aanstoot H, Christgau S et al. Identification of the 64K autoantigen in insulin dependent diabetes as the GABA-synthesizing enzyme glutamic acid decarboxylase. Nature 1990; 347: 151–6.
5. Pietropaolo M, Castano L, Babu S, Powers A, Eisenbarth GS. Molecular cloning and characterization of a novel neuroendocrine autoantigen (PM-1) related to type 1 diabetes. Diabetes 1992; 41 (suppl. 1): 98A (abstract).
6. Bleich D, Jackson RA, Soeldner JS, Eisenbarth GS. Analysis of metabolic progression to type 1 diabetes in islet cell antibody positive relatives of patients with type 1 diabetes. Diabetes Care 1990; 13: 111–18.
7. Hattori M, Buse JB, Jackson RA et al. The NOD mouse: recessive diabetogenic gene within the major histocompatibility complex. Science 1986; 231: 733–5.

8. Ghosh S, Palmer SM, Rodrigues NR et al. Polygenic control of autoimmune diabetes in non-obese diabetic mice. Nature Genet 1993; 4: 404–9.

9. Jacob HJ, Pettersson A, Wilson D, Mao Y, Lernmark A, Lander ES. Genetic dissection of autoimmune type 1 diabetes in the BB rat. Nature Genet 1992; 2: 56–60.

10. Nepom GT. Immunogenetics and IDDM. Diabet Rev 1993; 1: 93–103.

11. Erlich HA, Griffith RL, Bugawan TL, Ziegler R, Alper C, Eisenbarth GS. Implication of specific DQB1 alleles in genetic susceptibility and resistance by identification of IDDM siblings with novel HLA-DQB1 allele and unusual DR2 and DR1 haplotypes. Diabetes 1991; 40: 478–81.

12. Morel PA, Dorman JS, Todd JA, McDevitt HO, Trucco M. Aspartic acid at position 57 of the HLA-DQ beta chain protects against type 1 diabetes: a family study. Proc Natl Acad Sci USA 1988; 85: 8111–15.

13. Sheehy MJ, Scharf SJ, Rowe JR et al. A diabetes-susceptible HLA haplotype is best defined by a combination of HLA-DR and DQ alleles. J Clin Invest 1989; 83: 830–5.

14. Lucassen A, Julier C, Beressi J-P et al. Susceptibility to insulin dependent diabetes mellitus maps to a 4.1 kb segment of DNA spanning the insulin gene and associated VNTR. Nature Genet 1993; 4: 305–10.

15. Pugliese A, Bain SC, Todd JA, Awdeh ZL, Alper CA, Eisenbarth GS. INS polymorphisms on chromosome 11 in type 1 diabetes. Autoimmunity 1993; 15 (suppl.): 32 (abstract).

16. Rabinowe SL, Rubin L, George KL, Adri MNS, Eisenbarth GS. Trisomy 21 (Down's syndrome): autoimmunity, aging and monoclonal antibody defined T cell abnormalities. J Autoimmunity 1989; 2: 25–30.

17. Karasik A, O'Hara C, Srikanta S, Swift M et al. Genetically programmed selective islet beta-cell loss in diabetic subjects with Wolfram's syndrome. Diabetes Care 1989; 12: 135–8.

18. Eisenbarth GS, Jackson RA. The immunoendocrinopathy syndromes. In Wilson JD, Foster DW (eds) Williams textbook of endocrinology, 8th edn. Philadelphia: W.B. Saunders Company, 1992: pp 1555–66.

19. Maclaren NK, Riley WJ. Inherited susceptibility to autoimmune Addison's disease is linked to human leukocyte antigens-DR3 and/or DR4 except when associated with type 1 autoimmune polyglandular syndrome. J Clin Endocrinol Metab 1986; 62: 455–9.

20. Gianani R, Pugliese A, Bonner-Weir S et al. Prognostically significant heterogeneity of cytoplasmic islet cell antibodies in relatives of patients with type 1 diabetes. Diabetes 1992; 41: 347–53.

21. Genovese S, Bonifacio E, McNally JM et al. Distinct cytoplasmic islet cell antibodies with different risks for type 1 (insulin dependent) diabetes mellitus. Diabetologia 1992; 35: 385–8.

22. Rabinowe SL, George KL, Laughlin R, Soeldner JS, Eisenbarth GS. Congenital rubella: monoclonal antibody defined T cell abnormalities in young children. Am J Med 1986; 81: 779–82.

23. Wiggs J, Nordenskjold M, Yandell D et al. Prediction of the risk of hereditary retinoblastoma, using DNA polymorphisms within the retinoblastoma gene. New Engl J Med 1988; 318: 151–7.

24. Karjalainen J, Martin JM, Knip M et al. A bovine albumin peptide as a possible trigger of insulin-dependent diabetes mellitus. New Engl J Med 1992; 327: 302–7.

25. Colman PG, Nayak RC, Campbell IL, Eisenbarth GS. Binding of cytoplasmic islet cell antibodies is blocked by human pancreatic glycolipid extracts. Diabetes 1988; 37: 645–52.

26. Vardi P, Ziegler AG, Matthews JH et al. Concentration of insulin autoantibodies at onset of type 1 diabetes: inverse log-linear correlation with age. Diabetes Care 1988; 11: 736–9.

27. Greenbaum C, Palmer JP, Kuglin B, Kolb H and Participating Laboratories. Insulin autoantibodies measured by radioimmunoassay methodology are more related to insulin dependent diabetes mellitus than those measured by enzyme-linked immunosorbent assay: results of the fourth international workshop on the standardization of insulin autoantibody measurement. J Clin Endocrinol Metab 1992; 74: 1040–4.

28. Harrison LC, Honeyman MC, DeAizpurua HJ et al. Inverse relation between humoral and cellular immunity to glutamic acid decarboxylase in subjects at risk of insulin-dependent diabetes. Lancet 1993; 341: 1365–9.

29. Christie MR, Hollands JA, Brown TJ, Michelsen BK, Delovitch TL. Detection of pancreatic islet 64 000 Mr autoantigens in insulin-dependent diabetes distinct from glutamate decarboxylase. J Clin Invest 1993; 22: 240–8.

30. Vardi P, Crisa L, Jackson RA et al. Predictive value of intravenous glucose tolerance test insulin secretion less than or greater than the first percentile in islet cell antibody positive relatives of type 1 (insulin-dependent) diabetic patients. Diabetologia 1991; 34: 93–102.

31. Palmer JP, McCulloch DK. Prediction and prevention of IDDM–1991. Diabetes 1991; 40: 943–7.

32. McCulloch DK, Koerker DJ, Kahn SE, Bonner-Weir S, Palmer JP. Correlations of in vivo beta-cell function tests with beta-cell mass and pancreatic insulin content in streptozocin-treated baboons. Diabetes 1991; 40: 673–9.

33. Bingley PJ, Colman P, Eisenbarth GS et al. Standardization of IVGTT to predict IDDM. Diabetes Care 1992; 15: 1313–16.

34. Carel J-C, Boitard C, Bougneres P-F. Decreased insulin response to glucose in islet cell antibody-negative siblings of type 1 diabetic children. J Clin Invest 1993; 92: 509–13.

35. Burcelin RG, Eddouks M, Beylot M et al. Hypersensitivity to insulin during remissions in cyclosporin-treated IDDM patients. Diabetes Care 1993; 16: 881–8.

36. Shah SC, Malone JI, Simpson NE. A randomized trial of intensive insulin therapy in newly diagnosed insulin-dependent diabetes mellitus. New Engl J Med 1989; 320: 550–4.

37. Gottsfredsen CF, Buschard K, Frandsen EK. Reduction of diabetes incidence of BB Wistar rats by early prophylactic insulin treatment of diabetes-prone animals. Diabetologia 1985; 28: 933–5.

38. Keller RJ, Eisenbarth GS, Jackson RA. Insulin prophylaxis in individuals at high risk of type 1 diabetes. Lancet 1993; 341: 927–8.

39. Rabin DU, Pleasic SM, Shapiro JA et al. Islet cell antigen 512 is a diabetes-specific islet autoantigen related to protein tyrosine phosphatases. J Immunol 1994; 152: 3183–7.

40. Davies JL, Kawaguchi Y, Bennett ST et al. A genome-wide search for human type 1 diabetes susceptibility genes. Nature 1994; 371: 130-6.

41. Aaltonen J, Bjorses P, Sandkuijl L, Perheentupa J, Peltonen L. An autosomal locus causing autoimmune disease: autoimmune polyglandular disease type 1 assigned to chromosome 21. Nature Genet 1994; 8: 83-7.

42. Polymeropoulos MH, Swift RG, Swift M. Linkage of the gene for Wolfram syndrome to markers on the short arm of chromosome 4. Nature Genet 1994; 8: 95-7.

43. Owerbach D, Gabbay KH. The HOXD8 locus (2q31) is linked to type 1 diabetes: interaction with chromosome 6 and 11 disease susceptibility genes. Diabetes 1995; 44: 132-6.

44. Vandewalle CL, Falorni A, Svanholm S et al. High diagnostic sensitivity of glutamate decarboxylase autoantibodies in insulin-dependent diabetes mellitus with clinical onset between age 20 and 40 years. J Clin Endocrinol Metab 1995; 80: 846-51.

45. Kennedy GC, German MS, Rutter WJ. The minisatellite in the diabetes susceptibility locus IDDM2 regulates insulin transcription. Nature Genet 1995; 9: 293.

46. Bennett ST, Lucassen AM, Gough SCL et al. Susceptibility to human type 1 diabetes at IDDM2 is determined by tandem repeat variation at the insulin gene minisatellite locus. Nature Genet 1995; 9: 284.

6

Molecular Genetics of Type 1 Diabetes Mellitus

D.A. Cavan, M.A. Penny, S.C. Bain and A.H. Barnett

The University of Birmingham, UK

INTRODUCTION

Type 1 (insulin-dependent) diabetes mellitus is a T-cell-dependent autoimmune disease characterised by infiltration and destruction of the pancreatic islets, leading to absolute dependence on exogenous insulin [1]. It is most common in Europid populations, with highest prevalence rates in northern European countries [2]. Although only scanty data are available in some cases, evidence suggests that the prevalence is low in most other races including Asian Indians [3], Chinese [4], Japanese [2] and black Africans [2]. Differences in prevalence in migrant populations from those of their host country have also been described [5], as have marked temporal changes in incidence in well-defined areas [6]. Both genetic and environmental factors have been implicated to explain these inter- and intra-racial differences in prevalence.

As type 1 diabetes results from the autoimmune destruction of pancreatic B cells, both those genes involved in the immune response and those whose expression is islet B-cell-specific (e.g. the insulin gene) have been considered as candidate susceptibility determinants. An early clue to the nature of the genetic susceptibility was the demonstration that type 1 diabetes is associated with certain human leucocyte antigens (HLA) [7, 8]. These are cell surface molecules which present antigenic peptide to T cells. The heavy T cell infiltration of pancreatic islets in autoimmune diabetes suggests a role for T cells in disease development. Evidence from animal experiments suggests that both CD4+ (helper) and CD8+ (cytotoxic) T cells are required for development of insulitis but that CD4+ cells can also confer protection from the disease [9]. As CD8+ and CD4+ cells are stimulated following interaction with class I and class II HLA molecules respectively, these data may imply a role for HLA molecules in disease development. Antigen presentation, and hence disease susceptibility, may be influenced by particular HLA molecules and the genes encoding them have been extensively studied as candidate susceptibility genes for type 1 diabetes. Although strong disease associations have been demonstrated with HLA genes, these alone cannot account for the genetic susceptibility to the disease [10]. Non-HLA genes which may be implicated include the insulin gene, T cell receptor genes and immunoglobulin genes.

In this chapter we consider HLA associations with type 1 diabetes, mechanisms of HLA-associated susceptibility and other genes which may be involved in susceptibility to type 1 diabetes.

THE GENES OF THE MAJOR HISTOCOMPATIBILITY COMPLEX

HLA molecules are encoded by a cluster of genes within the major histocompatibility complex (MHC) (Figure 1). This region comprises about four megabases and is located on the short arm of chromosome 6. It is one of the most gene-dense areas of the human

International Textbook of Diabetes Mellitus, Second Edition. Edited by K.G.M.M. Alberti, P. Zimmet, R.A. DeFronzo, and H. Keen (Honorary)

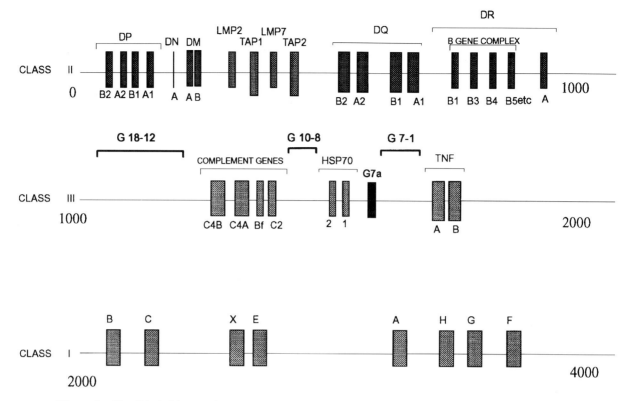

Figure 1 Simplified diagram of the major histocompatibility complex on the short arm of chromosome 6

genome and contains a number of genes involved in the immune response. The genes of the MHC are divided into class I, II and III loci and many exhibit considerable polymorphism with, in some cases, in excess of 40 distinct alleles (for example HLA-DRB1). This polymorphism has presumably arisen in response to the array of antigens encountered. Several other genes have recently been characterised, many of which are immune-response genes and may thus have an effect on disease development.

Class I Region

Class I HLA genes encode α-chains which combine with β_2-microglobulin (encoded by a gene on chromosome 15) to form the HLA-A, -B and -C molecules. Polymorphism at the respective class I locus determines the HLA-A, -B or -C type. Class I molecules are expressed by all nucleated cells where they bind antigen which has been processed intracellularly. The HLA–antigen complex then migrates to the cell surface, where it interacts with, and activates, CD8+ (cytotoxic) T cells [11]. The HLA molecule has cytoplasmic, transmembrane and extracellular portions. The latter is divided into first and second domains. The first domains are highly variable as a result of polymorphism of the second exon of class I genes; they enclose the cleft into which antigen is bound and are

potentially of functional significance in determining the binding affinity of a particular antigen.

Other class I genes include HLA-E, -F, and -G genes and the OCT (octomer binding protein) gene [12].

Class II Region

This region contains genes which encode class II HLA molecules as well as genes involved in antigen-processing and those with non-immune functions. The HLA-DR, -DQ and -DP genes are each subdivided into A and B loci. The DQA1 and DQB1 genes encode α and β chains respectively, which combine to form a DQ molecule (Figure 2). There is a high degree of polymorphism of both DQα and DQβ-chains. The DPA1 and DPB1 genes are analogous. The DRB1 gene encodes a β-chain which combines with the α-chain encoded by the non-polymorphic DRA gene. Class II HLA molecules enclose an antigen binding cleft and are expressed on certain cell types only (e.g. B lymphocytes, activated T cells, macrophages) which are collectively known as antigen presenting cells; they present antigen to CD4+ (helper) T cells [11].

Other class II genes include the DNA and DOB genes which are situated between the DQ and DP loci [13]. They are thought to express a pair of proteins analogous to the DQA1 and DQB1 genes but they have not been characterised. Eight further loci have been

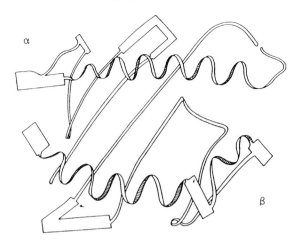

Figure 2 Structural model of a class II molecule. The α and β chains enclose an antigen binding cleft

identified between DNA and DOB. These were originally termed RING ('really interesting new genes') and several have now been characterised, including DM, TAP and LMP genes. DMA and DMB encode products which combine to form a heterodimer with about 30% homology with class I and class II molecules [14]. They are expressed by both B and T lymphocytes and may be focused on particular pathogens. TAP1 and TAP2 (transporter associated with antigen processing) genes are involved in transport of peptides across the membrane of the endoplasmic reticulum prior to binding with class I molecules [15, 16]. LMP2 and LMP7 (large molecular weight protein) map close to the TAP genes and encode products thought to be involved in producing peptides for transport by the TAP complex [17]. Class II genes with non-immune response functions include RING 3 with homology to *Drosophila* gene *Fsh* and the collagen gene IIA2 [17].

Class III Region

This region contains hundreds of genes, including both those involved in the immune response and those with non-immune functions. Class III immune-response genes include the complement genes Bf (encodes properdin factor B), C2, C4A and C4B [18], the genes encoding tumour necrosis factor (TNFA and TNFB) [19] and heat shock protein (HSP70) [20]. Complement molecules form part of the complement cascade which is important in causing lysis of cells, bacteria and enveloped viruses and the opsonisation of bacteria prior to phagocytosis. A further function is the generation of peptide fragments which regulate inflammatory and immune responses including, for example, vasodilatation at the site of inflammation [21]. TNFA and TNFB genes encode the cytokines TNFα and β respectively, which are secreted by many cell types.

Their effects include enhancement of interleukin-2 (IL-2) receptor expression on T cells and promotion of B lymphocyte proliferation and antibody production [21]. Heat shock proteins (HSP) are expressed in response to cellular damage. Their functions include induction of thermotolerance. They reduce IL-1β expression and may protect from the effects of TNF [22].

Class III genes with non-immune functions include the 21-β-hydroxylase gene, the valyl tRNA synthase gene (G7a). In addition, many recently discovered G genes have yet to be characterised [17].

In summary, many of the genes within the MHC are closely involved in the immune response, as suggested by the strong associations of many autoimmune diseases with particular HLA types. The elucidation of the functions of other HLA genes, including those of as yet unidentified genes, may increase our understanding of the pathogenesis of disorders such as type 1 diabetes.

HLA ASSOCIATIONS WITH TYPE 1 DIABETES

Several population studies have been performed to investigate HLA genes associated with type 1 diabetes. These association studies have demonstrated significant differences in the frequency of a number of alleles between diabetic and control subjects. There is strong linkage disequilibrium between HLA genes, both between class I and class II alleles and between different class II alleles. Linkage disequilibrium is defined as the co-occurrence of two or more alleles on the same chromosome more frequently than expected by chance, so that certain combinations of alleles at different loci (e.g. DRB1, DQA1 and DQB1) are often inherited together as a haplotype. Thus a significant disease association with a particular allele may either reflect a true association with that allele or may be secondary to linkage disequilibrium with the true susceptibility allele elsewhere on the haplotype. Such spurious secondary associations hinder accurate mapping of disease susceptibility within the MHC.

This problem has been partly overcome by studies of type 1 diabetes in ethnically distinct populations (transracial analysis). These exploit the interracial differences in patterns of linkage disequilibrium which result from rare recombination events during evolution, in an attempt to distinguish primary from secondary HLA disease associations. Assuming genetic susceptibility to the disease to be identical in all races, any allele consistently associated with disease in all races studied, despite differences in linkage disequilibrium, is likely to be a primary disease determinant. Transracial studies do, however, depend on accurate and consistent diagnostic criteria in all racial groups studied.

The study of HLA disease associations has been greatly facilitated by the development of molecular genotyping techniques such as restriction fragment length polymorphism analysis and oligonucleotide probing of genes amplified using the polymerase chain reaction. These techniques have clear advantages over the previously used serological typing methods in that all alleles can be distinguished and no allele will be missed as a 'blank' (as occurs with serological typing if reagents are not available to distinguish a particular antigen).

Early serological typing in man showed positive associations between the class I antigens HLA-B8 and B15 and type 1 diabetes [7, 8]. Studies in different races, however, showed little consistency in HLA-B associations (Table 1). Stronger disease associations were later shown with the class II antigens HLA-DR3 and -DR4 [23]. The alleles encoding these antigens are in linkage disequilibrium with those encoding B8 and B15 respectively in Europids. Class II HLA-DR associations are also more consistent across races (Table 1). This suggested that class II genes, or closely linked genes, may have a greater susceptibility effect than class I genes, whose associations with type 1 diabetes were thought to be secondary to linkage disequilibrium. A role for class I genes in determining susceptibility has not been excluded and it has also been proposed that both class I and class II genes have interdependent susceptibility effects when inherited together as an 'extended haplotype' [31].

Ninety-five per cent of Europid type 1 diabetic subjects possess one or both of DR3 or DR4, which are positively associated with disease in all races in which they are common [32]. DR3/4 heterozygosity confers even greater disease susceptibility and the genes encoding these types, or closely associated genes, may act synergistically in predisposing to disease. Type 1 diabetes does not follow a simple Mendelian pattern of inheritance and the synergistic effect of DR3 and DR4 suggests that more than one gene is involved in susceptibility. It has been suggested that DR3 is linked with a gene which acts recessively in the absence of DR4, and DR4 is linked with a gene which acts with dominant susceptibility in the absence of DR3 [33], although the dominance of DR4-associated susceptibility has been questioned in further studies [34, 35]. DR3 or DR4 occur, however, in up to 60% of non-diabetic Europids and are unlikely to be primary susceptibility determinants [34]. Attention has therefore focused on other class II genes, particularly the DQ loci, in the search for susceptibility genes [32].

DR4-associated Susceptibility to Type 1 Diabetes

The first evidence that DR4-associated susceptibility might be DQ-encoded was suggested by the finding that 90% of a Europid DR4-positive diabetic population possessed the DQB1*0302 allele and only 10% the DQB1*0301 allele, whereas both alleles were equally represented in a DR4-positive control population [36, 37]. The predominance of DQB1*0302 on DR4 haplotypes was also demonstrated in North Indian Asian [38], Afro-Caribbean [39] and Southern Chinese diabetic populations [40], but not in a Japanese population

Table 1 Associations between class I and class II HLA alleles and type 1 diabetes in different races

	Europid	Negroid	Asian	Chinese	Japanese
Class I					
B8	+[7, 8, 30]	+[24]	N+[25, 26]	R[27]	R[28, 29]
B15	+	N	N	N	N
Class II					
DR3	+	+	+	+	R
DR4	+	+	+	N+	+
DR7	N−	+	N	N	N
DR9	N	+	N	N	+
DR13	—	N−	N−	N	N−
DR15	—	—	—	N	N
DQA1*0102	—	—	N−	N−	N−
DQA1*0103	—	R	—	R	N−
DQA1*0201	—	N−	—	R	R
DQA1*0301	+	+	+	N	+
DQB1*0201	+	+	+	N	N
DQB1*0302	+	+	+	N+	N
DQB1*0602	—	—	—	R	N−
DQB1*0603	—	—	—	R	R

Key. + = positive association; − = negative association and N = neutral association. N+ and N− denote inconsistent positive and negative associations respectively. R = race in which antigen is rare or absent. References for class I associations are shown; class II references are cited in the text.

[41]. This suggests that if DQB1*0302 is a primary disease susceptibility determinant, its effect may be modified by other factors.

The DQA1 allele associated with DR4 is DQA1*0301. The demonstration that this allele also occurs on predisposing DR7 haplotypes in Negroids [42] suggested that the presence of DQA1*0301 may confer susceptibility to disease, despite its occurrence on different haplotypes in different races. DQA1*0301 also occurs on predisposing DR9 haplotypes in Negroid [39] and Japanese [41] populations. Such transracial susceptibility is consistent with a primary susceptibility effect of the gene. Although it was found to be positively associated with disease in Europid [43], North Indian Asian [44], Japanese [41] and Negroid [39] populations, its frequency in a Southern Chinese type 1 diabetic population was not significantly different from that in controls [40]. Furthermore, DQA1*0301 occurs on all DR4 haplotypes, whether or not they are associated with disease. These data suggest either that disease associations with this allele may be secondary to linkage disequilibrium with an as yet undetermined susceptibility allele or that DQA1*0301 interacts with, or its effect is modified by, a factor encoded at a distinct locus. One explanation, namely that DQA1*0301 may be a susceptibility allele whose effects are modified by differential levels of gene expression, has been examined by sequencing the DQA1*0301 promoter. This was found to be identical in Europid diabetic and control subjects [45]. While ultimate levels of expression are dependent on a number of factors, this finding suggests that differential expression of DQA1*0301 may not be important in determining disease susceptibility and questions the role of DQA1*0301 as a direct susceptibility determinant.

DR3-associated Susceptibility to Type 1 Diabetes

DR3 is associated with the DQA1 allele DQA1*0501 in many races. This allele is not consistently associated with type 1 diabetes in all races and is not, therefore, considered to be a susceptibility determinant. In Europids, DR3 is in strong linkage disequilibrium with the DQB1 allele DQB1*0201 which also occurs on disease-predisposing DR3 haplotypes in other races [32]. This suggests that DR3-associated susceptibility may be mediated by DQB1*0201. This allele also occurs on a proportion of Europid DR7 haplotypes which are not associated with disease and it has been suggested that another gene on the DR7 haplotype interacts to modify the predisposing effect of DQB1*0201 [35].

The DR7-DQB1*0201 haplotype is, however, positively associated with disease in Negroids. The Europid and Negroid DR7-DQB1*0201 haplotypes differ at the DQA1 locus: the Negroid haplotype possesses the predisposing DQA1*0301 allele whereas the Europid haplotype possesses the DQA1*0201 allele [42], thought to be protective [35]. It is possible, therefore, that it is the DQA1 locus which determines the disease association of DR7 haplotypes from these races.

Possible Mechanisms of Class II-associated Susceptibility to Type 1 Diabetes

There are a number of mechanisms by which class II HLA molecules may influence susceptibility to type 1 diabetes and thus explain the observed HLA associations. As they are critical to antigen presentation to CD4+ T cells, the different disease associations of class II alleles suggest that particular HLA molecules may be more effective either in binding antigen, or in interacting with the T-cell receptor, thereby influencing disease susceptibility. It has been postulated that the predisposing effect of DR3- and/or DR4-associated alleles arises as a result of more efficient binding of a particular 'diabetogenic peptide', consistent with a model of disease susceptibility whereby HLA molecules of differing affinity compete for peptide [46]. According to this model, peptide binds to the HLA molecule present with the highest affinity. If, in a given individual, this was a predisposing molecule, disease would ensue. This hypothesis requires that an additional property, apart from binding affinity, distinguishes predisposing and non-predisposing HLA molecules; it also has a competitive element which implies that the supply of antigen is limiting.

Evidence for a peripheral involvement of the DR molecule in the pathogenesis of type 1 diabetes in man has been suggested by the presence of DR-restricted CD4+ T cells specific for an islet B-cell antigen in diabetic subjects [47]. Whether these T cells are a primary factor in islet B-cell destruction, or whether they arise as a result of macrophage-induced islet B-cell destruction is unknown. The role of DQ-restricted T cell clones in the pathogenesis of type 1 diabetes is unclear. To date, no islet B-cell specific DQ-restricted T cells have been isolated from type 1 diabetic subjects. There is evidence that DQ-restricted T cells are involved in immunological suppression and it has been suggested that DQ molecules may present antigen to 'suppressor-inducer' T cells which, in turn, induce CD8+ suppressor T cells to bring about immunosuppression [48].

Polymorphism in class II HLA molecular structure has been demonstrated to have an effect on T-cell activation [49]. Thus, polymorphism in a region of the DQ molecule which is involved in T-cell activation might suggest a mechanism of disease susceptibility due to failure of activation of T cells. Sequence differences in the first exon of the DQB1*0201 gene have been identified, which distinguish the allele occurring on DR3 haplotypes from that on DR7 haplotypes [50]. This results in amino acid differences in the second (membrane-proximal) domain of the DQβ chain which has been implicated as a site of interaction between the CD4 and class II molecules and may be important in T cell activation (Figure 3) [51]. It is possible that the amino acid sequence of the second domain of the DQβ chain encoded by the predisposing DQB1*0201 allele results in failure of the DQ molecule to interact with and activate the CD4+ suppressor-inducer T cell, thus predisposing to disease because of a lack of immunosuppression. This would be consistent with a recessive mode of inheritance of the DR3-linked susceptibility allele.

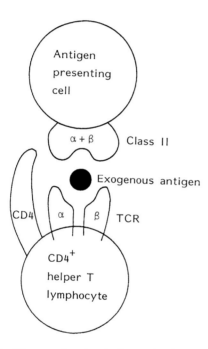

Figure 3 Diagram showing the interaction between a T cell receptor (TCR), class II HLA molecule and CD4 molecule. The CD4 molecule interacts with the HLA molecule membrane proximal to the antigen-binding site

The Role of DQβ-Asp 57 and Diabetogenic Heterodimers

Sequence studies of the DQB1 alleles led to the observation that those alleles negatively associated with disease in Europids encode aspartate at position 57 of the DQβ chain, whereas those positively associated with disease do not [52]. This position is at one end of the antigen binding cleft and it has been shown that a negatively charged residue such as aspartate at this position forms a salt bridge across the end of the binding cleft and thus may impede binding of 'diabetogenic' antigen [53]. Support for a role for

DQβ-Asp57 as a susceptibility determinant comes from an animal model of type 1 diabetes—the non-obese diabetic (NOD) mouse. The murine homologue of DQB1 is I-Aβ and the sequence of the NOD I-Aβ molecule is distinctive in having serine rather than aspartate at position 57 [54]. The demonstration that, in Europids, disease-associated DQA1 alleles encode arginine at position 52 has led to the hypothesis that disease susceptibility correlates with expression of a DQ molecule bearing Arg52 on the α chain and lacking Asp57 on the β chain, the so-called 'diabetogenic heterodimer' [43].

The high relative risk for disease of DR3/4 heterozygous subjects implies interaction between DR3 and DR4 haplotypes. DQ molecules may be encoded by DQA1 and DQB1 alleles on the same haplotype (in *cis* position) or on different haplotypes (in *trans* position) [55]. The increased disease risk of DR3/4 heterozygosity could be explained by a DQ molecule encoded in *trans* by, for example, the DQA1 allele on the DR3 haplotype (DQA1*0501) and the DQB1 allele on the DR4 haplotype (DQB1*0302). A unique ability of such a molecule to bind a diabetogenic peptide (or inability to bind a protective one) would thus confer susceptibility to disease over and above the effect of the *cis*-encoded DR3- and DR4-associated DQ molecules. This molecule would also occur in DR4/5 heterozygotes, although such genotypes are found in only about 4% of Europid populations [35] and are too rare for any disease association to be detected.

On the assumption that risk for disease correlates with the number of 'diabetogenic' heterodimers, attempts have been made to quantify disease susceptibility by calculating the number of possible 'diabetogenic' DQ heterodimers (i.e. DQA Arg52-positive and DQB Asp57-negative) that could be expressed in either *cis* or *trans* in individual subjects [56]. Although the maximum possible, four heterodimers, is associated with a high relative risk for disease, there is no consistent correlation between the number of possible 'diabetogenic' heterodimers and disease susceptibility [57, 58]. This is not unexpected, as genotyping data alone cannot take into account any differences in the level of expression between DQ molecules encoded in *cis* and *trans* or between different DQ molecules. Studies in mice have shown that molecules encoded in *cis* are expressed more efficiently than those encoded in *trans* [59] and there is evidence to suggest that certain combinations of DQα and DQβ chains are unable to form DQ molecules [49, 60].

It is significant that the only common Arg52-positive DQA1 alleles in Europids are those associated with DR3 and DR4 [57, 58]. While many studies have shown significant disease associations with Asp57-negative DQB1 alleles, both animal and human data cast doubt on the hypothesis that Asp57 is of primary importance as a disease susceptibility determinant. Transgenic mouse experiments suggest that Asp57-negative I-Aβ alleles may be protective [61]. In man, Asp57-positive alleles which predispose to disease [62] and Asp57-negative alleles which protect from type 1 diabetes have been described [35]. Data from Finland, where the prevalence of type 1 diabetes is amongst the highest in the world, showed a weaker disease association with 'diabetogenic' heterodimers [63], refuting both the Asp57 hypothesis and the putative quantitative effect of such heterodimers on disease susceptibility. Thus, while Asp57 may be a contributory factor in determining disease susceptibility, it is not the primary HLA-associated susceptibility determinant.

Similar arguments counter the Arg52 hypothesis: the Arg52-negative allele DQA1*0102, although strongly associated with protection in most cases, is positively associated with disease when it occurs with DQB1*0502 [64]. This suggests that, if the structure of the DQ molecule is important in determining disease susceptibility, it is likely that the tertiary structure of the whole DQ molecule, determined by the individual α and β chains, is important, rather than simply aspartate at position 57 of the β-chain (or arginine on the α-chain). Whether this is the case can only be determined by accurate structural models of all possible DQ heterodimers.

PROTECTIVE HLA ASSOCIATIONS WITH TYPE 1 DIABETES

In addition to a predisposing HLA effect, there is evidence that HLA genes may be important in conferring protection from type 1 diabetes. It is well established that DR15 (a subset of DR2) protects from type 1 diabetes in a number of races [35, 39, 43, 44]. Other DR types associated with protection include DR13 (a subset of DR6), which was found to be strongly protective in a large Europid population [35]. DR13 was positively associated with disease in another study which used serological typing [34], although confusion between DR3 and DR13 using older serological typing reagents may account for this discrepancy. There is also evidence that a DR7 haplotype has a weak protective effect in Europids [35].

Both DR13 and DR15 haplotypes carry DQA1*0102, which occurs on over 40% of non-diabetic haplotypes and was the single most frequent DQ allele in the Europid non-diabetic population in one study [35]. The occurrence of the same DQA1 allele on two distinct protective haplotypes suggests that the DQA1 locus may have a role in conferring protection from disease. DQA1*0102 is reduced in diabetic compared with control subjects in Afro-Caribbeans [39], North Indian

Asians [44] and Southern Chinese [40], as well as in Europids. The only haplotype carrying DQA1*0102 that has been shown to predispose to disease is DR16-DQA1*0102-DQB1*0502, which occurs in Ashkenazi Jews but is otherwise rare in Europid populations [64]. It is possible that the protective effect of DQA1*0102 is modified by a strong predisposing effect of the DQB1 allele on this haplotype. A structurally similar allele DQA1*0103 is associated with protection from disease in Europids [35], Japanese [41] and North Indian Asians [44]. The DQα-chains encoded by DQA1*0102 and DQA1*0103 are very similar, differing at only 2 amino acid residues [65].

Further evidence for the role of the DQA1 locus comes from the protective association of Europid DR7 haplotypes [35]. This is despite the occurrence on 70% of these haplotypes of DQB1*0201, which is positively associated with disease. Almost all Europid DR7 haplotypes carry DQA1*0201, which is significantly protective, in contrast to the negroid DR7 haplotype which carries DQA1*0301 and is positively associated with disease [42]. The protective effect of DQA1*0201, which may counter the predisposing effect of DQB1*0201 on DR7 haplotypes, is also seen in North Indian Asians [44], but this allele is rare in other races.

No single DQB1 allele occurs on both DR13 and DR15 haplotypes: DR13 is associated with DQB1*0603 and DQB1*0604 and DR15 with DQB1*0602. All have been shown to be significantly protective in Europids [35]. DQB1*0602 and DQB1*0603 are very similar alleles whose products differ at only two amino acid residues [65]. They are protective in Negroids and North Indian Asians. One study showed both alleles to be absent from a Southern Chinese diabetic population [40] and DQB1*0602 is reduced in Japanese diabetic subjects [41]. The protective effects of DQA1*0102 and/or DQA1*0103 and DQB1*0602 and/or DQB1*0603 are, therefore, consistent in many racial groups. If the minor structural differences between the DQ molecules encoded by these pairs of alleles are shown to be functionally insignificant, this would be strong evidence for HLA-associated protection as an influence on disease susceptibility, consistent with the experimental evidence of 'protective' CD4+ T cells in animal models.

HLA Molecules as Protective Determinants

The rarity, and in some cases absence, of protective DR and DQ types in diabetic populations contrasts with the high frequency of diabetes-predisposing types in healthy controls. This has been interpreted as suggesting that HLA status may be more important in conferring protection from disease rather than susceptibility to it. This is supported by the demonstration that the effect of a protective HLA type is dominant in subjects heterozygous for a protective and predisposing allele at either the DRB1, DQA1 or DQB1 locus [35].

There is strong animal evidence to support the concept of HLA-associated protection. In the diabetes-prone NOD mouse, the MHC I-E gene, analogous to DR, is not expressed. Insulitis is prevented, however, in transgenic mice which express I-E, suggesting that I-E expression protects from disease [66]. A number of immunological differences provide supportive evidence that disease is associated with deficient and not 'overactive' immune mechanisms [67, 68, 69]. Diabetes incidence is reduced in NOD mice by injection of TNFα and IL-2, both of which are associated with immune activation [70, 71]. These data suggest that disease prevention may be an active process which induces immunological tolerance, deficiency of which facilitates disease development. As the trigger for these immune responses is interaction of an HLA–peptide complex with a T cell receptor, these data are thus consistent with presentation of an HLA–peptide complex, whose effect is protective.

HLA molecules may protect from type 1 diabetes through their role in shaping T cell repertoire. Both positive and negative selection of T cell clones occur in the thymus. During negative selection, T cells which recognise HLA–self-antigen complexes are deleted in the thymic medulla; T cells which react with foreign antigen are selected in the thymic cortex. Autoreactive T cell clones which enter the peripheral circulation are thought to undergo clonal anergy or inactivation [72]. Failure to remove islet-B-cell specific T cells from the circulation may thus predispose to diabetes. Studies in the NOD mouse have provided conflicting data on the role of clonal deletion as a protective mechanism. While one effect of the protective I-E molecule was to facilitate the clonal deletion of autoreactive T cells [73], another study showed that apparently normal I-E expression in the thymic medulla was insufficient to prevent disease [74]. The protective CD4+ cells demonstrated in animal experiments are not, however, present in neonates [75], suggesting that they may have arisen following exposure to an environmental stimulus; the significant environmental effect on disease susceptibility may suggest a role for peripheral tolerance.

It has been suggested that protection from type 1 diabetes follows binding of protective antigenic peptide or 'tolerogen' by class II molecules and its subsequent presentation to suppressor T cells [69]. According to this model, the most protective DQ molecules, for example DQ6 (encoded by DQA1*0102 and DQB1*0602) are those which bind tolerogen most efficiently, possibly because of structural determinants.

The structure of some HLA molecules (for example DQ8, encoded by DQA1*0301 and DQB1*0302) may prevent binding of the tolerogen and hence predispose to insulitis. The model proposed by Nepom [46] suggests that protection would ensue in an individual in whom no high-affinity predisposing DQ molecules were expressed. As no common amino acid sequences consistently distinguish protective from predisposing DQ molecules, the mechanism by which structural effects influence peptide binding requires further elucidation.

The magnitude of response of MHC-restricted T cell clones is a function of the concentrations of both antigen and MHC molecules [76]. It is of interest that the promoter strength of the neutral DQB1*0301 allele (which encodes DQ7) is four times that of the predisposing DQB1*0302 allele (which encodes DQ8) [77]. It would be expected that antigen presented by DQ8 will induce a considerably reduced T cell response. The respective disease associations of these two alleles are consistent with the effect of tolerogen presentation to suppressor T cells. This may be evidence for a functional difference, rather than a structural one, between diabetes-predisposing and protective DQ alleles and it is possible that overall DQ molecular density, rather than specific DQ type alone, is important in determining disease susceptibility. Further studies are indicated to determine whether protective DQA1 and DQB1 alleles have increased promoter strengths compared to predisposing ones and to demonstrate the occurrence of DQ-restricted suppressor T cells.

OTHER MHC GENES

Other MHC genes have been considered as candidate susceptibility determinants for type 1 diabetes. The DPA1 and DPB1 loci (centromeric to the DQ loci) are polymorphic [78]. A positive association between a DPB1 polymorphism and type 1 diabetes was observed in a Europid population but not in other races [79]. The DP genes are not, therefore, thought to confer a susceptibility effect independent of DR or DQ. The TAP1 and TAP2 genes are polymorphic and a possible protective association of TAP2*0201 was suggested [80] although a subsequent study has provided conflicting data [81]. Susceptibility to type 1 diabetes has been associated with the C4A3 allele of the C4 complement locus (class III) and an increase in the frequency of C4AQ0/C4BQ0 (null) alleles [82,83]. It has been suggested that single gene copies of the C4 genes were a common feature of diabetes-associated haplotypes [84]. The HSP70 genes (1 and 2), also located in the class III region of the MHC, have been considered as susceptibility loci. Although restriction fragment length polymorphism (RFLP) analysis has demonstrated an increase in an 8.5 kb RFLP fragment of the HSP70 2 gene among patients, this allele occurred on DR3 haplotypes and it was suggested that the increase in the 8.5 kb RFLP merely reflected the disease association of DR3 [85].

RFLP analysis has demonstrated two polymorphisms of the TNFB gene which were detected by a TNFα cDNA probe [86]. Heterozygosity for the TNFB polymorphism has been associated with increased risk of type 1 diabetes in Europid subjects [87] but not in North Indian Asians [88] or Southern Chinese [89] and this association is probably secondary to linkage disequilibrium.

NON-HLA GENES AND TYPE 1 DIABETES

A significant component of inherited susceptibility to type 1 diabetes is encoded by genes outside the MHC. Until recently the search for non-HLA susceptibility genes was limited to candidate gene studies in human populations; these were generally unrewarding with few consistent disease associations. Subsequently the use of animal models of type 1 diabetes identified regions associated with disease susceptibility which could be tested in humans. This comparative mapping strategy has, however, been largely superseded by exclusion mapping of the human genome using highly polymorphic microsatellite markers and fluorescence-based genotyping technology.

Candidate Gene Studies

Insulin Gene Region (INS)

The autoimmune process leading to type 1 diabetes is highly specific to pancreatic B cells, the only cells which produce insulin. The insulin gene is, therefore, a plausible candidate susceptibility locus for type 1 diabetes; for example, insulin or insulin precursors may act as autoantigens targeting the islet B cells for destruction. Alternatively, levels of insulin secretion may modulate the interaction between the immune system and islet B cells. It is of note that intensive insulin therapy given at the time of diagnosis can reduce B cell loss, possibly by reducing insulin secretion [90]. Further, treatment of prediabetic NOD mice with insulin prevents onset of disease, suggesting that exogenous insulin protects islet B cells from autoimmune attack [91]. A pilot study of low-dose insulin therapy in high-risk siblings of type 1 diabetic patients has shown results consistent with these animal data [116].

The insulin gene region (INS) lies on the short arm of chromosome 11. A major polymorphism is located upstream (5') to the transcription region of the insulin gene in which alleles differ in their number of tandem repeats. This type of polymorphism, which is common throughout the human genome, is termed a variable number tandem repeat (VNTR). In Europids, the alleles of the INS VNTR can be assigned to two major groups; class 1 alleles are of approximately 40 repeats and the larger class 3 alleles of 170 repeats. Most population studies have shown a positive association between class 1 alleles within the INS region and type 1 diabetes in Europids [92, 93]. Early linkage analyses in multiplex families, however, failed to confirm this finding [94]. In a more recent study from France, analysis of a large group of unrelated subjects with type 1 diabetes confirmed an association with newly defined polymorphisms across the INS region. Direct evidence for linkage was then obtained by analysis of sibling pairs whose parents were heterozygous for the disease-associated INS polymorphisms [95]. Interestingly, in that study, linkage was observed only in male meioses, suggesting maternal imprinting of the INS region. In addition, the INS association was significant only in HLA-DR4-positive diabetic subjects, implying an interaction between HLA and INS susceptibility loci. A number of studies have since failed to confirm an interaction between INS and HLA-DR4 [96, 97, 98, 99]. Moreover, analysis using the British Diabetic Association–Warren Repository of multiplex families [100] found no evidence for maternal imprinting at INS [98].

The nature of any interaction between INS and HLA remains controversial, as does the existence of parent-of-origin effects on INS susceptibility. However, there is no doubt that susceptibility to type 1 diabetes is encoded by INS and the responsible polymorphisms reside within the VNTR itself. Bennett et al have shown that length polymorphism of the class 1 VNTR is associated with differing levels of risk of disease (from protection through to increased susceptibility) [117]. These polymorphisms are also causally related to variation in insulin gene expression (and hence insulin secretion), offering a putative mechanism for the genetic association.

T-Cell Receptor Genes

T cells recognise antigen when it is in combination with HLA molecules on the surface of antigen presenting cells (Figure 3). This recognition is facilitated by the T cell receptor (TCR), a heterodimeric cell surface molecule comprising an α and β chain, both with constant and variable regions. Since type 1 diabetes is T-cell mediated, the genes encoding the TCR are plausible candidates for disease susceptibility. The loci for TCR α and β chains (TCRA and TCRB) are located on chromosomes 14 and 7 respectively. Association and linkage analyses of polymorphisms of the gene encoding TCRA constant region and type 1 diabetes have been negative [101, 102]. Early association studies of polymorphisms within the TCRB constant region suggested that patients were more likely to be heterozygous at this locus than controls [103, 104]. Recent studies, however, using larger populations and linkage studies in families, have failed to confirm this observation [101, 102]. It should be noted that these studies are concerned only with susceptibility due to variation in germ-line TCR genes; somatic diversification mechanisms allow for random addition and deletion of nucleotides at junctions between TCR gene segments. For this reason, the TCR products expressed on the surface of peripheral T cells are not entirely encoded in the germ line and even monozygotic twins may differ in their repertoire of TCR specificities.

Immunoglobulin Heavy Chain (Gm) Regions

Antibody production against islet cell antigens, insulin and glutamic acid decarboxylase (GAD) is a feature of type 1 diabetes. Available data suggest that these antibodies are a secondary phenomenon, although anti-GAD antibodies may be primarily involved in disease susceptibility. The immunoglobulin heavy chain region (Gm) is found on the long arm of chromosome 14. Gm allotypes are serologically defined antigens located in the constant portion of the γ heavy chains of IgG immunoglobulins. There is evidence for associations between Gm allotypes and susceptibility to autoimmune disease; hence the Gm region is a candidate for genetic susceptibility to type 1 diabetes. Several studies have failed to demonstrate a direct disease association and linkage studies yielded negative results [105]. However, it has been proposed that genes encoding Gm allotypes, or in linkage disequilibrium with them, may contribute to susceptibility through interactions with HLA, TCRB and INS [105]. These complex proposals are based on small numbers of subjects taken from pooled data sets; replication is required from independent populations.

Comparative Mapping Using Animal Models of Type 1 Diabetes

Until recently the best evidence for the existence of susceptibility genes outside HLA and INS came from genetic analysis of the non-obese diabetic (NOD) mouse [106]. The NOD mouse is an inbred strain (i.e. individuals within a colony are genetically identical) that spontaneously develops diabetes which is very similar to human type 1 diabetes. Autoimmune islet-cell destruction is a shared characteristic, as are the appearance of autoantibodies to islet B cell components

and other endocrine tissues, defects in T cell activity, sensitivity to immunosuppression and the presence of a susceptibility locus within the MHC. Comparative mapping of the mouse and human has revealed extensive regions of homology (see Chapter 3). Prediction of the location of disease loci in man, given their location in the mouse, is a potentially powerful application of the mouse/human comparative map [107].

A linkage map of the mouse genome was generated using the polymerase chain reaction (PCR) to amplify microsatellite DNA markers [108]. Microsatellites are blocks of simple repetitive DNA (di-, tri- and tetra-nucleotide repeats) possessing length polymorphism that can be resolved on agarose or acrylamide gels, without the need for restriction enzyme digestion or radiolabelling [108, 109]. Analysis of the co-segregation of these randomly dispersed markers and disease in outcross and backcross experiments led to the discovery of three significant linkages in 1991 [106, 110]. *Idd-3* is located on mouse chromosome 3 (in mouse, the MHC susceptibility gene complex is *Idd-1* and a putative locus on chromosome 9 has been designated *Idd-2*), *Idd-4* on chromosome 11 and *Idd-5* on chromosome 1. Continuing studies of the NOD mouse suggest that at least 10 loci contribute to disease development. Syntenous conserved regions in the human are located on chromosomes 1 or 4, 17 and 2 respectively and are candidate susceptibility regions for human type 1 diabetes [111].

The comparative mapping strategy has now been used to investigate the human homologues of *Idd-2* and *Idd-5*. Data from the NOD mouse suggested that the Thy-1 gene on mouse chromosome 9 is linked to diabetes susceptibility at a recombination distance of 10–15% (*Idd-2*) [113]. In humans, the Thy-1 locus lies in a syntenous conserved linkage group on chromosome 11q. Eighty-one affected sib-pair families were analysed with 17 marker loci for linkage to type 1 diabetes [112]; there was no evidence to support the existence of a major susceptibility locus (roughly equivalent to HLA) within the region. In the same year as this study, another group examined alleles of the CD3 epsilon (ε) gene; this encodes the TCR-CD3 complex ε chain and is located on chromosome 11q23. They reported a significant difference between the frequency of a CD3ε 8 kb allele in male and female diabetic subjects and between female diabetics and controls (114). This led to the suggestion that a gene residing on chromosome 11q23 might cause susceptibility to type 1 diabetes in women and subsequently led to the designation of CD3ε as human '*IDDM 2*' by the Eleventh International Workshop on Human Gene Mapping [115]. Attempts have subsequently been made to confirm this finding using both association and linkage analyses in diabetic and control subjects from the same population as was studied by Wong et al [118]. In this larger data set, there was no evidence of a sex-specific effect at CD3ε and the designation '*IDDM2*' has subsequently been assigned to INS.

Examination of the homologue of *Idd*-5 on chromosome 2 has shown more promising data [119]. The region of chromosome 2q homologous with the location of *Idd*-5 is of specific interest since two potential candidate genes reside within this area; the interleukin-1 receptor gene (IL-1R1) and Lsh/Lty/Bcg, which influence macrophage activation and resistance to infection. Copeman et al examined allele sharing and linkage disequilibrium at 21 microsatellite marker loci and at 3 polymorphisms in the interleukin-1 gene region in six independent data sets. The marker D2S152 was associated with disease in three data sets (and showed evidence for linkage in one), localising a gene designated *IDDM7* to within 2 centiMorgans (cM) of this marker. More detailed linkage disequilibrium mapping of marker loci within this region will allow closer definition of the diabetogenic polymorphism(s).

Exclusion Mapping of the Human Genome

Until 1994, successful dissection of complex traits by genome-wide linkage mapping was restricted to experimental organisms such as mice and tomatoes. A number of technological advances allowed the application of these techniques to humans. Specifically, characterisation of PCR-analysed microsatellite marker loci [109]; construction of high resolution human genetic linkage maps [120]; and the application of fluorescence-based, automated DNA fragment sizing technology [121, 122] facilitated genome-wide exclusion mapping. The availability of large numbers of multiple-case pedigrees [100, 123] allowed type 1 diabetes to be the first complex disorder to be subjected to a methodical search for susceptibility loci using these advances. In contrast to the technological aspects of this approach, the statistics are relatively simple; a significant excess of alleles shared identical-by-descent (IBD) in affected sibling pairs (ASPs) versus that expected is taken as evidence of genetic linkage. This approach does not require prior knowledge of disease gene frequencies or mode of inheritance.

Davies et al employed a two-stage approach to map novel susceptibility genes for type 1 diabetes [124]. First, a genome screen was performed by testing 290 microsatellite marker loci in 96 UK ASPs. The fluorescence-based genome linkage map had an average spacing of 11 cM and the markers had a mean heterozygosity of 0.8. This gave 97% coverage of the human genome at a resolution of 20 cM. Those marker loci for which preliminary evidence of linkage was obtained (maximum lod score [MLS] ≥ 1; equivalent to $p <$

0.05) were then tested in two additional data sets comprising 102 UK ASPs and 84 sib-pair families collected from the USA. Confirmation of initial findings is essential given previous failures to replicate linkage data in other complex disorders. Finally, since the HLA region was known to be an important locus of disease susceptibility, ASPs were subdivided into two groups by IBD status at HLA; those sharing two HLA alleles or haplotypes IBD (i.e. families showing strongest evidence of linkage to HLA) and those sharing either one or zero alleles [125].

This landmark study confirmed the primacy of MHC-encoded susceptibility (designated *IDDM1*) to type 1 diabetes. The microsatellite marker locus used to analyse linkage to the MHC (TNFα) gave an MLS of 7.3; MLS values approaching this magnitude were not observed for any other chromosome. Furthermore, marker loci located up to 20 cM away from TNFα were found to have MLS values exceeding 1.0; by taking a 20 cM radius of all the other marker loci it was possible to exclude at least 97% of the genome for genes with effects equivalent to *IDDM1*. The INS region on chromosome 11p15 (*IDDM2*) also showed evidence of linkage to type 1 diabetes (MLS = 2.1). In addition, 18 other chromosome regions showed positive evidence of linkage to disease. Ten of these exceeded MLS value of 1.7 ($p < 0.005$): chromosomes 3q (D3S1303), 6q (ESR and D6S264), 7q (CFTR), 8q (D8S556), 10cen (D10S193), 11q (FGF3), 13q (D13S158) and X (DXS991 and DXS999). Some of these linked marker loci occur in regions containing candidate genes; notably, D10S193 is located close to the GAD2 gene which encodes the enzyme glutamic acid decarboxylase, a possible B cell autoantigen. The linkages to chromosomes 11q and 6q were confirmed by replication.

In all families, FGF3 on chromosome 11q was linked to disease; however, the most significant evidence of linkage was obtained in the subset of families sharing 1 or 0 alleles IBD at HLA. Six additional polymorphic microsatellite marker loci in the FGF3 region were analysed, giving a peak MLS of 3.4 at FGF3 ($p < 0.0001$). This implies that a disease locus, designated *IDDM4*, lies in the 14 cM region between D11S1253 and D11S1314. Independent analyses have also confirmed linkage in this region. Hashimoto et al performed genome-wide linkage analysis of 314 ASPs from 231 families of French, American and North African origin; linkage between FGF3 and disease was demonstrated and, once again, this effect was enhanced by subdivision of the dataset according to HLA [126]. Field et al identified *IDDM4* by candidate gene analysis of 250 pedigrees which included 100 families from the British Diabetic Association–Warren Repository

[100, 127] (also studied by Davies et al). Chromosome 11q13 was considered a candidate region following reports that it contained a locus influencing atopy [128].

In the 96 UK families, the MLS for the chromosome 6q marker locus ESR was 1.8 ($p < 0.005$), and MLS $= 2.5$ ($p < 0.001$) was obtained in the families sharing 2 alleles IBD at HLA. Linkage of chromosome 6q to disease was also obtained in the USA families, thereby replicating the initial finding. Although no evidence for linkage was seen in the second UK data set, this locus has been designated *IDDM* 5. Interestingly, *IDDM* 5 maps close to the gene SOD2, encoding superoxide dismutase, which may relate to the sensitivity of B cells to free radical damage. Preliminary data suggest an association between a SOD2 RFLP and type 1 diabetes [129].

The microsatellite locus D18S64, which in the 96 UK families showed evidence of linkage to type 1 diabetes, is in the same region of chromosome 18 as the Kidd blood group locus. Linkage to Kidd blood group was first reported in 1981 [130] and, although a second independent study failed to replicate this finding [131], a population-based association between Kidd blood group and type 1 diabetes has been observed [132]. Taken together with the linkage data on chromosome 18, these results suggest that a susceptibility gene may be located close to the Kidd blood group locus.

IDDM 3 (reported after *IDDM* 4 and 5) is located on chromosome 15q26. This locus was identified by Field et al following exclusion mapping of 250 families with more than one diabetic offspring [127]. This group also analysed affected–unaffected sibling pairs to provide additional evidence for involvement of this region. It is of note that the region of mouse chromosome 9 to which *Idd*-2 was mapped is homologous in humans to portions of both chromosome 11q and 15q [133]. A candidate for *IDDM* 3 is the insulin-like growth factor I receptor (IGF1R), since IGF-I levels and bioactivity have been reported to be reduced in children with type 1 diabetes [134] (see Chapter 20).

SUMMARY

The strongest genetic associations of type 1 diabetes are with HLA genes, and certain HLA alleles are good markers of disease risk. Modern DNA techniques have resulted in a rapid increase in our knowledge of these genes and of their associations with type 1 diabetes. Despite this, and the discovery of previously unknown genes, there has been little progress in mapping susceptibility to the disease more precisely within the MHC. Much attention has focused on the role of DQβ-Asp57 and specific heterodimers in disease susceptibility, but these have failed adequately to explain the observed HLA associations in different populations.

The contribution of HLA genes to protection from disease has been examined in this chapter. Preliminary evidence suggests that such protective effects may be more important than those of predisposing markers, and this may partly explain the difficulty in mapping HLA-associated susceptibility. The mechanism(s) by which HLA genes influence susceptibility to type 1 diabetes have yet to be established. Possible mechanisms of action of HLA molecules include differential effects on antigen binding, effects on T cell repertoire and activation of suppressor cells.

Recently, there have been considerable advances in the identification of non-HLA susceptibility genes. *IDDM* 2 has been mapped to the insulin VNTR and the fine mapping of at least five other susceptibility loci is under way. Ultimately, this research effort should facilitate genetic population screening for individuals at high risk of type 1 diabetes.

For large-scale screening, the use of genetic markers has a number of advantages over serological and physiological testing: a genetic screening test need only be performed once since the inherited genome is invariant; invasive procedures are not necessary as PCR analyses can be performed on buccal cell mouthwashes; and PCR methodologies are simple, robust and easily transferred between laboratories. A cohort of high-risk individuals, identified before any indication of disease pathogenesis (ideally at birth), would facilitate the prospective study of environmental influences on diabetes development. Early diagnosis of type 1 diabetes in this group would also provide an important reagent for testing therapies which may reduce or prevent the need for insulin.

Finally, the identification of genetic susceptibility markers will ultimately lead to the isolation of individual genes, and their responsible polymorphisms. This will allow insights into the pathophysiology of type 1 diabetes and ultimately lead to new therapeutic strategies.

ACKNOWLEDGEMENTS

The authors gratefully acknowledge financial support from the Medical Research Council (UK), The Wellcome Trust, The British Diabetic Association, Juvenile Diabetes Foundation International and Lilly Industries (UK). We would also like to thank Dr Cath Mijovic for useful discussion.

REFERENCES

1. Todd JA. Genetic control of autoimmunity in type 1 diabetes. Immunol Today 1990; 11: 122–9.

2. Karvonen M, Tuomilehto J, Libman I, LaPorte R for the WHO DIAMOND project group. A review of the recent epidemiologial data on the worldwide incidence of type 1 (insulin-dependent) diabetes mellitus. Diabetologia 1993; 36: 883–92.

3. Vaishnava H, Bashin RC, Galati PO. Diabetes mellitus with onset under 40 years in North India. J Assoc Physicians India 1974; 22: 879–88.

4. Shanghai Diabetes Research Cooperative Group. Diabetes mellitus survey in Shanghai. Chin Med J 1980; 93: 663–7.

5. Diabetes Epidemiology Research International. Preventing insulin-dependent diabetes mellitus: the environmental challenge. Br Med J 1987; 295: 479–81.

6. Rewers M, LaPorte RE, Walczak M, Dmochowski K, Bogaczynska E. An apparent 'epidemic' of youth onset insulin-dependent diabetes mellitus in Western Poland. Diabetes 1987; 36: 106–13.

7. Singal DP, Blajchman MA. Histocompatibility (HLA) antigens, lymphocytotoxic antibodies and tissue-specific antibodies in patients with diabetes mellitus. Diabetes 1973; 22: 429–32.

8. Nerup J, Platz P, Andersen OO et al. HLA antigens in diabetes mellitus. Lancet 1974; ii: 864–6.

9. Boitard C. The differentiation of the immune system towards anti-islet autoimmunity. Clinical prospects. Diabetologia 1992; 35: 1101–12.

10. Risch N. Assessing the role of HLA-linked and unlinked determinants of disease. Am J Hum Genet 1987; 40: 1–14.

11. Schwartz RH. T-lymphocyte recognition of antigen in association with gene products of the major histocompatibility complex. Ann Rev Immunol 1985; 3: 237–61.

12. Campbell RD, Trowsdale J. Map of Human MHC. Immunol Today 1993; 14: 349–52.

13. Bodmer JG, Marsh SGE, Parham P et al. Nomenclature for factors of the HLA system 1989. Tissue Antigens 1990; 35: 1–8.

14. Kelly AP, Manaco JJ, Cho SG, Trowsdale J. A new human HLA class II-related locus, DM. Nature 1991; 353: 571–3.

15. Powis SH, Mockridge I, Kerr LA et al. Polymorphism in a second ABC transporter gene located within the class II region of the human major histocompatibility complex. Proc Natl Acad Sci USA 1992; 89: 1463–7.

16. Carrington M, Colonna M, Spies T, Stephens JC, Mann DL. Haplotypic variation of the transporter-associated with antigen processing (TAP) genes and their extension of HLA class II region haplotypes. Immunogenetics 1993; 37: 266–73.

17. Trowsdale J. Genomic structure and function in the MHC. Trends Genet 1993; 9: 112–22.

18. Carroll MC. A molecular map of the human major histocompatibility complex class III region linking complement genes C4, C2 and factor B. Nature 1984; 307: 237–41.

19. Spies T, Morton CC, Nedospasor SA, Fiers W, Pious D, Strominger JL. Genes for the tumour necrosis factors α and β are linked to the human major histocompatibility complex. Proc Natl Acad Sci USA 1986; 86: 1968–72.

20. Sargant CA, Durham I, Trowsdale J, Campbell RD. Human major histocompatibility complex contains genes for the major heat shock protein HSP70. Proc Natl Acad Sci USA 1989; 86: 1968–72.

21. Schwartz BD. The human major histocompatibility human leukocyte antigen (HLA) complex. In Stites DP, Terr AI (eds) Basic and clinical immunology, 7th edn. Norwalk: Appleton & Lange, 1991: pp 45–60.

22. Winfield J, Janjour W. Do stress proteins play a role in arthritis and autoimmunity? Immunol Rev 1991; 121: 193–220.

23. Wolf E, Spencer KM, Cudworth AG. The genetic susceptibility to type 1 (insulin-dependent) diabetes: analysis of the HLA-DR association. Diabetologia 1983; 24: 224–30.

24. Hammond MG, Asmal AC, Omar MAK. HLA and insulin-dependent diabetes in South African Negroes. Diabetologia 1980; 19: 101–2.

25. Omar MAK, Hammond MG, Asmal MC. HLA-A, B, C and DR antigens in young South African blacks with type 1 (insulin-dependent) diabetes mellitus. Diabetologia 1984; 26: 20–3.

26. Srikanta S, Mehra NK, Vaidya MC, Malaviya AN, Amuja MMS. HLA antigens in type 1 (insulin-dependent) diabetes mellitus in North India. Metabolism 1981; 30: 992–3.

27. Lee BW, Chan SH, Tan SH et al. HLA-system in Chinese children with insulin-dependent diabetes mellitus: a strong association with DR3. Metabolism 1984; 33: 1102–5.

28. Moriuchi J, Katagiri M, Wakisaka A et al. Association of B cell alloantigen with juvenile onset diabetes mellitus in the Japanese. Hum Immunol 1980; 4: 357–62.

29. Wakisaka A, Aizawa M, Matsura N et al. HLA and juvenile diabetes mellitus in the Japanese. Lancet 1976; i: 970.

30. Patel R, Ansari A, Covarrubias CLP. Leucocyte antigens and disease. III: Association of HLA B8 and HLA B15 with insulin-dependent diabetes in three different population groups. Metabolism 1977; 26: 487–92.

31. Rich SS, Weitkamp LR, Barbosa J. Genetic heterogeneity of insulin-dependent (type 1) diabetes mellitus: evidence from a study of extended haplotypes. Am J Hum Genet 1984; 36: 1015–23.

32. Jenkins D, Mijovic C, Fletcher J, Jacobs KH, Bradwell AR, Barnett AH. Identification of susceptibility loci for type 1 (insulin-dependent) diabetes by trans-racial gene mapping. Diabetologia 1990; 33: 387–95.

33. Louis EJ, Thomson G. Three-allele synergistic mixed model for insulin-dependent diabetes. Diabetes 1986; 35: 958–63.

34. Thomson G, Robinson WP, Kuhner MK et al. Genetic heterogeneity, modes of inheritance and risk estimates for a joint study of Caucasians with insulin-dependent diabetes mellitus. Am J Hum Genet 1988; 43: 799–816.

35. Cavan DA, Jacobs KH, Penny MA et al. Both DQA1 and DQB1 genes are implicated in HLA-associated protection from type 1 (insulin-dependent) diabetes in a British Caucasian population. Diabetologia 1993; 35: 252–7.

36. Owerbach D, Lernmark A, Platz P, Ryder LP, Peterson PA, Ludvigsson J. HLA-D region β-chain DNA endonuclease fragments differ between HLA-DR-identical healthy and insulin-dependent diabetic individuals. Nature 1983; 303: 815–17.

37. Nepom BS, Palmer J, Kim SJ, Jansen JA, Holbeck SL, Nepom GT. Specific genomic markers for the HLA-DQ subregion discriminate between DR4+ insulin-dependent diabetes mellitus and DR4+ seropositive juvenile rheumatoid arthritis. J Exp Med 1986; 164: 345–50.

38. Fletcher J, Odugbesan O, Mijovic C, Mackay E, Bradwell AR, Barnett AH. Class II HLA DNA polymorphisms in type I (insulin-dependent) diabetic patients of North Indian origin. Diabetologia 1988; 31: 343–50.

39. Mijovic CH, Jenkins D, Jacobs KH, Penny MA, Fletcher J, Barnett AH. HLA-DQA1 and -DQB1 alleles associated with genetic susceptibility to IDDM in a black population. Diabetes 1991; 40: 748–53.

40. Penny MA, Jenkins D, Mijovic CH et al. Susceptibility to insulin-dependent diabetes mellitus in a Chinese population: role of HLA class II alleles. Diabetes 1992; 41: 914–19.

41. Jacobs KH, Jenkins D, Mijovic CH et al. An investigation of Japanese subjects maps susceptibility to type 1 (insulin-dependent) diabetes mellitus close to the DQA1 gene. Hum Immunol 1992; 33: 24–8.

42. Todd JA, Mijovic C, Fletcher J, Jenkins D, Bradwell AR, Barnett AH. Identification of susceptibility loci for insulin-dependent diabetes mellitus by transracial gene mapping. Nature 1989; 338: 587–9.

43. Khalil I, d'Auriol L, Gobet M et al. A combination of HLA-DQβ Asp 57-negative and HLA DQα Arg 52 confers susceptibility to insulin-dependent diabetes mellitus. J Clin Invest 1990; 85: 1315–19.

44. Jenkins D, Mijovic C, Jacobs KH, Penny MA, Fletcher J, Barnett AH. Allele-specific gene probing supports the DQ molecule as a determinant of inherited susceptibility to type 1 (insulin-dependent) diabetes mellitus. Diabetologia 1991; 34: 109–13.

45. Jacobs KH, Cavan DA, Penny MA, Barnett AH. DR4-associated susceptibility to type 1 diabetes mellitus does not result from DQA1 promoter region polymorphism. Diabetic Med 1993; 10 (suppl 1): S41.

46. Nepom GT. A unified hypothesis for the complex genetics of HLA associations with IDDM. Diabetes 1990; 39: 1153–7.

47. Roep BO, Kallan AA, De Vreis RRP. β-cell antigen-specific lysis of macrophages by CD4+ T-cell clones from newly diagnosed IDDM patient. A putative mechanism of T-cell-mediated autoimmune islet cell destruction. Diabetes 1992; 41: 1380–4.

48. Sasazuki T, Kikuchi K, Hirayama S, Matsushita S, Ohta N, Nishimura Y. HLA-linked immune suppression in humans. Immunology (suppl) 1989; 2: 21–4.

49. Kwok WW, Mickelson E, Masewicz, Milner ECB, Hansen J, Nepom GT. Polymorphic DQα and DQβ interactions dictate HLA class II determinants of allorecognition. J Exp Med 1990; 171: 85–95.

50. Seidl C, Lee JS. Expression of alternatively spliced HLA class II transcripts in lymphoid and non lymphoid tissues. Immunogenetics 1992; 35: 385–90.

51. Lombardi G, Barber L, Aichinger G, Heaton T, Sidhu S, Batchelor JR, Lechler RI. Structural analysis of anti-DR1 allorecognition by using DR1/H-2E^k hybrid molecules. Influence of the β2-domain correlates with C4-dependence. J Immunol 1991; 147: 2034–40.

52. Todd JA, Bell JI, McDevitt HO. HLA-DQβ gene contributes to susceptibility and resistance to insulin-dependent diabetes mellitus. Nature 1987; 329: 599–604.

53. Braun JH, Jardetzky TS, Garga JC, Stern LJ, Urban RG, Strominger JL, Wiley DC. Three-dimensional structure of the human class II histocompatibility antigen HLA-DR1. Nature 1993; 364: 33–9.

54. Achea-Orbea H, McDevitt HO. The first external domain of the non-obese diabetic mouse class II I-A beta-chain is unique. Proc Natl Acad Sci USA 1987; 84: 2435–9.

55. Nepom BS, Schwarz D, Palmer JP, Nepom GT. Transcomplementation of HLA genes in IDDM. Diabetes 1987; 36: 114–17.

56. Gutierrez-Lopez MD, Bertera S, Chantres MT, Vavassori C, Dorman JS, Trucco M, Serrano-Rios M. Susceptibility to type 1 (insulin-dependent) diabetes mellitus in Spanish patients correlates quantitatively with expression of HLA-DQα Arg52 and HLA-DQβ non-Asp 57 alleles. Diabetologia 1992; 35: 583–8.

57. Penny MA, Mijovic CH, Cavan DA, Jacobs KH, Jenkins D, Fletcher JA, Barnett AH. An investigation into the role of HLA-DQα Arg52-DQβ non-Asp57 heterodimers in susceptibility to type 1 (insulin-dependent) diabetes mellitus: studies in five racial groups. Hum Immunol 1993; 38: 179–83.

58. Buzzetti R, Nistico L, Osborn JF, Giovanni C, Chersi C, Sorrentino R. HLA-DQA1 and DQB1 gene polymorphism in type 1 diabetes patients from central Italy and their use for risk prediction. Diabetes 1993; 42: 1173–8.

59. Germain RN, Bentley DM, Quill H. Influence of allelic polymorphism on the assembly and surface expression of class II MHC (Ia) molecules. Cell 1985; 43: 233–42.

60. Kwok WW, Kovats S, Thurtle P, Nepom GT. HLA-DQ allelic polymorphisms constrain patterns of heterodimer formation. J Immunol 1993; 150: 2263–72.

61. Miyazaki T, Uno M, Uehira M et al. Direct evidence for the contribution of the unique I-A^{NOD} to the development of insulitis in non-obese diabetic mice. Nature 1990; 345: 722–4.

62. Awata T, Kuzuya T, Matsuda A, Iwamoto Y, Kanazawa Y, Okuyama M, Juji T. High frequency of aspartic acid at position 57 of HLA-DQ β-chain in Japanese IDDM patients and non-diabetic subjects. Diabetes 1990; 39: 266–9.

63. Tuomilehto-Wolf E, Tuomilehto J, Hitman GA. DQA1 and DQB1 heterodimers in IDDM: a genetic-epidemiological study in Finland. DiMe Study Group. Ann Med 1992; 24: 533–8.

64. Cohen N, Brautbar C, Font M-P et al. HLA-DR2-associated Dw subtypes correlate with RFLP clusters: most DR2 IDDM patients belong to one of these clusters. Immunogenetics 1992; 23: 84–9.

65. Marsh SGE, Bodmer JG. HLA Class II nucleotide sequences, 1991. Tissue Antigens 1991; 37: 181–9.

66. Lund T, O'Reilly L, Hutchings P et al. Prevention of insulin-dependent diabetes mellitus in non-obese diabetic mice transgenes encoding modified I-A β-chain or normal I-E α-chain. Nature 1990; 345: 727–9.

67. Baisch JM, Weeks T, Giles R, Hoover M, Stastny P, Capra JD. Analysis of HLA-DQ genotypes and

susceptibility in insulin-dependent diabetes mellitus. N Engl J Med 1990; 322: 1836–41.

68. Mordes JP, Desemone J, Rossini AA. The BB rat. Diabetes Metab Rev 1987; 3: 725–50.

69. Sheehy MJ. HLA and insulin-dependent diabetes. A protective perspective. Diabetes 1992; 41: 123–9.

70. Satoh J, Seino H, Abo T et al. Recombinant human tumour necrosis factor α suppresses autoimmune diabetes in NOD mice. J Clin Invest 1989; 84: 1345–8.

71. Serreze DV, Hamaguchi K, Leiter EH. Immuno-stimulation circumvents diabetes in NOD/Lt mice. J Autoimmunity 1989; 2: 759–76.

72. Rennie J. The body against itself. Sci Am 1990 (December); 263: 76–85.

73. Bill J, Kanagawa O, Woodland DL, Palmer E. The MHC molecule I-E is necessary but not sufficient for the clonal deletion of VβII-bearing T cells. J Exp Med 1989; 169: 1405–19.

74. Böhme J, Schuhbaur B, Kanagawa O, Benoist C, Mathis D. MHC-linked protection from diabetes dissociated from clonal deletion of T cells. Science 1990; 249: 293–5.

75. Boitard C, Yasunami R, Dardenne M, Bach JF. T-cell mediated inhibition of the transfer of autoimmune diabetes in NOD mice. J Exp Med 1989; 169: 1669–80.

76. Lechler RI, Norcross MA, Germain RN. Qualitative and quantitative studies of antigen-presenting cell function by using I-A-expressing L cells. J Immunol 1985; 135: 2914–22.

77. Andersen CL, Beaty JS, Nettles JW, Seyfried CE, Nepom GT, Nepom BS. Allelic polymorphism in transcriptional regulatory regions of HLA-DQB genes. J Exp Med 1991; 173: 181–92.

78. Al-Daccack R, Wang FQ, Theophille D, Lethiel-leux P, Colombani J, Loiseau P. Gene polymorphism of HLA-DPA1 and DPB1 loci in Caucasoid population: frequencies and DPA1-DPB1 associations. Hum Immunol 1991; 31: 277–85.

79. Easteal S, Kohonen-Corish MRJ, Zimmet P, Ser-jeantson SW. HLA-DP variation as additional risk factor in IDDM. Diabetes 1990; 39: 855–7.

80. Colonna M, Bresnahen M, Bahram S, Strominger J, Spies T. Allelic variants of the human putative peptide transporter involved in antigen processing. Proc Natl Acad Sci 1992; 89: 3932–6.

81. Ronningen KS, Undlien DE, Ploski R et al. Linkage disequilibrium between TAP2 variants and HLA class II alleles; no primary association between TAP2 variants and insulin dependent diabetes mellitus. J Immunol 1993; 23: 1050–6.

82. Thomsen M, Molvig J, Zerbib A et al. The susceptibility to insulin-dependent diabetes mellitus is associated with C4 allotypes independently of the association with HLA-DQ alleles in HLA-DR3/4 heterozygotes. Immunogenetics 1988; 28: 320–7.

83. White PC. Molecular genetics of the class III region of the HLA complex. In Dupont B (ed) Immunobiology of HLA, vol II. Immunogenetics and histocompatibility. New York: Springer-Verlag, 1989: pp 62–9.

84. Serguado OG, Giles CM, Iglesias-Casarrubios P, Co-rell A, Martinez-Laso J, Vicaro JL, Arnaiz-Villena A. A single C4 gene copy might be a marker of diabetogenic haplotypes. In Tsuji K, Aizawa M,

Sasazuki T (eds) Proceedings of the 11th international histocompatibility workshop and conference. Oxford: Oxford Scientific Publications 1992: pp 496–8.

85. Pugliese A, Awdeh ZL, Galluzo A, Yunis EJ, Alper CA, Eisenbarth GS. No independent association between HSP70 gene polymorphism and IDDM. Diabetes 1992; 41: 788–91.

86. Webb GC, Chaplin DD. Genetic variability at the human tumour necrosis factor loci. J Immunol 1990; 145: 1278–85.

87. Badenhoop K, Schwarz G, Trowsdale J et al. TNF-α polymorphism in type 1 (insulin-dependent) diabetes mellitus. Diabetologia 1989; 32: 445–8.

88. Jenkins D, Penny MA, Mijovic C, Jacobs KH, Fletcher J, Barnett AH. Tumor necrosis factor beta polymorphism is unlikely to determine susceptibility to type 1 (insulin-dependent) diabetes mellitus. Diabetologia 1991; 34: 576–8.

89. Mijovic CH, Jenkins D, Penny MA et al. Trans-racial analysis of tumor necrosis factor gene polymorphism and type 1 (insulin-dependent) diabetes. Diabetologia 1991; 34 (suppl 2): A65.

90. Shah SC, Malone JI, Simpson NE. A randomized trial of intensive insulin therapy in newly diagnosed insulin-dependent diabetes mellitus. New Engl J Med 1989; 320: 550–4.

91. Atkinson MA, Maclaren NK, Luchetta R. Insulitis and diabetes in NOD mice reduced by prophylactic insulin therapy. Diabetes 1990; 39: 933–7.

92. Bell GI, Horita S, Karam JH. A polymorphic locus near the human insulin gene is associated with insulin-dependent diabetes mellitus. Diabetes 1984; 33: 176–83.

93. Hitman GA, Tarn AC, Winter RM et al. Type 1 (insulin-dependent) diabetes and a highly variable locus close to the insulin gene on chromosome 11. Diabetologia 1985; 28: 218–22.

94. Field LL. Non-HLA region genes in insulin dependent diabetes mellitus. Baillière's Clinical Endocrinol Metab 1991; 5: 413–38.

95. Julier C, Hyer RN, Davies J et al. Insulin-IGF2 region on chromosome 11p encodes a gene implicated in HLA-DR4-dependent diabetes susceptibility. Nature 1991; 354: 155–9.

96. Donald JA, Barendse W, Cooper DW. Linkage studies of HLA and insulin gene restriction fragment length polymorphisms in families with IDDM. Genet Epidemiol 1989; 6: 77–81.

97. Raffel LJ, Vadheim CM, Klein R et al. HLA-DR and the 5′ insulin gene polymorphism in insulin-dependent diabetes. Metabolism 1991; 40: 1244–8.

98. Bain SC, Prins JB, Hearne CM et al. Insulin gene region-encoded susceptibility to type 1 diabetes is not restricted to HLA-DR4-positive individuals. Nature Genetics 1992; 2: 212–15.

99. Van der Auwea BJ, Heimberg H, Schrevens AF, Waayenberg CV, Flament J, Schuit FC. 5′ insulin gene polymorphism confers risk to IDDM independently of HLA-class II susceptibility. Diabetes 1993; 42: 851–4.

100. Bain SC, Todd JA, Barnett AH. The British Diabetic Association–Warren Repository. Autoimmunity 1990; 7: 83–5.

101. Concannon P, Wright JA, Wright LG, Sylvester DR, Spielman RS. T-cell receptor genes and insulin-dependent diabetes mellitus (IDDM): no evidence for

linkage from affected sib pairs. Am J Hum Genet 1990; 47: 45-52.

102. Hoover ML, Black KE, Ball E. Polymorphisms of the human T-cell receptor a and b chain genes and their relationship to insulin-dependent diabetes mellitus. In Dupont B (ed) Immunobiology of HLA. New York: Springer-Verlag, 1989: pp 411-12.

103. Hoover ML, Angelini G, Ball E et al. HLA-DQ and T-cell receptor genes in insulin dependent diabetes mellitus. Cold Spring Harbor symposia on quantitative biology 1986; 51: 803-9.

104. Millward BA, Welsh KI, Leslie RDG, Pyke DA. T-cell receptor beta chain polymorphisms are associated with insulin-dependent diabetes. Clin Exp Immunol 1987; 70: 152-7.

105. Field LL, McArthur RG. The genetics of susceptibility to insulin dependent diabetes mellitus—possible new markers. Clin Invest Med 1987; 10: 437-43.

106. Todd JA, Aitman TJ, Cornall RJ et al. Genetic analysis of autoimmune type 1 diabetes mellitus in mice. Nature 1991; 351: 542-7.

107. Nadeau JH. Maps of linkage and synteny homologies between mouse and man. Trends Genet 1989; 5: 82-6.

108. Love JM, Knight AM, McAleer AM, Todd JA. Towards construction of a high resolution map of the mouse genome using PCR-analysed microsatellites. Nucleic Acids Res 1990; 18: 4123-30.

109. Weber JL, May PE. Abundant class of human DNA polymorphisms which can be typed using the polymerase chain reaction. Am J Hum Genet 1989; 44: 388-96.

110. Cornall RJ, Prins JB, Todd JA, Pessey A, DeLarato NH, Wicker LS, Peterson LB. Type 1 diabetes in mice is linked to the interleukin-1 receptor and Lsh/Ity/Bcg genes on chromosome 1. Nature 1991; 353: 262-5.

111. Todd JA, Bain SC. A practical approach to the identification of susceptibility genes for type 1 diabetes. Diabetes 1992; 41: 1029-34.

112. Hyer RN, Julier C, Buckley JD et al. High-resolution linkage mapping for susceptibility for genes in human polygenic disease: insulin-dependent diabetes mellitus and chromosome 11q. Am J Hum Genet 1991; 48: 243-57.

113. Prochazka M, Leiter EH, Serreze DV, Coleman DL. Three recessive loci required for insulin-dependent diabetes in nonobese diabetic mice. Science 1987; 237: 286-9.

114. Wong S, Moore S, Orisio S, Millward A, Domaine AG. Susceptibility to type 1 diabetes in women is associated with the CD3 epsilon locus on chromosome 11. Clin Exp Immunol 1991; 83: 69-73.

115. Junien C, van Heyningen V. Report of the committee on the genetic constitution of chromosome 11. Cytogenet Cell Genet 1991; 58: 459-554.

116. Keller RJ, Eisenbarth GS, Jackson RA. Insulin prophylaxis in individuals at high risk of type 1 diabetes. Lancet 1993; 341: 927-8.

117. Bennett ST, Lucassen AM, Gough SCL et al. Susceptibility to human type 1 diabetes at IDDM2 is determined by tandem repeat variation at the insulin gene minisatellite locus. Nature Genet 1995; 9: 284-92.

118. Pritchard LE, Kawaguchi Y, Reed PW et al. Analysis of the CD3 gene region and type 1 diabetes; application of fluorescence-based technology to association studies. Hum Molec Genet 1995; 4: 197-202.

119. Copeman JB, Hearne CM, Cornall RJ et al. Fine localisation of a type 1 diabetes susceptibility gene to human chromosome 2q by linkage disequilibrium mapping. Nature Genet 1995; 9: 80-5.

120. Gyapay G, Morissette J, Vignal A et al. The 1993-94 Genethon human genetic linkage map. Nature Genet 1994; 7: 246-339.

121. Ziegle JS, Su Y, Corcoran KP et al. Application of automated DNA sizing technology for genotyping microsatellite loci. Genomics 1992; 14(4): 1026-31.

122. Reed PW, Davies JL, Copeman JB et al. Chromosome-specific microsatellite sites for fluorescence-based, semi-automated genome mapping. Nature Genet 1994; 7: 390-5.

123. Lernmark A, Ducat L, Eisenbarth G et al. Family cell lines available for research. Amer J Hum Genet 1990; 47: 1028-30.

124. Davies JL, Kawaguchi Y, Bennett ST et al. A genome-wide search for human type 1 diabetes susceptibility genes. Nature 1994; 371(6493): 130-6.

125. Morton NE, Green A, Dunsworth T et al. Heterozygous expression of insulin-dependent diabetes mellitus (IDDM) determinants in the HLA system. Amer J Hum Genet 1983; 35(2): 201-13.

126. Hashimoto L, Habita C, Beressi JP et al. Genetic mapping of a susceptibility locus for insulin-dependent diabetes mellitus on chromosome 11q. Nature 1994; 371(6493): 161-4.

127. Field LL, Tobias R, Magnus T. A locus on chromosome 15q26 (*IDDM 3*) produces susceptibility to insulin-dependent diabetes mellitus. Nature Genet 1994; 8: 189-94.

128. Cookson WOCM, Sharp PA, Faux JA, Hopkin JM. Linkage between immunoglobulin E responses underlying asthma and rhinitis and chromosome 11q. Lancet 1989; i: 1292-5.

129. Pociot F, Nerup J. A chromosome 2 susceptibility marker in familial IDDM: the IL-1 receptor antagonist (abstract). Diabetologia 1993; 36 (suppl 1): A17.

130. Hodge SE, Anderson CE, Neiswanger K et al. Close genetic linkage between diabetes mellitus and Kidd blood group. Lancet 1981; ii(8252): 893-5.

131. Dunsworth TS, Rich SS, Swanson J, Barbosa J. No evidence for linkage between diabetes and the Kidd marker. Diabetes 1982; 31(11): 991-3.

132. Barbosa J, Rich SS, Dunsworth TS, Swanson J. Linkage disequilibrium between insulin-dependent diabetes and the Kidd blood group Jkb. J Clin Endocrinol Metab 1982; 55(1): 193-5.

133. Ghosh S. Polygenic control of autoimmune diabetes in non-obese diabetic mice. Nature Genet 1993; 4: 404-9.

134. Cheetham TD, Jones J, Taylor AM, Holly J, Matthews DR, Dunger DB. The effects of recombinant insulin-like growth factor I administration on growth hormone levels and insulin requirements in adolescents with type 1 (insulin-dependent) diabetes mellitus. Diabetologia 1993; 36: 678-81.

7

Epidemiology of NIDDM in Europids

Timo Valle, Jaakko Tuomilehto and Johan Eriksson

National Public Health Institute, Diabetes and Genetic Epidemiology Unit, Department of Epidemiology and Health Promotion, Helsinki, Finland

Epidemiological studies carried out during the last decades have revealed major differences in the occurrence of diabetes between populations and among various ethnic groups. Diabetes in populations of European origin (Europids) shows a peculiar epidemiological pattern. It has been claimed that Europid people are the ethnic group which can be considered to be at a relatively low risk of NIDDM (Table 1) [1]. On the other hand, young-onset IDDM is much more common in most Europid populations than in other populations [2]. Nevertheless, adult-onset NIDDM accounts for 80–90% of all cases of diabetes in Europids. Like the risk of IDDM, the risk of NIDDM varies markedly among different Europid populations. There seems to be no correlation between the risk of IDDM and that of NIDDM among these populations.

Before accepting the claim on the low risk of NIDDM in Europids, it is necessary to have a careful look at the existing epidemiological data. Certainly, Europids are not protected against NIDDM. There are several problems that complicate epidemiological and aetiological studies of NIDDM, and make the interpretation of the results difficult (Table 2). Furthermore, in many non-Europid populations at very high risk for NIDDM, the levels of the common environmental risk factors for NIDDM (obesity and low physical activity) are also very prevalent, sometimes reaching extreme proportions, as in some American Indian or Pacific island populations (see Chapter 8). According to the WHO MONICA project, the mean body mass index (BMI) among middle-aged Europid populations is raised but not very high, ranging from 24.3 kg/m^2

in women and 25.3 kg/m^2 in men in Gothenburg, Sweden to 29.8 kg/m^2 in women and 27.7 kg/m^2 in men in Kaunas, Lithuania (Figure 1). It is much more difficult to estimate the variation in physical activity between populations and therefore similar comparisons cannot be made. In any case, it may be premature to claim that the potentially lower risk of NIDDM observed in Europids is due to a less strong genetic predisposition for NIDDM compared with other ethnic groups.

The basic parameters for the assessment of the epidemiology of a disease are the *incidence* (the number of new cases per year in the population) and the *prevalence* (the number of currently existing cases in the population). Thus, the prevalence of NIDDM depends both on the incidence of NIDDM and mortality among patients with NIDDM. While the incidence and prevalence are both important, the incidence is a better parameter in the assessment of the effect of risk factors and for the evaluation of the efficacy of primary prevention measures. Since a large proportion of NIDDM cases are symptomless, at least in the beginning, it is difficult or at least impractical to determine the incidence of NIDDM in the population accurately. Thus, the only practical way to study the frequency of NIDDM in the population is to determine its prevalence. Obviously, knowing the prevalence and mortality, the incidence can be computed.

The prevalence of NIDDM can be detected using cross-sectional study designs, and time trends can be determined by repeated surveys with independent random population samples at certain time intervals. The

---

International Textbook of Diabetes Mellitus, Second Edition. Edited by K.G.M.M. Alberti, P. Zimmet, R.A. DeFronzo, and H. Keen (Honorary)

interpretation of time trends is not easy, since the prevalence estimates also reflect mortality in NIDDM which cannot be assumed to be constant. Standards assuring the best possible comparability of survey results between populations and over time have been recommended by expert committees in 1979, 1980 and 1985 [3–5]. Data obtained by diabetes surveys before 1980 may not be fully comparable with these currently agreed standards. Many of them were carried out in Europid populations, including the first population-based diabetes survey, which was performed in Oxford, Massachusetts, USA in the mid-1940s [6].

Table 1 The risk of NIDDM in Europids and other ethnic groups living in the same country

Country	Ethnic group	
	Lower risk	Higher risk
Australia	Europids	Aboriginals
Canada	Europids	Native Indians
New Zealand	Europids	Maoris
UK	Europids	Asian Indians
		Caribbean Blacks
USA	Europids	African-Americans
		Native Americans
Russia (Siberia)	Native Mongoloids	Europids

Table 2 Problems complicating epidemiological studies of NIDDM and the interpretation of results from different studies

Genotypic heterogeneity of NIDDM, and age-related penetrance of NIDDM susceptibility genes
Phenotypic heterogeneity of abnormal glucose tolerance, and changes in phenotype over time and with aging
Late and varying age of onset of NIDDM
Long asymptomatic period and lack of specific early symptoms, except in severe cases and late stages of NIDDM
High mortality among subjects with NIDDM
Lack of standardization of measurements to determine NIDDM or abnormal glucose tolerance and their risk factors

The advent of commonly agreed criteria for diabetes and impaired glucose tolerance (IGT) resulted in widespread interest in determining the prevalence of NIDDM and IGT in various populations using diabetes surveys. Most of the surveys, however, have been carried out in other than Europid populations [7]. One of the major achievements of the WHO MONICA Project has been the introduction of independent cardiovascular risk factor surveys at regular intervals in well-defined populations in more than 20 countries which are all primarily Europid, except the one in Beijing, China [8]. Unfortunately, there is no similar multinational coordinated activity to determine the prevalence of NIDDM between populations and over time. Diabetes surveys in Europid populations have

been isolated, and at present there is no systematic long-term community surveillance of the prevalence of NIDDM and IGT in countries other than the USA.

HETEROGENEITY OF NIDDM IN EUROPIDS

The heterogeneity of NIDDM is one of the reasons why it is difficult to estimate the true prevalence of the disease. NIDDM is characterized by insulin resistance and hence by relative insulin deficiency. During the natural course of NIDDM the endogenous insulin secretion often diminishes and eventually leads to a requirement for exogenous insulin [9, 10]. This makes it difficult to distinguish NIDDM from adult-onset IDDM in epidemiological studies. Thus, in the NHANES II study in the USA, 32% of diabetic patients diagnosed over 30 years of age had used insulin at some time during the course of the disease. It was estimated that 7% of all diabetic patients diagnosed at 30–74 years of age were in fact adult-onset IDDM cases [11]. The current trend in the treatment of NIDDM [12, 13] has been to apply a more aggressive treatment with insulin which makes the estimation of the NIDDM prevalence even more difficult.

Age of onset, years free of insulin therapy after the diagnosis of diabetes, presence of overweight, serum C-peptide levels, and immune markers have often been used to separate IDDM and NIDDM cases [9, 14, 15]. Islet-cell antibodies (ICA) and, more recently, antibodies to glutamic acid decarboxylase (GAD) have been used to predict the progression to insulin dependence in adult-onset diabetes [16, 17]. However, since approximately 20% of adult-onset IDDM cases are anti-GAD negative [18], and 3–9% of elderly subjects with IGT or normal glucose tolerance are anti-GAD positive (J. Tuomilehto, unpublished), the inferences from anti-GAD values must be made with caution. A Finnish study [18] showed that almost one-third of the newly diagnosed NIDDM cases in young adults aged 20–39 years were anti-GAD positive. How many of them will actually become insulin-dependent and how long this will take, remains to be seen. Data from a Swedish study suggest that many young-onset NIDDM patients will be re-classified as IDDM within a few years of the first diagnosis of diabetes [19]. While it is premature to base the classification of IDDM and NIDDM on anti-GAD antibodies, they may be helpful when combined with other indicators suggesting IDDM. This is true in Europids but not in other populations, since IDDM cases in Mongoloids and Blacks are often anti-GAD and ICA-negative.

If IDDM is defined as a state where the patient has insulin-requiring diabetes from the onset of the

127

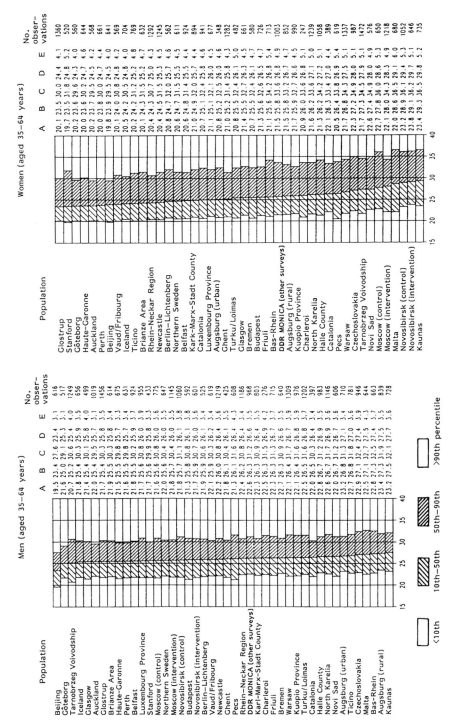

Figure 1 Body mass index in WHO MONICA Project. Age-standardized 10th(A), 50th(B) and 90th(C) percentiles, mean (D) and standard deviation (E) of body mass index (kg/m²) are given for men and women separately. Adapted from reference 8, with permission

disease and has a fasting C-peptide level below 0.2 nmol/l (0.6 ng/ml), and/or glucagon-stimulated C-peptide below 0.6 nmol/l (1.8 ng/ml), then age of onset $\geq$ 40 years has been shown to have a sensitivity of 97% and a specificity of 90% in correctly predicting NIDDM [9]. In most epidemiological studies age of onset $\leq$ 30 years has been used to distinguish IDDM and NIDDM [7, 20]. However, since the vast majority of diabetic patients in the total population have NIDDM, the overall prevalence of diabetes essentially reflects the prevalence of NIDDM.

Treatment for diabetes

Diet, exercise, oral hypoglycaemic agents (OHA) and insulin are the cornerstones for the treatment of NIDDM. However, the use of drug treatment for NIDDM varies in different countries. In the USA the use of OHA has been low compared with European countries since the results of the University Group Diabetes Program (UGDP) came out in the 1970s and biguanides were taken off the market. In 1989, of patients with NIDDM aged $\geq$ 18 years, 39% were treated with insulin, 52% with OHA, while 63% reported they were following a diet for their diabetes. Of insulin-treated NIDDM patients, 10% were using OHA in addition. Insulin therapy was more prevalent with longer duration of NIDDM, being used by 22% of patients within 4 years from diagnosis and by 58% of those with $\geq$ 20 years of NIDDM [21]. However, the situation in the USA may be changing due to the recent approval of metformin by the FDA, the introduction of α-glucosidase inhibitors for the treatment of NIDDM, and the current consensus statement for the pharmacological treatment of hyperglycaemia in NIDDM [13].

Even in Europe, where biguanides have been available, the patterns of use of insulin and OHA differ substantially between countries. A study in the Nordic countries (Denmark, Finland, Iceland, Norway and Sweden) showed that consumption of insulin and OHA measured as defined daily doses (DDD/1000 population/day) in Finland and Sweden was five times that in Iceland and twice that in Denmark and Norway [22]. More than half of these differences are possibly explained by the varying prevalence of diabetes in these countries. In Sweden the fact that a high proportion of the population is elderly accounts for part of the higher prevalence of diabetes. In Finland both men and women are considerably more obese than in the other Nordic countries and this is one likely explanation for the high prevalence. The rest of the variation is due to the prescribing traditions in the treatment of diabetes. The use of OHA was highest in Finland while the use of insulin was highest in Sweden.

There are some population-based surveys which show the spectrum of diabetes therapy in different European countries. In Malta, 43.5% of patients aged over 15 years with previously diagnosed diabetes used diet treatment alone, 43% received OHA therapy, and 13.5% insulin [23]. In Norway (diabetic patients $\geq$ 20 years old), the corresponding numbers were 41%, 39% and 20%, respectively [24]. In the Verona diabetes study in Italy, only 12% of previously diagnosed diabetic patients were on diet treatment alone, 78% were on OHA, 6% on insulin and 4% received a combination of insulin and OHA [25]. In a rural area in Austria, 37% of patients were on diet alone, 47% on OHA and 16% on insulin treatment [26].

PREVALENCE OF NIDDM

Table 3 summarizes the prevalence estimates obtained in epidemiological surveys in Europid populations reported during 1947–1995. For many countries with mainly Europid populations internationally published population-based data on NIDDM prevalence are not available. Since the methods and the age groups studied vary, direct comparison of prevalence between populations is not possible. Nevertheless, it seems that in all these populations studied the prevalence of NIDDM is less than 10% in middle-aged people under 65 or 75 years. In Europids aged $\leq$ 40 years NIDDM is relatively uncommon, the prevalence being approximately 1%.

It is more informative to compare age-specific data from studies carried out according to the WHO criteria for classification of glucose tolerance, but fewer than 20 such studies were identified (Tables 4 and 5). The prevalence increases steeply with age. In some populations the peak prevalence was reached around 75–80 years of age, whereas in several others the increase was seen over all age groups. Prevalence in the oldest age groups varied considerably among populations, the lowest being 10–15%, and the highest 30–50%.

Although far from being an ideal estimate, the prevalence among the oldest people may be taken as an approximation of the life-time risk of diabetes. According to this reasoning, we might propose that in Europid populations the risk of NIDDM is not low, and in several countries half or at least one-third of the population may be at risk of developing NIDDM. This assumption is based on past data, and it is important to note that the major environmental risk factors (obesity and physical inactivity) have markedly increased in most Europid populations during the past few decades [70–74]. Advances in treatment of hypertension and in prevention of premature deaths from coronary heart disease also increase the pool of elderly people potentially at risk for developing NIDDM. Thus,

Table 3 Prevalence of diabetes mellitus in Europid populations

Country	Prevalence (%)	Males (%)	Females (%)	Method	Age (years)	Reference
Australia						
Busselton	–	5.1	3.7	Survey, OGTT	25–	Glatthaar 1985 [27]
Belgium						
Whole country	1.6	–	–	Drug registers	All	Walckiers 1992 [28]
Denmark						
Fredericia	5.8	5.3	6.2	Survey, FBG >7.0 mmol/l	60–74	Damsgaard 1987 [14]
Finland						
Tampere	17	16	17	Survey, FBG >7.0 mmol/l	85–	Haavisto 1983 [29]
Kuopio	2.8	–	–	Medical record review	All	Laakso 1985 [30]
Kuopio	–	15.7	18.8	OGTT	65–74	Mykkänen 1990 [31]
Whole country	–	2.8	2.7	Drug register	30–	Laakso 1991 [32]
Whole country	3.3	3.5	3.1	Survey	30–	Laakso 1991 [32]
Three areas	–	5.7	4.6	OGTT × 2	45–64	Tuomilehto 1991 [33]
Närpes	2.1	1.9	2.4	Register	NIDDM	Eriksson 1992 [9]
East and West	–	16.6	–	OGTT	65–84	Stengård 1993 [34]
UK						
Poole	1.0	1.0	0.9	Multiple registers	All	Gatling 1985 [35]
Southall	1.1	1.1	1.0	Survey	All	Mather 1985 [36]
Islington	4.6	–	–	OGTT	40–	Forrest 1986 [37]
Oxford	1.0	1.1	1.0	Survey	All	Neil 1987 [38]
Leicester	6.6	–	–	Survey	16–	Samanta 1987 [39]
Melton Mowbray	9.3	–	–	Register, OGTT	65–85	Croxson 1991 [40]
London	–	3.4	2.6	Register	40–75	Yudkin 1993 [42]
Greece						
Aegaleo	4.3	–	–	Survey	All	Katsilambros 1993 [43]
Italy						
Laurino	–	10.7	9.8	OGTT	30–64	Verrillo 1983 [44]
Sanza	–	6.6	6.8	OGTT	18–	Verrillo 1985 [45]
Vicenza	2.1	–	–	Prescriptions, in-patient	All	Erle 1988 [46]
San Marino	–	1.8	1.9	Out-patient register	All	Simetovic 1990 [47]
Cas. Monferrato	2.1	1.9	2.3	Registers, capture/recapture	Onset 30–	Bruno 1992 [48]
Campania	2.5	1.7	3.4	Drug register	All	Vaccaro 1992 [49]
Cremona	–	11.0	11.3	OGTT	45–	Garancini 1995 [50]
Verona	2.5	2.5	2.5	Registers	All	Muggeo 1995 [25]
Israel						
Jerusalem	–	4.6	4.0	Survey, non-WHO OGTT	15–	Donchin 1984 [51]
The Netherlands						
Hoorn	8.4	7.9	8.7	OGTT	50–74	Mooy 1995 [41]
New Zealand						
Auckland	1.9	–	–	OGTT	40–64	Scragg 1991 [52]
Christchurch	14.9	17.2	12.5	OGTT	65–	Lintott 1992 [53]
Otara	2.8	–	–	Survey	20–	Simmons 1994 [54]
Malta						
Whole country	7.7	–	–	OGTT	15–	Katona 1986 [23]
Whole country	–	12.9	13.2	OGTT	35–69	Schranz 1989 [55]
Poland						
Wroclaw	3.5	3.5	3.5	OGTT	30–64	Szybinski 1989 [56]
Portugal						
Lisbon	9	–	–	50 g OGTT	25–64	Lisboa 1989 [57]
Romania						
Buda, rural	1.4	–	–	Non-WHO OGTT	17–70	Mincu 1972 [58]
Bucharest	4.7	5.9	3.7	Non-WHO OGTT	25–65	Mincu 1972 [58]
Russia						
Novosibirsk	–	1.8	3.6	OGTT	30–64	Shubnikov 1988, cited in King & Rewers, 1993 [7]
Spain						
Leon	5.6	–	–	OGTT	NIDDM	Franch 1992 [59]

continued overleaf

Table 3 (*continued*)

Country	Prevalence (%)	Males (%)	Females (%)	Method	Age (years)	Reference
Sweden						
Ystad	2.0	2.0	2.0	Registers	All	Sartor 1984 [60]
Gotland	3.1	–	–	Registers	All	Idman 1985 [61]
Kinda	3.3	–	–	Registers	All	Falkenberg 1987 [62]
Gothenburg	–	10.8	–	Survey, FBG	67	Ohlson 1987 [63]
Laxå	4.3	4.2	4.4	Registers, OGTT	All	Andersson 1991 [20]
USA						
Oxford	1.7	–	–	Survey, non-WHO criteria	All	Wilkerson 1947 [6]
Sudbury	1.9	2.4	1.3	Survey, FBG, non-WHO	15–	O'Sullivan 1967 [64]
Rochester	4.1	4.3	3.9	Register, non-WHO	40–	Palumbo 1976 [65]
San Antonio						
middle income	–	7.0	7.3	OGTT	25–64	Stern 1984 [66]
upper income	–	3.6	2.2	OGTT	25–64	Stern 1984 [66]
NHANES II	6.4	5.5	7.3	Survey, OGTT	20–74	Harris 1987 [67]
San Luis Valley	–	2.1	1.3	Registers, OGTT	20–74	Hamman 1989 [68]
Rancho Bernardo		16.5	12.7	Survey, OGTT	50–89	Wingard 1990 [69]

FBG, fasting blood glucose; OGTT, oral glucose tolerance test.

Table 4 Diabetes in the middle-aged and the elderly

	Age (years)	Prevalence (%)		
		Men	Women	Both
Using WHO criteria for OGTT				
Australia				
Busselton [27]	45–54	2.8	0.3	–
	55–64	5.1	4.2	–
	65–74	6.5	8.6	–
	75–	18.9	11.8	–
Finland				
Kuopio, Finland [31]	65–74	15.7	18.8	–
Three areas [33]	45–54	4.3	2.4	–
	55–64	6.9	7.5	–
Eastern and Western	65–74	14.5	–	–
Finland [34]	75–84	24.4	–	–
Oulu, Finland [99]	70–	22.0	28.2	–
UK				
Melton Mowbray [40]	65	–	–	6.3
	70	–	–	10.5
	75	–	–	9.7
	80	–	–	11.1
	85	–	–	13.8
Italy				
Sanza [45]	40–59	9.3	6.2	–
	60–	12.6	18.1	–
Cremona, Italy [50]	45–54	6.0	4.4	–
	55–64	13.1	9.5	–
	65–74	14.7	15.4	–
	75–	12.6	20.8	–
The Netherlands				
Twolle [100]	65–69	16	22	–
	70–74	27	26	–
	75–79	34	33	–
	80–	27	50	–
New Zealand				
Christchurch [53]	65–	17.2	12.5	–

Table 4 (*continued*)

	Age (years)	Prevalence (%)		
		Men	Women	Both
Sweden				
Gothenburg [63]	57	6.4	–	–
	67	10.8	–	–
Laxå [20]	45–54	3.9	2.0	–
	55–64	7.8	5.1	–
	65–74	12.8	15.0	–
	75–	14.7	17.2	–
USA				
NHANES II [67]	45–54	7.8	8.7	–
	55–64	9.4	15.2	–
	65–74	19.1	17.0	–
Rancho Bernardo [69]	50–59	8.6	3.9	–
	60–69	11.2	10.4	–
	70–79	20.7	13.7	–
	80–89	21.8	23.7	–
Using fasting blood glucose ≥ 7.0 mmol/l				
Denmark				
Fredericia, Denmark [14]	60–64	4.1	4.3	–
	65–69	5.1	7.2	–
	70–74	8.9	9.5	–

it is likely that the life-time risk of NIDDM in many Europid populations may be over 30%, possibly close to 50%.

INCIDENCE OF NIDDM

During the past decades the incidence of NIDDM has been found to be fairly stable in several European populations. In Sweden the incidence of NIDDM was estimated to be 3.3 cases per 1000 population.

Table 5 Age group-specific prevalence of diabetes in Europid populations

| | Prevalence (%) | | | | | | |
| | Age 55–64 years | | | Age 65–74 years | | | |
	Males	Females	All	Males	Females	All	Method
Poole, UK [35]	–	–	–	3.3	2.5	–	Registers
Southall, UK [36]	–	–	1.9	–	–	3.0	Survey
Fredericia, Denmark [14]	–	–	–	6.7	8.3	–	Survey, FBG >7.0 mmol/l
Busselton, Australia [27]	5.1	4.2	–	6.5	8.6	–	Survey, OGTT
Kinda, Sweden [62]	–	–	–	–	–	9	Registers
Verona, Italy [25]	7	5	–	10	9	–	Registers
Gotland, Sweden [61]	–	–	–	–	–	10	Registers
Wroclaw, Poland [56]	7.7	7.1	–	7.5	14.2	–	OGTT
Rancho Bernardo, USA [69]	11.4	4.9	–	11.9	12.9	–	OGTT
Laxå, Sweden [20]	7.8	5.1	–	12.8	15.0	–	Registers, OGTT
East and West Finland [34]	–	–	–	14.5	–	–	OGTT
Cremona, Italy [50]	13.1	9.5	–	14.7	15.4	–	OGTT
Kuopio, Finland [31]	–	–	–	15.7	18.8	–	OGTT
NHANES II, USA [67]	9.4	15.2	–	19.1	17.0	–	OGTT

Studies are arranged according to the ascending total prevalence of diabetes in the age group 65–74.

In Laxå community, in 1972–1987 there was a significant increase in the incidence of NIDDM in men aged 25–54 years, but in women and in older men no increase in incidence was found [20]. In Finland the incidence of drug-treated diabetes has been constant in 1970–1987 with only some year-to-year variation. In 1987 the incidence of drug-treated diabetes was 2.8 and 2.4 per 1000 population for men and women, respectively [32]. According to the National Health Interview Survey in the USA, the age-adjusted incidence of diabetes per 1000 population was 2.35 in 1980, 2.98 in 1983, 2.90 in 1986, 2.81 in 1989 [75] and 2.42 in 1990–1992 [76]. Incidence rates have been relatively constant since the late 1960s, with some year-to-year variation. Incidence has been higher for women than for men, and higher for the Black population than for Europids [75]. Since one-third to half of NIDDM cases in the community are undiagnosed (see below), the variation in incidence of NIDDM may well be due to changes in public awareness and methods of diagnosis rather than actual changes in the frequency of the disease.

DETERMINANTS OF NIDDM

Genetic Predisposition

Evidence for a genetic predisposition for the development of NIDDM has been known for a long time. The importance of the genetic contribution has been evaluated in a large number of family studies, assessing the prevalence of various degrees of glucose intolerance among family members of NIDDM subjects and studying early metabolic defects in NIDDM. For accurate estimates of prevalence of NIDDM among family members, physiological assessments are essential to detect asymptomatic undiagnosed disease.

The prevalence of NIDDM among family members of a known NIDDM proband vary. Cook and co-workers studied 20 consecutive nuclear families and observed that seven probands had neither parent affected with diabetes or glucose intolerance [77], while O'Rahilly et al reported a prevalence of 92% in 23 available parents of 13 NIDDM subjects with disease onset at 30–50 years of age [78]. Cheta noted a 33% prevalence of NIDDM among first-degree family members of 300 NIDDM subjects [79], while Baird noted that 10% of the diabetic patients had a diabetic sibling [80].

The cumulative risk of abnormal glucose tolerance or diabetes mellitus by the age of 60 years in offspring of conjugal diabetic parents has been found to be around 60% [81]. The family history of 311 German subjects with NIDDM was carefully documented, and the calculated prevalence of NIDDM among siblings and offspring of NIDDM subjects were 38% and 32%, respectively [82]. Köbberling and co-workers also followed the first-degree relatives of NIDDM patients, and the observation was that a relative with normal glucose tolerance had a 99% chance of not developing 'overt diabetes' over the course of 5 years [83].

A maternal effect of diabetes has been suggested. Among others, Alcolado et al reported that mothers were implicated in significantly more cases than fathers (36% vs. 15%) [84]. Dörner et al reported familial diabetes being 2.54-fold more frequent on the maternal side than on the paternal side [85]. The reason for this maternal preponderance is still unclear, but possible explanations have included the longer life expectancy of women in Europid populations and the impact of gestational diabetes or glucose intolerance on the fetus during the intrauterine period.

Defective insulin-dependent glucose uptake has been shown to be an independent predictor of NIDDM in offspring of NIDDM subjects. Insulin resistance is often accompanied by hyperinsulinaemia, and hyperinsulinaemia has been observed to precede the development of NIDDM in different ethnic groups, including Europids [86, 87]. Familial clustering of insulin sensitivity has been observed in 183 non-diabetic offspring who have both parents with NIDDM. Insulin sensitivity has an intraclass correlation coefficient of 0.26, suggesting that around 50% of the variability of insulin sensitivity is of familial origin [88].

The genetic predisposition for the development of NIDDM has been confirmed in twin studies which have been instrumental in establishing the proof for the strong genetic component in NIDDM. Most of the twin studies in NIDDM have been carried out in Europid populations. In monozygotic twins concordance rates are 50–80%, approximately twice those among dizygotic twins [89–91]. The high concordance for NIDDM in monozygotic twins results from both genetic and environmental effects [91]. Nevertheless, the genes that confer susceptibility to NIDDM, as well as the mode of inheritance in NIDDM, have thus far remained unclear.

A potentially useful way to assess the mode of inheritance of NIDDM and confirm a genetic role is to examine the risk ratio λ_R, which is defined as the disease risk to a relative (type R) of an index case compared with the population prevalence. Risch has shown that the rate of reduction of $(\lambda_R - 1)$ in first-, second- and third-degree relatives can be used to help identify the mode of inheritance for the disorder [92]. For NIDDM, λ_s (s = sibs) is about 3.5, assuming an average lifetime risk of 8% [93]. The values of λ_R for monozygotic twins, sibs and half-sibs (second-degree relatives) are 10, 3.5 and 1.5, respectively. This sharp decline in λ_R for successive degrees of relatives suggests that a multi-locus genetic model (as opposed to a single-locus model) would be the best one to fit the observed data for NIDDM [92]. Rich concludes that in NIDDM there may be a major locus with polygenes or a few multiplicative (epistatic) loci with polygenes [93]. However, both environmental and genetic factors contribute to NIDDM. The effect of the environment is evident from the lack of 100% disease concordance in monozygotic twins, and the increased frequency of obesity (which is, at least partially, environmentally induced) in the NIDDM population.

Sex and Age

Differences are found between men and women in the prevalence of NIDDM, but these differences vary in studies of Europid populations. In some studies there is a higher age-adjusted prevalence in women than in men [9, 14, 48, 55, 67] but there are also reports with opposite findings [27, 44, 45, 53, 58, 69]. Furthermore, in some communities there seems to be a trend towards a male excess in prevalence in people with a higher socioeconomic status [66]. In Finland, the age-specific prevalence of known diabetes is higher in men up to the age of 60 years, whereas in older groups the prevalence is higher in women [9]. However, when data based on an oral glucose tolerance test (OGTT) are used, the crossover in prevalence between men and women is found around the age of 55 years [33]. A similar trend was also seen in Italy [25, 50], but not in all populations. In Rancho Bernardo, California, the prevalence of diabetes was significantly higher for men than for women, even in the age group 50–89 years [69].

Glucose tolerance is known to decrease with age [94–98]. A progressive increase with age in 2-h glucose values following a 75-g OGTT has repeatedly been observed in Europids, being approximately 0.24–0.40 mmol/l per decade of life [95]. However, it is unclear whether this deterioration is independently caused by increased chronological age or whether it is secondary to age-related factors such as decrease in physical activity and lean body mass. Of interest is that fasting blood glucose seems to be relatively insensitive to the effect of age, but 1-h and 2-h post-challenge glucose values increase significantly with age [67]. This increase in post-challenge glucose values is due not to a shift of the entire blood glucose distribution to the higher levels, but rather to those in the upper part of the distribution showing a tendency for deterioration of glucose tolerance.

In most Western countries the peak in diabetes prevalence is found in the age-group 70–80 years (Table 4), although the peak prevalence has been observed in even older age groups in some studies, especially among women [20, 25, 69, 99, 100]. The decrease in prevalence after the age of 80 in several populations is probably due to higher mortality among diabetic than non-diabetic subjects [101]. Prevalence of IGT has been noted to show a similar rise with age (see below).

The age distribution of the prevalence of NIDDM in Europids seems to be different from that seen in populations with very high risk for NIDDM, such as Pima Indians, Nauruans and Asian Indians in whom the peak prevalence is at the age of 40–50 years.

Obesity

NIDDM is strongly associated with obesity. It has been estimated that 50–90% of NIDDM patients are obese. Joslin was one of the first to draw attention to the association. He noticed that of 1000 diabetic patients, 75% were clearly overweight [102]. Obesity is causally related to NIDDM, but it alone is not a sufficient cause of NIDDM. Since standardized diabetes surveys have been carried out only in a limited number of Europid populations, it is not easy to have a precise estimate of the extent to which differences in obesity may contribute to the variation in the prevalence of NIDDM.

The Nurses' Health Study in the USA showed that even in lean women (BMI $22.0-22.9$ kg/m^2) there was a three-fold increase in the age-adjusted relative risk compared with women with a BMI less than 22.0 kg/m^2. Women with BMI of $24.0-24.9$ kg/m^2 had a relative risk of 5.0 compared to the leanest group. BMI over 31 kg/m^2 increased the risk of diabetes over 40-fold. Overweight remained a strong risk factor for women even up to the age of 69 [103]. In the 5-year prospective follow-up study by Chan and co-workers, men with BMI over 35 kg/m^2 had a multivariate relative risk of 42, compared with men with a BMI under 23 kg/m^2. Relative risk was calculated controlling for smoking, family history of diabetes and age [104]. Ohlson and co-workers followed a randomly selected Swedish cohort of 54-year-old men for 13.5 years. Relative risk of diabetes in those above the top quintile vs. those below the lowest quintile of BMI was 21.7. The incidence of diabetes was 0.7% in those below the lowest BMI quintile and 15% in those above the top quintile. Those with larger waist-to-hip ratio for a given BMI had a higher incidence of NIDDM [105]. Not only the total fat mass but also body fat distribution (especially android fat distribution) has been associated with NIDDM [104–106]. The abdominal fat deposits also give us a possible pathogenetic model for NIDDM via elevated FFA concentrations in both systemic and portal circulations, leading to peripheral insulin insensitivity and reduced hepatic insulin action [107].

It is not known what duration of obesity is required for NIDDM to develop, but there is evidence that a longer duration of obesity increases the risk of NIDDM [103, 108]. In an Israeli study, BMI and total fat mass were associated with increased incidence of NIDDM, and the duration of obesity was also found to be important. In men aged 40–70 years with the same current BMI, a higher BMI measured 10 years earlier was associated with an increased risk of NIDDM [108]. Similar findings came out in the Nurses' Health Study, where the weight gain after the age of 18 was strongly associated with risk for diabetes. Women who lost weight after the age of 18 had a greatly reduced risk for diabetes. Such a trend was also seen in older age groups up to the age of 69 [103]. Holbrook et al saw a similar association with weight gain and diabetes in Rancho Bernardo. Weight gain of 10 pounds (4.5 kg) or more

between 40 and 60 years of age significantly increased the risk of diabetes in both men and women [109].

Physical Activity

Data on the relationship between physical activity and NIDDM have mainly been derived from Europid populations. They show unequivocally that the risk of NIDDM is temporally associated with physical inactivity and that there is a gradient between the exposure and the outcome. Thus, the risk of NIDDM associated with low physical activity is well documented among Europids [110–115], but fewer data are available for other ethnic groups. The only prospective study among non-Europids was carried out in Japanese-Hawaiian men and gave results similar to those in Europids [116].

Two studies thus far have evaluated whether an increase in physical activity has an effect on the incidence of NIDDM in people with IGT. One was carried out in Sweden [117] and the other in China [118], with very similar results: progression from IGT to NIDDM can be prevented by increased physical activity in both Europids and Chinese. Thus there is no evidence for differences between ethnic groups in the role of physical activity in the pathogenesis and prevention of NIDDM. Interestingly, in both studies it did not matter whether people with IGT reduced their body weight or increased physical activity, or did both, the effect on the reduction of NIDDM risk was the same (about 50%).

Fetal and Childhood Growth and Diabetes in Adult Life

Specific patterns of disproportionate fetal growth (e.g. low birth weight, thinness at birth, small size in relation to placental size) as well as factors associated with childhood growth (e.g. low weight at 1 year) have been implicated as important causes of chronic diseases such as hypertension, coronary heart disease and NIDDM in adult age. The 'Barker hypothesis' states that fetal and childhood malnutrition, by programming metabolism, predisposes to certain diseases in adult life. Both epidemiological data and animal studies have quite convincingly shown that undernutrition programs changes in several metabolic and physiological parameters. Since pancreatic B cells develop during fetal life, it is plausible that any lack of essential nutrients (proteins, amino acids, etc.) may result in a smaller B cell mass than required for remaining nondiabetic throughout life, especially in the presence of obesity.

Among 370 British males aged 64 years studied by Hales and co-workers, the percentage who had either NIDDM or IGT fell from 40% in those whose birth weight was < 2.50 kg to 14% in those whose birth weight was ≥ 4.31 kg [119]. Similar trends were observed with weight at 1 year of age. Findings confirming the association between disturbances in glucose tolerance and a low birth weight have been demonstrated in both men and women [120]. These associations have been suggested to be mediated through impairment of islet B cell function, but more recent work has suggested that they seem to be mediated through insulin resistance and to depend on interaction with obesity in adult life [121]. A Swedish study has also suggested that reduced fetal growth is associated with increased risk of diabetes mediated through insulin resistance [122]. A 'thrifty phenotype' has been proposed, in which inadequate nutrition programs the fetus to develop insulin resistance in adult life. Also, a genetically determined defect in insulin action could manifest itself *in utero* as reduced growth and later on as insulin resistance.

In addition to the associations observed between early growth and diabetes, correlations with lower birth weights have been found for increased rates of coronary heart disease and hypertension in adult life, as well as for the metabolic syndrome [123–125]. It has even been proposed that this syndrome be re-named 'the small baby syndrome'.

There is impressive epidemiological evidence supporting the association between early growth and diseases in adult life. However, we need to progress beyond epidemiological associations to understand the underlying mechanisms. Nevertheless, based on the vast epidemiological data available, the role of fetal malnutrition needs to be included as one of the major risk factors for NIDDM among Europid populations. It may be even more important for non-Europid populations in developing countries where malnutrition is a big health problem in general.

NATURAL HISTORY OF NIDDM

Impaired Glucose Tolerance

All individuals developing NIDDM pass through a phase of impaired glucose tolerance (IGT), which must therefore be considered an important part of the diabetes spectrum. IGT is a somewhat arbitrary category between normal glucose tolerance and diabetes and can be considered part of a continuum of glucose intolerance. Nevertheless, it is the first abnormal stage of the pathophysiological process which can be easily identified by biochemical methods. During the transition from normal glucose tolerance to IGT, fasting and postload insulin levels, obesity and insulin resistance increase [126, 127]. Individuals with IGT have

risk factors for diabetes, dyslipidaemia and cardiovascular disease that are in general intermediate between those observed in persons with normal glucose tolerance and those observed in persons with diabetes. Also, increased mortality has been associated with IGT [128–137].

The most widely employed criteria for the diagnosis and classification of IGT are those of the World Health Organization [4, 5] and the National Diabetes Data Group [3]. These criteria are based upon the results of an OGTT, which is considered as the 'gold standard' for the classification of glucose intolerance. The prevalence for IGT varies greatly between studies (Table 6) depending on study population and diagnostic criteria used, and IGT comprises around two-thirds of all cases with abnormal glucose tolerance. The frequency of IGT is known to increase with age (Table 6), and there is also a strong association with degree of physical activity/inactivity, prevalence of IGT being higher in physically inactive individuals [45, 138]. Results regarding the sex distribution of IGT are somewhat contradictory. Some studies have observed a higher prevalence among men, while others showed higher prevalence among women (Table 6).

Most studies indicate an increased risk for developing diabetes in individuals with IGT—the risk being related to the severity of IGT. Most frequently, a decompensation rate of 1–5%/year has been reported in Europid populations [55, 117, 130, 132, 133, 139–141].

Up to 34% of individuals with IGT have been found to have normal glucose tolerance when retested within 2–4 months, while 24–53% of individuals who initially have IGT have normal glucose tolerance within 10 years of follow-up [130, 131, 142]. However, a transient IGT state does seem to be of importance, indicating a predisposition to abnormal glucose tolerance, and should not be considered clinically unimportant [143]. The cause of this short-term variation or low reproducibility is unknown. A part of it is due to random variation, regression to the mean, and inaccuracy of the casual blood glucose determination. Diabetogenic drugs, changes in body weight and/or diet, and emotional and physical stress might influence glucose tolerance. Host factors like fluctuation in absorption, distribution and utilization of glucose might also be of importance.

The significance of identifying individuals with IGT relates to their increased risk for progression to manifest diabetes and their increased risk for macrovascular disease. Furthermore, individuals with IGT constitute a possible target group for intervention and subjects with this abnormality may benefit from interventions which may delay or prevent the development of diabetes (see Chapter 93).

Table 6   Prevalence of impaired glucose tolerance in Europid populations

	Age-group (years)	Males (%)	Females (%)	All (%)	Reference
Australia					
Busselton	35–44	1.8	1.3	1.5	
	45–54	3.6	2.3	2.9	
	55–64	5.1	3.7	4.3	
	65–74	7.8	5.9	6.8	
	≥ 75	7.9	11.8	9.8	Glatthaar 1985 [27]
Finland					
Kuopio	≥ 65	17.8	19.1	18.6	Mykkänen 1990 [31]
Three areas	45–54	2.1	3.8	3.0	
	55–64	3.9	7.4	5.7	Tuomilehto 1991 [33]
East and West	65–74	28.7	–	–	
	75–84	25.6	–	–	Stengård 1993 [34]
Italy					
Sanza	18–39	2.0	3.4	2.8	
	40–59	5.1	9.1	7.3	
	≥ 60	9.2	12.1	10.8	Verrillo 1985 [45]
Cremona	≥ 45	7.7	8.9	–	
	≥ 75	20.0	18.9	–	
	≥ 80	40.0	30.0	–	Garancini 1995 [50]
Malta	35–69	12.9	13.2	–	Schranz 1989 [55]
The Netherlands					
Twolle	65–69	12	32	23	
	70–74	15	35	27	
	75–79	20	33	27	
	≥ 80	38	29	32	Cromme 1991 [100]
Hoorn	50–54	5.7	5.9	–	
	55–59	6.8	7.1	–	
	60–64	11.1	10.6	–	
	65–69	9.0	16.4	–	
	70–74	16.3	18.1	–	Mooy 1995 [41]
New Zealand	40–44	–	–	1.0	
	45–49	–	–	1.9	
	50–54	–	–	2.0	
	≥ 55	–	–	3.2	Scragg 1991 [52]
USA					
NHANES II	20–44	4.6	6.5	5.6	
	45–54	12.6	14.5	13.6	
	55–64	17.2	13.7	15.3	
	65–74	22.8	23.0	23.0	Harris 1987 [67]

Undiagnosed NIDDM in Europid Populations

A large proportion of NIDDM cases are undiagnosed even in developed countries, due to the fact that NIDDM is relatively symptomless at the beginning of its natural course. The proportion of previously undiagnosed diabetes varies considerably in Europid populations (Table 7), being highest in Hoorn, The Netherlands, in rural Italy, and in the USA (where half of diabetes cases were undiagnosed in the 1980s) [41, 45, 67]. In most Europid populations the proportion of undiagnosed diabetes is higher in men than women (Table 7). Overall, about one-third to half of NIDDM cases are undiagnosed in Europid populations. Thus epidemiological studies based on questionnaire survey, hospital discharge registries, drug prescriptions or diabetic clinic out-patient registries markedly underestimate the true prevalence of NIDDM, and represent only the most severe cases of NIDDM who are at the most advanced stage in the natural history of the disease.

Secular Trends

NIDDM is an increasing problem in developing countries. Several studies have shown the increasing prevalence of NIDDM in the Pacific area, Africa, Asia and North American Indian populations [1]. However, NIDDM is not to be underestimated in populations originating from Europe. It has been shown that the prevalence of NIDDM increases with age in most populations up to the age of 70–80 years. With the increasing life expectancy and thus changing demography in Westernized countries, the number of diabetic patients

Table 7 The proportion of undiagnosed diabetes in Europid populations

			Prevalence of diabetes				
		Proportion undiagnosed (%)	Known (%)	New (%)	Method	Age	Reference
Three areas, Finland	Males	18	4.6	1.0	OGTT,	45–64	Tuomilehto 1991 [33]
	Females	32	3.4	1.6	>4-h fasting		
Malta	Males	20	10.6	2.6	OGTT	45–74	Schranz 1989 [55]
	Females	32	7.9	3.7			
Cremona, Italy	Males	23	8.5	2.5	OGTT	45–	Garancini 1995 [50]
	Females	30	7.9	3.4			
Fredericia, Denmark	Males	30	3.9	1.7	FBG	60–74	Damsgaard 1987 [14]
	Females	25	5.0	1.7			
	All	27	4.5	1.7			
Busselton, Australia	Males	33	3.5	1.7	OGTT	25–	Glatthaar 1985 [27]
	Females	27	2.7	1.0			
Melton Mowbray, UK	All	35	6.0	3.3	OGTT	65–85	Croxson 1991 [40]
Kuopio, Finland	Males	45	8.7	7.0	OGTT	65–74	Mykkänen 1990 [31]
	Females	38	11.7	7.1			
Auckland, New Zealand	All	43	1.1	0.8	OGTT	40–64	Scragg 1991 [52]
NHANES II, USA	Males	49	2.8	2.7	OGTT	20–74	Harris 1987 [67]
	Females	51	3.6	3.7			
	All	50	3.2	3.2			
Sanza, Italy	Males	67	2.3	4.7	OGTT	18–	Verrillo 1985 [45]
	Females	42	4.0	2.9			
	All	54	3.2	3.7			
Hoorn, The Netherlands	Males	61	3.1	4.8	OGTT	50–74	Mooy 1995 [41]
	Females	54	4.0	4.7			
	All	57	3.6	4.8			

Studies are arranged according to the ascending proportion of undiagnosed diabetes

Table 8 The estimates for current and future prevalence of NIDDM in Europid populations

	Year 1994		Year 2010 (prediction)	
	Prevalence of NIDDM (%)	No. of individuals with NIDDM	Prevalence of NIDDM (%)	No. of individuals with NIDDM
World	1.8	98 868 000	3.8	215 616 000
Europe	3.1	16 044 000	4.8	24 391 000
Northern Europe	2.5	2 340 000	4.9	4 543 000
Western Europe	3.2	5 624 000	4.9	8 713 000
Eastern Europe	2.4	2 297 000	4.5	4 371 000
Southern Europe	4.0	5 783 000	4.7	6 764 000
Former USSR	2.0	5 735 000	4.2	11 946 000
North America	4.7	13 402 000	5.9	16 787 000
Australia and New Zealand	2.9	613 000	3.2	892 000

The prevalence estimate for 2010 is based on the 1994 world population. Adapted from reference 157.

will grow considerably during the next two decades (Table 8). For instance in The Netherlands it has been calculated with a dynamic model that the number of diabetic patients will increase by 46% between 1990 and 2005 [144]. In the USA the prevalence of diabetes has increased by 360% from 1.0% in 1960 to 3.6% in 1980 [145]. In Sweden the prevalence has been calculated to be rising by 0.1% per year [20]. The prevalence has also increased in the Europid population in Australia. In the town of Busselton the prevalence of diabetes increased from 2.2% to 3.4% in 1966–1981 [27, 146]. The same trend is also seen in other Europid populations [32, 43, 147]. The increase in prevalence observed in these studies may to a large extent be due to the aging of the population, reduced mortality from diabetes and especially its cardiovascular complications, or to more effective case-finding and the increased public awareness of diabetes. According to the estimates by McCarty and Zimmet, the number of NIDDM patients in Europe will increase from 16 million in 1994 to 24.4 million in 2010 (a 52.5% increase) [57] (Table 8).

THE METABOLIC SYNDROME IN EUROPID POPULATIONS

The 'metabolic syndrome', or 'insulin resistance syndrome', which also has other names, has been defined by varying criteria (see Chapter 12). Typically the metabolic syndrome is described as a clustering of cardiovascular risk factors with hyperinsulinaemia as a marker for insulin resistance, abnormal glucose tolerance, hypertension, low levels of HDL-cholesterol, high levels of triglycerides, upper-body obesity, and hyperuricaemia. The prevalence of the metabolic syndrome is not known and WHO has strongly recommended that population-based studies should be performed to assess the true prevalence of the syndrome [149].

There are significant differences in the prevalence of individual cardiovascular risk factors among different ethnic groups. Insulin resistance or hyperinsulinaemia are more common in Blacks, Hispanics, and Native Americans than in Europids [150–152]. However, the combination of various cardiovascular risk factors depends to a considerable extent on the predisposition for, and levels of, these risk factors in the population. Even though obesity, diabetes and hyperinsulinaemia are common in many modernized non-Europid populations, they do not show the high levels of serum cholesterol seen in Europids [153]. Similarly, blood pressure levels are not particularly high in non-Europid populations [154], except in Blacks who are particularly susceptible to hypertension [155]. Against this background it is not surprising that Europid NIDDM patients will often develop coronary heart disease or stroke, unlike non-Europid NIDDM patients whose major late complication is diabetic renal disease.

In the Atherosclerosis Risk in Communities (ARIC) baseline study, a significant clustering of the cardiovascular risk factors (hypertension, diabetes, hyperuricaemia, hypertriglyceridaemia and low HDL-cholesterol) was seen in both African-American and Europid populations [156]. Overall, African-American subjects presented a greater number of abnormalities than did White subjects. In both ethnic groups men had more metabolic syndrome abnormalities than women. Individuals with three or more risk factors were observed more frequently than expected. Overall, 30% of abnormalities were concentrated in the 7% of individuals having three or more abnormalities. In Europids, hypertriglyceridaemia (≥ 2.26 mmol/l) was more prevalent than among African-Americans. Among Europids, hypertriglyceridaemia was the best single abnormality to predict clustering of two or more risk factors, followed by low HDL-cholesterol and diabetes. Of these metabolic abnormalities, hypertension was most commonly present as an isolated abnormality. After an adjustment for waist-to-hip ratio and BMI, high insulin levels were strongly related to the presence of clusters.

CONCLUSION

Good epidemiological data on Europid populations are limited. The prevalence of NIDDM has been estimated, using the standards recommended by WHO in 1980, in only a few European countries or Europid populations. It seems to be somewhat lower than in several non-Europid populations. To what extent this difference is due to differences in environmental risk factors or to different genetic predisposition cannot be determined for the time being. There is still a lack of longitudinal data to identify the risk factors for the development of NIDDM in Europid populations. Nevertheless it seems likely that the major determinants of NIDDM are the same in different ethnic groups. Obesity and physical inactivity play a significant role in the development of NIDDM in Europids. Studies to search for genes for NIDDM are ongoing in various populations (see Chapter 3), and the results will become available before the year 2000.

Epidemiological studies of NIDDM are particularly complicated in Europids because IDDM is common in many Europid populations, in contrast to non-Europids in whom IDDM is rare. Also the therapeutic traditions and their changes make epidemiological assessments, such as determination of interpopulation differences and time trends, difficult in NIDDM. In Europids, the risk of NIDDM increases exponentially with age, being relatively low before the age of 40 years. Based on available indirect data it can be estimated that the lifetime risk of NIDDM in most Europid populations is over 30%. The risk is much higher in subjects who have first-degree relatives with NIDDM. The estimated number of NIDDM patients in Europe in 1994 was 16 million, and by the year 2010 is predicted to be 24.4 million.

REFERENCES

1. Zimmet P. Kelly West Lecture 1991. Challenges in diabetes epidemiology—from West to the rest. Diabetes Care 1992; 15: 232–52.
2. Karvonen M, Tuomilehto J, Libman I, LaPorte R for the WHO DIAMOND Project Group. A review of the recent epidemiological data on the worldwide incidence of type 1 (insulin-dependent) diabetes mellitus. Diabetologia 1993; 36: 883–92.
3. National Diabetes Data Group. Classification and diagnosis of diabetes mellitus and other categories of glucose intolerance. Diabetes 1979; 28: 1038–57.
4. World Health Organization. WHO Expert Committee on Diabetes Mellitus, second report. Technical Report Series 646. Geneva: WHO, 1980; pp 1–80.

5. World Health Organization Study Group. Diabetes mellitus. Technical Report Series 727. Geneva: WHO, 1985; pp 1-113.

6. Wilkerson HLC, Krall LP. Diabetes in a New England town. JAMA 1947; 135: 209-16.

7. King H, Rewers M. Global estimates for prevalence of diabetes mellitus and impaired glucose tolerance in adults. Diabetes Care 1993; 16: 157-77.

8. The WHO MONICA Project. Geographical variation in the major risk factors of coronary heart disease in men and women aged 35-64 years. World Health Stat Q 1988; 41: 115-40.

9. Eriksson J, Forsen B, Häggblom M, Teppo AM, Groop L. Clinical and metabolic characteristics of type 1 and type 2 diabetes: an epidemiological study from the Närpes community in Western Finland. Diabet Med 1992; 9: 654-60.

10. Niskanen L, Karjalainen J, Siitonen O, Uusitupa M, Metabolic evolution of type 2 diabetes: a 10-year follow-up from the time of diagnosis. J Int Med 1994; 236: 263-70.

11. Harris MI, Robbins DC. Prevalence of adult-onset IDDM in the U.S. population. Diabetes Care 1994; 17; 1337-40.

12. Yki-Järvinen H, Kauppila M, Kujansuu E, Lahti J, Marjanen T, Niskanen L et al. Comparison of insulin regimens in patients with non-insulin-dependent diabetes mellitus. New Engl J Med 1992; 327: 1426-33.

13. Consensus statement. The pharmacological treatment of hyperglycemia in NIDDM. Diabetes Care 1995; 18: 1510-18.

14. Damsgaard EM, Faber OK, Fröland A, Green A, Hauge M, Holm NV, Iversen S. Prevalence of fasting hyperglycemia and known non-insulin-dependent diabetes mellitus classified by plasma C-peptide: Fredericia survey of subjects 60-74 years old. Diabetes Care 1987; 10: 26-32.

15. Madsbad S. Classification of diabetes in older adults. Diabetes Care 1990; 13 (suppl. 2): 93-6.

16. Tuomi TM, Groop LC, Zimmet PZ, Rowley MJ, Knowles W, Mackay IR. Antibodies to glutamic acid decarboxylase reveal latent autoimmune diabetes in adults with a non-insulin-dependent onset of disease. Diabetes 1993; 42: 359-62.

17. Niskanen LK, Tuomi TM, Karjalainen J, Groop LC, Uusitupa MIJ. GAD-antibodies in non-insulin-dependent diabetes. Ten-year follow-up from the diagnosis. Diabetes Care 1995; 18: 1557-65.

18. Tuomilehto J, Zimmet P, Mackay IR, Koskela P, Vidgren G, Toivanen L et al. Antibodies to glutamic acid decarboxylase as predictors of insulin-dependent diabetes before clinical onset of disease. Lancet 1994; 343: 1383-5.

19. Arnqvist HJ, Littorin B, Nyström L, Schersten B, Östman J, Blohme G et al. Difficulties in classifying diabetes at presentation in the young adult. Diabet Med 1993; 10: 606-13.

20. Andersson DKG, Svärdsudd K, Tibblin G. Prevalence and incidence of diabetes in a Swedish community 1972-1987. Diabet Med 1991; 8: 428-34.

21. National Center for Health Statistics. Current estimates from the National Health Interview Survey, 1989. Vital and Health Statistics, Series 10, no 176, 1990.

22. Groop PH, Klaukka T, Reunanen A, Bergman U, Borch-Johnsen K, Damsgaard EM et al. Anti-diabetic drugs in the Nordic countries. Reasons for variation in their use. Helsinki: Publications of the Social Insurance Institution, Finland, ML, 1991; p 105.

23. Katona G, Aganovic I, Vuksan V, Skrabalo Z, Hoet JJ, Grech A. National diabetes programme in Malta. Diabetologia Croat 1986; XV-2: 47-70.

24. Midthjell K, Holmen J, Björndal A. Types of diabetes treatment in a total, Norwegian, adult population. The Nord-Trondelag Diabetes Study. J Int Med 1994; 236: 255-61.

25. Muggeo M, Verlato G, Bonora E, Bressan F, Girotto S, Corbellini M et al. The Verona diabetes study: a population-based survey on known diabetes mellitus prevalence and 5-year all-cause mortality. Diabetologia 1995; 38: 318-25.

26. Mühlhauser I, Sulzer M, Berger M. Quality assessment of diabetes care according to the recommendations of the St. Vincent Declaration: a population-based study in a rural area of Austria. Diabetologia 1992; 35: 429-35.

27. Glatthaar C, Welborn TA, Stenhouse NS, Garcia-Webb P. Diabetes and impaired glucose tolerance. A prevalence estimate based on the Busselton 1981 survey. Med J Austr 1985; 143: 436-40.

28. Walckiers D, Van der Veken J, Papoz L, Stroobant A. Prevalence of drug-treated diabetes mellitus in Belgium. Results of a study with the collaboration of a network of pharmacies. Eur J Clin Pharmacol 1992; 43: 613-19.

29. Haavisto M, Mattila K, Rajala S. Blood glucose and diabetes mellitus in subjects aged 85 years or more. Acta Med Scand 1983; 214: 239-44.

30. Laakso M, Pyörälä K. Age of onset and type of diabetes. Diabetes Care 1985; 8: 114-17.

31. Mykkänen L, Laakso M, Uusitupa M, Pyörälä K. Prevalence of diabetes and impaired glucose tolerance in elderly subjects and their association with obesity and family history of diabetes. Diabetes Care 1990; 13: 1099-105.

32. Laakso M, Reunanen A, Klaukka T, Aromaa A, Maatela J, Pyörälä K. Changes in the prevalence and incidence of diabetes mellitus in Finnish adults, 1970-1987. Am J Epidemiol 1991; 133: 850-7.

33. Tuomilehto J, Korhonen HJ, Kartovaara L, Salomaa V, Stengård JH, Pitkänen M et al. Prevalence of diabetes mellitus and impaired glucose tolerance in the middle-aged population of three areas in Finland. Int J Epidemiol 1991; 20: 1010-17.

34. Stengård JH, Pekkanen J, Tuomilehto J, Kivinen P, Kaarsalo E, Tamminen M et al. Changes in glucose tolerance among elderly Finnish men during a five-year follow-up: the Finnish cohorts of the seven countries study. Diabète Métab 1993; 19: 121-9.

35. Gatling W, Houston AC, Hill RD. The prevalence of diabetes mellitus in a typical English community. J Roy Coll Phys 1985; 19: 248-50.

36. Mather HM, Keen H. The Southall diabetes survey. Br Med J 1985, 291: 1081-3.

37. Forrest RD, Jackson CA, Yudkin JS. Glucose intolerance and hypertension in North London: the Islington Diabetes Survey. Diabet Med 1986; 3: 338-42.

38. Neil HAW, Gatling W, Mather HM et al. The Oxford community diabetes study. Diabet Med 1987; 4: 539-43.

39. Samanta A, Burden AC, Fent B. Comparative prevalence of non-insulin-dependent diabetes mellitus in Asian and white Caucasian adults. Diabetes Res Clin Pract 1987; 4: 1–6.

40. Croxson SCM, Burden AC, Bodington M, Botha JL. The prevalence of diabetes in elderly people. Diabet Med 1991; 8: 28–31.

41. Mooy JM, Grootenhuis PA, de Vries H, Valkenburg HA, Bouter LM, Kostense PJ, Heine RJ. Prevalence and determinants of glucose intolerance in a Dutch population. The Hoorn Study. Diabetes Care 1995; 18: 1270–3.

42. Yudkin JS, Forrest RD, Jackson CA, Burnett SD, Gould MM. The prevalence of diabetes and impaired glucose tolerance in a British population. Diabetes Care 1993; 16: 1530.

43. Katsilambros N, Aliferis K, Darviri Ch, Tsapogas P, Alexiou Z, Tritos N, Arvanitis M. Evidence for an increase in the prevalence of known diabetes in a sample of an urban population in Greece. Diabet Med 1993; 10: 87–90.

44. Verrillo A, de Teresa A, Nunziata V, Rucco E. Epidemiology of diabetes mellitus in an Italian rural community. Diabète Métab 1983; 9: 9–13.

45. Verrillo A, de Teresa A, La Rocca S, Giarrusso PC. Prevalence of diabetes mellitus and impaired glucose tolerance in a rural area of Italy. Diabetes Res 1985; 2: 301–6.

46. Erle G, Gennaro R, Lora L, Basso A, Mingardi R, Piva I. Studio epidemiologico del diabete mellito nell'USL-Vicenza. Proposta di un nuovo metodo di indagine. G Ital Diabetol 1988; 8: 23–9.

47. Simetovic N, Devoti G, Stefanelli L, Valazzi C, Ferrari P, Prosperi R et al. Prevalenza del diabete mellito manifesto nella Repubblica di San Marino. G Ital Diabetol 1990; 10: 263–9.

48. Bruno G, Bargero G, Vuolo A, Pisu E, Pagano G. A population-based prevalence survey of known diabetes mellitus in Northern Italy based upon multiple independent sources of ascertainment. Diabetologia 1992; 35: 851–6.

49. Vaccaro O, Imperatore G, Ferrara A, Palombino R, Riccardi G. Epidemiology of diabetes mellitus in southern Italy: a case-finding method based on drug prescriptions. J Clin Epidemiol 1992; 45: 835–9.

50. Garancini MP, Calori G, Ruotolo G, Manara E, Izzo A, Ebbli E et al. Prevalence of NIDDM and impaired glucose tolerance in Italy: an OGTT-based population study. Diabetologia 1995; 38: 306–13.

51. Donchin M, Kark JD, Abramson JH, Epstein L, Hopp C. Prevalence of diabetes among ethnic groups in Jerusalem. The Kiryat Hayovel community health study. Israel J Med Sci 1984; 20: 578–83.

52. Scragg R, Baker J, Metcalf P, Dryson E. Prevalence of diabetes mellitus and impaired glucose tolerance in a New Zealand multiracial workforce. NZ Med J 1991; 104: 395–7.

53. Lintott CJ, Hanger HC, Scott RS, Sainsbury R, Frampton C. Prevalence of diabetes mellitus in an ambulant elderly New Zealand population. Diabetes Res Clin Pract 1992; 16: 131–6.

54. Simmons D, Gatland B, Fleming C, Leakehe L, Scragg R. Prevalence of known diabetes in a multiethnic community. NZ Med J 1994; 107: 219–22.

55. Schranz AG. Abnormal glucose tolerance in the Maltese. A population-based longitudinal study of the natural history of NIDDM and IGT in Malta. Diabetes Res Clin Pract 1989; 7: 7–16.

56. Szybinski Z, Zukowski W, Rita R, Sieradzki J, Turska-Karbowska I, Gizler M. Diabetes mellitus in urban population of Wroclaw. In Abstracts of the II Scientific Congress of the Polish Diabetological Association, Krakow: Polish Diabetological Association, 1989; p 225 (cited in reference [7]).

57. Lisboa PE, Duarte BS. Diabetes in Portugal. A contribution to epidemiology. Bull Del Health Care Diabet Worldwide 1989; 10: 5.

58. Mincu I, Dumitrescu C, Campeanu S, Mihalache N, Pirvulescu M, Covanov D et al. Epidemiological researches on diabetes mellitus in Roumanian urban and rural population. Diabetologia 1972; 8: 12–18.

59. Franch NJ, Alvarez TJC, Alvarez GF, Diego DF, Hernandez MR, Cueto EA. Epidemiology of diabetes mellitus in the province of Leon. Medicina Clinica 1992; 98: 607–11.

60. Sartor G. Prevalence of type 2 diabetes in Sweden. Acta Endocrinol 1984; 262 (suppl.): 27–9.

61. Idman I, Bergman U, Dahlen M, Martinsson L, Wessling A. Gotlandsstudie: Hög förskrivning av diabetesmedel men även hög morbiditet. Läkartidningen 1985; 82: 1051–4.

62. Falkenberg MGK. Diabetes mellitus: prevalence and local risk factors in a primary health care district. Scand J Soc Med 1987; 15: 139–44.

63. Ohlson LO, Larsson B, Eriksson H, Svärdsudd K, Welin L, Tibblin G. Diabetes mellitus in Swedish middle-aged men. Diabetologia 1987; 30: 386–93.

64. O'Sullivan JB, Williams RF, McDonald GW. The prevalence of diabetes mellitus and related variables—a population study in Sudbury, Massachusetts. J Chron Dis 1967; 20: 535–43.

65. Palumbo PJ, Elveback LR, Chu CP, Connolly DC, Kurland LT. Diabetes mellitus: incidence, prevalence, survivorship, and causes of death in Rochester, Minnesota, 1945–1970. Diabetes 1976; 25; 566–73.

66. Stern MP, Rosenthal M, Haffner SM, Hazuda HP, Franco LJ. Sex differences in the effects of sociocultural status on diabetes and cardiovascular risk factors in Mexican-Americans: the San Antonio Heart Study. Am J Epidemiol 1984; 120: 834–51.

67. Harris MI, Hadden WC, Knowler WC, Bennett PH. Prevalence of diabetes and impaired glucose tolerance and plasma glucose levels in US population aged 20–74 years. Diabetes 1987; 36: 523–34.

68. Hamman RF, Marshall JA, Baxter J, Kahn LB, Mayer EJ, Orleans M et al. Methods and prevalence of non-insulin-dependent diabetes mellitus in a biethnic Colorado population. Am J Epidemiol 1989; 129: 295–311.

69. Wingard DL, Sinsheimer P, Barrett-Connor EL, McPhillips JB. Community-based study of prevalence of NIDDM in older adults. Diabetes Care 1990; 13 (suppl. 2): 3–8.

70. Pietinen P, Vartiainen E, Männistö S. Trends in body mass index and obesity among adults in Finland from 1972 to 1992. Int J Obesity 1996; 20: 114–20.

71. Williamson DF. Descriptive epidemiology of body weight and weight gain in US adults. Ann Intern Med 1993; 119: 646–9.

72. Blokstra A, Kromhout D. Trends in obesity in young adults in The Netherlands from 1974 to 1986. Int J Obesity 1991; 15: 513–21.

73. Kuskowska-Wolk A, Bergström R. Trends in body mass index and prevalence of obesity in Swedish men, 1980–1989. J Epidemiol Comm Health 1993; 47: 103–8.

74. Marti B, Tuomilehto J, Salonen JT, Puska P, Nissinen A. Relationship between leisure-time physical activity and risk factors for coronary heart disease in middle-aged women. Acta Med Scand 1987; 222: 223–30.

75. Morbidity and Mortality Weekly Report. CDC Surveillance Summaries. Surveillance for diabetes mellitus United States, 1980–1989. US Dept of Health and Human Services, CDC, Atlanta, GA, 1993. MMWR 1993; 42: 1–20.

76. Kenny SJ, Aubert RE, Geiss LS. Prevalence and incidence of non-insulin-dependent diabetes. In Diabetes in America, NDDG. NIH publ no. 95–1468, 1995; pp 47–67.

77. Cook JTE, Hattersley AT, Levy JC, Patel P, Wainscoat JS, Hockaday TDR, Turner RC. The distribution of type 2 diabetes in nuclear families. Diabetes 1993; 42: 106–12.

78. O'Rahilly S, Spivey RS, Holman RR, Nugent Z, Clark A, Turner RC. Type II diabetes of early onset: a distinct clinical and genetic syndrome? Br Med J 1987; 294: 923–8.

79. Cheta D, Dimitrescu C, Georgescu M, Cocioaba G, Lichiardobol R, Stamoran M et al. A study on types of diabetes mellitus in first-degree relatives of diabetes patients. Diabète Métab 1990; 16: 11–15.

80. Baird JD. Diabetes mellitus and obesity. Proc Nutr Soc 1973; 32: 199–204.

81. Tattersall R, Fajans SS. Diabetes and carbohydrate intolerance in 199 offspring of 37 conjugal diabetic patients. Diabetes 1975; 24: 452–62.

82. Köbberling J, Tillil H. Empirical risk figures for the first-degree relatives of non-insulin dependent diabetics. In Köbberling J, Tattersall R (eds) The genetics of diabetes mellitus. London: Academic Press, 1982; pp 201–9.

83. Köbberling J, Kettermann R, Arnold A. Follow-up of 'non-diabetic' relatives of diabetics by retesting oral glucose tolerance after 5 years. Diabetologia 1975; 11: 451–6.

84. Alcolado JC, Alcolado R. Importance of maternal history of non-insulin-dependent diabetic patients. Br Med J 1991; 302: 1178–80.

85. Dörner G, Mohnike A, Steindel E. On possible genetic and epigenetic modes of diabetes transmission. Endokrinologie 1975; 66: 225–7.

86. Charles MA, Fontbonne A, Thibult N, Warnet JM, Rosselin GE, Eschwege E. Risk factors for NIDDM in white population: Paris prospective study. Diabetes 1991; 40: 796–9.

87. Warram JH, Martin BC, Krolewski AS, Soeldner JS, Kahn CR. Slow glucose removal rate and hyperinsulinemia precede the development of type II diabetes in the offspring of diabetic parents. Ann Intern Med 1990; 113: 909–15.

88. Martin BC, Warram JH, Rosner B, Rich SS, Soeldner JS, Krolewski AS. Familial clustering of insulin sensitivity. Diabetes 1992; 41: 850–4.

89. Barnett AH, Eff C, Leslie RDG, Pyke DA. Diabetes in identical twins: a study of 200 pairs. Diabetologia 1981; 20: 87–93.

90. Newman B, Selby JV, King MC, Slemenda C, Fabsitz R, Friedman GD. Concordance for type II (non-insulin-dependent) diabetes mellitus in male twins. Diabetologia 1987; 30: 763–8.

91. Kaprio J, Tuomilehto J, Koskenvuo M, Romanov K, Reunanen A, Eriksson J et al. Concordance for type 1 (insulin-dependent) and type 2 (non-insulin-dependent) diabetes mellitus in a population based cohort of twins in Finland. Diabetologia 1992; 35: 1060–7.

92. Risch N. Linkage strategies for genetically complex traits. I. Multilocus models. Am J Hum Genet 1990; 46: 222–8.

93. Rich SS. Mapping genes in diabetes: genetic epidemiological perspective. Diabetes 1990; 39: 1315–19.

94. Andres R. Aging and diabetes. Med Clin North Am 1971; 835–45.

95. Davidson MD. The effect of ageing on carbohydrate metabolism. A review of the English literature and a practical approach to the diagnosis of diabetes mellitus in the elderly. Metabolism 1979; 28: 688–705.

96. DeFronzo RA. Glucose intolerance and aging. Diabetes Care 1981; 4: 493–501.

97. Swerdloff RS, Pozefsky T, Tobin JD, Andres R. Influence of age on the intravenous tolbutamide response test. Diabetes 1967; 16: 161–70.

98. Shimokata H, Muller DC, Fleg JL, Sorkin J, Ziemba AW, Andres R. Age as independent determinant of glucose intolerance. Diabetes 1991; 40: 44–51.

99. Hiltunen L, Luukinen H, Koski K, Kivelä SL. Prevalence of diabetes mellitus in an elderly Finnish population. Diabet Med 1994; 11: 241–9.

100. Cromme PVM. Glucose tolerance in a typical Dutch community. Prevalence, determinants and diagnosis in the elderly. Academisch proefschrift. Amsterdam: Medicom Europe, 1991.

101. Stengård JH, Tuomilehto J, Pekkanen J, Kivinen P, Kaarsalo E, Nissinen A, Karvonen MJ. Diabetes mellitus, impaired glucose tolerance and mortality among elderly Finnish men: the Finnish cohorts of the Seven Countries Study. Diabetologia 1992; 35: 760–5.

102. Joslin EP. The prevention of diabetes mellitus. JAMA 1921; 76: 79–84.

103. Colditz GA, Willett WC, Rotnitzky A, Manson JE. Weight gain as a risk factor for clinical diabetes mellitus in women. Ann Intern Med 1995; 122: 481–6.

104. Chan JM, Rimm EB, Colditz GA, Stampfer MJ, Willett WC. Obesity, fat distribution, and weight gain as risk factors for clinical diabetes in men. Diabetes Care 1994; 17: 961–9.

105. Ohlson LO, Larsson B, Björntorp P, Eriksson H, Svärdsudd K, Welin L et al. Risk factors for type 2 (non-insulin dependent) diabetes mellitus: thirteen and one-half years of follow-up of the participants in a study of Swedish born men in 1913. Diabetologia 1988; 31: 798–805.

106. Hartz AJ, Rupley DC, Kalkhoff RD, Rimm AA. Relationship of obesity to diabetes: influence of obesity level and body fat distribution. Prev Med 1983; 12: 351–7.

107. Björntorp P. Metabolic implications of body fat distribution. Diabetes Care 1991; 14: 1132–43.

108. Modan M, Karasik A, Halkin H, Fuchs Z, Lusky A, Shitrit A, Modan B. Effect of past and concurrent body mass index on prevalence of glucose intolerance

and type 2 (non-insulin-dependent) diabetes and on insulin response. Diabetologia 1986; 29: 82–9.

109. Holbrook TL, Barrett-Connor E, Wingard TL. The association of lifetime weight and weight control patterns with diabetes among men and women in an adult community. Int J Obesity 1989; 13: 723–9.

110. Frisch RE, Wyshak G, Albright TE, Albright NL, Schiff I. Lower prevalence of diabetes in female former college athletes compared with non-athletes. Diabetes 1986; 35: 1101–5.

111. Schranz A, Tuomilehto J, Marti B, Jarrett JR, Grabauskas V, Vassallo A. Low physical activity and worsening of glucose tolerance: results from a 2-year follow-up of a population sample in Malta. Diabetes Res Clin Pract 1991; 11: 127–36.

112. Helmrich SP, Ragland DR, Ieung RW, Paffenberger RS Jr. Physical activity and reduced occurrence of non-insulin-dependent diabetes mellitus. New Engl J Med 1991; 325: 147–52.

113. Manson JE, Rimm EB, Stampfer MJ, Colditz GA, Willett WC, Krolewski AS et al. Physical activity and incidence of non-insulin-dependent diabetes mellitus in women. Lancet 1991; 338: 774–8.

114. Manson JE, Nathan DM, Krolewski AS, Stampfer MJ, Willett WC, Hennekens CH. A prospective study of exercise and incidence of diabetes among US male physicians. JAMA 1992; 268: 63–7.

115. Eriksson KF. Prevention of non-insulin-dependent diabetes mellitus. A population study with special reference to insulin secretion, skeletal muscle morphology and metabolic capacity (thesis). Skurup: Lidbergs Blankett AB, Sweden, 1992.

116. Burchfield CM, Sharp DS, Curb JD et al. Physical activity and incidence of diabetes; the Honolulu Heart Program. Am J Epidemiol 1995; 141: 360–8.

117. Eriksson KF, Lindgärde F. Prevention of type 2 (non-insulin-dependent) diabetes mellitus by diet and physical exercise: the six-year Malmö feasibility study. Diabetologia 1991; 34: 891–8.

118. Pan X, Li G, Hu Y, Bennett PH, Howard BV. Effect of dietary and/or exercise interventions on incidence of diabetes in subjects with IGT: the Da-Qing IGT and Diabetes Study. Abstract presented at the International Diabetes Federation Congress, Kobe, Japan, November, 1994.

119. Hales CN, Barker DJP, Clark PMS, Cox PMS, Fall C, Osmond C et al. Fetal and infant growth and impaired glucose tolerance at age 64. Br Med J 1991; 303: 1019–22.

120. Phipps K, Barker DJP, Hales CN, Fall CHD, Osmond C, Clark PMS. Fetal growth and impaired glucose tolerance in men and women. Diabetologia 1993; 36: 225–8.

121. Phillips DIW, Barker DJP, Hales CN, Hirst S, Osmond C. Thinness at birth and insulin resistance in adult life. Diabetologia 1994; 37: 150–4.

122. Lithell HO, Mckeigue PM, Berglund L, Mohsen R, Lithell UB, Leon DA. Relation of size at birth to non-insulin dependent diabetes and insulin concentrations in men aged 50–60 years. Br Med J 1996; 312: 406–10.

123. Barker DJP. Fetal origins of coronary heart disease. Br Med J 1995; 311: 171–4.

124. Barker DJP, Bull AR, Osmond C, Simmonds SJ. Fetal and placental size and risk of hypertension in adult life. Br Med J 1990; 301: 259–62.

125. Barker DJP, Hales CN, Fall CHD, Osmond C, Phipps K, Clark PMS. Type 2 (non-insulin-dependent) diabetes mellitus, hypertension and hyperlipidaemia (syndrome X): relation to reduced fetal growth. Diabetologia 1993; 36: 62–7.

126. Lillioja S, Mott DM, Howard BV et al. Impaired glucose tolerance as a disorder of insulin action: longitudinal and cross-sectional studies in Pima Indians. New Engl J Med 1988; 318: 1217–25.

127. Saad MF, Pettitt DJ, Mott DM, Knowler WC, Nelson RG, Bennett PH. Sequential changes in serum insulin concentration during development of non-insulin-dependent diabetes. Lancet 1989; i. 1356–9.

128. Harris MI. Impaired glucose tolerance in the US population. Diabetes Care 1989; 12: 464–74.

129. Modan M, Halkin H, Almog S et al. Hyperinsulinemia—a link between hypertension, obesity and glucose intolerance. J Clin Invest 1985; 75: 809–17.

130. Fuller JH, Shipley MJ, Rose G, Jarrett RJ, Keen H. Coronary heart disease risk and impaired glucose tolerance: the Whitehall study. Lancet 1980; i: 1373–6.

131. Jarrett RJ, McCartney P, Keen H. The Bedford survey: ten year mortality rates in newly diagnosed diabetics, borderline diabetics and normoglycaemic controls and risk indices for coronary heart disease in borderline diabetics. Diabetologia 1982; 22: 79–84.

132. Sartor G, Schersten B, Carlström S, Melander A, Norden Å, Persson G. Ten-year follow-up of subjects with impaired glucose tolerance: prevention of diabetes by tolbutamide and diet regulation. Diabetes 1980; 29: 41–9.

133. Keen H, Jarrett RJ, McCartney P. The ten-year follow-up of the Bedford survey (1962–1972): glucose intolerance and diabetes. Diabetologia 1982; 22: 73–8.

134. Annuzzi G, Vaccaro O, Caprio S, DiBonito P, Caso P, Riccardi G, Rivellese A. Association between low habitual physical activity and impaired glucose tolerance. Clin Physiol 1985; 5: 63–70.

135. Capaldo B, Tutino L, Patti L, Vaccaro O, Rivellese A, Riccardi G. Lipoprotein composition in individuals with impaired glucose tolerance. Diabetes Care 1983; 6: 575–8.

136. Vaccaro O, Rivellese A, Riccardi G, Capaldo B, Tutino L, Annuzzi G, Mancini M. Impaired glucose tolerance and risk factors for atherosclerosis. Atherosclerosis 1984; 4: 592–7.

137. Vaccaro O, Pauciullo P, Rubba P, Annuzzi G, Rivellese AA, Riccardi G, Mancini M. Peripheral arterial circulation in individuals with impaired glucose tolerance. Diabetes Care 1985; 8: 594–7.

138. Lindgärde F, Saltin B. Daily physical activity, work capacity and glucose tolerance in 115 lean and obese normoglycemic middle-aged men. Diabetologia 1981; 20: 134–8.

139. Birmingham Diabetes Survey Working Party. Ten-year follow-up report of the Birmingham diabetes survey of 1961. Br Med J 1976; 2: 35–7.

140. O'Sullivan JB, Mahan CM. Prospective study of 352 young patients with chemical diabetes. New Engl J Med 1968; 278: 1038–41.

141. Jarrett RJ, Keen H, Fuller JH, McCartney P. Worsening to diabetes in men with impaired glucose tolerance ('borderline diabetes'). Diabetologia 1979; 16: 25–30.

142. Yudkin JS, Alberti KGMM, McLarty DG, Swai ABM. Impaired glucose tolerance. Is it a risk factor for

diabetes or a diagnostic ragbag? Br Med J 1990; 301: 397–401.

143. Saad MF, Knowler WC, Pettitt DJ, Nelson RG, Bennett PH. Transient impaired glucose tolerance in Pima Indians: is it important? Br Med J 1988; 297: 1438.

144. Ruwaard D, Hoogenveen RT, Verkleij H, Kromhout D, Casparie AF, van der Veen AE. Forecasting the number of diabetic patients in The Netherlands in 2005. Am J Public Health 1993; 83: 989–95.

145. Harris MI. Prevalence of non-insulin-dependent diabetes and impaired glucose tolerance. In Diabetes in America: diabetes data compiled 1984. US Dept of Health and Human Services, publication no. (NIH) 85-1468; VI: 1–31. Washington, DC: US Government Printing Office, 1986.

146. Welborn TA, Curnow DH, Wearne JT et al. Diabetes detected by blood sugar measurement after a glucose load; report from the Busselton survey, 1966. Med J Aust 1968; 2: 778–83.

147. Reunanen A. Prevalence and incidence of type 2 diabetes in Finland. Acta Endocrinol 1984; suppl. 262: 31–5.

149. World Health Organization Scientific Group. Cardiovascular disease risk factors: new areas for research. Technical Report Series 841. Geneva: WHO, 1994.

150. Nabulsi AA, Folsom AR, Heiss G, Weir SS, Chambless LE, Watson RL, Eckfeldt JH. Fasting hyperinsulinemia and cardiovascular risk factors in nondiabetic adults: stronger associations in lean versus obese subjects. Metabolism 1995; 44: 914–22.

151. Boyko EJ, Keane EM, Marshall JA, Hamman RF. Higher insulin and C-peptide concentrations in Hispanic population at high risk for NIDDM: San Luis Valley Diabetes Study. Diabetes 1991; 40: 509–15.

152. Aronoff SL, Bennett PH, Gorden P, Rushforth N, Miller M. Unexplained hyperinsulinemia in normal and 'prediabetic' Pima Indians compared with Caucasians: an example of racial differences in insulin secretion. Diabetes 1977; 26: 827–40.

153. Li N, Tuomilehto J, Dowse G, Virtala E, Zimmet P. Prevalence of coronary heart disease indicated by ECG abnormalities and risk factors in developing countries. J Clin Epidemiol 1994; 47: 599–611.

154. Taylor R, Zimmet P, Tuomilehto J, Ram P, Hunt D, Sloman G. Blood pressure changes with age in two ethnic groups in Fiji. J Am Coll Nutr 1989; 8: 335–46.

155. Summerson JH, Bell RA, Konen JC. Coronary heart disease risk factors in Black and White patients with non-insulin-dependent diabetes mellitus. Ethnicity and Health 1996; 1: 9–20.

156. Schmidt MI, Duncan BB, Watson RL, Sharrett AR, Brancati FL, Heiss G. A metabolic syndrome in white and African-Americans. The Atherosclerosis Risk in Communities baseline study. Diabetes Care 1996; 19: 414–8.

157. McCarty D, Zimmet P. Diabetes 1994 to 2010: global estimates and projections. Leverkusen: Bayer, 1994: pp 1–46.

8

Epidemiology of NIDDM in Non-Europids

Maximilian de Courten*, Peter H. Bennett†, Jaakko Tuomilehto‡ and Paul Zimmet*

**International Diabetes Institute, Caulfield, Australia, †National Institute of Diabetes and Digestive and Kidney Diseases, Phoenix, AZ, USA, and ‡National Public Health Institute, Helsinki, Finland*

INTRODUCTION

Early in the history of the epidemiology of diabetes, the late Dr Kelly West drew attention to the higher prevalence of non-insulin dependent diabetes mellitus (NIDDM) in non-Europid populations in developing countries in Asia and South America [1] as well as amongst various American Indian tribes [2].

In the late 1960s the discovery of the Pima Indian population as a high prevalence group [3] led to a systematic and well-planned longitudinal study of the epidemiology and natural history of NIDDM. Subsequently, certain Pacific island populations were found to have high NIDDM prevalence [4], and a study was started of a number of island communities, with different ethnic backgrounds and varying degrees of acculturation.

With the standardization of the classification of diabetes by the 1980 World Health Organization (WHO) Expert Committee on Diabetes Mellitus [5] and new internationally accepted diagnostic criteria, a further major milestone was achieved in the epidemiology of NIDDM, leading to a better understanding of its aetiology and complications. These recommendations were updated by the 1985 WHO Study Group on Diabetes Mellitus [6] and are currently being revised.

Data compiled on estimates of NIDDM in adults from diverse populations worldwide have shown not only that diabetes is a global health problem [7] but also that the risk of diabetes is not uniform among populations. Non-Europid populations living in industrialized

societies seem to be at greatest risk. This increase is especially troubling since many high-risk migrant populations were traditionally believed to have low diabetes prevalence in their homeland.

This chapter reviews the epidemiology of NIDDM in non-Europids in the light of risk factors and determinants of this disease in these populations. Although not necessarily causal, a risk factor is defined as a characteristic which can be modified through intervention, whereas demographic characteristics such as age, sex and ethnicity are determinants of disease occurrence and cannot be modified. However, the lack of knowledge about the status of several factors (e.g. insulin resistance, genetic susceptibility, etc.), and the interaction of the different factors, limits the division into modifiable and non-modifiable factors. In addition, recent progress in understanding the aetiology of NIDDM has shown that it is a heterogeneous disease caused by several pathogenetic mechanisms, which are still largely unknown. Thus, not only the causes but also the means to prevent the disease may differ.

HETEROGENEITY OF NIDDM

NIDDM shows heterogeneity in numerous respects [8]. In the majority of cases, environmental factors unmask the disease to varying degrees, dependent on genetic susceptibility [9].

Our understanding of NIDDM is undergoing a radical change [10]. Previously, it was regarded as a relatively distinct disease entity, but in reality NIDDM

International Textbook of Diabetes Mellitus, Second Edition. Edited by K.G.M.M. Alberti, P. Zimmet, R.A. DeFronzo, and H. Keen (Honorary)
© 1997 John Wiley & Sons Ltd

(and its associated hyperglycaemia) is a descriptive term and a manifestation of a much broader underlying disorder [11, 12]. This includes a number of different aetiological entities which are discussed in other chapters. It probably also includes the Metabolic Syndrome [10, 12, 13], a cluster of cardiovascular disease (CVD) risk factors which, apart from hyperglycaemia (manifesting as NIDDM or impaired glucose tolerance, IGT), includes hyperinsulinaemia, dyslipidaemia, hypertension, and central obesity [14].

Social, behavioural and environmental risk factors [10, 15] appear to unmask the effects of genetic susceptibility with the result that NIDDM occurs on an epidemic scale in many countries, particularly developing and newly industrialized nations. This has occurred too quickly to be the result of altered gene frequencies [16] and the significance of this will be discussed in greater detail later. Oversecretion of insulin (hyperinsulinaemia) and insulin resistance characterize NIDDM in such populations, although islet B-cell failure occurs as the disease progresses [12].

During the last decade, research has shown that other forms of NIDDM do not fit the above pattern, and cases with decreased insulin secretion are seen [17, 18]. Some are cases of NIDDM where hyperinsulinaemia was present at an earlier stage and they have traversed the 'Starling curve of the pancreas' [19–21], resulting in secondary insulin secretory deficiency as the result of B-cell 'exhaustion'. However, other forms are associated with mutations of the insulin [22], insulin receptor [23] and glucokinase [18, 24] genes and mitochondrial DNA [25], while other cases are slow-onset IDDM, masquerading as NIDDM [26–28], a group now called (by some) latent autoimmune diabetes in adults (LADA).

It is for these reasons that the term NIDDM has inherent weaknesses. It reflects a mixture of genotype, phenotype and aetiology. Thus, it has become more difficult to define the limits of NIDDM or diabetes presenting in adult life [10, 29, 30]. An improved classification of individuals with, or at risk of, diabetes will help with the development of primary prevention strategies for a disorder which now affects over 100 million people world-wide and is likely to increase to affect over 230 million people by the year 2010 AD [31].

TIME TRENDS IN THE PREVALENCE AND INCIDENCE OF NIDDM

With the conquest of many infectious diseases and increasing life expectancy, the prevalence of NIDDM is expected to increase in most parts of the world because of changing demography and the ageing of populations. In developing countries demographic trends such as

decreasing birth rates and lower mortality from infectious causes will change age composition dramatically, and lead to populations where many more persons fall within the age range where chronic diseases such as NIDDM appear [32].

Apart from increases in frequency that result from changing demographic characteristics, there are many indications that the age-specific prevalence of NIDDM is increasing. In the USA, for example, the National Health Interview Survey provided data on the prevalence of diagnosed diabetes in persons aged 18–74 years since 1958 [33]. The observed increase was from about 1% in 1960 to 3% in 1991–93 [33]. Several factors have contributed to this increase. First, the average age of the US population has increased modestly; second, the criteria used to diagnose diabetes have become more sensitive and specific and the widespread use of automated methods for plasma glucose determination has contributed to increased recognition of previously undiagnosed diabetes. Furthermore, since 1970 mortality attributed to diabetes has decreased appreciably [34], as has mortality from cardiovascular disease, both of which probably result in increased survival among diabetics. The increase might also be explained by an increase in prevalence of risk factors for diabetes, such as obesity and physical inactivity, which still continue to rise in the USA. An increasing prevalence of diabetes has also been reported in Australia [35], and the UK [36].

Since 1964, annual age-specific incidence rates of diagnosed NIDDM have been available for the USA [33]. Incidence, i.e. the rate of development of newly detected cases, increased during the 1960s but was relatively stable from the early 1970s on, suggesting that the increasing prevalence since that time is largely the result of demographic changes and decreasing mortality.

While these studies leave some doubt as to whether or not there has been a true increase in the incidence of diabetes, there are population based studies which document a real increase. Among American Indians and a number of Polynesian and Micronesian populations, diabetes was reported to be rare before 1940 [37, 38]. On the other hand, by the mid-1960s diabetes was much more frequent. For example in 1967, the prevalence of NIDDM among the Pima Indians of Arizona was estimated to be 10 to 15 times that of the general US population [3], and over the next 10-year period the age-adjusted incidence of diabetes was about 20 times higher than in the predominantly Europid community of Rochester, Minnesota [39]. Between 1970 and 1980 the age–sex-adjusted prevalence of diabetes among the Pima increased 42%, primarily the result of a greater incidence of the disease, which increased by over 40% in the same interval. The study period from 1982 until

1990 showed further increases compared to the earlier period, with highest rates in young adults before the age of 55 years [40]. This study is unique in design in that the same systematic methods and criteria for assessing prevalence and incidence have been used since 1965.

Only environmental factors can explain such secular increases in the incidence of diabetes because gene frequencies cannot change enough in so short a period [16].

DETERMINANTS AND RISK FACTORS FOR NIDDM

Genetic Factors

Twin Studies

The earliest convincing evidence that familial aggregation of NIDDM is the result of genetic determinants arose from studies of monozygotic twins. Concordance rates for NIDDM in identical twins in reported series range from about 34 to 100% [41–51]. This frequency is at least twice that among non-identical twins, siblings or other first-degree relatives. Although twin studies indicate that genetic factors play a role in the aetiology of NIDDM, they provide no information about whether the disorder is caused by one or many genes, or about its mode of inheritance [52]. Furthermore, evidence of concordance from twin studies does not preclude the possibility that there are several distinct forms of NIDDM which result in similar phenotypic expression. Estimates of concordance also include some unknown components due to shared environment and support the influence of non-genetic factors if the rate of concordance is much less than 100%.

Populations of Mixed Ancestry

Other indirect evidence for genetic determinants of the susceptibility to NIDDM comes from studies of admixed populations, particularly where one group has a very high frequency of NIDDM compared to the other. Studies in Native Americans, Mexican-Americans, Pacific island populations, and Australian Aboriginals with European admixture have shown that the likelihood of developing NIDDM in offspring of mixed heritage is a function of the extent of genetic admixture [2, 53–58]. In these groups, the frequency of diabetes among subjects of mixed ancestry is intermediate between that in the high and low groups. In full-blooded Pima Indians, for example, the prevalence of NIDDM is twice that in those of half-Pima, half non-Indian ancestry, even though the subjects reside in the same community and are exposed to the same environment [55]. In an ecologic comparison of Mexican-Americans, the prevalence of diabetes correlated with

the degree of Native American admixture [56]. However predicting susceptibility to diabetes on an individual level according to the degree of admixture is not yet possible and is subject to methodological problems [59, 60].

Different Ethnic Groups Living in the Same Environment

Studies of different ethnic groups living in the same communities are thought to provide further evidence of the importance of genetic susceptibility in the aetiology of NIDDM [35, 38, 39, 61–75]. Major differences in the frequency of NIDDM were first described among the different ethnic groups resident in the state of Hawaii [61] and in Afro-Caribbeans and Indians living in Trinidad [62]. Subsequently, differences in prevalence in other ethnic groups have been shown in many countries, such as among Chinese, Indians and Malays residing in Singapore [63], Polynesians and Melanesians in the Loyalty Islands [64], Asian Indians and Melanesians living in Fiji [65], Indians and Europids in the UK [66]; between African-Americans and Europids [67], and Mexican-Americans and different groups of Native Americans [38, 39, 74–76] living in the USA and Canada. However, living in the same country or even community does not necessarily mean that the different ethnic groups share a similar environment. Differences in health-related behaviour may well exist between various groups in such communities, and attributing such differences to differences in genetic susceptibility may be spurious.

Familial Aggregation: Genetic Inheritance vs. Intra-uterine Environment

NIDDM has long been recognized as showing familial aggregation, but pedigree studies have been difficult to interpret largely because the age of onset of the disease is typically in older age groups, and it is difficult to find pedigrees where two or more generations have attained an age at which the disease is likely to be expressed. In addition, the disease may be asymptomatic and unless all relatives are tested, undiagnosed cases cannot be recognized. The incidence and prevalence of NIDDM in first-degree relatives of subjects with NIDDM, however, is much greater than that in the general population [77–79]. Because the disease is relatively frequent in the population and family members share environmental factors, the occurrence of NIDDM in relatives cannot necessarily be taken as evidence that susceptibility has arisen from the same genetic source, or even that affected relatives have the same form of NIDDM. Affected sib-pair studies do not require assumptions about the mode of inheritance like linkage analyses, but are also limited by the informativeness of the members of the pedigrees. Linkage and sib-pair studies of candidate NIDDM genes are extensively discussed in Chapter 3.

Many studies reporting familial aggregation of NIDDM have observed a predominantly maternal transmission of the disease [80–83]. One explanation for this observation is the effect of the intra-uterine environment on the risk of developing NIDDM in the offspring. In offspring of Pima Indian women who had diabetes during pregnancy, a higher prevalence of diabetes occurred than in offspring of mothers who did not have diabetes or who developed the disease after that pregnancy [84]. Relative fetal overnutrition during a diabetic pregnancy could produce metabolic effects on the fetus which convey a risk for NIDDM independent of the genetic susceptibility. A similar concept of the influence of the fetal and early postnatal nutrition contributing to the risk for NIDDM was deduced from studies showing that low birthweight babies are at higher risk for developing the disease [85] than normal weight babies. In each of these situations, an excess influence of the mothers over fathers contributing to the risk of NIDDM would be seen, without implying genetic inheritance [52]. Alternatively, linkage of NIDDM to mitochondrial mutations (which are inherited maternally) would also explain excess maternal transmission of NIDDM [86–88].

Genetic Markers

Recent efforts in molecular biology have increased our understanding of the pathophysiology of NIDDM (or some of its sub-types) and identified a growing number of candidate genes involved in glucose homeostasis.

A major difficulty in studying the genetics of NIDDM is the variability of its clinical manifestation. This is reflected in the current classification of diabetes, which was based on clinical criteria such as requirement for insulin treatment, proneness to ketosis and presence of obesity, rather than on aetiological determinants which are still largely unknown. Similar clinical presentations of cases of diabetes might be caused by different genetic mechanisms and/or environmental factors. Alternatively, the same genetic defect might be responsible for different phenotypic effects, so that the same aetiological entity might be allocated to different classes of diabetes. NIDDM in its current classification is thought to have a heterogeneous background and to be polygenic [8, 89], occurring at rates which are well above those observed for single-gene diseases [52]. Unlike single-gene diseases, where the expression of the disease is influenced by a mutant allele at one gene locus, alone or in

interaction with an environmental factor, NIDDM may depend on many gene loci with only small to moderate effects, which act in combination to create a genetic susceptibility. According to this model, predisposition to NIDDM could be determined by many different combinations of genotypes and environmental factors, while NIDDM will not necessarily develop in all predisposed individuals. For these reasons, classical gene mapping strategies are not readily applicable to the identification of diabetogenic genes [90] and the focus up to the present time has been on research with candidate genes, i.e. genes which encode proteins involved in physiological processes central to the pathogenesis of NIDDM. However, apart from some rare forms, candidate genes (reviewed in Chapter 3) have not been able to explain a substantial proportion of the prevalence of NIDDM.

Thrifty Gene Hypothesis

The extremely high prevalence and incidence of obesity and NIDDM in some non-Europid populations, points towards the involvement of genetic factors, in addition to the contributions of environmental and behavioural factors.

The thrifty genotype hypothesis [91–93], first proposed by Neel in 1962 [94], has been invoked to explain the persistence of obesity- and NIDDM-prone genotypes in human populations. The thrifty genotype, which is hypothesized to promote fat deposition and storage of calories in times of plenty, is presumed to have offered a survival advantage to individuals in early agricultural and hunter-gatherer societies during periods of food shortage and starvation [95]. Populations which were formerly most subject to such adverse circumstances would be those where the frequency of the thrifty genotype would be the highest, and also those which in times of uninterrupted food supply would be expected to have the highest incidence of NIDDM.

This is consistent with the natural history of obesity and NIDDM in Polynesians in Western Samoa and other Pacific islanders, where a metabolism suited to rapid weight gain through hyperinsulinaemia and selective tissue insulin resistance would have been an advantage under alternating conditions of feast or famine [92].

The concept of a thrifty gene is not without precedence. Genetic traits such as sickle cell anaemia and glucose-6-phosphate dehydrogenase deficiency are more frequent in populations where malaria exists [97] and can be regarded as examples of a selected genotype. The persistence of these potentially lethal single-gene disorders in certain parts of the world has been ascribed to the fact that heterozygote individuals are selectively protected against malaria, a major environmental hazard. There is no direct evidence that populations which are highly susceptible to NIDDM survive famine better than do other groups (other than anecdotal suggestions [98]), but experimental studies in diabetes- and obesity-prone rodents do show a survival advantage under fasting conditions [99].

In this context, the relatively low prevalence of NIDDM in European populations is of some interest [93]. It might be due to the fact that there has been less selection in favour of the thrifty genotype because there were not the repeated food shortages seen elsewhere. Thus, the prevalence of diabetes in the USA is about 7% overall [67] compared with over 50% in the Pima Indian population [40]. Similar differences are observed in the prevalence of obesity across ethnic groups.

Demographic Determinants

Sex

The relative frequency of NIDDM in men and women varies inconsistently in epidemiological studies. Comparisons of population-based studies in US adults with diabetes, subdivided by ethnic background, do not show any consistent sex preference in diabetes frequency in any of the ethnic groups studied [7, 101]. Much if not all of the difference in sex ratio of diabetes can be explained by male/female differences in the relative frequency of obesity and physical activity in different cultures and ethnic groups.

Age

The prevalence of NIDDM increases with age in most populations although some studies show a fall in the oldest age groups. Prevalence, however, represents the balance between the cumulative rate of development of new cases (cumulative incidence) and the effect of differential mortality among those with the disease. This limits the inferences that can be made when only prevalence figures are available. Furthermore, prevalence data can be considerably influenced by secular changes in incidence. To examine the effect of age on the occurrence of NIDDM from an aetiological point of view it is necessary to have incidence data.

Few studies of the age-specific incidence of diabetes have been conducted. In the USA, based on a diabetes diagnosis during the past 12 months, the National Health Interview Surveys have estimated the incidence of diabetes on a number of occasions [33]. These studies indicate that incidence increases up to ages 65–74 years, with no further rise in those aged 75 years and over. These findings are essentially consistent with

those from Rochester, Minnesota, USA, where the age-specific incidence of NIDDM shows a progressive increase with advancing age [102].

In contrast with these studies, the age-specific incidence of NIDDM in the Pima Indians peaks between 40 and 50 years, but then falls thereafter [40]. These peak incidence rates in the Pima, about 60/1000 person-years, are three times higher than in the older US population and in Edinburgh, Scotland, where the highest rates were approximately 20/1000 person-years [102]. The difference in these patterns is remarkable, but may relate to the extent of obesity among the Pima as well as their genetic susceptibility to the disease. When the age-sex specific incidence patterns are examined according to degree of obesity, incidence is extremely high at an early age in those who are extremely obese and then falls [77]. In those with lesser degrees of obesity the peak incidence occurs at a later age. This has two implications: First, it suggests that obesity may advance the onset of diabetes in those who are susceptible. If so, avoidance of obesity would delay the onset of diabetes. Second, if the majority of the obese susceptible persons develop the disease at a relatively early age, then older obese subjects may have less risk than equally obese younger persons. These findings illustrate the importance of genetic–environmental interaction in the causation of NIDDM. Unfortunately, similar data on the relationship of extreme obesity to incidence of diabetes in other ethnic groups are not available. However, it is also well known that many extremely obese subjects do not develop NIDDM.

In general, NIDDM in Europids is usually characterized by onset after the age of 50 years, whereas in Pacific islanders and the other high risk populations, onset in the 20–30-year age-group is common [103]. The socio-economic and health impact of the diabetes epidemic in such societies is therefore much greater.

Ethnicity

NIDDM has long been a problem in developed countries, but now it has become epidemic in many developing and newly industrialized nations. Currently, inter-population differences in the prevalence of diabetes are dramatic. The prevalence of adult diabetes in non-Europid populations varies from <1% in rural Bantu in Tanzania, and in Chinese in mainland China, to 40–50% in Pima Indians and in Micronesians in Nauru [7, 31]. This variation can be explained in part by underlying differences in obesity and other behavioural risk factors. Studies in the US comparing the Hispanic population with non-Hispanic whites [105, 106] and African-Americans with whites [107] show excess diabetes in these minorities even after differences in age, sex, obesity, fat distribution, family history of

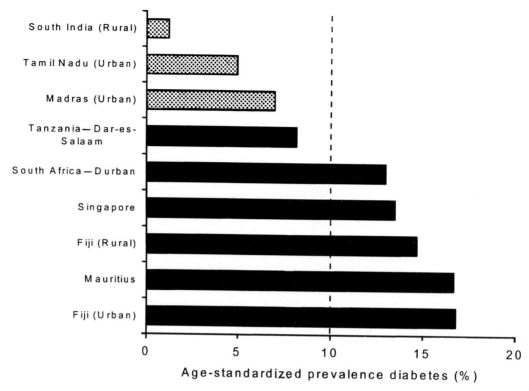

Figure 1 Age-standardized prevalence (Segi's world population) of NIDDM in ▨ native and ■ migrant Asian Indian populations. Adapted from reference 112

diabetes, and level of education or income, are taken into account. This points to genetic risk factors manifesting in such geographic and ethnic differences and/or to the existence of yet unknown or insufficiently measured known non-genetic risk factors.

The following section describes the epidemiology of NIDDM in different regions of the world, first in populations living in their home country and then in migrant populations.

Epidemiology of NIDDM in Native Non-Europid Populations

NIDDM in Asian Indians Asian Indians are defined here as people who originated in the Indian subcontinent (including India, Pakistan and Bangladesh). The prevalence of NIDDM in India was reported low in older studies, but geographical differences were noted. In Indians aged 15 years and over it has been estimated to be 2.1% in urban areas and 1.5% in rural populations [108]. However, in Indians living in an affluent suburb of New Delhi, diabetes prevalence was as high as 20% in men aged 45–74 years and somewhat lower in women [109]. Already in 1975 the Indian Council of Medical Research demonstrated rates of NIDDM in urban living populations of India that were more than three times greater than in rural areas

[111]. A recent study comparing the urban population of Madras with nearby rural areas reported age-adjusted rates of NIDDM of 7.0% in the urban population and of 1.2% in the rural area [110]. Figure 1 shows age-standardized prevalence data in Asian Indians from the most recent studies using WHO screening criteria for NIDDM [112]. The lowest prevalences on the Indian subcontinent were observed in Bangladesh with 0.2% [113], whereas a study in Pakistan reported a prevalence of NIDDM of 14.3% [114].

NIDDM in East and South-east Asia In East Asia the highest prevalence of diabetes reported is 10.2% in a 1993 study from Japan [115]. This compares with a prevalence of 5% which was seen a decade earlier in Tokyo [116] for persons over age 40. Recent reports from South Korea [117] and Taiwan [118] show intermediate rates, whereas the lowest rates in that region are observed in China [7, 119] (and X Pan, personal communication). In the late 1970s the overall prevalence of NIDDM among the Chinese population of Shanghai was estimated to be less than 1%, and 1.3% among those aged 20 years and over [121]. The prevalence was related to age, obesity and occupation. Among the occupational groups, farm workers had the lowest prevalence; workers in heavy industry and office workers had a higher prevalence. A recent study in the city of Da Qing in northern China using WHO

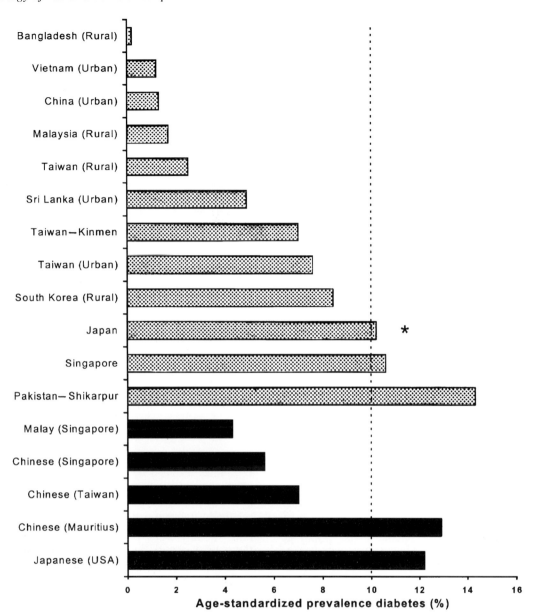

Figure 2 Age-standardized prevalence (Segi's world population) of NIDDM in ▧ native and ■ migrant non-Indian Asian populations. *Age 40–69 years. Subjects from Bangladesh and Pakistan are also shown for comparison. Adapted from reference 112

criteria showed that the prevalence of diabetes is 2.6% in those aged 25 and over, with similar prevalence in males and females, double that found ten years earlier (X Pan, personal communication). Published studies conducted in East and South-east Asia using WHO screening criteria are summarized in Figure 2 [112].

NIDDM in North American Indians and Alaska natives Native Americans are a diverse group of people whose ancestors lived in North America before the European settlement. Contemporary native American populations live in urban areas and on reservations or reserves in the USA and in Canada. In general,

the Native American populations of North America are young and disadvantaged both economically and educationally compared with the general US population. Few data exist on the health of urban Native Americans living outside areas served by the US Indian Health Service (IHS). However, prevalence estimates for diagnosed diabetes are available from health care facilities where care is provided to Native Americans, and age-adjusted prevalence of diabetes in the IHS Areas is 6.9% overall [122], ranging from 1.5% in the Alaska area to 12% in Native Americans living in Arizona, which includes the Pima Indians. In Canada, the highest prevalence of diabetes (8.7%)

was reported in the Atlantic Area serviced by the Medical Service Branch of the Department of National Health and Welfare, and the lowest (0.4%) in the Inuit population [122].

Striking increases in the prevalence of diabetes in recent years have been described in Pima Indians and other tribes [76, 123–126]. Moreover, in the Pima Indians who have participated in a longitudinal study of diabetes since 1965, the incidence of diabetes has increased [40]. The increase in prevalence in many tribes is therefore probably due to an increased incidence and cannot be attributed solely to longer survival of diabetic individuals [40].

NIDDM in African populations The estimated prevalence of NIDDM for the African continent was 4.7 million cases over the age of 20 in an estimated population of 698 million in 1994 [31]. However, epidemiologic studies are only available from very few countries and many of the older studies did not employ NIDDM screening methods recommended by the WHO. In a rural community in Northern Africa 1.3% of the population were reported to have fasting glucose levels over 7.8 mmol/l (140 mg/dl) [127], and in rural Tanzania the prevalence of NIDDM as assessed by WHO criteria was also low at 0.9% [128]. More recent data from Tanzania show an increase in the prevalence of NIDDM [129]. In rural Cameroon a similar prevalence of 0.8% in those over 25 has recently been reported, with 2.0% in an urban sample [104]. However, at present the prevalence of diabetes among African adults seems to be less than that reported for migrant African populations or migrant populations such as South Asians living in Africa [129].

NIDDM in Pacific islanders During the twentieth century, populations in the Pacific region have experienced the full scope of the health transition from predominance of infectious diseases to the present predominance of non-communicable diseases associated with modernization. The original incursions of European explorers, missionaries and traders introduced infectious diseases which in many instances devastated indigenous populations [130]. The accelerated modernization over the last decades has changed the disease profile towards non-communicable diseases, including obesity, NIDDM and cardiovascular diseases, as major health problems [103, 131–133].

The highest recent estimates of the prevalence (age-standardized) of NIDDM in Pacific islanders for adults 20 years and older are: Nauruans, 33% and 35% [134]; urban Samoans, 12% and 16% [135]; urban Wanigelas of Papua New Guinea, 31% and 40% [136] in men and women respectively. Figure 3 demonstrates the marked variability in prevalence in men from

recently studied populations [112]. The combined prevalence of NIDDM and impaired glucose tolerance (IGT) in urbanized Wanigela adults aged 30–64 years (60% in men and 67% in women) is close to that of Pima Indians (61% and 68%, respectively), which is the highest yet recorded in any population [40]. Furthermore, these studies have highlighted differences in the prevalence of NIDDM (and IGT) between rural and urban dwelling segments of the same population.

There is compelling evidence that the high frequency of NIDDM (like the high frequency of obesity) observed in these populations represents a modern epidemic. Old medical records, where these are available, even in the first half of this century when diabetes was readily diagnosed [137], do not mention diabetes. Only single cases of diabetes were recorded in Nauruan mortality data in 1925 and 1935, but no further cases were recorded until the 1950s when the current epidemic appears to have commenced [134].

Serial surveys in Polynesian Western Samoans [135] and Tokelauans [138], and Melanesian Wanigelas of Papua New Guinea [136] have clearly documented increases in prevalence in recent times. In urban Wanigelas there was a near doubling in prevalence of both NIDDM and IGT over 14 years up to 1991 [136]. In Western Samoans increases over 13 years up to 1991 were observed in both rural and urban locations, with the more dramatic increases in rural men (0.1% to 5.3% in rural and 2.3% to 7.0% in urban areas) and urban women (8.2% to 13.4%) [135]. In Nauruans, however, serial surveys have demonstrated a relatively stable prevalence of NIDDM over the period since 1975 [134], as was observed also for obesity. In this case it seems that the epidemic of NIDDM had already peaked by the time of the original survey.

Cross-sectional data from all Pacific populations which have been studied implicate obesity as the most important modifiable risk factor for NIDDM [103]. Even in Nauruans, who are almost uniformly obese, there is a graded relationship of overall adiposity (BMI) and abdominal fat distribution (WHR) with plasma glucose concentrations [139]. Similar cross-sectional studies in Western Samoans [135] have demonstrated BMI and WHR as independent risk factors for both IGT and NIDDM, after controlling for other factors including age, physical activity and family history of diabetes. Furthermore, longitudinal studies in Nauruans [20, 140], as in other populations, have shown BMI to predict future NIDDM.

Ecological comparisons of physical activity levels and NIDDM prevalence between urban and rural populations in the Pacific suggest a beneficial effect of exercise. More substantively, cross-sectional data from Melanesian and Indian Fijians [141], Micronesian i-Kiribati [142] and Polynesian Western Samoans

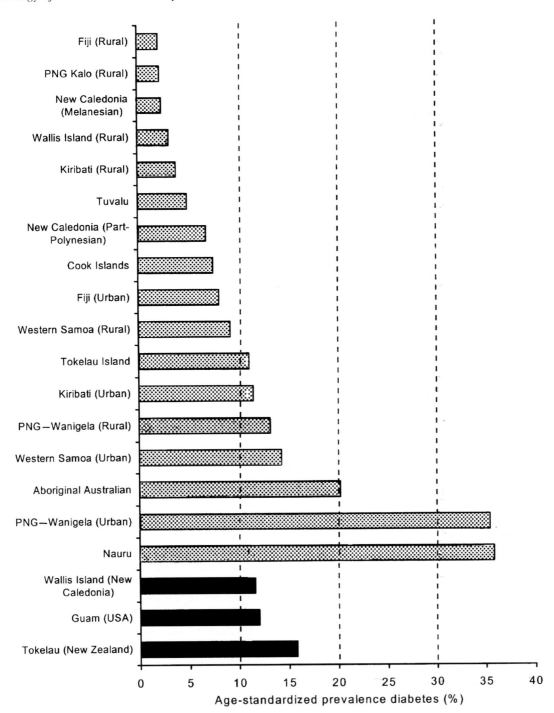

Figure 3 Age-standardized prevalence (Segi's world population) of NIDDM in ▒ native and ■ migrant Pacific Island populations, and Australian Aboriginals. PNG = Papua New Guinea. Adapted from reference 112

[135] have shown 'usual' physical activity to be independently associated with IGT and NIDDM, even after controlling for variables including age, BMI, WHR, rural/urban area and family history of diabetes.

There have been major changes in the diets of Pacific island populations since contact with Europeans, and it is clear that these changes are associated with increases in obesity [143–146] suggesting that diet is contributing to the epidemic of NIDDM. However, so far it has not been possible to detect a direct effect of any specific food or nutrient on risk of NIDDM within a Pacific population, including Nauruans [144] and Wanigelas of Papua New Guinea [147].

Overall adiposity, fat distribution and physical activity are important determinants of insulin sensitivity and insulin secretion in Pacific islander populations, and it is generally assumed that it is via effects on either or both of these that obesity and physical activity are related to NIDDM [139, 148–152]. However, longitudinal data from Nauruans [20], Western Samoans and Papua New Guineans and from the Indian Ocean nation of Mauritius [153], show obesity as an independent predictor of NIDDM, after controlling for glucose and insulin concentrations, suggesting that obesity may also cause NIDDM via other mechanisms.

NIDDM in Australian Aboriginals   Although many of the studies available on the prevalence of NIDDM in Australian Aboriginals and Torres Strait islanders were performed using older diagnostic criteria, reviews of the published data consistently report rates exceeding those observed in non-Aboriginal populations [154, 155]. Whereas the 1981 population-based diabetes survey in Busselton found that 3.7% of the female and 5.1% of the male Europid residents had diabetes, studies performed in Aboriginals living in several rural and urban regions of Australia showed 11.6% in women and 7.0% in men, age standardized to the 1981 Australian population [155]. A more recent study found an even higher prevalence of diabetes (29.6%) in Aboriginals aged 35 years and above living in a highly 'Westernized' community [156]. Pooled data from studies in south-eastern and central Australia furthermore showed a 12% prevalence of NIDDM in Australian Aboriginals aged 20–49 years, in contrast to only 1% in a country town sample of non-Aboriginal people in the same age range in the state of Victoria [155]. This highlights the higher age-specific prevalence of diabetes seen in many non-Europid populations at younger ages.

Epidemiology of NIDDM in Migrant Non-Europid Populations

Over the millennia, but especially during the last two centuries, human populations have moved from place to place. Migrants often move to an alien social, cultural, economic and geographic environment, and their way of life changes. The frequency of disease in migrants can be compared to that among persons who remained in the original environment, and differences can be examined in relation to the characteristics of the new and the original environment. Caution must be exercised in interpreting such studies, however, since those who migrate are not always identical to those who remain behind. Migration, itself, may be related to religion, health, socio-economic status and geography. Thus the migrants may differ from the majority of the original population. Conversely, migrants may continue to practise many of their traditional social, cultural and dietary habits, or they may adopt the characteristics of populations in their new environment to a varying degree. Over the course of a few generations

their genetic pool may change as a result of admixture, even though the group may retain its original nominal identity. Nevertheless, in spite of these difficulties, studies of migrant populations offer a unique opportunity to examine the effects of genetic–environmental interaction.

NIDDM in migrant Asian Indians   Populations of South Asian origin are found in many parts of the world. Although studies among native and migrant populations often employ different methodology, much higher frequencies of NIDDM are reported among expatriate Indians (Figure 1). Thus, in Singapore 13.5% of Asian Indians were reported to have diabetes [158]; in Asian Indians aged 15 years and over residing in South Africa it was 13% [159]; in Fiji 14% have been reported to have diabetes in both urban and rural areas [65]; and a similar high prevalence was found in Mauritius [71].

Previously diagnosed diabetes was found among 2.2% of Asian Indian residents of Southall in West London in the early 1980s. Among those aged 40–64 years prevalence was at least five times higher than among the Europeans [66]. While this figure does not account for undiagnosed diabetes, it does indicate a higher prevalence than in Europids in the same environment, and higher than generally reported from India. While the majority of expatriate Indians live in more affluent circumstances than the majority in their homeland, this excess frequency of NIDDM should perhaps not be entirely unanticipated since, as early as 1907, it was stated that 'What gout is to the nobility of England, diabetes is to the aristocracy of India' [160].

NIDDM in migrant African populations   The epidemiology of diabetes in African populations who migrated to the USA is much better documented than in African populations in their homelands. Differing degrees of European admixture exist today across African-American populations [161]. In addition, changes in culture have emerged that contribute to environmental and life-style factors that influence rates of diabetes differently to African populations living outside the USA. Data on diagnosed diabetes in African-Americans based on the 1993 National Health Interview Survey (NHIS) show a prevalence of 4.1%, about 1.4 times as frequent as in the Europid population living in the USA [162]. Over the past 30 years prevalence and incidence of NIDDM in African-Americans seem to have increased at a faster rate than in the White population of the USA. Data from the Follow-up Study of the 1971–75 NHANES I showed age-adjusted incidences of diagnosed diabetes of 10.9% for African-American men and 15% for women, whereas for White men and women 7.0% and 6.9% were reported, respectively [163].

Estimates of the prevalence of diabetes in the African-Caribbean population range widely from 0.7 to 14.5% [63, 164–170], but many of the studies were performed before the WHO criteria for NIDDM. Differing degrees of economic development in the Caribbean islands could at least partly explain such different rates. African-Caribbeans in Manchester, UK, showed a prevalence of 11.2% [104].

NIDDM in Japanese migrants Many Japanese migrated to the island of Hawaii from the Hiroshima prefecture in Japan and their offspring now constitute the majority of the Japanese population residing in Hawaii. Between 1973 and 1978 a survey of NIDDM was conducted using the same methods in Hiroshima and Hawaii, and in 1978 in Los Angeles [171–173]. The presence of diabetes was defined by a 2-hour post-load venous serum glucose level of at least 200 mg/dl (11.1 mmol/l) after a 50 g oral glucose load. The age–sex-adjusted prevalence of diabetes in Japanese aged 40 years and over in Hawaii and Los Angeles was similarly high at 13.9%, compared to 6.5% in Hiroshima. Although the Japanese in Hawaii were on average more obese, their total caloric intake was similar to those in Hiroshima, but the estimated level of physical activity was lower among the Hawaiian Japanese. In contrast, the consumption of animal fat and simple carbohydrates was at least twice as high in the Hawaiian as in the Hiroshima Japanese, whereas the Hiroshima Japanese consumed about twice as much complex carbohydrate. Even after adjustment for the degree of obesity, the prevalence of NIDDM in the Hawaiian Japanese remained almost twice that observed in Hiroshima, strongly suggesting that other determinants, perhaps related to diet or physical activity, were responsible for the differences. Analogous changes are found in Japanese residents of Seattle. Using a 75 g oral glucose load and WHO criteria, about 20% of second-generation Japanese men and 16% of the women in Seattle have NIDDM [116, 174], compared to 5% of men and 4% of women in the same age group living in Tokyo.

Diabetes in migrant Chinese populations Estimates of the prevalence of diabetes among Chinese emigrants vary considerably. The prevalence of known diabetes was reported in 1963 to be 1.8% among the Chinese in Hawaii [61], and more recently Thai and associates [63] found an age-standardized prevalence of 5.6% in the Chinese population of Singapore. On the other hand, West and Kalbfleish [1] found a prevalence of 7.4% among Chinese in Malaya, based on glucose tolerance testing with a diagnosis of diabetes made when plasma glucose level was 160 mg/dl (8.9 mmol/l) and over. A recent report from Taiwan showed a prevalence of 7.0% in urban Chinese individuals [118].

Another recent study conducted in Mauritius, using WHO criteria, reported that about 13% of those of Chinese origin aged 25 years and over have NIDDM [71]. Notably absent are recent estimates of the prevalence of diabetes among Chinese living in the USA. In Singapore, between the 1984 survey [63] and the most recent 1992 survey, there was a twofold secular increase in NIDDM in all three ethnic groups (Chinese, Malaysians, Asian Indians). Interestingly, in a recent study of adult Chinese in the UK the prevalence of diabetes of 4% was the same as in the local population [157].

NIDDM in migrant Pacific island populations
Studies of Polynesian migrants from Wallis Island to New Caledonia [175] and from the Tokelau Islands to New Zealand [138, 176] have also documented increased prevalence of NIDDM in the emigrant groups.

Early studies indicate that the frequency of glucose intolerance varies considerably in Pacific island populations. The prevalence of diabetes in Chamorros was 3% and 8% in males and females, respectively, on the more traditional Micronesian island of Rota, compared to 10% in males and 13% in females in Guam, and 10% in males and 14% in females who had migrated to California [177]. These differences suggested that 'Westernization' of lifestyle is associated with increasing prevalence of diabetes. (Although Guam is one of the traditional homelands of the Chamorros, it has undergone considerable Westernization since 1945.) Studies of migration in Polynesia have shown that in the late 1960s the inhabitants of Tokelau aged 25 years and over had a prevalence of diabetes of 1% in males and 3.3% in females, whereas those who migrated to New Zealand had an age-standardized prevalence of 5.6% in males and 8% in females [176]. The prevalence subsequently increased. By 1976, 3.7% of the males and 8.6% of females in Tokelau had diabetes, whereas 5.4% of males and 13.6% of females living in New Zealand now had the disease.

Other recent migrations have taken place in the Pacific. Between 1970 and 1980 many Polynesians from the Pacific Island of Wallis moved to the much more urbanized community of Noumea, New Caledonia. The way of life in Wallis is still relatively traditional, but the majority of the Wallisians who migrated were attracted to the occupational opportunities provided by the nickel industry in New Caledonia. In 1980 the age–sex-standardized prevalence of diabetes (by WHO criteria) in Wallis among those aged 20 years and over was 2.9% compared to 11.6% in New Caledonia [177, 178]. Even after adjustment for age and differences in obesity the prevalence was 6.6 times higher in men and 3.5 times higher in the women in New Caledonia compared to those in Wallis.

Studies of migrant populations have provided overwhelming evidence of the importance of environmental factors as determinants of NIDDM, but have yielded limited information about the role of specific factors. Socio-economic status almost invariably increases with migration; the type of occupational activity frequently changes, and the amount of physical activity often, although not invariably, decreases. While some elements of the traditional dietary patterns are often retained, the nutrients and dietary composition often change dramatically. Other factors, such as the consumption of alcohol, use of tobacco and other more subtle, yet perhaps important factors, may change. The change in most instances is towards a more 'Westernized' way of life. Typically, calorie, animal fat and refined carbohydrate consumption increase, but dietary fibre diminishes. There is reduced physical activity, with lower energy expenditure both for occupational activities and the requirements of daily living. Obesity is generally more frequent in migrants than in the traditional environment, but even after accounting for the increased obesity, an unexplained excess of NIDDM generally prevails. Unfortunately, few studies have used identical methods and assessed the components of change in a comprehensive way. It appears, however, that the increased frequency of diabetes seen among migrants cannot be wholly explained on the basis of increased obesity. The effect of changes in diet, and extent and type of physical activity (and possibly other factors) are potential reasons for the increased NIDDM prevalence among migrants.

Behavioural and Life-style-related Risk Factors

The development of NIDDM is influenced substantially by environmental factors. Several lines of epidemiological evidence can be cited. First, NIDDM develops at different frequencies when populations move to a different environment. Second, there is evidence of large secular changes in the prevalence and incidence of NIDDM. These are far greater and have occurred much more rapidly than can be explained on the basis of genetic drift. Third, the occurrence of NIDDM within a population is related to demographic and environmental characteristics such as age, the degree of obesity, physical activity, dietary habits, and degree of modernization. Finally, even the intra-uterine environment may alter the rate of development of NIDDM. The following section discusses behavioural and life-style-related risk factors of NIDDM such as obesity, physical inactivity, diet and Westernization of life-style.

Obesity

A relationship between obesity and diabetes has been recognized for centuries [37]. However, the nature of this relationship has been and remains controversial. Do obese subjects develop NIDDM more frequently, or do those prone to NIDDM develop obesity more frequently? Are genes that result in susceptibility to diabetes and obesity the same?

While there is clear evidence that obesity is an important risk factor for NIDDM, it is also apparent that only a proportion of obese subjects develop diabetes. Conversely, many non-obese subjects also develop NIDDM. Moreover, the relationship between the occurrence of NIDDM and obesity measured at one point in time is complicated by the fact that diabetes itself can lead to weight loss and that most patients with diabetes are specifically encouraged to lose weight. Given these problems, only limited inferences can be deduced from cross-sectional data which demonstrate associations between NIDDM and obesity. Far more relevant in the context of a possible causal relationship are incidence data. Recent research on the relationship of obesity and NIDDM has shown that not only the degree of overweight, but also weight change, duration and onset of obesity and the distribution of body fat are important contributors to the risk, and each of them might be of different relevance in different populations. These relationships are complicated by the effects of physical activity, genetic factors, and possibly fetal and early infant growth rate, all of which contribute to the risk of NIDDM by themselves, and modify the effect of fat mass *per se* [179].

Degree of overweight, weight changes Both cross-sectionally [105, 135, 149, 180–189] and in prospective studies [183, 190–198] there is clear evidence that the degree of obesity is an important risk factor for NIDDM. Weight loss associated with the onset of NIDDM in Pima Indians and in obese Micronesian Nauruans [196, 199] means that the association of obesity with NIDDM prevalence is generally weaker than its association with incidence. Results from a prospective study in Mauritius indicate clearly that subjects with newly diagnosed or known diabetes at baseline lost weight over the subsequent 5 years, while those with normal or impaired glucose tolerance at baseline gained weight [200]. Baseline body mass index (BMI) was also strongly related to the incidence of NIDDM in Pima Indians, but there was little association between diabetes prevalence and concurrent obesity [77]. In a small group of subjects with BMI data from 4 years before diagnosis to 2 years after, there was a clear pattern of weight gain in the 4 years preceding diagnosis, followed by a weight loss in the following 2 years. Older subjects developed diabetes at a lower BMI than younger individuals, suggesting that the age-related deterioration in insulin sensitivity enables the development of diabetes at lower levels of adiposity than that required for the development of diabetes in younger subjects [77]. In addition, populations which are more obese may show a greater weight loss in association with NIDDM. Stronger cross-sectional associations of obesity and NIDDM could also be expected in populations where diabetes is diagnosed earlier and better controlled, so as to minimize both hyperglycaemia and weight loss.

Evidence for a specific effect of weight gain on the development of NIDDM comes from two American cohort studies, where self-reported weight gain throughout adulthood or immediately prior to the study period was associated with increased risk of NIDDM independent of BMI in early adulthood [194, 195]. The deleterious effect of weight gain was shown to occur over a whole range of ages and in several populations [77, 196, 201, 202]. The association between weight gain and NIDDM could be explained in a number of ways. It is possible that weight gain in the short term could lead to worsening of insulin resistance, islet B-cell decompensation, glucose intolerance and NIDDM in already susceptible individuals, with the level or type of obesity at which this occurs determined by other factors such as genotype, age or physical activity. Alternatively, weight gain could be a result of the hyperinsulinaemia that precedes NIDDM [20, 203, 204]. Thirdly, behavioural factors resulting in weight gain, such as dietary changes or reduced physical activity, may also promote the development of NIDDM.

Onset and duration of obesity The duration of obesity influences the incidence of diabetes. West provided evidence that the maximum attained weight or weight at age 25 was a better predictor of the presence of diabetes than current weight [37]. Indirect evidence for the importance of duration of obesity in the development of NIDDM was found in a study of 2000 Israeli men [198]. Subjects who had lost weight to reach a specific BMI class had an increased risk of NIDDM relative to those who had remained stable within that class. Those with a stable BMI had, in turn, a greater risk of NIDDM than those who had increased their BMI class, indicating that weight gain *per se* was not associated with increased risk of NIDDM. Similar findings were provided in longitudinal studies of the multi-ethnic population of Mauritius [200]. For any level of BMI at follow-up, the greatest prevalence of NIDDM was associated with weight loss since baseline, and the least with weight gain. Subjects who gained weight to reach a specific BMI level would not have been at that level as long as those who had remained stable at that BMI, and who had a higher risk of NIDDM. Subjects who had lost weight to reach a specific BMI would have had some duration of an even greater degree of obesity which would contribute to the highest prevalence of NIDDM in this group. This suggests that the

duration of obesity, or the maximum attained degree of obesity may be important determinants of the risk of NIDDM.

Although the duration of obesity is considered important in determining the risk of obesity-associated conditions, including NIDDM, little information is available to quantify this relationship. Even in most prospective studies the actual onset of obesity is not measured and can only be obtained by recall. Moreover, if weight is changing it is difficult to differentiate between the effects of degree and duration of obesity. In one of the few reports to actually examine the levels of glucose tolerance associated with different durations of self-reported obesity, it took 5–18 years of obesity to develop glucose intolerance, and 12–38 years for diabetes to occur [206].

Distribution of obesity Not only the presence but also the distribution of adiposity determines incidence of diabetes. Anthropometric measures of body fat distribution are associated with risk of diabetes, both in longitudinal [190–193] and cross-sectional [135, 149, 180, 184–189] studies, and are generally independent of measures of overall fatness [135, 149, 184, 185, 187, 188, 190–193]. In fact, in many cases fat distribution appears more important [149, 184–188, 196] than general obesity. With increasing age, however, the associations with both waist-hip ratio (WHR) and BMI seem to be attenuated.

Longitudinal data are less consistent in showing fat distribution (as reflected by WHR) as a stronger predictor of both NIDDM and IGT than BMI [190, 191, 193] although there is interaction between BMI and WHR. The tendency for markers of fat distribution to be more strongly associated with NIDDM prevalence than is BMI could be explained if a fall in BMI but not WHR was associated with the onset of diabetes. Furthermore, some studies suggest sex differences in the relative importance of overall fatness and fat distribution. In Mauritius, where WHR and BMI are independently associated with NIDDM [149], the effect of WHR was greater than that of BMI in women, while in men the converse was found. In Brazilian and Chinese adults BMI and WHR are independently associated with NIDDM in women but only WHR remained significant in multivariate analysis in men [184, 185]. In Mexican-American and non-Hispanic White men and women [207], overall obesity was independently associated with NIDDM prevalence, but the association with central obesity was only significant in women. This could be explained by assuming a plateau effect of central body fat distribution, whereby above a certain level of central obesity, which might have been reached by most men, there would be no further increase in rates of NIDDM independent of the effects of overall obesity.

Fat deposition in men is generally abdominal, so that waist circumference or WHR can be expected to correlate strongly with overall obesity. In women there is more variation in fat distribution, so measures such as WHR would be expected to differentiate between higher- and lower-risk individuals at a given level of overall fat mass, and are therefore more likely to be independently significant in multivariate analysis.

An interaction between general and central obesity must be considered. In extremely obese subjects with a tendency to abdominal adipose distribution, further increases in adiposity may result in fat being accumulated in other areas, leading to a proportional reduction in abdominal fat in association with increasing BMI. The risk of NIDDM may continue to increase as body fat content rises, weakening the association between fat distribution and NIDDM. Biochemical aspects of obesity and fat distribution are discussed in Chapter 29.

In summary, overall obesity, duration of obesity and fat distribution all contribute to the risk of NIDDM. Their apparent relative importance varies according to whether incidence or prevalence of NIDDM is assessed, the gender of the individuals, or their degree of obesity.

The incidence of diabetes and its relationship to obesity is related to other factors, in particular, the interaction of genetic susceptibility and obesity. Studies of family history of diabetes as a predictor of diabetes in offspring suggest that a higher level of obesity is required for the development of diabetes in individuals with lower genetic predisposition to NIDDM [208, 209]. Patients with NIDDM with a definite history of obesity had a lower prevalence of family history of diabetes than those who had not been obese [210]. In Pima Indians the prevalence of NIDDM is higher in relatives of leaner NIDDM cases than in relatives of more obese cases [211].

In Pima Indians, a clear interaction between family history and BMI in relation to the incidence of NIDDM is present, such that subjects with a parent with diabetes have a much higher incidence of NIDDM than those who are equally obese, but whose parents do not have diabetes [77].

Physical Activity

The relationship of NIDDM and physical activity in observational and ecological studies is discussed in detail in Chapter 35. Ecological studies suggest that NIDDM prevalence is lower in populations with higher levels of physical activity [101]. Data from the US 1971–75 NHANES I [212] demonstrate a cross-sectional association between a lower prevalence of NIDDM and higher levels of physical activity. An epidemiological study of Melanesian and Indian men in

Fiji reported the prevalence of diabetes to be twice as high in those considered sedentary or undertaking only light activities, as compared to those performing moderate or heavy exercise, differences which remain when the confounding effects of age and obesity are taken into account [141].

In a longitudinal study of Pima Indians, historical physical activity was related to NIDDM, even after differences in age, sex and current obesity are taken into account [213]. This finding suggests that physical activity may protect against the development of NIDDM.

Several mechanisms by which exercise and physical training increase insulin sensitivity have been proposed [215]. Changes in glucose uptake and transport into muscle cells and adipose tissue are observed in response to insulin stimulation, but the relation of insulin levels to exercise seems to vary between studies [101]. Genetic differences in muscle structure associated with diabetes and obesity, as well as different responses of insulin secretion to physical activity according to the glucose tolerance status of the persons tested, could be responsible for the heterogeneity of these findings.

At least six large prospective studies measuring physical activity levels prior to the onset of NIDDM show a preventive effect [216–221]. Several risk factors emerged from these prospective studies which were independent of the protective effect of physical exercise, such as age, parental history of diabetes and current obesity. The age-related decline in insulin sensitivity could therefore be related to declining physical activity with older age [222], which could also partly explain higher rates of NIDDM with the ageing of populations [223]. On the other hand, the findings of the prospective studies emphasize the critical role of obesity in the risk of NIDDM. Prevention of NIDDM has therefore to include treatment or prevention of obesity through dietary restrictions and increased energy expenditure, which in turn can be expected to be beneficial for those at risk not only for NIDDM but also for hypertension and hyperlipidaemia [224].

Diet

Diet has long been suspected to play a role in the development of diabetes. As early as the sixth century Hindu physicians attributed diabetes to an overindulgence in rich foods. By 1875 Bouchardat had clearly described what we now call NIDDM as being associated with obesity, and he also observed that the rates of diabetes declined during the siege of Paris and attributed this to food shortages [225]. Subsequently, Himsworth showed that diabetes mortality declined markedly during the 1914–18 war in Berlin and Paris, both cities with severe food shortages, whereas in New York and Tokyo, where there were no food shortages, mortality from diabetes remained constant or even increased [226]. These findings were confirmed during severe food shortages in World War II [227, 228] but can only provide indirect evidence for a role of diet, since the effects are confounded by rapid weight loss and other changes during those times.

However, unbiased retrospective estimates of diet are largely unobtainable, and the different methods used to detect differences in average intake of nutrients between groups contain errors which can be in the same order of magnitude as the differences to be detected [229]. This has an important implication for the ability of the methods to detect effects of diet on the development of NIDDM. Furthermore, unless dietary records for epidemiological studies can be validated, findings of associations or, more importantly, non-associations, with certain dietary factors remain largely a matter for debate.

Nevertheless, a beneficial effect of a traditional diet on glucose homeostasis has been demonstrated in a study in which Polynesian Hawaiians were placed on a pre-European-contact diet which was low in fat (7%) and high in complex carbohydrates (78%), and encouraged to eat to satiety [230]. Average energy intakes decreased by 40%, and after only 21 days there was significant weight loss and significant improvement in serum lipids, fasting glucose and blood pressure. Similarly, weight loss and normalization of metabolic parameters were observed in a group of Australian Aborigines who reverted to a hunter-gatherer lifestyle involving increased physical activity and a traditional diet [231].

High caloric intake A high caloric intake can result in an increased frequency of diabetes. For example, Japanese Sumo wrestlers consume 4500–6500 kcal per day, compared to a typical Japanese diet of about 2500 kcal [232]. The Sumo, after several years of training, which includes dietary manipulation to attain the body mass necessary to be effective, become active wrestlers for about 10 years before they retire in their late 30s. Many develop diabetes even while still competing and more than 40% of the retired wrestlers have NIDDM. The high frequency of diabetes in Sumo wrestlers, especially after their retirement, may be primarily attributable to their high caloric intake, which leads to obesity and then to NIDDM.

Studies in Nauru, where there is a high prevalence of NIDDM and obesity, have documented total energy intakes 15–35% greater than recommended for maintenance of a healthy weight, with simple sugar intake double, alcohol consumption (in men) triple, and fibre intake only 27–30% of recommended levels [144]. Together with a sedentary lifestyle, it is clear that such

a diet leads to a positive energy balance, promotes obesity and poses a risk for diabetes. Analyses comparing the diets of Nauruan men with those of urban, but relatively less affluent, Kiribati (also Micronesians) demonstrate that mean total energy and fat intake, and the prevalence of obesity, are almost twice as high in the Nauruans [133].

Dietary composition: carbohydrate, fat and fibre content Dietary studies in a number of Pacific populations have demonstrated the change from high-fibre, low-fat traditional diets to modern diets which are characteristically made up of low-fibre, high-energy foods such as sugar, white bread, polished rice, and tinned meats [143–145]. It is likely that large quantities of these processed foods must be eaten to achieve the same degree of satiety associated with traditional foods, hence leading to relative caloric excess [200].

A positive association between high-fat, low-carbohydrate diets and the occurrence of NIDDM has been shown in several ecological studies [171, 181, 182, 226, 227]. This association was shown among Japanese participating in the Hiroshima–Hawaii migrant study [171]. In Hawaii the prevalence of diabetes is about twice that found in Hiroshima, Japan, but obesity is also considerably more frequent. Nevertheless, in spite of the higher prevalence of obesity, the number of calories consumed by the Hawaiian-Japanese was similar to that of the inhabitants of Hiroshima. On the other hand, the Hawaiian-Japanese consumed approximately twice as much fat, less complex carbohydrate and almost three times as much simple carbohydrate as their counterparts in Hiroshima. This study suggests that if diet plays a role in the development of diabetes, its effect may be mediated by dietary composition, which in turn determines both the level of obesity and the incidence of NIDDM. However, interpretation of studies based on interpopulation comparisons is confounded by differences in genetic susceptibility, physical activity, obesity, etc., in the respective countries, and the results may not reflect a causal effect of diet on the occurrence of NIDDM. Cross-sectional and retrospective studies have also shown a positive relationship [233–235]. Himsworth pioneered case-control studies of nutrition and diabetes and reported that before the onset of symptoms, diabetics consumed diets of greater calorie content and greater fat composition [233]. However, the case-control approach to investigating the role of diet in the development of NIDDM is particularly difficult because dietary interventions are used in the treatment of NIDDM. In Papua New Guinea a case-control study was carried out in a population with high prevalence of NIDDM [147]. Cases were individuals with NIDDM who had been diagnosed in the concurrent survey and completed the diet study before being informed of their diagnosis. Thus dietary changes associated with diabetes were minimized. However, the study was not able to find any specific nutrients that were associated with NIDDM [147].

Prospective studies of the incidence of NIDDM in relation to diet show less consistent results [101, 144]. Among Israeli men participating in a prospective study of heart disease, no effect of diet or its composition was found on the incidence of diabetes in a 5-year period [236]. Other European studies and the US Nurses Health Study following participants over longer periods of time also did not find any association [190, 194, 237]. Among 187 non-diabetic Pima Indian women aged 25–44 years of whom 87 developed diabetes in the subsequent decade, total carbohydrate intake and complex carbohydrate intake were positively related to the incidence of NIDDM [237], before adjusting for obesity. On the other hand the intake of simple carbohydrate (sugar) bore no relationship to the incidence of the disease. As carbohydrate intake, fat consumption and total caloric intake are strongly related to each other, this study, while suggesting that carbohydrate intake is perhaps the most important, cannot be taken to implicate only this component of the diet in the pathogenesis of the NIDDM. Preliminary data on the effects of omega-3 fatty acids [238] offer new prospects in the search for single dietary components which may have protective properties against the development of NIDDM.

Alcohol Alcohol consumption has been implicated as a possible independent risk factor for NIDDM [101]. Mechanisms could include its effects on increasing weight [239, 240], in particular abdominal fat tissue, or its effects on the liver and pancreas (see Chapter 11). Studies in men [241] report higher incidence of NIDDM with high alcohol intake, and a proportion of the excess mortality seen in French men with NIDDM or IGT might be due to alcohol-related worsening of glucose tolerance [242]. Available data in women are less consistent [101]. The incidence of NIDDM in women who had a moderate alcohol intake was reported to be lower than in those who drank less [243]. However, obesity was less common in such women and the strength of the relationship was reduced, but not obliterated, after adjusting for obesity. Other dietary factors were not assessed. A recent epidemiological study investigated the associations of alcohol intake with the prevalence and incidence of NIDDM in three populations at high risk for NIDDM [244]. No consistent relation of alcohol intake to NIDDM was seen, in either the prevalence or the prospective study. Alcohol consumption was, however, related to other metabolic parameters associated with cardiovascular disease.

The complex interrelationship between dietary intake, obesity and energy expenditure, all of which are implicated to one degree or another in the pathogenesis of NIDDM, certainly suggests that there may be more than a casual role of diet in the pathogenesis of the disease. More extensive prospective studies in which all three of these related variables (diet, physical activity, and obesity) are adequately measured, and taken into account in the analysis, will be necessary to assess their relative importance to the development of NIDDM.

Westernization, Urbanization, Modernization

Secular trends in the epidemiology of NIDDM, urban–rural gradients, and migration to a more modern lifestyle are all indicators that environmental change promotes obesity and the epidemic of NIDDM seen in many non-Europid populations. It is assumed that indicators of socio-economic status and 'modernity', such as duration of residence in an urban environment, duration of paid employment, type of housing and educational achievement, are in fact surrogate measures for dietary factors and aspects of physical activity not discerned by measures applied in epidemiological studies.

Many studies show a higher prevalence of NIDDM in urban than in rural environments [65, 142, 175, 245, 246, 248, 249]. Although there is little difference in the prevalence of NIDDM between urban and rural environments in developed countries such as the USA, studies in several developing countries show a threefold or greater prevalence of NIDDM in urban than in rural populations. Reasons for these differences are uncertain, but in developing countries many features of the urban and rural environment differ. In urban areas occupational activities are more often sedentary than in rural areas where agriculture is usually the predominant occupation. Urban dwellers are usually more obese due to reduced physical activity and/or increased caloric intake. The diet in urban areas often contains a greater proportion of refined carbohydrates, less fibre and more fat than in the rural environment. Urbanization is also often associated with increased alcohol consumption and increased smoking. The differences between rates of NIDDM in urban and rural populations in developing countries suggest that the combined effects of reduced physical activity, increased dietary intake and increasing obesity are important factors in determining the risk of diabetes. Other concomitant changes usually include increases in blood pressure and serum total cholesterol levels in the urban groups.

The secular changes in NIDDM prevalence, the higher prevalence among those living in an urban environment, and the extraordinary prevalence of NIDDM in populations such as the Nauruans and Pima Indians, have been attributed to increasing 'Westernization'. The rates of NIDDM seen in populations such as the Asian Indians, Japanese living in a Western environment, many tribes of American Indians, including the Pima, and several groups of Micronesians and Polynesians, however, far exceed the rates of NIDDM observed in western Europe and the USA. The epidemic of NIDDM (and obesity) in these populations who are exposed to a new environment may represent a first stage in adaptation to this new environment. Future generations of these populations may modify their way of life and adapt to these new environments to the extent that their rates of NIDDM may eventually approach those of the host country. This appears to have occurred for some other diseases and there is one report suggesting that this may occur in NIDDM [250].

On the other hand, some other populations who now have a 'Western' lifestyle have not experienced epidemics of NIDDM to the same extent. Examples include the Eskimos [75], the non-Austronesian Melanesian populations of the Solomon Islands and Papua New Guinea [251], and perhaps some native African tribes [248]. Whether or not such groups have a reduced genetic susceptibility to NIDDM is unknown. Certainly NIDDM is now recognized more frequently among them than earlier in the century, but it is still less common than in Europid populations. This may be because changes in life-style have occurred for many only very recently, and exposure to the new environment has not yet been sufficient to lead to full expression of the diabetic genotype. Alternatively, such populations may not have been exposed historically to periodic famines and may therefore never have developed high frequencies of the 'thrifty gene'.

Metabolic Determinants and Intermediate Risk Categories of NIDDM

Impaired Glucose Tolerance

Diagnosed NIDDM is only the tip of the iceberg of an epidemic of glucose intolerance. Subjects with impaired glucose tolerance (IGT), characterized by current WHO criteria as having hyperglycaemia between normal and overtly diabetic levels [6], are at high risk of developing NIDDM, and are at least as prevalent as subjects with NIDDM. Among Europid populations the prevalence of IGT and NIDDM has been found to be almost equal [67, 252], and some studies from non-Europid populations have shown the prevalence of IGT to be much higher than that of NIDDM [7]. Subjects with IGT on one occasion may subsequently develop diabetes, may return to normal or retain impaired glucose tolerance. Approximately 30–40% of persons identified as having IGT eventually develop NIDDM,

and the annual rate of progression from IGT to NIDDM is estimated to be 1–5% [20, 120, 253–257]. Increased risk for the development of diabetes in persons with IGT is related to higher levels of fasting or postprandial glycaemia within the IGT category; family history of NIDDM; greater degree of obesity [201]; higher fasting and post-load insulin levels and a greater degree of insulin resistance [258, 259], and may also differ between populations. As is the case for NIDDM, age is a strong determinant for IGT, and on the basis of the continuing growth of the fraction of elderly people in many populations, the overall prevalence of NIDDM and IGT will continue to increase. In addition to being a major risk factor for the development of NIDDM, IGT is associated with an increased risk of macrovascular disease [67, 254, 260–268]. However, IGT is not associated with diabetes-specific complications such as retinopathy, nephropathy or neuropathy [120].

There is little information on factors that lead to the development of IGT. Among Nauruans obesity, age and a higher 2-hour post-load insulin concentration were the only measures that predicted transition from normal glucose tolerance to IGT [20]. Similar findings have been observed in the Pima Indians, in whom higher 2-hour insulin levels relative to the glucose level predicted worsening of glucose tolerance among those with normal glucose tolerance [257, 269].

As prevention of NIDDM is now increasingly being tested, individuals with IGT constitute a high-risk group where possible interventions might be targeted first to demonstrate their effectiveness.

Insulin Resistance

Decreased peripheral glucose uptake because of decreased sensitivity to insulin action, as seen in subjects with IGT, led to the concept of insulin resistance. Accordingly, the risk of developing NIDDM in those with normal or impaired glucose tolerance is strongly related to circulating insulin levels [20, 256, 257, 269]. Populations with a high incidence of NIDDM are characterized by relative hyperinsulinaemia. Studies among the Pima Indians [270], Nauruans [271, 272], Australian Aborigines [273], Mexican-Americans [274] and Asian Indians [275] have shown that average fasting and stimulated insulin levels, even in subjects with normal glucose tolerance, are greater than in non-diabetic Europid controls with identical degrees of glucose tolerance. This observation suggests that insulin resistance is a characteristic of populations at high risk of developing NIDDM [276]. Longitudinal studies in Nauruans [20, 140, 277] have shown that baseline glucose and insulin concentrations are powerful predictors of deterioration in glucose tolerance. In subjects with

IGT, declining 2-hour insulin secretion, indicative of islet B-cell exhaustion, is associated with the strongest risk of progression to NIDDM [20]. Unpublished longitudinal data relating baseline insulin and glucose concentrations for Western Samoans and Papua New Guineans demonstrate the general applicability of the pancreatic decompensation theory in the pathogenesis of NIDDM.

Insulin resistance is associated with several other abnormalities: obesity, particularly central obesity, glucose intolerance, hypertension, dyslipidaemia, hyperuricaemia and perhaps hyperleptinaemia. The strength of these relationships, however, varies from one population to another. Epidemiological studies show significant differences in the prevalence of individual cardiovascular risk factors and insulin resistance or hyperinsulinaemia among different ethnic groups. Hyperinsulinaemia is observed more often in Hispanics, African-Americans and Native Americans than in Europids [270, 278, 279]. Even though obesity, diabetes and hyperinsulinaemia are common in many modernized non-Europid populations, levels of serum cholesterol are generally lower than those seen in Europids [280]. Conversely, a greater clustering of multiple cardiovascular risk factors (hypertension, diabetes, hyperuricaemia, hypertriglyceridaemia and low HDL-cholesterol) was seen in the African-American than in the Europid population [281], in whom hypertriglyceridaemia was the most frequent single cardiovascular risk factor. Similarly, blood pressure levels are relatively low in non-Europid populations [282], except in African-Americans who are particularly susceptible to hypertension [283]. This observation is reflected in the predominance of cardiovascular disease and stroke amongst Europid NIDDM patients, whereas in non-Europid NIDDM patients diabetic renal disease is one of the major late complications. The estimated prevalence of end-stage renal disease in persons with diabetes is 160% greater in African-Americans than in Europids [284].

Recent studies, discussed in detail in Chapter 12, have shown that insulin resistance has a genetic basis in several populations and represents a syndrome with a common pathogenetic outcome. In addition, and increasing the difficulty of investigation, insulin resistance modifies the expression of other—perhaps also genetically determined—factors involved in the aetiology of NIDDM.

Pregnancy and NIDDM

Parity Early reports that death from diabetes was more commonly recorded among married or widowed women than single women [285, 286], led to the conclusion that parity and diabetes were associated. Subsequent studies demonstrated higher frequency of diabetes with increasing parity [287–290], an association which could not be explained entirely by the greater body mass of parous compared to non-parous women [291]. In 1978, however, West [37, 292] reviewed the literature and concluded that there was little evidence to support an independent relationship between parity and NIDDM. This review, and other more recent studies in several populations including Pacific islanders [293, 294], led to the consensus position that parity conveyed little or no risk of NIDDM [37, 96, 294]. This is supported by observations of low prevalence of NIDDM in underdeveloped countries where multiparity is common and yet the prevalence of NIDDM is similar in men and women [37, 101].

Gestational diabetes Glucose tolerance is often tested and gestational diabetes mellitus [6] (GDM) discovered during pregnancy. The likelihood of abnormal glucose tolerance is greatest towards the end of the second and during the third trimester. The mild nature and transience of the glucose intolerance, which following delivery usually returns to normal, is associated with a high risk of developing NIDDM in the mother. Untreated GDM may also have adverse effects on the offspring, such as increased birthweight and pre- and perinatal mortality. Approximately 30–50% of women with a history of gestational diabetes progress to NIDDM within 5–10 years [295–297].

GDM varies considerably in the severity of hyperglycaemia but whether mild GDM is different from IGT in non-pregnant subjects is still unclear (see Chapter 57). Risk factors that increase the development from GDM to post-partum NIDDM include a higher degree of pre-pregnancy obesity and antepartum blood glucose level, requirement for insulin during pregnancy, low insulin secretion during pregnancy, recurrent GDM in subsequent pregnancies and higher post-partum glucose levels [298–303]. Nevertheless, impairment of glucose tolerance, whether it occurs in the pregnant or non-pregnant state, is a strong predictor of the subsequent occurrence of diabetes.

Gestational diabetes has also been shown to be more common in certain non-Europid populations [304–307] than in Europids, but differences in obesity and increased maternal age seem not to explain this finding [308, 309]. A recent study, comparing pregnant women with GDM who had different ethnic origins but were living in Australia, confirmed these observations and related the more frequent occurrence in some ethnic groups to the earlier onset of NIDDM observed in ethnically similar comparison groups of non-gestational patients of the diabetes clinic [309].

Diabetes in offspring of women with diabetes during pregnancy NIDDM in women before or during their childbearing age seems to be more frequent in non-Europid populations, often complicates pregnancy, and influences the occurrence of NIDDM in their offspring. Furthermore, diabetes can be associated with failure to conceive or menstrual irregularities, although mechanisms are still unclear [205]. Almost 50% of Pima Indian offspring aged 20–24 years had NIDDM when their mothers had diabetes at the time of the pregnancy [40]. Such offspring have a much higher risk of NIDDM than those whose fathers have NIDDM or whose mothers eventually developed diabetes but were not diabetic at the time of their pregnancy. As genetic susceptibility to diabetes can come from either the mother or father, the particular risk associated with the diabetic pregnancy implicates a contribution of the intra-uterine environment as influencing the development of NIDDM in offspring of diabetic women, as already discussed at the beginning of this chapter. The high rate of diabetes in the offspring of diabetic mothers may in addition be mediated by their unusually high frequency of obesity in childhood and adolescence [247].

CONCLUSION

There is little doubt that many non-Europid populations have a genetic susceptibility to NIDDM which, in parallel with the decrease in mortality from infectious causes, is expressed when they adopt modern life-styles characterized by decreased physical activity, and qualitative and quantitative changes in diet. Cultural and socio-economic factors influencing nutrition are also important determinants of obesity. Physical inactivity and generalized and abdominal obesity act to modulate risk of NIDDM, at least in part via effects on insulin action and secretion.

Both natural selection and genetic drift are thought to have contributed to the emergence of obesity and NIDDM genotypes in many non-Europid populations, but it is likely that there are a number of variants of the 'thrifty genotype' within and between populations, with different components of the genotype contributing to either or both the obesity and NIDDM phenotypes.

Attempts to develop large-scale life-style intervention programs, aimed at changing diet and increasing physical activity, to decrease obesity and NIDDM, are now under way. So far, small and uncontrolled short-term studies in non-Europid populations have indicated the contribution of modern lifestyle to the metabolic maladies of formerly traditional populations, and indirectly have highlighted the potential for prevention. While it would be naive to expect populations to reverse the tide of modernization, the challenge lies in integrating old and new lifestyles to optimize health.

REFERENCES

1. West KM, Kalbfleisch JM. Glucose tolerance, nutrition and diabetes in Uruguay, Venezuela, Malaya and East Pakistan. Diabetes 1966; 19: 656–63.
2. Stein JH, West KM, Robey JM, Tirador DF, McDonald GW. The high prevalence of abnormal glucose tolerance in the Cherokee Indians of North Carolina. Arch Intern Med 1965; 116: 843–5.
3. Bennett PH, Burch TA, Miller M. Diabetes mellitus in American (Pima) Indians. Lancet 1971; 2: 125–8.
4. Zimmet P, Taft P, Guinea A, Guthrie W, Thoma K. The high prevalence of diabetes mellitus on a central Pacific island. Diabetologia 1977; 13: 111–15.
5. World Health Organization. WHO Expert Committee on Diabetes Mellitus, Second Report. Technical Report Series 646. Geneva: WHO, 1980; pp 1–80.
6. World Health Organization Study Group. Diabetes mellitus. Technical Report Series 727. Geneva: WHO, 1985; pp 1–113.
7. King H, Rewers M. World Health Organization Ad Hoc Diabetes Reporting Group: global estimates for prevalence of diabetes mellitus and impaired glucose tolerance in adults. Diabetes Care 1993; 16: 157–77.
8. Zimmet P. The pathogenesis and prevention of diabetes in adults: genes, autoimmunity and demography. Diabetes Care 1995; 18: 1050–64.
9. Zimmet P. Kelly West Lecture 1991. Challenges in diabetes epidemiology—from West to the rest. Diabetes Care 1992; 15: 232–52.
10. Zimmet P. Non-insulin-dependent (type 2) diabetes mellitus—does it really exist? Diabet Med 1989; 6: 728–35.
11. Zimmet P. Diabetes care and prevention—around the world in 80 days. In Rifkin H, Colwell JA, Taylor SI (eds) Diabetes 1991. Amsterdam: Elsevier, 1991; pp 721–9.
12. Zimmet P. Hyperinsulinaemia—how innocent a bystander? Diabetes Care 1993; 16: 56–70.
13. Reaven GM. Role of insulin resistance in human disease. Diabetes 1988; 37: 1595–1607.
14. Zimmet PZ, McCarty DJ, de Courten M. The global epidemiology of non-insulin dependent diabetes mellitus and the metabolic syndrome. J Diabet Compl 1996; in press.
15. Zimmet P. Type 2 (non-insulin-dependent) diabetes—an epidemiological overview. Diabetologia 1982; 22: 399–411.
16. Diamond JM. Diabetes running wild. Nature 1992; 357: 362–3.
17. Temple RC, Carrington CA, Luzio SD et al. Insulin deficiency in non-insulin-dependent diabetes. Lancet 1989; 1: 293–5.
18. Velho G, Froguel P, Clement K et al. Primary pancreatic beta-cell secretory defect caused by mutations in glucokinase gene in kindreds of maturity onset diabetes of the young. Lancet 1992; 340: 444–8.
19. De Fronzo RA. Lilly Lecture 1987: The triumvirate: B-cell, muscle, liver: a collusion responsible for NIDDM. Diabetes 1988; 37: 667–87.
20. Sicree RA, Zimmet PZ, King HOM, Coventry JS. Plasma insulin response among Nauruans: prediction

of deterioration in glucose tolerance over 6 years. Diabetes 1987; 36: 179–86.

21. Reaven G, Miller R. Study of the relationship between glucose and insulin responses to an oral glucose load in man. Diabetes 1968; 17: 560–69.

22. Bell GI. Lilly Lecture 1990. Molecular defects in diabetes mellitus. Diabetes 1991; 40: 413–22.

23. Taylor SI, Cama A, Accili D et al. Mutations in the insulin receptor gene. Endocr Rev 1992; 13: 566–95.

24. Vionnet N, Stoffel M, Takeda J et al. Nonsense mutation in the glucokinase gene causes early-onset non-insulin-dependent diabetes mellitus. Nature 1992; 356: 721–2.

25. Alcolado JC, Majid A, Brockington M et al. Mitochondrial gene defects in patients with NIDDM. Diabetologia 1994; 37: 372–6.

26. Gleichmann H, Zörcher B, Greulich B et al. Correlation of islet cell antibodies and HLA-DR phenotypes with diabetes mellitus in adults. Diabetologia 1984; 27: 90–92.

27. Groop LC, Bottazzo GF, Doniach D. Islet cell antibodies identify latent type 1 diabetes in patients aged 35–75 years at diagnosis. Diabetes 1986; 35: 237–41.

28. Tuomi T, Groop LC, Zimmet PZ, Rowley MJ, Knowles W, Mackay IR. Antibodies to glutamic acid decarboxylase reveal latent autoimmune diabetes mellitus in adults with a non-insulin dependent onset of disease. Diabetes 1993; 42: 359–62.

29. Orchard TJ. From diagnosis and classification to complications and therapy. Diabetes Care 1994; 17: 326–38.

30. Harris MI, Zimmet P. Classification of diabetes mellitus and other categories of glucose intolerance. In Keen H, DeFronzo R, Alberti KGMM, Zimmet P (eds). International textbook of diabetes mellitus, 1st edn. Chichester: John Wiley, 1992; pp 3–18.

31. McCarty D, Zimmet P. Diabetes 1994 to 2010: global estimates and projections. Melbourne: International Diabetes Institute, 1994.

32. Omran AR. The epidemiologic transition theory: a preliminary update. J Trop Pediat 1983; 29: 305–16.

33. Kenny SJ, Aubert RE, Geiss LS. Prevalence and incidence of non-insulin dependent diabetes. In National Diabetes Data Group, Diabetes in America, 2nd edn. Washington DC: NIH publication no. 95–1468, 1995: pp 47–68.

34. Nelson RG, Everhart JE, Knowler WC, Bennett PH. Incidence, prevalence, and risk factors for non-insulin-dependent diabetes mellitus. Primary Care 1988; 15: 227–50.

35. Glatthaar C, Welborn TA, Stenhouse NS, Garcia-Webb P. Diabetes and impaired glucose tolerance. A prevalence estimate based on the Busselton 1981 survey. Med J Aust 1985; 143: 436–40.

36. Neil HAW, Gatling W, Mather HM, Thompson AU, Thorogood M, Fowler GH et al. The Oxford Community Diabetes Study: evidence for an increase in the prevalence of known diabetes in Great Britain. Diabet Med 1987; 4: 539–43.

37. West KM. Epidemiology of diabetes and its vascular lesions. New York: Elsevier, 1978.

38. West KM. Diabetes in American Indians and other native populations of the New World. Diabetes 1974; 23: 841–55.

39. Knowler WC, Bennett PH, Hamman RF et al. Diabetes incidence and prevalence in Pima Indians: a 19-fold greater incidence than in Rochester, Minnesota. Am J Epidemiol 1978; 108: 497–505.

40. Knowler WC, Nelson RG, Saad M, Bennett PH, Pettitt DJ. Determinants of diabetes mellitus in the Pima Indians. Diabetes Care 1993; 16: 216–27.

41. Serjeantson S, Zimmet P. Diabetes in the Pacific: evidence for a major gene. In Baba S, Gould MK, Zimmet P (eds) Diabetes mellitus: recent knowledge on aetiology, complications and treatment. Sydney: Academic Press, 1984; pp 23–30.

42. O'Rahilly S, Wainscoat JS, Turner RC. Type 2 (non-insulin-dependent) diabetes mellitus: new genetics for old nightmares. Diabetologia 1988; 31: 407–14.

43. Newman B, Selby JV, King MC, Slemenda C, Fabsitz R, Friedman GD. Concordance for type 2 (non-insulin-dependent) diabetes mellitus in male twins. Diabetologia 1987; 30: 763–8.

44. Lo SS, Tun RY, Hawa M, Leslie RD. Studies of diabetic twins. Diabetes Metab Rev 1991; 7: 223–38.

45. Harvald B, Hauge M. Selection in diabetes in modern society. Acta Med Scand 1963; 173: 459–65.

46. Gottlieb MS, Root HF. Diabetes mellitus in twins. Diabetes 1968; 17: 693–704.

47. Tattersall RB, Pyke DA. Diabetes in identical twins. Lancet 1972; ii: 1120–25.

48. Barnett AH, Eff C, Leslie RD, Pyke DA. Diabetes in identical twins. A study of 200 pairs. Diabetologia 1981; 20: 87–93.

49. Newman B, Selby JV, King MC, Slemenda C, Fabsitz R, Friedman GD. Concordance for type 2 (non-insulin-dependent) diabetes mellitus in male twins. Diabetologia 1987; 30: 763–8.

50. Committee on Diabetic Twins, Japan Diabetes Society. Diabetes mellitus in twins: a cooperative study in Japan. Diabetes Res Clin Pract 1988; 5: 271–80.

51. Kaprio J, Tuomilehto J, Koskenvuo M et al. Incidence of diabetes in the nationwide panel of 13 888 twin pairs in Finland. Diabetologia 1990; 33 (suppl.): A57.

52. Valsania P, Micossi P. Genetic epidemiology of non-insulin-dependent diabetes. Diabetes Metab Rev 1994; 10: 385–405.

53. Serjeantson SW, Owerbach D, Zimmet P, Nerup J, Thoma K. Genetics of diabetes in Nauru: effects of foreign admixture, HLA antigens and insulin-gene-linked polymorphism. Diabetologia 1983; 25: 13–17.

54. Gardner LI, Stern MP, Haffner SM et al. Prevalence of diabetes in Mexican Americans—relationship to percent of gene pool derived from Native American sources. Diabetes 1984; 33: 86–92.

55. Knowler WC, Williams RC, Pettitt DJ, Steinberg AG. $Gm^{3;5,13,14}$ and type 2 diabetes mellitus: an association in American Indians with genetic admixture. Am J Hum Genet 1988; 43: 520–26.

56. Stern MP, Haffner SM. Type II diabetes and its complications in Mexican Americans. Diabetes Metab Rev 1990; 6: 29–45.

57. King H, Zimmet P, Bennett P, Taylor R, Raper LR. Glucose tolerance and ancestral genetic admixture in six semitraditional Pacific populations. Genet Epidemiol 1984; 1: 315–28.

58. Williams DRR, Moffitt PS, Fisher JS, Bashir HV. Diabetes and glucose tolerance in New South Wales

coastal Aborigines. Possible effects of non-Aboriginal genetic admixture. Diabetologia 1987; 30: 72–7.

59. Hanis CL, Chakraborty R, Ferrell RE, Schull WJ. Individual admixture estimates: disease associations and individual risk of diabetes and gallbladder disease among Mexican-Americans in Starr County, Texas. Am J Phys Anthropol 1986; 70: 433–41.

60. Chakraborty R, Ferrell RE, Stern MP, Haffner SM, Hazuda HP, Rosenthal M. Relationship of prevalence of non-insulin-dependent diabetes mellitus to Amerindian admixture in the Mexican Americans of San Antonio, Texas. Am J Phys Anthropol 1986; 3: 433–41.

61. Sloan NR. Ethnic distributions of diabetes mellitus in Hawaii. JAMA 1963; 183: 123–8.

62. Poon-King T, Henry MV, Rampersad F. Prevalence and natural history of diabetes in Trinidad. Lancet 1968; 1: 155–60.

63. Thai AC, Yeo PB, Lun KC et al. Changing prevalence of diabetes mellitus in Singapore over a ten-year period. J Med Assoc Thailand 1987; 70 (suppl. 2): 63–7.

64. Zimmet P, Canteloube D, Genelle B et al. The prevalence of diabetes mellitus and impaired glucose tolerance in Melanesians and part-Polynesians in rural New Caledonia and Ouvea (Loyalty Islands). Diabetologia 1982; 23: 393–8.

65. Zimmet P, Taylor R, Ram P et al. Prevalence of diabetes and impaired glucose tolerance in the biracial (Melanesian and Indian) population of Fiji: a rural–urban comparison. Am J Epidemiol 1983; 118: 673–88.

66. Mather HM, Keen H. The Southall diabetes survey: prevalence of diabetes in Asians and Europeans. Br Med J 1985; 291: 1081–4.

67. Harris MI, Hadden WC, Knowler WC, Bennett PH. Prevalence of diabetes and impaired glucose tolerance and plasma glucose levels in US population aged 20–74 years. Diabetes 1987; 36: 523–34.

68. Flegal KM, Ezzati TM, Harris MI et al. Prevalence of diabetes in Mexican-Americans, Cubans, and Puerto Ricans from the Hispanic health and nutrition examination survey 1982–1984. Diabetes Care 1991; 14: 628–38.

69. Schaad JDG, Terpstra J et al. Diabetes prevalence in the three main ethnic groups in Surinam (South America). Population survey. Neth J Med 1985; 28: 17–22.

70. Eason RJ, Pada J, Wallace R et al. Changing patterns of hypertension, diabetes, obesity and diet among Melanesians and Micronesians in the Solomon Islands. Med J Aust 1987; 146: 465–73.

71. Dowse G, Gareeboo H, Zimmet P et al. The high prevalence of glucose intolerance in Indian, Creole and Chinese Mauritians. Diabetes 1990; 39: 390–96.

72. Cameron WI, Moffitt PS, Williams DRR. Diabetes mellitus in the Australian Aborigines of Bourke, New South Wales. Diabetes Res Clin Pract 1986; 2: 307–14.

73. King H, Heywood P, Zimmet P et al. Glucose tolerance in a Highland population in Papua New Guinea. Diabetes Res 1984; 1: 45–51.

74. Sievers ML, Fisher JR. Diabetes in North American Indians. In Diabetes in America: diabetes data compiled 1984. US Department of Health and Human Services, publication no. (NIH) 85-1468: X-1–20.

75. Schraer CD, Lanier AP, Boyko EJ, Gohdes D, Murphy NJ, Prevalence of diabetes in Alaskan Eskimos, Indians and Aleuts. Diabetes Care 1988; 11: 693–700.

76. Godhes D. Diabetes in North American Indians and Alaska natives. In National Diabetes Data Group. Diabetes in America, 2nd edn. Washington DC: NIH publication no. 95-1468, 1995; pp 683–701.

77. Knowler WC, Pettitt DJ, Savage PJ, Bennett PH. Diabetes in Pima Indians: contributions of obesity and parental diabetes. Am J Epidemiol 1981; 113: 144–56.

78. O'Sullivan JB, Mahan CM. Blood sugar levels, glycosuria, and body weight related to development of diabetes mellitus. J Am Med Assn 1965; 194: 117–22.

79. Baird JD. Diabetes mellitus and obesity. Proc Nutr Soc 1973; 32: 199–204.

80. Dorner G, Mohnike A, Steindel E. On possible genetic and epigenetic modes of diabetes transmission. Endokrinologie 1975; 66: 225–7.

81. Alcolado JC, Alcolado R. Importance of maternal history of non-insulin dependent diabetic patients. Br Med J 1991; 302: 1178–80.

82. Korugan U, Yilmaz MT, Sipahioglu F et al. The Istanbul family study. Diabetologia 1991; 34 (suppl. 1): A177.

83. Thomas F, Balkau B, Vauzelle-Kervroedan F, Papoz L, and the CODIAB-INSERM-ZENECA Group. Material effect and familial aggregation in NIDDM: the CODIAB Study. Diabetes 1994; 43: 63–7.

84. Pettitt DJ, Aleck KA, Baird HR, Carraher MJ, Bennett PH, Knowler WC. Congenital susceptibility to NIDDM: role of intrauterine environment. Diabetes 1988; 37: 622–8.

85. Hales CN, Barker DJP. Type 2 (non-insulin-dependent) diabetes mellitus: the thrifty phenotype hypothesis. Diabetologia 1992; 35: 595–601.

86. Gerbitz KD. Does the mitochondrial DNA play a role in the pathogenesis of diabetes? Diabetologia 1992; 35: 1181–6.

87. Reardon W, Ross RJM, Sweeney MG et al. Diabetes mellitus associated with a pathogenic point mutation in mitochondrial DNA. Lancet 1992; 340: 1376–9.

88. Cox NJ. Maternal component in NIDDM transmission: how large an effect? Diabetes 1994; 43: 166–8.

89. Hamman RF. Genetic and environmental determinants of non-insulin-dependent diabetes mellitus (NIDDM). Diabetes Metab Rev 1992; 8: 287–338.

90. Lander ES, Schork NJ. Genetic dissection of complex traits. Science 1994; 265: 2037–48.

91. Neel JV. The thrifty genotype revisted. In Kobberling J, Tattersall R (eds) The genetics of diabetes mellitus. Proceedings of the Serono symposium. London: Academic Press, 1982; pp 283–93.

92. Dowse G, Zimmet P. The thrifty genotype in non-insulin-dependent diabetes. The hypothesis survives. Br Med J 1993; 306: 532–3.

93. Swinburn BA. The thrifty genotype hypothesis: how does it look after 30 years? Diabet Med 1996; 13: 695–9.

94. Neel JV. Diabetes mellitus: a thrifty genotype rendered detrimental by 'progress'? Am J Hum Genet 1962; 14: 353–62.

Washington DC: US Government Printing Office, 1985.

95. O'Dea K, Zimmet P. Thrifty genotypes. In Leslie RDG (ed.) Causes of diabetes. Chichester: Wiley, 1993: pp 269–90.

96. Charles MA, Pettitt DJ, McCance DR, Hanson RL, Bennett PH, Knowler WC. Gravidity, obesity and non-insulin-dependent diabetes among Pima Indian women. Am J Med 1994; 97: 250–5.

97. Weatherall D. The Harveian Oration. The role of nature and nurture in common diseases. Garrod's Legacy. London: Royal College of Physicians, 1992; pp 1–21.

98. Fabricius W. Nauru 1888–1900. An account in German and English based on official records of the Colonial Section of the German Foreign Office held by the Deutsches Zentralarchiv in Potsdam, Clark D, Firth S (eds) Canberra: Australian National University Press, 1992.

99. Coleman DL. Obesity genes: beneficial effects in heterozygous mice. Science 1979; 203: 663–5.

100. Nabarro J. Diabetes in the United Kingdom: some facts and figures. Diabet Med 1988; 5: 816–17.

101. Rewers M, Hamman RF. Risk factors for non-insulin dependent diabetes. In National Diabetes Data Group. Diabetes in America, 2nd edn. Washington DC: NIH Publication No. 95-1468, 1995; pp 179–220.

102. Palumbo PJ, Elveback LR, Chu C-P, Connolly DC, Kurland LT. Diabetes mellitus: incidence, prevalence, survivorship, and causes of death in Rochester, Minnesota, 1945–1970. Diabetes 1976; 25: 566–73.

103. Zimmet P, Dowse G, Finch C, Serjeantson S, King H. The epidemiology and natural history of NIDDM—lessons from the South Pacific. Diabetes Metab Rev 1990; 6: 91–124.

104. Cruickshank JK, Riste L, Jackson M et al. Standardized comparison of glucose tolerance and diabetes prevalence in four African/African-Caribbean populations in Britain, Jamaica and Cameroon. Diabet Med 1997; in press.

105. Marshall JA, Hamman RF, Baxter J et al. Ethnic differences in risk factors associated with the prevalence of non-insulin dependent diabetes mellitus. The San Luis Valley Diabetes Study. Am J Epidemiol 1993; 137: 706–18.

106. Haffner SM, Hazuda HP, Mitchell BD, Patterson JK, Stern MP. Increased incidence of type 2 diabetes mellitus in Mexican Americans. Diabetes Care 1991; 14: 102–8.

107. Cowie CC, Harris MI, Silverman RE, Johnson EW, Rust KF. Effect of multiple risk factors on differences between blacks and whites in the prevalence of non-insulin-dependent diabetes mellitus in the United States. Am J Epidemiol 1993; 137: 719–32.

108. Ahuja MMS. Epidemiological studies on diabetes mellitus in India. In Ahuja MMS (ed.) Epidemiology of diabetes in developing countries. New Delhi: Interprint, 1979; pp 29–38.

109. Verma NPS, Mehta SP, Madhu S, Mather HM, Keen H. Prevalence of known diabetes in an urban Indian environment: the Darya Ganj diabetes survey. Br Med J 1986; 293: 423–4.

110. Ramachandran A, Dharmaraj D, Snehalatha C, Viswanathan M. Prevalence of glucose intolerance in Asian Indians: urban–rural difference and significance of upper body adiposity. Diabetes Care 1992; 15: 1348–55.

111. Gupta OP, Joshi MH, Dave SK. Prevalence of diabetes in India. In Levine R, Luft R (eds) Advances in metabolic disorders, vol 9. New York: Academic Press, 1978; pp 147–65.

112. Coughlan A, McCarty D, Jorgensen LN, Zimmet P. Diabetes in Asian and Pacific Island populations. Horm Metab Res 1996 (in press).

113. Sayeed MA, Banu A, Khan AR, Hussian MZ. Prevalence of diabetes and hypertension in a rural population of Bangladesh. Diabetes Care 1995; 18: 555–8.

114. Shera AS, Rafique G, Khwaja IA, Ara J, Baqai S, King H. Pakistan National Diabetes Survey: prevalence of glucose intolerance and associated factors in Shikarpur, Sindh Province. Diabet Med 1995; 12: 1116–21.

115. Ohmura T, Ueda K, Kiyohara Y et al. Prevalence of type 2 (non-insulin dependent) diabetes mellitus and impaired glucose tolerance in the Japanese general population: the Hisayama study. Diabetologia 1993; 36: 1198–1203.

116. Kitazawa Y, Murakami K, Goto Y, Hamazski S. Prevalence of diabetes mellitus detected by 75 g GTT in Tokyo. Tohoku J Exp Med 1983; 141 (suppl. 1): 229–34.

117. Park Y, Lee H, Koh C, Min H, Yoo K, Kim Y, Shin Y. Prevalence of diabetes and IGT in Yonchon County, South Korea. Diabetes Care 1995; 18: 545–8.

118. Chou P, Liao M, Kuo H, Hsiao K, Tsai S. A population survey on the prevalence of diabetes in Kin-Hu, Kinmen. Diabetes Care 1994; 17: 1055–8.

119. Hong-ding X, Zhi-sheng C. A survey of diabetes and impaired glucose tolerance in 44 747 persons of Shanxi, Beijing and Liaoning, North China 1989. In Mimura G, Qian R, Murakami K (eds) Current status of diabetes mellitus in East Asia. Amsterdam: Elsevier, 1994; pp 33–6.

120. Alberti KGMM. The clinical implications of impaired glucose tolerance. Diabet Med 1996; 13: 927–37.

121. Shanghai Diabetes Research Cooperative Group, Diabetes Mellitus Survey in Shanghai. Chinese Med J 1980; 93: 663–72.

122. Valway S, Freeman W, Kaufman S, Welty T, Helgerson SD, Gohdes D. Prevalence of diagnosed diabetes among American Indians and Alaska Natives, 1987: estimates from a national outpatient data base. Diabetes Care 1993; 16: 271–6.

123. Hall T, Hickey M, Young T. Evidence for recent increases in obesity and non-insulin dependent diabetes mellitus in a Navajo community. Am J Human Biol 1992; 4: 547–53.

124. Farrell MA, Quiggins PA, Eller JD, Owle PA Miner KM, Walkingstick ES. Prevalence of diabetes and its complications in the eastern band of Cherokee Indians. Diabetes Care 1993; 16 (suppl. 1): 253–6.

125. Knowler WC, Saad MF, Pettitt DJ, Nelson RC, Bennett PH. Determinants of diabetes mellitus in the Pima Indians. Diabetes Care 1993; 16 (suppl. 1): 216–27.

126. Brousseau DJ. Increasing prevalence of diabetes among the three affiliated tribes. Diabetes Care 1993; 16 (suppl. 1): 248–9.

127. Papoz L, Ben Khalifa F, Eschwege E, Ben Ayed H. Diabetes mellitus in Tunisia: description in urban and rural populations. Int J Epidemiol 1988; 17: 419–22.

128. McLarty DG, Swai ABM, Kitange HM et al. Prevalence of diabetes and impaired glucose tolerance in rural Tanzania. Lancet 1989; i: 871–5.

129. McLarty DG, Pollitt C, Swai ABM. Diabetes in Africa. Diabet Med 1990; 7: 670–84.

130. Moorehead A. The fatal impact: the invasion of the South Pacific 1767–1840. London: Hamish Hamilton, 1966.

131. Zimmet P. Epidemiology of diabetes and its macrovascular manifestations in Pacific populations: the medical effects of social progress. Diabetes Care 1979; 2: 144–53.

132. Taylor R, Lewis ND, Levy S. Societies in transition: mortality patterns in Pacific island populations. Int J Epidemiol 1989; 18: 634–46.

133. Dowse GK, Hodge AM, Zimmet PZ. Paradise lost: obesity and diabetes in Pacific and Indian Ocean populations. In Angel A et al (eds) Progress in obesity research '94. London: John Libbey & Co, 1995; pp 227–38.

134. Dowse GK, Zimmet PZ, Finch CF, Collins V. Decline in incidence of epidemic glucose intolerance in Nauruans: implications for the 'thrifty genotype'. Am J Epidemiol 1991; 133: 1093–104.

135. Collins VR, Dowse GK, Toelupe PM et al. Increasing prevalence of NIDDM in the Pacific island population of Western Samoa over a 13-year period. Diabetes Care 1994; 17: 288–96.

136. Dowse GK, Spark RA, Mavo B et al. Extraordinary prevalence of non-insulin-dependent diabetes mellitus and bimodal plasma glucose distribution in the Wanigela people of Papua New Guinea. Med J Aust 1994; 160: 767–74.

137. Grant AMB. A medical survey of the island of Nauru. Med J Aust 1933: 113–18.

138. Ostbye T, Welby TJ, Prior IAM, Salmond CE, Stokes YM. Type 2 (non-insulin-dependent) diabetes mellitus, migration and Westernization. The Tokelau Island Migrant study. Diabetologia 1989; 32: 585–90.

139. Hodge AM, Dowse GK, Zimmet PZ. Association of body mass index and waist–hip circumference ratio with cardiovascular disease risk factors in Micronesian Nauruans. Int J Obesity 1993; 17: 399–407.

140. Balkau B, King H, Zimmet P, Raper LR. Factors associated with the development of diabetes in the Micronesian population of Nauru. Am J Epidemiol 1985; 122: 594–605.

141. Taylor R, Ram P, Zimmet P, Raper LR, Ringrose H. Physical activity and prevalence of diabetes in Melanesian and Indian men in Fiji. Diabetologia 1984; 27: 578–82.

142. King H, Taylor R, Zimmet P et al. Non-insulin-dependent diabetes (NIDDM) in a newly independent Pacific nation—the Republic of Kiribati. Diabetes Care 1984; 7: 409–15.

143. Taylor R, Badcock J, King H et al. Dietary intake, exercise, obesity and noncommunicable disease in rural and urban populations of three Pacific island countries. J Am Coll Nutr 1992; 11: 283–93.

144. Hodge AM, Dowse GK, Zimmet PZ. Diet does not predict incidence or prevalence of non-insulin-dependent diabetes in Nauruans. Asia Pacific J Clin Nutr 1993; 2: 35–41.

145. Bindon JR. Breadfruit, banana, beef, and beer: modernization of the Samoan diet. Ecol Food Nutr 1982; 12: 49–60.

146. Hanna JM, Pelletier DL, Brown VJ. The diet and nutrition of contemporary Samoans. In Baker PT, Hanna JM, Baker TS (eds) The changing Samoans: behaviour and health in transition. New York: Oxford University Press, 1986; pp 275–96.

147. Hodge AM, Montgomery J, Dowse GK, Mavo B, Watt T, Zimmet PZ. A case-control study of diet in newly diagnosed non-insulin-dependent diabetes mellitus in the Wanigela people of Papua New Guinea. Diabetes Care 1996; 19: 457–62.

148. Zimmet PZ, Collins VR, Dowse GK et al. The relation of physical activity to cardiovascular disease risk factors in Mauritians. Am J Epidemiol 1991; 134: 862–75.

149. Dowse GK, Zimmet PZ, Gareeboo H et al. Abdominal obesity and physical inactivity as risk factors for NIDDM and impaired glucose tolerance in Indian, Creole and Chinese Mauritians. Diabetes Care 1991; 14: 271–82.

150. Saad MF, Knowler WC, Pettitt DJ, Nelson RG, Mott DM, Bennett PH. The natural history of impaired glucose tolerance in the Pima Indians. New Engl J Med 1988; 319: 1500–1506.

151. Dowse GK, Zimmet PZ, Alberti KGMM et al. Serum insulin distributions and reproducibility of the relationship between 2-hour insulin and plasma glucose levels in Asian Indian, Creole and Chinese Mauritians. Metabolism 1993; 42: 1232–41.

152. Devlin JT, Horton ES. Effects of prior high-intensity exercise on glucose metabolism in normal and insulin-resistant men. Diabetes 1985; 34: 973–9.

153. Hodge AM, Dowse GK, Gareeboo H, Tuomilehto J, Alberti KGMM, Zimmet PZ. Incidence, increasing prevalence, and predictors of change in obesity and fat distribution over 5 years in the rapidly developing population of Mauritius. Int J Obesity 1996; 20: 137–46.

154. McGrath M, Collins V, Zimmet P, Dowse G, Lifestyle disorders in Australian Aborigines. Diabetes and cardiovascular disease risk factors. A review. Melbourne: International Diabetes Institute, 1991.

155. Guest CS. Diabetes in Aborigines and other Australian populations. Aus J Public Health 1992; 16: 340–49.

156. O'Dea K, Hopper J, Patel M, Traianedes K, Kubisch D. Obesity, diabetes, and hyperlipidemia in a Central Australian Aboriginal community with a long history of acculturation. Diabetes Care 1993; 16: 1004–10.

157. Unwin N, Harland J, White M et al. Body mass index, waist circumference, waist:hip ratio and glucose intolerance in Chinese and Europid adults in Newcastle upon Tyne. J Epidemiol Commun Health 1996, in press.

158. Thai AC, Yeo PPB, Lun KC et al. Changing prevalence of diabetes mellitus in Singapore over a ten year period. In Vannasaeng S, Nitiannt W, Chandraprasert S (eds) Epidemiology of diabetes mellitus: proceedings of the International Symposium on Epidemiology of Diabetes Mellitus. Bangkok: Crystal House Press, 1987; pp 63–7.

159. Omar MAK, Seedat MA, Dyer RB, Motala AA, Knight LT, Becker PJ. South African Indians show a high prevalence of NIDDM and bimodality in plasma glucose distribution patterns. Diabetes Care 1994; 17: 70–3.

160. Bose CL. Some observations on diabetes in India. J Trop Med Hyg 1907; 10: 320.

161. Tull ES, Roseman JM. Diabetes in African Americans. In National Diabetes Data Group. Diabetes in America, 2nd edn. Washington DC: NIH Publ. 95-1468, 1995; 613–30.

162. National Center for Health Statistics: current estimates from the National Health Interview Survey, 1993. Vital and Health Statistics, Series 10, no. 190, 1994.

163. Lipton RB, Liao Y, Cao G, Cooper RS, McGee D. Determinants of incident non-insulin dependent diabetes mellitus among blacks and whites in a national sample: the NHANES I Epidemiologic Follow-up Study. Am J Epidemiol 1993; 138: 826–39.

164. Tulloch JA, Johnson HM. A pilot survey of the incidence of diabetes in Jamaica. W Ind Med 1958; 7: 134–6.

165. Wright HB, Taylor B. The incidence of diabetes in a sample of the adult population in South Trinidad. W Ind Med 1958; 7: 123.

166. Tulloch JA. The prevalence of diabetes in Jamaica. Diabetes 1961; 10: 286–88.

167. Ashcroft MT, Beadnell HM, Bell R, Miller GJ. Characteristics relevant to cardiovascular disease among adults of African and Indian origin in Guyana. WHO Bull 1970; 42: 205.

168. Florey CV, McDonald HJ, Miall WE. The prevalence of diabetes in a rural population of Jamaican adults. Int J Epidemiol 1972; 1: 157–66.

169. Patrick AL, Boyd HA. Blood sugar levels, weights and heights of Tobagonians. W Ind Med 1985; 34: 114.

170. Beckles GLA, Kirkwood BR, Carson DC, Miller SJ, Alexis SD, Byam NTA. High total cholesterol and cardiovascular disease mortality in adults of Indian descent in Trinidad, unexplained by major coronary risk factors. Lancet 1986; 1: 1298–9.

171. Kawate R, Kamakido M, Nishimoto Y, Bennett PH, Hamman RF, Knowler WC. Diabetes mellitus and its vascular complications in Japanese migrants on the island of Hawaii. Diabetes Care 1979; 2: 161–70.

172. Kawate R, Yamakido M, Nishimoto Y. Migrant studies among the Japanese in Hiroshima and Hawaii. In Waldhausl WK (ed.) Diabetes 1979, Proceedings of the 10th Congress of the International Diabetes Federation. The Netherlands: Excerpta Medica, 1980; pp 526–31.

173. Hara H, Egusa G, Yamane K, Yamakido M. Diabetes and diabetic macroangiopathy in Japanese-Americans. In Roberts DF, Fujiki N, Torizuka K (eds) Isolation, migration and disease. SSHB Monograph Series 33, Cambridge, UK: Cambridge University Press, 1992; pp 219–32.

174. Fujimoto WY, Leonetti DL, Bergstrom RW, Kinyoun JL, Stolov WC, Wah PW. Glucose intolerance and diabetic complications among Japanese-American women. Diabetes Res Clin Prac 1991; 13: 119–30.

175. Taylor R, Bennett P, Uili R et al. Diabetes in Wallis Polynesians: a comparison of residents of Wallis Island and first generation migrants to Nourmea, New Caledonia. Diabetes Res Clin Pract 1985; 1: 169–78.

176. Stanhope JM, Prior IAM. The Tokelau Island Migrant Study: prevalence and incidence of diabetes mellitus. NZ Med J 1980; 92: 417–21.

177. Reed D, Labarthe D, Stallones R, Brody J. Epidemiological studies on serum glucose levels among Micronesians. Diabetes 1973; 22: 129–36.

178. Taylor R, Bennett P, Uili R et al. The prevalence of diabetes mellitus in a traditional-living Polynesian population. The Wallis Island survey. Diabetes Care 1983; 6: 333–40.

179. Barrett-Connor E. Epidemiology, obesity, and non-insulin-dependent diabetes mellitus. Epidemiol Rev 1989; 11: 172–81.

180. Haffner SM, Stern MP, Hazuda HP, Pugh J, Paterson JK. Do upper-body and centralized adiposity measure different aspects of regional body-fat distribution? Relationship to non-insulin dependent diabetes mellitus, lipids, and lipoproteins. Diabetes 1987; 36: 43–51.

181. Skarfors ET, Selinus KI, Lithell HO. Risk factors for developing non-insulin dependent diabetes: a 10-year follow-up of men in Uppsala. Br Med J 1991; 303: 755–60.

182. Shaten BJ, Smith GD, Kuller LH, Neaton JD. Risk factors for the development of type 2 diabetes among men enrolled in the Usual Care group of the Multiple Risk Factor Intervention Trial. Diabetes Care 1993; 16: 1331–9.

183. Tai T-Y, Chuang L-M, Wu H-P, Chen C-J. Association of body build with non-insulin-dependent diabetes mellitus and hypertension among Chinese adults: a 4-year follow-up study. Int J Epidemiol 1992; 21: 511–17.

184. Chou P, Liao M-J, Shih-Tzer T. Associated risk factors of diabetes in Kin-Hu, Kinmen. Diabetes Res Clin Pract 1994; 26: 229–35.

185. Schmidt MI, Duncan, BB, Canani LH, Karohl C, Chambless L. Associations of waist–hip ratio with diabetes mellitus. Strength and possible modifiers. Diabetes Care 1992; 15: 912–14.

186. Van Noord PAH, Seidell JC, Den Tonkelaar I, Baanders-Van Halewiin EA, Ouwehand IJ. The relationship between fat distribution and some chronic diseases in 11 825 women participating in the DOM-Project. Int J Epidemiol 1990; 19: 564–70.

187. Shelgikar KM, Hockaday TDR, Yajnik CS. Central rather than generalized obesity is related to hyperglycaemia in Asian Indian subjects. Diabet Med 1991; 8: 712–17.

188. McKeigue PM, Pierpoint T, Ferrie JE, Marmot MG. Relationship of glucose intolerance and hyperinsulinaemia to body fat pattern in South Asians and Europeans. Diabetologia 1992; 35: 785–91.

189. Hartz AJ, Rupley DC, Kalkhoff RD, Rimm AA. Relationship of obesity to diabetes: influence of obesity level and body fat distribution. Preventive Med 1983; 12: 351–7.

190. Ohlson L-O, Larsson B, Svardsudd K et al. The influence of body fat distribution on the incidence of diabetes mellitus. 13.5 years of follow-up of the participants in the study of men born in 1913. Diabetes 1985; 34: 1055–8.

191. Lundgren H, Bengtsson C, Blohme G, Lapidus L, Sjöstrom L. Adiposity and adipose tissue distribution in relation to incidence of diabetes in women: results from a prospective population study in Gothenburg, Sweden. Int J Obesity 1989; 13: 413–23.

192. Haffner SM, Stern MP, Mitchell BD, Hazuda HP, Patterson JK. Incidence of type 2 diabetes in Mexican Americans predicted by fasting insulin and glucose levels, obesity, and body-fat distribution. Diabetes 1990; 39: 283–8.

193. Cassano P, Rosner B, Vokonas PS, Weiss ST. Obesity and body fat distribution in relation to the incidence of non-insulin-dependent diabetes mellitus. Am J Epidemiol 1992; 136: 1474–86.

194. Colditz GA, Willett WC, Stamper MJ et al. Weight as a risk factor for clinical diabetes in women. Am J Epidemiol 1990; 132: 501–13.

195. Chan JM, Rimm EB, Colditz GA, Stampfer MJ, Willett WC. Obesity, fat distribution, and weight gain as risk factors for clinical diabetes in men. Diabetes Care 1994; 17: 961–9.

196. Knowler WC, Pettitt DJ, Saad MF, Charles MA, Nelson RG, Howard BV. Obesity in the Pima Indians: its magnitude and relationship with diabetes. Am J Clin Nutr 1991; 53: 1543S–51S.

197. Charles MA, Fontbonne A, Thibult N, Warnet J-M, Rosselin GE, Eschwege E. Risk factors for NIDDM in white population. Paris Prospective Study. Diabetes 1991; 40: 796–9.

198. Modan M, Karasik A, Halkin H et al. Effect of past and concurrent body mass index on prevalence of glucose intolerance and type 2 (non-insulin-dependent) diabetes and on insulin response. The Israel study of glucose intolerance, obesity and hypertension. Diabetologia 1986; 29: 82–9.

199. Sicree RA, Zimmet PZ, King H, Coventry J. Weight change amongst Nauruans over 6.5 years: extent, and association with glucose intolerance. Diabetes Res Clin Pract 1987; 3: 327–36.

200. Hodge AM, Collins VR, Zimmet PZ, Dowse GK. Non-insulin-dependent diabetes mellitus and obesity. In Zimmet P, Ekoe JM, Williams R (eds) The epidemiology of diabetes mellitus—an international perspective. Chichester: Wiley, 1996.

201. Harris MI. Impaired glucose tolerance in the US population. Diabetes Care 1989; 12: 464–74.

202. DiPietro L, Mossberg H-O, Stunkard AJ. A 40-year history of overweight children in Stockholm: life-time overweight, morbidity, and mortality. Int J Obesity 1994; 18: 585–90.

203. Hansen BC, Bodkin NL. β-cell hyperresponsiveness: earliest event in development of diabetes in monkeys. Am J Physiol 1990; 259: R612–17.

204. Bogardus C, Lillioja S, Bennett PH. Pathogenesis of NIDDM in Pima Indians. Diabetes Care 1991; 14 (suppl. 3): 685–90.

205. Roumain J, Charles MA, de Courten MP, Hanson RL, Pettitt DJ, Knowler WC. Menstrual irregularity is associated with non-insulin-dependent diabetes mellitus in Pima Indian women. Am J Med 1996 (in press).

206. Ogilvie RF. Sugar tolerance in obese subjects. A review of sixty-five cases. Q J Med 1935; series 2,4: 345–58.

207. Haffner SM, Stern MP, Hazuda HP, Rosenthal M, Knapp JA, Malina RM. Role of obesity and fat distribution in non-insulin-dependent diabetes mellitus in Mexican Americans and non-Hispanic whites. Diabetes Care 1986; 9: 153–61.

208. Fujimoto WY, Leonetti DL, Newell-Morris L, Shuman WP, Wahl PW. Relationship of absence or presence of a family history of diabetes to body weight and body fat distribution in type 2 diabetes. Int J Obesity 1991; 15: 111–20.

209. Lemieux S, Després J-P, Nadeau A, Prud'homme D, Tremblay A, Bouchard C. Heterogeneous glycaemic and insulinaemic responses to oral glucose in non-diabetic men: interactions between duration of obesity, body fat distribution and family history of diabetes mellitus. Diabetologia 1992; 35: 653–9.

210. Kuzuya T, Matsuda A. Family histories of diabetes among Japanese patients with type 1 (insulin-dependent) and type 2 (non-insulin-dependent) diabetes. Diabetologia 1982; 22: 372–4.

211. Hanson RL, Pettitt DJ, Bennett PH et al. Familial relationships between obesity and NIDDM. Diabetes 1995; 44: 418–22.

212. Chen MK, Lowenstein FW. Epidemiology of factors related to self-reported diabetes amongst adults. Am J Prev Med 1986; 2: 14–19.

213. Kriska AM, LaPorte RE, Pettitt DJ et al. The association of physical activity with obesity, fat distribution and glucose intolerance in Pima Indians. Diabetologia (in press).

214. Despres J-P, Pouliot M-C, Moorjani S et al. Metabolic effects of aerobic exercise training-induced loss of abdominal fat in obese woman. Med Sci Sports Exercise 1990; 22: 5128 (abstr 768).

215. Tuomilehto J, Knowler WC, Zimmet P. Primary prevention of non-insulin dependent diabetes mellitus. Diabetes Metab Rev 1992; 8: 339–53.

216. Eriksson KF, Lindgarde F. Prevention of type 2 (non-insulin-dependent) diabetes mellitus by diet and physical exercise. The 6-year Malmö feasibility study. Diabetologia 1991; 34: 891–8.

217. Frisch RE, Wyshak G, Albright TE, Albright NL, Schiff I. Lower prevalence of diabetes in female former college athletes compared with non-athletes. Diabetes 1986; 35: 1101–5.

218. Schranz A, Tuomilehto J, Marti B, Jarrett RJ, Grabauskas V, Vassallo A. Low physical activity and worsening of glucose tolerance: results from a 2-year follow-up of a population sample in Malta. Diabetes Res Clin Pract 1991; 11: 127–36.

219. Helmrich SP, Ragland DR, Leung RW, Paffenbarger RS Jr. Physical activity and reduced occurrence of non-insulin dependent diabetes mellitus. New Engl J Med 1991; 325: 147–52.

220. Manson JE, Rimm EB, Stampfer MJ et al. Physical activity and incidence of non-insulin dependent diabetes mellitus in women. Lancet 1991; 338: 774–8.

221. Manson JE, Nathan DM, Krolewski AS, Stampfer MJ, Willett WC, Hennekens CH. A prospective study of exercise and incidence of diabetes among US male physicians. J Am Med Assoc 1992; 268: 63–7.

222. Rewers M, Wagenknecht L, Watanabe RM. Insulin sensitivity in non-diabetic Blacks, Hispanics and non-Hispanic whites: the Insulin Resistance Arteriosclerosis Study (IRAS). Diabetes 1994; 43 (suppl. 1): 151A.

223. Laws A, Reaven GM. Effect of physical activity on age-related glucose intolerance. Clin Geriatr Med 1990; 6: 849–63.

224. Horton E. Exercise and decreased risk of NIDDM. New Engl J Med 1991; 325: 147–52.

225. Bouchardat A. De la glycosurie ou diabète sucré, vol 2. Paris: Germer-Baillière, 1875.

226. Himsworth HP. Diet and the incidence of diabetes mellitus. Clin Sci 1935; 2: 117–48.

227. Mann JI, Houston A. The aetiology of non-insulin dependent diabetes mellitus. In Mann JL, Pyorala K,

Teuscher A (eds) Diabetes in epidemiological perspective. Edinburgh: Churchill Livingstone, 1983; pp 122–64.

228. Westlund K. Incidence of diabetes mellitus in Oslo, Norway, 1925–1954. Br J Prev Soc Med 1966; 20: 105.

229. Bingham SA. The dietary assessment of individuals; methods, accuracy, new techniques and recommendations. Nutr Abs Reviews 1987; 57: 705–42.

230. Shintani TT, Hughes CK, Beckham S, O'Connor HK. Obesity and cardiovascular risk intervention through the ad libitum feeding of traditional Hawaiian diet. Am J Clin Nutr 1991; 53: 1647–51S.

231. O'Dea K. Marked improvement in carbohydrate and lipid metabolism in diabetic Australian Aborigines after temporary reversion to a traditional lifestyle. Diabetes 1984; 33: 596–603.

232. Irie M, Hyodo T, Togane T. Summary of previous studies on Sumo wrestlers. In Abe H, Hoshi M (eds) Diabetic microangiopathy. Tokyo: University of Tokyo, 1983; Japan Medical Research Foundation Publication no. 20; pp 397–402.

233. Himsworth HP, Marshall EM. The diet of diabetics prior to the onset of disease. Clin Sci 1935; 2: 95–115.

234. Tsunehara CH, Leonetti DL, Fujimoto WY. Diet of second generation Japanese-American men with and without non-insulin dependent diabetes. Am J Clin Nutr 1990; 52: 731–8.

235. Marshall JA, Hamman RF, Baxter J. High fat, low carbohydrate diet and the etiology of non-insulin-dependent diabetes mellitus: the San Luis Valley Diabetes Study. Am J Epidemiol 1991; 134: 590–603.

236. Medalie JH, Herman JB, Goldbourt U, Papier CM. Variations in incidence of diabetes among 10 000 adult Israeli males and the factors related to their development. In Levine R, Luft R (eds) Advances in metabolic disorders. New York: Academic Press, 1978; pp 93–110.

237. Bennett PH, Knowler WC, Baird HR et al. Diet and development of non-insulin-dependent diabetes: an epidemiological perspective. In Pozza G et al (eds) Diet and atherosclerosis. New York: Raven Press, 1984; pp 109–19.

238. Malasanos TH, Stacpoole PW. Biological effects of omega-3 fatty acids in diabetes mellitus. Diabetes Care 1991; 14: 1160–79.

239. Colditz GA, Giovannucci E, Rimm EB et al. Alcohol intake in relation to diet and obesity in women and men. Am J Clin Nutr 1991; 54: 49–55.

240. Rissanen AM, Heliovaara M, Knekt P, Reunanen A, Aromaa A. Determinants of weight gain and overweight in adult Finns. Eur J Clin Nutr 1991; 45: 419–30.

241. Holbrook TL, Barrett-Connor E, Wingard DL. A prospective population-based study of alcohol use and non-insulin-dependent diabetes mellitus. Am J Epidemiol 1990; 132: 902–9.

242. Balkau B, Eschwege E, Fontbonne A, Claude J-C, Warnet J-M. Cardiovascular and alcohol-related deaths in abnormal glucose tolerant and diabetic subjects. Diabetologia 1992; 35: 39–44.

243. Stampler MJ, Colditz GA, Willett WC et al. A prospective study of moderate alcohol drinking and risk of diabetes in women. Am J Epidemiol 1988; 128: 549–58.

244. Hodge AM, Dowse GK, Collins VC, Zimmet PZ. Abnormal glucose tolerance and alcohol consumption in three populations at high risk of non-insulin-dependent diabetes mellitus. Am J Epidemiol 1993; 137: 178–89.

245. Tai T-Y, Yang C-L, Chang C-J et al. Epidemiology of diabetes mellitus in Taiwan ROC—comparison between rural and urban areas. In Vanesaeng S, Nitianant W, Chandraprasert S (eds) Epidemiology of diabetes mellitus: proceedings of the International Symposium on Epidemiology of Diabetes Mellitus. Bangkok: Crystal House Press, 1987; pp 49–58.

246. Fatani HH, Mira SA, El-Zubier AG. Prevalence of diabetes mellitus in rural Saudi Arabia. Diabetes Care 1987; 10: 180–83.

247. Pettitt DJ, Baird HR, Aleck KA, Bennett PH, Knowler WC. Excessive obesity in offspring of Pima Indian women with diabetes during pregnancy. New Engl J Med 1983; 308: 242–5.

248. Papoz L, Ben Khalifa F, Eschwege E, Ben Ayed H. Diabetes mellitus in Tunisia: description in urban and rural populations. Int J Epidemiol 1988; 17: 419–22.

249. Patel M, Jamrozik K, Allen O et al. A high prevalence of diabetes in a rural village in Papua New Guinea. Diabetes Res Clin Pract 1986; 2: 97–103.

250. Hazuda HP, Haffner SM, Stern MP, Eifler CW. Effects of acculturation and socio-economic status on obesity and diabetes in Mexican Americans. Am J Epidemiol 1988; 128: 1289–1301.

251. Martin FIR, Wyatt GB, Griew AR, Haurahelia L, Higginbotham L. Diabetes mellitus in urban and rural communities in Papua New Guinea. Diabetologia 1980; 18: 369–74.

252. Garancini MP, Calori G, Ruotolo G et al. Prevalence of NIDDM and impaired glucose tolerance in Italy: an OGTT-based population study. Diabetologia 1995; 38: 306–13.

253. Jarrett RJ, Keen H, Fuller JH, McCartney P. Worsening to diabetes in men with impaired glucose tolerance (borderline diabetes). Diabetologia 1979; 16: 25–30.

254. Keen H, Jarrett RJ, McCartney P. The ten-year follow-up of the Bedford Survey (1962–1972): glucose tolerance and diabetes. Diabetologia 1982; 22: 154–7.

255. Sasaki A, Suzuki T, Horiuchi N. Development of diabetes in Japanese subjects with impaired glucose tolerance: a seven-year follow-up study. Diabetologia 1982; 22: 154–7.

256. Kadowaki T, Miyake Y, Hagura R et al. Risk factors for worsening to diabetes in subjects with impaired glucose tolerance. Diabetologia 1984; 26: 44–9.

257. Saad MF, Knowler WC, Pettitt DJ et al. The natural history of impaired glucose tolerance in the Pima Indians. New Engl J Med 1988; 319: 1500–06.

258. Savage PJ, Dippe SE, Bennett PH et al. Hyperinsulinemia and hypoinsulinemia. Insulin responses to oral carbohydate over a wide spectrum of glucose tolerance. Diabetes 1975; 24: 362–8.

259. Lillioja S, Mott DM, Howard BV et al. Impaired glucose tolerance as a disorder of insulin action: longitudinal and cross-sectional studies in Pima Indians. New Engl J Med 1988; 318: 1217–25.

260. Modan M, Halkin H, Almog S et al. Hyperinsulinemia—a link between hypertension, obesity and glucose intolerance. J Clin Invest 1985; 75: 809–17.

261. Fuller JH, Shipley MJ, Rose G, Jarrett RJ, Keen H. Coronary heart disease risk and impaired glucose tolerance: the Whitehall study. Lancet 1980; i: 1373-6.

262. Jarrett RJ, McCartney P, Keen H. The Bedford survey: ten-year mortality rates in newly diagnosed diabetics, borderline diabetics and normoglycaemic controls and risk indices for coronary heart disease in borderline diabetics. Diabetologia 1982; 22: 79-84.

263. Sartor G, Schersten B, Carlström S, Melander A, Norden Å, Persson G. Ten-year follow-up of subjects with impaired glucose tolerance: prevention of diabetes by tolbutamide and diet regulation. Diabetes 1980; 29: 41-9.

264. Annuzzi G, Vaccaro O, Caprio S et al. Association between low habitual physical activity and impaired glucose tolerance. Clin Physiol 1985; 5: 63-70.

265. Capaldo B, Tutino L, Patti L, Vaccaro O, Rivellese A, Riccardi G. Lipoprotein composition in individuals with impaired glucose tolerance. Diabetes Care 1983; 6: 575-8.

266. Vaccaro O, Rivellese A, Riccardi G et al. Impaired glucose tolerance and risk factors for atherosclerosis. Atherosclerosis 1984; 4: 592-7.

267. Vaccaro O, Pauciullo P, Rubba P et al. Peripheral arterial circulation in individuals with impaired glucose tolerance. Diabetes Care 1985; 8: 594-7.

268. Eriksson KE, Saltin B, Lindgarde F. Increased skeletal muscle capillary density precedes diabetes development in men with impaired glucose tolerance. Diabetes 1994; 43: 805-8.

269. Saad MF, Pettitt DJ, Mott DM, Knowler WC, Nelson RG, Bennett PH. Sequential changes in serum insulin concentration during development of non-insulin-dependent diabetes. Lancet 1989; i: 1356-9.

270. Aronoff SL, Bennett PH, Gorden P, Rushforth N, Miller M. Unexplained hyperinsulinemia in normal and prediabetic Pima Indians compared with normal Caucasians. Diabetes 1977; 26: 827-40.

271. Zimmet P, Whitehouse S, Kiss J. Ethnic variability in the plasma insulin response to oral glucose in Polynesian and Micronesian subjects. Diabetes 1979; 28: 624-8.

272. Zimmet P, Whitehouse S, Alford F, Chisholm D. The relationship of insulin to a glucose stimulus over a wide range of glucose tolerance. Diabetologia 1978; 15: 23-7.

273. O'Dea K, Traianedes K, Hopper JL, Larkins RG. Impaired glucose tolerance, hyperinsulinemia and hypertriglyceridemia in Australian Aborigines from the desert. Diabetes Care 1988; 11: 23-9.

274. Haffner SM, Stern MP, Hazuda HP, Pugh JA, Patterson JK. Hyperinsulinemia in a population at high risk for non-insulin-dependent diabetes. New Engl J Med 1986; 315: 220-24.

275. Mohan V, Sharp PS, Cloke HR, Schumer B, Kohner EM. Serum immunoreactive insulin responses to a glucose load in Asian Indian and European type 2 (non-insulin-dependent) diabetic patients and control subjects. Diabetologia 1986; 29: 235-7.

276. Nagulesparan M, Savage PJ, Knowler WC, Johnson GC, Bennett PH. Increased *in vivo* insulin resistance in non-diabetic Pima Indians compared with Caucasians. Diabetes 1982; 31: 952-6.

277. Zimmet PZ, Collins VR, Dowse GK, Knight LT. Hyperinsulinaemia in youth is a predictor of type 2 (non-insulin-dependent) diabetes mellitus. Diabetologia 1992; 35: 534-41.

278. Nabulsi AA, Folsom AR, Heiss G et al. Fasting hyperinsulinemia and cardiovascular risk factors in non-diabetic adults: stronger associations in lean versus obese subjects. Metabolism 1995; 44: 914-22.

279. Boyko EJ, Keane EM, Marshall JA, Hamman RF. Higher insulin and C-peptide concentrations in Hispanic population at high risk for NIDDM: San Luis Valley Diabetes Study. Diabetes 1991; 40: 509-15.

280. Li N, Tuomilehto J, Dowse G, Virtala E, Zimmet P. Prevalence of coronary heart disease indicated by ECG abnormalities and risk factors in developing countries. J Clin Epidemiol 1994; 47: 599-611.

281. Schmidt MI, Duncan BB, Watson RL, Sharrett AR, Brancati FL, Heiss G. A metabolic syndrome in white and African-Americans. The Atherosclerosis Risk in Communities baseline study. Diabetes Care 1996; 19: 414-18.

282. Taylor R, Zimmet P, Tuomilehto J, Ram P, Hunt D, Sloman G. Blood pressure changes with age in two ethnic groups in Fiji. J Am Coll Nutr 1989; 8: 335-46.

283. Summerson JH, Bell RA, Konen JC. Coronary heart disease risk factors in Black and White patients with non-insulin-dependent diabetes mellitus. Ethnicity and Health 1996; 1: 9-20.

284. Cowie CC, Port FK, Wolfe RA, Savage PJ, Moll PP, Hawthorne VM. Disparities in incidence of diabetic end-stage renal disease according to race and type of diabetes. New Engl J Med 1989; 321: 1074-9.

285. Mosenthal HO, Boluan C. Diabetes mellitus—problems of present day treatment. Am J Med Sci 1933; 186: 605.

286. Joslin EP, Dublin LI, Marks HH. Studies in diabetes mellitus. IV. Etiology. Am J Med Sci 1936; 191: 759-75.

287. Pyke DA. Parity and incidence of diabetes. Lancet 1956; 270: 818-21.

288. Fitzgerald MG, Malins JM, O'Sullivan DJ, Wall M. The effect of sex and parity on the incidence of diabetes mellitus. Q J Med 1961; 30: 57.

289. Middleton GD, Caird FI. Parity and diabetes mellitus. Br J Prev Soc Med 1968; 22: 100-104.

290. Kritz-Silverstein D, Barrett-Connor E, Wingard D. The effect of parity on the later development of non-insulin-dependent diabetes mellitus or impaired glucose tolerance. New Engl J Med 1989; 321: 1214-19.

291. Pyke DA, Please NW. Obesity, parity and diabetes. J Endocrinol 1957; 15: 26-33.

292. West KM, Kalbfleisch JM. Diabetes in Central America. Diabetes 1970; 19: 656-63.

293. Sicree R, Hoet J, Zimmet P, King H, Coventry J. The association of non-insulin-dependent diabetes with parity and still-birth occurrence amongst five Pacific populations. Diabetes Res Clin Pract 1986; 2: 113-22.

294. Collins VR, Dowse GK, Zimmet PZ. Evidence against association between parity and NIDDM from five population groups. Diabetes Care 1991; 14: 975-81.

295. O'Sullivan JB, Mahan CM. Blood sugar levels, glucosuria and body weight related to development of diabetes mellitus. J Am Med Assn 1965; 194: 117-22.

296. Harris MI. Gestational diabetes may represent discovery of pre-existing glucose intolerance. Diabetes Care 1988; 11: 402–11.

297. O'Sullivan JB. Diabetes mellitus after GDM. Diabetes 1991; 40: 131–5.

298. Metzger BE, Bybee DE, Freinkel N, Phelps RL, Radvany RM, Vaisrub N. Gestational diabetes mellitus. Correlations between the phenotypic and genotypic characteristics of the mother and abnormal glucose tolerance during the first year post partum. Diabetes 1985; 34: 115.

299. Grant PT, Oats JN, Beischer NA. The long-term follow-up of women with gestational diabetes. Aust NZ J Obstet Gynaecol 1986; 16: 17–22.

300. Lam KS, Li DF, Lauder IJ, Lee CP, Kung AWC, Ma JTC. Prediction of persistent carbohydrate intolerance in patients with gestational diabetes. Diabetes Res Clin Prac 1991; 12: 181–6.

301. Coustan DR, Carpenter MW, O'Sullivan PS, Carr SR. Gestational diabetes: predictors of subsequent disordered glucose metabolism. Am J Obstet Gynecol 1993; 168: 1139–44.

302. Damm P, Kuhl C, Hornnes P, Molsted-Pedersen L. A longitudinal study of plasma insulin and glucagon in women with previous gestational diabetes. Diabetes Care 1995; 18: 654–64.

303. Kjos SL, Peters RX, Xiang A, Henry OA, Montoro M, Buchanan TA. Predicting future diabetes in Latino women with gestational diabetes. Utility of early postpartum glucose tolerance testing. Diabetes 1995; 44: 586–91.

304. Samanta A, Burden ML, Burden AC, Jones GR. Glucose tolerance during pregnancy in Asian women. Diabetes Res Clin Pract 1989; 7: 127–35.

305. Fraser D, Weitzman S, Leiberman JR, Zmora E, Laron E, Karplus M. Gestational diabetes among Bedouins in southern Israel: comparison of prevalence and neonatal outcomes with the Jewish population. Acta Diabetol 1994; 31: 78–81.

306. Hollingsworth DR, Vaucher Y, Yamamoto TR. Diabetes in pregnancy in Mexican Americans. Diabetes Care 1991; 14: 695–705.

307. Oats JN, Beischer NA. Gestational diabetes. Progr Obstet Gynaecol 1984; 3: 101–16.

308. Dornhost A, Paterson CM, Nicholls JSD et al. High prevalence of gestational diabetes in women from ethnic miniority groups. Diabet Med 1992; 9: 820–25.

309. Yue DK, Molyneaux LM, Ross GP, Constantino MI, Child AG, Turtle JR. Why does ethnicity affect prevalence of gestational diabetes? The underwater volcano theory. Diabet Med 1996; 13: 748–52.

9

Diabetes in the Tropics

V. Mohan* and K.G.M.M. Alberti†

*M.V. Diabetes Specialities Centre, Madras, India, and †University of Newcastle upon Tyne, UK

Interest in the study of diabetes in the tropics was first generated after a 1907 symposium which drew attention to the peculiarities of diabetes in tropical countries [1]. Tulloch's book [2] also evoked considerable interest in this subject. It was the late Professor Kelly West who renewed the interest of Western scientists in tropical forms of diabetes [3, 4]. The recent World Health Organization (WHO) Study Group Report on diabetes mellitus [5] included malnutrition-related diabetes mellitus (MRDM) as an entity distinct from insulin dependent diabetes mellitus (IDDM) and non-insulin dependent diabetes mellitus (NIDDM). This has led to increased awareness of and interest in diabetes of tropical countries. Several reviews [4–14, 161] have highlighted the differences between diabetes in tropical countries and that seen in Western countries.

TERMINOLOGY

The two main forms of primary diabetes seen in developed countries of the temperate region, namely IDDM and NIDDM, are also seen in tropical countries but there are some differences in their clinical profiles. In addition, there are special forms of diabetes confined to the tropical belt which are presumed to have a common denominator—protein–energy malnutrition. For this reason, they have been designated 'malnutrition-related diabetes mellitus' (MRDM) [5], based on a review by Bajaj [13]. The category of MRDM has been divided into two subtypes [5, 13]: fibrocalculous pancreatic diabetes (FCPD) and protein deficient diabetes mellitus (PDDM). Earlier terms used for these special

types of diabetes, such as 'tropical diabetes', 'tropical pancreatic diabetes', 'pancreatic diabetes', 'J-type diabetes', 'ketosis resistant diabetes', 'juvenile tropical pancreatitis syndrome' and 'Z-type diabetes', have been replaced by 'MRDM'. It must be stressed, however, that MRDM is not the most common form of diabetes seen in tropical countries. The frequency of the different forms of diabetes in the tropics as seen at the MV Diabetes Specialities Centre, Madras, is summarized in Figure 1. Similar low prevalences of MRDM are found in many other tropical countries. The Madras figures show that NIDDM is the most common type of diabetes, followed by IDDM and MRDM. Although this review covers all forms of diabetes seen in the tropics, special emphasis is given to MRDM. It should be noted that recently a consensus statement from an International Workshop in Cuttack has suggested that PDDM be replaced by the term 'malnutrition-modulated diabetes mellitus' (MMDM) and that low BMI NIDDM be added to the spectrum of MRDM [172].

IDDM IN THE TROPICS

Classical juvenile-onset IDDM is believed to be less common in tropical countries [9–13, 173]. The possibility exists, of course, that early death or undiscovered diabetes accounts for some, if not all, of this low frequency of IDDM in tropical countries. Moreover, there are few well-conducted epidemiological studies in tropical countries and hence the prevalence of IDDM in the population still remains largely unknown. Patel

International Textbook of Diabetes Mellitus, Second Edition. Edited by K.G.M.M. Alberti, P. Zimmet, R.A. DeFronzo, and H. Keen (Honorary)

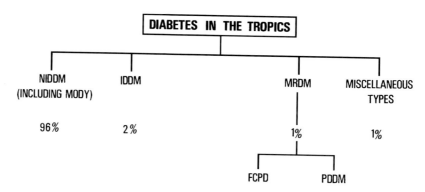

Figure 1 Classification of diabetes in the tropics. Relative frequencies of the various forms of diabetes as seen at the MV Diabetes Specialities Centre, Madras

et al [15] and Guptha [16] have shown that IDDM is uncommon in northern India. Krishnaswami and Chandra [17] reported that the prevalence of juvenile diabetes in southern India was 0.8% of all diabetics. Zimmet [18] has stated that IDDM is rare in certain ethnic groups including the Filipinos, Sri Lankans, South African blacks, Polynesians, Micronesians and Melanesians. Observations in East Africa suggest a low prevalence, even allowing for a low detection rate. IDDM is also reported to be rare in Korea, Singapore, Pakistan, Bangladesh and Thailand [19].

HLA studies have shown some differences in the profile of IDDM in tropical countries. Among the Chinese, HLA-DR3 was significantly increased whereas DR4 was absent [20, 21]. Similar increases in DR3 were reported from Thailand [19]. Interestingly, some differences in the association with HLA and other genetic markers were seen between IDDM in north and south India [22–24]: in north India [22] there was an association with DR3, BW21 and the properdin system BFS1; in south India, on the other hand, the association was seen with HLA-DR3 and DR4, B8 and the properdin system BFF [23, 24]. Similar differences have been noted between northern Indian and southern Indian IDDM patients in South Africa [25]. A recent study [26] showed that the strong association seen with the HLA-DQ β gene among European IDDM patients is also seen among southern Indian IDDM patients. The prevalence of islet cell antibodies (ICA) appears to be low in Indian patients and in Tanzanian blacks [27]. GAD antibodies are also positive in less that 20% of apparent IDDM subjects in Tanzanians (Zimmet, McLarty, Alberti et al, unpublished observations). Again, some differences were observed between northern and southern Indian patients [28, 29]. In southern Indians, the ICA appeared to persist for a shorter time, and by the end of 6 months the prevalence of ICA positivity came down sharply [29]. A study from South Africa also showed that the ICA in Indians had a shorter duration than in the Africans [30].

However, a study in migrant Indian IDDM subjects in the UK could not confirm these findings [31].

One point that seems to be common to IDDM in many tropical countries is that it occurs at a slightly older age [32–34, 78]. Tropical IDDM patients also appear to be relatively ketosis resistant compared with the IDDM patients seen in the West, which may reflect some residual B-cell function.

NIDDM IN THE TROPICS

Prevalence

A number of prevalence studies on NIDDM have been published (see also Chapter 8). Ramachandran et al [35] performed oral glucose tolerance tests (OGTT: WHO criteria) in patients in an iron ore factory township (Kudremukh) in south India. The overall prevalence of diabetes was high at 5%, and in those older than 40 years it rose to 21%. Higher socio-economic status and obesity were associated with increased risk. As with the Darya Ganj survey [36], this study emphasizes the very high prevalence of diabetes in Indians in Asia. These studies show that the prevalence of diabetes is now very much higher in the Indian subcontinent than the figure of 2% reported by the Indian Council of Medical Research (ICMR) multicentric study in 1975 [37].

Omar et al [38] studied the prevalence of diabetes (diagnosed by OGTT) in South African Indians, and also reported a high prevalence of diabetes (9%). Simmons et al [39] have also shown higher prevalence of diabetes in Asians compared with Europids. A recent survey of diabetes from Madras [40] looked at two Dravidian populations with considerable socio-economic differences living in urban and rural areas. The study showed that the age-adjusted prevalence of diabetes in the rural population was 2.4%, compared with a prevalence of 8.2% in the urban population. Age, body mass index (BMI) and waist:hip ratio (WHR) showed positive association with diabetes in both urban and rural populations. Another important observation made in the Madras survey was that although prevalence of diabetes was four times lower in the rural population, the prevalence of impaired glucose tolerance (IGT) was similar in urban (8.7%) and rural (7.8%) populations.

It thus appears that Asians are genetically more susceptible to develop NIDDM either at home or abroad. Ramachandran et al [41] have demonstrated a very high risk of diabetes in the south Indian families with one diabetic parent. Native Africans, on the other hand, seem less prone to develop NIDDM. A study in rural Mali [42] found only 0.92% of the population with fasting glucose levels over 7.0 mmol/l; Europids and Fulanis were more susceptible than Negroes. In rural Tanzania, using WHO criteria, the prevalence of NIDDM was only 0.7% in those aged 16 years and above [43]. Prevalence in urban dwellers was twofold higher, whilst in higher socio-economic groups 4–10% had diabetes (unpublished observations). The high prevalence of diabetes in Asians was also found in Tanzania [44].

Reversal of Sex Ratio

Unlike most Western countries, where a female predominance is seen, in many tropical countries there is a male predominance [4]. Interpretation of this finding is difficult because in developing countries women are less likely to seek medical attention.

Younger Age at Onset

Several studies [37, 45–47] have shown that NIDDM patients are younger at diagnosis, with the peak prevalence occurring at least a decade earlier in Indian patients. Similar observations have been made in Ethiopia [48]. This could either be attributable to the fact that the form of diabetes known as maturity onset diabetes of the young (MODY) is more common, or it could be a reflection of the younger age structure of these populations.

MODY Among Indians

Studies on Indian diabetic patients in south India [46, 49–51] and in South Africa [47, 52–54] have shown that MODY is common among Indian subjects. MODY was first described by Tattersall and Fajans, but it is not a common entity among Europeans [55–58]. As the frequency of MODY is much higher among Indians compared with the black and white communities in South Africa [47] this could represent an ethnic variation. Studies on the clinical profile, insulin secretion,

insulin resistance in MODY and B-cell function studies in offspring of MODY patients have been reported from India and South Africa [46, 47, 49–54, 59]. An important finding that has emerged from these studies, which disproves Tattersall's earlier findings [58] but supports Fajans's findings [57], is that patients with MODY do develop specific diabetic complications, just like patients with classic NIDDM.

Genetic Factors in NIDDM

There are several lines of evidence to show that genetic mechanisms are very strong in Indian patients [60]. Firstly, the prevalence of diabetes in migrant Indians has been shown to be higher than that in the local host populations of these countries [45, 61–63]. Recently, the prevalence of diabetes among Indians in India has also been shown to be high [36]. Secondly, the prevalence of diabetes among the offspring of conjugal diabetic parents, which varies from 3% to 25% among Europeans [64], was 62% among Indians [65]. Finally, the high prevalence of autosomal dominant diabetes among Indians [46, 47] also suggests that genetic factors could be stronger in Indian patients.

Hyperinsulinaemia and Insulin Resistance in NIDDM

Hyperinsulinaemia leading to insulin resistance could be one of the mechanisms responsible for the high prevalence of diabetes among Indian patients. In one study, it was found that immunoreactive insulin responses to an oral glucose load were higher among Asian Indians than among Europeans [66]. Euglycaemic clamp studies showed that Asian Indian patients were more insulin resistant than Europeans [67]. More studies are needed to determine whether this insulin resistance has a genetic basis or is due to the influence of environmental factors. By contrast, we have recently shown that Tanzanian blacks appear to be less insulin-resistant than Europids, although still much more resistant than control non-diabetic subjects (Ramaiya et al, unpublished).

Complications in NIDDM

The WHO Multinational Study [68] reported wide differences in the prevalence of macrovascular and microvascular disease in NIDDM subjects from different countries. Reports have now appeared from Africa, the continent not represented in the WHO study [14]. Lester and Keen [69] found low rates of macrovascular disease in Ethiopian diabetic patients from Addis Ababa, as did Rolfe [70–73] in Zambian Africans.

Hypertension was fairly common in both these populations (20% and 40%, respectively) and did show an association with the macrovascular disease. Other risk factors, such as elevated blood lipids, smoking and obesity, were relatively uncommon. Both studies noted a moderate prevalence of background retinopathy, peripheral neuropathy and proteinuria. Proliferative retinopathy was rare. The main cause of visual loss was cataracts. Microvascular disease was associated with hypertension but not with HbA_1 concentrations. Dietary habits have been described in an Ethiopian study: low energy intake and a high ratio of polyunsaturated to saturated fatty acids seems to have favourably affected blood lipids and atherogenesis.

By contrast, migrant Indian Asians show very high rates of morbidity and mortality from coronary artery disease [74–76]. At least part of this seems to be related to the high prevalence of diabetes in these populations. Bangladeshis in East London [74] have three times the prevalence of diabetes and higher plasma triglyceride and insulin concentrations than those found in Europids. The authors hypothesize that insulin resistance may be the basic metabolic abnormality in Indian Asians, leading to hyperinsulinaemia, diabetes and abnormalities of lipoprotein metabolism, culminating in atherosclerotic coronary artery disease. This is, however, pure speculation.

Several excellent reports have been published on the clinical features and epidemiological characteristics of diabetes in Africa, with particular reference to Tanzania [43, 77–80]. There is evidence that diabetes in Africa is on the increase [77]. In a prospective study, Swai et al [78] noted that most patients in Tanzania do not require insulin. McLarty et al [79] showed that diabetes in sub-Saharan Africa is a serious disease with a poor prognosis, although most deaths are due to preventable causes. McLarty et al [80] have also reported on an interesting seasonal pattern of presentation of both insulin-requiring and non-insulin-requiring diabetes.

MALNUTRITION-RELATED DIABETES MELLITUS, PROTEIN-DEFICIENT DIABETES MELLITUS

In 1955, Hugh-Jones [81] described a form of diabetes with certain unique features, which he called 'J-type' diabetes because it was reported from Jamaica. The characteristics of this type of diabetes are: (a) onset in youth (usually between 15 years and 40 years of age); (b) insulin requirement with evidence of insulin resistance, as shown by the large amounts of insulin needed (more than 1.5 U/kg body weight); (c) ketosis resistance, i.e. absence of ketoacidosis even when insulin injections are withdrawn for long periods; and (d) extreme leanness with present evidence, or

a childhood history, of protein–energy malnutrition. The WHO Study Group report designated this form of diabetes as protein deficient diabetes mellitus (PDDM). The occurrence of a similar clinical syndrome has been reported from several tropical countries in Asia and Africa [3–5, 8–13]. Excellent studies by Tripathy and colleagues [82–84], Ahuja et al [85–89], Vaishnava et al [90] and others [91] have provided valuable data on the clinical and biochemical features of PDDM. There is usually no family history of diabetes in patients with PDDM. The onset of diabetes is abrupt with symptoms of severe hyperglycaemia, but apart from polyuria, polydipsia and polyphagia, affected individuals are not seriously ill. Blood glucose levels can be very high, ranging from 20 mmol/l to 30 mmol/l (360–540 mg/dl), but ketosis is rare. There is no response to sulphonylureas and insulin is required for maintenance of euglycaemia.

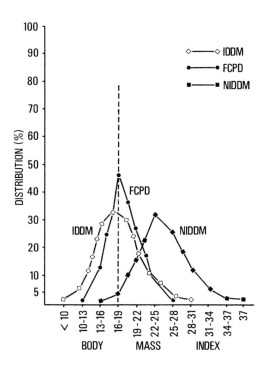

Figure 2 Distribution of patients with IDDM, FCPD and NIDDM, based on the body mass indices

One of the problems with PDDM is that it lacks a specific diagnostic marker [92]. The commonly suggested criteria [93], such as body mass index (BMI) below 19 kg/m² (some authors specify 18 or 17 kg/m² [172]), ketosis resistance or requirement of large doses of insulin, are not specific enough. Low BMI is seen in 70% of classic IDDM patients and not infrequently among NIDDM patients [32]. Figure 2 shows the distribution of BMI of the patients seen at the MV Diabetes Specialities Centre, Madras. If BMI below 19 kg/m² is used as a diagnostic criterion, several

IDDM and NIDDM patients would be classified as MRDM; conversely, about half of the patients with FCPD would be excluded from the diagnosis. Low BMI is thus of very little diagnostic value.

Ketosis resistance is a useful clinical clue, but it is not universal and does not always distinguish between patients with PDDM and those with IDDM, because even in the latter a slower progression of the disease to a ketosis-prone stage may occur in some patients. Moreover, with earlier diagnosis and intensive treatment of IDDM, the use of immunosuppressive drugs and other treatment modalities, there is better preservation of B-cell function. Ketoacidosis is therefore becoming less common in IDDM in Western societies [94]. At the Joslin Clinic, of a group of 127 newly diagnosed IDDM patient, 10% were in diabetic ketoacidosis, 49% had significant acetonuria, and 15% had minor acetonuria while the remaining 26% had hyperglycaemia and glycosuria without acetonuria [94]. Thus, even among IDDM patients seen in Western countries, absence of ketosis is not uncommon. It has also been shown that when IDDM sets in at an older age, ketosis is present only infrequently [94].

The large insulin doses required may be due to the use of impure insulins in tropical countries although insulin antibodies have not been demonstrated in this group of patients [95]. The role of ICA in distinguishing IDDM from PDDM is also limited, because ICA are present only in 30% of Indian IDDM patients (and few Africans) at the time of diagnosis, and this figure declines rapidly with increasing duration of diabetes [29]. Moreover, one study found ICA in 37% of PDDM cases [96]. Antibodies to Coxsackie B virus have also been found by the same group in PDDM patients [97].

From the above description it is obvious that the distinction of J-type diabetes from IDDM and PDDM is not as clear as was first thought. It is of interest that follow-up of the original J-type cases showed that many patients had reduced their insulin dose and could be controlled by oral agents, some had subsequently become ketoacidotic, and several had gained weight [98]. Some of Ahuja's patients also became ketoacidotic [86]. Lester [99], reported from Ethiopia that those of her patients who were initially diagnosed as having PDDM later were found to have classic features of IDDM. Abdulkadir et al [100] have reported similar findings.

Some authors have questioned the very existence of PDDM [8, 101]. It is worth emphasizing that studies in Tanzania showed no relation between NIDDM and current malnutrition (BMI < 19 kg/m^2) [174]. These subjects came from areas where infantile malnutrition was endemic. The overall prevalence of NIDDM was only 0.7% in adults aged over 16, suggesting that undernutrition was not important in the pathogenesis of diabetes

in these subjects. The evidence available to date neither dismisses nor establishes the presence of PDDM. The recent suggestion that this should be renamed malnutrition-modulated diabetes mellitus (MMDM) is probably wise [172]. In summary, clinicians in tropical countries frequently encounter young, lean, insulin-requiring diabetic patients who do not readily become ketotic. However, with the available markers, it is difficult to distinguish between an IDDM patient who is in a preketotic phase, and a patient with PDDM.

FIBROCALCULOUS PANCREATIC DIABETES

Diabetes secondary to pancreatic disorders is classified under 'other types' in the 1985 WHO classification of diabetes [5]. All forms of pancreatic disorders are associated with diabetes. However, acute pancreatitis only rarely leads to permanent diabetes, and other causes such as pancreatic carcinoma are rare. Diabetes secondary to pancreatic disorders is therefore usually due to chronic pancreatitis. In Western countries the most common cause of chronic pancreatitis is alcoholism [102]. Alcoholic pancreatitis with diabetes is a disease of middle age, and a history of alcoholism is present for several years before the onset of the disease. In the last two decades it has become increasingly apparent that there is a youth-onset form of chronic, non-alcoholic pancreatitis that is widely prevalent in several tropical countries. This type of chronic pancreatitis is termed 'tropical calcific pancreatitis (TCP) [103, 104], and the diabetes secondary to this form of pancreatitis has been referred to as 'pancreatic diabetes' [105] and 'tropical pancreatic diabetes' [106]. The WHO report [5] renamed this entity 'fibrocalculous pancreatic diabetes' (FCPD), as the two characteristic pathological features of the disease are fibrosis of the pancreas and the presence of pancreatic calculi. The rest of this chapter deals with the present state of knowledge regarding FCPD.

Historical Perspective

In 1959, Zuidema from Indonesia [107] was the first to describe cases of pancreatic calculi in association with diabetes. The report of Shaper from Kampala, Uganda, followed soon thereafter [108]. Subsequent reports from several tropical developing countries including Brazil, Congo, Nigeria, Madagascar, Kenya, Zimbabwe, Zambia, Thailand, Sri Lanka, Bangladesh, Singapore, New Guinea and India firmly established FCPD as a distinct form of diabetes [8]. In India, FCPD is more common in south India (situated within the tropical belt) than in north India (outside the tropics). The largest numbers of patients have been reported from the southwestern state of Kerala, where Geevarghese, one of the pioneers in this field, has seen over 1700 cases [109]. Large series have also been reported from the states of Tamil Nadu [110, 111], Orissa [112] and Karnataka [113]. Reports of FCPD have also been published from Andhra Pradesh [114], Bombay [115], Pune [116], Nagpur [117], Tripura [118] and New Delhi [119]. Figure 3 shows the distribution of FCPD in India.

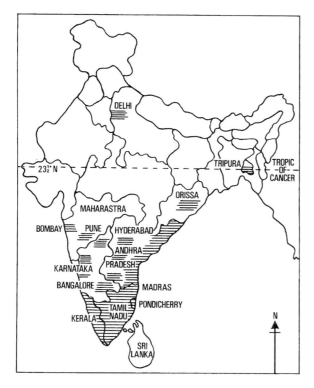

Figure 3 Map of India, with shaded areas showing the places where FCPD has been reported

Prevalence and Incidence of FCPD

There is only one population-based study on the prevalence of tropical chronic pancreatitis. Balaji [120] made a systematic survey of 6079 families in Quilon district, Kerala. A population of 28 507 was interviewed and 518 subjects identified who had one of the following three characteristics: abdominal pain suggestive of pancreatitis; diabetes mellitus; or a history of weight loss (malnutrition). Using a combination of abdominal radiographs, ultrasound and the N-benzoyl-L-tyrosyl-para-aminobenzoic acid (PABA) test, twenty-eight cases of chronic calcific pancreatitis (CCP) and eight cases of non-calcific pancreatitis (NCP) were identified. Thus 1 in 1020 subjects had CCP (0.09%). The prevalence of FCPD in diabetic clinic populations varies widely. Reports from Africa showed that in Zimbabwe 1% of diabetic patients had FCPD [121] and in Nigeria 8.6% of patients had FCPD [122]. In South

Africa, FCPD was found to be rare [123]. In Thailand, 14 of 253 (5.5%) of young diabetic patients, defined as those with age at diagnosis below 30 years, had FCPD [33]. Another 16 patients had signs of malnutrition but did not have pancreatic calculi. In Kerala, FCPD constituted 29.3% of the total diabetic cases registered and 1.3% of all inpatient admissions at the Kottayam Medical College in 1964. However, the latter rate came down to 0.03% in 1971 and 0.009% in 1980 [109]. It is not clear whether this is due to a true decline in the incidence of FCPD or merely represents a change in the priorities for admission at this hospital. In Indonesia also there has been a decline in the incidence of FCPD, but some centres continue to report new cases [124]. At the MV Diabetes Specialities Centre, Madras, we currently register 50–60 new patients with FCPD every year, which represents about 1% of all diabetics and 4% of 'young' diabetics, defined as those with age at diagnosis below 30 years [32].

Clinical Features

In Zuidema's original description [107], 18 cases of disseminated pancreatic calcification were described, of whom 16 had diabetes. All patients were poor and consumed diets deficient in proteins and energy. Emaciation, parotid gland enlargement and skin and hair changes resembling those of kwashiorkor were some of the striking clinical features. Twenty-seven other patients were also described with similar clinical features but without calcification of the pancreas. Most patients were young and steatorrhoea was not a prominent feature. In Shaper's report also [108], the patients were young and poor. A history of recurrent abdominal pain was present in over 50% of cases. In Kinnear's series from Nigeria [125], steatorrhoea was a prominent feature but abdominal pain was less common.

In its classic form, FCPD has several distinct characteristics. Diagnosis of diabetes is made in the majority of patients between the ages of 10 years and 40 years. There is a marked male predominance. Extreme emaciation, peculiar cyanotic hue of the lips, bilateral parotid enlargement and distended abdomen are some of the classic clinical features [103–105, 126]. Recently, however, there appears to be a change in the clinical features of the disease, perhaps because of people's better nutritional status. In one series, malnutrition was observed in only 25% of patients, although 70% were lean [106]. Nowadays, patients are seen from the middle and upper strata of society as well [106, 127]. Many patients give a past history of abdominal pain in childhood or adolescence, but this is rarely the main symptom for which they come to the diabetologist. This is because, in the natural history of the disease, painful abdomen usually occurs several years before the onset of diabetes and it usually disappears by the time that diabetes manifests. In a minority of patients the abdominal pain may persist or, indeed, may start after the onset of diabetes. The pain is usually severe, epigastric in location and characterized by periods of remission and exacerbation. It radiates to the back on either side and is typically relieved by stooping forward or lying in a prone position. About one-third of patients complain of passing bulky or oily stools. The low frequency of steatorrhoea has been attributed to the low fat content of the diet. When the fat content of the diet was experimentally increased, steatorrhoea occurred in over 90% of patients [128]. Other endocrine abnormalities such as absence of secondary sexual characteristics and sterility are not infrequently seen in these patients.

Nature of Diabetes

The diabetes is usually severe. Most patients require insulin for control of their diabetes. It is of interest, however, that despite requiring insulin for control of diabetes, patients with FCPD rarely develop ketoacidosis even if the insulin injections are withdrawn for prolonged periods [105, 110]. The authors [129] have recently observed a spectrum of glucose intolerance in tropical calcific pancreatitis. Although the majority of patients with TCP ultimately develop overt diabetes, in earlier stages of the disease a stage of impaired glucose tolerance may be seen and, at a still earlier stage, the OGTT can be normal (Figure 4). Even among those with overt diabetes, there is a spectrum ranging from those who can be treated with diet and oral agents to the occasional patient who is ketotic (Figure 5). There appears to be a good correlation between the response to treatment and the pancreatic B-cell function assessed by serum C-peptide levels [106]. Yajnik et al [116] have reported on the spectrum of pancreatic endocrine and exocrine function in TCP and confirmed the existence of an impaired glucose tolerance phase in the pathogenesis of FCPD. These features are very similar to those found in the chronic pancreatitis of developed countries.

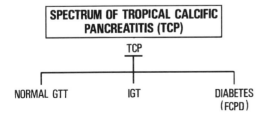

Figure 4 The clinical spectrum of tropical calcific pancreatitis with respect to glucose tolerance

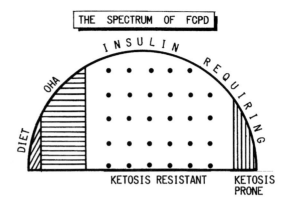

Figure 5 The wide spectrum of FCPD with respect to the type of treatment and proneness to ketosis

Radiological Features

The classic radiological finding in FCPD is the presence of pancreatic calculi on a plain X-ray of the abdomen [106, 110]. The calculi are mostly situated to the right of the first or second lumbar vertebrae, but may occasionally overlap the spine. In some patients the whole pancreas may be studded with calculi (Figure 6). It is extremely rare to find isolated calculi to the left of the vertebrae [109].

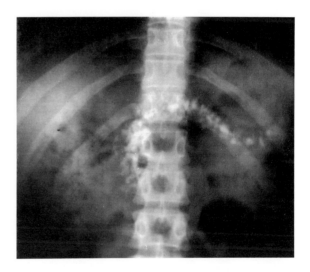

Figure 6 Plain X-ray of the abdomen showing multiple pancreatic calculi distributed throughout the whole of the pancreas

Ultrasonographic and ERCP Findings

Ultrasonography is a useful tool in the diagnosis of FCPD. Structural changes such as fibrosis and shrinkage of the gland, increased echogenicity and ductal dilatation can be made out in these patients [130]. Figure 7 shows the ultrasound scan of a patient with FCPD showing marked ductal dilatation. Ultrasonography also helps to localize the calculi to the pancreas and to document other features of chronic pancreatitis, e.g. ductal dilation. Endoscopic retrograde cholangiopancreatography (ERCP) studies were performed by Balakrishnan and colleagues in patients with tropical chronic pancreatitis [131]: it was seen that the patients with pancreatic calculi had marked ductal changes; in the non-calcific patients, ductal changes were minimal to moderate, and two patients had normal pancreatograms. Figure 8 shows the ERCP of a patient with FCPD showing a grossly dilated pancreatic duct.

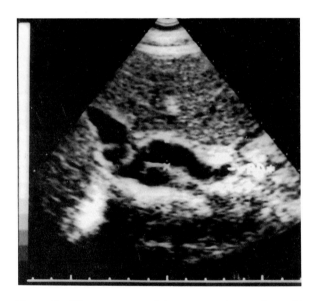

Figure 7 Ultrasonogram of the pancreas in a patient with FCPD showing markedly dilated pancreatic duct

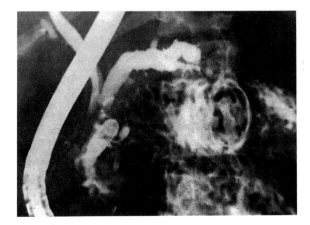

Figure 8 Endoscopic retrograde cholangiopancreatogram (ERCP) of a patient with FCPD showing grossly dilated and irregular pancreatic duct (courtesy of Dr Raja Sambandam and Dr Raghuram)

Lipid Studies

In the authors' experience, total cholesterol, low-density lipoprotein cholesterol and very low-density lipoprotein cholesterol were significantly lower among FCPD patients compared with NIDDM patients or non-diabetic control subjects [106]. However, serum triglyceride levels were normal.

Specific Diabetic Complications in FCPD

It was formerly believed that, as FCPD is a secondary form of diabetes, specific diabetic complications were uncommon. It has been shown more recently that the sight-threatening forms of retinopathy, namely proliferative retinopathy and maculopathy, do develop in FCPD when followed for long periods [132]. Neuropathy [133], nephropathy [106] and left ventricular dysfunction [134] also occurred in these patients. By contrast, macrovascular complications were less common [135], perhaps owing to the relative youth of the patients, their leanness and the low cholesterol levels [106]. Other complications frequently seen in FCPD are tuberculosis, urinary infections and cataract [103–105].

Ketosis Resistance

Earlier studies to explain the ketosis resistance in MRDM had suggested a number of mechanisms such as low adipose tissue mass and delayed mobilization of free fatty acids from adipose tissue [136, 137]. More recent studies have offered other explanations. In one study it was shown that although the plasma glucagon levels in IDDM patients rose after administration of oral glucose, in patients with MRDM (PDDM variety) there was a paradoxical fall in the glucagon levels [138]: thus low glucagon levels were suggested as one of the mechanisms for the resistance to ketosis. It has been reported that pancreatic A-cell function is defective in FCPD patients and the lack of glucagon response may be one of the factors responsible for protection against ketoacidosis [139]. Studies of pancreatic B-cell function have shown that FCPD patients have some residual function [140]. Figure 9 shows that the C-peptide levels in FCPD are intermediate between those seen in patients with NIDDM and IDDM. Thus, FCPD patients appear to have sufficient insulin to protect them from developing ketosis. These findings have subsequently been confirmed by other workers [141–143]. Yajnik et al [144] recently reported that the diminished B-cell function in FCPD may be at least partly reversible after treatment of diabetes.

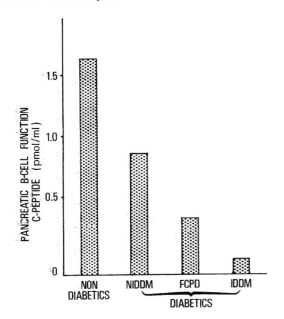

Figure 9 Stimulated serum C-peptide responses in non-diabetic control subjects and in patients with NIDDM, FCPD and IDDM (from reference 9, with permission)

Pathology of the Pancreas

The pathological findings in FCPD are quite striking [145, 146]. The pancreas is small, atrophic and fibrosed. There is extensive atrophy of the acini with replacement by sheets of fibrous tissue. Periductal fibrosis is a characteristic finding. The ducts are dilated and usually contain multiple calculi in the major ducts or its tributaries. Sometimes putty-like material or debris may be seen. There may be degeneration of the epithelium lining the duct. Inflammatory cells may be seen occasionally. The islets of Langerhans are usually normal or atrophic, but may be hypertrophied. The calculi are composed of carbonates, with traces of phosphates, oxalates, magnesium and proteins. The calculi vary greatly in size and shape, but are usually hard. The parotid glands show hypertrophy of the acini and sometimes cirrhotic changes may occur.

Recently it has been observed that whereas some patients may show extensive pathology in the pancreas, in some others there appears to be an arrested form of the disease with localized and minimal changes in the pancreas (S.J. Nagalotimath, personal communication). This might explain, at least in part, the heterogeneity noted with reference to the B-cell function, the response to therapy, as well as the proneness to ketosis referred to earlier (Table 1). Pitchumoni and colleagues [103, 147] have analysed the composition of pancreatic stones from FCPD patients by X-ray diffractiometry, scanning electron microscopy and energy dispersive X-ray fluorescence: they found that the stones are rich in $CaCO_3$ and many other elements. It was also shown that the nidus of the stone contained only iron, chromium and nickel, whereas the outer shell contained calcium and 17 other elements. These authors postulate that the formation of the pancreatic calculi takes place in numerous layers and stages. Formation of the inner protein nidus in the form of a cobweb is the first stage, then the calcite is deposited on this fibrous network as tiny crystals. Because of the large surface area and high surface activity of the calculi, other metallic ions are incorporated through coprecipitation, adsorption and/or lattice substitution. It is fascinating that, irrespective of the aetiology of chronic pancreatitis, the structure and

Table 1 Heterogeneity in tropical chronic pancreatitis

1. Symptoms	Asymptomatic	
	Marked symptoms	[109, 110]
2. Carbohydrate intolerance	Normal OGTT	
	IGT	
	Overt diabetes	[116, 129]
3. B-cell reserve	Good	
	Poor	
	Negligible	[106]
4. Response to therapy	Diet alone	
	Oral agents	
	Insulin	[106]
5. Proneness to ketosis	Ketosis-resistant	
	Ketosis-prone	[106, 109]
6. Exocrine dysfunction	Only after provocative tests	
	Clinical steatorrhoea	[103, 105]
7. ERCP	Absent to mild ductal changes	
	Marked ductal changes	[131]
8. Histopathology	Mild changes: calculi absent or small	
	Marked changes:	
	extensive fibrosis	
	ductal dilatation	
	multiple calculi	[145]

composition of pancreatic calculi are the same, suggesting that there could be a final common pathway for lithogenesis in tropical and alcoholic pancreatitis.

Exocrine Pancreatic Function

Several reports on exocrine pancreatic function tests in TCP have been published [109, 110]. Punnose et al [148] reported the usefulness of the Lundh meal test. Using a cut-off point of 2 IU/ml, 93% of the calcific TCP cases compared with 27% of the non-calcific variety had low tryptic activity. Secretin–pancreozymin tests done by Balakrishnan's group in collaboration with the Marseille group showed that the lactoferrin level of the duodenal juice was considerably higher in Indian patients and controls than in their European counterparts [149]. Yajnik et al [150], using serum immunoreactive trypsin levels to assess exocrine pancreatic function, found that 93% of FCPD patients compared with about 30% of IDDM patients and 15% of NIDDM patients had subnormal immunoreactive trypsin levels. It has been shown that the faecal chymotrypsin test is a simple, reliable and inexpensive test of exocrine pancreatic function, and 87% of FCPD patients had low faecal chymotrypsin levels [151].

Management of Chronic Pancreatitis in FCPD

Steatorrhoea, when present, can be reduced, but not totally alleviated, by the use of pancreatic extracts and various enzyme preparations [104]. Pain, if severe and intractable, may require surgical intervention. A variety of surgical procedures have been employed, reflecting the inadequacy of the available techniques [105, 110]. Sphincterotomy is of limited benefit. Side-to-side pancreaticojejunostomy has been tried, with varied results [104, 105]. Surgery does not influence the course of the disease or the insulin requirement [104]. Many patients have recurrence of pain.

Pathogenesis

The aetiology of FCPD is still far from clear. The following have been suggested as pathogenic factors.

Undernutrition

The clinical evidence of protein–energy malnutrition in FCPD patients has often been used to cite undernutrition as an aetiological factor. However, this could well be the effect rather than the cause, in that chronic pancreatitis with consequent maldigestion and malabsorption could itself lead to protein–energy malnutrition. The presence of large pockets of malnutrition with relative infrequency of FCPD, e.g. in Ethiopia [99], also suggests that malnutrition by itself is unlikely to have an aetiological role. It is of interest that Kerala State, with the highest literacy rate and lowest infant mortality rate, has the highest prevalence of FCPD in India [103]. The exact role of malnutrition in the pathogenesis of FCPD is thus far from clear. It is also possible that subclinical malnutrition (e.g. micronutrient deficiency) may contribute to pancreatic tissue damage in FCPD (see below).

Cassava Hypothesis

McMillan and Geevarghese [152] put forward the 'cassava hypothesis' to explain the occurrence of FCPD. The geographic distribution of FCPD coincides with the areas of consumption of cassava. Cassava is known to contain cyanogenic glycosides, linamarin and lotaustralin. Cyanide is normally detoxified in the body by conversion to thiocyanate. This detoxification requires sulphur which is derived from sulphur-containing amino acids. Experiments in rats [152] showed that ingestion of cyanide led to transient hyperglycaemia. It was therefore concluded that cyanide played a part in the pathogenesis of FCPD. It must, however, be noted that none of the rats in the above experiments developed permanent diabetes. Moreover, the effects were seen only with potassium cyanide and not with cassava; thus, the relevance of these experiments to the human situation is far from clear [103]. Doubts regarding the cassava hypothesis are raised by a study in which rats fed on a diet containing cassava did not show significant pancreatic damage, irrespective of whether they were malnourished or not [153]. Two other studies are contrary to the hypothesis: a study from the Ivory Coast [154] has shown that the chronic pancreatitis seen in that region was not related to either kwashiorkor or cassava ingestion. More important, a study was reported in a rural area of Tanzania where nerve damage secondary to cassava consumption is endemic [175]. The prevalence of diabetes and IGT were low and not different from other parts of the country despite high plasma cyanide and thiocyanate levels. Finally, although the cassava hypothesis might explain the occurrence of FCPD in areas where the tuber is consumed, it does not explain its occurrence in other areas (e.g. Madras) where it is not. The possibility exists that other foodstuffs such as sorghum, ragi, jowar or certain varieties of peas may contain cyanide.

Other Dietary Factors

Studies on the dietary intake of FCPD patients have been done by Balakrishnan's group in collaboration with that of Sarles in Marseille [149, 155]. The mean protein intake in the diet was 53 g per day in FCPD patients, which was not different from that of the controls. However, the fat intake of the diet of both FCPD patients and controls in India was very low (27 g per day). It is possible that a low fat intake could be one of the factors responsible for the occurrence of FCPD. Durbec and Sarles [156] have shown that a low-fat diet increases susceptibility to alcoholic pancreatitis.

Familial and Genetic Factors

Familial occurrence of FCPD is not uncommon and Pitchumoni [157] was the first to report on a large series of familial cases of FCPD. Familial aggregation has also been noted by Geevarghese [109] and Balakrishnan [155]. In a recent report the authors showed that about 10% of FCPD cases have a familial aggregation [158]. It is of interest that, whereas aggregation of FCPD occurs in some families, in others FCPD overlaps with NIDDM, and in the remaining families FCPD occurs in a sporadic manner. Familial occurrence suggests—but does not necessarily prove—a hereditary aetiology for FCPD. Several family members could be exposed to the same environmental factors that could produce the disease. However, support for a genetic predisposition to FCPD comes from a recent study of gene markers using the restriction fragment length polymorphism technique (RFLP) [159]. It was found that FCPD shares susceptibility genes in common with NIDDM (class 3 of the insulin gene) and IDDM patients (HLA-DQ β gene). This provides evidence for the first time of a genetic basis for FCPD.

Micronutrient Deficiency and Oxidant Stress

Chronic pancreatitis in Europids has been linked to 'heightened oxidative detoxification reactions' conducted by cytochrome $P450_1$ within the pancreas and/or liver [160]. Several factors may be involved, including chronic induction of cytochrome $P450_1$ subfamily of monoxygenases by xenobiotics (cigarettes, alcohol, occupational chemicals, dietary corn oil, etc.); concurrent exposure to a chemical that undergoes metabolic activation, and suboptimal intake of micronutrient antioxidants, especially those that defend cells against non-biological reactive intermediaries. Collaborative studies between our centre and Dr Braganza's group at the University of Manchester, UK, have revealed low intake of fat-soluble antioxidants, and this suggests low bioavailability of ascorbic acid [162]. Furthermore, theophylline clearance (a measure of cytochrome $P450_1$ activity *in vivo*) was faster in patients with FCPD than in controls [163]. These studies suggest, for the first time, that common aetiological factors may operate in tropical and temperate-zone pancreatitis.

Miscellaneous Theories

Nwokolo and Oli [164] suggested that FCPD could result from stasis caused by prolonged starvation leading to blockage of the pancreatic duct by inspissated mucous plugs. The viral aetiology has not been fully explored. One study [165] showed significantly raised antibody titres against mumps virus, cytomegalovirus and *Mycoplasma pneumoniae*. Various immunological changes have been described, such as reduction in T lymphocytes, elevation of IgG and IgM, and presence of pancreatic haemagglutinating antibodies [104, 155]. These changes may well be secondary, but their role in perpetuation of an already existing injury merits study.

Heterogeneity in Tropical Chronic Pancreatitis

The studies mentioned above highlight the heterogeneous nature of the chronic pancreatitis seen in developing countries.

Table 1 summarizes the evidence for the heterogeneity which is seen with respect to the clinical, biochemical, ERCP and histopathological features of tropical chronic pancreatitis. Indeed, the presence or absence of diabetes is in itself an evidence of the heterogeneous nature of this disease.

Criteria for FCPD

Despite excellent clinical descriptions of the disease, no definite criteria have been laid down as yet for the diagnosis of FCPD. Mohan et al [166] have proposed the following criteria for the diagnosis of FCPD, based on their own studies and an extensive review of the literature:

(1) Diabetes must be present according to the National Diabetes Data Group [167] or the WHO Study Group report criteria [5].
(2) There must be evidence of chronic pancreatitis. For this, the single most important diagnostic criterion is the presence of pancreatic calculi on plain X-ray of the abdomen. In cases where calculi are absent, at least three of the following must be present: (a) presence of structural pathology in the pancreas such as fibrosis, ductal dilation, etc., as demonstrated by ultrasound, computed tomographic scan, ERCP or on histopathology; (b) history of recurrent abdominal pain from childhood; (c) history of steatorrhoea; or (d) abnormal exocrine pancreatic function demonstrated by tests such as the secretin–pancreozymin or Lundh meal test, or tubeless tests such as the PABA test.
(3) Other causes of chronic pancreatitis, such as alcoholism, must be excluded.

The following are helpful clinical pointers to FCPD, but are not diagnostic criteria in themselves: (a) onset at young age; (b) leanness, i.e. body mass index below 19; (c) insulin-requiring diabetes (often requiring large doses) but absence of ketosis on withdrawal of insulin; and (d) present or past evidence of protein energy malnutrition.

Other Causes of Chronic Pancreatitis in Developing Countries

Although FCPD is the major form of chronic pancreatitis associated with diabetes in tropical countries, recent reports have suggested that alcoholic pancreatitis is becoming increasingly common. In a series of 200 patients with chronic pancreatitis in Brazil, 93% were reported to be alcoholic and there was no evidence of protein deficiency in the diets of these patients [168]. In another study in South African blacks, alcoholism was reported to be the cause of almost every case of chronic pancreatitis [169]. Pancreatic damage and diabetes may follow an epidemic of viral hepatitis [170]. In 7% of a consecutive series of African diabetic subjects aged 40 years or more, Seftel and co-workers found haemochromatosis associated with pancreatic fibrosis [171]. Rare causes of chronic pancreatitis in the tropics include roundworm infestations, schistosomiasis, etc. [105].

UNRESOLVED ISSUES IN DIABETES IN THE TROPICS

Future studies would help to determine the exact prevalence of IDDM in tropical countries and thus to determine whether IDDM is indeed as uncommon as it is now believed to be. Similarly, studies on NIDDM would help to prove or disprove the hypothesis that MODY is a syndrome distinct from classic NIDDM. Studies aimed at looking for possible explanations for the high prevalence of NIDDM in certain ethnic groups might lead to a better understanding of the pathogenesis of NIDDM. Finally, more studies are urgently needed on MRDM. Specific markers must be found in order to establish PDDM as a separate entity. With regard to FCPD, studies aimed at establishing the prevalence and incidence patterns in different tropical countries are needed. The role of malnutrition should be more clearly defined. The role of environmental and toxic factors needs to be explored. Further studies on the oxidant stress hypothesis certainly seem justified. Knowledge regarding the causative factors of this enigmatic problem might lead not only to possible prevention of this disease, but also to better understanding of other forms of diabetes.

REFERENCES

1. Havelock-Charles R. Discussion on diabetes mellitus in the tropics. Br Med J 1907; 2: 1051-64.
2. Tulloch JA. Diabetes mellitus in the tropics. Edinburgh: Livingstone, 1962.
3. West KM. Diabetes in the tropics: some lessons for western diabetology. In Podolsky S, Viswanathan M (eds) Secondary diabetes. The spectrum of the diabetic syndromes. New York: Raven Press, 1980; pp 249-56.
4. West KM. Epidemiology of diabetes and its vascular lesions. New York: Elsevier, 1978.
5. WHO Study Group Report on Diabetes Mellitus. WHO Technical Report Series 727. Geneva: WHO, 1985.
6. Yajnik CS. Diabetes in tropical developing countries. In Alberti KGMM, Krall LP (eds) Diabetes annual 6. Amsterdam: Elsevier, 1991; pp 62-81.
7. Ahuja MMS. Diabetes in the tropics—perspectives of research. Tohuku J Exp Med 1983; 141 (suppl): 65-72.
8. Abu-Bakare A, Taylor R, Gill GV, Alberti KGMM. Tropical or malnutrition related diabetes: a real syndrome? Lancet 1986; i: 1135-8.
9. Mohan V, Ramachandran A, Viswanathan M. Tropical diabetes. In Alberti KGMM, Krall LP (eds) Diabetes annual 1. Amsterdam: Elsevier, 1985; pp 82-92.
10. Mohan V, Ramachandran A, Viswanathan M. Tropical diabetes. In Alberti KGMM, Krall LP (eds) Diabetes annual 2. Amsterdam: Elsevier, 1986; pp 30-8.
11. Mohan V, Ekoe JM, Ramachandran A, Snehalatha C, Viswanathan M. Diabetes in the tropics: differences from diabetes in the west. Acta Diab Lat 1986; 23: 91-100.
12. Keen H, Ekoe JM. The geography of diabetes mellitus. Br Med Bull 1986; 40: 339-65.
13. Bajaj JS. Diabetes mellitus, the third dimension. In Mngola EN (ed.) Diabetes 1982. International Congress Series 600. Amsterdam: Excerpta Medica, 1983; pp 11-17.
14. Yajnik CS. Diabetes in tropical developing countries. In Alberti KGMM, Krall LP (eds) Diabetes annual 5. Amsterdam: Elsevier, 1990; pp 72-87.
15. Patel JC, Dhirawani MK, Kadekar SG. Analysis of 5481 subjects with diabetes mellitus. In Patel JC, Talwalkar NG (eds) Diabetes mellitus in the tropics. Bombay: Diabetic Association of India, 1966; pp 94-100.
16. Guptha OP. The study of juvenile diabetes in Ahmedabad. J Assoc Phys Ind 1964; 12: 89-93.
17. Krishnaswami CV, Chandra P. The significance of certain epidemiological variants in the genesis of juvenile insulin dependent diabetes. The need for a global programme of cooperation. Tohuku J Exp Med 1983; 141 (suppl): 161-70.
18. Zimmet P. Epidemiology of diabetes. In Ellenburg M, Rifkin H (eds) Diabetes mellitus theory and practice. New York: Medical Examination, 1983; pp 451-68.
19. Thadanand S, Vannasaeng S, Nitiyanant W, Vichayanrat A. Diabetes in developing countries in 1985—present situation in Asia. IDF Bull 1986; 7: 3-8.

20. Lee TD, Zhaio T, Chi Z, Wong H, Shen M, Rochey G. HLA-A and B and DR phenotypes in mainland Chinese patients with diabetes mellitus. Tissue Antigens 1984; 22: 92–4.

21. Gen-yao Y, Fan-hua K, Chang-yu P, Shi-min W, Dong-lin L, Wei-gin W, Xin-yun Z. HLA study of insulin dependent diabetes mellitus amongst Chinese. In Proceedings of the 2nd Asian Symposium on Childhood and Juvenile Diabetes Mellitus, Tokyo. Amsterdam: Excerpta Medica, 1985; pp 106–110.

22. Bhatia E, Mehra NK, Taneja V, Vaidya MC, Ahuja MMS. HLA-DR antigen frequencies in a North Indian type 1 population. Diabetes 1985; 34: 565–7.

23. Kirk RL, Ranford PR, Serjeantson SW et al. HLA, complement C2, C4, properdin factor B and glyoxalase types in South Indian diabetics. Diabetes Res Clin Pract 1985; 1: 41–7.

24. Serjeantson SW, Ranford PR, Kirk RL et al. HLA DR and DQ DNA genotyping in insulin dependent diabetes patients in South India. Disease Markers 1987; 5: 101–8.

25. Hammond MG, Asmal AC. HLA and insulin dependent diabetes in South African Indians. Tissue Antigens 1980; 15: 244–8.

26. Hitman GA, Karir PK, Sachs JA, Ramachandran A, Snehalatha C, Mohan V, Viswanathan M. HLA-D region RFLPs indicate that susceptibility to insulin dependent diabetes in south India is located in the HLA-DQ region. Diabet Med 1988; 5: 57–60.

27. McLarty DG, Athaide I, Bottazzo GF, Swai ABM, Alberti KGMM. Islet cell antibodies are not specifically associated with insulin-dependent diabetes in Tanzanian Africans. Diabetes Res Clin Pract 1990; 9: 219–24.

28. Srikantia S, Malaviya NK, Mehra MC, Vaidya PJ, Geevarghese PJ, Ahuja MMS. Autoimmunity in type 1 (insulin dependent) diabetes mellitus in North India. J Clin Immunol 1981; 1: 169–73.

29. Ramachandran A, Rosenbloom AL, Mohan V et al. Autoimmunity in South Indian patients with IDDM. Diabetes Care 1985; 9: 435.

30. Omar MAK, Bottazzo GF, Asmal AC. Islet cell antibodies and other autoantibodies in South African Blacks and Indians with insulin dependent diabetes mellitus (IDDM). Horm Metab Res 1986; 18: 126–8.

31. Odugbesan O, Fletcher JA, Sanders A et al. Autoantibodies in Indian Asians with insulin dependent diabetes in the UK. Postgrad Med J 1988; 64: 357.

32. Ramachandran A, Mohan V, Snehalatha C, Bharani G, Chinnikrishnudu M, Mohan R, Viswanathan M. Clinical features of diabetes in the young as seen at a diabetes centre in south India. Diabetes Res Clin Pract 1988; 4: 117–25.

33. Vannasaeng S, Nitiyanant W, Vichayanrat A, Ploybutr S. Characteristics of diabetes with onset under 30 years in Thailand. In Mimura G (ed.) Childhood and juvenile diabetes mellitus. Amsterdam: Excerpta Medica, 1985; pp 75–9.

34. Mustaffa B, Ngan A. Youth onset diabetes in a Malaysian population. In Mimura G (ed.) Childhood and juvenile diabetes mellitus. Amsterdam: Excerpta Medica, 1985; pp 49–54.

35. Ramachandran A, Jali MV, Mohan V et al. High prevalence of diabetes in an urban population in South India. Br Med J 1988; 297: 587.

36. Verma NPS, Mehta SP, Madhu S, Mather HM, Keen H. Prevalence of known diabetes in an urban Indian environment. The Darya Ganj survey. Br Med J 1986; 293: 423–4.

37. Ahuja MMS. Epidemiological studies in diabetes mellitus in India. In Ahuja MMS (ed.) Epidemiology of diabetes mellitus in developing countries. New Delhi: Interprint, 1979.

38. Omar MAK, Seedat MA, Dyer RB et al. Diabetes and hypertension in South African Indians. A community study. S Afr Med J 1988; 73: 635.

39. Simmons D, Williams DRR, Powell MJ. Prevalence of diabetes in a predominantly Asian community: preliminary findings of the Coventry diabetes study. Br Med J 1989; 298: 18.

40. Ramachandran A, Snehalatha C, Dharmaraj D, Viswanathan M. Prevalence of glucose intolerance in Asian Indians: urban–rural difference and significance of upper body adiposity. Diabetes Care 1992; 15: 1348–55.

41. Ramachandran A, Mohan V, Snehalatha C et al. Prevalence of non-insulin dependent diabetes mellitus in Asian Indian families with a single diabetic parent. Diabetes Res Clin Pract 1988; 4: 241.

42. Fisch A, Pichard E, Prazuck T et al. Prevalence and risk factors of diabetes mellitus in the rural region of Mali (West Africa). A practical approach. Diabetologia 1987; 30: 859.

43. McLarty DG, Kitange HM, Mtinangi BL et al. Prevalence of diabetes and impaired glucose tolerance in rural Tanzania. Lancet 1989; i: 871–5.

44. Swai ABM, McLarty DG, Sherrif F et al. Diabetes and impaired glucose tolerance in an Asian community in Tanzania. Diabetes Res Clin Pract 1990; 8: 227–34.

45. Mather HM, Keen H. The Southall diabetes survey: prevalence of known diabetes in Asians and Europeans. Br Med J 1985; 291: 1081–4.

46. Mohan V, Ramachandran A, Snehalatha C, Mohan R, Bharani G, Viswanathan M. High prevalence of maturity onset diabetes of the young (MODY) among Indians. Diabetes Care 1985; 8: 371–4.

47. Asmal AC, Dayal B, Jialal I et al. Non-insulin dependent diabetes mellitus with young age at onset in Blacks and Indians. S Afr Med J 1981; 60: 93–6.

48. Belcher DW. Diabetes mellitus in Northern Ethiopia. Ethiop Med J 1970; 8: 73–84.

49. Mohan V, Ramachandran A, Snehalatha C, Jayashree R, Viswanathan M. C-peptide responses to glucose load in maturity onset diabetes of young (MODY). Diabetes Care 1985; 8: 69–72.

50. Mohan V, Snehalatha C, Ramachandran A, Viswanathan M. Abnormalities of insulin secretion in healthy offspring of Indian patients with maturity onset diabetes of the young. Diabetes Care 1986; 9: 53–6.

51. Mohan V, Sharp PS, Aber VR, Mather HM, Kohner EM. Insulin resistance in maturity onset diabetes of the young. Diabète Métab 1987; 13: 193–7.

52. Jialal I, Joubert SM, Asmal AC et al. The insulin and glucose responses to an oral glucose load in non-insulin dependent diabetes of the young. S Afr Med J 1982; 61: 351–4.

53. Jialal I, Joubert SM. Obesity does not modulate insulin secretion in patients with non-insulin dependent diabetes in the young. Diabetes Care 1984; 7: 77–9.

54. Naidoo C, Jialal I, Joubert SM. Arginine stimulated acute phase of insulin secretion in non-insulin

dependent diabetes in the young. Diabetes Res Clin Pract 1986; 3: 127–9.

55. Tattersall RB, Fajans, SS. A difference between the inheritance of classical juvenile diabetes and maturity onset type diabetes of young people. Diabetes 1975; 24: 44–53.

56. Tattersall RB. The present status of maturity onset diabetes of young people (MODY). In Kobberling J, Tattersall RB (eds) Genetics of diabetes mellitus. London: Academic Press, 1982; pp 261–70.

57. Fajans SS. Heterogeneity between various families with non-insulin dependent diabetes of the MODY type. In Kobberling J, Tattersall RB (eds) Genetics of diabetes mellitus. London: Academic Press, 1982; pp 251–60.

58. Tattersall RB. Mild familial diabetes with dominant inheritance. Q J Med 1974; 43: 339–57.

59. Ramachandran A, Snehalatha C, Mohan V, Viswanathan M. Vascular complications in Asian Indian non-insulin dependent diabetic patients. In Proceedings of the International Symposium on Epidemiology of Diabetes Mellitus. J Med Assoc Thai 1987; 70 (suppl 2): 180–4.

60. Mohan V, Ramachandran A, Viswanathan M. Southall Diabetes Survey (letter). Br Med J 1986; 292: 58–9.

61. Marine N, Edelstein O, Jackson WPU, Vinik AI. Diabetes, hyperglycaemia and glycosuria among Indians, Malayas and Africans (Bantus) in Cape Town, South Africa. Diabetes 1969; 18: 840–57.

62. Zimmet P, Taylar R, Ram P et al. Prevalence of diabetes and impaired glucose tolerance in the bi-racial (Melanesian and Indian) population of Fiji: urban–rural comparison. Am J Epidemiol 1983; 118: 673–8.

63. Poon-King T, Henry MV, Rampersad F. Prevalence and natural history of diabetes in Trinidad. Lancet 1968; i: 155–60.

64. Tattersall RB. Diabetes in offspring of conjugal diabetic parents. In Creutzfeldt W, Neel JV (eds) Genetics of diabetes mellitus. Berlin: Springer, 1976; pp 181–5.

65. Viswanathan M, Mohan V, Snehalatha C, Ramachandran A. High prevalence of type 2 (non-insulin dependent) diabetes among offspring of conjugal type 2 diabetic parents in S. India. Diabetologia 1985; 28: 907–10.

66. Mohan V, Sharp PS, Cloke HR, Burrin JM, Schumer B, Kohner EM. Serum immunoreactive insulin responses to glucose load in Asian Indian and European type 2 (non-insulin dependent) diabetic patients and control subjects. Diabetologia 1986; 29: 235–7.

67. Sharp PS, Mohan V, Levy JC, Mather HM, Kohner EM. Insulin resistance in patients of Asian Indian and European origin with non-insulin dependent diabetes. Horm Metab Res 1987; 19: 84–5.

68. Diabetes Drafting Group. Prevalence of small vessel and large vessel disease in diabetic patients from 14 centres. The WHO Multinational Study of Vascular Disease in Diabetics. Diabetologia 1985; 28 (suppl): 615.

69. Lester FT, Keen H. Macrovascular disease in middle-aged diabetic patients in Addis Ababa, Ethiopia. Diabetologia 1988; 31: 361.

70. Rolfe M. Macrovascular disease in diabetics in Central Africa. Br Med J 1988; 296: 1522.

71. Rolfe M. The neurology of diabetes mellitus in Central Africa. Diabet Med 1988; 5: 399.

72. Rolfe M. Diabetic eye disease in Central Africa. Diabetologia 1988; 31: 88.

73. Rolfe M. Diabetic renal disease in Central Africa. Diabet Med 1988; 5: 630.

74. McKeigue PM, Marmot MG, Syndercombe Court YD et al. Diabetes, hyperinsulinaemia and coronary risk factors in Bangladeshis in East London. Br Heart J 1988; 60: 390.

75. Editorial. Coronary heart disease in Indians overseas. Lancet 1986; i: 1307.

76. Tuomilehto J, Zimmet P, Kankaanpaa J et al. Prevalence of ischaemic ECG abnormalities according to the diabetes status in the population of Fiji and their associations with other risk factors. Diabetes Res Clin Pract 1988; 5: 205.

77. McLarty DG, Pollitt C, Swai ABM. Diabetes in Africa. Diabet Med 1990; 7: 670–84.

78. Swai ABM, Lutale J, McLarty DG. Diabetes in tropical Africa: a prospective study, 1981–7. I. Characteristics of newly presenting patients in Dar es Salaam, Tanzania, 1981–7. Br Med J 1990; 300: 1103–6.

79. McLarty DG, Kinabo L, Swai ABM, II. Course and prognosis. Br Med J 1990; 300: 1107–10.

80. McLarty DG, Yusafali A, Swai ABM. Seasonal incidence of diabetes mellitus in tropical Africa. Diabet Med 1989; 6: 762–5.

81. Hugh-Jones P. Diabetes in Jamaica. Lancet 1955; ii: 891–7.

82. Tripathy BB, Kar BC. Observations on the clinical profile of diabetes mellitus in India. Diabetes 1965; 14: 404–12.

83. Tripathy BB, Samal KC, Tej SC. Clinical profile of young onset diabetes in Orissa, India. In Bajaj JS (ed.) Diabetes mellitus in developing countries. New Delhi: Interprint, 1984; pp 159–64.

84. Kar BC, Tripathy BB. Observations on type 'J' diabetes. J Assoc Phys Ind 1965; 13: 181–7.

85. Ahuja MMS. Ketosis resistant young diabetics. Lancet 1965; i: 1254–5.

86. Ahuja MMS, Talwar GP, Verma VM, Kumar R. Diabetes mellitus in young Indians. Ind J Med Res 1965; 53: 1138–43.

87. Krishna Ram B, Ahuja MMS. A study of intermediary metabolism in different clinical types of diabetes mellitus in India (with reference to pyruvate, lactate, glycerol and plasma insulin). Ind J Med Res 1970; 58: 456–67.

88. Ahuja MMS, Umashankar P, Gary VK. Different clinical types of Indian diabetics, characterisation based on response of immunoreactive plasma insulin responses to glucose and tolbutamide load. Ind J Med Res 1972; 60: 123–31.

89. Ahuja MMS. Profile of young Indian diabetics: biochemical studies. Acta Diabet Lat 1972; 60: 123–31.

90. Vaishnava H, Bhasin RC, Gulati PD. Diabetes mellitus with onset under 40 years in northern India. J Assoc Phys Ind 1974; 22: 879–88.

91. Patney NL, Wahal PK, Paharoi SB, Sharma BB. Observations on clinical profile of diabetes in young Indian subjects. In Bajaj JS (ed.) Diabetes mellitus in developing countries. New Delhi: Interprint, 1984; pp 180–5.

92. Mohan V, Ramachandran A, Snehalatha C, Viswanathan M. Malnutrition related diabetes mellitus (letter). J Assoc Phys Ind 1987; 35: 671.

93. Ahuja MMS. Heterogeneity in tropical pancreatic diabetes (letter). Diabetologia 1985; 28: 708.

94. Krolewski AS, Warram JA, Christlieb AR. Onset, course, complications and prognosis of diabetes mellitus. In Marble A, Krall LP, Bradley RF, Christlieb AR, Soeldner JS (eds) Joslin's diabetes mellitus, 12th edn. Philadelphia: Lea & Febiger, 1985; pp 251–77.

95. Rao H. The role of undernutrition in the pathogenesis of diabetes mellitus. Diabetes Care 1984; 7: 595–600.

96. Hazra DK, Singh R, Singh B, Gupta MK, Agarwal P, Mittal S. Autoantibodies in tropical, ketosis-resistant but insulin dependent diabetes mellitus. In Bajaj JS (ed.) Diabetes mellitus in developing countries. New Delhi: Interprint, 1984; pp 165–8.

97. Hazra DK, Singh R, Wahal PK et al. Coxsackie antibodies in young Asian diabetics (letter). Lancet 1980; i: 877.

98. Tulloch JA, Macintosh D. J type diabetes. Lancet 1961; ii: 119–21.

99. Lester FT. A search for malnutrition related diabetes in an Ethiopian diabetic clinic. IDF Bull 1984; 29: 14–16.

100. Abdulkadir J, Mengesha B, Welde Gebriel Z et al. The clinical and hormonal (C-peptide and glucagon) profile and liability to ketoacidosis during nutritional rehabilitation in Ethiopian patients with malnutrition-related diabetes mellitus. Diabetologia 1990; 33: 222–7.

101. Oli JM. Diabetes mellitus in Africans. J Roy Coll Phys 1983; 17: 224–7.

102. Singer MV, Sarles H. Chronic pancreatitis in western Europe. In Podolsky S, Viswanathan M (eds) Secondary diabetes. New York: Raven Press, 1980; pp 89–104.

103. Pitchumoni CS. 'Tropical' or 'nutritional pancreatitis' —an update. In Gyr KE, Singer MV, Sarles H (eds) Pancreatitis—concepts and classification. Amsterdam: Elsevier, 1984; 359–63.

104. Balakrishnan V. Chronic calcifying pancreatitis in the tropics. Ind J Gastroenterol 1984; 3: 65–7.

105. Geevarghese PJ. Pancreatic diabetes. Bombay: Popular Prakashan, 1968.

106. Mohan V, Mohan R, Susheela L et al. Tropical pancreatic diabetes in South India: heterogeneity in clinical and biochemical profile. Diabetologia 1985; 28: 229–32.

107. Zuidema PJ. Cirrhosis and disseminated calcification of the pancreas in patients with malnutrition. Trop Geo Med 1959; 11: 70–4.

108. Shaper AG. Chronic pancreatic disease and protein malnutrition. Lancet 1960; ii: 1223–4.

109. Geevarghese PJ. Calcific pancreatitis. Bombay: Varghese, 1985.

110. Viswanathan M. Pancreatic diabetes in India: an overview. In Podolsky S, Viswanathan M (eds) Secondary diabetes. The spectrum of the diabetic syndromes. New York: Raven Press, 1980; pp 105–16.

111. Moses SGP, Kannan V. The clinical profile of undernourished diabetics aged 30 years or less with associated complications in Madras, India. In Baba S, Goto Y, Fukui I (eds) Diabetes mellitus in Asia. Amsterdam: Excerpta Medica, 1976; pp 259–62.

112. Tripathy BB. Diabetes with exocrine pancreatic disease. In Bajaj JS (ed.) Diabetes in developing countries. New Delhi: Interprint, 1984; pp 135–42.

113. Hedge JS, Jituri KH, Channappa NK. Pancreatic diabetes in Hubli area (N. Karnataka). J Assoc Phys Ind 1976; 24: 305–7.

114. Rao SV, Choudhurani CPD, Sathyanarayana S. Pancreatic calculi with diabetes. In Patel JC, Talwakar NG (eds) Diabetes in the tropics. Bombay: Diabetic Association of India, 1966; pp 234–8.

115. Ratnam VS, Bhandarkar SJ, Bapar RD, Rais N, Rao PN. Diabetes with pancreatic calcification. In Bajaj JS (ed.) Diabetes in developing countries. New Delhi: Interprint, 1984; pp 147–9.

116. Yajnik CS, Shelgikar KM, Sahasrabudhe RA et al. The spectrum of pancreatic exocrine and endocrine (beta-cell) function in tropical calcific pancreatitis. Diabetologia 1990; 33: 417–21.

117. Pendsey SP, Doongaji SK, Vaidya MG. Clinical profile of fibrocalculous pancreatic diabetes (FCPD) from Vidarbha region. J Diabet Assoc Ind 1990; 30: 7–10.

118. Bhattacharyya PK, Mohan V, Ramachandran A, Viswanathan M. Fibrocalculous pancreatic diabetes in Tripura. Antiseptic 1990; 87: 161–5.

119. Ahuja MMS, Sharma GP. Serum C-peptide content in nutritional diabetes. Horm Metab Res 1985; 17: 267–8.

120. Balaji LN. The problem of chronic calcific pancreatitis. PhD Thesis. All India Institute of Medical Sciences, New Delhi, 1988.

121. Gefland M, Forbes J. Diabetes mellitus in the Rhodesian African. S Afr Med J 1953; 32: 1208–13.

122. Osuntokun BO, Akinkugbe FM, Francis TI, Reddy S, Osuntokun O, Taylor GOL. Diabetes mellitus in Nigerians. A study of 832 patients. W Afr Med J 1971; 20: 295–312.

123. Omar MAK, Asmal AC. Patterns of diabetes mellitus in young Africans and Indians in Natal. Trop Geog Med 1984; 36: 133–8.

124. Kariadi SHKS. Diabetes with pancreatic calcification. In Baba S, Iwai S, Sukaton U (eds) Diabetes mellitus as related to over- and under-nutrition. Kobe: International Center for Medical Research, Kobe University School of Medicine, 1984; pp 125–30.

125. Kinnear TWA. Patterns of diabetes in a Nigerian teaching hospital. W Afr Med J 1963; 40: 228–33.

126. Viswanathan M, Sampath KS, Sarada S, Krishnaswami CV. Etiopathological and clinical profile of pancreatic diabetes from Madras. J Assoc Phys Ind 1973; 21: 753–9.

127. Narendranathan M. Chronic calcific pancreatitis of the tropics. Trop Gastroenterol 1981; 2: 40–5.

128. Ramachandran M, Pai KN. Clinical features and management of pancreatic diabetes. In Bhaskar Rao M (ed.) Diabetes mellitus. New Delhi: Arnold Heinemann, 1977; pp 239–46.

129. Mohan V, Chari S, Viswanathan M, Madanagopalan N. Tropical calcific pancreatitis in southern India. Proc Roy Coll Phys Edin 1990; 20: 34–42.

130. Mohan V, Sreeram D, Ramachandran A, Viswanathan M, Doraiswamy KRI. Ultrasonography of the pancreas in tropical pancreatic diabetes. Acta Diabetol Lat 1985; 22: 143–8.

131. Balakrishnan V, Hariharan M, Rao VRK, Anand BS. Endoscopic pancreatography in chronic pancreatitis of the tropics. Digestion 1985; 32: 128–31.

132. Mohan R, Rajendran B, Mohan V, Ramachandran A, Viswanathan M. Retinopathy in tropical pancreatic diabetes. Arch Ophthalmol 1985; 103: 1487–9.

133. Ramachandran A, Mohan V, Kumaravel TS et al. Peripheral neuropathy in tropical pancreatic diabetes. Acta Diabetol Lat 1986; 23: 135–40.

134. Ramachandran A, Mohan V, Snehalatha C et al. Left ventricular function in fibrocalculous pancreatic diabetes. Acta Diabetol Lat 1987; 24: 81–4.

135. Mohan V, Ramachandran A, Viswanathan M. Two case reports of macrovascular complications in fibrocalculous pancreatic diabetes. Acta Diabetol Lat 1989; 26: 345–9.

136. Hagroo AA, Verma NPS, Datta P, Ajmani NK, Vaishnava H. Observations on lipolysis in ketosis resistant growth onset diabetes. Diabetes 1974; 23: 268–75.

137. Ahuja MMS, Viswanathan K. Differential mobilisation of non-esterified fatty acids and insulin reserve in various types of diabetes mellitus in India. Ind J Med Res 1967; 55: 870–83.

138. Rao RH, Vigg BL, Rao KSJ. Suppressible glucagon secretion in young ketosis resistant, type 'J' diabetic patients in India. Diabetes 1983; 32: 1168–71.

139. Mohan V, Snehalatha C, Ramachandran A, Chari S, Madanagopalan N, Viswanathan M. Plasma glucagon responses in tropical fibrocalculous pancreatic diabetes. Diabetes Res Clin Pract 1990; 9: 97–101.

140. Mohan V, Snehalatha C, Jayashree R, Ramachandran A, Viswanathan M. Pancreatic beta cell function in tropical pancreatic diabetes. Metabolism 1983; 32: 1091–2.

141. Sood R, Ahuja MMS, Karmarkar MG. Serum C-peptide levels in young ketosis resistant diabetics. Ind J Med Res 1983; 78: 661–4.

142. Vannasaeng S, Nitiyanant W, Vachayanrat A, Ploybutr S, Harnthong S. C-peptide secretion in calcific tropical pancreatic diabetes. Metabolism 1986; 35: 814–17.

143. Samal KC, Das S, Parija CR, Tripathy BB. C-peptide response to glycaemic stimuli. J Assoc Phys Ind 1987; 37: 362–4.

144. Yajnik CS, Kanitkar SV, Shelgikar KM, Naik SS, Alberti KGMM, Hockaday D. Pancreatic C-peptide response to oral glucose in fibrocalculous pancreatic diabetes: improvement after treatment. Diabetes Care 1990; 13: 525–7.

145. Nagalotimath SJ. Pancreatic pathology in pancreatic calcification with diabetes. In Podolsky S, Viswanathan M (eds) Secondary diabetes: the spectrum of the diabetic syndromes. New York: Raven Press, 1980; pp 117–45.

146. Ramachandran P, Saraswathy B, Ramachandran M, Thangavelu M. Endemic pancreatic syndrome of Kerala—etiopathology. Ind J Med Res 1969; 57: 2075–82.

147. Pitchumoni CS, Viswanathan KV, Geevarghese PJ, Banks PA. Ultrastructure and elemental composition of human pancreatic calculi. Pancreas 1987; 2: 152–8.

148. Punnose J, Balakrishnan V, Bhadran A. Exocrine pancreatic function in chronic pancreatitis with and without calcification. Ind J Gastroenterol 1987; 6: 85–6.

149. Balakrishnan V, Sauniere JH, Hariharan M et al. Diet, pancreatic function and chronic pancreatitis in South India and France. Pancreas 1988; 3: 30–5.

150. Yajnik CS, Katrak A, Kanitkar SV et al. Serum immunoreactive trypsin in tropical pancreatic diabetes syndrome. Ann Clin Biochem 1989; 26: 69–73.

151. Mohan V, Snehalatha C, Ahmed MR et al. Exocrine pancreatic function in tropical fibrocalculous pancreatic diabetes. Diabetes Care 1989; 12: 145–7.

152. McMillan D, Geevarghese PJ. Dietary cyanide and tropical malnutrition diabetes. In Podolsky S, Viswanathan M (eds) Secondary diabetes. The spectrum of the diabetic syndromes. New York: Raven Press, 1980; pp 239–48.

153. Pushpa M. Chronic cassava toxicity: an experimental study. MD (Pathology) Thesis, University of Kerala, 1980.

154. Sarles H, Sauniere JF, Atia Y et al. Pancreatic function in children and chronic calcific pancreatitis in the Ivory Coast. The tropical form of CCP is not due to kwashiorkor or cassava. In Gyr KE, Singer MV, Sarles H (eds) Pancreatitis: concepts and classification. Amsterdam: Elsevier, 1984; pp 365–6.

155. Balakrishnan V. Tropical pancreatitis (pancreatite tropicale). In Bernades P, Hugier M (eds) Maladies du pancreas exocrine. Paris: Doin, 1987.

156. Durbec JP, Sarles H. Multicentric survey of the etiology of pancreatic disease: relationship between the relative risk of developing chronic pancreatitis and alcohol, protein and lipid consumption. Digestion 1978; 18: 337–70.

157. Pitchumoni CS, Geevarghese PJ. Familial pancreatitis and diabetes mellitus. In Patel JC, Talwalkar NG (eds) Proceedings of the World Congress on Diabetes in the Tropics. Bombay: Diabetic Association of India, 1966; pp 240–1.

158. Mohan V, Chari S, Hitman GA et al. Familial aggregation in tropical fibrocalculous pancreatic diabetes. Pancreas 1989; 4: 690–3.

159. Kambo PK, Hitman GA, Mohan V et al. The genetic predisposition to fibrocalculous pancreatic diabetes. Diabetologia 1989; 32: 45–7.

160. Braganza JM. Free radicals and pancreatitis. In Rice-Evans C, Dormandy T (eds) Free radicals: chemistry, pathology and medicine. London: Richelieu Press, 1988; pp 357–81.

161. Yajnik CS. Malnutrition-related diabetes mellitus: diagnosis and treatment. IDF Bulletin 1992; 37: 11–73.

162. Braganza JM, John S, Padmalayam I et al. Xenobiotics and tropical chronic pancreatitis. Int J Pancreatol 1990; 5: 231–45.

163. Chaloner C, Sandle LN, Mohan V, Snehalatha C, Viswanathan M, Braganza JM. Evidence for induction of cytochrome P-450 I in patients with tropical chronic pancreatitis. Int J Clin Pharm Ther Toxicol 1990; 28: 235–40.

164. Nwokolo C, Oli J. Pathogenesis of juvenile tropical pancreatitis syndrome. Lancet 1980; i: 456–8.

165. Shenoy KT, Shanmugham J, Balakrishnan V. Viral and *Mycoplasma pneumoniae* antibodies in chronic pancreatitis of tropics. Ind J Med Res 1986; 84: 22–6.

166. Mohan V, Ramachandran A, Viswanathan M. Diabetes secondary to tropical pancreatopathy. In Tiengo A, Alberti KGMM, Del Prato S, Vranic M (eds) Diabetes secondary to pancreatopathy. Amsterdam: Elsever, 1988: pp 215–26.

167. National Diabetes Data Group. Classification of diabetes and other categories of glucose intolerance. Diabetes 1979; 28: 1039–59.

168. Mot CB, Guarita DR, Machado MCC, Bettarello A. Epidemiology and etiology of chronic pancreatitis in Sao Paulo (Brazil): a prospective study of 200 cases. In Gyr KE, Singer MV, Sarles H (eds) Pancreatitis: concepts and classification. Amsterdam: Elsevier, 1984; pp 355–8.

169. Segal I, Lerios M, Grieve T. The emergence of chronic calcific pancreatitis in a developing country. In Gyr KE, Singer MV, Sarles H (eds) Pancreatitis: concepts and classification. Amsterdam: Elsevier, 1984; pp 417–20.

170. Oli JM, Nwokolo C. Diabetes after infectious hepatitis: a follow-up study. Br Med J 1979; 1: 926–7.

171. Seftel HC, Keeley KJ, Isaacson C, Bothwell TH. Siderosis in the Bantu: the clinical incidence of haemochromatosis in diabetic subjects. J Lab Clin Med 1961; 58: 837–44.

172. Workshop Report. Consensus statement from the International Workshop on Types of Diabetes Peculiar to the Tropics, 17–19 October 1995, Cuttack, India. Acta Diabetol 1996; 33: 62–4.

173. Swai ABM, Lutale J, McLarty DG. Prospective study of incidence of juvenile diabetes in Dar es Salaam, Tanzania. Br Med J 1993; 306: 1570–2.

174. Swai ABM, Kitange HM, Masuki G, Kilima PM, Alberti KGMM, McLarty DG. Is diabetes related to undernutrition in rural Tanzania? Br Med J 1992; 305: 1057–62

175. Swai ABM, McLarty DG, Mtinangi BL et al. Diabetes is not caused by cassava toxicity. A study in a Tanzanian community. Diabetes Care 1992; 15: 1378–85

10

Diabetes Secondary to Acquired Disease of the Pancreas

Stefano Del Prato and Antonio Tiengo

University of Padua, Italy

INTRODUCTION

Secondary diabetes is a condition of persistent disturbance of glucose metabolism (hyperglycemia) which develops after the destruction of the pancreas by an acquired disease and, as such, it results from damage to both anatomic acinar and endocrine tissues. Although high plasma glucose concentration is the common hallmark of all diabetic conditions, pancreatic diabetes presents such peculiar features as to prompt the National Diabetes Data Group to classify it as a distinct form of diabetes.

Diabetes secondary to acquired disease of the pancreas represents approximately 0.5% of all cases of diabetes mellitus. However, its frequency is likely to be twice as high in populations with heavy alcohol consumption. In the tropics, the prevalence of diabetes secondary to fibrocalculous pancreatitis can be as high as 10–20% [1].

Table 1 Major causes of diabetes secondary to pancreatic disease

---

1. Infection
2. Pancreatitis
   (a) Acute
   (b) Chronic
3. Infiltration
   (a) Primary hemochromatosis
   (b) Secondary hemochromatosis
4. Neoplasia
5. Surgical resection
6. Cystic fibrosis

Any disease of the pancreas can be associated with glucose intolerance or overt diabetes (Table 1). The peculiar metabolic and hormonal features of diabetes secondary to acquired diseases of the pancreas also lead to specific clinical aspects, and the diabetologist should be aware of these to ensure appropriate diagnostic and therapeutic management. The epidemiology and the hormonal, metabolic and clinical implications of these forms of diabetes will be presented and discussed in this chapter.

HISTORY

Secondary diabetes was first described in 1788, when Sir Thomas Cawley reported the case of a man 'aged 34 years, strong, healthy and corpulent, accustomed to free living and strong corporeal exertions in the pursuit of country amusements . . . in December 1787, was seized with diabetes.' The patient gradually became emaciated and, despite treatment, eventually died. At necropsy 'the pancreas was full of calculi, which were firmly impacted in its substance. They were of various sizes, not exceeding that of a pea, . . . which made their surface rough, like mulberry stones. The right extremity of the pancreas was very hard, and appeared to be scirrhous' [2]. However, more than 100 years passed before Minkowski's [3] demonstration that experimental pancreatectomy in dogs caused diabetes. With this discovery, the association between glycosuria and acute pancreatitis became clear, and in 1940 Schumacker [4]

International Textbook of Diabetes Mellitus, Second Edition. Edited by K.G.M.M. Alberti, P. Zimmet, R.A. DeFronzo, and H. Keen (Honorary)
© 1997 John Wiley & Sons Ltd

estimated that at least 2% of all cases of acute pancreatitis were followed by overt clinical diabetes. In spite of the appreciation that acute pancreatitis was infrequently followed by overt diabetes, clinicians began to recognize chronic pancreatitis or relapsing acute pancreatitis as a common cause of glucose intolerance. Total pancreatectomy in humans was first performed in 1942 [5] and has since been used for the surgical treatment of various pancreatic lesions. Extensive use of this procedure proved that more than 80–90% of the pancreas had to be removed before overt diabetes mellitus would ensue. An association between hemochromatosis and diabetes was also recognized at the beginning of the century, and the high incidence of diabetes in this rare metabolic disorder was subsequently confirmed [6]. Further information on the different characteristics of diabetes secondary to the various pancreatic diseases continues to be collected.

ETIOLOGY OF PANCREATIC DIABETES

Any pathologic process of the pancreatic acinar tissue results in an insult to its endocrine diffuse component, leading to some degree of hormone insufficiency. The main causes of pancreatic diabetes are listed in Table 1, while Table 2 summarizes the frequency of association between the various pathologic conditions and diabetes mellitus.

Table 2 Frequency of diabetes secondary to pancreatic diseases

Total pancreatectomy	100%
Partial pancreatectomy	
pancreatoduodenectomy	20–40%
distal pancreatectomy	20–40%
40–80% resection	40%
80–90% resection	> 60%
Pancreatitis	
acute	~ 2%
chronic calcifying	60–70%
chronic non-calcifying	15–30%
Hemochromatosis	
primary	~ 75%
secondary	~ 16%
Carcinoma of the pancreas	40–50%
Cystic fibrosis	~ 10%

INFECTIOUS DISEASES

The possibility that viruses such as mumps, rubella, Coxsackie B4, Epstein–Barr and hepatitis may cause diabetes by direct involvement of the pancreatic tissue has been suggested by a number of investigators. As such, diabetes might be seen as an acquired disease. Nevertheless, definite proof of a viral etiology of diabetes mellitus is still lacking. The evidence that viruses may precipitate insulin dependent diabetes mellitus in immunologically predisposed individuals is discussed in Chapter 5.

ACUTE PANCREATITIS

Acute pancreatitis is characterized by an acute inflammatory response of the pancreatic tissue, followed by complete clinical and biological restitution of the pancreas [7]. Transient hyperglycemia and glycosuria are found in about 50% of patients with acute pancreatitis. The degree of glucose intolerance is an indicator of the severity of pancreatitis. The incidence of glucose intolerance in acute pancreatitis ranges from 9% to 70% [8]. This wide range is related to the definition of impaired glucose tolerance used in the different surveys, as well as to the cause of the acute inflammatory process. Alcohol, for example, is associated with more severe injury of pancreatic tissue, and alcoholic pancreatitis is complicated by a higher incidence of glucose intolerance [9]. The transient hyperglycemia accompanying the bout of pancreatitis is influenced by the pancreatic damage and the concomitant severe stress condition. Both the severity and the duration of the disturbance in carbohydrate metabolism are related to the extent of pancreatic tissue damage. Hyperglycemia and glycosuria usually subside within 3–6 weeks, but about 10% of patients will continue to exhibit impaired glucose tolerance [10]. Although early surveys suggested that overt diabetes developed in only 1–2% of individuals with a single episode of acute pancreatitis [4, 11], this proportion increases to 15–18% when the National Diabetes Data Group criteria are applied [12].

Hormone Secretion

In patients with acute pancreatitis, the plasma insulin concentration is lower than in healthy individuals with or without a comparable degree of stress [13]. Secretion of insulin in response to glucose or glucagon is also impaired. On the other hand, infusion of alanine results in a significant increase in plasma insulin levels. With the amelioration of the acute process, a normal insulin response is usually recovered [14]. In acute pancreatitis, plasma glucagon concentration is increased and tends to remain high for at least 1 week [15]. The combination of hyperglucagonemia and hypoinsulinemia is sufficient to account for the development of ketoacidosis and the rare occurrence of diabetic coma. Basal levels of plasma pancreatic polypeptide (PP) are normal, but fail to increase in response to hyperglycemia or secretin infusion.

CHRONIC PANCREATITIS

Chronic pancreatitis is defined as the presence of chronic inflammatory lesions characterized by the destruction of exocrine parenchyma and fibrosis and, at least in the late stage, destruction of endocrine parenchyma. There are several forms of chronic pancreatitis. Chronic calcifying pancreatitis (or pancreatic lithiasis) is by far the most frequent form. Chronic obstructive pancreatitis, recurrent acute pancreatitis and idiopathic pancreatitis represent less frequent subsets of inflammatory processes of the pancreas [16].

The frequency of diabetes secondary to chronic pancreatitis depends on the regional frequency of chronic pancreatitis, the type of lesion and the duration of the disease [16]. In a series collected at the Mayo Clinic in 1947, Sprague [17] found that diabetes secondary to chronic pancreatitis represented 0.5% of all cases of diabetes. A higher incidence of diabetes mellitus is associated with fibrocalculous pancreatitis in the tropics. In 1985, this form of diabetes was classified by WHO as a subclass of malnutrition related diabetes mellitus (MRDM) [18], and it has now been described in more than 15 different tropical regions. Its prevalence is variable, ranging from 0.5% to 4.0% of all diabetic patients in India, and perhaps up to 80% of young insulin-treated patients in Nigeria [19] (see Chapter 9).

Diabetes is an almost universal late complication of chronic calcifying pancreatitis, and it correlates better with the patient's age than with duration of the disease [20]. Nevertheless, actuarial studies show that after 15 years 80% of patients with chronic pancreatitis have diabetes. Specific precipitating etiological factors contribute to carbohydrate intolerance. Hypertriglyceridemia, for instance, is associated with insulin resistance and commonly leads to overt diabetes mellitus. Alcohol impairs insulin action and leads to glucose intolerance through direct effects on the liver. Chronic pancreatitis secondary to alcohol and/or malnutrition is more often associated with diabetes mellitus [9]. By contrast, the idiopathic form of chronic pancreatitis is associated with a lower incidence of diabetes. In hereditary pancreatitis, a rare autosomal dominant disease [21], diabetes may develop at a late stage and long-term diabetic complications may ensue.

Whatever the cause, it can be calculated that, in the western hemisphere, 60–70% of patients with calcific pancreatitis develop overt diabetes mellitus; 20% have impaired glucose tolerance and a further 5–8% exhibit abnormalities in insulin secretion. Among patients without pancreatic calcification, 30% are affected by diabetes mellitus, 25% show impaired glucose tolerance and 25% present a defect in insulin secretion [22].

A positive family history of diabetes might predispose patients with chronic pancreatitis to develop diabetes at a younger age [16]. The prevalence of diabetes without any association with pancreatitis is, indeed, higher in families of those patients who develop diabetes. However, no apparent increase in the frequency of HLA antigens B8, DR3, DR4 and DR3/DR4 has been demonstrated in patients with diabetes secondary to chronic pancreatitis [23–25]. It has been suggested that autoimmunity may contribute to the development of diabetes secondary to chronic pancreatitis, because islet cell antibodies (ICA) were found in some patients before the onset of diabetes [26]. However, this is a controversial issue. Other investigators were unable to demonstrate ICA in patients with either acute or chronic pancreatitis [24, 25, 27–29]. In our own series, ICA could be detected in only one of 88 patients, and the presence of organ-specific antibodies did not differ from that in the general population [23].

Pathology

As pointed out in the definition of chronic pancreatitis, involvement of the endocrine tissue represents a late stage of the disease, due to the relative resistance of the islets of Langerhans to the destructive process. Sometimes the pancreas can assume an adenomatous aspect due to the complete loss of exocrine tissue as opposed to persistence of its endocrine component. Within the remaining islets, a rearrangement of the endocrine cell population takes place, with a proportionally greater loss of B cells than of A cells, leading to a reversal of the normal 2:1 ratio. The number of D cells is usually normal, and there is some increase in PP cells. Islets surrounded by normal acinar tissue tend to exhibit a normal cytological composition, suggesting a trophic effect of the exocrine pancreas.

Hormone Secretion

In chronic pancreatitis, fibrosis leads to destruction of the B-cell mass. The fibrotic process may alter pancreatic capillary circulation, leading to diminished islet perfusion which may account for impaired delivery of secretagogues to the B cells and reduced outflow of pancreatic hormones. Chronic pancreatitis is associated with a loss of functioning B cells, which accounts for reduced insulin secretion: the greater the loss of pancreatic endocrine tissue, the greater the impairment in insulin secretion and the greater the degree of glucose intolerance [22]. In patients with diabetes secondary to chronic pancreatitis with mild-to-moderate fasting hyperglycemia, the basal plasma insulin concentration is either normal or moderately elevated [30, 31].

Fasting insulin level tends to decrease as a function of the duration of the pancreatitic process, and it is deficient whenever pancreatic calcification and steatorrhea are apparent [10, 32–36, 38, 39]. Exocrine and endocrine functions are correlated, suggesting a direct cause and effect relationship between the inflammatory process of the exocrine pancreas and the development of diabetes mellitus. A good correlation has been found between insulin response to oral glucose and the concentration of pancreatic enzymes in the duodenal juice after intravenous cholecystokinin-pancreozymin (CCK-PZ) [38, 39]. Patients with steatorrhea have lower C-peptide secretion than patients with less severe impairment of the exocrine function [39]. Although fasting plasma insulin concentration may be normal or even increased, there is an almost universal impairment in insulin secretion following an oral glucose load [30–36, 38, 39]. A reduction in the maximal insulin secretory capability [33] is readily demonstrated in these patients, indicating reduced insulin reserve. When fasting plasma glucose levels exceed 10 mmol/l (180 mg/dl), plasma insulin and C-peptide concentrations are often undetectable [34]. The B-cell response to amino acids is also reduced as a function of the degree of pancreatic B-cell destruction and severity of glucose intolerance [22]. Arginine-stimulated C-peptide secretion (Figure 1) can be normal in patients with chronic pancreatitis and impaired glucose tolerance, but is always reduced in patients with fasting hyperglycemia [34, 40].

incretin factors—CCK-PZ, gastrin, enteroglucagon, gastric inhibitory polypeptide (GIP) and vasoactive intestinal polypeptide (VIP)—is impaired. In patients with diabetes secondary to chronic pancreatitis, the insulin response to CCK-PZ is proportional to the degree of hyperglycemia [41]. In contrast, insulin secretion in response to GIP is reduced. It remains unclear whether, in diabetes secondary to chronic pancreatitis, there is an unbalanced enteropancreatic axis or a simultaneous alteration in the secretion of gut and pancreatic hormones. The plasma concentration of GIP is elevated in diabetic patients with chronic pancreatitis, particularly following insulin withdrawal [42]. On the other hand, the meal-related increase in plasma CCK is reduced when compared with non-diabetic subjects or non-diabetic individuals with chronic pancreatitis [43].

In patients with chronic pancreatitis the greater the loss of pancreatic endocrine tissue, the greater the impairment in insulin secretion and the greater the degree of glucose intolerance. It is likely that these factors are linked in a vicious cycle through the negative effect of chronic hyperglycemia, a phenomenon also known as 'glucose toxicity' [44]. Figure 2 summarizes the changes in plasma insulin and glucose concentrations as a function of residual B-cell mass [22]. In patients with chronic pancreatitis, normal fasting plasma glucose concentrations are maintained until 20–40% of the B-cell mass has been lost. Nonetheless, this degree of loss of B-cell mass is associated with a

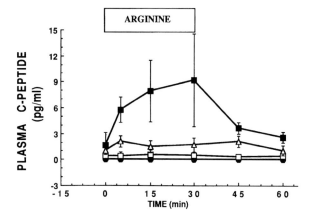

Figure 1 Plasma C-peptide concentration following IV infusion of L-arginine (25 g per 30 min) in normal subjects (■) and individuals with impaired glucose tolerance (△) or diabetes mellitus secondary to chronic pancreatitis (□) and diabetic subjects with total pancreatectomy (●)

In normal subjects, glucose ingestion elicits a greater insulin secretion than does the intravenous infusion of an equivalent amount of glucose as a consequence of the activation of the enteropancreatic axis. In chronic pancreatitis, the secretion of the

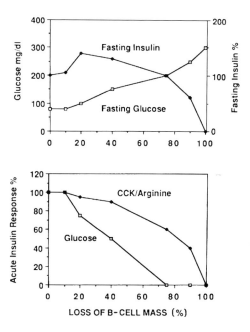

Figure 2 Diagram of changes in the plasma concentration of insulin and glucose, and insulin secretory response to glucose, gastrointestinal factors and arginine expressed as a function of residual B-cell mass in patients with chronic pancreatitis (from reference 22 with permission)

marked impairment in glucose-mediated insulin release [31], even though the response to CCK and arginine is still normal. An altered response to incretin factors and amino acids becomes apparent when 40–60% of B-cell mass has been lost. Finally, when the B-cell mass is reduced by more than 80–90%, there is both fasting hyperglycemia and an inability to secrete insulin in response to all secretagogues. Residual B-cell function in diabetes secondary to chronic pancreatitis can be evaluated using the glucagon test [14, 39, 45].

Glucagon secretion in these patients is heterogeneous, and two main conditions are recognized [46]. While some patients present a combined defect in insulin and glucagon secretion, others may exhibit severe hypoinsulinemia and high plasma glucagon concentrations. Similarly, the glucagon response to arginine or alanine stimulation is blunted in only 50% of patients with impaired glucose tolerance (Figure 3). With the progression of the pancreatic disease, the ability of A cells to respond to insulin-induced hypoglycemia wanes [47]. Nevertheless, the ingestion of an oral glucose load can be followed by a paradoxical rise in plasma glucagon levels, whereas the glucagon response to secretin and CCK-PZ is either normal or increased [33].

Controversy exists about the molecular nature and source of circulating glucagon in patients with diabetes secondary to chronic pancreatitis [48]. At least four varieties of immunoreactive glucagon ($M_r > 50\,000$, 9000, 3500 and 2000, respectively) have been identified in the plasma of normal individuals [49]. The 3500 M_r glucagon is of pancreatic origin and possesses full biological activity. This is the only form that responds to stimulation by arginine and suppression by somatostatin. Functional studies and gel chromatography analysis support the pancreatic origin of the circulating glucagon in chronic pancreatitis [50, 51], but a major contribution of enteropancreatic glucagon to the circulating plasma concentration measured by radioimmunoassay is also likely. Consistent with this, the basal concentration of gastrointestinal glucagon is increased in patients with pancreatic diabetes [52].

In chronic pancreatitis patients with residual insulin secretion, fasting plasma levels of PP are normal [14]. However, when residual B-cell function is severely impaired, a marked PP secretory defect is evident, as shown by the inability of arginine infusion, meal ingestion or insulin-induced hypoglycemia to evoke any rise in plasma PP concentration [14, 53]. A strong relationship between pancreatic enzyme secretion and stimulated plasma PP concentration has been reported [54, 55]. In patients with chronic pancreatitis without steatorrhea, PP response to CCK is reduced, but when steatorrhea ensues this response is no longer elicited [56]. Therefore, evaluation of PP secretion

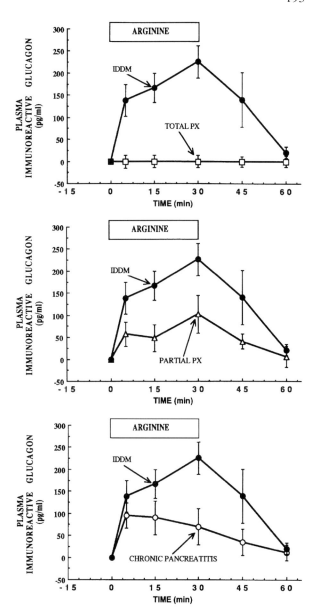

Figure 3 Increment above baseline of plasma immunoreactive glucagon (IRG) following IV infusion of L-arginine (25 g per 30 min) in IDDM patients (●), and individuals with diabetes secondary to total pancreatectomy (□), partial pancreatectomy (△) and chronic pancreatitis (○)

represents a reliable index of endocrine function in these patients [14]. Plasma somatostatin concentration is increased both in the basal state and following stimulation by glucagon, arginine, mixed meal and hyperglycemia [14].

PANCREATIC INFILTRATIVE DISEASES

Primary Hemochromatosis

In 1865 Trousseau first reported the association between diabetes mellitus and hemochromatosis.

Six years later, Troisier described the association of diabetes with pigmentation of the liver and pancreas. The pigment was subsequently identified as iron by von Recklinghausen, who coined the term 'hemochromatosis'. It is now recognized that diabetes mellitus occurs in over 75% of patients with hemochromatosis [57, 58]. Even though concomitant liver cirrhosis *per se* can affect glucose metabolism, this does not fully account for the diabetic condition. In contrast to chronic pancreatitis, in patients with hemochromatosis, diabetes mellitus is an early complication. Thus, more often than not, diabetes precedes the clinical recognition of hemochromatosis. On average, diabetes mellitus is diagnosed approximately 1 year before hemochromatosis [59]. It is rarely associated with obesity and it affects males 10 times more frequently than females.

In primary hemochromatosis, diabetes was initially explained as a classic infiltrative disorder with destruction of endocrine tissue. More recently, it has become recognized that diabetes and hemochromatosis have independent genetic transmission [58]. Thus, the diabetes associated with primary hemochromatosis results from the interaction of a diabetic genetic predisposition and pancreas infiltration by iron excess. Iron infiltration/destruction may be considered an environmental factor capable of unmasking the diabetic predisposition.

Pathology

Inspection of pancreas shows a firm light-brown tissue, with focal fibrotic lesions. Microscopic examination reveals atrophy of the acini, with a marked increase in interstitial collagen. The deposition of hemosiderin is extensive. The iron deposits are more evident in the acinar tissue rather than in the islets of Langerhans, many of which appear histologically normal. A quantification of the endocrine cell population is still lacking.

Hormone Secretion

The basal plasma insulin concentration and the plasma insulin response to oral glucose are often altered, while the plasma glucagon concentration is usually increased [60]. Most of the circulating glucagon, however, is represented by high M_r species that do not possess full biological activity. Hypoinsulinemia reflects a primary defect in B-cell function. Insulin resistance is common in hemochromatosis, possibly due to the coexisting hepatic cirrhosis. Impaired glucose uptake assessed by the euglycemic insulin clamp technique suggests insulin resistance in muscle tissue as well.

Secondary Hemochromatosis

Excessive iron deposition occurs in a variety of conditions (other than primary hemochromatosis) that are unlikely to be genetically linked to diabetes mellitus, including thalassemia major [61] and other hemoglobin disorders associated with iron overload [62]. In thalassemia major, frequent blood transfusions are required and this leads to massive iron overload. The duration of the disease and the number of transfusions are highly correlated with the degree of glucose intolerance [63]. Therefore, the relationship between iron excess and diabetes mellitus is even more striking than in primary hemochromatosis where quantification of iron overload is less accurate. The development of diabetes in individuals receiving multiple chronic blood transfusions is a negative prognostic sign and usually precedes death by about 2 years [63]. The reported prevalence of diabetes in treated thalassemia major is about 16%, while the incidence of impaired glucose tolerance is approximately 60%. Although insulin secretion may be only moderately impaired, hyperglucagonemia is almost universally encountered.

A different model of iron infiltration of the pancreas is found in rural male Bantus. Many Bantus ingest in excess of 100 mg of iron per day in alcoholic drinks which are brewed in iron containers. In such individuals, the prevalence of diabetes is 10 times higher than in Bantus who do not consume such alcoholic beverages [62].

PANCREATIC TUMORS

In 1833, Bright reported the case of a 49-year-old man who initially presented chronic symptoms of diabetes and subsequently became jaundiced. Twelve months following the onset of diabetes he died from complications of cancer of the head of the pancreas [64]. Following this original description, an association between carcinoma of the pancreas and diabetes mellitus was recognized. Hyperglycemia and pancreatic neoplasia are usually diagnosed within 1–2 years of each other [65], suggesting that the neoplastic process may directly affect the endocrine pancreas. The incidence of hyperglycemia at the time of diagnosis of the pancreatic cancer ranges between 40 and 50% [66]. However, when challenged by an oral glucose tolerance test, impaired glucose tolerance can be diagnosed in about 80% of the patients [67]. Although it has been suggested that carcinoma of the pancreas tends to be more prevalent in the diabetic population [66], a recent survey has concluded that diabetes in patients with pancreatic cancer is probably caused by the tumor, and that diabetes is not a risk factor for neoplasia of the pancreas

[193]. The mechanism(s) involved in the pathogenesis of diabetes in this condition are multiple and include: disruption of the islets of Langerhans; occlusion of the pancreatic duct with consequent cell degeneration; tumor-related pancreatitis; and fibrosclerosis with compression of blood vessels and autonomic nerve fibers. However, factors such as inactivity, stress, weight loss and low caloric intake may contribute to impaired glucose tolerance and to insulin resistance. More recently, insulin resistance of patients with pancreatic cancer and diabetes has been attributed to overproduction of islet amyloid polypeptide (IAPP), a hormonal factor secreted from the B cell [68].

Pathology

A 50% reduction of B-cell number has been reported, and the residual B-cell mass is inversely correlated with fasting plasma glucose concentration [69]. The reduction of B-cell mass is related to the degree of fibrosis. Fibrosis may lead to a diminished supply of trophic factors to islets. In spite of the reported increase in circulating IAPP, its pancreatic concentration is reduced [68]. The number of A cells may be normal or reduced, while the D-cell population tends to be reduced. Conversely, intra- as well as extra-insular PP-cell hyperplasia is often observed along the front line of the carcinoma.

Hormone Secretion

Both insulin and C-peptide responses to oral glucose are frequently decreased and/or delayed. Peripheral insulin resistance has been reported [67, 68]. The fasting plasma glucagon concentration can be either normal or increased, while a paradoxical rise has been observed following an oral glucose load [67].

PANCREATECTOMY

In 1889, Minkowski demonstrated that ablation of the pancreas in dogs was associated with development of diabetes mellitus [3]. In humans, after sporadic attempts, total pancreatectomy was not performed until insulin became available. That early experience showed that more than 80–90% of the pancreas had to be removed to produce diabetes. Nevertheless, the post-operative onset of diabetes can be unpredictable and is not always directly related to the extent of pancreatic ablation. Preceding history of chronic pancreatitis is, indeed, associated with greater incidence of diabetes mellitus.

Total pancreatectomy is invariably followed by diabetes. Following subtotal pancreatectomy, the post-operative development of diabetes mellitus is directly related to the amount of pancreatic tissue that is removed (Table 2). In the initial weeks following pancreaticoduodenectomy, the incidence of diabetes mellitus ranges from 20 to 40%; however, incidence approaches 70% during prolonged follow-up. Some differences exist between distal and proximal pancreatectomy [70]. Distal pancreatectomy is not followed by appreciable changes in exocrine function although it may result in an insulin-dependent diabetic condition. By contrast, following proximal pancreatectomy there is a sharp decline in the exocrine secretion without significant impairment of the endocrine function [70]. Preservation of the duodenum has been claimed to preserve hormone secretion and glucose tolerance [71]. Nevertheless, it can be estimated that, on average, resection of 40–80% of the pancreas is associated with an approximately 40% incidence of diabetes, whereas following 80–95% pancreatectomy, the incidence exceeds 60% [72–75]. These figures are comparable with the incidence of diabetes (about 60%) observed in patients with chronic pancreatitis who received medical treatment alone [76].

Hormone Secretion

As already discussed, the insulin secretory response is related to residual B-cell mass. This is not true in patients who had partial pancreatectomy performed for chronic pancreatitis, because extensive disruption of the remaining pancreatic parenchyma is already present. In patients undergoing pancreatic resection for carcinoma of the pancreas, secretion of pancreatic hormones closely resembles that observed in patients with chronic pancreatitis receiving medical treatment (Figure 2), although medial pancreatectomy in patients with tumors of the neck of the pancreas does not seem to be associated with diabetes mellitus [77]. Similarly, when hemipancreatectomy is carried out in healthy individuals for the purpose of donation to a family member with IDDM, a deterioration of insulin and glucagon secretion is evident in spite of persistent normal glucose homeostasis [78, 79]. It has been suggested that in otherwise normal, healthy individuals, undefined mechanisms must compensate for diminished insulin secretion following hemipancreatectomy [80].

Total pancreatectomy is always followed by complete insulin deficiency, as evidenced by the absence of insulin or C-peptide in the circulation (Figure 1). Measurement of stimulated plasma C-peptide concentration can be used to confirm completeness of the surgical removal of the pancreas [46]. Figure 1 shows the time course of plasma C-peptide concentration during arginine stimulation. Although no response is elicited in totally pancreatectomized patients, a blunted endogenous insulin secretion can be provoked in patients with chronic pancreatitis and also in those with partial pancreatectomy.

The basal concentration of immunoreactive glucagon can be normal or even increased [81]. The source and nature of measurable immunoreactive glucagon has been a matter of argument for many years. In pancreatectomized dogs and other animal species, including humans, total pancreatectomy does not affect the plasma levels of immunoreactive glucagon. In dogs, A cells have been identified in the gastrointestinal tract and these cells secrete glucagon molecules that are biologically and immunologically indistinguishable from 3500 M_r pancreatic glucagon [82]. In rats, the salivary glands produce biologically active glucagon [83]. In humans, no such alternative sites of glucagon production are operative, so that total pancreatectomy might be expected to result in a complete loss of pancreatic glucagon and thus to lead to aglucagonemic diabetes [84–86]. Nevertheless, even when specific antisera are used, normal or increased levels of circulating glucagon have been reported in pancreatectomized patients [14, 52, 81, 85–94]. However, challenging glucagon secretion by stimulatory or suppressive maneuvers is never followed by appreciable changes in plasma immunoreactive glucagon concentration [81, 87–89, 92, 95], suggesting absolute lack of active pancreatic or extrapancreatic sources of 3500 M_r glucagon in humans after total pancreatectomy. Persistence of measurable basal levels of immunoreactive glucagon depends on the cross-reactivity, even with supposedly specific antibodies, of glucagon-like molecules of uncertain biological activity. Secretion of gastrointestinal glucagon-like polypeptides is increased after total pancreatectomy [96], and glucagon-related peptides arising from the gut are responsible for the paradoxical response to oral glucose load reported in some pancreatectomized subjects [94]. Standard chromatographic analysis could not demonstrate significant amounts of circulating 3500 M_r glucagon in the plasma of patients with total pancreatectomy. By further improvement in the sensitivity of the method of analysis, some pancreatic glucagon activity in patients with total pancreatectomy was detected [93]. Nevertheless, the magnitude of the ectopic 3500 M_r glucagon secretion is trivial compared with the pancreatic secretion of healthy subjects. Thus, chromatographic analysis of plasma taken from the portal vein in patients undergoing total pancreatectomy demonstrated negligible amounts of pancreatic glucagon, even after arginine infusion (Figure 4) [97]. In summary, it is likely that, after total pancreatectomy, some 'pancreatic' glucagon may be measured in the circulation, but pancreatectomy does result in a chronic deficiency of 3500 M_r

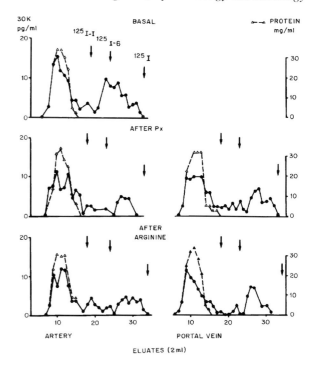

Figure 4 Chromatographic analysis (gel filtration on Bio-Gel P30) of the plasma immunoreactive glucagon assessed by C-terminal antibody (30 K) in a subject who underwent total pancreatectomy. Blood specimens were collected at different phases of the surgical procedure from a radial artery and portal vein. Broken line indicates protein concentration in eluates. Elution times for ^{125}I-labelled insulin (^{125}I-I), ^{125}I-labelled glucagon (^{125}I-G) and ^{125}I are indicated by the arrows. Arterial basal profile of glucagon immunoreactivity obtained 60 min before pancreas removal is shown in the upper panel. Fifteen minutes after pancreatectomy, the peak of pancreatic glucagon (3500 M_r) eluting with ^{125}I-labelled glucagon is markedly reduced both in the arterial and portal circulation (middle panel). Injection of 12.5 g L-arginine does not elicit any change in the chromatographic glucagon profile (from reference 97, with permission)

glucagon, leading to a diabetic condition in which deficiencies in insulin and glucagon secretion coexist.

Basal plasma levels of somatostatin are normal or slightly increased following pancreatectomy, and the response to a mixed meal is normal [98], whereas no PP is detectable in plasma [96]. Among other gastrointestinal hormones, gastrin is increased, while plasma levels of neurotensin and motilin are within the normal range [96]. Both gastrointestinal inhibitory polypeptide and enteroglucagon concentrations are normal in pancreatectomized individuals; their response to glucose is preserved, while a supranormal increase follows a mixed meal [52].

The absence of significant amounts of pancreatic glucagon may account for diabetes 'brittleness'. In patients with diabetes secondary to total pancreatectomy, insulin sensitivity is diminished when compared to normal subjects but higher than in IDDM individuals

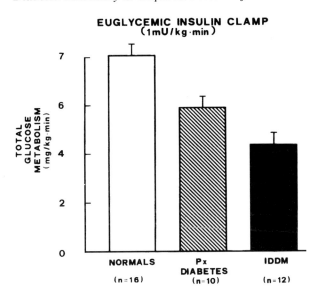

EUGLYCEMIC INSULIN CLAMP
(1mU/kg·min)

Figure 5 Whole body glucose utilization during euglycemic (90 mg/dl, 5.0 mmol/l) insulin (1 mU/kg·min) clamp studies in 16 normal subjects (open column), 10 patients with diabetes secondary to total pancreatectomy (crosshatched column) and 12 IDDM individuals (closed column) (from reference 97, with permission)

(Figure 5) [97]. This observation has been confirmed by some [99–101] but not all [102, 103] investigators. Conversely, in normal subjects, long-term physiologic hyperglucagonemia induces a modest degree of insulin resistance [104]. Similarly in pancreatectomized patients, replacement of basal glucagon concentration leads to a worsening of the insulin resistance [103]. The liver, in particular, seems to be more sensitive to insulin in the absence of glucagon. Thus, in pancreatectomized patients the rate of hepatic glucose production is similar to that of IDDM subjects, even though plasma insulin concentrations are much lower [102], whereas, when comparable plasma insulin levels are attained, individuals with total pancreatectomy have a much lower rate of hepatic glucose production [105].

CYSTIC FIBROSIS

An increased incidence of diabetes mellitus has long been recognized in patients with cystic fibrosis. With the increase in life expectancy brought about by improved medical therapy, the prevalence of diabetes mellitus has dramatically increased. Recent figures show that overt hyperglycemia occurs in 4–10% of the patients with cystic fibrosis, whereas impaired glucose tolerance is found in 8–75% [106–108].

The development of diabetes mellitus has classically been looked upon as a complication of the fibrotic process of the pancreas. However, diabetes can occur at any age, and no correlation exists between the duration of disease and the severity of glucose intolerance [109]. This suggests that etiological factors other than pancreatic fibrosis may contribute to the development of glucose intolerance and diabetes. A genetic linkage between cystic fibrosis and diabetes mellitus is unlikely since there is no increased incidence of cystic fibrosis in families with diabetes mellitus. Recent investigations have reported that diabetic patients with cystic fibrosis have an increased incidence of the HLA-DR3 and HLA-DR4 antigens [110]. An increased incidence of islet cell antibodies has been reported as well [110]. These findings suggest that in genetically predisposed patients, cystic fibrosis may damage the pancreatic tissue and result in a mounting autoimmune response which contributes to B cell destruction and development of diabetes mellitus. It is also possible that different genotypes may be associated with different clinical manifestations. Thus, patients with the R117H Δ F508 genotype are likely to maintain long-term pancreatic function so that development of glucose intolerance is delayed [111].

Pathology

The volume and weight of the pancreas is severely reduced in patients with cystic fibrosis and diabetes and the pancreatic tissue is disrupted by thick, collagenous bands which surround and separate clusters of islets of Langerhans. The number of B cells is reduced by 40–50% even in patients with normoglycemia, and this reduction is sufficient to explain the impairment in insulin secretion. A cells are normally represented, while somatostatin-producing cells are increased.

Hormone Secretion

Insulin and C-peptide responses to oral and intravenous glucose, arginine, tolbutamide and glucagon are reduced in patients with cystic fibrosis with or without overt fasting hyperglycemia (112–114). The reduction in insulin secretion is a function of the loss of B-cell mass. Patients with no exocrine insufficiency have normal insulin secretion, whereas exocrine-insufficient patients without diabetes present a significant impairment in insulin secretion and oral glucose intolerance [115]. Alteration of islet cell microcirculation by fibrosis, and/or inhibition of insulin secretion by a somatostatin paracrine effect, may contribute to hypoinsulinemia. The defect in insulin secretion is associated with increased tissue sensitivity to insulin, possibly through an increase in insulin receptor number [116], although controversy exists on this issue. Some studies have reported increased insulin sensitivity [113, 116, 117], whereas others have shown decreased [107, 118] or normal insulin action [119, 120].

Arginine-stimulated glucagon response is altered in diabetic patients with cystic fibrosis [112, 121]. Following an oral glucose load, plasma glucagon concentrations decline in non-diabetic patients, whereas they fail to be suppressed in diabetic individuals. Reduction in insulin reserve may cause an exaggerated hyperglycemic response during exacerbation of pulmonary infections in patients with cystic fibrosis [109]. In contrast, ketoacidosis is rare, because of some residual B-cell function and impaired glucagon secretion. The GIP response following oral glucose is normal, suggesting that enteropancreatic axis function is preserved [122].

METABOLIC PROFILE

Glucose Metabolism

In contrast to IDDM, all endocrine cell types are involved in the inflammatory process in pancreatic diabetes, and defects in both B- and A-cell function are characteristic. Impairment in insulin secretion is a function of the destruction of B cells and it accounts for the different degree of fasting and post-prandial hyperglycemia. It is the concomitant impairment in glucagon secretion that is mainly responsible for the peculiar metabolic and clinical features of diabetes secondary to pancreatic diseases (Tables 3 and 4): the more profound the defect in A cell function, the more pronounced these features [97]. Thus, chronic pancreatitis and pancreatectomy are more likely to develop the full picture of pancreatogenic diabetes (Table 4). In the extreme condition of diabetes secondary to total pancreatectomy or insulin-deficient pancreatitis, the blood levels of alanine, lactate, pyruvate and glycerol are 50–100% higher than in IDDM patients (Table 5). This metabolic pattern is not affected by insulin therapy [123] or its withdrawal [91, 92, 97, 124]. Furthermore, in these patients, blood concentrations of gluconeogenic precursors and glucose are not affected by infusion of somatostatin (an inhibitor of glucagon secretion) or arginine (a stimulant of glucagon secretion) [92]. Conversely,

Table 3 Clinical differences between diabetes secondary to chronic pancreatitis/pancreatectomy and insulin dependent diabetes mellitus (IDDM)

	Pancreatic diabetes	IDDM
Glycemic instability	+ + ++	++
Insulin requirement	+	+ + +
Hypoglycemia	+ + ++	++
Ketoacidosis	+	+ + +
Vascular complications	+	+ + +

Table 4 Hormonal and metabolic differences between diabetes secondary to chronic pancreatitis/pancreatectomy and insulin dependent diabetes mellitus (IDDM)

	Pancreatic diabetes	IDDM
Insulin secretion	↓	↓
Glucagon secretion	↓	↑
Hepatic glucose production	↓	↑
Gluconeogenic amino acids	↑	↓
Lactate and pyruvate	↑	↑↓
Ketone bodies	↓	↑
Insulin sensitivity	↑↓	↓

exogenous glucagon infusion causes a significant drop in blood lactate, pyruvate and alanine levels [97, 105]. Patients with diabetes secondary to chronic pancreatitis or partial pancreatectomy with residual glucagon secretion, exhibit blood levels of gluconeogenic substrates that are similar to those of IDDM patients, but much lower than those of patients with total pancreatectomy (Figure 6 and Table 5) [97, 123]. Amongst the gluconeogenic precursors, alanine is particularly elevated in patients with pancreatectomy (Figure 6). Such metabolic specificity is supported by the immediate increase in blood alanine concentration that follows pancreatic resection [125].

Glucagon exerts a major stimulatory action on hepatic glucose production and gluconeogenesis [126]. In the absence of significant amounts of pancreatic glucagon, insulin exerts an enhanced inhibitory effect on the liver, causing a marked reduction in post-absorptive plasma glucose concentration [105]. The combined increase in hepatic [102, 105, 127] and

Table 5 Mean 24-hour blood concentration (μmol/l) of gluconeogenic precursors during intensive subcutaneous insulin therapy

	Totally pancreatectomized patients	Partially pancreatectomized patients	IDDM patients
Lactate	1073 ± 105	792 ± 76	707 ± 49
Pyruvate	82 ± 8	47 ± 5	56 ± 5
Alanine	437 ± 62	226 ± 14	216 ± 10
Glycerol	60 ± 8	33 ± 6	35 ± 4

Adapted from reference 123, with permission.

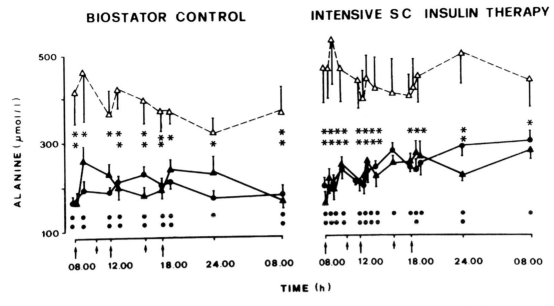

Figure 6   Blood alanine concentration during 24-hour glucose controlled insulin infusion (artificial endocrine pancreas–Biostator GCIIS) and intensive subcutaneous insulin therapy in patients with diabetes secondary to total (△-△) compared with patients with diabetes secondary to partial pancreatectomy (▲-▲) ($^{*}p < 0.05$; $^{**}p < 0.005$) and with IDDM individuals (●-●) ($^{*}p < 0.05$; $^{**}p < 0.005$) (reproduced from reference 123 by permission of Springer-Verlag)

peripheral [97, 99–101, 128] insulin sensitivity may contribute to frequent hypoglycemic episodes in patients with total pancreatectomy or severe pancreatitis.

When evaluating the overall metabolic status of a patient with total pancreatectomy, factors other than glucagon and insulin lack should be considered. Nutrition, malabsorption, changes in dietary behavior, abnormalities in gastrointestinal hormone secretion, local recurrence of tumor, and distant metastases can affect intermediary metabolism. Nevertheless, the available data suggest that a major metabolic difference exists between IDDM patients, who retain the ability to secrete glucagon (i.e. who have either absolute or relative hyperglucagonemia), and glucagon-deficient totally pancreatectomized patients. This difference is explained by a diminished rate of hepatic gluconeogenesis, due to the lack of pancreatic glucagon [105]. This leads to the progressive accumulation in blood of gluconeogenic precursors, especially alanine.

Lipid Metabolism

In a minority of patients with acute pancreatitis and no previous history of hyperlipidemia, serum concentration of lipids may be elevated. Following an attack of acute pancreatitis, however, the rise in plasma triglyceride and cholesterol does not always occur [13], and indeed a reduction in the cholesterol levels may be observed similar to that noted in response to non-specific stress. Plasma free fatty acid (FFA) concentrations are elevated following acute pancreatitis

as a consequence of both impaired insulin secretion and concomitant increase in glucagon and cortisol secretion [13]. Although the hormonal milieu that follows acute pancreatitis may account for ketoacidosis, this is an unusual metabolic event in patients with secondary diabetes [10, 129]. This is due to the persistence of residual endogenous insulin secretion that inhibits both lipolysis and ketogenesis, and to deficient glucagon secretion. In patients with total pancreatectomy and marked glucagon deficiency, insulin withdrawal is followed by a significant increment in plasma FFA and blood ketone body concentrations (Figure 7). However, the rise above baseline is less pronounced than in IDDM individuals [130–132]. By contrast, the rate of increase in blood ketones in patients with diabetes secondary to chronic pancreatitis or partial pancreatectomy with residual insulin secretion, is lower than in pancreatectomized and IDDM patients (Figure 7) [37, 131]. These observations suggest that insulin deficiency is the primary factor in promoting ketogenesis, whereas hyperglucagonemia can accelerate the process.

In IDDM individuals, especially those who are poorly controlled, high plasma levels of FFA and triglycerides are common. Although raised fasting plasma FFA concentrations have been reported in insulin-treated pancreatectomized patients, this elevation occurs in the presence of much lower plasma free-insulin concentrations [102]. In diabetes secondary to acquired disease of the pancreas, plasma lipid levels are variable. Low serum levels of cholesterol,

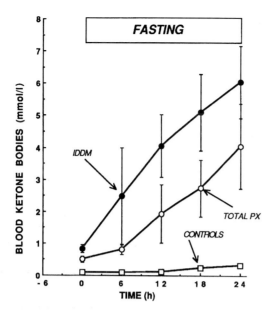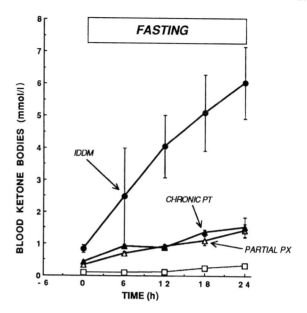

Figure 7   Blood ketone body concentration after insulin withdrawal and 24-hour fasting in normal individuals (□), patients with IDDM (●), and patients with diabetes secondary to total (○) and partial (△) pancreatectomy, and chronic pancreatitis (▲)

phospholipids and triglycerides have been reported in patients with diabetes secondary to chronic pancreatitis [133]. More recent surveys have found normal serum triglycerides and cholesterol [134]. In particular, plasma lipid concentrations do not seem to be related to duration of disease, the patient's age or type of therapy. Conflicting results have been reported in patients with total pancreatectomy [127, 135, 136]. In these patients, glucagon replacement is not associated with significant effects on plasma lipid levels [135]. In summary, the plasma lipid and lipoprotein profile in patients with diabetes secondary to acquired disease of the pancreas is heterogeneous. It is likely that this variability reflects the impact of other factors that affect lipid metabolism, including changes in the nutritional status, diet, malabsorption and alcohol intake.

Amino Acid Metabolism

Alteration in the plasma amino acid profile seems to be a characteristic of diabetes secondary to total pancreatectomy, whereas less information is available for other forms of pancreatogenic diabetes. Glucagon deficiency that follows total pancreatectomy is associated with elevation in blood concentrations of gluconeogenic and urea cycle amino acids [137]. In particular, alanine, asparagine, cystine, aspartate, glycine, proline, serine, citrulline, ornithine, phenylalanine, taurine, threonine and tyrosine are all increased in patients with glucagon deficiency (Figure 8). Similar changes in amino acid levels can be induced by inhibition of glucagon secretion with somatostatin [91], whereas restoration of

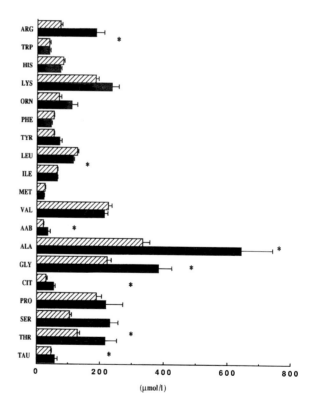

Figure 8   Basal plasma concentration of amino acids in patients with diabetes secondary to total pancreatectomy (closed columns) and normal individuals (crosshatched columns) $*p < 0.05$ v. normal individuals (adapted from reference 137 with permission)

physiologic plasma glucagon concentrations in pancreatectomized patients returns the plasma amino acid profile to normal [90, 91, 105, 135]. In contrast to the elevated plasma concentrations of gluconeogenic amino acids, plasma levels of branched-chain amino acids are not altered in pancreatectomized individuals [91, 135, 138]. In patients with chronic pancreatitis or partial pancreatectomy under strict metabolic control, blood alanine concentration is similar to that observed in IDDM patients [123]. The available data suggest that glucagon deficiency causes an impairment in the rates of both gluconeogenesis and ureagenesis, with secondary increases in the plasma concentrations of gluconeogenic but not branched-chain amino acids.

CLINICAL MANIFESTATIONS

In general, patients with secondary forms of diabetes develop symptoms similar to those exhibited by patients with primary diabetes. The diabetic condition develops immediately after total pancreatectomy, whereas in patients with chronic diseases of the pancreas it tends to develop gradually over several (1–12) years.

In primary hemochromatosis, the diagnosis of diabetes is often made before the disturbance in iron metabolism is recognized. The mean age of diagnosis for diabetes in patients with primary hemochromatosis ranges between 47 and 50 years [59], which is much younger than for NIDDM in Europid patients. A short interval usually occurs between the diagnosis of diabetes mellitus and that of carcinoma of the pancreas. In cystic fibrosis, the onset of diabetes can occur at any age and bears no relationship to the initial diagnosis of the primary disease.

Patients with pancreatogenic diabetes are prone to frequent, severe and unpredictable hypoglycemic events once started on insulin therapy. This complication is related to preserved peripheral tissue (muscle) sensitivity to insulin and enhanced inhibition of hepatic glucose production by insulin. The only exception seems to be diabetes mellitus associated with hemochromatosis, where insulin resistance has been found.

Patients with chronic pancreatitis may experience hypoglycemia either after the initial dose of insulin or, unexpectedly, after maintenance insulin or oral antidiabetic therapy [10] has been established. These episodes tend to be severe and prolonged, and represent a frequent cause of hospital admission for coma, and of death in these patients [139, 140]. Hypoglycemia is even more frequent after pancreatectomy [141–146], being a cause of death in 20–50% of the patients [142, 147, 148]. The severity of these hypoglycemic episodes is the consequence of impaired counter-regulation and glucose recovery [149, 150]. The inability of the organism to respond promptly to a drop in plasma glucose concentration is due to deficient glucagon secretion and blunted catecholamine response [151, 152] associated

with impaired activation of hepatic glucose production [153]. Increased frequency of hypoglycemic episodes is associated with metabolic instability characterized by erratic fluctuation of plasma glucose concentrations [154, 155]. Thus, it is not uncommon to observe early postprandial hyperglycemic peaks followed by severe hypoglycemia even after small doses of regular insulin (Figure 9). Frequent hypoglycemic reactions during insulin therapy have also been described in patients with diabetes secondary to cystic fibrosis.

The difficulty in maintaining satisfactory, stable metabolic control in patients with diabetes secondary to acquired disease of the pancreas has prompted the inclusion of this group of disorders under the category of 'brittle diabetes' [155]. Several factors are responsible for the unstable control in pancreatogenic diabetes (Table 6). The effects of glucagon deficiency have been discussed. Exocrine pancreatic insufficiency with malabsorption can contribute to the instability of glucose control [156]. Steatorrhea may cause glucose malabsorption, thus contributing to postprandial hypoglycemic reactions and altered insulin secretion [157]. The development of diabetes in patients with pancreatic disease can be associated with dramatic weight loss, which is difficult to correct even with appropriate insulin therapy. Furthermore, weight loss *per se* can markedly alter insulin sensitivity.

Table 6 Factors contributing to excessive glucose fluctuation

1. Hypoglycemia
   (a) Glucagon deficiency
   (b) Impaired catecholamine secretion
   (c) Malabsorption
   (d) Low carbohydrate intake
   (e) Alcohol
   (f) Non-compliance with therapy and diet
   (g) Increased insulin sensitivity
2. Hyperglycemia
   (a) Antral resection
   (b) Non-compliance with therapy and diet

Chronic alcohol consumption is a frequent cause of pancreatitis, and it is associated with an increased frequency of carbohydrate intolerance [16]. Persistence of ethanol abuse after medical or surgical therapy of pancreatitis may affect the metabolic control of diabetic patients. Alcohol inhibits gluconeogenesis [158], affects hypothalamic–pituitary secretion of adrenocorticotropic hormone and growth hormone [159, 160], and induces insulin resistance [161]. Hypoglycemia may be particularly troublesome if nutrient intake is reduced and liver glycogen stores are depleted. Alcohol abuse after pancreatectomy is a major factor in hypoglycemia and death [145, 147]. In these patients, poor compliance with the insulin regimen frequently

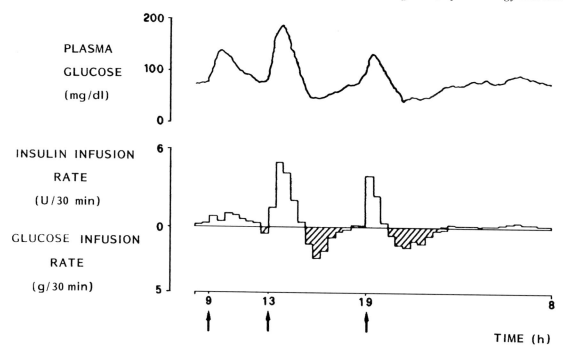

Figure 9 The 24-hour plasma glucose profile and insulin/dextrose requirement in a patient with diabetes secondary to total pancreatectomy under control with a glucose controlled insulin infusion system (artificial endocrine pancreas – Biostator GCIIS) illustrating postprandial tendency to hypoglycemia (from reference 97, with permission)

contributes to metabolic instability. Finally, ethanol-induced liver disease will affect both hepatic glucose production and peripheral glucose metabolism [157].

In contrast to the frequent occurrence of hypoglycemia and the wide fluctuations in plasma glucose levels, development of ketoacidosis and diabetic coma in pancreatic diabetes is uncommon [10, 129, 145, 147]. When these problems do occur, they are almost always associated with stress, such as infection or surgery.

The persistence of insulin secretion largely accounts for the resistance to ketosis [131]. However, even in patients without residual C-peptide secretion, ketoacidosis is quite rare. The rarity of diabetic ketoacidosis may be related to depletion of fat stores and to decreased rate of lipolysis [10]. A similar resistance to ketosis has been observed in diabetes of the tropics, where malnutrition and very low intake of unsaturated fat contribute to the rarity of ketoacidosis [162] (see Chapter 9).

The role of glucagon deficiency in protecting pancreatectomized diabetic patients from ketoacidosis is controversial. Barnes et al [130] suggested that glucagon lack in these subjects mitigates against the development of ketoacidosis. In IDDM individuals, suppression of glucagon secretion with somatostatin prevents a rise in blood ketone concentrations [163]. Although insulin withdrawal in pancreatectomized patients causes a rise in plasma FFA and ketone

bodies, this increase is significantly lower than in IDDM subjects [130, 131]. Therefore, it is likely that, even though glucagon may not be essential for the development of ketosis, its deficiency can delay or slow down progression towards diabetic ketoacidosis.

DIABETIC COMPLICATIONS

The pathogenesis of long-term diabetic complications remains a subject for debate, with the genetic hypothesis and the metabolic hypothesis each receiving support and criticism. It has been assumed by some that a genetic predisposition must be necessary [164], although the Diabetes Control and Complications Trial (DCCT) results strongly support the over-riding importance of hyperglycemia for the 'specific' complications (see Chapter 67). Evaluation of the incidence of microvascular and macrovascular complications in diabetes secondary to acquired pancreatic disease is of interest because it may shed light on the relative contributions of heredity and hyperglycemia. In animals, experimental pancreatectomy is associated with development of vascular changes similar to those found in spontaneous genetic diabetes [165]. In humans with pancreatogenic diabetes, controversy exists concerning the incidence of diabetic complications. Since the late 1950s, the general idea has been that diabetes secondary to chronic pancreatitis or hemochromatosis is not associated with vascular complications [166–169]. Several factors have been claimed for this apparent reduced frequency of diabetic complications in pancreatogenic diabetes, including absent or less penetrant genetic predisposition, exocrine pancreatic insufficiency, low serum cholesterol levels, low caloric intake, etc. However, with the improved life expectancy of these patients, more and more cases of diabetic angiopathy have been reported [23, 134, 170, 171]. Caution is required in drawing conclusions on the unique role of hyperglycemia, because patients with pancreatogenic diabetes frequently have a family history of diabetes, and because the duration of their disease is still relatively short [12].

Retinopathy

The prevalence of diabetic retinopathy in patients with diabetes secondary to chronic pancreatitis or pancreatectomy was initially reported to vary considerably (Table 7). During the last 10 years a more accurate assessment of diabetic lesions of the retina has yielded an incidence of 30–40%, a figure similar to that found in IDDM subjects [134, 177, 179, 180]. Incidence of retinopathy is correlated with the duration of the hyperglycemia [23, 134] (Figure 10). By contrast, no apparent relationship exists between the presence of retinopathy and a positive family history of diabetes mellitus, frequency of HLA antigens, presence of islet cell antibodies or plasma C-peptide level [23, 134]. In spite of early observations suggesting that diabetes associated with primary hemochromatosis was relatively complication-free [169], all diabetic complications have been shown to occur at a rate comparable to that for primary diabetes after a 5-year duration of diabetes [181]. Similar findings have been reported

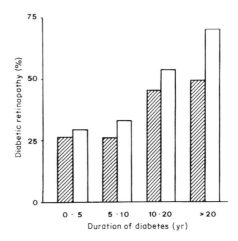

Figure 10 Prevalence of diabetic retinopathy in a cohort of 88 patients with pancreatogenic diabetes (crosshatched columns) and in a population of IDDM individuals (open columns) (from reference 23, with permission)

in patients with diabetes secondary to cystic fibrosis [109]. It is noteworthy that retinopathy in secondary diabetes is usually 'background' in nature, while proliferative lesions are more rarely described [23, 109, 134, 177].

Nephropathy

There is still controversy about the incidence of diabetic nephropathy in secondary diabetes. Calwell et al [166] stated that they were 'unable to find any one who knows about a case, verified at autopsy, of intercapillary glomerulosclerosis due to hemochromatosis or pancreatitis'. However, more and more cases of nodular glomerulosclerosis in patients with diabetes secondary to hemochromatosis

Table 7 Prevalence of microangiopathy in pancreatic diabetes

Author	Year	Number of patients	Diabetes duration (years)	Retinopathy		Nephropathy	
				No.	%	No.	%
Sprague [17]	1947	24		1/24	4	1/24	4
Deckert [170]	1960	26	0–12	7/26	26		7
Dettwyler [129]	1964	28		2/28	7	2/28	
Tutin [171]	1966	31		4/31	12		
Ennis [172]	1969	14	> 3	5/14	35		
Sevel [173]	1971	27	3–15	2/27	7		
Verdonk [174]	1975	168	0–36	24/168	14	2/168	2
Maekawa [175]	1978	47	0–15	8/47	17		
Moinade [176]	1979	20	2–17	8/20	40	3/20	1.5
Tiengo [134]	1983	54	0–15	17/54	31		
Couet [177]	1985	88	1–26	36/88	41		
Mohan [178]	1985	40	4–18	13/40	32		
Tiengo [23]	1987	86	0–25	32/86	37	19/86	22#
Gullo [179]	1990	40	1–15	19/40	47	–	–
Larsen [180]	1990	25	10*	5/25	20	1/25	4#
Tiengo [185]	1992	33	11*	9/33	27	10/33	30#

*mean value; #microalbuminuria > 40 mg/24 h

[183] and pancreatitis [174] have been described. Sporadic cases of diabetic glomerulopathy have been reported in patients with total pancreatectomy [23]. The overall lower prevalence of diabetic nephropathy may be due to the shorter duration of diabetes, which does not allow the full appearance of clinically significant nephropathy. Furthermore, most of the studies have looked for patients with late-stage diabetic kidney involvement, but early functional alterations can be detected several years before the appearance of albuminuria. In a series of 86 patients with diabetes secondary to pancreatopathy [23], urinary albumin excretion > 40 mg/24 h was found in 23% of the patients (Figure 11). Albuminuria is related to diabetes duration and arterial blood pressure, but not to family history of diabetes mellitus, HLA antigens or plasma C-peptide levels [23, 180, 182]. Incidence of retinopathy was almost twice as high in patients with microalbuminuria, suggesting that the oculorenal syndrome described in IDDM may occur in pancreatogenic diabetes as well. Glomerular hyperfiltration, another early sign of renal dysfunction,

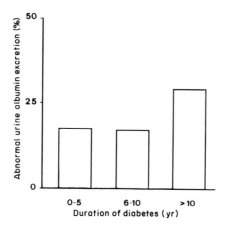

Figure 11 Prevalence of abnormal rate of urine albumin excretion (> 40 mg/24 h) in pancreatogenic diabetes expressed as a function of duration of hyperglycemia (from reference 23, with permission)

can be detected in pancreatogenic diabetes [184] with a prevalence that is similar to that of IDDM patients [185]. In spite of the demonstration of diabetic kidney involvement in these patients, albumin excretion rate > 0.5 g/day or overt renal failure is unusual, in agreement with the rarity of reports of glomerulosclerosis in secondary diabetes.

Diabetic Neuropathy

Neuropathy is a common complaint in pancreatogenic diabetes. A 10–20% incidence of distal polyneuropathy or mononeuropathy is reported [174],

and electrophysiologic signs of impaired motor conduction velocity are found in > 80% of patients with diabetes secondary to pancreatic disease [23]. Vibration threshold was found to be similar to that of matched IDDM patients [180]. At variance with both retinopathy and nephropathy, there is no relationship with the duration of diabetes. This may be because diabetic neuropathy is an early complication of diabetes mellitus, and/or to the concurrent effect of factors other than hyperglycemia (smoking, alcohol, malabsorption). Alterations of autonomic nervous function occur as well. Impaired cardiovascular reflexes have been found in 8% of a population with diabetes secondary to chronic pancreatitis, while a borderline defect was observed in an additional 13% of these patients [23]. However, some caution should be used in relating hyperglycemia to diabetic somatic and autonomic neuropathy, because alcohol consumption is common in these individuals. Therefore, the true pathogenetic mechanism(s) of neuropathy in diabetic patients with pancreatic disease is difficult to define.

Macroangiopathy

Macroangiopathy, in particular myocardial infarction, is uncommon in pancreatogenic diabetes, although in one report [148] 25% of patients with diabetes secondary to chronic pancreatitis were found to be affected by vascular complications, and some required amputations or vascular bypass operations. The relatively short duration of diabetes and the underlying disease of the pancreas make it difficult to estimate the prevalence of macrovascular complications in pancreatogenic diabetes. When long enough follow-up has proved possible, cardiovascular complications have been found to account for 16% of deaths in chronic pancreatitis patients [76].

THERAPY

Diabetes secondary to acquired pancreatic disease has been included in so-called 'brittle diabetes' because of marked instability of metabolic control [155]. Appropriate therapy must be defined on an individual basis to avoid the risk of severe hypoglycemic reactions as well as exaggerated hyperglycemia.

In diabetes associated with cystic fibrosis, sulfonylurea therapy can be used in patients with moderate hyperglycemia [109]. Insulin is, however, needed during hyperglycemic exacerbation related to recurrent pulmonary infections [109]. The incidence of insulin-treated diabetes mellitus in cystic fibrosis patients is about 1% [186]. In these individuals insulin requirement ranges between 0.6 and 3.3 U/kg body weight per day, with an average of 1.45 U/kg per day [187].

Table 8 Insulin requirement (U/day) in patients with pancreatic diabetes and IDDM during intensive subcutaneous insulin therapy and glucose controlled insulin infusion (artificial endocrine pancreas – Biostator GCIIS)

	Total pancreatectomy patients	Partial pancreatectomy patients	IDDM patients
Intensive subcutaneous therapy	47 ± 7	60 ± 1	66 ± 6
Artificial endocrine pancreas	44 ± 12	70 ± 8	62 ± 5

Adapted from reference 123, with permission

Development of diabetes and subsequent need for insulin therapy do not worsen the natural history of cystic fibrosis [186]. The short life-expectancy of these patients does not justify the effort and potential risks of aggressive antidiabetic therapy aimed at achieving meticulous glycemic control.

Most patients with diabetes secondary to hemochromatosis are treated with insulin [57]. Although oral antidiabetic agents can be successfully employed, the presence of concomitant liver cirrhosis requires caution in their use. The removal of excess iron deposits by phlebotomy is usually associated with an improvement in glucose tolerance and a reduction in insulin requirement.

Acute pancreatitis is associated with significant hyperglycemia in 50% of patients with secondary diabetes and occasionally ketosis or diabetic coma may develop [10, 13]. In these cases, close monitoring of the plasma glucose concentration, electrolytes, ketones and other aspects of metabolism is required, along with intravenous insulin infusion according to classic guidelines for treatment of diabetic ketoacidosis. Glucose tolerance should be assessed 3–6 months after an episode of acute pancreatitis. In the treatment of patients with acute fulminant pancreatitis conservative therapy rather than tissue resection should be advised, as the latter is associated with much higher incidence of diabetes [188].

The treatment of diabetes secondary to chronic pancreatitis or pancreatectomy is more complex. In patients with chronic pancreatitis or partial pancreatectomy, oral hypoglycemic agents may be introduced in those individuals who still retain a satisfactory C-peptide response to glucagon or a meal [10]. Short- rather than long-acting sulfonylureas are preferred, in order to minimize the risk of severe hypoglycemia [189]. Nevertheless, care should be used when employing sulfonylurea agents in patients with altered liver function tests, and biguanides should be avoided in such patients. Insulin therapy is mandatory following total pancreatectomy, although insulin requirements are lower than in IDDM patients, particularly at night [190]. In contrast, post-prandial insulin requirement may be more pronounced. This is particularly true in patients with total pancreatectomy, while

insulin-dependent patients with chronic pancreatitis or partial pancreatectomy usually have insulin requirements which are similar to those of IDDM individuals (Table 8) [123].

Whatever the chosen therapy, hypoglycemia remains the main concern [154, 155]. The increased frequency and severity of hypoglycemic events is the likely consequence of the concurrence of several factors, including insulin excess, insulin sensitivity, impaired counterregulation, deficient diet or nutrient absorption, alcohol intake, and liver diseases [10, 155, 156]. The risk of lethal hypoglycemia is particularly high in totally pancreatectomized patients, and this has prompted the search for safer surgical and medical approaches. Thus, preservation of the duodenum and pylorus seems to ensure more stable metabolic control and fewer hypoglycemic episodes [191]. Finally, islet autotransplantation may be an effective adjunct to extensive pancreatic resection for preventing development of diabetes in patients with severe chronic pancreatitis [192]. Rigorous home glucose monitoring and multiple administration of small doses of insulin, along with intensive education programs, may result in good, stable metabolic control in these patients as well [146, 189]. However, this must be associated with a number of specific steps (Table 9). Correction of the patient's nutritional status must be pursued. Alcohol withdrawal is essential; often, it is the primary cause of the pancreatic inflammation, and it may precipitate hypoglycemia [158–160]. Excessive alcohol intake also causes progressive liver damage, which *per se* may worsen metabolic control [157]. Malabsorption with steatorrhea contributes to the development of hypoglycemic events. Steatorrhea may also impair insulin secretion through derangement of the enteropancreatic axis [156]. In patients with pancreatic diabetes, pancreatic digestive enzymes should be replaced to reduce stool fat excretion below 20 g/day. Concomitant treatment with H_2-receptor antagonists should be considered, because reduction in gastric acid output may reduce pancreatic enzyme degradation. Acid-resistant preparations of pancreatic enzymes are recommended.

A high energy diet (> 2500 kcal/day) with a high complex carbohydrate and low fat content is advisable. In patients with chronic pancreatitis, high-fat meals

Table 9   Therapeutic approaches to the patient with
diabetes secondary to pancreatic disease

1. Diet:
     High-energy diet (2200–3000 kcal/day)
     Small and frequent meals
     Alcohol withdrawal
     Low intake of neutral fat
     Increased intake of complex carbohydrates
2. Pancreatic digestive enzyme replacement
3. Electrolytes, calcium, vitamins D and K
4. Sulfonylureas
     If stimulated C-peptide > 2 ng/mg
5. Insulin:
     Small doses of regular insulin before each meal
     Caution in the use of long-acting insulin
       preparations
     Continuous subcutaneous infusion only in highly
       motivated and educated patients

may increase the frequency and intensity of abdominal
pain. Therefore, limitation of fat calories to 20–25% of
total caloric intake is recommended. Meals should be
small and frequent, with three principal meals and two
or three intervening snacks. If needed, the diet should
be supplemented with electrolytes, calcium, vitamin D
and potassium. The accelerated intestinal transit and
dumping syndrome that occurs after gastrectomy may
also contribute to malabsorption and unstable metabolic
control.

In defining a strategy for insulin treatment in patients
with marked glycemic fluctuations, it is necessary to
be cognizant of the lower insulin requirements in such
patients, as well as the lower incidence and slower
progression of diabetic complications (Table 10). The
use of small doses of regular insulin administered
before each meal is most effective in preventing
excessive postprandial hyperglycemia while avoiding
hypoglycemia [146, 189, 190]. A night-time dose
of intermediate insulin should be employed to control overnight and fasting hyperglycemia. The use
of two injections per day of long-acting insulin has
been advocated to achieve better glycemic stability [8]. In highly motivated and educated patients,
insulin treatment by continuous subcutaneous infusion
has been successfully employed to achieve meticulous
metabolic control while avoiding hypoglycemia and
ketosis [146, 189].

Table 10   Management goals in diabetes
secondary to pancreatic disease

Improve nutritional condition
Avoid steatorrhea and malabsorption
Maintain an adequate diet and energy intake
Avoid excessive fluctuations in blood glucose
Avoid hypoglycemia

Hypoglycemic reactions, if they occur, must be
treated aggressively and their cause(s) and mech-
anism(s) carefully evaluated and explained to the
patient. Even though ketoacidosis is uncommon in
pancreatogenic diabetes, it can develop under conditions of stress (infection, surgery, etc.) and it requires
appropriate adjustment of the insulin dose. Because
of the extreme brittleness of patients with pancreatogenic diabetes, patient education and self-monitoring of
blood glucose are extremely important. Lastly, in some
patients with diabetes secondary to acquired disease
of the pancreas it may be difficult to achieve optimal
metabolic control because of the high risk of hypoglycemia. The maintenance of plasma glucose levels
slightly above the normal range may be necessary to
avoid frequent hypoglycemic reactions and to improve
the quality of life. It should be remembered that many
of these patients have a reduced life-expectancy and
are at lower risk of developing diabetic complications.

REFERENCES

1. Yajnik CS. Diabetes secondary to tropical calcific
    pancreatitis. Baillières Clin Endocrinol Metab 1992;
    6: 777–96.
2. Cawley T. A singular case of diabetes, consisting
    entirely in the quality of the urine: with an inquiry
    into the different theories of that disease. Lond Med J
    1788; 9: 286–308.
3. Minkowski O. De l'estirpation du pancreas chez les
    animaux et du diabète expérimentale. Semaine Med
    1889; 9: 175–80.
4. Schumacker HS Jr. Acute pancreatitis and diabetes.
    Ann Surg 1940; 112: 177–200.
5. Priestly JT, Comfort MW, Randcliff J. Total pancrea-
    tectomy for hyperinsulinism due to an islet cell ade-
    noma. Ann Surg 1944; 199: 211–21.
6. Finch SC, Finch CA. Idiopathic hemochromatosis. An
    iron storage disease. Medicine 1955; 34: 361–430.
7. Singer MV, Sarles H. Chronic pancreatitis in west-
    ern Europe. In Podolsky S, Viswanathan M (eds)
    Secondary diabetes. New York: Raven Press, 1980:
    pp 89–103.
8. Thow J, Samad A, Alberti KGMM. Epidemiology
    and general aspects of diabetes secondary to
    pancreatopathy. In Tiengo A, Alberti KGMM, Del
    Prato S, Vranic M (eds) Diabetes secondary to
    pancreatopathy. Amsterdam: Excerpta Medica, 1988:
    pp 7–20.
9. Sarles H, Cros RC, Bidart JM. International Group for
    the Study of Pancreatic Diseases: a multicenter inquiry
    on the etiology of pancreatic diseases. Digestion 1979;
    19: 110–25.
10. Bank S, Marks IN, Vinik AL. Clinical and hormonal
    aspects of pancreatic diabetes. Am J Gastroenterol
    1975; 64: 13–22.
11. Warren KW, Fallis LS, Barron J. Acute pancreatitis
    and diabetes. Ann Surg 1950; 132: 1103–10.
12. Scuro LA, Angelini G, Cavallini G, Vantini I. The
    late outcome of acute pancreatitis. In Gyr KL,
    Singer MV, Sarles H (eds) Pancreatitis: concepts and

classification. Amsterdam: Excerpta Medica, 1984: pp 403–8.

13. Drew SI, Joffe B, Vinik AI, Seften H, Singer F. The first 24 hours of acute pancreatitis. Changes in biochemical and endocrine homeostasis in patients with pancreatitis compared with those in control subjects undergoing stress for reasons other than pancreatitis. Am J Med 1978; 64: 795–803.

14. Larsen S, Hilsted J, Tronier B, Worning H. Metabolic control and B cell function in patients with insulin-dependent diabetes mellitus secondary to chronic pancreatitis. Metabolism 1987; 36: 964–7.

15. Donowitz M, Hendler R, Spiro HM, Binder H, Felig P. Glucagon secretion in acute and chronic pancreatitis. J Intern Med 1975; 83: 778–81.

16. Sarles H. Chronic pancreatitis and diabetes. Baillières Clin Endocrinol Metab 1992; 6: 745–75.

17. Sprague RG. Diabetes mellitus associated with chronic relapsing pancreatitis. Proc Mayo Clin 1947; 22: 553–8.

18. World Health Organisation. Diabetes mellitus: report of a WHO study group. Technical Report Series 727. Geneva: WHO, 1985.

19. Mohan V, Alberti KGMM. Diabetes in the tropics. In Alberti KGMM, Keen H, Zimmet P (eds) International textbook of diabetes mellitus. Chichester: Wiley, 1992: pp 177–96.

20. Sarles H, Sahel J, Satub JL, Bourry J, Laugier R. Chronic pancreatitis. In Howatt HT, Sarles H (eds) The exocrine pancreas. London: W.B. Saunders, 1979: pp 402–39.

21. Gross JB. Hereditary pancreatitis. In Go VLN (ed.) The exocrine pancreas: biology, pathology and diseases. New York: Raven Press, 1986; pp 541–75.

22. Vinik AI. Insulin secretion in chronic pancreatitis. In Tiengo A, Alberti KGMM, Del Prato S, Vranic M (eds) Diabetes secondary to pancreatopathy. Amsterdam: Excerpta Medica, 1988: pp 35–50.

23. Tiengo A, Briani G, Riva F, et al. Microangiopathic complications in diabetes secondary to pancreatopathy. In Tiengo A, Alberti KGMM, Del Prato S, Vranic M (eds) Diabetes secondary to pancreatopathy. Amsterdam: Excerpta Medica, 1988: pp 245–57.

24. Rummesen JJ, Marner B, Pedersen NT et al. Autoantibodies in chronic pancreatitis. Scand J Gastroenterol 1985; 20: 966–70.

25. Larsen S, Hilsted J, Jacobsen BK, Svejgaard A, Marner B, Worning H. Insulin-dependent diabetes mellitus secondary to chronic pancreatitis is not associated with HLA or the occurrence of islet-cell antibodies. J Immunogenet 1990; 17: 189–93.

26. Scuro LA, Bovo P, Sandrini T, Angelini G, Cavellini G, Mirakian R. Autoimmunity and diabetes associated with chronic pancreatitis. Lancet 1983; 1: 424–7.

27. Marner B, Bille G, Christy M, Damsgaard EM, Garne S, Heinze E et al. Islet cell cytoplasmic antibodies (ICA) in diabetes and disorders of glucose tolerance. Diabet Med 1991; 8: 812–16.

28. Colman PG, Begley CG, Tait BD, Roberts-Thompson IC, Harrison LC. Evidence against an immunogenetic basis for diabetes in chronic pancreatitis. Aust NZ J Med 1987; 17: 392–5.

29. Lendrum R, Walker G. Serum antibodies in human pancreatic disease. Gut 1975; 16: 365–71.

30. Keller P, Bank S, Marks IN, O'Reilly IG. Plasma insulin levels in pancreatic diabetes. Lancet 1965; 2: 1211–14.

31. Bonora E, Rizzi C, Lesi C, Berra P, Coscelli C, Butturini U. Insulin and C-peptide plasma levels in patients with severe chronic pancreatitis and fasting normoglycemia. Dig Dis Sci 1988; 33: 732–6.

32. Peters N, Dick AP, Hales CN, Orrell DH, Sarner M. Exocrine and endocrine pancreatic function in diabetes mellitus and chronic pancreatitis. Gut 1966; 7: 277–81.

33. Vinik AE, Jackson WPU. Endocrine secretion in chronic pancreatitis. In Podolsky S, Viswanathan M (eds) Secondary diabetes: the spectrum of the diabetic syndromes. New York: Raven Press, 1980: pp 165–89.

34. Kalk WJ, Vinik AI, Bank S, Keller P, Jackson WPU. Selective loss of beta cell response to glucose in chronic pancreatitis. Horm Metab Res 1974; 6: 95–8.

35. Joffe BI, Bank S, Jackson WPU, Keller P, O'Reilly TG, Vinik AI. Insulin reserve in patients with chronic pancreatitis. Lancet 1968; 2: 121–4.

36. McKiddie MT, Buchanan KD, McBain GC, Bell G. The insulin response to glucose in patients with pancreatic disease. Postgrad Med J 1969; 45: 726–30.

37. Larsen S, Hilsted J, Philipsen EK, Tronier B, Nielsen MD, Worning H. The effect of insulin withdrawal on intermediary metabolism in patients with diabetes secondary to chronic pancreatitis. Acta Endocrinol 1991; 124: 510–15.

38. Kalk WJ, Vinik AI, Jackson WPU, Bank S. Insulin secretion and pancreatic exocrine function in patients with chronic pancreatitis. Diabetologia 1979; 16: 355–8.

39. Nyboe Andersen B, Krarup T, Thorsgaard Pedersen N, Faber OK, Hagen C, Worning H. B cell function in patients with chronic pancreatitis and its relation to exocrine pancreatic function. Diabetologia 1982; 23: 86–9.

40. Duckworth WC, Solomon SS, Jallepalli P, Iyer R, Bobal MA. Hormonal response to intravenous glucose and arginine in patients with pancreatitis. Horm Res 1983; 17: 65–73.

41. Kalk WJ, Vinik AI, Botha JL, Keller P, Jackson WPU. Insulin responses to crude cholecystokinin pancreozymin in normal subjects, in patients with chronic pancreatitis and patients with mild maturity onset diabetes. J Clin Endocrinol Metab 1975; 41: 172–6.

42. Botha JL, Vinik AI, Child PT. GIP in acquired pancreatic diabetes: effects of insulin treatment. J Clin Endocrinol Metab 1978; 47: 543–9.

43. Nakano I, Funakoahi A, Shinozaki H, Sakai K. Plasma cholecystokinin and pancreatic polypeptide response after ingestion of a liquid test meal rich in medium-chain fatty acids in patients with chronic pancreatitis. Am J Nutr 1989; 49: 247–51.

44. Rossetti L, Shulman GI, Zawalich W, DeFronzo RA. Effect of chronic hyperglycemia on in vivo insulin secretion in partially pancreatectomised rats. J Clin Invest 1987; 80: 1037–44.

45. Tiengo A, Del Prato S, Meneghel A. C-peptide values in diabetes following pancreatectomy. Giorn Ital Chim Clin 1979; 4 (Suppl 1): 169–70.

46. Kalk WJ, Vinik AI, Bank S, Buchanan KD, Keller P, Jackson WPU. Glucagon responses to arginine in

chronic pancreatitis: possible pathogenic significance in diabetes. Diabetes 1974; 23: 257–63.

47. Persson I, Gyntelberg F, Heding LG, Ross Nielsen J. Pancreatic glucagon-like immunoreactivity after IV insulin in normal and chronic pancreatitis patients. Acta Endocrinol 1971; 67: 401–4.

48. Holst JJ. Sources and molecular moieties of glucagon in diabetes secondary to pancreatopathy. In Tiengo A, Alberti KGMM, Del Prato S, Vranic M (eds) Diabetes secondary to pancreatopathy. Amsterdam: Excerpta Medica 1988: pp 63–70.

49. Valverde I, Rigolopoulou D, Marco J, Faloona GR, Unger RH. Molecular size of extractable glucagon and glucagon-like immunoreactivity (GLI) in plasma. Diabetes 1970; 19: 624–9.

50. Assan R, Tiengo A. Comparaison des sécrétions de glucagon chez le diabète sucré avec ou sans pathologie organique acquis. Path Biol 1973; 21: 17–24.

51. Larsen S. Pancreatic hormone secretion in diabetes mellitus secondary to chronic pancreatitis. In Tiengo A, Alberti KGMM, Del Prato S, Vranic M (eds) Diabetes secondary to pancreatopathy. Amsterdam: Excerpta Medica 1988: pp 203–7.

52. Botha JL, Vinik AI, Child PT, Paul M, Jackson WPU. Pancreatic glucagon-like immunoreactivity in a pancreatectomised patient. Horm Metab Res 1977; 9: 199–205.

53. Nealon WH, Townsend CM, Thompson JC. The time course of beta cell dysfunction in chronic ethanol-induced pancreatitis: a prospective analysis. Surgery 1988; 104: 1074–9.

54. Adrian TE, Basferman HS, Mallison CN et al. Impaired pancreatic polypeptide release in chronic pancreatitis with steatorrhea. Gut 1979; 20: 98–101.

55. Owyang C, Scarpello JH, Vinik AI. Correlation between pancreatic enzyme secretion and plasma concentration of human pancreatic polypeptide in health and chronic pancreatitis. Gastroenterology 1982; 83: 55–62.

56. Anagnostides AA, Cox TM, Adrian TE, Christfides ND, Maton PN, Bloom SR, Chadwick VS. Pancreatic exocrine and endocrine response in chronic pancreatitis. Am J Gastroenterol 1984; 79: 206–12.

57. Saudek CD. Diabetes and diseases of iron excess. In Podolsky S, Viswanathan M (eds) Secondary diabetes: the spectrum of the diabetic syndrome. New York: Raven Press, 1980: pp 165–89.

58. Milman N. Hereditary haemochromatosis in Denmark 1950–1985. Clinical, biochemical, and histological features in 179 patients and 13 preclinical cases. Dan Med Bull 1991; 38: 385–93.

59. Saddi R, Feingold J. Idiopathic haemochromatosis and diabetes mellitus. Clin Genet 1974; 5: 242–7.

60. Nelson LR, Baldus WP, Rubenstein AH, Gov LW, Service FJ. Pancreatic cell function in diabetic hemochromatic subjects. J Clin Endocrinol Metab 1979; 48: 412–15.

61. Ellis JT, Schulman I, Smith CH. Generalized siderosis with fibrosis of liver and pancreas in Cooley's (Mediterranean) anemia. With observations on the pathogenesis of the siderosis and fibrosis. Am J Pathol 1953; 30: 287–309.

62. Isaacson C, Seftel SC, Keeley KJ, Bothwell TH. Siderosis in the Bantu: the relationship between iron overload and cirrhosis. J Lab Clin Med 1961; 58: 845–53.

63. Saudek CD, Hemm RM, Peterson CM. Abnormal glucose tolerance in B-thalassemia major. Metabolism 1977; 26: 43–52.

64. Bright R. Cases and observations connected with disease of the pancreas and duodenum. Med Chir Tr 1833; 18: 1–16.

65. Karmody AJ, Kyle J. The association between carcinoma of the pancreas and diabetes mellitus. Br J Surg 1969; 56: 362–4.

66. Kessler II. Cancer and diabetes mellitus. A review of the literature. J Chron Dis 1971; 23: 579–600.

67. Schwartz SS, Zeidler A, Moossa AR, Kuku SF, Rubenstein AH. A prospective study of glucose tolerance, insulin, C-peptide, and glucagon responses in patients with pancreatic carcinoma. Dig Dis Sci 1978; 23: 1107–14.

68. Permert J, Larsson J, Westermark GT, Herrington MK, Christmanson L, Pour PM, Westermark P, Adrian TE. Islet amyloid polypeptide in patients with pancreatic cancer and diabetes. New Engl J Med 1994; 330: 313–18.

69. Hayashida CY, Suzuki K, Fujika H, Koizumi M, Toyota T, Goto Y. Morphometrical quantitation of pancreatic endocrine cells in patients with carcinoma of the pancreas. Tohoku J Exp Med 1983; 141: 311–22.

70. Jalleh RP, Williamson RCN. Pancreatic exocrine and endocrine function after operations for chronic pancreatitis. Ann Surg 1992; 216: 656–62.

71. Bittner R, Butters M, Buchler M, Nagele S, Roscher R, Beger HG. Glucose homeostasis and endocrine pancreatic function in patients with chronic pancreatitis before and after surgical therapy. Pancreas 1994; 9: 47–53.

72. Morrow CE, Cohen JI, Sutherland DER, Najarian JS. Chronic pancreatitis: long-term surgical results of pancreatic duct drainage, pancreatic resection, and near-total pancreatectomy and islet transplantation. Surgery 1984; 90: 608–15.

73. Morel PH, Rohner A. Surgery for chronic pancreatitis. Surgery 1987; 101: 130–5.

74. Rossi RL, Rothschild J, Braash JW, Munson JL, ReMine SG. Pancreatoduodenectomy in the management of chronic pancreatitis. Arch Surg 1987; 122: 416–20.

75. Keith RG, Saibil FG, Sheppard RH. Treatment of chronic alcoholic pancreatitis by pancreatic resection. Am J Surg 1989; 157: 156–62.

76. Ammann RW, Akovbiantz A, Largiader G, Schueler G. Course and outcome of chronic pancreatitis. Longitudinal study of a mixed medical-surgical series of 245 patients. Gastroenterology 1984; 86: 820–8.

77. Rotman N, Sastre B, Fagniez PL. Medial pancreatectomy for tumors of the neck of the pancreas. Surgery 1993; 113: 532–5.

78. Kendall DM, Sutherland DER, Najarian JS, Goetz FC, Robertson RP. Effects of hemipancreatectomy on insulin secretion and glucose tolerance in healthy humans. New Engl J Med 1990; 322: 898–903.

79. Seaquist ER, Robertson RP. Effects of hemipancreatectomy on pancreatic alpha and beta cell function in healthy human donors. J Clin Invest 1992; 89: 1761–6.

80. Seaquist ER, Pyzdrowski K, Moran A, Teuscher AU, Robertson RP. Insulin-mediated and glucose-mediated uptake following hemipancreatectomy in healthy human donors. Diabetologia 1994; 37: 1036–43.

81. Valverde I, Alercon C, Ruiz-Grande C, Rovira A. Plasma glucagon and glucagon-like immunoreactivity in totally pancreatectomised humans. In Tiengo A, Alberti KGMM, Del Prato S, Vranic M (eds) Diabetes secondary to pancreatopathy. Amsterdam: Excerpta Medica, 1988: pp 51–62.

82. Doi K, Prentki M, Yip C, Muller WA, Jeanrenaud B, Vranic M. Identical biological effects of pancreatic glucagon and a purified moiety of canine gastric immunoreactive glucagon. J Clin Invest 1979; 63: 525–31.

83. Lawrence AM, Kristins L, Hoguat S et al. Submaxillary gland hyperglycemic factor in man and animals: an extrapancreatic glucagon. Clin Res 1976; 24: 364–7.

84. Barnes AJ, Bloom RS. Pancreatectomised man: a model for diabetes without glucagon. Lancet 1976; 1: 219–21.

85. Geric JE, Karam JH, Lorenzi M. Diabetes without glucagon. Lancet 1976; 1: 855 (letter).

86. Donowitz M, Felig P. Diabetes without glucagon. Lancet 1976; 1: 855–6 (letter).

87. Muller WA, Brennan MF, Tan MH, Aoki TT. Studies of glucagon secretion in pancreatectomised patients. Diabetes 1974; 23: 512–16.

88. Werner PL, Palmer JP. Immunoreactive glucagon response to oral glucose, insulin infusion and deprivation, and somatostatin in pancreatectomised man. Diabetes 1978; 27: 1005–12.

89. Bringer J, Mirouze J, Marchal G, Pham TC, Luyckx A, Lefebvre P, Orsetti A. Glucagon immunoreactivity and antidiabetic action of somatostatin in the totally pancreatectomised and gastrectomised human. Diabetes 1981; 30: 851–6.

90. Muller WA, Berger M, Suter P, Cuppers JH et al. Glucagon immunoreactivities and amino acid profile in plasma of duodenopancreatectomized patients. J Clin Invest 1979; 63: 820–7.

91. Boden G, Master RW, Rezvani I, Palmer JP, Lobe TE, Owen OE. Glucagon deficiency and hyperaminoacidaemia after total pancreatectomy. J Clin Invest 1980; 65: 706–16.

92. Tiengo A, Bessioud M, Valverde I, Tabbi-Anneni A, Del Prato S et al. Absence of alfa cell function in pancreatectomized patients. Diabetologia 1982; 22: 25–32.

93. Holst JJ, Pederson JH, Baldissera F, Stadil F. Circulating glucagon after total pancreatectomy in man. Diabetologia 1983; 25: 396–9.

94. Bajorunas DR, Fortner JG, Jaspan JB. Glucagon immunoreactivity and chromatography pattern in pancreatectomised humans. Paradoxical response to glucose. Diabetes 1986; 35: 886–93.

95. Villanueva ML, Hedo JA, Marco J. Plasma glucagon immunoreactivity in a totally pancreatectomized man. Diabetologia 1976; 12: 613–16.

96. Dammann HG, Bestirman HS, Bloom SR, Schreiber H. Gut-hormone profile in totally pancreatectomised patients. Gut 1981; 22: 103–7.

97. Del Prato S, Vigili de Kreutzenberg S, Lisato G et al. Glucose and intermediary metabolism in diabetes following total pancreatectomy. In Tiengo A, Alberti KGMM, Del Prato S, Vranic M (eds) Diabetes secondary to pancreatopathy. Amsterdam: Excerpta Medica, 1988: pp 143–162.

98. Gutniak M, Grill V, Wiechel K-L, Efendic S. Basal and meal-induced somatostatin-like immunoreactivity in healthy subjects and IDDM and totally pancreatectomised patients. Effect of acute blood glucose normalization. Diabetes 1987; 36: 802–7.

99. Yasida H, Harano Y, Ohgaku S, Kosugi K, Hideka H, Kashiwagi A, Shigeta Y. Insulin sensitivity in pancreatitis, liver diseases, steroid treatment and hyperthyroidism assessed by glucose, insulin, and somatostatin infusion. Horm Metab Res 1984; 16: 3–6.

100. Ginsberg H, Kimmerling G, Olefsky JM, Reaven GM. Demonstration of insulin resistance in untreated adult onset diabetic subjects with fasting hyperglycemia. J Clin Invest 1975; 55: 454–61.

101. Nosadini R, Del Prato S, Tiengo A, Duner E, Toffolo G, Cobelli C, Faronato PP, Moghetti P, Muggeo M. Insulin sensitivity, binding and kinetics in pancreatogenic diabetes. Diabetes 1982; 31: 346–55.

102. Yki-Jarvinen H, Kiviluoto T, Taskinen M-R. Insulin resistance is a prominent feature of patients with pancreatogenic diabetes. Metabolism 1986; 35: 718–21.

103. Bajorunas DR, Dressler CM, Horowitz GD, McDermott K, Jeevanandam M, Fortner JG, Brennan MF. Basal glucagon replacement in chronic glucagon-deficiency increases insulin resistance. Diabetes 1986; 35: 556–62.

104. Del Prato S, Castellino P, Simonson DC, DeFronzo RA. Hyperglucagonemia and insulin-mediated glucose metabolism. J Clin Invest 1987; 79: 547–56.

105. Vigili de Kreutzenberg S, Maifreni L, Lisato G, Riccio A, Trevisan R, Tiengo A, Del Prato S. Glucose turnover and recycling in diabetes secondary to total pancreatectomy: effect of glucagon infusion. J Clin Endocrinol Metab 1990; 70: 1023–9.

106. Finkelstein SM, Wielinski CL, Elliott GR, Warwick WJ, Barbosa J, Wu SC, Klein DJ. Diabetes mellitus associated with cystic fibrosis. J Pediatr 1988; 112: 373–7.

107. Lanng S, Thorsteinsson F, Erichsen G, Nerup J, Koch C. Glucose tolerance in cystic fibrosis. Arch Dis Child 1991; 66: 612–16.

108. Reisman J, Corey M, Canny G, Levison H. Diabetes mellitus in patients with cystic fibrosis. Pediatrics 1990; 86: 374–9.

109. Rodman HM, Doezshuk CF, Roland JM. The interaction of 2 diseases: diabetes mellitus and cystic fibrosis. Medicine 1986; 65: 389–97.

110. Stutchfield PR, O'Halloran SM, Smith CS, Woodrow JC, Bottazzo GF, Heaf D. HLA type, islet cell antibodies and glucose intolerance in cystic fibrosis. Arch Dis Child 1988; 63: 1234–9.

111. The cystic fibrosis genotype–phenotype consortium. Correlation between genotype and phenotype in patients with cystic fibrosis. New Engl J Med 1993; 329: 1308–13.

112. Stahl M, Girard J, Rutishauser M, Nars PW, Zuppinger K. Endocrine function of the pancreas in cystic fibrosis: evidence for an impaired glucagon and insulin response following arginine infusion. J Pediatr 1974; 84: 821–4.

113. Wilmshurst EG, Soeldner JS, Holsclaw DS et al. Endogenous and exogenous insulin responses in patients with cystic fibrosis. Pediatrics 1975; 55: 75–82.

114. Moran A, Diem P, Klein DJ, Levitt MD, Robertson RP. Pancreatic endocrine function in cystic fibrosis. J Pediatr 1991; 118: 715–23.

115. Moran A, Pyzdrowski KL, Weinreb J et al. Insulin sensitivity in cystic fibrosis. Diabetes 1994; 43: 1020–6.

116. Lippe BM, Kaplan SA, Neufeld ND et al. Insulin receptors in cystic fibrosis: increased receptor number and altered affinity. Pediatrics 1980; 65: 1018–22.

117. Anderson O, Garne S, Heilmann C, Petersen KE, Petersen W, Koch C. Glucose tolerance and insulin receptor binding to monocytes and erythrocytes in patients with cystic fibrosis. Acta Pediatr Scand 1988; 77: 67–71.

118. Holl RW, Wolf A, Rank N, Heinze E. Reduced pancreatic release and impaired insulin sensitivity contribute to high incidence of diabetes mellitus in young adults with cystic fibrosis. Diabetes 1993; 42: 60A.

119. Cucinotta D, Nibali SC, Arigo T et al. Beta cell function and peripheral sensitivity to insulin and islet cell autoimmunity in cystic fibrosis patients with normal glucose tolerance. Horm Res 1990; 34: 33–8.

120. Austin A, Kalhan SC, Orenstein D, Nixon P, Arslanian S. Roles of insulin resistance and β-cell dysfunction in the pathogenesis of glucose intolerance in cystic fibrosis. J Clin Endocrinol Metab 1994; 79: 80–5.

121. Lippe BM, Sperling MA, Dooley RR. Pancreatic alpha and beta cell function in cystic fibrosis. J Pediatr 1977; 90: 751–5.

122. Geffner ME, Lippe BM, Kaplan SA, Itami RM, Gaillard BK, Levin SR, Taylor IL. Carbohydrate tolerance in cystic fibrosis is closely linked to pancreatic exocrine function. Pediatr Res 1984; 18: 1107–11.

123. Del Prato S, Tiengo A, Baccaglini U et al. Effect of insulin replacement on intermediary metabolism in diabetes secondary to pancreatectomy. Diabetologia 1983; 25: 252–9.

124. Barnes AJ, Bloom SR, Mashiter K, Alberti KGMM. Persistent metabolic abnormalities in diabetes in the absence of glucagon. Diabetologia 1977; 13: 71–5.

125. Del Prato S, Vigili de Kreutzenberg S, Trevisan R et al. Hyperalaninemia is an early feature of diabetes secondary to total pancreatectomy. Diabetologia 1985; 28: 277–81.

126. Cherrington AD. Gluconeogenesis: its regulation by insulin and glucagon. In Brownlee M (ed) Diabetes mellitus, vol 3. New York: Sarland SPIM Press, 1981: pp 49–117.

127. Kiviluoto T, Yki-Jarvinen H, Taskinen M-R. Metabolic characteristics in patients with pancreatogenic diabetes. In Tiengo A, Alberti KGMM, Del Prato S, Vranic M (eds) Diabetes secondary to pancreatopathy. Amsterdam: Excerpta Medica, 1988: pp 137–42.

128. Muggeo M, Moghetti P, Faronato PP, Valerio A, Del Prato S, Nosadini R. Insulin receptors on circulating blood cells from patients with pancreatogenic diabetes and normal subjects. J Endocrinol Invest 1987; 10: 311–19.

129. Dettwyler W. Le diabete des pancreatopathies. Sem Hop Paris 1964; 40: 1676–82.

130. Barnes AJ, Bloom SD, Alberti KGMM, Smythe P, Alford FP, Chisholm DJ. Ketoacidosis in pancreatectomised man. New Engl J Med 1977; 296: 1250–3.

131. Del Prato S, Nosadini R, Riva F, Fedele D, Devide A, Tiengo A. Glucagon levels and ketogenesis in human diabetes following total or partial pancreatectomy and severe chronic pancreatitis. Acta Diabetol Lat 1980; 117: 111–18.

132. Santeusanio F, Massi-Benedetti M, Angeletti G, Calabrese G, Bueti A, Brunetti P. Glucagon and carbohydrate disorder in a totally pancreatectomised man. A study with the aid of an artificial endocrine pancreas. J Endocrinol Invest 1981; 4: 93–6.

133. Joffe B, Kurt L, Bank S, Marks IN, Keller P. Serum lipid levels in diabetes secondary to chronic pancreatitis. Metabolism 1970; 19: 87–9.

134. Tiengo A, Segato T, Briani G et al. The presence of retinopathy in patients with secondary diabetes following pancreatectomy or chronic pancreatitis. Diabetes Care 1983; 6: 570–8.

135. Muller WA, Cuppers HJ, Zimmerman-Telschow H, Micheli H, Wyss T, Renold AE, Berger M. Amino acid and lipoproteins in plasma of duodenopancreatectomized patients: effects of glucagon in physiological amounts. Eur J Clin Invest 1983; 13: 141–9.

136. Kiviluoto T, Schröder T, Karonen S-L, Kuusi T, Lempinen M, Taskinen M-R. Glycemic control and lipoproteins after total pancreatectomy. Ann Clin Res 1985; 17: 110–15.

137. Boden G. Amino acid metabolism in diabetes secondary to pancreatopathy. In Tiengo A, Alberti KGMM, Del Prato S, Vranic M (eds) Diabetes secondary to pancreatopathy. Amsterdam: Excerpta Medica, 1988: pp 179–86.

138. Trevisan R, Marescotti C, Avogaro A, Tessari P, Del Prato S, Tiengo A. Effects of different insulin administrations on plasma amino acid profile in insulin-dependent diabetic patients. Diabetes Res 1989; 12: 57–62.

139. Sinha SK. Pancreatic diabetes in man: clinical features and management. In Podolsky S, Viswanathan M (eds) Secondary diabetes. New York: Raven Press 1980: pp 197–214.

140. Linde J, Nilsson LH, Baramy F. Diabetes and hypoglycemia in chronic pancreatitis. Scand J Gastroenterol 1977; 12: 369–73.

141. Ishe I, Lilja P, Arnesjo B, Bengmark S. Total pancreatectomy for cancer. Ann Surg 1977; 186: 675–80.

142. Braasch JW, Vito L, Nugent FW. Total pancreatectomy for end-stage chronic pancreatitis. Ann Surg 1978; 188: 317–22.

143. Trede M, Schwall G. The complications of pancreatectomy. Ann Surg 1988; 207: 39–47.

144. Pliam MB, ReMine WH. Further evaluation of total pancreatectomy. Arch Surg 1975; 110: 506–12.

145. Frey C, Child CG, Fry W. Pancreatectomy for chronic pancreatitis. Ann Surg 1976; 184: 403–14.

146. Dressler CM, Fortner JG, McDermott K, Bajorunas DR. Metabolic consequences of (regional) total pancreatectomy. Ann Surg 1991; 214: 131–40.

147. Gall FP, Guhe E, Gebhardt C. Results of partial and total pancreaticoduodenectomy in 117 patients with chronic pancreatitis. World J Surg 1981; 5: 269–75.

148. Assan R, Alexander HH, Tiengo A, Marre M, Costauoilleres L, Lhomme C. Survival and rehabilitation after total pancreatectomy. A follow-up of 36 patients. Diabète Métab 1983; 11: 303–9.

149. Joffe BI, Bank S, Marks IN. Hypoglycemia in pancreatitis. Lancet 1968; 2: 1038.

150. Larsen S, Hilsted J, Philipsen EK, Tronier B, Christensen NJ, Damkjear Nielsen M, Worning H. Glucose counterregulation in diabetes secondary to chronic pancreatitis. Metabolism 1990; 39: 138–43.

151. Horie H, Matsuyama T, Namba M et al. Responses of catecholamines and other counterregulatory hormones

to insulin-induced hypoglycemia in totally pancreatectomised patients. J Clin Endocrinol Metab 1984; 59: 1193-6.

152. Polonski KS, Herold KC, Gilden JL, Bergenstal RM, Faug US, Moossa AR, Jaspan JB. Glucose counterregulation in patients after pancreatectomy. Diabetes 1984; 33: 1112-19.

153. Del Prato S, Vigili de Kreutzenberg S, Riccio A, Duner E, Lisato G, Valerio A, Tiengo A. Insulininduced hypoglygemia in patients with diabetes secondary to total pancreatectomy; mechanisms of impaired counterregulation. Diabet Nutr Metab 1990; 3: 111-21.

154. Bajorunas DR. Insulin action and sensitivity in diabetes secondary to pancreatopathy. In Tiengo A, Alberti KGMM, Del Prato S, Vranic M (eds) Diabetes secondary to pancreatopathy. Amsterdam: Excerpta Media, 1988: pp 123-36.

155. Alberti KGMM. Diabetes secondary to pancreatopathy: an example of brittle diabetes. In Tiengo A, Alberti KGMM, Del Prato S, Vranic M (eds) Diabetes secondary to pancreatopathy. Amsterdam: Excerpta Medica, 1988: pp 211-14.

156. Ebert R, Creutzfeldt W. Reversal of impaired GIP and insulin secretion in patients with pancreatogenic steatorrhea following enzyme substitution. Diabetologia 1980; 19: 198-204.

157. Petrides A, DeFronzo RA. Glucose metabolism in cirrhosis: a review with some perspective for the future. Diabetes Metab Rev 1989; 5: 691-709.

158. Avogaro A, Tiengo A. Alcohol, glucose metabolism, and diabetes. Diabetes Metab Rev 1993; 9: 129-46.

159. Emanuele MA, Kirsteins L, Reda D, Emanuele NV, Lawrence AM. The effect of in vivo ethanol exposure on basal growth hormone secretion. Endocr Res 1989; 14: 283-91.

160. Jenkins JS, Connolly J. Adrenocortical response to ethanol in man. Br Med J 1968; 2: 804-5.

161. Avogaro A, Fontana P, Valerio A et al. Alcohol impairs insulin sensitivity in normal subjects. Diabetes Res 1987; 5: 23-7.

162. Mohan V, Ramachandran A, Viswanathan M. Diabetes secondary to pancreatopathy. In Tiengo A, Alberti KGMM, Del Prato S, Vranic M (eds) Diabetes secondary to pancreatopathy. Amsterdam: Excerpta Medica, 1988: pp 215-26.

163. Gerich JE, Lorenzi M, Bier DM, Schneider V, Tsalikian E, Karam JH, Forsham J. Prevention of human ketoacidosis by somatostatin: evidence for an essential role of glucagon. New Engl J Med 1975; 292: 985-9.

164. Raskin P, Rosenstock J. Blood glucose control and diabetic complications. Ann Intern Med 1986; 105: 254-62.

165. Dulin WE, Gerritsen GC, Chang AY. Experimental and spontaneous diabetes in animals. In Ellenberg M, Rifkin H (eds) Diabetes mellitus: theory and practice. New York: Medical Examiners Publishers 1983: pp 361-408.

166. Calwell AR, Alpert LK, Becker B, Kendall FE, LeCompte PM, Vascular disease. Panel discussion. Diabetes 1957; 6: 180-6.

167. Bell ET. Pancreatitis. Surgery 1958; 43: 527-37.

168. Siperstein MD, Unger RH, Madison LL. Studies of muscle capillary basement membranes in normal subjects, diabetic and prediabetic patients. J Clin Invest 1968; 47: 1973-99.

169. Pirart J, Barbier S. Effect protecteur de l'hémochromatose vis-à-vis des lésions vasculaires séniles ou diabétiques. Diabetologia 1971; 7: 227-36.

170. Deckert T. Late complications in pancreatogenic diabetes mellitus. Acta Med Scand 1960; 168: 439-44.

171. Tutin M, Bour H. Le diabete des pancreatites chroniques. Rev Prat Paris 1966; 16: 3355-63.

172. Ennis G, Miller M, Unger FM, Unger L. Intercapillary glomerulosclerosis in diabetes secondary to chronic relapsing pancreatitis. Diabetes 1969; 18: 333.

173. Sevel D, Bristow JH, Bank S, Marks I, Jackson P. Diabetic retinopathy in chronic pancreatitis. Arch Ophthalmol 1971; 86: 245-50.

174. Verdonk CA, Palumbo PJ, Gharib H, Bartholomew LG. Diabetic microangiopathy in patients with pancreatic diabetes mellitus. Diabetologia 1975; 11: 395-400.

175. Maekawa N, Ohneda A, Kai Y, Saito Y, Koseki S. Secondary diabetic retinopathy in chronic pancreatitis. Am J Ophthalmol 1978; 85: 835-40.

176. Moinade S, Meyrand G. Diabète et pancréatite chronique: à propos de 20 cas. Sem Hop Paris 1979; 55: 1883-6.

177. Couet C, Genton P, Pointel JP et al. The prevalence of retinopathy is similar in diabetes mellitus secondary to chronic pancreatitis with or without pancreatectomy and in idiopathic diabetes mellitus. Diabetes Care 1985; 8: 323-8.

178. Mohan V, Mohan R, Susheela L, Snehalatha C, Bharani G, Mahajan VK, Ramachandran A. Tropical pancreatic diabetes in South India: heterogeneity in clinical and biochemical profile. Diabetologia 1985; 28: 229-32.

179. Gullo L, Parenti M, Monti L, Pezzilli R, Barbara L. Diabetic retinopathy in chronic pancreatitis. Gastroenterology 1990; 98: 1577-81.

180. Larsen S, Hilsted J, Philipsen EK, Lund-Anderson H, Parving HH, Worning H. A comparative study of microvascular complications in patients with secondary and type 1 diabetes. Diabet Med 1990; 7: 815-18.

181. Griffiths JD, Dymock IW, Davies EWG, Hill DW, Williams R. Occurrence and prevalence of diabetic retinopathy in hemochromatosis. Diabetes 1971; 20: 766-70.

182. Briani G, Riva F, Midena E et al. Prevalence of microangiopathic complications in hyperglycemia secondary to acquired pancreatic disease. J Diabet Compl 1988; 2: 50-2.

183. Becker D, Miller M. Presence of diabetes glomerulosclerosis in patients with hemochromatosis. New Engl J Med 1960; 263: 367-73.

184. Marre M, Hallab M, Roy J, Lejeune JJ, Jallet P, Fressinaud P. Glomerular hyperfiltration in type I, type II, and secondary diabetes. J Diabet Compl 1992; 6: 19-24.

185. Tiengo A, Briani G, Scaldaferri E et al. Renal hemodynamics and albumin excretion rate in patients with diabetes secondary to acquired pancreatic disease. Diabetes Care 1992; 15: 1591-7.

186. Green OC. Endocrinological complication associated with cystic fibrosis. In Lloyd Stoll JD (ed.) Textbook of cystic fibrosis. Bristol: John Wright, 1983: pp 329-50.

187. Rosnan RC, Shwachman H, Kulczycki L. Diabetes mellitus and cystic fibrosis of the pancreas. Am J Dis Child 1962; 104: 625-34.

188. Eriksson WJ, Doepel M, Widen E, Halme L, Ekstrand A, Groop L, Hockerstedt K. Pancreatic surgery, not pancreatitis, is the primary cause of diabetes after acute fulminant pancreatitis. Gut 1992; 33: 843-7.

189. Starke AAR, Cuppers HJ, Berger M. Therapeutic problems. In Tiengo A, Alberti KGMM, Del Prato S, Vranic M (eds) Diabetes secondary to pancreatopathy. Amsterdam: Excerpta Medica, 1988: pp 227-33.

190. Beyer J, Schulz G, Cordes U. A glucose-controlled insulin infusion system (Biostator) in pancreatectomised patients. In Brunetti P, Alberti KGMM, Albisser M, Hepp KD, Massi Benedetti M (eds) Artificial systems for insulin delivery. New York: Raven Press, 1983: pp 535-42.

191. Easter DW, Cuschieri A. Total pancreatectomy with preservation of the duodenum and pylorus for chronic pancreatitis. Ann Surg 1990; 214: 575-80.

192. Farney AC, Najarian JS, Nakheleh RE, Loveras G, Field MJ, Gores PF, Sutherland DE. Autotransplantation of dispersed pancreatic islet tissue combined with total or near-total pancreatectomy for treatment of chronic pancreatitis. Surgery 1991; 110: 427-37.

193. Gullo L, Pezzilli R, Morselli-Labate AM, and the Italian Pancreatic Cancer Study Group. Diabetes and the risk of pancreatic cancer. New Engl J Med 1994; 331: 81-4.

11

Drug Effects on Glucose Homeostasis

Peter Bressler and Ralph A. DeFronzo

Diabetes Division, University of Texas Health Science Center, San Antonio, TX, USA

INTRODUCTION

The onset of non-insulin dependent diabetes mellitus (NIDDM) usually occurs after the age of 40–50 years (at least in Europids), so many individuals with NIDDM have multiple medical conditions that are associated with the aging process. It has become recognized recently that NIDDM is part of a complex metabolic–cardiovascular syndrome comprising hypertension, dyslipidemia, obesity, and atherosclerosis [1–4]. It is therefore hardly surprising that most diabetic patients are on multiple drug combinations in addition to their standard diabetic medications. The purpose of the present chapter is, first, to review those medicines which are known to affect glucose homeostasis adversely in diabetic and non-diabetic subjects; and second, where evidence exists, to examine the mechanism(s) via which these drugs exert their deleterious effect(s) on carbohydrate metabolism. The emphasis will be on antihypertensive and related drugs (as in a previous review by us [5]), and on sex steroids. Table 1 lists the drugs discussed, together with some other drugs which may have adverse effects on glucose homeostasis.

DIURETICS

It is now well recognized that use of diuretics is associated with the development of impaired glucose metabolism. In acknowledgment of the potential adverse side effects of classical antihypertensive agents, the Canadian Hypertension Consensus Conference has recommended that thiazides and β-blockers

Table 1 Drugs with potential adverse effects on glucose homeostasis

Diuretics
β-adrenergic blockers
Calcium channel blockers
α-agonists—clonidine
β-adrenergic agonists
Nicotinic acid
Alcohol
Pentamidine
Encainide
Dilantin
Rifampin
Isoniazid
Phenothiazines
Cyclosporine
Lithium
Aspirin
Estrogens and progestogens
Anabolic steroids
Testosterone
Glucocorticoids
Thyroid hormones
Librium [358]
Dapsone [359]
Amoxapine [360]
Indomethacin [361]
Theophylline [362]
Cimetidine [363]
Nalixidic acid [364]
Fish oil (omega-3 fatty acids) [365]
Tricyclic antidepressants
Asparginase

Drugs are listed in the order in which they are discussed in this chapter. Reports on drugs not discussed here are indicated by reference numbers.

be relegated to second-line therapy in the treatment of hypertension in diabetic patients [6]. Nonetheless, in the most recent US Joint National Committee Report

---

International Textbook of Diabetes Mellitus, Second Edition. Edited by K.G.M.M. Alberti, P. Zimmet, R.A. DeFronzo, and H. Keen (Honorary)

(V) (JNC-V) on Hypertension [7], diuretics (along with β-blockers) were recommended as first-line therapy for the treatment of patients with hypertension, on the basis that these are the only class(es) of drugs that have been shown to decrease cardiovascular morbidity and mortality in long-term, prospective intervention trials in *non-diabetic* subjects [8–10]. It should be noted, however, that meta-analyses of these major primary prevention studies [8–10] have failed to demonstrate the expected decline in coronary artery morbidity and mortality following effective lowering of the blood pressure with diuretics (and/or β-blockers), the observed decrease being less than half of that predicted (in contrast to stroke morbidity and mortality, where findings matched predictions). Moreover, three recent studies [11–13] have shown an increase in cardiovascular morbidity and mortality in hypertensive *diabetic* patients who received diuretic therapy (Figure 1). Using the newer, more stringent JNC-V guidelines [14], the prevalence of hypertension has been estimated to be 51% in IDDM and a staggering 80% in NIDDM; and in NIDDM patients with any degree of nephropathy it rises to 90%. In newly diagnosed NIDDM patients the prevalence of hypertension (using the WHO definition of SBP ≥ 160 mmHg and/or DBP ≥ 90 mmHg) is approximately 40% [15]. This raises significant concern about the use of diuretics in this population because of their potential to impair glucose metabolism (see below) and to promote a more atherogenic plasma lipid profile (reviewed in ref. [16]).

Shortly after their institution in the 1950s, it quickly became clear that many hypertensive patients who were treated with thiazide diuretics developed impaired glucose tolerance or overt diabetes mellitus [17–28]. Consistent with these early observations, a number of longitudinal studies [29–42] have suggested a link between glucose intolerance and use of diuretics. However, many of these studies lacked appropriate controls and must therefore be viewed with caution, since there is an age-related decline in glucose tolerance [43] that results from the development of insulin resistance [44]. Murphy et al [29] followed 34 non-diabetic hypertensive patients over a 14-year period and found a 28% increase in the fasting blood glucose concentration and a 45% increase in the 2 h post-glucose load blood glucose concentration in thiazide-treated patients; 10 of the patients developed new-onset impaired glucose tolerance or frank diabetes mellitus after starting treatment. Seven months after cessation of the thiazide, plasma glucose values had decreased modestly but remained significantly above pretreatment levels. In a longitudinal study carried out in Sweden, 1462 women were followed-up for 12 years [30]; those receiving diuretics had a 3.4 greater relative risk of developing diabetes compared to those who were normotensive and were not receiving diuretics (Figure 2). In the Framingham study, the relative risk of developing diabetes was increased by 2.1 in males and by 2.5 in women treated with diuretics [31]. The European Working Party on High Blood Pressure in the Elderly (EWPHE) [32, 33] in a 3-year follow-up of 270 patients treated with hydrochlorothiazide plus triamterene, showed significant increases in both the fasting and 2 h postprandial plasma glucose concentrations in the treatment group, compared with controls. Similar results have been reported in

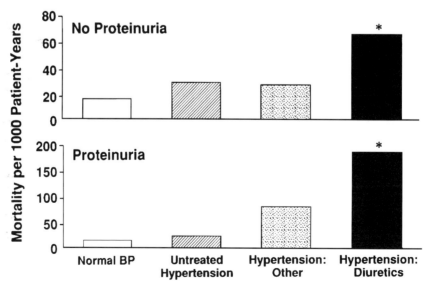

Figure 1 Effect of diuretic therapy on cardiovascular mortality in hypertensive diabetic patients with and without proteinuria. Effective lowering of the blood pressure was associated with a twofold increase in coronary artery disease mortality. *p < 0.01 vs. all other groups. Drawn from the data presented in reference 11

the Medical Research Council (MRC) trial [34, 35], the VA cooperative study [36, 37], and other studies [38–40]. With a few exceptions, these long-term studies, although subject to methodological differences and carried out in different patient populations, have demonstrated a deterioration in glucose tolerance in non-diabetic subjects treated with thiazide diuretics.

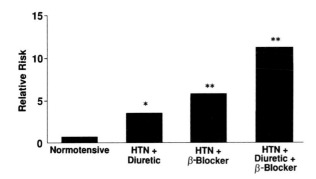

Figure 2 Relative risk of developing diabetes mellitus following the institution of diuretic and β-blocker therapy for the treatment of hypertension (HTN) in a 12-year prospective study of women in Sweden. *$p < 0.01$ and **$p < 0.001$ vs. the normotensive group. Drawn from the data presented in reference 30

The effect of diuretic therapy on glycemic control has been studied extensively in diabetic subjects. Following initial case reports which demonstrated a worsening of diabetic control following the institution of diuretic therapy [45–47], numerous long-term studies

carried out in larger numbers of NIDDM patients have confirmed this observation. Plavnik et al [48] examined the effect of 25 mg chlorthalidone in 21 non-diabetic hypertensive and 9 NIDDM hypertensive patients before and after 4 weeks of therapy. A significant deterioration in the OGTT was found in the diabetic group and similar results were observed in the subgroup of non-diabetic subjects who experienced a decline in the serum potassium concentration (see below) (Figure 3). In a short-term study Rapoport and Hurd [49] studied 16 patients with either mild diabetes or a positive family history of diabetes, who received an OGTT before and after 8 days of chlorothiazide. Seven of the 16 experienced a deterioration in glucose tolerance, which returned to baseline in all subjects after discontinuation of the diuretic. Conrad et al [50] treated 20 NIDDM patients with 50 mg/day of hydrochlorothiazide for 4 weeks, and noted a 1.4 mmol/l (25 mg/dl) rise in fasting plasma glucose concentration. A number of other studies have shown that doses of thiazide diuretics ranging from 25 to 50 mg/day cause a similar deterioration in glycemic control in NIDDM patients [24, 51–54]. A cross-sectional study of 434 insulin-treated diabetic patients found significantly higher HbA$_{1c}$ in those receiving hydrochlorothiazide treatment than in those not receiving diuretic therapy [55]. Because the thiazide diuretics have been in use for a long time and have been employed in most of the large, long-term prospective antihypertensive trials, their diabetogenic action is well established. However, it is now clear that most, if not

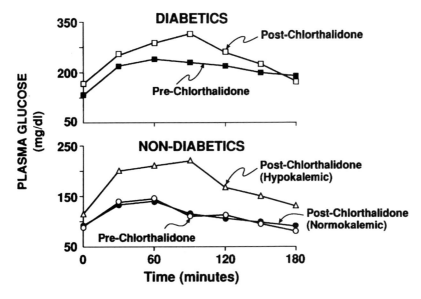

Figure 3 Plasma glucose concentration during an OGTT in NIDDM hypertensive subjects (upper panel) and non-diabetic hypertensive subjects (lower panel) following 4 weeks of therapy with chlorthalidone (25 mg/day). Glucose tolerance declined significantly in the diabetic group, irrespective of changes in plasma potassium concentration. In the subgroup of non-diabetics who developed hypokalemia, a deterioration in glucose tolerance was observed. Redrawn from the data presented in reference 48

all, of the oral diuretic agents also have the potential to impair glucose tolerance.

The loop diuretics, including furosemide and ethacrynic acid, have been shown to increase the fasting glucose concentration and to impair oral glucose tolerance [56–63]. Indeed, the loop diuretics, along with the thiazides, have been implicated in precipitation of hyperosmolar hyperglycemic non-ketotic coma [61, 62] (see Chapter 61). Several reports have demonstrated that triamterene, a potassium sparing diuretic, also causes an impairment in glucose tolerance [62, 65, 66]. Indapamide has been reported to have no significant adverse effects on glucose tolerance [67–69], but these studies were small and the follow-up was short. One study [70] however, extended these observations over a 3-year period and demonstrated that indapamide, 2.5 mg/day, had no adverse effect on fasting glucose concentration, post-prandial hyperglycemia, or HbA$_{1c}$. Additional long-term, carefully controlled studies are needed to confirm the observation that indapamide is metabolically neutral with respect to glucose homeostasis.

Most of the studies described above employed doses of thiazides which would be considered to be high ($\geq$ 50 mg of hydrochlorothiazide or the equivalent) by current therapeutic standards. In the VA Cooperative Study [36, 37], which included both diabetic and non-diabetic subjects, large doses of hydrochlorothiazide (up to 200 mg/day) were compared with propranolol. The study followed 683 patients for up to 48 weeks and found a significant increase in the fasting plasma glucose concentration, as well as an excessive rise in the plasma glucose response during the OGTT with hydrochlorothiazide (as well as propranolol). In the hydrochlorothiazide treated group, 10% developed overt NIDDM, while a further 10% manifested impaired glucose tolerance, and there was a clear dose–response relationship between the daily dose of hydrochlorothiazide and the deterioration in glucose tolerance. Studies such as this, suggesting that the effect of thiazides on glucose tolerance is dose related, have led investigators to look at lower doses of thiazides. Most recently, it has been suggested that 12.5–25 mg/day of hydrochlorothiazide is effective in lowering blood pressure, is devoid of any adverse effects on glucose metabolism in non-diabetic hypertensive individuals [71–75, 79], and does not worsen glycemic control in non-insulin dependent diabetic subjects [76]. Reducing the dosage of chlorthalidone from 25 to 15 mg/day negated the hyperglycemic effect induced by the higher (25 mg/day) dosage [77]. In a subset of the MRFIT trial [78], 140 patients were treated with either 50 or 100 mg/day of chlorthalidone. The higher dosage produced a non-significant 3 mg/dl (0.2 mmol/l) increase in fasting glucose; the lower dose

had no effect on glucose levels. Using cyclopenthiazide in dosages ranging from 125 to 500 μg/day, no changes in glucose or insulin values during an OGTT were observed [80]. In a 2-year trial with low dose bemetizide no improvement in glycemia was noted when the dosage was decreased from 20 to 10 mg/day [81].

However, there are an equal number of reports in which low-dose diuretic therapy has either caused an overt impairment in glucose tolerance or has induced insulin resistance. In the study of Berglund et al [75], 53 hypertensive subjects were followed for 1, 2, 4, 6 and 10 years. Low doses of bendroflumethiazide, 2.5–5.0 mg/day, caused significant increases in both fasting glucose and insulin concentrations and a deterioration in the oral glucose tolerance test (Figure 4). In an earlier study they had shown that low doses of hydrochlorothiazide, 12.5–25.0 mg/day, for 6 weeks also caused a significant rise in fasting glucose concentration [74] by contrast with many others (see above). McKenney confirmed these results, demonstrating a 10 mg/dl (0.56 mmol/l) increase in fasting glucose with very low doses of hydrochlorothiazide, 12.5 mg/day [83]. Harper et al [84] examined the effects of bendrofluazide (5 vs. 1.25 mg/day) in non-diabetic hypertensive patients with the insulin clamp. Although no difference in insulin-mediated whole body glucose uptake was observed between dosages, higher fasting plasma insulin concentrations and an elevated rate of basal glucose production were observed with the 5 mg/day dose, which would be considered low-dose diuretic therapy. These results indicate that, even when administered in low doses, thiazides may have

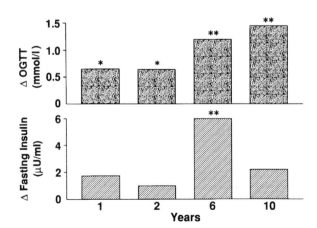

Figure 4 Effect of bendroflumethiazide on plasma glucose and insulin concentrations during the OGTT. Low doses of bendroflumethiazide, 2.5–5.0 mg/day (equivalent to 12.5–25.0 mg/day of hydrochlorothiazide), caused significant rises in both the plasma glucose and insulin concentrations in non-diabetic individuals with essential hypertension. $^*p < 0.01$, $^{**}p < 0.001$. Redrawn from the data presented in reference 75

the potential to cause abnormalities in glucose tolerance, at least in some individuals. It is also important to remember that both insulin resistance and hyperinsulinemia, which were not measured in most of these earlier reports, have been implicated as important etiologic factors in the development of atherosclerosis [1–4]. Since thiazides cause insulin resistance and hyperinsulinemia (see below), changes in glucose tolerance will underestimate the true deleterious impact of diuretic therapy on atherosclerotic cardiovascular complications. Glucose tolerance may not in fact decline at all if the compensatory increase in insulin secretion is sufficient to offset the defect in insulin action. In this context, it is disturbing that increases in fasting insulin levels (an index of worsening insulin sensitivity) have been noted even with low-dose diuretic therapy [74, 75]. Even if low-dose diuretics were to be shown to be free of adverse side effects on glucose (and lipid) metabolism, they would still be contraindicated in the treatment of non-diabetic hypertensive patients according to JNC-V guidelines, because there would still be no long-term studies showing that they are efficacious in preventing atherosclerotic cardiovascular events.

Even though a multitude of studies have demonstrated a deterioration in glucose tolerance in both non-diabetic and diabetic patients receiving diuretic therapy, the mechanism(s) underlying the impairment in carbohydrate homeostasis have yet to be clearly delineated. Following ingestion of glucose, insulin secretion is stimulated and the combination of hyperinsulinemia plus hyperglycemia enhances glucose uptake by peripheral tissues, primarily muscle, and suppresses hepatic glucose production. In the most general sense, a deterioration in glucose tolerance might be explained either

by a defect in insulin secretion or by diminished tissue (muscle and/or liver) sensitivity to insulin [85, 86].

Effects on tissue sensitivity to insulin, which have been demonstrated for diuretics (and for other antihypertensive drugs discussed later), are shown in Figure 5. Pollare, Lithell and colleagues [87–89], using the hyperinsulinemic euglycemic clamp technique, demonstrated a decrease in peripheral (muscle) insulin sensitivity in patients with essential hypertension who were treated with hydrochlorothiazide, 40 mg/day, for 4 months. The impairment in insulin sensitivity was associated with higher fasting plasma insulin and glucose concentrations and a rise in HbA_{1c} levels. Mean serum potassium fell in the diuretic-treated group, but no correlation was found between the potassium concentration and degree of insulin resistance. Kageyama et al, using similar methods, noted a 12% decrease in insulin sensitivity after 12 weeks of trichlormethiazide treatment [90]. Swislocki et al [91] showed that hypertensive patients who were treated with a thiazide diuretic developed impaired glucose tolerance despite a twofold increase in the plasma insulin response during an OGTT, indicating an impairment in insulin sensitivity. They then used the insulin suppression test to provide direct evidence for the presence of insulin resistance (Figure 6).

In a study of reversibility of the deleterious effect of diuretics, Ames and Hill [92] withdrew thiazides from 23 hypertensive patients for an average of 7.5 weeks and noted improvements in fasting glucose and HbA_{1c} levels and in the OGTT. The plasma insulin response during the OGTT also declined following cessation of the thiazide, suggesting reversal of the underlying insulin resistance. Rooney et al [93], using the euglycemic insulin clamp, studied control subjects

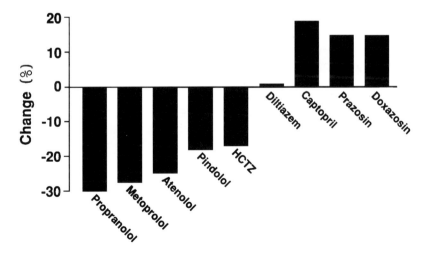

Figure 5 Effect of antihypertensive drugs on tissue sensitivity to insulin. Diuretics and both non-specific and specific β-adrenergic antagonists were shown to be associated with the development of insulin resistance. HCTZ = hydrochlorothiazide. Drawn from the data presented in references 87–89

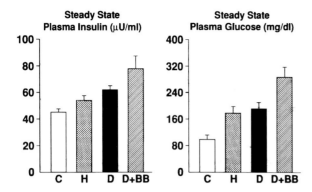

Figure 6 Effect of thiazide diuretics and combined diuretic/β-blocker therapy on the steady-state plasma glucose (SSPG) and steady-state plasma insulin concentrations (SSPI) during the insulin suppression test in hypertensive subjects. Higher SSPG in the presence of higher SSPI levels indicates the presence of insulin resistance in the groups treated with diuretics and β-blockers. C = control; H = untreated hypertensives; D = hypertensive subjects treated with thiazide diuretic; D + BB = hypertensives treated with a diuretic plus a β-blocker (propranolol). Redrawn from reference 91, with permission

and patients with untreated hypertension before and after 12 weeks of treatment with cyclopenthiazide (500 µg/day). Although no change in peripheral insulin sensitivity was seen in either group, increases in fasting glucose and insulin concentrations and basal hepatic glucose production were observed after treatment. Consistent with these *in vivo* observations, chlorothiazide has been shown to inhibit insulin-mediated glucose uptake by the rat hemidiaphragm and epididymal fat in some [94] but not all studies [95]. Somewhat inconsistent with these findings is the report that short-term (2 weeks) thiazide therapy did not impair insulin sensitivity (insulin clamp technique) in insulin dependent diabetic patients [96]. Using the tolbutamide tolerance test, both Beardwood et al [97] and Chazan and Boshell [24] demonstrated a similar decline in plasma glucose concentration before and after 3 days of chlorothiazide treatment. However, neither group measured plasma insulin levels during the tolbutamide tolerance test, so one cannot be certain that the stimulus for glucose uptake was the same before and after chlorothiazide treatment. Chazan and Boshell [24] also failed to observe an impaired hypoglycemic action of insulin during the insulin tolerance test in hypertensive subjects who developed impaired glucose tolerance following treatment with hydrochlorothiazide.

A number of studies have examined the effect of thiazides on insulin secretion *in vitro*. They have demonstrated either no effect [94, 98] or a stimulatory effect [100] of thiazides on insulin secretion. Infusion of large doses of chlorothiazide into dogs failed to alter glucose-stimulated insulin release into the pancreatic

vein [101]. By contrast, several studies in man have shown that chronic thiazide administration can lead to impairment of insulin secretion [25, 45, 102]. However, at least one study has shown a deterioration in glucose tolerance without any change in insulin secretion [26].

In some patients the defect in insulin secretion following thiazide treatment can be related to the presence of hypokalemia. Rowe et al [103] examined the effect of total body potassium depletion and hypokalemia on glucose homeostasis in seven healthy young subjects. Using Kayexalate, total body potassium stores were decreased by 4.9% over an 8-day period, and this was associated with a decline in plasma potassium concentration from 3.7 to 3.3 meq/l. Insulin sensitivity, measured with the insulin clamp technique, remained unchanged. Insulin secretion, measured with the hyperglycemic clamp technique, declined by 26%, and the decrease in insulin response correlated well with the severity of total body potassium depletion and degree of hypokalemia. The development of hypokalemia has also been reported to be associated with an increased proportion of proinsulin [104]. Consistent with the results of Rowe et al [103] are the results of an early study by Sagild et al [105], who failed to demonstrate any deleterious effect of hypokalemia on insulin sensitivity in healthy subjects.

In agreement with the deleterious effects of hypokalemia on glucose tolerance and insulin secretion, potassium repletion has been shown to reverse thiazide-induced hyperglycemia in several studies [36, 106]. Helderman et al [107] studied seven healthy subjects with the hyperglycemic clamp before and after 10 days of hydrochlorothiazide treatment (100 mg/day). Five of the subjects received supplemental potassium replacement which was sufficient to maintain normokalemia, and no changes in insulin secretion or insulin sensitivity were observed. In the two subjects who received no supplemental potassium, hypokalemia was associated with impaired glucose tolerance and a decrease in insulin secretion. By contrast, Fajans et al [102] showed that in healthy volunteers treated with large doses of thiazides, glucose tolerance and insulin secretion were impaired, but that these abnormalities could not be corrected by potassium repletion. These results suggest the presence of an insulin secretory defect which is independent of potassium depletion or hypokalemia.

In summary, a large number of studies have shown consistently that diuretic therapy can cause a significant impairment in glucose tolerance in non-diabetic individuals and a deterioration in glycemic control in NIDDM patients. The deleterious effect on glucose tolerance is observed with all classes of diuretics and is seen even in the lower dose ranges. Defects in both insulin sensitivity and insulin secretion contribute to the deterioration in glucose homeostasis. The pancreatic defect may be related to the development of total body potassium depletion and hypokalemia.

BETA-BLOCKERS

β-Adrenergic blockers, along with diuretics, were recommended by the most recent US JNC-V report on hypertension as first-line drug therapy in non-diabetic and diabetic subjects [7]. However, the Committee added a precautionary statement about the use of β-blockers in patients with diabetes. When considering the use of these drugs in diabetic patients, one also must take into account many factors other than glucose tolerance. In particular, the β-blockers, especially the non-selective β-1 and β-2 antagonists, are known: (a) to cause dyslipidemia [18]; (b) to promote hypoglycemia, both by directly inhibiting hepatic glucose production and by blocking the counter-regulatory hormonal response to hypoglycemia; (c) to interfere with the recognition of hypoglycemic symptoms; (d) to exacerbate peripheral vascular disease; (e) to induce hyperkalemia; and (f) to cause sexual dysfunction. On the other hand, coronary artery disease occurs with increased frequency in diabetic patients, and β-blockers are the only class of drugs that have been shown to decrease the incidence of sudden death in the post-myocardial infarction period. Moreover, in diabetic patients with angina pectoris, β-adrenergic antagonists and calcium channel blockers represent the primary therapeutic options for the control of chest pain.

Many long-term studies in non-diabetic hypertensive subjects have demonstrated that β-blockers can effectively lower blood pressure [34, 36, 108], but diabetic patients have generally been excluded from these large, population-based intervention trials. Numerous small studies have, however, demonstrated the efficacy of β-blockers for treating hypertension in NIDDM and in IDDM subjects [109–115].

The β-blockers were recommended as first-line agents by JNC-V, based upon their proven efficacy to reduce cardiovascular morbidity and mortality. However, few of the large, long-term, prospective studies have in fact employed β-blockers as monotherapy for treatment of essential systolic/diastolic hypertension in non-diabetic subjects [34, 116–121]. Moreover, the results of these trials are not necessarily in agreement. In the Medical Research Council trial [34], which involved over 17 000 hypertensive individuals, β-blockers had absolutely no protective effect on morbidity or mortality from cardiac disease, while the beneficial effect on stroke was largely lost after 7 years. The Heart Attack Primary Prevention in Hypertension (HAPPHY) trial [117] and its continuation, the Metoprolol Atherosclerosis

Prevention in Hypertension (MAPHY) trial [118], have also provided conflicting results about the use of β-blockers in the treatment of essential hypertension. In the HAPPHY trial [117] β-blockers (atenolol or metoprolol) were compared with thiazides in 6500 male subjects with moderately severe hypertension who were followed for 4.2 years. Total and cardiovascular mortality was similar in both groups. The MAPHY trial was a 14-month extension of the HAPPHY trial, in which the atenolol patients were dropped from follow-up. After 4.2 years, patients treated with metoprolol displayed a 58% reduction in cardiovascular mortality, but by 5.4 years this had decreased to 27% which was no longer significantly different from the diuretic-treated group. Moreover, when the 4.2 year follow-up results of β-blocker therapy (both metoprolol and atenolol) from the HAPPHY trial are compared with the 4.2 year follow-up of the MAPHY trial, it is clear that the group treated with atenolol must have done significantly worse than the groups treated with metoprolol or thiazides. In the International Prospective Primary Prevention Study in Hypertension (IPPPHS), β-blockers were compared with other antihypertensive drugs (diuretics, sympatholytics, vasodilators). No difference in myocardial infarction, stroke, or total/cardiovascular mortality was observed between the two treatment groups [119]. Unfortunately, there was no true control group (i.e. placebo only).

It is therefore possible to make a strong argument that the efficacy of β-blockers in the treatment of young to middle-aged patients with combined systolic/diastolic hypertension has not been irrefutably established. It is noteworthy that these equivocal results stand in contrast to the consistent reduction in cardiovascular events observed in elderly (>60 years) patients with isolated systolic hypertension [116, 120–122]. However, elderly hypertensives by definition represent a selected population who have avoided atherosclerotic complications, and are therefore unlikely to have the insulin resistance syndrome [1–4]. They would then be less susceptible to the deleterious effects of β-blockers (and diuretics) on carbohydrate and lipid metabolism.

Diabetic subjects have generally been excluded from hypertension intervention trials or, when included, have not been analyzed separately. Only two studies, the Hypertension Detection Follow-up Program (HDFP) [123, 124] and the Hypertension–Stroke Cooperative Study Group (HSCSG) [125] have presented separate data on diabetic and control subjects but β-blocker therapy was not employed in either of these studies. Interestingly, antihypertensive therapy failed to decrease total mortality in diabetic subjects in the HDFP [123, 124] and did not decrease the recurrence of stroke or myocardial infarction in hypertensive diabetic patients who previously had suffered a myocardial infarction or stroke in the HSCSG [125]. In both of these studies diuretics were employed as the primary antihypertensive agent. A long-term prospective study would seem to be needed to define what role, if any, β-blockers and diuretics have in the treatment of the hypertensive diabetic patient in the absence of renal disease and/or sodium retention.

Despite the lack of clear-cut data to support their efficacy in preventing long-term atherosclerotic cardiovascular complications, and despite their many potential adverse side effects (Table 2), especially in diabetics, the β-blockers have gained widespread use in the treatment of hypertension. Their potential to cause impaired glucose tolerance and/or to precipitate overt diabetes in non-diabetic individuals and to worsen glycemic control in established diabetic patients has long been recognized.

Both *in vitro* and *in vivo* studies [126, 127] have established that stimulation of the β-2 adrenergic receptor stimulates insulin secretion and, conversely, that β-2 adrenergic blockade inhibits insulin release [126–128]. Infusion of propranolol has been shown to impair glucose-stimulated [129, 130], as well as sulfonylurea-stimulated [131, 132] insulin release. In 1462 Swedish women followed for over 12 years, Bengtsson [133] reported that the incidence of diabetes mellitus was increased 5.7-fold in hypertensive individuals treated with β-adrenergic blockers and a similarly high incidence has been reported in men by Skarfors et al [134]. Other studies have found modest increases, 0.5–1.0 mmol/l (9–18 mg/dl), in fasting and postprandial plasma glucose concentrations in non-diabetic hypertensive individuals treated with non-selective β-adrenergic blockers [35, 36, 136–138]. In the VA cooperative study [36, 37] a significant

worsening of both fasting and postprandial glucose was found after 48 weeks of treatment with propranolol in NIDDM patients. In the MRC trial [34, 35] a trend towards worsened glucose tolerance was observed with propranolol treatment, although this did not reach statistical significance. Mohler et al [139] treated 40 non-diabetic patients with propranolol in doses ranging from 160 to 320 mg/day, and found that over half of them developed either impaired glucose tolerance or overt diabetes mellitus. Most of these patients returned to normoglycemia after discontinuation of the drug. Cardioselective β-adrenoreceptor blockers appear to have a less deleterious impact on glucose homeostasis in non-diabetic individuals than non-selective β-blockers [140].

It was to be expected, in view of the findings in non-diabetic subjects, that diabetic patients treated with β-adrenergic blockers would experience a deterioration in glucose tolerance. Wright et al [110], using a cross-over design to examine the effect of propranolol vs. metoprolol therapy in 20 hypertensive NIDDM patients, found significant elevations (1.0–1.5 mmol/l, 18–27 mg/dl) in the fasting glucose concentration with both drugs. Groop et al [142] in a similar study showed a significant rise in the fasting glucose concentration with propranolol together with deterioration in oral glucose tolerance, but no significant change with metoprolol. Whitcroft et al [143] examined 27 NIDDM patients after 3 months of treatment with either propranolol, nadolol or atenolol, and found significant increases in HbA$_{1c}$ in all three groups compared with the placebo period. In the Norwegian multicenter [144] trial, timolol was administered to diabetic and non-diabetic subjects following a myocardial infarction. Compared with a placebo-treated group, there was a significant increase in fasting glucose concentration in

Table 2 Effects of β-adrenergic blockers, diuretics and other antihypertensive drugs in hypertensive diabetic individuals

	Diuretics	β-Adrenergic blockers	Converting enzyme inhibitors	Calcium channel blockers	α-Adrenergic blockers
Insulin secretion	⇓	⇓	0	0	0
Insulin action	⇓	⇓	0,⇑	0	⇑
Hepatic glucose production	0	⇓	0	0	0
Counter-regulatory hormone response	0	⇓	0	0	0
Recognition of hypoglycemia	0	⇓	0	0	0
Dyslipidemia	⇓	⇓	0,⇑	0	⇑
Preservation of renal function*	0	0	⇑	⇑	0,⇑
Antiatherogenic**	0	0	⇑	⇑	?
Potassium					
Hyperkalemia	0	⇑	⇑	0	0
Hypokalemia	⇓	0	0	0	0
Impotence	⇓	⇓	0	0	0
Aggravation of PVD	0	⇓	0	0	0

⇓ = worsened; ⇑ = improved; 0 = neutral.
*Specific effect, independent of blood pressure.
**Animal studies.

both diabetic and non-diabetic groups who received timolol. An important feature of this study was the significant reduction in sudden death in patients treated with timolol compared with placebo. Thus, β-blockers are indicated for the prevention of sudden death in the post-myocardial infarction period [144–146]. However, the protective effect of the β-blockers against sudden death is lost after 14–18 months and, if angina is not a problem, the β-blocker can be discontinued 1–1.5 years after the myocardial infarction (see also Chapter 64).

The combination of a diuretic plus a β-adrenoreceptor blocker appears to act synergistically to worsen glucose tolerance. Fuh et al [147] found a 20 mg/dl (1.1 mmol/l) greater increase in fasting blood glucose concentration in NIDDM subjects treated with hydrochlorothiazide plus propranolol than in those treated with hydrochlorothiazide or propranolol alone. Similarly, in 14 NIDDM patients reported by Dornhorst et al [148], propranolol *or* hydrochlorothiazide alone caused only a small increase in fasting glucose concentrations, whereas the combination of hydrochlorothiazide plus propranolol resulted in a significantly greater rise in both fasting glucose and in HbA$_{1c}$ values. Swislocki et al [91], in studies discussed above, showed that combination therapy with a β-blocker plus a diuretic causes a much greater impairment in glucose tolerance and in insulin sensitivity (Figure 6) than either agent alone. The long-term population based studies of Bengtsson [133, 136] and Skarfors et al [134], as well as the Oslo Study [40], also indicate that thiazide diuretics plus a β-blocker act synergistically to impair glucose tolerance.

Currently available β-blockers differ widely in both their selectivity (β-1 vs. β-2) and in their lipophilicity, and it has been suggested that these differences may account for some of the variability in the results that have been reported with different β-blockers [127]. In addition to the above-mentioned study by Groop et al [142], a study by Micossi et al [109] has provided evidence that the selective β-1 blocker metoprolol has less of a deleterious effect on oral glucose tolerance than the non-selective propranolol. Metoprolol also caused less impairment in glucose tolerance than alprenolol (another non-selective β-adrenergic blocker) in NIDDM patients, when the two drugs were given in equipotent β-blocking dosages [149]. Further support for the importance of β-adrenergic selectivity comes from a recent study using celiprolol, a selective β-1 blocker. After 3 months of treatment, NIDDM subjects showed no worsening in fasting glucose or postprandial glucose concentrations, or in 24-h urinary glucose excretion [150]. Similarly, no adverse effect on the IVGTT was observed when celiprolol was given

to young healthy subjects [151]. Waal-Mannig [152] found an improvement in the OGTT in a group of 15 hypertensive patients with impaired glucose tolerance, after metoprolol was substituted for a variety of non-selective β-blockers. Further evidence for the importance of β-receptor selectivity comes from a study comparing metoprolol (a β-1 blocker) with dilevalol, a β-1 blocker with both β-2 antagonist and agonist properties [153]. In this trial equipotent blood pressure-lowering dosages were employed for 24 weeks to treat 50 hypertensive subjects. In the metoprolol group insulin sensitivity decreased significantly and the HbA$_{1c}$ level rose slightly. By contrast, the dilevalol group showed a small increase in insulin sensitivity.

Whitcroft et al [143] suggested that it might not be the β-adrenergic selectivity, but rather the lipophilicity, that determined the differing effects of β-blockers on glucose tolerance. They compared propranolol (non-selective and lipophilic) vs. nadolol (non-selective and non-lipophilic) vs. atenolol (β-1 selective and non-lipophilic). HbA$_{1c}$ was significantly greater in the propranolol-treated group than in both the nadolol group and the atenolol group when equipotent doses were compared. However, it is important to note that HbA$_{1c}$ levels worsened in all three groups. Results with celiprolol [150], which is both non-lipophilic and β-selective, also support the concept that the degree of lipophilicity may be an important determinant of the effect of β-blockers on glucose tolerance.

Fewer studies have examined the impact of β-blockers on glucose control in IDDM patients. Kolendorf et al [111] found no change in fasting blood glucose concentrations in 12 IDDM subjects after 3 months of treatment with β-adrenergic blockers. Östman et al [155], Lager et al [156] and Viberti et al [157] showed no change in fasting glucose concentrations in IDDM patients following short-term treatment with metoprolol.

The mechanism(s) via which the β-adrenergic antagonists impair glucose tolerance in normal subjects and worsen glycemic control in NIDDM patients are related to their action in inhibiting insulin secretion and causing insulin resistance. NIDDM subjects have coexisting defects in both insulin secretion and insulin sensitivity [85, 86], and overt NIDDM does not occur until the augmented islet B-cell response can no longer keep up with the severity of insulin resistance [85, 86]. At this point in the natural history of NIDDM, even a small decrease in insulin secretion can have a profound effect on glucose homeostasis. Moreover, if insulin resistance declines, albeit slightly, at a time when islet B-cell function cannot increase to offset the defect in insulin action, glycemic control will deteriorate markedly.

A number of studies have examined the effect of treatment with various β-adrenergic blockers on insulin secretion and insulin sensitivity. In one study [110] both metoprolol and propranolol therapy were associated with significant rises in fasting and postprandial plasma glucose levels, but hyperglycemia failed to elicit the appropriate increase in either fasting or meal-stimulated insulin secretion, indicating the presence of a defect in insulin secretion. Groop et al [142] also failed to observe any change in plasma insulin levels following treatment with selective or non-selective β-blockers, and Holm et al [149] demonstrated a worsening of glycemic control on alprenolol (a non-selective β-blocker) without an appropriate increase in plasma insulin levels. These observations are consistent with those of Dornhorst et al [148], who used the mean 24 h urinary C-peptide excretion to provide a measure of the integrated daily insulin secretory rate. Despite the development of significant fasting and postprandial hyperglycemia, urinary C-peptide excretion failed to increase, indicating the presence of an insulin secretory defect. Micossi et al [109], who also found increased postprandial plasma glucose levels following the institution of propranolol therapy, actually observed a decrease in insulin secretion compared with diabetic patients receiving placebo therapy (Figure 7).

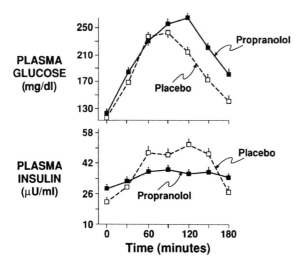

Figure 7 Effect of propranolol on glucose tolerance and insulin secretion in non-insulin dependent diabetic subjects. The deterioration in glycemic control was associated with the inhibition of insulin secretion. Drawn from the data presented in reference 109

These long-term clinical intervention trials have been supported by acute studies examining the effect of β-blockers on insulin secretion. Porte [126] demonstrated a rise in insulin secretion in healthy subjects following infusion of the β-adrenergic agonist, isoproterenol, and this was completely reversed with the addition of

propranolol. Cerasi et al [129], again in healthy subjects, showed that both early and late plasma insulin responses to glucose were impaired following the administration of β-adrenergic blocking agents. Hedstrand et al [128] showed that propranolol inhibited the late, although not the early, plasma insulin response to glucose in normal subjects. In anesthetized dogs, propranolol was found to inhibit insulin secretion, while practolol (a β-1 adrenergic blocker) had only a minimal effect on insulin secretion [127]. *In vitro* studies using isolated islets have also demonstrated an inhibitory effect of β-adrenergic antagonists on insulin secretion [158] (see also Chapters 14 and 15). Thus, *in vivo* and *in vitro* studies carried out in humans and animals have consistently demonstrated an inhibitory effect of β-adrenoreceptor antagonists on insulin secretion, and have shown that this effect is mediated via the β-2 receptor. Since it is clear that α-agonists also inhibit insulin secretion, β-blockers will additionally impair insulin release by causing unopposed α-stimulation.

In NIDDM subjects who are started on β-adrenergic blockers, especially non-specific β-1, β-2 antagonists, the typical picture is of deterioration in glycemic control without any change in fasting or meal-stimulated plasma insulin levels [141, 142, 148, 149], implying a significant impairment in insulin sensitivity. Pollare, Lithell and co-workers [87–89, 161] have used the euglycemic insulin clamp technique to address this issue systematically, and have demonstrated a consistent decline in insulin sensitivity, which was greatest with the non-specific β-adrenergic blockers and which averaged about 30% (Figure 5). Haenni and Lithell [153] have speculated that the effect may be mediated through a reduction in peripheral blood flow and subsequent decrease in glucose availability, since it could be offset with the addition of a vasodilator. It is noteworthy that the 'specific' β-blockers also significantly impaired insulin sensitivity, although the decrease was somewhat less than that observed with propranolol. Swislocki et al [91] have also provided evidence that propranolol causes a decline in insulin sensitivity (Figure 6), and Tötterman et al [162] found a decreased glucose disappearance rate with β-blockers during the insulin tolerance test. By contrast, neither Deibert and DeFronzo [163] nor Ferrara et al [164] observed any deleterious effect of propranolol on insulin action, although the latter study [164] employed a pharmacologic level of insulin and this may have obscured the presence of insulin resistance.

β-Adrenergic blocking drugs have been associated with the development of hypoglycemia in both diabetic [165] and non-diabetic [166, 167] subjects. This can be particularly severe in insulin dependent patients [156, 169]. The hypoglycemic action of the β-blockers is mediated through an inhibition of hepatic glucose production. Epinephrine infusion [163, 170] and sympathetic nervous system stimulation [171] augment hepatic glucose production, while β-blockade inhibits glucose release by the liver. β-Adrenergic drugs also inhibit glucagon secretion [157, 173]. Since catecholamines and glucagon represent the most important counter-regulatory hormones in the defense against hypoglycemia, and since their secretion is often impaired in diabetes, it is not surprising that the use of β-blockers in diabetic patients is not uncommonly associated with hypoglycemia. β-Antagonists also interfere with hypoglycemia awareness by blocking the sympathetic response to hypoglycemia [169]. Most [157], but not all studies have shown that the inhibitory effects of the β-adrenergic antagonists on the counter-regulatory hormone response to hypoglycemia and on hypoglycemia awareness are less marked with the specific β-adrenoreceptor blockers.

In summary, the β-adrenergic blockers have been shown to worsen glycemic control in NIDDM subjects and to impair glucose tolerance or even precipitate overt diabetes mellitus in non-diabetic individuals. The deleterious effect of β-blockers on glucose tolerance is more pronounced with the non-specific β-1, β-2 adrenergic antagonists. Impaired glucose tolerance has also been reported with the specific β-2 antagonists, although this is less common. Combination therapy with a β-blocker plus a diuretic has an additive, perhaps even a synergistic, effect to cause glucose intolerance. The deleterious effect of the β-blockers on glucose homeostasis is related to their ability both to inhibit insulin secretion and to induce insulin resistance. By inhibiting the counter-regulatory response to hypoglycemia and by impairing hypoglycemia awareness, β-blockers also predispose to the development of hypoglycemia, especially in insulin dependent diabetic patients. Because of these adverse effects on glucose metabolism and because of their propensity to promote a more atherogenic plasma lipid profile [18], we believe that the β-adrenergic antagonists should not be considered first-line agents for the treatment of hypertension in diabetic patients.

CALCIUM CHANNEL BLOCKERS

The calcium channel blockers are a pharmacologically diverse group of drugs which have assumed increasing importance in the treatment of patients with essential hypertension and coronary artery disease. Since the incidence of both hypertension and coronary artery disease in diabetes mellitus is two- to threefold that in the normal population, these drugs are commonly prescribed for diabetic patients. There is controversy in the literature regarding the effect(s) of the calcium channel blockers on glucose homeostasis. Some of this

is explicable by differences in study design and drug dosage, some to the fact that the drugs in this category are chemically diverse. Trost and Weidmann [174], in an excellent summary of this topic, concluded that when all of the studies on calcium channel blockers are reviewed collectively, this class of drugs does not appear to have any adverse effect on glucose metabolism. In the present chapter, we will examine the major classes of the calcium channel blockers individually to see if any differences between them can be discerned.

Dihydropyridines (Nifedipine)

Nifedipine is the calcium channel blocker most commonly stated to be associated with the development of impaired glucose tolerance. It belongs to the dihydropyridine class of calcium channel blockers, which are powerful peripheral vasodilators. Nicardipine, isradipine and felodipine are the other dihydropyridines which have been available in the USA, but these have been less extensively studied than nifedipine, at least with respect to effects on glucose metabolism. In NIDDM patients treated with nifedipine for 10 days, increases in both the fasting plasma glucose concentration and the glucose area under the curve (AUC) during an OGTT were observed and these changes were associated with decreased plasma insulin levels, indicating an impairment in insulin secretion [175]. Similar results were found in NIDDM patients treated for as little as 3 days with either nifedipine or nicardipine [176]. Ferlito et al [177] studied 10 hypertensive NIDDM subjects after two doses of nifedipine and found an increase in the plasma glucose concentration at the third hour during an OGTT, but no significant change in the insulin response. An increase in the fasting glucose concentration, but no change in the glucose AUC during an OGTT, occurred in both control and NIDDM subjects after 2 weeks of nifedipine treatment in a study by Deedwania et al [178].

In contrast to the deleterious effects on glucose tolerance observed with short-term administration of dihydropyridines, most longer-term therapeutic trials have failed to reveal any effect on glucose tolerance or insulin secretion [179–181]. Gill et al [182] examined the effect of 1 month of nifedipine therapy on six NIDDM and six non-diabetic hypertensive subjects, and found no changes in fasting glucose or insulin levels, glucose tolerance or insulin response during an OGTT in either group. Lastly, several studies in non-diabetic hypertensive subjects have shown no deleterious effect on either oral or intravenous glucose tolerance tests after 4–6 weeks of treatment with either felodipine or nifedipine [183, 184].

Studies with the newer-generation dihydropyridines have yielded mixed results, although the overall trend appears to be favorable, with no deterioration in either glucose or insulin values during an OGTT after 8 months of amlodipine treatment in subjects with hypertension and diabetes [185], and even an improvement in non-diabetic hypertensive patients [186]. These same authors showed similar results with nifedipine [187]. In hypertensive rats amlodipine has been shown to lower the fasting glucose concentration and increase muscle glucose uptake [188]. By contrast belodipine, in a 4-week study in hypertensive diabetic subjects, was associated with a slight increase in HbA_{1c} values [189]. Longer-term trials (up to 2 years) with isradipine in hypertensive patients revealed a decrease in insulin sensitivity and an increase in HbA_{1c} [190]. However, this study is difficult to interpret because of significant (2.2 kg) weight increase in the isradipine-treated group.

There is some *in vitro* evidence to suggest that dihydropyridines inhibit insulin secretion. Malaisse and Sener [191] demonstrated a dose-related inhibition of insulin secretion in isolated rat islets with nifedipine and four other dihydropyridine compounds. However, the majority of *in vivo* studies have failed to demonstrate a significant inhibitory effect of the dihydropyridines on insulin secretion. One *in vitro* study has shown that nifedipine decreases insulin-stimulated but not hypoxia-stimulated glucose transport in rat muscle [192]. Giordano and DeFronzo [193] failed to find any changes in fasting glucose and insulin levels, glucose and insulin AUC, and HbA_{1c} after 3 months of nifedipine therapy in hypertensive diabetic patients. In summary, most of the evidence points to little or no impairment in glucose tolerance or insulin secretion in patients who are treated with dihydropyridines.

Diltiazem

Diltiazem is a benzothiazepine calcium antagonist which exerts its primary antihypertensive effect via a decrease in peripheral vascular resistance; it also appears to have a small negative ionotrophic effect. In humans, three long-term studies [194–196] have examined the effect of diltiazem on metabolic control and none found any adverse effects on glucose homeostasis. Pollare et al [194], using both the IVGTT and the euglycemic clamp technique, found no significant changes in glucose tolerance, insulin secretion or insulin sensitivity (Figure 5). Nagai et al [195] confirmed these neutral results in a long-term (1-year) study using the OGTT. Andrén et al [196] found no change in fasting glucose, HbA_{1c} or urinary glucose excretion during 3 weeks of diltiazem vs. placebo, and

Jones et al [197] found no change in glucose tolerance after 1 week of diltiazem treatment. Like the dihydropyridines, diltiazem has been shown to inhibit both first- and second-phase insulin release *in vitro* and this inhibitory effect is reversible with increasing concentrations of extracellular calcium [198]. However, as with the dihydropyridines, it is unlikely that the high doses of diltiazem used in these *in vitro* studies have any clinical relevance. Overall there appear to be no deleterious effects of diltiazem on glycemic control in diabetic or non-diabetic individuals.

Verapamil

Verapamil is a phenylalkamine calcium antagonist whose primary antihypertensive effect is mediated via peripheral vasodilation, but it also exerts significant negative ionotrophic and chronotrophic actions, leading to modest reduction in cardiac output. There have been a small number of reports which have examined the effects of verapamil on glucose metabolism. In both acute and long-term studies, verapamil has been shown to produce no change in glucose tolerance in diabetic subjects [112, 113, 199, 200]. Several studies [199–204] have even demonstrated a slight improvement in glucose tolerance in NIDDM patients. Verapamil, like the other calcium channel blockers, has been shown to inhibit glucose-stimulated insulin release *in vitro* in the rat pancreas [205]. However, an inhibitory effect of verapamil on insulin secretion has not been reported *in vivo* [203], and studies examining the effect of verapamil on insulin sensitivity have yet to be reported.

In summary, with the possible exception of short-term worsening of glucose control with nifedipine, the calcium channel blockers do not appear to exert any negative effect on glucose homeostasis in either diabetic or non-diabetic subjects. Although all classes of calcium channel blockers inhibit insulin secretion *in vitro* [191, 198, 205], this effect has not been observed with doses that are normally employed to treat patients with hypertension. None of the calcium channel blockers has been shown to exert any deleterious effect on insulin sensitivity, or to aggravate the plasma lipid profile.

ALPHA-AGONISTS—CLONIDINE

Clonidine is a centrally acting α-2 agonist that is used to treat patients with hypertension. In normal subjects it has been shown to impair glucose tolerance and to decrease insulin secretion, especially the first phase of insulin release [206, 207]. Consistent with this observation, clonidine has been shown to inhibit insulin secretion in a dose-dependent manner in isolated islets and perfused pancreatic tissue [208]. It has been demonstrated that stimulation of α-2 pancreatic receptors leads to the inhibition of insulin secretion [160, 209] and that this effect can be completely reversed by the administration of an α-2 but not an α-1 antagonist [160, 210].

The results of the only two studies to examine the effect of clonidine in diabetic subjects have been somewhat disparate. Guthrie et al [211] treated 10 hypertensive diabetic patients with clonidine 0.1 mg for 10 weeks, and found an increase in the glucose AUC during an IVGTT, but no changes in fasting glucose, HbA$_{1c}$ or 24 h urine glucose. Plasma insulin levels failed to increase despite the increase in plasma glucose response during the IVGTT. Nilsson-Ehle et al [212], in 20 NIDDM patients who were treated with clonidine for 3 months, found no change in fasting glucose and only a small but insignificant increase in HbA$_{1c}$. Similarly, Sung et al [213] found no change in OGTT during 6 weeks of clonidine treatment in a group of non-diabetic subjects.

In summary, clonidine may exert a small deleterious effect on glucose metabolism in some patients, through inhibition of insulin secretion.

BETA-ADRENERGIC AGONISTS

Since the β-blockers inhibit insulin secretion, one might expect that stimulation of the pancreatic β-receptor would augment insulin release. It is therefore somewhat surprising that treatment with β-adrenergic agonists can lead to carbohydrate intolerance. There are a number of studies, mostly from the obstetrics literature, showing that β-2 agonists impair glucose metabolism in normal and diabetic subjects. These drugs are frequently used to induce premature labor late in pregnancy, a physiological condition that is characterized by insulin resistance. Moreover, gestational diabetes is not uncommon during the third trimester of pregnancy in the general population.

Wager et al [214] showed that acute administration of salbutamol, a selective β-2 agonist, caused significant hyperglycemia in normal subjects and in patients with IDDM and NIDDM, the largest increase in glucose levels being observed in IDDM. Fredholm et al [215] gave intravenous salbutamol to pregnant women during the third trimester, and found that the plasma glucose concentration increased by 72 mg/dl (4.0 mmol/l) in both NIDDM and IDDM compared to 32 mg/dl (1.8 mmol/l) in non-diabetic women. Main et al [216] looked at more chronic treatment with 1 week of oral terbutaline in 247 control and 30 pre-term patients at similar stages in late pregnancy and found that 53% of the pre-term patients (compared with

16% in the control group) had an abnormal OGTT. In a large series of 86 non-diabetic women the combination of oral/intravenous ritodrine (a selective β-2 agonist) led to a 12% incidence of gestational diabetes mellitus in the treated group compared with 2.3% in the group not receiving β-agonist therapy [217]. Similar increases in blood glucose concentrations have been observed with all routes of administration (oral, intravenous, subcutaneous) in IDDM, NIDDM, and non-diabetic women [214–227]. Only oral ritodrine has failed to show any significant hyperglycemic action when given to pregnant women [218, 219].

Despite the deterioration in glucose tolerance observed with the β-2 agonists, most studies have shown that insulin secretion increases, although obviously not enough to prevent the rise in glucose levels. Lipschitz and Vinik [220] demonstrated a rise in plasma insulin concentration prior to any increase in plasma glucose levels, which is consistent with the known stimulatory action of β-2 agonists on insulin secretion, and suggests that the rise in plasma insulin was not simply a compensatory response to the development of hyperglycemia. Gündogdu et al [221] studied six control and six IDDM subjects with intravenous salbutamol, using tritiated glucose to follow glucose kinetics. They documented an increase in hepatic glucose production without any change in peripheral glucose disposal. These results suggest that the β-2 agonists have two distinct effects. First, they stimulate release of glucose by the liver. Second, they induce peripheral insulin resistance, since one would have expected the combination of hyperinsulinemia plus hyperglycemia to have augmented glucose disappearance. β-Agonist administration has been shown to lead to a rise in both plasma FFA and glycerol, suggesting that lipolysis was stimulated [226, 227]. A significant rise in plasma glucagon has also been reported with β-2 agonists [220]. Although providing only indirect evidence, these observations suggest that the rise in hepatic glucose production reflects the stimulation of both glycogenolysis and gluconeogenesis by hyperglucagonemia and increased gluconeogenic substrate delivery. It also is likely that β-agonists directly stimulate hepatic glucose output.

In summary, there is considerable evidence that β-2 agonists cause hyperglycemia, especially in the later stages of pregnancy. There have been case reports of diabetic ketoacidosis [228] following infusion of β-2 agonists, and IDDM patients appear to be especially prone to the hyperglycemic effect of these agents, since they lack the endogenous insulin secretory capacity to counteract the increase in plasma glucose concentration. The hyperglycemia appears to be due to stimulation of hepatic glucose production and induction of peripheral tissue resistance to insulin.

NICOTINIC ACID

Nicotinic acid lowers plasma triglyceride and LDL-cholesterol and raises HDL-cholesterol levels [229], and has also been shown to decrease morbidity and mortality from cardiovascular disease [230]. It would therefore appear, at first glance, to be an ideal drug for the treatment of diabetic dyslipidemias. However, its use in diabetic patients is limited by its adverse effects on glucose metabolism. There are numerous case reports of worsened glycemic control in patients with established diabetes mellitus and of precipitation of diabetes in non-diabetic individuals.

It was initially suggested, on the basis of animal studies that nicotinic acid might improve glucose tolerance. In an insulin-deficient rat model, Gross and Carlson [231] showed that an acute infusion of nicotinic acid led to a decline in blood glucose concentration for up to 6 hours; this hypoglycemic action was associated with a decrease in plasma free fatty acid levels. In streptozocin diabetic rats Reaven et al [232] demonstrated that acute intravenous administration of nicotinic acid lowered the elevated plasma glucose concentration and that this beneficial effect was closely correlated with the drug's antilipolytic and plasma FFA lowering effects. When acutely administered in non-diabetic subjects [233, 234] nicotinic acid enhanced insulin sensitivity and glucose tolerance. These beneficial effects result from inhibition of the glucose–fatty acid cycle in muscle [235] and a reduction in hepatic gluconeogenesis [236].

Although these short-term studies demonstrated a beneficial effect, long-term therapeutic trials have overwhelmingly demonstrated worsening glycemic control in both diabetic and non-diabetic patients. Garg and Grundy [237] treated 13 NIDDM patients with nicotinic acid 4.5 g/day over an 8-week period, and noted a 16% increase in the mean plasma glucose concentration and a 21% increase in HbA_{1c}. Molnar et al [238] found a deterioration in glucose control in both IDDM and NIDDM patients who took nicotinic acid for several months to 2 years in dosages ranging from 1–3 g/day. In a study on heart transplant patients, 88% of diabetic subjects had to discontinue nicotinic acid because of worsened glycemic control, while 33% of non-diabetic patients developed diabetes during treatment with nicotinic acid [239]. Lithell et al [240] followed 66 non-diabetic patients who were treated with nicotinic acid for a variety of dyslipidemias and found significant increases in blood glucose levels and a 40% decrease in the K value during an IVGTT. In a study of 28 hypertriglyceridemic patients treated with nicotinic acid, fasting glucose levels increased by 13% and the K value during the IVGTT decreased by 26% after only 4 weeks of treatment [241]. Kahn et al [242] treated 11 normal male volunteers with nicotinic acid (2 g/day) for 2 weeks and found significant increases in both the fasting plasma glucose and insulin concentrations. The fractional rate of glucose decline (K value) during the IVGTT was markedly reduced (Figure 8) despite the presence of hyperinsulinemia, indicating the presence of severe insulin resistance, but there were no changes in plasma cortisol, epinephrine, norepinephrine or glucagon. In parallel studies performed in baboons, the same authors [243, 244] demonstrated that insulin resistance induced by nicotinic acid was associated with a markedly hyperinsulinemic response to both hyperglycemia and arginine infusion. Miettinen et al [245] performed both oral and intravenous glucose tolerance tests on normal subjects before and after 2 weeks of treatment with nicotinic acid. They found higher blood glucose levels with increased insulin concentrations during the OGTT, and diminished K values during the IVGTT, consistent with the induction of insulin resistance. Since nicotinic acid has no direct stimulatory effect on insulin secretion and since elevated (not decreased) FFA levels augment insulin secretion, the hyperinsulinemia seen during treatment of patients with nicotinic acid must represent a compensatory response to the development of insulin resistance.

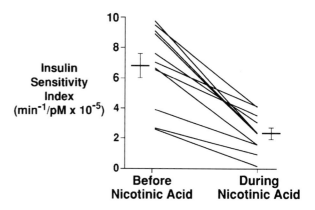

Figure 8 Effect of nicotinic acid ingestion for 2 weeks on insulin sensitivity, as measured with the modified intravenous glucose tolerance test in 11 healthy subjects. From reference 242, with permission

The deterioration in glucose control and development of insulin resistance in patients treated with nicotinic acid is related to the rebound increase in plasma FFA concentration that occurs when the antilipolytic effect of the drug wears off [246, 247]. After ingestion of nicotinic acid, plasma FFA levels decline by 30–40% during the first 4–6 hours, but then rebound to 50–100% above baseline concentrations. This increase in plasma FFA concentration is associated with an augmented rate of FFA oxidation [248]. According to the glucose–fatty acid cycle proposed by Randle and colleagues [249] accelerated FFA oxidation consumes NAD, decreasing the redox potential of the cell, and this leads to an inhibition of the tricarboxylic acid (TCA) cycle and decreases the activity of pyruvate dehydrogenase, with a resultant decrease in glucose oxidation. The accumulation of citrate inhibits phosphofructokinase, leading to product inhibition of the early steps of glucose metabolism. As glucose-6-phosphate accumulates, glucose transport is inhibited and this leads to a decline in glycogen formation. The fatty acyl-CoA derivatives have also been shown to have a direct inhibitory effect on glycogen synthase [250]. At the level of the liver, increased fatty acid oxidation augments gluconeogenesis and, secondarily, total hepatic glucose production [251–253].

Acipimox, a long-acting nicotinic acid-like drug which has recently become available, causes a sustained reduction in plasma FFA concentration without any rebound effect. In over 3000 diabetic subjects treated for at least 2 months, the plasma lipid profile improved (LDL-cholesterol and triglycerides decreased and HDL-cholesterol increased) without any deleterious effect on the fasting plasma glucose concentration, oral glucose tolerance, plasma insulin levels, insulin sensitivity, or HbA$_{1c}$ [254]. Similar results were reported by Tornvall and Walldius in 31 non-diabetic patients after 6 weeks of treatment [255].

ALCOHOL

The effects of ethanol consumption on glucose metabolism in diabetic subjects are varied and highly dependent on the amount and chronicity, and the type of diabetes that is involved [256]. The relation of chronic liver disease, often alcohol-induced, to diabetes mellitus is not considered in the present chapter (see Petrides [64]). Cases of profound hypoglycemia associated with excessive alcohol intake can be found together with reports describing a marked deterioration in glucose control. Ethanol also has adverse effects on triglyceride metabolism and this takes on added importance in the diabetic patient, who has an accelerated rate of atherosclerosis.

When ingested acutely, alcohol has been associated with hypoglycemia, due to inhibition of gluconeogenesis [256, 257]. This is most commonly seen in fasted individuals, who have depleted glycogen stores and therefore depend on gluconeogenesis to maintain hepatic glucose output. When ethanol is metabolized to acetaldehyde and thence to acetate, two molecules of NADH are formed for each molecule of ethanol metabolized. The decline in NAD/NADH (intracellular redox

potential) inhibits the TCA cycle, limiting the supply of precursors for gluconeogenesis (lactate, alanine, and other gluconeogenic amino acids) (Figure 9). Oxaloacetate is a key intermediate in the gluconeogenic pathway, and can be formed not only via the TCA cycle, but also by direct carboxylation of pyruvate by the enzyme pyruvate carboxylase.

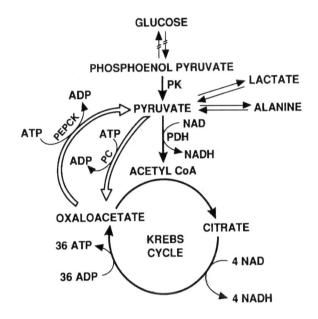

Figure 9 Effect of alcohol on hepatic gluconeogenesis. Metabolism of ethanol causes the intracellular depletion of NAD and subsequent inhibition of the Krebs (TCA) cycle. This leads to a deficiency in energy supply (ATP), resulting in an inhibition of the two key enzymes (PC = pyruvate carboxylase and PEPCK = phosphoenolpyruvate carboxykinase) which regulate flux through the gluconeogenic pathway. See text for a more detailed discussion. PK = pyruvate kinase; PDH = pyruvate dehydrogenase

Both this step, and the conversion of oxaloacetate to phosphoenolpyruvate (PEP) by the enzyme PEP carboxykinase, require ATP, which is primarily derived from the oxidation of pyruvate in the TCA cycle. When the TCA cycle is inhibited by ethanol, ATP is deficient within the cell and both pyruvate carboxylase and PEP carboxykinase are inhibited, leading to a reduction in the rate of gluconeogenesis. If glycogen stores have been depleted by diminished food intake, hepatic glucose output is critically dependent upon gluconeogenesis. Thus, in the glycogen-depleted state acute ethanol ingestion has the potential to induce hypoglycemia by inhibiting gluconeogenesis.

By contrast, chronic ethanol consumption has been associated with a worsening of glycemic control. In one large epidemiological study a strong association was found between elevated plasma glucose levels and alcohol consumption [258]. An inpatient study of chronic alcoholics found that 75% had abnormal glucose tolerance tests, and 25% were classified as diabetic [259]. After 1 week of abstinence these figures were reduced by half, but remained much higher than in the general population. Several studies have examined the effect of short-term ingestion of modest amounts of alcohol in diabetic patients. Early reports suggested that alcohol unmasked glucose intolerance in individuals predisposed to develop diabetes [260], but Singh et al [261], examining the effect of the equivalent of two glasses of wine in NIDDM individuals, found no changes in either fasting plasma glucose or insulin concentrations or in glucose tolerance in an acute short-term study. Walsh and O'Sullivan [262] reported similar findings in NIDDM subjects, but again the dose of ethanol was low and the study was relatively short-term. Ben et al [263], in a study of over 80 NIDDM subjects, found higher fasting and postprandial plasma glucose concentrations, and HbA$_{1c}$ levels, in those (roughly half the group) who consumed moderate amounts of alcohol (45 g/day) than in those who consumed no alcohol. Plasma glucose values decreased to control levels after only 3 days of abstinence. A similar deterioration in glycemic control with moderate alcohol intake has also been reported in insulin dependent diabetic subjects [264, 265]. Nikkilä and Taskinen [266] observed impaired IVGTTs and OGTTs in normal subjects after only 1 week of moderate alcohol use (25% of total daily calories), and a similar deleterious effect of ethanol on glucose tolerance has been reported by others [267, 268].

Several studies have examined the effect of acute ethanol infusion on tissue sensitivity to insulin. When alcohol was infused in normal subjects for 5 h to raise the blood levels to 8.4–17.1 mmol/l (151–308 mg/dl), peripheral tissue muscle sensitivity was reduced by 20–30% [269], and it was demonstrated that ethanol also interfered with the normal inhibitory effect of insulin on hepatic glucose production. Similar results were obtained by Yki-Jarvinen and colleagues, who found a 23% decrease in insulin sensitivity in normal subjects [270, 271]. Using the combined leg/splanchnic balance technique, Jorfeldt and Juhlin-Dannfelt [272] were able to confirm that ethanol inhibited muscle glucose uptake and decreased splanchnic glucose production, and to show that the decline in splanchnic glucose output was associated with decreased lactate and alanine uptake, consistent with an inhibition of gluconeogenesis. Other studies have confirmed these observations. Thus, ethanol administration caused a 70% inhibition of lactate and glycerol conversion to glucose, although no change in total hepatic glucose output was noted. This finding indicates that the observed glucose intolerance must be secondary to peripheral insensitivity to insulin [273]. Consistent with these observations, administration of ethanol in conjunction with a glucose load has been shown to cause a significant shift in fuel metabolism, leading to marked decreases in fat, protein, and carbohydrate oxidation [274]. *In vitro* studies have shown that ethanol, as well as its metabolites (2,3 butanediol and 1,2 propanediol), are potent inhibitors of insulin-stimulated glucose oxidation and lipogenesis [275]. Several studies have suggested that in addition to its effects on muscle and liver, ethanol may also have an inhibitory action on insulin secretion by the pancreatic B cells [276–278].

Although cortisol levels increase acutely with ethanol ingestion [279], no long-term elevation has been observed in chronic alcoholics [280]. In addition, no change in plasma growth hormone, cortisol or glucagon levels were seen following ethanol infusion, even though insulin-mediated glucose disposal declined significantly [281].

In summary, chronic, excessive alcohol consumption even in the absence of cirrhosis is associated with moderate to severe insulin resistance and glucose intolerance. Acute administration of large amounts of ethanol causes insulin resistance in peripheral tissues, primarily muscle. In short-term studies, the consumption of small to modest amounts of alcohol (1–2 glasses of wine/day) does not appear to acutely worsen glycemic control in most diabetic patients. In diabetic subjects whose glycogen stores are depleted (for instance, after a prolonged fast) excessive alcohol consumption can result in hypoglycemia by inhibitory effects on gluconeogenesis.

PENTAMIDINE

It has been known for over 40 years that pentamidine can lead to the development of impaired glucose tolerance and overt diabetes mellitus [282–284]. With the onset of the AIDS epidemic, the use of pentamidine for the treatment of *Pneumocystis carinii* infections has increased dramatically and the development of glucose intolerance and overt diabetes mellitus has become an increasing problem in AIDS patients [285]. It has been estimated that 6–27% of AIDS patients who receive treatment with pentamidine develop impaired glucose tolerance or diabetes [286, 287]. Higher doses of pentamidine have been associated with more severe hyperglycemia [284, 287].

Pentamidine appears to have a direct toxic effect on the islet B-cell, similar in nature to that seen with streptozotocin [288]. Following initial exposure to pentamidine, B-cell injury is associated with the release of insulin secondary to B-cell lysis, but with prolonged exposure, permanent B-cell damage may ensue, resulting in an irreversible B-cell insulin secretory defect [288]. *In vitro* studies have demonstrated that the toxic effect of pentamidine on the B-cell is dose response-related [289]. The clinical picture of pentamidine toxicity closely parallels the histological and pathophysiological change in islet B-cell morphology and function [289]. Hypoglycemia is common during the initial phase of treatment, occurring in 10–38% of individuals [286]. B-cell degranulation and cell lysis are prominent [289] and the very high insulin levels measured during this period [290] can fully account for the development of hypoglycemia. Days to months later, persistent hyperglycemia ensues and B-cell destruction is evident [290]. However, not all pentamidine-treated patients who eventually develop impaired glucose tolerance or diabetes have documented hypoglycemia in the earlier stages of treatment.

Pentamidine isoethionate is an aromatic diamidine and Boillot et al [289] have shown that six other chemically related compounds have similar toxic effects on the islet B cell. Pentamidine mesylate has been reported to be more cytotoxic than pentamidine isoethionate, which is the main compound used in the USA, but in several cases hyperglycemia with pentamidine mesylate has been found to be reversible when the patient was switched to pentamidine isoethionate [291].

In summary, pentamidine appears to have a multi-phasic effect on the islet B-cell, causing cytolysis and degranulation initially (with insulin release and hypoglycemia), and B-cell destruction later (resulting in impaired insulin release, hyperglycemia and even diabetic ketoacidosis [292]). Patients who experience hypoglycemia and renal insufficiency during pentamidine treatment are especially prone to develop glucose intolerance and/or overt diabetes mellitus. Interestingly, pentamidine has been employed in at least one patient with malignant insulinoma to control hypoglycemia [293].

ENCAINIDE

The anti-arrhythmic drug Encainide has been implicated in the case of a patient who developed overt diabetes mellitus, which resolved after the drug was stopped [294]. Plasma insulin and C-peptide levels were significantly increased in this patient. In a larger series of 23 patients, Salerno et al [295] failed to observe any cases of diabetes or impaired glucose tolerance after one month of treatment in the non-diabetic subjects, but found a substantial rise in blood glucose in four diabetic patients. Although the data are sparse, there appears to be sufficient evidence to implicate Encainide in the development of worsened glucose tolerance, especially in individuals with established NIDDM.

DILANTIN

The older literature contains a number of case reports of hyperglycemia following treatment with phenytoins [296–299], but Fariss and Lutcher [300] were the first to document the induction of diabetes following initiation of dilantin therapy and the reversibility of hyperglycemia following withdrawal of the medication. The onset of diabetes was associated with a markedly blunted insulin response to both oral and intravenous glucose, while cessation of the drug resulted in restoration of normal B-cell function [300]. However, long-term, prospective studies which have employed therapeutic doses of dilantin have failed to show any worsening of glucose tolerance after 1 year [301]. Interestingly, although there was no deterioration of glucose tolerance during dilantin therapy, fasting and post-glucose levels declined significantly after the drug was discontinued.

Dilantin has been shown to inhibit both first and second phases of insulin release in the isolated perfused pancreas and in isolated islets [302, 303], and to inhibit both glucose- and arginine-stimulated insulin secretion [302–304]. Kizer et al [302], using isolated pancreatic tissue, showed that the inhibition of insulin release was related to stimulation of the Na-K-Mg ATPase with subsequent lowering of the intracellular sodium concentration, but other groups have suggested that calcium influx is the major determinant of inhibition [302, 304]. In isolated islet cells, phenytoin was shown to inhibit glucose-induced calcium uptake, which is necessary for insulin release [303], and Herschuelz et al [304] confirmed these observations, while Pace et al [305] proposed defects in both sodium and calcium transport. The *in vitro* studies correlate well with the short-term *in vivo* studies carried out by Malherbe et al in humans [306]. Six normal subjects treated with dilantin for 3 days showed a significantly higher rise in plasma glucose concentration and an impaired rate of glucose decline, associated with a decrease in both first- and second-phase insulin responses [306]. From a historical perspective, it is of interest that the inhibitory effect of dilantin on B-cell function was employed to detect early insulin secretory defects in patients with mild glucose intolerance [307]. That test has now fallen from favor, but dilantin has been used successfully to inhibit insulin secretion in patients with insulinomas [308, 309].

In summary, dilantin has been shown to precipitate diabetes in isolated reports, but the individuals involved probably had underlying insulin resistance, so were critically dependent upon intact islet B-cell function to compensate for the defect in insulin action. The incidence of impaired glucose tolerance and/or frank diabetes mellitus in individuals who are treated with dilantin on a chronic basis appears to be quite small.

ANTI-TUBERCULOSIS MEDICATIONS

Certain antituberculosis drugs have been associated with elevated fasting plasma glucose concentrations. Takasu et al [310] demonstrated a deterioration in the OGTT in patients who were treated with rifampicin. This effect was independent of other tuberculosis medications or activity of disease. An augmented plasma insulin response during the OGTT suggested the presence of underlying insulin resistance [310]. Following cessation of rifampicin, glucose tolerance reverted to normal, and none of the patients developed overt diabetes mellitus. Rifampicin has also been reported to accelerate the hepatic metabolism of oral hypoglycemic agents, leading to a worsening of glycemic control in NIDDM patients [311]. Isolated case reports of isoniazid-induced glucose intolerance have been described [312], but neither the frequency nor the mechanism has been defined. With the recent increase in the number of reported cases of tuberculosis, especially those which are resistant to INH, more cases of hyperglycemia following institution of antituberculosis therapy can be expected, and more work is clearly needed in this field.

PHENOTHIAZINES

Although phenothiazines (particularly chlorpromazine) have long been implicated in the development of impaired glucose tolerance [313–316], controlled studies which systematically examine the effect of phenothiazines on glucose metabolism are difficult to find. Erle et al found no change in either the OGTT or IVGTT following 7 days of treatment with chlorpromazine in 10 normal subjects, but the IVGTT was significantly impaired in NIDDM subjects who received intravenous chlorpromazine [317]. In mice, it has been shown that chlorpromazine causes hyperglycemia via an effect on the α-adrenergic receptor, since its diabetogenic action can be blocked by yohimbine, an α-2-blocker [318]. In rats chlorpromazine has been shown to impair glucose utilization in peripheral tissues, specifically muscle [319, 320]. Other groups have reported inhibition of insulin secretion by chlorpromazine both *in vitro* and *in vivo* [321, 322]. In the absence of conclusive data, caution should be exercised when using this class of medication in patients predisposed to develop glucose intolerance.

CYCLOSPORIN

This immunosuppressive drug (commonly used to prevent organ rejection after transplantation) has recently been implicated in the development of impaired glucose tolerance, but findings in transplant patients are confounded by the concomitant use of other medications, including high dose steroids [323–327]. Studies comparing the incidence of overt diabetes mellitus in individuals treated with cyclosporin plus steroids vs. azathioprine plus steroids, have found a twofold greater incidence of diabetes in the patients receiving cyclosporin despite lower dosages of steroids in the cyclosporin group [325]. Onset of diabetes is usually within several months after initiation of cyclosporin therapy, and is often severe enough to require insulin treatment. Reported incidence of impaired glucose tolerance and/or diabetes mellitus in transplant patients treated with cyclosporin ranges from 13% to 47% [326]. Interestingly, a group of 13 patients with multiple sclerosis who were treated with cyclosporin for 1 year showed no evidence of adverse effects on plasma glucose or insulin levels during an IVGTT performed before and after treatment, and there were no differences between these patients and an appropriately matched group of control subjects [327]. It should be noted that the patients with multiple sclerosis were not receiving other immunosuppressive agents, in particular steroids. It may be that the combination of cyclosporin plus glucocorticoids is especially dangerous in the precipitation of diabetes mellitus.

A combination of defects in insulin secretion and peripheral tissue sensitivity to insulin seems to be involved in cyclosporin-induced glucose intolerance. Yale et al [328] found a significant increase in the postprandial glucose levels in rats treated with cyclosporin for 12 weeks. During the first 4 weeks of cyclosporin treatment, the plasma glucose concentration increased without any change in insulin secretion, suggesting the development of insulin resistance with an inappropriate compensatory islet B-cell response. During the last 8 weeks of cyclosporin treatment, there was an absolute decrease in the amount of insulin that was secreted, clearly indicating the presence of a B-cell defect, as has been confirmed by other investigators [329]. Cyclosporin has been shown to inhibit the stimulatory action of the oral sulfonylurea agents on insulin secretion [330, 331]. This toxic effect of cyclosporin on B-cell function appears to be enhanced by administration of prostaglandin inhibitors [332]. Consistent with this observation, the prostaglandin analog, risoprostil, partially protects against the toxic effects of cyclosporin on the B cell [333].

In summary, defects in both insulin secretion and insulin sensitivity [334] are responsible for the impairment in glucose homeostasis often found in cyclosporin-treated transplant recipients. However, cyclosporin cannot be withheld in transplant patients, so it is important to use the lowest possible dose of cyclosporin which is adequate to prevent rejection of the transplanted organ.

LITHIUM

Lithium therapy has been variously associated with improved [335], impaired [336] and no change [337] in glucose tolerance. Interpretation of these results is confounded by the observation that the manic depressive disorder may itself be associated with a higher incidence of impaired glucose tolerance [338], and also by the fact that the lithium treatment is not uncommonly associated with weight gain [336], which of itself may be associated with the development of insulin resistance.

Significant weight gain was noted in a group of 49 patients treated with lithium for 1 year, in whom there was a threefold increase in the incidence of impaired glucose tolerance compared with a normal control group [336]. Higher plasma glucose levels in lithium-treated patients were also reported by Mellerup et al [339], but other reports have described either no change or an improvement in glucose tolerance following lithium treatment. Treatment with lithium for 1 week resulted in lower plasma glucose and insulin concentrations in six NIDDM patients [335], and a significant improvement in the fractional rate of glucose decline (K value) during the IVGTT in 8 normal subjects [340]. The apparent discrepancy in results may be related to opposing actions of the element on islet B-cell function and tissue sensitivity to insulin. Studies in isolated islets *in vitro* [341] have demonstrated an inhibitory effect of lithium on B-cell function which appears to be limited to glucose-induced insulin release, since there was no change in glucagon-induced insulin secretion. By contrast, lithium has been shown to augment insulin sensitivity and to enhance glucose tolerance in diabetic rats [342].

In summary, since published studies have shown both improvement and deterioration in glycemic control, close observation is warranted following the institution of lithium treatment in all diabetic patients.

ASPIRIN

Low dose aspirin therapy has been associated with the development of hypoglycemia [343]. This is related to the well known stimulatory effect of aspirin on the islet B cell [344–347], which is mediated via an inhibition of prostaglandin synthesis [348–350]. In larger doses salicylates can lead to development of impaired glucose tolerance or even frank diabetes mellitus [351–353], and this is related to the ability of salicylates to inhibit oxidative phosphorylation [354], leading to an impairment in glucose oxidation [355]. Acetyl-CoA cannot

enter the TCA cycle to be oxidized, so it is shunted into the ketone pathway and serum ketone levels rise. Because salicylate intoxication is often associated with the development of an anion gap metabolic acidosis, the presence of hyperglycemia and hyperketonemia may be mistakenly diagnosed as diabetic ketoacidosis [355]. One systematic study has examined the effect of chronic aspirin administration in NIDDM patients. Bratusch-Marrain et al [356], using the insulin clamp technique, found a decrease in insulin sensitivity in both NIDDM patients and healthy control subjects, but in both groups plasma insulin levels also rose, so there was no deterioration in glucose tolerance. Newman and Brodows [357] have also reported an impairment in insulin sensitivity in non-diabetic subjects who were treated with aspirin.

In summary, aspirin has a biphasic effect on glucose tolerance. In low doses, glucose tolerance improves and hypoglycemia may occur secondary to a stimulation of insulin secretion, but in higher doses, aspirin impairs insulin sensitivity by uncoupling oxidative phosphorylation, and this may lead to a decline in glucose tolerance.

ESTROGENS

The effect of estrogens on glucose homeostasis has been clouded by their frequent co-administration with progestins. There are, however, a number of studies which have examined the effects of estrogens alone. When all studies are viewed collectively, there appears to be some small negative effect of estrogens on glucose homeostasis, but this is more than outweighed by their beneficial effect on plasma lipids.

The majority of the studies which have demonstrated a deleterious effect of estrogens on glucose metabolism used higher doses of synthetic estrogens than the low doses of naturally-occurring estrogens currently in use. Goldman and Ovadia [366] were amongst the first to examine the effect of estrogens on glucose tolerance in women. They studied two groups: one group, immediately post-partum, was treated with diethylstilbestrol (15 mg/day for 10 days), and another postmenopausal group received Premarin (1.25 mg/day for 3 months). Using the IVGTT, they found a significant impairment in the rate of decline in plasma glucose in both estrogen-treated groups compared with controls. The study included women with both normal and impaired glucose tolerance; the deterioration in glucose tolerance was seen in both groups. Similar results were found in 50 postmenopausal females who were treated with Premarin (1.25 mg/day) [367]. In a study of 29 surgically induced postmenopausal females, glucose tolerance was found to deteriorate after 2 years of treatment with relatively high doses (up to 80 µg) of Mestranol

[368]. Talaat et al [369] reported that short-term estrogen administration caused a worsening of glucose tolerance in diabetic patients due to a decrease in insulin sensitivity. Using high doses of estrogen (Premarin, 1.25 mg twice daily), Aguilo et al found that 23% of women developed diabetes while on treatment [370]. In another group of postmenopausal women treated with either Premarin (1.25 mg/day) or Enovid (5 mg/day), 40% showed a deterioration in glucose tolerance without compensatory hyperinsulinemia [371]. Polderman et al examined 18 trans-sexuals (male to female) before and after 4 months of ethinyl estradiol (0.1 mg/day) [372]. Using the insulin clamp technique, they found decreases in insulin sensitivity and glucose tolerance after treatment. A number of other short-term studies have shown a similar worsening of glucose tolerance with estrogen therapy [373–376]. All of the preceding studies which demonstrated an impairment in glucose tolerance used oral estrogen replacement. Blum et al [377], using vaginal estrogen cream in postmenopausal women, showed a staggering increase in HbA_{1c} from 6.4% to 14.8% and a corresponding decrease in oral glucose tolerance. This deterioration in glucose tolerance is well beyond that seen in any other study. Whether this represents an aberrant response or is in some way related to the vaginal route of administration remains unclear.

A minority of studies have demonstrated either no effect or even a beneficial effect of estrogen treatment on glucose tolerance. In the Rancho Bernardo study, 260 women who were taking estrogen were compared with women who were not taking estrogen [378]. In this epidemiological study estrogen users had a slightly lower fasting blood glucose concentration. The Cardiovascular Health Study [379], which included almost 3000 women aged >65, examined multiple risk factors and their association with coronary artery disease. Insulin and glucose were slightly lower in estrogen users vs. non-estrogen users. These epidemiologic studies are difficult to interpret, since subjects did not serve as their own control. Spellacy et al [380] examined 36 women before and after 1 year of Premarin (1.25 mg/day) treatment and found only a small elevation in the 1 h postprandial glucose level. In a larger study by the same author, a variety of estrogens (Premarin, Mestranol, ethinyl estradiol) were studied in pre- and post-menopausal females [381]. In both groups, only minimal increases in blood glucose levels were observed. In 20 healthy postmenopausal females receiving standard replacement therapy with Premarin (0.625 or 1.25 mg/day) for 2 months, no effects on OGTT were seen [382] and similar results have been reported by Notelovitz [383]. In a study by Cagnacci et al [384], transdermal estradiol was shown to have no deleterious effect on glucose levels.

In summary, the studies reviewed above indicate that estrogens, if given in *high* doses, have a modest negative effect on glucose tolerance.

A number of studies have attempted to define the mechanism(s) of these effects. Using the minimal model method, Elkhind-Hirsch et al [385] examined six women with premature ovarian failure during different phases of their hormone replacement cycle. No change in insulin sensitivity was observed with estrogen alone, but a decrease in insulin action was observed with estrogen plus progesterone therapy. Similarly, Caprio et al [386] found no difference in insulin sensitivity using the insulin clamp in patients with Turner's syndrome who were treated with estrogen therapy. In contrast to these studies, Polderman et al [372] demonstrated that estrogen treatment in trans-sexual men caused a decrease in insulin sensitivity (Figure 10). Several studies suggest that estrogens may impair insulin secretion. Thus, monkeys chronically treated with estrogen exhibited a decrease in the plasma insulin response during an IVGTT and a slower rate of glucose disappearance [387]. Faure et al [388] demonstrated a similar decrease in glucose-stimulated insulin secretion in estrogen-treated rats.

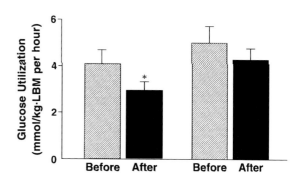

Figure 10 Whole body insulin-mediated glucose utilization in six healthy young men during a two-step euglycemic insulin clamp—≃400 (left panel) and ≃940 (right panel) pmol/l—before (cross-hatched bars) and after (solid bars) treatment with ethinyl estradiol. *$p < 0.01$. LBW = lean body weight. From reference 372, with permission

Finally, oral estrogens may induce significant counter-regulatory hormonal responses which could lead to impaired glucose tolerance. Estrogens have been shown to decrease IGF-I and this could lead to a secondary increase in plasma levels of growth hormone, an insulin antagonistic hormone [389]. No significant effect of estrogen on hepatic glucose production has been observed in estrogen-treated Turner's patients and in trans-sexuals [372, 386, 390].

In conclusion, high doses of synthetic estrogens clearly can cause glucose intolerance. However, the lower doses of naturally occurring estrogens, which currently are employed for menopausal replacement therapy, appear to have no or only a small adverse effect on glucose homeostasis. To place the above studies in perspective, it should be remembered that a dosage of 0.625 mg of Premarin is equivalent to 5–10 μg of ethinyl estradiol, and this is 4–5 times greater than most preparations used in oral contraceptive therapy today [391]. Most importantly, estrogen therapy has a very beneficial effect in reducing plasma cholesterol and triglyceride levels and in decreasing cardiovascular morbidity and mortality [392]. Whatever small deterioration in glucose tolerance occurs with estrogen therapy is more than offset by the beneficial effect on plasma lipids and prevention of atherosclerosis.

PROGESTOGENS

Progesterone has marked and important effects on carbohydrate metabolism. From the long- and well-established changes seen in pregnancy to the more recently identified more subtle changes during various stages of the menstrual cycle, progesterone clearly does have a deleterious influence on glucose metabolism. In this section we will focus primarily on those studies that have looked at progesterone alone, although the combination of estrogen and progesterone (see subsequent section) may have an additive or even synergistic adverse effect on glucose homeostasis.

Spellacy et al [393] examined 89 females who were treated for more than 1 year with norgestrel (0.75 mg/day) and found elevated glucose and insulin values during an OGTT, although only 10% had an abnormal test. As in many of the studies which will be discussed, there was a small, approximately 1 kg, increase in body weight. These same authors [394] found similar results using ethynodiol acetate (0.25 mg/day) in 36 women, with 17% of the OGTTs becoming frankly abnormal. Subsequently, they confirmed these observations [395]. Kalkoff et al [396], using high doses of medroxyprogesterone (300–400 mg/day for 5 days), found a consistent elevation in plasma insulin levels without any change in glucose tolerance, suggesting the presence of insulin resistance. In an 18-month study, 50 women taking norgestrel (0.075 mg/day) experienced a significant increase in plasma glucose and insulin levels [397] and 16% developed a frankly abnormal OGTT. Similar results were reported by the same authors [398] with medroxyprogesterone (150 mg i.m. for 3–12 months). In this later study [398], the fasting glucose concentration rose from 86 to 96 mg/dl (4.8–5.3 mmol/l) and the areas under both the glucose and insulin curves increased. Essentially identical results were found with depomedroxyprogesterone, 400 mg i.m. for

6 months [399]. Leis et al [400], using large doses of medroxyprogesterone acetate to treat endometrial cancer, found elevated plasma glucose concentrations and markedly increased insulin levels during an OGTT after only 3 weeks of treatment. With lower doses of medroxyprogesterone (400 mg i.m. every 6 months for 15 months), no change in plasma glucose levels was observed during an OGTT; however, this was at the expense of modest hyperinsulinemia, indicating the presence of insulin resistance [401]. Levonorgestrel treatment [402] has also been shown to cause IGT, despite an increase in plasma insulin levels. In women with gestational diabetes small increases in the fasting glucose were observed with ethynodiol acetate [403] and similar results were seen with norethindrone in women with IGT or a history of large babies [404]. Although the great majority of studies have demonstrated an impairment in glucose tolerance and/or hyperinsulinemia, some studies with medroxyprogesterone, norethindrone, and ethynodiol [405–407] have failed to find any adverse effects on glucose tolerance.

Impaired insulin secretion cannot explain the deterioration in glucose tolerance observed during progesterone treatment. On the contrary, the great majority of women receiving progesterone demonstrate hyperinsulinemia [393–402, 408, 409], while in some the plasma insulin response remains unchanged [410–412]. These findings strongly suggest that impaired tissue sensitivity to insulin is responsible for development of impaired glucose tolerance following progesterone treatment. It has been suggested that the relative androgenicity of the progestational agent accounts for the development of glucose intolerance. Some progesterone derivatives also possess small amounts of glucocorticoid activity, although the clinical significance of this remains uncertain.

The effect of endogenously produced progesterone on insulin sensitivity has also been examined by studying women in various parts of the menstrual cycle, when progesterone levels are very high. Diamond et al [413] studied eight women in the mid-follicular (high estrogen) and mid-luteal (high progesterone) phases of menstrual cycles with the hyperglycemic clamp technique. They consistently found a decrease in the amount of glucose metabolized per unit of insulin secreted during the luteal compared with the follicular phase of the menstrual cycle (Figure 11). Because the defect in insulin-mediated glucose disposal was observed under hyperglycemic [413] but not euglycemic [414] conditions, the authors suggested that impaired glucose transport was responsible for the insulin resistance. Valdes et al [415], using the tolbutamide IVGTT, also found decreased insulin sensitivity during the luteal vs. the follicular phase.

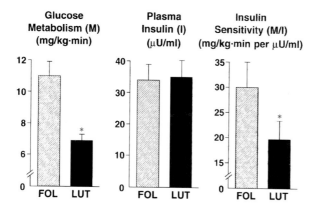

Figure 11 Effect of the menstrual cycle on total body glucose metabolism (M), insulin secretion (I), and tissue sensitivity to insulin (M/I × 100). A significant decline in insulin sensitivity was observed during the luteal (LUT) phase (high progesterone) of the menstrual cycle, compared to the follicular (FOL) phase. *$p < 0.01$. From reference 413, with permission

In vivo and *in vitro* studies in animals have consistently demonstrated the development of insulin resistance following progesterone administration. [416–422]. Ryan and Enns [422] have reported a decrease in maximal insulin binding and decreased glucose transport in rat adipocytes after progesterone treatment. Sutter-Dub and Vergnaud [418] also found that progesterone impaired insulin action in rat fat cells, but observed no decrease in insulin binding. This latter observation indicates a postreceptor abnormality in insulin action and is consistent with a defect in glucose transport.

In summary, progesterone derivatives have consistently been shown to cause insulin resistance and impair glucose tolerance. The newer progesterone derivatives may have a less deleterious effect on glucose homeostasis. However, any woman, especially if diabetic, should have her plasma glucose levels checked within 2–3 months after being started on any progesterone derivative.

COMBINED ESTROGEN/PROGESTERONE ADMINISTRATION

The effects of estrogen alone or progesterone alone on glucose homeostasis were discussed in preceding sections. In this section we shall examine the effect of combination estrogen/progesterone oral contraceptive preparations, which have long been known to impair glucose tolerance [423]. It should be pointed out, however, that much of the older literature is not applicable, since the strength of the individual components has been decreased progressively with time to minimize side effects, and synthetic estrogens/progesterones have been replaced by naturally occurring equivalents. In

general, the more recently developed oral contraceptive formulations have fewer adverse effects with respect to glucose and insulin metabolism because of their lower dosage.

Several large epidemiological studies have demonstrated the adverse effects of oral contraceptive pills (OCP) on glucose homeostasis. In the Telecom experience [424], a retrospective study with 1290 women, OCP users ($n = 431$) had higher postprandial glucose levels and fasting hyperinsulinemia compared to women who were not taking OCPs. Data from NHANES (National Health and Nutrition Examination Survey) [425] showed that 734 female OCP users had elevated 1-h and 2-h plasma glucose values and the overall rate of impaired glucose tolerance was almost twice as high as in non-OCP users (13% vs. 7%). The Walnut Creek Contraception Drug Study [426], a 10-year prospective trial in over 2000 women, found a twofold greater incidence of impaired glucose tolerance (16% vs. 8%) and a 13 mg/dl (0.7 mmol/l) increase in postprandial glucose values in 354 OCP users. In a more recent study employing lower-dose formulations, Godsland et al [427] studied 296 women on various OCP regimens. All estrogen/progesterone combinations were associated with an elevated glucose AUC during the IVGTT. The same group confirmed these observations in over 1000 women in whom the AUC for glucose increased by 50% without change in the fasting glucose [428].

A number of smaller short-term studies have attempted to define which component, i.e. estrogen vs. progesterone, is responsible for the glucose intolerance in women treated with OCPs. Godsland et al [429] examined the effect of desogestrel (150 µg) with the minimum dose of ethinyl estradiol (20 µg) in the treatment of 83 women for 3 months. Despite the lower dose of ethinyl estradiol, the glucose AUC during the OGTT increased by almost 60%; this was similar to results obtained with the same dose of desogestrel plus a higher dosage of ethinyl estradiol (30 µg) [430]. Jandrain et al [431], using 30–35 µg of ethinyl estradiol and varying doses of progesterones, found increases in the fasting glucose concentration and the glucose AUC at 12 months. Similar findings have been reported by a number of investigators who have employed relatively low doses of ethinyl estradiol (30–35 µg) in combination with a variety of progesterone derivatives [432–438]. These results suggest that it is the progesterone alone, or acting synergistically with a low dose of estrogen, that is responsible for the impairment in glucose tolerance. In contrast to these studies [8–16], in a trial comparing progesterone alone vs. combination OCPs, the HbA$_{1c}$ rose from 5.4% to 8.7% after 6 months of combination treatment, while no change was seen in the progesterone only group [439].

In contrast to the above studies, a number of investigators, using the newer OCP formulations, have shown no adverse effects of OCPs on glucose tolerance. Van der Vange et al [440] followed 70 women over 6 months and found no changes in HbA$_{1c}$ or in the AUC for glucose, although an upward trend in the latter was observed. Spellacy et al [441] tested ethinyl estradiol (0.035 mg) with 0.4 mg norethindrone (considerably lower than previous doses) and found no deterioration in glucose tolerance in 24 women after 6 months of treatment. The same authors reported similar negative findings with a triphasic OCP [442]. Scheen et al [443] also failed to find any deterioration in OGTT after 1 year of a low dose OCP. Even though these studies [441–443] have not found any changes in glucose tolerance, some caution in their interpretation is warranted since the plasma insulin concentrations were not measured. Thus, several studies have shown that, even though glucose tolerance may remain unchanged, there is a significant increase in the plasma insulin response during the glucose challenge [444–445]. The maintenance of normal glucose tolerance at the expense of hyperinsulinemia indicates the presence of insulin resistance.

The development of peripheral insulin resistance has been shown after short-term usage of OCPs. Kasdorf et al [446], using the insulin clamp technique, demonstrated a decrease in insulin-mediated glucose metabolism after 3 months of OCP treatment, although insulin sensitivity tended to return to normal at 6 months. No changes in basal or insulin-mediated suppression of HGP were seen. In a larger study of 296 women who received a lower dosage formulation, the K value during the IVGTT was decreased by 30–40% with four different OCPs [427]. By contrast, Scheen et al [443] failed to find any change in insulin sensitivity using the insulin clamp technique. Thornton et al [447] also failed to find any effect of low doses of naturally occurring micronized estradiol (2 mg three times a day) alone, micronized progesterone (200 mg three times a day) alone, or combined micronized estradiol/progesterone on insulin secretion (hyperglycemic clamp) or insulin sensitivity (euglycemic insulin clamp) in normally menstruating women. There is some evidence that transdermally administered estrogen has less of an effect on glucose tolerance than orally administered estrogen [444]. In 61 postmenopausal women studied with either Premarin or transdermal estrogen, no changes were seen in the transdermal group, while an increase in the glucose AUC occurred in the patients treated with oral Premarin [444].

Most of the studies reviewed above have excluded women with a predisposition to diabetes or overt diabetes mellitus. Skouby et al [448], using a low-dose triphasic OCP (ethinyl estradiol and levonorgestrel 50/75/125), found no change in plasma glucose or insulin levels after 6 months in six women with a history of gestational diabetes. However, there was a significant decrease in insulin sensitivity using the insulin clamp. In a follow-up study in women with a history of gestational diabetes, they again found no worsening of glucose tolerance, although this was at the expense of mild hyperinsulinemia [449, 450]. Other investigators have reported more pronounced effects of OCPs in women with gestational diabetes mellitus (GDM). Radberg et al [451] found a 27% decrease in the K value during an IVGTT in women with GDM who were treated with ethinyl estradiol (50 mg/day) and lynesternol (2.5 mg/day) for 6 months. Other investigators [452, 453] also have reported the development of impaired glucose tolerance in women who are treated with OCPs.

Few studies have examined the effect of combined estrogen/progesterone therapy in patients with diabetes mellitus. In a small group of women with IDDM, Wiese and Osler [454] reported a deterioration in glucose control in 4 out of 11 IDDM patients who were placed on oral contraceptive pills. However, other investigators [455–457], using a variety of OCPs, have not observed any deterioration in fasting glucose or HbA$_{1c}$ or any change in insulin requirements.

In summary, it would appear that in women with normal glucose tolerance, as well as in women with gestational diabetes and IDDM, there may be a modest deterioration in glucose tolerance due to a worsening in insulin sensitivity. However, these effects on glucose metabolism are seldom clinically significant and seem to occur less frequently when low doses of naturally occurring estrogens and progesterones are used.

ANABOLIC STEROIDS

Anabolic steroids have been estimated to be used by one million or more athletes. The exact incidence is difficult to ascertain since most of these drugs are obtained illegally. Initial studies carried out in small numbers of subjects suggested that anabolic steroids improved glucose tolerance in diabetic patients [458]. However, more recent studies have yielded conflicting results. In several studies a decline in fasting glucose concentration has been observed in diabetic subjects. However, in both diabetic and non-diabetic individuals, the areas under the plasma glucose and insulin curves have been shown to increase, indicating the presence of insulin resistance.

Cohen et al [459] examined 15 powerlifters, 8 of whom used anabolic steroids for up to 7 years. The steroid-using group had higher glucose and insulin levels during an OGTT, suggesting the presence of underlying insulin resistance. In a study by Small et al [460] stanzolol administration for 8 weeks in 12 non-insulin dependent diabetic patients caused a decrease in the fasting glucose from 10.9 to 9.0 mmol/l (196 to 162 mg/dl) with a concomitant fall in HbA_{1c}. Unfortunately, there was no control group in this study. Similar results have been reported with methandienone [461]; most subjects had a fall in fasting glucose, but the area under the oral glucose tolerance curve increased significantly, and the K value during an IVGTT fell in seven out of nine subjects [461]. Using the tolbutamide tolerance test, Landon et al [462] demonstrated that anabolic steroid users had a similar decline in fasting plasma glucose concentration compared to controls; however, this occurred at the expense of a three-fold elevation in plasma insulin levels, indicating the presence of steroid-induced insulin resistance. This insulin antagonistic effect was limited to steroids with a 17 α-alkyl group. In patients receiving oxymetholone for aplastic anemia [463], glucose tolerance remained unchanged but plasma insulin levels rose fourfold. In another group of patients receiving a variety of anabolic steroids for aplastic anemia, glycosuria was present in all subjects [463]. In seven patients receiving long-term oxymethodone for aplastic anemia, both the insulin and glucose areas under the OGTT curve were clearly and progressively increased by treatment [464].

In the most comprehensive study, Godsland et al [465] examined nine non-diabetic patients who were receiving dianabol to improve body weight. Although the fasting glucose concentration decreased, both the glucose and insulin concentrations during the OGTT increased. Using the minimal model technique, they demonstrated a decrease in peripheral tissue sensitivity to insulin. The site of the insulin resistance was not determined. Post-mortem studies performed on anabolic steroid users have demonstrated islet cell hypertrophy, consistent with the presence of insulin resistance [466]. Interestingly, several recent studies have shown that anabolic steroids decrease HDL levels and elevate LDL and triglyceride levels [467, 468]. This pattern of dyslipidemia is typical of that observed in the insulin resistance syndrome.

The studies reviewed above indicate that anabolic steroids have two distinct effects on glucose metabolism: (a) a decrease or no change in fasting glucose concentration, and (b) impaired glucose tolerance and induction of insulin resistance. The mechanism of this paradox is unknown, although anabolic steroids have been shown to block the hyperglycemic effect of glucagon [461, 465]. This could lead to a decrease in hepatic glucose production and explain the decline in fasting glucose concentration. With regard to insulin resistance,

anabolic steroid users consistently demonstrate an increase in body weight, which is primarily confined to lean body, i.e. muscle, mass [469]. Therefore, it is possible that a change in muscle fiber type is responsible for the development of insulin resistance. In addition, some anabolic steroids can be converted to estradiol, and levels of the latter have been reported to rise sevenfold above control values [470]. Recently, Diamond and DeFronzo (unpublished observations) have used the euglycemic insulin clamp to study insulin sensitivity in 8 healthy women who received methyl testosterone (5 mg thrice daily for 10 days). Insulin sensitivity decreased consistently in each subject by a mean of 19%. All of the defect in insulin action was in the non-oxidative pathway (which primarily represents glycogen synthesis) of glucose disposal. The finding of islet cell hypertrophy in anabolic steroid users also suggests the presence of insulin resistance [464] and is consistent with the presence of peripheral insulin resistance. Lastly, anabolic steroids have a number of other organ system effects, including the induction of hepatic dysfunction, which may contribute to the disturbance in glucose homeostasis. In summary, the effect of anabolic steroids on glucose metabolism has been poorly studied and this area warrants further investigation.

ANDROGENS

Clinical endocrinologists who take care of female patients with polycystic ovary syndrome (PCO) [471–475] have long been aware of the association between insulin resistance and hyperandrogenemia. Although part of the insulin resistance can be attributed to obesity, even lean subjects with PCO have been shown to be severely insulin resistant. However, epidemiological and investigative studies have yielded conflicting results regarding the causality of this association.

In the Rancho Bernardo study of 848 non-diabetic females, the free plasma testosterone concentration was positively correlated with the fasting plasma glucose concentration, while sex hormone binding globulin displayed a negative association with glucose levels [476]. However, this correlation was lost in males. In contrast, in the Telecom study [477], hyperinsulinemia was negatively related to the plasma testosterone concentration in over 1200 males after accounting for age. Clinical studies in humans also have failed to demonstrate a clear-cut causal association between increased androgen levels and insulin resistance. In female trans-sexuals treated with testosterone for 4 months, a decrease in insulin sensitivity was seen at physiological but not at pharmacological levels of hyperinsulinemia [372]. In contrast, Marin et al [478] failed to observe any change in insulin sensitivity in 23 middle-aged males after testosterone replacement. Similar negative results were found by Byerly et al [479], who suppressed testosterone levels in normal males with a GnRH agonist and replaced them with either high or normal levels of testosterone. No change in insulin sensitivity was observed in either group using the insulin clamp technique. Dunaif et al [480] treated nine PCO patients with a GnRH agonist to suppress plasma testosterone and androgen levels and found no change in plasma insulin levels in response to a glucose load, in whole body insulin sensitivity, or in insulin-mediated suppression of hepatic glucose production, suggesting that hyperandrogenemia was not responsible for the insulin resistance. Similarly, in 30 males treated with testosterone or 19-nortestosterone decanate, no worsening of glucose tolerance or increase in plasma insulin levels during an OGTT was found [481]. Herbert et al [482] also failed to find any difference in insulin or glucose levels during an IVGTT in non-obese hyperandrogenemic females compared to an appropriately matched control group. In a study by Haffner et al [483] a decrease in plasma testosterone concentration was correlated with a decrease in total and non-oxidative glucose disposal during the euglycemic insulin clamp.

Despite the negative studies reviewed above, much evidence favors an association between elevated androgen levels and insulin resistance. In a group of hyperprolactinemic females, the plasma free testosterone concentration correlated positively with insulin values during an oral glucose challenge, indicating the presence of insulin resistance [484]. Consistent with this, elevated plasma insulin and C-peptide levels have been demonstrated during an OGTT in both lean and obese females with PCO, compared to weight-matched controls [472, 474]. Increased plasma free testosterone and/or decreased sex hormone binding globulin levels have been shown to correlate with elevated insulin levels, or the areas under the glucose and insulin curves during an OGTT [473, 484–486].

Animal data also have been inconsistent in their support for an association between hyperandrogenemia and insulin resistance. In rats, Hulmang et al [487, 488] demonstrated that testosterone administration decreased insulin sensitivity specifically by inhibiting glycogen synthesis in muscle. However, in dogs [489] and monkeys [387], hyperandrogenemia did not affect plasma glucose or insulin levels.

In examining the potential sites of impaired glucose metabolism Peiris et al [490] demonstrated a decrease in insulin-mediated peripheral glucose uptake without any change in hepatic glucose production in hyperandrogenic females. Consistent with this observation, we have also shown that testosterone administration to healthy male subjects leads to the development of insulin resistance (M Diamond and RA DeFronzo, unpublished results). It has also been suggested that androgens cause a shift in muscle morphology, with an increase in type IIB fibers which are less insulin-responsive [487]. Thus, the increase in lean body mass that is associated with testosterone administration [491, 492] may adversely affect glucose metabolism by enhancing the formation of muscle fibers that are intrinsically resistant to insulin. In summary, the available data suggest that androgens, especially testosterone, can induce insulin resistance and impaired glucose tolerance. However, more studies are needed to define the mechanism(s) via which androgens exert their deleterious effect on glucose metabolism.

GLUCOCORTICOIDS

Glucocorticoid excess, whether of exogenous or endogenous origin, has been recognized for over 50 years to adversely affect glucose tolerance in both non-diabetic and diabetic individuals [493, 494]. Impaired glucose tolerance or overt diabetes mellitus are characteristic features of patients who present with Cushing's disease [495]. Moreover, non-diabetic individuals who are treated with high doses of glucocorticoids not uncommonly develop overt diabetes mellitus [496] or hyperosmolar non-ketotic coma [497].

Perley and Kipnis [498] administered high doses of dexamethasone for 3 days to normal volunteers and noted a significant increase in fasting blood glucose (78–93 mg/dl, 4.3–5.2 mmol/l), despite a fivefold increase in plasma insulin concentration. Shamoon et al [499] demonstrated that infusion of cortisol (to reproduce levels seen in mild to moderate stress) for as little as 5 hours caused a 15–20 mg/dl (0.8–1.1 mmol/l) increase in basal glucose levels in normal subjects. Acute administration of a single dose of cortisone (200–400 mg) caused an increase in fasting glucose concentration and markedly impaired glucose tolerance [500]. More chronic (1 week) treatment with cortisone caused a further elevation in fasting glucose and impairment in IVGTT, both of which returned to normal after discontinuation of the steroids [500]. West [501], using a cortisone–glucose tolerance test, found a significant impairment in the OGTT after two doses of cortisone acetate, and Conn and Fajans [502] reported impaired glucose tolerance in 25% of normal volunteers after only two doses of hydrocortisone. These studies clearly indicate that short-term administration (hours to days) of high doses of glucocorticoids can lead to elevated fasting plasma glucose levels and impaired glucose tolerance.

In addition to these short-term studies in normal individuals, there exists a large amount of data on patients who are given steroids for a variety of inflammatory diseases or for immunosuppressive purposes. Although these studies are somewhat inherently flawed by the underlying medical disorder and the fact that the dosing schedules vary greatly, there is a clear-cut deterioration in glucose tolerance while the patients are on steroid therapy. McKiddie et al [503] examined 36 patients with rheumatoid arthritis, 20 of whom were receiving chronic steroid therapy. One-third of those on steroids had an abnormal OGTT compared with only one of 16 in the control group who were not being treated with steroids. In patients who were treated with steroids for a variety of disorders, Shi and Zhang [496] found 'overt' diabetes in approximately 10%. Since this percentage only reflected individuals who were symptomatic, i.e. showing polyuria, polydipsia or nocturia, it most likely represents a gross underestimation of the actual incidence of diabetes mellitus. Bookman et al [504] reported a 5% incidence of overt diabetes in a large number of patients who were receiving either cortisone or ACTH therapy. Bastenie et al [505] found a consistent worsening of the K value during the IVGTT in patients with connective tissue disorders or with asthma who were treated with cortisone.

Patients with Cushing's syndrome provide an excellent model for examining the effects of chronic glucocorticoid excess on glucose homeostasis, independent of other associated medical conditions. Plotz et al [506] reported an impaired glucose tolerance curve in 31 of 33 patients with Cushing's syndrome, and five of these 31 had frank diabetes. Ross et al [507] reported a 50% incidence of either overt diabetes mellitus or impaired OGTT in 70 patients with Cushing's disease, and a similar incidence (45%) of impaired glucose tolerance was reported by Urbanic et al [508]. These results indicate that impaired glucose tolerance occurs in approximately half of all individuals who are chronically exposed to high levels of steroids, and that as many as 5–10% may develop overt diabetes mellitus. Moreover, it would appear that the incidence of glucose intolerance is similar whether the steroids are secreted endogenously or given exogenously.

In the most general sense the impairment in glucose tolerance in subjects exposed to high doses of glucocorticoids could result from: (a) diminished insulin secretion; (b) peripheral tissue (muscle) resistance to insulin; or (c) elevated basal rates of hepatic glucose production which fail to suppress normally in response to insulin. Each of these mechanisms has been extensively studied both *in vivo* and *in vitro* in man and animals.

During short-term administration (days to weeks) of glucocorticoids, the fasting insulin concentration and both glucose-stimulated and sulfonylurea-stimulated plasma insulin responses are significantly enhanced (Figure 12) [509, 510]. Therefore, a defect in insulin secretion cannot account for the steroid-induced glucose intolerance. However, in patients who are exposed to excess glucocorticoids for prolonged periods (months to years) and who eventually develop overt NIDDM, insulin secretion becomes impaired, the islet B cells can no longer maintain their high rate of insulin secretion, and plasma insulin levels decline [493, 494]. Even though they may remain hyperinsulinemic compared to controls, the magnitude of hyperinsulinemia is no longer sufficient to offset the steroid-induced insulin resistance (see below) and overt diabetes mellitus ensues. The cause of this late B-cell failure is not known.

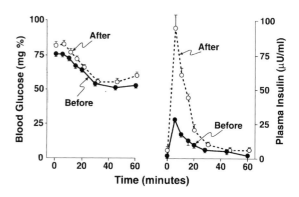

Figure 12 Blood glucose and plasma insulin responses in healthy young subjects to intravenous tolbutamide before (solid circles and solid lines) and after (open circles and dashed lines) dexamethasone ingestion (2 mg every 6 hours) for 2 days. Redrawn from reference 498, with permission

A number of studies have examined peripheral and hepatic sensitivity to insulin in subjects receiving short-term glucocorticoid administration [511–514] and in patients with Cushing's disease [515] (Figures 13 and 14). All investigators have shown consistently that short-term steroid administration in man decreases peripheral tissue (both muscle and adipose) sensitivity to insulin [511–514]. Similar results have been reported in patients with Cushing's disease [515] and in animals which are exposed to high circulating levels of glucocorticoids [516, 517]. The defect in insulin action cannot be explained by a decrease in the number of insulin receptors or by a decrease in the affinity of insulin for its receptor [518]. Several studies have examined glucose transport in adipocytes and muscle [512, 519, 520] following glucocorticoid administration and all have demonstrated a defect in this key step in insulin action. In addition, defects in both glucose oxidation and glycogen synthesis have been demonstrated in muscle and adipocytes [493, 494, 520].

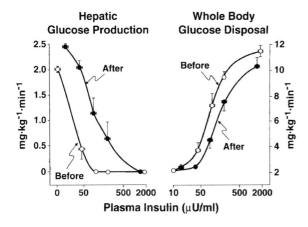

Figure 13 Insulin dose-response curves for the suppression of hepatic glucose production (left) and stimulation of whole body glucose disposal (right) in healthy young subjects before (solid circles and solid lines) and after (open circles and interrupted lines) a 24 h infusion of cortisol at 2 μg/kg min. From reference 511, with permission

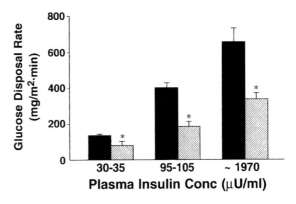

Figure 14 Whole body glucose disposal rates during a three-step euglycemic insulin clamp performed in patients with Cushing's syndrome (cross hatched bars) and in healthy control subjects (solid bars). $^*p < 0.01$. Redrawn from reference 515, with permission

Abnormalities in hepatic glucose production also contribute to the impairment in glucose homeostasis. Following short-term administration of glucocorticoids, basal hepatic glucose production has been reported to be increased [511] or normal [499] in the face of markedly increased fasting insulin levels. Similar results have been reported in patients with Cushing's disease [516]. In response to physiological levels of hyperinsulinemia, suppression of hepatic glucose production is markedly impaired in the presence of glucocorticoid excess [511] (Figure 13). The disturbance in hepatic glucose production can be explained by a number of metabolic abnormalities. First, glucocorticoids increase the activity of a number of key enzymes involved in gluconeogenesis [82, 521, 522]. Second, glucocorticoids increase proteolysis and lipolysis, leading to increased circulating levels of alanine, lactate, glycerol and free fatty acids [99, 135, 141, 154, 159]. Alanine, lactate and glycerol supply the substrate for gluconeogenesis, while increased oxidation of free fatty acids provides the energy. Third, glucocorticoids act synergistically with glucagon and epinephrine to augment hepatic glucose production [160, 168, 172]. Fourth, glucocorticoids augment secretion of glucagon [135], a potent stimulator of hepatic gluconeogenesis and glycogenolysis.

In summary, glucocorticoid excess, whether created endogenously or exogenously, impairs glucose tolerance. In adult patients receiving chronic high-dose steroids and in patients with Cushing's disease, approximately 40–50% will develop impaired glucose tolerance and, of these, 5–10% will become overtly diabetic. The glucose intolerance results from peripheral tissue resistance to insulin, an elevated basal rate of hepatic glucose production, and an impaired suppression of hepatic glucose production in response to insulin.

REFERENCES

1. Ferrannini E, Haffner SM, Mitchell BD, Stern MP. Hyperinsulinaemia: the key feature of a cardiovascular and metabolic syndrome. Diabetologia 1991; 34: 416–22.
2. DeFronzo RA, Ferrannini E. Insulin resistance. A multifaceted syndrome responsible for NIDDM, obesity, hypertension, dyslipidemia, and atherosclerotic cardiovascular disease. Diabetes Care 1991; 14: 173–94.
3. Reaven G. Banting Lecture. Role of insulin resistance in human disease. Diabetes 1988; 37: 1595–1607.
4. DeFronzo RA. Insulin resistance, hyperinsulinemia, and coronary artery disease: a complex metabolic web. Coronary Art Dis 1992; 3: 11–25.
5. Bressler P, DeFronzo RA. Drugs and diabetes. Diabetes Rev 1994; 2: 53–84.
6. Dawson KG, McKenzie JK, Ross SA, Chiasson JL, Hamel P. Report of the Canadian Hypertension Society and Consensus Conference: 5. Hypertension and diabetes. Can Med Assoc J 1993; 149: 821–6.
7. The Fifth Report of the Joint National Committee on Detection, Education, and Treatment of High Blood Pressure (JNC V). Arch Intern Med 1993; 153: 154–83.
8. Collins R, Peto R, MacMahon S. Blood pressure, stroke, and coronary heart disease. Part 2. Short-term reductions in blood pressure: overview of randomized drug trials in the epidemiological context. Lancet 1990; 335: 827–38.
9. Davidson RA, Caranos GS. Should the elderly hypertensive be treated? Evidence from clinical trials: Arch Intern Med 1987; 147: 1933–97.
10. MacMahon SW, Cutler JA, Furberg CD, Payne GH. The effects of drug treatment for hypertension on morbidity and mortality from cardiovascular disease: a review of randomized controlled trials. Prog Cardiovasc Dis 1986; 3 (suppl. 1): 99–118.

11. Warram JH, Laffel LMB, Valsania P, Christlieb AR, Krolewski AS. Excess mortality associated with diuretic therapy in diabetes mellitus. Ann Intern Med 1991; 151: 1380–85.

12. Klein R, Moss SE, Klein BE, De Mets DL. Relation of ocular and systemic factors to survival in diabetes. Arch Intern Med 1989; 149: 266–72.

13. Multiple Risk Factor Intervention Trial Research Group. Relationship among baseline resting ECG abnormalities, antihypertensive treatment, and mortality in the Multiple Risk Factor Intervention Trial. Am J Cardiol 1985; 55: 1–15.

14. Tarnow L, Rossing P, Gall MA, Nielsen FS, Parving HH. Prevalence of arterial hypertension in diabetic patients before and after the JNC-V. Diabetes Care 1994; 17: 1247–51.

15. The Hypertension in Diabetes Study Group. Hypertension in diabetes study (HDS): I. Prevalence of hypertension in newly presenting type 2 diabetic patients and the association with risk factors for cardiovascular and diabetic complications. J Hypertens 1993; 11: 309–17.

16. Elliott WJ, Stein PP, Black HR. Drug treatment of hypertension in patients with diabetes mellitus. Diabetes Rev 1995; 3: 477–509.

17. Freis ED. Critique of the clinical importance of diuretic-induced hypokalemia and elevated cholesterol levels. Arch Intern Med 1989; 149: 2640–48.

18. Stein PP, Black HR. Drug treatment of hypertension in patients with diabetes mellitus. Diabetes Care 1991; 14: 425–48.

19. Hollis WC. Aggravation of diabetes mellitus during treatment with chlorothiazide. JAMA 1961; 176: 947–9.

20. Wilkins RN. New drugs for the treatment of hypertension. Ann Intern Med 1959; 50: 1–10.

21. Runyan JW. Influence of thiazide diuretics on carbohydrate metabolism in patients with mild diabetes. New Engl J Med 1962; 267: 541–3.

22. Goldner MG, Zarowitz M. Hyperglycemia and glycolysis due to thiazide derivatives administered in diabetes mellitus. New Engl J Med 1960; 262: 403–5.

23. Zatuchni J, Kordasz F. The diabetogenic effect of thiazide diuretics. Am J Cardiol 1961; 7: 565–7.

24. Chazan JA, Boshell BR. Etiological factors in thiazide-induced or aggravated diabetes mellitus. Diabetes 1965; 14: 132–6.

25. Breckenridge A, Welborn TA, Dollery CT, Fraser R. Glucose tolerance in hypertensive patients on long-term diuretic therapy. Lancet 1967; 1: 61–4.

26. Shapiro AP, Benedek TG, Small JL. Effect of thiazides on carbohydrate metabolism in patients with hypertension. New Engl J Med 1961; 265: 1028–33.

27. Wolff FW, Parmley WW, White K, Okun R. Drug-induced diabetes. Diabetogenic activity of long-term administration of benzothiadiazines. JAMA 1963; 185: 568–74.

28. Wolff FW, Parmley WW. Further observations concerning the hyperglycemic activity of benzothiadiazines. Diabetes 1964; 13: 115–21.

29. Murphy MB, Kohner E, Lewis PJ, Schumer B, Dollery CT. Glucose intolerance in hypertensive patients treated with diuretics; a fourteen-year follow-up. Lancet 1982; 2: 1293–5.

30. Bengtsson C, Blohmé G, Lapidus L et al. Do antihypertensive drugs precipitate diabetes? Br Med J 1984; 289: 1495–7.

31. Donahue R, Abbott R, Wilson P. Effect of diuretics on the development of diabetes mellitus: the Framingham study. Horm Metab Res 1990; 22 (suppl.): 46–8.

32. Amery A, Birkenhager W, Brixko P et al. Glucose intolerance during diuretic therapy in elderly hypertensive patients. A second report from the European Working Party on high blood pressure in the elderly (EWPHE). Postgrad Med J 1986; 62: 919–24.

33. Amery A, Bulpitt C, DeSchaepdryver, Fagard R et al. Glucose intolerance during diuretic therapy. Results of trial by the European Working Party on Hypertension in the Elderly. Lancet 1978; 1: 681–3.

34. Medical Research Council Working Party: MRC trial of treatment of mild hypertension: principal results. Br Med J 1985; 291: 97–104.

35. Report of Medical Research Council Working Party on Mild to Moderate Hypertension; adverse reactions to bendrofluazide and propranolol for the treatment of mild hypertension. Lancet 1981; 2: 539–43.

36. Veterans Administration Cooperative Study Group on Antihypertensive Agents. Propranolol or hydrochlorothiazide alone for the initial treatment of hypertension. IV. Effect on plasma glucose and glucose tolerance. Hypertension 1985; 7: 1008–16.

37. Veterans Cooperative Administration Study Group on Antihypertensive Agents. Comparision of propranolol and hydrochlorthiazide for the initial treatment of hypertension. II. Results of long-term therapy. JAMA 1982; 248: 2004–11.

38. Lewis P, Petrie A, Kohner E, Dollery C. Deterioration of glucose tolerance in hypertensive patients on prolonged diuretic treatment. Lancet 1976; 2: 564–6.

39. Wilhelmsen L, Berglund G, Elmfeldz D et al. The multifactor primary prevention trial in Goteborg, Sweden. Eur Heart J 1986; 7: 278–88.

40. Helgeland A, Leren P, Per Foss O, Hjermann I, Holme I, Lund-Larsen PG. Serum glucose levels during long-term observation of treated and untreated men with mild hypertension. The Oslo study. Am J Med 1984; 76: 802–5.

41. Wales J, Viktora J, Wolff F. The effect of hydrochlorthiazide in normal subjects receiving high fat or high carbohydrate diets. Am J Med Sci 1967; 252: 133–9.

42. Robinson D, Nilsson C, Leonard R, Horton E. Effects of loop diuretics on carbohydrate metabolism and electrolyte excretion. J Clin Pharmacol 1981; 21: 637–46.

43. Andres R. Aging and diabetes. Med Clin North Am 1971; 55: 835–45.

44. DeFronzo RA. Glucose intolerance and aging; evidence for tissue insensitivity to insulin. Diabetes 1979; 28: 1095–101.

45. Samaan N, Alexandria DM, Dollery CT, Fraser R. Diabetogenic action of benzothiadiazines. Serum-insulin-like activity in diabetes worsened or precipitated by thiazide diuretics. Lancet 1963; 1: 1244–6.

46. Lowder NK, Bussey HI, Sugarek NJ. Clinically significant diuretic-induced glucose intolerance. Drug Intell Clin Pharm 1988; 22: 969–71.

47. Goldner MG, Zarowitz H, Akgun S. Hyperglycemia and glycosuria due to thiazide derivative administered in diabetes mellitus. Med Intelligence 1960; 262: 403–5.

48. Plavnik FL, Rodrigues CIS, Zanella MT, Ribeiro AB. Hypokalemia, glucose intolerance, and hyperinsulinemia during diuretic therapy. Hypertension 1992; 19(II): 26–9.

49. Rapoport M, Hurd H. Thiazide-induced glucose intolerance treated with potassium. Arch Intern Med 1964; 113: 405–8.

50. Conrad K, Fagan T, Lee S, Simons J. Effect of tripamide on glucose tolerance in patients with hypertension. Clin Pharmacol Ther 1986; 40: 476–9.

51. Gall M, Rossing P, Skott P et al. Placebo-controlled comparison of captopril, metoprolol, and hydrochlorothiazide therapy in non-insulin dependent diabetic patients with primary hypertension. Am J Hypertension 1992; 5: 257–65.

52. Kansal P, Buse J, Buse M. Thiazide diuretics and control of diabetes mellitus. South Med J 1969; 62: 1274–9.

53. Runyan JW Jr. Influence of thiazide diuretics on carbohydrate metabolism in patients with mild diabetes. New Engl J Med 1962; 267: 541–3.

54. Hicks BH, Ward JD, Jarrett RJ, Keen H, Wise P. A controlled study of clopamide, clorexolone, and hydrochlorothiazide in diabetics. Metabolism 1973; 22: 101–9.

55. Bloomgarden Z, Ginsberg-Fellner F, Rayfield EJ, Bookman J, Brown WV. Elevated hemoglobin A_{1c} and low-density lipoprotein cholesterol levels in thiazide-treated diabetic patients. Am J Med 1984; 77: 823–7.

56. Wales JK, Grant A, Wolff FW. Studies on the hyperglycaemic effects of non-thiazide diuretics. J Pharmacol Exp Ther 1968; 159: 229–35.

57. Breckenridge A, Dollery CT, Welborn TA, Fraser R. Glucose tolerance in hypertensive patients on long-term diuretic therapy. Lancet 1967; 1: 61–4.

58. Hutcheon DE, Leonard G. Diuretic and antihypertensive effects of furosemide. J Clin Pharmacol 1967; 7: 26–33.

59. Jones IG, Pickens PT. Diabetes mellitus following oral diuretics. Practitioner 1967; 199: 209–10.

60. Weller JM, Borondy PE. Effects of benzothiadiazine drugs on carbohydrate metabolism. Metabolism 1967; 16: 532–6.

61. Lavender S, McGill RJ. Non-ketotic hyperosmolar coma and furosemide therapy. Diabetes 1974; 23: 247–8.

62. Tasker P. Non-ketotic diabetic precoma associated with high-dose frusemide therapy. Br Med J 1976; 1: 626–7.

63. Andersen O, Persson I. Carbohydrate metabolism during treatment with chlorthalidone and ethacrynic acid. Br Med J 1968; 2: 798–801.

64. Petrides AS. Liver disease and diabetes mellitus. Diabetes Rev 1994; 2: 2–18.

65. Manzino BE, Salviolo JE, Castelleto R, De Mario O. Hyperglycemic effects of diuretics. Rev Clin Esp 1966; 101: 349–55.

66. Grant AM, Wolff FW. The hyperglycemic activity of triamterene. Pharm Res Commun 1969; 1: 224–30.

67. Harrower AD, McFarlane G. Antihypertensive therapy in diabetic patients: the use of indapamide. Am J Med 1988; 84 (suppl. 1B): 89–91.

68. Harrower A, McFarlane G, Donnelly T, Gray C. Effect of indapamide on blood pressure and glucose tolerance in non-insulin dependent diabetes. Hypertension 1985; 7 (suppl. II): 161–3.

69. Raggi U, Palumbro P, Moro B, Bevilacqua M, Norbiato G. Indapamide in the treatment of hypertension in non-insulin dependent diabetes. Hypertension 1985; 7 (suppl. II): II–157–160.

70. Gambardella S, Frontoni S, Lala A et al. Regression of microalbuminuria in type II diabetic hypertensive patients after long-term indapamide treatment. Am Heart J 1991; 122: 1232–8.

71. Kaplan NM. The case for low-dose diuretic therapy. Am J Hypertens 1991; 4: 970–1.

72. McVeigh G, Galloway D, Johnston D. The case for low-dose diuretics in hypertension: comparison of low and conventional doses of cyclopenthiazide. Br Med J 1988; 297: 95–8.

73. Carlsen JE, Kober L, Torp-Pedersen C, Johansen P. Relation between dose of bendrofluazide, antihypertensive effect, and adverse biochemical effects. Br Med J 1990; 300: 975–8.

74. Berglund G, Andersson O. Low doses of hydrochlorothiazide in hypertension. Antihypertensive and metabolic effects. Eur J Clin Pharmacol 1976; 10: 177–82.

75. Berglund G, Andersson O, Widgren B. Low-dose antihypertensive treatment with a thiazide diuretic is not diabetogenic. A 10-year controlled trial with bendroflumethiazide. Acta Med Scand 1986; 220: 419–24.

76. Prince M, Stuart C, Padia M, Bandi Z, Holland O. Metabolic effects of hydrochlorthiazide and enalapril during treatment of the hypertensive diabetic patient. Arch Intern Med 1988; 148: 2363–8.

77. Vardan S, Mehrota KG, Mookherjee S, Willsey GA, Gens JD, Green DE. Efficacy and reduced metabolic side effects of a 15 mg chlorthalidone formulation in the treatment of mild hypertension. JAMA 1987; 258: 484–8.

78. Grimm RH, Neaton JD, McDonald M et al for the Multiple Risk Factor Intervention Trial Research Group. Beneficial effects from systematic dosage reduction of the diuretic, chlorthalidone: randomized study within a clinical trial. Am Heart J 1985; 109: 858–63.

79. Holzgrave M, Distler A, Michaels J, Phillip T, Welleck S on behalf of the Verapamil vs. Diuretic (VERDI) Trial Research Group. Verapamil vs. hydrochlorothiazide in the treatment of hypertension: results of long-term double-blind comparative trial. Br Med J 1989; 299: 881–6.

80. McVeigh GE, Dulie EB, Ravenscroft A, Galloway DB, Johnson DB. Low and conventional dose cyclopenthiazide on glucose and lipid metabolism in mild hypertension. Br J Clin Pharmacol 1989; 27: 523–6.

81. Weisser B, Ripka O. Long-term diuretic therapy: effects of dose reduction on antihypertensive efficacy and counter-regulatory systems. J Cardiovas Pharmacol 1992; 19: 361–6.

82. Granner D, O'Brien R, Imai E, Forest C, Mitchell J, Lucas P. Complex hormone response unit regulating transcription of the phosphoenolpyruvate carboxykinase gene: from metabolic pathways to molecular biology. In Recent progress in hormone research, vol. 47. New York: Academic Press, 1991; pp 319–48.

83. McKenney JM, Goodman RP, Wright Jr JT, Ritui N, Aycock DG, King ME. The effect of low-dose hydrochlorothiazide on blood pressure, serum potassium, and lipoproteins. Pharmacol 1986; 6: 179–84.

84. Harper R, Ennis LN, Sheridan B, Atkinson AB, Johnston DG, Bell PM. Effects of low-dose vs. conventional dose thiazide diuretics on insulin action in essential hypertension. Br Med J 1994; 309: 226–30.

85. DeFronzo RA. The triumvirate: β-cell, muscle, liver: a collusion responsible for NIDDM. Diabetes 1988; 37: 667–87.

86. DeFronzo RA, Bonadonna RC, Ferrannini E. Pathogenesis of NIDDM: a balanced overview. Diabetes Care 1992; 15: 318–68.

87. Pollare T, Lithell H, Berne C. A comparison of the effects of hydrochlorothiazide and captopril on glucose and lipid metabolism in patients with hypertension. New Engl J Med 1989; 321: 868–73.

88. Lithell HO, Pollare T, Berne C. Insulin sensitivity in newly detected hypertensive patients: influence of captopril and other antihypertensive agents on insulin sensitivity and related biological parameters. J Cardiovasc Pharmacol 1990; 15 (suppl. 5): S46–52.

89. Lithell HO. Effect of antihypertensive drugs on insulin, glucose, and lipid metabolism. Diabetes Care 1991; 14: 203–9.

90. Kageyama S, Yamomoto J, Mimura A et al. Comparison of effects of nicardepine and trichlormethiazide on insulin sensitivity in hypertensive patients. Am J Hypertens 1994; 7: 474–7.

91. Swislocki AL, Hoffman BB, Reaven GM. Insulin resistance, glucose tolerance and hyperinsulinemia in patients with hypertension. Am J Hypertens 1989; 2: 419–23.

92. Ames RP, Hill P. Improvement of glucose tolerance and lowering of glycohemoglobin and serum lipid concentrations after discontinuation of antihypertensive drug therapy. Circulation 1982; 65: 899–904.

93. Rooney DP, Neely RDG, Ennis CN et al. Insulin action and hepatic glucose cycling in essential hypertension. Metabolism 1992; 41: 317–24.

94. Barnett CA, Whitney JE. The effect of diazoxide and chlorothiazide on glucose uptake *in vitro*. Metabolism 1966; 15: 88–93.

95. Field JB, Mandell S. Effects of thiazides on glucose uptake and oxidation in rat muscle and adipose tissue. Metabolism 1964; 13: 959–63.

96. Schmitz O, Hermansen K, Nielsen OH et al. Insulin action in insulin-dependent diabetics after short-term thiazide therapy. Diabetes Care 1986; 9: 631–6.

97. Beardwood DM, Alden JS, Graham CA, Beardwood Jr JT, Marble A. Evidence for a peripheral action of chlorothiazide in normal man. Metabolism 1965; 14: 561–7.

98. Malaisse W, Malaisse-Lagae F. Effect of thiazides upon insulin secretion in vitro. Arch Int Pharmacodyn 1968; 171: 235–9.

99. Louard RJ, Bhushan R, Gelfand RA, Barrett EJ, Sherwin RS. Glucocorticoids antagonize insulin's antiproteolytic action on skeletal muscle in humans. J Clin Endocrinol Metab 1994; 79: 278–84.

100. Hermansen K, Schmitz O, Mogensen CE. Effects of a thiazide diuretic (hydroflumethiazide) and a loop diuretic (bumetanide) on the endocrine pancreas: studies *in vitro*. Metabolism 1985; 34: 784–9.

101. Seltzer HB, Crout JR. Insulin secretory blockage by benzothiadiazines and catecholamines: reversal by sulfonylureas. Ann NY Acad Sci 1968; 150: 309–21.

102. Fajans SS, Floyd JC Jr, Knopf RF, Rull J, Guntsche EM, Conn JW. Benzothiadiazine suppression of insulin release from normal and abnormal islet tissue in man. J Clin Invest 1966; 45: 481–92.

103. Rowe JW, Tobin JD, Rosa RM, Andres R. Effects of experimental potassium deficiency on glucose and insulin metabolism. Metabolism 1980; 29: 493–502.

104. Gorden P, Sherman BM, Simopoulos AP. Glucose intolerance with hypokalemia: an increased proportion of circulating proinsulin-like component. J Clin Endocrinol 1972; 34: 235–40.

105. Sagild U, Andersen V, Buch Andreasen P. Glucose tolerance and insulin responsiveness on experimental potassium depletion. Acta Med Scand 1961; 169: 243–51.

106. MacFarland K, Carr A. Changes in the fasting blood sugar after hydrochlorthiazide and potassium supplementation. J Clin Pharmacol 1977; 17: 13–17.

107. Helderman JH, Elahi D, Andersen DK et al. Prevention of the glucose intolerance of thiazide diuretics by maintenance of body potassium. Diabetes 1983; 32: 106–11.

108. Berglund G, Andersson O. Beta-blockers or diuretics in hypertension? A six-year follow-up of blood pressure and metabolic side effects. Lancet 1981; 1: 744–7.

109. Micossi P, Pollavini G, Raggi U, Librenti M, Garimberti B, Beggi P. Effects of metoprolol and propranolol on glucose tolerance and insulin secretion in diabetes mellitus. Horm Metab Res 1984; 16: 59–63.

110. Wright A, Barber S, Kendall M, Poole P. Beta-adrenoceptor-blocking drugs and blood sugar control in diabetes mellitus. Br Med J 1979; 1: 159–61.

111. Kølendorf K, Bonnevie-Nielsen V, Broch-Møller B. A trial of metoprolol in hypertensive insulin-dependent diabetic patients. Acta Med Scand 1982; 211: 175–8.

112. Chellingsworth M, Kendall M, Wright A, Singh B, Pasi J. The effects of verapamil, diltiazem, nifedipine and propranolol on metabolic control in hypertensives with non-insulin dependent diabetes mellitus. J Hum Hypertens 1989; 3: 35–9.

113. Cruickshank J, Anderson N, Wadsworth J, McHardy Young S, Jepson E. Treating hypertension in black compared with white non-insulin dependent diabetics: a double-blind trial of verapamil and metoprolol. Br Med J 1988; 297: 1155–9.

114. Elving L, deNobel E, van Lier J, Thien T. A comparison of the hypotensive effects of captopril and atenolol in the treatment of hypertension in diabetic patients. J Clin Pharmacol 1989; 29: 316–20.

115. Parving HH, Andersen AR, Smidt UM, Svendsson PAA. Early aggressive antihypertensive treatment reduces rate of decline in kidney function in diabetic nephropathy. Lancet 1983; 1: 1175–9.

116. Dahlöf B, Lindholm LH, Hansson L, Scherstén B, Ekbom T, Wester P.-O. Morbidity and mortality in the Swedish Trial in old patients with hypertension (STOP-Hypertension). Lancet 1991; 338: 1281–5.

117. Wilhelmsen L, Berglund G, Elmfeldt D et al. Beta-blockers vs. diuretics in hypertensive men: main results from the HAPPHY trial. J Hypertens 1987; 5: 561–72.

118. Wikstrand J, Warnold I, Olsson G, Tuomilehto J, Elmfeldt D, Berglund G. Primary prevention with metoprolol in patients with hypertension: mortality results from the MAPHY study. JAMA 1988; 259: 1976–82.

119. The IPPPSH Collaborative Group. Cardiovascular risk and risk factors in a randomized trial of treatment based on the beta-blocker oxprenolol: the International Prospective Primary Prevention Study in Hypertension (IPPPSH). J Hypertens 1985; 3: 379–92.

120. SHEP Cooperative Research Group. Prevention of stroke by antihypertensive drug treatment in older persons with isolated systolic hypertension. JAMA 1991; 265: 3255–64.

121. Coope J, Warrender TS. Randomized trial of treatment of hypertension in elderly patients in primary care. Br Med J 1986; 293: 1145–51.

122. Management Committee. Treatment of mild hypertension in the elderly. Med J Australia 1981; 2: 398–402.

123. Hypertension Detection and Follow-up Program Cooperative Group. Five-year findings of the hypertension detection and follow-up program. I. Reduction in mortality of persons with high blood pressure, including mild hypertension. JAMA 1979; 242: 2562–71.

124. Hypertension Detection and Follow-up Program Cooperative Group. The effect of treatment on mortality in mild hypertension: results of the hypertension detection and follow-up program. New Engl J Med 1982; 307: 976–80.

125. Hypertension–Stroke Cooperative Study Group. Effect of antihypertensive treatment on stroke recurrence. JAMA 1974; 229: 409–18.

126. Porte D. Beta-adrenergic stimulation of insulin release in man. Diabetes 1967; 16: 150–5.

127. Loubatieres A, Mariani M, Sorel G, Savi L. The action of β-adrenergic blocking and stimulating agents on insulin secretion: characterization of the type of β-receptor. Diabetologia 1971; 7: 127–32.

128. Hedstrand H, Aberg H. Insulin response to intravenous glucose during long-term treatment with propranolol. Acta Med Scand 1974; 196: 39–40.

129. Cerasi E, Luft R, Efendic S. Effect of adrenergic blocking agents on insulin response to glucose infusion in man. Acta Endocrinol 1972; 69: 335–46.

130. Imaru H, Kato Y, Ikeda M, Morimoto M, Yawata M. Effect of adrenergic-blocking or stimulating agents on plasma growth hormone, immunoreactive insulin and blood free fatty acid levels in man. J Clin Invest 1971; 50: 1069–78.

131. Massara F, Strumia E, Camanni F, Molinatti G. Depressed tolbutamide-induced insulin response in subjects treated with propranolol. Diabetologia 1971; 7: 287–9.

132. Sirek O, Sirek A, Policova Z. Inhibition of sulphonylurea-stimulated insulin secretion by beta-adrenergic blockade. Diabetologia 1975; 11: 269–72.

133. Bengtsson C. Impairment of glucose metabolism during treatment with antihypertensive drugs. Acta Med Scand (suppl.) 1979; 628: 63–7.

134. Skarfors E, Lithell H, Selinus I, Aberg H. Do antihypertensive drugs precipitate diabetes in predisposed men? Br Med J 1989; 298: 1147–52.

135. Wise JK, Hendler R, Felig P. Influence of glucocorticoids on glucagon secretion and plasma amino acid concentrations in man. J Clin Invest 1973; 52: 2774–82.

136. Bengtsson C, Blohmé G, Lapidus L, Lundgren H. Diabetes in hypertensive women: an effect of antihypertensive drugs or the hypertensive state *per se*? Diabet Med 1988; 5: 261–4.

137. Captopril Research Group of Japan: Clinical effects of low-dose captopril plus a thiazide diuretic on mild to moderate essential hypertension: a multicenter double-blind comparison with propranolol. J Cardiovasc Pharmacol 1985; 7 (suppl.): S77–81.

138. Cressman MD, Vidt DG, Mohler H, Gifford RW Jr. Glucose tolerance during chronic propranolol treatment. J Clin Hypertens 1985; 2: 138–44.

139. Mohler MM, Bravo EL, Tasazi RC. Glucose intolerance during chronic β-adrenergic blockade in man. Clin Pharmacol Ther 1979; 25: 237.

140. Pollare T, Lithell H, Selinus I, Berne C. Sensitivity to insulin during treatment with atenolol and metoprolol: a randomized, double-blind study of effects on carbohydrate and lipoprotein metabolism in hypertensive patients. Br Med J 1989; 298: 1152–7.

141. Divertie GD, Jensen MD, Miles JM. Stimulation of lipolysis in humans by physiological hypercortisolemia. Diabetes 1991; 40: 1228–32.

142. Groop L, Tötterman KG, Harno K, Gordin A. Influence of beta-blocking drugs on glucose metabolism in patients with non-insulin dependent diabetes mellitus. Acta Med Scand 1982; 211: 7–12.

143. Whitcroft IA, Thomas J, Rawsthorne A, Wilkinson N, Thompson H. Effects of alpha- and beta-adrenoceptor blocking drugs and ACE inhibitors on long-term glucose and lipid control in hypertensive non-insulin dependent diabetics. Horm Metab Res 1990; 22 (suppl.): 42–6.

144. The Norwegian Multicenter Study Group. Timolol induced reduction in mortality and reinfarction in patients surviving acute myocardial infarction. New Engl J Med 1985; 313: 1055–8.

145. Beta Blocker Heart Attack Trial Research Group. A randomized trial of propranolol in patients with acute myocardial infarction. I. Mortality results. JAMA 1981; 247: 1707–14.

146. Hjalmasson A, Elmfeldt D, Helitz J. Effect on mortality of metoprolol in acute myocardial infarction. Lancet 1981; 2: 823–6.

147. Fuh MMT, Sheu WHH, Shen DC, Wu DA, Chen YDI, Reaven GM. Metabolic effects of diuretic and beta-blocker treatment of hypertension in patients with non-insulin-dependent diabetes mellitus. Am J Hypertens 1990; 3: 387–90.

148. Dornhorst A, Powell SH, Pensky J. Aggravation by propranolol of hyperglycaemic effect of hydrochlorothiazide in type II diabetics without alteration of insulin secretion. Lancet 1985; 1: 123–6.

149. Holm G, Johansson S, Vedin A, Wilhelmsson C, Smith U. The effect of beta-blockade on glucose tolerance and insulin release in adult diabetes. Acta Med Scand 1980; 208: 187–91.

150. Fogari R, Lazzari P, Zoppi A, Tettamanti F, Malamani G, Boari L. The effects of celiprolol in the short-term treatment of hypertensive patients with type 2 diabetes. Curr Ther Res 1990; 47: 879–88.

151. Bohlen LM, de Courten M, Hafezi F, Shaw S, Riesen W, Weidmann P. Insulin sensitivity and atrial natriuretic factor during beta-receptor modulation with celiprolol in normal subjects. J Cardiovas Pharmacol 1994; 23: 877–83.

152. Waal-Mannig HJ. Metabolic effects of β-adrenoreceptor blockers. Drugs 1976; 11 (suppl. 1): 121–6.

153. Haenni A, Lithell M. Treatment with a beta-blocker with beta-2 agonism improves glucose and lipid

metabolism in essential hypertension. Metabolism 1994; 43: 455–461.

154. Darmaun D, Matthews DE, Bier DM. Physiological hypercortisolemia increases proteolysis, glutamine, and alanine production. Am J Physiol 1988; 255: E366–73.

155. Östman J, Arner P, Haglund K, Julin-Dannfelt A, Novac J, Wennlund A. A cardio-selective beta-blocker (metoprolol) in hypertensive, insulin-dependent diabetics. Acta Med Scand (suppl.) 1980; 639: 29–32.

156. Lager I, Blohmé G, Smith U. Effect of cardioselective and non-selective β-blockade on the hypoglycaemic response in insulin-dependent diabetes. Lancet 1979; 1: 458–62.

157. Viberti GC, Keen H, Bloom SR. Beta blockade and diabetes mellitus. Effect of oxprenolol and metoprolol on the metabolic, cardiovascular, and hormonal response to insulin-induced hypoglycemia in insulin-dependent diabetics. Metabolism 1980; 29: 873–9.

158. Bia MJ, DeFronzo RA. Extrarenal potassium homeostasis. Editorial Review. Am J Physiol 1981; 240: F257–68.

159. Tessari P, Inchiostro SS, Biolo G et al. Leucine kinetics and the effects of hyperinsulinemia in patients with Cushing's syndrome. J Clin Endocrinol Metab 1989; 68: 256–62.

160. Exton J, Corbin J, Parck C. Control of gluconeogenesis in liver. J Biol Chem 1969; 244: 4095–4102.

161. Andersson PE, Johnson J, Berne C, Lithell H. Effects of selective alpha 1 and beta-1 adrenoreceptor blockade on lipoprotein and carbohydrate metabolism in hypertensive subjects, with special emphasis on insulin sensitivity. J Human Hypertens 1994; 8: 219–26.

162. Tötterman K, Groop L, Groop PH, Kala R, Tolppanen EM, Fyhrquist F. Effect of beta-blocking drugs on beta-cell function and insulin sensitivity in hypertensive non-diabetic patients. Eur J Clin Pharmacol 1984; 26: 13–17.

163. Deibert DC, DeFronzo RA. Epinephrine-induced insulin resistance in man. J Clin Invest 1980; 65: 717–21.

164. Ferrara LA, Capaldo B, Rivellese AA et al. Effects of B-receptor blockade on carbohydrate metabolism. J Hypertension 1985; 3 (suppl. 2): S199–201.

165. Verschoor L, Wolffenbuttel BH, Weber RF. Beta-blockade and carbohydrate metabolism: theoretical aspects and clinical implications. J Cardiovasc Pharmacol 1986; 11(suppl. 8): S92–5.

166. Abramson EA, Arky RA. Role of beta-adrenergic receptor in counterregulation to insulin-induced hypoglycemia. Diabetes 1964; 17: 141–6.

167. Mikhailidis DP, Barradas MA, Hutton RA, Jeremy JY, Sabur M, Dandona P. The effect of non-specific beta-blockade on metabolic and hemostatic variables during hypoglycaemia. Diabetes Res 1985; 2: 127–34.

168. Le Cavalier L, Bolli G, Gerich J. Glucagon-cortisol interactions on glucose turnover and lactate gluconeogenesis in humans. Am J Physiol 1990; 258: E569–75.

169. Cryer PE, White NH, Santiago JV. The relevance of glucose counter-regulatory systems to patients with insulin-dependent diabetes mellitus. Endocr Rev 1986; 7: 131–9.

170. Gerich GE, Lorerzi M, Tsaklian E, Karan JM. Studies on the mechanism of epinephrine-induced hyperglycemia in man. Diabetes 1976; 25: 65–71.

171. Shimazu T. Neuronal regulation of hepatic glucose metabolism in mammals. Diabetes Metab Rev 1987; 3: 185–206.

172. Shamoon H, Hendler R, Sherwin R. Altered responsiveness to cortisol, epinephrine, and glucagon in insulin-infused juvenile-onset diabetes. Diabetes 1980; 29: 284–91.

173. Popp DA, Tse TF, Shah SD, Clutter WE, Cryer PE. Oral propranolol and metoprolol impair glucose recovery from insulin-induced hypoglycemia in insulin-dependent diabetes mellitus. Diabetes Care 1984; 7: 243–7.

174. Trost BN, Weidmann P. Effects of calcium antagonists on glucose homeostasis and serum lipids in non-diabetic and diabetic subjects. A review. J Hypertension 1987; 5 (suppl. 4): S81–104.

175. Giugliano D, Torella R, Cacciapuoti F, Gentile S, Verza M, Varricchio M. Impairment of insulin secretion in man by nifedipine. Eur J Clin Pharmacol 1980; 18: 395–8.

176. Sando M, Katagiri M, Okura R et al. The effect of nifedipine and nicardipine on glucose tolerance, insulin and C-peptide. Diabetes 1983; 32 (suppl. 1): 66A.

177. Ferlito S, Fichera C, Carra G, Puleo F, Calafato M, Volpicelli D. Effect of nifedipine on blood sugar, insulin and glucagon levels after an oral glucose load. Panminerva Med 1981; 23: 75–80.

178. Deedwania P, Shah S, Robison C, Watson P, Hurks C. Effects of nifedipine on glucose tolerance and insulin release in man. J Am Coll Cardiol 1984; 3: 577.

179. Tentorio A, Ghilardi G, Pedroncelli A et al. Insulin secretion and glucose tolerance in non-insulin dependent diabetic patients after nifedipine treatment. Eur J Clin Pharmacol 1989; 36: 311–13.

180. Collins WCJ, Cullen MJ, Feely J. Calcium channel blocker drugs and diabetic control. Clin Pharmacol Ther 1987; 42: 420–3.

181. Winocour PH, Waldek S, Cohen H, Anderson DC, Gordon C. Glycaemic control and exercise tolerance in hypertensive insulin-treated diabetes during nifedipine therapy. Br J Clin Pract 1987; 41: 772–8.

182. Gill JS, Al-Hussary N, Zezulka AV, Pasi J, Atkins TW, Beevers DG. Effect of nifedipine on glucose tolerance, serum insulin, and serum fructosamine in diabetic and non-diabetic patients. Clin Ther 1987; 9: 304–10.

183. Palumbo G, Barantani E, Pozzi F, Azzolini V, Gronda D, Ronchi E. Long-term nifedipine treatment and glucose homeostasis in hypertensive patients. Curr Ther Res 1988; 43: 171–9.

184. Ramirez LC, Koffler M, Arauz C, Schnurr-Breen L, Raskin P. Effect of nifedipine GITS on blood pressure, glucose metabolism, and lipid levels in hypertensive patients. Curr Ther Res 1992; 52: 468–77.

185. Zanetti-Elshater F, Pingitore R, Beretta-Piccoli C, Riesen W, Heinen G. Calcium antagonists for treatment of diabetes-associated hypertension. Metabolic and renal effects of amlodipine. Am J Hyper 1994; 7: 36–45.

186. Beer NA, Jakubowicz DJ, Beer RM, Nestler JE. The calcium channel blocker amlodipine raises dehydroepiandrosterone sulfate and androstenedione, but lowers serum cortisol in insulin-resistant obese and hypertensive men. J Clin Endocrinol Metab 1993; 76: 1464–9.

187. Beer NA, Jakubowicz DJ, Beer RM, Arocha IR, Nestler JE. Effects of nitrendipine on glucose tolerance and serum insulin and dehydroepiandrosterone sulfate levels in insulin-resistant obese and hypertensive men. J Clin Endocrinol Metab 1993; 76: 178–83.

188. Bursztyn M, Raz I, Mekler J, Ben-Ishay D. Nitrendipine improves glucose tolerance and deoxyglucose uptake in hypertensive rats. Hypertension 1994; 23: 1051–3.

189. Kjellstrom T, Blychert E, Lindgarde F. Short-term effects of felodipine in hypertensive type II diabetic males on sulfonylurea treatment. J Intern Med 1994; 236: 51–6.

190. Lind L, Berne C, Pollare T, Lithell H. Metabolic effects of isradipine as monotherapy or in combination with pindolol during long-term antihypertensive treatment. J Intern Med 1994; 236: 37–42.

191. Malaisse WJ, Sener A. Calcium-antagonists and islet function—comparison between nifedipine and chemically related drugs. Biochem Pharmacol 1981; 30: 1039–41.

192. Cartee GD, Briggs-Tung C, Holloszy JO. Diverse effects of calcium channel blockers on skeletal muscle glucose transport. Am J Physiol 1992; 263: R70–75.

193. Giordano M, Sanders LR, DeFronzo RA. Effects of captopril, nifedipine, and doxazosin on blood pressure and renal function in non-insulin dependent diabetic hypertensive patients. J Am Soc Nephrol 1993; 4: 533.

194. Pollare T, Lithell H, Mörlin C, Präntare H, Hvarfner A, Ljunghall S. Metabolic effects of diltiazem and atenolol: results from a randomized, double-blind study with parallel groups. J Hypertens 1989; 7: 551–9.

195. Nagai K, Takeda N, Endo Y et al. Effects of diltiazem hydrochloride in diabetics. Int J Clin Pharmacol Ther Tox 1986; 24: 602–8.

196. Andrén L, Höglund P, Dotevall A et al. Diltiazem in hypertensive patients with type II diabetes mellitus. Am J Cardiol 1988; 62: 114–20G.

197. Jones BJ, McKenney JM, Wright JT Jr, Goodman RP. Effects of diltiazem hydrochloride on glucose tolerance in persons at risk for diabetes mellitus. Clin Pharm 1988; 7: 235–8.

198. Yamaguchi I, Akimoto Y, Nakajima H, Kiyomoto A. Effect of diltiazem on insulin secretion. II. Experiments on perfused rat pancreas, anesthetized dogs and conscious rats. Japan J Pharmacol 1979; 29: 375–86.

199. Whitcroft I, Thomas I, Davies I, Wilkinson N, Rawthorne A. Calcium antagonists do not impair long-term glucose control in hypertensive non-insulin dependent diabetes. Br J Clin Pharmacol 1986; 22: 208P.

200. Andersson D, Rojdmark S. Improvement of glucose tolerance by verapamil in patients with non-insulin dependent diabetes mellitus. Acta Med Scand 1981; 210: 27–33.

201. Fessies C, Ferrari P, Weidmann P, Keller U, Beretta-Piccoli C, Riesen WF. Antihypertensive therapy with Ca^{++} antagonist verapamil and/or ACE inhibitor enalapril in NIDDM patients. Diabetes Care 1991; 14: 911–14.

202. Röjdmark S, Andersson DEH, Hed R, Sundblad L. Calcium-antagonistic effects on glucose response to glucagon in patients with non insulin-dependent diabetes mellitus and in normoglycemic subjects. Horm Metab Res 1981; 13: 664–7.

203. Röjdmark S, Andersson DEH, Hed R, Nordlund A, Sundblad L, Wiechel KL. Does verapamil influence glucose-induced insulin release in man? Acta Med Scand 1981; 210: 501–5.

204. Ferlito S, Modica L, Romano F et al. Effect of verapamil on glucose, insulin and glucagon levels after oral glucose load in normal and diabetic subjects. Panminerva Med 1982; 24: 221–6.

205. Devis G, Somers G, Van Obberghen E, Malaisse WJ. Calcium antagonists and islet function I. Inhibition of insulin release by verapamil. Diabetes 1975; 24: 574–81.

206. Metz SA, Halter JB, Robertson RP. Induction of defective insulin secretion and impaired glucose tolerance by clonidine. Selective stimulation of metabolic alpha-adrenergic pathways. Diabetes 1978; 27: 554–62.

207. Webster Jr WB, McConnaughey MM. Clonidine and glucose intolerance. Drug Intell Clin Pharm 1982; 16: 325–8.

208. Leclercq-Meyer V, Herchuelz A, Valverde I, Couturier E, Marchand J, Malaisse WJ. Mode of action of clonidine upon islet function: dissociated effects upon the time-course and magnitude of insulin release. Diabetes 1980; 29: 193–200.

209. Hsu WH, Hummel SK. Xylazine-induced hyperglycemia in cattle: a possible involvement of alpha 2-adrenergic receptors regulating insulin release. Endocrinology 1981; 109: 825–9.

210. Nakadate T, Nakaki T, Muraki T, Kato R. Adrenergic regulation of blood glucose levels: possible involvement of postsynaptic alpha-2 type adrenergic receptors regulating insulin release. J Pharmacol Exp Ther 1980; 215: 226–30.

211. Guthrie Jr GP, Miller RE, Kotchen TA, Koenig SH. Clonidine in patients with diabetes and mild hypertension. Clin Pharm Ther 1983; 34: 713–17.

212. Nilsson-Ehle P, Ekberg M, Fridström P, Ursing D, Lins LE. Lipoproteins and metabolic control in hypertensive type II diabetics treated with clonidine. Acta Med Scand 1988; 224: 131–4.

213. Sung PK, Samet P, Yeh BK. Effects of clonidine and chlorthalidone on blood pressure and glucose tolerance in hypertensive patients. Curr Ther Res 1971; 13: 280–85.

214. Wager J, Fredholm BB, Lunell NO, Persson B. Metabolic and circulatory effects of oral salbutamol in the third trimester of pregnancy in diabetic and non-diabetic women. Br J Obstet Gynaecol 1981; 88: 352–61.

215. Fredholm BB, Lunell NO, Persson B, Wager J. Actions of salbutamol in late pregnancy: plasma cyclic AMP, insulin and C-peptide, carbohydrate and lipid metabolites in diabetic and non-diabetic women. Diabetologia 1978; 14: 235–42.

216. Main EK, Main DM, Gabbe SG. Chronic oral terbutaline tocolytic therapy is associated with maternal glucose intolerance. Am J Obstet Gynecol 1987; 157: 644–7.

217. Angel JL, O'Brien WF, Knuppel RA, Morales WJ, Sims CJ. Carbohydrate intolerance in patients receiving oral tocolytics. Am J Obstet Gynecol 1988; 159: 762–6.

218. Main DM, Main EK, Strong SE, Gabbe SG. The effect of oral ritodrine therapy on glucose tolerance in pregnancy. Am J Obstet Gynecol 1985; 152: 1031–3.

219. Caritis SN, Toig G, Heddinger LA, Ashmead G. A double-blind study comparing ritodrine and terbutaline in the treatment of preterm labor. Am J Obstet Gynecol 1984; 150: 7–12.

220. Lipschitz J, Vinik AI. The effects of hexoprenaline, a beta 2-sympathomimetic drug, on maternal glucose, insulin, glucagon and free fatty acid levels. Am J Obstet Gynecol 1978; 130: 761–4.

221. Gündogdu AS, Juul S, Brown PM, Sachs L, Sönksen PH. Comparison of hormonal and metabolic effects of salbutamol infusion in normal subjects and insulin-requiring diabetics. Lancet 1979; 2: 1317–21.

222. Westgren M, Carlsson C, Lindholm T, Thysell H, Ingemarsson I. Continuous maternal glucose measurements and fetal glucose and insulin levels after administration of terbutaline in term labor. Acta Obstet Gynecol Scand 1982; suppl. 108: 63–65.

223. Cotton DB, Strassner HT, Lipson LG, Goldstein DA. The effects of terbutaline on acid base, serum electrolytes, and glucose homeostasis during the management of preterm labor. Am J Obstet Gynecol 1981; 141: 617–24.

224. Bassett JM, Burks AH, Levine DH, Pinches RA, Visser GHA. Maternal and fetal metabolic effects of prolonged ritodrine infusion. Obstet Gynecol 1985; 66: 755–61.

225. Bengtsson B, Fagerstrom PO. Extrapulmonary effects of terbutaline during prolonged administration. Clin Pharmacol Ther 1982; 31: 726–32.

226. Spellacy WN, Cruz AC, Buhi WC, Birk SA. The acute effects of ritodrine infusion on maternal metabolism: measurements of levels of glucose, insulin, glucagon, triglycerides, cholesterol, placental lactogen, and chorionic gonadotropin. Am J Obstet Gynecol 1978; 131: 637–42.

227. Lunell NO, Joelsson I, Larsson A, Persson B. The immediate effect of a beta-adrenergic agonist (salbutamol) on carbohydrate and lipid metabolism during the third trimester of pregnancy. Acta Obstet Gynecol Scand 1977; 56: 475–8.

228. Leslie D, Coetz PM. Salbutamol induced diabetic ketoacidosis. Br Med J 1977; 768: 70.

229. Saloranta C, Taskinen M-R, Widén E, Härkönen M, Melander A, Groop L. Metabolic consequences of sustained suppression of free fatty acids by acipimox in patients with NIDDM. Diabetes 1993; 42: 1559–66.

230. Cunner PL, Beige KG, Wenger NK, Stamler J, Friedman L, Prineas RJ, Friedwald W. Fifteen-year mortality in coronary drug projects patients: long-term benefit with niacin. J Am Coll Cardiol 1986; 8: 1245–55.

231. Gross RC, Carlson LA. Metabolic effects of nicotinic acid in acute insulin deficiency in the rat. Diabetes 1968; 17: 353–61.

232. Reaven GM, Chang H, Hoffman BB. Additive hypoglycemic effects of drugs that modify free-fatty acid metabolism by different mechanisms in rats with streptozocin-induced diabetes. Diabetes 1988; 37: 28–32.

233. Davidson MB, Bernstein JM. The effect of nicotinic acid on growth hormone-induced lipolysis and glucose intolerance. J Lab Clin Med 1973; 81: 568–76.

234. Gomez F, Jequier E, Chabot V, Felber JP. Carbohydrate and lipid oxidation in normal human subjects: its influence on glucose tolerance and insulin response to glucose. Metabolism 1972; 21: 381–91.

235. Randle PJ, Garland PB, Hales CN, Newsholme EA. The glucose–fatty acid cycle: its role in insulin

236. Saloranta C, Franssila-Kallunki A, Ekstrand A, Taskinen M-R, Groop L. Modulation of hepatic glucose production by non-esterified fatty acids in type II (non-insulin-dependent) diabetes mellitus. Diabetologia 1991; 34: 409–15.

237. Garg A, Grundy SM. Nicotinic acid as therapy for dyslipidemia in non-insulin-dependent diabetes mellitus. JAMA 1990; 264: 723–6.

238. Molnar GD, Berge KG, Rosevear JW, McGuckin WF, Achor RWP. The effect of nicotinic acid in diabetes mellitus. Metabolism 1964; 13: 181–9.

239. Henkin Y, Oberman A, Hurst DC, Segrest JP. Niacin revisited: clinical observations on an important but underutilized drug. Am J Med 1991; 91: 239–46.

240. Lithell H, Vessby B, Hellsing K. Changes in glucose tolerance and plasma insulin during lipid-lowering treatment with diet, clofibrate and niceritrol. Atherosclerosis 1982; 43: 177–84.

241. Wahlberg G, Walldios G, Efendic S. Effects of nicotinic acid on glucose tolerance and glucose incorporation into adipose tissue in hypertriglyceridemia. Scand J Clin Lab Invest 1992; 52: 537–45.

242. Kahn SE, Beard JC, Schwartz MW et al. Increased β-cell secretory capacity as mechanism for islet adaptation to nicotinic acid-induced insulin resistance. Diabetes 1989; 38: 562–8.

243. McCulloch DK, Kahn SE, Schwartz MW, Koerker DJ, Palmer JP. Effect of nicotinic acid-induced insulin resistance on pancreatic B cell function in normal and streptozocin-treated baboons. J Clin Invest 1991; 87: 1395–1401.

244. Kahn SE, McCulloch DK, Schwartz MW, Palmer JP, Porte D Jr. Effect of insulin resistance and hyperglycemia on proinsulin release in a primate model of diabetes mellitus. J Clin Endocrinol Metab 1992; 74: 192–7.

245. Miettinen TA, Taskinen MR, Pelkonen R, Nikkilä EA. Glucose tolerance and plasma insulin in man during acute and chronic administration of nicotinic acid. Acta Med Scand 1969; 186: 247–53.

246. Pereira JN. The plasma free fatty acid rebound induced by nicotinic acid. J Lipid Res 1967; 8: 239–44.

247. Pinter ES, Patter CT. Biphasic nature of blood glucose and free fatty acid changes following intravenous nicotinic acid in man. J Clin Endocrinol Metab 1967; 27: 440–3.

248. Felber JP, Ferrannini E, Golay A et al. Role of lipid oxidation in the pathogenesis of insulin resistance of obesity and type II diabetes. Diabetes 1987; 36: 1341–50.

249. Randle PJ, Newsholme EA, Garland PB. Regulation of glucose uptake by muscle. Biochem J 1964; 93: 652–65.

250. Wittsuwannakul D, Kin KH. Mechanism of palmitoyl coenzyme A inhibition of liver glucagon synthase. J Biol Chem 1971; 252: 7802–7.

251. Gonzalez-Manchon C, Martin-Requero A, Ayuso MS, Parrilla R. Role of endogenous fatty acids in the control of hepatic gluconeogenesis. Arch Biochem Biophys 1992; 29: 95–101.

252. Draye JP, Vamecq J. The gluconeogenicity of fatty acids in mammals. Trends Biochem Sci 1989; 14: 478–9.

253. Veech RL, Gitomer WL, King MT, Balaban RS, Costa JL, Eanes ED. The effect of short chain fatty acid administration on hepatic glucose, phosphate, magnesium and calcium metabolism. Adv Exp Med Biol 1986; 194: 617–46.

254. Lavezzasi M, Milaneri G, Ozzioni E, Pumparana F. Results of a phase IV study carried out in type II diabetic patients with concomitant hyperlipoproteinemia. J Int Med Res 1989; 17: 373–80.

255. Tornvall P, Walldius G. A comparison between nicotinic acid and acipimox in hypertriglyceridaemia—effects on serum lipids, lipoproteins, glucose tolerance and tolerability. J Intern Med 1991; 230: 415–21.

256. Adler RA. Clinically important effects of alcohol on endocrine function. J Clin Endocrinol Metab 1992; 74: 957–60.

257. Freinkel N, Arby RA, Singer DL et al. Alcohol hypoglycemia IV. Current concepts about its pathogenesis. Diabetes 1965; 14: 350–61.

258. Gerard MJ, Klatsky AL, Siegeluub AB, Friedman GD, Feldman R. Serum glucose levels and alcohol consumption habits in a large population. Diabetes 1977; 26: 780–85.

259. Sereny G, Endrenyl L. Mechanism and significance of carbohydrate intolerance in chronic alcoholism. Metabolism 1978; 27: 1041–6.

260. Philips GB, Safrit HF. Alcoholic diabetes. J Am Med Assn 1971; 217: 1513–19.

261. Singh SP, Kumar Y, Snyder AK, Ellyin FE, Gilden JL. Effect of alcohol on glucose tolerance in normal and non-insulin-dependent diabetic subjects. Clin Exp Res 1988; 12: 727–30.

262. Walsh CH, O'Sullivan DJ. Effect of moderate alcohol intake on control of diabetes. Diabetes 1974; 23: 440–2.

263. Ben G, Gnudi L, Maran A et al. Effects of chronic alcohol intake on carbohydrate and lipid metabolism in subjects with type II (non-insulin-dependent) diabetes. Am J Med 1991; 90: 70–6.

264. Avogaro A, Duner E, Marescotti C et al. Metabolic effects of moderate alcohol intake with meals in insulin-dependent diabetics controlled by artificial endocrine pancreas and in normal subjects. Metabolism 1983; 32: 463–70.

265. Feingold KR, Siperstein MD. Normalization of fasting blood glucose levels in insulin-requiring diabetes: the role of ethanol abstention. Diabetes Care 1983; 6: 186–8.

266. Nikkilä EA, Taskinen MR. Ethanol-induced alterations of glucose tolerance, postglucose hypoglycemia, and insulin secretion in normal, obese, and diabetic subjects. Diabetes 1975; 24: 933–43.

267. Dornhorst A, Quyang A. Effect of alcohol on glucose tolerance. Lancet 1971; 3: 957–9.

268. McDonald J. Alcohol and diabetes. Diabetes Care 1980; 3: 629–37.

269. Avogaro A, Fontana P, Valerio A et al. Alcohol impairs insulin sensitivity in normal subjects. Diabetes Res 1987; 5: 23–7.

270. Yki-Jarvinen H, Nikkila EA. Ethanol decreases glucose utilization in healthy man. J Clin Endocrinol Metab 1985; 61: 941–5.

271. Yki-Jarvinen H, Koivisto VA, Ylikahri R, Taskinen MR. Acute effects of ethanol and acetate on glucose kinetics in normal subjects. Am J Physiol 1988; 254: E175–80.

272. Jorfeldt L, Juhlin-Dannfelt A. The influence of ethanol on splanchnic and skeletal muscle metabolism in man. Metabolism 1978; 27: 97–106.

273. Puhakainen I, Koivisto VA, Yki-Jarvinen H. No reduction in total hepatic glucose output by inhibition of gluconeogenesis with ethanol in NIDDM patients. Diabetes 1991; 10: 1319–27.

274. Shelmet JJ, Reichard GA, Skutches CL, Hoeldtke RD, Owen OE, Boden G. Ethanol causes acute inhibition of carbohydrate, fat, and protein oxidation and insulin resistance. J Clin Invest 1988; 81: 1137–45.

275. Lomeo F, Khokher MA, Dandona P. Ethanol and its novel metabolites inhibit insulin action on adipocytes. Diabetes 1988; 37: 912–15.

276. Holley DC, Bagby GJ, Curry DL. Ethanol–insulin interrelationships in the rat studied *in vitro* and *in vivo*: evidence for direct ethanol inhibition of biphasic glucose-induced insulin secretion. Metabolism 1981; 30: 894–9.

277. Tiengo A, Valerio A, Molinari M, Meneghel A, Lapolla A. Effect of ethanol, acetaldehyde, and acetate on insulin and glucagon secretion in the perfused rat pancreas. Diabetes 1981; 30: 705–9.

278. Patel DG, Singh SP. Effect of ethanol and its metabolites on glucose mediated insulin release from isolated islet of rats. Metab Clin Exp 1979; 28: 85–9.

279. Fazekas G. Hydrocortisone content of human blood and alcohol content of blood and urine after wine consumption. Q J Stud Alcohol 1966; 27: 439–46.

280. Merry J, Marks V. Plasma hydrocortisone response to ethanol in chronic alcoholics. Lancet 1969; 1: 921–3.

281. Avogaro A, Tiengo A. Alcohol, glucose metabolism and diabetes. Diabetes Metab Rev 1993; 9: 129–46.

282. Zuger A, Wolf BZ, El-Sadr W, Simberkotl MS, Rahal JJ. Pentamidine-associated fatal acute pancreatitis. JAMA 1986; 256: 2383–5.

283. Bryceson A, Woodstock L. The cumulative effects of pentamidine dimethanesulphonate on the blood sugar. East Afr Med J 1969; 46: 170–3.

284. Jha Tk, Sharma VK. Pentamidine-induced diabetes mellitus. Trans R Soc Trop Med Hyg 1984; 78: 252–3.

285. Podolsky S, Zimelman A. Diabetes and AIDS. Clin Diabet 1993; 11: 29–35.

286. Stahl-Bayliss CM, Kalman CM, Laskin OL. Pentamidine-induced hypoglycemia in patients with the acquired immune deficiency syndrome. Clin Pharmacol Ther 1986; 39: 271–5.

287. Perronne C, Bricaire F, Leport C, Assan D, Vilde JL, Assan R. Hypoglycaemia and diabetes mellitus following parenteral pentamidine mesylate treatment in AIDS patients. Diabet Med 1990; 7: 585–9.

288. Sai P, Boillot D, Boitard C, Debray-Sachs M, Reach G, Assan R. Pentamidine, a new diabetogenic drug in laboratory rodents. Diabetologia 1983; 25: 418–23.

289. Boillot D, Veld P, Sai P, Feutren G, Gepts W, Assan R. Functional and morphological modifications induced in rat islets by pentamidine and other diamidines *in vitro*. Diabetologia 1985; 28: 359–64.

290. Bouchard P, Sai P, Reach G, Caubarrère I, Ganeval D, Assan R. Diabetes mellitus following pentamidine-induced hypoglycemia in humans. Diabetes 1982; 31: 40–5.

291. Belehu A, Naafs B. Diabetes mellitus associated with pentamidine mesylate. Lancet 1982; 1: 1463–4.

292. Lambertus MW, Murthy AR, Nagami P, Bidwell G, Goetz M. Diabetic ketoacidosis following pentamidine therapy in a patient with the acquired immunodeficiency syndrome. West J Med 1988; 149: 602-4.

293. Osei K, Falko JM, Nelson KP, Stephens R. Diabetogenic effect of pentamidine: *in vitro* and *in vivo* studies in a patient with malignant insulinoma. Am J Med 1984; 77: 41-6.

294. Winter WE, Funahashi M, Koons J. Encainide-induced diabetes: analysis of islet cell function. Res Comm Chem Path Pharmacol 1992; 76: 259-68.

295. Salerno DM, Fifield J, Krejci J, Hodges M. Encainide-induced hyperglycemia. Am J Med 1988; 84: 39-44.

296. Sanbar SG, Conway FJ, Zweifler AJ, Smef G. Diabetogenic effect of dilantin. Diabetes 1967; 16: 533.

297. Klein JP. Diphenylhydantoin intoxication associated with hyperglycemia. J Pediatrics 1966; 69: 463-5.

298. Goldberg EM, Sanbar SS. Hyperglycemic nonketotic coma following administration of dilantin. Diabetes 1969; 18: 101-6.

299. Dahl JR. Diphenylhydantoin toxic psychosis with associated hyperglycemia. Calif Med 1967; 107: 345-7.

300. Fariss BL, Lutcher CL. Diphenylhydantoin-induced hyperglycemia and impaired insulin release: effect of dosage. Diabetes 1971; 20: 177-81.

301. Perry-Keene DA, Larkins RG, Heyma P, Peter CT, Ross D, Solman JG. The effect of long-term diphenylhydantoin therapy on glucose tolerance and insulin secretion: a controlled trial. Clin Endo 1980; 12: 575-80.

302. Kizer SJ, Vargas-Cordon M, Brendel K, Bressler R. The *in vitro* inhibition of insulin secretion by diphenylhydantoin. J Clin Invest 1970; 49: 1942-8.

303. Siegel EG, Janjic D, Wollheim CB. Phenytoin inhibition of insulin release—studies on the involvement of Ca^{++} fluxes in rat pancreatic islets. Diabetes 1982; 31: 265-9.

304. Herschuelz A, Lebrun P, Stenor A, Malaisse WS. Ionic mechanism of diphenylhydantoin action on glucose-induced insulin release. Eur J Pharmacol 1981; 73: 189-97.

305. Pace CS, Livingston E. Ionic basis of phenytoin solution inhibition of insulin secretion in pancreatic islets. Diabetes 1979; 28: 1077-82.

306. Malherbe C, Burrill KC, Levin SR, Karan JM, Forsham PM. Effect of diphenylhydantoin on insulin secretion in man. New Engl J Med 1972; 286: 339-42.

307. Levin SR, Reed JW, Ching KN, Davis JW, Blum R, Forsham PH. Diphenylhydantoin: its use in detecting early insulin secretory defects in patients with mild glucose intolerance. Diabetes 1973; 22: 194-201.

308. Holfeldt FD, Pippe SE, Levin STL, Kasam JM, Blum MR, Forsham PM. Effect of diphenylhydantoin upon glucose-induced insulin secretion in three patients with insulinoma. Diabetes 1974; 23: 192-8.

309. Vaisrub S. Diphenylhydantoin and insulin secreting tumors. JAMA 1973; 223: 553-4.

310. Takasu N, Yamada T, Miura H et al. Rifampicin-induced early phase hyperglycemia in humans. Am Rev Respir Dis 1982; 125: 23-7.

311. Baciewicz AM, Self TM. Rifampin drug interactions. Arch Intern Med 1984; 144: 1667-71.

312. Dickson I. Glycosuria and diabetes following INH therapy. Med J Aust 1962; 1: 325-6.

313. Waitzki LA. A survey for unknown diabetes in a mental hospital. Diabetes 1966; 15: 164-72.

314. Hiler B. Hyperglycemia and glycosuria following chlorpromazine therapy. JAMA 1956; 162: 1651.

315. Van Praag HM, Leijnse B. Depression, glucose tolerance, peripheral glucose uptake and their alterations under the influence of anti-depressive drugs of the hydrazine type. Psychopharm 1965; 8: 67-78.

316. Arneison GA. Phenothiazine derivatives and glucose metabolism. J Neuropsych 1964; 5: 181-5.

317. Erle G, Basso M, Federspil G, Sicolo N, Scandellari C. Effect of chlorpromazine on blood glucose and plasma insulin in man. Eur J Clin Pharmacol 1977; 11: 15-18.

318. Nakadate T, Muraki T, Kato R. Effect of alpha and beta-adrenergic blockers on chlorpromazine-induced elevation of plasma glucose and cyclic AMP in fed mice. Japan J Pharmacol 1980; 30: 199-206.

319. Bhide MB, Tiwari NM, Balwani JH. Effect of chlorpromazine on peripheral utilization of glucose. Arch Int Pharmacodyn 1965; 156: 166-71.

320. Rafaelsen OJ. Action of phenothiazine derivatives on carbohydrate uptake of isolated rat diaphragm and isolated rat spinal cord. Psychopharmacologia 1961; 2: 185-96.

321. Ammon M, Steinke J. Apparent biphasic effect of chlorpromazine on insulin release from isolated rat pancreatic islets. Diabetes 1971; 20 (suppl.): 345-6.

322. Lambert A, Menquin JL, Ori L. Chlorpromazine in malignant insulinoma. Br Med J 1972; III: 701.

323. Yamamoto M, Akazuwa S, Yamaguchi Y et al. Effects of cyclosporin A and low dosages of steroid on post-transplantation diabetes in kidney transplant recipients. Diabetes Care 1991; 14: 867-70.

324. Yoshimura N, Nakia I, Ohmori Y et al. Effect of cyclosporine on the manic-melancholic patients. Acta Psychiatr Scand 1979; 59: 306-16.

325. Boudreaux JP, McHugh L, Cunetax DM et al. The impact of cyclosporin and combination immunosuppression on the incidence of post-transplant diabetes in renal allograft recipients. Transplantation 1987; 44: 376-81.

326. Öst L, Tydén G, Fehrman I. Impaired glucose tolerance in cyclosporine-prednisolone-treated renal graft recipients. Transplantation 1988; 46: 370-2.

327. Robertson RP, Franklin G, Nelson L. Glucose homeostasis and insulin secretion during chronic treatment with cyclosporin in non-diabetic humans. Diabetes 1989; 38 (suppl. 1): 99-100.

328. Yale JF, Chamelian M, Courchesne S, Vigeant C. Peripheral insulin resistance and decreased insulin secretion after cyclosporine. Transplant Proc 1988; 20 (suppl. 3): 985-8.

329. Sestior C, Odert-Pogo S, Bonneville M, Murel C, Leng F, Sai P. Cyclosporin enhances diabetes induced by low-dose streptozotocin treatment in mice. Immunol Lett 1985; 10: 57-60.

330. Pollock SM, Reichbaum MI, Collies BM, D'Souza M. Inhibitory effect of cyclosporin A on the activity of oral hypoglycemic agents in rats. J Pharmacol Exp Ther 1991; 258: 8-12.

331. Mopps V, Galione A, Vetri P, Vaccaso F. Sorrentino ML, Woodrow ME. Glibenclamide and cyclosporin A: an interaction on glucose metabolism. Transplant Proc 1988; 20: 979-84.

332. Runzi M, Peskar BM, von Schonfield S, Muller MK. Importance of endogenous prostaglandins for the

toxicity of cyclosporin A to rat endocrine and exocrine pancreas. Gut 1992; 33: 1572-7.

333. Muller MK, Wojzck M, Runzi M, von Schonfield S, Goebell M, Singer MV. Cytoprotection and dose-dependent inhibitory effects of prostaglandin E1 on rat pancreas treated with cyclosporin A. Digestion 1991; 50: 2-9.

334. Wahlstrom ME, Akimoto R, Endres D, Kolterman O, Moossa AR. Recovery and hypersecretion of insulin and reversal of insulin resistance after withdrawal of short term cyclosporin treatment. Transplantation 1992; 53: 1190-5.

335. Jones GR, Lazarus JH, Davies CJ, Greenwood RH. The effect of short-term lithium carbonate in type II diabetes mellitus. Horm Metab Res 1983; 15: 422-4.

336. Müller-Oerlinghausen B, Passoth PM, Poster W, Pudel V. Impaired glucose tolerance in long-term lithium-treated patients. Int Pharmacopsychiatry 1979; 14: 350-62.

337. Vestergaard P, Schou M. Does long-term lithium treatment induce diabetes mellitus? Neuropsychobiol 1987; 17: 130-32.

338. Lillikes SL. Prevalence of diabetes in a manic-depressive population. Compr Psychiatry 1985; 21: 270-5.

339. Mellerup ET, Dam H, Wildschidotz G, Rafaelsen OJ. Diurnal variation of blood glucose during lithium treatment. J Affect Disord 1983; 5: 341-7.

340. Vendsborg PB. Lithium treatment and glucose tolerance in manic-melancholic patients. Acta Psychiatr Scand 1979; 59: 306-16.

341. Anderson JH Jr, Blackard WG. Effect of lithium on pancreatic islet insulin release. Endocrinology 1978; 102: 291-5.

342. Rossetti L. Normalization of insulin sensitivity with lithium in diabetic rats. Diabetes 1989; 38: 648-52.

343. Black MB, Rubenstein AM. Aspirin induced hypoglycemia. Lancet 1971; 2: 1315.

344. Field JB, Royle C, Remer A. Effect of salicylate infusion on plasma insulin and glucose tolerance in healthy persons and mild diabetics. Lancet 1967; 1: 1191-4.

345. Micossi P, Pontiroli AE, Baron SH et al. Aspirin stimulates insulin and glucagon secretion and increases glucose tolerance in normal and diabetic subjects. Diabetes 1978; 27: 1176-1204.

346. Garcia J, Arata M, Fernandez ME, Astolfi E, Basabe JL. Salicylate intoxication and glucose-induced insulin secretion in the rat. Horm Metab Res 1982; 14: 553-4.

347. Giugliano D, Torella R, Siniscalchi N, Impronta L, D'Onofrio F. The effect of acetylsalicylic acid on insulin response to glucose and arginine in normal man. Diabetologia 1978; 14: 359-62.

348. Metz SA, Robertson RP, Fujimoto WY. Inhibition of prostaglandin E synthesis augments glucose-induced insulin secretion in cultured pancreas. Diabetes 1981; 30: 551-7.

349. Chen M, Robertson RP. Effects of prostaglandin synthesis inhibitors on human insulin secretion and carbohydrate tolerance. Prostaglandins 1979; 18: 557-67.

350. Robertson RP. Prostaglandins, glucose homeostasis, and diabetes mellitus. Med Clin North Am 1981; 65: 759-77.

351. Secmo Y, Usami M, Nakahasa M et al. Effect of acetylsalicylic acid on blood glucose and glucose regulatory hormones in mild diabetes. Prost Leuk Med 1982; 8: 49-53.

352. Segar WE, Holliday MA. Physiologic abnormalities of salicylate intoxication. New Engl J Med 1958; 259: 1191-8.

353. Buchanan N. Salicylate intoxication in infancy. S Afr Med J 1975; 49: 349-52.

354. Jorgensen TG, Weis-Fogh UT, Nielsen MM, Olesen MP. Salicylate and aspirin induced uncoupling of oxidative phosphorylation in mitochondria isolated from the mucosal membrane of the stomach. Scan J Clin Lab Inv 1976; 36: 649-54.

355. Berg KJ, Berger A. Effects of different doses of acetylsalicylic acid on renal oxygen consumption. Scand J Clin Lab Inv 1977; 37(3): 238-41.

356. Bratusch-Marrain PR, Vierhapper H, Komjati M, Waldhäusl WK. Acetyl-salicylic acid impairs insulin-mediated glucose utilization and reduces insulin clearance in healthy and non-insulin dependent diabetic man. Diabetologia 1985; 28: 671-6.

357. Newman WP, Brodows RG. Aspirin causes tissue insensitivity to insulin in normal man. J Clin Endocrinol Metab 1983; 57: 1102-6.

358. Zumott B, Mellmen L. Aggravation of diabetic hyperglycemia by chlordiazepoxide. JAMA 1977; 237: 1960-1.

359. Asensio AS, Caticha-Alfonso OS, Bieguelman B, Magna LA. Diabetogenic effect of dapsone. Int J Lepr Myco Dis 1987; 55: 357-8.

360. Tollefson G, Lejar T. Nonketototic hyperglycemia associated with loxapine and amoxapine. Case report. J Clin Psych 1983; 44: 347-8.

361. Tkach JR. Indomethacin-induced hyperglycemia in psoriatic arthritis. J Am Acad Derm 1982; 7: 802-3.

362. Hall KW, Dobson KE, Dalton JG, Ghignone MC, Penner SB. Metabolic abnormalities associated with intentional theophylline overdose. Ann Intern Med 1984; 101: 457-62.

363. Reddy J. Hyperglycemia and renal failure related to use of cimetidine. NZ Med J 1981; 93: 354-5.

364. Fraser AG, Harrower AD. Convulsions and hyperglycemia associated with nalidixic acid. Br Med J 1977; 2: 1518-19.

365. Malasanos TH, Stacpoole PW. Biological effects of omega-3 fatty acids in diabetes mellitus. Diabetes Care 1991; 14: 1160-79.

366. Goldman JA, Ovadia JL. The effect of estrogen on intravenous glucose tolerance in women. Am J Obstet Gynecol 1969; 103: 172-80.

367. Notelovitz M. Metabolic effect of conjugated oestrogens on glucose tolerance. S Afr Med J 1971; 48: 2599-603.

368. Spellacy WN, Buhi WC, Birk SA. The effects of two years of mestranol treatment on carbohydrate metabolism. Metabolism 1982; 31: 1006-8.

369. Talaat M, Habib YA, Higazy AM, Abdel Naby S, Mulek AY, Ibraham ZA. Effect of sex hormones on the carbohydrate metabolism in normal and diabetic women. Arch Int Pharmacodyn 1965; 154: 402-10.

370. Aguilo F, Robles T, Gandala JR, Huddock L. Effect of estrogen therapy on glucose tolerance in Sheehan's syndrome. Clin Res 1970; 18: 672.

371. Ajabor LN, Tsai CC, Vela P, Yen SS. Effect of exogenous estrogen on carbohydrate metabolism in postmenopausal women. Am J Obstet Gynecol 1972; 113: 383-7.

372. Polderman KH, Gooren LJ, Asscheman H, Bakker A, Heine RJ. Induction of insulin resistance by androgens and estrogens. J Clin Endocrinol Metab 1994; 79: 265-71.

373. Yen SSC, Vela P. Carbohydrate metabolism and long-term use of oral contraceptives. J Reprod Med 1969; 3: 6-18.

374. Pyorala K, Pyorala T, Lampinen V. Sequential oral contraceptive treatment and intravenous glucose tolerance. Lancet 1967; 2: 776-7.

375. Carter AC, Slivko B, Feldman EB. Metabolic effects of mestranol in high dosage. Steroids 1970; 16: 5-13.

376. Javier Z, Gershberg H, Hulse M. Ovulatory suppressants, estrogens, and carbohydrate metabolism. Metabolism 1968; 17: 443-56.

377. Blum M, Pery J, Gelenter I. Increase in glycosylated hemoglobin (HbAlc) in menopausal women treated with vaginal estrogen cream. Clin Exp Obstet Gynecol 1985; 12: 72-5.

378. Saxman KA, Barrett-Connor EL, Morton DJ. Thiazide-associated metabolic abnormalities and estrogen replacement therapy: an epidemiological analysis of postmenopausal women in Rancho Bernardo, California. J Clin Endocrinol Metab 1994; 78: 1059-63.

379. Manolio TA, Furberg CD, Shemanski L et al. Associations of postmenopausal estrogen use with cardiovascular disease and its risk factors in older women. The CHD Collaborative Research Group. Circulation 1993; 88: 2163-71.

380. Spellacy WN, Buhi WC, Birk SA. Effect of estrogen treatment for one year on carbohydrate and lipid metabolism in women with normal and abnormal glucose tolerance test results. Glucose, insulin, growth hormone, triglycerides, and Premarin. Am J Obstet Gynecol 1978; 131: 87-90.

381. Spellacy WN, Buhi WC, Birk SA. The effect of estrogens on carbohydrate metabolism: glucose, insulin, and growth hormone studies on 171 women ingesting Premarin. Am J Obstet Gynecol 1972; 114: 378-83.

382. De Cleyn K, Buytaert P, Coppens M. Carbohydrate metabolism during hormonal substitution therapy. Maturitas 1989; 11: 235-42.

383. Notelovitz M. The effect of long-term oestrogen replacement therapy on glucose and lipid metabolism in postmenopausal women. S Afr Med J 1976; 50: 2001-3.

384. Cagnacci A, Soldani R, Carriero PL, Paoletti AM, Fioretti P, Melis GB. Effects of low doses of transdermal 17 beta-estradiol on carbohydrate metabolism in postmenopausal women. J Clin Endocrinol Metab 1992; 74: 1396-1400.

385. Elkind-Hirsch KE, Sherman LD, Malinak R. Hormone replacement therapy alters insulin sensitivity in young women with premature ovarian failure. J Clin Endocrinol Metab 1993; 76: 472-5.

386. Caprio S, Boulware S, Diamond M et al. Insulin resistance: an early metabolic defect of Turner's syndrome. J Clin Endocrinol Metab 1991; 72: 832-6.

387. Billiar RB, Richardson D, Schwartz R, Posner B, Little B. Effect of chronically elevated androgen or estrogen on the glucose tolerance test and insulin response in female rhesus monkeys. Am J Obstet Gynecol 1987; 157: 1297-1302.

388. Faure A, Haouari M, Sutter BC. Oestradiol and insulin secretion in the rat: when does oestradiol start stimulating the insulin release? Horm Res 1987; 27: 225-30.

389. Weissberger AJ, Ho KK, Lazarus L. Contrasting effects of oral and transdermal routes of estrogen replacement therapy on 24-hour growth hormone (GH) secretion, insulin-like growth factor I, and GH-binding protein in postmenopausal women. J Clin Endocrinol Metab 1991; 72: 374-81.

390. Matute ML, Kalkhoff RK. Sex steroid influence on hepatic gluconeogenesis and glycogen formation. Endocrinol 1973; 92: 762-8.

391. Mandel FP, Geola FL, Lu JK et al. Biologic effects of various doses of ethinyl estradiol in postmenopausal women. Obstet Gynecol 1982; 59: 673-9.

392. Stampfer MJ, Willett WC, Colditz GA, Rosner B, Speizer FE, Hennekens CH. A prospective study of postmenopausal estrogen therapy and coronary heart disease. New Engl J Med 1985; 313: 1044-9.

393. Spellacy WN, Buhi WC, Birk SA. Norgestrel and carbohydate-lipid metabolism: glucose, insulin and triglyceride changes during six months time of use. Contraception 1974; 9: 615-25.

394. Spellacy WN, Buhi WC, Birk SA. Carbohydrate and lipid metabolic studies before and after one year of treatment with ethynodiol diacetate in 'normal' women. Fertil Steril 1976; 27: 900-4.

395. Spellacy WN, Buhi WC, Birk SA. The effect of the progestogen ethynodiol diacetate on glucose, insulin and growth hormone after six months treatment. Acta Endocrinol 1972; 70: 373-84.

396. Kalkhoff RK, Jacobson M, Lemper D. Progesterone, pregnancy and the augmented plasma insulin response. J Clin Endocrinol Metab 1970; 31: 24-8.

397. Spellacy WN, Buhi WC, Birk SA. Prospective studies of carbohydrate metabolism in 'normal' women using norgestrel for eighteen months. Fertil Steril 1981; 35: 167-71.

398. Spellacy WN, McLeod AG, Buhi WC, Birk SA. The effects of medroxyprogesterone acetate on carbohydrate metabolism: measurements of glucose, insulin, and growth hormone after twelve months' use. Fertil Steril 1972; 23: 239-44.

399. Spellacy WN, McLeod AG, Buhi WC, Birk SA, McCreary SA. Medroxyprogesterone acetate and carbohydrate metabolism: measurement of glucose, insulin, and growth hormone during 6 months' time. Fertil Steril 1970; 21: 457-63.

400. Leis D, Botterman P, Ermler R, Henderkott U, Gluck H. The influence of high doses of oral medroxyprogesterone acetate on glucose tolerance, serum insulin levels and adrenal response to ACTH. A study of 17 patients under treatment for endometrial cancer. Arch Gynecol 1980; 230: 9-13.

401. Tuttle S, Turkington VE. Effects of medroxyprogesterone acetate on carbohydrate metabolism. Obstet Gynecol 1974; 43: 685-92.

402. Konje JC, Otolorin EO, Ladipo OA. The effect of continuous subdermal levonorgestrel (Norplant) on carbohydrate metabolism. Am J Obstet Gynecol 1992; 166: 15-19.

403. Pyorala T, Vahapassi J, Huhtala M. The effect of lynestrenol and norethindrone on the carbohydrate and lipid metabolism in subjects with gestational diabetes. Ann Chir Gynaecol 1979; 68: 69-74.

404. Goldman JA, Eckerling B. Blood glucose levels and glucose tolerance in prediabetic and subclinical

diabetic women on a low dose progestogen contraceptive. Israel J Med Sci 1970; 6: 703-7.

405. Dhall K, Kumar M, Rastogi GK, Devi PK. Short-term effects of norethisterone oenanthate and medroxyprogesterone acetate on glucose, insulin, growth hormone, and lipids. Fertil Steril 1977; 28: 156-8.

406. Larsson-Cohn U, Tengstrom B, Wide L. Glucose tolerance and insulin response during daily continuous low-dose oral contraceptive treatment. Acta Endocrinol 1969; 62: 242-50.

407. Basdevant A, Pelissier C, Conard J, Degrelle H, Guyene TT, Thomas JL. Effects of nomegestrol acetate (5 mg/d) on hormonal, metabolic and hemostatic parameters in premenopausal women. Contraception 1991; 44: 599-605.

408. Kalkhoff RK. Metabolic effects of progesterone. Am J Obstet Gynecol 1982; 142: 735-8.

409. Nielson JH. Direct effect of gonadal and contraceptive steroids on insulin release from mouse pancreatic islets in organ culture. Acta Endocrinol Copenh 1984; 105: 245-50.

410. Sorenson RL, Brelje TC, Roth C. Effects of steroid and lactogenic hormones on islets of Langerhans: a new hypothesis for the role of pregnancy steroids in the adaptation of islets to pregnancy. Endocrinol 1993; 133: 2227-34.

411. Khatim MS, Gumaa KA. Islet cell growth and function. A reappraisal of the role of progesterone and prednisolone. Biochem Pharmacol 1987; 36: 2795-8.

412. Sutter-Dub MT. Effects of pregnancy and progesterone and/or oestradiol on the insulin secretion and pancreatic insulin content in the perfused rat pancreas. Diabète Métab 1979; 5: 47-56.

413. Diamond MP, Simonson DL, DeFronzo RA. Menstrual cyclicity has a profound effect on glucose homeostasis. Fertil Steril 1989; 52: 204-8.

414. Diamond MP, Jacob RA, Connally-Diamond M, DeFronzo RA. Glucose metabolism during the menstrual cycle: assessment with the euglycemic hyperinsulinemic clamp. J Reprod Med 1993; 38: 417-21.

415. Valdes CT, Elkind-Hirsch KE. Intravenous glucose tolerance test-derived insulin sensitivity changes during the menstrual cycle. J Clin Endocrinol Metab 1991; 72: 642-6.

416. Sutter-Dub MT, Dazey B, Vergnaud MT, Madec AM. Progesterone and insulin-resistance in the pregnant rat. I. *In vivo* and *in vitro* studies. Diabète Métab 1981; 7: 97-104.

417. Sutter-Dub MT, Dazey B, Hamdan E, Vergnaud MT. Progesterone and insulin-resistance: studies of progesterone action on glucose transport, lipogenesis and lipolysis in isolated fat cells of the female rat. J Endocrinol 1981; 88: 455-62.

418. Sutter-Dub MT, Vergnaud MT. Progesterone and insulin resistance. III. Time-course study of progesterone action on differentially labelled ^{14}C-glucose utilization by adipose tissue and isolated adipocytes of the female rat. J Physiol 1981; 77: 797-802.

419. Renauld A, Sverdlik RC, Aguero A, Perez RL. Influence of estrogen-progesterone sequential administration on pancreas cytology. Serum insulin and metabolic adjustments in female dogs. Acta Diab Latina 1990; 27: 315-27.

420. Sugiyama Y. The role of insulin in reproductive endocrinology and perinatal medicine. Acta Obstet Gyn Jap 1990; 42: 791-9.

421. Ri K. Study on insulin resistance in rats treated with estrogen and progesterone—assessment with the euglycemic glucose clamp technique. Folia Endocrinol Jap 1987; 63: 798-808.

422. Ryan EA, Enns L. Role of gestational hormones in the induction of insulin resistance. J Clin Endocrinol Metab 1988; 67: 341-7.

423. Waine H, Frieden EH, Caplan HI, Cole T. Metabolic effects of enovid in rheumatoid patients. Arthritis Rheum 1963; 6: 796.

424. Simon D, Senan C, Garner P et al. Effects of oral contraceptives on carbohydrate and lipid metabolism in a healthy population: the Telecom Study. Am J Obstet Gynecol 1990; 163: 382-7.

425. Russell-Briefel R, Ezzati TM, Perlman JA, Murphy RS. Impaired glucose tolerance in women using oral contraceptives: United States 1976-1980. J Chron Dis 1987; 40: 3-11.

426. Perlman JA, Russell-Briefel R, Ezzati T, Lieberknecht G. Oral glucose tolerance and the potency of contraceptive progestins. J Chronic Dis 1985; 38: 857-64.

427. Godsland IF, Waton LC, Felton C, Proudler A, Patel A, Wynn V. Insulin resistance, secretion, and metabolism in users of oral contraceptives. J Clin Endocrinol Metab 1992; 74: 64-70.

428. Godsland IF, Crook D, Simpson R et al. The effects of different formulations of oral contraceptive agents on lipid and carbohydrate metabolism. New Engl J Med 1990; 323: 1375-81.

429. Godsland IF, Crook D, Worthington M et al. Effects of a low-estrogen, desogestrel-containing oral contraceptive on lipid and carbohydate metabolism. Contraception 1993; 48: 217-27.

430. Crook D, Godsland IF, Worthington M, Felton CV, Proudler AJ, Stevenson JC. A comparative metabolic study of two low-estrogen-dose oral contraceptives containing desogestrel or gestodene progestins. Am J Obstet Gynecol 1993; 169: 1183-9.

431. Jandrain BJ, Humblet DM, Jaminet CB, Scheen AJ, Gaspard UJ, Lefebvre PJ. Effects of ethinyl estradiol combined with desogestrel and cyproterone acetate on glucose tolerance and insulin response to an oral glucose load: a one-year randomized, prospective, comparative trial. Am J Obstet Gynecol 1990; 163: 378-81.

432. Luyckx AS, Gaspard UJ, Romus MA, Grigorescu F, De Meyts P, Lefebvre PJ. Carbohydrate metabolism in women who used oral contraceptives containing levonorgestrel or desogestrel: a 6-month prospective study. Fertil Steril 1986; 45: 635-42.

433. Gershbert H, Javier Z, Hulse M. Glucose tolerance in women receiving an ovulatory suppressant. Diabetes 1964; 13: 378-82.

434. Halling GR, Michals EL, Paulsen CA. Glucose intolerance during ethynodiol diacetate-mestranol therapy. Metabolism 1967; 16: 465-8.

435. Peterson WF, Steel MW Jr, Coyne RV. Analysis of the effect of ovulatory suppressants on glucose tolerance. Am J Obstet Gynecol 1966; 95: 484-8.

436. Posner NA, Silverstone FA, Pomerance W, Baumgold D. Oral contraceptives and intravenous glucose tolerance. I. Data noted early in treatment. Obstet Gynecol 1967; 29: 79-86.

437. Spellacy WN, Carlson KL, Birk SA, Schade SL. Glucose and insulin alterations after one year of combination-type oral contraceptive treatment. Metabolism 1968; 17: 496–501.

438. Wynn V, Doar JW. Some effects of oral contraceptives on carbohydrate metabolism. Lancet 1966; 2: 715–19.

439. Blum M, Rusecky Y, Gelernter I. Glycohemoglobin (HbA1) levels in oral contraceptive users. Eur J Obstet Gynecol Reprod Biol 1983; 15: 97–101.

440. Van der Vange N, Kloosterboes MJ, Haspels AA. Effect of seven low dose combined oral contraceptive preparations on carbohydrate metabolism. Am J Obstet Gynecol 1987; 156: 918–22.

441. Spellacy WN, Buhi WC, Birk SA. Carbohydrate metabolism prospectively studied in women using low-estrogen oral contraceptive for six months. Contraception 1979; 20: 137–48.

442. Spellacy WN, Ellingson AB, Kotlik A, Tsibris JC. Prospective study of carbohydrate metabolism in women using a triphasic oral contraceptive containing norethindrone and ethinyl estradiol for 3 months. Am J Obstet Gynecol 1988; 159: 877–9.

443. Scheen AJ, Jandrain BJ, Humblet DM, Jaminet CB, Gaspard UJ, Lefebvre PJ. Effects of a 1-year treatment with a low-dose combined oral contraceptive containing ethinyl estradiol and cyproterone acetate on glucose and insulin metabolism. Fertil Steril 1993; 59: 797–802.

444. Godsland IF, Gargas K, Walton C et al. Insulin resistance, secretion, and elimination in postmenopausal women receiving oral or transdermal hormone replacement therapy. Metabolism 1993; 42: 846–53.

445. Skouby SO, Andersen O, Saurbrey N, Kuhl C. Oral contraception and insulin sensitivity: *in vivo* assessment in normal women and women with previous gestational diabetes. J Clin Endocrinol Metab 1987; 64: 519–23.

446. Kasdorf G, Kalkhoff RK. Prospective studies of insulin sensitivity in normal women receiving oral contraceptive agents. J Clin Endocrinol Metab 1988; 66: 846–52.

447. Thornton KL, DeFronzo RA, Sherwin RS, Diamond MP. Micronized estradiol and progesterone: effects on carbohydrate metabolism in reproductive aged women. J Soc Gyn Invest (submitted).

448. Skouby SO, Molsted-Pedersen L, Kuhl C. Low dosage oral contraception in women with previous gestational diabetes. Obstet Gynecol 1982; 59: 325–8.

449. Rubeck Petersen K, Skouby SO, Dreisler A, Kuhl C, Svenstrup B. Comparative trial of the effects on glucose tolerance and lipoprotein metabolism of two new oral contraceptives containing gestoden and desogestrel. Acta Obstet Gynecol Scand 1988; 67: 37–41.

450. Skouby SO, Kuhl C, Molsted-Pedersen L, Petersen K, Christensen MS. Triphasic oral contraception: metabolic effects in normal women and those with previous gestational diabetes. Am J Obstet Gynecol 1985; 153: 495–500.

451. Radberg T, Gustafson A, Karlsson K, Skryten A. Metabolic effects of different types of oral contraception in insulin dependent and latent diabetes. Acta Obstet Gynecol Scand 1978; 93 (suppl.): 70–1.

452. Szabo AJ, Cole HS, Grimaldi RD. Glucose tolerance in gestational diabetic women during and after treatment with a combination-type oral contraceptive. New Engl J Med 1970; 282: 646–50.

453. Kung WC, Ma JT, Wong VC et al. Glucose and lipid metabolism with triphasic oral contraceptives in women with history of gestational diabetes. Contraception 1987; 35: 257–69.

454. Wiese J, Osler M. Contraception in diabetic patients. Acta Endocrinol 1974; 182 (suppl.): 87–9.

455. Radberg T, Gustafson A, Skryten A, Karlsson K. Oral contraception in diabetic women. Horm Metab Res 1982; 14: 61–5.

456. Skouby SO, Molsted-Pedersen L, Kuhl C, Bennet P. Oral contraceptives in diabetic women: metabolic effects of four compounds with different estrogen/progestogen profiles. Fertil Steril 1986; 46: 858–64.

457. Skouby SO, Jensen BM, Kuhl C, Molsted-Pedersen L, Svenstrup B, Nielsen J. Hormonal contraception in diabetic women: acceptability and influence on diabetes control and ovarian function of a nonalkylated estrogen–progestogen compound. Contraception 1985; 32: 23–31.

458. Tainter ML. Anabolic steroids in the management of the diabetic patient. New York State J Med 1965; 65: 519–30.

459. Cohen JC, Hickman A. Insulin resistance and diminished glucose tolerance in powerlifters ingesting anabolic steroids. J Clin Endocrinol Metab 1987; 64: 960–63.

460. Small M, Forbes CD, MacCuish AC. Metabolic effects of stanozolol in type II diabetes mellitus. Horm Metab Res 1986; 18: 647–8.

461. Landon J, Wynn V, Cooke JNL, Kennedy A. Effects of anabolic steroid methandienone on carbohydrate metabolism in man. Metabolism 1962; 11: 501–11.

462. Landon J, Wynn V, Sands E. The effect of anabolic steroids on blood sugar and plasma insulin levels in man. Metabolism 1963; 12: 924–34.

463. Williams G, Ghatei M, Burrin J, Bloom S. Severe hyperglucagonaemia during treatment with oxymetholone. Br Med J Clin Res 1986; 292: 1637–8.

464. Woodard TL, Burghen GA, Kitabchi AE, Wilimas JA. Glucose intolerance and insulin resistance in aplastic anemia treated with oxymetholone. J Clin Endocrinol Metab 1981; 53: 905–8.

465. Godsland IF, Shennan NM, Wynn V. Insulin action and dynamics modelled in patients taking the anabolic steroid methandienone (Dianabol). Clin Sci 1986; 71: 665–73.

466. Novak R, Wilimas J, Johnson W. Hypertrophy and hyperplasia of islets of Langerhans associated with androgen therapy. Arch Pathol Lab Med 1979; 103: 483–5.

467. Glazer G. Atherogenic effects of anabolic steroids on serum lipid levels. A literature review. Arch Intern Med 1991; 151: 1925–33.

468. Hurley BF, Seals DR, Hagberg JM et al. High-density-lipoprotein cholesterol in bodybuilders vs. powerlifters. Negative effects of androgen use. JAMA 1984; 252: 507–13.

469. Wilson JD. Androgen abuse by athletes. Endocr Rev 1988; 9: 181–99.

470. Alen M, Reinila M, Vihko R. Response of serum hormones to androgen administration in power athletes. Med Sci Sports Exerc 1985; 17: 354–9.

471. Burghen GA, Givens JR, Kitabchi AE. Correlation of hyperandrogenism with hyperinsulinism in polycystic

ovarian disease. J Clin Endocrinol Metab 1980; 50: 113–16.

472. Mahabeer S, Jialal I, Norman RJ, Naidoo C, Reddi K, Joubert SM. Insulin and C-peptide secretion in non-obese patients with polycystic ovarian disease. Horm Metab Res 1989; 21: 502–6.

473. Chang RJ, Nakamura RM, Judd HL, Kaplan SA. Insulin resistance in non-obese patients with polycystic ovarian disease. J Clin Endocrinol Metab 1983; 57: 356–9.

474. Tropeano G, Lucisano A, Liberale I et al. Insulin, C-peptide, androgens, and beta-endorphin response to oral glucose in patients with polycystic ovary syndrome. J Clin Endocrinol Metab 1994; 78: 305–9.

475. Golland IM, Vaughan-Williams CA, Shalet SM, Laing I, Elstein M. Glucagon in women with polycystic ovary syndrome (PCO): relationship to abnormalities of insulin and androgens. Clin Endocrinol 1990; 33: 645–51.

476. Khaw KT, Barrett-Connor E. Fasting plasma glucose levels and endogenous androgens in non-diabetic postmenopausal women. Clin Sci 1991; 80: 199–203.

477. Simon D, Preziosi P, Barrett-Connor E, Roger M, Saint-Paul M, Nahoul K, Papoz L. Interrelation between plasma testosterone and plasma insulin in healthy adult men: the Telecom Study. Diabetologia 1992; 35: 173–7.

478. Marin P, Holmang S, Jonsson L et al. The effects of testosterone treatment on body composition and metabolism in middle-aged obese men. Int J Obesity 1992; 16: 991–7.

479. Byerly L, Swerdloff RJ, Lee WP et al. Effects of manipulating testosterone levels in the normal male range on protein carbohydrate and lipid metabolism in man: implications for testosterone replacement therapy. Clin Sci 1993; 41: 84A.

480. Dunaif A, Green G, Futterweit W, Dobrjansky A. Suppression of hyperandrogenism does not improve peripheral or hepatic insulin resistance in the polycystic ovary syndrome. J Clin Endocrinol Metab 1990; 70: 699–704.

481. Friedel KE, Jones RE, Hannan CJ, Plymate SR. The administration of pharmacological doses of testosterone or 19-nortestosterone to normal men is not associated with increased insulin secretion or impaired glucose tolerance. J Clin Endocrinol Metab 1989; 68: 971–5.

482. Herbert CM, Hill GA, Diamond MP. The use of the intravenous glucose tolerance test to evaluate nonobese hyperandrogenic women. Fertil Steril 1990; 53: 647–53.

483. Haffner SM, Karhapaa P, Mykkanen L, Laakso M. Insulin resistance, body fat distribution, and sex hormones in men. Diabetes 1994; 43: 212–19.

484. Kim SY, Sung YA, Ko KS. Direct relationship between elevated free testosterone and insulin resistance in hyperprolactinemic women. Korean J Intern Med 1993; 8: 8–14.

485. Shoupe D, Lobo RA. The influence of androgens on insulin resistance. Fertil Steril 1984; 41: 385–8.

486. Rajkhowa M, Bicknell J, Jones M, Clayton RN. Insulin sensitivity in women with polycystic ovary syndrome: relationship to hyperandrogenemia. Fertil Steril 1994; 61: 605–12.

487. Holmang A, Larsson BM, Brzezinska Z, Bjorntorp P. Effects of short-term testosterone exposure on insulin sensitivity of muscles in female rats. Am J Physiol 1992; 262: E851–5.

488. Holmang A, Svedberg J, Jennische E, Bjorntorp P. Effects of testosterone on muscle insulin sensitivity and morphology in female rats. Am J Physiol 1990; 259: E555–60.

489. Renauld A, Sverdlik RC. Influence of testosterone on blood sugar, serum insulin and free fatty acid responses to glucose in normal male dog. Acta Physiol Latino 1975; 25: 423–9.

490. Peiris AN, Aiman EJ, Drucker WD, Kissebah AH. The relative contributions of hepatic and peripheral tissues to insulin resistance in hyperandrogenic women. J Clin Endocrinol Metab 1989; 68: 715–20.

491. Forbes GB, Porta CR, Herr BE, Griggs RC. Sequence of changes in body composition induced by testosterone and reversal of changes after drug is stopped. JAMA 1992; 267: 397–9.

492. Welle S, Jozefowicz R, Forbes G, Griffs RC. Effect of testosterone on metabolic rate and body composition in normal men and men with muscular dystrophy. J Clin Endocrinol Metab 1992; 74: 332–5.

493. Boyle PJ. Cushing's disease, glucocorticoid excess, glucocorticoid deficiency and diabetes. Diabetes Rev 1993; 1: 301–8.

494. McMahon M, Gerich J, Rizza R. Effects of glucocorticoids on carbohydrate metabolism. Diabetes Metab Rev 1988; 4: 17–30.

495. Miller WL, Tyrrell J Blake. The adrenal cortex. In Felig P, Baxter JD, Frohman LA (eds) Endocrinology and Metabolism. New York: McGraw-Hill, 1995; pp 665–7.

496. Shi MZ, Zhang SF. Steroid diabetes: an analysis of 28 years. Chinese J Intern Med 1985; 28: 139–41.

497. Umpierrez GE, Khajavi M, Kitabchi AE. Review: diabetic ketoacidosis and hyperglycemic hyperosmolar nonketotic syndrome. Am J Med Sci 1996; 311: 225–33.

498. Perley M, Kipnis D. Effect of glucocorticoids on plasma insulin. New Engl J Med 1966; 274: 1237–41.

499. Shamoon M, Soman V, Sherwin R. The influence of acute physiological increments of cortisol on fuel metabolism and insulin binding to monocytes in normal humans. J Clin Endocrinol Metab 1980; 50: 495–500.

500. Burns TW, Engel FL, Viau A, Scott JL, Hollingsworth DR, Werk E. Studies on the interdependent effects of stress and the adrenal cortex on carbohydrate metabolism in man. J Clin Invest 1953; 32: 781–91.

501. West KW. Response to cortisone in prediabetes, glucose and steroid–glucose tolerance in subjects whose parents are both diabetic. Diabetes 1960; 9: 379–84.

502. Conn JW, Fajans SS. Influence of adrenal cortisol steroids on carbohydrate metabolism in man. Metabolism 1956; 5: 114–27.

503. McKiddie MT, Jasani MK, Buchanan KD, Boyle JA, Buchanan WW. The relationship between glucose tolerance, plasma insulin, and corticosteroid therapy in patients with rheumatoid arthritis. Metabolism 1968; 17: 730–39.

504. Bookman JT, Drachman SR, Schaefer LI, Adlersberg D. Steroid diabetes occurring during cortisone and adrenocorticotropin (ACTH) therapy. J Clin Invest 1952; 31: 619–20.

505. Bastenie PA, Conard V, Franckson JRM. Effect of cortisone on carbohydrate metabolism measured by

the 'glucose assimilation coefficient'. Diabetes 1954; 3: 205–9.

506. Plotz CM, Knowlton AI, Ragan C. The natural history of Cushing's syndrome. Am J Med 1952; 13: 597–614.

507. Ross EJ, Linch DC. Cushing's syndrome—killing disease: discriminatory value of signs and symptoms aiding early diagnosis. Lancet 1982; 2: 646–9.

508. Urbanic RC, George JM. Cushing's disease—18 years' experience. Medicine 1981; 60: 14–24.

509. Perley M, Kipnis D. Effect of glucocorticoids on plasma insulin. New Engl J Med 1966; 274: 1237–41.

510. Kitabchi A, Jones G, Duckworth W. Effect of hydrocortisone and corticotropin on glucose induced insulin and pro-insulin secretion in man. J Clin Endocrinol Metab 1973; 37: 79–84.

511. Rizza RA, Mandarino LJ, Gerich JE. Cortisol-induced insulin resistance in man: impaired suppression of glucose production and stimulation of glucose utilization due to a postreceptor defect of insulin action. J Clin Endocrinol Metab 1982; 54: 131–8.

512. Olfesky J, Kimmerling G. Glucocorticoids in carbohydrate metabolism. Am J Med Sci 1976; 271: 203–10.

513. Yasuda K, Hines III E, Kitabchi AE. Hypercortisolism and insulin resistance: comparative effects of prednisone, hydrocortisone, and dexamethasone on insulin binding of human erythrocytes. J Clin Endocrinol Metab 1982; 55: 910–15.

514. Clerc D, Wick H, Keller U. Acute cortisol excess results in unimpaired insulin action on lipolysis and branched chain amino acids, but not on glucose kinetics and C-peptide concentration in man. Metabolism 1986; 35: 404–10.

515. Nosadini R, Del Prato S, Tiengo A et al. Insulin resistance in Cushing's syndrome. J Clin Endocrinol Metab 1983; 57: 529–36.

516. Munck A, Koritz SB. Studies on the mode of action of glucorticoids in rats. I. Early effects of cortisol on blood glucose entry into muscle, liver, and adipose tissue. Biochim Biophys Acta 1962; 57: 310–18.

517. Vann Bennett GV, Cuatrecasas P. Insulin receptor of fat cells in insulin-resistant metabolic states. Science 1972; 176: 805–6.

518. Shamoon H, Soman V, Sherwin RS. The influence of acute physiological increments of cortisol on fuel metabolism and insulin binding to monocytes in normal humans. J Clin Endocrinol Metab 1980; 50: 495–501.

519. Okuno Y, Nishizawa Y, Kawagishi T, Morii M. *In vivo* and *in vitro* effects of glucocorticoids on glucose transport in human polymorphonuclear leukocytes. Horm Metab Res 1993; 25: 165–9.

520. Olefsky JM. Effect of dexamethasone on insulin binding, glucose transport, and glucose oxidation of isolated rat adipocytes. J Clin Invest 1975; 56: 1499–1508.

521. Exton J, Mallettie L, Jefferson L et al. The hormonal control of hepatic gluconeogenesis. Recent Prog Horm Res 1970; 26: 411–57.

522. Kraus-Friedmann N. Hormonal regulation of hepatic gluconeogenesis. Physiol Rev 1984; 64: 170–259.

12

The Insulin Resistance Syndrome

Michael P. Stern

University of Texas Health Science Center, San Antonio, Texas, USA

A large number of epidemiologic and clinical studies have firmly established consistent correlations between certain anthropometric, metabolic and hemodynamic variables. These variables include obesity, unfavorable body fat distribution, glucose intolerance or type 2 diabetes, hyperinsulinemia, hypertriglyceridemia, low levels of high density lipoprotein (HDL) cholesterol, and hypertension. It is also well established that patients exhibiting these features are at increased risk of atherosclerotic disease. While not the first to report these correlations, Modan and colleagues in the early 1980s were the first to call attention to the central role of insulin resistance and hyperinsulinemia, thereby stimulating renewed interest in this field. These investigators studied 2475 men and women randomly drawn from the Israel Central Population Registry [1]. Strong correlations were observed between obesity, glucose intolerance, hypertension and hyperinsulinemia, leading the investigators to conclude that 'insulin resistance is a common pathophysiologic feature of (these conditions), explaining their ubiquitous association'.

The literature on this cluster of disorders is vast. Most of the available studies, however, are cross-sectional and have been reviewed previously [2]. This chapter will therefore concentrate primarily on prospective studies, since these tend to be more recent and constitute a stronger experimental design for elucidating cause and effect. An exception will be studies in which insulin resistance was measured by a direct method such as the euglycemic clamp or the intravenous glucose tolerance test, almost all of which are cross-sectional.

Two developments in the 1980s contributed to the emergence of a specific hypothesis regarding the underlying mechanism responsible for this cluster of abnormalities. The first was the appearance of three prospective epidemiologic studies which were widely interpreted as showing that circulating insulin concentration was an independent risk factor for cardiovascular disease [3–5]. The second development was the demonstration that lean patients with hypertension were insulin-resistant relative to lean subjects without hypertension [6–8]. It was primarily these findings which led Reaven in his 1988 Banting Lecture to propose a syndrome which he labeled 'syndrome X' and which consisted of resistance to insulin-stimulated glucose uptake, glucose intolerance, hyperinsulinemia, increased very-low density lipoprotein triglyceride, decreased high-density lipoprotein cholesterol, and hypertension [9]. However, beyond merely describing a syndrome, Reaven put forth a specific hypothesis about its pathogenesis, viz. that insulin resistance was the underlying metabolic defect which caused all of the other manifestations. For this reason the syndrome has also become known as the insulin resistance syndrome (IRS) which is the terminology that is used in this chapter.

It should be noted that the syndrome described by Reaven was observed in *lean* individuals. While it is undoubtedly true that the IRS can occur in such individuals, epidemiologic studies have indicated that the great majority of individuals having the syndrome are, in fact, obese, and moreover have an unfavorable distribution of body fat. It should also be noted that, although the studies linking circulating insulin

International Textbook of Diabetes Mellitus, Second Edition. Edited by K.G.M.M. Alberti, P. Zimmet, R.A. DeFronzo, and H. Keen (Honorary)

concentrations to future cardiovascular disease (CVD) were prospective, all of the studies linking insulin resistance, measured by a direct method, to hypertension were cross-sectional. While it has been widely assumed that it is the insulin resistance which causes the hypertension and not the reverse, it bears mention that cross-sectional data, by themselves, cannot definitively distinguish between cause and effect. Thus, in the absence of other types of evidence, it is equally possible that it is the hypertension which causes the insulin resistance. As we shall see, this point of view has its advocates.

This chapter will first explore the IRS as an antecedent of type 2 diabetes and atherosclerotic disease. Next, the relationship between insulin resistance and other manifestations of the IRS will be critically evaluated, followed by a discussion of several factors which, although not part of the original description of the IRS, may nevertheless deserve to be included. Specifically, these include small dense LDL (low-density lipoproteins), microalbuminuria, sex hormones and platelet activator inhibitor 1. Although little is known about the genetics of the IRS, information is available on a variety of apparently related conditions, and the genetic determinants of the most important of these will be discussed. Finally, the chapter concludes with a discussion of early life exposures, i.e. those operating during fetal life and infancy, which may influence the development of the IRS in later life.

DEFINITION OF THE INSULIN RESISTANCE SYNDROME (IRS)

It is useful to make a distinction between those elements which are *features* of the IRS and those conditions which are *outcomes*. For purposes of this chapter we will regard the disorders of lipid and insulin metabolism described above as features of the syndrome. Similarly, hypertension will be regarded as a feature of the IRS, although, as will be discussed, there is significant controversy on this point. This concerns the extent to which it is *caused* by insulin resistance. Although the IRS was initially described in lean individuals [9], since the majority of patients with this syndrome are obese and have an unfavorable distribution of body fat, I will include these attributes as features of the IRS as well. By contrast, type 2 diabetes mellitus and atherosclerotic disease, especially coronary artery disease, will be viewed as outcomes of the IRS. These conditions are pictured as the consequences of having had the IRS for many years or perhaps decades. As will be seen, the evidence that type 2 diabetes is an outcome of the IRS is stronger than the evidence for atherosclerotic disease. It should

also be noted that, with the possible exception of obesity, the IRS itself is asymptomatic and it is the long-term outcomes of the IRS that produce morbidity, functional disability and ultimately excess mortality.

It is important to emphasize that, although the elements of the IRS can be specified, there is as yet no consensus on either the optimum cut-off points or the manner of combining the various IRS components in such a way as to generate an operational definition or diagnostic criteria for the syndrome. This deficiency sharply limits our ability to define the epidemiology and genetics of the IRS. Despite this limitation, some progress has been made on characterizing the genetic features of several related conditions, if not the IRS itself.

THE IRS AS AN ANTECEDENT OF TYPE 2 DIABETES

A widely accepted theory of the pathogenesis of type 2 diabetes may be referred to as the 'insulin resistance/islet cell exhaustion' theory. According to this concept, insulin resistance is a fundamental lesion which compels the pancreatic islet cells to hypersecrete insulin in order to maintain glucose homeostasis. After many years or decades of this obligatory hypersecretion, the islet cells eventually fail and clinical diabetes supervenes. There are a large number of cross-sectional studies which have reported inverted U-shaped relationships between circulating insulin concentrations and glucose tolerance, i.e. low levels of insulin in subjects with normal glucose tolerance, higher levels in those with mild or moderate glucose tolerance, and low levels again in those with severe hyperglycemia [10, 11]. Since these results are cross-sectional, they do not necessarily prove that each individual progresses through these several stages as he or she develops diabetes. Recently, however, it has been demonstrated in a longitudinal study of Pima Indians that individuals who are destined to develop diabetes do in fact progress through these stages of first rising and then falling insulin levels [12]. The 'insulin resistance/islet cell exhaustion' theory implies that, at a certain stage, hyperinsulinemia will be an antecedent of type 2 diabetes. There are now at least six prospective epidemiological studies which document this phenomenon [13–18]. The generalizability of these findings is indicated by the broad spectrum of populations in which they have been observed, including Europids, native Americans, Mexican Americans, Japanese Americans and Micronesians from the south Pacific. In further support of the 'insulin resistance/islet cell exhaustion' theory is the fact that insulin resistance, when directly measured, is also a risk factor for the development of type 2 diabetes. This has been demonstrated in Pima Indians using the euglycemic clamp technique [19] and in Europid offspring of two diabetic parents in whom insulin resistance was measured by an intravenous glucose tolerance test [20].

Granted that insulin resistance is an antecedent of type 2 diabetes, the question arises whether the other elements of the IRS are also antecedents of diabetes. There is, of course, an extensive literature indicating that obesity is a risk factor for type 2 diabetes [13–15, 17, 18, 21–25]. There are also a large number of cross-sectional studies which indicate that diabetic patients have a more central and more upper-body distribution of adipose tissue [2]. Moreover, there is now mounting evidence from prospective studies that unfavorable body fat distribution is an antecedent of type 2 diabetes [15–18, 24]. A variety of indices have been used to characterize body fat distribution. Thus, the subscapular-to-triceps skinfold ratio, a measure of truncal adiposity, has been found to be predictive of future diabetes in Mexican Americans [15]. The ratio of waist circumference to hip circumference, a measure of upper body adiposity, has been found to be predictive in Europids (Swedes and Finns) [18, 24] and visceral fat, measured by CT-scan, has been found to be predictive in Japanese Americans [16]. Again, the wide spectrum of populations represented by these results supports the generalizability of the role of unfavorable body fat distribution as an antecedent of type 2 diabetes.

If insulin, obesity and unfavorable body fat distribution are 'traditional' risk factors for diabetes, abnormal lipids and high blood pressure, which are also features of the IRS, may be regarded as 'non-traditional' risk factors for diabetes. Although it is well-known that hypertension is common in patients with diabetes, it is perhaps less well appreciated that the hypertension can precede the diabetes. This was first pointed out by Pell and d'Alonzo in 1967 [21] and has since been confirmed in several other prospective studies [15, 18, 22, 25]. One mechanism which has been suggested whereby hypertension might increase the risk of diabetes is through the action of certain antihypertensive drugs such as thiazide diuretics and/or β-blockers, which can produce insulin resistance and glucose intolerance. However, it has been shown that the risk of diabetes is increased even in hypertensives who are not receiving these drugs. In one study from Sweden, although hypertensives treated with thiazide diuretics and/or β-blockers had an increased incidence of diabetes relative to hypertensives not on these agents, both groups had an elevated incidence relative to normotensive subjects [26]. In the San Antonio Heart Study, the incidence of diabetes was the same in hypertensives on thiazides and/or β-blockers and those on other antihypertensive agents or on no treatment, and both groups had an elevated incidence of diabetes relative to normotensives [27].

Serum triglyceride concentration has also been found to be a risk factor for diabetes in five out of five prospective studies [13, 15, 18, 25, 28]. Again, the generalizability of these findings is indicated by the fact that they have been reported in Micronesians from the south Pacific [13], Mexican Americans [15] and non-Hispanic Europids from Finland, USA, and UK [18, 25, 28]. HDL cholesterol has been studied prospectively in only two studies, both of which confirmed that low levels of this lipoprotein are a significant predictor of diabetes [15, 18].

The results of 12 prospective studies of diabetes risk factors are summarized in Table 1. Taken in aggregate, these studies provide impressive evidence that all of the elements of the IRS are consistent risk factors for type 2 diabetes across a broad spectrum of racially and ethnically diverse populations.

An important consideration is the extent to which the above-mentioned diabetes risk factors are independent of one another. It could be, for example, that since they are all correlated with obesity, their association with diabetes reflects nothing more than the fact that obesity itself is a well-known diabetes risk factor. One way to approach the question of independence is to attempt systematically to develop optimum predicting models. This has been done in the San Antonio Heart Study [29]. In this study, 19 variables including age, gender, ethnic group, body mass index (BMI), subscapular-to-triceps skinfold ratio, fasting and 2-hour glucose and fasting insulin levels, systolic and diastolic blood pressure, LDL and HDL cholesterol, triglyceride concentration and cigarette smoking were allowed to compete in a stepwise multiple logistic regression analysis to see which combination of variables generated the optimum predicting models. A number of models were examined including models for Mexican Americans, non-Hispanic whites, men, women, and for the overall population. A series of 'reduced' models were also tested. In these latter models only variables which are commonly used in clinical practice were allowed to compete. Thus, insulin levels, skinfold measurements, and blood glucose measurements 2 hours after an oral glucose load were excluded. Several models are presented in Table 2. These equations can be solved for P, the probability that an individual will develop diabetes over 8 years, by entering his or her risk factor values, multiplying them by the appropriate coefficients, and summing across risk factors. As can be seen in Table 2, glucose concentration and body mass index (weight divided by height squared, a common index of obesity in epidemiologic studies) entered all of the models. All models also contained a representative from both the

Table 1 Risk factors for type 2 diabetes

Risk factor	Positive studies/total studies	Populations	References
Obesity	10/11	Europid, Mexican American, native American, Micronesian	13–15, 17, 18, 21–25, 28*
Unfavorable fat distribution	5/5	Europid, Mexican American, Japanese American	15–18, 24
Glycemia	9/9	Europid, Mexican American, native American, Japanese American, Micronesian	13–18, 23, 25, 28
Insulinemia	6/6	Europid, Mexican American, native American, Japanese American, Micronesian	13–18
Blood pressure	5/7	Europid, Mexican American	13*, 15, 18, 21, 22, 25, 28*
Triglyceride	5/5	Europid, Mexican American, Micronesian	13, 15, 18, 25, 28
Low HDL	2/2	Europid, Mexican American	15, 18

*Negative study.
By permission of The American Diabetes Association. From Stern MP, Perspectives in Diabetes. Diabetes and cardiovascular disease: the "common soil" hypothesis. Diabetes 1995; 44: 369–74.

lipid and the hemodynamic category of variables. Thus, the question of independence can be viewed from the following perspective: although the specific risk factors which independently predict diabetes will vary depending on the population under study and the particular combination of risk factors examined, they will most likely contain representatives from each of the four major categories of IRS-related variables,

viz. anthropometric variables, variables reflecting carbohydrate and lipid metabolism, and hemodynamic variables.

Historically, impaired glucose tolerance (IGT) has been regarded as the main predictor of future diabetes. Table 3 indicates that the sensitivity, specificity, and positive predictive value of the models is at least as good, if not better than, the corresponding parameters

Table 2 Equations for optimum and reduced* predicting models for type 2 diabetes

1. Optimal model, overall population ($n = 1272$):
   $\ln(P/1 - P) = -16.8547 + (0.0909 \times \text{FPG}) + (0.0237 \times 2\text{-hPG}) + (0.0966 \times \text{BMI}) + (-0.0397 \times \text{HDL}) + (0.0318 \times \text{PPr})$

2. Reduced model, overall population ($n = 1453$):
   $\ln(P/1 - P) = -15.6863 + (0.1120 \times \text{FPG}) + (0.1008 \times \text{BMI}) + (-0.0477 \times \text{HDL}) + (0.0433 \times \text{PPr}) + (-0.8659 \times \text{sex})$

3. Reduced model, men ($n = 612$):
   $\ln(P/1 - P) = -12.9642 + (0.0936 \times \text{FPG}) + (0.0614 \times \text{PPr}) + (-0.0443 \times \text{HDL}) + (0.8707 \times \text{HT})$

4. Reduced model, women ($n = 841$):
   $\ln(P/1 - P) = -19.6987 + (0.1295 \times \text{FPG}) + (0.1029 \times \text{BMI}) + (-0.0519 \times \text{HDL}) + (0.0382 \times \text{SBP}) + (-1.1159 \times \text{HT})$

5. Reduced model, Mexican American ($n = 825$):
   $\ln(P/1 - P) = -19.1121 + (0.1107 \times \text{FPG}) + (0.0983 \times \text{BMI}) + (-0.9800 \times \text{sex}) + (0.6915 \times \ln \text{TG})$

6. Reduced model, non-Hispanic white ($n = 628$):
   $\ln(P/1 - P) = -22.6261 + (0.1170 \times \text{FPG}) + (0.0691 \times \text{SBP}) + (-0.0605 \times \text{HDL}) + (0.0982 \times \text{BMI})$

where $P/1 - P$ = odds of developing diabetes in 8 years; FPG = fasting plasma glucose (mg/dl); 2-hPG = 2-hour plasma glucose (mg/dl); BMI = body mass index (kg/m^2); HDL = high density lipoprotein cholesterol (mg/dl); PPr = pulse pressure (mmHg); HT = hypertension (1 = present, 2 = absent); SBP = systolic blood pressure (mmHg); sex: 1 = male, 0 = female; lnTG = natural log of triglyceride concentration (mg/dl).

*For definition of optimum and reduced models see text.
From reference 29, by permission of the American Diabetes Association.

Table 3 Sensitivity, specificity, predictive value, and relative risks (RR) of reduced* predicting models compared with impaired glucose tolerance (IGT) as predictors of type 2 diabetes

	Overall population	Men	Women	Mexican American	Non-Hispanic white
IGT models					
n	1419	604	815	796	623
Sensitivity (%)	59.2	62.1	57.4	60.4	56.5
Specificity (%)	87.3	88.3	86.6	86.1	88.8
Percentage correctly classified	85.8	87.1	84.9	84.4	87.6
Predictive value of a positive test (%)	20.9	21.2	20.8	23.7	16.3
Predictive value of a negative test (%)	97.4	97.9	97.1	96.8	98.2
RR	8.04	10.0	7.11	7.46	8.82
*Reduced models***					
n	1453	612	841	825	628
Sensitivity (%)	69.6	67.7	81.3	72.7	83.3
Specificity (%)	88.1	88.0	88.0	87.0	89.9
Percentage correctly classified	87.1	86.9	87.6	86.1	89.6
Predictive value of a positive test (%)	25.2	23.1	29.1	28.6	24.7
Predictive value of a negative test (%)	98.1	98.1	98.7	97.8	99.3
RR	13.26	12.16	22.38	13.00	35.29

*n for IGT models slightly smaller than for corresponding reduced models, as a result of missing values for 2-hour plasma glucose concentrations. **For definition of reduced models see text.
From reference 29, by permission of the American Diabetes Association.

for IGT. (The model parameters were calculated based on defining the top 15% of the risk score continuum as 'high risk' to correspond to the 15% prevalence of IGT.) This is true even for the 'reduced' models which require a fasting blood draw only.

It is noteworthy that insulinemia, the variable most closely linked to insulin resistance, did not enter any of the optimum predicting models, even though it is a highly significant univariate predictor of diabetes [29]. It should be emphasized, however, that these models are 'optimum' only in their ability to *predict* future disease, not necessarily in their ability to shed light on pathogenesis. There are a number of reasons why variables which play an important role in pathogenesis may fail to appear in optimum predicting models. Thus, if two variables lie in the same causal pathway—as might obesity and hyperinsulinemia—only one might survive the multivariate analysis and appear in the final model. Nor is the survivor necessarily the one which bears the most proximate relationship to the disease. If one of the two candidate variables can be measured with greater precision (e.g. body mass index compared with serum insulin), the more precisely measured variable may well win a place in the final model even if it is less closely linked to the disease.

THE IRS AS AN ANTECEDENT OF CARDIOVASCULAR DISEASE (CVD)

At the outset it should be emphasized that the principal risk factors for atherosclerotic disease, and the ones which would invariably be included in any optimum predicting model which might be developed, are LDL cholesterol, cigarette smoking, and hypertension. Of these, only one, hypertension, is part of the IRS. Neither LDL nor cigarette smoking has ever been identified as a risk factor for type 2 diabetes. Thus, although the IRS may be an antecedent of CVD, clearly it cannot be the only antecedent, or even the most important one.

It must also be acknowledged that, whereas in the case of diabetes insulin resistance measured by a direct method has been demonstrated to be a risk factor in two prospective studies [19, 20], no similar demonstration has ever been reported in the case of cardiovascular disease. The Insulin Resistance/Atherosclerosis Study (IRAS), currently in progress, should help to clarify the situation. In this study diabetic and non-diabetic participants of three racial/ethnic groups (non-Hispanic white, African American, and Mexican American) are undergoing measurements of insulin resistance by the minimal model technique developed by Bergman [30]. These measurements will be correlated with various non-invasive measures of atherosclerosis, such as carotid ultrasound. Although this study is currently cross-sectional, it could readily be converted into a prospective study.

For the present, the case for insulin resistance as a risk factor for cardiovascular disease can only be supported indirectly and rests on studies in which insulinemia, rather than insulin resistance, was assessed. The evidence, which includes data from animal studies, *in vitro* studies and prospective epidemiologic studies, has been summarized by Stout [31]. The earliest evidence that insulin might be atherogenic came from studies of alloxan-induced diabetes in cholesterol-fed rabbits. These animals failed to develop the expected degree of aortic atherosclerosis that normally follows cholesterol-feeding, unless insulin was administered [32, 33]. Similarly, alloxan-induced diabetic monkeys developed more atherosclerosis in response to high cholesterol feeding if they were treated with insulin than if they were not [34]. Also, in chickens insulin administration prevented the regression of arterial lesions that normally follows withdrawal of a high-cholesterol diet [35]. Finally, injection of insulin directly into one femoral artery of an alloxan-induced diabetic dog resulted in more medial thickening and a higher cholesterol content than in the contralateral femoral artery, injected with saline [36].

Insulin has also been shown to cause *in vitro* proliferation of smooth muscle cells from a number of experimental animals [31] including primates [37] and also from man [38]. It has also been shown to stimulate sterol synthesis in cultured smooth muscle cells [39] as well as the binding of LDL to both smooth muscle cells [40] and fibroblasts [41]. Insulin also stimulates cholesterol synthesis and the binding of LDL to cell membranes in monocytes [42, 43]. Thus, insulin may promote atherogenesis by a direct effect on the arterial wall.

The epidemiologic evidence that insulinemia is a risk factor for CVD rests on three prospective studies which appeared in 1979–80, the Helsinki Policeman Study [3], the Paris Prospective Study [4] and the Busselton Study [5]. Only the Busselton Study included women, among whom insulin was *not* predictive of future CVD. Thus, there has never been any evidence that insulin is a cardiovascular risk factor in women. With respect to the data in men, a number of inconsistencies have been pointed out [2, 44]: in the Helsinki study only the 2-hour post-oral glucose load insulin value was significantly predictive of future CVD in multivariate analysis [3], whereas in the original 5-year follow-up of the Paris Prospective Study only the fasting value remained significant in multivariate analyses [4]. In the 11-year Paris follow-up the fasting insulin value remained predictive of coronary heart disease (CHD) mortality, but this time only in obese individuals (BMI $\geq$ 26 kg/m^2) [45]. In a subsequent 15-year follow-up, however, the fasting value ceased to be predictive and the 2-hour value emerged as significant [46], although only when analyzed as a categorical variable (top quintile vs. lower four quintiles), and not when analyzed as a continuous variable. It should also be noted that, whereas in the original 5-year follow-up of the Paris Study both fatal and non-fatal coronary events were reported, in subsequent reports only mortality data were available. The Busselton study implicated 1-hour post-load insulin as a

risk factor for CVD incidence in men only, in univariate analyses only, and only in one of the three age groups studied (60–69 years). In multivariate analyses insulin was a significant risk factor for cardiovascular mortality in men of all ages, but not for CVD incidence (i.e. fatal and non-fatal events combined). Thus, except for the early and intermediate results from the Paris Prospective Study, these results tend to implicate the post-oral glucose load insulin values rather than the fasting values. Thus it is difficult to infer from these results the role of insulin resistance as an underlying risk factor, since there are conflicting data over whether fasting [47] or post-load insulin values [48] are more highly correlated with insulin resistance.

More recently, two additional studies have appeared, neither of which gives strong support to the theory that insulin is a cardiovascular risk factor. In the Gothenberg Study of men born in 1913, the fasting but not the 1-hour insulin value showed a borderline significant trend with incidence of CHD, but this trend disappeared in multivariate analyses [49]. Using a case–control design, 94 participants of the Multiple Risk Factor Intervention Trial (MRFIT) who had died of CHD and 114 who had experienced non-fatal myocardial infarction were matched to 414 participants who had remained free of CHD throughout the follow-up period. No difference in fasting insulin levels between the two groups was observed [50]. It should be noted, however, that MRFIT participants were selected to be at high risk of CHD based on their total cholesterol, blood pressure and cigarette smoking status, which could have overwhelmed any effect of insulin.

Before dismissing insulin as a cardiovascular risk factor, however, it should be recalled that even in the case of diabetes, insulin, although it was independently predictive in several studies [13, 14, 17, 51], did not win a place in the optimum predicting model [29]. On the other hand, the role of hyperinsulinemia as a diabetes risk factor does not rest solely on statistical arguments. It is also strongly supported by the biological plausibility of the insulin resistance/compensatory hypersecretion/islet cell exhaustion theory described above. Although, as we have seen, arguments can be made for the biological plausibility of hyperinsulinemia as a risk factor for atherosclerosis, these arguments do not seem as compelling as in the case of diabetes.

The role of obesity as a cardiovascular risk factor has been controversial for many years. It is not usually considered as one of the 'big three', i.e. cholesterol, blood pressure and cigarette smoking. The reason seems to be that, although there is evidence that obesity is a univariate predictor of future CVD, it often fails to retain statistical significance in multivariate analyses and is therefore said not to be an 'independent' cardiovascular risk factor: but one may well ask, independent of what? The variables which tend to displace it in multivariate analyses are blood pressure, high triglyceride and low HDL levels, which may lie in the same causal pathway. This type of lack of independence does not of itself refute the biological importance of a risk factor as a disease antecedent.

Obesity or overweight has been shown to be a univariate predictor of cardiovascular mortality in some impressively large studies. Thus, the American Cancer Society Study presented mortality data according to relative weight in 750 000 men and women. This study revealed a stepwise increase in mortality due to CHD in both sexes as relative weight increased from 20% below the average for the population as a whole to 40% above [52]. Similar results were reported from the Build Study 1979, involving 106 000 deaths among 4.2 million life insurance policy holders from 1950 to 1971. CHD mortality was more than twice as high in men who were 55–65% overweight compared to those who were 25–35% underweight [53]. Again, a clear dose–response effect was noted. The findings in women were similar, except that there was a modest excess CHD mortality in the two leanest groups relative to the next leanest group, after which there was a stepwise increase in CHD mortality with rising relative weight.

One of the earliest studies suggesting that obesity did not make an independent contribution to CHD once other risk factors were taken into account was the Seven-Country Study, in which a univariate effect of obesity ceased to be statistically significant once hypertension was considered in a multivariate model [54]. Early results from the Framingham Study gave similar results [55, 56], but in a subsequent report reflecting 26 years of follow-up, relative weight predicted the incidence of CHD independently of age, cholesterol, blood pressure, cigarette smoking, left ventricular hypertrophy and glucose intolerance [57]. The British Regional Heart Study also reported that the rate of major CHD events rose with increasing body mass index in both hypertensive and normotensive individuals, independently of age and cigarette smoking [58]. The Pooling Project which involved 6 major prospective epidemiologic studies in the USA found that relative weight predicted CHD incidence independently of cholesterol, blood pressure and cigarette smoking in men of 40–49 years of age, but not in older men [59]. It should be noted that triglyceride and high density lipoprotein (HDL) levels, both strong correlates of obesity, were not measured at baseline in any of these studies and thus could not be adjusted for in the analyses. The importance of triglyceride and HDL as cardiovascular risk factors is discussed below. It should also be noted that there are a number of studies which have failed to find obesity to be a CVD risk factor

even in univariate analyses [46, 49]. It is of interest that the studies which have given the strongest support for obesity as a univariate predictor of CHD have been mortality studies, whereas those studies which have included non-fatal CHD events have, in general, provided weaker evidence. These findings are compatible with the possibility that obesity influences case fatality rates as much as, or perhaps even more than, CHD incidence.

Visceral fat as measured by CAT scan has been correlated with CVD in a cross-sectional study of Japanese Americans [60]. There are only two prospective studies in which the distribution of body fat was documented as a risk factor for CVD [61, 62]. Both used the waist-to-hip ratio (WHR) as an indicator of upper body distribution of adiposity. In a 12-year follow-up of 38–60-year-old Swedish women, WHR was significantly predictive of myocardial infarction, stroke and all cause mortality independently of age, BMI, cigarette smoking, cholesterol, systolic blood pressure and, in the case of myocardial infarction, triglyceride level [61]. WHR was also predictive of angina pectoris independently of age and cholesterol, but not of the other covariates. In 54-year-old Swedish men, of the anthropometric variables studied which included BMI, three skinfolds and waist and hip circumference, only the WHR was significantly associated with 13-year incidence of ischemic heart disease or stroke [62]. This effect, however, was not independent of cholesterol, systolic blood pressure or cigarette smoking. In the Framingham Study subscapular skinfold was strongly predictive of 22-year coronary heart disease (CHD) incidence in both men and women independently of BMI and other conventional CVD risk factors [63]. In fact, in men it was more highly predictive than any other risk factor except cholesterol. Waist circumference was also independently predictive of CHD incidence in men. Hip circumference was not measured. However, since subscapular skinfold and waist circumference reflect adiposity at one site only, they are not, strictly speaking, indices of body fat *distribution*.

Like obesity, the role of triglyceride as a CVD risk factor has also been controversial for many years. Apart from statistical questions of independence, there is the heterogeneity of various hypertriglyceridemic syndromes and of the composition of triglyceride-bearing lipoproteins. Thus, familial combined hyperlipoproteinemia, a disorder characterized by overproduction of apolipoprotein B [64] and often presenting with hypertriglyceridemia, is associated with an increased risk of atherosclerosis, whereas familial hypertriglyceridemia, at least in some families, does not appear to be associated with increased atherosclerotic risk [65]. There are also differences in the atherogenic potential of various subclasses of very low density lipoprotein (VLDL), the lipoprotein which transports the majority of circulating triglycerides. Thus, large buoyant VLDL particles are considered to be less atherogenic than smaller VLDL particles which have a relatively higher cholesterol content [65, 66]. Intermediate density lipoprotein (IDL), which is produced by the action of lipoprotein lipase on VLDL resulting in the hydrolysis of a portion of its triglyceride, is an intermediate product on the pathway from VLDL to LDL (low density lipoprotein). This particle, which is thought to be highly atherogenic, is present in high concentrations in the rare disorder known as type III hyperlipoproteinemia, but may also play a role in promoting atherogenesis in other hypertriglyceridemic states [67, 68]. Hypertriglyceridemia is also associated with increased concentrations of small dense LDL particles, which are thought to be more atherogenic than ordinary LDL. This lipoprotein is discussed in further detail in a subsequent section of this chapter.

In view of this heterogeneity, it is not surprising that triglyceride concentration often fails to emerge as an independent CVD risk factor in multivariate analyses. In the Paris Prospective Study, triglyceride levels were independent predictors of CVD in patients with glucose intolerance after adjusting for age, total cholesterol, cigarette smoking, systolic blood pressure, BMI, and fasting and 2-hour insulin values [69]. However, HDL was not measured at baseline in this study and so it was not possible to test for independence from this lipoprotein. In those studies such as the Lipid Research Clinics (LRC) Follow-up Study, where HDL was measured at baseline, although triglyceride was a univariate predictor of cardiovascular endpoints, it was displaced by HDL in multivariate analyses [70]. Similar findings have been reported in diabetic patients by Laakso et al [71]. Again, HDL but not VLDL emerged as the more robust CVD risk factor.

Because of the consistent, strong correlations between high triglyceride levels and low HDL it makes sense to consider these two variables jointly as CVD risk factors. In general, HDL has proven to be a more consistent, independent predictor of CVD than triglyceride. The earliest demonstration that HDL was protective against CVD was based on ultracentrifuge measurements [72]. These measurements were technically demanding and expensive, and it was not until cheaper and more convenient precipitation techniques were developed that HDL underwent extensive evaluation as an inverse CVD risk factor. The Framingham study was one of the earliest to demonstrate the protective effects of HDL as measured by the precipitation technique [73]. More recently, low HDL levels have been confirmed to be strong inverse risk factors for CVD independently of

age, cigarette smoking, systolic blood pressure, BMI, total or LDL cholesterol and, in particular, VLDL cholesterol in four large multicenter studies in the USA [74]. It would seem reasonable to conclude that, even though we still lack precise knowledge of mechanisms, the high triglyceride–low HDL complex is almost certainly an important marker for increased atherosclerotic risk.

What conclusions can we draw about the CVD risk factor status of the IRS from the above discussion? Clearly, several important elements of the IRS are themselves CVD risk factors. These include blood pressure, the high triglyceride–low HDL complex, obesity and probably unfavorable body fat distribution. Whether or not insulin resistance itself or its accompanying hyperinsulinemia are CVD risk factors is less clear. It is possible to take the view that the IRS is a CVD risk factor only because several of its elements are CVD risk factors, wholly unrelated to their association with insulin resistance.

Of course, diabetes itself is a CVD risk factor. A recent dramatic demonstration of this is provided by the follow-up of nearly 350 000 men screened for participation in the Multiple Risk Factor Intervention Trial (MRFIT), over 5000 of whom were self-reported diabetic patients. Cardiovascular mortality in the latter was 2–4 times higher than in the non-diabetic men, even after stratifying on total cholesterol concentration, systolic blood pressure or cigarette smoking [75]. The results stratified on total cholesterol are depicted in Figure 1. One could therefore argue that, since the IRS is a risk factor for diabetes (see previous section), and since diabetes is a risk factor for cardiovascular disease, the IRS is itself a risk factor for CVD. However, this begs the question of the mechanisms by which diabetes increases cardiovascular risk. Plasma glucose itself is an inconsistent cardiovascular risk factor in diabetic patients [76, 77]. In some studies the risk of CVD appears to be no greater in subjects with established

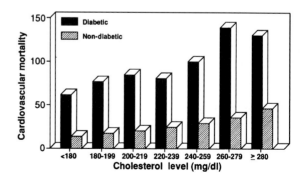

Figure 1 Age-adjusted cardiovascular mortality (per 10 000 person-years) in diabetic and non-diabetic men according to serum cholesterol level. Adapted from reference 75, by permission of the American Diabetes Association

diabetes than in those with impaired glucose tolerance [78] and among those with overt diabetes, neither disease duration nor severity of hyperglycemia have correlated well with atherosclerotic risk [78–81]. This has not been a universal finding, however; for example, Laakso et al found that disease duration and glycated hemoglobin levels were univariate predictors of several cardiovascular endpoints in diabetic patients [71]. Nevertheless, the lackluster performance of hyperglycemia as a CVD risk factor has focused attention on the lipid and hemodynamic concomitants of diabetes as explanations for the enhanced CVD risk associated with the diabetic state. This brings us full circle back to the IRS. Since these concomitants all precede the diabetes, it has been postulated that, rather than regarding CVD as a 'complication' of diabetes, it is more appropriate to regard both conditions as 'springing from the same soil'. This concept has been summarized by the 'ticking clock' metaphor which states that, '... unlike microvascular complications, where the "clock starts ticking" with the onset of clinical diabetes (i.e. hyperglycemia), in the case of macrovascular disease, the clock may start ticking decades earlier' [15].

DOES INSULIN RESISTANCE CAUSE THE OTHER MANIFESTATIONS OF THE IRS?

Obesity and Unfavorable Body Fat Distribution

It should be reiterated that, as originally described by Reaven [9], neither obesity nor unfavorable body fat distribution was included in the IRS and it is clear that the syndrome can exist in lean individuals [82]. On the other hand, as noted above, most individuals with the IRS are obese and have unfavorable body fat distribution. Regardless of whether one wishes to include these anthropometric features as 'official' elements of the syndrome, the evidence is rather persuasive that obesity is *not* caused by insulin resistance, but rather the other way around. Thus, acute weight change studies have consistently demonstrated that experimental weight gain leads to rising serum insulin concentrations [83–85] and weight loss results in falling concentrations [86, 87]. Moreover, an amelioration of insulin resistance in response to weight loss has been directly demonstrated using the euglycemic hyperinsulinemic clamp technique [86, 88, 89]. Further evidence that insulin resistance does not cause obesity comes from studies in the Pima Indians, which demonstrated that insulin-resistant subjects gained less weight over a 3.5-year follow-up period than insulin-sensitive subjects [90]. It has been postulated that insulin resistance develops as a defense against continuing unchecked weight gain. Compatible with this idea are recent data

from the San Antonio Heart Study showing that, among the obese but not among the lean, higher insulin values predict weight loss, rather than weight gain, 8 years later [91]. In any case, none of these data is compatible with the idea that insulin resistance causes obesity, but rather with the reverse.

With respect to unfavorable body fat distribution and insulin resistance, there are few if any data on which is the cause and which the effect, but that unfavorable fat distribution causes the insulin resistance seems more likely than the converse.

Hypertension

In 1987 Ferrannini et al studied 13 normal-weight, hypertensive patients (BMI = 26 kg/m^2) and 11 age- and weight-matched controls (BMI = 25 kg/m^2) and found that, compared to controls, hypertensive patients had decreased insulin sensitivity as determined by the euglycemic hyperinsulinemic clamp technique [6]. This decrease was almost entirely due to diminished non-oxidative glucose disposal (i.e. glycogen synthesis), since glucose oxidation was essentially normal, as were suppression of hepatic glucose production and lipolysis. Swislocki et al subsequently characterized insulin sensitivity using the insulin-suppression test in 14 untreated and 17 treated hypertensive patients and confirmed that both groups were insulin-resistant compared to 16 controls matched for age and BMI [92]. Moreover, the insulin resistance persisted even among those whose blood pressure had been partially restored towards normal with antihypertensive agents. Those who had been treated with both diuretics and β-blockers were even more insulin-resistant than those who had been treated with diuretics alone or who were untreated. These patients were also relatively lean, with the average BMIs of the different patient groups ranging from 25.7 to 26.2 kg/m^2. One might well have anticipated an association between hypertension and insulin resistance among obese subjects as well, since such individuals have been shown to have impaired glucose tolerance and an exaggerated insulin response to an oral glucose load compared to obese normotensive patients [93]. However, direct measurement of insulin resistance using the insulin clamp technique has indicated that, although obese subjects (BMIs ranging from 32.2 to 34.7 kg/m^2) are insulin resistant, hypertension was not associated with a further increase in insulin resistance relative to normotensive obese subjects [94–96]. This was true for both obese non-diabetic [94, 95] and obese diabetic [95, 96] subjects (see Figure 2). By contrast, among lean diabetic patients (BMIs ranging from 23 to 24 kg/m^2) hypertension was associated with a greater degree of insulin

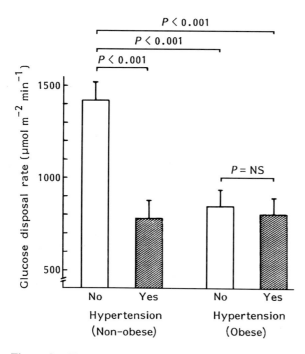

Figure 2 Glucose disposal rates during euglycemic clamp studies in non-obese and obese type 2 diabetic subjects with and without hypertension. From reference 96, by permission of Blackwell Scientific Publications, Ltd.

resistance than was observed among normotensive lean subjects [96].

Saad et al reported that the association between insulin resistance and hypertension was present in Europids, but absent or markedly attenuated in Pima Indians and Blacks [97] (see Figure 3). These data have been interpreted as suggesting racial and ethnic differences in the insulin resistance–hypertension relationship. However, the Blacks included in the report by Saad et al were obese with a mean BMI of 33.0 kg/m². A subsequent study of lean Blacks with and without hypertension (BMI = 23 kg/m²) revealed that lean hypertensive Blacks were indeed more insulin-resistant than lean normotensive Blacks [98]. Since Pima Indians are also very obese, it is unclear whether the racial and ethnic differences that have been reported are real or rather reflect differences between lean and obese hypertensives. Apart from Europids [6, 92–96] and Blacks [97, 98], there is limited information on the insulin resistance–hypertension relationship encompassing both lean and obese members of other racial and ethnic groups.

Since all these studies are cross-sectional, they do not distinguish cause and effect. Prospective studies relevant to this issue have depended, not on measurements of insulin resistance *per se*, but rather on serum insulin measurements as a surrogate variable. In the San Antonio Heart Study, among individuals who were normotensive at baseline, fasting insulin was

a weak, univariate predictor of hypertension 8-year later [99, 100]. Specifically, whereas an increase in the baseline fasting insulin level from 50 to 100 pmol/l was associated with a more than two-fold increase in the 8-year odds of developing diabetes ($p = 0.001$), the same insulin gradient was associated with only a 21% increase in the odds of hypertension ($p < 0.05$) (unpublished data). Moreover, insulin was not a significant risk factor for hypertension in multivariate analyses which adjusted for age, sex, ethnic group, BMI and the ratio of subscapular to triceps skinfold (STR). Of importance was the finding of a significant interaction between insulin and BMI, implying that insulin was a risk factor for hypertension only among lean individuals (lowest tertile of BMI) [99]. The CARDIA (Coronary Artery Risk Development in Young Adults) study also reported that insulin was a risk factor for hypertension [101].

The case for insulin resistance as a *cause* of hypertension rests, however, primarily on arguments of biological plausibility and on the results of pharmacologic interventions. A number of mechanisms have been postulated to explain the link between insulin resistance or hyperinsulinemia and hypertension. Thus, exogenous intravenous administration of insulin under euglycemic clamp conditions has been shown to induce a 30–40% reduction in urinary sodium excretion, an effect that has been localized to both the proximal and distal tubules [102]. Insulin has also been shown to stimulate the release of norepinephrine [103–105]. On the other hand, insulin has a direct vasodilatory effect [105] (see below). It has been postulated that the net effect of insulin on blood pressure represents the balance between its direct vasodilatory effect and the indirect vasoconstrictor effect mediated through adrenergic stimulation [105]. Increased intracellular concentrations of both sodium and calcium ions sensitize vascular smooth muscle to pressor substances such as norepinephrine and angiotensin [106, 107]. These ion fluxes are controlled by various 'pumps' such as the sodium–hydrogen exchanger, the sodium–potassium ATPase pump and the calcium–ATPase pump, all of which are insulin-sensitive [106, 107]. Depending on the direction of the ion fluxes induced by each pump, one may postulate either that the pump shares in a generalized insulin resistance or, conversely, that it remains insulin-sensitive, thereby becoming an 'innocent victim' of the hyperinsulinemia. Although attractive as theoretical mechanisms, the full details of the function of these pumps in various insulin-resistant states remain to be worked out (see also reviews by DeFronzo and Ferrannini [106] and DeFronzo [107]). Finally, as mentioned above, insulin is a growth factor which has been shown to stimulate smooth muscle

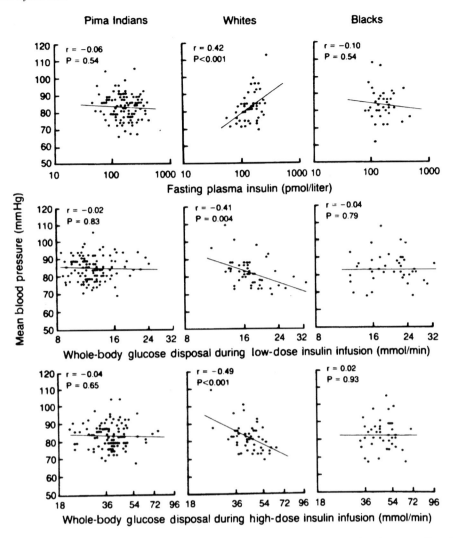

Figure 3 Relation between mean blood pressure and fasting plasma insulin concentration (top panel) and insulin-mediated glucose disposal during low-dose (middle panel) and high-dose (bottom panel) insulin infusions in Pima Indians, whites and blacks, after adjustment for age, sex, body weight and percentage of body fat. From reference 97, by permission of The New England Journal of Medicine

proliferation *in vitro* [31, 37, 38] and could thus cause hypertension by producing hypertrophy of vascular walls.

A number of pharmacological interventions which enhance insulin sensitivity, both in animals and man, have also been reported to lower blood pressure. Thus, the administration of metformin to lean, non-diabetic, hypertensive men both increased insulin sensitivity and lowered blood pressure [108]. This study, however, was not a controlled, double-blind trial, although the blood pressure tended to return to baseline following withdrawal of metformin. Also, pioglitazone and ciglitazone, both of which agents are known to reduce insulin resistance, have been shown to lower blood pressure in various rat models [109, 110]. Similar effects have been reported with metformin in spontaneously hypertensive rats [111].

The principal argument against hyperinsulinemia as a cause of hypertension is that insulin, when infused intravenously together with glucose to preserve euglycemia, generally produces vasodilation and fails to raise blood pressure. Both systemic [112, 113] and local arterial [114] infusions of insulin have been reported to produce decreased vascular resistance and increased leg and forearm blood flow, representing primarily blood flow to skeletal muscles. Moreover, in most human studies euglycemic insulin infusions have failed to raise blood pressure despite increases in circulating norepinephrine concentrations [105, 115, 116]. In one study insulin infusion failed to raise blood pressure when physiologic levels of insulinemia were achieved (44–154 µU/ml), but did when supraphysiological levels were achieved (600 µU/ml) [103]. It appears, however, that euglycemic insulin infusions do elevate blood pressure in rats [117], suggesting species differences. All of the above studies were relatively acute and, even though Hall et al failed to induce hypertension in dogs with insulin infusions lasting up to 28 days [118], the effects of long-term hyperinsulinemia lasting for years or decades are unknown.

In addition to vasodilation insulin increases cardiac output [103, 112], causes tachycardia [103, 112, 118] and increases myocardial contractility [119, 120]. There is also evidence suggesting that fixed high peripheral resistance hypertension is preceded by labile high cardiac output hypertension [121]. In view of the similarity of these hemodynamic effects of insulin and the hemodynamic alterations of early essential hypertension, Stern et al postulated that the primary effect of hyperinsulinemia might be to produce a hyperdynamic state which only after many years resulted in fixed hypertension. In other words, they suggested that hypertension was a relatively late manifestation of the IRS [122]. They defined a hyperdynamic state in terms of a widened pulse pressure and tachycardia (top quartile of the respective distributions for these variables) and showed that individuals who met these criteria displayed many of the features of the IRS [122]. Contrary to the hypothesis, however, the hyperdynamic state did not predict future hypertension, although it did predict future diabetes, itself a *bona fide* IRS outcome [29, 122].

Laakso et al, noting that most muscle capillaries are unperfused in the resting state, proposed that by 'recruiting' such capillaries, the mean intercapillary distance would be decreased, resulting in a decreased insulin concentration gradient between capillary vessels and muscle cell membranes [113]. This would lead to the delivery of a higher concentration of insulin to the muscle cell membrane. If insulin induces increased glucose uptake in part by augmenting muscle blood flow, clearly an impairment in this effect could contribute to insulin resistance. Using the Fick Principle it is possible to estimate the proportion of insulin-induced augmentation of glucose uptake which can be attributed to increased blood flow. Since glucose uptake is equal to the product of the arteriovenous (A-V) glucose difference × the blood flow to the vascular bed in question, one can subtract out the glucose uptake that would have occurred, given the new, insulin-stimulated A-V difference, had the blood flow remained constant, i.e. at its pre-insulin flow rate [113]. Using this approach, Laakso et al demonstrated that, whereas in lean individuals the contribution of increased blood flow to insulin-induced augmentation of glucose uptake reached a plateau of approximately 40% at serum insulin levels of 300 pmol/l and above, in obese individuals increased blood flow made almost no contribution to insulin-induced augmentation of glucose

uptake at 300 pmol/l and rose to a maximum of only 25% at 800 pmol/l (see Figure 4) [113]. These results strongly suggest that failure to augment regional blood flow in response to insulin could be at least one factor that contributes to insulin-resistant states. On the other hand, this is clearly not the sole mechanism for insulin resistance in obesity. Laakso et al also showed that, although the insulin concentration/muscle blood flow dose response curve was shifted to the right in obesity, augmentation of muscle blood flow ultimately reached the same level in the obese as in the lean, albeit at a higher insulin concentration [113]. However, even at insulin concentrations and muscle blood flow rates comparable to those attained in lean subjects, the femoral A-V glucose difference widened less in the obese than in the lean [113], indicating that impairment in glucose extraction by leg muscles also made a contribution to insulin resistance.

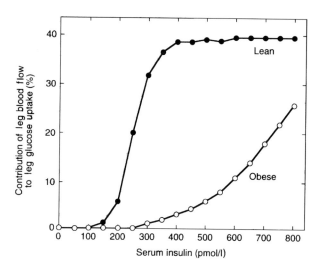

Figure 4 Contribution of increased leg blood flow to increased glucose uptake at various insulin concentrations in lean and obese subjects, calculated from the formula: $100 \times (AVG_{obs} \times F_{obs} - AVG_{obs} \times F_{fixed})/(AVG_{obs} \times F_{obs})$, where AVG_{obs} = the observed femoral artery A-V glucose difference during insulin infusion, F_{obs} = the observed femoral artery blood flow during insulin infusion, and F_{fixed} = femoral artery blood flow prior to insulin infusion. From reference 113, by permission of the Journal of Clinical Investigation, by copyright permission of the American Society for Clinical Investigation

Julius et al have proposed a mechanism whereby hypertension could cause insulin resistance rather than the reverse [123]. They have suggested that in hypertension, '... closure of small vessels by vascular hypertrophy could lead to vascular rarefaction', i.e. a reduction in the capillary density of skeletal muscle [123]. This would limit the ability of insulin to increase blood flow by recruiting new capillaries, thereby eliminating one of its means of increasing glucose uptake. This concept has received support recently from the work of Baron et al, who showed in 19 lean, normotensive subjects that mean arterial blood pressure at baseline was inversely correlated with insulin-mediated glucose uptake in both whole body ($r = -0.63$, $p < 0.01$) and leg ($r = -0.47$, $p < 0.05$) [124]. Baseline blood pressure was also inversely correlated with the increment in leg blood flow following insulin administration ($r = -0.59$, $p < 0.01$) [124]. There was no association between blood pressure and A-V glucose difference, indicating that the relationship between blood pressure and glucose uptake was not caused by an inhibitory effect of blood pressure on glucose extraction by muscle.

Muscle fibers are of two types: slow twitch (type 1), which have a rich capillary blood supply and a high oxidative capacity; and fast twitch (type 2b), which are capillary-poor and have a high glycolytic, but low oxidative, capacity [125]. The former are relatively insulin-sensitive and the latter are relatively insulin-resistant, as would be predicted by the capillary recruitment/insulin gradient concept described above. A shift in the distribution towards more slow-twitch fibers has been reported to accompany the improvement in insulin sensitivity that occurs as a result of physical training [125]. Moreover, Lillioja et al have demonstrated direct correlations between insulin-stimulated glucose uptake, capillary density and the percentage of slow-twitch fibers [126]. Finally, there are two reports of decreased numbers of slow-twitch fibers in hypertensive patients [127, 128]. What role, if any, is played by muscle fiber type in the IRS is at present unknown, but it is tempting to postulate a shift away from slow-twitch, insulin-sensitive fibers in this condition.

Dyslipidemia

Elevations of fasting levels of very low density lipoprotein (VLDL), the principal triglyceride-bearing lipoprotein in the fasting state, are the result of either increased hepatic production and secretion of VLDL, decreased removal of VLDL from the circulation, or some combination of both. There is evidence that VLDL production by the liver is stimulated by insulin and is further determined by the supply of substrates for triglyceride synthesis, glucose and free fatty acids (FFAs) [129, 130]. Thus, the increased concentrations of insulin observed in the IRS would be expected to augment VLDL production and secretion. There is considerable evidence that insulin concentration is highly correlated with VLDL concentration and secretion rate [131–133] and also that these variables co-vary in response to various perturbations such as high carbohydrate diets (increases all three variables) [132] and weight loss (decreases all three) [134]. A

number of *in vitro* studies have demonstrated that perfusion of rat livers with insulin stimulates VLDL production rates [135, 136]. On the other hand, there are also *in vivo* studies suggesting an acute inhibitory effect of insulin on VLDL production [137–139]. These contrary *in vivo* results could be explained by an insulin-induced suppression of FFA flux, although in one case [137] the insulin was infused directly into the portal vein and the inhibition was judged to be independent of FFA concentrations.

FFA levels are elevated in the IRS, since such elevations are a feature of obesity, especially abdominal obesity [130, 140, 141], and result from an impairment in insulin-mediated suppression of lipolysis in adipocytes [142, 143]. We need to hypothesize that the machinery for VLDL synthesis and secretion retains normal sensitivity to insulin and is overdriven by the hyperinsulinemia, but that the machinery for shutting down lipolysis in the adipocyte participates in the generalized insulin resistance which is the defining feature of the IRS. The available evidence suggests that precisely this pattern of insulin resistance and retained insulin sensitivity does, in fact, exist [142, 143].

Removal of VLDL from the circulation is controlled by lipoprotein lipase (LPL), which is found in the vascular endothelium, particularly in adipose tissue and skeletal muscle [144]. The triglyceride content of the VLDL is hydrolyzed and removed by this enzyme, and the lipoprotein is transformed into IDL and LDL [145], both of which are atherogenic [67, 68, 146, 147]. Adipose tissue LPL is also insulin-sensitive, although skeletal muscle LPL may not be [144]. There is suggestive evidence that LPL levels may be resistant to insulin action in subjects who are either obese or diabetic and the plasma levels of this enzyme are either normal or low in diabetic patients [144]. These changes could thus contribute to hypertriglyceridemia by impairing VLDL clearance.

The inverse association between serum triglyceride and HDL cholesterol concentration is one of the most consistently observed of all metabolic and epidemiologic correlations. The exact mechanisms underlying this inverse relationship are not known, but certain elements of the relationship are reasonably clear. Nascent HDL particles are produced primarily in the liver, then transformed in the plasma first into HDL_3 and then into HDL_2 particles [145]. This maturation process is the result of the acquisition by the nascent HDL particles of various apolipoprotein and lipid components, especially surface components, from VLDL as the latter is metabolized (see Bagdade [148]). One of the VLDL components which is transferred to HDL is free cholesterol which is subsequently esterified

Table 4 Relation of fasting insulin concentration at baseline to IRS-related disorders 8 years later*

Number of metabolic disorders 8 years later	Observed	Expected	Observed/ expected	Baseline fasting insulin (pmol/l)
None	502	422	1.19	57
One	385	481	0.81	78
LHDL	191	208	0.92	70
HGluc	98	128	0.77	72
HBP	74	91	0.82	75
HTG	22	54	0.41	87
Two	158	190	0.83	102
LHDL × HGluc	47	63	0.75	128
LHDL × HBP	30	45	0.70	85
LHDL × HTG	31	27	1.17	86
HGluc × HBP	32	28	1.16	100
HGluc × HTG	15	16	0.92	105
HBP × HTG	3	12	0.26	107
Three	61	20	3.08	117
LHDL × HGluc × HBP	24	14	1.77	118
LHDL × HGluc × HTG	20	8	2.48	126
LHDL × HBP × HTG	10	6	1.75	90
HGluc × HBP × HTG	7	3	2.00	133
Four				
HDL × HGluc × HBP × HTG	19	1.7	11.0	149

LHDL = low high-density lipoprotein; HGluc = impaired glucose tolerance or non-insulin dependent diabetes mellitus; HBP = hypertension; HTG = hypertriglyceridemia.
*Adapted from reference 154, by permission of the American Diabetes Association. See reference 154 for definition of disorders.

under the influence of lecithin:cholesterol acyltransferase (LCAT). If the acquisition of free cholesterol by nascent HDL is impaired, the serum level of HDL, measured as its cholesterol content as is usually done in clinical practice, would presumably fall. Since, as noted above, LPL-mediated catabolism of VLDL is impaired in obesity and diabetes, this impairment could provide an explanation for the low levels of HDL cholesterol typically seen in these conditions. This appears to be the explanation for the low HDL concentrations seen in various insulin-deficient states (e.g. streptozotocin-treated rats), since under these conditions VLDL-triglyceride turnover is decreased [149, 150], as is adipose tissue, skeletal muscle and plasma post-heparin LPL activity [151, 152]. Also compatible with this idea is the fact that in well-controlled type 1 diabetic patients both HDL and LDL levels tend to be increased [148]. It is a little more difficult, however, to see how this mechanism could explain the low HDL levels seen in insulin-resistant, hyperinsulinemic states, since, even allowing that LPL activity may be resistant to insulin action, VLDL turnover is nevertheless generally thought to be elevated [153].

Finally, there is also evidence that apo-A1 catabolism is accelerated in diabetic subjects, leading to low plasma concentrations [148]. Thus, the low HDL cholesterol concentrations seen in diabetic patients result both from cholesterol-depleted HDL particles and from fewer particles.

INSULIN RESISTANCE AND MULTIPLE METABOLIC DISORDERS

The argument for insulin resistance as a cause of the full-blown IRS would be bolstered if it could be shown that insulin resistance *precedes* the other manifestations of the syndrome. This has not been demonstrated using direct measures of insulin resistance. However, Haffner et al, using fasting insulin as a proxy for insulin resistance, showed that among individuals free of metabolic and hemodynamic disorders (hyperglycemia, hypertriglyceridemia, low HDL and hypertension) at baseline, increasing insulinemia was predictive of a stepwise increase in the number of disorders which developed over 8 years of follow-up (see Table 4) [154]. Although suggestive, this paper did not specifically examine the alternative hypothesis, viz. that the various metabolic and hemodynamic disorders performed equally well as predictors of follow-up insulin concentrations.

'APPLICANTS' FOR MEMBERSHIP IN THE IRS

Ferrannini (personal communication) has used the term 'applicants' to refer to a number of variables which have been proposed for membership in the IRS cluster. These applicants include small dense LDL, microalbuminuria, sex hormones and plasminogen activator inhibitor 1 (PAI-1). The evidence for including each of these as a component of the IRS is discussed in this section.

Small Dense LDL

Gradient gel electrophoresis of the low density lipoprotein (LDL) fraction has revealed the presence of multiple bands (up to seven) having different electrophoretic mobilities [156]. These subfractions differ from one another in percentage composition, density and average particle size. Austin et al have proposed that the LDL spectrum can be subdivided into two distinct patterns, type A and type B, the former having a major peak of large buoyant particles and the latter having a major peak of small dense particles [157]. These workers have also suggested 255 Å as a convenient cut-off point for distinguishing between the two patterns; the mean particle diameter of the principal LDL subfraction peak exceeds this cut-off point in subjects with the type A pattern and falls below this cut-off point in subjects with the type B pattern. A small percentage of subjects (13%) could not be readily classified into one or the other of these two categories and were labeled as having an 'intermediate' pattern. A large number of papers have consistently reported strong correlations between small dense LDL and serum triglyceride and insulin levels, and also inverse correlations with HDL [158–162]. Thus, it is hardly surprising that small dense LDL would be statistically associated with the IRS. Indeed, it has recently been demonstrated that, compared to subjects with LDL pattern A, subjects with pattern B are more insulin resistant as measured by the insulin suppression test [163].

The reason that the IRS–small dense LDL association is of more than just statistical interest is the claim that these particles are more atherogenic than large buoyant LDL particles. In fact, it is possible that the increased atherosclerotic risk associated with elevated triglyceride concentration is explained, either wholly or in part, by its association with small dense LDL. There have been several case–control studies of small dense LDL and coronary artery disease, assessed either by history of a myocardial infarction [164] or by coronary arteriography [165, 166]. These studies have all indicated that the LDL profile was shifted towards small dense particles in coronary cases compared to controls. In none of the studies, however, was this difference statistically independent of triglyceride or HDL concentrations. This begs the question of which of these three risk factors is most directly involved in the pathogenesis of atherosclerosis, a question which is not fundamentally statistical in nature. A more pertinent question is whether the effect of small dense LDL is independent of the overall LDL concentration, since this question bears on the issue of whether

or not the atherogenicity of LDL is enhanced when its size distribution is shifted downward. In one study [164] the association of small dense LDL with coronary disease was independent of LDL level, whereas in another study [165] it was not. It should be noted that there are as yet no prospective studies assessing small dense LDL as an independent cardiovascular risk factor. Finally, it has been reported that small dense LDL is more readily oxidized than large buoyant LDL [167], which could further enhance its atherogenicity [168].

Microalbuminuria

The term microalbuminuria has been used to describe an amount of albumin in the urine which is less than can be detected by ordinary clinical tests, such as Albustix, but which nevertheless is associated with future disease (see also Chapter 70). Several reports have indicated that early morning 'spot' urines are usually sufficient for defining the presence of microalbuminuria [169, 170]. A common definition for microalbuminuria is a urinary albumin concentration greater than 30 mg/l but less than 300 mg/l, the level which defines 'clinical proteinuria', i.e. an Albustix test of 1+ or greater.

It is well established that microalbuminuria is a precursor of diabetic nephropathy in both type 1 [171–173] and type 2 [174] diabetic subjects. Microalbuminuria has also been associated with elevated blood pressure and dyslipidemia [175–178] and has been identified as an independent risk factor for mortality in patients with type 2 diabetes [174, 179]. Of significance is the fact that CVD, and not uremia, is the principal cause of death in these patients.

A number of studies have suggested that microalbuminuria may be part of the prediabetic state. Thus, an increased prevalence of microalbuminuria has been reported in patients with impaired glucose tolerance (IGT) [180–183] and in non-diabetic subjects with a parental history of diabetes [183]. Among non-diabetic subjects from two ethnic groups (Mexican Americans and non-Hispanic whites), microalbuminuria has been associated with most of the features of the IRS including high blood pressure, hypertriglyceridemia, hyperinsulinemia and low HDL cholesterol [184, 185]. Most of these abnormalities were found to accompany microalbuminuria even in the absence of hypertension. Moreover, several recent studies have reported that subjects with microalbuminuria are more insulin-resistant than subjects without microalbuminuria [186–188]. Although these studies were performed on diabetic patients and need to be repeated in non-diabetic subjects, the results are compatible with an association between microalbuminuria and the central underlying feature of the IRS, viz. insulin resistance.

Another finding which tends to link microalbuminuria and insulin resistance is the action of angiotensin converting enzyme inhibitors which have been reported to decrease both insulin resistance [189] and microalbuminuria [190].

Another argument supporting the candidacy of microalbuminuria for membership in the IRS is provided by prospective studies which indicate that microalbuminuria is predictive of the two principal outcomes of the IRS, namely, type 2 diabetes and CVD. Thus, Mykkänen et al reported that microalbuminuria predicted the development of type 2 diabetes in elderly Finns followed for 3.5 years [185]. This effect was independent of baseline blood pressure level, although not of plasma glucose and insulin levels. Yudkin et al reported both cross-sectional and prospective associations between microalbuminuria, coronary mortality and peripheral vascular disease in both diabetic and non-diabetic subjects [191]. In this study the effect of microalbuminuria was independent of age, BMI, smoking status and systolic and diastolic blood pressure.

The mechanisms linking microalbuminuria to the metabolic and hemodynamic features of the IRS and to its subsequent outcomes, namely diabetes and CVD, are still not entirely clear. Micropuncture studies [192] and studies of isolated perfused rat kidneys [193] have indicated that insulin has important renal hemodynamic effects. Specifically, insulin dilates afferent and efferent arterioles, thereby increasing renal plasma flow, glomerular hydrostatic pressure and glomerular filtration rate. These effects could produce greater leakage of albumin, thereby directly linking microalbuminuria to insulin resistance and hyperinsulinemia. It has also been postulated that microalbuminuria is a marker for a generalized increase in vascular permeability [194] which might facilitate the entry of atherogenic lipoproteins into the arterial wall.

Sex Hormones

A role for sex hormones in the pathogenesis of the IRS is implied by the well-established sexual dimorphism for certain of the features of the IRS. Thus, upper body obesity is unquestionably more common in men than women, and men have been consistently shown to have higher triglyceride and lower HDL levels than women [2]. On the other hand, there do not seem to be consistent sex differences in the other cardinal features of the IRS, namely, insulin resistance, hyperinsulinemia and hypertension.

Endogenous androgenization has most often been assessed by total or percentage free testosterone (T or %FT) and by sex hormone binding globulin (SHBG), low levels of which usually indicate androgenization, at least in women [195]. Using one or more of these indicators, increased endogenous androgenization in premenopausal women has been found in cross-sectional studies to correlate with upper body obesity [141, 196, 197], increased glucose and insulin concentrations [198, 199] and hypertriglyceridemia and low HDL [200–202]. Low levels of SHBG also predict future diabetes in premenopausal women [203, 204]. Similar metabolic abnormalities have been described in women with polycystic ovarian disease who are known to be androgenized [201, 205].

Although relatively less information is available on postmenopausal women, most of the above correlations have been replicated in this group [206, 207], including the ability of low SHBG levels to predict future diabetes [203].

Paradoxically, most of the above associations between sex hormones and IRS features are either not present or in the opposite direction in men. Thus, both castrated male rats and men with abdominal obesity and relative hypogonadism show insulin resistance which is *improved* by testosterone replacement [208]. Consistent with these findings are the observations that in men endogenous levels of both total T and %FT as well as DHEA-SO$_4$ (dehydroepiandrosterone sulfate) are inversely correlated with insulinemia [209–211]. There are also data indicating that in men insulin sensitivity, as measured by the euglycemic clamp technique, is positively correlated with total T, although not with %FT, and with low levels of SHBG [212]. Total T and %FT have also been found to be *inversely* correlated with upper body obesity in men [210, 211], rather than directly correlated as in women (see above). The associations between DHEA-SO$_4$ and upper body obesity in men, however, have been inconsistent [209–211]. Inverse associations between total T and %FT and the characteristic dyslipidemia of the IRS (high triglyceride and low HDL) have also been reported in men [213, 214]. Finally, in prospective studies of men, low total T is a risk factor for future diabetes [215], although the evidence for SHBG as a risk factor is mixed [204, 215]. It should also be mentioned that low levels of DHEA-SO$_4$ predict cardiovascular mortality in men [216], but not in postmenopausal women [217].

It may be that the unexpected effects of testosterone in men are dose-related since, even though testosterone replacement therapy in castrated rats and in men with abdominal obesity appears to ameliorate insulin resistance [208], higher testosterone doses in rats worsen insulin resistance [218], as do pharmacological doses of anabolic steroids in men [219, 220]. Nevertheless, in view of the opposite effects in men and women of sex hormones in the physiological range, it is hard to assign them a primary role in the pathogenesis of the IRS. This conclusion is reinforced by the fact that the cause-and-effect relationship between sex hormones and insulin resistance is unclear. Although most of the pharmacologic studies imply that sex hormone administration *causes* the changes in insulin sensitivity, there is contrary evidence as well. For example, there is evidence that exogenous insulin infusions can increase androgen output in women [221].

Plasminogen Activator Inhibitor-1 (PAI-1)

A number of studies, mostly cross-sectional, have revealed positive correlations between PAI-1 and various features of the IRS including fasting insulin concentration [222–224], triglyceride levels [224–226], and upper body obesity [223, 224, 227]. Elevated PAI-1 levels have also been reported in type 2 diabetes [228] and in untreated mild hypertension [229, 230]. Moreover, insulin resistance itself has been reported to be positively correlated with PAI-1 [223, 226]. In addition, PAI-1 levels are reduced by interventions which improve the IRS such as weight loss [231, 232], physical conditioning [233, 234] and metformin treatment [235].

The reasons for believing that these correlations represent more than just statistical associations are twofold: first, there is evidence that insulin may stimulate PAI-1 production; and second, PAI-1 is believed to play a role in the pathogenesis of atherothrombosis. PAI-1 is produced by endothelial cells and hepatocytes [224]. Insulin has been shown to increase PAI-1 production *in vitro* in the hepatocyte cell line HepG2 [236] and in cultured human hepatocytes [237], although not in endothelial cells [236]. Whether insulin influences PAI-1 concentrations *in vivo*, however, is less certain, since even though PAI-1 levels rise acutely after oral glucose administration [238], no effect has been observed following intravenous insulin administration under hyperinsulinemic, euglycemic clamp conditions, either short-term [239, 240] or for as long as 24 hours [241].

Diminished fibrinolysis is thought to play an important role in the pathogenesis of the atherosclerotic plaque [224]. Tissue plasminogen activator (t-PA) catalyzes the conversion of plasminogen to plasmin, which in turn catalyzes fibrinolysis. There is evidence to suggest that PAI-1, by inhibiting t-PA, is the main determinant of deficient fibrinolysis which, in turn, favors thrombus formation [224]. A number of case–control studies have documented that patients with coronary artery disease, identified either by a past history of myocardial infarction or by coronary arteriography, have higher PAI-1 levels than normal controls [242–245]. There is, however, at least one negative case–control study which failed to confirm

higher PAI-1 levels in patients with angiographically documented CAD compared to controls [225]. There are also prospective studies which indicate that PAI-1 predicts recurrent infarction in patients who survived an initial myocardial infarction [246, 247]. The effect of PAI-1 appears to be independent of other risk factors for reinfarction, such as dyslipidemia (high VLDL and low HDL) [246].

The data summarized above suggest a further mechanism in addition to those described earlier, whereby insulin, by contributing to elevated PAI-1 levels, could influence the development of atherosclerotic disease.

GENETIC DETERMINANTS OF THE IRS

Little is known about the genetic determinants of the IRS. This is hardly surprising inasmuch as there is no generally agreed definition of the IRS phenotype. There are, however, a number of genetic studies of traits which overlap with the IRS and since these studies may shed light on the genetics of the IRS itself, they will be reviewed in this section.

In a population-based study of Hispanics from southern Colorado, subjects were classified as having the IRS if they were simultaneously in the upper tertile of both the triglyceride and fasting insulin distribution and also in the lowest tertile of the HDL cholesterol distribution [248]. A total of 890 normoglycemic subjects were studied, of whom 370 were classified as having the IRS. The remaining 520 were treated as controls. A statistically significant association was found between a *Hind*III restriction fragment length polymorphism of the lipoprotein lipase (LPL) gene and the IRS. Such population associations do not, however, necessarily imply genetic linkage, particularly in a genetically admixed population such as Hispanics. If, for example, the frequency of both the allele and the phenotype co-varied in the ancestral populations (although for unrelated reasons), a significant but spurious association between the marker and the trait may appear in the admixed population even in the absence of genetic linkage.

Family studies are required to establish both the mode of inheritance of a trait and linkage of the trait to a particular marker. A number of family studies have been carried out on phenotypes related to the IRS, especially lipid and lipoprotein phenotypes. In many such studies major genes influencing the trait of interest are not directly characterized, but are statistically inferred from the pattern of segregation of the trait in families. However, in the absence of direct information about the gene itself, the relationship between the inferred gene and the phenotype under study may represent a pleiotropic effect. Pleiotropy refers to secondary effects which a gene may have on various traits other than the one which it directly determines. For example, a major gene whose presence is inferred by the segregation of a lipid or lipoprotein phenotype may affect these phenotypes only indirectly, while its principal biochemical effect could be to produce insulin resistance by a direct mechanism. If the insulin resistance is the *cause* of the lipoprotein abnormality, then the latter might tend to segregate in a Mendelian fashion and appear linked to the insulin resistance marker, provided that the chain of causality is not excessively long and/or extraneous genetic and environmental influences on the lipoprotein abnormality do not overwhelm the effect. It is because of these possible pleiotropic effects that genetic studies on lipids, lipoproteins and other phenotypes have the potential to contribute to our understanding of the genetics of the IRS.

An early study of the genetics of hyperlipidemia was carried out by Goldstein et al on 2520 relatives and spouses of 176 survivors of a myocardial infarction [249]. Five types of hyperlipidemia were identified, mainly on the basis of the familial pattern of age- and sex-adjusted cholesterol and/or triglyceride values in excess of the 95th percentile values as computed among the spouse controls. Since most of the non-lipid features of the IRS were not described in this study, it is difficult to assess the extent to which any of these types of hyperlipidemia overlaps with the IRS. The greatest likelihood of overlap is probably with familial hypertriglyceridemia, familial combined hyperlipidemia and sporadic hypertriglyceridemia, rather than with the two hypercholesterolemic types. Although there is evidence, at least in some families, that familial hypertriglyceridemia is not associated with an increased risk of CHD [65], this is evidently not universal, since in the study by Goldstein et al [249] all probands were survivors of a myocardial infarction.

A number of studies have been carried out on the mode of inheritance of LDL subclass patterns [157, 250–252] (recently reviewed by Austin [253]). In these studies LDL subclasses have been characterized in several different ways, including dichotomization into pattern A and pattern B [157, 250] and as a continuous quantitative trait, e.g. a weighted average of the three major LDL subclasses [251] or LDL peak particle diameter [252]. Each of these studies provided evidence for a major autosomal gene, usually with a dominant mode of inheritance with or without additive polygenic factors, contributing to the inheritance of LDL subclasses. One of these studies was carried out in pedigrees in which the familial combined hyperlipidemia (FCHL) trait was also segregating [250]. Although evidence was found for an autosomal gene with either a dominant or an additive mode of inheritance influencing LDL subclass pattern B, it is not clear whether this is the same gene that determines

the FCHL trait itself. Individuals with pattern B tended to display the lipid and lipoprotein features of FCHL, but the estimated frequency of the pattern B allele was 0.3, essentially similar to the 0.25 allele frequency estimated in families not selected for FCHL [157]. These similar allele frequencies suggest that the allele for LDL subclass pattern B is a common one and segregates in FCHL families just as it does in non-FCHL families, without necessarily being in any way related to the FCHL trait. Which of these two traits—FCHL or LDL subclass pattern B—is most closely related to the IRS is unclear. It is entirely possible, of course, that neither is.

Twin studies have also provided evidence for genetic determinants of LDL subclass pattern with heritability estimates ranging from 0.39 to 0.55 [254, 255]. On the other hand, among monozygotic twins discordant for the trait, those with subclass pattern B had higher BMI, waist-to-hip ratios, blood pressures and triglyceride and insulin levels, and lower HDL levels than those with pattern A [161]. These findings imply that significant environmental influences are also at play.

A number of studies have been performed to evaluate the possibility of linkage between LDL subclass phenotypes and various candidate genes. Strong evidence against linkage with the *apo*-B gene has been reported, both in families with FCHL [256] and those without [257]. On the other hand, there is evidence for tight linkage between LDL subclass pattern and the LDL receptor gene on the short arm of chromosome 19 [258]. Additional linkage was also noted with the insulin receptor gene, also located on the short arm of chromosome 19. This latter finding raises the possibility of a direct connection between the inheritance of LDL subclass patterns and the IRS. The evidence for linkage with the insulin receptor gene, however, was considerably weaker than for the LDL receptor.

Finally, preliminary evidence for linkage between LDL subclass pattern B and the *apo*-AI-CIII-AIV locus has been reported in 24 pedigrees using sib-pair analysis [260]. Interestingly, evidence for linkage has also been reported between *apo*-AI-CIII-AIV and FCHL in one study [261], although evidence against such linkage was reported in another [262].

Williams et al studied 131 individuals from 58 families residing in the state of Utah in which at least two siblings were concordant for essential hypertension diagnosed prior to 60 years of age [263]. They found that in 48% of these sibships the hypertensive siblings were also concordant for one or more of three lipid abnormalities: LDL cholesterol or triglyceride levels in excess of the 90th percentile or HDL cholesterol less than the 10th percentile, according to the Lipid Research Clinics guidelines. They labeled this entity familial dyslipidemic hypertension (FDH) and estimated that it affected approximately 12% of all patients with so-called essential hypertension [263]. In a subsequent report they noted that 8 of the 27 FDH sibships also had familial combined hyperlipidemia (FCHL) [264]. Apolipoprotein B levels were found to be higher in FDH patients with FCHL than in those without, but were higher than normal in both groups [264]. Fasting insulin levels were similarly elevated in both groups of FDH patients relative to normal controls. Also, in both FDH groups the LDL size distribution was shifted towards small dense particles relative to normal controls.

Turning to the genetics of insulin resistance itself, there is evidence that insulin resistance as measured by the euglycemic clamp technique is trimodally distributed in Pima Indians (see Figure 5) [265]. A similar trimodal distribution has also been observed for serum insulin levels [265]. Although a variety of interpretations can be advanced to account for these observations, they are compatible with an autosomal co-dominant mode of inheritance of insulin resistance. In a study from Utah involving 206 family members and 65 spouses from 16 large Europid pedigrees ascertained through two or more diabetic siblings, complex segregation analysis was used to seek evidence for a major gene determining insulin levels [266]. The results suggested the presence of a major gene which accounted for 33.1% of the variance in fasting insulin concentration. Autosomal recessive inheritance was suggested, with an estimated allele frequency for the recessive allele of 0.25. Fasting insulin levels in the 6.25% of the population predicted to be homozygous for the recessive allele were estimated to be 211.1 pmol/l compared to 70.3 pmol/l in the rest of the population. These investigators also presented evidence for a major gene controlling the 1-hour post-oral glucose load insulin

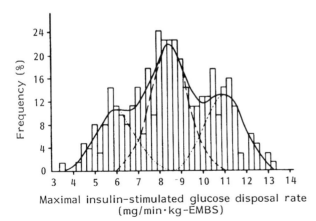

Figure 5 Frequency distribution of maximal insulin-stimulated glucose disposal rates among non-diabetic Pima Indians. EMBS, estimated metabolic body size. From reference 265, by permission of the American Diabetes Association

value, for which the mode of inheritance appeared to be autosomal co-dominant.

It is difficult to synthesize all of these results into a satisfactory whole. Conceivably, the IRS represents some kind of 'final common pathway' for several unrelated genetic disorders. Alternatively, there may be a more or less homogeneous underlying genetic disorder accounting for the IRS.

FETAL AND INFANT INFLUENCES ON THE IRS

Recently, there has been interest in the possibility that early exposures during fetal life and infancy exert an important influence on the occurrence of various adult diseases and conditions, among them the IRS. This idea has become known as the programming hypothesis. Barker is the main instigator and promoter of this hypothesis. He has gathered together 31 of his unit's publications on this topic in a single volume [267]. The initial observation was that mortality for various chronic conditions in the UK, including ischemic heart disease, chronic bronchitis and stroke, varied from region to region in parallel with variations in infant mortality in the same regions 4 to 5 decades earlier [268]. The hypothesis advanced to explain these findings was that the same adverse conditions which contributed to a high infant mortality also contributed to various diseases in adult life among those who survived infancy. Later it was shown that various indicators of inadequate nutrition in early life, e.g. low birthweight and slow weight gain in the first year of life, were predictive of a wide variety of subsequent health outcomes. Thus, low birthweight and low weight at 1 year of age were predictive of increased mortality from CHD and chronic obstructive lung disease many years later [269]. Similar inverse associations were found between birthweight and weight at 1 year of life and the subsequent development of hypertension and diabetes [270]. Also, adult blood levels of apolipoprotein B [271], fibrinogen and factor VII [272], and 32–33 split proinsulin [270] (the latter thought to be a marker for failing insulin secretion) were found to increase with decreasing weight at 1 year of life. Finally, lower birthweight and lower weight at 1 year of age were also associated with increased amounts of visceral fat in adult life as measured by the waist-to-hip ratio [273]. In the case of diabetes it was postulated that poor fetal and early postnatal nutrition might impair the development of the pancreatic islets, limiting their ability to hypersecrete insulin indefinitely in response to stresses such as obesity, particularly abdominal obesity, which produce insulin resistance [274]. Of particular relevance to this chapter is the observation that lower birthweights and weights at 1 year of life predicted the IRS as defined by a 2-hour plasma glucose of 7.8 mmol/l (140 mg/dl) or greater, a systolic blood pressure of 160 mmHg or greater, and a fasting serum triglyceride concentration of 1.4 mmol/l (125 mg/dl) or greater [155]. These effects were independent of a number of potential confounding variables including cigarette and alcohol consumption and current social class.

Our group recently had the opportunity to examine the birth certificates of 564 individuals who were 25–39 years of age at the time of their participation in the San Antonio Heart Study. The IRS was defined in this cohort as any two of the following: hypertension; diabetes or impaired glucose tolerance; triglyceride concentration greater than 250 mg/dl (2.8 mmol/l); or HDL concentration less than 35 mg/dl (0.9 mmol/l) in men and less than 45 mg/dl (1.2 mmol/l) in women. As shown in Figure 6, the prevalence of the IRS declined significantly with increasing birthweight in both Mexican Americans and non-Hispanic whites [259]. These results thus confirm the findings of Barker and associates in Europids and extend them to Mexican Americans.

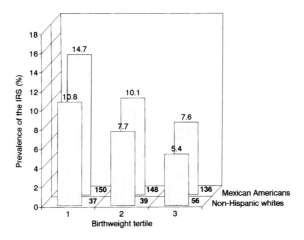

Figure 6 Prevalence of IRS in Mexican Americans and non-Hispanic whites according to increasing birthweight tertile. From reference 259, by permission of Springer-Verlag

CONCLUSIONS

It is well documented that many patients display a cluster of findings which include insulin resistance, hyperinsulinemia, impaired glucose tolerance, hypertension, hypertriglyceridemia and low HDL cholesterol levels. The concept that insulin resistance is the underlying defect accounting for this cluster, first advanced by Reaven [9], has considerable merit, since plausible mechanisms can be advanced to explain how insulin resistance and compensatory hyperinsulinemia could produce all of the other manifestations. If this formulation is correct, it seems reasonable to use the term insulin resistance syndrome (IRS) to describe this cluster. On the other hand, alternative scenarios have also been advanced, particularly in the case of blood pressure, to account for the cluster. Thus, it has been proposed that hypertension, by producing vascular rarefaction in skeletal muscle [123], actually *causes* insulin resistance, rather than being its result.

Although the IRS can occur in lean individuals, most patients with the syndrome are at least mildly obese, usually with visceral obesity, which undoubtedly contributes to their insulin resistance.

Long-term consequences of the IRS are the development of type 2 diabetes and CVD. It is well established that insulin resistance is a precursor of diabetes [19], but this is less clear in the case of CVD. Although a variety of mechanisms have been proposed whereby insulin might promote atherogenesis [31], the epidemiologic evidence for insulin as a CVD risk factor is weak. An intriguing possibility, which has received considerable attention recently, is that insulin may stimulate production of plasminogen activator inhibitor-1 (PAI-1) which could contribute to thrombus formation by inhibiting fibrinolysis [224]. In any case, whatever the role of insulin *per se*, the IRS is almost surely an antecedent of CVD, since several of its individual components, e.g. blood pressure, low HDL, etc., are themselves established CVD risk factors.

In addition to PAI-1, there are several other 'applicants' for membership in the IRS. Most of these, however, are not readily measured in ordinary clinical practice. If any of them are subsequently confirmed to play a more critical role in the pathogenesis of the IRS than the classical features of the syndrome—for example, small dense LDL in place of triglycerides—this would enhance the desirability of developing more readily available clinical tools for measuring these new 'players'.

A major limitation in studying the IRS is the lack of generally agreed diagnostic criteria for the syndrome. Such criteria, if they were available, would facilitate prospective epidemiologic studies which could confirm the extent to which the IRS is a precursor of CVD. They would also facilitate genetic studies of the IRS itself, instead of having to rely on proxies such as the familial hyperlipidemias which overlap with, but which are not identical to, the IRS.

Finally, there is evidence that nutritional and perhaps other factors operating in fetal life and infancy may contribute to the development of the IRS in adult life [259, 267].

REFERENCES

1. Modan M, Halkin H, Almog S, Lusky A, Eshkol A, Shefi M, Shitrit A, Fuchs Z. Hyperinsulinemia: a

link between hypertension, obesity, and glucose intolerance. J Clin Invest 1985; 75: 809-17.

2. Stern MP, Haffner SM. Body fat distribution and hyperinsulinemia as risk factors for diabetes and cardiovascular disease. Arteriosclerosis 1986; 6: 123-30.

3. Pyörälä K. Relationship of glucose tolerance and plasma insulin to the incidence of coronary heart disease: results from two population studies in Finland. Diabetes Care 1979; 2: 131-41.

4. Ducimetiere P, Eschwege E, Papoz L, Richard JL, Claude JR, Rosselin G. Relationship of plasma insulin levels to the incidence of myocardial infarction and coronary heart disease mortality in a middle-aged population. Diabetologia 1980; 19: 205-10.

5. Welborn TA, Wearne K. Coronary heart disease incidence and cardiovascular mortality in Busselton with reference to glucose and insulin concentrations. Diabetes Care 1979; 2: 154-60.

6. Ferrannini E, Buzzigoli G, Bonadona R, Giorico MA, Oleggini M, Graziadei L, Pedrinelli R, Grandi L, Bevilacqua S. Insulin resistance in essential hypertension. New Engl J Med 1987; 317: 350-7.

7. Laakso M, Sarlund H, Mykkänen L. Essential hypertension and insulin resistance in non-insulin-dependent diabetes. Eur J Clin Invest 1989; 19: 518-26.

8. Shen D-C, Sheih S-M, Fuh M, Chen Y-DI, Reaven GM. Resistance to insulin-stimulated glucose uptake in patients with hypertension. J Clin Endocrinol Metab 1988; 66: 580-3.

9. Reaven GM. Banting lecture 1988: Role of insulin resistance in human disease. Diabetes 1988; 37: 1595-607.

10. Reaven GM, Miller R. Study of the relationship between glucose and insulin responses to an oral glucose load in man. Diabetes 1968; 17: 560-9.

11. Savage PJ, Dippe SE, Bennett PH, Gorden P, Roth J, Rushforth NB, Miller M. Hyperinsulinemia and hypoinsulinemia. Insulin responses to oral carbohydrate over a wide spectrum of glucose tolerance. Diabetes 1975; 24: 362-8.

12. Saad MF, Pettitt DJ, Mott DM, Knowler WC, Nelson RG, Bennett PH. Sequential changes in serum insulin concentration during development of non-insulin-dependent diabetes. Lancet 1989; 1: 1356-9.

13. Sicree RA, Zimmet PZ, King HOM, Coventry JS. Plasma insulin response among Nauruans. Prediction of deterioration in glucose tolerance over 6 years. Diabetes 1987; 36: 179-86.

14. Knowler WC, Pettitt DJ, Saad MF, Bennett PH. Diabetes mellitus in the Pima Indians: incidence, risk factors and pathogenesis. Diabet Metab Rev 1990; 6: 1-27.

15. Haffner SM, Stern MP, Hazuda HP, Mitchell BD, Patterson JK. Cardiovascular risk factors in confirmed prediabetic individuals. Does the clock for coronary heart disease start ticking before the onset of clinical diabetes? JAMA 1990; 263: 2893-8.

16. Bergstrom RW, Newell-Morris LL, Leonetti DL, Shuman WP, Wahl PW, Fujimoto WY. Association of elevated fasting C-peptide level and increased intra-abdominal fat distribution with development of NIDDM in Japanese-American men. Diabetes 1990; 39: 104-11.

17. Charles MA, Fontbonne A, Thibult N, Warnet JM, Rosselin GE, Eschwege E. Risk factors for NIDDM in white population. Paris Prospective Study. Diabetes 1991; 40: 796-9.

18. Mykkänen L, Kuusisto J, Pyörälä K, Laakso M. Cardiovascular disease risk factors as predictors of type 2 (non-insulin-dependent) diabetes mellitus in elderly subjects. Diabetologia 1993; 36: 553-9.

19. Lillioja S, Mott DM, Spraul M, Ferraro R, Foley JE, Ravussin E, Knowler WC, Bennett PH, Bogardus C. Insulin resistance and insulin secretory dysfunction as precursors of non-insulin-dependent diabetes mellitus. Prospective Study of Pima Indians. New Engl J Med 1993; 329: 1988-92.

20. Warram JH, Martin BC, Krolewski AS, Soeldner JS, Kahn R. Slow glucose removal rate and hyperinsulinemia precede the development of type 2 diabetes in the offspring of diabetic parents. Ann Intern Med 1990; 113: 909-15.

21. Pell S, D'Alonzo CA. Some aspects of hypertension in diabetes mellitus. JAMA 1967; 202: 104-10.

22. Medalie JH, Papier CM, Goldbourt U, Herman JB. Major factors in the development of diabetes mellitus in 10 000 men. Arch Intern Med 1975; 135: 811-17.

23. Keen H, Jarrett RJ, McCartney P. The ten-year follow-up of the Bedford survey (1962-1972): glucose tolerance and diabetes. Diabetologia 1982; 22: 73-8.

24. Ohlson LO, Larsson B, Svärdsudd K, Welin L, Eriksson H, Wilhelmsen L, Björntorp P, Tibblin G. The influence of body fat distribution on the incidence of diabetes mellitus. 13.5 years of follow-up of the participants in the study of men born in 1913. Diabetes 1985; 34: 1055-8.

25. McPhillips JB, Barrett-Connor E, Wingard DL. Cardiovascular disease risk factors prior to the diagnosis of impaired glucose tolerance and non-insulin-dependent diabetes mellitus in a community of older adults. Am J Epidemiol 1990; 131: 443-53.

26. Bengtsson C, Blohme G, Lapidus L, Lundgren H. Diabetes in hypertensive women: an effect of antihypertensive drugs or the hypertensive state *per se*? Diabet Med 1988; 5: 261-4.

27. Morales PA, Mitchell BD, Valdez RA, Hazuda HP, Stern MP, Haffner SM. Incidence of NIDDM and impaired glucose tolerance in hypertensive subjects. The San Antonio Heart Study. Diabetes 1993; 42: 154-61.

28. Jarrett RJ, Keen H, McCartney P. The Whitehall Study: ten-year follow-up report on men with impaired glucose tolerance with reference to worsening to diabetes and predictors of death. Diabet Med 1984; 1: 279-83.

29. Stern MP, Morales PA, Valdez RA, Monterrosa A, Haffner SM, Mitchell BD, Hazuda HP. Predicting diabetes. Moving beyond impaired glucose tolerance. Diabetes 1993; 42: 706-14.

30. Bergman R, Prager R, Volund A, Olefsky J. Equivalence of the insulin sensitivity index derived by the minimal model and the euglycaemic clamp. J Clin Invest 1987; 79: 790-800.

31. Stout RW. Insulin and atheroma, 20-year perspective. Diabetes Care 1990; 13: 631-54.

32. McGill HC Jr, Holman RL. The influence of alloxan diabetes on cholesterol atheromatosis in the rabbit. Proc Soc Exp Biol Med 1949; 72: 72-3.

33. Duff GL, Brechin DJH, Findelstein WE. The effect of alloxan diabetes on experimental cholesterol atherosclerosis in the rabbit. IV. The effect of insulin

therapy on the inhibition of atherosclerosis in the alloxan-diabetic rabbit. J Exp Med 1954; 100: 371–80.

34. Lehner NDM, Clarkson TB, Lofland HB. The effect of insulin deficiency, hypothyroidism and hypertension on atherosclerosis in the squirrel monkey. Exp Mol Pathol 1971; 15: 230–44.

35. Stamler J, Pick R, Katz LN. Effect of insulin in the induction and regression of atherosclerosis in the chick. Circ Res 1960; 8: 572–6.

36. Cruz AB Jr, Amatuzio DS, Grande F, Hay LJ. Effect of intra-arterial insulin on tissue cholesterol and fatty acids in alloxan-diabetic dogs. Circ Res 1961; 9: 39–43.

37. Stout RW, Bierman EL, Ross R. Effect of insulin on the proliferation of cultured primate arterial smooth muscle cells. Circ Res 1975; 36: 319–27.

38. Pfeifle B, Ditschuneit H. Effect of insulin on growth of cultured human arterial smooth muscle cells. Diabetologia 1981; 20: 155–8.

39. Stout RW. The effect of insulin and glucose on sterol synthesis in cultured rat arterial smooth muscle cells. Atherosclerosis 1977; 27: 271–8.

40. Young IR, Stout RW. Effects of insulin and glucose on the cells of the arterial wall: interaction of insulin with dibutyryl cyclic AMP and low density lipoprotein in arterial cells. Diabète Métab 1987; 13: 301–6.

41. Oppenheimer MJ, Sundquist K, Bierman EL. Down-regulation of high-density lipoprotein receptor in human fibroblasts by insulin and IGF-I. Diabetes 1987; 38: 117–22.

42. Krone W, Greten H. Evidence for post-transcriptional regulation by insulin of 3-hydroxy-3-methylglutaryl coenzyme A reductase and sterol synthesis in human mononuclear leukocytes. Diabetologia 1984; 26: 366–9.

43. Krone W, Nagele H, Behnke B, Greten H. Opposite effects of insulin and catecholamines on LDL-receptor activity in human mononuclear leukocytes. Diabetes 1988; 37: 1386–91.

44. Jarrett RJ. Is insulin atherogenic? Diabetologia 1988; 31: 71–5.

45. Fontbonne A, Tchobroutsky G, Eschwege E, Richard JL, Claude JR, Rosselin GE. Coronary heart disease mortality risk: plasma insulin level is a more sensitive marker than hypertension or abnormal glucose tolerance in overweight males. The Paris Prospective Study. Int J Obesity 1988; 12: 557–65.

46. Fontbonne A, Charles MA, Thibult N, Richard JL, Claude JR, Warnet JM, Rosselin GE, Eschwege E. Hyperinsulinemia as a predictor of coronary heart disease mortality in a healthy population: the Paris Prospective Study, 15-year follow-up. Diabetologia 1991; 34: 356–61.

47. Laakso M. How good a marker is insulin level for insulin resistance? Am J Epidemiol 1993; 137: 959–65.

48. Hollenbeck CB, Chen N, Chen Y-DI, Reaven GM. Relationship between the plasma insulin response to oral glucose and insulin-stimulated glucose utilization in normal subjects. Diabetes 1984; 33: 460–3.

49. Welin L, Eriksson H, Larsson B, Ohlson LO, Svärdsudd K, Tibblin G. Hyperinsulinemia is not a major coronary risk factor in elderly men. The study of men born in 1913. Diabetologia 1992; 35: 766–70.

50. Orchard TJ, Eichner J, Kuller LH, Becker DJ, McCallum LM, Grandits GA. Insulin as a predictor of coronary heart disease: interaction with apo-E phenotype. A report from MRFIT. Ann Epidemiol 1994; 4: 53–8.

51. Haffner SM, Stern MP, Mitchell BD, Hazuda HP, Patterson JK: Incidence of type 2 diabetes in Mexican Americans predicted by fasting insulin and glucose levels, obesity, and body-fat distribution. Diabetes 1990; 39: 283–8.

52. Lew EA, Garfinkel L. Variations in mortality by weight among 750 000 men and women. J Chron Dis 1974; 32: 563–76.

53. Build Study, 1979. Chicago, IL: Society of Actuaries and Association of Life Insurance Medical Directors, 1980.

54. Keys A, Aravanis C, Blackburn H et al. Coronary heart disease: overweight and obesity as risk factors. Ann Intern Med 1972; 77: 15–27.

55. Truett J, Cornfield J, Kannel W. A multivariate analysis of the risk of coronary heart disease in Framingham. J Chronic Dis 1967; 20: 511.

56. Kannel WB, Gordon T: Obesity and cardiovascular disease. The Framingham Study. In Burland WL, Samuel PD, Yudkin J (eds) Obesity Symposium. Proceedings of a Servier Research Institute Symposium. Edinburgh: Churchill Livingstone, 1974: p. 24.

57. Hubert HB, Feinleib M, McNamara PM, Castelli WP. Obesity as an independent risk factor for cardiovascular disease: a 26-year follow-up of participants in the Framingham Heart Study. Circulation 1983; 67: 968–77.

58. Phillips A, Shaper AG. Relative weight and major ischemic heart disease events in hypertensive men. Lancet 1989; 1: 1005–8.

59. The Pooling Project Research Group. Relationship of blood pressure, serum cholesterol, smoking habit, relative weight and ECG abnormality to incidence of major coronary events. Final report of the Pooling Project. J Chronic Dis 1978; 31: 201–306.

60. Bergstrom RW, Leonetti DL, Newell-Morris LL, Shuman WP, Wahl PW, Fujimoto WY. Association of plasma triglyceride and C-peptide with coronary heart disease in Japanese-American men with a high prevalence of glucose intolerance. Diabetologia 1990; 33: 489–96.

61. Lapidus L, Bengtsson C, Larsson B, Pennert K, Rybo E, Sjöström L. Distribution of adipose tissue and risk of cardiovascular disease and death: a 12-year follow up of participants in the population study of women in Gothenburg, Sweden. Br Med J 1984; 289: 1257–61.

62. Larsson B, Svärdsudd K, Welin L, Wilhelmsen L, Björntorp P, Tibblin G. Abdominal adipose tissue distribution, obesity and risk of cardiovascular disease and death: a 13-year follow-up of participants in the study of men born in 1913. Br Med J 1984; 288: 1401–4.

63. Stokes J, Garrison RJ, Kannel WB. The independent contributions of various indices of obesity to the 22-year incidence of coronary heart disease: the Framingham Heart Study. In Vague J, Björntorp P, Guy-Grand B, Rebuffé-Scrive M, Vague P (eds) Proceedings of the international symposium on the metabolic complications of human obesities, Marseille, France May 30–June 1, 1985 (ICS No. 682). Amsterdam: Elsevier, 1985: pp. 49–57.

64. Janus ED, Nicoll AM, Turner PR, Magill P, Lewis B. Kinetic bases of the primary hyperlipidaemias: studies of apolipoprotein-B turnover in genetically defined subjects. Eur J Clin Invest 1980; 10: 161–72.

65. Brunzell JD, Schrott HG, Motulsky AG, Bierman EL. Myocardial infarction in the familial forms of hypertriglyceridemia. Metab Clin Exp 1976; 25: 313–20.

66. Brunzell JD, Albers JJ, Chait A, Grundy SM, Groszek E, McDonald GB. Plasma lipoproteins in familial combined hyperlipidemia and monogenic familial hypertriglyceridemia. J Lipid Res 1983; 24: 147–55.

67. Krauss RM, Williams PT, Brensike J, Detre KM, Lindgren FT, Kelsey SF, Vranizan K, Levy RI. Intermediate density lipoproteins and progression of coronary artery disease in hypercholesterolaemic men. Lancet 1987; 2: 62–6.

68. Steiner G, Schwartz L, Shumak S, Poapst M. The association of increased levels of intermediate density lipoproteins with smoking and with coronary artery disease. Circulation 1987; 75: 124–30.

69. Fontbonne A, Thibult N, Eschwege E, Ducimetiere P. Body fat distribution and coronary heart disease mortality in subjects with impaired glucose tolerance or diabetes mellitus: the Paris Prospective Study, 15-year follow-up. Diabetologia 1992; 35: 464–8.

70. Criqui MH, Heiss G, Cohn R, Cowan LD, Suchindran CM, Bangdiwala S et al. Plasma triglyceride level and mortality from coronary heart disease. New Engl J Med 1993; 328: 1220–5.

71. Laakso M, Lehto S, Penttilä I, Pyörälä K. Lipids and lipoproteins predicting coronary heart disease mortality and morbidity in patients with non-insulin-dependent diabetes. Circulation 1993; 88 (I): 1421–30.

72. Gofman JW, Young W, Tandy R. Ischemic heart disease, atherosclerosis and longevity. Circulation 1966; 34: 679–97.

73. Gordon T, Castelli WP, Hjortland MC, Kannel WB, Dawber TR. Diabetes, blood lipids, and the role of obesity in coronary heart disease for women. The Framingham Study. Ann Intern Med 1977; 87: 393–7.

74. Gordon DJ, Probstfield JL, Garrison RJ, Neaton JD, Castelli WP, Knoke JD, Jacobs DR, Bangdiwala S, Tyroler HA. High-density lipoprotein cholesterol and cardiovascular disease. Four prospective American studies. Circulation 1989; 79: 8–15.

75. Stamler J, Vaccaro O, Neaton JD, Wentworth D. Diabetes, other risk factors, and 12-year cardiovascular mortality for men screened in the Multiple Risk Factor Intervention Trial. Diabetes Care 1993; 16: 434–44.

76. West KM, Ahuja MMS, Bennett PH, Czyzyk A, Mateo de Acosta O, Fuller JH et al. The role of circulating glucose and triglyceride concentrations and their interactions with other 'risk factors' as determinants of arterial disease in nine diabetic population samples from the WHO Multinational Study. Diabetes Care 1983; 6: 361–9.

77. Nielsen NV, Ditzel J. Prevalence of macro- and microvascular disease as related to glycosylated hemoglobin in type 1 and 2 diabetic subjects: an epidemiologic study in Denmark. Horm Metab Res 1985; suppl. 15: 19–23.

78. Fuller JH, Shipley MJ, Rose G, Jarrett RJ, Keen H. Coronary heart disease risk and impaired glucose tolerance: the Whitehall Study. Lancet 1980; 1: 1373–6.

79. Herman JB, Medalie JH, Goldbourt U. Differences in cardiovascular morbidity and mortality between previously known and newly diagnosed adult diabetics. Diabetologia 1977; 13: 229–34.

80. Morrish NJ, Stevens LK, Head J, Fuller JH, Jarrett RJ, Keen H. A prospective study of mortality among middle aged diabetic patients (the London cohort of the World Health Organization Multinational Study of Vascular Disease in Diabetics). II. Associated risk factors. Diabetologia 1990; 33: 542–8.

81. Jarrett RJ, Shipley MJ. Type 2 (non-insulin-dependent) diabetes mellitus and cardiovascular disease – putative association via common antecedents; further evidence from the Whitehall Study. Diabetologia 1988; 31: 737–40.

82. Zavaroni I, Bonora E, Pagliara M, Dall'Aglio E, Luchetti L, Buonanno G et al. Risk factors for coronary artery disease in healthy persons with hyperinsulinemia and normal glucose tolerance. New Engl J Med 1989; 320: 702–6.

83. Sims EAH, Horton ES. Endocrine and metabolic adaptation to obesity and starvation. Am J Clin Nutr 1968; 21: 1455–70.

84. Wing RR, Matthews KA, Kuller LH, Meilahn EN, Plantinga PL. Weight gain at the time of menopause. Arch Intern Med 1991; 151: 97–102.

85. Oppert J-M, Nadeau A, Tremblay A, Déprés J-P, Thériault G, Dériaz O, Bouchard C. Plasma glucose, insulin and glucagon before and after long-term overfeeding in identical twins. Obesity Res 1993; 1 (suppl. 2): 74S (abstr).

86. Hale PJ, Singh BM, Crase J, Baddeley RM, Nattrass M. Following weight loss in massively obese patients correction of the insulin resistance of fat metabolism is delayed relative to the improvement in carbohydrate metabolism. Metabolism 1988; 37: 411–17.

87. Henry RR, Wiest-Kent TA, Scheaffer L, Kolterman OG, Olefsky JM. Metabolic consequences of very-low-calorie diet therapy in obese non-insulin-dependent diabetic and nondiabetic subjects. Diabetes 1986; 35: 155–64.

88. Henry RR, Wallace P, Olefsky JM. Effects of weight loss on mechanisms of hyperglycemia in obese non-insulin-dependent diabetes mellitus. Diabetes 1986; 35: 990–8.

89. Friedman JE, Dohm GL, Leggett-Frazier N, Elton CW, Tapscott EB, Porles WP, Caro JF. Restoration of insulin responsiveness in skeletal muscle of morbidly obese patients after weight loss. Effect on muscle glucose transport and glucose transporter GLUT4. J Clin Invest 1992; 89: 701–5.

90. Swinburn BA, Nyomba BL, Saad MF, Zurlo F, Raz I, Knowler WC, Lillioja S, Bogardus C, Ravussin E. Insulin resistance associated with lower rates of weight gain in Pima Indians. J Clin Invest 1991; 88: 168–73.

91. Valdez RA, Mitchell BD, Haffner SM, Hazuda HP, Morales PA, Monterrosa A, Stern MP. Predictors of weight change in a bi-ethnic population. The San Antonio Heart Study. Int J Obesity 1994; 18: 85–91.

92. Swislocki AL, Hoffman BB, Reaven GM. Insulin resistance, glucose intolerance and hyperinsulinemia in patients with hypertension. Am J Hypertens 1989; 2: 419–23.

93. Manicardi V, Camellini L, Bellodi G, Coscelli C, Ferrannini E. Evidence for an association of high blood pressure and hyperinsulinemia in obese man. J Clin Endocrinol Metab 1986; 62: 1302-4.

94. Bonora E, Moghetti P, Zenere M, Tosi F, Travia D, Muggeo M. B cell secretion and insulin sensitivity in hypertensive and normotensive obese subjects. Int J Obesity 1990; 14: 735-42.

95. Bonora E, Bonadonna RC, Del Prato S, Gulli G, Solini A, Matsuda M, DeFronzo RA. *In vivo* glucose metabolism in obese and type 2 diabetic subjects with or without hypertension. Diabetes 1993; 42: 764-72.

96. Laakso M, Sarlund H, Mykkänen L. Essential hypertension and insulin resistance in non-insulin-dependent diabetes. Eur J Clin Invest 1989; 19: 518-26.

97. Saad MF, Lillioja S, Nyomba BL, Castillo C, Ferraro R, DeGregorio M et al. Racial differences in the relation between blood pressure and insulin resistance. New Engl J Med 1991; 324: 733-9.

98. Falkner B, Hulman S, Tannenbaum J, Kushner H. Insulin resistance and blood pressure in young black men. Hypertension 1990; 16: 706-11.

99. Haffner SM, Ferrannini E, Hazuda HP, Stern MP. Clustering of cardiovascular risk factors in confirmed prehypertensive individuals. Hypertension 1992; 20: 38-45.

100. Mitchell BD, Haffner SM, Hazuda HP, Valdez R, Stern MP. The relation between serum insulin levels and 8-year changes in lipid, lipoprotein, and blood pressure levels. Am J Epidemiol 1992; 136: 12-22.

101. Flack JM, Liu K, Savage P et al. Baseline fasting insulin predicts 2 year blood pressure change in young adults: the CARDIA Study. Circulation 1991; 83: 724 (abstr).

102. DeFronzo RA, Goldberg M, Agus ZS. The effects of glucose and insulin on renal electrolyte transport. J Clin Invest 1976; 58: 83-90.

103. Rowe JW, Young JB, Minaker KL, Stevens AL, Pallotta J, Landsberg L. Effect of insulin and glucose infusions on sympathetic nervous system activity in normal man. Diabetes 1981; 30: 219-25.

104. Troisi RJ, Weiss ST, Parker DR, Sparrow D, Young JB, Landsberg L. Relation of obesity and diet to sympathetic nervous system activity. Hypertension 1991; 17: 669-77.

105. Anderson EA, Hoffman RP, Balon TW, Sinkey CA, Mark AL. Hyperinsulinemia produces both sympathetic neural activation and vasodilation in normal humans. J Clin Invest 1991; 87: 2246-52.

106. DeFronzo RA, Ferrannini E. Insulin resistance: a multifaceted syndrome responsible for NIDDM, obesity, hypertension, dyslipidemia, and atherosclerotic cardiovascular disease. Diabetes Care 1991; 14: 173-94.

107. DeFronzo RA. Insulin resistance, hyperinsulinemia, and coronary artery disease: a complex metabolic web. Coronary Art Dis 1992; 3: 11-25.

108. Landin K, Tengborn L, Smith U. Treating insulin resistance in hypertension with metformin reduces both blood pressure and metabolic risk factors. J Intern Med 1991; 229: 181-7.

109. Dubey RK, Kotchen TA, Boegehold MA, Zhang HY. Pioglitazone (PIO) attenuates hypertension and inhibits growth of arteriolar smooth muscle cells (ASMC). FASEB J 1992; 6: A1251 (abstr).

110. Pershadsingh HA, Kurtz TW. Pharmacologic reversal of hyperinsulinemia is associated with a reduction in blood pressure: a novel approach to treatment of hypertension. Hypertension 1992; 20: 410 (abstr).

111. Morgan DA, Ray CA, Balon TW, Mark AL. Metformin increases insulin sensitivity and lowers arterial pressure in spontaneously hypertensive rats. Hypertension 1992; 20: 421 (abstr).

112. Liang C-S, Doherty JU, Faillace R, Maekawa K, Arnold S, Gavras H, Hood WB. Insulin infusion in conscious dogs: effects on systemic and coronary hemodynamics, regional blood flows, and plasma catecholamines. J Clin Invest 1982; 69: 1321-36.

113. Laakso M, Edelman SV, Brechtel G, Baron AD. Decreased effect of insulin to stimulate skeletal muscle blood flow in obese man: a novel mechanism for insulin resistance. J Clin Invest 1990; 85: 1844-52.

114. Creager MA, Liang C-S, Coffman JD. Beta-adrenergic-mediated vasodilator response to insulin in the human forearm. J Pharmacol Exp Ther 1985; 235: 709-14.

115. Berne C, Fagius J, Pollare T, Hjemdahl P. The sympathetic response to euglycaemic hyperinsulinaemia. Diabetologia 1992; 35: 873-9.

116. Gans ROB, Toorn LVD, Bilo HJG, Nauta JJP, Heine RJ, Doner AJM. Renal and cardiovascular effects of exogenous insulin in healthy volunteers. Clin Sci 1991; 80: 219-225.

117. Brands MW, Hildebrandt DA, Mizelle HL, Hall JE. Sustained hyperinsulinemia increases arterial pressure in conscious rats. Am J Physiol 1991; 260: R764-8.

118. Hall JE, Coleman TG, Mizelle HL. Does chronic hyperinsulinemia cause hypertension? Am J Hypertens 1989; 2: 171-3.

119. Lucchesi BR, Medina M, Kniffen FJ. The positive inotropic action of insulin in the canine heart. Eur J Pharmacol 1972; 18: 107-15.

120. Lee JC, Downing SE. Effects of insulin on cardiac muscle contraction and responsiveness to norepinephrine. Am J Physiol 1976; 230: 1360-5.

121. Lund-Johansen P. Hemodynamic alterations in early essential hypertension: recent advances. In Gross F, Strasser T (eds) Mild hypertension: recent advances. New York: Raven Press, 1993; pp 237-49.

122. Stern MP, Morales PA, Haffner SM, Valdez RA. Hyperdynamic circulation and the insulin resistance syndrome ('Syndrome X'). Hypertension 1992; 20: 802-8.

123. Julius S, Gudbrandsson T, Jamerson K, Tariq Shahab S, Andersson O. The hemodynamic link between insulin resistance and hypertension. J Hypertens 1991; 9: 983-6.

124. Baron AD, Brechtel-Hook G, Johnson A, Hardin D. Skeletal muscle blood flow. A possible link between insulin resistance and blood pressure. Hypertension 1993; 21: 129-35.

125. Krotkiewski M, Bylund-Fallenius A-C, Holm J, Björntorp P, Grimby G, Mandroukas K. Relationship between muscle morphology and metabolism in obese women: the effects of long-term physical training. Eur J Clin Invest 1983; 13: 5-12.

126. Lillioja S, Young AA, Culter CL, Ivy JL, Abbott WGH, Zawadzki JK, et al. Skeletal muscle capillary density and fiber type are possible determinants of *in vivo* insulin resistance in man. J Clin Invest 1987; 80: 415-24.

127. Juhlin-Dannfelt A, Frisk-Holmberg F, Karlsson J, Tesch P. Central and peripheral circulation in relation

to muscle-fibre composition in normo- and hypertensive man. Clin Sci 1979; 56: 335-40.

128. Karlsson J, Smith HJ. Muscle fibers in human skeletal muscle and their metabolic and circulatory significance. In Hunyor S, Ludbrook JL, Shaw J, McGrath M (eds) The peripheral circulation. Amsterdam: Elsevier, 1984: pp 67-77.

129. Ginsberg HN. Very low density lipoprotein metabolism in diabetes mellitus. Diabet Metab Rev 1987; 3: 571-89.

130. Björntorp P. Regional fat distribution—implications for type 2 diabetes. Int J Obesity 1992; 16 (suppl. 4): S19-S27.

131. Reaven GM, Lerner RL, Stern MP, Farquhar JW. Role of insulin in endogenous hypertriglyceridemia. J Clin Invest 1967; 46: 1756-67.

132. Olefsky JM, Farquhar JW, Reaven GM. Reappraisal of the role of insulin in hypertriglyceridemia. Am J Med 1974; 57: 551-60.

133. Toby TA, Greenfield M, Kraemer F, Reaven GM. Relationship between insulin resistance, insulin secretion, very low density lipoprotein kinetics and plasma triglyceride levels in normotriglyceridemic man. Metabolism 1981; 30: 165-71.

134. Olefsky JM, Reaven GM, Farquhar JW. Effect of weight reduction on obesity. Studies of lipid and carbohydrate metabolism in normal and hyperlipoproteinemic subjects. J Clin Invest 1973; 53: 64-76.

135. Topping DL, Mayes PA. The immediate effects of insulin and fructose on the metabolism of the perfused liver. Changes in the lipoprotein secretion, fatty acid oxidation and esterification, lipogenesis and carbohydrate metabolism. Biochem J 1972; 126: 295-311.

136. Raman M, Steiner G. Effect of insulin on VLDL-triglyceride secretion and glucose production in the perfused rat liver. Diabetes 1990; 39 (suppl. 1): 45A (abstr).

137. Vogelberg KH, Gries FA, Moschinski D. Hepatic production of VLDL-triglycerides. Dependence on portal substrate and insulin concentration. Horm Metab Res 1980; 12: 688-94.

138. Pietri AO, Dunn FL, Grundy SM et al. The effect of continuous subcutaneous insulin infusion on very-low-density lipoprotein triglyceride metabolism in type 1 diabetes mellitus. Diabetes 1983; 32: 75-81.

139. Lewis G, Uffelman K, Steiner G. Acute hyperinsulinemia decreases VLDL triglyceride and VLDL apolipoprotein B production *in vivo* in humans. Diabetes 1992; 41 (suppl. 1): 25A.

140. Kissebah AH, Evans DJ, Peiris A, Wilson CR. Endocrine characteristics in regional obesities: role of sex steroids. Proceedings of the international symposium on the metabolic complications of human obesities, Marseille, France, May 30-June 1, 1985. Amsterdam: Elsevier, 1985: pp 115-30.

141. Kissebah AH, Vydelingum N, Murray R, Evans DJ, Hartz AJ, Kalfhoff RK, Adams PW. Relation of body fat distribution to metabolic complications of obesity. J Clin Endocrinol Metab 1982; 54: 254-60.

142. Golay A, Swislocki ALM, Chen Y-DI, Jaspan JB, Reaven GM. Effect of obesity on ambient plasma glucose, free fatty acid, insulin, growth hormone, and glucagon concentrations. J Clin Endocrinol Metab 1986; 63: 481-4.

143. Kissebah AH, Alfarsi S, Adams PW, Wynn V. Role of insulin resistance in adipose tissue and liver in

pathogenesis of endogenous hypertriglyceridemia in man. Diabetologia 1976; 12: 563-71.

144. Taskinen M-R. Lipoprotein lipase in diabetes. Diabet Metab Rev 1987; 3: 551-70.

145. Howard BV. Lipoproteins: structure and function. In Draznin B, Eckel RH (eds) Diabetes and atherosclerosis. Molecular basis and clinical aspects. New York: Elsevier, 1993: pp 3-15.

146. Goldstein JL, Brown MS. The low-density lipoprotein pathway and its relation to atherosclerosis. Annu Rev Biochem 1977; 46: 897-930.

147. Schwartz CJ, Valente AJ, Sprague EA, Kelley JL, Nerem RM. The pathogenesis of atherosclerosis: an overview. Clin Cardiol 1991; 14(I): 1-16.

148. Bagdade JD. High-density lipoprotein transport in diabetes mellitus. In Draznin B, Eckel RH (eds) Diabetes and atherosclerosis. Molecular basis and clinical aspects. New York: Elsevier, 1993: pp 59-76.

149. Weiland D, Mondon CE, Reaven GM. Evidence for multiple causality in the development of diabetic hypertriglyceridemia. Diabetologia 1980; 18: 335-40.

150. Chen Y-DI, Jeng C-Y, Reaven GM. HDL metabolism in diabetes. Diabet Metab Rev 1987; 3: 653-68.

151. Taskinen M-R, Nikkilä EA. Lipoprotein lipase activity of adipose tissue and skeletal muscle in insulin-deficient human diabetes. Diabetologia 1979; 17: 351-6.

152. Nikkilä EA, Huttunen JK, Ehnholm C. Postheparin plasma lipoprotein lipase and hepatic lipase in diabetes mellitus: relationship to plasma triglyceride metabolism. Diabetes 1977; 26: 11-21.

153. Lewis GF, Steiner G. Triglyceride-rich lipoproteins in diabetes. In Draznin B, Eckel RH (eds) Diabetes and atherosclerosis. Molecular basis and clinical aspects. New York: Elsevier, 1993: pp 3-15.

154. Haffner SM, Valdez RA, Hazuda HP, Mitchell BD, Morales PA, Stern MP. Prospective analysis of the insulin resistance syndrome (Syndrome X). Diabetes 1992; 41: 715-22.

155. Barker DJP, Hales CN, Fall CHD, Osmond C, Phipps K, Clark PMS. Type 2 (non-insulin-dependent) diabetes mellitus, hypertension, and hyperlipidaemia (syndrome X): relation to reduced fetal growth. Diabetologia 1993; 36: 62-7.

156. Krauss RM, Burke DJ. Identification of multiple subclasses of plasma low density lipoproteins in normal humans. J Lipid Res 1982; 23: 97-104.

157. Austin MA, King MC, Vranizan KM, Newman B, Krauss RM. Inheritance of low density lipoprotein subclass patterns: results of complex segregation analysis. Am J Hum Genet 1988; 43: 838-46.

158. Barakat HA, Carpenter JW, McLendon VD, Khazarie P, Leggett N, Heath J, Marks R. Influence of obesity, impaired glucose tolerance, and NIDDM on LDL structure and composition: possible link between hyperinsulinemia and atherosclerosis. Diabetes 1990; 39: 1527-33.

159. McNamara JR, Campos H, Ordovas JM, Peterson RM, Wilson PWF, Schaefer EJ. Effect of gender, age and lipid status on low density lipoprotein subfraction distribution: results of the Framingham Offspring Study. Arteriosclerosis 1987; 7: 483-90.

160. Swinkels DW, Demacker PNM, Hendriks JCM, Van't Laar A. Low-density lipoprotein subfractions and relationship of other risk factors for coronary artery disease in healthy individuals. Arteriosclerosis 1989; 9: 604-13.

161. Selby JV, Austin MA, Newman B, Zhang D, Quesenberry CP, Mayer EJ, Krauss RM. LDL subclass phenotypes and the insulin resistance syndrome in women. Circulation 1993; 88: 381-7.

162. Haffner SM, Mykkänen L, Valdez RA, Paidi M, Stern MP, Howard BV. LDL size and subclass pattern in a biethnic population. Arterioscler Thromb 1993; 13: 1623-30.

163. Reaven GM, Chen Y-DI, Jeppesen J, Maheux P, Krauss RM. Insulin resistance and hyperinsulinemia in individuals with small, dense, low density lipoprotein particles. J Clin Invest 1993; 92: 141-6.

164. Austin MA, Breslow JL, Hennekens CH, Buring JE, Willett WC, Krauss RM. Low density lipoprotein subclass patterns and risk of myocardial infarction. JAMA 1988; 260: 1917-21.

165. Campos H, Genest JJ, Blijlevens E, McNamara JR, Jenner JL, Ordovas JM, Wilson PWF, Schaefer EJ. Low-density lipoprotein particle size and coronary artery disease. Arteriosclerosis 1992; 12: 187-95.

166. Crouse JR, Parks JS, Schey HM, Kahl FR. Studies of low density lipoprotein molecular weight in human beings with coronary artery disease. J Lipid Res 1985; 26: 566-74.

167. Tribble DL, Hull LG, Wood PD, Krauss RM. Variations in oxidative susceptibility among six low-density lipoprotein subfractions of different density and particle size. Atherosclerosis 1992; 93: 189-94.

168. Steinberg D, Parthasarathy S, Carew TE, Khou JC, Witztum JL. Beyond cholesterol: modifications of low density lipoprotein that increase its atherogenicity. New Engl J Med 1989; 320: 913-24.

169. Gatling W, Knight C, Hill RD. Screening for early diabetic nephropathy: which sample to detect microalbuminuria? Diabetic Med 1985; 2: 451-5.

170. Cowell CT, Rodgers S, Silkink M. First morning urinary albumin concentration is a good predictor of 24-hour urinary albumin excretion in children with type 1 (insulin-dependent) diabetes. Diabetologia 1986; 29: 97-9.

171. Parving HH, Oxenboll B, Svendsen PA, Sandahl-Christensen J, Andersen AR. Early detection of patients at risk of developing diabetic nephropathy. A longitudinal study of urinary albumin excretion. Acta Endocrinol 1982; 100: 550-5.

172. Viberti GC, Jarrett RJ, Mahmud U, Hill RD, Argyropoulos A, Keen H. Microalbuminuria as a predictor of clinical nephropathy in insulin-dependent diabetes mellitus. Lancet 1982; 1: 1430-2.

173. Mogensen CE, Christensen CK. Predicting diabetic nephropathy in insulin dependent patients. New Engl J Med 1984; 311: 89-93.

174. Mogensen CE. Microalbuminuria predicts clinical proteinuria and early mortality in maturity-onset diabetes. New Engl J Med 1984; 310: 356-60.

175. Christensen CK, Mogensen CE. The course of incipient diabetic nephropathy: studies of albumin excretion and blood pressure. Diabetic Med 1985; 2: 97-102.

176. Wiseman M, Viberti G, Mackintosh D, Jarrett RJ, Keen H. Glycemia, arterial pressure and microalbuminuria in type 1 (insulin-dependent) diabetes mellitus. Diabetologia 1984; 26: 401-5.

177. Jensen T, Stender S, Deckert T. Abnormalities in plasma concentrations of lipoproteins and fibrinogen in type 1 (insulin-dependent) diabetic patients with increased urinary albumin excretion. Diabetologia 1988; 31: 142-5.

178. Niskanen L, Uusitupa M, Sarlund H, Siitonen O, Voutilainen E, Penttilä I, Pyörälä K. Microalbuminuria predicts the development of serum lipoprotein abnormalities favoring atherogenesis in newly diagnosed type 2 (non-insulin-dependent) diabetic patients. Diabetologia 1990; 33: 237-43.

179. Mattock MB, Morrish NJ, Viberti GC, Keen H, Fitzgerald AP, Jackson G Prospective study of microalbuminuria as predictor of mortality in NIDDM. Diabetes 1992; 41: 736-41.

180. Collins VR, Dowse GK, Finch CF, Zimmet PZ, Linnane AW. Prevalence and risk factors for micro- and macroalbuminuria in diabetic subjects and entire population of Nauru. Diabetes 1989; 38: 1602-10.

181. Nelson RG, Runzelman CL, Pettitt DJ, Saad MF, Bennett PH, Knowler WC. Albuminuria in type 2 (non-insulin-dependent) diabetes mellitus and impaired glucose tolerance in Pima Indians. Diabetologia 1989; 32: 870-6.

182. Keen H, Chouverakis C, Fuller J, Jarrett RJ. The concomitants of raised blood sugar: studies in newly-detected hyperglycaemics. II. Urinary albumin excretion, blood pressure and their relationship to blood sugar levels. Guy's Hosp Rep 1969; 118: 247-54.

183. Haffner SM, González C, Valdez RA, Mykkänen L, Hazuda HP, Mitchell BD, Monterrosa A, Stern MP. Is microalbuminuria part of the prediabetic state? The Mexico City Diabetes Study. Diabetologia 1993; 36: 1002-6.

184. Haffner SM, Stern MP, Gruber MK, Hazuda HP, Mitchell BD, Patterson JK. Microalbuminuria. Potential marker for increased cardiovascular risk factors in non-diabetic subjects? Arteriosclerosis 1990; 10: 727-31.

185. Mykkänen L, Haffner SM, Kuusisto J, Pyörälä K, Laakso M. Microalbuminuria precedes the development of NIDDM. Diabetes 1994; 43: 552-7.

186. Nosadini R, Solini A, Sambataro M, Cipollina MR, Trevisan R, Duner E, Strazzabosco M, Barzon I, Brocco E, Velussi M, Crepaldi G. Relationships among insulin resistance, hypertension and microalbuminuria in non-insulin-dependent diabetes. Role of cell ion handling. Diabetes 1992; 41 (suppl. 1): 62A (abstr).

187. Groop L, Ekstrand A, Forsblom C, Widén E, Groop P-H, Teppo A-M, Eriksson J. Insulin resistance, hypertension and microalbuminuria in patients with type 2 (non-insulin-dependent) diabetes mellitus. Diabetologia 1993; 36: 642-7.

188. Niskanen L, Laakso M. Insulin resistance is related to albuminuria in patients with type 2 (non-insulin-dependent) diabetes mellitus. Metabolism 1993; 42: 1541-5.

189. Pollare T, Lithell H, Berne C. A comparison of the effects of hydrocholorothiazide and captopril on glucose and lipid metabolism in patients with hypertension. New Engl J Med 1989; 321: 868-73.

190. Marre M, Leblanc M, Suarez L, Guyenne TT, Menard J, Passa P. Converting enzyme inhibition and kidney function in normotensive diabetic subjects with persistent microalbuminuria. Br Med J 1987; 294: 1484-8.

191. Yudkin JS, Forrest RD, Jackson CA. Microalbuminuria as a predictor of vascular disease in non-diabetic

subjects. Islington Diabetes Survey. Lancet 1988; 2: 530-3.

192. Tucker BJ, Anderson CM, Thies RS, Collins RC, Blantz RC. Glomerular hemodynamic alterations during acute hyperinsulinemia in normal and diabetic rats. Kidney Int 1992; 42: 1160-8.

193. Cohen AJ, McCarthy DM, Stoff JS. Direct hemodynamic effect of insulin in the isolated perfused kidney. Am J Physiol 1989; 257: F580-85.

194. Deckert T, Feldt-Rasmussen B, Borch-Johnsen K, Jensen T, Kofoed-Enevoldsen A. Albuminuria reflects widespread vascular damage: the Steno hypothesis. Diabetologia 1989; 32: 219-26.

195. Anderson DC. Sex hormone binding globulin. Clin Endocrinol 1974; 3: 69-96.

196. Peiris AN, Mueller RA, Struve MF, Smith GA, Kissebah AH. Relationship of androgenic activity to splanchic insulin metabolism and peripheral glucose utilization in premenopausal women. J Clin Endocrinol Metab 1987; 64: 162-9.

197. Haffner SM, Katz MS, Stern MP, Dunn JF. Relationship of sex hormone binding globulin to overall adiposity and body fat distribution in a biethnic population. Int J Obesity 1989; 13: 1-9.

198. Evans DJ, Hoffmann RG, Kalkhoff RK et al. Relationship of androgenic activity to body fat topography, fat cell morphology, and metabolic aberrations in premenopausal women. J Clin Endocrinol Metab 1983; 57: 304-10.

199. Haffner SM, Katz MS, Stern MP. The relationship of sex hormones to hyperinsulinemia and hyperglycemia. Metabolism 1988: 37: 683-8.

200. Haffner SM, Katz MS, Stern MP, Dunn JF. The association of decreased sex hormone binding globulin and cardiovascular risk factors. Arteriosclerosis 1989; 9: 136-43.

201. Wild RA, Applebaum-Bowden D, Demers LM et al. Lipoprotein lipids in women with androgen excess: independent associations with increased insulin and androgen. Clin Chem 1990; 36: 283-9.

202. Gorbach SL, Schaefer EJ, Woods M et al. Plasma lipoprotein cholesterol and endogenous sex hormones in healthy young women. Metabolism 1989; 38: 1077-81.

203. Lindstedt G, Lundberg PA, Lapidus L, Lundgren H, Bengtsson C, Björntorp P. Low sex-hormone-binding globulin concentration as independent risk factor for development of NIDDM. Twelve-year follow-up of population study of women in Gothenburg, Sweden. Diabetes 1991; 40: 123-8.

204. Haffner SM, Valdez RA, Morales PA, Hazuda HP, Stern MP. Decreased sex hormone binding globulin predicts non-insulin dependent diabetes mellitus in women but not in men. J Clin Endocrinol Metab 1993; 77: 56-60.

205. Smith S, Ravnikar VA, Barbieri RL. Androgen and insulin response to an oral glucose challenge in hyperandrogenic women. Fertil Steril 1987; 48: 72-7.

206. Soler JT, Folsom AR, Kaye SA et al. Associations of abdominal adiposity, fasting insulin, sex hormone binding globulin, and estrone with lipids and lipoproteins in postmenopausal women. Atherosclerosis 1989; 79: 21-7.

207. Haffner SM, Dunn JF, Katz MS. Relationship of sex hormone-binding globulin to lipid, lipoprotein, glucose, and insulin concentrations in postmenopausal women. Metabolism 1992; 41: 278-87.

208. Björntorp P. Androgens, the metabolic syndrome, and non-insulin-dependent diabetes mellitus. Ann NY Acad Sci 1993; 676: 242-52.

209. Pasquali R, Casimirri F, Cantobelli S, Melchionda N, Labate AMM, Fabbri R, Capelli M, Bortozoli L. Effect of obesity and body fat distribution on sex hormones and insulin in men. Metabolism 1991; 40: 101-4.

210. Phillips G. Relationship between sex hormones and the glucose-insulin-lipid defect in men with obesity. Metabolism 1993; 42: 116-20.

211. Haffner SM, Valdez RA, Mykkänen L, Stern MP, Katz MS. Decreased testosterone and dehydroepiandrosterone sulfate concentrations are associated with increased glucose and insulin concentrations in non-diabetic men. Metabolism 1994; 43: 599-603.

212. Birkeland KI, Hanssen KF, Torjesen PA, Vader S. Low level of sex-hormone-binding globulin is positively correlated with insulin sensitivity in men with type 2 diabetes. J Clin Endocrinol Metab, 1993; 76: 275-8.

213. Dai WS, Gutai JP, Kuller LH, LaPorte RE, Falvo-Gerard L, Caggiula A. Relation between plasma high-density lipoprotein cholesterol and sex hormone concentrations in men. Am J Cardiol 1984; 53: 1259-63.

214. Haffner SM, Mykkänen L, Valdez RA, Katz MS. Relationship of sex hormones to lipids and lipoproteins in non-diabetic men. J Clin Endocrinol Metab 1993; 77: 1610-15.

215. Shaten J, Haffner S, Smith GD, Kuller L, for the MRFIT Research Group. Low levels of sex hormone binding globulin and testosterone predict the incidence of non-insulin dependent diabetes mellitus in men. The Multiple Risk Factor Intervention Trial. Amer J Epidemiol (in press).

216. Barrett-Connor E, Khaw KT, Yen SSC. A prospective study of dehydroepiandrosterone sulfate, mortality and cardiovascular disease. New Engl J Med 1986; 315: 1519-24.

217. Barrett-Connor E, Khaw KT, Yen SSC. Absence of an inverse relation of dehydroepiandrosterone sulfate with cardiovascular mortality in postmenopausal women. New Engl J Med 1987; 317: 711 (letter).

218. Holmäng A, Björntorp P. The effects of testosterone on insulin sensitivity in male rats. Acta Physiol Scand 1992; 146: 505-10.

219. Cohen JC, Hickman R. Insulin resistance and diminished glucose tolerance in power lifters ingesting anabolic steroids. J Clin Endocrinol Metab 1987; 64: 960-3.

220. Woodard TL, Burghen GA, Kitabchi AE, Wilmas JA. Glucose intolerance and insulin resistance in aplastic anemia treated with oxymethalone. J Clin Endocrinol Metab 1981; 53: 905-8.

221. Barbieri RL, Ryan KJ. Hyperandrogenism, insulin resistance and acanthosis nigricans syndrome: a common endocrinopathy with distinct pathophysiologic features. Am J Obstet Gynecol 1983; 147: 90-101.

222. Vague P, Juhan-Vague I, Aillaud MF, Badier C, Viard R, Alessi MC, Collen D. Correlation between blood fibrinolytic activity, plasminogen activator inhibitor level, plasma insulin level, and relative body weight in normal and obese subjects. Metabolism 1986; 35: 250-3.

223. Landin K, Stigendal L, Eriksson E, Krotkiewski M, Risberg B, Tengborn L, Smith U. Abdominal obesity

is associated with an impaired fibrinolytic activity and elevated plasminogen activator inhibitor 1. Metabolism 1990; 39: 1044-8.

224. Juhan-Vague I, Alessi MC, Vague P. Increased plasma plasminogen activator inhibitor 1 levels. A possible link between insulin resistance and atherothrombosis. Diabetologia 1991; 34: 457-62.

225. Mehta J, Mehta P, Lawson D, Saldeen T. Plasma tissue plasminogen activator inhibitor levels in coronary artery disease: correlation with age and serum triglyceride concentrations. J Am Coll Cardiol 1987; 9: 263-8.

226. Asplund-Carlson A, Hamsten A, Wiman B, Carlson LA. Relationship between plasma plasminogen activator inhibitor-1 activity and VLDL triglyceride concentration, insulin levels and insulin sensitivity: studies in randomly selected normo- and hypertriglyceridaemic men. Diabetologia 1993; 36: 817-25.

227. Sundell IB, Nilsson TK, Hallmans G, Hellsten G, Dahlen GH. Interrelationships between plasma levels of plasminogen activator inhibitor, tissue plasminogen activator, lipoprotein (a), and established cardiovascular risk factors in a North Swedish population. Atherosclerosis 1989; 80: 9-16.

228. Juhan-Vague I, Roul C, Alessi MC, Ardissone JP, Heim M, Vague P. Increased plasminogen activator inhibitor activity in non-insulin dependent diabetic patients. Relationship with plasma insulin. Thromb Haemostas 1989; 61: 370-3.

229. Nordby G, Haaland A, Os I. Evidence of decreased fibrinolytic activity in hypertensive premenopausal women. Scand J Clin Lab Invest 1992; 52: 275-81.

230. Landin K, Tengborn L, Smith U. Elevated fibrinogen and plasminogen activator inhibitor (PAI-1) in hypertension are related to metabolic risk factors for cardiovascular disease. J Intern Med 1990; 227: 273-8.

231. Mehrabian M, Peter JB, Barnard RJ, Lusis AJ. Dietary regulation of fibrinolytic factors. Atherosclerosis 1990; 84: 25-32.

232. Huisveld IA, Leenen R, v d Kooy K, Hospers JEH, Seidell JC, Deurenberg P, Koppeschaar HPF, Mosterd WL, Boupma BN. Body composition and weight reduction in relation to antigen and activity of plasminogen activator inhibitor (PAI-1) in overweight individuals. Fibrinolysis 1990; 4: 84-5.

233. Estelles A, Aznar J, Tormo G, Sapena P, Tormo V, Espana F. Influence of a rehabilitation sports program on the fibrinolytic activity of patients after myocardial infarction. Thromb Res 1989; 55: 203-12.

234. Gris JC, Schved JF, Aguilar-Martinez P, Arnaud A, Sanchez N. Impact of physical training on plasminogen activator inhibitor activity in sedentary men. Fibrinolysis 1990; 4: 97-8.

235. Vague P, Juhan-Vague I, Alessi MC, Badier C, Valadier J. Metformin decreases the high plasminogen activator inhibitor capacity, plasma insulin and triglyceride levels in non diabetic obese subjects. Thromb Haemostas 1987; 57: 326-8.

236. Alessi MC, Juhan-Vague I, Kooistra T, Declerck PJ, Collen D. Insulin stimulates the synthesis of plasminogen activator inhibitor 1 by the human hepatocellular cell line HepG2. Thromb Haemostas 1988; 60: 491-4.

237. Kooistra T, Bosma P, Tons H, van den Berg A, Meyer P, Princen H. Plasminogen activator inhibitor 1: biosynthesis and mRNA levels are increased by insulin in cultured human hepatocytes. Thromb Haemostas 1989; 62: 723-8.

238. Medvescek M, Keber D, Stegnar M, Borovnicar A. Plasminogen activator inhibitor 1 response to a carbohydrate meal in obese subjects. Fibrinolysis 1990; 4: 89-90.

239. Grant PJ, Kruithof EKO, Felley CP, Felber JP, Bachmann F. Short-term infusions of insulin, triacylglycerol and glucose do not cause acute increases in plasminogen activator inhibitor 1 concentrations in man. Clin Sci 1990; 79: 513-16.

240. Vuorinen-Markkola H, Puhakainen I, Yki-Järvinen H. No evidence for short-term regulation of plasminogen activator inhibitor activity by insulin in man. Thromb Haemostas 1992; 67: 117-20.

241. Juhan-Vague I, Vague P. Hypofibrinolysis and insulin resistance. Diabète Metab 1991; 17 (suppl. 2): 96-100.

242. Nilsson TK, Johnson O. The extrinsic fibrinolytic system in survivors of myocardial infarction. Thromb Res 1987; 48: 621-30.

243. Hamsten A, Wiman B, Defaire U, Blomback M. Increased plasma level of a rapid inhibitor of tissue plasminogen activator in young survivors of myocardial infarction. New Engl J Med 1985; 313: 1557-63.

244. Francis RB, Kawanishi D, Baruch T, Mahrer P, Rahimtoola S, Feinstein DI. Impaired fibrinolysis in coronary artery disease. Am Heart J 1988; 115: 776-80.

245. Olofsson BO, Dahlen G, Nilsson TK. Evidence for increased levels of plasminogen activator inhibitor and tissue plasminogen activator in plasma of patients with angiographically verified coronary artery disease. Eur Heart J 1989; 10: 77-82.

246. Hamsten A, Defaire U, Walldius G, Dahlen G, Szamosi A, Landou C, Blomback M, Wiman B. Plasminogen activator inhibitor in plasma: risk factor for recurrent myocardial infarction. Lancet 1987; 2: 3-9.

247. Gram J, Jespersen J, Kluft C, Rijken DC. On the usefulness of fibrinolysis variables in the characterization of a risk group for myocardial reinfarction. Acta Med Scand 1987; 221: 149-53.

248. Ahn YI, Ferrell RE, Hamman RF, Kamboh IM. Association of lipoprotein lipase gene variation with physiological components of the insulin-resistance syndrome in the population of the San Luis Valley, Colorado. Diabetes 1993; 16: 1502-6.

249. Goldstein JL, Schrott HG, Hazzard WR, Bierman EL, Motulsky AG. Hyperlipidemia in coronary artery disease. II. Genetic analysis of lipid levels in 176 families and delineation of a new inherited disorder, combined hyperlipidemia. J Clin Invest 1973; 52: 1544-68.

250. Austin MA, Brunzell JD, Fitch WL, Krauss RM. Inheritance of low density lipoprotein subclass patterns in familial combined hyperlipidemia. Arteriosclerosis 1990; 10: 520-30.

251. de Graaf J, Swinkels DW, de Haan AF, Demacker PN, Stalenhoef AF. Both inherited susceptibility and environmental exposure determine the low-density lipoprotein-subfraction pattern distribution in healthy Dutch families. Am J Hum Genet 1992; 51: 1295-310.

252. Austin MA, Jarvik GP, Hokanson JE, Edwards KE. Complex segregation analysis of low-density lipoprotein peak particle diameter. Genet Epidemiol 1993; 10: 599-604.

253. Austin MA. Genetics of low-density lipoprotein subclasses. Curr Opin Lipidol 1993; 4: 125–32.

254. Lamon-Fava S, Jimenez D, Christian JC, Fabsitz RR, Reed T, Carmelli D, Castelli WP, Ordovas JM, Wilson PW, Schaefer EJ. The NHLBI Twin Study: heritability of apolipoprotein A-I, B, and low density lipoprotein subclasses and concordance for lipoprotein (a). Atherosclerosis 1991; 91: 97–106.

255. Austin MA, Newman B, Selby JV, Edwards K, Mayer EJ, Krauss RM. Genetics of LDL subclass phenotypes in women twins. Concordance, heritability and commingling analysis. Arterioscler Thromb 1993; 13: 687–95.

256. Austin MA, Wijsman E, Guo SW, Krauss RM, Brunzell JD, Deeb S. Lack of evidence for linkage between low-density lipoprotein subclass phenotypes and the apolipoprotein B locus in familial combined hyperlipidemia. Genet Epidemiol 1991; 8: 287–97.

257. LaBelle M, Austin MA, Rubin E, Krauss RM. Linkage analysis of low-density lipoprotein subclass phenotypes and the apolipoprotein B gene. Genet Epidemiol 1991; 8: 269–75.

258. Nishina PM, Johnson JP, Naggert KJ, Krauss RM. Linkage of atherogenic lipoprotein phenotype to the low density lipoprotein receptor locus on the short arm of chromosome 19. Proc Natl Acad Sci USA 1992; 89: 708–12.

259. Valdez R, Athens MA, Thompson GH, Bradshaw BS, Stern MP. Birthweight and adult health outcomes in a biethnic U.S. population. Diabetologia 1994; 37: 624–31.

260. Bu X, Krauss RM, DeMeester C, Lopez R, Daneshma S, Puppione D, Gray R, Lusis AJ, Rotter JI. Multigenic control of LDL particle size in 24 coronary artery disease (CAD) pedigrees. Circulation 1992; 86 (suppl. I): 1552 (abstr).

261. Wojciechowski AP, Farrall M, Cullen P, Wilson TME, Bayliss JD, Farren B et al. Familial combined hyperlipidemia linked to the apolipoprotein AI-CIII-AIV gene cluster on chromosome 11q23-q24. Nature 1991; 349: 161–4.

262. Wijsman EM, Motulsky AG, Guo W, Yang M, Austin MA, Brunzell JD, Deeb S. Evidence against linkage of familial combined hyperlipidemia to the AI-CIII-AIV gene complex. Circulation 1992; 86 (suppl. I): 1420 (abstr).

263. Williams RR, Hunt SC, Hopkins PN, Stults BM, Wu LL, Hasstedt SJ, Barlow GK, Stephenson SH, Lalouel JM, Kuida H. Familial dyslipidemic hypertension. Evidence from 58 Utah families for a syndrome present in approximately 12% of patients with essential hypertension. JAMA 1988; 259: 3579–86.

264. Hunt SC, Wu LL, Hopkins PN, Stults BM, Kuida H, Ramirez ME, Lalouel JM, Williams RR. Apolipoprotein, low density lipoprotein subfraction, and insulin associations with familial combined hyperlipidemia: study of Utah patients with familial dyslipidemic hypertension. Arteriosclerosis 1989; 9: 335–44.

265. Bogardus C, Lillioja S, Nyomba BL, Zurlo F, Swinburn B, Eposito-del Puente A, Knowler WC, Ravussin E, Mott DM, Bennett PH. Distribution of *in vivo* insulin action in Pima Indians as mixture of three normal distributions. Diabetes 1989; 38: 1423–32.

266. Schumacher MC, Hasstedt SJ, Hunt SC, Williams RR, Elbein SC. Major gene effect for insulin levels in familial NIDDM pedigrees. Diabetes 1992; 41: 416–23.

267. Medical Research Council Environmental Epidemiology Unit. In DJP Barker (ed.) Fetal and infant origins of adult disease. London: British Medical Journal, 1992.

268. Barker DJP, Osmond C. Infant mortality, childhood nutrition, and ischaemic heart disease in England and Wales. Lancet 1986; 1: 1077–81.

269. Barker DJP, Winter PD, Osmond C, Margetts B, Simmonds SJ. Weight in infancy and death from ischaemic heart disease. Lancet 1989; 2: 577–80.

270. Hales CN, Barker DJP, Clark PMS, Cox LJ, Fall C, Osmond C, Winter PD. Fetal and infant growth and impaired glucose tolerance at age 64. Br Med J 1991; 303: 1019–22.

271. Fall CHD, Barker DJP, Osmond C, Winter PD, Clark PMS, Hales CN. Relation of infant feeding to adult serum cholesterol concentration and death from ischaemic heart disease. Br Med J 1992; 304: 801–5.

272. Barker DJP, Meade TW, Fall CHD, Lee A, Osmond C, Phipps K, Stirling Y. Relation of fetal and infant growth to plasma fibrinogen and factor VII concentrations in adult life. Br Med J 1992; 304: 148–52.

273. Law CM, Barker DJP, Osmond C, Fall CHD, Simmonds SJ. Early growth and abdominal fatness in adult life. J Epidemiol Community Health 1992; 46: 184–6.

274. Hales CN, Barker DJP. Type 2 (non-insulin-dependent) diabetes mellitus: the thrifty phenotype hypothesis. Diabetologia 1992; 35: 595–601.

Biochemistry and Pathophysiology
of Diabetes

13

Morphology of the Pancreas in Normal and Diabetic States

G. Klöppel*‡ and P.A. In't Veld†

*Vrije Universiteit, Brussels, Belgium, and †Erasmus University, Rotterdam, The Netherlands

THE NORMAL ENDOCRINE PANCREAS

Islets of Langerhans

The human pancreas is basically composed of two types of secretory cells that are both involved in nutrient handling: 98% of the cells—the exocrine type—secrete a food-processing enzyme–bicarbonate mixture into the duodenum, while the remaining 2%—the endocrine type—have a metabolic function and secrete a mixture of nutrient-generated hormones into the portal vein. The small-endocrine part is of vital importance in maintaining glucose homeostasis, mainly through the action of the 51-amino acid peptide insulin. In the human the endocrine part consists of $10^5 - 10^6$ cellular aggregates scattered throughout the exocrine parenchyma, each aggregate containing approximately a thousand endocrine cells. Morphologically these structures were first described by Paul Langerhans (1849–88) in his doctoral thesis of 1869. He was unable to determine their function but suggested a close connection with the nervous system, as he observed nerve fibres and ganglion cells in close proximity to the islet cells. It was not until 1889 that an endocrine function could be ascribed to the pancreas, when Minkowski and von Mering performed their classic pancreatectomy experiments and established the relation of the gland to carbohydrate metabolism and diabetes [1].

‡ *Present address: Department of Pathology, University of Kiel, Germany*

The adult human islet is characterized by an average diameter of 140 µm [2]. It consists of a compact mass of epithelial cells pervaded by a dense network of anastomosing capillaries [3]. Around the islet a thin collagen capsule is often present, separating endocrine from exocrine tissue. Mean endocrine mass present in the total adult pancreas is estimated at 1395 mg [4], corresponding to roughly 2% of the mean pancreatic weight of 68 g [5] (range 45–120 g). Adult islets incorporate more than 90% of all pancreatic endocrine cells; the remaining cells occur singly or in small clusters. Four endocrine cell types can be distinguished: A cells (alpha; formerly called A_2), B cells (beta), D cells (delta; formerly called A_1) and PP cells (pancreatic polypeptide; formerly also called F or D_1). The A and B cells were both first described by Lane in 1907 [6] on the basis of their different histochemical staining characteristics, while the D cell was identified by Bloom in 1931 [7]. The most recent addition is the PP cell, discovered immunocytochemically using an antibody raised against impurities found in insulin preparations [8, 9].

Embryology and Fetal Development

The pancreas is derived from three diverticula of the primitive gut. At 3–4 weeks of age one dorsal primordium and two ventral primordia can be recognized at the level of the hepatic duct. The left-side ventral primordium normally disappears, leaving only the small right-side ventral primordium

International Textbook of Diabetes Mellitus, Second Edition. Edited by K.G.M.M. Alberti, P. Zimmet, R.A. DeFronzo, and H. Keen (Honorary)
© 1997 John Wiley & Sons Ltd

to fuse with the larger dorsal one at 7 weeks. At this stage the gland consists of unbranched tubules with columnar epithelium surrounded by mesenchymal tissue. Endocrine cells are immunocytochemically recognized at 8–9 weeks, albeit not in islets but lying isolated at the basal side of the cells lining the tubules. Islet hormone mRNA expression is found much earlier in development, with insulin and glucagon mRNA being present before pancreatic primordia can be recognized. At 10–12 weeks exocrine acini with zymogen granules are formed and primitive islets are located in the acinar interstitium [10–12, 215]. Growth of the endocrine cell mass during fetal life follows that of total gland volume (Figure 1), with endocrine tissue forming 2–5% of the combined exocrine/endocrine cell mass [13]. During development, the relative proportion of endocrine cell types changes: glicentin/glucagon-containing A cells form approximately 50% of the endocrine volume at a fetal age of 8 weeks but make up only 15–20% in adults [13, 14]. Similarly, the somatostatin-containing D cells form 20–25% of the total endocrine volume in neonates, but only 5% in adults [15, 16]. Exact estimates of endocrine volumes in the fetal pancreas are complicated by the apparent co-expression of different hormones in a single endocrine cell. Insulin, glucagon and somatostatin have been found to co-localize within the same granule, indicating the existence of multihormone precursor cells [21, 216, 217, 218, 219].

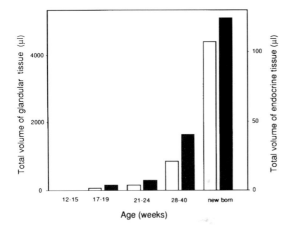

Figure 1 Fetal growth of the pancreatic gland. Open bars show the total volume of glandular tissue, closed bars the total volume of endocrine tissue (based on reference 13)

Whether B-cell neogenesis is primarily based on division of differentiated cells or on differentiation from uncommitted stem cells is not known. Indeed, it has never been unequivocally established whether the endocrine cells derive from the same endodermal precursor cells as the exocrine cells or are derived from the neural crest, as suggested by Pearse in his APUD concept [17]. Close functional relationships between pancreatic endocrine cells and neurons are suggested by the similarity in enzyme profiles of endocrine cells and adrenergic neurons [18, 19]. Endocrine cells are found to contain enzymes like tyrosine hydroxylase [220], neuron-specific enolase [221] and glutamic acid decarboxylase [208], involved in the production of neurotransmitters, as well as the neurotransmitters dopamine [206], serotonin [207] and γ-aminobutyric acid (GABA) [208]. In addition, mature B cells display electrophysiologic characteristics usually only found in neuronal tissue [20]. Whether these functional relationships imply a developmental relationship with neuronal tissue, or point to the existence of a developmental pathway in which endodermal cells can acquire neuronal traits, is not known.

Evolutionary Origin of the Pancreatic Islet

Insulin and other biologically active peptides are remarkably well preserved in evolution. Already in unicellular organisms peptides have an important role in intercellular communication. In invertebrates, insulin is found in giant neurons of the nervous system associated with growth [22]. In higher invertebrates the peptides are no longer confined to the nervous system, but are also found in endocrine cells dispersed in the alimentary channel. Islets of Langerhans are first encountered in primitive vertebrates where they are still partly embedded in the gut mucosa and consist of aggregates of B and D cells. These primitive islets are not accompanied by any exocrine tissue and do not contain any A or PP cells. Later in evolution, endocrine cells are found between the exocrine cells, together forming the pancreatic organ. At this stage A cells join the islet, followed by PP cells, which latter cell type therefore constitutes the latest addition to this micro-organ. It is only in the higher vertebrates, especially in mammals, that a regional variation in the composition of the islets is noted, with PP cells being most abundant in the pancreatic region closest to the gut. In general, it appears that in evolution the peptidergic peripheral nerve cells involved in nutrient-related regulatory functions change into specialized endocrine cells that at first have a diffuse localization in the alimentary tract, but later are concentrated in islets of Langerhans. Their presence in the exocrine pancreas may be related to trophic effects of pancreatic hormones on exocrine cells, possibly creating a positive feedback mechanism in which increased nutrient availability results in increased pancreatic mass.

Endocrine Cell Types

Adult islets of Langerhans are mainly composed of four endocrine cell types whose characteristics are

Table 1 Cell types in the endocrine pancreas

	Cell type			
	A	B	D	PP
Peptide hormone	Glucagon	Insulin	Somatostatin	Pancreatic polypeptide
Molecular weight	3500	5800	1500	4200
Number of amino acids	29	51	14	36
Volume % (adult)				
Dorsal	15–20	70–80	5–10	<1
Ventral	<1	10–20	2	80
Total	15–20	70–80	5–10	15–25

briefly summed up in Table 1 and whose ultrastructural appearance [23], apart from PP cells, is illustrated in Figure 2; other types of endocrine cells may occasionally be present but their frequency in the normal adult gland is below 0.5% and they are not discussed here.

A Cell

The pancreatic A cell contains glucagon, a 29-amino acid peptide whose hyperglycaemic action was discovered in 1923 [24] and whose cellular location was immunocytochemically established by Baum et al in 1962 [25]. The A cells form 15–20% of the total endocrine mass and contain typical glucagon secretory granules with an electron-dense core and a paler peripheral mantle (Figure 2a) [23, 26]. Glucagon is derived

from a 180-amino acid precursor, proglucagon, through proteolytic cleavage. Other cleavage products from the same precursor include two glucagon-like peptides (GLPs) and glicentin [27, 28]. Glucagon is primarily found in the electron-dense core of the A cell secretory granule, while other proglucagon-derived peptides are preferentially located in the peripheral rim [29].

B Cell

Pancreatic B cells form 70–80% of the endocrine cell mass. They contain insulin (Latin *insula*, islet), first isolated by Banting and Best [30, 31] and immunocytochemically located to the B cell by Lacy [32]. Like other pancreatic hormones, insulin is formed via proteolytic cleavage from a precursor

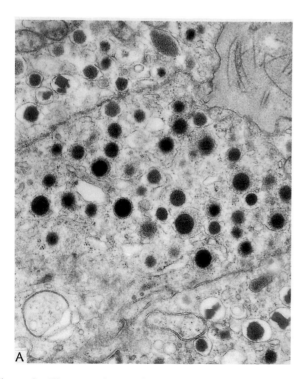 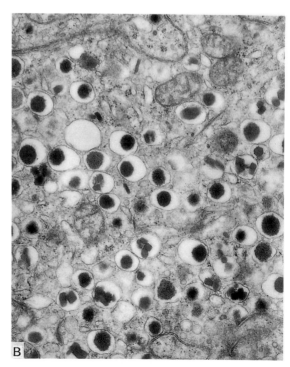

Figure 2 Electron-microscopic appearance of endocrine cells of the adult human pancreas demonstrating the secretory vesicle morphology of A cells (Figure 2A) and B cells (Figure 2B) (×20 000)

molecule, proinsulin. The resulting byproduct, C-peptide (connecting peptide), is secreted together with insulin in a 1:1 molar ratio [33]. B cells store up to 13 000 secretory granules, some of which fuse with the plasma membrane after an appropriate secretory stimulus and release their content into the extracellular space. If one assumes a daily insulin dose of 40 IU it can be estimated that 10^{12} insulin secretory granules are needed each day to meet the physiological demand [34]. These granules display characteristic crystalline inclusions consisting of insulin crystals made up of zinc–insulin hexamers (Figure 2b). In addition, secretory granules contain calcium, adenine nucleotides, biogenic amines and enzymes [203]. Most endocrine cells, including B cells, have been found to contain chromogranin A, an acidic 48 kDa protein containing a sequence homology to the putative peptide hormone pancreastatin [35]. Also present in B-cell secretory granules is IAPP, a 37-amino acid peptide with a 46% sequence homology to calcitonin gene-related peptide (CGRP) [36]. The function of both chromogranin A and IAPP is unknown, although the former is suggested to represent a prohormone that may give rise to other biologically active peptides in the B cell, such as pancreastatin and betagranin [37], while the latter is primarily known for its fibril-forming capability which may lead to islet amyloidosis in type 2 diabetes (see section on type 2 diabetes, below).

D Cell

The D cell (5–10% v/v) secretes somatostatin, formerly called somatotropin release inhibiting factor (SRIF), first isolated from the hypothalamus in 1973 [38] and later immunocytochemically located in the pancreatic D cell [39]. The hormone is a potent inhibitor of both insulin and glucagon secretion and exists in both a 14 (S14) and a 28 (S28) amino acid form [40]. D cells may form long, slender cell processes that end with a knob-like structure in the pericapillary space; these structures are rich in secretory granules, suggesting a localized secretion [41].

PP Cells

Although it is the major endocrine cell type in the ventrally derived pancreatic lobule, the function of the pancreatic polypeptide-containing PP cell (15–25% v/v) is relatively poorly understood. The peptide has been found immunocytochemically in two morphologically distinct cell types: PP immunoreactive cells (formerly designated as F cells), characterized by round to angular secretory granules, were found in the ventrally derived head of the pancreas, while cells with small granules, formerly called D_1 cells, were found in the dorsally derived part.

Islet Anatomy

Human islets of Langerhans are not uniformly sized: their distribution resembles an inverse Gauss curve with a mean value of 140 μm and a maximum diameter of 250 μm [2]. Traditionally, the islets are considered to be more frequent in the tail of the pancreas (adjoining the spleen) than in the duodenal part of the gland [42]. Precise morphometric studies using immunocytochemical staining for islet hormones failed to corroborate this; in contrast, these studies suggest a higher relative endocrine mass in the ventrally derived posterior head (PP-rich part) than in the A-cell-rich dorsal part of the pancreas [4, 14].

In non-human species, islets of Langerhans are characterized by a precise localization of the endocrine cell types: in rodents a core of B cells is surrounded by a mantle of A, D and PP cells, while in monkey, cat and horse the reverse situation is true and a core of non-B cells is surrounded by a mantle of B cells [43]. Although in neonatal human islets a rodent-type organization can be observed [44], this pattern is less evident in the adult organ (Figure 3). Careful three-dimensional reconstructions [41, 45] have shown that the human islet consists of one continuous B-cell mass, part of which is in direct contact with non-B cells, while other B cells only contact homologous cells. Such a topography resembles the situation found in experimental animals and supports the hypothesis of a functional subdivision of the islet based on paracrine, endocrine or junctional interactions [46, 49, 227].

A functional heterogeneity within the islet of Langerhans is not only based on topographical data: it has long since been accepted that marked differences in granulation exist between B cells within the same islet [42]. Long-term stimulation of insulin release in rodents has shown a stronger degranulation of B cells located in the islet center than in the islet periphery [47]. Moreover, B cells appear markedly heterogeneous in their expression of several key enzymes like glucokinase [225] as well as in their response to glucose. Electrophysiologic, metabolic and biosynthetic studies have indicated a differential glucose sensitivity of individual B cells, each cell becoming active above an individual glucose threshold value [48, 49, 223, 224].

The topography and relative frequency of islet cells is not identical for all parts of the gland. The posterior part of the pancreatic head contains islets with a cellular composition that differs from those in the rest of the gland. As the posterior head is derived from the ventral pancreatic primordium, and the anterior head, body and tail from the dorsal primordium, the different cellular

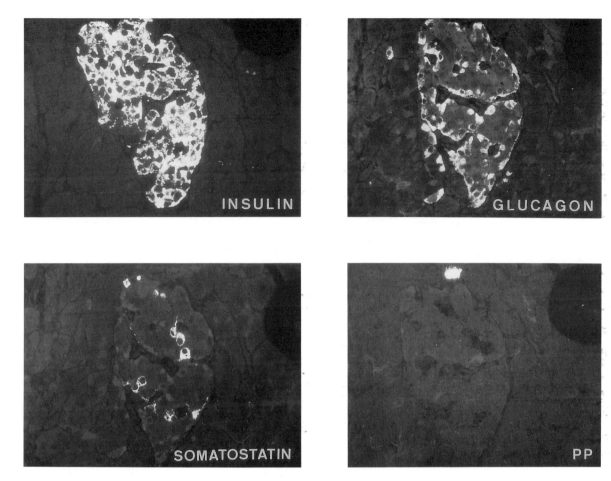

Figure 3 Human islet of Langerhans from the dorsal pancreatic lobe: consecutive 1 μm plastic sections stained for the four pancreatic hormones (×310)

composition of the islets seems to have its basis in a different ontogeny. Ventral islets are reported to contain up to 80% PP cells and <0.5% A cells, whereas dorsal islets contain 15–20% A cells and <0.5% PP cells [50, 51]. The endocrine pancreas is thus found to contain both PP-rich and glucagon-rich islets that may be characterized by different secretory characteristics. In spite of the relatively small size of the ventral pancreas (5–15% of the total gland), its high content of PP cells results in an overall frequency of this cell type, in the total gland, of 15–25% of the endocrine volume (Table 1).

Blood Flow in the Islets

The ventrally derived part of the pancreas is drained of exocrine secretions by the duct of Santorini and is supplied with blood via the superior mesenteric artery. The dorsally derived part is drained by the duct of Wirsung and irrigated by the coeliac artery. Islets are directly supplied with arterial blood via one or more arterioles that branch into a dense capillary network within the islets. Capillaries either directly fuse into venules, which ultimately drain into the portal vein, or first leave the islet and pass through the exocrine tissue [222]. Anastomoses therefore exist between the blood supply to the exocrine part of the gland and the endocrine pancreas, permitting exposure of the peri-insular exocrine tissue to pancreatic hormones.

In comparison to the exocrine component of the gland, islets receive 5–10 times more blood per volume of tissue [52]. This is caused by the large number of capillaries per volume of B cells; in vascular casts of the pancreas, islets of Langerhans are easily recognized as dense capillary clusters. The large number of blood vessels results in a topography in which B cells are often bordered by two or more capillaries [53] (Figure 4). Polarity of B cells has been described, with most secretory granules located near the apical pole of the cell bordered by one of the capillaries [226]. The endothelial cells lining these capillaries are characterized by numerous 95-nm fenestrations closed by a diaphragm and arranged in sieve-plates. The structure of the diaphragm closing the fenestration appears to be

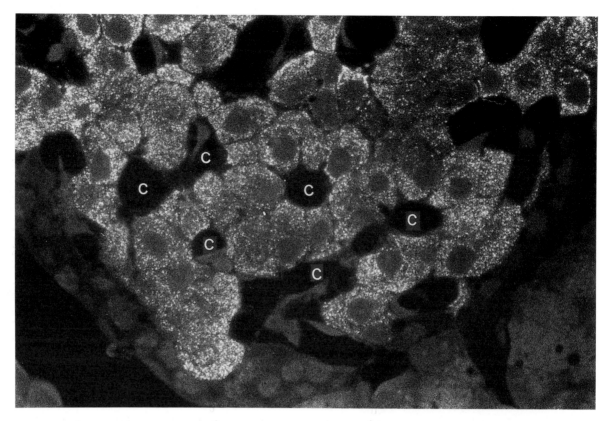

Figure 4   Immunofluorescent staining for insulin on a 1 μm plastic section from a perfusion-fixed rat islet illustrating the dense capillary network within the islet. Individual B cells are often bordered by two capillaries (×1000)

such that small molecules pass unhindered but large serum proteins are stopped [54]. Fenestrated endothelial cells may be found in many endocrine organs and presumably mediate a fast exchange of metabolites and hormones between blood and intracellular space.

The islet capillaries are separated from the endocrine cells by a double basement membrane composed of collagen fibers. In general the B-cell surface adjoining the capillaries is devoid of microvilli, but a limited number of villi are located at sites where neighboring B cells and capillaries meet, forming a network resembling canaliculi [55]. It has been suggested that these canaliculi are preferential sites of exocytosis, the microvilli resulting from excess membrane inserted through the fusion of secretory vesicles with the plasma membrane.

Two models for the direction of blood flow within the islet exist: according to the model of Fujita [56], the afferent arteries branch in the non-B cell zone before reaching the B cells. This model is based on the observation that in species where a central core of B cells is surrounded by a mantle of non-B cells the arterioles branch in the islet periphery, whereas in species in which a core of non-B cells is surrounded by a mantle of B cells, the reverse situation is found

and the arterioles branch in the islet center. In the currently favored alternative model of Bonner-Weir and Orci [57] it is proposed that arterioles enter the islets, and give off branches, in areas of the islet periphery devoid of non-B cells (in the case of a B-cell core type islet). The afferent vessels would thus branch in the B-cell zone and subsequently irrigate the A, D and PP cells. The major difference between these two models is that, in the former, islet B cells would be exposed to the secretory products of the non-B cells, secretory products that have been shown to alter B-cell function [58], whereas in the second model they would only be exposed to such secretory products after their passage through the liver and the general circulation. It should be noted that the two models outlined above are based upon studies in experimental animals in which the various islet cell types have a clear topography. The situation in the human islets, with their much less evident topographical distribution, may be quite different. Moreover, light-microscopy studies *in vivo* of the islet blood flow have suggested that flow in islet capillaries displays a marked temporal and directional variability [53], complicating any model based on histological data alone.

Innervation

The islets of Langerhans are innervated by both sympathetic and parasympathetic nerve fibers, consisting of adrenergic, cholinergic and peptidergic neurons entering the islet alongside the blood vessels. The sympathetic fibers of the splanchnic nerve synapse outside the pancreas on adrenergic ganglion cells located either in the celiac ganglion, when innervating the dorsal pancreas, or in the superior mesenteric ganglion, when innervating the ventral pancreas. In contrast, the parasympathetic fibers of the vagus nerve synapse on intrapancreatic cholinergic ganglion cells. Peptidergic neurons are found in both sympathetic and parasympathetic fibers, while peptidergic ganglion cells are present within the pancreatic gland. The peptidergic neurons contain vasoactive intestinal peptide (VIP), galanin or cholecystokinin-like immunoreactivity; these peptides are reported to alter B-cell function [59, 60]. None of the three classes of neurons mentioned above has synapses on endocrine cells. Most nerve fibers end blindly in the pericapillary space or near the endocrine cell surface. Cholinergic fibers have been reported to show a preferential islet topography forming a peri-insular network and a preferential association with A cells. However, the three types of neurons do not appear to be associated with only one particular cell type [61–63]. All intrapancreatic neuronal fibers are accompanied by non-myelinating Schwann cells, which also appear to encapsulate the whole islet with thin sheets of cellular processes [64].

Non-endocrine Islet Cells

Apart from endothelial cells, neurons and Schwann cells, islets of Langerhans contain approximately 1% of other cell types. Among them are monocytic cells with a small, elongated cell body and long, branching cellular processes. These dendritic cells present major histocompatibility complex (MHC) class II molecules on their cell surfaces and are thought to play a role in the immune response through phagocytosis and antigen presentation [205]. They are thought to correspond to the 'passenger leukocytes' of transplantation biology, involved in the initiation of graft rejection.

DIABETES-RELATED ISLET CHANGES

Diabetes Classification and Islet Morphology

The current classification of diabetes considers the clinical, genetic and immunological heterogeneity of the disease and distinguishes on this basis between insulin dependent type 1 diabetes (IDDM), non-insulin dependent type 2 diabetes (NIDDM), diabetes secondary to pancreatic diseases and hormone overproduction, and gestational diabetes [65] (see also Chapter 1). The heterogeneous islet lesions observed in the diabetic pancreas confirm the heterogeneity of the disease. From a morphological point of view, the islet changes associated with the various types of diabetes can be divided into those with and those without severe (to absolute) B-cell loss. While severe B-cell loss is found in type 1 diabetes and some uncommon forms of diabetes such as virus-related diabetes and congenital diabetes, islets without a severe loss of B cells are encountered in type 2 diabetes and in the secondary forms of diabetes.

Classic Type 1 Diabetes

Macroscopy

Pancreases from patients with recent onset type 1 diabetes (duration less than 1 year) are normal in appearance, size and weight [66–68]. Occasionally, diabetic ketoacidotic coma may be complicated by acute pancreatitis [69], probably resulting from circulatory failure.

Patients with chronic type 1 diabetes display a considerable reduction in weight and volume of the pancreas [4, 66, 70, 71] (Figure 5). This volume reduction results from severe atrophy of the acinar cells (Figure 6), involving either the whole gland [71] or only the part poor in PP cells [72]. Pancreatic atrophy is attributed to the lack of trophic effect of insulin on the acinar cells [68, 73, 74]; its extent, however, varies considerably from patient to patient. Correlations between the number of surviving insulin cells in these pancreases, duration of diabetes, age at onset of the disease or degree of microangiopathy, do not seem to exist [71].

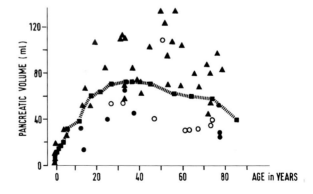

Figure 5 Volume of the pancreas in 18 patients with chronic type 1 diabetes (○ insulin negative. ● insulin positive) compared with that of 45 control subjects (▲) and the means in 600 non-diabetic subjects according to Rössle (from reference 71, with permission of Springer-Verlag)

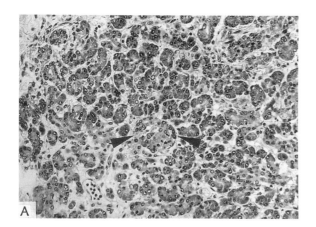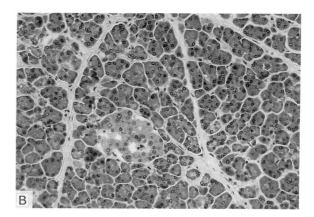

Figure 6   Severe atrophy of the pancreatic acinar cells in long-lasting type 1 diabetes (A) compared with acinar cell morphology of a normal pancreas (B). Note also the islet with small cells and blurred outlines (arrows) in the diabetic pancreas and the well-demarcated islet in the normal pancreas. H&E (×175)

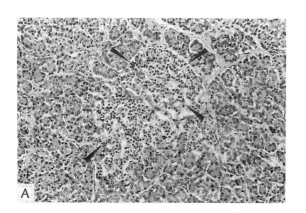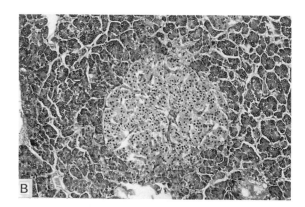

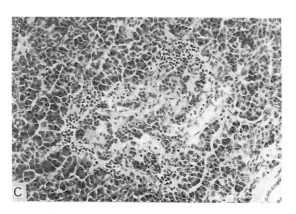

Figure 7   Islet changes in type 1 diabetes of recent onset. (A) Islet with small cells and irregular outlines (arrows): this so-called pseudoatrophic islet is always insulin deficient. (B) Normal-appearing islet: this islet type always contains B cells. (C) Islet showing insulitis; insulitis islets still contain B-cells. H&E (×90)

Microscopy

In pancreases of patients dying of recent onset type 1 diabetes, the majority of islets have lost their B cells and contain only A, D and some rare PP cells

[66–68, 75] (Figure 7A). In a minority of islets, however, B cells and non-B cells are still present in the usual numbers (Figure 7B). Occasionally, the B cells of these islets may show nuclear hypertrophy and sparse granulation. The key finding of type 1 diabetes of short clinical duration, a lymphocytic peri-insular and intrainsular infiltrate termed insulitis [66, 76], is usually restricted to individual islets (Figure 7C). The islet infiltrate consists primarily of T lymphocytes with only sparse B lymphocytes and macrophages [77]. As a rule, insulitis affects only islets that still contain B cells. It is usually seen in individuals younger than 15 years [68, 69, 75, 78, 234] and is particularly common in very young diabetics. Insulitis is infrequent in the pancreas of diabetics with longer than 6–12 months survival [234], but in exceptional cases it may be observed up to 6 years after diagnosis [75]. Insulin-immunoreactive islets are unevenly distributed in the pancreas, but may be confined to individual lobules (Figure 8).

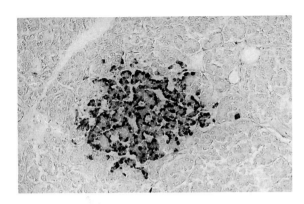

Figure 9 Chronic type 1 diabetes: insulin-deficient islet immunostained for glucagon. Note the relative hyperplasia of A (glucagon) cells (×175)

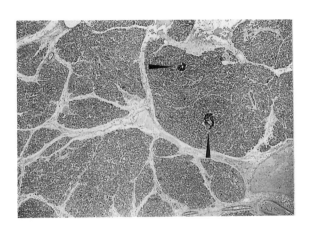

Figure 8 Insulin-positive islets in recent onset type 1 diabetes, restricted to one lobule of the pancreas (arrows). Immunostaining for insulin (×25)

Quantitative evaluation of the immunocytochemically stained islet tissue reveals a reduction in total B-cell volume to about one-third to one-seventh of that of non-diabetics [67, 234].

In chronic type 1 diabetes with a duration of more than one year, islets are often difficult to recognize in routinely stained sections. This is due to their irregular outlines and the small size of their cells, which can barely be distinguished from the atrophic acinar cells (Figure 6). Immunocytochemistry and electron microscopy reveal that the vast majority of islets are devoid of B cells and consist almost entirely of A and D cells (Figure 9) or, within the PP lobe, of PP cells [67, 79]. Quantitatively, these changes result in a relative hyperplasia of the non-B cells. An absolute hyperplasia of D cells, as has been suggested [80], seems not to occur. PP cells can be more numerous than normal, but the extreme PP cell hyperplasia that has been reported in type 1 diabetics [81] is most probably related to the subsequently reported uneven

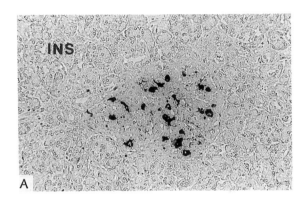

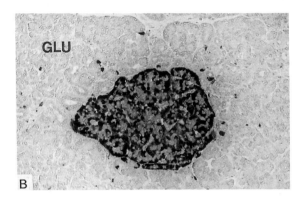

Figure 10 Chronic type 1 diabetes of 21 years duration: few surviving B (insulin) cells in an islet with relative hyperplasia of A cells. Immunostaining for insulin (INS) and glucagon (GLU) (×170)

distribution of PP cells in the pancreas [51] and not to diabetes itself. It is now also known that, in a number of patients, insulin cells do not disappear completely [4, 82] (Figure 10), but are still present in most patients with a disease duration of less than 10 years, and in about 40% of patients with a disease duration between 11 and 40 years [71]. There appears to be no clear correlation between the age at onset of diabetes and survival of insulin cells.

Islet amyloidosis is also an exceptional finding in type 1 diabetics [78], because the formation of islet amyloid requires insulin-producing cells (see type 2 diabetes). Islet calcification or fibrosis are equally rare lesions [83]. Mitosis, as an unequivocal sign of cell replication and regeneration, has not been observed in surviving B cells of type 1 diabetics.

All acinar cells show considerable atrophy. The perilobular spaces, and to some degree also the interacinar spaces, are enlarged and contain loosely arranged connective tissue. In some cases, fibrosis of the exocrine tissue is associated with a sparse and unevenly distributed lymphocytic infiltration [71, 75]. The large arteries are often affected by arteriosclerosis, while the small arterial vessels show diabetic microangiopathy.

Etiology and Pathogenesis

Insulitis and selective loss of B cells are pathognomonic of type 1 diabetes [66, 75, 234]. The largely lymphocytic nature of insulitis, its restriction to islets still containing B cells, and the lack of correlation between extent of insulitis and clinical severity of the disease [234] suggest an autoimmune process gradually destroying the insulin-producing cells of the pancreas.

Other findings lending support to the autoimmune theory of B-cell destruction are:

(1) demonstration of autoantibodies to islet cells (ICA, islet cell antibodies; ICSA, islet cell surface antibodies), insulin (IAA, insulin autoantibodies) and the GABA-synthesizing enzyme glutamic acid decarboxylase of the B-cells (64 K autoantigen) which can be present for several years before clinical onset of diabetes [84, 85, 209–211];

(2) association of type 1 diabetes with some well-known autoimmune diseases such as Hashimoto's thyroiditis, idiopathic Addison's disease, and pernicious anemia [86–88];

(3) recurrence of insulitis in pancreatic isografts from HLA-identical donors in pancreas-transplanted patients with longstanding type 1 diabetes [89];

(4) experimental production of insulitis by active immunization of rabbits (Figure 11A), cows or sheep against homologous or heterologous insulin [90];

(5) immune-related B-cell destruction in BB rats (Figure 11B) [91] and NOD mice [92] which serve as models for human type 1 diabetes.

The mechanisms and factors initiating autoimmune responses towards B cells are still obscure. However, it

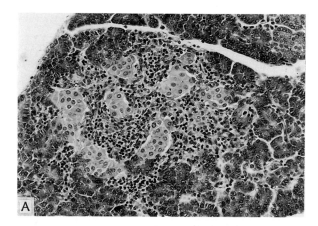

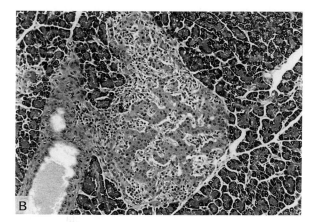

Figure 11 Experimental insulitis. (A) Lymphoid cellular insulitis in a rabbit immunized with insulin and Freund's adjuvant. (B) Insulitis consisting of macrophages and lymphocytes in a BB rat aged 65 days H&E (×85)

can be postulated that there is a B-cell specific protein which, for yet unknown reasons, acquires autoantigenic properties and eventually becomes the target for the autoimmune reaction. According to the hypothesis of Bottazzo and Foulis, autoimmune destruction is initiated by aberrant expression of class II MHC molecules on B cells, which would then allow the presentation of self or altered-self antigens to T-helper lymphocytes [93]. This assumption has been based on the immunocytochemical demonstration of class II MHC expression on insulin-containing cells in patients with recent onset type 1 diabetes [77, 94], an observation which has still to be confirmed [234]. In light microscopy, the cells staining for insulin and HLA-DR did not appear to represent HLA-DR-positive monocytes engulfing remnants of damaged B cells, a finding recently described in experimental animals [95], but showed the features of endocrine cells. No HLA-DR immunoreactivity was found on B cells of pancreases from patients with chronic type 1 diabetes of more than 4 years [71], type 2 diabetes, chronic pancreatitis, cystic fibrosis, graft-versus-host disease, and Coxsackie B viral pancreatitis [77]. Because of the almost exclusive expression of class II MHC in islets that were unaffected by insulitis, the epithelial expression of class II MHC (epitopes) is thought to precede the stage in which heavy lymphocytic infiltration of the islets occurs. Thus class II MHC expression appears not to be secondary to the secretion of lymphokines such as γ-interferon and tumour necrosis factor by inflammatory cells.

In addition to class II MHC, the same islets, i.e. islets with no evidence of insulitis, were found to hyperexpress class I MHC [96], which is normally involved in antigen presentation to cytotoxic T lymphocytes. However, in contrast to the findings with class II MHC, hyperexpression of class I MHC involved not only the B cells but also the adjacent A and D cells. In addition, all the islet cells hyperexpressing class I MHC also stained for immunoreactive α-interferon [97], a lymphokine that can cause the hyperexpression of class I MHC on B cells *in vitro*.

On the basis of these findings, Foulis proposed a tentative sequence of events leading to autoimmune B-cell destruction [98]. One of the earliest events in type 1 diabetes may be a process that induces α-interferon secretion from B cells, thereby causing these B cells and the adjacent non-B cells to hyperexpress class I MHC. In a second stage, the same process might then initiate aberrant class II MHC expression on some B cells and/or insulitis. Finally, class II MHC-positive B cells presenting a specific antigen undergo apoptotic destruction by autoreactive T lymphocytes and macrophages. Once initiated, this process may also involve B cells not expressing class II MHC. This latter assumption is needed as class II MHC expression was not seen on B cells in transplanted pancreas isografts, affected and destroyed by insulitis within weeks after transplantation to diabetics with longstanding type 1 diabetes [89]. On the other hand, there are, presumably, mechanisms that protect B cells from immune-mediated destruction, as surviving insulin-producing and insulin-secreting cells were detected in up to 40% of patients with longstanding type 1 diabetes, even decades after disease onset [71, 99].

If an autoimmune mechanism accounts for the selective B-cell loss in type 1 diabetes, what is its cause? Is it of infectious or genetic origin, or both? Studies in monozygotic twins with type 1 diabetes revealed that genetic factors may not be the only cause of type 1 diabetes: half the twin pairs were found to be discordant (i.e. only one twin diabetic) and remained so throughout their life [100]. This stresses the important role of environmental factors in the pathogenesis of type 1 diabetes. Toxic drugs and viral infections have been implicated in the origin of type 1

diabetes; although drugs may be rare causes, viruses seem more likely to be involved. Foulis observed that pancreases affected by viral (Coxsackie B) pancreatitis contained α-interferon positive B cells [97]. As none of the other pancreases examined (including those from patients with chronic pancreatitis, type 2 diabetes and graft-versus-host disease) contained α-interferon positive B cells, viral infections of B cells may be a possible trigger for a specific autoimmune reaction. Further and earlier indications of such a concept are the temporal relationships between common childhood viral infections (such as mumps, rubella, cytomegalovirus and Coxsackie B) and the subsequent development of diabetes [101], and the experimental production of B-cell necrosis, insulitis and diabetes in mice infected with EMC virus [102]. In addition, Coxsackie B virus infections have been demonstrated in children dying in ketoacidotic coma and displaying insulitis [103, 104]. However, review of the pancreatic pathology of Yoon's and Gladisch's cases by Gepts has revealed that they showed the altered islet-cell composition typical of type 1 diabetes. As these are long-term changes, and as these patients had an encephalitis and myocarditis in addition to diabetes, a Coxsackie B infection was probably superimposed on a classic type 1 diabetes. If viruses or other environmental factors have a decisive role in the initiation of type 1 diabetes, they must affect the B cells as non-cytopathic agents long before the clinical onset of the disease [212].

A prerequisite of a diabetes-inducing viral interaction with pancreatic B cells may be a specific immunogenetic environment. From experimental EMC virus infection it is obvious that diabetes develops only in certain strains of mice [105]. In humans, susceptibility to type 1 diabetes is closely linked to the HLA antigens DR3 and/or DR4 [106, 107] and more specifically to certain DR4 haplotypes in association with DQw8. As the D region of the HLA complex on chromosome 6 contains immune response genes that may facilitate immune responses against autoantigens, it is conceivable that an individual who possesses such genes would be at great risk of developing autoimmune diabetes.

In summary, the classic type 1 diabetes appears to be an autoimmune-mediated process determined by defects in immune regulatory genes and triggered by environmental factors. These mechanisms in concert lead to a gradual B-cell loss, that becomes clinically manifest only when the B-cell mass is reduced to a critical point in terms of metabolic compensation [67] and when, in addition, B-cell function is overstressed by an incidental event such as an infection. The presence of ICA has been used to predict the onset of type 1 diabetes and to estimate its preclinical period [108]. However, the time-course of this autoimmune phenomenon (ICA have even disappeared from some subjects in long-term trials [109]), the nature of the antigens recognized by ICA [110], their role in the disease process and their relation to B-cell destruction are not well understood [84]. This is also the case for the other autoantibodies, including the autoantibody directed against the enzyme glutamic acid decarboxylase (64K autoantigen) which synthesizes the neuroendocrine transmitter GABA [211].

Late-onset Type 1 Diabetes

Patients with late-onset diabetes and progressive deterioration of B-cell function frequently exhibit the immunological and genetic characteristics of classic type 1 diabetes, i.e. ICA and HLA-DR3/DR4 [111, 112]. Among these patients are those who suffer from polyendocrinopathy [113]. Diabetes associated with polyglandular autoimmunity occurs preferentially in middle-aged women, is strongly related to HLA-DR3 only and has an insidious clinical onset and persisting islet cell antibodies [114, 115]. In this diabetes type, histological changes have been described similar to those in classic type 1 diabetes [87, 88, 116, 117]. In addition, the same abnormalities of MHC expression have been documented [87]. The only difference with respect to the MHC expression seems to be a quantitative one, as fewer islets were found to be affected than in classic type 1 diabetes. This finding is compatible with the slow clinical evolution of the late onset type 1 diabetes.

Islet Lesions in Pancreas Grafts

The pathology of pancreas grafts transplanted to type 1 diabetics is complex and differs from one patient to another [118]. The morphological abnormalities include infarction, pancreatitis, rejection, CMV infection and insulitis. Inflammatory infiltration of the islets, mainly consisting of T8 lymphocytes and macrophages, was noted in 25% of the grafts [118]. Whether this form of insulitis was due to rejection or to recurrent type 1 diabetes, was difficult to decide. The most intense insulitis with evidence of selective B-cell loss (and class I MHC expression on islet cells) was observed in the grafts of HLA-identical recipients [89, 118]. In these patients recurrent diabetes was therefore thought to be the consequence of the destruction of the B cells due to an anamnestic cytotoxic T-lymphocyte-mediated autoimmune response. However, graft dysfunction was also noted in patients without signs of acute rejection or islet damage. The pathophysiology of the recurrent diabetes in these patients remains to be explained.

Type 2 Diabetes

Macroscopy

There are no gross abnormalities of the pancreas—qualitative or quantitative—that are specific for type 2 diabetes.

Microscopy

Qualitatively, the islets of type 2 diabetics are either indistinguishable from those of non-diabetics or show islet amyloidosis. Other changes, such as islet fibrosis or B-cell degranulation and hydropic degeneration, are unspecific. Islet fibrosis is more closely related to pancreatic fibrosis than to diabetes.

Immunocytochemically, the islets in type 2 diabetes (unlike those in type 1) always contain B cells in regular distribution and in considerable numbers. Significant B-cell degranulation is lacking and can only be observed in patients dying in diabetic coma with sustained high glucose levels. In these patients, the B cells also display hydropic change of the cytoplasm due to glycogen accumulation (Figure 12), a reversible lesion that can be experimentally produced by prolonged hyperglycemia [119, 120]. Ever since diabetes has been treated with insulin, hydropic degeneration of B cells has been a rare lesion.

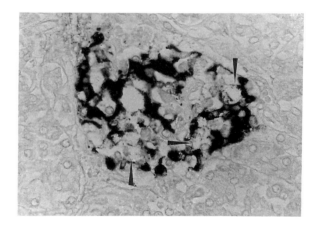

Figure 12   Islets of type 2 diabetic dying in diabetic coma with long-lasting hyperglycemia. Apart from well-granulated B cells there are degranulated B cells with hydropic transformation of the cytoplasm (arrows). Immunostaining for insulin (×170)

Islet amyloidosis (islet hyalinization) is a form of localized amyloidosis restricted to the islets [121]. It is not specific to diabetes, because it has also been observed in subjects who did not suffer from overt diabetes [122]. However, it is far more frequent and usually also more severe in type 2 diabetics than non-diabetics [123, 124]. In addition, there is an even more marked relationship with the age of the patients [125]: whereas in patients younger than 50 years amyloidosis is uncommon, it affects about 80% of diabetics older than 60 years [126, 213].

Islet amyloid occurs only in islets containing insulin-producing cells. Here it is deposited between the capillaries and the endocrine cells (Figure 13). It stains brightly with thioflavin T, but weakly with Congo red. Electron-microscopic studies have shown that amyloid consists of thin, branching fibrils with a diameter of 7.5–10 nm, which run into deep plasma-membrane pockets of the B cells [127]. Recently, it was found that the major constituent of the amyloid fibrils is a previously unknown peptide, designated islet amyloid polypeptide (IAPP) [128, 204] or amylin [129] (Figure 14). Immunocytochemically, IAPP has also been demonstrated in normal B-cell secretory granules [36]. Islet amyloidosis affects the islets unevenly and in only a small percentage of patients are all islets involved; in these patients, amyloidosis may be

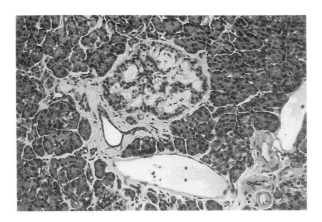

Figure 13 Islet amyloidosis. Perisinusoidal deposits of amyloid replacing endocrine cells H&E (×180)

associated with a reduced islet volume [130]. There is no relation between islet amyloidosis and the presence of human megalovirus which was demonstrated in

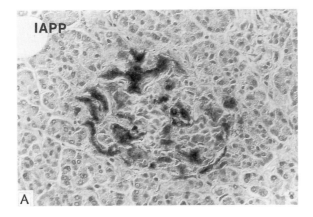

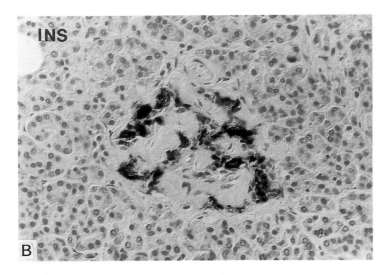

Figure 14 Islet amyloidosis. (A) Islet amyloid immunostained with antiserum to islet amyloid polypeptide (IAPP): the antiserum against IAPP was a gift of Dr Per Westermark. (B) Islet with amyloid immunostained for insulin (INS) (×110)

the pancreas of about half of patients with type 2 diabetes [231].

Quantitative data on the number and total area of islets in pancreases of type 2 diabetics indicate a range from normal to a distinct reduction [131, 132] (Figure 15). Similar findings have emerged from studies using immunocytochemistry combined with morphometry [4, 14, 133]. Although there is a marked overlap of the data in diabetics with the findings in non-diabetics, a mean decrease up to the order of 50% may be found. This variability of the quantitative changes of the endocrine pancreas in type 2 diabetes has been interpreted as being due to the obvious heterogeneity of the disease, because it includes patients differing in age, disease duration, weight and B-cell function.

In our own pilot study in obese and non-obese subjects with or without diabetes, obese non-diabetics were found to have a greater pancreatic parenchymal volume and islet volume than non-obese non-diabetics [134]. Diabetics showed a decrease in pancreatic parenchymal volume and endocrine tissue volume. This was much more pronounced in lean patients than in obese patients. With respect to the non-diabetics, these findings seemed to confirm Ogilvie's study reported over 55 years earlier [135], in which obese subjects were found to have a greater percentage of islet tissue and a greater islet size than controls. However, these preliminary results could not be confirmed in a larger study which correlated the quantitative data of 71 subjects to five clinical parameters: obesity, age, sex, disease duration and type of therapy (Klöppel G, Bergström B and Löhr M: unpublished observations). In this investigation, which was based on computerized morphometric evaluation of immunostained sections and statistically analysed with the test of variance and co-variance, obesity lacked any clear association with an increased B-cell volume, either in diabetics or non-diabetics (Table 2). However, the study revealed that patients who had received insulin showed a significantly ($P < 0.045$) lower endocrine cell volume (mean 0.67 ml), and especially B-cell volume (mean 0.41 ml, $P < 0.0027$), than those treated with oral compounds and diet (mean endocrine cell volume 0.81 ml, mean B-cell volume 0.52 ml) or diet alone

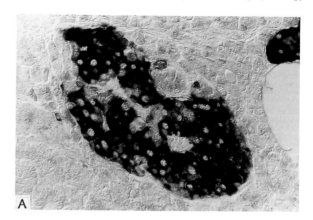

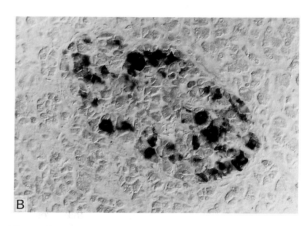

Figure 15 Type 2 diabetes. (A) Islet with normal B-cell content. (B) Islet with distinctly reduced B-cell number. Immunostaining for insulin ($\times 170$)

(mean endocrine cell volume 1.26 ml, mean B-cell volume 0.8 ml). Sex, age, body weight and disease duration had no significant effect on these variables. This suggests that the B-cell failure of those type 2 diabetics who have to be treated with insulin therapy is, at least in part, due to a decreased B-cell volume (see below). As the patients in our retrospective study were not checked regarding their HLA-DR and ICA status, the possibility cannot be excluded that some of the patients who were treated with insulin represented late onset type 1 diabetics [111]. However, as the observed B-cell reduction in these patients did not exceed the

Table 2   Results of pancreatic morphometry in obese and non-obese diabetics and non-diabetic controls

	Body weight (kg)	Pancreatic volume* (ml)	Parenchymal volume (%)	B-cell volume (ml)
Normal weight non-diabetics ($n = 17$)	61.2 ± 10.0	79.3 ± 16.6	70.8 ± 14.0	0.737 ± 0.478
Obese non-diabetics ($n = 7$)	77.0 ± 15.4	108.7 ± 24.6	77.4 ± 8.9	0.592 ± 0.461
Normal weight type 2 diabetics ($n = 31$)	61.7 ± 8.8	86.7 ± 29.3	65.4 ± 12.8	0.516 ± 0.321
Obese type 2 diabetics ($n = 16$)	74.5 ± 11.9	91.6 ± 34.2	55.9 ± 13.2	0.549 ± 0.477

Morphometry was done by measuring the immunostained area with a computerized device (Zeiss Vidas 2). The stereological data are calculated according to the principles of Weibel.
*The volume of the PP lobe amounting to 10% of the total pancreatic volume was excluded.

50% reduction that is characteristically seen in type 1 diabetics (even in those with late onset type 1 diabetes), it is likely that all these patients had type 2 diabetes.

Etiology and Pathogenesis

Type 2 diabetes mellitus or NIDDM is a complex disease of the endocrine pancreas and the insulin-requiring tissues, which is caused by endogenous factors as well as environmental influences.

In contrast to type 1 diabetes mellitus (IDDM), there is no association with autoimmune phenomena and certain HLA antigens in type 2 diabetes. Moreover, even in type 2 diabetic subjects with long-standing and severe disease the islets are never devoid of B cells, although the B-cell mass may be reduced to one-half the average value of non-diabetic subjects. Consequently, these patients always have some endogenous insulin production and thus never develop an absolute insulin deficiency. This raises the question why the patients' endogenous insulin production is insufficient to maintain normoglycemia.

The most relevant factors which seem to play a key role in the pathogenesis of type 2 diabetes are a positive family history, obesity-associated insulin resistance and impaired B-cell function [136]. This is discussed in detail in Chapters 7 and 8.

Obesity is the most important factor that promotes the manifestation of type 2 diabetes. Population-based studies have shown that obese subjects have a greater incidence of diabetes and countries with the greatest prevalence of obesity have the highest incidence of the disease. Type 2 diabetes is therefore a disease of the 'developed' countries and is rare in developing countries. This strong influence of obesity on the manifestation of diabetes is best explained by the fact that weight gain is associated with a marked reduction in insulin sensitivity (i.e. reduced insulin-mediated glucose uptake by muscle and fat tissues) and a concomitant rise in serum insulin levels [136]. Obesity, however, needs an additional, probably inherited, factor to precipitate diabetes. An attractive hypothesis is that the conditions which lead to insulin resistance, such as obesity or pregnancy, unmask a primary B-cell defect which under normal circumstances would not have occurred.

To date nothing is known about the precise nature of the assumed B-cell defect in type 2 diabetes. Theoretically, B-cell failure could be due to a reduced B-cell mass which is either already present at birth or in the neonatal period, or develops later in life. Alternatively, or in addition, B-cell failure could be the consequence of a programmed abnormality of insulin secretion.

Referring to our morphometric findings in type 2 diabetes, described in the preceding paragraph on the microscopic changes of the endocrine pancreas, it seems that the severity of the B-cell defect correlates with the B-cell volume. Studying the relationship between B-cell volume and such variables as age, duration and type of therapy, we were able to distinguish between two groups of diabetic subjects. The first group comprised diabetic patients whose hyperglycemia was controlled by diet or antidiabetic compounds. These patients were found to have an almost normal or only slightly reduced B-cell volume compared to that of non-diabetic subjects. The second group consisted of patients who had received insulin treatment, suggesting that their insulin secretion was strongly impaired. They showed a significantly reduced B-cell volume approximating 50% of the average value found in non-diabetic subjects. Since in both groups neither the patients' age nor the duration of the disease were significantly correlated with the morphometric data, it is possible that we are dealing with two pathogenetically different populations of type 2 diabetic patients: one, in which diabetes never becomes severe because the only underlying defect which is unmasked by obesity is a functional defect at the level of the B cells [137], and another in which the diabetes, when unmasked by obesity, progresses to insulin dependency because it is based on a structural defect, i.e. a reduction in the number of B cells. The pancreases of type 2 diabetic patients belonging to the second group are probably also those that were found to contain a reduced amount of extractable insulin [138]. Causes or mechanisms leading to a diminished B-cell mass in type 2 diabetic patients are not known. One possibility is an inherited reduced capacity for B-cell replication. This assumption is supported by some animal studies suggesting that the genetic background is of importance for the growth response of B cells to hyperglycemia [139]. Another possibility is a damage to the endocrine pancreas in the fetal or early postnatal period which may result in a diminished B-cell mass throughout life, because the regenerative capacity of the B cell seems to be very limited [140]. The latter assumption fits the 'thrifty phenotype' hypothesis which suggests that poor fetal and early postnatal nutrition results in reduced development of B cells, which therefore later in life are not able to compensate adequately for insulin resistance [141]. Conversely, it has been suggested that sustained hyperglycemia *per se* is toxic to the B cell and thus exacerbates insulin deficiency [142, 143], conceivably through a negative influence not only on B-cell function but also on B-cell replication.

Although a reduction in B-cell mass may have a decisive influence on the severity of type 2 diabetes, it is probably not the sole cause of the disturbed insulin secretion. Considering the enormous variability of the

B-cell mass in non-diabetic subjects [4, 134] and the fact that experimentally more than 80% of a normal pancreas has to be removed in order to induce glucose intolerance [142, 144], it remains doubtful whether a decline in the B-cell mass in the range 10–50% fully explains a severely insufficient insulin secretion. The development of severe type 2 diabetes therefore seems to require not only a significantly reduced B-cell mass but also a separate functional defect of the B cells.

The functional defect of the B cells is characterized by a delayed and diminished insulin secretion in response to glucose. Morphological indications of this functional defect are lack of signs of B-cell hyperactivity, i.e. degranulation and compensatory cell hypertrophy with an enlarged Golgi apparatus [145]. Another finding that also points to a functional abnormality of the B cells in type 2 diabetes is the precipitation of islet amyloid polypeptide (IAPP) [126, 204] or amylin [129] outside the B cells, which leads to islet amyloidosis (see also Chapter 19). IAPP is a 37-amino acid peptide with an approximately 50% homology with human calcitonin gene-related peptide. It is a normal component of B cells in non-diabetic and diabetic humans and animals, which is localized in the secretory granules and co-secreted with insulin [214]. Its effects as a hormone are as yet unclear. In particular, there is no evidence that IAPP acts as a physiologically relevant modulator of insulin secretion or inducer of insulin resistance [228]. No diabetes-associated abnormalities have been identified in the IAPP gene, which is located on the short arm of chromosome 12. In type 2 diabetic subjects, and rarely also in obviously non-diabetic subjects, IAPP forms amyloid fibrils in the B cells and these are then deposited between the B cells and the capillaries. The cause of amyloid formation is not known, but it indicates abnormalities within the cell. Considering the impaired insulin secretion in type 2 diabetes, it seems obvious to relate amyloid deposition to disturbances in the rates of synthesis, conversion and secretion of IAPP which are linked to altered insulin secretion [215]. It is unclear whether the precipitation of amyloid in the islet has in turn an effect on the function of the B cell, because in humans the extent of islet amyloid in the islets is very variable and therefore difficult to correlate to the severity and duration of the disease [213, 214]. However, it has been shown that in some type 2 diabetic patients amyloid deposition may lead to a 30% reduction in the B-cell population [229] and that in monkeys the degree of amyloid formation and the number of islets affected increases with the progression of diabetes [230]. This could suggest that progressive amyloid deposition around islet capillaries impairs islet function by creating a perivascular diffusion barrier that affects glucose recognition and insulin secretion by the B cells.

In summary, it seems that on the background of strong family history two factors are important for the pathogenesis of type 2 diabetes: peripheral insulin resistance, often induced by obesity, and B-cell failure. How these defects relate in the individual patient to islet changes such as reduced B-cell number or deposition of amyloid remains speculative.

Uncommon Forms of Diabetes

Permanent diabetes mellitus in newborns (congenital diabetes) is extremely rare. Except for aplasia of the pancreas (see later), its pathological basis has not been well established. In some cases congenital absence of the islets [146, 147] or of the B cells [148] has been suggested; in other cases the cause has remained entirely obscure [149]. Recently, a novel autoantibody reacting with interstitial tissue antigens of the pancreas has been described in a sibship with permanent neonatal diabetes, who were ICA-negative but HLA-Dw3/4-positive [150].

Foulis and co-workers described 4 children aged 18 months or less (including a female with neonatal diabetes) who died of diabetes, but showed no apparent pancreatic abnormalities [97]. There were no insulin-deficient islets nor was there insulitis. An intact, though somewhat hyperplastic, islet system mainly composed of B cells was also observed in a diabetic aged 22 years with IDDM of 14 years [151]. In addition, a diffuse glomerulosclerosis was present in this patient. The pathogenesis of these special cases of IDDM is still not clear.

Viral infections such as mumps, herpes simplex, cytomegalovirus and varicella have been reported to affect the exocrine pancreas [152, 153]. Acute islet cell damage (varying from clusters of cells with pyknotic nuclei to total islet necrosis) in addition to or without pancreatitis was observed in infants dying of culture-proven Coxsackie virus encephalomyocarditis [97, 153, 154]. In Foulis's series two Coxsackie-affected pancreases showed striking infiltration by eosinophils. As a similar inflammatory pattern in association with a massive and recent B-cell necrosis was also found in the pancreas of a 22-year-old man who died in diabetic coma, this patient's diabetes may also be of viral origin [155].

Diabetes Associated with Pancreatic Diseases

Aplasia

Congenital aplasia of the pancreas is extremely rare [156, 157]. Often it is combined with other malformations such as gallbladder aplasia, diaphragmatic hernia and cardiac defects [158, 159]. The pancreatic parenchyma is replaced by soft tissue, mainly consisting of fatty tissue and nerve fibres. Because of the absence of exocrine and endocrine pancreatic tissue, maldigestion, diabetes and growth retardation are the leading clinical symptoms.

Pancreatitis

In *acute pancreatitis* temporary hyperglycemia may occur, depending on the extent of pancreatic necrosis. Permanent diabetes as a consequence of a single attack of acute pancreatitis is a rare event. Diabetic coma is associated with acute pancreatitis in about 10% of cases [160].

Overt diabetes mellitus as a result of *chronic pancreatitis* is found in about 10–30% of patients, while another 10–30% show impaired glucose tolerance [161]. Higher rates of diabetes are reported when only longstanding chronic pancreatitis with distinct exocrine insufficiency and calcification is considered. In India, as well as in other third world countries, chronic calcifying pancreatitis in adolescents is one of the most frequent causes of diabetes in this age group [162]. Causally, Indian pancreatic fibrosis is most probably related to severe undernutrition.

Chronic pancreatitis, with only focally accentuated perilobular fibrosis, leaves the distribution and architecture of the islets largely unchanged. Distinct qualitative and quantitative changes of the endocrine pancreas occur only in advanced chronic pancreatitis, when the acinar parenchyma is extensively replaced by connective tissue. This entails clustering and embedding of islets in sclerosed tissue [163] (Figure 16A). The islets are of various size and may form 'adenoma-like' complexes. Close to the islets ductular proliferation often develops, occasionally displaying budding-off of endocrine cells from duct cells. When peri-insular fibrosis progresses it is, in most instances, accompanied by insular fibrosis, with distinct perisinusoidal sclerosis [163].

Immunocytochemistry combined with morphometry has revealed that the ratio of A to B cells in the islets entrapped in fibrotic tissue is often changed in favour of the A cells [163]; this suggests a gradual loss of B cells (Figure 16B). In advanced scarring of the pancreatic head there may also be a reduction of PP cells, as in those cases only remnants of PP islets are encountered in the PP lobe. This finding correlates well with an impaired PP secretion observed in these cases [164]. No data are currently available relating to the behaviour of the total endocrine cell volume in severe chronic pancreatitis, but it can be assumed that in advanced scarring of the gland a reduction of the endocrine cell volume may occur. Ultrastructurally, there is no

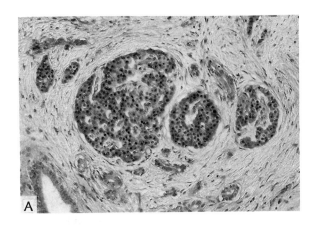

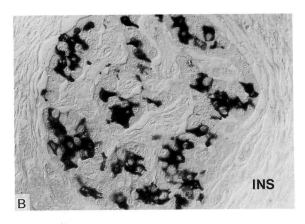

Figure 16 Pancreas in advanced chronic pancreatitis. (A) Clustering and embedding of islets in fibrous tissue. H&E (×90). (B) Islet with B-cell reduction. Immunostaining for insulin (×175)

evidence of cellular damage to the remaining B cells or to other islet cells [163].

The morphological and functional features of chronic pancreatitis suggest that the islet system develops a functional defect, once it has been invaded by fibrotic tissue. As possible causes of this defect, circulatory disturbances due to scarring in connection with functional changes of the entero–insular axis, in particular of gastrin inhibitory peptide secretion under conditions of maldigestion, may be relevant [163, 165]. Another possibility may be that a gradual reduction of the B-cell volume secondary to exocrine tissue loss below a critical value impairs B-cell function and finally leads to overt diabetes.

Pancreatic Carcinoma

Pancreatic carcinoma is frequently associated with diabetes mellitus. This association is best explained by the development of chronic obstructive pancreatitis due to the frequent localization of the tumor in the head of the pancreas where it obstructs the pancreatic duct.

This in turn leads to atrophy and fibrosis of the body and tail of the pancreas and to the same changes of the islet system as in chronic pancreatitis [163]. Impaired insulin secretion in this condition is therefore probably due to factors similar to those operative in chronic pancreatitis. Whether malignancy-related insulin resistance [232], possibly induced by IAPP hypersecretion [233], also plays a role, remains to be clarified.

Cystic Fibrosis

Diabetes mellitus occurring in conjunction with cystic fibrosis used to be rare (1–2%); however, presumably as a consequence of the increasing survival of cystic fibrosis patients, a rising incidence (8–13%) of overt diabetes has been reported in young adults with advanced cystic fibrosis [166, 167]. The clinical and functional features of this type of diabetes are essentially the same as those in chronic pancreatitis. The longstanding duct occlusion by inspissated secretions, with subsequent acinar atrophy, focal fibrosis and lipomatosis, leads to qualitative and quantitative islet changes similar to those in chronic pancreatitis [168–170] (Figure 17). It is therefore concluded that the pathogenesis of these islet changes and of diabetes in cystic fibrosis is the same as in chronic pancreatitis [171, 172].

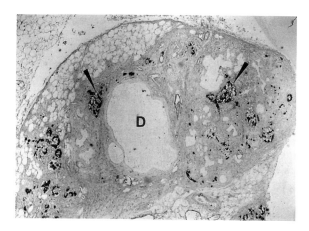

Figure 17 Pancreas in end-stage cystic fibrosis: islets entrapped in fibrous tissue with reduced number of B cells (arrows). Note the dilated duct (D). Immunostaining for insulin (×25)

Diabetes in Hemochromatosis

Diabetes is a well-known feature of primary hemochromatosis, but may also be observed in secondary hemochromatosis [173]. At the onset, this diabetes can often be controlled without insulin; later on, however, it is usually an insulin-dependent diabetes. Iron deprivation or phlebotomy can improve the insulin dependency in some patients. In patients with secondary hemochromatosis due to thalassemia, glucose intolerance correlates with the number of transfusions received. The last two observations emphasize that iron overload has a specific role in hemochromatotic diabetes. Recent immunocytochemical and ultrastructural studies support this view [174]. It was found that iron deposits were restricted to B cells. Moreover, in diabetic patients requiring insulin, iron deposition in B cells was associated with a loss of their insulin granules. This suggests that iron overload of B cells affects insulin biosynthesis, thereby leading to diabetes. As B-cell destruction does not occur, this type of diabetes differs from type 1 diabetes. It remains to be explained how iron interferes with B-cell function and why it does not affect the non-B cells.

Diabetes Associated with Overproduction of Hormones

Hormones with an insulin-antagonistic effect, such as growth hormone, glucocorticoids, catecholamines, thyroxin and glucagon, cause impaired glucose tolerance or even overt diabetes, when produced in excess due to a tumor or hyperplasia of their respective gland of origin [175]. Endocrine syndromes frequently associated with carbohydrate abnormalities of variable intensity are acromegaly, Cushing's syndrome, pheochromocytoma syndrome, glucagonoma syndrome and hyperthyroidism, Conn's syndrome and carcinoid syndrome. Whereas no changes of the islets can be observed in syndromes with mild glucose intolerance and caused by hormones that inhibit insulin secretion, hypertrophic islets with signs of B-cell stimulation may be found in syndromes leading to manifest diabetes due to insulin resistance. This has been observed in some cases of Cushing's disease [126].

Diabetes Associated with Miscellaneous Diseases

The most important syndromes, which are frequently genetically determined, are the syndromes of Prader–Labhart–Willi, Werner, Mauriac, Lawrence–Moon–Biedl–Bardet, the syndrome of optic atrophy combined with diabetes and the diabetes associated with ataxia telangiectasia. Although in some of these syndromes a genetic defect may account for the B-cell insufficiency, in others hyperinsulinism due to insulin insensitivity may be operative. In none of the syndromes have special islet lesions been described [126, 168].

Diabetes mellitus is an integral part of the disease entities termed generalized lipodystrophia and leprechaunism [176]. The syndromes are characterized by hyperinsulinism due to a decrease in insulin receptors. No constant changes of the islet system, in particular no unequivocal evidence of islet hyperplasia, have been reported, except in children with leprechaunism.

Patients with acanthosis nigricans and diabetes can be divided into two categories [177]. In the first group, insulin resistance due to a primary decrease in receptor numbers seems to be the primary event. The other group shows antibodies against the insulin receptor and may develop islet hyperplasia [178].

The high coincidence of cirrhosis and diabetes was established a long time ago (Naunyn's diabetcs) [179]. As possible causes of hepatogenic diabetes, reduced insulin degradation by the cirrhotic liver with subsequent hyperinsulinism and insulin resistance have been suggested [180, 181].

Diabetes due to Chemical Compounds

Two groups of drugs causing glucose intolerance can be distinguished: (a) substances with a cytotoxic effect on B cells, and (b) substances inducing transient hyperglycemia without destruction of B cells. The first group includes alloxan, glyoxal, streptozotocin, oxine, dithizone and recently asparaginase, pentamidine isothionate and *N*-3-pyridylmethyl-*N'*-*p*-nitrophenyl urea (PNU) [182–184]. Diazoxide, diphenylhydantoin, cyproheptadine and mannoheptulose form the second group. The majority of these drugs have been used for the induction of a temporary or permanent diabetic syndrome in laboratory animals [185]. However, some of these compounds serve as therapeutic agents.

The B-cell destructive properties of alloxan and streptozotocin have been used in the treatment of malignant insulinomas and other malignant endocrine tumors. Whereas alloxan appeared to be largely ineffective and showed many side-effects, the successful administration of streptozotocin has been reported in many cases with inoperable pancreatic endocrine tumors. However, there are as yet no observations reported on the effects of streptozotocin on normal human B cells. In animals, streptozotocin, like alloxan [186] (Figure 18), causes B-cell cytolysis within 4–8 hours [187]. This effect is probably attributable to an interaction with protein systems associated with the cell membrane and may be mediated by a depression of nicotinamide adenine dinucleotide (NAD) levels in the B cells. The selective action of streptozotocin on the B cells may be related to the region of the streptozotocin molecule displaying structural similarities to glucose.

Recently, ketotic insulin-requiring diabetes has been reported in several individuals who attempted suicide with rat poison containing PNU [188]. PNU, which is

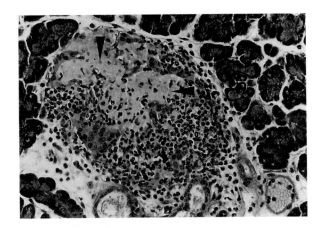

Figure 18 Islet with acute B-cell necrosis (arrows) and polymorphocellular infiltration in alloxan-treated mouse. Aldehyde fuchsin (×170)

structurally related to alloxan and streptozotocin in that it contains a urea group, selectively destroys B cells [189]. Apart from diabetes, PNU induces a severe sensory and mild motor neuropathy.

Diazoxide, diphenylhydantoin, cyproheptadine and mannoheptulose are inhibitors of insulin secretion and partly also of insulin biosynthesis, with a reversible dose-dependent effect [185, 190, 191]. The B cells remain intact, and in the case of diazoxide and diphenylhydantoin, are well granulated, but show crinophagy (Figure 19). Regarding the mechanisms of diazoxide action it seems that they are closely related to sulfonylureas, as sulfonylureas abolish in a dose-dependent manner the diazoxide-induced inhibition of insulin secretion [185].

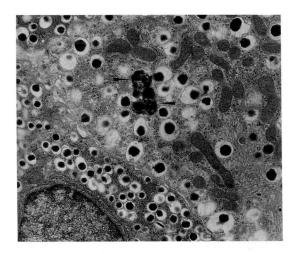

Figure 19 Pancreatic B cell of a mouse with diazoxide-induced hyperglycemia. Cytoplasm shows granulolysis and crinophagy (arrows) (×10 800)

Islet Changes in Embryopathia Diabetica

Infants of mothers with untreated or poorly controlled diabetes have a significantly increased mortality rate due to respiratory distress disease. Moreover, they show other characteristic features such as high birthweight, macrosomia, increased amount of pancreatic endocrine tissue and greater prevalence of congenital malformations.

Pathogenetically, all fetal changes are best explained by the sustained effects of maternal hyperglycemia on fetal tissues. As glucose passively passes through the placenta, the elevated blood glucose levels of the mother stimulate fetal insulin production, thereby causing B-cell hyperplasia and hypertrophy [192]. The insulin released, on the other hand, cannot cross the placenta and thus promotes utilization of glucose in the fetus and, in addition, exerts growth-enhancing anabolic effects. This results in enlargement of the subcutaneous fat depots, in glycogen storage and in hypertrophy of visceral organs. For these reasons, islet volume correlates with birthweight and maternal blood glucose levels [193].

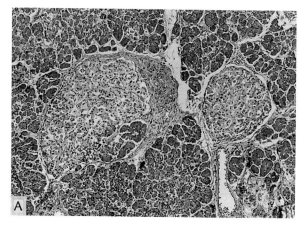

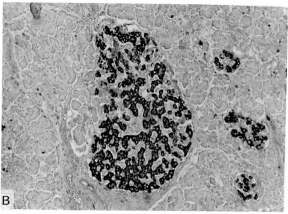

Figure 20 Pancreas of newborn of diabetic mother. (A) Islets with distinct hypertrophy (×25). (B) Hypertrophic islet with B-cell hyperplasia. Immunostaining for insulin (×85)

The gross appearance of the pancreas is normal and its weight unchanged. Histologically, the most conspicuous feature is the increased size of many islets (mean islet diameter 120–180 μm vs. 60–100 μm in controls) [194, 195] (Figure 20A). An increased islet number is not invariably present and seems to be of minor importance as an indicator of maternal diabetes. Quantitatively, the absolute volume may be doubled [193], and this increase is due to hypertrophy and hyperplasia of the B cells [196] (Figure 20B). The qualitative islet changes are therefore dominated by pleomorphism and hyperchromasia of the B-cell nuclei. These B-cell changes may be accompanied by a considerable infiltration by lymphocytes and especially eosinophilic leukocytes [197, 198], surrounding large islets and infiltrating the interstitial septa. Eosinophilic infiltration is frequently associated with peri-insular fibrosis and the deposition of Charcot–Leyden crystals. Its degree appears to be positively correlated with volume and size of the islets and with the severity of maternal diabetes [186]. Apart from eosinophilic infiltration there may be considerable numbers of hemopoietic cells associated with extramedullary hemopoiesis. The cause of the eosinophilic infiltration is not known but immunologic mechanisms are strongly suspected [199].

ISLET CHANGES UNRELATED TO DIABETES

Damage to the pancreatic islets can be observed in young infants dying of profound shock [200]. These shock-related lesions are characterized by islet cell necrosis devoid of cellular inflammatory response, fibrin thrombi, and hemosiderin. The non-islet endocrine cells and the acinar tissue of the pancreas are not involved. It is not clear why such islet changes have not yet been seen in adults.

B-cell degranulation and hydropic transformation are reversible changes occurring in connection with sustained hyperglycemia (see type 2 diabetes). Hypertrophy of the B-cell nuclei can be observed in normal adults and is thought to be the expression of polyploidy [201]. B-cell hypertrophy with hyperplasia, as a true sign of functional hyperactivity, particularly occurs in the pancreas of newborns of diabetic mothers.

Regeneration of islet cells, and particularly of B cells, during adult life can, in principle, be achieved in two ways: replication of functionally active islet cells by mitotic division (for review see reference 202), or neoformation of islet cell complexes by budding-off of endocrine cells from progenitor cells in the ductal epithelium. The latter process, also called nesidioblastosis, is seen in all diseases leading to pancreatic fibrosis. It is not clear whether this process can really contribute to increasing the islet mass.

Acknowledgments

We thank Nicole Buelens, Marleen Berghmans, Christiane Arijs and Suzanne Peters for expert technical assistance and Hilde Lox for secretarial help. This work was supported by a grant of the Belgian Fund for Medical Research (30059.86).

REFERENCES

1. Volk BW, Wellman KF. Historical review. In Volk BW, Arquilla ER (eds) The diabetic pancreas. New York: Plenum, 1985: pp 1–16.
2. Hellman B, Hellerström C. Histology and histophysiology of the islets of Langerhans in man. In Pfeiffer EF (ed) Handbook of diabetes mellitus. Munich: Lehmanns, V, 1969: pp 90–118.
3. Goldstein MB, Davis EA. The three dimensional architecture of the islets of Langerhans. Acta Anat 1968; 71: 161–71.
4. Rahier J, Goebbels RM, Henquin JC. Cellular composition of the human diabetic pancreas. Diabetologia 1983; 24: 366–71.
5. Ogilvie RF. A quantitative study of the pancreatic islet tissue. Quart J Med 1937; 6: 287.
6. Lane MA. The cytological characteristics of the areas of Langerhans. Am J Anat 1907; 7: 409–22.
7. Bloom W. A new type of granular cell in the islets of Langerhans of man. Anat Record 1931; 49: 363–71.
8. Larsson LS, Sundler F, Håkansson R, Pollock HG, Kimmel JR. Localization of APP, a postulated new hormone to a pancreatic endocrine cell type. Histochemistry 1974; 42: 377.
9. Kimmel JR, Pollock HG, Hazelwood RL. A new pancreatic polypeptide. Fed Proc (USA) 1971; 30: 1318 (abstr.).
10. Pictet R, Rutter WJ. Development of the embryonic endocrine pancreas. In Steiner DF, Freinkel N (eds) Handbook of Physiology. Section 7: Endocrinology. Vol. I: Endocrine pancreas. Baltimore: Williams & Wilkins, 1972: pp 25–66.
11. Clark A, Grant AM. Quantitative morphology of endocrine cells in human fetal pancreas. Diabetologia 1983; 25: 31–5.
12. Like AA, Orci L. Embryogenesis of the human fetal pancreatic islets: a light and electron microscopic study. Diabetes 1972; 21: 511–34.
13. Stefan Y, Grasso S, Perrelet A, Orci L. A quantitative immunofluorescent study of the endocrine cell populations in the developing human pancreas. Diabetes 1983; 32: 293–301.
14. Stefan Y, Orci L, Malaisse-Lagae F, Perrelet A, Patel Y, Unger RH. Quantitation of endocrine cell content in the pancreas of non-diabetic and diabetic humans. Diabetes 1982; 31: 694–700.
15. Rahier J, Wallon J, Henquin JC. Cell populations in the endocrine pancreas of human neonates and infants. Diabetologia 1981; 20: 540–6.
16. Orci L, Stefan Y, Malaisse-Lagae F, Perrelet A. Instability of pancreatic endocrine cell population throughout life. Lancet 1979; 1: 615–6.
17. Pearse AGE. Islet cell precursors are neurones. Nature 1982; 295: 96–7.
18. Le Douarin NM. On the origin of pancreatic endocrine cells. Cell 1988; 53: 169–71.
19. Teitelman G, Joh TH, Reis DJ. Transformation of catecholaminergic precursors into glucagon (A) cells in mouse embryonic pancreas. Proc Natl Acad Sci USA 1981; 78: 5225–9.
20. Dean PM, Matthews EK. Glucose-induced electrical activity in pancreatic islet cells. J Physiol (Lond.) 1970; 210: 255–64.
21. Alpert S, Hanahan D, Teitelman G. Hybrid insulin genes reveal a developmental lineage for pancreatic endocrine cells and imply a relationship with neurons. Cell 1988; 53: 295–308.
22. Smit AB, Vreugdenhil E, Ebberink RHM, Geraerts WPM, Klootwijk J, Joosse J. Growth-controlling molluscan neurons produce the precursor of an insulin-related peptide. Nature 1988; 331: 535–8.
23. Deconinck JF, Potvliege PR, Gepts W. The ultrastructure of the human pancreatic islets. I. The islets of adults. Diabetologia 1971; 7: 266–82.
24. Murlin JR, Clough HG, Gibbs CB, Stokes AM. Aqueous extracts of pancreas. I. Influence on the carbohydrate metabolism of depancreatized animals. J Biol Chem 1923; 56: 253.
25. Baum J, Simmons BE, Unger RH, Madison LL. Localization of glucagon in the A-cells in the pancreatic islet by immunofluorescence. Diabetes 1962; 11: 371.
26. Orci L, Bordi C, Unger RH, Perrelet A. Glucagon- and glicentin-producing cells. In Lefèbvre P (ed) Glucagon. Berlin: Springer, 1983; pp 57–79.
27. Bell GI, Santerre RF, Mullenbach GT. Hamster preproglucagon contains the sequence of glucagon and two related peptides. Nature 1983; 302: 716–8.
28. Vaillant CR, Lund PK. Distribution of glucagon-like peptide I in canine and feline pancreas and gastrointestinal tract. Histochem Cytochem 1986; 34: 1117–21.
29. Ravazzola M, Orci L. Glucagon and glicentin immunoreactivity are topographically segregated in the alpha granule of the human pancreatic A cell. Nature 1980; 284: 66–7.
30. Banting FG, Best CH. The internal secretion of the pancreas. J Lab Clin Med 1922; 7: 465–80.
31. Bliss M. The discovery of insulin. University of Chicago Press, 1982.
32. Lacy PE. Electron microscopic and fluorescent antibody studies on islets of Langerhans. Exp Cell Res 1959; 7: 296–308.
33. Orci L. The insulin cell: its cellular environment and how it processes (pro)insulin. Diabetes Metab Rev 1986; 2: 71–106.
34. Howell SJ. The mechanism of insulin secretion. Diabetologia 1984; 26: 319–27.
35. Eiden LE. Is chromogranin a prohormone? Nature 1987; 325: 301.
36. Johnson KH, O'Brien TD, Hayden DW, Jordan K, Ghobrial HKG, Mahoney WC, Westermark P. Immunolocalization of islet amyloid polypeptide (IAPP) in pancreatic beta cells by means of peroxidase-antiperoxidase (PAP) and protein A-gold techniques. Am J Pathol 1988; 130: 1–8.
37. Hutton JC, Peshavaria M, Johnston CF, Ravazzola M, Orci L. Immunolocalization of betagranin: a chromogranin A-related protein of the pancreatic B-cell. Endocrinology 1988; 122: 1014–20.
38. Brazeau P, Vale W, Burgus R, Ling N, Butcher M, Rivier J, Guillemin R. Hypothalamic polypeptide that

inhibits the secretion of immunoreactive pituitary growth hormone. Science 1973; 1979: 77–9.

39. Luft R, Efendic S, Hökfelt T, Johansson O, Azimura A. Immunohistochemical evidence for the localization of somatostatin-like immunoreactivity in a cell population of the pancreatic islets. Med Biol 1974; 52: 428–30.

40. Bloom SR, Polak JM. Somatostatin. Br Med J 1987; 295: 288–9.

41. Grube D, Bohn R. The microanatomy of human islets of Langerhans with special reference to somatostatin (D-) cells. Arch Histol Jap 1983; 46: 327–53.

42. Lazarus SS, Volk BW. The pancreas in human and experimental diabetes. New York: Grune & Stratton, 1962.

43. Ferner H. Das Inselsystem des Pankreas. Stuttgart: Thieme, 1952.

44. Orci L, Stefan Y, Bonner Weir S, Perrelet A, Unger R. 'Obligatory' association between A and D cells demonstrated by bipolar islets in neonatal pancreas. Diabetologia 1981; 21: 73–4.

45. Grube D, Eckert I, Speck PT, Wagner HJ. Immunohistochemistry and microanatomy of the islets of Langerhans. Biomed Res 1983: 4 (suppl.): 25–36.

46. Orci L, Unger RH. Functional subdivision of islets of Langerhans and possible role of D-cells. Lancet 1975; ii: 1243–4.

47. Stefan Y, Meda P, Neufeld M, Orci L. Stimulation of insulin secretion reveals heterogeneity of pancreatic B cells in vivo. J Clin Invest 1987; 80: 175–83.

48. Schuit F, In't Veld PA, Pipeleers DG. Glucose recruits pancreatic B-cells to proinsulin biosynthesis. Proc Natl Acad Sci USA 1988; 85: 3865–9.

49. Pipeleers DG. The biosociology of pancreatic B-cells. Diabetologia 1987; 30: 277–91.

50. Bencosme SA, Liepa E. Regional differences of the pancreatic islet. Endocrinology 1955; 57: 588–93.

51. Orci L, Malaisse-Lagae F, Baetens D, Perrelet A. Pancreatic-polypeptide-rich regions in human pancreas. Lancet 1978; ii: 1200–1.

52. Lifson N, Kramlinger KG, Mayrand RR, Lender EJ. Blood flow to the rabbit pancreas with special reference to the islets of Langerhans. Gastroenterology 1980; 79: 466–73.

53. McCuskey RS, Chapman TS. Microscopy of the living pancreas in situ. Am J Anat 1969; 126: 395–408.

54. Bearer EL, Orci L. Endothelial fenestral diaphragms: a quick-freeze, deep-etch study. J Cell Biol 1985; 100: 418–28.

55. Yamamoto M, Kataoka K. A comparative study on the intercellular canalicular system and intercellular junctions in the pancreatic islets of some rodents. Arch Histol Jap 1984; 47: 485–93.

56. Fujita T. Insulino-acinar portal system in the horse pancreas. Arch Histol Jap 1973; 35: 161–71.

57. Bonner-Weir S, Orci L. New perspectives on the microvasculature of the islets of Langerhans. Diabetes 1982; 31: 883–9.

58. Samols E, Bonner-Weir S, Weir GC. Intra-islet insulin-glucagon-somatostatin relationships. Clin Endocrinol Metab 1986; 15: 33–58.

59. Sundler F, Alumets J, Håkanson R, Fahrenkrug J, Schaffalitzky de Muckadell O. Peptidergic (VIP) nerves in the pancreas. Histochemistry 1978; 55: 173–6.

60. Rehfeld JF, Larsson LI, Goltermann NR, Schwartz TW, Holst JJ, Jensen SL, Morley JS. Neural regulation of pancreatic hormone secretion by the C-terminal tetrapeptide of CCK. Nature 1980; 284: 33–8.

61. Tominaga M, Marayuma H, Vasko MR, Baetens D, Orci L, Unger RH. Morphologic and functional changes in sympathetic nerve relationships with pancreatic alpha-cells after destruction of beta-cells in rats. Diabetes 1987; 36: 365–73.

62. Richens CA. The innervation of the pancreas. J Comp Neurol 1945; 83: 223–36.

63. Fujita T. Histological studies on the neuroinsular complex in the pancreas of some mammals. Z. Zellforsch 1959; 50: 94–109.

64. Smith PH. Structural modification of Schwann cells in the pancreatic islets of the dog. Am J Anat 1975; 144: 513–7.

65. WHO Expert Committee on Diabetes Mellitus. Second report. Technical report series. Geneva: WHO, 1980.

66. Gepts W. Pathologic anatomy of the pancreas in juvenile diabetes mellitus. Diabetes 1965; 14: 619–33.

67. Klöppel G, Drenck CR, Oberholzer M, Heitz PhU. Morphometric evidence for a striking B-cell reduction at the clinical onset of type 1 diabetes. Virchows Arch (Pathol Anat) 1984; 403: 441–52.

68. Foulis AK, Stewart JA. The pancreas in recent-onset Type 1 (insulin-dependent) diabetes mellitus: insulin content of islets, insulitis and associated changes in the exocrine acinar tissue. Diabetologia 1984; 26: 456–61.

69. LeCompte PM. 'Insulitis' in early juvenile diabetes. Arch Path 1958; 66: 450–7.

70. MacLean N, Ogilvie RF. Observations on the pancreatic islet tissue of young diabetic subjects. Diabetes 1959; 8: 83–91.

71. Löhr M, Klöppel G. Residual insulin positivity and pancreatic atrophy in relation to duration of chronic Type 1 (insulin-dependent) diabetes mellitus and microangiopathy. Diabetologia 1987; 30: 757–62.

72. Rahier J, Wallon J, Loozen S, Lefevre A. Gepts W, Haot J. The pancreatic polypeptide cells in the human pancreas: the effect of age and of diabetes. J Clin Endocrinol Metab 1983; 56: 441–4.

73. Henderson JR, Daniel PM, Fraser PA. The pancreas as a single organ: the influence of the endocrine upon the exocrine part of the gland. Gut 1981; 22: 158–67.

74. Korc M, Owerbach D, Quinto C, Rutter WJ. Pancreatic islet-acinar cell interaction: amylase messenger RNA levels are determined by insulin. Science 1981; 213: 351–3.

75. Foulis AK, Liddle CN, Farquharson MA, Richmond JA, Weir RS. The histopathology of the pancreas in Type 1 (insulin-dependent) diabetes mellitus: a 25-year review of deaths in patients under 20 years of age in the United Kingdom. Diabetologia 1986; 29: 267–74.

76. Von Meyenburg H, Über 'Insulitis' bei Diabetes. Schweiz Med Wschr 1940; 21: 554–7.

77. Bottazzo GF, Dean BM, McNally JM, MacKay EH, Swift PGF, Gamble DR. In situ characterisation of autoimmune phenomena and expression of HLA molecules in the pancreas in diabetic insulitis. New Engl J Med 1985; 313: 353–60.

78. Junker K, Egeberg J, Kromann H, Nerup J. An autopsy study of the islets of Langerhans in acute-onset juvenile diabetes mellitus. Acta Pathol Microbiol Scand 1977; 85: 699–706.

79. Cossel L, Schade J, Verlohren HJ, Lohmann D, Mättig H. Ultrastructural, immunohistological, and clinical findings in the pancreas in insulin-dependent

diabetes mellitus (IDDM) of long duration. Zbl Pathol Anat 1983; 128: 147–59.

80. Orci L, Baetens D, Rufener C, Amherdt M, Ravazzola M, Studer P, Malaisse-Lagae F, Unger RH. Hypertrophy and hyperplasia of somatostatin-containing D-cells in diabetes. Proc Natl Acad Sci USA 1976; 73: 1338–42.

81. Gepts W, De Mey J, Marichal-Pipeleers M. Hyperplasia of 'pancreatic polypeptide' cells in the pancreas of juvenile diabetics. Diabetologia 1977; 13: 27–34.

82. Gepts W, De Mey J. Islet cell survival determined by morphology. An immunocytochemical study of the islets of Langerhans in juvenile diabetes mellitus. Diabetes 1978; 27 (suppl. 1): 251–61.

83. Ogilvie RF. The endocrine pancreas in human and experimental diabetes. In Cameron MP, O'Connor M (eds) The aetiology of diabetes mellitus, and its complications. Ciba Foundation Colloquia on Endocrinology, vol. 15, London: Churchill, 1964: pp 49–74.

84. Lernmark A. Islet cell antibodies. Diabet Med 1987; 4: 285–92.

85. Gorsuch AN, Lister J, Dean BM, Spencer KM, McNally JM, Bottazzo GF, Cudworth AG. Evidence for a long prediabetic period in type I (insulin-dependent) diabetes mellitus. Lancet 1981; ii: 1363–5.

86. Handwerger BS, Fernandes G, Brown DM. Immune and autoimmune aspects of diabetes mellitus. Hum Pathol 1980; 11: 338–52.

87. Foulis AK, Jackson R, Farquharson MA. The pancreas in idiopathic Addison's disease—a search for a prediabetic pancreas. Histopathology 1988; 12: 481–90.

88. Löhr M, Schmitt P, Klöppel G. Inselveränderungen beim Insulin-abhängigen Diabetes im Alter. Immunzytochemische Pankreasuntersuchungen bei einer diabetischen Patientin mit Hypothyreose. Pathologe 1988; 9: 103–8.

89. Sibley RK, Sutherland DER, Goetz FC, Michael AF. Recurrent diabetes mellitus in the pancreatic iso- and allograft period. A light and electronmicroscopic and immunohistochemical analysis of four cases. Lab Invest 1985; 53: 132–44.

90. Klöppel G. Experimental insulitis. In Volk B, Arquilla E, Allen R (eds) The diabetic pancreas, 2nd edn. New York: Plenum, 1985: pp 467–92.

91. Like AA, Weringer EJ. Autoimmune diabetes in the Bio Breeding/Worcester rat. In Lefèbvre P, Pipeleers DG (eds) The pathology of the endocrine pancreas in diabetes. Berlin: Springer, 1988: pp 269–84.

92. Kolb H. Mouse models of insulin dependent diabetes: low-dose streptozocin-induced diabetes and nonobese diabetic (NOD) mice. Diabetes Metab Rev 1987; 3: 751–78.

93. Bottazzo GF, Pujol-Borrell, Gale E. Etiology of diabetes: the role of autoimmune mechanisms. In Alberti KGMM, Krall LP (eds) Diabetes Annual 1. Amsterdam: Elsevier, 1985: pp 16–52.

94. Foulis AK, Farquharson MA. Aberrant expression of HLA-DR antigens by insulin-containing B-cells in recent-onset type I diabetes mellitus. Diabetes 1986; 35: 1215–24.

95. Pipeleers DG, In't Veld PA, Pipeleers-Marichal MA, Gepts W, Van de Winkel M. Presence of pancreatic hormones in islet cells with MHC-Class II antigen expression. Diabetes 1987; 36: 872–6.

96. Foulis AK, Farquharson MA, Hardman R. Aberrant expression of Class II major histocompatibility complex molecules by B cells and hyperexpression of Class I major histocompatibility complex molecules by insulin containing islets in Type 1 (insulin-dependent) diabetes mellitus. Diabetologia 1987; 30: 333–43.

97. Foulis AK, Farquharson MA, Meager A. Immunoreactive alpha-interferon in insulin-secreting B cells in type 1 diabetes mellitus. Lancet 1987; ii: 1423–8.

98. Foulis, AK. The pathogenesis of beta cell destruction in type 1 (insulin-dependent) diabetes mellitus. J Pathol 1987; 152: 141–8.

99. Madsbad S. Prevalence of residual B cell function and its metabolic consequences in type 1 (insulin-dependent) diabetes. Diabetologia 1983; 24: 141–7.

100. Barnett AH, Epp C, Leslie RDG, Pyke DA. Diabetes in identical twins. A study of 200 pairs. Diabetologia 1981; 20: 87–93.

101. Rayfield EJ, Yoon IW. Role of viruses in diabetes. In Cooperstein SJ, Watkins D (eds) The islets of Langerhans. New York: Academic Press, 1981: pp 427–51.

102. Craighead JE, Steinke J. Diabetes mellitus-like syndrome in mice infected with encephalomyocarditis virus. Am J Pathol 1971; 63: 119–34.

103. Gladisch R, Hofmann W, Waldherr R. Myokarditis und Insulitis nach Coxsackie-Virus-Infekt. Zeitschr Kardiol 1976; 65: 849–55.

104. Yoon JW, Austin M, Onodera T, Notkins AL. Virus-induced diabetes mellitus. Isolation of a virus from the pancreas of a child with diabetic ketoacidosis. New Engl J Med 1979; 300: 1173–9.

105. Craighead JE, Higgins DA. Genetic influences affecting the occurrence of a diabetes mellitus-like disease in mice infected with the encephalomyocarditis virus. J Exp Med 1974; 139: 414–26.

106. Cudworth AG, Festenstein H. HLA genetic heterogeneity in diabetes mellitus. Br Med Bull 1978; 34: 285–9.

107. Wolf E, Spencer KM, Cudworth AG. The genetic susceptibility to type 1 (insulin-dependent) diabetes: analysis of the HLA-DR association. Diabetologia 1983; 24: 224–30.

108. Gorsuch AN, Spencer KM, Lister J, Wolf E, Bottazzo GF, Cudworth AG. Can future type 1 diabetes be predicted? A study in families of affected children. Diabetes 1982; 31: 862–6.

109. Millward BA, Alviggi L, Hoskins PJ, Johnston C, Heaton D, Bottazzo GF, Vergani D, Leslie RDG, Pyke DA. Immune changes associated with insulin dependent diabetes may remit without causing the disease: a study in identical twins. Br Med J 1986; 292: 793–6.

110. Baekkeskov S, Nielson JH, Marner B, Bilde T, Ludvigsson J, Lernmark A. Autoantibodies in newly diagnosed diabetic children immunoprecipitate specific human pancreatic islet cell protein. Nature 1982; 298: 167–9.

111. Gleichmann H, Zörcher B, Greulich B, Gries FA, Henrichs HR, Bertrams J, Kolb H. Correlation of islet cell antibodies and HLA-DR phenotypes with diabetes mellitus in adults. Diabetologia 1984; 27: 90–2.

112. Groop L, Miettinen A, Groop PH, Meri S, Koskimies S, Bottazzo GF. Organ-specific autoimmunity and HLA-DR antigens as markers for B-cell destruction in patients with Type II diabetes. Diabetes 1988; 37: 99–103.

113. Bottazzo GF, Florin-Christensen A, Doniach D. Islet-cell antibodies in diabetes mellitus with autoimmune polyendocrine deficiencies. Lancet 1974; ii: 1279–83.
114. Doniach D, Bottazzo GF. Autoimmunity and the endocrine pancreas. Pathol Ann 1977; 7: 327–46.
115. Ludvigsson J, Samuelsson U, Beauforts C, Deschamps I, Dorchy H, Drash A, Francois R, Herz G, New M, Schober E. HLA-DR3 is associated with a more slowly progressive form of Type 1 (insulin-dependent) diabetes. Diabetologia 1986; 29: 207–10.
116. Masi AT, Hartmann WH, Hahn BN, Abbey H, Shulman LE. Hashimoto's disease—a clinicopathological study with matched controls. Lancet 1965; i: 123–6.
117. Susman W. Atrophy of the adrenals associated with Addison's disease. J Pathol Bact 1930; 33: 749–60.
118. Sibley RK, Sutherland DER. Pancreas transplantation: an immunohistologic and histopathologic examination of 100 grafts. Am J Pathol 1987; 128: 151–70.
119. Kern H, Logothetopoulos J. Steroid diabetes in the guinea pig. Studies on islet-cell structure and regeneration. Diabetes 1970; 19: 145–54.
120. Toreson WE. Glycogen infiltration (so-called hydropic degeneration) in the pancreas in human and experimental diabetes mellitus. Am J Pathol 1951; 27: 327–47.
121. Westermark P, Johnson KH. The polypeptide hormone-derived amyloid forms: nonspecific alterations or signs of abnormal peptide-processing? Acta Pathol Microbiol Immunol Scand 1988; 96: 475–83.
122. Bell ET. Hyalinization of the islets of Langerhans in nondiabetic individuals. Am J Pathol 1959; 35: 801–5.
123. Seifert G. Die pathologische Morphologie der Langerhansschen Inseln besonders beim Diabetes mellitus des Menschen. Verh Dtsch Ges Path 1959; 18: 50–84.
124. Maloy AL, Longnecker DS, Greenberg ER. The relation of islet amyloid to the clinical type of diabetes. Hum Pathol 1981; 12: 917–22.
125. Bell ET. Hyalinization of the islets of Langerhans in diabetes mellitus. Diabetes 1952; 1: 341–4.
126. Westermark P, Wilander E, Westermark GT, Johnson KH. Islet amyloid polypeptide-like immunoreactivity in the islet B cells of Type 2 (non-insulin-dependent) diabetic and non-diabetic individuals. Diabetologia 1987; 30: 887–92.
127. Westermark P. Fine structure of islets of Langerhans in insular amyloidosis. Virchows Arch (A) 1973; 359: 1–18.
128. Westermark P, Wernstedt C, O'Brien TD, Hayden DW, Johnson KH. Islet amyloid in Type 2 human diabetes mellitus and adult diabetic cats contains a novel putative polypeptide hormone. Am J Pathol 1987; 127: 414–17.
129. Cooper GJS, Willis AC, Clark A, Turner RC, Sim RB, Reid KBM. Purification and characterization of a peptide from amyloid-rich pancreases of Type 2 diabetic patients. Proc Natl Acad Sci USA 1987; 84: 8628–32.
130. Westermark P, Wilander E. The influence of amyloid deposits on the islet volume in maturity onset diabetes mellitus. Diabetologia 1978; 15: 417–21.
131. MacLean N, Ogilvie RF. Quantitative estimation of the pancreatic islet tissue in diabetic subjects. Diabetes 1955; 4: 367–76.
132. Gepts W. Contribution à l'étude morphologique des îlots de Langerhans au cours du diabète. Ann Soc Roy Sci Med Nat 1957; 10: 1.
133. Klöppel G, Drenck CR. Immunzytochemische Morphometrie beim Type-I und Type-II Diabetes mellitus. Dtsch Med Wschr 1983; 108: 188–9.
134. Klöppel G, Löhr M, Habich K, Oberholzer M, Heitz PhU. Islet pathology and the pathogenesis of type 1 and type 2 diabetes mellitus revisited. Surv Synth Path Res 1985; 4: 110–25.
135. Ogilvie RF. The islands of Langerhans in 19 cases of obesity. J Pathol Bact 1933; 37: 473–81.
136. DeFronzo RA. Pathogenesis of type 2 (non-insulin dependent) diabetes mellitus: a balanced overview. Diabetologia 1992; 35: 389–97.
137. Yki-Järvinen H. Pathogenesis of non-insulin-dependent diabetes mellitus. Lancet 1994; 343: 91–5.
138. Wrenshall GA, Bogoch A, Ritchie RC. Extractable insulin of pancreas: correlation with pathological and clinical findings in diabetic and non-diabetic cases. Diabetes 1952; 1: 87–107.
139. Andersson A. The influence of hyperglycaemia, hyperinsulinaemia and genetic background on the fate of intrasplenically implanted mouse islets. Diabetologia 1983; 25: 269–72.
140. Wang RN, Bouwens, L, Klöppel G. Beta-cell proliferation in normal and streptozotocin-treated newborn rats: site, dynamics and capacity. Diabetologia 1994; 37: 1088–96.
141. Hales CN, Barker DJ. Type 2 (non-insulin-dependent) diabetes mellitus: the thrifty phenotype hypothesis. Diabetologia 1992; 35: 595–601.
142. Weir GC, Leahy JL, Bonner-Weir S. Experimental reduction of B-cell mass: implications for the pathogenesis of diabetes. Diabetes Metab Rev 1986; 2: 125–61.
143. Rossetti L, Shulman GI, Zawalich W, DeFronzo RA. Effect of chronic hyperglycemia on *in vivo* insulin secretion in partially pancreatectomized rats. J Clin Invest 1987; 80: 1037–44.
144. Löhr M, Lübbersmeyer J, Otremba B, Klapdor R, Grossner D, Klöppel G. Increase in B-cells in the pancreatic remnant after partial pancreatectomy in pigs. An immunocytochemical and functional study. Virchows Archiv B (Cell Pathol) 1989; 56: 277–86.
145. Kawanishi H, Akazawa Y, Machii B. Islet of Langerhans in normal and diabetic humans. Ultrastructure and histochemistry with specific reference to hyalinosis. Acta Pathol Jap 1966; 16: 117–96.
146. Moore RA. Congenital aplasia of islands of Langerhans with diabetes mellitus. Am J Dis Child 1936; 52: 627–32.
147. Dodge JA, Laurence KM. Congenital absence of islets of Langerhans. Arch Dis Child 1977; 52: 411–13.
148. Wong KC, Tse K, Chan JKC. Congenital absence of insulin-secreting cells. Histopathology 1988; 12: 541–5.
149. Hattevig G, Kjellman B, Fallstrom SP. Congenital permanent diabetes mellitus and coeliac disease. J Paed 1982; 101: 955–7.
150. Ivarsson SA, Marner B, Lernmark A, Nilsson KO. Nonislet pancreatic autoantibodies in sibship with permanent neonatal insulin-dependent diabetes mellitus. Diabetes 1988; 37: 347–50.
151. Evans DJ. Generalized islet hypertrophy and beta-cell hyperplasia in a case of long-term juvenile diabetes. Diabetes 1972; 21: 114–16.
152. Bostrom K. Patho-anatomical findings in a case of mumps, with pancreatitis, myocarditis, orchitis,

epididymitis and seminal vesiculitis. Virchows Arch 1968; 344: 111-7.

153. Ujevich MM, Jaffe R. Pancreatic islet cell damage. Its occurrence in neonatal Coxsackie-virus encephalomyocarditis. Arch Path Lab Med 1980; 104: 438-41.

154. Ahmad A, Abraham AA. Pancreatic isleitis with Coxsackie virus B5 infection. Hum Pathol 1982; 13: 661-2.

155. Foulis AK, Francis ND, Farquharson MA, Boylston A. Massive synchronous B-cell necrosis causing Type 1 (insulin-dependent) diabetes; a unique histopathological case report. Diabetologia 1988; 31: 46-50.

156. Dourov M, Buyl-Strouvens ML. Agénésie du pancréas. Observation anatomoclinique d'un cas de diabète sucré, avec stéatorrhée et hypotrophie, chez un nouveau-né. Arch Franc Pédiat 1969; 26: 641-50.

157. Sherwood WC, Chance GW, Hill DE. A new syndrome of familial pancreatic agenesis: the role of insulin and glucagon in somatic and cell growth. Paed Res 1974; 8: 360.

158. Töpke B, Menzel K. Die Pankreasagenesie des Neugeborenen; ein seltenes, klinisch aber charakteristisches Krankheitsbild. Acta Paed Acad Sci Hungar 1976; 17: 147-51.

159. Wöckel W, Scheibner K. Aplasie des Pankreas mit Diabetes mellitus, intrahepatische Gallengangsaplasie und weitere Missbildungen bei einem hypotrophen Neugeborenen. Zbl Pathol Anat 1977; 121: 186-94.

160. Dürr GH-K. Acute pancreatitis. In Howat HT, Sarles H (eds) The exocrine pancreas. Philadelphia: W.B. Saunders, 1979: pp 352-401.

161. Nyboe Andersen B, Krarup T, Thorsgaard Pedersen N, Faber OK, Hagen C, Worning H. B cell function in patients with chronic pancreatitis and its relation to exocrine pancreatic function. Diabetologia 1982; 23: 86-9.

162. Harsha Rao R. Diabetes in the undernourished: coincidence or consequence? Endocr Rev 1988; 9: 67-87.

163. Klöppel G, Bommer G, Commandeur G, Heitz PhU. The endocrine pancreas in chronic pancreatitis. Immunocytochemical and ultrastructural studies. Virchows Arch A (Path Anat Histol) 1978; 377: 157-74.

164. Adrian TE, Bestermann HS, Mallinson CH, Garalotis C, Bloom SR. Impaired pancreatic polypeptide release in chronic pancreatitis with steatorrhoea. Gut 1979; 20: 98-101.

165. Ebert R, Creutzfeldt W. Reversal of impaired GIP and insulin secretion in patients with pancreatogenic steatorrhea following enzyme substitution. Diabetologia 1980; 19: 198-204.

166. Lippe BM, Sperling MA, Dooley RR. Pancreatic alpha and beta cell functions in cystic fibrosis. J Pediatr 1977; 90: 751-5.

167. Lebenthal E, Lerner A, Heitlinger L. The pancreas in cystic fibrosis. In Go VLW, Gardner JD, Brooks FP, Lebenthal E, DiMagno EP, Scheele GA (eds) The exocrine pancreas. New York: Raven Press, 1986: pp 783-817.

168. Klöppel G. Islet histopathology in diabetes mellitus. In Klöppel G, Heitz PhU (eds) Pancreatic pathology. Edinburgh: Churchill Livingstone, 1984: pp 154-92.

169. Iannucci A, Mukai K, Johnson D, Burke B. Endocrine pancreas in cystic fibrosis: an immunohistochemical study. Hum Pathol 1984; 15: 278-84.

170. Abdul-Karim FW, Dahms BB, Velasco ME, Rodman HM. Islets of Langerhans in adolescents and adults with cystic fibrosis. A quantitative study. Arch Pathol Lab Med 1986; 110: 602-6.

171. Handwerger S, Roth J, Gorden P, Di Sant'Agnese P, Carpenter DF, Peter G. Glucose intolerance in cystic fibrosis. New Engl J Med 1969; 281: 451-61.

172. Löhr M, Goertchen P, Nizze H, Gould NS, Gould VE, Oberholzer M, Heitz PhU, Klöppel G. Cystic fibrosis associated islet changes may provide a basis for diabetes. An immunocytochemical and morphometrical study. Virchows Arch A (Path Anat) 1989; 414: 179-85.

173. Saudek CD. Diabetes and the diseases of iron excess. In Podolsky S, Viswanathan M (eds) Secondary diabetes: the spectrum of the diabetic syndromes. New York: Raven Press, 1980: pp 257-68.

174. Rahier J, Loozen S, Goebbels RM, Abrahem M. The haemochromatotic human pancreas: a quantitative immunohistochemical and ultrastructural study. Diabetologia 1987; 30: 5-12.

175. Harrison LC, Flier JS. Diabetes associated with other endocrine diseases. In Podolsky S, Viswanathan M (eds) Secondary diabetes: the spectrum of the diabetic syndromes. New York: Raven Press, 1980: pp 269-86.

176. Podolsky S. Lipoatrophic diabetes and leprechaunism. In Podolsky S, Viswanathan M (eds) Secondary diabetes: the spectrum of the diabetic syndromes. New York: Raven Press, 1980: pp 335-52.

177. Kahn CR, Flier JS, Bar RS, Archer JA, Gordon P, Martin MM, Roth J. The syndromes of insulin resistance and acanthosis nigricans. Insulin receptor disorders in man. New Engl J Med 1976; 294: 739-45.

178. Jennette JC, Wilman AS, Bagnell CR. Insulin auto-antibody-induced pancreatic islet beta (B) cell hyperplasia. Arch Pathol Lab Med 1982; 106: 218-20.

179. Creutzfeldt W, Sickinger K, Frerichs H. Diabetes und Lebererkrankungen. In Pfeiffer EF (ed.) Handbuch des Diabetes mellitus. Pathophysiologie und Klinik, Vol. II. Munich: Lehmanns, 1971: pp 807-59.

180. Johnston DG, Alberti KGMM, Faber OK, Binder C, Wright R. Hyperinsulinism of hepatic cirrhosis: diminished degradation or hypersecretion? Lancet 1977; i: 10-12.

181. Shankar TP, Solomon SS, Duckworth WC, Hummelstein S, Gray S, Jerkins T, Bobal MA, Iyer RS. Studies of glucose intolerance in cirrhosis of the liver. J Lab Clin Med 1983; 102: 459-69.

182. Chang AY, Diani AR. Chemically and hormonally induced diabetes mellitus. In Volk BW, Arquilla ER (eds) The diabetic pancreas, 2nd edn. New York: Plenum, 1985: pp 415-38.

183. Khan A, Adachi M, Hill JM. Diabetogenic effect of L-asparaginase. J Clin Endocrinol Metab 1969; 29: 1373-6.

184. Bryceson A, Woodstock L. The accumulative effect of pentamidine dimethane sulfonate on the blood sugar. East Afr Med J 1969; 46: 170-3.

185. Creutzfeldt W, Creutzfeldt C, Frerichs H, Pekings E, Sickinger K. The morphological substrate of the inhibition of insulin secretion by diazoxide. Horm Metab Res 1969; 1: 53-64.

186. Boquist L. The endocrine pancreas in early alloxan diabetes. Acta Pathol Microbiol Scand 1977; 85A: 219-29.

187. Wilander E, Boquist L. Streptozotocin-diabetes in the chinese hamster. Blood glucose and structural changes during the first 24 hours. Horm Metab Res 1972; 4: 426-33.

188. Prosser PR, Karam JH. Diabetes mellitus following rodenticide ingestion in man. JAMA 1978; 239: 1148–50.

189. Kenney RM, Michaels IAL, Flomenbaum NE, Yu GSM. Poisoning with *N*-3-pyridylmethyl-*N'*-*p*-nitrophenylurea (Vacor). Immunoperoxidase demonstration of B-cell destruction. Arch Pathol Lab Med 1981; 105: 367–70.

190. Bommer G, Schäfer HJ, Klöppel G. Morphologic effects of diazoxide and diphenylhydantoin on insulin secretion and biosynthesis in B-cells of mice. Virchows Arch A (Path Anat Histol) 1976; 371: 227–41.

191. Bommer G, Joost HG, Klöppel G. Subcellular B-cell calcium and insulin secretion *in vitro*. Comparative ultracytochemical studies after glucose stimulation and cyproheptadine inhibition. Virchows Arch A (Path Anat Histol) 1978; 379: 203–17.

192. Pedersen J. Diabetes and pregnancy. In Pfeiffer EF (ed.) Handbook of diabetes mellitus, vol. 2. Munich: Lehmann, 1971: pp 503–36.

193. Hultquist GT, Olding LB. Endocrine pathology of infants of diabetic mothers. Acta Endocrinol 1981; 241 (suppl.): 97.

194. Borchard F, Müntefering H. Beitrag zur quantitativen Morphologie der Langerhansschen Inseln bei Frühgeborenen und Neugeborenen. Virchows Arch A (Path Anat Histol) 1969; 346: 178–98.

195. Naeye RL. Infants of diabetic mothers: a quantitative morphologic study. Pediatrics 1965; 35: 980–9.

196. Milner RDG, Wirdnam PK, Tsanakas J. Quantitative morphology of B, A, D and PP cells in infants of diabetic mothers. Diabetes 1981; 30: 271–4.

197. Mölsted-Pedersen L, Tygstrup P. Cell infiltration in the pancreas of newborn infants of diabetic mothers. Acta Pathol Microbiol Scand 1968; 73: 537–48.

198. Silverman JL. Eosinophilic infiltration in the pancreas of infants of diabetic mothers. A clinicopathologic study. Diabetes 1963; 12: 528–37.

199. Freytag G, Klöppel G. Insulitis: a morphological review. Curr Top Pathol 1973; 58: 49–90.

200. Seemayer TA, Osborne C, De Chadarévian JP. Shock-related injury of pancreatic islets of Langerhans in newborn and young infants. Hum Pathol 1985; 16: 1231–4.

201. Pohl MN, Swartz FJ, Carstens PHB. Polyploidy in islets of normal and diabetic humans. Hum Pathol 1981; 12: 184–6.

202. Hellerström C, Swenne J, Andersson A. Islet cell replication and diabetes. In Lefèbvre PJ, Pipeleers DG (eds) The pathology of the endocrine pancreas in diabetes. Berlin: Springer, 1988; pp 141–70.

203. Hutton JC. The insulin secretory granule. Diabetologia 1989; 32: 271–81.

204. Johnson KH, O'Brien TD, Betsholtz C, Westermark P. Islet amyloid, islet-amyloid polypeptide, and diabetes mellitus. New Engl J Med 1989; 321: 513–18.

205. In't Veld PA, Pipeleers DG. In situ analysis of pancreatic islets in rats developing diabetes. J Clin Invest 1988; 82: 1123–8.

206. Feldman JM, Chapman B. Characterization of pancreatic islet monoamine oxidase. Metabolism 1975; 24: 581–8.

207. Lundquist I, Sundler F, Hakanson R, Larsson LI, Heding LG. Differential changes in the 5-hydroxytryptamine and insulin content of guinea-pig B-cells. Endocrinology 1975; 97: 937–47.

208. Okada Y, Taniguchi H, Shimada C. High concentration of GABA and high glutamate decarboxylase activity in rat pancreatic islets and human insulinoma. Science 1976; 194: 620–2.

209. Wilkin TJ. Insulin autoantibodies as markers for type I diabetes. Endocr Rev 1990; 11: 92–104.

210. Solimena M, Folli F, Aparisi R, Pozza G, De Camilli P. Autoantibodies to GABA-ergic neurons and pancreatic beta cells in Stiff-Man syndrome. New Engl J Med 1990; 322: 1555–60.

211. Baekkeskov S, Aanstoot HJ, Christgau S, Reetz A, Solimena M, Cascalho M, Folli F, Richter-Olesen H, De Camilli P. Identification of the 64 K autoantigen in insulin-dependent diabetes as the GABA-synthesizing enzyme glutamic acid decarboxylase. Nature 1990; 347: 151–6.

212. Foulis AK, Farquharson MA, Cameron SO, McGill M, Schönke H, Kandolf R. A search for the presence of the enteroviral capsid protein VP 1 in pancreases of patients with type 1 (insulin-dependent) diabetes and pancreases and hearts of infants who died of Coxsackie-viral myocarditis. Diabetologia 1990; 33: 290–8.

213. Clark A, Saad MF, Nezzer T, Uren C, Knowler WC, Bennet PH, Turner RC. Islet amyloid polypeptide in diabetic and non-diabetic Pima Indians. Diabetologia 1990; 33: 285–9.

214. Westermark GT, Christmanson L, Terenghi G, Permerth J, Betsholtz C, Larsson J, Polak JM, Westermark P. Islet amyloid polypeptide: demonstration of mRNA in human pancreatic islets by *in situ* hybridization in islets with and without amyloid deposits. Diabetologia 1993; 36: 323–8.

215. Gittes GK, Rutter WJ. Onset of cell-specific gene expression in the developing mouse pancreas. Proc Natl Acad Sci (USA) 1992; 89: 1128–32.

216. Teitelman G, Alpert S, Polak JM, Martinez A, Hanahan D. Precursor cells of mouse endocrine pancreas co-express insulin, glucagon and the neuronal proteins tyrosine hydroxylase and neuropeptide Y, but not pancreatic polypeptide. Development 1993; 118: 1031–9.

217. Lukinius A, Ericsson JLE, Grimelius L, Korsgren O. Ultrastructural studies of the ontogeny of fetal human and porcine endocrine pancreas, with special reference to colocalization of the four major islet hormones. Dev Biol 1992; 153: 376–85.

218. De Krijger RR, Aanstoot HJ, Kranenburg G, Reinhard M, Visser WJ, Bruining GJ. The midgestational human fetal pancreas contains cells coexpressing islet hormones. Dev Biol 1992; 153: 368–75.

219. Upchurch BH, Aponte GW, Leiter AB. Expression of peptide YY in all four cell types in the developing mouse pancreas suggests a common peptide YY-producing progenitor. Development 1994; 120: 245–52.

220. Teitelman G, Lee GK, Alpert S. Cell lineage analysis of pancreatic exocrine and endocrine cells. Cell Tissue Res 1987; 250: 435–9.

221. Polak JM, Bloom SR, Marango PJH. Neuron-specific enolase, a marker for neuroendocrine cells. In Steiner DF, Frenkel M (eds) Evolution and tumor pathology of the neuroendocrine system. Washington: American Physiological Society, 1984: vol. 1; pp 25–66.

222. Henderson JR, Daniel PM. A comparative study of the portal vessels connecting the endocrine and exocrine pancreas, with a discussion of some functional implications. Quart J Exp Phys 1979; 64: 267–75.

223. Kiekens R, In't Veld PA, Mahler T, Schuit F, Van De Winkel M, Pipeleers DG. Differences in glucose recognition by individual rat pancreatic B cells are associated with intercellular differences in glucose-induced biosynthetic activity. J Clin Invest 1992; 89: 117-25.

224. Hiriart M, Ramirez-Medeles MC. Functional subpopulations of individual pancreatic B-cells in culture. Endocrinology 1991; 128: 3193-8.

225. Jetton TJ, Magnuson MA. Heterogeneous expression of glucokinase among pancreatic beta cells. Proc Natl Acad Sci USA 1992; 89: 2619-23.

226. Bonner-Weir S. Morphological evidence for pancreatic polarity of beta cell within islets of Langerhans. Diabetes 1988; 37: 616-21.

227. In't Veld PA. Insulin release and islet cell junctions. In: Lefebvre PJ, Pipeleers DG (eds) The pathology of the endocrine pancreas in diabetes. Berlin: Springer Verlag, 1988: pp 233-48.

228. Steiner DF, Ohagi S, Nagamatsu S, Bell GI, Nishi M. Is islet amyloid polypeptide a significant factor in pathogenesis or pathophysiology of diabetes? Diabetes 1991; 40: 305-9.

229. Clark A, Wells CA, Duley ID, Cruickshank JK, Vanhegan RI, Matthews DR, Cooper GJS, Holman RR, Turner RC. Islet amyloid, increased A-cells, reduced B-cells and exocrine fibrosis: quantitative changes in the pancreas in type 2 diabetes. Diabet Res 1988; 9: 151-9.

230. de Koning EJP, Bodkin NL, Hansen BC, Clark A. Diabetes mellitus in *Macaca mulatta* monkeys is characterised by islet amyloidosis and reduction in beta-cell population. Diabetologia 1993; 36: 378-84.

231. Löhr M, Bergstrome B, Maekawa R, Oldstone MBA, Klöppel G. Human cytomegalovirus in the pancreas of patients with type 2 diabetes: is there a relation to clinical features, mRNA and protein expression of insulin, somatostatin, and MHC class II? Virchows Archiv A (Pathol Anat) 1992; 421: 371-8.

232. Cersosimo E, Pisters PWT, Pesola G, McDermott K, Bajorunas D, Brennan MF. Insulin secretion and action in patients with pancreatic cancer. Cancer 1991; 67: 486-93.

233. Permert J, Larsson J, Westermark GT, Herrington MK, Christmanson L, Pour PM, Westermark P, Adrian TE. Islet amyloid polypeptide in patients with pancreatic cancer and diabetes. New Engl J Med 1994; 330: 313-18.

234. Lernmark Å, Klöppel G, Stenger D, Vathanaprida C, Fält K, Landin-Olsson M et al. Heterogeneity of islet pathology in two infants with recent onset diabetes mellitus. Virchows Archiv 1995; 425; 631-40.

14

Insulin Biosynthesis and Secretion *In Vitro*

W.J. Malaisse

Laboratory of Experimental Medicine, Brussels Free University, Belgium

The output of insulin from the endocrine pancreas needs to be continuously adjusted; this is in order to maintain fuel homeostasis despite acute or sustained changes in both energy supply and expenditure occurring in situations such as growth, fasting, feeding, exercise, pregnancy, lactation or ageing. Insulin has a critical role in the mobilization and utilization of nutrients in several extrapancreatic organs. The regulation of insulin release is ensured by a series of factors which exert either immediate or delayed effects upon the pancreatic B cell [1]; among these factors, D-glucose has a prominent role. A rise in extracellular D-glucose concentration stimulates the release of insulin, which itself reduces glycaemia. Thus, in a simplified scheme, the secretion of insulin could be viewed as part of a control loop. However, in several situations, e.g. during muscular exercise, the output of insulin from the pancreatic gland is modified without any major change in glycaemia, indicating the participation of factors other than D-glucose in the control of insulin secretion.

Our understanding of the regulation of insulin secretion in the intact organism has gained considerably over the last 30 years from experiments carried out *in vitro* with either the isolated perfused pancreas, pieces of pancreatic tissue, isolated islets of Langerhans or purified islet B cells [2]. The technique of the isolated perfused pancreas provides an opportunity to monitor the secretion of insulin under conditions in which the administration of secretagogues and release of insulin occur through the physiological pathway of the vascular bed. This may be important in view of the proposal that pancreatic endocrine cells display a receptor–secretion polarity [3]. Moreover, in

the model of the isolated perfused pancreas, possible interactions between the acinar and insular moieties of the pancreatic gland would be normally operative. Compared with this method, the incubation or perifusion of pieces of pancreatic tissue offer little advantage, unless the size of the pancreatic gland hinders perfusion. A direct comparison between insulin secretion and associated metabolic and ionic events requires the incubation or perifusion of isolated pancreatic islets. Even so, it should be realized that each islet consists of a heterogeneous collection of cells, including those secreting insulin, glucagon, somatostatin and pancreatic polypeptide, not to mention non-endocrine cells [4]. Hence, whereas the measurement of insulin release specifically concerns the functional response of the B cell, metabolic and ionic data derived from isolated islets reflect the integrated behaviour of all islet cell types. Suitable techniques are now available to isolate purified populations of insulin-producing or glucagon-producing cells [5]. However, the secretory behaviour of isolated B cells differs from that of intact pancreatic islets, indicating the significance of intercellular interactions. Clearly, there is as yet no single method that could be considered optimal for the simultaneous or parallel investigation of metabolic, ionic and secretory events in the pancreatic B cell, when the latter is investigated *in situ*.

Despite such limitations, the experimental work carried out *in vitro* has facilitated characterization both of the major steps in the secretory sequence and of the mode of action of distinct agents involved in the regulation of insulin secretion [6]. This chapter reviews the information currently available on these two topics.

International Textbook of Diabetes Mellitus, Second Edition. Edited by K.G.M.M. Alberti, P. Zimmet, R.A. DeFronzo, and H. Keen (Honorary)
© 1997 John Wiley & Sons Ltd

FUNCTIONAL ORGANIZATION OF THE B CELL

Before considering the regulation of insulin secretion, an overall picture of the functional organization of the B cell is presented, with emphasis on proinsulin biosynthesis and conversion, the mechanism of insulin release, the interaction between distinct cells within each islet and the bioelectrical activity of the B cell.

Proinsulin Biosynthesis and Conversion

The synthesis of insulin occurs through a precursor, proinsulin. The biosynthesis of proinsulin occurs in ribosomes attached to the cisternae of the rough endoplasmic reticulum (RER). After removal of the signal sequence, proinsulin is transferred from the lumen of the RER cisternae to the Golgi apparatus via vesicles originating from transitional elements of the RER. This first type of motile event seems to involve the same structural and biochemical determinants as those discussed below for the intracellular translocation of secretory granules [7].

Proinsulin is then converted into insulin and C-peptide by enzymes which act outside the Golgi apparatus, in immature secretory granules. In parallel with changes in the pH within the secretory granules, insulin is deposited in microcrystalline form in the lumen of these granules. At the exocytotic site, insulin is released together with an equimolar amount of C-peptide. Normally, only a small fraction of the secretory products is released as proinsulin. Newly synthesized proinsulin and insulin may be released in preference to the preformed hormone.

The biosynthesis of proinsulin is stimulated by nutrient secretagogues to a greater relative extent than that of other islet proteins. Although cyclic AMP may, within limits, simulate the stimulant action of nutrient secretagogues upon proinsulin biosynthesis, most non-nutrient insulinotropic agents stimulate insulin release without affecting the biosynthesis of its precursor.

The stimulation of proinsulin biosynthesis by nutrient secretagogues occurs first at the translation level and later through an increase in the cell content of the messenger RNA [8]. The latter content may be affected by both transcription of the insulin gene and degradation of messenger RNA. The threshold value for stimulation of proinsulin synthesis at increasing concentrations of D-glucose is lower than the minimal concentration of the hexose required to stimulate insulin release. In a teleological perspective, this difference may prevent depletion of the hormonal stores whenever insulin release is stimulated by agents failing to affect the biosynthesis of the hormone. If the biosynthetic rate exceeds that of insulin release, excess insulin may undergo lysosomal degradation in a process of granulolysis [9].

The stimulation of proinsulin biosynthesis by glucose and other nutrient secretagogues is closely connected with the capacity of these nutrients to augment the rate of ATP generation in islet cells. The precise nature of the coupling between metabolic and biosynthetic events remains unknown. It is conceivable that an increase in the intracellular concentration of K^+, secondary to a decreased efflux of this cation, participates in such a coupling process [10].

Insulin Release

As already mentioned, stimulation of insulin release may occur independently of any change in the rate of proinsulin biosynthesis. Hence, an increase in insulin output results mainly from the mobilization of secretory granules.

Effector System for Insulin Release

It is currently believed that a sustained stimulation of insulin secretion implies both the translocation of secretory granules to the cell periphery and their access to exocytotic sites at the plasma membrane. The latter process may be sufficient to account for the early secretory response that often occurs as an initial peak in insulin output. These mechanical events are placed under the control of a microtubular–microfilamentous system [11]. Microtubules, which are formed through tubulin polymerization, may act as a guiding cytoskeleton for the intracellular translocation of secretory granules (Figure 1). The latter undergo back-and-forth saltatory movements along microtubular pathways oriented towards or along the cell surface. A microfilamentous cell web located beneath the plasma membrane is thought to act as a sphincter and to control the final access of the secretory granules to their exocytotic site. Agents which increase cytosolic Ca^{2+} concentration stimulate the contractile activity of the microfilamentous network [12]. At the exocytotic site, the fusion of the granule-limiting and plasma membranes may lead, through an anion-osmotic process, to the fission of the membrane and the dissolution of the insulin microcrystal in the extracellular fluid. Thus, the insertion at the site of fusion of an anionic transport system, presumably derived from the granule-limiting membrane, may allow for the inflow of extracellular anions into the lumen of the secretory granule and, consequently, the fission of membrane by osmotic lysis. This process may also account for the chain release of several secretory granules at the same exocytotic site, a phenomenon known as compound exocytosis [13].

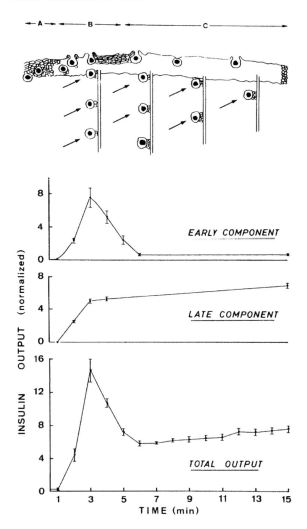

Figure 1 Schematic view for the participation of the microtubular–microfilamentous system in the process of glucose-induced insulin release. In the unstimulated B cell, the granules are kept away from the plasma membrane by the cell web (A). During the first phase of the secretory response (B), the release of insulin corresponds, in part, to the extrusion of granules that were already located in close vicinity to the cell web/plasma membrane complex (early component). During the later phase (C), the release of insulin is largely dependent on the provision of secretory granules transported to the cell web along microtubular pathways (late component). Data for insulin output are expressed as a percentage of the total amount of insulin released over the entire period of stimulation

Role of Protein Kinases

The mechanical events just described may also be explained in biochemical terms. For instance, the contractile activity of microfilaments may be triggered by an increase in the cytosolic concentration of ionized calcium at the intervention of a Ca–calmodulin-responsive protein kinase catalysing the phosphorylation of myosin light chains [14]. Each constituent of this system has been identified in islet cells, as follows.

An increase in the concentration of cytosolic Ca^{2+} is observed in islet cells labelled with fluorescent Ca^{2+} probes and stimulated by a number of secretagogues. Such measurements may disclose a twofold to fourfold increase in cytosolic Ca^{2+} activity above a basal value close to 0.1 μmol/l. Such overall measurements, which may reveal oscillations in the cytosolic Ca^{2+} activity of individual B cells, do not shed light on the heterogeneity of Ca^{2+} concentrations in distinct cytoplasmic domains within the same cell.

The Ca^{2+}-binding regulatory protein calmodulin is present in islet cells and may regulate the activity of several enzymes, including adenylate cyclase, cyclic AMP phosphodiesterase, a plasma membrane-associated Ca^{2+}-ATPase and selected protein kinases, such as the myosin light chain kinase [15]. The presence of actin, too, in the microfilamentous cell web of islet cells, has been detected by histoimmunological methods.

It should be realized that stimulus–secretion coupling for insulin release involves a number of distinct kinases responsive to distinct regulatory factors [16]. For instance, the cyclic AMP-responsive protein kinase A, as well as the phospholipid-dependent, Ca^{2+}-responsive and diacylglycerol-activated protein kinase C, and their respective protein substrates, have all been identified in islet cells. Moreover, other enzymatic activities may participate in the control of mechanical events in the islet cells. A Ca^{2+}-responsive transglutaminase could be cited as an example, inhibition of this enzyme being associated with impairment of translocation both of proinsulin from its site of biosynthesis to its site of conversion and of insulin from its site of storage to its site of release [17].

Recently, several components of the exocytotic fusion machinery have been identified in pancreatic islets. For instance, a functional role has now been proposed for proteins involved in the docking of secretory vesicles to the plasma membrane, such as a soluble *N*-ethylmaleimide-sensitive factor (NSF) attachment protein (SNAP) and its receptor (SNARE) [88].

Dynamics of the Secretory Process

In response to a step-wise increase in glucose concentration from an initial non-stimulant level, the release of insulin (the time-course of which from a single B cell has not yet been measured) displays a biphasic pattern when examined in the isolated perfused rat pancreas, isolated islets or dispersed islet cells [18]. An initial secretory peak is followed by a slow and progressive resurgence of insulin output. This time-course resembles closely that observed for the bioelectrical activity of each B cell [19]. Indeed, in the latter case, a first long phase of continuous spike activity is followed by a repolarization without spike, and, eventually, by the development of slow waves of electrical activity. This analogy strongly suggests that the major determinant of the phasic pattern of the secretory response coincides with those factors that regulate the gating and closing of Ca^{2+}-channels located at the plasma membrane (Figure 2). This is not to deny that such a setting may coexist with other functional aspects relevant to the time-course of the secretory response. For instance, it remains conceivable that the secretory granules mobilized during the initial peak and late secretory phase, respectively, originate from distinct storage sites in each B cell. Similarly, slow oscillations in insulin release with a periodicity of several minutes (e.g. 6–15 minutes), as observed in the perfused pancreas or in perifused islets, may be under the control of a pacemaker mechanism distinct from that involved in the regulation of bioelectrical activity, being conceivably associated with slow oscillations in glycolytic flux.

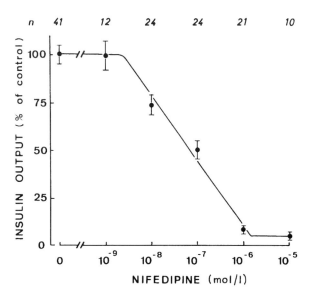

Figure 2 Effect of nifedipine (concentrations shown on a logarithmic scale) upon insulin release evoked by D-glucose (16.7 mmol/l) in isolated islets. Mean values (± SEM) are expressed as a percentage of the mean control value and refer to the number of individual determinations (*n*) shown at the top of the figure. The inhibitory action of the organic calcium antagonist supports the idea that Ca^{2+} enters the B cell through L-type Ca^{2+} channels

Cellular Interaction, Heterogeneity and Recruitment

The pancreatic B cell is located in the islets of Langerhans, where it is surrounded by both other B cells and non-B islet cells, including cells producing glucagon, somatostatin and pancreatic polypeptide. It is conceivable that the local release of the latter hormones affects,

in a paracrine process, the secretory activity of adjacent B cells [20]. The organization of the microvasculature within each islet is also relevant. The influence of pancreatic hormones such as glucagon and somatostatin upon the secretory activity of the B cell is considered later in this chapter. At this point, however, it should be mentioned that the existence of a feedback inhibitory action of insulin upon its own rate of secretion remains the subject of an apparently endless debate. Recent findings suggest that islet cells may contain the membrane glycophospholipid which, in extrapancreatic target cells for insulin, acts as the precursor of a phospho-oligosaccharide currently considered as the insulin second messenger, and that the latter phospho-oligosaccharide might inhibit insulin secretion [21]. However, there is as yet no evidence that insulin promotes, in the B cell, the generation of this messenger. This seems unlikely, because islet B cells are apparently devoid of high-affinity receptors for insulin, the binding of the latter hormone being restricted to a limited interaction with receptors for the type 1 insulin-like growth factor [22].

In addition to the possible intra-islet hormonal control of insulin release either by a paracrine process or via the microcirculation, B cells and non-B islet cells may interact through gap junctions and bioelectrical intercellular coupling [23]. Hence, it may be unwise to consider the B cell as an isolated secretory unit. Instead, all cells within the same islet could be viewed as a functional syncytium displaying coordinated and synchronized secretory activity. This concept may have several implications. To cite only one example, one could question whether the difference in the kinetics of D-glucose transport into B and non-B islet cells, respectively, as documented in purified populations of isolated islet cells, is operative in intact islets, when D-glucose could move from the cytosol of one cell to another.

At variance with the latter considerations, there is evidence that distinct B cells, whether isolated or distributed within the same islet, may display vastly different levels of metabolic, biosynthetic and secretory activity at any given concentration of D-glucose. The latter finding suggests that the graded functional response of the endocrine pancreas to increasing concentrations of D-glucose might involve a phenomenon of cell recruitment. The mathematical modelling of such a phenomenon indicates that it may also have a role in the phasic and oscillatory time-course of insulin release [24].

Bioelectrical Activity

In addition to its biosynthetic and secretory responses, the pancreatic B cell also displays bioelectrical activity when stimulated by suitable secretagogues [19]. This bioelectrical activity can be dissociated from the process of insulin release, for instance by a lowering of the temperature. Therefore, it does not merely represent an epiphenomenon of insulin release, but instead seems to play a crucial part in the secretory response.

In the absence of glucose or at low concentrations of the hexose the membrane potential of B cells is stable, between −60 and −70 mV. When the glucose concentration is raised to a stimulatory value, an initial and slow depolarization is thought to reflect the closing of K$^+$-channels, and brings the membrane potential to a threshold value from which a fast depolarization leads to a plateau potential, onto which spike activity is superimposed. At the end of each burst of spikes, the membrane repolarizes to a level slightly more negative than the threshold potential. The phasic pattern of bioelectrical activity is replaced by continuous spike activity with persistent depolarization at the plateau potential at very high glucose concentrations. The fast process of depolarization at the onset of each burst of spikes and the ascending segment of each spike are thought to reflect mainly the facilitated entry of Ca^{2+} into the B cell. Conversely, the descending segment of each spike and the repolarization process at the end of each burst are attributed mainly to an increase in K$^+$ permeability. The latter may result from activation of Ca^{2+}-sensitive or voltage-dependent K$^+$ channels.

The monitoring of electrical activity in an impaled B cell is most informative in that it enables identification of rapidly occurring events located at the plasma membrane in individual B cells. When combined with sophisticated electrophysiological measurements, such as the permeability ratio P_{Na}/P_K and input resistance, such monitoring may help to identify the cationic determinants of the changes in plasma membrane potential. Moreover, by use of the patch clamp technique in its different forms, it has recently been possible to identify the various channels mediating the passive flux of cations across the B-cell plasma membrane [25].

Thus, ATP-sensitive K$^+$ channels, calcium-activated K$^+$ channels, delayed rectifier K$^+$ channels, voltage-gated Ca^{2+} channels, non voltage-gated Ca^{2+} channels and Na$^+$ channels have all been described in islet cells [89].

NUTRIENT PATHWAY FOR INSULIN RELEASE

Circulating nutrients, especially D-glucose, have a critical role in the control of insulin release. The stimulation of insulin secretion by these secretagogues is currently considered within the framework of a 'fuel' concept for insulin release. According to this concept, the response of the B cell to nutrient secretagogues reflects their

capacity to augment oxidative fluxes and, hence, ATP generation in the same cell [26, 27].

Identification of Nutrient Secretagogues

The 'fuel' concept, as just defined, differs from a previous hypothesis, according to which the stimulation of insulin release by D-glucose and other nutrient secretagogues would be attributable to the activation of stereospecific receptors, possibly located at the B-cell plasma membrane [28]. The selection of one of these two theories required the elucidation of such points as the anomeric specificity of the secretory response to D-glucose and D-mannose (Figure 3), and the insulinotropic action of a non-metabolized analogue of L-leucine, 2-aminobicyclo[2,2,1]-heptane-2-carboxylic acid (BCH) (Figure 4) as reviewed elsewhere [29, 30]. In all cases, it was eventually established that the magnitude of insulin release could

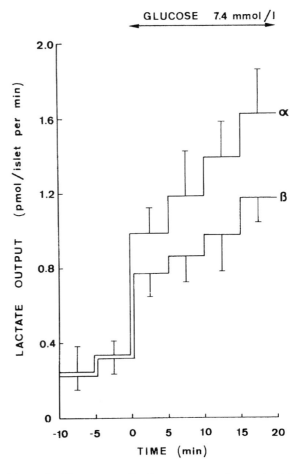

Figure 3 Time-course for lactate output from rat islets before and after the addition of either α or β D-glucose (7.4 mmol/l) to the incubation medium. Mean values ($\pm$ SEM) refer to 6 individual measurements in each case. The higher rate of glycolysis in islets exposed to α D-glucose reflects the greater insulinotropic efficiency of this anomer

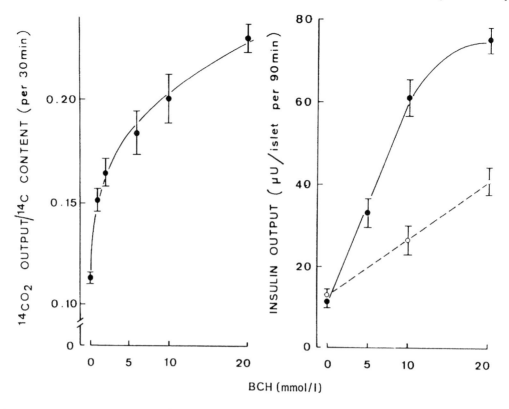

Figure 4 Concentration–response relationship for the effect of BCH upon $^{14}CO_2$ output from islets prelabelled with L-[U-^{14}C]glutamine (left panel) and upon insulin release from islets incubated in the absence (open circles and dashed line) or presence (closed circles and solid line) of 1.0 mmol/l L-glutamine (right panel). Mean values ($\pm$ SEM) refer to five or more individual observations. These findings illustrate that BCH, a non-metabolized analogue of L-leucine, may, by activating glutamate dehydrogenase, accelerate the oxidative metabolism of L-glutamine and by doing so stimulate insulin release

be accounted for by the metabolic response of the islet cells. For instance, the greater efficiency of the α-anomers of both D-glucose and D-mannose to stimulate insulin release coincides with a higher rate of glycolysis in the islet cells. Similarly, the insulinotropic action of BCH was found to be attributable to the activation of glutamate dehydrogenase, resulting in the accelerated catabolism of endogenous amino acids.

The 'fuel' concept for insulin release stresses the importance of such phenomena as the regulation of nutrient catabolism in the islet cells, the generation of those second messengers conceivably coupling the metabolism of nutrients to more distal cellular events in the secretory sequence, and the implicit alignment between the rate of ATP generation and hydrolysis in both resting and stimulated islet cells.

Regulation of Glucose Metabolism

Hexose Transport

Several features of glucose metabolism in islet B cells are well suited to their glucostatic function [31]. For instance, in normal B cells, the carrier system

for D-glucose transport is quite efficient, so that the extracellular and intracellular concentrations of D-glucose are virtually in instantaneous equilibrium. Other hexoses, including D-mannose, D-fructose and D-galactose, are also rapidly equilibrated across the B-cell plasma membrane. Incidentally, this does not appear to be the case in either normal non-B islet cells or tumoral islet cells [32].

Glucose Phosphorylation

The rapid equilibration of D-glucose concentration across the B-cell plasma membrane allows for the participation of both a high K_m glucokinase and a low K_m hexokinase in the phosphorylation of the hexose (Figure 5). In intact islet cells, the low K_m enzyme is thought to be largely inhibited by endogenous glucose 6-phosphate and, to a lesser extent, glucose 1,6-bisphosphate. Hence, glucokinase may have a predominant role in D-glucose phosphorylation in the B cell. It has even been suggested that glucokinase represents the key component of the B-cell glucose sensor device and, as such, should be considered as a glucoreceptor. This proposal is misleading, however, for both semantic and

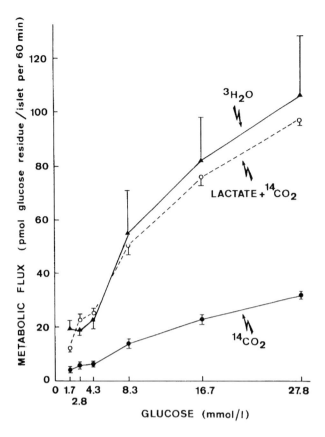

Figure 5 Concentration dependency for the production of ^3H_2O from D-[5-^{3}H]glucose (closed triangles and solid line), the oxidation of D-[U-^{14}C]glucose (closed circles and solid line) and the production of both lactate and $^{14}CO_2$ (open circles and dashed line) by rat pancreatic islets. Mean values ($\pm$ SEM) refer to five or more individual determinations. The figure illustrates the sigmoidal pattern of the metabolic response at increasing concentrations of hexose, a situation attributable in part to the participation of both hexokinase and glucokinase in the phosphorylation of D-glucose

biological reasons [33]. Incidentally, pancreatic islets are virtually devoid (at least in the rat) of specific glucose 6-phosphatase.

The affinity of both hexokinase and glucokinase for ATP is sufficiently low to postulate that the changes in cytosolic ATP concentration, as encountered in glucose-stimulated islets, exert a positive feedback effect on D-glucose phosphorylation, which would thus be the object of a sequential synarchistic regulation. Furthermore, the recent demonstration that hexokinase isoenzymes are largely bound to mitochondria in islet cells opens new perspectives for the regulation of glucose metabolism. Thus, the ubiquity of these enzymes, the preferential utilization of mitochondrial ATP as a substrate for D-glucose phosphorylation by the bound enzymes, the lesser inhibition by glucose 6-phosphate of bound compared with free hexokinase, and the direct coupling between hexose phosphorylation and mitochondrial respiration all need now to

be integrated into the regulatory pattern of glucose catabolism [34].

The activity of glucokinase can be modulated by a regulatory protein that confers on the enzyme the property of being inhibited by D-fructose 6-phosphate and relieved from such an inhibition by D-fructose 1-phosphate [90]. There is also recent evidence to suggest that a translocation of glucokinase to the periphery of the B cell takes place in glucose-stimulated islets, and that the enzyme needs to interact with a yet unidentified target protein to fully express its catalytic activity [91, 92]. The perturbation of these processes in islets which have undergone cross-linking of intracellular proteins causes a preferential impairment of D-glucose metabolism at high, as distinct from low, concentrations of the hexose [93].

Further Glycolytic Events

The utilization of glucose in islet cells is also regulated at sites distal to the level of hexose phosphorylation. First, the channelling of hexose 6-phosphate into distinct metabolic pathways does not display an invariable pattern. For instance, in both normal and tumoral islet cells, the β anomer of D-glucose 6-phosphate is channelled preferentially into the pentose shunt, whereas the corresponding α anomer is channelled preferentially into the glycolytic pathway [35]. The expression of the anomeric specificity of glycolytic enzymes is apparently favoured by the enzyme-to-enzyme channelling of hexose 6-phosphates in the sequence of reactions catalysed by phosphoglucoisomerase and phosphofructokinase [94]. Second, phosphofructokinase is (and needs to be) suitably activated in order for the rate of fructose 6-phosphate phosphorylation to keep pace with its rate of generation from glucose 6-phosphate. Both fructose 2,6-bisphosphate and glucose 1,6-bisphosphate participate in such an activation of phosphofructokinase [36].

Mitochondrial Oxidative Events

In normal islets, an increase in glucose concentration causes preferential stimulation of mitochondrial oxidative events such as the transfer of NADH into the mitochondria, as apparently mediated by the glycerol phosphate shuttle, the decarboxylation of pyruvate and the oxidation of acetyl residues in the tricarboxylic acid (TCA) cycle [37]. The glucose-induced increment in the rate of these mitochondrial oxidative events is, indeed, more marked, in relative terms, than the corresponding increment in the overall rate of glucose utilization. Such a situation is quite unusual, the opposite picture being observed in either non-glucose-responsive secretory cells (e.g. parotid cells) or in some models of B-cell dysfunction (e.g. tumoral cells of the RINm5F line). It is obviously well suited to favour the generation of ATP at increasing concentrations of glucose, in which case the preferential stimulation of mitochondrial oxidative events represents a concentration-related and time-related phenomenon. This phenomenon coincides with the stimulation by D-glucose of ATP-consuming functional processes, including the biosynthesis of proinsulin and the active transport of Ca^{2+} by Ca^{2+}-ATPases located at either the plasma membrane or endoplasmic reticulum [38].

The preferential stimulation of mitochondrial oxidative events in islets exposed to a high concentration of D-glucose appears attributable to the activation by either cytosolic or mitochondrial Ca^{2+} of key mitochondrial dehydrogenases including FAD-linked glycerophosphate dehydrogenase (the key enzyme of the glycerol phosphate shuttle), NAD-isocitrate dehydrogenase and the 2-ketoglutarate dehydrogenase complex [95].

The regulation of metabolic events in the TCA cycle may also involve the enzyme-to-enzyme channelling of symmetric intermediates in the sequence of reactions catalysed by succinate thiokinase, succinate dehydrogenase and fumarase [96].

Metabolism of Endogenous Nutrients

If the assumption is correct that the secretory response of the B cell to nutrient secretagogues is causally linked to an increase in ATP generation rate and oxygen consumption, it follows that equal attention should be paid to the metabolic fate of the exogenous nutrient

used to stimulate insulin release and its effect upon the catabolism of endogenous nutrients in the islet cells [39]. The basal oxygen uptake by islets, which is close to the maximal increment in oxygen consumption evoked by potent nutrient secretagogues, can be accounted for mainly by the catabolism of endogenous amino acids and that of fatty acids derived from endogenous triglycerides. A sparing action of certain exogenous nutrients, e.g. pyruvate or L-glutamine, upon the utilization of endogenous nutrients may account for the absence of any sizeable increase in insulin output. Conversely, certain non-metabolized nutrient analogues, e.g. phenylpyruvate and BCH, may stimulate insulin release by accelerating the catabolism of endogenous nutrients.

Coupling of Metabolic to Distal Events

The identity of the second messengers coupling metabolic to more distal events in the secretory sequence remains to be fully elucidated [40]. One of the difficulties encountered in such an investigation is the selection, from a great number of distal events, of those that may be directly regulated by metabolic events. In this respect, emphasis is currently given to a decrease in K^+ conductance resulting from the closure of a class of K^+ channels located at the B-cell plasma membrane (Figure 6). Several coupling factors could be considered. Indeed, an increase in nutrient oxidation usually coincides with an increase in the generation rate of reducing equivalents (NADH and NADPH), high-energy phosphate intermediates (ATP) and protons (H^+). Alternatively, metabolites generated

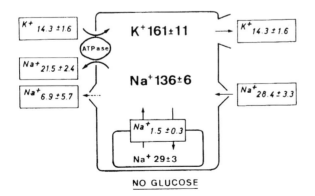

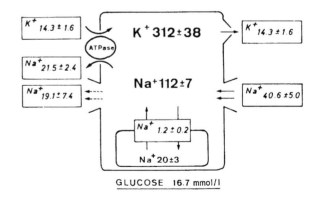

Figure 6 Schematic view of the handling of monovalent cations by pancreatic islets incubated in the absence or presence of D-glucose (16.7 mmol/l). Steady-state values for pool sizes are expressed as pmol per islet (intracellular water space: 2 to 3 nl per islet). Fluxes are given in the rectangles as pmol per islet per min. The opening or closing of the gates reflects changes in permeability, as judged from either the inflow rate or fractional outflow rate of each cation. Also depicted is the existence of a small and possibly organelle-bound pool of Na^+ characterized by a low turnover rate. A 3/2 stoichiometry is postulated for Na^+/K^+ transport by the membrane-associated ATPase, and all influent K^+ is assumed to be transported by such an ATPase. The figure illustrates that a rise in glucose concentration, by causing the closure of ATP-responsive K^+ channels while failing to affect the activity of the Na^+, K^+-ATPase, decreases the fractional outflow rate of K^+ and hence increases its intracellular concentration. This coincides with a decrease in Na^+ cell content, itself attributable to a greater increase in Na^+ outflow than inflow rate

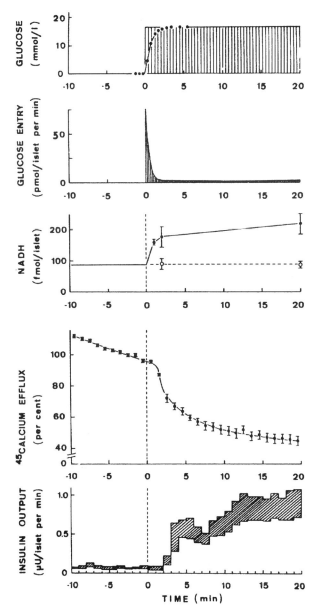

Figure 7 Sequential events in the process of glucose-induced insulin release. The upper panel depicts the square-wave increase in extracellular D-glucose concentration of incubation media (hatched area) or progressive increase in hexose concentration of the effluent in a system of perifused islets (closed circles). The second panel refers to the time-course for the net uptake of D-glucose by the islets. The third panel illustrates the changes in NADH content of glucose-stimulated islets (closed circles and solid line) as distinct from glucose-deprived islets (open circles and dashed line). The fourth panel documents the glucose-induced decrease in $^{45}Ca^{2+}$ efflux from islets perifused in the absence of extracellular Ca^{2+}, the results being expressed as a percentage of the mean basal value found over the 5 min preceding glucose administration. The lowest panel provides the pattern of insulin release obtained after depriving the islets of glucose for 45 min. This figure emphasizes the chronological hierarchy for changes in selected metabolic, ionic and secretory variables

in suitable catabolic pathways may act as coupling factors. It is also conceivable that the coupling between metabolic and more distal events in the secretory sequence represents a multifactorial process, distinct coupling factors acting separately or in concert to affect distinct distal targets (Figure 7).

Metabolic Intermediates

A few years ago, when it was still a matter of debate whether glucose needed to be metabolized in islet cells in order to stimulate insulin release, the view had been taken into consideration that an early metabolite of glucose, e.g. glucose 6-phosphate, might act as a signal for insulin release. Now that it seems evident that distinct nutrient secretagogues—which are metabolized by vastly different pathways—owe their insulinotropic capacity to their ability to act as a fuel in islet cells, the idea that a critical metabolite acts as the major coupling factor is received with greater scepticism. Nevertheless, such an idea should not be ruled out. For instance, phosphoenol-pyruvate may affect the mitochondrial handling of Ca^{2+} or the activity of enzymes such as adenylate cyclase and protein kinase [41, 42].

Reducing Equivalents and Protons

The possible role of either increased generation of reducing equivalents, such as NADH, NADPH and reduced glutathione, or the changes in intracellular pH evoked by nutrient secretagogues in the coupling of metabolic to distal events, has been examined in detail in two reviews [40, 43]. Recent findings have cast some doubt on the view that either of these two processes would represent the key second messenger in nutrient-induced insulin release. As far as the redox state is concerned, no parallelism could be found between the changes in cytosolic $NADH/NAD^+$ and $NADPH/NADP^+$ ratios evoked by distinct nutrient secretagogues and their insulinotropic action. With regard to the role of intracellular pH, it has been emphasized [44] that intracellular alkalinization may provoke insulin release at a very low glucose concentration (1.0 mmol/l). As D-glucose does, indeed, increase intracellular pH, this would be compatible with a role for such a pH in stimulus–secretion coupling. However, the increase in cellular pH evoked by D-glucose does not, apparently, represent a primary consequence of the acceleration in glucose catabolism but, instead, may result from the secondary activation of processes such as Na^+/H^+ and HCO_3^-/Cl^- exchange. Hence, it might be unwise to consider the rise in cell pH as a coupling factor immediately generated through the catabolism of nutrients in islet cells.

ATP

Over the last few years, considerable attention has been paid to the possible role of a rise in cytosolic ATP concentration as the major factor coupling the catabolism of nutrients to ionic events in the secretory sequence. This concept is based mainly on the following three series of findings.

First, electrophysiological studies by the patch clamp technique have identified in the islet cell membrane a class of K^+ channels that can be inhibited by intracellular ATP [45–47]. In islet cells stimulated by D-glucose or D-glyceraldehyde, the closure of these channels is thought to cause membrane depolarization, which is required for opening the voltage-gated Ca^{2+} channels and, hence, facilitated influx of Ca^{2+}. In excised inside-out membrane patches, a concentration of 1.0 mmol/l ATP is largely sufficient to abolish all K^+ channel activity. As the resting cytosolic ATP concentration is not lower than 1.0 mmol/l, it may appear unlikely that a nutrient-induced increase in the latter concentration would indeed affect the probability of the open state of the ATP-sensitive K^+ channels. However, a recent study suggests that, in saponin-permeabilized insulin-secreting cells of the RINm5F line, ADP (0.1–0.5 mmol/l) markedly activates K^+ channels, as judged from single-channel current recording [48]. The effect of ADP (0.5 mmol/l) to activate K^+ channels was also operative in the presence of ATP

(0.5 mmol/l). Hence, the probability of these K^+ channels opening or closing may be dependent on changes in ATP/ADP ratio, rather than being determined solely by the ATP concentration.

Second, we have recently indicated [49] that D-glucose does indeed markedly increase the cytosolic ATP/ADP ratio in normal pancreatic islets, whereas previous studies had been restricted to measuring the total cellular concentrations of adenine nucleotides.

Last, exposure of tumoral islet cells of the RINm5F line to the non-metabolized analogue of L-leucine, BCH, provided a unique opportunity to distinguish between changes in cytosolic redox state and ATP availability (or ATP/ADP ratio) as a determinant of nutrient-stimulated insulin release [50]. In these cells, BCH unexpectedly inhibited insulin release, despite the induction of a more reduced cytosolic redox state. The inhibition of insulin release by BCH coincided with a decrease in O_2 uptake and a lowering of ATP concentration and ATP/ADP ratio (Figure 8), and was accompanied by an increase in ^{86}Rb outflow from prelabelled cells. Thus, in this system, the changes in ATP generation rate, which were found to be attributable to a sparing action on the catabolism of endogenous fatty acids [51], were apparently responsible (rather than the changes in cytosolic redox state) for the functional response of these tumoral cells.

Another, additional, mechanism by which ATP could affect insulin release may consist of the exocytotic

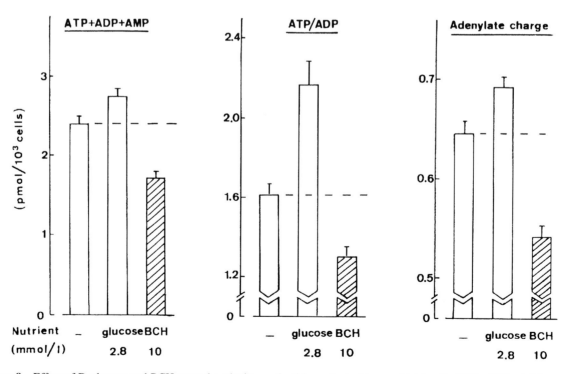

Figure 8 Effect of D-glucose and BCH upon the adenine nucleotide content of tumoral islet cells (RINm5F line). Mean values (± SEM) were recorded after 30 min incubation and refer to eight or more individual determinations. The figure illustrates the opposing effects of the hexose and the non-metabolized analogue of L-leucine, respectively, in this model of B-cell dysfunction

release of the adenine nucleotide, which is present in the secretory granules, leading (at the intervention of purinergic receptors) to a further amplification of the secretory response [52] (Figure 9). It should again be stressed that, although only the role of ATP has been considered in detail in this chapter, the participation of other factors generated through the catabolism of nutrients, e.g. reducing equivalents and protons, in the coupling of metabolic to distal events should not be entirely neglected.

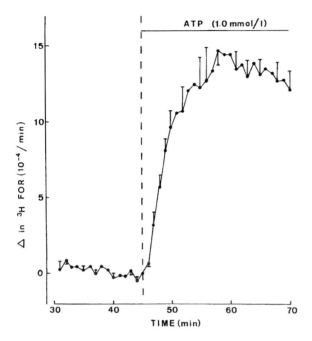

Figure 9 Effect of exogenous ATP (1.0 mmol/l), administered from min 46 onwards, upon the ^{3}H fractional outflow rate (FOR) from islets prelabelled with myo-[2-^{3}H]inositol and perifused in the presence of 7.0 mmol/l D-glucose. Mean values ($\pm$ SEM) refer to the paired differences from the control readings recorded at the 45th min of perifusion and are derived from four individual experiments. This figure indicates that exogenous ATP may, at the intervention of purinergic receptors, stimulate the hydrolysis of phosphoinositides, this coinciding with an enhancement of insulin release

Amplification Devices

Later in this chapter emphasis is placed on two modalities for the modulation of nutrient-stimulated insulin release by non-nutrient environmental agents, namely the activation of either adenylate cyclase or phospholipase C. It should be realized, however, that in intact pancreatic islets exposed solely to D-glucose, the generation of cyclic AMP and hydrolysis of phosphoinositides are apparently also involved in the secretory response to this hexose. As a working hypothesis, it could be proposed that the effect of D-glucose upon such processes represents a suitable device for amplification of the functional response to nutrient secretagogues.

D-glucose and other nutrient secretagogues do apparently augment the rate of cyclic AMP generation in islet cells [53]. This is best demonstrated in the presence of phosphodiesterase inhibitors. The modelling of cyclic AMP turnover suggests, however, that the activation of adenylate cyclase by nutrients is not dependent on the presence of such inhibitors. The nutrient-induced increase in cyclic AMP formation is considerably impaired when the islets are incubated in the absence of extracellular Ca^{2+} [54]. This raises the possibility that the effect of nutrients upon adenylate cyclase is secondary to the increase in cytosolic Ca^{2+} activity observed in glucose-stimulated islet cells exposed to a normal concentration of extracellular Ca^{2+} [55]. The discovery that, in a subcellular particulate fraction prepared from isolated islets, calmodulin causes, in a calcium-dependent manner, activation of adenylate cyclase, provides such a pathway for the acceleration of cyclic AMP generation in nutrient-stimulated islet cells [56].

A somewhat comparable proposal was recently advanced to account for the stimulation by nutrient secretagogues of the hydrolysis of inositol-containing phospholipids. This effect was documented in islets exposed to such nutrient secretagogues as D-glucose, 2-ketoisocaproate, 3-phenylpyruvate and 2-*endo*-aminonorbornane-2-carboxylic acid [57]. The response to D-glucose is abolished in the presence of mannoheptulose. These findings indicate that the activation of phospholipase C in islets exposed to nutrient secretagogues is closely dependent on the integrity of their metabolic effects. The effect of these nutrients upon the hydrolysis of inositol-containing lipids is abolished at extracellular Ca^{2+} concentrations equal or below 10^{-5} mol/l, and can be duplicated by a rise in extracellular K^+ concentration (from 5 mmol/l to 30 mmol/l or more), which is known to cause cell membrane depolarization and, hence, facilitated Ca^{2+} inflow into islet cells [58]. Moreover, in digitonin-permeabilized islets, a marked stimulation of phosphoinositide hydrolysis is observed when the Ca^{2+} concentration of the medium is raised from 10^{-7} mol/l to 10^{-5} mol/l. All these data are consistent with the view that the effect of nutrient secretagogues upon phospholipase C in islet cells is secondary to an increase in cytosolic Ca^{2+} activity.

The two examples just mentioned do not exhaust the list of cellular mechanisms possibly involved in the stimulus–secretion coupling for nutrient-induced insulin release. For instance, the activation of phospholipase A$_2$ and the resulting generation of eicosanoids in the arachidonate cascade, the influence of a change in both redox state and cytosolic Ca^{2+} concentration upon the activity of transglutaminase, or a decrease in plasma membrane fluidity, could be cited as further cytophysiological processes participating in the stimulation of islet cells by D-glucose. In this respect, it remains a challenge to assess the relative importance, in both qualitative and quantitative terms, of each of these coupling processes, when considering the overall magnitude—and time-course—of the secretory response to D-glucose and other nutrient secretagogues.

Semantic Games

In the light of the above considerations on the coupling of metabolic to more distal events in the secretory sequence, it is not surprising that suitable manipulations of the B-cell environment may reveal coupling modalities that are not necessarily obvious under physiological conditions. This approach has led, over recent years, to a kind of semantic game in which distinct pathways for stimulation of insulin release by D-glucose are arbitrarily defined.

The first of these pathways is currently described as the K_{ATP}-channel-dependent pathway. It includes the closure of the ATP-sensitive K^+ channels, with resultant depolarization of the plasma membrane, increased influx of Ca^{2+} via L-type voltage-dependent Ca^{2+} channels and elevated intracellular Ca^{2+} concentration.

A second Ca^{2+}-dependent pathway by which D-glucose increases insulin secretion is referred to as the K_{ATP}-channel-independent pathway. For example, when the ATP-sensitive K^+ channels are kept in their open configuration by diazoxide, and when a high extracellular concentration of K^+ is used to nevertheless cause plasma membrane depolarization, D-glucose still causes a concentration-related enhancement of insulin release, the mechanism of which remains to be elucidated.

Quite recently, a third pathway, namely a Ca^{2+}-independent effect of D-glucose to augment insulin release from islets deprived of extracellular Ca^{2+} but exposed to activators of protein kinases A and C, was proposed as a novel branch of stimulus–secretion coupling [97]. Since findings similar to those quoted in support of this third modality have been available for more than 20 years, such semantic games merely reinforce the view that the coupling between the metabolic and functional response to D-glucose represents a multifactorial process.

NON-NUTRIENT SECRETAGOGUES
The Cholinergic Pathway

It has been known for more than two decades that cholinergic agents exert an immediate and direct stimulatory effect upon insulin release by the pancreatic

B cell [59], and vagal stimulation of insulin secretion has long been postulated to participate in the response of the endocrine pancreas to food intake, including a cephalic phase of insulin release [60]. However, it is only relatively recently that the cytophysiologic events mediating the response to cholinergic neurotransmitters have been elucidated [61].

Muscarinic Receptors and Activation of Phospholipase C

Islet cells are equipped with muscarinic receptors. In membranes isolated from dispersed islet cells, carbamylcholine causes a concentration-related decrease in the amount of ^{32}P-labelled phosphatidylinositol 4-phosphate and phosphatidylinositol 4,5-bisphosphate. In these experiments, the polyphosphoinositides were prelabelled by exposing the isolated membranes to $[\gamma\text{-}^{32}P]ATP$, and carbamylcholine was then added 10 s before lipid extraction [62]. The formation of diacylglycerol was documented by preincubating the islet cells with $[U\text{-}^{14}C]$arachidonate. These experiments support the view that activation of a plasma membrane-associated phospholipase C directed against polyphosphoinositides represents an early event in the cholinergic stimulation of insulin release. Moreover, the modulation of the response to carbamylcholine by atropine, calcium chelators and calcium antagonists in the isolated membranes points to a key role for membrane-bound Ca^{2+} in the coupling between muscarinic receptor occupancy and polyphosphoinositide hydrolysis. It was recently proposed that a GTP-binding regulatory protein participates in the activation of phospholipase C by cholinergic agents in islet cells [63]. This regulatory protein is apparently distinct from either Ns or Ni. Thus, none of the agents acting at the intervention of the latter two regulatory proteins (glucagon, clonidine, cholera toxin) affects the hydrolysis of inositol-containing phospholipids, whether in resting or carbamylcholine-stimulated normal or tumoral islet cells. It should be noted, however, that clonidine suppresses the insulin secretory response of the islets to cholinergic agents.

Hydrolysis of Polyphosphoinositides in Intact Islet Cells

In intact islets, carbamylcholine also stimulates the hydrolysis of polyphosphoinositides [64]. This coincides with a rise in the production of inositol 1,4,5-triphosphate, myo-inositol 1,4-bisphosphate and myo-inositol 1-phosphate. The carbamylcholine-induced hydrolysis of phosphoinositides appears to be tightly coupled with their resynthesis from phosphatidic acid. Moreover, cholinergic stimuli apparently also favor the *de novo* synthesis of phosphatidic acid and phosphatidylinositol. The enhanced turnover of inositol-containing phospholipids caused by cholinergic agents in islet cells represents a calcium-dependent process, though apparently not triggered by an increase in Ca^{2+} fluxes into the islet cells.

The effect of cholinergic agents on phospholipid metabolism in islet cells is not restricted to the turnover of phosphoinositides. Carbamylcholine also apparently causes activation of phospholipase A_2. By analogy with findings obtained in other tissues, the suggestion has been made that such an activation may be mediated, in part at least, through the hydrolysis of polyphosphoinositides. The activation of phospholipase A_2 being more marked in response to cholinergic agents than to D-glucose, the liberation of arachidonate and the generation of messengers in the arachidonate cascade could have a greater role in the cholinergic stimulation of the B cell than in nutrient-induced insulin release.

Activation of Protein Kinase C

As reviewed in greater detail elsewhere [61], there are a number of mechanisms by which the above-mentioned changes in phospholipid metabolism could participate in the secretory response of the B cell to cholinergic neurotransmitters. A current hypothesis postulates that diacylglycerol and inositol 1,4,5-triphosphate, which are liberated from phosphatidylinositol 4,5-bisphosphate, may lead respectively to activation of protein kinase C and mobilization of Ca^{2+} from non-mitochondrial organelles.

The presence of a phospholipid-dependent, Ca^{2+}-responsive and diacylglycerol-activated protein kinase activity in islet homogenates has been documented by several investigators. The sensitivity of this enzyme to increasing concentrations of Ca^{2+} is modulated by the extent of activation by either diacylglycerol or its substitute 12-*O*-tetradecanoylphorbol-13-acetate. It is conceivable, therefore, that activation of the enzyme leads to stimulation of insulin release even at a resting level of cytosolic Ca^{2+} activity. This is supported by comparison between the cationic and secretory responses, respectively, to such agents as tumor-promoting phorbol esters and the membrane-accessible diglyceride 1-oleyl-2-acetylglycerol [65, 66]. A selective inhibitor of protein kinase C (H-7) was used to establish further the participation of this enzyme in the secretory response to cholinergic agents.

Mobilization of Intracellular Ca^{2+}

The ionic response of islet cells to cholinergic agents differs in several respects from that evoked by nutrient secretagogues. For instance, whereas the latter usually decrease ^{86}Rb outflow from prelabelled islets, carbamylcholine increases ^{86}Rb outflow. This effect persists in the absence of extracellular Ca^{2+} and at low glucose concentrations, under which conditions the neurotransmitter does not change the B-cell membrane potential.

Cholinergic agents also provoke a rapid increase in ^{45}Ca outflow from prelabelled islets. This effect, which is blocked by atropine, is seen both in the absence and the presence of either D-glucose or extracellular Ca^{2+}. It is thought, therefore, to reflect mobilization of ^{45}Ca from cellular sites by inositol 1,4,5-triphosphate in a manner comparable to that described in rat insulinoma microsomes.

Modulation of the Secretory Response to Cholinergic Agents

In the light of the information so far reviewed, the stimulation of insulin release by cholinergic agents could be viewed as resulting from a dual mechanism, namely the activation of protein kinase C and mobilization of intracellular Ca^{2+}. According to some authors [67], such a dual mechanism may account for the biphasic pattern of insulin release. It should be stressed, however, that cholinergic agents fail to stimulate insulin release in the absence of exogenous nutrient or at low concentrations of D-glucose. The permissive role of D-glucose was tentatively ascribed to the capacity of the sugar to cause membrane depolarization and, hence, to allow for stimulation of Ca^{2+} inflow by the cholinergic agent. Incidentally, cholinergic agents fail to exert any obvious effect upon glucose oxidation, although they may increase the NADH content of islet cells. The secretory response to acetylcholine is amplified by physostigmine (eserine), simulated by muscarine, and abolished by atropine or methylscopolamine.

In conclusion, the cholinergic pathway for stimulation of insulin release apparently involves a sophisticated sequence of cellular events, starting with the occupation of muscarinic receptors, followed by the activation of phospholipase C and the liberation of diacylglycerol and inositol phosphate from membrane phosphoinositides. These biochemical processes eventually lead to a remodelling of ionic fluxes, induction of bioelectrical activity and the activation of enzymes such as protein kinase C and phospholipase A_2.

Although the functional response of the pancreatic B cell to cholinergic agents differs in some respects from that evoked by insulinotropic nutrients, these two types of secretagogues may act synergistically upon insulin release. This may be essential for the anabolic disposal of nutrients in extrapancreatic tissues at the time of food intake.

The Adrenergic Pathway

Adrenergic agents either increase or inhibit glucose-stimulated insulin release. The enhancing action, e.g. that provoked by isoprenaline (isoproterenol), appears to be mediated by β-adrenoreceptors and hence may be linked to increased production of cyclic AMP. It is not further considered in this report. The inhibitory and prevailing action of catecholamines is thought to have a role in the control of insulin release during stress and exercise. It is mediated by α_2-adrenoreceptors. There is no convincing evidence for the presence of α_1-adrenoreceptors in the pancreatic B cell.

Activation of Adrenergic Receptors

The presence of adrenergic receptors in islet cells has been documented. Studies based on the use of selected adrenergic agonists and antagonists indicate that α_2-adrenergic receptors mediate the inhibitory action of catecholamines on insulin release. Such an inhibitory action is suppressed when the islets are exposed *in vitro* or *in vivo* to the islet-activating protein isolated from the culture medium of *Bordetella pertussis*. This treatment results in typical changes in the activity of adenylate cyclase in islet homogenates or subcellular fractions. In addition to a decrease in basal enzyme activity, these changes include an increased responsiveness to GTP relative to stable GTP analogues, such as GTPγS, and resistance to the inhibitory action of α_2-adrenergic agonists. These findings suggest the presence in islet cells of the regulatory protein Ni. This was confirmed by the demonstration that the islet-activating protein catalyses in islet cell membrane the ADP-ribosylation of a single protein with an M_r close to 41 kDa, which corresponds to the α subunit of Ni [68].

Changes in Cyclic AMP Generation

Several studies have shown that adrenergic agents inhibit islet adenylate cyclase in acellular systems. This effect is best seen in crude homogenates and in the presence of NaCl [69]. It coincides with a decreased production of cyclic AMP in intact islets. In purified B cells exposed to both D-glucose (20 mmol/l) and glucagon (10 nmol/l), the lowering action of adrenaline (epinephrine) upon the cell content of cyclic AMP is dose-related in the range 0.1 nmol/l to 0.1 μmol/l [70]. The effect of adrenaline is reproduced by noradrenaline and clonidine but not by isoprenaline or methoxamine, and is prevented by yohimbine and phentolamine, but not by prazosin or propanolol.

Apart from their effects upon cyclic AMP content and insulin release, adrenergic agents do not cause any obvious change in other functional variables such as the oxidation of glucose and the net uptake of ^{45}Ca by intact islets. Similarly, clonidine fails to prevent the rapid changes in ^{45}Ca efflux evoked by D-glucose in prelabelled islets and, although severely decreasing insulin output, does not alter the biphasic time-course of the secretory response to the hexose. These negative findings suggest that the primary site of action of adrenergic agents is located distally to those metabolic and ionic events involved in the secretory response to nutrient secretagogues.

Interference with Distal Events in the Secretory Sequence

In the light of the experimental data reviewed so far, the most naïve hypothesis concerning the interference of adrenergic agents with the secretory sequence would be a lowering of the cyclic AMP content of islet cells. As adrenergic agents abolish the release of insulin evoked by virtually all secretagogues, this hypothesis would imply that an adequate cell content of cyclic AMP has a permissive role in insulin release. This proposal is compatible with a recent mathematical model for the interaction between Ca^{2+} and cyclic AMP in the control of insulin release [71]. Indeed, in this model, it was postulated that the cyclic AMP concentration must exceed a critical threshold value in order to allow stimulation of insulin release. The threshold value was taken as that found in glucose-stimulated islets incubated for 90 min in the absence of $CaCl_2$ and EGTA. Moreover, it has recently been proposed that the ample secretory response to D-glucose, as observed in intact islets, could only be duplicated in purified B cells when the latter are concomitantly exposed to exogenous glucagon which markedly augments cyclic AMP content of glucose-stimulated cells [70].

A number of observations, however, strongly suggest that the inhibitory effect of adrenergic agents upon insulin release cannot be accounted for solely by a change in the cyclic AMP content of the B cell. This is best illustrated by the two following series of observations. First, in 1970, it was first reported that exogenous dibutyryl cyclic AMP, when used at a concentration (0.2 mmol/l) sufficient to double insulin release evoked by D-glucose (16.7 mmol/l) in rat pancreatic islets, failed to prevent the inhibitory action of adrenaline (10 μmol/l) upon insulin release [72]. Second, quite recently, it was reported that adrenaline (0.1 μmol/l) suppresses insulin release evoked in purified B cells by the tumour-promoting phorbol ester tetradecanoylphorbol acetate (TPA, 10 nmol/l), whether at low (1.0 mmol/l) or high (20 mmol/l) concentration of D-glucose, although the cyclic AMP content of the cells was identical in the presence of TPA alone and both TPA and adrenaline [70]. Thus, in the first instance, adrenaline blocked insulin release despite the provision of exogenous dibutyryl cyclic AMP, while in the second instance, adrenaline again abolished secretion despite unaltered cyclic AMP cell content.

The possibility must thus be considered that catecholamines affect insulin release through a mechanism distal to the generation of cyclic AMP. This proposal is not incompatible with the postulated role of Ni in the response to adrenergic agents, since the regulatory protein could conceivably affect the activity of enzyme(s) other than adenylate cyclase. This proposal is also consistent with the view that the α subunits released from GTP regulatory proteins can act as programmable messengers. Distal events possibly affected by catecholamines may include the subcellular distribution of Ca^{2+} or the responsiveness to the latter cation of target systems involved in the function of the effector system for insulin release.

The Peptidergic Pathway

Several peptide hormones affect insulin release in an immediate and direct fashion [73]. The effect of these hormones may correspond to either stimulation or inhibition of insulin release.

With regard to the physiological regulation of insulin release *in vivo*, emphasis has been placed, for the past few decades, on the effect of gastrointestinal hormones which may be released as a consequence of food intake and would increase insulin release, e.g. in response to prandial hyperglycaemia, to a greater extent than is observed when a comparable hyperglycaemic profile is achieved by intravenous administration of the hexose. It is currently believed that these positive insulinotropic hormonal agents, which would participate in the function of a so-called enteroinsular axis, may act upon the B cell in a manner comparable to that seen with pancreatic glucagon, which also enhances insulin release from isolated islets or purified B cells. A crucial feature of the insulinotropic action of glucagon is the failure (except under unusual experimental conditions) of the hormone to affect insulin output, as recorded at low extracellular concentrations of D-glucose, whereas glucagon efficiently augments insulin release evoked by higher concentrations of the hexose or other secretagogues. Such a situation, which was previously defined as glucose potentiation, is shared by all secretagogues, including forskolin or phosphodiesterase inhibitors, which are supposed to act in the B cell by specifically augmenting its cyclic AMP content.

The potentiation of nutrient-stimulated insulin release by one of the gastrointestinal hormones, namely GLP-1 (glucagon-like peptide 1), is presently considered as a possible modality for the treatment of patients with non-insulin dependent diabetes. In this respect, it

was recently proposed that, in order to optimize the secretory response to GLP-1, advantage could be taken of the effect of concomitant administration of exogenous non-glucidic nutrients [98]. Like D-glucose, these nutrients allow expression of GLP-1 insulinotropic potential. Since, in type 2 diabetes, the B cell often suffers from a kind of blindness to D-glucose, the non-glucidic nutrients would indeed allow GLP-1 to exert its full insulinotropic action, thanks to their capacity to bypass those site-specific defects in D-glucose transport, phosphorylation or further metabolism responsible for the preferential impairment of the B-cell response to the hexose.

The classic example of a peptide with inhibitory action on insulin release is somatostatin. Both somatostatin-14 and somatostatin-28, as well as several other somatostatin analogues, efficiently inhibit insulin release in various experimental models. Dose–action relationships for the inhibition of insulin release from purified B cells by the two somatostatins and their analogues suggest somatostatin receptor heterogeneity [70]. The physiological relevance of the inhibitory action of somatostatin upon insulin release remains to be documented; current speculations concern a possible paracrine effect of the hormone released by the islet D cells upon adjacent B cells.

Both the enhancing action of glucagon and inhibitory action of somatostatin upon insulin release coincide with parallel changes in the cyclic AMP content of purified B cells. Hence, we restrict discussion of the peptidergic pathway in this review to the modality of cyclic AMP generation and action in these cells. It should be noted, however, that, as is the case with adrenergic agents, somatostatin has been suggested to inhibit insulin release by both cyclic AMP-dependent and independent mechanisms.

Generation of Cyclic AMP

It has already been mentioned in this report that nutrient secretagogues exert a modest effect upon cyclic AMP generation in islet cells, this effect being possibly secondary to a cytosolic Ca^{2+} accumulation and mediated by Ca-calmodulin. The effect of nutrients to increase the cyclic AMP content of the islet cell is much less marked than that seen in response to suitable activators of adenylate cyclase, such as forskolin or glucagon.

In the case of the latter hormone, the occupancy of the glucagon receptor is thought to be coupled with the activation of adenylate cyclase at the intervention of the GTP-regulatory protein Ns. In rat pancreatic islet membrane exposed to $[\alpha\text{-}^{32}P]NAD$, cholera toxin stimulates the labelling of both the light and heavy forms of the α subunit of Ns, with predominance of the heavy form [74]. When intact islets are preincubated with cholera toxin, the adenylate cyclase activity of a subcellular particulate fraction is increased. The responsiveness of adenylate cyclase to GTP, but not GTPγS, is also augmented, but that to NaF is decreased. In intact islets, the production of cyclic AMP and the glucose-stimulated release of insulin are both enhanced after pretreatment with cholera toxin. These findings thus indicate the presence in pancreatic islets of the guanyl nucleotide regulatory protein Ns, which mediates the hormonal activation of adenylate cyclase. We have already indicated in this review that islet cells are also equipped with the regulatory protein Ni.

Mode of Action of Cyclic AMP

The mode of action of cyclic AMP in the pancreatic B cell has been reviewed in detail [53]. The essential information can be summarized as follows.

It is currently assumed, but remains to be proved, that the functional effects of cyclic AMP are linked to the activation of a cyclic AMP-responsive protein kinase; this has been identified in islet homogenates [16].

The bulk of the evidence suggests that (especially at high glucose concentrations) the enhancing action of cyclic AMP upon insulin release is not attributable to any marked facilitation of nutrient catabolism in islet cells. An exceptional situation should be mentioned, however, in this respect. When pancreatic tissue is removed from rats maintained hyperglycaemic by infusion of exogenous glucose, or when pancreatic islets are first cultured at a very high concentration of the hexose, the B cells—which are normally free of glycogen—accumulate significant amounts of glycogen judged by both ultrastructural and chemical criteria. In these preparations, agents that augment the islet cell content of cyclic AMP, e.g. phosphodiesterase inhibitors, stimulate insulin release even in the absence of exogenous nutrient. The secretory response coincides with, and seems attributable to (in part at least), stimulation of glycogenolysis and acceleration of glycolysis [75].

An increase in cyclic AMP content may affect either the intracellular distribution or net uptake of Ca^{2+} in islet cells. The intracellular redistribution of Ca^{2+} was first postulated in the light of findings indicating that agents raising the islet cell content of cyclic AMP tend to restore, at least to a limited extent, the secretory response to glucose of islets incubated in the nominal absence of Ca^{2+}. When forskolin was used as an activator of adenylate cyclase, such a partial restoration was even observed in islets incubated in the absence of Ca^{2+} and presence of EGTA. The view that cyclic AMP

may exert a modest effect upon Ca^{2+} net uptake by islet cells is based mainly on the bioelectrical effects of forskolin or dibutyryl cyclic AMP in mouse pancreatic B cells.

A last, but possibly most important, modality for the insulinotropic action of endogenous cyclic AMP could be increased responsiveness to Ca^{2+} of the effector system for insulin release. This view is supported by findings suggesting that a rise in cyclic AMP content may coincide with an unaltered cytosolic Ca^{2+} activity in these cells [76]. It is also consistent with a model for the mathematical simulation of stimulus–secretion coupling in the B cell. Indeed, in this model, the major mode of action of cyclic AMP is precisely to augment the output of insulin at any given concentration of cytosolic Ca^{2+}, provided that the latter concentration exceeds the threshold value required for stimulation of insulin output. Last, forskolin augments Ca^{2+}-induced insulin release in rat islets permeabilized with digitonin, again suggesting a mode of action of cyclic AMP distal to the provision of Ca^{2+} [77].

Cationic Amino Acids

The cationic amino acid L-arginine is one of the most commonly used insulin secretagogues in experiments carried out either *in vivo*, e.g. in human subjects, or *in vitro*, e.g. in the isolated perfused rat pancreas. However, the mechanism responsible for the insulinotropic action of L-arginine seems to differ from that involved in the secretory response to other nutrient or non-nutrient secretagogues. The functional response to L-arginine in fact differs from that evoked by glucose in several respects, including the absence of a phosphate flush, an increase rather than a decrease in K^+ permeability, and the failure to stimulate proinsulin biosynthesis. Although L-arginine (or L-ornithine) is efficiently metabolized and represents the precursor of polyamines in islet cells, the secretory response to this amino acid may be merely attributable to its accumulation in islet cells. Thus, the uptake of this positively charged amino acid, like that of its catabolite (L-ornithine) or non-metabolized analogue (L-homoarginine) coincides with depolarization of the plasma membrane and, hence, with the gating of voltage-sensitive Ca^{2+} channels [78, 79].

Hypoglycaemic and Hyperglycaemic Sulphonamides

Hypoglycaemic sulphonylureas and the hyperglycaemic agent diazoxide represent the most common tools used in the treatment of non-insulin dependent diabetic subjects and patients presenting with insulinoma, respectively, in order to interfere with the secretion of insulin. It was soon recognized that the positive and negative insulinotropic actions of these drugs coincide with either stimulation or inhibition of Ca^{2+} inflow into the B cell [80]. However, the molecular determinants of such a cationic change long remained elusive (Figure 10). It was recently observed, by the patch clamp technique, that hypoglycaemic sulphonylureas cause the closing of a class of K^+ channels which happen to coincide with the ATP-responsive K^+ channels involved in the functional response of the B cell to nutrient secretagogues. Diazoxide exerts an effect opposite to that of hypoglycaemic sulphonylureas upon these K^+ channels. It was proposed, therefore, that the direct and immediate interference of these pharmacological agents with K^+ permeability represents their primary mode of action in the B cell. The K^+ channel or a closely related structure could be viewed, therefore, as a receptor for these agents. The vastly different concentration–action relationships observed with distinct sulphonylureas of the so-called first and second generations might conceivably reflect differences in the affinity of the receptor. Alternatively, the insulinotropic efficiency of distinct hypoglycaemic sulphonylureas may be linked to differences in their capacity to be inserted in the phospholipid domain of the plasma membrane and/or in the stoichiometry of the complexes that they form with cations such as Ca^{2+}. It should also be stressed that the closure of ATP-sensitive K^+ channels may not be sufficient to account fully for all the effects of hypoglycaemic sulphonylureas upon biophysical and biochemical variables in the islet cells. For instance, it hardly accounts for the decrease in Na^+ cell content or the inhibition of K^+ inflow by an ouabain-resistant process, as observed in islets exposed to hypoglycaemic sulphonylureas. Moreover, certain of these agents, e.g. glibenclamide, are thought to be internalized into the B cell. Last, the current hypothesis does not readily explain the stimulation of bioelectrical activity, Ca^{2+} inflow and insulin release observed in response to the hypoglycaemic agents in islets exposed to a physiological concentration of D-glucose, namely when the vast majority of ATP-responsive K^+ channels are already closed and when the sulphonylurea enhances rather than decreases K^+ outflow from perifused islets [81].

LONG-TERM CONTROL OF INSULIN RELEASE

The complex sequence of metabolic, ionic and mechanical events forming the main axis for stimulus–secretion coupling in the B cell and the heterogeneous participation of each B cell in the overall response of the endocrine pancreas provide a suitable framework for the understanding of the long-term regulation of insulin release by ontogenic, nutritional and hormonal environmental factors, as well as the perturbation of islet function encountered in certain pathological situations. For instance, a change in the number of secretory units (hyperplasia or hypoplasia), in their intercellular coupling or in their functional efficiency may play a part in the ontogeny of insulin release in the process of growth and ageing. In this chapter, this topic is restricted to a few illustrative situations, in which site-specific changes in the secretory sequence have been identified as the major long-term regulatory mechanism.

Pregnancy and Lactation

During pregnancy there is a marked increase in the secretory responsiveness of isolated pancreatic islets to a number of nutrient and non-nutrient secretagogues. Such an increase cannot be accounted for solely by an increase in the number of cells and in insulin content of each islet; it coincides with increased activity of several enzymes involved in the secretory process, such as adenylate cyclase and distinct protein kinases. These enzymic changes may reflect the delayed but direct influence of placental hormones upon islet function.

After delivery, the restoration of normal secretory behaviour seems accelerated, at least in rats, when the postpartum period coincides with lactation. In this case,

HYPOGLYCEMIC SULFONYLUREA

↓

BINDING TO THE PLASMA MEMBRANE

↓

CLOSING OF ATP-SENSITIVE K^+ CHANNELS

↓

PLASMA MEMBRANE DEPOLARIZATION

↓

GATING OF VOLTAGE-SENSITIVE Ca^{2+} CHANNELS

↓

FACILITATED Ca^{2+} INFLUX INTO THE B-CELL

↓

INCREASE IN CYTOSOLIC Ca^{2+} ACTIVITY

↓

STIMULATION OF INSULIN RELEASE

Figure 10 Current hypothesis for the stimulus–secretion coupling of insulin release provoked by hypoglycemic sulfonylurea in the pancreatic islet B cell

however, the difference in secretory behaviour between islets removed from lactating and non-lactating animals, respectively, may be attributable mainly to a lower calcium content of the islet cells during lactation [82].

Starvation and Obesity

In islets removed from fasting rats, the secretory response to D-glucose is severely impaired whereas other secretagogues evoke insulin release at a near-normal rate. Once again, the impaired response to the hexose is not attributable solely to a change in the insulin content of the islet cells. Instead, it appears primarily due to a decreased islet content of glucokinase and, possibly, phosphofructokinase (Figure 11). The former enzyme, which is known to be insulin-inducible in the liver, indeed appears to be glucose-inducible in the B cell, the absence of prandial hyperglycaemic waves being held responsible for the repression of islet glucokinase during starvation. In addition, the rate of glycolysis in islets removed from fasting rats is further decreased as a result of impaired activation of phosphofructokinase in response to a rise in hexose concentration [83]. Incidentally, a low islet glucokinase content may also play a part in the poor insulinotropic action of glucose observed in fetal islets.

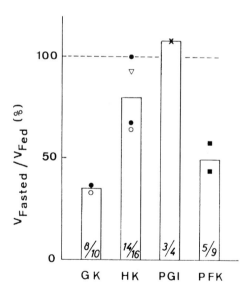

Figure 11 Effect of fasting upon the activity of glycolytic enzymes (GK glucokinase; HK hexokinase; PGI phosphoglucoisomerase; PFK phosphofructokinase) in islet homogenates. Values observed in islets from fasted rats are expressed as a percentage of the paired control value found in fed animals. The symbols correspond each to a different set of experiments. The mean value for each enzyme activity is indicated by the open columns. The total number of homogenates in fasted/fed rats is shown in each column. This figure illustrates that a 48-h fast affects preferentially the activity of glucokinase and phosphofructokinase

In obese human subjects or animals, the secretory activity of the B cells is often increased. This may be due, in part at least, to excessive carbohydrate intake, the elevated secretory activity not being found in rats made obese by administration of a high-fat diet.

Vitamin D Deficiency

In addition to ontogenic and nutritional factors, a number of humoral or hormonal agents such as pituitary growth hormone or adrenal and gonadal steroids exert long-term control of islet function [1]. It is often difficult to decide whether the changes in the secretory behaviour of the endocrine pancreas, observed in response to the hyposecretion or hypersecretion of these hormones, result from a direct or indirect effect. This also applies to the decrease in insulin release found in islets removed from vitamin D-deficient animals. Nevertheless, in the latter case, the secretory defect coincides with altered handling of $^{45}Ca^{2+}$ by isolated islets, and hence could conceivably be attributable to a decreased calbindin content of the islet cells [84, 85]. This vitamin D-inducible calcium-binding protein has recently been identified in both normal and tumoral islet cells. Although vitamin D deficiency is certainly not a common cause of impaired insulin secretion in human subjects, this example is purposely cited here to illustrate the wide spectrum of environmental factors liable to interfere with the functional behaviour of pancreatic B cells.

CONCLUSION

This chapter has attempted to illustrate (although far from exhaustively) the information gained from *in vitro* experiments about both the functional organization of the pancreatic B cell and the multifactorial regulation of insulin release. It is the author's firm belief that this information, albeit still fragmentary, provides a possible explanation for the heterogeneity in distinct models of B-cell dysfunction. As a matter of fact, virtually each step in the secretory sequence could conceivably be affected by a site-specific defect: examples of such defects could be the biosynthesis of proinsulin with an abnormal amino acid sequence, a defect in its conversion to insulin and C-peptide, delayed equilibration of D-glucose concentration across the B-cell plasma membrane, an abnormal pattern of hexokinase isoenzymes, perturbed channelling of hexose 6-phosphates into distinct metabolic pathways, insufficient activation by glucose of phosphofructokinase, failure of the hexose to preferentially stimulate mitochondrial oxidative events, primary anomalies in either K^+ or Ca^{2+} movements across the plasma membrane, and an inherited defect in the B-cell microtubular apparatus [86]. Moreover, as reviewed elsewhere, the biochemical organization of the B cell may also account for its sensitivity to specific cytotoxic aggressions [87]. Lastly, further progress in this field may provide both an explanation for the unfavourable consequences of sustained hyperglycaemia upon B-cell secretory potential, and the tools to prevent such a phenomenon of glucotoxicity.

REFERENCES

1. Malaisse WJ. Hormonal and environmental modification of islet activity. In Steiner DF, Freinkel N (eds) Handbook of physiology 7, vol. 1: endocrine pancreas. Washington: American Physiological Society, 1972: pp 237–60.
2. Malaisse WJ. The use of perifused pancreatic islets to study insulin secretion and associated metabolic and ionic events. In Poisner AM, Trifaro JM (eds) *In vitro* methods for studying secretion. New York: Elsevier, 1987: pp 63–78.
3. Lombardi T, Montesano R, Wohlhwend AL, Amherdt M, Vassalli JD, Orci L. Evidence for polarization of plasma membrane domains in pancreatic endocrine cells. Nature 1985; 313: 694–6.
4. Orci L. Macro- and microdomains in the endocrine pancreas. Diabetes 1982; 31: 538–65.
5. Pipeleers DG. Islet cell purification. In Larner J, Pohl SL (eds) Diabetes research, vol. I. Laboratory methods. Chichester: Wiley, 1984: pp 185–211.
6. Malaisse WJ. Stimulus–secretion coupling in the pancreatic B cell. In Ganten D, Pfaff D (eds) Current topics in neuroendocrinology. Heidelberg: Springer, 1988: pp 231–51.
7. Orci L. The insulin factory: a tour of the plant surroundings and a visit to the assembly line. Diabetologia 1985; 28: 528–46.
8. Welsh M, Sherberg N, Gilmore R, Steiner DF. Translational control of insulin biosynthesis. Evidence for regulation of elongation, initiation and signal-recognition-particle-mediated translational arrest by glucose. Biochem J 1986; 235: 459–67.
9. Halban PA, Wollheim CB. Intracellular degradation of insulin stores by pancreatic islets *in vitro*: an alternative pathway for homeostasis of pancreatic insulin content. J Biol Chem 1980; 255: 6003–6.
10. Sener A, Malaisse WJ. The stimulus–secretion coupling of glucose-induced insulin release. XXXIX. Long term effects of K^+ deprivation upon insulin biosynthesis and release. Endocrinology 1980; 106: 778–85.
11. Malaisse WJ, Orci L. The role of the cytoskeleton in pancreatic B cell function. In Gabbiani G (ed.) Methods of achievements in experimental pathology, vol. 9. Basel: Karger, 1979: pp 112–36.
12. Somers B, Blondel B, Orci L, Malaisse WJ. Motile events in pancreatic endocrine cells. Endocrinology 1979; 104: 255–64.
13. Orci L, Malaisse WJ. Hypothesis: single and chain release of insulin secretory granules is related to anionic transport at exocytotic sites. Diabetes 1980; 29: 943–4.
14. Howell SL, Tyhurst M. Insulin secretion: the effector system. Experientia 1984; 40: 1098–105.
15. Valverde I, Malaisse WJ. Calmodulin and pancreatic B cell function. Experientia 1984; 40: 1061–8.
16. Harrison DE, Ashcroft SJH, Christie MR, Lord JM. Protein phosphorylation in the pancreatic B cell. Experientia 1984; 40: 1075–84.
17. Alarcon C, Valverde I, Malaisse WJ. Transglutaminase and cellular motile events: retardation of proinsulin conversion by glycine methylester. Biosci Rep 1985; 5: 581–7.
18. Gold G, Grodsky GM. Kinetic aspects of compartmental storage and secretion of insulin and zinc. Experientia 1984; 40: 1105–14.
19. Henquin JC, Meissner HP. Significance of ionic fluxes and changes in membrane potential for stimulus–secretion coupling in pancreatic B cells. Experientia 1984; 40: 1043–52.
20. Pipeleers DG. Islet cell interactions with pancreatic B cells. Experientia 1984; 40: 1114–26.
21. Malaisse WJ. Dual role of lipids in the stimulus–secretion coupling for insulin release. Biochem Soc Trans 1989; 17: 59–60.
22. Van Schravendijk CFH, Foriers A, Van den Brande JL, Pipeleers DG. Evidence for the presence of type I insulin-like growth factor receptors on rat pancreatic A and B cells. Endocrinology 1987; 121: 1784–8.
23. Orci L. A portrait of the pancreatic B cell. Diabetologia 1974; 10: 163–87.
24. Malaisse WJ, Owen A. Mathematical modelling of stimulus–secretion coupling in the pancreatic B cell. VI. Cellular heterogeneity and recruitment. Appl Math Mod 1989; 13: 41–6.
25. Ashcroft FM. Adenosine 5′-triphosphate-sensitive potassium channels. Ann Rev Neurosci 1988; 11: 97–118.
26. Malaisse WJ, Sener A, Herchuelz A, Hutton JC. Insulin release: the fuel hypothesis. Metabolism 1979; 28: 373–86.
27. Malaisse WJ. Insulin secretion: multifactorial regulation for a single process of release. Diabetologia 1973; 9: 163–7.
28. Matschinsky FM, Ellerman J, Stillings S, Raybaud F, Pace C, Zawalich W. Hexoses and insulin secretion. In Hasselblatt A, Bruchhausen FV (eds) Insulin, part 2. Heidelberg: Springer, 1975: pp 79–114.
29. Malaisse WJ, Malaisse-Lagae F, Sener A. Anomeric specificity of hexose metabolism in pancreatic islets. Physiol Rev 1983; 63: 773–86.
30. Malaisse WJ, Sener A, Malaisse-Lagae F. Insulin release: reconciliation of the receptor and metabolic hypotheses. Nutrient receptors in islet cells. Mol Cell Biochem 1981; 37: 157–65.
31. Sener A, Malaisse WJ. Nutrient metabolism in islet cells. Experientia 1984; 40: 1026–35.
32. Malaisse WJ. Possible sites for deficient glucose recognition in islet cells. In Lefèbvre PJ, Pipeleers DG (eds) The pathology of the endocrine pancreas in diabetes. Heidelberg: Springer, 1988: pp 219–32.
33. Malaisse WJ. Insulin release: the glucoreceptor myth. IRCS Med Sci Res 1987; 15: 65–7.
34. Malaisse WJ. Metabolic signals to insulin release. Excerpta Medica ICS 1989; 800: 387–90.
35. Malaisse WJ, Malaisse-Lagae F, Sener A. Channeling of α-D-glucose 6-phosphate in tumoral islet cells exposed to D-galactose. J Biol Chem 1987; 262: 11746–51.
36. Malaisse WJ, Malaisse-Lagae F, Sener A. The glycolytic cascade in pancreatic islets. Diabetologia 1982; 23: 1–5.

37. Sener A, Malaisse WJ. Stimulation by D-glucose of mitochondrial oxidative events in islet cells. Biochem J 1987; 246: 89–95.

38. Malaisse WJ, Sener A. Hexose metabolism in pancreatic islets. Feedback control of D-glucose oxidation by functional events. Biochim Biophys Acta 1988; 971: 246–54.

39. Malaisse WJ, Best L, Kawazu S, Malaisse-Lagae F, Sener A. The stimulus–secretion coupling of glucose-induced insulin release. Fuel metabolism in islets deprived of exogenous nutrient. Arch Biochem Biophys 1982; 224: 102–10.

40. Malaisse WJ, Malaisse-Lagae F, Sener A. Coupling factors in nutrient-induced insulin release. Experientia 1984; 40: 1035–43.

41. Capito K, Hedeskov CJ. Effects of glucose, glucose metabolites and calcium ions on adenylate cyclase activity in homogenates of mouse pancreatic islets. Biochem J 1977; 162: 569–73.

42. Sugden MC, Ashcroft SJH. Effects of phosphoenolpyruvate, other glycolytic intermediates and methylxanthines on calcium uptake by a mitochondrial fraction from rat pancreatic islets. Diabetologia 1978; 15: 173–80.

43. Malaisse WJ, Sener A. The redox potential. In Akkerman JWN (ed.) Boca Raton: CRC Press, 1988: pp 29–43.

44. Lindström P, Sehlin J. Effect of intracellular alkalinization on pancreatic islet calcium uptake and insulin secretion. Biochem J 1986; 239: 199–204.

45. Cook DL, Hales CN. Intracellular ATP directly blocks K^+ channels in pancreatic B cells. Nature 1984; 311: 271–3.

46. Ashcroft FM, Harrison DE, Ashcroft SJH. Glucose induces closure of single potassium channels in isolated rat pancreatic B cells. Nature 1984; 312: 446–8.

47. Rorsman P, Trube G. Glucose dependent K^+-channels in pancreatic B cells are regulated by intracellular ATP. Pflügers Arch 1985; 405: 305–9.

48. Dunne MJ, Petersen OH. Intracellular ADP activates K^+ channels that are inhibited by ATP in an insulin-secreting cell line. FEBS Lett 1986; 208: 59–62.

49. Malaisse WJ, Sener A. Glucose-induced changes in cytosolic ATP content in pancreatic islets. Biochim Biophys Acta 1987; 927: 190–5.

50. Sener A, Leclercq-Meyer V, Giroix M-H, Malaisse WJ, Hellerström C. Opposite effects of D-glucose and a non-metabolized analogue of L-leucine on respiration and secretion in insulin-producing tumoral cells (RINm5F). Diabetes 1987; 36: 187–92.

51. Blachier F, Sener A, Malaisse WJ. Interference of a non-metabolized analog of L-leucine with lipid metabolism in tumoral pancreatic islet cells. Biochim Biophys Acta 1987; 921: 494–501.

52. Blachier F, Malaisse WJ. Effect of exogenous ATP upon inositol phosphate production, cationic fluxes and insulin release in pancreatic islet cells. Biochim Biophys Acta 1988; 970: 222–9.

53. Malaisse WJ, Malaisse-Lagae F. The role of cyclic AMP in insulin release. Experientia 1984; 40: 1068–75.

54. Valverde I, Garcia-Morales P, Ghiglione M, Malaisse WJ. The stimulus–secretion coupling of glucose-induced insulin release. III. Calcium dependency of the cyclic AMP response to nutrient secretagogue. Horm Metab Res 1983; 15: 62–8.

55. Deleers M, Mahy M, Malaisse WJ. Glucose increases cytosolic Ca^{2+} activity in pancreatic islet cells. Biochem Int 1985; 10: 97–103.

56. Valverde I, Vandemeers A, Anjaneyulu R, Malaisse WJ. Calmodulin activation of adenylate cyclase in pancreatic islets. Science 1979; 206: 225–7.

57. Best L, Malaisse WJ. Effects of nutrient secretagogues upon phospholipid metabolism in rat pancreatic islets. Mol Cell Endocrinol 1983; 32: 205–14.

58. Best L. A role for calcium in the breakdown of inositol phospholipids in intact and digitonin-permeabilized pancreatic islets. Biochem J 1986; 238: 773–9.

59. Malaisse WJ, Malaisse-Lagae F, Wright PH, Ashmore J. Effects of adrenergic and cholinergic agents upon insulin secretion *in vitro*. Endocrinology 1967; 80: 975–8.

60. Malaisse WJ. Insulin secretion and food intake. Proc Nutr Soc 1972; 31: 213–17.

61. Malaisse WJ. Stimulus–secretion coupling in the pancreatic B cell: the cholinergic pathway for insulin release. Diabet Metab Rev 1986; 2: 243–59.

62. Dunlop ME, Malaisse WJ. Phosphoinositide phosphorylation and hydrolysis in pancreatic islet cell membrane. Arch Biochem Biophys 1986; 244: 421–9.

63. Blachier F, Malaisse WJ. Phospholipase C activation via a GTP-binding protein in tumoral islet cells stimulated by carbamylcholine. Experientia 1987; 43: 601–2.

64. Best L, Malaisse WJ. Nutrient and hormone-neurotransmitter stimuli induce hydrolysis in polyphosphoinositides in rat pancreatic islets. Endocrinology 1984; 115: 1814–20.

65. Malaisse WJ, Sener A, Herchuelz A, Carpinelli AR, Poloczek P, Winand J, Castagna M. Insulinotropic effect of the tumor promoter 12-O-tetradecanolyl-phorbol-13-acetate in rat pancreatic islets. Cancer Res 1980; 40: 3827–31.

66. Malaisse WJ, Dunlop ME, Mathias PCF, Malaisse-Lagae F, Sener A. Stimulation of protein kinase C and insulin release by 1-oleyl-2-acetyl-glycerol. Eur J Biochem 1985; 149: 23–7.

67. Zawalich W, Brown C, Rasmussen H. Insulin secretion: combined effects of phorbol ester and A23187. Biochem Biophys Res Comm 1983; 117: 448–55.

68. Malaisse WJ, Svoboda M, Dufrane SP, Malaisse-Lagae F, Christophe J. Effect of *Bordetella pertussis* toxin on ADP-ribosylation of membrane proteins, adenylate cyclase activity and insulin release in rat pancreatic islets. Biochem Biophys Res Comm 1984; 124: 190–6.

69. Garcia-Morales P, Dufrane SP, Sener A, Valverde I, Malaisse WJ. Inhibitory effect of clonidine upon adenylate cyclase activity, cyclic AMP production and insulin release in rat pancreatic islets. Biosci Rep 1984; 4: 511–21.

70. Schuit FC, Pipeleers DG. Differences in adrenergic recognition by pancreatic A and B cells. Science 1986; 232: 875–7.

71. Owen A, Malaisse WJ. Mathematical modelling of stimulus–secretion coupling in the pancreatic B cell. V. Threshold phenomenon for the response to cyclic AMP. Diabète Métab 1987; 13: 514–19.

72. Malaisse WJ, Brisson G, Malaisse-Lagae F. The stimulus–secretion coupling of glucose-induced insulin release. I. Interaction of epinephrine and alkaline earth cations. J Lab Clin Med 1970; 76: 895–902.

73. Ahren B, Taborsky GJ Jr, Porte D Jr. Neuropeptidergic versus cholinergic and adrenergic regulation of islet hormone secretion. Diabetologia 1986; 29: 827–36.

74. Svoboda M, Garcia-Morales P, Dufrane SP, Sener A, Valverde I, Christophe J, Malaisse WJ. Stimulation by cholera toxin of ADP-ribosylation of membrane proteins, adenylate cyclase and insulin release in pancreatic islets. Cell Biochem Funct 1985; 3: 25–32.

75. Malaisse WJ, Sener A, Koser M, Ravazzola M, Malaisse-Lagae F. The stimulus–secretion coupling of glucose-induced insulin release. XXV. Insulin release due to glycogenolysis in glucose-deprived islets. Biochem J 1977; 164: 447–54.

76. Wollheim CB, Ullrich S, Pozzan T, Glyceraldehyde, but not cyclic AMP-stimulated insulin release is preceded by a rise in cytosolic free Ca^{2+}. FEBS Lett 1984; 177: 17–22.

77. Tamagawa T, Niki H, Niki A. Insulin release independent of a rise in cytosolic free Ca^{2+} by forskolin and phorbol ester. FEBS Lett 1985; 183: 430–2.

78. Henquin JC, Meissner HP. Effects of amino acids on membrane potential and $^{86}Rb^{+}$ fluxes in pancreatic β-cells. Am J Physiol 1981; 240: E245–E252.

79. Blachier F, Mourtada A, Sener A, Malaisse WJ. Stimulus–secretion coupling of arginine-induced insulin release. Uptake of metabolized and non-metabolized cationic amino acids by pancreatic islets. Endocrinology 1989; 124: 134–41.

80. Gylfe E, Hellman B, Sehlin J, Täljedal I-B. Interaction of sulfonylureas with the pancreatic B cell. Experientia 1984; 40: 1126–34.

81. Malaisse WJ, Lebrun P. Mechanisms of sulfonylurea-induced insulin secretion. Diabetes Care 1990; 13 (suppl 2): 9–17.

82. Hubinont CJ, Dufrane SP, Garcia-Morales P, Valverde I, Sener A, Malaisse WJ. Influence of lactation upon pancreatic islet function. Endocrinology 1986; 118: 687–94.

83. Giroix M-H, Dufrane SP, Malaisse-Lagae F, Sener A, Malaisse WJ. Fasting-induced impairment of glucose 1,6-bisphosphate synthesis in pancreatic islets. Biochem Biophys Res Comm 1984; 119: 543–8.

84. Billaudel B, Labriji-Mestaghamni H, Sutter BCJ, Malaisse WJ. Vitamin D and pancreatic islet function. II. Dynamics of insulin release and cationic fluxes. J Endocrinol Invest 1988; 11: 585–93.

85. Pochet R, Pipeleers DG, Malaisse WJ. Calbindin-D 27 kDa: preferential localization in non-B islet cells of the rat pancreas. Biol Cell 1987; 61: 155–61.

86. Malaisse WJ. Insulin release: physiology and patho-physiology of nutrient metabolism in pancreatic islet cells. In Grill V (ed.) Pathogenesis of non-insulin dependent diabetes mellitus. New York: Raven Press, 1988: pp 27–38.

87. Malaisse WJ. Alloxan toxicity to the pancreatic B cell. A new hypothesis. Biochem Pharmacol 1982; 31: 3527–34.

88. Kiraly-Borri CE, Morgan A, Burgyone RD, Weller U, Wollheim CB, Lang J. Soluble *N*-ethylmaleimide-sensitive-factor attachment protein and N-ethylmaleimide-insensitive factors are required for Ca^{2+}-stimulated exocytosis of insulin. Biochem J 1996; 314: 199–203.

89. Atwater I, Kukuljan M, Perez-Armendasiz EM. Molecular biology of the ion channels in the pancreatic B cell. In Draznin B, LeRoith D (eds) Molecular biology of diabetes. Totowa: Humana Press, 1994: pp 303–32.

90. Malaisse WJ, Malaisse-Lagae F, Davies DR, Vandercammen A, Van Schaftingen E. Regulation of glucokinase by a fructose-1-phosphate-sensitive protein in pancreatic islets. Eur J Biochem 1990; 190: 539–45.

91. Noma Y, Bonner-Weir S, Latimer JB, Davalli AM, Weir GC. Beta cell glucokinase is translocated by acute glucose stimulation. Diabetologia 1995; 38 (suppl 1): A107.

92. Becker TC, Noel RJ, Johnson JH, Lynch RM, Hirose H, Tokuyama Y et al. Differential effects of overexpressed glucokinase and hexokinase I in isolated islets. Evidence for functional segregation of the high and low K_m enzymes. J Biol Chem 1996; 271: 390–4.

93. Vanhoutte C, Malaisse-Lagae F, Malaisse WJ. D-glucose metabolism in cross-linked pancreatic islets. Biochem Biophys Res Commun 1995; 217: 561–5.

94. Malaisse WJ, Bodur H. Hexose metabolism in pancreatic islets. Enzyme-to-enzyme tunnelling of hexose 6-phosphate. Int J Biochem 1991; 23: 1471–81.

95. Malaisse WJ. Glucose-sensing by the pancreatic B cell: the mitochondrial part. Int J Biochem 1992; 24: 693–701.

96. Malaisse WJ, Ladrière L, Zhang T-M, Verbruggen I, Willem R. Enzyme-to-enzyme channelling of symmetric Krebs cycle intermediates in pancreatic islet cells. Diabetologia 1996; 39: 990–2.

97. Komatsu M, Schermerhorn T, Aizawa T, Sharp GWG. Glucose stimulation of insulin release in the absence of extracellular Ca^{2+} and in the absence of any increase in intracellular Ca^{2+} in rat pancreatic islets. Proc Natl Acad Sci USA 1995; 92: 10728–32.

98. Leclercq-Meyer V, Malaisse WJ. Potentiation of glucagon-like peptide 1 insulinotropic action by succinic acid dimethyl ester. Life Sciences 1996; 58: 1195–9.

15

Insulin Secretion in the Normal and Diabetic Human

Steven E. Kahn*, David K. McCulloch †and Daniel Porte, Jr*

*University of Washington and V A Medical Center, Seattle, USA, and †University of Washington and Virginia Mason Medical Center, Seattle, USA

Recent advances in techniques to study human islet function have improved our understanding of the normal physiology of insulin secretion and have provided further evidence that impaired islet cell function is an important contributor to hyperglycemia in both insulin dependent diabetes mellitus (IDDM, type 1 diabetes) and non-insulin dependent diabetes mellitus (NIDDM, type 2 diabetes) [1, 2]. In addition, islet cell function studies in predisposed individuals have demonstrated that an early lesion in many IDDM and NIDDM patients is impaired secretion of insulin [3, 4]. In this chapter, we review the physiology of insulin secretion in normal and diabetic humans, and discuss the role of impaired insulin secretion in the overall carbohydrate tolerance of individuals with preclinical and overt diabetes mellitus.

PHYSIOLOGY OF NORMAL BASAL INSULIN SECRETION

The B cell of the pancreas secretes approximately equimolar quantities of C-peptide and insulin, with resulting plasma venous or arterial concentrations of insulin in normal lean individuals of 3–15 μU/ml (18–90 pmol/l). Approximately 60% of the insulin secreted by the pancreas into the portal system is removed during its initial passage through the liver (first-pass effect) which leads, in part, to a 2.5–3 times greater concentration of insulin in the portal vein

compared with a peripheral vein [5]. Insulin clearance also occurs in the kidney with the normal kidney removing nearly 40% of the insulin presented to it [6].

Basal insulin secretion is critical to the maintenance of basal euglycemia. Quantitatively, pancreatic insulin secretion in the basal state varies from 0.25 to 1.5 U/h in normal subjects and accounts for 50% or more of the 24-hour integrated insulin secretion. Both basal insulin secretion and meal-related insulin secretion are regulated by glucose, although other nutrients, hormones and neural factors affect insulin release. In turn, the glucose level is regulated by insulin and glucagon secretion. The maintenance of this steady state glucose level is determined by the sensitivity of liver and peripheral tissues to insulin and the sensitivity of the islet to glucose. Thus, a classic feedback loop is created which maintains glucose concentrations relatively constant in the basal state (Figure 1).

PHYSIOLOGY OF NORMAL MEAL-RELATED INSULIN SECRETION

Carbohydrate Regulation of Insulin Secretion

The remarkably narrow range of basal plasma glucose found in most individuals is largely accounted for by the moment-to-moment regulation of insulin and glucagon secretion by plasma glucose. During meals, direct glucose regulation of the B cell is also a key

International Textbook of Diabetes Mellitus, Second Edition. Edited by K.G.M.M. Alberti, P. Zimmet, R.A. DeFronzo, and H. Keen (Honorary)
© 1997 John Wiley & Sons Ltd

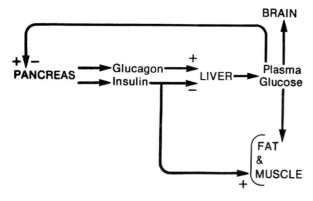

Figure 1 A model for normal steady-state regulation of plasma glucose. Plasma glucose has direct effects on the pancreas to increase insulin and decrease glucagon secretion during hyperglycemia, and to increase glucagon and decrease insulin secretion during hypoglycemia. Glucagon stimulates glucose production, and insulin suppresses glucose production from the liver and increases glucose uptake in muscle and fat. Glucose uptake is not insulin dependent in the brain. Any change in hormone secretion or hormone sensitivity will be modulated by this loop to minimize the change in glucose concentration and maintain peripheral glucose utilization (from reference 75, with permission)

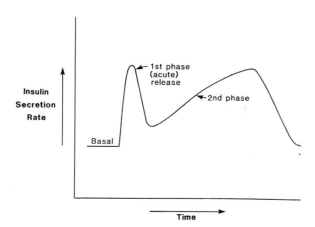

Figure 2 The biphasic insulin response to a constant glucose stimulus. A theoretical response to a square-wave (constant) change in glucose level is shown. The peak of the first phase in humans is between 3 and 5 min and lasts 10 min. The second phase begins at 2 min but is not evident until 10 min have passed. It continues to increase slowly for at least 60 min or until the stimulus stops (from reference 73, with permission)

factor in islet function. However, the response pattern is highly non-linear. In response to intravenous (IV) glucose, insulin is released in a biphasic pattern [7, 8] (Figure 2). The first phase (acute) insulin response to glucose begins within 1 minute after an IV glucose bolus, peaks between 3 and 5 minutes, and lasts for up to 10 minutes. The quantitative insulin response depends upon two factors. First, the rate and

amount of glucose, with a 20-g IV bolus given in less than 3 minutes representing a maximal stimulus in the human [9]. Second, the degree of insulin sensitivity, with larger responses occurring in insulin resistant individuals [80]. The insulin released from the pancreas during this first phase has already been synthesized and stored in the secretory granules of the B cell. The second phase insulin response to glucose begins just after the glucose bolus but is not evident until 10 minutes later and lasts as long as the hyperglycemia persists [10, 11]. This second phase insulin response depends primarily on insulin stores, but is also regulated by new protein synthesis within the B cell [12]. Unlike the first phase, the second phase insulin release is directly proportionate to the steady state glucose concentration immediately preceding the glucose bolus [10, 11]. Thus, when evaluating second phase insulin responses it is critical to achieve comparable pre-stimulus glucose concentrations in the study and control subjects.

Oral glucose tolerance testing is not a precise or reproducible method of measuring insulin secretion as the results of such tests can be quite variable, even within the same individual [13]. One reason for this variability is that the insulin response to oral glucose is influenced by hormones such as gastroenteropancreatic (GEP) polypeptides, and neuroregulators such as acetylcholine, which are released during the ingestion of glucose. Second, the absorption of an oral glucose load varies due to differences in gastric emptying and gastrointestinal motility. Third, much of the insulin is secreted long after the glucose is ingested. Thus, the level of glycemia later in the oral test depends on the ability of the islet to produce insulin and the peripheral tissues and liver to respond to it earlier in the test. Therefore, an oral glucose tolerance test in glucose-intolerant individuals may falsely appear to produce normal insulin secretion when compared with glucose-tolerant subjects, due to a greater glycemic stimulus later in the test producing higher insulin levels. Thus, while the oral test is a good measure of overall glucose tolerance, the intravenous glucose tolerance test (IVGTT) is preferable for evaluating glucose-regulated insulin secretion and B-cell function.

Amino Acid Regulation of Insulin Secretion

Amino acids are important regulators of insulin release. Arginine is a powerful amino acid stimulus of insulin secretion and is commonly used in research because of its safety and potency [14]. As with the second phase of IV glucose, arginine-stimulated insulin release is proportionate to the steady state glucose concentration immediately preceding the arginine challenge (Figure 3). The magnitude of the acute (2–10 minutes after injection) insulin response (AIR) to arginine is a linear function of plasma glucose between 60 and 250 mg/dl (3.3 and 13.9 mmol/l) [15]. Thus, if one determines two or more AIRs to arginine at plasma glucoses in this linear range, one can calculate the slope of the least squares regression line relating these insulin responses to the glucose level. This measurement, termed the glucose potentiation slope, is an index of the ability of hyperglycemia to potentiate the AIR to arginine and thus provides a measure of B-cell modulation by glucose. A maximum potentiation of the AIR to arginine (AIR$_{max}$) occurs at a plasma glucose level of 450 mg/dl and above, and is a measure of the maximal responsiveness of the system to glucose [2]. From this value and the slope of potentiation the glucose level at half-maximal response can be calculated. This is termed the PG$_{50}$ and is a measure of the islet's sensitivity to glucose. Other non-glucose stimulants such as the β-adrenergic agonist isoproterenol or the gut hormone secretin can be used to derive the same information, as there appears to be parallel regulation of their responses by glucose. In summary, the glucose potentiation slope, AIR$_{max}$ and PG$_{50}$ are useful indices which permit functional characterization of the B cell (Figure 3).

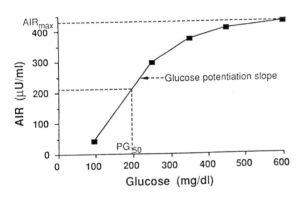

Figure 3 Acute insulin responses (AIR) to IV arginine at five different glucose levels in a normal individual. The magnitude of the AIRs is a linear function of plasma glucose level between 60 and 250 mg/dl (3.3 and 13.9 mmol/l) and the least squares regression line relating these two functions, termed the glucose potentiation slope, is a measure of B-cell modulation by glucose. Maximal potentiation of the AIR by glucose (AIR$_{max}$) is a measure of B-cell secretory capacity and occurs at a glucose level above 450 mg/dl (25 mmol/l). From the glucose potentiation slope and AIR$_{max}$, the glucose level at half-maximal response can be calculated and this level, termed PG$_{50}$, provides an assessment of islet sensitivity to glucose

Fat Regulation of Insulin Secretion

A small increase in insulin secretion occurs following the ingestion of medium-chain triglycerides. In obese subjects acetoacetate leads to an increase in insulin secretion, but cholesterol and fatty acids have no effect on insulin secretion. Thus, fat-derived products appear

to have a modest role (if any) in regulating human insulin secretion.

Gastroenteropancreatic Polypeptide Regulation of Insulin Secretion

Glucagon, which is secreted by the A cells of the pancreas, increases insulin secretion [16, 17], while somatostatin-14, which is secreted by the pancreatic D cells, decreases insulin secretion [18]. These effects may contribute to B-cell function by a paracrine regulatory control of B-cell insulin release. Hormonal effects of gut somatostatin-28 may also lead to a decrease in insulin secretion. Such effects include diminished absorption of glucose and protein, decreased gastrointestinal motility, decreased splanchnic blood flow, and suppression of insulin and glucagon secretion. Glucagon-like peptide 1 (GLP-1) [93, 101], gastric inhibitory polypeptide (GIP) [19], gastrin [20, 21], cholecystokinin [21] and secretin [21–23] lead to a glucose-dependent increase in insulin secretion. These gut hormones are presumably important to normal oral nutrient tolerance. Other hormones that affect insulin secretion are listed in Table 1.

Neural Regulation of Insulin Secretion

Alpha-adrenergic receptor activation inhibits [35] whereas β-adrenergic receptor activation stimulates insulin secretion [22]. Generally, α-adrenergic activation predominates, resulting in a net inhibition of insulin secretion during sympathetic activation. During stress the combination of systemic epinephrine release from the adrenal gland and/or local norepinephrine release from the pancreatic nerves leads to a significant suppression of insulin release, contributing to the development of hyperglycemia.

Parasympathetic cholinergic stimulation, on the other hand, results in an increase in insulin secretion [34]. Such release occurs during meal ingestion and appears to be mediated by vagal nerve stimulation. Neuropeptides are also found in pancreatic neurons. Infusion of neuropeptides such as vasoactive intestinal peptide (VIP), calcitonin gene-related peptide (CGRP), cholecystokinin-pancreozymin (CCK), neuropeptide Y (NPY), galanin, substance P and enkephalins have been shown to regulate insulin release, providing evidence for peptidergic regulation of insulin secretion [27]. Hypothalamic control centers are believed to be the central input for these neural effects on insulin secretion. Stimulation of the ventromedial nucleus suppresses insulin release whereas stimulation of the lateral hypothalamus increases it. The complete role of these neural systems in metabolic regulation is still being actively investigated [100].

Table 1 Non-glucose regulators of insulin secretion. Adapted from reference 73, with permission

Nutrients	Effect on B cell	Reference
Amino acids	Stimulatory	14
Ketones*		24
Hormones		
Growth hormone	Stimulatory†	25
Glucagon	Stimulatory	16, 17
Glucagon-like peptide 1 (GLP-1)	Stimulatory	93, 101
GIP	Stimulatory	19
Secretin	Stimulatory	21, 22, 23
Cholecystokinin	Stimulatory	21
Gastrin	Stimulatory	20, 21
VIP	Stimulatory	26
Gastrin-releasing peptide (GRP)	Stimulatory	27
Adrenocorticosteroids	Inhibitory‡	28
Somatostatin	Inhibitory	18
Epinephrine	Inhibitory§	29
Norepinephrine	Inhibitory§	30
Galanin	Inhibitory	31
NPY	Inhibitory	27
Calcitonin gene-related peptide (CGRP)	Inhibitory	27
Prostaglandin E	Inhibitory	32, 33
Enkephalins	Variable¶	27
Substance P	Variable¶	27
Neural mechanisms		
Beta-adrenergic	Stimulatory	22
Parasympathetic (vagal)	Stimulatory	34
Alpha-adrenergic	Inhibitory	35

*Ketones (i.e. acetoacetate) stimulate insulin secretion in dogs but not significantly in humans.

†Inhibitory effects have also been reported.

‡Although the direct B-cell effect is inhibitory, corticosteroids may indirectly stimulate insulin secretion by causing insulin resistance and hyperglycemia.

§α (inhibitory) effects usually predominate over β (stimulatory) effects.

¶ Effects are stimulatory or inhibitory depending on dose, species studied and experimental conditions.

INSULIN RESISTANCE AS A REGULATOR OF INSULIN SECRETION

Obesity is the most common cause of insulin resistance in humans. The pancreatic islets of obese individuals have a greater mass and diameter than those of lean individuals, suggesting enhanced insulin synthesis by the B cell in obese individuals [36], while the existence of a positive correlation between basal plasma insulin levels and percentage ideal body weight suggests enhanced insulin secretion [37]. Elevated plasma insulin levels also occur during stimulation by glucose, non-glucose secretagogues and meal ingestion, resulting in significant elevations of the 24-hour integrated insulin levels in obese individuals. Insulin levels vary as adiposity changes during interventions such as dieting (decreased insulin levels) and forced overfeeding (increased insulin levels), suggesting that hyperinsulinemia is a consequence of obesity. The slope of glucose potentiation is also increased in obesity, suggesting an increased responsiveness to glucose [38].

This increase in islet B-cell efficiency minimizes the development of hyperglycemia in obese individuals, and appears to be an adaptive response to insulin resistance. This adaptive response has now been quantified [80]. These studies show that the product of B-cell function and insulin sensitivity (B-cell function × insulin sensitivity) is a constant in normally tolerant humans. Thus, as obesity and insulin resistance develops, there is a reciprocal increase in insulin secretion to maintain tolerance. If this adaptive mechanism fails, hyperglycemia develops [102].

In contrast to these findings, the B cell does not appear to adapt to the insulin resistance of aging. Individuals over the age of 60 years are not only insulin resistant but also have a diet-dependent decrease in B-cell responsiveness to the potentiating effects of glucose when compared with younger subjects matched for weight and sex [39]. The frequency of glucose intolerance in older individuals may therefore be determined in part by an alteration in the set point for the feedback loop between the insulin sensitive tissues and the islet B cell.

Steroids such as dexamethasone and the B-group vitamin nicotinic acid have been exploited to study the effect of experimentally induced insulin resistance on B-cell function. Whereas normal individuals given steroids or nicotinic acid are capable of increasing their B-cell responsiveness to glucose [40, 103], individuals with NIDDM fail to increase their insulin secretory capacity as an adaptation to experimentally induced insulin resistance [41]. Former gestational diabetics also demonstrate this defect, and this suggests that abnormal islet function is present in women with former gestational diabetes mellitus (GDM) and may be causally related to the pregnancy-associated hyperglycemia [42]. This subclinical defect, when combined with an increase in insulin secretory demand in response to the insulin resistance of aging and obesity, provides a possible explanation for the development of diabetes later in life.

The mechanism for the regulation of islet B-cell function by insulin resistance is not known. However, glucose probably participates in a significant way. The administration of even a relatively modest 20-hour glucose infusion results in a similar enhancement of the responsiveness of the B cell to arginine [15]. Both A and B cells appear to adapt their responsiveness to glucose in an attempt to minimize the degree of hyperglycemia. This ability to adapt may explain why states of insulin resistance are characterized by hyperinsulinemia with little hyperglycemia. Patients with NIDDM fail to show this adaptation to glucose [97]. In summary, insulin resistance is usually accompanied by hyperinsulinemia. Hyperglycemia is minimal in individuals with responsive B cells, but develops when this adaptive mechanism fails. This finding suggests that insulin resistance is a regulator of insulin secretion and that a component of this regulatory mechanism involves enhanced B-cell responsiveness to glucose which fails in NIDDM.

DRUGS THAT AFFECT INSULIN SECRETION

A number of drugs affect islet function and are listed in Table 2.

Sympathomimetic agents have an inhibitory effect on insulin secretion and some of these, such as ephedrine and phenylpropanolamine, are constituents of common 'over the counter' preparations. Amphetamines, epinephrine and norepinephrine, although less commonly prescribed, also inhibit islet B-cell function [29, 30]. Glucocorticoids have been demonstrated to have a direct suppressive effect on the B cell [28] and this, along with the other effects that these agents have

Table 2 Drugs affecting insulin secretion

A. *Inhibitory*
Sympathomimetic agents
Glucocorticoids
Diuretics—potassium-depleting
β-Blockers
Diazoxide
Phenytoin
Ethanol
Cytotoxics: streptozotocin, alloxan

B. *Stimulatory*
Sulfonylureas
Non-steroidal anti-inflammatory agents
α-Adrenergic blockers

on glucose metabolism, contributes to steroid-impaired glucose tolerance, especially in those individuals predisposed to the development of diabetes. Normal islet function is dependent on an adequate plasma potassium concentration, so that any drug that depletes potassium will impair insulin secretion. Many of the more commonly used diuretics have this side-effect, and may have a clinically significant effect if plasma potassium levels are not carefully monitored [43]. Beta blockers, although of more importance in diabetes for their ability to blunt the normal counter-regulatory response to hypoglycemia, are also inhibitors of B-cell secretion and can occasionally lead to hyperglycemia [44, 45]. The more potent antihypertensive agent diazoxide has a significant inhibitory effect on insulin secretion, and this effect has been of value in counteracting the hypoglycemia occurring in patients with B-cell hyperplasia or insulinomas [46]. Large doses of phenytoin may also depress islet B-cell function [47]. Thus, thought should be given to the use of any of these medications when treating individuals with impaired glucose tolerance, especially when alternatives are available.

Other agents not commonly prescribed by most physicians may suppress insulin release. Ethanol in large doses can reduce insulin secretion, but hypoglycemia may still occur in some subjects due to the concurrent inhibition of gluconeogenesis [48]. The cytotoxics streptozotocin and alloxan are used to induce experimental diabetes in animals and the former is also used in the treatment of pancreatic islet cell tumors in humans. The toxic effect of these two drugs can result in mild to total impairment of insulin secretion [49].

Increased insulin release occurs with a few medications. The sulfonylurea agents, which are discussed in more detail later, improve glucose tolerance by a number of mechanisms but mainly because of an enhancement of insulin secretion. Salicylates and some other non-steroidal anti-inflammatory agents also increase insulin release by the B cell, and the effect is probably mediated by prostaglandin synthesis inhibition [32,

33]. Alpha-adrenergic blockade improves insulin secretion and may prove to have a role in the treatment of NIDDM [45, 50].

PATHOPHYSIOLOGY OF INSULIN SECRETION IN IDDM

The majority of patients who have had insulin dependent diabetes (also known as juvenile onset or type 1 diabetes) for more than 5 years have essentially no endogenous insulin secretion either in the basal state or in response to meals. It is this complete insulin deficiency that makes such patients totally dependent on exogenous insulin therapy to prevent the rapid development of hyperglycemia, ketosis, coma and death.

While the clinical onset of IDDM is usually abrupt and dramatic, it is now known that the underlying autoimmune destructive process may take place over months or years before the overt clinical presentation [1, 51, 104]. During this time the individuals are asymptomatic and have normal glucose tolerance. Animal studies have suggested that over 90% of the functioning B cells need to be destroyed before clinical diabetes will develop [52]. However, more recent data in animals has suggested that 40–50% of functioning B cells may still be present and viable at a time when insulin-requiring diabetes has developed (Figure 4); [126]. In support of this, when the pancreas is examined in humans with recently diagnosed IDDM, the pancreatic insulin content is about one-third of normal, with over 20% of the islets still containing insulin-positive cells on staining [127]. Therefore, lesser degrees of B-cell destruction may be present prior to clinical diabetes than previously thought. It seems likely that 20–50% of B cells may be potentially viable at the clinical onset of IDDM, but that they are functionally impaired due to the metabolic upset and the local release of cytokines from the ongoing autoimmune process in the islets. Recent studies indicate that there are changes in the patterns of B-cell secretion which appear to be predictable and progressive in a variety of experimental models [52–54]. The earliest marker of impaired B-cell function appears to be a loss of the ability of glucose to potentiate non-glucose secretagogues [54]. The next detectable abnormality is loss of the acute (or first phase) insulin response to IV glucose ($AIR_{glucose}$) [1, 55]. Thus, individuals who are progressing towards clinical IDDM can be found to have a complete loss of the glucose potentiation slope and a total absence of $AIR_{glucose}$ at a time when other measures of B-cell function and glucose tolerance are almost completely normal [1, 54]. By the time that clinical IDDM is present the usual pattern of B-cell function is for individuals to have no potentiation slope,

lack of a first and second phase insulin response to glucose, low to normal fasting insulin, and a reduced but detectable insulin response to IV glucagon or arginine [55] (Figures 5 and 6).

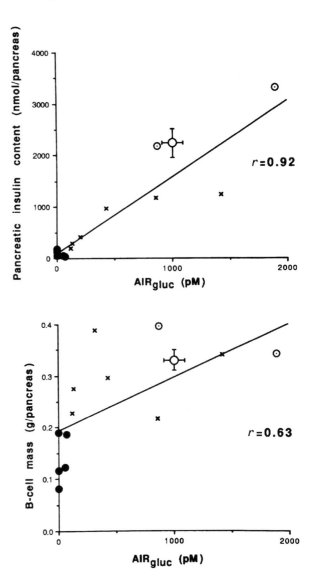

Figure 4 Relationship between acute insulin response to intravenous glucose (AIR_{gluc}) and pancreatic insulin content (upper panel) and B-cell mass (lower panel) in non-diabetic animals (⊙) and streptozocin-administered animals that were insulin-requiring (●) and non-insulin-requiring (x). O, mean ± SEM in non-diabetic animals for AIR_{gluc} ($n = 36$), pancreatic insulin content ($n = 9$), and B-cell mass ($n = 5$) (from reference 126, with permission)

Once individuals are treated with exogenous insulin injections, it becomes more difficult to follow endogenous B-cell function. However, the discoveries (a) that when insulin is secreted from the B cells into the portal circulation equimolar amounts of C-peptide are also released, and (b) that C-peptide is not extracted

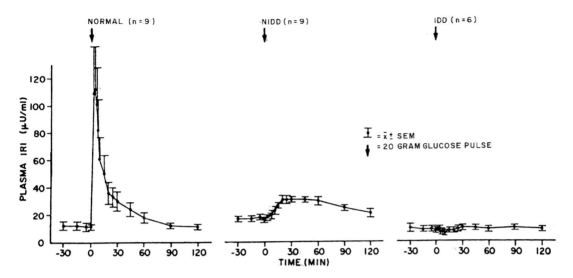

Figure 5 Insulin release in response to the intravenous administration of glucose in normal and diabetic subjects. Mean fasting plasma glucose concentrations: normal subjects 85 ± 3 mg/dl; non-insulin dependent diabetic subjects (NIDD) 160 ± 10 mg/dl; and insulin-dependent diabetic subjects (IDD) 325 ± 33 mg/dl. Note the lack of first-phase insulin response and the relative preservation of second-phase insulin response in non-insulin dependent diabetic subjects and the total lack of any response to glucose in the insulin dependent diabetic subjects (from reference 75, with permission)

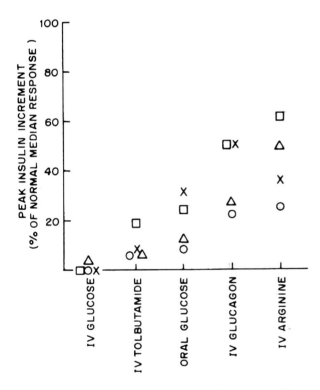

Figure 6 Summary of peak insulin increments (above basal) to all secretagogues for four IDDM patients. Results for each patient are expressed as the percentage of respective insulin increment compared with the median response in normal controls for the corresponding test. Patient 1, □; patient 2, △; patient 3, ×; patient 4, ○ (from reference 55, with permission)

significantly by the liver, have allowed investigators to study residual B-cell function by measuring C-peptide

after the onset of clinical IDDM. Several studies confirm that although some endogenous insulin secretion is usually present at the onset of clinical diabetes, the variations in the amount present and its subsequent rate of decline vary considerably [56, 57]. In general, stimulated C-peptide is about 20% of normal at the onset of clinical IDDM. The rate of decline is much faster in children and adolescents than it is in adults [56, 57, 105]. This loss may be slowed to some extent by attention to strict metabolic control using insulin infusion pumps or multiple daily insulin injections and home blood glucose monitoring [57, 58]. Following initiation of insulin therapy, more than 40% of patients undergo a partial remission, during which insulin therapy can be withdrawn completely and management continued with oral hypoglycemic agents or no treatment at all [59]. This so-called 'honeymoon period' occurs largely because of a transient improvement in B-cell function [58, 59] along with an improvement in insulin sensitivity [60]. However, this phase rarely lasts more than a few months. Even after treatment with exogenous insulin is once again instituted, the presence of some endogenous insulin secretion has been shown to reduce glycemic swings and improve the overall metabolic control [57]. Attempts have therefore been made to preserve endogenous insulin secretion in newly diagnosed insulin dependent diabetics using various immunosuppressive or other techniques, but so far success has been limited [59, 61–64]. In subjects with newly diagnosed IDDM treated with cyclosporin, clinical remission was associated with an increase in endogenous insulin secretion and an increase in insulin sensitivity.

Interestingly, loss of remission to an insulin-requiring state was associated with a decrease in insulin sensitivity rather than insulin secretion, despite continuing cyclosporin [128].

PATHOPHYSIOLOGY OF INSULIN SECRETION IN NIDDM

Basal Insulin Secretion

Basal insulin concentrations in patients with NIDDM have been reported as either elevated [65, 66], reduced [67] or normal [37, 68–70]. However, it is difficult to compare the insulin levels of different individuals unless they are matched for both the steady state glucose concentration and degree of insulin sensitivity. When such matching is performed, it is evident that there is a marked insulin secretory defect in patients with NIDDM, be they lean or obese [2, 71, 98]. For example, in studies in which an insulin infusion is administered to diabetic subjects in order to match their preceding steady state glucose levels to the fasting glucose level in weight-matched controls, basal insulin levels are less than those in control subjects [72]. Thus, it is clear that NIDDM individuals have a major defect in basal or steady state insulin secretion. As basal insulin secretion is critical to the maintenance of overall carbohydrate tolerance, this defect in basal insulin secretion is an important feature of NIDDM.

The glucose islet feedback loop which comprises the B cell, liver and peripheral tissues is depicted in Figure 7. As noted in Figure 7A, the basal glucose concentration is regulated by a feedback loop in which the endocrine pancreas acts as a glucose sensor to balance hepatic glucose delivery to the rate of insulin dependent and insulin independent glucose uptake. Any change in

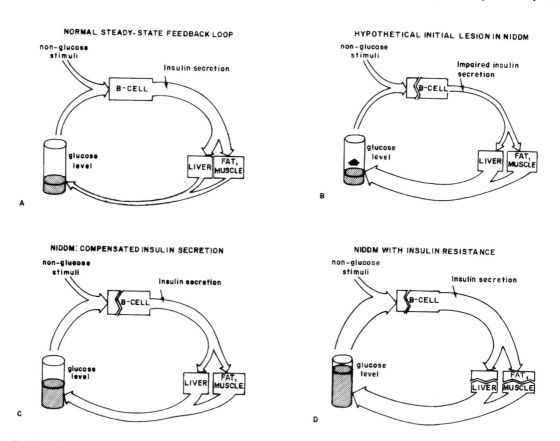

Figure 7 How islet dysfunction and insulin resistance interact to produce hyperglycemia in NIDDM. (A) Normal basal feedback loop for insulin and glucose. Insulin secretion, through effects on liver, fat and muscle, modulates blood glucose. Blood glucose level, via interaction with non-glucose stimuli, feeds back to the islet to maintain insulin output. (B) Hypothetical initial B-cell lesion of NIDDM. The impairment of insulin output would tend to lead to overproduction and underutilization of glucose, which would cause the glucose level to rise. A major reduction of insulin level would only be observed in this situation if glucose level remained normal. (C) Effect of hyperglycemia to compensate for the B-cell defect in NIDDM. Insulin deficiency from an initial islet lesion leads to hyperglycemia, which in turn stimulates insulin secretion. Thus, resulting basal insulin output is partially restored, and insulin levels are only slightly diminished. As a result of increased insulin output, glucose production and utilization return towards normal. (D) Interaction of B-cell function in NIDDM and tissue insensitivity to insulin. Further hyperglycemia is needed to compensate. Under these conditions the islet may secrete normal or even supranormal amounts of insulin despite the presence of impaired B-cell function (from reference 73, with permission)

glucose production by the liver or glucose utilization by fat and muscle is sensed by the islet and leads to changes in insulin and glucagon secretion in order to achieve a new steady state. The next panel (Figure 7B) illustrates the hypothetical initial lesion in NIDDM in which the existence of a defect in B-cell insulin secretion is postulated. Inadequate plasma insulin levels fail to suppress hepatic glucose production and also prevent normal glucose utilization by fat and muscle. Consequently, fasting glucose levels rise. This situation is only transient because, as depicted in Figure 7C, the elevation in the fasting plasma glucose level leads to increased B-cell stimulation along with increased A-cell suppression. The resultant improved insulin secretion and suppressed glucagon secretion produce more 'normal' basal plasma insulin and glucagon levels. Glucose production and utilization then return towards normal, but remain elevated in proportion to the glucose level. In the presence of insulin resistance, such as obesity, as shown in Figure 7D, further elevations in fasting plasma glucose occur and lead to enhanced stimulation of insulin secretion by the B cell in an attempt to overcome tissue insensitivity to insulin at both the liver and periphery. Thus, glycemia is very sensitive to insulin resistance in an individual with reduced islet function, and a much greater degree of hyperglycemia must result before compensation can occur. It is therefore apparent that regardless of whether insulin levels are normal or elevated, islet dysfunction is always present in NIDDM and hyperglycemia is the compensation that occurs to overcome the islet secretory defect [73]. Thus, NIDDM can be characterized as a reregulated steady state hyperglycemia. When the glycemia needed exceeds the renal threshold, unregulated metabolic decompensation occurs. These important concepts have been recently reviewed [98].

Defects in Postprandial Regulation of Insulin Secretion

NIDDM is characterized by an absent first phase insulin response to IV glucose [74] (Figure 5). In contrast, the second phase insulin response is still sensitive to glucose and therefore partially maintained in patients with compensated NIDDM. These responses are maintained by hyperglycemia until plasma glucose can no longer rise sufficiently to compensate for impaired insulin secretion. Decompensation occurs in patients with fasting plasma glucose levels greater than 250 mg/dl (13.9 mmol/l), although an elevated renal glucose threshold may preserve this compensation until glucose rises to over 350 mg/dl (19.4 mmol/l). Whenever significant glycosuria is found such individuals have been termed decompensated NIDDMs, because

hyperglycemia cannot develop to sufficient levels to compensate for the impaired insulin secretion [75].

The mechanism for the defect in glucose regulation of insulin secretion in NIDDM subjects is not known. One theory is that the B cell of the pancreas has a glucose-sensing defect and therefore does not respond as effectively to a given level of plasma glucose [76]. Another hypothesis is that NIDDMs possess intrinsic abnormalities to other modulators of insulin secretion. Support for this theory comes from the improvement in carbohydrate tolerance noted in patients with NIDDM who are treated with α-adrenergic blocking agents or non-steroidal anti-inflammatory agents [33, 45, 50]. Thirdly, some data suggest that the islet mass is reduced and therefore the capacity of the pancreas to secrete insulin is diminished in NIDDM. This is suggested by the reduction in maximal glucose-stimulated insulin release in subjects with NIDDM compared with age-matched and weight-matched controls [2], and by autopsy studies suggesting the existence of a decreased B-cell mass in patients with NIDDM [77, 78] which in part appears to be related to the deposit of amyloid composed largely of a new B-cell peptide called amylin or islet amyloid polypeptide (IAPP) [99].

Support for a major loss of islet functional capacity in NIDDMs comes from studies of the non-glucose regulation of insulin secretion as shown in Figure 8. In normal individuals, when the steady state glucose level is elevated, an increase in the AIR to the non-glucose secretagogues such as arginine or isoproteronol is observed [71]. However, in NIDDM subjects, the AIR to arginine is reduced at matched glucose levels. At glucose levels greater than 450 mg/dl (25 mmol/l), the AIR to arginine is normally maximal (AIR_{max}), but this AIR_{max} is also markedly reduced in patients with NIDDM compared with controls [2]. As mentioned previously, from the relationship between glucose and the AIR to arginine can be derived the glucose level at which the half-maximal response occurs, and this value—called PG_{50}—is a measure of B-cell sensitivity to glucose. Although there is a major reduction in AIR_{max} in NIDDM, the PG_{50} remains normal [2]. Such a finding supports the concept that the impaired capacity of the B cell to respond to glucose potentiation constitutes a major islet abnormality in patients with NIDDM [98].

Relationship between Islet Function and Insulin Resistance

Evaluation of the relationship of islet function to insulin sensitivity has demonstrated that there is a reciprocal relationship between B-cell insulin output and insulin sensitivity [80] (Figure 9). Studies in normal volunteers have shown that after 2 days

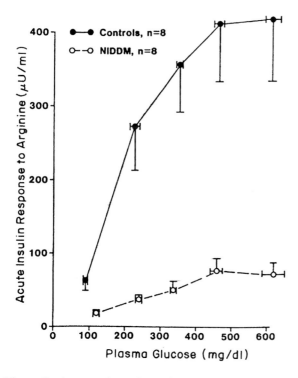

Figure 8 A comparison of acute insulin responses to 5 g IV arginine (mean 2–5 min insulin increment) at five matched plasma glucose levels in 8 patients with NIDDM and in 8 controls of similar age and body weight. Note that the maximal insulin response, a measure of insulin secretory capacity, is much lower in the diabetic group. The lowest glucose level in diabetic subjects was attained by an insulin infusion (from reference 2, with permission)

of dexamethasone-induced [40] or 2 weeks of nicotinic acid-induced [103] insulin resistance, normal islet B cells increase their responsiveness to glucose by increasing the slope of glucose potentiation. In contrast, studies of NIDDM patients suggest that they are unable to adapt their insulin secretion in response to 3 days of dexamethasone-induced insulin resistance. These NIDDM subjects demonstrate a marked reduction in maximal glucose-stimulated insulin release (AIR$_{max}$) following dexamethasone treatment when compared with matched, normal controls [41]. Such an inability of the B cell to adapt to increased insulin demand may contribute to the development of hyperglycemia when insulin resistance develops during weight gain and aging in individuals predisposed to NIDDM.

Etiology of NIDDM

While it is well recognized that NIDDM is an inherited disorder characterized by impaired insulin secretion and insulin resistance, the genetic basis for the disorder has not been identified. What is clear is that a fundamental abnormality of the pancreatic B cell is present prior to the onset of fasting hyperglycemia. This

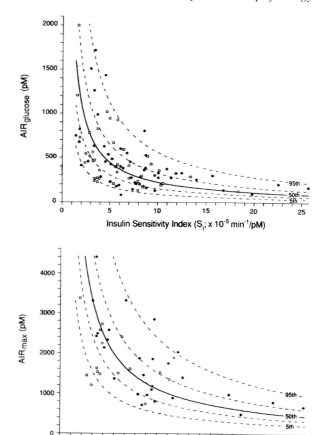

Figure 9 Relationship between first phase (acute) insulin response to glucose (AIR$_{glucose}$) (upper panel), and maximal acute insulin response to arginine (AIR$_{max}$) (lower panel) and insulin sensitivity (S$_I$) in normal subjects. A reduction in insulin action, measured by a decreased S$_I$, results in enhancement of glucose-induced insulin secretion and an increase in insulin secretory capacity. These compensatory changes in islet function contribute to the maintenance of euglycemia in normal individuals (from reference 80, with permission)

observation is based on studies done in subjects at high risk of subsequently developing NIDDM.

Obese former gestational diabetics have a 10-fold increased risk of developing NIDDM when compared with obese controls. When studied following pregnancy at a time when they are euglycemic, these subjects demonstrate a reduction in B-cell function measured as a reduction in first-phase insulin release and B-cell secretory capacity (AIR$_{max}$) compared to age-matched and weight-matched controls [79]. This same group have also been demonstrated to have disproportionately increased proinsulin release when compared to controls providing further evidence for altered islet function at a time when their diabetes has resolved [106]. The significance of this latter finding is related to the observation that in NIDDM, the proportion of immunoreactive insulin comprised of proinsulin (PI/IRI ratio) is increased, compatible with altered B-cell function [107–110].

Individuals with impaired glucose tolerance (IGT) comprise a group who have a high rate of conversion to NIDDM. As would be predicted, a number of the secretory abnormalities observed in NIDDM can be demonstrated in these subjects. In recent studies of carefully weight, sex and age-matched groups, lower insulin levels are seen in response to glucose in the early time points of the oral test [111]. Studies of the oscillatory nature of insulin release, which occurs every 105–120 minutes, demonstrate disturbances in insulin oscillations including a lack of entrainment by glucose [112, 113]. Recently, an increased PI/IRI ratio has been found to be present in Japanese-American subjects with IGT who subsequently progress on to develop NIDDM over a 5-year follow-up period, when compared to IGT subjects who either remain IGT or revert to normal glucose tolerance over the same follow-up period [114].

Based on the familial nature of NIDDM, first-degree relatives of NIDDM subjects with normal glucose tolerance represent another high risk group. As a group, these relatives can be demonstrated to have a reduction in insulin secretion prior to developing NIDDM. Offspring of two NIDDM parents demonstrate reduced glucose potentiation of insulin secretion when compared with controls matched for age, weight and insulin resistance [85]. In addition to this study which has demonstrated impaired insulin release under conditions when the prevailing glucose level is raised, alterations in insulin secretion have also been demonstrated at the basal glucose level. Under euglycemic conditions, pulsatile insulin release, which occurs every 12–15 minutes, has also been shown to be deranged in non-diabetic siblings of subjects with NIDDM [115].

As alluded to above, it has been demonstrated that alterations in pancreatic B-cell function are a feature of the preclinical disease state but the mechanism underlying these changes has not been determined. However, recent studies of families with an autosomal dominant form of NIDDM known as maturity onset diabetes of the young (MODY), have provided the first definitive description of the genetic basis for NIDDM. First, in a group of French MODY families, some 60% of subjects were found to have 16 different mutations in the coding region of the glucokinase gene [116, 117], a gene which encodes an enzyme critical to glucose metabolism in the pancreatic B cell and the hepatocyte. As would be predicted for an abnormality of this enzyme which is vital for glucose sensing by the B cell, affected subjects have been demonstrated to have impaired B-cell function [118]. In further studies these mutant enzymes have been expressed *in vitro* and all have been shown to have little or no biological

activity [119]. However, it is important to recognize that these gene mutations are not the explanation for the altered insulin secretion seen in the vast majority of subjects with NIDDM, based on screening studies done in a variety of population groups. In a recent report of former GDM, the prevalence of mutations in this gene in this high risk group has been estimated at 5% [120].

In summary, recent studies using sophisticated measures of B-cell function have demonstrated that alterations in pancreatic B-cell function are an integral component of the pathophysiology of NIDDM and are present in subjects at high risk of developing the clinical syndrome at a time when they are still euglycemic. While coding mutations in glucokinase appear to be the explanation for the islet dysfunction in a large proportion of MODY subjects, this does not seem to be so for most NIDDM individuals. Nevertheless, it represents an example of what is undoubtedly the first of many genetic abnormalities that will be associated with the disease.

OTHER SYNDROMES THAT AFFECT INSULIN SECRETION

Acromegaly

Acromegaly is characterized by insulin resistance due to the counter-regulatory effects from the excessive growth hormone present in this condition [86]. This usually leads to compensatory hyperinsulinemia. In many subjects, almost complete compensation occurs and glucose tolerance remains normal. In some, compensation is inadequate and carbohydrate intolerance develops. In others (about 25%), clinical hyperglycemia occurs and gross islet dysfunction is evident. This alteration in islet function results from the effects of both growth hormone *per se* [121] and insulin-like growth factor I (IGF-I) [122, 123]. There is a significant family history of diabetes in those who develop overt decompensation, suggesting that the variability of compensation may be on a genetic basis. However, it is also possible that varying degrees of growth hormone hypersecretion and variations in the insulin resistance and islet dysfunction in response to excess growth hormone may contribute.

Cushing's Syndrome

Cushing's syndrome is also characterized by glucose intolerance. Although carbohydrate intolerance is common, fasting euglycemia is maintained in most individuals. Approximately 25% of patients with Cushing's syndrome develop clinical hyperglycemia. The mechanism clearly is partially related to insulin resistance, but steroids have been shown to impair islet B-cell function *in vivo* [28, 107, 121] and are also known to stimulate glucagon secretion [87].

Glucagonoma

Glucose intolerance is observed in patients with glucagonoma. Because of compensatory hyperinsulinemia, severe hyperglycemia is unusual despite the immense hyperglycemic potential of hyperglucagonemia. An interesting observation is that many patients with glucagonoma have hypoaminoacidemia as a result of the intense gluconeogenesis stimulated by glucagon [88].

Pheochromocytoma

The glucose intolerance associated with pheochromocytoma is multifactorial. As catecholamines have a direct α-inhibitory effect on the islet, most patients with pheochromocytoma have hypoinsulinemia [29, 30]. However, insulin resistance also occurs, because of simultaneous β-adrenergic insulin resistance and glycogenolysis [89].

IMPLICATIONS FOR TREATMENT

Improvement of Glucose Tolerance with Insulin Treatment

Insulin resistance, a common finding in patients with diabetes, may be secondary to hypoinsulinemia which is present in individuals with both IDDM and NIDDM. It has been demonstrated that insulin treatment for a period as short as 7 days improves insulin sensitivity [83]. However, this treatment did not completely reverse the insulin resistance in patients with NIDDM. The improvement in insulin sensitivity may even be somewhat greater than observed in this particular study, due to the fact that the NIDDM patients were somewhat older and heavier than the control subjects and it is well known that aging and obesity are associated with insulin resistance. Other groups have also demonstrated this improvement in insulin action in NIDDM patients following treatment with insulin [84, 90]. Approximately 40% of patients with IDDM undergo a partial remission ('honeymoon period') following insulin treatment, which occurs partly through improvement in insulin sensitivity [60]. Thus, the use of insulin treatment leads to an improvement of insulin sensitivity in patients with either IDDM or NIDDM.

An improvement of islet function is also observed with insulin treatment. In carefully controlled trials, obese patients with NIDDM increased their integrated

plasma insulin response to glucagon more than three-fold after insulin treatment [84]. This effect persisted for at least 2 weeks after insulin withdrawal and was associated with a significant reduction in both the fasting and postprandial plasma glucose concentrations. Improvements in islet function with insulin treatment also include increased C-peptide secretion and enhanced second phase insulin response to IV glucose. Lean patients with IDDM may also demonstrate an improvement in insulin secretion after insulin treatment [58]. In addition, a partial remission permitting the complete withdrawal of insulin therapy or its replacement with oral agents has been demonstrated in up to 40% of newly diagnosed patients with IDDM [59, 105]. Thus, the use of insulin treatment leads to improvements of insulin secretion in patients with IDDM and NIDDM.

Improvement of Glucose Tolerance with Sulfonylurea Treatment

Sulfonylurea agents improve glucose tolerance through a number of mechanisms. The most important mechanism responsible for a decrease in fasting plasma glucose is a reduction in hepatic glucose production due to improved islet B-cell function. Patients with NIDDM who show the greatest improvement in glucose level during treatment with sulfonylurea agents are those who have the greatest reduction in hepatic glucose production rates [91, 92]. Sulfonylurea agents may also lead to an improvement in insulin action but only when the islet B cell is intact (see Chapter 36). Long-term treatment with sulfonylureas often results in insulin levels that return to pretreatment control values. However, islet function is still markedly improved [75]. As shown in Figure 10, when plasma glucose during sulfonylurea treatment is matched by a glucose clamp, β-adrenergically stimulated insulin secretion can be shown to be markedly enhanced. Insulin secretion in response to the non-glucose secretagogue arginine and the second phase insulin response to glucose also increase, indicating that stimulation of the B cell by sulfonylurea agents is always an important mechanism of their effect, regardless of whether insulin levels are increased [75].

Recently, interest in combining sulfonylurea agents with insulin for the treatment of NIDDM has been advocated. The theoretical advantage is an improvement in postreceptor insulin sensitivity and a lowering of plasma insulin levels. However, plasma levels of insulin achieved in patients treated with insulin plus sulfonylurea agents are very similar to, or higher than, those observed when sulfonylureas and insulin are used alone [94, 124, 125].

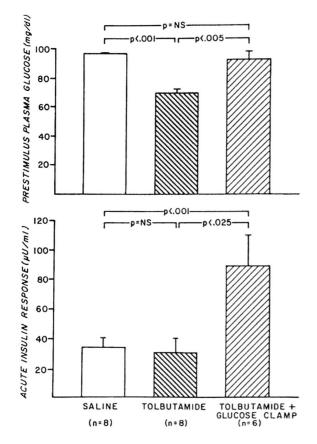

Figure 10 Importance of the prestimulus glucose concentration to the effect of tolbutamide on the insulin response to 12 μg of isoproterenol. The tolbutamide infusion (7 mg/m² · min) caused a significant decrease in glucose levels but no change in insulin response to isoproterenol. When the decrease in plasma glucose during tolbutamide was prevented by a concomitant glucose infusion, augmentation of the insulin response was observed. Thus, the decrease in glucose masked the insulinotrophic effects of the tolbutamide (from reference 75, with permission)

Improvement of Glucose Tolerance with Weight Loss

When weight reduction is successful in NIDDM, an improvement in glucose tolerance can usually be demonstrated. This is illustrated by the results obtained in one study in which a subset of 36 patients who achieved weight loss to within 6% of ideal body weight demonstrated an improvement in the oral glucose tolerance test, with the fasting plasma glucose returning to normal in 25 of the 36 patients. Residual hyperglycemia after weight reduction was demonstrable in only six of the 36 patients [95]. Unfortunately, achieving this degree of success is rare. However, dietary programs that combine a hypocaloric diet and behavior modification have demonstrated some success with weight reduction [96]. Thus, long-term weight reduction may be possible in some obese

individuals and lead to an improvement in glucose tolerance.

The mechanism for this improved glucose tolerance with weight loss has been thought to be related to an improvement in insulin sensitivity. However, in subjects with poor islet function and severe hyperglycemia, a clear-cut increase in insulin levels has also been observed [81, 82]. Unfortunately, the greatest effect on glucose level is found during the period of reduced caloric intake. When weight stabilizes, even at the lower level, glucose levels will tend to rise. Therefore, the reduced glucose levels after a weight plateau is reached are often much more modest.

CONCLUSION

Studies of healthy normal individuals with widely varying insulin sensitivity have provided important new data to evaluate the regulation of islet B-cell function. These studies have clearly demonstrated that islet B-cell dysfunction is an integral component of the pathophysiology of hyperglycemia in IDDM and NIDDM. While insulin replacement therapy is a requirement for individuals with IDDM, interventions such as reduced caloric intake and weight loss which aim to decrease the demand on the islet B cell can have important effects to reduce hyperglycemia in subjects with NIDDM. However, dietary therapy is often unsuccessful. In this setting, sulfonylureas, which can directly enhance B-cell function, may be useful. Ultimately, however, a progressive reduction in insulin secretion, possibly in part due to the replacement of the islet by amyloid, results in further deterioration in glucose control and the eventual need for insulin therapy in the majority of NIDDM.

REFERENCES

1. Srikanta S, Ganda OP, Jackson RA et al. Type 1 diabetes mellitus in monozygotic twins: chronic progressive beta cell dysfunction. Ann Intern Med 1983; 99: 320–6.
2. Ward WK, Bolgiano DC, McKnight B, Halter JB, Porte D Jr. Diminished B cell secretory capacity in patients with noninsulin-dependent diabetes mellitus. J Clin Invest 1984; 74: 1318–28.
3. Johnston C, Raghu P, McCulloch DK et al. B-cell function and insulin sensitivity in non-diabetic HLA-identical siblings of insulin-dependent diabetics. Diabetes 1987; 36: 829–37.
4. Ward WK, Johnston CL, Beard JC, Benedetti TJ, Porte D Jr. Abnormalities of islet B-cell function, insulin action, and fat distribution in women with histories of gestational diabetes: relationship to obesity. J Clin Endocrinol Metab 1985; 61: 1039–45.
5. Ferrannini E, Cobelli C. The kinetics of insulin in man. II. Role of the liver. Diabetes Metab Rev 1987; 3: 365–97.

6. Rabkin R, Simon NM, Steiner S, Colwell JA. Effect of renal disease on renal uptake and excretion of insulin in man. New Engl J Med 1970; 282: 182–7.

7. Porte D Jr, Pupo AA. Insulin responses to glucose: evidence for a two pool system in man. J Clin Invest 1969; 48: 2309–19.

8. Bennett LL, Grodsky GM. Multiphasic aspects of insulin release after glucose and glucagon. In Ostman J (ed.) Diabetes. Proceedings of the Sixth Congress of the International Diabetes Federation. Amsterdam: Excerpta Medica, 1969: pp 462–9.

9. Chen M, Porte D Jr. The effect of rate and dose of glucose infusion on the acute insulin response in man. J Clin Endocrinol Metab 1976; 42: 1168–75.

10. Karam JH, Grodsky GM, Ching KN, Schmid F, Burrill K, Forsham PH. 'Staircase' glucose stimulation of insulin secretion in obesity. Measure of beta-cell sensitivity and capacity. Diabetes 1974; 23: 763–70.

11. DeFronzo RA, Tobin JD, Andres R. Glucose clamp technique: a method for quantifying insulin secretion and resistance. Am J Physiol 1979; 237: E214–23.

12. Curry DL, Bennett LL, Grodsky GM. Dynamics of insulin secretion by the perfused rat pancreas. Endocrinology 1968; 83: 572–84.

13. Elrick H, Stimmler L, Hlad CJ Jr, Arai Y. Plasma insulin response to oral and intravenous glucose administration. J Clin Endocrinol 1964; 24: 1076–82.

14. Floyd JC Jr, Fajans SS, Conn JW, Knopf RF, Rull J. Stimulation of insulin secretion by amino acids. J Clin Invest 1966; 45: 1487–502.

15. Ward WK, Halter JB, Beard JC, Porte D Jr. Adaptation of B- and A-cell function during prolonged glucose infusion in human subjects. Am J Physiol 1984; 246: E405–11.

16. Samols E, Marri G, Marks V. Promotion of insulin secretion by glucagon. Lancet 1965; ii: 415–6.

17. Asplin CM, Paquette TL, Palmer JP. *In vivo* inhibition of glucagon secretion by paracrine beta cell activity in man. J Clin Invest 1981; 68: 314–8.

18. Chideckel EW, Palmer J, Koerker DJ, Ensinck J, Davidson MB, Goodner CJ. Somatostatin blockade of acute and chronic stimuli of the endocrine pancreas and the consequences of this blockade on glucose homeostasis. J Clin Invest 1975; 55: 754–62.

19. Verdonk CA, Rizza RA, Nelson RL, Go VL, Gerich JE, Service FJ. Interaction of fat-stimulated gastric inhibitory polypeptide on pancreatic alpha and beta cell function. J Clin Invest 1980; 65: 1119–25.

20. Rehfeld JF, Stadil F. The effect of gastrin on basal and glucose-stimulated insulin secretion in man. J Clin Invest 1973; 52: 1415–26.

21. Dupre J, Cutris JD, Unger RH, Waddell RW, Beck JC. Effects of secretin, pancreozymin, or gastrin on the response of the endocrine pancreas to administration of glucose or arginine in man. J Clin Invest 1969; 48: 745–57.

22. Halter JB, Porte D Jr. Mechanisms of impaired acute insulin release in adult onset diabetes: studies with isoproterenol and secretin. J Clin Endocrinol Metab 1978; 46: 952–60.

23. Lerner RJ, Porte D Jr. Studies of secretin-stimulated insulin responses in man. J Clin Invest 1972; 51: 2205–10.

24. Fajans SS, Floyd JC Jr, Knopf RF, Conn JW. A comparison of leucine and acetoacetate-induced hypoglycemia in man. J Clin Invest 1964; 43: 2003–8.

25. Felig P, Marliss EB, Cahill GF Jr. Metabolic response to human growth hormone during prolonged starvation. J Clin Invest 1971; 50: 411–21.

26. Schebalin M, Said SI, Makhlouf GM. Stimulation of insulin and glucagon secretion by vasoactive intestinal peptide. Am J Physiol 1977; 232: E197–200.

27. Ahren B, Taborsky GJ Jr, Porte D Jr. Neuropeptidergic versus cholinergic and adrenergic regulation of islet hormone secretion. Diabetologia 1986; 29: 827–36.

28. Kalhan SC, Adam PAJ. Inhibitory effect of prednisone on insulin secretion in man: model for duplication of blood glucose concentration. J Clin Endocrinol Metab 1975; 41: 600–10.

29. Beard JC, Weinberg C, Pfeifer MA, Best JD, Halter JB, Porte D Jr. Interaction of glucose and epinephrine in the regulation of insulin secretion. Diabetes 1982; 31: 802–7.

30. Porte D Jr, Williams RH. Inhibition of insulin release by norepinephrine in man. Science 1966; 152: 1248–50.

31. Dunning BE, Ahrén B, Veith RC, Böttcher G, Sundler F, Taborsky GJ Jr. Galanin: a novel pancreatic neuropeptide. Am J Physiol 1986; 251: E127–33.

32. McRae JR, Metz SA, Robertson RP. A role for endogenous prostaglandins in defective glucose potentiation of nonglucose insulin secretagogues in diabetics. Metabolism 1981; 30: 1065–75.

33. Robertson RP, Chen M. A role for prostaglandin E in defective insulin secretion and carbohydrate intolerance in diabetes mellitus. J Clin Invest 1977; 60: 747–53.

34. Kajinuma H, Kaneto A, Kuzuya T, Nakao K. Effects of methacholine on insulin secretion in man. J Clin Endocrinol Metab 1968; 28: 1384–8.

35. Robertson RP, Halter JB, Porte D Jr. A role for alpha-adrenergic receptors in abnormal insulin secretion in diabetes mellitus. J Clin Invest 1976; 57: 791–5.

36. Ogilvie RF. The islands of Langerhans in 19 cases of obesity. J Pathol Bacteriol 1933; 37: 473–81.

37. Bagdade JD, Bierman EL, Porte D Jr. The significance of basal insulin in the evaluation of the insulin response to glucose in diabetic and non-diabetic subjects. J Clin Invest 1967; 46: 1549–57.

38. Beard JC, Ward WK, Halter JB, Wallum BJ, Porte D Jr. Relationship of islet function to insulin action in human obesity. J Clin Endocrinol Metab 1987; 65: 59–64.

39. Chen M, Bergman RN, Pacini G, Porte D Jr. Pathogenesis of age-related glucose intolerance in man: insulin resistance and decreased beta-cell function. J Clin Endocrinol Metab 1985; 60: 13–20.

40. Beard JC, Halter JB, Best JD, Pfeifer MA, Porte D Jr. Dexamethasone-induced insulin resistance enhances B cell responsiveness to glucose level in normal men. Am J Physiol 1984; 247: E592–6.

41. LaCava EC, Halter JB, Porte D Jr. Failure of islet B-cell adaptation to insulin resistance in NIDDM. Diabetes 1985; 34 (suppl. 1): 45A.

42. Wallum BJ, Benedetti TJ, Porte D Jr. Predisposition to NIDDM identifiable by a lack of B-cell adaptation to insulin resistance. Diabetes 1985; 34 (suppl. 1): 297A.

43. Amery A, Berthaux P, Bulpitt C et al. Glucose intolerance during diuretic therapy. Results of trial by the European Working Party on Hypertension in the Elderly. Lancet 1978; i: 681–3.

44. Robertson RP, Porte D Jr. Adrenergic modulation of basal insulin secretion in man. Diabetes 1973; 22: 1–8.

45. Broadstone VL, Pfeifer MA, Bajaj V, Stagner JI, Samois E. Alpha-adrenergic blockade improves glucose-potentiated insulin secretion in non-insulin-dependent diabetes mellitus. Diabetes 1987; 36: 932–7.

46. Graber AL, Porte D Jr, Williams RH. Clinical use of diazoxide and mechanism for its hyperglycemic effects. Diabetes 1966; 15: 143–8.

47. Malherbe C, Burrill KC, Levin SR, Karam JH, Forsham PH. Effect of diphenylhydantoin on insulin secretion in man. New Engl J Med 1972; 286: 339–42.

48. Singh SP, Patel DG. Effects of ethanol on carbohydrate metabolism. I. Influence on oral glucose tolerance. Metabolism 1976; 25: 239–43.

49. Dulin WE, Soret MG. Chemically and hormonally induced diabetes. In Volk BW, Wellman KF (eds) The diabetic pancreas. New York: Plenum, 1977: pp 425–65.

50. Kashiwagi A, Harano Y, Suzuki M, Kojima H, Harada M, Nishio Y, Shigeta Y. New alpha$_2$-adrenergic blocker (DG-5128) improves insulin secretion and *in vivo* glucose disposal in NIDDM patients. Diabetes 1987; 35: 1085–9.

51. Gorsuch AN, Spencer KM, Lister J, McNally JM, Dean BM, Bottazzo GF, Cudworth AG. Evidence for a long prediabetic period in type I (insulin-dependent) diabetes mellitus. Lancet 1981; ii: 1363–5.

52. Bonner-Weir S, Trent DF, Weir GC. Partial pancreatectomy in the rat and subsequent defect in glucose-induced insulin release. J Clin Invest 1983; 71: 1544–53.

53. Leahy JL, Bonner-Weir S, Weir GC. Abnormal glucose regulation of insulin secretion in models of reduced B-cell mass. Diabetes 1984; 33: 667–73.

54. McCulloch DK, Raghu PK, Johnston C, Klaff LJ, Kahn SE, Beard, JC, Ward WK, Benson EA, Koerker DJ, Bergman RN, Palmer JP. Defects in β-cell function and insulin sensitivity in normoglycemic streptozocin-treated baboons: a model of preclinical insulin-dependent diabetes. J Clin Endocrinol Metab 1988; 67: 785–92.

55. Ganda OP, Srikanta S, Brink SJ, Morris MA, Gleason RE, Soeldner JS, Eisenbarth GS. Differential sensitivity to beta-cell secretagogues in 'early' type I diabetes mellitus. Diabetes 1984; 33: 516–21.

56. Madsbad S, Faber OK, Binder C, McNair P, Christiansen C, Transbol I. Prevalence of residual beta-cell function in insulin-dependent diabetics in relation to age at onset and duration of diabetes. Diabetes 1978; 27 (suppl. 1): 262–4.

57. DCCT Research Group. Effects of age, duration and treatment of insulin-dependent diabetes mellitus on residual beta-cell function: observations during the eligibility testing for the Diabetes Control and Complications Trial (DCCT). J Clin Endocrinol Metab 1987; 65: 30–6.

58. Perlman K, Ehrlich RM, Filler RM, Albisser AM. Sustained normoglycemia in newly diagnosed type I diabetic subjects: short-term effects and one-year follow-up. Diabetes 1984; 33: 995–1001.

59. Koivisto VA, Aro A, Cantell K et al. Remissions in newly diagnosed type I (insulin-dependent) diabetes: influence of interferon as an adjunct to insulin therapy. Diabetologia 1984; 27: 193–7.

60. Lager I, Lönnroth P, von Schenck H, Smith U. Reversal of insulin resistance in type I diabetes after treatment with subcutaneous continuous insulin infusion. Br Med J 1983; 287: 1661–4.

61. Stiller CR, Dupre J, Gent M et al. Effects of cyclosporine immunosuppression in insulin-dependent diabetes mellitus of recent onset. Science 1984; 223: 1362–7.

62. Feutren G, Papoz L, Assan R et al. Cyclosporin increases the rate and length of remissions in insulin-dependent diabetes of recent onset. Results of a multicentre double-blind trial. Lancet 1986; ii: 119–24.

63. Harrison LC, Colman PG, Dean B, Baxter R, Martin FI. Increase in remission rate in newly diagnosed type I diabetic subjects treated with azathioprine. Diabetes 1985; 34: 1306–8.

64. Culler FL, O'Connor R, Kaufmann S, Jones KL, Roth JC. Immunospecific therapy for type I diabetes mellitus. New Engl J Med 1985; 313: 695–6.

65. Felig P, Wahren J, Hendler R. Influence of maturity-onset diabetes on splanchnic glucose balance after oral glucose ingestion. Diabetes 1978; 27: 121–6.

66. Hollenbeck CB, Chen YD, Reaven GM. A comparison of the relative effects of obesity and non-insulin-dependent diabetes mellitus on *in vivo* insulin-stimulated glucose utilization. Diabetes 1984; 33: 622–6.

67. Holman RR, Turner RC. Maintenance of basal plasma glucose and insulin concentrations in maturity-onset diabetes. Diabetes 1979; 28: 227–30.

68. Lerner RL, Porte D Jr. Acute and steady-state insulin responses to glucose in nonobese diabetic subjects. J Clin Invest 1972; 51: 1624–31.

69. Goodner CJ, Conway MJ, Werrbach JH. Control of insulin secretion during fasting hyperglycemia in adult diabetics and in non-diabetic subjects during infusion of glucose. J Clin Invest 1969; 48: 1878–87.

70. Perley MJ, Kipnis DM. Plasma insulin responses to oral and intravenous glucose: studies in normal and diabetic subjects. J Clin Invest 1967; 46: 1954–62.

71. Halter JB, Graf RJ, Porte D Jr. Potentiation of insulin secretory responses by plasma glucose levels in man: evidence that hyperglycemia in diabetes compensates for impaired glucose potentiation. J Clin Endocrinol Metab 1979; 48: 946–54.

72. Turner RC, McCarthy ST, Holman RR, Harris E. Beta-cell function improved by supplementing basal insulin secretion in mild diabetes. Br Med J 1976; 1: 1252–4.

73. Ward WK, Beard JC, Halter JB, Pfeifer MA, Porte D Jr. Pathophysiology of insulin secretion in non-insulin-dependent diabetes mellitus. Diabetes Care 1984; 7: 491–502.

74. Brunzell JD, Robertson RP, Lerner RL, Hazzard WR, Ensinck JW, Bierman EL, Porte D Jr. Relationships between fasting glucose levels and insulin secretion during intravenous glucose tolerance tests. J Clin Endocrinol Metab 1976; 42: 222–9.

75. Pfeifer MA, Halter JB, Porte D Jr. Insulin secretion in diabetes mellitus. Am J Med 1981; 70: 579–88.

76. Ward WK, Halter JB, Best JD, Beard JC, Porte D Jr. Hyperglycemia and beta-cell adaptation during prolonged somatostatin infusion with glucagon replacement in man. Diabetes 1983; 32: 943–7.

77. Westermark P, Wilander E. The influence of amyloid deposits on the islet volume in maturity onset diabetes mellitus. Diabetologia 1978; 15: 417–21.

78. Saito K, Yaginuma N, Takahashi T. Differential volumetry of A, B and D cells in the pancreatic islets of diabetic and nondiabetic subjects. Tohoku J Exp Med 1979; 129: 273–83.

79. Ward WK, Johnston CL, Beard JC, Benedetti TJ, Halter JB, Porte D Jr. Insulin resistance and impaired insulin secretion in subjects with histories of gestational diabetes mellitus. Diabetes 1985; 34: 861–9.

80. Kahn SE, Prigeon RL, McCulloch DK, Boyko EJ, Bergman RN, Schwartz MW et al. Quantification of the relationship between insulin sensitivity and B-cell function in human subjects. Evidence for a hyperbolic function. Diabetes 1993; 42: 1663–72.

81. Stanik S, Marcus R. Insulin secretion improves following dietary control of plasma glucose in severely hyperglycemic obese patients. Metabolism 1989; 29: 346–50.

82. Kosaka K, Kuzuya T, Akanuma Y, Hagura R. Increase in insulin response after treatment of overt maturity-onset diabetes is independent of the mode of treatment. Diabetologia 1980; 18: 23–8.

83. Andrews WJ, Vasquez B, Nagulesparan M, Klimes I, Foley J, Unger R, Reaven GM. Insulin therapy in obese, non-insulin-dependent diabetes induces improvements in insulin action and secretion that are maintained for two weeks after insulin withdrawal. Diabetes 1984; 33: 634–42.

84. Garvey WT, Olefsky JM, Griffin J, Hamman RF, Kolterman OG. The effect of insulin treatment on insulin secretion and insulin action in type II diabetes mellitus. Diabetes 1985; 34: 222–34.

85. Johnston C, Ward WK, Beard JC, McKnight B, Porte D Jr. Islet cell function and insulin sensitivity in the non-diabetic offspring of conjugal type 2 diabetic patients. Diabet Med 1990; 7: 119–25.

86. Muggeo M, Bar RS, Roth J, Kahn CR, Gorden P. The insulin resistance of acromegaly: evidence for two alterations in the insulin receptor on circulating monocytes. J Clin Endocrinol Metab 1979; 48: 17–25.

87. Wise JK, Hendler R, Felig P. Influence of glucocorticoids on glucagon secretion and plasma amino acid concentrations in man. J Clin Invest 1973; 52: 2774–82.

88. Stacpoole PW. The glucagonoma syndrome: clinical features, diagnosis, and treatment. Endocr Rev 1981; 2: 347–61.

89. Deibert DC, DeFronzo RA. Epinephrine-induced insulin resistance in man. J Clin Invest 1980; 65: 717–21.

90. Ginsberg H, Rayfield EJ. Effect of insulin therapy on insulin resistance in type II diabetic subjects. Evidence for heterogeneity. Diabetes 1981; 30: 739–45.

91. Best JD, Judzewitsch RG, Pfeifer MA, Beard JC, Halter JB, Porte D Jr. The effect of chronic sulfonylurea therapy on hepatic glucose production in non-insulin-dependent diabetics. Diabetes 1982; 31: 333–8.

92. Simonson DC, Ferrannini E, Bevilacqua S, Smith D, Barrett E, Carlson R, DeFronzo RA. Mechanism of improvement in glucose metabolism after chronic glyburide therapy. Diabetes 1984; 33: 838–45.

93. Kreymann B, Williams G, Ghatei MA, Bloom SR. Glucagon-like peptide-1 7–36: a physiological incretin in man. Lancet 1987; 2: 1300–4.

94. Vigili De Kreutzenberg S, Listato G, Riccio A, Valerio A, Tiengo A. Effects of sulfonylurea and insulin therapy on glucose control and insulin secretion in type 2 diabetics (NIDDM). Diabetes 1987; 36 (suppl. 1): 226A.

95. Newburgh LH. Control of the hyperglycemia of obese 'diabetics' by weight reduction. Ann Intern Med 1942; 17: 935–42.

96. Wing RR. Behavioral treatment of obesity: its application to type 2 diabetes. Diabetes Care 1993; 16: 193–9.

97. Johnston CLW, Ward WK, Beard JC, Halter JB, Porte D Jr. Lack of B- and A-cell adaptation to hyperglycemia in non-insulin dependent diabetes mellitus. Diabet Nutr Metab Clin Exp 1989; 2: 17–26.

98. Porte D Jr. The B-cell in type-II diabetes mellitus. Diabetes 1991; 40: 166–80.

99. Porte D Jr, Kahn SE. Perspectives in diabetes. Hyperproinsulinemia and amyloid in type II diabetes: clues to the etiology of islet B-cell dysfunction? Diabetes 1989; 38: 1333–6.

100. Porte D Jr, Woods SC. Neural regulation of islet hormones and its role in energy balance and stress hyperglycemia. In Rifkin H, Porte D Jr (eds) Diabetes mellitus: theory and practice. New York: Elsevier, 1990; pp 175–97.

101. Nauck MA, Heimesaat MM, Orskov C, Holst JJ, Ebert R, Creutzfeldt W. Preserved incretin activity of glucagon-like peptide 1 [7–36 amide] but not of synthetic human gastric inhibitory polypeptide in patients with type 2 diabetes mellitus. J Clin Invest 1993; 91: 301–7.

102. McCulloch DK, Kahn SE, Schwartz MW, Koerker DJ, Palmer JP. Effect of nicotinic acid-induced insulin resistance on pancreatic B cell function in normal and streptozocin-treated baboons. J Clin Invest 1991; 87: 1395–1401.

103. Kahn SE, Beard JC, Schwartz MW, Ward WK, Ding HL, Bergman RN, Taborsky GJ Jr, Porte D Jr. Increased β-cell secretory capacity as mechanism for islet adaptation to nicotinic acid-induced insulin resistance. Diabetes 1989; 38: 562–8.

104. McCulloch DK, Klaff LJ, Kahn SE, Schoenfeld SL, Greenbaum CJ, Mauseth RS et al. Non-progression of subclinical β-cell dysfunction among first-degree relatives of IDDM patients: 5-year follow up of the Seattle family study. Diabetes 1990; 39: 549–56.

105. Shah SC, Malone JI, Simpson NE. A randomized trial of intensive insulin therapy in newly diagnosed insulin-dependent diabetes mellitus. New Engl J Med 1989; 320: 550–4.

106. Persson B, Hanson U, Hartling SG, Binder C. Follow-up of women with previous GDM: insulin, C-peptide, and proinsulin responses to oral glucose load. Diabetes 1991; 40 (suppl. 2): 136–41.

107. Ward WK, LaCava EC, Paquette TL, Beard JC, Wallum BJ, Porte D Jr. Disproportionate elevation of immunoreactive proinsulin in type 2 (non-insulin-dependent) diabetes mellitus and experimental insulin resistance. Diabetologia 1987; 30: 698–702.

108. Yoshioka N, Kuzuya T, Matsuda A, Taniguchi M, Iwamoto Y. Serum proinsulin levels at fasting and

after oral glucose load in patients with type 2 (non-insulin-dependent) diabetes mellitus. Diabetologia 1988; 31: 355–60.

109. Temple RC, Carrington CA, Luzio SD, Owens DR, Schneider AE, Sobey WJ, Hales CN. Insulin deficiency in non-insulin-dependent diabetes. Lancet 1989; 1: 293–5.

110. Saad MF, Kahn SE, Nelson RG, Pettitt DJ, Knowler WC, Schwartz MW et al. Disproportionately elevated proinsulin in Pima Indians with non-insulin-dependent diabetes mellitus. J Clin Endocrinol Metab 1990; 70: 1247–53.

111. Mitrakou A, Kelley D, Mokan M, Veneman T, Pangburn T, Reilly J, Gerich J. Role of reduced suppression of glucose production and diminished early insulin release in impaired glucose tolerance. New Engl J Med 1992; 326: 22–9.

112. Polonsky KS, Given BD, Hirsch LJ, Tillil H, Shapiro ET, Beebe C et al. Abnormal patterns of insulin secretion in non-insulin-dependent diabetes mellitus. New Engl J Med 1988; 318: 1231–9.

113. O'Meara NM, Sturis J, Van Cauter E, Polonsky KS. Lack of control by glucose of ultradian insulin secretory oscillations in impaired glucose tolerance and in non-insulin-dependent diabetes mellitus. J Clin Invest 1993; 92: 262–71.

114. Kahn SE, Leonetti DL, Prigeon RL, Boyko EJ, Bergstrom RW, Fujimoto WY. Proinsulin as a marker for the development of non-insulin dependent diabetes mellitus in Japanese-American men. Diabetes 1995; 44: 173–9.

115. O'Rahilly S, Turner RC, Matthews DR. Impaired pulsatile secretion of insulin in relatives of patients with non-insulin-dependent diabetes. New Engl J Med 1988; 318: 1225–30.

116. Froguel P, Vaxillaire M, Sun F, Velho G, Zouali H, Butel MO, et al. Close linkage of glucokinase locus on chromosome 7p to early-onset non-insulin-dependent diabetes mellitus. Nature 1992; 356: 162–4.

117. Froguel P, Zouali H, Vionnet N, Velho G, Vaxillaire M, Sun F, et al. Familial hyperglycemia due to mutations in glucokinase. Definition of a subtype of diabetes mellitus. New Engl J Med 1993; 328: 697–702.

118. Velho G, Froguel P, Clement K, Pueyo ME, Rakotoambinina B, Zouali H, et al. Primary pancreatic beta-cell secretory defect caused by mutations in glucokinase gene in kindreds of maturity onset diabetes of the young. Lancet 1992; 340: 444–8.

119. Gidh-Jain M, Takeda J, Xu LZ, Lange AJ, Vionnet N, Stoffel M et al. Glucokinase mutations associated with non-insulin-dependent (type 2) diabetes mellitus have decreased enzymatic activity: implications for structure/function relationships. Proc Natl Acad Sci USA 1993; 90: 1932–6.

120. Stoffel M, Bell KL, Blackburn CL, Powell KL, Seo TS, Takeda J et al. Identification of glucokinase mutations in subjects with gestational diabetes mellitus. Diabetes 1993; 42: 937–40.

121. Kahn SE, Horber FF, Prigeon RL, Haymond MW, Porte D Jr. Effect of glucocorticoid and growth hormone treatment on proinsulin levels in humans. Diabetes 1993; 42: 1082–5.

122. Mauras N, Horber FF, Haymond MW. Low dose recombinant human insulin-like growth factor-I fails to affect protein anabolism but inhibits islet cell secretion in humans. J Clin Endocrinol Metab 1992; 75: 1192–7.

123. Rennert NJ, Caprio S, Sherwin RS. Insulin-like growth factor I inhibits glucose-stimulated insulin secretion but does not impair glucose metabolism in normal humans. J Clin Endocrinol Metab 1993; 76: 804–6.

124. Simpson HC, Sturley R, Stirling CA, Reckless JP. Combination of insulin with glipizide increases peripheral glucose disposal in secondary failure type 2 diabetic patients. Diabet Med 1990; 7: 143–7.

125. Pugh JA, Wagner ML, Sawyer J, Ramirez G, Tuley M, Friedberg SJ. Is combination sulfonylurea and insulin therapy useful in NIDDM patients? A meta-analysis. Diabetes Care 1992; 15: 953–9.

126. McCulloch DK, Koerker DJ, Kahn SE, Bonner-Weir S, Palmer JP. Correlations of *in vivo* β-cell function tests with β-cell mass and pancreatic insulin content in streptozocin-administered baboons. Diabetes 1991; 40: 673–9.

127. Conget I, Fernandez-Alvarez J, Ferrer J, Sarri Y, Novials A, Somoza N et al. Human pancreatic islet function at the onset of type 1 (insulin-dependent) diabetes mellitus. Diabetologia 1993; 36: 358–60.

128. Hramiak IM, Dupre J, Finegood DT. Determinants of clinical remission in recent-onset IDDM. Diabetes Care 1993; 16: 125–32.

16

C-peptide and Proinsulin

Sten Madsbad*, Svend G. Hartling*† and Ole K. Faber‡

*Hvidovre University Hospital, Denmark; *†University of Copenhagen, Herlev Hospital, Denmark; and ‡Øresund Hospital, Denmark

Proinsulin is the precursor or prohormone for insulin. In 1967 it was shown that formation of insulin is preceded by the biosynthesis of a single-chain insulin-containing peptide about 1.5 times the size of insulin itself [1, 2]. By translation of the mature mRNA on the ribosomes of the rough endoplasmic reticulum, preproinsulin is synthesized. The preproinsulin contains a 24-amino acid extension on the B chain. Proinsulin is then formed by removal of the 'leader' sequence of preproinsulin before translocation to the Golgi apparatus [3], where proinsulin is packed into vacuoles derived from the Golgi tubules, forming secretory granules. The conversion of proinsulin takes place in the secretory granules [4]. Proinsulin contains the insulin A chain, a connecting peptide including C-peptide, and the insulin B chain. There are two main conversion pathways (Figure 1). The conversion process is energy-dependent; it requires a pH close to 5.5, and the ionic composition in the granules is critical (reviewed in reference 5). To date, the biosynthesis and secretion of proinsulin has been found only in the B cell of the pancreas. The conversion of proinsulin into insulin, C-peptide and four amino acids is not complete: about 3–5% escapes the complete cleavage process, and thus a relatively small amount of proinsulin immunoreactive material (PIM) can be detected in the portal circulation [6, 7]. The secretory output from the pancreatic B cells consists of insulin, C-peptide and proinsulin [6], insulin and C-peptide being secreted in equimolar amounts [6, 8]. Human C-peptide is composed of 31 amino acids and has a molecular weight of 3021.

The measurement of insulin secretion, especially in patients with diabetes mellitus, is of great importance. The great interest in C-peptide is due to the limitations of the use of serum insulin as a measure of insulin secretion. After its secretion into the portal vein, insulin passes through the liver where approximately 50% of the insulin delivered is extracted [9]. The fractional hepatic insulin extraction may vary considerably among individuals and in the same individual under different conditions [10–12]. It has been suggested that the extraction of insulin by the liver may be altered by oral glucose, sulphonylurea treatment or obesity, and in patients with impaired glucose tolerance and diabetes mellitus [10–13]. Peripheral insulin concentrations, therefore, reflect posthepatic insulin delivery rather than the actual secretory rates of insulin. Until the development of C-peptide assays, evaluation of B-cell function in insulin-treated patients was impossible as the insulin assay is unable to discriminate between secreted and injected insulin. Further, C-peptide determinations are disturbed to a lesser degree than insulin measurements by the presence of insulin-binding antibodies. Since the 1970s, C-peptide measurements have been used extensively to evaluate the insulin secretion and hepatic insulin extraction of insulin (reviewed in references 14–19).

Until recently, there have been few detailed studies of the secretion and metabolic actions of proinsulin, because of assay problems and scarcity of human proinsulin for metabolic studies. The main interest in proinsulin has been as a marker of qualitative B-cell

International Textbook of Diabetes Mellitus, Second Edition. Edited by K.G.M.M. Alberti, P. Zimmet, R.A. DeFronzo, and H. Keen (Honorary)
© 1997 John Wiley & Sons Ltd

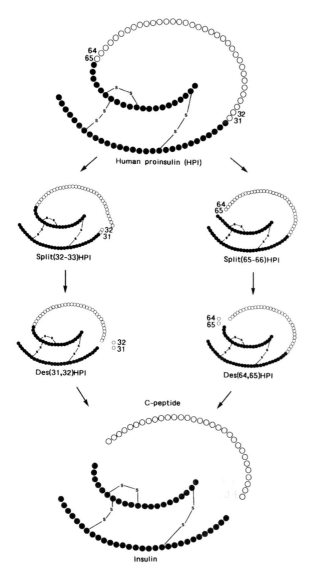

Figure 1 The conversion of human proinsulin to insulin (solid circles) and C-peptide (open circles) via split and des-proinsulin intermediates. Amino acid 64 is lysine; 31, 32 and 65 are arginine

defects in prediabetic and diabetic states, and in the diagnosis of insulinoma.

In this chapter the following are reviewed: (a) methodological aspects of the measurement of C-peptide; (b) physiological effects of C-peptide; (c) the kinetics and validity of plasma C-peptide as a marker of insulin secretion; (d) C-peptide as a measure of hepatic insulin extraction; (e) urinary C-peptide excretion as a measure of insulin secretion; and (f) the clinical application of C-peptide measurements, especially in relation to evaluation of residual B-cell function and its metabolic consequences in insulin dependent diabetes mellitus (IDDM), and in the classification of patients with diabetes mellitus. In relation to proinsulin, the following are discussed: (a) methodological aspects

of the measurement of proinsulin; (b) the kinetics and metabolism of proinsulin; (c) human proinsulin secretion; and (d) the clinical applications of proinsulin.

C-PEPTIDE

Radioimmunoassay of C-peptide

C-peptide is measured by radioimmunoassay [20–28]. Standardization of assays presents a problem, and it is difficult to compare results from different assay systems [21, 25, 28]. The variation in normal fasting C-peptide values between assay systems is explained by several factors, including non-specific displacement of the tracer, differences in antibodies which are known to differ in their antigenic domains, differences in labelled C-peptide, and in standards used [20–22]. Gel filtration studies have shown that immunoreactive C-peptide exists in more than one form, which may also explain some of the different concentrations of C-peptide measured with different assay systems [27]. An international reference preparation of synthetic human C-peptide (human proinsulin fragment 33–63) has been developed and shown to be suitable for use in some (but not all) radioimmunoassay systems [25]. As heterogeneity of serum C-peptide exists, it cannot necessarily be equated quantitatively with the use of a human synthetic C-peptide as standard [25, 27]. Even the use of identical standards in various C-peptide radioimmunoassays does not ensure the equivalence of C-peptide results obtained from the same blood sample in different laboratories [25].

The most important problems related to the C-peptide radioimmunoassay are (a) degradation of C-peptide in the serum, (b) non-specific displacement of the tracer by serum proteins, and (c) cross-reactivity of proinsulin with the insulin antibodies as well as with the C-peptide antibodies.

Degradation of C-peptide in Plasma

C-peptide immunoreactivity in plasma samples declines considerably with time, depending upon the storage temperature [22, 23]. The reactivity of the degradation products with various anti-C-peptide sera ranges from zero to 100% [22, 23]. The degradation of C-peptide may be inhibited by the addition of trasylol in a concentration of approximately 500 kIU/ml serum or plasma [22]. At a storage temperature below −20°C, C-peptide is stable in serum for months [22].

Non-specific Displacement of Tracer

Falsely high C-peptide values may occur as a consequence of non-specific binding of serum proteins to the C-peptide antiserum, causing tracer displacement [20–22]. Non-specific displacement varies greatly with the antiserum employed [20–22]. Antisera have to be selected to give the lowest value of C-peptide immunoreactivity in patients without B-cell function. A major part of the variation in normal fasting C-peptide values between different assay systems is probably attributable to non-specific displacement of the tracer [20–22, 25].

Proinsulin Interference

Because the C-peptide sequence is contained within the proinsulin molecule, antisera against C-peptide also react against proinsulin. The contribution of the serum proinsulin to the total serum C-peptide immunoreactivity depends on the molar concentration of proinsulin compared with that of C-peptide, and on the cross-reactivity of proinsulin with the antisera employed in the assay [20–22]. Hitherto 8% cross-reactivity on a molar basis has been the lowest reported [28]. The cross-reactivity in many assays may be in the 50–75% range [22]. The proinsulin interference is negligible in sera from normal subjects because of the relatively low serum proinsulin concentrations compared with C-peptide concentrations. Insulin treatment may cause formation of insulin binding antibodies, which also bind proinsulin by its insulin moiety and thereby delay its clearance, leading to elevated proinsulin concentrations. In insulin-treated patients proinsulin may account for up to 90% of the total C-peptide immunoreactivity in plasma [29]. In order to measure C-peptide specifically, therefore, proinsulin must be removed from the serum either by binding to anti-insulin antibodies coupled to Sepharose or by polyethylene glycol (PEG) precipitation [20, 24]. An alternative approach to this problem is to remove proinsulin by insulin antibodies bound to a solid phase [20]. This method involves a preliminary acid extraction of the serum samples to release proinsulin from endogenous antibodies. The procedure is time-consuming and requires large amounts of insulin antibodies.

The conventional C-peptide assay is a two-step assay, which runs over 24–28 hours. The standard or sample is incubated with the antiserum first and the tracer added later. This long assay time may, in some situations, be too long and limits its clinical application. A rapid (4–5 hours) assay has been developed as a one-step assay which displays the same intra-assay and interassay precision as the conventional assay [26]. Its wide working range makes it suitable for studies of subjects with non-insulin dependent diabetes mellitus (NIDDM) or for monitoring B-cell function after pancreas transplantation [26].

Physiological Effects of C-peptide

C-peptide has previously been considered to be without intrinsic physiological effects [237–239]. However, recent *in vitro* studies have suggested that C-peptide in physiological concentrations increases glucose transport and glycogen content in skeletal muscle [240]. In IDDM patients, short-term (2-hour) infusion of C-peptide to a physiological steady-state plasma level of 0.81 nmol/1 (2.45 ng/ml) significantly increased whole body glucose uptake by about 25% [241]. A further increase of 15% in glucose uptake was observed when the plasma C-peptide level was increased to 2.1 nmol/1 (6.34 ng/ml) [241]. Glomerular hyperfiltration was reduced by 7% [241]. Whether the effect on glucose metabolism reflects increased glucose utilization or a suppression of endogenous hepatic glucose production is unknown, but enhanced peripheral glucose uptake seems to be one possible explanation, since glucose uptake increased in the forearm during C-peptide infusion [242]. C-peptide infusion in IDDM has also been shown to reduce forearm vascular resistance with a parallel increase in skeletal muscle blood flow, capillary diffusion capacity and oxygen uptake [242]. Also pulmonary oxygen uptake increased in exercising IDDM patients during C-peptide infusion [243]. After subcutaneous injection of C-peptide (60 nmol), plasma C-peptide increased to 1.8 nmol/1 (5.43 ng/ml) at 53 minutes and glucose utilization increased by 48% during a 6-hour period after injection [244]. In a randomized double-blind study carried out for 1 month, in which young IDDM patients were treated with either fast-acting insulin mixed with equimolar amounts of biosynthetic C-peptide or insulin alone, improvements in glycaemic control, renal function (reduced glomerular hyperfiltration and normalized albumin excretion) and blood–retinal barrier function were only observed in the C-peptide-treated group [245]. The findings suggest that C-peptide is of physiological importance for the maintenance of normal blood flow and capillary function and that C-peptide may have a role in the regulation of carbohydrate metabolism. The primary structure of C-peptide, unlike that of insulin, varies considerably between species, which implies that C-peptide would not be expected to have any metabolic effects of major importance. Further studies from independent groups are therefore needed to define the metabolic actions of C-peptide.

Kinetics and the Validity of C-peptide as a Marker of Insulin Secretion

Plasma C-peptide concentrations can be used to determine insulin secretion rates. In addition, the relationship between the endogenous secretion rate of insulin and peripheral insulin concentration provides insight into endogenous insulin clearance [18, 30–33]. The validity of C-peptide measurements as an indicator of B-cell secretion depends on the following assumptions: (a) C-peptide and insulin are secreted in equimolar quantities; (b) hepatic extraction of C-peptide is negligible, and (c) the overall kinetics of C-peptide are known under the conditions studied, or the behaviour of C-peptide in the systemic circulation is such that its rate of appearance can be predicted from its plasma concentrations.

Equimolar Secretion of C-peptide and Insulin

The equimolar secretion of insulin and C-peptide has been demonstrated in dogs, both in the basal state and after various stimuli such as intravenous and oral glucose and intravenous arginine [17, 18]. In humans, the C-peptide:insulin ratio has been demonstrated to be approximately 1.0 [17, 18].

Hepatic Extraction of C-peptide

In dogs the hepatic extraction of C-peptide has been shown to be indistinguishable from zero in the basal state, and up to 6–7% during stimulation with intravenous or oral glucose [34]. The metabolic clearance rate of C-peptide was similar after intravenous and intraportal infusion of C-peptide [35]. In pigs it has been demonstrated that the C-peptide flux across the liver never falls by more than 12% [36]. Hence, it cannot be excluded that C-peptide is extracted in the liver, at least in some animals, but most results suggest that the hepatic extraction of C-peptide is negligible, both in the basal state and after stimulation with intravenous or oral glucose. In IDDM patients no hepatic C-peptide extraction has been detected [246]. As C-peptide is sampled in the systemic circulation, the transit time of C-peptide through the liver should also be considered. The pathways followed through the liver by C-peptide molecules are not all equal. This leads to staggering of the appearance in the hepatic vein of a bolus of C-peptide injected into the portal vein. This staggering has been well characterized using indicator dilution techniques and it has been demonstrated that the mean transit time through the liver is less than 30 seconds [37]. This time lag is so short that it is generally neglected. Consequently, the rate of appearance of C-peptide in peripheral blood is assumed to coincide with the B-cell (prehepatic) secretion rate.

Kinetics and Metabolic Clearance Rate of C-peptide

In normal individuals and patients with type 1 diabetes (IDDM), analysis of the decay curves after a bolus

injection of C-peptide in the fasting state and during a meal has revealed similar metabolic clearance rate (MCR) values [38, 39]. Furthermore, the MCR of C-peptide was independent of its plasma concentration over a wide range of concentrations [33, 38]. In contrast, recent data have demonstrated that during a six-fold increase of C-peptide infusion rate no more than a three-fold increase in plasma level was observed, indicating that the tissue uptake of C-peptide increased following the increased infusion rate [241]. The C-peptide MCR shows great interperson variability [33, 38]. Determination of C-peptide kinetics in individual subjects, therefore, increases the accuracy with which the insulin secretion rate can be calculated from the peripheral C-peptide concentration. The MCR values reported vary between 3.5 ml/kg per minute and 5.5 ml/kg per minute in normal and diabetic subjects [33, 38]. The average half-life in plasma was significantly longer in IDDM patients (42.5 minutes) than in normal subjects (33.5 minutes) [38]. This difference in half-life in the plasma suggests different kinetics of the disappearance of the C-peptide. The volume of distribution in normal-weight and obese subjects is, on average, $2.21/m^2$ [30].

In the basal state 30–50% of the secreted C-peptide is removed in the kidney, about 20% in skeletal muscle and the rest elsewhere [40, 41, 242, 246]. Release of C-peptide from muscle was found during exercise, suggesting that C-peptide is reversibly retained under resting conditions [242]. In patients with even a modest elevation in serum creatinine, a reduction in both plasma and urinary C-peptide clearance has been observed, together with elevated plasma C-peptide concentrations [18, 40, 247]. As a consequence, estimation of C-peptide kinetics in individual patients with renal disease is necessary for accurate assessment of insulin secretion. The C-peptide clearance rate has been demonstrated to be increased in hyperthyroidism [248].

In the fasting state, C-peptide accurately reflects the B-cell secretory activity, and the secretion rate of insulin can be estimated as the product of the peripheral C-peptide concentration and the MCR of C-peptide [38]. The total amount of C-peptide secreted in response to a stimulus can be calculated as the product of the integrated plasma C-peptide concentration and MCR [38]. Under most physiological non-steady state conditions, after stimulation of the B cells, the peripheral concentration of C-peptide does not change directly in proportion to its secretion rate, because C-peptide is distributed outside the plasma compartment and because C-peptide has a half-life in excess of 30 minutes (Figure 2) [42, 43]. During increasing secretion rates the concentration of C-peptide in the plasma compartment is considerably greater than the concentration in the extravascular compartment, and

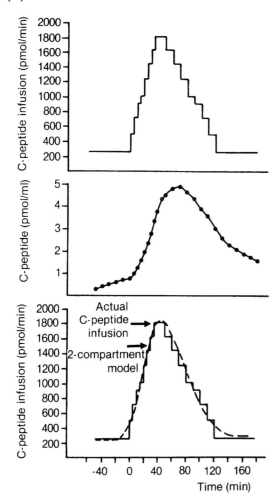

Figure 2 Variable infusions of biosynthetic human C-peptide in 10 normal volunteers and 7 IDDM subjects. The infusion rate of C-peptide is shown in the top panel and mean plasma concentrations are shown in the middle panel. The bottom panel depicts the actual infusion rate of C-peptide (solid line) in comparison with mean infusion rates calculated according to a two-compartment model using the deconvolution method on plasma C-peptide values in the middle panel (dashed line). The accuracy of the two-compartment model is evident from the close match between actual and calculated C-peptide infusion rates. The peripheral concentration of C-peptide does not change directly in proportion to the infusion rate of C-peptide, as C-peptide is distributed outside the plasma compartment (reproduced from reference 33 by copyright permission of The Rockefeller University Press)

C-peptide in the plasma moves into the extravascular compartment. The peripheral concentration, therefore, increases less than would be predicted from the actual secretion rate of insulin (Figure 2) [33, 34]. On the other hand, when the secretion rate is slowing, the amount of C-peptide in the plasma compartment falls, but now C-peptide is transferred from the extravascular to the plasma compartment and the plasma concentration falls more slowly than predicted (Figure 2)

[42, 43]. The plasma C-peptide (and insulin) profiles, therefore, give a distorted representation of B-cell secretion in situations with changes in insulin secretion rate. The faster the changes, the less accurate is the estimation of insulin secretion rates directly from C-peptide concentrations (Figures 2 and 3). This has been very convincingly demonstrated during calculation of the first-phase and second-phase insulin responses after intravenous glucose (Figure 3). Evaluated from the direct measurements of C-peptide, the first-phase insulin response is minimal compared with the second-phase response. When calculating the true prehepatic insulin secretion rates, the maximal secretion rate occurs during the first-phase insulin response in normal subjects, and the first-phase response accounted for about 66% of the total incremental insulin secretion

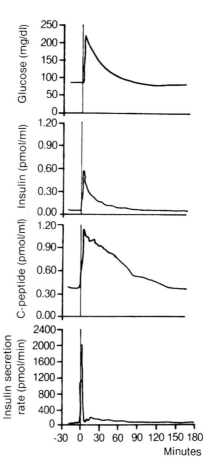

Figure 3 Average time-course of plasma glucose, insulin, C-peptide and calculated insulin secretion rates after glucose injection. Glucose (0.3 g/kg) was injected at time zero. The plasma insulin and C-peptide profiles give a distorted representation of insulin secretion rates. Evaluated from the C-peptide profile the first-phase insulin response is minimal. When calculating true insulin secretion rate (bottom panel) the maximal secretion rate is found during the first-phase insulin response, which accounted for 66% of the total incremental insulin secretion (reproduced with permission from reference 44, © 1989 The Endocrine Society)

during an intravenous glucose bolus (Figure 3) [44]. Thus, the images of prehepatic insulin secretion evaluated directly from the C-peptide curves and after mathematical calculation may be strikingly different (Figures 2 and 3) [44].

To estimate the insulin secretion rate at distinct time points, a more complete mathematical analysis of the peripheral plasma C-peptide concentration is necessary. Most studies have used the deconvolution method and the two-compartment model proposed by Eaton and his colleagues (Figure 4) [31]. According to this model, C-peptide distributes into two compartments: a central compartment consisting of plasma and tissues in rapid equilibration, and a peripheral extravascular compartment. The compartmental distribution of C-peptide is in accordance with the previously mentioned temporal discrepancy between changes in C-peptide secretion rate and in plasma C-peptide concentration.

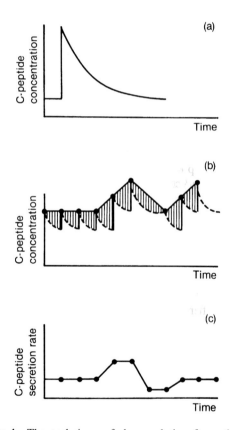

Figure 4 The technique of deconvolution for estimation of insulin secretion rates. (a) The disappearance curve of C-peptide after a bolus dose. (b) The C-peptide concentration curve during the study day. The dotted lines represent the course that C-peptide concentration would have followed at different sampling times if no C-peptide had been added to the system. The dotted lines follow the pattern of the disappearance curve of C-peptide after a bolus dose. The shaded area is then proportional to the amount of C-peptide secreted between two C-peptide measurements. (c) C-peptide secretion rate is derived from the shaded area in (b) (from reference 285, with permission)

The compartmental distribution of C-peptide is responsible for the observations that the same C-peptide secretion rate results in a higher peripheral C-peptide concentration when the overall direction of secretion is falling than when it is increasing [42].

The two-compartment model of C-peptide kinetics has been exploited by Polonsky and colleagues, who have also provided extensive and compelling validation of the Eaton deconvolution model [32–35, 43, 45–48]. This approach necessitates that C-peptide kinetics are studied on a separate day by an infusion of somatostatin to reduce endogenous insulin secretion followed by an intravenous bolus of C-peptide (Figure 4) [31]. The plasma C-peptide is used to construct decay curves, from which the metabolic clearance rate (MCR), the volume of distribution and fractional rate constants are calculated by application of the two-compartment model of C-peptide distribution [31]. The fractional rate constants and the distribution volume of C-peptide for each individual are then applied to the endogenous plasma C-peptide measured during a specific study, and individual insulin secretion rates are derived (Figure 4) [31].

It has been demonstrated that the model allows accurate estimates of insulin secretion rates to be derived even under non-steady state conditions (Figure 2) [33, 43]. Using this model, Polonsky and colleagues have demonstrated that hypersecretion of insulin appears to be the most important factor in the pathogenesis of the peripheral hyperinsulinaemia of obesity when compared with diminished insulin clearance [46]. Reduced hepatic insulin extraction may, however, have a contributory role in the hyperinsulinaemia of obesity [11, 46]. When the amount and temporal pattern of insulin secretion in patients with untreated NIDDM were studied using this model, the basal insulin secretion was slightly higher than, but not significantly different from, that in control subjects [45]. Similarly, the total quantities of insulin secreted during a 24-hour period did not differ significantly in the patients and the controls [45]. As both the basal and the 24-hour glucose concentrations were significantly higher in the patients, these findings indicate that insulin secretion is relatively reduced in NIDDM patients. Furthermore, the increase in insulin in relation to meals was reduced and delayed in these patients [45]. The Eaton concept has also been applied to assessment of oscillatory insulin secretion patterns in patients with NIDDM and in IDDM patients after pancreas transplantation [45, 247]. To use the model it is necessary to assess, in each subject, the disappearance kinetics of C-peptide on a separate day (Figure 4) [32–35, 43, 45–48]. This procedure gives the most accurate determination of B-cell secretory activity in humans, but it is cumbersome, laborious and expensive. Against this background it is of interest that it has been possible to estimate insulin secretion rates accurately using standard parameters for C-peptide kinetics, rather than individually derived parameters, if effects of sex, body surface area and age are taken into account [249]. This circumvents the need for obtaining a decay curve for C-peptide in each individual. The approach with standard parameters is not applicable in patients with altered renal function [249].

Another method ('combined model') for calculating insulin secretion rates has been proposed by Vølund et al [49]. Their method allows determination of prehepatic insulin secretion rates from simultaneous measurements of peripheral insulin and C-peptide concentrations, without separate kinetic studies of either peptide, which reduces the procedure to a single study day. The 'combined model' also provides estimates of insulin extraction by the liver, fractional clearance rate of C-peptide, and kinetics of insulin and C-peptide [44, 49, 250]. The method has been evaluated in dogs, where the appearance of secreted insulin was calculated with acceptable accuracy [49]. The 'combined model' also assumes equimolar rates of secretion of insulin and C-peptide, no C-peptide extraction by the liver, and first-order kinetics of each peptide in plasma, including constancy of the kinetic parameters of the model during the measurement periods. This last assumption is probably reasonable as long as the concentrations of insulin and C-peptide stay within physiological limits. However, because hepatic insulin extraction may vary when metabolism is disrupted, the model requires further validation. Another assumption of the model is that the insulin and C-peptide kinetics can be described by a single-compartment model: this may be an oversimplification. Recently, the 'combined model' has been successfully modified by incorporation of two-compartment C-peptide kinetics [251]. Lastly, the calculated secretion rates do not represent the mass rate of appearance of insulin, but the relative rate of appearance per unit volume of distribution of C-peptide (V_d) in pmol/ml per minute. As there is good correlation between V_d and body weight, the absolute secretion rate may be calculated by multiplying body weight and V_d.

Cobelli and Pacini have also provided data on a minimal model for estimation of the time-course of insulin secretion and hepatic insulin extraction by modelling C-peptide and insulin kinetics [50]. Their model also provides a direct prehepatic measure of B-cell sensitivity to glucose. Because of the non-invasiveness of this procedure, such minimal models may prove useful in the clinical investigation of many pathophysiological states.

C-peptide as a Measure of Hepatic Insulin Extraction

The liver has a dominant role in insulin metabolism [51]. It receives the newly secreted hormone via the portal circulation and extracts insulin during its first passage, before distribution into the systemic vascular compartments, as well as each time it undergoes splanchnic recirculation. Hepatic insulin extraction is not constant and varies according to the physiological conditions [10–12, 32, 48]. However, it is difficult to measure hepatic insulin extraction *in vivo* [52]. Intraportal insulin administration and hepatic vein catheterization are invasive and can be used for investigative purposes under steady state conditions only [52]. These technical difficulties have encouraged the use of the C-peptide/insulin molar ratio as a measure of hepatic insulin extraction *in vivo*. This ratio is determined by the complex relationship between the overall kinetics of the two peptides [12, 32, 42, 43]. The ratio is only valid, therefore, as an indirect measure of hepatic insulin extraction in situations where all other aspects of kinetics of the two peptides are constant. Thus, the molar C-peptide/insulin ratio may be used under steady state conditions in the fasting state as well as after B-cell stimulation, provided that the concentration curves of the peptides are followed until they return to the basal level, and that the areas under the concentration curves are used in the calculation [10, 18, 32].

A more precise method has been introduced by Polonsky and co-workers [32]. After calculating the insulin secretion rates, as described above, they calculated hepatic insulin extraction by employing the relationship between insulin secretion rates and peripheral insulin concentrations [32, 48]. Under basal steady state conditions, hepatic insulin extraction is calculated as the ratio of the insulin secretion rates and the simultaneously measured peripheral insulin concentration. After B-cell stimulation, the total area under the insulin secretion rate curve and the area under the peripheral plasma insulin curve are calculated, and the endogenous insulin clearance is calculated as the ratio between the area under the insulin secretion rate curve and the area under the peripheral insulin concentration curve [32, 48]. The method gives only an integrated expression of insulin extraction following insulin stimulation, and does not provide insight into any time-dependent changes in hepatic insulin extraction. An alternative approach, which can encompass transient changes in hepatic insulin extraction at specific time points, has therefore been proposed [32, 48]. The poststimulatory insulin secretion rates and simultaneously measured peripheral insulin concentrations are expressed as the percentage of their respective mean basal values. Because insulin has a high metabolic clearance rate, a similar increase in the relative insulin secretion rate and the peripheral insulin concentration is taken as evidence that no change in the clearance of endogenous insulin has occurred [32, 48]. A relatively greater increase in the peripheral insulin concentration than in the insulin secretion rate is assumed to indicate a reduction in the clearance of secreted insulin [32, 48]. By this method it has been demonstrated that reduced insulin clearance contributes to hyperinsulinaemia after both oral and intravenous glucose [32]. Oral glucose seems to have a more pronounced effect than intravenous glucose on hepatic insulin extraction. Thus, the hepatic insulin extraction decreases after doses of oral glucose over 25 g, whereas changes in insulin extraction were first observed after 100 g intravenous glucose [32]. Furthermore, during hyperglycaemic clamping a reduction in insulin clearance occurred, both with increasing incremental hyperglycaemia above 120 mg/dl (6.7 mmol/l) and with the time-course of the clamp [48]. It should, however, be emphasized that it is changes in the total MCR of endogenous insulin that are calculated, and that this measure of hepatic insulin extraction is valid only with the assumption that the liver is the site at which a change in the MCR of endogenous insulin occurs.

Urinary C-peptide as a Measure of Insulin Secretion

Evaluation of insulin secretion over a period of time by plasma C-peptide measurements requires multiple blood sampling, which is difficult and time-consuming, and in most clinical situations impractical or possible only over relatively short periods. Urinary C-peptide measurement has been proposed as an indication of endogenous insulin secretion because, in both lean and obese non-diabetic subjects and in most studies of patients with NIDDM, urinary C-peptide has been found to correlate with plasma C-peptide levels [53–65]. Furthermore, in children with IDDM urinary C-peptide excretion may be the parameter of choice, as it can be measured by non-invasive procedures, and can be used to follow endogenous insulin production at frequent intervals [66–69]. Several studies also indicate that urinary C-peptide estimation may be a more sensitive indicator of residual B-cell function in patients with IDDM of long duration [64, 66, 68, 69]. Thus, prevalence of residual B-cell function after 10–15 years of IDDM has been estimated to be 15% from plasma C-peptide estimations, but 84% when evaluated from urinary C-peptide measurements [64].

The relatively high urinary clearance of C-peptide, and the absence of significant hepatic uptake, suggest that urinary C-peptide might be a reliable indicator of the amount of insulin secreted over specific time intervals [40, 42, 246]. C-peptide is freely filtered across the glomerular barrier and thereafter removed by tubular reabsorption and degradation, and urinary excretion [40, 61, 246]. C-peptide probably is also metabolized in the kidney by peritubular uptake [40, 61, 246]. In the basal state 30–50% of the secreted C-peptide is removed in the kidney [40, 61, 246]. In fasting normal subjects the fractional renal extraction of arterial C-peptide is 0.20–0.25 [40]. Renal plasma clearance is about 90 ml/minute [40]. Urinary C-peptide clearance is substantially lower (10–20 ml/min) indicating that renal metabolism is the dominating process for C-peptide elimination [40]. On average, urinary excretion of C-peptide accounts for only 15–20% of the total renal elimination [40], and the urinary excretion of C-peptide is approximately 2–10% of the total amount secreted per day [18, 40, 246]. In fasting IDDM patients the renal uptake of C-peptide was found to be 124 ± 18 pmol/minute at a plasma level of 0.81 nmol/l (2.45 ng/ml) and 155 ± 21 pmol/min at 2.3 nmol/l (6.95 ng/ml) [246]. The proportion of infused C-peptide taken up by the kidney was 39% at 0.81 nmol/l and 9% at 2.3 nmol/l, indicating a limit to the capacity of the kidney for C-peptide uptake. C-peptide fractional renal extraction was 20% and 8%, respectively. Urinary excretion of C-peptide corresponded to 3% and 2% of the amounts infused, and to 8% and 19% of the uptake of C-peptide over the kidney, respectively, on the low and high C-peptide concentrations [246]. Therefore, about 80–90% of that filtered through the glomeruli is reabsorbed and metabolized, so that 10–20% of filtered C-peptide is excreted in the urine [40, 61, 246]. Thus, the renal uptake of C-peptide is 6–7 times greater than its urinary excretion. A wide range of urinary C-peptide values under various conditions have been published by different authors (Table 1).

The use of urinary C-peptide, as an index of B-cell activity, is primarily based on the assumption that the arterial and urinary C-peptide levels are correlated. As C-peptide in urine is derived by glomerular filtration of plasma C-peptide, a correlation between the two variables might be expected to exist. However, correlation alone does not imply that urinary C-peptide reflects insulin secretion accurately. Thus, for C-peptide in urine to be a valid marker of insulin secretion, the clearance of secreted C-peptide must vary within a narrow range between subjects, and should remain constant in the same subject during different physiological conditions and disease states. Horwitz et al have observed that C-peptide urinary clearance remains constant over a wide range of values for creatinine clearance from 6–190 ml/minute [55], while others have demonstrated a reduction in urinary C-peptide secretion in patients with moderately impaired renal function [58, 70]. In accordance with these results, patients with impaired

Table 1 Studies that have evaluated urinary C-peptide excretion

Author	Subjects	Urinary C-peptide clearance (ml/min)	C-peptide excreted/ C-peptide secreted (%)
Meistas [56]	NIDDM	10.5 ± 3.9	4.0 ± 1.5
Kajinuma [70]	Non-diabetic	8.7 ± 3.0	
Kaneto [53]			5.0
Kuzuja [54]			13–20
Meistas [50]	Non-diabetic, lean		2.8 ± 0.7
	Non-diabetic, obese		2.4 ± 1.0
	NIDDM		2.3 ± 1.4
Blix [57]	Non-diabetic, fasting	16.2	
	Non-diabetic, exercise	11.8	
	Non-diabetic, meal	22.3	
Horwitz [55]	Normal	5.1	
Brodows [63]	Normal, basal		3.0 ± 0.75
	Normal, 72 hour fasting		0.38
Garvey [73]	Untreated NIDDM	38.1 ± 7.8	
	Treated NIDDM	26.0 ± 4.6	
	Normal	20.4 ± 1.7	
Tillil [74]	NIDDM	23.8 ± 3.0	11.3 ± 1.6
	Normal	16.5 ± 2.7	8.0 ± 1.7
Zavaroni [61]	Normal	19.2 ± 11.1	13.5 ± 7.8
Henriksen [40]	Normal	12.0	
Sjøberg [246]	Normal		3.4 ± 0.7[a]
	Normal		1.9 ± 0.3[b]

[a] Arterial C-peptide concentration 0.81 nmol/l (2.45 ng/ml).
[b] Arterial C-peptide concentration 2.30 nmol/l (6.95 ng/ml).

renal function displayed elevated plasma C-peptide levels in the fasting state [71, 72]. During long-term fasting, and during and after exercise, a constant urinary clearance rate of C-peptide was observed, whereas a 50% increase was observed after a meal [57, 63]. It is noteworthy, however, that although urinary C-peptide excretion and plasma C-peptide concentration are highly correlated, the magnitude of the relative changes in plasma and urinary C-peptide may differ. Thus, during prolonged fasting a 3-fold decrease in urinary C-peptide against a 1.5-fold fall in plasma C-peptide was observed [63]. After a meal, plasma C-peptide increased by 250%, whereas urinary excretion of C-peptide was 570% above baseline [57].

In patients with NIDDM in poor glycaemic control, urinary C-peptide clearance was 82% higher than in control subjects [73]. Insulin treatment partially reversed this abnormality in urinary C-peptide clearance [73]. When controlling for differences in glomerular filtration rate by expressing urinary C-peptide clearance as a fraction of the creatinine clearance, the increased clearance was explained by a reduction in tubular reabsorption of C-peptide [73]. Unfortunately, no clinical or metabolic markers exist for selecting patients with abnormal urinary clearance of C-peptide. Other authors have demonstrated similar urinary clearance of C-peptide in NIDDM patients and control subjects (Table 1). In children with IDDM, a higher urinary C-peptide clearance has been found

in patients with duration of the disease of less than 1 year, compared with patients with longer disease duration and with normal subjects [66, 67]. These studies demonstrate (Table 1) that changes in urinary clearance of C-peptide may occur during disease states and different physiological conditions, and, therefore, urinary C-peptide measurements should be considered with caution as an index of insulin secretion. This was further emphasized in a study that allowed precise calculation of the amount of C-peptide secreted in individual subjects [74]. By simultaneous measurement of urinary C-peptide excretion, determination of the accuracy of urinary C-peptide values as a measure of endogenous insulin secretion was possible. No significant differences in the various urinary C-peptide measurements were found between the patients with NIDDM and the control subjects, although both C-peptide clearance and fractional C-peptide excretion tended to be higher in the diabetic subjects. The correlations between total urinary C-peptide excretion and total daily C-peptide secretion in the NIDDM patients ($r = 0.58$) and the control subjects ($r = 0.62$) were rather weak. The fraction of secreted C-peptide that was excreted in the urine varied between 1% and 28%, both in NIDDM subjects and in normal subjects. Meistas et al also found a 10-fold range in fractional C-peptide excretion during a 24-hour period in patients with NIDDM [60]. The coefficient of variation of the fractional 24-hour urinary C-peptide excretion in both control and diabetic subjects, and that of urinary C-peptide clearance, is approximately 30% [54, 55, 57, 59–62, 65, 74].

The practical implications of these findings are that when the individual fractional urinary C-peptide clearance rate is not known, comparison of insulin secretion rates, based purely on urinary C-peptide excretion, is subject to considerable error, and may be of limited value as a quantitative marker of insulin secretion. The changes in urinary C-peptide may not necessarily reflect changes in B-cell function, but may merely be attributable to variability in renal handling of C-peptide. One advantage of urinary C-peptide determinations may be the detection of residual B-cell function in IDDM when the plasma C-peptide is below the detection limit of the plasma assay [64, 66, 68, 69].

Clinical Application of C-peptide

Insulin Secretion in IDDM Patients

C-peptide has been the most important research tool in the study of the natural course of B-cell destruction in IDDM patients and of therapeutic interventions to arrest or delay this process [14, 15, 75–148]. Most IDDM patients have residual B-cell function at the onset of their disease and all continue to secrete insulin during the first 2 years of the disease (Figures 5 and 6) [75–94, 117–142]. Thereafter, the prevalence of residual B-cell function declines to about 10–15% after approximately 5 years and remains at this level in patients with up to 40 years' disease duration (Figure 6) [14, 15, 77–80, 87, 90, 91, 93]. Age at onset is the most important variable in predicting the duration and magnitude of residual B-cell function [75–93]. Thus, B-cell survival is shorter the younger the subjects are at disease onset [75–93]. During the first 2 years after diagnosis, a faster reduction in residual B-cell function has been demonstrated in patients remaining islet cell antibody-positive [78, 79, 82, 83, 94, 252] and in males as opposed to females [79, 81]. In other studies, no difference in B-cell function was observed between patients persistently positive and those negative for islet cell antibodies several years after diagnosis [14, 91]. Neither the presence of insulin autoantibodies at the time of onset, nor the subsequent formation of antibodies after start of insulin therapy, were correlated to B-cell function [78, 79, 92, 93, 98]. No association has been demonstrated between HLA antigens and B-cell function, except that a more rapid loss of B-cell function has been observed in the first months after remission in patients who lacked HLA-DR3 and -DR4 [89, 93, 253].

After initiation of insulin therapy and subsequent metabolic stabilization, most diabetic subjects experience an improvement in B-cell function (Figure 5)

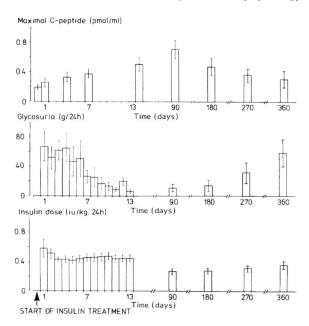

Figure 5 Average maximal C-peptide concentrations obtained in 12 IDDM patients during test meal (top panel), average glycosuria (middle panel), and average daily dose of insulin during the first year of conventional insulin treatment (bottom panel). Most IDDM patients have B-cell function at onset corresponding to about 20% of the maximal values seen in normal subjects. The maximal B-cell function is observed 1–6 months after start of insulin therapy. Thereafter, B-cell function declines. The best degree of glycaemic control is observed in periods with maximal B-cell function, despite treatment with only a minimal daily dose of insulin (from reference 286)

[75–96, 117–142]. On average, B-cell function doubles in magnitude after 7–14 days of conventional insulin treatment (Figure 5) [76,119,122]. In most patients, maximal B-cell function is observed after 1–6 months of insulin treatment (Figure 5); thereafter, B-cell function declines (Figure 5) [75–96, 117–142]. The patients with the highest C-peptide concentrations at onset will display the best degree of B-cell function during the first 1–2 years after diagnosis [75–96]. The residual B-cell function is highly correlated to the degree of remission [75–95, 117–142]. After remission, the patients with the greatest increase in insulin dose also have the most pronounced decrease in B-cell function (Figure 5) [75–95, 117–142]. Another factor of importance in relation to remission is insulin resistance [96]. Thus, clinical remission is a result of both an improvement in endogenous insulin secretion and an enhancement in insulin sensitivity [96]. During the remission period, 10–20% of patients can be taken off insulin, and about 10% of these patients can be managed without insulin at the end of the first year of disease [75, 117–142].

In IDDM patients beyond the remission period, when the B-cell function in most patients is absent or

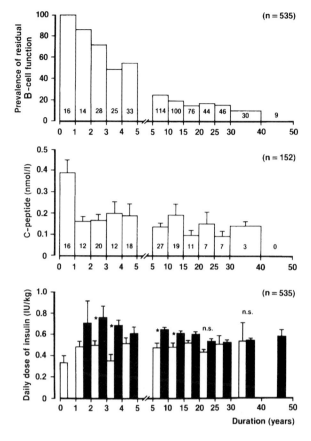

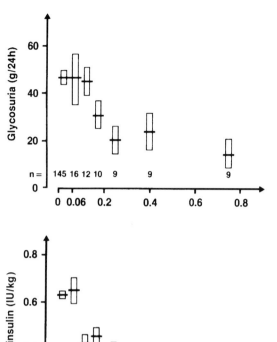

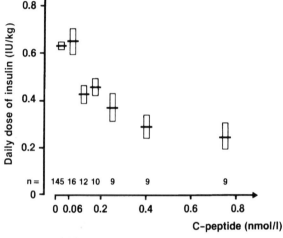

Figure 6 Prevalence of residual B-cell function in 535 IDDM patients with up to 50 years' duration of disease (upper panel). Middle panel: average maximal C-peptide concentration after 1 mg of glucagon given intravenously in the 152 patients with residual B-cell function (mean value in normal subjects 1.3 nmol/l, 3.92 ng/ml). Daily dose of insulin in patients with (open columns) or without (solid columns) B-cell function (bottom panel). Nearly 100% of IDDM patients have residual B-cell function for the first 2 years after diagnosis. Thereafter, the prevalence of residual B-cell function declines to about 10–15% after 5 years and remains at this level in patients with up to 40 years' duration of disease. The magnitude of residual B-cell function (maximal C-peptide concentration) declines from a mean of 0.39 nmol/l (1.18 ng/ml) in patients who have had diabetes for less than 1 year to about 0.15 nmol/l (0.45 ng/ml) in patients with more than 1 year of diabetes duration. *indicates significant difference in daily dose of insulin between the two groups; n.s., not significant (from reference 286)

Figure 7 Correlation between maximal C-peptide concentration (after intravenous administration of 1 mg of glucagon) and glycosuria (g per 24 hours) in 210 IDDM patients (upper panel), and between maximal C-peptide concentration and daily dose of insulin (lower panel); 145 patients were without B-cell function. Patients with residual B-cell function need a smaller daily dose of insulin than those without B-cell function, to obtain the same degree of glycaemic control (from reference 286)

minimal, the effect on metabolic control is of minor importance (Figure 6) [97–108]. In most studies no major difference in the degree of metabolic control has been demonstrated between patients with or without B-cell function [97–108]. In patients with B-cell function, an inverse correlation has been shown between variables of metabolic control and B-cell function, but it is evident that the B-cell function must be considerable before it has any effect on glycaemic control (Figure 7) [107]. Most patients with residual B-cell function need a smaller daily dose of insulin

than those without B-cell function, to obtain the same degree of control, and often only one daily dose of insulin is needed to obtain acceptable metabolic control in patients with B-cell function (Figures 6 and 7) [90, 107]. This indicates that minimal B-cell function is not without effect on metabolic control, but that the influence of low endogenous insulin secretion can be overridden by the quality of insulin treatment and other factors of importance for glucose regulation. Moreover, the tendency to severe ketoacidosis is reduced in patients with residual B-cell function [109, 110]. IDDM patients with B-cell function also display a relatively more normal glucagon response during hypoglycaemia than do patients without B-cell function [104, 105, 108, 111]. The glucagon response to a mixed meal is similar in patients with and without B cell function [112].

In most studies it has not been possible to observe any effect of preserved B-cell function on the development of late diabetic complications [87, 113–116]. On the other hand, remaining B-cell function has been found to protect the blood–retinal barrier function more effectively than good metabolic control [254, 255]. A significant inverse relationship between residual B-cell function (C-peptide) and degree of retinopathy has been observed [254, 255].

Different therapeutic approaches to preserve B-cell function, and thereby to prolong the temporary remission period, have been attempted, including strict metabolic control and immunosuppressive therapy. In two studies using intensive insulin treatment by an external artificial pancreas for up to 14 days after diagnosis, improved B-cell function and also better metabolic control were observed during the subsequent year when compared with the conventionally treated group [117, 118]. In four other randomized prospective studies in which the experimental group was treated with multiple daily injections of insulin or insulin pumps (subcutaneous continuous insulin infusion) for up to 2 years after diagnosis, the experimental group displayed a more prompt improvement in B-cell function, but the effect was transient [119–122]. No difference could be demonstrated in residual B-cell function after 3 months and throughout the follow-up period between the conventionally and experimentally treated groups [119–122]. In patients past the initial remission period, strict metabolic control for 1 week can also cause a functional improvement in B-cell function [123, 124]. However, the improvement has been reported to disappear a few weeks after strict metabolic control has ended [123, 124]. These results indicate that B-cell function in IDDM patients is related to the degree of glycaemic control, but short periods of strict control do not appear to influence the long-term outcome of B-cell function, although they promote maximal function of the B cells on a temporary basis.

The hypothesis that autoimmune phenomena are involved in the pathogenesis of IDDM has encouraged the use of immunosuppressive therapy to stop B-cell destruction. Investigations with prednisolone [125, 126], plasmapheresis [127], γ-globulin [128], methisoprinol [129], interferon [130], antithymocyte globulin and prednisone [131], and azathioprine alone [132, 133] or in combination with prednisone [134], have shown little or no long-term effect on B-cell function, except for those regimens including corticosteroids [125, 126, 134].

With the introduction of the more powerful immunosuppressant cyclosporin A, interest in this mode of treatment in IDDM heightened [135–142]. Cyclosporin therapy induces high rates of remission, with 50–55% of patients not requiring insulin, and with 20–40% still off insulin after 1 year [135–142]. The remission is associated with a greater improvement in and maintenance of B-cell function in the cyclosporin groups [135–142]; the sooner immunosuppression is started the better the results [135–142]. After withdrawal of cyclosporin, B-cell function declines, with relapse of diabetes [135–142]. The results of short-term cyclosporin trials are interesting and promising, but do not justify long-term treatment with cyclosporin because of the side-effects of the drug [135–142]. Another major problem is that the intervention is usually started too late, when it is generally believed that about 90% of the B cells have been lost, and when the remaining 10% are insufficient to maintain normal metabolism [143].

Experiments *in vitro* and *in vivo* in animals have demonstrated that nicotinamide enhances the regeneration of B cells, and retards or arrests diabetes induced by streptozotocin or immune processes, e.g. diabetes in non-obese diabetic (NOD) mice [144–166]. Nicotinamide has been used in several studies in newly diagnosed IDDM and in prediabetes. The results have been heterogeneous, with some studies showing a marginal beneficial effect of nicotinamide on B-cell function and others showing no effect [47, 48, 256–261].

Use of C-peptide in the Classification and Prediction of Insulin Requirement in Diabetic Patients

It is important, both for scientific and for therapeutic purposes, to monitor B-cell function in diabetic patients [14, 15, 149, 150]. The classification of newly diagnosed patients with diabetes mellitus is normally without problems in young patients with ketoacidosis [14, 15, 83, 150–157]. There are, however, patients with less straightforward classification, usually middle-aged or elderly patients [87, 150–157]. Even when these patients present with hyperglycaemia and ketoacidosis, some can be managed without insulin after treatment of the initial metabolic decompensation [83, 150–158]. Other patients may progress toward insulin dependency, but cannot initially be distinguished from other NIDDM patients [150–162]. A group of NIDDM patients may need insulin to control symptomatic hyperglycaemia. In other patients starting insulin treatment during periods with intercurrent disease, insulin is often continued unnecessarily. This heterogeneity, and the fact that many patients are unable to comply with dietary recommendations, make it difficult to classify patients according to clinical criteria, especially in the outpatient clinic [150–162]. Determination of islet cell antibodies (ICA) may be of some help [159–161];

patients positive for ICA will become insulin dependent [159–161].

Measurement of C-peptide after B-cell stimulation appears to be a useful aid for decisions regarding diabetes classification and clinical management [83, 149, 150, 158, 163–167]. The glucagon test has become the most widely used B-cell test [168]; it is rapid, simple, convenient, with high reproducibility, and the results are easy to interpret [55, 168, 169, 170]. The predictive value, as to how the B cells respond during everyday life, is high [168]. However, the outcome of the glucagon test is dependent on the prevailing blood glucose concentration [169, 170]. At fasting blood glucose concentrations greater than 7 mmol/l (125 mg/dl), maximal plasma C-peptide concentration after intravenous glucagon correlates with the maximum concentration during a mixed meal, whereas the C-peptide response at lower blood glucose values is underestimated [169, 170]. The test has been simplified by the demonstration that little information is lost by using only the fasting and the 6-minute C-peptide concentrations after intravenous injection of glucagon [168].

At the time of diagnosis it is possible to classify diabetic patients into insulin-requiring or non-insulin-requiring [167]. All patients with a plasma C-peptide level over 0.6 nmol/l (1.8 ng/ml) 6 minutes after 1 mg of intravenous glucagon were not insulin-requiring after 1 year of diabetes [167]. All insulin-requiring patients and 7% of the non-insulin-requiring patients had C-peptide values below 0.6 nmol/l [167]. In 268 patients up to 70 years of age, with IDDM or NIDDM of varying duration (0–30 years), a C-peptide value of 0.6 nmol/l after intravenous glucagon had a high degree of accuracy in categorizing patients as insulin-requiring or non-insulin-requiring (Figure 8) [150]. Several other studies have demonstrated the value of C-peptide measurements in the classification of patients with diabetes mellitus [83, 158, 163–167]. The test is especially useful in the outpatient clinic to estimate the potential success of various treatments: a low C-peptide value in an insulin-treated patient suggests that the patient is truly insulin-requiring; a high C-peptide level suggests the possibility of discontinuing insulin treatment without risk.

Fasting C-peptide concentration is not reliable for classification of patients as being without B-cell function. Some patients will display B-cell function after stimulation with a meal-test or a glucagon test [169].

PROINSULIN

Measurement of Proinsulin

As proinsulin contains the sequence of both insulin and C-peptide and is present in much lower concentrations than either of these, cross-reactivity becomes a major problem in the immunoassay for proinsulin. This problem has been solved by separation of proinsulin from the other components by gel filtration, taking advantage of differences in molecular weight and shape [171–173], with subsequent insulin radioimmunoassay on each elution fraction. The method is fairly laborious. The formerly used 'insulin-specific protease' method [174] has been shown to be unreliable, because degradation of insulin was incomplete and some proinsulin could also be degraded [173, 175]. Now that large quantities of biosynthetic human proinsulin have become available [176], different kinds of immunoassays [177–184, 262–266] have replaced such cumbersome methods. The most sensitive assays can now detect a minimum proinsulin immunoreactive material (PIM) concentration in serum from fasting normal subjects [262, 264–266]. The assays use mainly monoclonal antibodies and some also use enzyme amplification. However, it is a problem that most proinsulin immunoassays measure both intact proinsulin and the major conversion intermediates (Figure 1) equally well. No assay has proven 100% specific for intact proinsulin or one of the conversion intermediates; the cross-reactivities are summarized

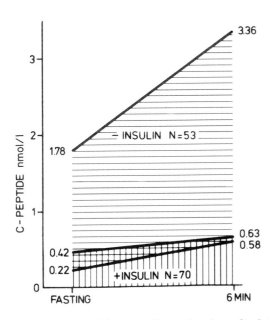

Figure 8 Fasting and 6-minute C-peptide values after intravenous administration of 1 mg of glucagon grouped according to therapy after evaluation: diet or diet and oral antidiabetic therapy (horizontal shading) and insulin (vertical shading). Only 3 patients were found to have 6-minute C-peptide values in the overlap range (0.58–0.63 nmol/l). A C-peptide value of 0.6 nmol/l after intravenous administration of glucagon had a high degree of accuracy in classifying the patients into insulin-requiring and non-insulin-requiring groups (from reference 150, with permission)

Table 2 Proinsulin immunoreactive material (PIM) assays, showing their sensitivity and cross-reactivity[a] with the other PIM products

Author	Reference	Antibodies[b]	Year	Sensitivity (pmol/l)	PI (%)	Spl(65–66) (%)	Des (64,65) (%)	Spl (32–33) (%)	Des (31,32) (%)
Cohen et al	186	poly 18D	1986	Extraction	100	80–100	80–100	2–3	0.5
		poly 11E			100	10		38	
Deacon/Conlon	179	poly	1985	4	100		100		0.1
Ward et al	181	poly	1986	3	100	100	100	100	100
Cohen et al	178	poly	1985	Extraction	100	60–80		10–33	
Hampton et al	184	poly	1988	4	100				
Naylor et al	182	poly	1987	9	100				
Heding	177	poly	1977	2	100				
Yoshioka et al	183	poly	1988	2	100	46	51	2	0.7
Gray et al	187	mono 3B1/2E6	1987	1	100	55	55	0	0
Hartling et al	180	poly GP102 M1227	1986 1992	1.2	100	91	94	57	73
Sobey et al	189	mono 14B/A6	1989	0.8	6	100	100	0	0
		3B1/PEP001		2.5	84	60		100	100
		3B1/A6		1.8	100	66		0	
Alpha et al	265	3B1/A6	1992	0.8	100			2.3	
Dhahir et al	262	PEP001/	1992	0.1	100	68		200	
Bowsher et al	263	poly IA	1992	3.5	100	3	<1	46	44
Kjems et al	264	PEP001/ HUI001	1993	0.25	100	78	99	74	65
Cook & Self	266	poly/PEP001	1993	0.017	100				

[a]The cross-reactivity is given for major conversion intermediates where information is available.

[b]Antibodies are either polyclonal (poly) or monoclonal (mono and code).

Table 3 Fasting values of blood glucose, insulin, C-peptide, proinsulin immunoreactive material (PIM) and ratio of PIM to insulin

Disease/condition	Fasting values				
	BG	I	C-P	PIM	PIM:I
B-cell hyperactivity					
IDDM at onset	++	−−	−−	+	++
NIDDM	+	+	+	++	+
IGT	(+)	≈	≈	+	+
Newborn	≈	−	−	+	++
Thyrotoxicosis	≈	≈	≈	+	+
Obesity	≈	+	+	+	≈
Kinetic					
Cirrhosis	≈	+	(+)	+	≈
Renal failure	≈	+	++	+++	++
Tumour					
Insulinoma	−	+	+	++	+
Mutants					
Familial hyperproinsulinaemia	−	(+)	(+)	++	++
	(+)	+	+	++	++
Genetic					
Siblings of DM	≈	≈	0	++	++
Identical twins	≈	≈	≈	+	+

BG, blood glucose; I, insulin; C-P, C-peptide; PIM, proinsulin immunoreactive material; IGT, impaired glucose tolerance; DM, diabetes mellitus. +, ++, increased; ≈, no change; −, −−, decreased; 0, no measurement.

in Table 2. Therefore, unless specified, a proinsulin assay measures proinsulin-like material or proinsulin immunoreactive material. The matter is important because at least some of the intermediates can be found in peripheral blood [185–187], and clinically relevant differences in the PIM composition between NIDDM patients and healthy controls have been reported [188].

Still the only system that separates all the components is the chromatographic method [190, 236], but this is cumbersome and large-scale studies are impossible, as 10–50 ml of serum are required. Reaven et al [267] using an HPLC system could demonstrate all four conversion products along with intact proinsulin in some normal subjects. In NIDDM patients and subjects with impaired glucose tolerance only intact proinsulin and the *des*-forms were found, of which *des* (31, 32)-proinsulin seemed the most important. This is consistent with studies based upon the 'specific' immunochemical assays [189], where *des* (31,32)-proinsulin is the major conversion product [188, 268], remembering that both *des* (31,32)- and split (32–33)-proinsulin are measured together. The major conversion intermediates have different kinetics and biological potencies [191]; one cannot, therefore, quantitate precisely the biological potency or the secretion pattern of PIM in a patient without knowing the composition of the PIM. In Table 3 only the PIM levels in the fasting state are presented. In this steady state condition it can be relevant to calculate the ratio of PIM to insulin. In dynamic situations the secretion pattern of the B cells cannot be evaluated because neither the kinetics of the proinsulin conversion intermediates nor the composition of the PIM are known. The serum concentrations of insulin, C-peptide and PIM after intravenous bolus injection of glucose (0.5 g/kg body weight) given over 3 minutes are shown in Figure 9. Even after 3 hours, the PIM level is still above the starting value.

Kinetics and Metabolism of Proinsulin

Studies in which pharmacological amounts of proinsulin were infused have indicated that the fractional hepatic extraction of proinsulin is less than 5% under steady state concentrations of proinsulin [192, 193]. The concentrations attained (1.4–40 nmol/l) were 100–1000 times greater than the normal fasting level. Proinsulin seems mainly to be cleared by the kidney [193, 194], which is consistent with the finding of very marked increases in proinsulin levels in chronic renal failure [71, 195]. Although proinsulin and the conversion intermediates *in vitro* can be shown to bind to the insulin receptor and undergo internalization [191, 196–198], it is not known whether the degradation takes place via a receptor-binding mechanism. The metabolic clearance

rate (MCR) calculated from constant infusion studies or single bolus injections varied from 1.6 ml/kg per minute to 3.5 ml/kg per minute [192, 199–202]. The differences in the results obtained are not related to dosages or plasma concentration achieved, but are most likely to be due to methodological problems. One factor could be differences in specificity of the assays used; another, that the evaluation methods differ (incompatible models). Conversion of proinsulin after intravenous administration is of little significance as it has been demonstrated that conversion intermediates comprised less than 1% of proinsulin immunoreactivity after intravenous infusion of supraphysiological amounts of proinsulin [190]. In contrast, intermediates comprised up to 11% of proinsulin immunoreactivity after subcutaneous administration of proinsulin. Further conversion to significant amounts of circulating insulin could not be demonstrated for either route of administration [190]. Recently 64/65 split proinsulin (*des* + split) was found to comprise 13% of proinsulin immunoreactivity [284] after subcutaneous administration of intact proinsulin. This is much higher than expected since the ratio of *des* (32,33) to *des* (64,65) was 3:1 in the earlier study by Given et al [190]. Unfortunately *des* (32,33)-proinsulin was not measured in this study [284].

As previously mentioned, proinsulin binds to the same receptor as insulin, and insulin and proinsulin can mutually displace their radiolabelled ligands from the receptor, but the concentration of proinsulin needed to compete is 10 times higher than that of insulin [196]. The lower receptor affinity has been demonstrated in human monocytes [203], in IM-9 lymphocytes and in purified rat liver membranes [191]. The binding properties correspond well with the biological activity of proinsulin, which is 8–12% of that of insulin, both in normal subjects and in IDDM patients [199, 200]. The dose needed to maintain normal fasting blood glucose in IDDM was 14 times that of insulin, resulting in concentrations more than 100 times higher than fasting proinsulin levels in normal subjects [200]. Normal concentrations of proinsulin, could not protect against the development of ketoacidosis in IDDM [200]. As proinsulin and insulin-like growth factor I (IGF-I) are similar in both primary and tertiary structure, it has been proposed that proinsulin could bind to the IGF-I receptor. This seems, however, not to be the case, as Gruppuso et al [204], using placental membrane IGF-I receptors, found that insulin was approximately 0.5% as potent as IGF-I and proinsulin only 2% as potent as insulin. The conversion intermediates had potencies between those of insulin and proinsulin. Burguera et al [269] used IGF-I receptors purified from liver, muscle, and adipose tissue and found binding of

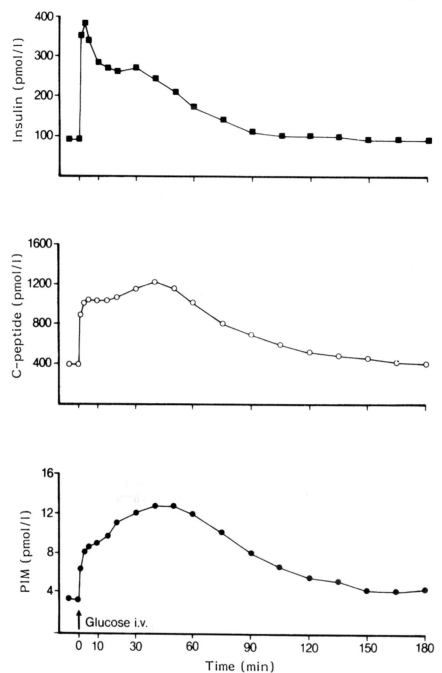

Figure 9   Dynamic patterns of serum insulin (squares), C-peptide (open circles) and proinsulin immunoreactive material (PIM) (solid circles) concentrations in 9 healthy subjects after glucose (0.5 g/kg body weight) had been administered intravenously over the course of 3 minutes. Insulin concentration falls back to basal values in 60–90 minutes and C-peptide concentration in 150–180 minutes, whereas the PIM concentration at 180 minutes is still above the initial fasting value

human proinsulin virtually non-existent. Thus, proinsulin effects in humans are not mediated via the IGF-I receptor.

By combining proinsulin and insulin it was shown that they had additive and not synergistic effects on glucose disposal in the normal human [205]. Pretreatment with proinsulin did not enhance insulin and proinsulin action on glucose disposal [206]. In all these studies the proinsulin dose (concentration) has been extremely high. The possibility can therefore not be ruled out that proinsulin in physiological or slightly elevated concentrations could have a synergistic effect on hepatic glucose production or glucose disposal. In this context is should be borne in mind that the proinsulin intermediates have higher receptor binding affinities and biological potencies than proinsulin itself [198].

Proinsulin Secretion in Humans

Elevated proinsulin levels have been found in various conditions and diseases. Table 3 lists the most frequently described conditions in which proinsulin immunoreactive material (PIM) is increased. Formerly, all findings of elevated PIM except in tumours and renal failure were explained by an increased B-cell drive. This can either be caused by a direct glucose stimulus, or by non-specific increased demands. Increased B-cell stimulation could then result in release of immature granules with a higher PIM to insulin ratio. This hypothesis is questionable.

In hyperglycaemia, as in patients with newly diagnosed IDDM, the increased PIM is accompanied by a low or undetectable insulin concentration [206, 207]. Patients with NIDDM have elevated fasting PIM concentrations or PIM:insulin (PIM:C-peptide) ratios [183, 188, 208–210, 272, 273]. Ward et al [210] showed that when the insulin demand was increased as a result of dexamethasone treatment, the proinsulin response to arginine was exaggerated in patients with NIDDM, as well as in normal subjects. However, it should be noted that corticosteroids may themselves have an inhibitory effect on insulin secretion [274, 275]. Nicotinic acid inducing insulin resistance did not result in a changed PIM:insulin ratio in baboons [276]. However, Kahn et al [276] showed that, when streptozotocin was administered in a dose producing subclinical (no hyperglycaemia) impairment of B-cell function, a significant increase in both the basal and the stimulated (arginine) PIM:insulin ratio was observed. When nicotinic acid was subsequently introduced, hyperglycaemia developed but the PIM:insulin ratio tended to decrease. In dogs where 60% of the pancreas was removed the PIM:insulin ratio was unchanged and diabetes did not develop [277]. Therefore, increased demand on the B cells cannot be solely responsible for PIM elevation. This is also emphasized by the fact that the PIM:insulin ratio is unchanged in obese subjects. They secrete more insulin as well as PIM [218, 219, 273]. As suggested by Porte and Kahn [277] the increased PIM in NIDDM patients seems therefore to be a feature of B-cell dysfunction. Further supporting this was the finding of a normal to low PIM:insulin ratio in first-degree relatives of NIDDM patients, whereas the diabetic patients had high PIM and high PIM:insulin ratios [278]. Glaser et al [209] showed that, following near-normalization of blood glucose (reducing insulin demand) in NIDDM subjects, proinsulin levels declined but did not return to normal. Not only relatives with normal glucose tolerance but also those with impaired glucose tolerance seem to have normal fasting PIM levels and high insulin levels [213, 278]; but in other studies elevated PIM concentrations have been found in patients with impaired glucose tolerance [211, 212, 279].

The elevated PIM:C-peptide ratio in the newborn offspring of normal subjects, compared with adults [214, 270] could be caused by release of immature granules in the perinatal period. Newborn children of IDDM mothers, compared with those of normal mothers [214], have the same ratio but at a higher level of hormones. In patients with hyperthyroidism, proinsulin is elevated both absolutely and relatively to insulin and C-peptide. Insulin and C-peptide have been found to be unchanged [215, 216] or slightly elevated [217].

The mechanism leading to elevated insulin immunoreactive material found in liver cirrhosis is not clear. Both normal proinsulin levels accompanied by insulin and C-peptide elevation [220], and markedly elevated proinsulin concentrations [221], explaining most of the increased insulin immunoreactivity, have been demonstrated. These discrepancies probably are explicable in terms of differences in the selection of patients, and thereby differences in the kinetics of PIM, together with differences in the methods applied. The elevated C-peptide and PIM levels in renal failure [71, 195] are an effect of diminished clearance of these.

A unique situation is found in patients with insulinoma [186, 219, 222]. In this condition the blood glucose value is low or normal; insulin and C-peptide levels are often high but can be normal; in contrast, PIM levels have always been found to be increased. Whether the secreted PIM mainly comprises intact proinsulin or intermediates is not known. The reason that the adenoma preferentially secretes PIM instead of insulin could be related to maturation of the adenoma cells.

In families with inherited hyperproinsulinaemia, first described by Gabbay et al [223], blood glucose levels have been found to be low, normal or slightly elevated. The defect, later also found in other families (at the moment five different pedigrees) [271], was the result of a point mutation, substituting arginine with histidine at amino acid position 65, leading to incomplete conversion. The AC-intermediate (C-peptide attached to the insulin A-chain) accounted for more than 80% of the immunoreactive insulin [224–226]. In another kindred with familial hyperproinsulinaemia, circulating PIM accounted for 60% of immunoreactive insulin and was shown to be intact proinsulin [227]. Subsequently, it was demonstrated that the defect was in the insulin gene itself [228] and that histidine at B10 had been substituted by aspartic acid [229]. This change interferes with the packaging of proinsulin into granules, so that proinsulin escapes conversion.

In a study of healthy siblings of IDDM patients [230], all had normal fasting blood glucose and insulin concentrations, but 30% had an increased fasting PIM concentration. Similar results have been found in identical twins with IDDM, discordant for more than 11 years [231]. In these cases the increased ratio of PIM to insulin cannot be explained by a hyperreactivity of the B cell. The meaning of the elevated PIM concentrations in healthy relatives of IDDM patients is still a matter of speculation. It could reflect B-cell dysfunction, indicating an increased risk of developing diabetes. This is, however, probably not the case as the siblings and the twins [230, 231] were all discordant for several years and therefore probably would not develop diabetes. In fact, the three siblings who later presented with diabetes had proinsulin concentrations in the normal range. Also arguing against this hypothesis is the finding that there were no differences in proinsulin levels between HLA-identical, HLA-haploidentical and HLA-non-identical subjects [230]. Other immunological markers also seem to bear no relation to the elevated proinsulin concentration in relatives of IDDM patients [232]. The finding could represent a family trait, mirroring a B cell more vulnerable to destruction, or it could reflect previous B-cell damage that has not led to diabetes. In a study by Lindgren et al [270] of cord blood from neonate siblings of type 1 diabetic children (but with normal mothers), proinsulin levels were comparable to levels in neonates unrelated to type 1 diabetic patients. Both groups had higher PIM concentrations than adults, confirming previous studies [214]. The finding of no difference among the neonates at birth indicates that the difference shown in older first-degree relatives occurs later in life and that an exogenous event is needed. For further clarification, longitudinal studies are awaited. That proinsulin or PIM values reflect altered B-cell function has been supported by the finding of higher concentrations in IDDM patients responding to cyclosporin induction of remission [207], even though differences in kinetics or composition cannot be excluded as an explanation. Nagi et al [280] reported a significant correlation between *des* (31,32)-proinsulin and total cholesterol, triglyceride, plasminogen activator inhibitor-1 (PAI-1), and diastolic blood pressure in 51 NIDDM patients. HDL-cholesterol correlated negatively. In an intervention study with insulin, Jain et al [281] showed a fall in PAI-1, but no change in other cardiovascular risk factors. The fall could be attributed to the reduction in proinsulin molecules. These findings suggest an association between PIM and increased cardiovascular risk, but this remains a matter for debate. Drexel et al [282], for instance, found a favourable effect of proinsulin on lipid status in NIDDM patients compared with NPH insulin.

An interesting observation was made by Hales et al [283] studying 468 men born in 1920–30, whose birthweight and weight at 1 year were known. They found a relationship between reduced growth in early life and impaired glucose tolerance and NIDDM. Reduced early growth was also related to raised split (32–33)-proinsulin concentrations and systolic blood pressure, so could be linked with syndrome X, hypertension, diabetes mellitus and hyperlipidaemia.

Clinical Application of Proinsulin

Measurements of plasma proinsulin concentrations are clinically relevant in the evaluation of patients with hypoglycaemia. In patients with insulinomas, the plasma proinsulin concentration is elevated irrespective of the prevailing blood glucose concentration, whereas the concentrations of insulin and C-peptide may be within the normal range or slightly elevated [186, 219, 222]. In a patient presenting with fasting hypoglycaemia, the initial test is measurement of plasma insulin, proinsulin and C-peptide, as well as blood glucose concentrations. Increased concentrations of the three peptides, especially of proinsulin, is highly indicative of an insulinoma. The final diagnosis is established on the basis of lack of suppression of insulin, C-peptide and proinsulin during prolonged fasting, insulin-induced hypoglycaemia or euglycaemic hyperinsulinaemic clamp [186, 219, 233]. Factitious hypoglycaemia caused by surreptitious injection of insulin will be detected with this diagnostic strategy: such patients will, like insulinoma patients, have fasting hypoglycaemia with elevated insulin concentrations, but their C-peptide and proinsulin concentrations will be low, in contrast to those of the insulinoma patient [234].

It is still not clear whether proinsulin will ultimately have a role in predicting the risk of developing diabetes, the prognosis, or the chance to achieve insulin-free remission during immunosuppressive therapy.

Proinsulin has been suggested as a therapeutic agent, but it has been withdrawn from the market because of an unexpected increased incidence of coronary heart disease in diabetic patients treated with human proinsulin. In the clinical use of proinsulin, the serum concentration of proinsulin was 100–150 times higher than physiological concentrations, which might be the explanation for the accelerated macrovascular disease. The clinical use of proinsulin and the suspension of clinical trials in February 1988, has been thoroughly evaluated in a review by Galloway et al [235], and in spite of thorough investigations in major prospective clinical trials, it has not been proved that proinsulin itself was the causative agent.

REFERENCES

1. Steiner DF, Oyer PE. The biosynthesis of insulin and a probable precursor of insulin by a human islet cell adenoma. Proc Natl Acad Sci USA 1967; 57: 473–80.

2. Steiner DF, Cunningham D, Spigelman L, Aten B. Insulin biosynthesis: evidence for a precursor. Science 1967; 157: 697–700.

3. Robbins DC, Tager HS, Rubenstein AH. Biological and clinical importance of proinsulin. New Engl J Med 1984; 310: 1165–75.

4. Sørensen RI, Steffes MW, Lindall AW. Subcellular localization of proinsulin to insulin conversion in isolated rat islets. Endocrinology 1970; 86: 88–96.

5. Hutton JC. The insulin secretory granule. Diabetologia 1989; 32: 271–81.

6. Horwitz DL, Starr JI, Mako ME, Blackard WG, Rubenstein AH. Proinsulin, insulin and C-peptide concentrations in human portal and peripheral blood. J Clin Invest 1975; 55: 1278–83.

7. Gutman RA, Lazarus NR, Recant L. Electrophoretic characterization of circulating human proinsulin and insulin. Diabetologia 1972; 8: 136–40.

8. Rubinstein AH, Clark JL, Melani F, Steiner DF. Secretion of proinsulin, C-peptide by pancreatic beta-cells and its circulation in blood. Nature 1969; 209: 697–9.

9. Rubinstein AH, Pottienger LA, Mako M, Getz CS, Steiner DF. The metabolism of proinsulin and insulin by the liver. J Clin Invest 1972; 51: 912–21.

10. Madsbad S, Kehlet H, Hilsted J, Tronier B. Discrepancy between plasma C-peptide and insulin response to oral and intravenous glucose. Diabetes 1983; 32: 436–8.

11. Faber OK, Christensen K, Kehlet H, Madsbad S, Binder C. Decreased insulin removal contributes to hyperinsulinemia in obesity. J Clin Endocrinol Metab 1981; 53: 618–21.

12. Bonora E, Zavaroni I, Coscilli C, Buttuvini V. Decreased hepatic insulin extraction in subjects with mild glucose intolerance. Metabolism 1983; 32: 438–46.

13. Scheen AJ, Lefèbvre PJ, Luyckx AS. Glipizide increases plasma insulin but not C-peptide level after a standardized breakfast in Type 2 diabetic patients. Eur J Clin Pharmacol 1984; 26: 471–4.

14. Madsbad S. Prevalence of residual beta-cell function and its metabolic consequences in Type 1 (insulin-dependent) diabetics. Diabetologia 1983; 24: 141–7.

15. Madsbad S. Factors of importance for residual beta-cell function in type 1 diabetics. A review. Acta Med Scand 1983; 671: 61–7.

16. Bonser AM, Garcia-Webb P. C-peptide measurement and its clinical usefulness: a review. Ann Clin Biochem 1981; 18: 200–6.

17. Polonsky KS, Rubinstein AH. Current approaches to measurement of insulin secretion. Diabetes Metab Rev 1986; 2: 315–29.

18. Polonsky KS, Rubinstein AH. C-peptide as a measure of the secretion and hepatic extraction of insulin. Pitfalls and limitations. Diabetes 1984; 33: 486–94.

19. Malmquist J, Birgerstam G. Assays of pancreatic B-cell secretory products: utility in investigative and clinical diabetology. Scand J Lab Invest 1986; 46: 705–13.

20. Heding L. Radioimmunological determination of human C-peptide in serum. Diabetologia 1975; 11: 541–8.

21. Faber OK, Markussen J, Naithani VK, Binder C. Production of antisera to synthetic benzylooxycarbonyl-c-peptide of human proinsulin. Hoppe-Seyler Z Physiol Chem 1976; 357: 751–7.

22. Faber OK, Binder C, Markussen J et al. Characterization of seven C-peptide antisera. Diabetes 1978; 27 (suppl. 1): 170–7.

23. Garcia-Webb P, Bonser A. Decrease in measured C-peptide immunoreactivity on storage. Clin Chem 1979; 95: 139–41.

24. Kuzuya H, Blix PM, Horwitz DL, Steiner DF, Rubinstein AH. Determination of free and total insulin and C-peptide in insulin-treated diabetics. Diabetes 1977; 26: 22–9.

25. Caygill CPJ, Gaines Das RE, Bangham DR. Use of a common standard for comparison of insulin and C-peptide measurements by different laboratories. Diabetologia 1980; 18: 197–204.

26. Saelsen L, Tronier B, Madsbad S, Christensen NJ. A rapid method for determination of human C-peptide in plasma. Clin Chem Acta 1991; 196: 1–6.

27. Kuzuya H, Blix PM, Horwitz DL, Rubinstein AH, Steiner DF, Binder C, Faber OK. Heterogeneity of circulating C-peptide. J Clin Endocrinol Metab 1977; 44: 952–62.

28. Koskinen P. Nontransferability of C-peptide measurements with various commercial radioimmunoassay reagents. Clin Chem 1988; 34: 1575–8.

29. Heding LG, Ludvigsson J. Human proinsulin in insulin-treated juvenile diabetics. Acta Paediatr Scand 1979 (suppl. 270): 48–52.

30. Polonsky KS, Given BD, Hirsch L, Shapiro ET, Tillil H, Beebe C, Galloway JA. Quantitative study of insulin secretion and clearance in normal and obese subjects. J Clin Invest 1988; 81: 435–41.

31. Eaton RP, Allen RC, Shade DS, Erichson KM, Standefer J. Prehepatic insulin production in man. Kinetic analyses using connecting peptide behaviour. J Clin Endocrinol Metab 1980; 51: 520–8.

32. Tillil H, Shapiro ET, Miller MA et al. Dose-dependent effects of oral and intravenous glucose on insulin secretion and clearance in normal humans. Am J Physiol 1988; 254: E349–57.

33. Polonsky KS, Licinio-Paixao J, Given BD et al. Use of biosynthetic human C-peptide in the measurement of insulin secretion rates in normal volunteers and Type 1 diabetic patients. J Clin Invest 1986; 77: 98–105.

34. Polonsky K, Jaspan JB, Pugh W et al. The metabolism of C-peptide in the dog. *In vivo* demonstration of the absence of hepatic extraction. J Clin Invest 1983; 72: 1114–23.

35. Polonsky KS, Pugh W, Jaspan JB, Cohon DM, Karrison T, Tager HS, Rubinstein AH. C-peptide and insulin secretion. Relationship between peripheral concentrations of C-peptide and insulin and their secretion rates in dog. J Clin Invest 1984; 74: 1821–9.

36. Kühl C, Faber OK, Hornes P, Jensen SL. C-peptide metabolism and the liver. Diabetes 1978; 27 (suppl. 1): 197–200.

37. Norwich RH, Pinto C, March JE, Zelin S. A practical method for removing catheter distortions from

indicator dilution curves. Cardiovasc Res 1974; 8: 430–8.

38. Faber OK, Hagen C, Binder C et al. Kinetics of human connecting peptide in normal and diabetic subjects. J Clin Invest 1978; 62: 197–203.

39. Licinio-Paixao J, Polonsky KS, Given BD, Pugh W, Ostrega D, Frank BH, Rubinstein AH. Ingestion of a mixed meal does not affect the metabolic clearance rate of biosynthetic human C-peptide. J Clin Endocrinol Metab 1986; 63: 401–3.

40. Henriksen JH, Tronier B, Bülow JB. Kinetics of circulating endogenous insulin, C-peptide, and proinsulin in fasting nondiabetic man. Metabolism 1987; 36: 463–8.

41. Madsbad S, Jeppesen J, Krarup T, Boesgaard S, Tronier B. The importance of arterial versus venous blood sampling for calculation of insulin secretion, insulin clearance and 'incretin' effect. Diabetes 1989; 38 (suppl. 2): 207A.

42. Faber OK, Kehlet H, Madsbad S, Binder C. Kinetics of human C-peptide in man. Diabetes 1978; 27 (suppl. 1): 207–9.

43. Polonsky K, Frank B, Pough W et al. The limitations to and valid use of C-peptide as a marker of the secretion of insulin. Diabetes 1986; 35: 379–86.

44. Watanabe RM, Vølund A, Roy S, Bergman RN. Prehepatic B-cell secretion during the intravenous glucose tolerance test in humans: application of a combined model of insulin and C-peptide kinetics. J Clin Endocrinol Metab 1989; 69: 790–7.

45. Polonsky KS, Given BD, Hirsch LJ et al. Abnormal patterns of insulin secretion in non-insulin-dependent diabetes mellitus. New Engl J Med 1988; 318: 1231–9.

46. Polonsky KS, Given BD, Hirsch L, Shapiro ET, Tillil H, Beebe C, Galloway JA. Quantitative study of insulin secretion and clearance in normal and obese subjects. J Clin Invest 1988; 81: 435–41.

47. Shapiro ET, Tillil HT, Miller MA, Frank BH, Galloway JA, Rubinstein AH, Polonsky KS. Insulin secretion and clearance. Comparison after oral and intravenous glucose. Diabetes 1987; 36: 1367–71.

48. Tillil H, Shapiro ET, Rubinstein AH, Galloway JA, Polonsky KS. Reduction of insulin clearance during hyperglycemic clamp. Dose–response study in normal humans. Diabetes 1988; 37: 1351–7.

49. Vølund A, Polonsky KS, Bergman RN. Calculated pattern of intraportal insulin appearance without independent assessment of C-peptide kinetics. Diabetes 1987; 36: 1195–1202.

50. Cobelli C, Pacini G. Insulin secretion and hepatic insulin extraction in humans by minimal modelling of C-peptide and insulin kinetics. Diabetes 1988; 37: 223–31.

51. Field JB. Extraction of insulin by liver. Ann Rev Med 1973; 24: 309–14.

52. Ferannini E, Cobelli C. The kinetics of insulin in man. 2. Role of the liver. Diabetes Metab Rev 1987; 3: 365–97.

53. Kaneko T, Meinemura M, Oka H et al. Demonstration of C-peptide immunoreactivity in various body fluids and clinical evaluation of the determination of urinary C-peptide immunoreactivity. Endocrinol Jpn 1975; 22: 207–22.

54. Kuzuya T, Matsuda A, Saito T, Yoshida S. Human C-peptide immunoreactivity (CPR) in blood and urine—evaluation of a radioimmunoassay method and its clinical application. Diabetologia 1976; 12: 511–18.

55. Horwitz DL, Rubinstein AH, Katz AI. Quantitation of human pancreatic beta-cell function by immunoassay of C-peptide in urine. Diabetes 1977; 26: 30–5.

56. Meistas MT, Zadik Z, Margolis S, Kowarski AA. Correlation of urinary extraction of C-peptide with the integrated concentration and secretion rates of insulin. Diabetes 1981; 30: 639–43.

57. Blix PM, Boddie WC, Landau RL, Rochman H, Rubinstein AH. Urinary C-peptide: an indicator of beta-cell secretion under different metabolic conditions. J Clin Endocrinol Metab 1982; 54: 574–80.

58. Kuzuya T, Matsuda A, Sakamota Y, Tanabshi S, Kajinuma H. C-peptide immunoreactivity (CPR) in urine. Diabetes 1978; 27 (suppl. 1): 210–15.

59. Hoogwerf B, Goetz FC. Urinary C-peptide: a simple measure of integrated insulin production with emphasis on the effects of body size, diet and corticosteroids. J Clin Endocrinol Metab 1983; 56: 60–7.

60. Meistas MT, Rendell M, Margolis S, Kowarski AA. Estimation of the secretion rate of insulin from the urinary excretion rate of C-peptide. Study in obese and diabetic subjects. Diabetes 1982; 31: 449–53.

61. Zavaroni I, Deferrari G, Lugari R et al. Renal metabolism of C-peptide in man. J Clin Endocrinol Metab 1987; 65: 494–8.

62. Yale JF, Leiter LA, Marliss EB. Urine C-peptide as index of integrated insulin secretion in hypocaloric states in obese human subjects. Diabetes 1987; 36: 447–53.

63. Brodows RG. Use of urinary C-peptide to estimate insulin secretion during starvation. J Clin Endocrinol Metab 1985; 61: 654–7.

64. Gjessing HJ, Matzen LE, Faber OK, Frøland A. Sensitivity and reproducibility of urinary C-peptide as estimate of islet B-cell function in insulin-treated diabetes. Diabet Med 1988; 6: 329–33.

65. Gjessing HJ, Damsgaard EM, Matzen LE, Frøland A, Faber OK. Reproducibility of B-cell function estimates in non-insulin-dependent diabetes mellitus. Diabetes Care 1987; 10: 558–62.

66. Huttenen NP, Knip M, Käär ML, Puukka R, Åkerblom HK. Clinical significance of urinary C-peptide excretion in children with insulin-dependent diabetes mellitus. Acta Paediatr Scand 1989; 78: 271–7.

67. Ivarsson SA, Johansson E, Nilsson KO, Thorell JL. Urinary C-peptide excretion at onset of insulin dependent diabetes mellitus in children. Acta Paediatr Scand 1987; 76: 608–11.

68. Sjøberg S, Gunnarsson R, Østman J. Residual C-peptide production in type 1 diabetes mellitus: a comparison of different methods of assessment and influence on glucose control. Acta Med Scand 1983; 214: 231–7.

69. Sjøberg S, Gunnarssen R, Gjötterberg M, Lefvert AK, Persson A, Östman J. Residual insulin production, glycaemic control and prevalence of microvascular lesions and polyneuropathy in long-term type 1 (insulin-dependent) diabetes mellitus. Diabetologia, 1987; 30: 208–13.

70. Kajinuma H, Tanabashi S, Ishiwata K, Kuzuya N. Urinary excretion of C-peptide in relation to renal function. In Baba S, Koneko T, Yanahaira N (eds) Proinsulin, C-peptide. Amsterdam: Excerpta Medica, 1979: pp 183–9.

71. Jaspan JB, Mako ME, Kuzuya H, Blix PM, Horwitz DL, Rubinstein AH. Abnormalities in circulating beta-cell peptides in chronic renal failure: comparison of C-peptide, proinsulin and insulin. J Clin Invest 1977; 45: 441–7.

72. Regeur L, Faber OK, Binder C. Plasma C-peptide in uraemic patients. J Clin Lab Invest 1978; 38: 771–5.

73. Garvey WT, Olefsky JM, Rubinstein AH, Kolterman OG. Day-long integrated serum insulin and C-peptide profiles in patients with NIDDM. Correlation with urinary C-peptide excretion. Diabetes 1988; 37: 590–9.

74. Tillil H, Shapiro T, Given BD, Rue P, Rubinstein AH, Galloway JA, Polonsky KS. Reevaluation of urine C-peptide measure of insulin secretion. Diabetes 1988; 37: 1195–1201.

75. Agner T, Damm P, Binder C. Remission in IDDM: prospective study of basal C-peptide and insulin dose in 268 consecutive patients. Diabetes Care 1987; 10: 164–9.

76. Madsbad S, Krarup T, Regeur L, Faber OK, Binder C. Insulin secretory reserve in insulin dependent patients at time of diagnosis and the first 180 days of insulin treatment. Acta Endocrinol 1980; 95: 359–63.

77. Madsbad S, Faber OK, Binder C, McNair P, Christiansen C, Transbøl I. Prevalence of residual beta-cell function in insulin-dependent diabetics in relation to age at onset and duration of diabetes. Diabetes 1978; 27 (suppl. 1): 262–4.

78. Wallensteen M, Dahlquist G, Persson B, Landin-Olsson M, Lernmark Å, Sundkvist G, Thalme B. Factors influencing the magnitude, duration and the rate of fall of B-cell function in type 1 (insulin-dependent) diabetic children followed for two years from their clinical diagnosis. Diabetologia 1988; 31: 664–9.

79. Chiffrin A, Suissa S, Poussier P, Guttmann R, Weitzner C. Prospective study of predictors of B-cell survival in Type 1 diabetes. Diabetes 1988; 37: 920–5.

80. DCCT Research Group. Effects of age, duration and treatment of insulin-dependent diabetes mellitus on residual B-cell function: observations during eligibility testing for the Diabetes Control and Complications Trial (DCCT). J Clin Endocrinol Metab 1987; 30: 30–6.

81. Sochett EB, Daneman D, Ehrlich RM. Factors affecting and patterns of residual insulin secretion during the first year of Type 1 (insulin-dependent) diabetes mellitus in children. Diabetologia 1987; 30: 453–9.

82. Marner B, Agner T, Binder C, Lernmark Å, Nerup J, Mandrup-Poulsen T, Waldorff S. Increased reduction in fasting C-peptide is associated with islet cell antibodies in Type 1 (insulin-dependent) diabetic patients. Diabetologia 1985; 28: 875–80.

83. Landin-Olson M, Nilsson KO, Lernmark Å, Sundkvist G. Islet cell antibodies and fasting C-peptide predict insulin requirement at diagnosis of diabetes mellitus. Diabetologia 1990; 33: 561–8.

84. Knip M, Puukka R, Kääar M-L, Åkerblom H. Remission phase, endogenous insulin secretion and metabolic control in diabetic children. Acta Diab Lat 1982; 19: 243–51.

85. Mustonen A, Knip M, Huttenen N-P, Puukka R, Kääar M-L, Akerblom, H. Evidence of delayed B-cell destruction in Type 1 (insulin-dependent) diabetic patients with persisting complement fixing cytoplasmic islet cell antibodies. Diabetologia 1984; 27: 421–6.

86. Ludvigsson J. Insulin antibodies in diabetic children treated with monocomponent porcine insulin from the onset: relationship to B-cell function and partial remission. Diabetologia 1984; 26: 138–41.

87. Madsbad S, Lauritzen E, Faber OK, Binder C. The effect of residual beta-cell function on the development of diabetic retinopathy. Diabet Med 1986; 3: 42–5.

88. Block MB, Rosenfield RL, Mako ME, Steiner DF, Rubinstein AH. Sequential changes in B-cell function in insulin treated diabetic patients assessed by C-peptide immunoreactivity. New Engl J Med 1973; 288: 1144–8.

89. Ludvigsson J, Heding LG. C-peptide in children with diabetes. Diabetologia 1976; 12: 627–30.

90. Hendriksen C, Faber OK, Drejer J, Binder C. Prevalence of residual B-cell function in insulin treated diabetics evaluated by the plasma C-peptide response to intravenous glucagon. Diabetologia 1977; 13: 615–19.

91. Madsbad S, Bottazzo GF, Cudworth AG, Dean B, Faber OK, Binder C. Islet cell antibodies and beta-cell function in insulin dependent diabetics. Diabetologia 1980; 18: 45–7.

92. Sochett E, Daneman D. Relationship of insulin autoantibodies to presentation and early course of IDDM in children. Diabetes Care 1989; 12: 517–23.

93. Canevet B, Harter M, Viot G, Balarac N, Krebs BP. Residual B cell function in insulin-dependent diabetes: evaluation by circadian determination of C-peptide immunoreactivity. J Endocrinol Invest 1980; 3: 107–11.

94. Peig M, Gomis P, Ercilla G, Casamitjana R, Bottazzo GF, Pujol-Borrell R. Correlation between residual B-cell function and islet cell antibodies in newly diagnosed Type 1 diabetes. Diabetes 1989; 38: 1396–1401.

95. Faber OK, Binder C. B-cell function and blood glucose control in insulin-dependent diabetics within the first months of insulin treatment. Diabetologia 1977; 13: 263–8.

96. Yki-Järvinen H, Koivisto VA. Natural course of insulin resistance in type 1 diabetes. New Engl J Med 1986; 315: 224–30.

97. Grajwer LA, Pildes RS, Horwitz DL, Rubinstein AH. Control of juvenile diabetes mellitus and its relationship to endogenous insulin secretion as measured by C-peptide immunoreactivity. J Pediatr 1977; 90: 42–8.

98. Ludvigsson J, Säfwenberg J, Heding LG. HLA-types, C-peptide and insulin antibodies in juvenile diabetes. Diabetologia 1977; 13: 13–17.

99. Gerbitz K-D, Kemmler W, Edelmann A, Summer J, Mehnert H, Wieland OH. Free insulin, bound insulin, C-peptide and the metabolic control in juvenile onset diabetics: comparisons of C-peptide secretors and nonsecretors during 24 hours conventional insulin therapy. Eur J Clin Invest 1979; 9: 475–83.

100. Yue DK, Baxter RC, Turtle JR, C-peptide secretion and insulin antibodies as determinants of stability in diabetes mellitus. Metabolism 1978; 27: 35-44.

101. Gonen B, Goldman J, Baldwin D et al. Metabolic control in diabetic patients. Effects of insulin secretory reserve (measured by plasma C-peptide levels) and circulating insulin antibodies. Diabetes 1979; 28: 749-53.

102. Asplin CM, Hartog M, Goldie DJ, Alberti KGMM, Binder C, Faber OK. Diurnal profiles of serum insulin, C-peptide and blood intermediary metabolites in insulin treated diabetics, their relationship to the control of diabetes and the role of endogenous insulin secretion. Quart J Med 1979; 48: 343-60.

103. Madsbad S, Faber OK, Binder C, Alberti KGMM, Lloyd B. Diurnal profiles of intermediary metabolites in insulin-dependent diabetes and their relationship to different degrees of residual beta-cell function. Acta Diab Lat 1981; 18: 115-21.

104. Shima K, Tanaka R, Morishita S, Tarui S, Kamahara Y, Nishikawa M. Studies on the etiology of brittle diabetes. Relationship between diabetic instability and insulinogenic reserve. Diabetes 1977; 26: 717-25.

105. Raynolds C, Molnar GD, Horwitz DL, Rubinstein AH, Taylor WF, Jiang N-S. Abnormalities of endogenous glucagon and insulin in unstable diabetes. Diabetes 1977; 267: 36-45.

106. Ikeda Y, Ando N, Minami N, Ide Y. B-cell function of insulin-dependent young onset diabetics assessed by C-peptide immunoreactivity. Diabetologia 1975; 11: 351-2.

107. Madsbad S, McNair P, Faber OK, Binder C, Christiansen C, Transbøl I. Beta-cell function and metabolic control in insulin treated diabetics. Acta Endocrinol 1980; 93: 196-200.

108. Fukuda M, Tanaka A, Tahara Y, Ikegami H, Yamamoto Y, Kumahara Y, Shima K. Correlation between minimal secretory capacity of pancreatic B-cells and stability of diabetic control. Diabetes 1988; 37: 81-8.

109. Madsbad S, Alberti KGMM, Binder C, Burrin JM, Faber OK, Krarup T, Regeur L. Role of residual insulin secretion in protecting against ketoacidosis in insulin-dependent patients. Br Med J 1979; 2: 1257-9.

110. Madsbad S, Faber OK, Kurtz A et al. The significance of the portal insulin secretion in insulin dependent patients with residual B-cell function. A safeguard against hormonal and metabolic derangement. Clin Endocrinol 1982; 16: 605-13.

111. Madsbad S, Hilsted J, Krarup T, Sestoft L, Christensen NJ, Faber OK, Tronier B. Hormonal, metabolic and cardiovascular responses to hypoglycaemia in type 1 (insulin-dependent) diabetes with and without B-cell function. Diabetologia 1982; 23: 499-504.

112. Tronier B, Madsbad S, Krarup T, Faber OK. Lack of influence of the residual B-cell function on the glucagon and pancreatic polypeptide secretion in type 1 (insulin-dependent) diabetic patients. Diabète Métab 1987; 13: 141-3.

113. Smith RBW, Pyke DA, Watkins PJ, Binder C, Faber OK. C-peptide response to glucagon in diabetics with and without complications. NZ Med J 1979; 89: 304-6.

114. Bodansky HJ, Medbak S, Drury PL, Cudworth AG. Plasma C-peptide in long-standing type 1 diabetes with and without microvascular disease. Diabète Métab 1981; 7: 265-9.

115. Sjöberg S, Gunnarsson R, Gjötterberg M, Lefvert AK, Persson A, Östman J. Residual insulin production, glycaemic control and prevalence of microvascular lesions and polyneuropathy in long-term Type 1 (insulin-dependent) diabetes mellitus. Diabetologia 1987; 30: 208-13.

116. Klein R, Moss SE, Klein BEK, Davis MD, DeMets D. Wisconsin epidemiologic study of diabetic retinopathy. XII. Relationship of C-peptide and diabetic retinopathy. Diabetes 1990; 39: 1445-50.

117. Mirouze J, Selam JL, Pham TC, Mendoza E, Orsetti A. Sustained insulin-induced remissions of juvenile diabetes by means of an external artificial pancreas. Diabetologia 1978; 14: 223-7.

118. Shah SC, Malone JI, Simpson NE. A randomized trial of intensive insulin therapy in newly diagnosed insulin-dependent diabetes mellitus. New Engl J Med 1989; 320: 550-4.

119. Madsbad S, Krarup T, Faber OK, Binder C, Regeur L. The transient effect of strict metabolic control on B-cell function in newly diagnosed type 1 (insulin-dependent) diabetic patients. Diabetologia 1982; 22: 16-22.

120. Perlman K, Ehrlich RM, Filler RM, Albisser AM. Sustained normoglycemia in newly diagnosed Type 1 diabetic subjects. Short-term effects and one-year follow-up. Diabetes 1984; 33: 995-1001.

121. Beaufort CE, Houtzagers CMGJ, Bruining GJ et al. Continuous subcutaneous insulin infusion (CSII) versus conventional injection therapy in newly diagnosed diabetic children: two-year follow-up of a randomized, prospective trial. Diabet Med 1989; 6: 766-71.

122. Damsbo P, Madsbad S, Edsberg B, Krarup T, Buschard K. B-cell function during two years of pump treatment. Diabetes Res Clin Pract 1988; 5 (suppl. 1): 508.

123. Madsbad S, Krarup T, Regeur L, Faber OK, Binder C. Effect of strict blood glucose control on residual B-cell function in insulin-dependent diabetes. Diabetologia 1981; 20: 530-4.

124. Krarup T, Madsbad S. Effect of two periods with intensified insulin treatment on B-cell function during the first 18 months of Type 1 (insulin-dependent) diabetes mellitus. Diabète Métab 1986; 12: 156-60.

125. Elliott RB, Crossby JR, Bergman CC, James AG. Partial preservation of pancreatic B-cell function in children with diabetes. Lancet 1981; ii: 1-4.

126. Mistura L, Beccaria L, Meschi F, D'Arcais AF, Pellini C, Puzzovio M, Chiumello G. Prednisone treatment in newly diagnosed Type 1 diabetic children: 1-year follow-up. Diabetes Care 1987; 10: 39-43.

127. Ludvigsson J, Heding L, Liedén G, Marner B, Lernmark A. Plasmapheresis in the initial treatment of IDDM in children. Br Med J 1983; 286: 176-8.

128. Heinze E, Thon A, Vetter U, Gaedicke G, Zuppinger K. Gamma-globulin therapy in 6 newly diagnosed diabetic children. Acta Paediatr Scand 1985; 74: 605-6.

129. Mirouze J, Rodier M, Richard JL, Lashkar H, Monnier L. Trial of mild immunosuppression by methisoprinol in acute onset diabetes mellitus: effects on rate and duration of remission. Diabetes Res 1986; 3: 359-62.

130. Koivisto VA, Aro A, Cantell K et al. Remissions in newly diagnosed Type 1 (insulin-dependent) diabetes:

influence of interferon as an adjunct to insulin therapy. Diabetologia 1984; 27: 193–7.

131. Eisenbarth GS, Srikanta S, Jackson R, Rabinowe S, Dolinar R, Aoki T, Morris MA. Anti-thymocyte globulin and prednisone immunotherapy of recent onset type 1 diabetes mellitus. Diabetes Res 1985; 2: 271–6.

132. Harrison LC, Colman PG, Dean B, Baxter R, Martin FIR. Increase in remission rate in newly diagnosed Type 1 diabetic subjects treated with azathioprine. Diabetes 1985; 34: 1306–8.

133. Cook JJ, Hudson I, Harrison LC et al. Double-blind controlled trial of azathioprine in children with newly diagnosed Type 1 diabetes. Diabetes 1989; 38: 779–83.

134. Silverstein J, Maclaren N, Riley W, Spiller R, Radjenovic D, Johnson S. Immunosuppression with azathioprine and prednisolone in recent-onset insulin-dependent diabetes mellitus. New Engl J Med 1988; 319: 599–604.

135. Stiller CR, Dupre J, Gent M et al. Effects of cyclosporine immunosuppression in insulin-dependent diabetes mellitus of recent onset. Science 1984; 223: 1362–7.

136. Assan R, Feutren G, Depray-Sachs M et al. Metabolic and immunological effects of cyclosporin in recently diagnosed Type 1 diabetes mellitus. Lancet 1985; i: 67–71.

137. Feutren G, Papoz L, Assan R et al. Cyclosporin increases the rate and length of remission in insulin-dependent diabetes of recent onset. Lancet 1986; ii: 119–24.

138. Stiller CR, Dupre J, Gent M et al. Effects of cyclosporine in recent-onset juvenile Type 1 diabetes: impact of age and duration of disease. J Pediatr 1987; 111: 1069–72.

139. Bougnères PF, Carel JC, Castano L et al. Factors associated with early remission of Type 1 diabetes in children treated with cyclosporine. New Engl J Med 1988; 318: 663–70.

140. Canadian–European Randomized Control Trial Group. Cyclosporine-induced remission of IDDM after early intervention. Association of 1 year of cyclosporine treatment with enhanced insulin secretion. Diabetes 1988; 37: 1574–82.

141. Chase HP, Butler-Simon N, Garg SK, Hayward A, Klingensmith GJ, Hamman RF, O'Brien D. Cyclosporine A for the treatment of new-onset insulin-dependent diabetes mellitus. Pediatrics 1990; 85: 241–5.

142. Assan R, Feutren G, Sirmai J et al. Plasma C-peptide levels and clinical remission in recent-onset type 1 diabetic patients treated with cyclosporin A and insulin. Diabetes 1990; 39: 768–74.

143. Eisenbarth GH. Type 1 diabetes mellitus: a chronic autoimmune disease. New Engl J Med 1986; 314: 360–8.

144. Yonemura Y, Takashima T, Miwa K, Miyazadi I, Yamamoto H, Okamoto H. Amelioration of diabetes mellitus in partially depancreatized rats by poly(ADP-ribose) synthetase inhibitors. Evidence of islet cell regeneration. Diabetes 1984; 33: 401–4.

145. Stauffacher W, Burr I, Gutzeit A, Beaven D, Velinsky J, Renold AE. Streptozotocin diabetes: time course of irreversible B-cell damage; further observations on prevention by nicotinamide. Proc Soc Exp Biol Med 1970; 133: 194–200.

146. Yamada K, Nonaka K, Hanafusa T, Miyazaki A, Toyoshima H, Tarvis S. Prevention and therapeutic effects of large dose nicotinamide injections on diabetes associated with insulinitis. An observation in non obese diabetic (NOD) mice. Diabetes 1982; 31: 749–53.

147. Vague P, Picq R, Bernal M, Lassmann-Vague V, Vialettes B. Effect of nicotinamide treatment on the residual insulin secretion in type 1 (insulin-dependent) diabetic patients. Diabetologia 1989; 32: 316–21.

148. Pozzilli P, Visalli N, Ghirlanda G, Manna R, Andreani D. Nicotinamide increases C-peptide secretion in patients with recent onset Type 1 diabetes. Diabet Med 1989; 6: 568–72.

149. Madsbad S. Classification of diabetes in older adults. Diabetes Care 1990; 13 (suppl. 2): 93–6.

150. Madsbad S, Krarup T, McNair P, Christiansen C, Faber OK, Transbøl I, Binder C. Practical clinical value of the C-peptide response to glucagon stimulation in the choice of treatment in diabetes mellitus. Acta Med Scand 1981; 210: 153–6.

151. National Diabetes Data Group. Classification and diagnosis of diabetes mellitus and other categories of glucose intolerance. Diabetes 1979; 28: 1039–57.

152. Green A, Hougaard P. Epidemiological studies of diabetes mellitus in Denmark. IV. Clinical characteristics of insulin treated patients. Diabetologia 1983; 25: 231–4.

153. Laakso M, Pyörälä K. Age of onset and type of diabetes. Diabetes Care 1985; 8: 114–17.

154. Wilson BM, Van der Minne P, Deverill J, Heller SR, Getsthope K, Reevers WG, Tattersall RB. Insulin dependence: problems with classification of 100 consecutive patients. Diabet Med 1985; 2: 167–72.

155. Nathans DM, Singer DE, Godine JE, Perlmuter LC. Non insulin-dependent diabetes in older patients: complications and risk factors. Am J Med 1986; 81: 837–42.

156. Kilvert A, Fitzgerald MG, Wright AD, Nattrass M. Clinical characteristics and aetiological classification of insulin-dependent diabetes in the elderly. Quart J Med 1986; 60: 865–72.

157. Melton LJ, Palumbo PJ, Chu C-P. Incidence of diabetes mellitus by clinical type in the elderly. Diabetes Care 1983; 6: 75–86.

158. Rendell M, Zarriello J, Drew HM, Dranbauer B, Wilson G, Waud J, Ross D. Recovery from decompensated non-insulin-dependent diabetes mellitus: studies of C-peptide secretion. Diabetes Care 1981; 4: 354–9.

159. Irvine WJ, Gray RS, McCallum CS, Duncan LPJ. Clinical and pathogenic significance of pancreatic islet cell antibodies in diabetics treated with oral hypoglycaemic drugs. Lancet 1977; i: 1025–7.

160. Groop L, Bottazzo GF, Doniach D. Islet cell antibodies identify latent type 1 diabetes in patients aged 35–75 years at diagnosis. Diabetes 1986; 35: 237–41.

161. Groop L, Miettinen A, Groop P-H, Meri S, Koskimies S, Bottazzo GF. Organ-specific autoimmunity and HLA-DR antigens as markers for B-cell destruction in patients with Type 2 diabetes. Diabetes 1988; 37: 99–103.

162. Lyons TJ, Kennedy L, Atkinson AB, Buchanan KD, Hadden DR, Weaver JA. Predicting the need for insulin therapy in late onset (40–69 years) diabetes mellitus. Diabet Med 1984; 1: 105–7.

163. Welborn TA, Garcia-Webb P, Bonser AM. Basal C-peptide in the discrimination of type 1 from type 2 diabetes. Diabetes Care 1981; 4: 616-19.

164. Hoekstra JBL, Van Rijn HJM, Thijssen JHH, Erkelens DW. C-peptide reactivity as a measure of insulin dependency in obese patients treated with insulin. Diabetes Care 1982; 5: 585-91.

165. Rendell M. C-peptide levels as a criterion in treatment of maturity-onset diabetes. J Clin Endocrinol Metab 1983; 57: 1198-1206.

166. Koskinen P, Viikari J, Irjala K, Kaihola H-L, Seppälä P. C-peptide determination in the choice of treatment in diabetes mellitus. Scand J Clin Invest 1985; 45: 589-97.

167. Hother-Nielsen O, Faber O, Sørensen NS, Beck-Nielsen H. Classification of newly diagnosed diabetic patients as insulin-requiring or non-insulin-requiring based on clinical and biochemical variables. Diabetes Care 1988; 11: 531-7.

168. Faber OK, Binder C. C-peptide response to glucagon. A test for the residual B-cell function in diabetes mellitus. Diabetes 1977; 26: 605-10.

169. Arnold-Larson S, Madsbad S, Kühl C. Reproducibility of the glucagon test. Diabet Med 1987; 4: 299-303.

170. Madsbad S, Sauerbrey N, Møller-Jensen B, Krarup T, Kühl C. Outcome of the glucagon test depends upon the prevailing blood glucose concentration in Type 1 (insulin-dependent) diabetic patients. Acta Med Scand 1987; 222: 71-4.

171. Gorden P, Roth J. Plasma insulin: fluctuations in the 'big' insulin component in man after glucose and other stimuli. J Clin Invest 1969; 48: 2225-34.

172. Melani F, Rubenstein AH, Oyer PE, Steiner DF. Identification of proinsulin and C-peptide in human serum by a specific immunoassay. Proc Natl Acad Sci USA 1970; 67: 148-55.

173. Cresto JC, Lavine RL, Fink G, Recant L. Plasma proinsulin. Comparison of insulin specific protease and gel filtration assays. Diabetes 1974; 23: 505-11.

174. Kitabchi AE, Duckworth WC, Brush JS, Heinemann M. Direct measurement of proinsulin in human plasma by use of an insulin-degrading enzyme. J Clin Invest 1971; 50: 1792-9.

175. Starr JI, Juhn DD, Rubenstein AH, Kitabchi AE. Degradation of insulin in serum by insulin-specific protease. J Lab Clin Med 1975; 86: 631-7.

176. Frank BH, Pettee JM, Zimmerman RE, Burck PJ. The production of human proinsulin and its transformation to human insulin and C-peptide. In Rich DH, Gross E (eds) Peptides, structure and biological function. Rockford, IL: Pierce Chemical Co. 1981: pp 729-38.

177. Heding LG. Specific and direct radioimmunoassay for human proinsulin in serum. Diabetologia 1977; 13: 467-74.

178. Cohen RM, Nakabayashi T, Blix PM et al. A radioimmunoassay for circulating human proinsulin. Diabetes 1985; 34: 84-91.

179. Deacon CF, Conlon JM. Measurement of circulating human proinsulin concentrations using a proinsulin-specific antiserum. Diabetes 1985; 34: 491-7.

180. Hartling SG, Dinesen B, Kappelgård A-M, Faber OK, Binder C. ELISA for human proinsulin. Clin Chim Acta 1986; 156: 289-97.

181. Ward WK, Paquette TL, Frank BH, Porte D Jr. A sensitive radioimmunoassay for human proinsulin with sequential use of antisera to C-peptide and insulin. Clin Chem 1986; 32: 728-33.

182. Naylor BA, Matthews DR, Turner RC. A soluble-phase proinsulin radioimmunoassay and its use in diagnosis of hypoglycemia. Ann Clin Biochem 1987; 24: 352-63.

183. Yoshioka N, Kuzuya T, Matsuda A, Taniguchi M, Iwamoto Y. Serum proinsulin levels at fasting and after oral glucose load in patients with Type 2 (non-insulin-dependent) diabetes mellitus. Diabetologia 1988; 31: 355-60.

184. Hampton SM, Beyzavi K, Teale D, Marks V. A direct assay for the proinsulin in plasma and its applications in hypoglycemia. Clin Endocrinol 1988; 29: 9-16.

185. De Haën C, Little SA, May JM, Williams RH. Characterization of proinsulin-insulin intermediates in human plasma. J Clin Invest 1978; 62: 727-37.

186. Cohen RM, Given BD, Licinio-Paixao J et al. Proinsulin radioimmunoassay in the evaluation of insulinomas and familial hyperproinsulinemia. Metabolism 1986; 35: 1137-46.

187. Gray IP, Siddle K, Frank BH, Hales CN. Characterization and use in immunoradiometric assay of monoclonal antibodies directed against human proinsulin. Diabetes 1987; 36: 684-8.

188. Temple RC, Luzio SD, Schneider AE, Carrington CA, Owens DR, Sobey WJ, Hales CN. Insulin deficiency in non-insulin-dependent diabetes. Lancet 1989; i 293-5.

189. Sobey WJ, Beer SF, Carrington CA et al. Sensitive and specific two-site immunoradiometric assays for human insulin, proinsulin, 65-66 split and 32-33 split proinsulins. Biochem J 1989; 260: 535-41.

190. Given BD, Cohen RM, Shoelson SE, Frank BH, Rubenstein AH, Tager HS. Biochemical and clinical implications of proinsulin conversion intermediates. J Clin Invest 1985; 76: 1398-405.

191. Peavy DE, Brunner MR, Duckworth WC, Hooker CS, Frank BH. Receptor binding and biological potency of several split forms (conversion intermediates) of human proinsulin. J Biol Chem 1985; 260: 13989-94.

192. Waldhäusl WK, Bratusch-Marrain P, Gasic S, Komjati M, Heding L. Inhibition by proinsulin of endogenous C-peptide release in healthy man. Am J Physiol 1986; 251: E139-45.

193. Sodoyez-Goffaux F, Sodoyes J-C, Koch M, De Vos CJ, Frank BH. Scintigraphic distribution of ^{123}I labelled proinsulin, split conversion intermediates and insulin in rats. Diabetologia 1988; 31: 848-54.

194. Katz AI, Rubenstein AH. Metabolism of proinsulin, insulin and C-peptide in the rat. J Clin Invest 1973; 52: 1113-21.

195. Zilker TR, Rebel CH, Kopp KF et al. Kinetics of biosynthetic human proinsulin in patients with terminal renal insufficiency. Horm Metab Res 1988 (suppl. 18): 43-8.

196. Podlecki DA, Frank BH, Olefsky JM. *In vitro* characterization of biosynthetic human proinsulin. Diabetes 1984; 33: 111-18.

197. Ciaraldi TP, Brady D, Olefsky JM. Kinetics of biosynthetic human proinsulin action in isolated rat adipocytes. Diabetes 1986; 35: 318-23.

198. Peavy DE, Abram JD, Frank BH, Duckworth WC. *In vitro* activity of biosynthetic human proinsulin. Diabetes 1984; 33: 1062-7.

199. Revers RR, Henry R, Schmeiser L et al. The effects of biosynthetic human proinsulin on carbohydrate metabolism. Diabetes 1984; 33: 762-70.

200. Bergenstal RM, Cohen RM, Lever E et al. The metabolic effects of biosynthetic human proinsulin in individuals with type I diabetes. J Clin Endocrinol Metab 1984; 58: 973–9.

201. Nauck MA, Stöckmann F, Thiery J, Ebert R, Creutzfeldt W. Effects of single and combined infusions of human biosynthetic proinsulin and insulin on glucose metabolism and on plasma hormone concentrations in euglycaemic clamp experiments. Horm Metab Res 1988 (suppl. 18): 60–8.

202. Zilker TR, Gray IP, Hales CN et al. Pharmacokinetics of biosynthetic human proinsulin following intravenous and subcutaneous administration in metabolically healthy volunteers. Horm Metab Res 1988 (suppl. 18): 37–43.

203. Yu SS, Kitabchi AE. Biological activity of proinsulin and related polypeptides in the fat tissue. J Biol Chem 1973; 248: 3753–61.

204. Gruppuso PA, Frank BH, Schwartz R. Binding of proinsulin and proinsulin conversion intermediates to human placental insulin-like growth factor I receptors. J Clin Endocrinol Metab 1988; 67: 194–7.

205. Revers RR, Henry R, Schmeiser L et al. Biosynthetic human insulin and proinsulin have additive but not synergistic effects on total body glucose disposal. J Clin Endocrinol Metab 1984; 58: 1094–8.

206. Heding LG, Ludvigsson J, Kasperska-Czyzykowa T. B-cell secretion in non-insulin and insulin-dependent-diabetics. Acta Med Scand 1981 (suppl. 656): 5–9.

207. Snorgaard O, Hartling SG, Binder C. Proinsulin and C-peptide at onset and during 12 months cyclosporin treatment of Type 1 (insulin-dependent) diabetes mellitus. Diabetologia 1990; 33: 36–42.

208. Mako ME, Starr JI, Rubenstein AH. Circulating proinsulin in patients with maturity onset diabetes. Am J Med 1977; 63: 865–9.

209. Glaser B, Leibowich G, Nesher R, Hartling SG, Binder C, Cerasi E. Improved beta-cell function after intensive insulin treatment in severe non-insulin-dependent diabetes. Acta Endocrinol (Copenh) 1988; 118: 365–73.

210. Ward WK, LaCava EC, Paquette TL, Beard JC, Wallum BJ, Porte D Jr. Disproportionate elevation of immunoreactive proinsulin in type 2 (non-insulin-dependent) diabetes mellitus and in experimental insulin resistance. Diabetologia 1987; 30: 698–702.

211. Gorden P, Sherman BM, Simopoulos AP. Glucose intolerance with hypokalemia: an increased proportion of circulating proinsulin-like component. J Clin Endocrinol Metab 1972; 34: 235–40.

212. Hartling SG, Garne S, Binder C, Heilman C, Petersen W, Petersen KE, Koch C. Proinsulin, insulin and C-peptide in cystic fibrosis after an oral glucose tolerance test. Diabetes Res 1988; 7: 165–9.

213. Rosenbloom AL, Starr JI, Juhn D, Rubenstein AH. Serum proinsulin in children and adolescents with chemical diabetes. Diabetes 1975; 24: 753–7.

214. Heding LG, Persson B, Stangenberg M. B-cell function in newborn infants of diabetic mothers. Diabetologia 1980; 19: 427–32.

215. Sestoft L, Heding LG. Hypersecretion of proinsulin in thyrotoxicosis. Diabetologia 1981; 21: 103–7.

216. Hartling SG, Koivisto V, Binder C. Proinsulin secretion in hyperthyroid and hypothyroid patients. First European Congress of Endocrinology, Copenhagen, 1987, 26–725A.

217. Rovira A, Valdivielso L, Ortega R, Valverde I, Herrera Pombo JL. Plasma glucose, insulin, proinsulin, C-peptide and glucagon before and after a carbohydrate-rich meal in hyperthyroid patients. Diabète Métab 1987; 13: 431–5.

218. Melani F, Rubenstein AH, Steiner DF. Human serum proinsulin. J Clin Invest 1970; 49: 497–507.

219. Koivisto VA, Yki-Järvinen H, Hartling SG, Pelkonen R. The effect of exogenous hyperinsulinemia on proinsulin secretion in normal man, obese subjects and patients with insulinoma. J Clin Endocrinol Metab 1986; 63: 1117–20.

220. Ballmann M, Hartmann H, Deacon CF, Schmidt WE, Conlon JM, Creutzfeldt W. Hypersecretion of proinsulin does not explain the hyperinsulinaemia of patients with liver cirrhosis. Clin Endocrinol 1986; 25: 351–61.

221. Kasperska-Czyzykowa T, Heding LG, Czyzyk A. Serum levels of true insulin, C-peptide and proinsulin in peripheral blood of patients with cirrhosis. Diabetologia 1983; 25: 506–9.

222. Heding LG, Faber O, Kasperska-Czyzykowa T, Sestoft L, Turner R. Radioimmunoassays of proinsulin and hyperproinsulinemic states. In Baba S, Kaneko T, Yanaibara N (eds) Proinsulin, insulin, C-peptide. Amsterdam: Excerpta Medica, 1978: pp 254–61.

223. Gabbay KH, DeLuca K, Fisher JN, Mako ME, Rubenstein AH. Familial hyperproinsulinemia. An autosomal dominant defect. New Engl J Med 1976; 294: 911–15.

224. Robbins DC, Blix PM, Rubenstein AH, Kanazawa Y, Kosaka K, Tager HS. A human proinsulin variant at arginine 65. Nature 1981; 291: 679–81.

225. Shibasaki Y, Kawakami T, Kanazawa Y, Akanuma Y, Takaku F. Posttranslational cleavage of proinsulin is blocked by a point mutation in familial hyperproinsulinemia. J Clin Invest 1985; 76: 378–80.

226. Robbins DC, Shoelson SE, Rubenstein AH, Tager HS. Familial hyperproinsulinemia. Two cohorts secreting indistinguishable Type II intermediates of proinsulin conversion. J Clin Invest 1984; 73: 714–19.

227. Gruppuso PA, Gorden P, Kahn CR, Cornblath M, Zeller WP, Schwartz R. Familial hyperproinsulinemia due to a proposed defect in conversion of proinsulin to insulin. New Engl J Med 1984; 311: 629–34.

228. Elbein SC, Gruppuso PA, Schwartz R, Skolnick M, Permutt MA. Hyperproinsulinemia in a family with a proposed defect in conversion is linked to the insulin gene. Diabetes 1985; 34: 821–4.

229. Chan SJ, Seino S, Gruppuso PA, Schwartz R, Steiner DF. A mutation in the B chain coding region is associated with impaired proinsulin conversion in a family with hyperproinsulinemia. Proc Natl Acad Sci USA 1987; 84: 2194–7.

230. Hartling SG, Lindgren F, Dahlqvist G, Persson B, Binder C. Elevated proinsulin in healthy siblings of IDDM patients independent of HLA identity. Diabetes 1989; 38: 1271–4.

231. Heaton DA, Millward BA, Gray P, Tun Y, Hales CN, Pyke DA, Leslie RDG. Evidence of beta-cell dysfunction which does not lead to diabetes: a study of identical twins of insulin dependent diabetics. Br Med J 1987; 294: 145–6.

232. Spinas GA, Hartling SG, Wilkin TJ, Berger W. Immunologic markers and proinsulin secretion in subjects at risk for Type 1 (insulin-dependent) diabetes: results of a 6-years follow-up study. Diabetes Care 1992; 15: 632–7.

233. Service FJ, Horwitz DL, Rubenstein AH, Kuzuya H, Mako ME, Reynolds C, Molnar GD. C-peptide suppression test for insulinoma. J Lab Clin Med 1977; 90: 180–6.

234. Faber OK, Kehlet H. Strategy in the diagnosis of insulinoma. Scand J Gastroenterol 1979; 14 (suppl. 53): 45–8.

235. Galloway JA, Hooper SA, Spradlin CT, Howey DC, Frank BH, Bowsher RR, Anderson JH. Biosynthetic human proinsulin. Diabetes Care 1992; 15: 666–92.

236. Linde S, Røder ME, Hartling SG, Binder C, Welinder BS. Separation and quantitation of serum proinsulin and proinsulin intermediates in humans. J Chromatogr 1991; 548: 371–80.

237. Kitabchi AE. The biological and immunological properties of pork and beef insulin, proinsulin and connecting peptides. J Clin Invest 1970; 49: 979–87.

238. Hoogwerf BJ, Bantle JP, Gaenslen HE et al. Infusion of synthetic human C-peptide does not affect plasma glucose, serum insulin, or plasma glucagon in healthy subjects. Metabolism 1986; 35: 122–5.

239. Hagen C, Faber OK, Binder C, Alberti KGMM. Lack of metabolic effects of C-peptide in normal subjects and juvenile diabetic patients. Acta Endocrinol 1977; 85 (suppl. 209): 29A.

240. Zierath J, Galuska D, Johansson B-L, Wallberg-Henriksson H. Effect of human C-peptide on glucose transport in *in vitro* incubated human skeletal muscle. Diabetologia 1991; 34: 899–901.

241. Johansson B-L, Sjöberg S, Wahren J. The influence of human C-peptide on renal function and glucose utilization in type 1 (insulin-dependent) diabetic patients. Diabetologia 1992; 35: 121–8.

242. Johansson B-L, Linde B, Wahren J. Effect of C-peptide on blood flow, capillary diffusion capacity and glucose utilization in the exercising forearm of type 1 (insulin-dependent) diabetic patients. Diabetologia 1992; 35: 1151–8.

243. Johansson B-L, Brundin T, Wahren J. Human C-peptide stimulates exercise-induced oxygen uptake in type 1 diabetic patients. Diabetologia 1993; 36 (suppl. 1): A22.

244. Johansson B-L, Forbes E, Linde B, Wahren J. Absorption kinetics and glucose utilization after subcutaneous injection of combined C-peptide and insulin in IDDM patients. Diabetes 1993; 42 (suppl. 1): 35A.

245. Johansson B-L, Kernell A, Sjöberg S, Wahren J. Influence of combined C-peptide and insulin administration on renal function and metabolic control in diabetes type 1. J Clin Endocrinol Metab 1993; 77: 976–81.

246. Sjöberg S, Johansson B-L, Östman J, Wahren J. Renal and splanchnic exchange of human biosynthetic C-peptide in type 1 (insulin-dependent) diabetes mellitus. Diabetologia 1991, 34: 423–8.

247. Blackman JD, Polonsky KS, Jaspan JB, Sturis J, Cauter EV, Thistlethwaite JR. Insulin secretory profiles and C-peptide clearance kinetics at 6 months and 2 years after kidney–pancreas transplantation. Diabetes 1992; 41: 1346–54.

248. O'Meara NM, Blackman JD, Sturis J, Polonsky KS. Alterations in the kinetics of C-peptide and insulin secretion in hyperthyroidism. J Clin Endocrinol Metab 1993; 76: 79–84.

249. Cauter EV, Mestrez F, Sturis J, Polonsky KS. Estimation of insulin secretion rates from C-peptide levels. Comparison of individual and standard kinetic parameters for C-peptide clearance. Diabetes 1992; 41: 368–77.

250. Christiansen E, Andersen HB, Rasmussen K et al. Pancreatic β-cell function and glucose metabolism in human segmental pancreas and kidney transplantation. Am J Physiol 1993; 264 (Endocrinol Metab 27): E441–9.

251. Watanabe RM, Steil GM, Kruszynska Y. Accurate assessment of prehepatic insulin secretion from a single protocol using a combined model with 2-compartment C-peptide kinetics. Diabetes 1993; 42 (suppl. 1): 172A.

252. Schiffrin A, Suissa S, Weiltzner G, Poussier P, Lalla D. Factors predicting course of β-cell function in IDDM. Diabetes Care 1992; 15: 997–1001.

253. Martin S, Pawlowski B, Greulich B, Ziegler AG, Mandrup-Poulsen T, Mahon J. Natural course of remission in IDDM during 1st year after diagnosis. Diabetes Care 1992; 15: 66–74.

254. Sjöberg S, Gjötterberg M, Berglund L, Möller E, Östman J. Residual C-peptide excretion is associated with better long-term glycemic control and slower progress of retinopathy in type 1 (insulin-dependent) diabetes mellitus. J Diab Compl 1991; 5: 18–22.

255. Kernell A, Ludvigsson J, Finnström K. Vitreous fluorophotometry in juvenile diabetics with and without retinopathy in relation to metabolic control, insulin antibodies and C-peptide levels. Acta Ophthalmologica 1990; 68: 415–20.

256. Mendola G, Casamitgana R, Gomis R. Effects of nicotinamide therapy upon B-cell function in newly diagnosed type 1 (insulin-dependent) diabetes mellitus patients. Diabetologia 1989; 32: 160–2.

257. Chase HP, Butler-Simon N, Garg S et al. A trial of nicotinamide in newly diagnosed patients with type 1 (insulin-dependent) diabetes mellitus. Diabetologia 1990; 33: 444–6.

258. Lewis MC, Canafax DM, Sprafka JM, Barbosa JJ. Double-blind randomized trial of nicotinamide on early-onset diabetes. Diabetes Care 1992; 15: 121–3.

259. Dumont-Herskowitz R, Jackson RA, Soeldner JS, Eisenbarth GS. Pilot trial to prevent type 1 diabetes: progression to overt IDDM despite oral nicotinamide. J Autoimmun 1989; 2: 733–7.

260. Elliott RB, Chase HP. Prevention or delay of type 1 (insulin-dependent) diabetes mellitus in children using nicotinamide. Diabetologia 1991; 34: 362–5.

261. Elliott RB, Pilcher CC. Prevention of diabetes in normal school children. Diabet Res Clin Pract 1991; 14 (suppl. 1): S85.

262. Dhahir JF, Cook DB, Self CH. Amplified enzyme-linked immunoassay of human proinsulin in serum (detection limit: 0.1 pmol/l). Clin Chem 1992; 38: 227–32.

263. Bowsher RR, Wolny JD, Frank BH. A rapid and sensitive radioimmunoassay for the measurement of proinsulin in human serum. Diabetes 1992; 41: 1084–90.

264. Kjems LL, Røder ME, Dinesen B, Hartling SG, Jørgensen PN, Binder C. Highly sensitive enzyme immunoassay of proinsulin immunoreactivity with use of two monoclonal antibodies. Clin Chem 1993; 39: 2146–50.

265. Alpha B, Cox L, Crowther N, Clark PMS, Hales CN. Sensitive amplified immunoenzymometric assays

(IEMA) for human insulin and intact proinsulin. Eur J Clin Chem Clin Biochem 1992; 30: 27–32.

266. Cook DB, Self CH. Determination of one thousandth of an attomole (1 zeptomole) of alkaline phosphatase: application in an immunoassay of proinsulin. Clin Chem 1993; 39: 965–71.

267. Reaven GM, Chen YDI, Hollenbeck CB, Sheu WHH, Ostrega D, Polonsky KS. Plasma insulin, C-peptide, and proinsulin concentrations in obese and non-obese individuals with varying degrees of glucose tolerance. J Clin Endocrinol Metab 1993; 76: 44–8.

268. Clark PM, Levy JC, Cox L, Burnett M, Turner RC, Hales CN. Immunoradiometric assay of insulin, intact proinsulin and 32–33 split proinsulin and radioimmunoassay of insulin in diet-treated type 2 (non-insulin-dependent) diabetic subjects. Diabetologia 1992; 35: 469–74.

269. Burguera B, Frank BH, DiMarchi R, Long S, Caro JF. The interaction of proinsulin with insulin-like growth factor-I receptor in human liver, muscle, and adipose tissue. J Clin Endocrinol Metab 1991; 72: 1238–41.

270. Lindgren F, Hartling SG, Persson B, Røder ME, Snellman K, Dahlquist G, Binder C. Proinsulin levels in newborn siblings of type 1 (insulin-dependent) diabetic children and mothers. Diabetologia 1993; 36: 560–3.

271. Oohashi H, Ohgawara H, Nanjo K, Tasaka Y, Cao Q-P, Chan SJ et al. Familial hyperproinsulinemia associated with NIDDM. Diabetes Care 1993; 16: 1340–6.

272. Deacon CF, Schleser-Mohr S, Ballmann M, Willms B, Conlon JM, Creutzfeldt W. Preferential release of proinsulin relative to insulin in non-insulin-dependent diabetes mellitus. Acta Endocrinol 1988; 119: 549–54.

273. Saad MF, Kahn SE, Nelson RG, Pettitt DJ, Knowler WC, Schwartz MW et al. Disproportionately elevated proinsulin in Pima indians with non-insulin-dependent diabetes mellitus. J Clin Endocrinol Metab 1990; 70: 1247–53.

274. Barseghian G, Levine R. Effect of corticosterone on insulin and glucagon secretion by the isolated perfused rat pancreas. Endocrinology 1980; 106: 547–52.

275. Kalhan SC, Adam PAJ. Inhibitory effect of prednisone on insulin secretion in man: model for duplication of blood glucose concentration. J Clin Endocrinol Metab 1975; 41: 600–10.

276. Kahn SE, McCulloch DK, Schwartz MW, Palmer JP, Porte D Jr. Effect of insulin resistance and hyperglycemia on proinsulin release in a primate model of diabetes mellitus. J Clin Endocrinol Metab 1992; 74: 192–7.

277. Porte D Jr, Kahn SE. Hyperproinsulinemia and amyloid in NIDDM. Clues to etiology of islet β-cell dysfunction? Diabetes 1989; 38: 1333–6.

278. Røder ME, Eriksson J, Hartling SG, Groop L, Binder C. Proportional proinsulin responses in first-degree relatives of patients with type 2 diabetes mellitus. Acta Diabetol 1993; 30: 132–7.

279. Davies MJ, Rayman G, Gray IP, Day JL, Hales CN. Insulin deficiency and increased plasma concentration of intact and 32/33 split proinsulin in subjects with impaired glucose tolerance. Diabetic Medicine 1993; 10: 313–20.

280. Nagi DK, Hendra TJ, Ryle AJ, Cooper TM, Temple RC, Clark PMS et al. The relationships of concentrations of insulin, intact proinsulin, and 32–33 split proinsulin with cardiovascular risk factors in type 2 (non-insulin-dependent) diabetic subjects. Diabetologia 1990; 33: 532–7.

281. Jain SK, Nagi DK, Slavin BM, Lumb PJ, Yudkin JS. Insulin therapy in type 2 diabetic subjects suppresses plasminogen activator inhibitor (PAI-1) activity and proinsulin-like molecules independently of glycaemic control. Diabet Med 1993; 10: 27–32.

282. Drexel H, Hopferwieser Th, Braunsteiner H, Patsch JR. Effect of biosynthetic human proinsulin on plasma lipids in type 2 diabetes mellitus. Klin Wschr 1988; 66: 1171–4.

283. Hales CN, Barker DJP, Clark PMS, Cox LJ, Fall C, Osmond C, Winter PD. Fetal and infant growth and impaired glucose tolerance at age 64. Br Med J 1991; 303: 1019–22.

284. Davis SN, Piatti PM, Monti L, Brown M, Hetherington C, Antsiferov M et al. The effects of subcutaneous human proinsulin on the production of 64/65 split proinsulin, glucose turnover and intermediary metabolism in non-insulin-dependent diabetic man. Diabet Res Clin Pract 1993; 19: 103–13.

285. Ferner RE, Alberti KGMM. Why is there still disagreement over insulin secretion in non-insulin-dependent diabetes? Diabet Med 1986; 3: 13–17.

286. Madsbad S. The clinical significance of residual beta-cell function in patients with diabetes mellitus. Pract Cardiol 1985; 11: 101–16.

17

Biosynthesis, Secretion and Action of Glucagon

Pierre J. Lefèbvre

Department of Medicine, University of Liège, Belgium

Glucagon, discovered in 1923 as a contaminant of early insulin preparations, has long been a neglected hormone. Our knowledge of the physiology of glucagon is based on the work of Stahl, Foà, Sutherland and de Duve and on the work performed since the late 1950s in Dallas by Unger and his co-workers, joined in the seventies by Orci and his team in Geneva. Glucagon was among the very first polypeptide hormones to be isolated, purified, sequenced and synthesized. Thanks to the pioneer work of Unger, it was the second polypeptide hormone to become measurable by radioimmunoassay, only a few months after insulin. It has served as a valuable tool, which permitted Sutherland and his associates to discover cyclic AMP, and Rodbell and his co-workers to investigate polypeptide hormone cell-membrane receptors. More recently the nucleotide sequence of the glucagon gene has been determined and, consequently, the structure of the human glucagon precursor (preproglucagon) has been deduced. This discovery has been fundamental for clarifying the relationships of glucagon itself with various other peptides derived from the same common precursor, and originating from both the pancreas and the gut. A comprehensive bibliography on glucagon, up to 1983, has been edited by Lefèbvre [1] and recently updated [62, 63].

AMINO ACID COMPOSITION, EXTRACTION, SYNTHESIS AND BIOSYNTHESIS

As reviewed by Bromer [2], the amino acid sequence is identical for glucagon isolated from the pancreas of pigs, cattle and humans. Guinea-pig glucagon is different from all other glucagons that have been isolated, while avian glucagons differ from the predominant mammalian glucagon only by a few conservative replacements. This extreme conservation of primary structure exhibited by glucagon has been considered 'at least unusual and, at most, extraordinary' [2]. Mammalian glucagon contains 29 amino acid residues and has a molecular mass of 3485 daltons (Figure 1). Glucagon can be synthesized *in vitro* by either classic solution synthesis or solid-phase synthesis; in both cases, two substrategies can be used—either fragment assembly or stepwise assembly [3]. All procedures have given highly purified materials that are homogeneous and indistinguishable from natural glucagon by a range of sensitive analytic methods. The *glucagon gene* has been extensively investigated by Habener and his co-workers [review in 4]. The gene for glucagon encodes for a preprohormone of 180 amino acids that contains not only glucagon but several other

International Textbook of Diabetes Mellitus, Second Edition. Edited by K.G.M.M. Alberti, P. Zimmet, R.A. DeFronzo, and H. Keen (Honorary)
© 1997 John Wiley & Sons Ltd

H-His-Ser-Gln-Gly-Thr-Phe-Thr-Ser-Asp-Tyr-Ser-Lys-Tyr-Leu-Asp-
  1   2   3   4   5   6   7   8   9   10   11   12   13   14   15

Ser-Arg-Arg-Ala-Gln-Asp-Phe-Val-Gln-Trp-Leu-Met-Asn-Thr-OH
16   17   18   19   20   21   22   23 24 25   26   27   28   29

Figure 1 The primary structure of human–porcine glucagon

peptides including two glucagon-like peptides whose amino acid structures are distinct from, but closely resemble, that of glucagon and other members of the glucagon superfamily of peptides. The glucagon gene is expressed in both the A cells of the islets of Langerhans and the intestinal L cells. Interestingly, processing of proglucagon into its bioactive peptides differs markedly in the pancreas and in the gut (Figure 2).

In the pancreas glucagon is the predominant peptide produced, together with glucagon-related polypeptide (GRPP), while the glucagon-like peptides remain in an incompletely processed prohormone fragment. *In the gut* two glucagon-like peptides are produced, while glucagon remains in part as a prohormone fragment, glicentin. However, glicentin can be further processed to oxyntomodulin and GRPP. Of these peptides of the glucagon superfamily, oxyntomodulin and possibly glicentin are implicated in the physiological negative control of gastric acid secretion [5]. On the other hand, the glucagon-like peptide GLP-1-(7-37), a peptide of 31 amino acids, or the equally potent isopeptide GLP-1-(7-36) amide of 30 amino acids, has major insulinotropic action on pancreatic B cells [6, 40, 61]. This peptide binds to specific receptors on

islet B cells, stimulating cyclic AMP formation, insulin release, proinsulin gene transcription and proinsulin biosynthesis, all in a glucose-dependent manner [7]. It has recently been suggested that GLP-1-(7-36) amide has an antidiabetogenic effect and that it may therefore be useful in the treatment of patients with non-insulin dependent diabetes mellitus [8, 9].

Studies by Bataille and his co-workers [10, 41] have shown that both glucagon and oxyntomodulin are further processed into N-terminal and C-terminal fragments by cleavage at a dibasic site (Arg 17-Arg 18). The C-terminal fragments are of particular interest: glucagon-(19-29) modulates the plasma membrane calcium in the nanomolar range, whereas oxyntomodulin-(19-37) inhibits gastric acid secretion, as does oxyntomodulin itself. Finally, studies performed by Pavoine et al [11] have shown that glucagon processing to glucagon-(19-29) (miniglucagon) is probably essential for the positive inotropic effect of glucagon on heart contraction. Thus, the concept has emerged that glucagon and oxyntomodulin are first released into the blood and secondarily processed at the level of their respective targets into the corresponding biologically active C-terminal fragments.

PHYSIOLOGICAL EFFECTS OF GLUCAGON

Glucagon acts through binding to specific receptors located at the target cell plasma membrane. The major

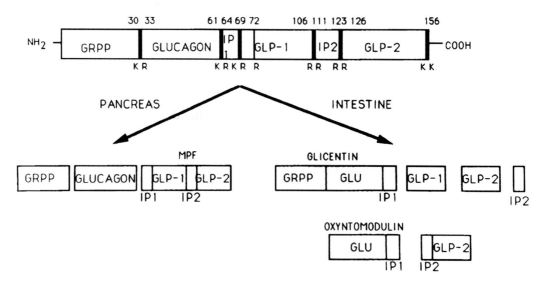

Figure 2 Differential processing of proglucagon in the pancreas and large intestine. Peptides released from the pancreas are glucagon, and the amino- and carboxy-terminal ends of the precursor, respectively. Very small amounts of GLP-1 are also liberated. Glicentin (GRPP + glucagon + IP1), GLP-1, GLP-2, IP2 and oxyntomodulin (glucagon + IP1) are secreted from the intestinal L cells. The amino- and carboxy-terminal ends of proglucagon are indicated by NH₂ and COOH, respectively. Numbers refer to the first and last amino acids of processed peptides, starting from the first amino acid of proglucagon. K (lysine) and R (arginine) indicate basic amino acids where processing sites have been localized. IP, intervening peptide (from reference 4, with permission, © 1991, The Endocrine Society)

common effect of glucagon is to activate adenylate (also called adenylyl) cyclase and to increase the intracellular production of cyclic AMP. As reviewed by Rodbell [12], there is now considerable evidence that binding of glucagon to its receptor activates an intermediate transduction process which involves the participation of guanosine triphosphate (GTP), divalent cations and adenosine (or other similar natural substances). The glucagon receptor has been characterized; it is a 62 kDa glycoprotein that contains at least four N-linked oligosaccharide chains and intramolecular disulfide bonds [51, 52]. Using various monoclonal antibodies, Iwanij and Vincent [53] have identified the location of the glucagon binding site near to the COOH-terminal domain of the receptor.

The hepatocyte is a major target cell of glucagon. The main effect of glucagon on the liver is to increase glucose output, an effect that results from inhibition of glycogen synthesis, stimulation of liver glycogenolysis and gluconeogenesis [13, 14]. The recent studies of Cherrington and his colleagues [54, 55] have established the importance of basal glucagon in maintaining hepatic glucose production during a prolonged fast and have shown that gluconeogenesis and glycogenolysis are equally sensitive to stimulation by glucagon *in vivo* [56]. There is ample evidence that most of these effects are mediated by cyclic AMP but the possibility has been raised that part of the glycogenolytic effect of glucagon may occur by a cAMP-independent mechanism, the nature of which has not yet been established [13]. *In vitro* studies performed by Weigle et al [42–44] and Komjati et al [45] have shown that pulsatile delivery of glucagon is more efficient than continuous exposure to stimulate hepatic glucose production. Similarly, pulsatile delivery of glucagon in humans has greater effects in stimulating endogenous glucose production than continuous infusion [46]. Furthermore, when both insulin and glucagon are delivered intermittently and out of phase, the greater effect of glucagon in stimulating glucose production prevails over the greater effect of insulin in inhibiting this parameter [46]. Another major effect of glucagon on the liver is to stimulate ketogenesis. The elegant studies of McGarry and Foster [15] have convincingly shown that liver ketogenesis depends upon both the flux of free fatty acids (FFA) into the liver and the pathway status of this organ, which is influenced in a crucial manner by the glucagon/insulin ratio in the blood perfusing the liver. The studies of these authors have shown that a high glucagon/insulin ratio increases the intracellular level of cAMP, reduces glycogenolysis and acetyl-CoA carboxylase activity, and reduces the intracellular concentration of malonyl-CoA. This fall in malonyl-CoA brings fatty acid synthesis to a halt and causes derepression of the enzyme carnitine acyltransferase such

that incoming fatty acids (made abundant through stimulation of lipolysis) are efficiently converted into the ketone bodies, acetoacetate and 3-hydroxybutyrate.

The effects of glucagon on the adipocyte markedly depend upon the species considered. Although glucagon is a potent lipolytic hormone in birds and in rodents, its effects on the human adipose cell have long been disputed [16]. Recent investigations have shown that glucagon is, indeed, strongly lipolytic in the human adipocyte *in vitro*, but that this effect is difficult to demonstrate using incubation of adipose cells or adipose tissue pieces because glucagon is rapidly destroyed by a proteolytic activity associated with those cells [17]. When perifusion techniques are used, the lipolytic effect of glucagon on human adipocytes can easily be demonstrated [17], an effect confirmed using an advanced *in vitro* system, pH stat titration [47]. A recent study performed by Paolisso et al [48] in man has shown that, in the presence of somatostatin-induced insulin deficiency, pulsatile glucagon exerts greater effects than its continuous delivery not only on blood glucose (see above) but also on plasma FFA, glycerol and 3-hydroxybutyrate levels. Interestingly, in the elderly, the lipolytic and ketogenic, but not the hyperglycemic, responses to pulsatile glucagon are significantly reduced [48]. Recent observations of Carlson et al [57] have convincingly shown, in healthy volunteers, that moderate hyperglucagonemia undoubtedly stimulates the rate of appearance in the plasma of both glycerol and free fatty acids.

All these effects of glucagon (stimulation of liver glucose output, hepatic ketogenesis and adipose tissue lipolysis) qualify it as a 'hormone of energy need' [18].

OTHER EFFECTS OF GLUCAGON

Other metabolic effects of glucagon include modification of the circulatory pattern of plasma amino acids (partly due to the stimulation of gluconeogenesis) and a reduction in circulating levels of cholesterol and triglycerides [19]. Glucagon also stimulates insulin release [20, 21]. It has a major role, together with insulin, in liver regeneration [22]. Under certain circumstances, glucagon increases renal blood flow and glomerular filtration rate, and promotes renal loss of sodium and other ions [23, 58]. At pharmacological doses, glucagon stimulates adrenal catecholamine release, an effect which has been used for the diagnosis of pheochromocytoma [24]. Combining glucagon stimulation and clonidine suppression testing has given a sensitivity of 100% and a specificity of 79% for the diagnosis of pheochromocytoma [59]. As reviewed by Farah [25] glucagon also exerts positive inotropic and chronotropic effects on the heart, effects that might be useful, for instance, in treating

Table 1 Stimulants of glucagon release

Substrates	Hypoglycemia or cytoglycopenia (2-deoxyglucose) Low circulating levels of free fatty acids (FFA) Most amino acids Fumarate and glutamate
Neural factors	Stimulation of adrenergic and cholinergic nervous systems; stimulation of ventromedial (and ventrolateral?) hypothalamus
Local transmitters or factors	Epinephrine, norepinephrine, acetylcholine, dopamine, vasoactive intestinal peptide (VIP), neurotensin, bombesin, substance P, prostaglandins, cyclic AMP, β-endorphin
Hormones	Gastrin, cholecystokinin-pancreozymin (CCK-PZ), gastric inhibitory peptide (GIP), growth hormone
Ions	Total absence of calcium; lack of phosphate; lack of magnesium; presence of potassium (?)
Pharmacological	Furosemide, scorpion venom, phospholipase A_2, L-dopa, clonidine, oxymetazoline, clonbuterol
Environmental factors	Starvation, exercise, stress, balanced meal

Table 2 Inhibitors of glucagon release

Substrates	Hyperglycemia (also fructose and xylitol) High circulating levels of FFA (and ketone bodies)
Local transmitters or factors	Serotonin, somatostatin
Hormones	Insulin, secretin, glucagon-like peptide 2(GLP-2), estrogens
Ions	Calcium, magnesium
Pharmacological	Atropine, β-receptor blocking agents, α_2-receptor blocking agents, indomethacin, meclofenemate, ibuprofen, diphenylhydantoin, procaine, diazepam, phenformin, various somatostatin analogs, diazoxide (?), sulfonylureas (?)
Environmental factors	Carbohydrate meal, pregnancy

the cardiodepressive manifestations of poisoning by β-receptor blocking agents; glucagon and several of its analogs (like glucagon 1–21, which is devoid of metabolic effects) exert a potent smooth-muscle spasmolytic action, largely used for various diagnostic procedures or for therapeutic applications [26].

CONTROL OF GLUCAGON RELEASE

Table 1 lists the factors and conditions demonstrated as stimulants of glucagon secretion. The main physiological or pathophysiological stimulants of glucagon release are hypoglycemia (insulin-induced, associated with starvation or intense muscular exercise), hyperaminoacidemia (the rise in plasma glucagon levels after a balanced meal is probably due mainly to amino acid-induced glucagon release), stimulation of the adrenergic system (stress, exercise), and stimulation of the vagal system (which together with hormones like GIP and CCK-PZ probably participate in the mixed meal-induced glucagon rise). The factors and conditions associated with inhibition of glucagon release are listed in Table 2. The main physiological inhibitors of glucagon release are probably hyperglycemia and hyperinsulinemia (in a glucose-rich or carbohydrate-rich meal) and high

circulating levels of FFA. Recent data suggest that glucose inhibition of glucagon secretion involves activation of $GABA_A$-receptor chloride channels [49]. Pharmacological inhibition of glucagon release may participate in various drug-induced hypoglycemic syndromes. Samols and his co-workers [27] have emphasized the delicate mechanisms by which intra-islet insulin, glucagon and somatostatin release may be interrelated. In those paracrine mechanisms, recent data have suggested that the oscillatory pattern of islet hormone release may be particularly important [28].

SOME ASPECTS OF GLUCAGON PHYSIOLOGY AND PATHOPHYSIOLOGY

Glucagon as a Counter-regulatory Hormone

Numerous studies, reviewed by Gerich [29] and Lickley et al [30], have shown that 'the liver is the main site at which moment-to-moment control of glucose homeostasis takes place and that in normal humans glucagon is the major glucose counter-regulatory hormone; by antagonizing the suppressive effects of insulin on glucose production and by stimulating glucose production when appropriate, glucagon not only defends the organism against hypoglycemia, but also restores normoglycemia if hypoglycemia occurs' [29]. Perturbation of the mechanisms controlling hypoglycemia-induced glucagon release in some diabetic patients markedly increases the risk of severe hypoglycemia in these subjects [31]. Other hormones, such as epinephrine (acutely) and growth hormone and cortisol (more slowly), participate in the counter-regulation of the effects of insulin, but careful clinical observations suggest that indeed glucagon is the first line of defense against hypoglycemia [32].

Glucagon in Exercise

Glucagon levels increase progressively during prolonged exercise [33], during which blood glucose remains relatively constant thanks to a fine balance between muscle glucose uptake and liver glucose production. Although a rise in plasma glucagon does not appear to be essential for increased glucose production during exercise, the presence of glucagon does appear to be necessary [30].

Glucagon in Stress

Hyperglucagonemia is a classic feature of stress [34]. It occurs mainly as a result of the β-adrenergic stimulation associated with stress [30] and undoubtedly contributes to the hyperglycemia classic in this condition.

Glucagon in Starvation

Starvation is accompanied by a decline in circulating insulin and a moderate rise in plasma glucagon [35]. The main effects of glucagon during starvation are at the liver, where it contributes to the maintenance of continuous liver glucose output (initially by stimulating glycogenolysis, later by promoting gluconeogenesis) and the induction of ketogenesis [36]. Whether glucagon contributes to the stimulation of adipose tissue lipolysis during starvation has been disputed, but recent observations made on human perifused adipocytes, as well as *in vivo* [57], make this plausible [17].

Glucagon and Adaptation to Extrauterine Life

A significant rise in plasma glucagon occurs soon after birth in all the species investigated so far [37], which suggests that glucagon has a crucial role in neonatal glucose homeostasis. Furthermore, an important role of glucagon in thermogenic regulation has been suggested [60].

Glucagon and Diabetes

Glucagon plasma levels are increased in both type 1 and type 2 diabetes mellitus [38]. This disturbance undoubtedly contributes to the hyperglycemia, excessive lipolysis and excessive ketogenesis of the disease [39]. It is now generally considered that the raised glucagon levels of diabetes are largely the consequence of the absolute or relative insulin deficiency that characterizes this syndrome [39]. An extensive review on glucagon and diabetes has been published elsewhere [50].

CONCLUSION

Glucagon is an important hormone exerting numerous metabolic effects, including stimulation of hepatic glycogenolysis and gluconeogenesis, inhibition of liver glycogen synthesis, stimulation of adipose tissue lipolysis and of hepatic ketogenesis. All these effects of glucagon are strongly antagonized by insulin. Glucagon originates in the A cells of the islets of Langerhans of the pancreas, where it is synthesized in the form of a large precursor, preproglucagon. Several peptides derive from the preproglucagon molecule; they include glicentin, oxyntomodulin, glucagon, and glucagon-like peptides 1 and 2. Glucagon release is stimulated in various physiological situations including hypoglycemia, low circulating levels of free fatty acids, high levels of numerous amino acids, stimulation of both vagal and adrenergic nervous systems, etc. Prolonged starvation, long-duration exercise and adaptation to the extrauterine life are also associated with high circulating levels of glucagon. All these effects of glucagon make it above all a hormone of energy need. Diabetes is characterized by excessive glucagon circulating levels which are now considered to stem largely from the absolute or relative insulin deficiency that is observed in this syndrome.

ACKNOWLEDGMENTS

I acknowledge the expert secretarial help of E. Vaessen-Petit.

REFERENCES

1. Lefèbvre PJ (ed.). Glucagon. Handbook of Experimental Pharmacology 66, vols I and II. Berlin: Springer, 1983.
2. Bromer WW. Chemical characteristics of glucagon. In Lefèbvre PJ (ed.) Glucagon, vol. I. Berlin: Springer, 1983: pp 1–22.
3. Merrifield RB, Mojsov S. The chemical synthesis of glucagon. In Lefèbvre PJ (ed.) Glucagon, vol. I. Berlin: Springer, 1983: pp 23–5.
4. Philippe J. Structure and pancreatic expression of the insulin and glucagon genes. Endocr Rev 1991; 12: 252–71.
5. Dubrasquet M, Bataille D, Gespach C. Oxyntomodulin (glucagon-37 or bioactive enteroglucagon): a potent

inhibitor of pentagastrin-stimulated acid secretion in rat. Biosci Rep 1982; 2: 151–5.

6. Göke R, Fehmann H-C, Göke B. Glucagon-like peptide-1(7-36) amide is a new incretin/enterogastrone candidate. Eur J Clin Invest 1991; 21: 135–44.

7. Ørskov C. Glucagon-like peptide-1, a new hormone of the entero-insular axis. Diabetologia 1992; 35: 701–11.

8. Gutniak M, Ørskov C, Holst JJ, Ahren B, Efendic S. Antidiabetogenic effect of glucagon-like peptide-1 (7-36) amide in normal subjects and patients with diabetes mellitus. New Engl J Med 1992; 326: 1316–22.

9. Ensinck JW, D'Alessio DA. The enteroinsular axis revisited. A novel role for an incretin. New Engl J Med 1992; 326: 1352–3.

10. Blache P, Kervran A, Dufour M et al. Glucagon-(19-29), a Ca^{2+} pump inhibitory peptide, is processed from glucagon in the rat liver plasma membrane by a thiol endopeptidase. J Biol Chem 1990; 265: 21514–19.

11. Pavoine C, Brechler V, Kervran A et al. Miniglucagon glucagon-(19-29) is a component of the positive inotropic effect of glucagon. Am J Physiol 1991; 260 (Cell Physiol 29): C993–9.

12. Rodbell M. The actions of glucagon at its receptor: regulation of adenylate cyclase. In Lefèbvre PJ (ed.) Glucagon, vol. I. Berlin: Springer, 1983: pp 263–90.

13. Stalmans W. Glucagon and liver glycogen metabolism. In Lefèbvre PJ (ed.) Glucagon, vol. I. Berlin: Springer, 1983: pp 291–314.

14. Claus TH, Park CR, Pilkis SJ. Glucagon and gluconeogenesis. In Lefèbvre PJ (ed.) Glucagon, vol. I. Berlin: Springer, 1983: pp 315–60.

15. McGarry JD, Foster DW. Glucagon and ketogenesis. In Lefèbvre PJ (ed.) Glucagon, vol. I. Berlin: Springer, 1983: pp 383–98.

16. Lefèbvre PJ. Glucagon and adipose tissue lipolysis. In Lefèbvre PJ (ed.) Glucagon, vol. I. Berlin: Springer, 1983: pp 419–40.

17. Korànyi L. Lipolytic effect of glucagon on perifused isolated human fat cells. Diabetologia 1983; 25: 172.

18. Lefèbvre PJ. Commentary: glucagon and adipose tissue. Biochem Pharmacol 1975; 24: 1261–6.

19. Tiengo A, Nosadini R. Glucagon and lipoprotein metabolism. In Lefèbvre PJ (ed.) Glucagon, vol. I. Berlin: Springer, 1983: pp 441–51.

20. Samols E, Marri G, Marks V. Promotion of insulin secretion by glucagon. Lancet 1965; ii: 415–16.

21. Samols E. Glucagon and insulin secretion. In Lefèbvre PJ (ed.) Glucagon, vol. I. Berlin: Springer, 1983: pp 485–518.

22. Leffert HL, Koch KS, Lad PJ, De Hemptinne B, Skelly H. Glucagon and liver regeneration. In Lefèbvre PJ (ed.) Glucagon, vol. I. Berlin: Springer, 1983: pp 453–84.

23. Kolanowski J. Influence of glucagon on water and electrolyte metabolism. In Lefèbvre PJ (ed.) Glucagon, vol. II. Berlin: Springer, 1983: pp 525–36.

24. Lefèbvre PJ, Luyckx AS. Glucagon and catecholamines. In Lefèbvre PJ (ed.) Glucagon, vol. II. Berlin: Springer, 1983: 537–43.

25. Farah AH, Glucagon and the heart. In Lefèbvre PJ (ed.) Glucagon, vol. II. Berlin: Springer, 1983: pp 553–609.

26. Diamant D, Picazo J. Spasmolytic action and clinical use of glucagon. In Lefèbvre PJ (ed.) Glucagon, vol. II. Berlin: Springer, 1983: pp 611–43.

27. Samols E, Weir GC, Bonner-Weir S. Intra-islet insulin-glucagon–somatostatin relationships. In Lefèbvre PJ

28. Paolisso G, Sgambato S, Passariello N, Varrichio M, Scheen A, D'Onofrio F, Lefèbvre PJ. Pulsatile insulin delivery is more efficient than continuous infusion in modulating islet-cell function in normal subjects and in patients with type-1 diabetes. J Clin Endocrinol Metab, 1988; 66: 1220–6.

29. Gerich JE. Glucagon as a counter-regulatory hormone. In Lefèbvre PJ (ed.) Glucagon, vol. II. Berlin: Springer, 1983: pp 275–95.

30. Lickley HLA, Kemmer FW, Wasserman DH, Vranic M. Glucagon and its relationship to other glucoregulatory hormones in exercise and stress in normal and diabetic subjects. In Lefèbvre PJ (ed.) Glucagon, vol. II. Berlin: Springer, 1983: pp 297–350.

31. White NH, Skor DA, Cryer PE, Levandorsky LA, Bier DM. Identification of type-1 diabetic patients at increased risk for hypoglycemia during intensive therapy. New Engl J Med 1983; 308: 485–91.

32. Gerich J, Davis J, Lorenzi M et al. Hormonal mechanisms of recovery from insulin-induced hypoglycemia in man. Am J Physiol 1979; 236: 380–5.

33. Luyckx AS, Pirnay F, Lefèbvre PJ. Effect of glucose on plasma glucagon and free fatty acids during prolonged exercise. Eur J Appl Physiol 1978; 39: 53–61.

34. Lindsey CA, Faloona GR, Unger RH. Plasma glucagon levels during rapid exsanguination with and without adrenergic blockade. Diabetes 1975; 24: 313–19.

35. Cahill GF Jr. Starvation in man. New Engl J Med 1970; 282: 668–75.

36. Gelfand RA, Sherwin RS. Glucagon and starvation. In Lefèbvre PJ (ed.) Glucagon, vol. II. Berlin: Springer, 1983: pp 223–37.

37. Girard J, Sperling M. Glucagon in the fetus and the newborn. In Lefèbvre PJ (ed.) Glucagon, vol. II. Berlin: Springer, 1983: pp 251–74.

38. Unger RH, Orci L. Glucagon and the A-cell. Physiology and pathophysiology. New Engl J Med 1981; 304: 1518–24, 1575–80.

39. Lefèbvre PJ, Luyckx AS. Glucagon and diabetes: a reappraisal. Diabetologia 1979; 16: 347–54.

40. D'Alessio DA, Fujimoto WY, Ensinck JW. Effects of glucagonlike peptide I-(7-36) on release of insulin, glucagon, and somatostatin by rat pancreatic islet cell monolayer cultures. Diabetes 1989; 38: 1534–8.

41. Bataille D, Jarrousse C, Blache P et al. Oxyntomodulin and glucagon: are the whole molecules and their C-terminal fragments different biological entities? Biomed Res 1988; 9 (suppl. 3): 169–79.

42. Weigle DS, Goodner CJ. Evidence that the physiological pulse frequency of glucagon secretion optimizes glucose production by perifused rat hepatocytes. Endocrinology 1986; 118: 1606–13.

43. Weigle DS, Koerker DJ, Goodner CJ. Pulsatile glucagon delivery enhances glucose production by perifused rat hepatocytes. Am J Physiol 1984; 247 (Endocrinol Metab 10): E564–8.

44. Weigle DS, Koerker DJ, Goodner CJ. A model for augmentation of hepatocyte response to pulsatile glucagon stimuli. Am J Physiol 1985; 248 (Endocrinol Metab 11): E681–6.

45. Komjati M, Bratusch-Marrain P, Waldhausl W. Superior efficacy of pulsatile versus continuous hormone exposure on hepatic glucose production in vitro. Endocrinology 1986; 118: 312–19.

46. Paolisso G, Scheen AJ, Albert A, Lefèbvre PJ. Effects of pulsatile delivery of insulin and glucagon in humans. Am J Physiol 1989; 257 (Endocrinol Metab 20): E686-96.

47. Richter WO, Robl W, Schwandt P. Human glucagon and vasoactive intestinal polypeptide (VIP) stimulate free fatty acid release from human adipose tissue in vitro. In Peptides, vol. 10. Oxford: Pergamon Press, 1989: pp 333-5.

48. Paolisso G, Buonocore S, Gentile S et al. Pulsatile glucagon has greater hyperglycaemic, lipolytic and ketogenic effects than continuous hormone delivery in man: effect of age. Diabetologia 1990; 33: 272-7.

49. Rorsman P, Berggren P-O, Bokvist K et al. Glucose-inhibition of glucagon secretion involves activation of $GABA_A$-receptor chloride channels. Nature 1989; 341: 233-6.

50. Lefèbvre PJ. Abnormal secretion of glucagon. In Samols E (ed.) The endocrine pancreas. New York: Raven Press, 1991: pp 191-205.

51. Iyengar R, Herberg JT. Structural analysis of the hepatic glucagon receptor. Identification of a guanine nucleotide-sensitive hormone-binding region. J Biol Chem 1984; 259: 5222-9.

52. Iwanij V, Hur KC. Direct cross-linking of ^{125}I-labeled glucagon to its membrane receptor by UV irradiation. Proc Natl Acad Sci USA 1985; 82: 325-9.

53. Iwanij V, Vincent AC. Characterization of the glucagon receptor and its functional domain using monoclonal antibodies. J Biol Chem 1990; 265: 21302-8.

54. Hendrick GT, Wasserman DH, Tyler Frizzel R et al. Importance of basal glucagon in maintaining hepatic glucose production during a prolonged fast in conscious dogs. Am J Physiol 1992; 263 (Endocrinol Metab 26): E541-9.

55. Steiner KE, Williams PE, Lacy WW, Cherrington AD. Effects of insulin on glucagon-stimulated glucose production in the conscious dog. Metabolism 1990; 39: 1325-33.

56. Stevenson RW, Steiner KE, Davis MA et al. Similar dose responsiveness of hepatic glycogenolysis and gluconeogenesis to glucagon *in vivo*. Diabetes 1987; 36: 382-9.

57. Carlson MG, Snead WL, Campbell PJ. Regulation of free fatty acid metabolism by glucagon. J Clin Endocrinol Metab 1993; 77: 11-15.

58. Ahloulay M, Bouby N, Machet F, Kubrusly M, Coutaud C, Bankir L. Effects of glucagon on glomerular filtration rate and urea and water excretion. Am J Physiol 1992; 263 (Renal Fluid Electrolyte Physiol 32): F24-36.

59. Grossman E, Goldstein DS, Hoffman A, Keiser HR. Glucagon and clonidine testing in the diagnosis of pheochromocytoma. Hypertension 1991; 17: 733-41.

60. Billington CJ, Briggs JE, Link JG, Levine AS. Glucagon in physiological concentrations stimulates brown fat thermogenesis *in vivo*. Am J Physiol 1991; 261 (Regulatory Integrative Comp Physiol 30): R501-7.

61. Fehmann HC, Göke R, Göke B. Glucagon-like peptide-1(7-37)/(7-36)amide is a new incretin. Mol C Endocr 1992; 85: C39-44.

62. Lefèbvre PJ (ed.) Glucagon III. Handbook of Experimental Pharmacology 123. Berlin: Springer, 1996.

63. Lefèbvre PJ. Glucagon and its family revisited. Diabetes Care 1995; 18: 715-30.

18

The Hypothalamus, Neuropeptides and Diabetes

David Hopkins and Gareth Williams

Diabetes & Endocrinology Research Group, University of Liverpool, UK

INTRODUCTION

The importance of the central nervous system in glucose homeostasis was first recognised more than half a century before the discovery of insulin when, in the 1850s, Claude Bernard demonstrated the experimental induction of diabetes in dogs by transfixing the medulla with a metal probe [1]. This discovery was subsequently overshadowed by work implicating the pancreas in the aetiology of diabetes, but in the last two decades there has been a gradual renaissance of interest in the interplay between diabetes and abnormalities in the central nervous system (CNS).

This increased interest has been fuelled by the discovery of a growing number of peptides with effects on metabolism mediated at various levels. It now seems likely that some of these peptides are important in the control of food intake, energy expenditure and body weight in animals, and some show striking changes in models of insulin dependent and/or non-insulin dependent diabetes.

Neuropeptides can be defined as any peptides thought to act physiologically as neurotransmitters, and the importance of such peptides is highlighted by the estimate that only about 10% of the synapses in the mammalian brain are served by the classical non-peptide transmitters. This broad definition embraces not only brain peptides but also peptides first isolated from the gut, and probably even insulin, which in addition to its classical role as a metabolic hormone is increasingly recognised as a potential regulatory peptide within the brain.

A clear understanding of the physiological role of neuropeptides is complicated by their great diversity. In the hypothalamus alone, some 40 different peptides have so far been identified, and new candidate peptides continue to be discovered. Any review of this complex area must therefore be selective, and in this chapter we shall discuss primarily those peptides whose experimental effects are particularly relevant to diabetes. In particular, we shall review the role of neuropeptides in the hypothalamic control of energy balance and blood glucose regulation, and discuss the possible relevance of neuroendocrine abnormalities to human diabetes.

THE HYPOTHALAMUS AND METABOLIC REGULATION

Although Claude Bernard's original paper on neurogenic diabetes reported the effects of lesioning the medulla, subsequent work has clearly placed the hypothalamus at the centre of metabolic regulation. The hypothalamus is well adapted for such a role as it receives and integrates diverse regulatory signals. It has a rich afferent input from other parts of the CNS, and is in close proximity to the 'circumventricular organs', discrete areas around the ventricular system where the blood–brain barrier is deficient and where circulating substances including metabolites, hormones and regulatory peptides can gain direct

International Textbook of Diabetes Mellitus, Second Edition. Edited by K.G.M.M. Alberti, P. Zimmet, R.A. DeFronzo, and H. Keen (Honorary)
© 1997 John Wiley & Sons Ltd

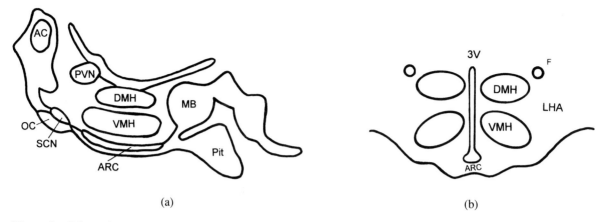

(a)　　　　　　　　　　　　　　　　　(b)

Figure 1　Schematic diagram of the rat hypothalamus in longitudinal section (A) and in transverse section at the mid-point of the arcuate nucleus (B), showing key nuclei discussed in text, VMH = ventromedial nucleus; DMH = dorsomedial nucleus; PVN = paraventricular nucleus; SCN = suprachiasmatic nucleus; ARC = arcuate nucleus; LHA = lateral hypothalamic area; AC = anterior commissure; F = fornix; MB = mamillary body; OC = optic chiasm; 3V = third ventricle; Pit = pituitary

access to neuronal tissue [2]. The hypothalamus can exert effects on metabolism through its output to the autonomic nervous system, and also by regulating pituitary secretion via regulatory peptides secreted into the hypothalamo–hypophyseal circulation.

Basic Anatomy

The structure of the hypothalamus is complex, with many histologically distinct areas. The detailed neuroanatomy has been most precisely characterised in the rat [3], and the most important features are illustrated

schematically in Figure 1. Anteriorly, the paraventricular nucleus (PVN) projects laterally from the apex of the third ventricle, whilst the ventromedial (VMH) and dorsomedial (DMH) nuclei lie in the lateral wall of the ventricle, comprising together about one-third of the medial hypothalamus. Lying lateral to these and separated by the fornix, a band of fibres running between the septum and mamillary bodies, is the lateral hypothalamic area (LHA). In the floor of the third ventricle, the suprachiasmatic nucleus (SCN) lies in the midline immediately above the optic chiasm, and posterior to this, the long thin arcuate nucleus (ARC)

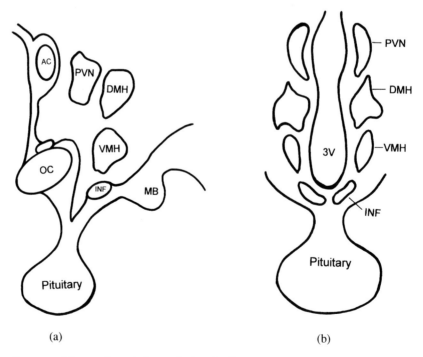

(a)　　　　　　　　　　　　　　　　　(b)

Figure 2　Schematic diagram of human hypothalamus in longitudinal (A) and transverse (B) sections. INF = infundibular nucleus: other abbreviations as Figure 1

runs for much of the length of the third ventricle, directly overlying the median eminence. Anterior to the third ventricle, the preoptic area lies between the optic chiasm and the anterior commissure, a transverse bundle of fibres that delineates the rostral boundary of the hypothalamus.

In man, the general arrangement of nuclei is broadly similar (Figure 2), the infundibular nucleus in the base of the third ventricle being equivalent to the arcuate nucleus in the rat [4].

Energy Homeostasis

Feeding behaviour in animals is largely controlled by the hypothalamus, interacting with various other brain regions including the olfactory cortex, amygdala and nucleus accumbens. Early studies suggested that selective stimulation or lesioning of specific hypothalamic areas could have profound effects on feeding [5], and led to the hypothesis that feeding behaviour was under the reciprocal control of the VMH and LHA. The VMH appeared to act as a 'satiety' centre, whose stimulation could terminate feeding, while LHA stimulation initiated feeding [5–7]. However, the true situation is much more complex, and these areas are now best thought of as forming part of a complex system regulating feeding. Current evidence suggests that there are no discrete 'satiety' or 'feeding' centres as such, although the PVN has emerged as a site of particular importance in the integration of various signals regulating food intake.

The hypothalamus, particularly the VMH and LHA, can also influence energy expenditure. In rats, stimulation of the VMH activates sympathetic outflow to brown adipose tissue (BAT) leading to increased energy expenditure through the uncoupling of oxidative phosphorylation in mitochondria, and resultant heat production. Conversely, LHA stimulation reduces BAT activity [8–10]. The relevance of this adaptive thermogenesis to human metabolism is uncertain, as adult man lacks significant amounts of brown adipose tissue [11].

Glucose Homeostasis

The hypothalamus can influence peripheral blood glucose control through autonomic afferents to the liver and pancreas [12, 13], and through changes in the secretion of ACTH and growth hormone from the anterior pituitary. The islets of Langerhans have a rich autonomic innervation, receiving parasympathetic afferents from the vagus, and sympathetic afferents from the splanchnic nerves; islet secretion is also influenced by circulating catecholamines.

Sympathetic activation results in an increase in glucagon secretion, with reciprocal inhibition of insulin secretion. The latter effect appears to be mediated by circulating catecholamines, and can be abolished by adrenalectomy [14, 15]. Parasympathetic inputs evoke both insulin and glucagon secretion, although the effect on insulin secretion predominates. These responses of the islet cells to autonomic stimulation are, however, dependent on local factors within the pancreas, and in particular on glucose availability.

The liver receives afferents from the vagus and the splanchnic sympathetic system, which can influence the activity of glycogen synthase and glycogen phosphorylase, the enzymes regulating glycogen turnover. Vagal stimulation increases glycogen synthase activity and thus glycogen formation, while sympathetic activation increases glycogen phosphorylase activity and glucose release [16].

Experimentally, the VMH and LHA have reciprocal effects on peripheral blood glucose; VMH stimulation leads to sympathetic activation and hyperglycaemia, whereas LHA stimulation increases vagal activity, with a subsequent increase in insulin secretion [13–15, 17]. Both nuclei have been shown to contain glucose-sensitive neurones [18], and may also receive afferents from putative glucoreceptors in other parts of the brain [19], or even from outside the CNS [20, 21]. These autonomic pathways could allow the hypothalamus to modulate peripheral blood glucose concentrations in response to changes in CNS glucose availability, and may be important in maintaining CNS glucose homeostasis.

THE ROLE OF NEUROPEPTIDES

The regulation of energy balance and glucose metabolism by the hypothalamus is thus an extremely complex process involving many discrete nuclei and undoubtedly mediated in part by both classical non-peptide neurotransmitters and peptides. Thus, noradrenaline acting on the PVN strongly stimulates eating, whilst adrenaline acting in the LHA inhibits feeding [22]. Of the monoamine transmitters, serotonin has attracted particular attention as a potential signal of satiety, as its injection into the PVN potently inhibits feeding in rats, an effect shared by serotonergic drugs such as fenfluramine and fluoxetine. This complex area has recently been extensively reviewed [23, 24].

Many of the peptides identified in the hypothalamus can influence feeding in experimental situations, but often in supraphysiological doses and in a non-specific fashion (Table 1). Similarly, many peptides can affect blood glucose levels when injected intracerebroventricularly (ICV), but the significance of these effects remains uncertain (Table 2). In the case of most peptides (e.g. β-endorphin, CRF and glucagon), ICV injection leads to hyperglycaemia and

Table 1 Major neuropeptides with experimental effects on feeding

	Peptide	Comments	References
Stimulate feeding	Neuropeptide Y	Most potent central appetite stimulant yet discovered. Enhances carbohydrate and fat ingestion	33, 34, 186
	Galanin	Potent appetite stimulant. Selectively enhances fat ingestion	49, 50, 187
	Dynorphin, β-endorphin	Stimulate feeding after injection into PVN and other sites. Increase protein and fat intake	71, 77
Inhibit feeding	Insulin	ICV administration induces satiety. May act by inhibiting NPY synthesis in the hypothalamus	107–109
	CRF	Potent anorexic agent. Attenuates feeding responses to noradrenaline, NPY and opioid peptides	62, 63
	Neurotensin	Inhibits feeding after injection into PVN. Reduces hypothalamic levels in obese rodents	117, 165
	CCK	Acts at peripheral (CCK A) and central (CCK B) receptors to terminate feeding. Weak effect at physiological doses	125, 126
	Bombesin	Inhibits food intake after both central and peripheral administration	128, 132

Table 2 Neuropeptides with central effects on blood glucose

	Peptide	Comments	References
Elevate blood glucose	Bombesin	Hyperglycaemia after both central and peripheral administration	130, 131
	β-endorphin	Hyperglycaemia after central administration. Effects mediated by sympathetic nervous system	118
	CRF		69, 70
	TRH		187
	Glucagon		188
	CCK		189
	Galanin	Suppresses insulin secretion after injection into PVN	57
	Neuropeptide Y	Stimulates both insulin and glucagon secretion after ICV administration, resulting in mild transient hyperglycaemia	40
	Neurotensin	Stimulates glucagon release after peripheral administration. No effect on blood glucose after central administration	118
Lower blood glucose	Insulin	Stimulates pancreatic insulin secretion after ICV administration with resultant hypoglycaemia	107, 190
	Somatostatin	Blocks hyperglycaemic responses to bombesin and β-endorphin	118, 120

in many cases, it is likely that this represents a non-specific effect leading to central sympathetic activation (Table 2).

Of the many peptides identified, only a few are likely to be of physiological significance in normal or diabetic animals, and these will be discussed further below. Of particular interest are neuropeptide Y (NPY) and galanin, which stimulate feeding; corticotrophin-releasing factor (CRF) which has potent central appetite-suppressant properties; the opioid peptides which have complex effects on both energy and glucose homeostasis; and insulin, which may act in the brain as an important regulatory peptide with actions distinct from its classical metabolic functions in other tissues.

NEUROPEPTIDE Y

Neuropeptide Y (NPY) is a 36-amino-acid peptide rich in tyrosine (='Y') which was first isolated from pig brain in 1982 [25]. It is one of the most plentiful of the peptidergic transmitters in the brain, and its possible metabolic functions have come under intense scrutiny.

The hypothalamus is particularly rich in NPY [26–28]. Within the hypothalamus, mRNA studies have localised NPY synthesis mainly to the arcuate nucleus [29, 30], and neurones originating here project through the LHA to terminate in the PVN and DMH [31]. The ratio of NPY mRNA to NPY in the hypothalamus is relatively low, suggesting that a significant proportion of the NPY found in the hypothalamus is synthesised elsewhere, and reaches the hypothalamus in axons projecting to the hypothalamic nuclei. One such projection consists of neurones originating in the medulla which terminate in the PVN [32].

When injected centrally into the third ventricle or PVN of rats, NPY is one of the most potent stimulators of feeding known [33–35], being over 100 times more potent on a molar basis than noradrenaline. Food intake can be increased several-fold even in previously satiated animals, and with repeated injections there is no attenuation of this effect, the animals eventually becoming obese [36]. In rats, NPY also affects energy balance by reducing energy expenditure, probably by reducing sympathetic outflow and thus thermogenesis in brown adipose tissue [37, 38]. As a consequence, weight gain in rats with NPY-induced obesity is greater than would be expected from the increased food consumption alone. These effects of NPY on energy balance are probably mediated predominantly via receptors in the PVN, although autoradiographic studies have revealed a surprisingly low density of NPY-binding sites within the hypothalamus when compared with the abundance of the peptide itself [39].

NPY has many other actions relevant to peripheral metabolism and diabetes. When injected into the PVN, NPY stimulates vagally-mediated pancreatic islet secretion, resulting in increased insulin and glucagon release [40]. The net effect of these changes is to produce mild transient hyperglycaemia, but the physiological relevance of this observation is unknown. Injection into the PVN also stimulates release of ACTH and thus leads to increased circulating glucocorticoids. This effect is probably brought about by stimulating the release of CRF from neurones originating in the PVN which project to the median eminence and thus have access to the hypothalamo–hypophyseal portal vessels [41]. Experimentally, NPY has many other complex effects on pituitary function, inhibiting growth hormone, prolactin and thyrotropin secretion [42], increasing vasopressin release [43] and modulating LH secretion in a manner dependent on circulating sex steroid levels [44, 45]. As discussed below, there is strong evidence that NPY may be involved in some of the abnormalities of hypothalamo–pituitary function seen in rodent models of both IDDM and NIDDM.

GALANIN

Galanin, a 29-amino-acid peptide, was first isolated from porcine intestine [46], and has subsequently been identified in central and peripheral neurones from many species. It is present in greatest concentration in the hypothalamus, particularly in the PVN [47], where galanin-binding sites have also been demonstrated [48]. Like neuropeptide Y, galanin potently induces feeding when injected into the hypothalamus of either fasted or satiated rats [49–51] and also inhibits BAT thermogenesis [52]. This effect appears to be mediated primarily by the PVN, although feeding responses have been elicited after injection into the VMH and LHA also [51].

Although both NPY and galanin induce feeding in rats, the effects of the two peptides are quite distinct. Galanin preferentially stimulates fat ingestion, in contrast to the preference for carbohydrate observed after NPY administration [53]. The effects of galanin on food intake appear closely linked with those of noradrenaline, and can be blocked by α-2-adrenergic receptor antagonists [48].

Further evidence that endogenous galanin plays a role in the normal control of food intake has been provided by recent studies using specific galanin receptor antagonists. These not only block the effects of galanin administration on food intake, but also markedly inhibit fat ingestion when injected alone, raising the possibility that galanin antagonists could be developed for the treatment of obesity [54, 55].

Galanin has many other experimental effects relevant to metabolism. When injected systemically in dogs, galanin produces mild hyperglycaemia due to inhibition of pancreatic insulin secretion [56]. In rats, similar experiments have been inconclusive, but injection of galanin into the PVN resulted in suppression of insulin secretion in a cyclical manner, suggesting a possible effect in the circadian control of metabolism [57].

CORTICOTROPHIN-RELEASING FACTOR

CRF is synthesised in many brain regions including the PVN. From here, neurones project to the median eminence, where CRF is released into the hypothalamo–hypophyseal portal circulation to evoke ACTH release from corticotrophs in the anterior pituitary. CRF synthesis is under potent negative feedback from circulating corticosteroids, and is also regulated by other neurotransmitters including serotonin [58] and NPY [59, 60], which stimulates its release when injected into the PVN [61].

Experimentally, CRF has a pronounced anorectic effect when administered centrally [62, 63], which is powerful enough to override the stimulatory effect of NPY on feeding [64]. CRF also increases energy expenditure in rats by increasing the sympathetic outflow to BAT, thus activating thermogenesis [65, 66]. Abnormalities of CRF may be important in animal models of obesity and NIDDM, in which obesity develops because of both reduced energy expenditure and increased food intake (see below). Furthermore, the pituitary–adrenocortical axis appears to be important in several of the rodent models of obesity and NIDDM as adrenalectomy prevents the development of the obese state [67, 68]. This may partly reflect central effects of CRF, the release of which increases after adrenalectomy in response to the loss of glucocorticoid negative feedback.

Central administration of CRF also increases plasma concentrations of glucagon, adrenaline and noradrenaline, resulting in hyperglycaemia. These responses occur independently of pituitary ACTH release and appear to be mediated by the sympathetic nervous system [69, 70].

OPIOID PEPTIDES

Before the endogenous opioid peptides and their receptors were identified, it was recognised that morphine and its antagonist naloxone could modulate feeding behaviour [71]. It now seems likely that the endogenous opioid peptides may act on various opioid receptors at several sites to play a physiological role in the control of food intake. To date most interest has focused on the possible role of dynorphin and β-endorphin, which bind to κ- and μ-receptors respectively [72, 73]. ICV injection of dynorphin or β-endorphin potently enhances feeding, while antibodies to β-endorphin and other endogenous opiates significantly reduce feeding when injected into the hypothalamus [74].

It is likely that opioids exert their effect on feeding behaviour both within the hypothalamus and at other sites. Within the hypothalamus, micro-injection studies have suggested a key role for the PVN in κ-receptor mediated feeding by dynorphin and other opioid peptides [75], although opiate action in other hypothalamic areas including the DMH and arcuate nucleus may be important. Outside the hypothalamus, feeding responses to opiate agonists have been demonstrated in the nucleus accumbens and ventral striatum [76]. These responses appear to be mediated primarily by the μ-receptor, and it has been suggested that β-endorphin-containing neurones projecting to the nucleus accumbens from the hypothalamus may play a role in regulating feeding at this site.

Abnormalities of opioid peptides have been noted in various animal models of obesity and diabetes (see below). In man, various anecdotal reports have purported to show evidence that opioid peptides may be involved in the development of human obesity; these include observations made on patients with the Prader–Willi syndrome, and traumatic hypothalamic damage [77, 78].

INSULIN

Prior to the discovery of insulin in the rat CNS in 1978 [79], the brain had been considered to be an insulin-independent organ. Previous studies had established that altering circulating insulin levels did not affect total brain glucose utilisation, and it was considered unlikely that insulin would cross the blood–brain barrier in significant amounts.

When first identified in rat brain, concentrations of immunoreactive insulin appeared to be higher than in plasma, and to vary considerably between different areas, suggesting that insulin might be synthesised locally within the brain [79, 80]. However, later work showed insulin concentrations to be close to plasma levels, in keeping with a peripheral origin of insulin [81]. The source of the insulin found in brain remains controversial, although most evidence favours uptake from plasma. *In vivo* autoradiographic studies in rats show rapid penetration of intravenously-injected radiolabelled insulin into the circumventricular organs, notably the median eminence and ARC [82]. Insulin can also penetrate into the cerebrospinal fluid of both animals and man [83–85], and may undergo active receptor-mediated transport across the blood–brain barrier [86, 87].

It is possible that at least some of the insulin found in brain is produced locally. In tissue culture, rat neurones synthesise and release insulin [88, 89]. In intact brain, mRNA hybridising with an insulin probe has been reported in the periventricular hypothalamus [90], but other studies have failed to confirm this, even when using the polymerase chain reaction to amplify the signal [91, 92].

Insulin receptors are widely distributed in rat brain, with particularly high receptor densities in the olfactory bulbs and hypothalamus, especially the ARC [93–95]. The CNS contains two distinct sub-types of insulin receptor, localised to neuronal and glial cells respectively. The neuronal receptors have a lower molecular weight than the glial receptors and appear unique to the CNS, whereas the glial receptors appear to be identical to those found in other tissues [96–98]. This difference results from reduced glycation of both α and β subunits of the neuronal receptor and appears to involve the insulin-binding site [99], but the significance of these changes is not known. Both types of insulin receptor have similar binding properties [100] and tyrosine kinase activity [101], but glial and neuronal cell cultures respond differently to insulin. Thus, glial cells demonstrate increased glucose uptake and Glut-1 mRNA expression in response to insulin binding [102–103]. In contrast, neurones show no change in glucose uptake but there are marked alterations in monoamine transport, with increased serotonin and decreased noradrenaline uptake [104]. Insulin could therefore exert a distinct neuromodulatory effect in the CNS.

Although insulin stimulates glucose entry in glial cells *in vitro*, *in vivo* studies using labelled 2-deoxyglucose (2-DOG) support the classical view that brain glucose uptake is largely independent of insulin [105]. Localised increases in glucose uptake in response to insulin have, however, been demonstrated in the VMH, DMH and anterior hypothalamic nuclei [106]. As these areas have been shown to contain glucose-responsive neurones, it has been postulated that insulin may act at these sites to modulate the response of the hypothalamus to neuroglycopenia, and may thus play a role in glucose homeostasis.

The most studied actions of insulin in the CNS are its effects on food intake and body weight [107]. In several species, direct injection of insulin into the third ventricle or VMH results in a rapid and prolonged suppression of feeding and weight loss [108, 109]; conversely, increased food intake has been demonstrated following the injection of antibodies to insulin into the VMH [110]. Central administration of insulin also leads to activation of the sympathetic nervous system, increased BAT thermogenesis and increased total energy expenditure which may contribute to the observed weight loss [111].

As peripheral insulin levels generally reflect body fat content, and circulating insulin appears able to reach the hypothalamus, it is postulated that insulin may function as a satiety signal involved in the regulation of body weight [107]. Consistent with this, systemic insulin administration does indeed inhibit feeding, provided that hypoglycaemia is avoided [112]. It has been suggested that insulin may induce satiety by inhibiting NPY neurones in the arcuate nucleus, as prepro-NPY mRNA levels fall in the ARC following ICV infusion of insulin [113]. However, conflicting evidence has been derived from studies of systemic insulin administration in which arcuate NPY levels were either unchanged or increased [114–116].

OTHER PEPTIDES

Neurotensin, a peptide first isolated from bovine hypothalamus, has attracted interest as a possible mediator of satiety and as a putative glucoregulatory peptide. It induces anorexia when injected into the PVN [117] and reduced hypothalamic neurotensin may be implicated in the development of obesity in animal models (see below). Systemic administration of neurotensin causes transient hyperglycaemia, but at present there is no convincing evidence that neurotensin within the CNS participates in glucose regulation [118].

Somatostatin has been extensively studied as a putative glucoregulatory peptide in both its paracrine inhibitory actions on insulin and glucagon secretion

within the pancreas, and its effects within the hypothalamus. When injected into the third ventricle, somatostatin blocks the hyperglycaemic effect of many other peptides, and also blocks the sympathetic and pituitary responses to neuroglycopenia [119]. It has been suggested that central administration of somatostatin can itself invoke hypoglycaemia, but experimental evidence has been conflicting, with an increase in blood glucose being observed by some investigators. In animal models of IDDM, there are marked changes in circulating somatostatin levels (originating from the gut), but no consistent changes in hypothalamic somatostatin levels [120].

Cholecystokinin (CCK) terminates feeding when injected peripherally or centrally in many species [121–123], although at physiological concentrations its anorectic effect is weak, and may in part result from local effects on gastric motility [124]. CCK may also produce satiety by acting at peripheral (CCK-A) receptors on vagal afferents which project to the PVN and other brain regions, where they may trigger the release of locally synthesised CCK, which then activates central (CCK-B) receptors [125, 126]. Within the PVN, CCK may induce satiety by antagonising the appetite-stimulating action of noradrenaline [127].

Bombesin, first isolated from frog skin, has potent metabolic effects when administered centrally or peripherally. ICV administration in rats causes hypophagia [128], reduced energy expenditure [129], stimulation of insulin and glucagon secretion, and hyperglycaemia [130, 131]. Peripheral administration reduces food intake in many species, including man [132, 133]. Neuromedin B, a mammalian neuropeptide structurally related to bombesin, can antagonise the inhibitory effects of bombesin on food intake, but does not affect food intake when administered by itself [134]. Hypothalamic neuromedin B levels are elevated in obese Zucker rats, but the central actions of this peptide, and its relevance to the development of the obesity syndrome in Zucker rats have yet to be elucidated [135].

NEUROENDOCRINE DISTURBANCE IN ANIMAL MODELS OF DIABETES

Insulin Dependent Diabetes Mellitus

Early in the development of insulin dependent diabetes, unopposed catabolism of carbohydrate and fat together with urinary glucose losses leads to a state of negative energy balance and weight loss. As a compensatory reaction to this, a dramatic increase in food intake with a preference for carbohydrate-rich foods, accompanied by a reduction in BAT energy expenditure, is seen in animal models of IDDM [136]. Similar changes are

Table 3 Neuropeptide abnormalities in animal models of IDDM

Peptide	Model	Comments	References
Neuropeptide Y	STZ, BB	Elevated NPY levels in ARC, PVN and other hypothalamic areas	144–146
	STZ, BB	Elevated NPY mRNA in hypothalamus	142
	STZ	Increased NPY release from PVN	143, 146
	STZ	Downregulation of hypothalamic NPY receptors	147
Galanin Bombesin Neurotensin Somatostatin Neuromedin B	STZ	Unchanged levels in lateral or medial hypothalamic blocks	144

STZ = streptozotocin-induced diabetic rat; BB = spontaneously diabetic BB rat.

difficult to document in man, but hunger is a common early symptom of IDDM, and many patients volunteer that they have noted a preference for sweet foods prior to diagnosis.

Pituitary secretion is also profoundly altered in insulin-deficient diabetic rats, with reduced secretion of growth hormone, gonadotrophins, TSH and prolactin [137, 138]; ACTH secretion increases, leading to elevated corticosterone levels and loss of the normal diurnal glucocorticoid cycle [139]. All of these changes are obviously secondary to insulin deficiency and are reversed by treatment with insulin.

The possible role of hypothalamic neuropeptides, notably NPY, in mediating these changes has been extensively studied in rats with streptozotocin-induced diabetes and in spontaneously-diabetic BB rats [140, 141, Table 3]. Although most other key peptides are unchanged, both models show increased activity of the ARC–PVN NPY-ergic projection, with increased NPY synthesis in the arcuate nucleus [142], increased NPY secretion in the PVN [143], significant elevations of NPY in several other hypothalamic areas [144–146], and secondary down-regulation of hypothalamic NPY receptors [147]. This increase in NPY activity could play a key role in the behavioural and endocrine responses to IDDM, given the peptide's recognised effects on energy balance and pituitary secretion: indeed, central injection of NPY to healthy animals closely simulates the pituitary dysfunction typical of IDDM. It seems likely that the stimulus that leads to increased NPY synthesis in the ARC is hypoinsulinaemia itself, rather than hyperglycaemia; as discussed earlier, insulin may normally inhibit NPY synthesis in the ARC.

NIDDM and Obesity

When interpreting data from animal studies of NIDDM, it is important to consider the differences between human diabetes and the available animal models. While obesity and insulin resistance are prominent features in human and rodent NIDDM, it has recently become clear that relative insulin deficiency is essential for the development of NIDDM in man. Obese diabetic rodents have grossly raised insulin levels, as measured by conventional radioimmunoassay (RIA), although it is not yet known whether this represents 'true' hyperinsulinaemia or reflects raised concentrations of other proinsulin derived molecules.

The most extensively studied model is the fatty Zucker rat, homozygous for the *fa* gene, which develops profound obesity and insulin resistance but is only mildly glucose-intolerant rather than frankly diabetic [148]. Impaired thermogenesis can be demonstrated in very young *fa/fa* rats compared with lean littermates, and is considered the major cause of obesity, although weight gain is accentuated by hyperphagia after weaning [149]. *fa/fa* rats also display insulin hypersecretion [150] and marked insulin resistance in skeletal muscle and liver [151]. The primary genetic defect in this syndrome has yet to be defined, but most features can be explained by defective autonomic regulation [152], and dramatic changes have been observed in several neuropeptides in the hypothalamus. Particular interest has focused on the possible role of NPY in the development of obesity in fatty Zucker rats as chronic ICV administration of this peptide produces a similar obesity syndrome in normal rats [153].

Elevated NPY levels have been demonstrated throughout the ARC–PVN projection of obese animals and also occur in the SCN [154–156], where they may contribute to observed changes in circadian feeding patterns that occur early in the development of obesity. Fatty Zucker rats also demonstrate increased NPY mRNA expression in the ARC [157], down-regulation of hypothalamic NPY receptors and attenuated feeding responses to intrahypothalamic injection of NPY [158].

Table 4 Changes in hypothalamic neuropeptides in animal models of NIDDM

Model	Peptide	Comments	References
Zucker rat	Neuropeptide Y	Elevated levels throughout ARC–PVN projection	154–156
		Increased NPY mRNA expression in the arcuate nucleus	157
		Downregulation of hypothalamic NPY receptors	158
	Neurotensin	Reduced levels in ARC, PVN and SCN	156, 165
	CRF	Reduced hypothalamic levels	166
	CCK	Impaired hypophagic response to CCK. Hypothalamic levels unchanged	168 169
	Insulin	Reduced brain insulin content. Impaired hypophagic response to ICV insulin	164 159
ob/ob mouse	Neuropeptide Y	Increased hypothalamic NPY mRNA expression	171
	Neurotensin	Reduced levels in central and lateral hypothalamic blocks	172
		Reduced hypothalamic neurotensin mRNA expression	171
	Bombesin Galanin Somatostatin	Unchanged levels in central and lateral hypothalamic blocks	172

These changes are all consistent with overactivity of hypothalamic NPY neurones, which could be due to hypothalamic 'resistance' to insulin's normal inhibitory action. Fatty Zucker rats given ICV insulin display neither the hypophagic response nor the reduction in hypothalamic NPY mRNA seen in normal Wistar and lean Zucker rats [159, 160]. This apparent resistance may reflect an abnormality of hypothalamic insulin receptors, although data are conflicting [161, 162]. Insulin concentrations are reportedly reduced in CSF and various brain regions including hypothalamus, despite peripheral hyperinsulinaemia [163, 164].

Reduced activity of anorectic peptides may also contribute to hyperphagia and obesity in the fatty Zucker rat. Reduced neurotensin concentrations have been observed in several key hypothalamic regions including the ARC, PVN and SCN [165, 156], but it has been suggested that, at least in the SCN, changes in neurotensin occur later than those in NPY, and thus may represent a secondary phenomenon. CRF is reduced in the hypothalamus of obese Zucker rats [166], and infusion of CRF suppresses body weight gain by both reducing food intake and activating BAT thermogenesis [167]. The satiety response to CCK appears blunted in weanling fatty Zucker rats [168], although hypothalamic levels of this peptide appear unchanged [169]. An as yet unexplained observation is the increased concentration of neuromedin B in the central hypothalamus of obese Zucker rats [170].

An obesity syndrome also develops in mice homozygous for the *ob* (obesity) gene. Like the fatty Zucker rat, the *ob/ob* mouse displays defective thermogenesis, hyperphagia and peripheral insulin resistance, but this model resembles human NIDDM more closely, in that hyperglycaemia and frank diabetes are more consistent features [152]. As in the Zucker rat, abnormalities of hypothalamic neuropeptide Y and neurotensin have been observed, *ob/ob* mice having increased hypothalamic NPY mRNA and decreased neurotensin mRNA compared to lean littermates [171]. Consistent with this, neurotensin levels are reduced in both the central and lateral hypothalamus of *ob/ob* mice [172]. Surprisingly, no increase has been observed in hypothalamic NPY levels, but the limited dissection method employed in these studies could miss significant regional changes in NPY. No convincing changes in the levels of other anorectic neuropeptides have been observed (Table 4), although CCK levels have been variably reported to be reduced or unchanged [169, 173].

Abnormalities of the opioid peptides have also been observed in these obesity/NIDDM syndromes. Pituitary β-endorphin levels are increased in both *ob/ob* mice and *fa/fa* rats compared with lean controls [174]. Dynorphin levels are increased in various brain regions of fatty Zucker rats, and in the posterior pituitary of *ob/ob* mice [175]. Both models demonstrate increased sensitivity to the suppressant effect of naloxone on food intake [174], whilst another opiate antagonist, naltrexone, can prevent *ob/ob* mice from becoming obese [176]. *ob/ob* mice also show increased sensitivity to κ-agonists, which stimulate feeding more than in lean mice [175].

In conclusion, many peptidergic systems are disturbed in these NIDDM-like syndromes, but it is not yet possible to identify which abnormalities are of primary importance.

THE CNS, OBESITY AND NIDDM IN MAN

Obesity is a well established risk factor in human NIDDM, though its precise aetiological significance remains controversial [177]. In extending observations from animal experiments to man, it should be noted that there are important differences between human and animal obesity. In rodents, obesity results primarily from reduced energy expenditure, and particularly from impaired thermogenesis in brown adipose tissue. In adult man, adaptive thermogenesis is probably not significant: brown fat is obvious in neonates but lacking in adults, and skeletal muscle, the main thermogenic tissue in man, has only a limited capacity for adaptive thermogenesis [178]. Furthermore it has been demonstrated that obese patients have *increased* resting and total energy expenditure compared with normal-weight controls, in contrast to the situation seen in animals [179]. Studies of Pima Indians (who have a high incidence of obesity and NIDDM) indicate that young individuals with relatively low energy expenditure are more prone to develop obesity in later life [180], but on balance, excessive consumption is probably more important in the development of human obesity. It can be postulated that hypothalamic dysregulation could contribute to this by driving appetite beyond energy requirements.

As yet, very little is known about the role of hypothalamic neuropeptides in human NIDDM and obesity. Post-mortem studies have established that NPY and other key neuropeptides are present in human brain in generally similar distributions to those found in animals [181], but no systematic post-mortem studies comparing neuropeptide levels from obese, diabetic and normal subjects have been conducted. Insulin is present in significant amounts in human brain [182] and insulin receptors have been demonstrated in human cerebral cortex, retina and hypothalamus [183–185]. As in other species, the human neuronal insulin receptor shows specific structural features different from the peripheral type of receptor, suggesting that it may have a specific central role analogous to that postulated in the rat, but as yet there have been no systematic studies of its distribution or properties.

It is evident that a great deal more work will be required, both to further clarify the primary hypothalamic abnormalities in the animal models of diabetes, and to extend these observations to apply to man. Hopefully, a fuller understanding of the role of the hypothalamus in metabolic regulation will provide new insights into the aetiology of human obesity and diabetes. One possible reward for this understanding will be the development of new anti-obesity drugs which could have the potential to revolutionise the management of NIDDM [186].

REFERENCES

1. Bernard C. Leçons de physiologie expérimentale appliquée à la médecine. vol. 1. Paris: Baillière, 1855.
2. Van Houten M, Posner BI. Circumventricular organs: receptors and mediators of direct peptide action on brain. Adv Metab Disord 1983; 10: 269–89.
3. Bleier R, Byne W. Forebrain and midbrain. In Paxinos G (ed.) The rat nervous system, 1st edn, vol. 1. Sydney: Academic Press, 1985: 87–118.
4. Morgane PJ, Panskepp J (eds) The handbook of the hypothalamus. vol. 1. New York: Dekker, 1979.
5. Hetherington AW, Ranson SW. The spontaneous activity and food intake of rats with hypothalamic lesions. Am J Physiol 1942; 136: 609–17.
6. Anand BK, Brobeck JR. Localisation of a feeding centre in the hypothalamus of the rat. Proc Soc Exp Biol Med 1951; 77: 323–4.
7. Grossman SP. Role of the hypothalamus in the regulation of food and water intake. Psychol Rev 1975; 82: 200–24.
8. Nicholls DG, Locke RM. Thermogenic mechanisms in brown fat. Physiol Rev 1984; 64: 1–45.
9. Rothwell NJ. Central control of brown adipose tissue. Proc Nutr Soc 1989; 48: 197–206.
10. Perkins MN, Rothwell NJ, Stock MJ, Stone TW. Activation of brown adipose tissue thermogenesis by the ventromedial hypothalamus. Nature 1981; 289: 401–2.
11. Sims EAH, Danforth E. Expenditure and storage of energy in man. J Clin Invest 1987; 79: 1019–25.
12. Woods SC, Porte D. Neural control of the endocrine pancreas. Physiol Rev 1974; 54: 596–619.
13. Benzo CA. The hypothalamus and blood glucose regulation. Life Sci 1983; 32: 2509–15.
14. Rohner-Jeanrenaud F, Bobbioni E, Ionescu E, Sauter JF, Jeanrenaud B. Central nervous system regulation of insulin secretion. Adv Metab Disord 1983; 10: 193–220.
15. Steffens AB, Strubbe JH. CNS regulation of glucagon secretion. Adv Metab Disord 1983; 10: 221–57.
16. Shimazu T. Neuronal regulation of hepatic glucose regulation in mammals. Diabetes Metab Rev 1987; 3: 185–206.
17. Shimazu T, Fukuda A, Ban T. Reciprocal influences of the ventromedial and lateral hypothalamic nuclei on blood glucose level and liver glycogen content. Nature 1960; 210: 1178–9.
18. Oomura Y, Ono T, Ooyama H, Wayner MJ. Glucose and osmosensitive neurones in the rat hypothalamus. Nature 1969; 222: 282–4.
19. Ritter RC, Slusser PG, Stone S. Glucoreceptors controlling feeding and blood glucose: location in the hindbrain. Science 1981; 213: 451–3.
20. Donovan CM, Cane P, Bergman RN. Search for the hypoglycaemia receptor using the local irrigation approach. In Vranic M et al (eds) Fuel homeostasis and the nervous system. New York: Plenum Press, 1991: 185–96.
21. Cane P, Artal R, Bergman RN. Putative hypothalamic glucoreceptors play no essential role in the response to moderate glycemia. Diabetes 1986; 35: 268–77.
22. Leibowitz S.F. Brain monoamines and peptides: role in the control of eating behavior. Fed Proc 1986; 45: 1396–403.

23. Leibowitz SF, Weiss GF, Shor-Posner G. Medial hypothalamic serotonin in the control of eating behaviour. Int J Obesity 1987; 11 (suppl. 3): 97–108.

24. Curzon G. Serotonin and appetite. Ann NY Acad Sci 1990; 600: 521–30.

25. Tatemoto K, Carlquist M, Mutt V. Neuropeptide Y: a novel brain peptide with structural similarities to PYY and pancreatic polypeptide. Nature 1982; 296: 659–60.

26. Allen YS, Adrian TE, Tatemoto K, Crow TJ, Bloom SR, Polak JM. Neuropeptide Y distribution in the rat brain. Science 1983; 221: 877–9.

27. De Quidt ME, Emson PC. Distribution of NPY-like immunoreactivity in the rat CNS II: immunohisto-chemical analysis. J Neurosci 1986; 18(3): 545–618.

28. Williams G, Steel JH, Polak JM, Bloom SR. Neuropeptide Y in the hypothalamus. In Mutt V, Hökfelt T, Fuxe K, Lundberg JM (eds) Neuropeptide Y, 1st edn. New York: Raven Press, 1989: pp 243–51.

29. Morris B.J. Neuronal localisation of neuropeptide Y gene expression in rat brain. J Comp Neurol 1989; 290: 358–68.

30. Chronwall BM. Anatomical distribution of NPY and NPY messenger RNA in rat brain. In Mutt V, Hökfelt T, Fuxe K, Lundberg JM (eds) Neuropeptide Y, 1st edn. New York: Raven Press, 1989: pp 51–9.

31. Bai FL, Yamano M, Shiotani Y et al. An arcuato-paraventricular and dorsomedial hypothalamic neuropeptide Y containing system which lacks noradrenalin in the rat. Brain Res 1985; 331: 172–5.

32. Sawchenko PE, Swanson LW, Grzanna R, Howe PRC, Bloom SR, Polak JM. Colocalization of neuropeptide Y immunoreactivity in brainstem catecholaminergic neurons that project to the paraventricular nucleus of the hypothalamus. J Comp Neurol 1985; 241: 138–53.

33. Levine AS, Morley JE. Neuropeptide Y: a potent inducer of consumatory behavior in rats. Peptides 1984; 5: 1025–9.

34. Stanley BG, Leibowitz SF. Neuropeptide Y injected into the paraventricular hypothalamus: a powerful stimulant of feeding behavior. Proc Natl Acad Sci USA 1985; 82: 3940–3.

35. Stanley BG, Chin AS, Leibowitz SF. Feeding and drinking elicited by central injection of neuropeptide Y: evidence for a hypothalamic site of action. Brain Res Bull 1985; 14: 521–4.

36. Stanley BG, Krykouli SE, Lampert S, Leibowitz SF. NPY chronically injected into the hypothalamus: a powerful neurochemical inducer of hyperphagia and obesity. Peptides 1986; 7: 1189–92.

37. Egawa M, Yoshimatsu H, Bray GA. Neuropeptide Y suppresses sympathetic activity into the intercapsular brown adipose tissue in rats. Am J Physiol 1991; 260: R328–34.

38. Billington CJ, Briggs JE, Grace M, Levine AS. Effects of intracerebroventricular injection of neuropeptide Y on energy metabolism. Am J Physiol 1991; 260: R321–7.

39. Dumont Y, Fournier A, St-Pierre S, Schwartz TW, Quirion R. Differential distribution of neuropeptide Y1 and Y2 receptors in the rat brain. Eur J Pharmacol 1990; 191: 501–3.

40. Moltz JH, McDonald JK. Neuropeptide Y: direct and indirect action on insulin secretion in the rat. Peptides 1985; 6: 1155–9.

41. Wahlestedt C, Skagerberg G, Eikman R, Heilig M, Sundler F, Harkanson R. Neuropeptide Y in the area of the hypothalamic paraventricular nucleus activates the pituitary-adrenocortical axis in the rat. Brain Res 1987; 417: 33–8.

42. McCann SM, Rettori L, Milenkovic M, Riedel M, Aguilla C, McDonald JK. The role of NPY in control of anterior pituitary hormone release in the rat. In Mutt V, Hökfelt T, Fuxe K, Lundberg JM (eds) Neuropeptide Y, 1st edn. New York: Raven Press, 1989: 215–27.

43. Willoughby JO, Blessing WW. Neuropeptide Y injected into the supraoptic nucleus causes secretion of vasopressin in the unanaesthetised rat. Neurosci Lett 1989; 75: 17–22.

44. Kalra SP, Sahu A, Kalra PS. Hypothalamic neuropeptide Y: a circuit in the regulation of gonadotrophin secretion and feeding behaviour. Ann NY Acad Sci 1990; 611: 273–83.

45. Kalra SP, Clark JT, Sahu A, Kalra PS, Crowley WR. Hypothalamic NPY: a local circuit in the control of reproduction and behaviour. In Mutt V, Hökfelt T, Fuxe K, Lundberg JM (eds) Neuropeptide Y, 1st edn. New York: Raven Press, 1989: 229–41.

46. Tatemoto K, Rökaeus Å, Jornvall H, McDonald TJ. Galanin—a novel biologically active peptide from porcine intestine. FEBS Lett 1983; 164: 124–8.

47. Palkovits M, Rökaeus Å, Antoni FA, Kiss A. Galanin in the hypothalamo-hypophyseal system. Neuroendocrinology 1987; 46: 417–23.

48. Kyrkouli SE, Stanley BG, Hutchinson R, Seirafi RD, Leibowitz SF. Peptide-amine interactions in the hypothalamic paraventricular nucleus: analysis of galanin and neuropeptide Y in relation to feeding. Brain Res 1990; 521: 185–91.

49. Kyrkouli SE, Stanley BG, Leibowitz SF. Galanin: stimulation of feeding induced by medial hypothalamic injection of this novel peptide. Eur J Pharmacol 1986; 122: 159–60.

50. Kyrkouli SE, Stanley BG, Seirafi RD, Leibowitz SF. Stimulation of feeding by galanin: anatomical localization and behavioral specificity of this peptide's effects in the brain. Peptides 1990; 11: 995–1001.

51. Schick RR, Samsami S, Zimmermann JP et al. Effect of galanin on food intake in rats: involvement of lateral and ventromedial hypothalamic sites. Am J Physiol 1993; 264: R355–61.

52. Menendez JA, Atrens DM, Leibowitz SF. Metabolic effects of galanin injections into the paraventricular nucleus of the hypothalamus. Peptides 1992; 13: 323–7.

53. Tempel DL, Leibowitz KJ, Leibowitz SF. Effects of PVN galanin on macronutrient selection. Peptides 1988; 9: 309–14.

54. Leibowitz SF, Kim T. Impact of a galanin antagonist on exogenous galanin and natural patterns of fat ingestion. Brain Res 1992; 599: 148–52.

55. Crawley JN, Robinson JK, Langel U, Bartfai T. Galanin receptor antagonists M40 and C7 block galanin-induced feeding. Brain Res 1993; 600: 268–72.

56. Dunning BE, Ahren B, Veith RC, Bottcher G, Sundler F, Taborsky GJJ. Galanin: a novel pancreatic neuropeptide. Am J Physiol 1986; 251: E127-33.

57. Tempel DL, Leibowitz SF. Galanin inhibits insulin and corticosterone release after injection into the PVN. Brain Res 1990; 536: 353-7.

58. Holmes MC, Renzo GD, Beckford U, Gillham B, Jones MJ. Role of serotonin in the secretion of CRF. J Endocrinol 1982; 93: 151-60.

59. Haas DA, George SR. Neuropeptide Y administration acutely increases hypothalamic CRF immunoreactivity: lack of effect in other brain regions. Life Sci 1987; 41: 2725-31.

60. Suda T, Towaza F, Iwai I, Sata Y, Sumitomo T, Nakano Y, Yamada M, Demura H. Neuropeptide Y increases the corticotrophin-releasing factor mRNA level in the rat. Mol Brain Res 1993; 18: 311-15.

61. Tsagarakis S, Rees LH, Besser GM, Grossman A. Neuropeptide Y stimulates CRF-41 release from rat hypothalami *in vitro*. Brain Res 1989; 502: 167-70.

62. Hotta M, Shibasaki T, Yamauchi N, Ohno H, Benoit R, Ling N, Demura H. Effects of chronic central administration of CRF on food intake, body weight and hypothalamic pituitary adrenocortical hormones. Life Sci 1991; 48: 1483-91.

63. Morley JE, Levine AS. CRF grooming and ingestive behaviour. Life Sci 1982; 31: 1459-64.

64. Heinrichs SC, Menzaghi F, Pich EM, Hauger RL, Koob GF. Corticotrophin-releasing factor in the paraventricular nucleus modulates feeding induced by neuropeptide Y. Brain Res 1993; 611: 18-24.

65. Arase K, York DA, Shimazu H, Shargill N, Bray GA. Effect of CRF on food intake and brown adipose tissue thermogenesis in rats. Am J Physiol 1988; 255: E225-59.

66. Le Feuvre RA, Rothwell NJ, Stock MJ. Activation of brown fat thermogenesis in response to central injection of corticotropin releasing hormone in the rat. Neuropharmacology 1987; 26: 1217-21.

67. Bruce BK, King BM, Phelps GR, Veitia MC. Effects of adrenalectomy and corticosterone administration on hypothalamic obesity in rats. Am J Physiol 1982; 243: E152-7.

68. Rothwell NJ. Central effects of CRF on metabolism and energy balance. Neurosci Biobehav Rev 1990; 14: 263-71.

69. Brown MR, Fisher LA, Speiss J, Rivier C, Rivier J, Vale W. Corticotropin-releasing factor: actions on the sympathetic nervous system and metabolism. Endocrinology 1982; 111: 928-31.

70. Brown MR, Fisher LA. Corticotrophin-releasing factor: effects on the autonomic nervous system and visceral system. Fed Proc 1985; 44(1): 243-8.

71. Morley JE, Levine AS, Yim GK, Lowy MT. Opioid modulation of appetite. Neurosci Biobehav Rev 1983; 7: 281-305.

72. Morley JE, Levine AS. Involvement of dynorphin and the kappa opioid receptor in feeding. Peptides 1983; 4: 797-800.

73. McKay LD, Kenney NJ, Edens NK, Williams RH, Woods SC. ICV beta-endorphin increases food intake of rats. Life Sci 1981; 29: 1429-34.

74. Morley JE. Neuropeptide regulation of appetite and weight. Endocrinol Rev 1987; 8(3): 256-87.

75. McLean S, Hoebel BG. Feeding induced by opiates injected into the paraventricular nucleus. Peptides 1983; 4: 287-92.

76. Bashki VP, Kelley AE. Feeding induced by opioid stimulation of the ventral striatum: role of opiate receptor subtypes. J Pharmacol Exp Ther 1993; 265: 1253-60.

77. Morley JE, Levine AS. The role of the endogenous opiates as regulators of appetite. Am J Clin Nutr 1982; 35: 757-61.

78. Kyriakides MT, Silverstone T, Jeffcoate W, Laurance B. Effect of naloxone on hyperphagia in the Prader-Willi syndrome. Lancet 1980; 1: 876-7.

79. Havrankova J, Schmechel D, Roth J, Brownstein M. Identification of insulin in rat brain. Proc Natl Acad Sci USA 1978; 75: 5737-41.

80. Havrankova J, Roth J, Brownstein M. Concentrations of insulin in the brain are independent of peripheral insulin levels. Studies of obese and streptozotocin treated rodents. J Clin Invest 1979; 64: 632-42.

81. Yalow RS, Eng G. Insulin in the Central Nervous System. Adv Metab Disord 1983; 10: 341-54.

82. van Houten M, Posner BI, Kopriwa BM, Brawer JR. Insulin-binding sites in the rat brain: *in vivo* localisation to the circumventricular organs by quantitative radioautography. Endocrinology 1979; 105: 666-73.

83. Baskin DG, Woods SC, West DB et al. Immunocytochemical detection of insulin in rat hypothalamus and its possible uptake from cerebrospinal fluid. Endocrinology 1983; 113: 1818-25.

84. Woods SC, Porte DJ. Relationship between plasma and cerebrospinal fluid insulin levels of dogs. Am J Physiol 1977; 233: E331-4.

85. Wallum BJ, Taborsky GJ, Porte DJ et al. CSF insulin levels increase during intravenous insulin infusions in man. J Clin Endocrinol Metab 1987; 64: 190-4.

86. Pardridge WM. Receptor mediated peptide transport through the blood-brain barrier. Endocrine Rev 1986; 7: 314-30.

87. Pardridge WM, Eisenberg J, Yang J. Human blood-brain barrier insulin receptor. J Neurochem 1985; 44: 1771-8.

88. Schechter R, Holtzclaw L, Sadiq F, Kahn A, Devaskar S. Insulin synthesis by isolated rabbit neurones. Endocrinology 1988; 123; 505-13.

89. Clarke DW, Mudd L, Boyd FT, Fields M, Raizada MK. Insulin is released from rat brain neuronal cells in culture. J Neurochem 1986; 47: 831-6.

90. Young WS. Periventricular hypothalamic cells in the rat brain contain insulin mRNA. Neuropeptides 1986; 8: 93-7.

91. Giddings SJ, Chirgwin J, Permutt MA. Evaluation of rat insulin messenger RNA in pancreatic and extrapancreatic tissues. Diabetologia 1985; 28: 343-7.

92. Coker GT, Studelska D, Harmon S, Burke W, O'Malley KL. Analysis of tyrosine hydroxylase and insulin transcripts in human neuroendocrine tissues. Mol Brain Res 1990; 8: 93-8.

93. Havrankova J, Roth J, Brownstein M. Insulin receptors are widely distributed in the central nervous system of the rat. Nature 1978; 272: 827-9.

94. Pacold ST, Blackard WG. Central nervous system insulin receptors in normal and diabetic rats. Endocrinology 1979; 105: 1452-7.

95. Unger J, McNeil TH, Moxley TR, White M, Moss A, Livingston JN. Distribution of insulin receptor-like immunoreactivity in the rat forebrain. Neuroscience 1989; 31: 143-57.

96. Heidenreich KA, Zanheiser NR, Berhanu P, Brandenburg D, Olfesky JM. Structural differences between insulin receptors in the brain and peripheral target tissues. J Biol Chem 1983; 258: 8527–30.

97. Hendricks SA, Agardh CD, Taylor SI, Roth J. Unique features of the insulin receptor in rat brain. J Neurochem 1984; 43: 1302–9.

98. LeRoith D, Rojeski M, Roth J. Insulin receptors in brain and other tissues: similarities and differences. Neurochem Int 1988; 12: 419–23.

99. Yip CC, Moule ML, Yeung CWT. Characterisation of insulin receptor subunits in brain and other tissues by photo-affinity labelling. Biochem Biophys Res Commun 1980; 96: 1671–8.

100. Zanheiser NR, Goens MB, Hanaway PJ, Vinych JV. Characterisation and regulation of insulin receptors in rat brain. J Neurochem 1984; 42: 1354–62.

101. Gammeltoft S, Kowalski A, Fehlmann M, van-Obberghen E. Insulin receptors in rat brain: insulin stimulates phosphorylation of its receptor beta-subunit. FEBS Lett 1984; 172(1): 87–90.

102. Clarke DW, Boyd FTJ, Kappy MS, Raizada MK. Insulin binds to specific receptors and stimulates 2-deoxyglucose uptake in cultured glial cells from rat brain. J Biol Chem 1984; 259: 11672–5.

103. Werner H, Raizada MK, Mudd LM et al. Regulation of rat brain/HepG2 glucose transporter gene expression by insulin and IGF-1 in primary cultures of neuronal and glial cells. Endocrinology 1989; 125: 1458–63.

104. Boyd FTJ, Clarke DW, Muther TF, Raizada MK. Insulin receptors and insulin modulation of norepinephrine uptake in neuronal cultures from rat brain. J Biol Chem 1985; 260: 15880–4.

105. Hom FG, Goodner CJ, Berrie MA. A (3H)2-deoxyglucose method for comparing rates of glucose metabolism and insulin responses among rat tissues *in vivo*. Diabetes 1984; 33: 141–52.

106. Lucignani G, Namba H, Nehlig A, Porrino LJ, Kennedy C, Sokoloff L. Effects of insulin on local cerebral glucose utilisation in the rat. J Cerebr Blood Flow Metab. 1987; 7: 309–14.

107. Schwartz MW, Figlewicz DP, Baskin DG, Woods SC, Porte DJ. Insulin in the brain: a hormonal regulator of energy balance. Endocrine Rev 1992; 13: 387–414.

108. Brief DJ, Davis JD. Reduction of food intake and body weight by chronic intraventricular insulin infusion. Brain Res Bull 1984; 12: 571–5.

109. Plata-Salamán CR, Oomura Y, Shimizu N. Dependence of food intake on acute and chronic ventricular administration of insulin. Physiol Behav 1986; 37: 717–34.

110. Strubbe JH, Mein CG. Increased feeding in response to bilateral injections of insulin antibodies in the VMH. Physiol Behav 1977; 19: 309–13.

111. Rothwell NJ, Stock MJ. Insulin and thermogenesis. Int J Obesity 1988; 12: 93–102.

112. Nicolaidis S, Rowland N. Metering of intravenous versus oral nutrients and the regulation of energy balance. Am J Physiol 1976; 231: 661–8.

113. Schwartz MW, Marks JL, Baskin DG, Woods SC, Kahn SE, Porte D Jnr. Central insulin administration decreases neuropeptide Y mRNA expression in the arcuate nucleus of food deprived lean (*fa/fa*) but not obese Zucker rats. Endocrinology 1991; 5: 2645–7.

114. Malabu UH, Cotton SJ, Kruszynska YT, McCarthy HD, Williams G. Acute hyperinsulinemia increases neuropeptide Y concentrations in the hypothalamic arcuate nucleus of fasted rats. Life Sci 1993; 52: 1407–16.

115. Malabu UH, McCarthy HD, McKibbin PE, Williams G. Peripheral insulin administration attenuates the increases in NPY levels in the hypothalamic arcuate nucleus of starved rats. Peptides 1992; 13: 1097–102.

116. Dryden S, Cusin I, Wang Q, Rohner-Jeanrenaud F, Jeanrenaud B, Williams G. Effect of sustained physiological hyperinsulinaemia on hypothalamic NPY and NPY mRNA levels in the rat. Diabet Med 1994; 11 (suppl. 1): S32.

117. Stanley BG, Hoebel BG, Leibowitz SF. Neurotensin: effects of hypothalamic and intravenous injections on eating and drinking in rats. Peptides 1983; 4: 493–500.

118. Frohman LA. CNS peptides and glucoregulation. Ann Rev Physiol 1983; 45: 95–107.

119. Olchovsky D, Bruno JF, Wood TL et al. Altered pituitary growth hormone (GH) regulation in streptozotocin-diabetic rats: a combined effect of hypothalamic somatostatin and GH-releasing factor. Endocrinology 1990; 126: 53–61.

120. Williams G, Bloom SR. Regulatory peptides, the hypothalamus and diabetes. Diabet Med 1989; 6: 472–85.

121. Gibbs J, Smith GP. Cholecystokinin and satiety in rats and rhesus monkeys. Am J Clin Nutr 1977; 30: 758–61.

122. Silver AJ, Flood JF, Song AM, Morley JE. Evidence for a physiological role for CCK in the regulation of food intake in mice. Am J Physiol 1989; 256: R646–51.

123. Kissilef HR, Pi-Sunyer FX, Thornton J. C-terminal octapeptide of cholecystokinin decreases food intake in man. Am J Clin Nutr 1981; 34: 154–60.

124. McHugh PR, Moran TH. The stomach, cholecystokinin, and satiety. Fed Proc 1986; 45: 1384–90.

125. Innis RB, Snyder SH. Distinct cholecystokinin receptors in brain and pancreas. Proc Natl Acad Sci USA 1980; 77: 6917–21.

126. Dourish CT, Rycroft W, Ivesen SD. Postponement of satiety by blockade of brain cholecystokinin (CCK-B) receptors. Science 1989; 245: 1509–11.

127. Tsai SH, Passaro E, Lin MT. Cholecystokinin acts through catecholaminergic mechanisms in the hypothalamus to influence ingestive behaviour in the rat. Neuropharmacology 1984; 23: 1351–6.

128. Kyrkouli SE, Stanley BG, Leibowitz SF. Bombesin-induced anorexia: sites of action in the rat brain. Peptides 1987; 8: 237–41.

129. Lin KS, Lin MT. Effects of bombesin on thermoregulatory responses and hypothalamic neuronal activities in the rat. Am J Physiol 1986; 251: R303–9.

130. Brown M, Tach Y, Fisher D. Central nervous system action of bombesin: mechanism to induce hyperglycaemia. Endocrinology 1979; 105: 660–5.

131. Iguchi A, Sakamoto N, Burleson PD. The effects of neuropeptides on glucoregulation. Adv Metab Disord 1983; 10: 421–34.

132. Gibbs J, Fauser DJ, Rowe EA, Rolls BJ, Rolls ET, Maddison SP. Bombesin suppresses feeding in rats. Nature 1979; 282: 208–10.

133. Muurhainen NE, Kissileff HR, Pi-Sunyer FX. Intravenous infusion of bombesin reduces food intake in humans. Am J Physiol 1993; 264: R350–4.

134. Morley JE, Levine AS, Gosnell BA, Mitchell JE, Krahn DD, Nizielski SE. Peptides and feeding. Peptides 1985; 6 (suppl. 2): 181–5.

135. Williams G, Cardoso HM, Lee YC et al. Hypothalamic regulatory peptides in obese and lean Zucker rat. Clin Sci 1991; 80: 419–26.

136. Koopman HS, Pi-Sunyer FX. Large changes in food intake in diabetic rats fed high-fat and low-fat diets. Brain Res Bull 1986; 17: 861–71.

137. Gonzalez C, Montoya E, Jolin T. Effect of STZ diabetes on the hypothalamo–pituitary and thyroid axis of the rat. Endocrinology 1980; 107: 2099–103.

138. Katayama S, Brownscheidle CM, Wootten V, Lee JB, Shimaoka K. Absent or delayed pre-ovulatory LH surge in experimental diabetes. Diabetes 1983; 33: 324–7.

139. Oster MH, Castonguay TW, Keen CL, Stern JS. Circadian rhythm of corticosterone in diabetic rats. Life Sci 1989; 43: 1643–5.

140. Frankish HM, Dryden S, Hopkins D, Wang Q, Williams G. Neuropeptide Y, the hypothalamus and diabetes. Peptides 1995: in press.

141. Williams G, McCarthy HD, McKibbin PE, Malabu UH, Leitch HF. Neuroendocrine disturbances in diabetes: role for hypothalamic regulatory peptides. Shafrir E (ed.) Less Animal Diabetes IV 1993; 18: 203–17.

142. Jones PM, Pierson AM, Williams G, Ghatei MA, Bloom SR. Increased hypothalamic neuropeptide Y messenger RNA levels in two rat models of diabetes. Diabet Med 1992; 9: 76–80.

143. Sahu A, Sninsky CA, Phelps CP, Dube MG, Kalra PS, Kalra SP. Neuropeptide Y release from the paraventricular nucleus increase in association with hyperphagia in streptozocin-induced diabetic rats. Endocrinology 1992; 131: 2979–85.

144. Williams G, Steel JH, Cardoso HM, Ghatei MA, Lee YC, Gill JS, Burrin JM, Polak JM, Bloom SR. Increased hypothalamic neuropeptide Y concentrations in diabetic rat. Diabetes 1988; 37: 763–72.

145. Williams G, Lee YC, Ghatei MA, Cardoso HM, Ball JA, Bone AJ, Baird JD, Bloom SR. Elevated neuropeptide Y concentrations in the central hypothalamus of the spontaneously diabetic BB/E Wistar rat. Diabet Med 1989; 6: 601–7.

146. Sahu A, Sninsky CA, Kalra PS, Kalra SP. NPY concentrations in microdissected regions and *in vitro* release from the medial basal hypothalamus-preoptic area of streptozocin diabetic rats with and without insulin substitution therapy. Endocrinology 1990; 126: 192–8.

147. Frankish HM, McCarthy HD, Dryden S, Kilpatrick A, Williams G. Reduced hypothalamic neuropeptide Y receptor numbers in streptozocin diabetic and food deprived rat. Peptides 1993; 14: 941–8.

148. Bray GA. The Zucker-fatty rat: a review. Fed Proc 1977; 36: 148–53.

149. Cleary MP, Vasselli JR, Greenwood MRC. Development of obesity in the Zucker obese (*fa/fa*) rat in absence of hyperphagia. Am J Physiol 1980; 238: E284–92.

150. Lee HC, Curry DL, Stern JS. Direct effect of CNS on insulin hypersecretion in obese Zucker rats: involvement of vagus nerve. Am J Physiol 1989; 256: E439–44.

151. Penicaud L, Ferre P, Terretez J, Kinebanyan MF, Lecturque A, Dore E, Girard J, Jeanrenaud B, Picon L. Development of obesity in Zucker rats: early insulin resistance in muscles but normal sensitivity in white adipose tissue. Diabetes 1987; 36: 626–31.

152. Bray GA, York DA. Hypothalamic and genetic obesity in experimental animals: an autonomic and endocrine hypothesis. Physiol Rev 1979; 59: 719–809.

153. Zarjevski N, Cusin I, Vettor R, Rohner-Jeanrenaud F, Jeanrenaud B. Chronic intracerebroventricular neuropeptide Y administration to normal rats mimics hormonal and metabolic changes of obesity. Endocrinology 1993; 133: 1753–8.

154. Beck B, Burlet A, Nicolas J-P, Burlet C. Hypothalamic neuropeptide Y in obese Zucker rats: implications in feeding and sexual behaviours. Physiol Behav 1990; 47: 449–53.

155. McKibbin PE, Cotton SJ, McMillan S, Holloway B, Mayers R, McCarthy HD, Williams G. Altered neuropeptide Y concentrations in specific hypothalamic regions of obese Zucker rats: possible relationship to obesity and neuroendocrine disturbances. Diabetes 1991; 40: 1423–9.

156. Beck B, Burlet A, Bazin R, Nicolas J-P, Burlet C. Early modification of neuropeptide Y but not neurotensin in the suprachiasmatic nucleus of the obese Zucker rat. Neurosci Lett 1992; 136: 185–8.

157. Sanacora G, Kershaw M, Finklestein JA, White JD. Increased hypothalamic content of preproneuropeptide Y mRNA in genetically obese Zucker rats and its regulation by food deprivation. Endocrinology 1990; 127: 730–7.

158. McCarthy HD, McKibbin PE, Holloway B, Mayers R, Williams G. Hypothalamic neuropeptide Y receptor characteristics and NPY-induced feeding responses in lean and obese Zucker rats. Life Sci 1991; 49: 1491–7.

159. Ikeda H, West DB, Pustek JJ, Figlewicz DP, Greenwood MRC, Porte D, Woods SC. Intraventricular insulin reduces food intake and body weight of lean but not obese Zucker rats. Appetite 1986; 7: 381–6.

160. Schwartz MW, Marks JL, Baskin DG, Woods SC, Kahn SE, Porte D Jr. Central insulin administration decreases neuropeptide Y mRNA expression in the arcuate nucleus of food deprived lean (*fa/fa*) but not obese Zucker rats. Endocrinology 1991; 128(5): 2645–7.

161. Wilcox BJ, Corp ES, Dorsa DM et al. Insulin binding in the hypothalamus of lean and genetically obese Zucker rats. Peptides 1989; 10: 1159–64.

162. Figlewicz DP, Dorsa DM, Stein LJ et al. Brain and liver insulin binding is decreased in Zucker rats carrying the *fa* gene. Endocrinology 1985; 117: 1537–43.

163. Stein LJ, Dorsa DM, Baskin DG, Figlewicz DP, Porte D, Woods SC. Reduced effect of experimental peripheral hyperinsulinemia to elevate CSF insulin concentrations of obese Zucker rats. Endocrinology 1987; 121: 1611–15.

164. Baskin DG, Stein LJ, Ikeda H et al. Genetically obese Zucker rats have abnormally low brain insulin content. Life Sci 1985; 36: 627–33.

165. Beck B, Burlet A, Nicolas JP, Burlet C. Neurotensin in microdissected brain nuclei and in the pituitary of the lean and obese Zucker rats. Neuropeptides 1989; 13: 1–7.

166. Nakaishi S, Nakai Y, Naito Y, Hsui T, Imura H. Immunoreactive CRH levels in brain regions of

genetic obese Zucker rats. Int J Obesity 1991; 14: 951-5.

167. Rohner-Jeanrenaud F, Greco-Perotta R, Jeanrenaud B. Central CRF administration prevents excess body weight gain in genetic obese rats. Endocrinology 1989; 124(2): 733-9.

168. McLaughlin CL, Baile CA, Della-Fera MA, Kasser TG. Meal-stimulated increased concentrations of CCK in the hypothalamus of Zucker obese and lean rats. Physiol Behav 1985; 35: 215-20.

169. Schneider BS, Monahan JW, Hirsch J. Brain CCK and nutritional status in rats and mice. J Clin Invest 1979; 64: 1348-56.

170. Williams G, Cardoso HM, Lee YC et al. Hypothalamic regulatory peptides in obese and lean Zucker rat. Clin Sci 1991; 80: 419-26.

171. Wilding JPH, Gilbey SG, Bailey CJ et al. Increased neuropeptide Y mRNA and decreased neurotensin mRNA in the hypothalamus of the obese (ob/ob) mouse. Endocrinology 1993; 132: 1939-44.

172. Williams G, Cardoso HM, Lee YC et al. Hypothalamic neurotensin concentrations in the genetically obese diabetic (ob/ob) mouse: possible relationship to obesity. Metabolism 1991; 41: 1112-16.

173. Straus E, Yalow RS. CCK in the brains of obese and non-obese mice. Science 1979; 203: 68-9.

174. Margules DL, Moisset B, Lewis MJ, Shibuya H, Pert CB. β-endorphin is associated with overeating in genetically obese mice (ob/ob) and rats (fa/fa). Science 1978; 202: 988-91.

175. Ferguson-Segall M, Flynn JJ, Walker J, Margules DL. Increased immunoreactive dynorphin and leu-enkephalin in posterior pituitary of obese mice (ob/ob) and super-sensitivity to drugs that act at kappa receptors. Life Sci 1982; 31: 2233-6.

176. Recant L, Voyles NR, Luciano M, Pert CB. Naltrexone reduces weight gain, alters β-endorphin, and reduces insulin output from pancreatic islets of genetically obese mice. Peptides 1980; 1: 309-13.

177. Yki-Järvinen H, Pathogenesis of non-insulin dependent diabetes mellitus. Lancet 1994; 343: 91-5.

178. Sims EAH, Danforth E. Expenditure and storage of energy in man. J Clin Invest 1987; 79: 1019-25.

179. Prentice AM, Black AE, Coward WA et al. High levels of energy expenditure in obesity. Br Med J 1986; 292: 983-7.

180. Zurlo F, Ferraro RT, Fontvielle AM, Rising R, Bogardus C, Ravussin E. Spontaneous physical activity and obesity: cross-sectional and longitudinal studies in Pima Indians. Am J Physiol 1992; 263: E296-300.

181. Adrian TE, Allen JM, Bloom SR et al. NPY in human brain—high concentrations in basal ganglia. Nature 1983; 306: 584-6.

182. Dorn A, Rinne A, Bernstein HG, Hahn HJ, Ziegler M. Insulin and C-peptide in human brain neurons. J Hirnforsch 1983; 24: 495-9.

183. Roth RA, Morgan DO, Beaudoin J, Sara V. Purification and characterisation of the human brain insulin receptor. J Biol Chem 1986; 261: 3753-7.

184. Rosenzweig SA, Zetterstrom C, Benjamin A. Identification of retinal insulin receptors using site-specific antibodies to a carboxy-terminal peptide of the human insulin a-subunit. J Biol Chem 1990; 265: 18030-4.

185. Hopkins DFC, Williams G. Insulin receptors are widely distributed in human brain and bind human and porcine insulin with equal affinity. Diabet Med 1994; 11 (suppl. 1): S6.

186. Dryden S, Frankish HM, Wang Q, Williams G. Neuropeptide Y and energy balance: one way ahead for the treatment of obesity? Eur J Clin Invest 1994; 24: 293-308.

187. Brown M. Thyrotropin-releasing factor: a putative CNS regulator of the autonomic nervous system. Life Sci 1981; 28: 1789-95.

188. Amir S. Central glucagon-induced hyperglycaemia is mediated by combined action of the adrenal medulla and sympathetic nerve endings. Physiol Behav 1986; 37: 563-6.

189. Morley JE, Levine AS. Intraventricular cholecystokinin octapeptide produces hyperglycaemia in rats. Life Sci 1981; 28: 2187-97.

190. Taborsky GJJ, Bergman RN. Effect of insulin, glucose and 2-DOG infusion into the third ventricle of conscious dogs on plasma insulin, glucose and free fatty acids. Diabetes 1980; 29: 278-83.

19

Islet Amyloid Polypeptide and Islet Amyloid

Anne Clark and Eelco J.P. de Koning

Radcliffe Infirmary and Department of Human Anatomy, University of Oxford, UK

Islet amyloid polypeptide (IAPP), also known as 'amylin', is a 37-amino acid peptide which was identified in 1987 in extracts of amyloid-containing pancreas and insulinoma [1, 2]. IAPP is the major constituent of amyloid fibrils which occur in pancreatic islets of type 2 diabetic patients and in 50% of human insulinomas [3]. IAPP is a normal component of B cells in non-diabetic and diabetic man and animals and is co-secreted with insulin [4, 5, 6]. The factors involved in amyloid formation are largely unknown and considerable controversy exists regarding possible physiological functions of the peptide.

STRUCTURE OF IAPP

IAPP is synthesised in islet B cells [7] and has been identified in all species so far examined [8, 9, 10, 11, 12, 13, 14, 15]. The amino acid sequence of IAPP and its propeptide varies according to the animal species. IAPP is derived from a larger precursor, proIAPP, by proteolytic cleavage at both the C- and N-terminus [7]. The structure of IAPP has close homologies with calcitonin gene-related peptides (CGRP): human IAPP (hIAPP) has a 46% homology with human CGRP-2 [3]. This is a neuropeptide produced largely by the C-cells of the thyroid as a result of alternate splicing of the calcitonin genes (CALC genes) [1, 2, 3] located on chromosome 11. The gene for islet amyloid polypeptide is located on the short arm of chromosome 12 and is a single copy gene [18]. It is possible that there has been a single common ancestral gene for the genes for CALC and IAPP since chromosomes 11 and 12 are thought to be related in evolution.

The IAPP gene consists of 3 exons (Figure 1): exon 1, (104 bp) encodes most of the 5′ untranslated part of the mRNA; exon 2 (95 bp) encodes 15 untranslated nucleotides, the nucleotides for the signal sequence (22 amino acid residues) and the mRNA for the first nine amino acids of the N-terminal flanking peptide (N-IAPP); exon 3 (1059 bp) encodes the mRNA for the dibasic processing site between N-IAPP and IAPP$_{1-37}$, the C-terminal peptide and the remainder of the 3′ untranslated region [19]. Three polyadenylation signals have been identified in the human IAPP gene and two IAPP mRNAs are always expressed in man and in animals [20].

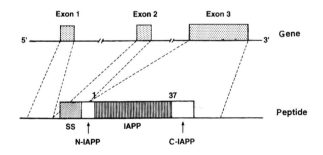

Figure 1 Diagrammatic representation of the IAPP gene. Exons and introns of the gene are shown in relation to the prepropeptide sequence. 1 and 37 indicate the position of IAPP 1–37; SS, signal sequence; N-IAPP, C-IAPP are the flanking peptides

International Textbook of Diabetes Mellitus, Second Edition. Edited by K.G.M.M. Alberti, P. Zimmet, R.A. DeFronzo, and H. Keen (Honorary)
© 1997 John Wiley & Sons Ltd

Whereas the amino acid sequences in the IAPP$_{1-37}$ domain show a high degree of conservation between species, there are considerable differences in the regions of the N- and C-terminal flanking peptides (Figure 2). In man, monkey and cat the N-terminal flanking peptide consists of 11 residues but in rat, mouse and guinea-pig, three additional residues are encoded by nucleotides at the junction of exon 2 and the adjacent intron.

Biosynthesis of IAPP

The promoter region of the gene shows several similarities with the insulin gene promoter, having both enhancer and inhibitory regions [21, 22]. However, there is no evidence for abnormalities in the 5' region of the IAPP gene which could be linked to type 2 diabetes [23]. PreproIAPP is expressed in islet B cells and comparison of biosynthesis of insulin and IAPP in mouse tumour cells indicates that IAPP is less efficiently translated than insulin and that conversion of proIAPP to the mature peptide occurs more quickly in these cells than the conversion of proinsulin to insulin [24]. Cleavage of proIAPP is likely to occur in the B cell granules, possibly utilising the granule peptidases involved in the conversion of proinsulin to insulin [25]. Immunoreactivity for both the C- and N-terminal flanking peptides of IAPP have been identified in the B cell granules [26, 27]. Type 2 diabetic subjects secrete an increased proportion of proinsulin to insulin compared to non-diabetic subjects [28]. If abnormalities in processing of granule peptides exist in type 2 diabetes, there

could be increased secretion of incompletely processed proIAPP.

Structure of IAPP in Relation to Amyloid Formation

Some other forms of amyloidosis are associated with genetic abnormalities resulting in single or multiple amino acid substitutions and production of an amyloidogenic peptide [29, 30]. Extensive genetic analyses have shown no variations in the IAPP gene linked to type 2 diabetes [31, 32]. Furthermore, the amino acid sequence for human IAPP (hIAPP) deduced from cDNA is identical to the peptide structure identified in extracts of amyloid [1]. This suggests that there is no post-translational structural change in the molecule resulting in fibril formation.

IAPP has been identified in every species so far examined: in the monkey [9], dog [14], cat [13], hamster [10], cougar [11], rat, mouse, guinea-pig and degu [8, 12, 17] (Figure 2). The sequence of IAPP$_{1-37}$ is highly conserved with a minimum of 78% homology between the human sequence and that of the guinea-pig or degu (Figure 2). Aggregation of IAPP *in vivo* is critically dependent upon the amino acid sequence of IAPP$_{25-28}$ which varies between species [13, 33, 34]. IAPP also aggregates to form fibrils *in vitro* [13, 33], a feature shared by other amyloidogenic proteins [35]. The sequence Ala–Ile–Lys–Ser (hIAPP$_{25-28}$) appears to be critical for fibrillogenesis *in vitro* [13, 33]. This sequence is also important for amyloid formation *in vivo* since it is common to man and domestic cat (Figure 2), species in which diabetes

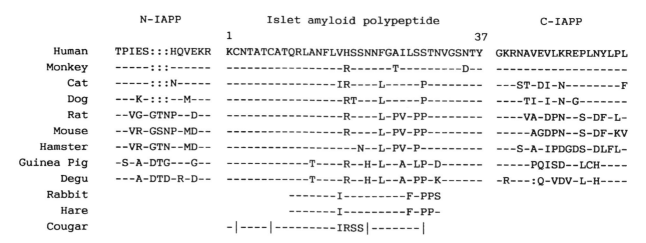

	N-IAPP	Islet amyloid polypeptide	C-IAPP
		1 37	
Human	TPIES:::HQVEKR	KCNTATCATQRLANFLVHSSNNFGAILSSTNVGSNTY	GKRNAVEVLKREPLNYLPL
Monkey	-----:::------	----------------R------T---------D--	-------------------
Cat	-----:::N-----	----------------IR----L-----P-------	---ST-DI-N--------F
Dog	---K-:::--M---	----------------RT---L-----P-------	----TI-I-N-G-------
Rat	--VG-GTNP--D--	----------------R----L-PV-PP-------	----VA-DPN--S-DF-L-
Mouse	--VR-GSNP-MD--	----------------R----L-PV-PP-------	-----AGDPN--S-DF-KV
Hamster	--VR-GTN--MD--	----------------N--L-PV-P---------	---S-A-IPDGDS-DLFL-
Guinea Pig	-S-A-DTG---G--	------------T----R--H-L--A-LP-D------	-----PQISD--LCH----
Degu	---A-DTD-R-D--	------------T----R--H-L--A-PP-K------	-R---:Q-VDV-L-H----
Rabbit		-------I---------F-PPS	
Hare		-------I---------F-PP-	
Cougar		-|----|---------IRSS|-------|	

Figure 2 The amino acid sequence of proIAPP in 9 species of mammal and partial sequence of IAPP in an additional three species. The amino acid sequence which is critical for fibrillogenesis, hIAPP$_{24-28}$ (GAILS), is conserved in species in which amyloid develops in islets or insulinomas (human, cat and dog) and has only one substitution in monkey. Synthetic fragments of rabbit and hare IAPP will form fibrils *in vitro*. Amino acids are indicated by a single letter code: A, alanine; C, cysteine; D, aspartic acid; E, glutamic acid; F, phenylalanine; G, glycine; H, histidine; I, isoleucine; K, lysine; L, leucine; M, methionine; N, asparagine; P, proline; Q, glutamine; R, arginine; S, serine; T, threonine; V, valine; Y, tyrosine

develops later in life and amyloid is present in the pancreatic islets. Diabetes-related amyloid also occurs in older non-human primates [36, 37]. IAPP in macaque monkeys (*Macaca nemestrina*) differs from hIAPP and feline IAPP in having threonine at position 25 [9], but since islet amyloid is present in other closely related Macaque species (*Macaca mulatta* and *M. nigra*) [36, 37], this substitution is unlikely to affect the potential for amyloid formation. Residue 25 is proline in mice, rats and hamsters. Westermark and colleagues [33] have suggested that this particular residue is a critical determinant for fibrillogenesis. However, analysis of canine IAPP has shown that the amino acid sequence cannot be the only determining factor for islet amyloid formation: whereas feline and canine IAPP$_{25-28}$ sequence is identical, islet amyloid is associated with diabetes in the cat, but not in the dog, even though amyloid formed from IAPP is present in some canine insulinomas [14, 38]. This suggests that, in addition to the IAPP sequence, physiological and/or biochemical factors are involved in amyloid formation.

Localisation of IAPP

Islet B cells are the major site of IAPP expression in the body. Immunoreactivity for IAPP$_{1-37}$ is present in the secretory granules but the highest density of IAPP is found in secondary lysosomes of both diabetic and non-diabetic man and monkeys (Figure 3) [4]. IAPP does not accumulate in the lysosomes of rodents [39]. The origin of this IAPP is unknown but is likely to result from incorporation of B cell granules into lysosomes

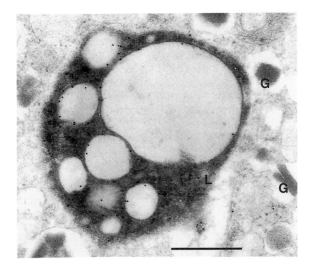

Figure 3 B cell lysosome from a human pancreas immuno-labelled for IAPP. Immunogold labelling is localised to the electron-dense parts of the lysosome (L) in a pancreatic B cell of a non-diabetic man. G = insulin granules. Scale bar 0.5 μm

(crinophagy) [40] and less efficient degradation of primate IAPP compared to rodents.

Expression of IAPP during embryogenesis may not be limited to B cells. During human fetal development, IAPP appears in the pancreas at 10 weeks gestation together with insulin [41]. Immunoreactivity for IAPP has been identified in pluripotent fetal islet cells [42] and IAPP can be co-expressed with glucagon (A cells) or somatostatin (D cells) in cell lines transformed from neonatal rat islet cells [43]. In adult rodents, IAPP has been identified in D cells [44].

IAPP has been identified in the stomach and duodenum of man and the rat; IAPP mRNA in extracts of rat stomach is approximately 5% of that found in the pancreas of rats [45], and cells immunoreactive for IAPP but not for insulin have been localised to the mucosa of the pyloric antrum in rat and man [46]. The function of IAPP in the intestinal tract is unknown.

Expression and Release of IAPP

Expression of mRNA and secretion of IAPP and insulin are closely linked in most conditions. In the rat pancreas, the amount of pancreatic IAPP mRNA is approximately 5–10% of insulin mRNA and is reduced in parallel with insulin in streptozotocin-induced diabetes, hypoglycaemia [12, 45, 47] and in spontaneously diabetic (BB) Wistar rats [48].

IAPP is co-secreted with insulin in response to glucose, arginine and other B cell secretagogues. Studies on isolated B cells, islets and perfused pancreas have indicated that, under most conditions, changes in IAPP secretion parallel changes in insulin secretion and represent 1–20% of the insulin production on a molar basis [6, 49, 50, 51, 52, 53, 54, 55]. It has been suggested that changes in the molar ratio of insulin to IAPP could be involved in type 2 diabetes. Experiments with long-term stimulation with high glucose concentrations on human islets and rat pancreas have suggested that secretion of the two peptides is not tightly coupled [56, 57].

Circulating Concentrations of IAPP

In non-diabetic man and animals, plasma IAPP concentrations are low in comparison with insulin: basal levels in normal weight individuals vary from 2 to 13 pmol/l and are elevated in parallel with insulin secretion to 5–17 pmol/l after a glucose load [53, 54, 58, 59, 60, 61]. Type 1 diabetic subjects with severely reduced C-peptide secretion have little or no measurable IAPP in the circulation [61]. Obese individuals in whom basal and stimulated insulin levels are elevated have higher plasma concentrations of IAPP than normal weight subjects [62, 63, 64]. However, there is no evidence for elevation or reduction of basal or stimulated IAPP concentrations in type 2 diabetic subjects which could be related to the deposition of islet amyloid [62, 63].

Plasma concentrations of IAPP higher than in obese subjects (25 pmol/l) have been reported in patients with chronic renal insufficiency. Following dialysis, the IAPP levels in these patients were reduced by 50% suggesting that, like C-peptide, IAPP is normally excreted via the kidney [65, 66].

The measurement of IAPP in plasma samples by radioimmunoassay is difficult. The iodinated IAPP tracer is relatively unstable and the assays currently available are relatively insensitive for the low plasma concentrations of IAPP [67]. Furthermore, more than one molecular form of IAPP has been detected in the circulation: both intact $IAPP_{1-37}$ and a shorter form, $IAPP_{17-37}$ have been identified, in variable ratios, in rat and human plasma [58].

AMYLOID AND TYPE 2 DIABETES

Diabetes-associated amyloid is found only in humans, non-human primates and cats [68]. Islet amyloid is not found in rodent models of obesity and diabetes even though the physiological parameters may be similar to that of the syndrome of type 2 diabetes in man. Amyloid deposits can be detected before the onset of hyperglycaemia in the course of development of spontaneous diabetes in cats [69, 70] and monkeys [37]. In these animal models of type 2 diabetes, the amyloid deposits in the 'prediabetic' period are relatively small and restricted to a few islets (Plate 1a,b). However, the degree of amyloid formation and the number of islets affected increases with the progression of symptoms which precede the onset of diabetes (Plate 1c,d) [36, 37, 69]. In monkeys (and possibly in man) the onset of hyperglycaemia could be closely related to the degree of loss of B cells (or B cell function) due to amyloid deposition (Plate 1). The critical mass of actively secreting B cells required to maintain normoglycaemia in man is unknown. In monkeys, a reduction of the B cell population by 30% is enough to induce hyperglycaemia [71]. The extent of islet amyloid at post mortem in type 2 diabetic subjects is very variable: these patients have 5–90% of islets affected with up to 30% reduction in B cell population (Plate 1e) [72]. Thus, relatively small deposits of amyloid could be involved in the onset of type 2 diabetes. Although the extent of amyloidosis is relatively small the localisation of the amyloid adjacent to the B cells and between the islet cells and capillaries (Figure 4a) could severely impair islet function: the dynamics of glucose signalling and the resultant insulin release could be affected by the perivascular diffusion barrier created by the amyloid deposits. In addition, the cell border of

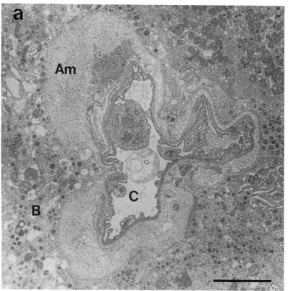

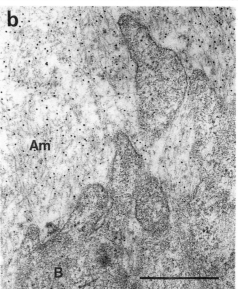

Figure 4 Amyloid deposits in islets of 'prediabetic' monkeys. (a) Amyloid (Am), immunogold-labelled for IAPP, surrounds an islet capillary (C), creating a barrier between the vessel and the adjacent B cell (B). Scale bar = 5 μm. (b) Amyloid fibrils immunogold-labelled for IAPP (Am) at the edge of a B cell (B). The irregular borders of the B cell suggest that amyloid deposition disrupts the normal architecture of the cell. Scale bar = 0.5 μm

B cells adjacent to amyloid deposits is often very irregular (Figure 4b), suggesting interaction of the B cell with amyloid.

If amyloid formation is initiated by abnormalities within the cell, this could have a considerable effect on the normal function of the B cell. In severe islet amyloidosis in type 2 diabetic man, amyloid deposits can be found in up to 90% of the pancreatic islets, occupying up to 80% of the islet space (Plate 1e) [72], and, in diabetic cats and monkeys, 60–100% of islets

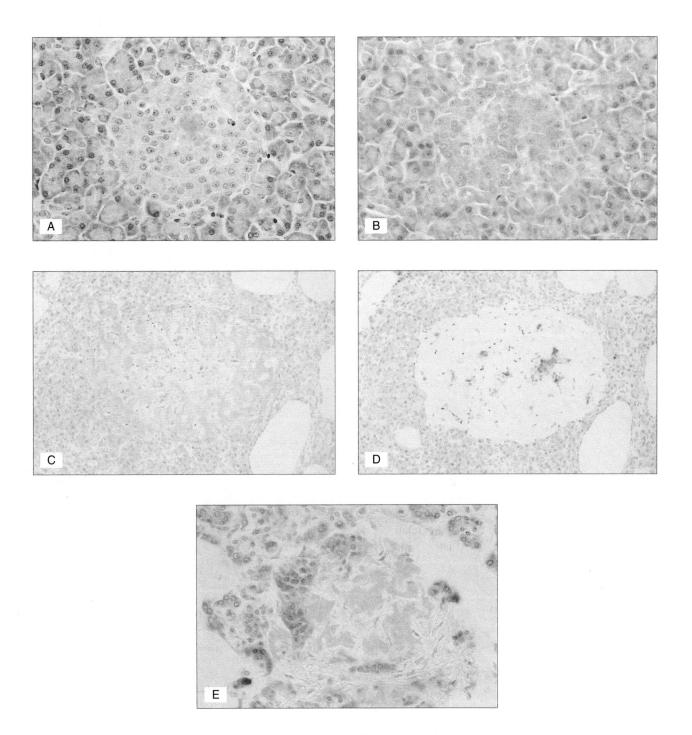

Plate 1 Amyloid deposits in (a-d) islets of *Macaca mulatta* monkeys and (e) pancreatic islet of a type 2 diabetic patient. (a,b) Adjacent sections of a pancreatic islet from an obese, hyperinsulinaemic, normoglycaemic monkey immunoperoxidase-labelled for IAPP (a) and insulin (b): two small patches of amyloid immunolabelled for IAPP (brown colour) are present in the islet which contains largely insulin-producing B cells. (x235). (c,d) Adjacent sections of an islet from a diabetic monkey immunoperoxidase labelled for IAPP (c) and insulin (d). Amyloid deposits immunoperoxidase-labelled for IAPP occupy most of the islet whilst B cells are severely reduced in number and surrounded by amyloid. (x94). (e) Amyloid deposits stained pink with Congo red fill the centre of the islet in a type 2 diabetic patient. The B cells (immunoperoxidase-labelled for insulin—brown colour) are severely reduced in number and occupy only a small proportion of the islet space. (x235)

are affected [37, 70]. In this severe pathological state the few remaining islet cells are completely enclosed within the mass of amyloid (Plate 1c,d). Glucose stimuli and the resulting insulin release in such conditions are likely to be severely compromised. In type 2 diabetic man, the extent of islet amyloidosis has been shown to relate to the severity of the diabetic symptoms as defined by the need for insulin therapy [73]. The clinically undetectable process of amyloid formation disrupts the islet and destroys the B cells, resulting in diminished islet function.

Amyloid Fibril Formation

The mechanisms by which IAPP molecules are converted into a β-sheet conformation and subsequently polymerise to form fibrils are unknown. The primary and secondary structures of IAPP are determining factors for fibril formation [68]. Human IAPP is relatively insoluble and polymerises to form fibrils in concentrated solution at neutral or alkaline pH *in vitro* [13, 33]. Hence, overproduction and accumulation of IAPP at intra- or extracellular sites combined with other unidentified biochemical factors (such as pH) could induce fibril formation. Amyloid formed from IAPP is present in human insulinomas [74]: hypersecretion of IAPP from the tumour cells and incomplete clearance from the extracellular space could result in accumulation of the peptide and fibrillogenesis. Amyloid deposition is a progressive phenomenon and it is likely that the first IAPP fibrils to be formed would act as a nidus for subsequent polymerisation of IAPP [75]. Hence, IAPP secreted from the islet B cells in response to B cell secretagogues, such as glucose or sulphonylurea drugs, would continue to polymerise onto fibrils forming amyloid.

In addition, IAPP fibrils are present within some insulinoma B cells suggesting that abnormal intracellular handling of the peptide leads to fibril formation [74]. IAPP fibrils within the cell could lead to disruption of metabolism and cell death. It is possible that, once initiated, the process of amyloid formation proceeds via more than one route: extracellular amyloid could be derived from (a) secreted IAPP, (b) cells dying as a result of IAPP accumulation, (c) extrusion from islet B cells of lysosomes containing high concentrations of IAPP [4, 39].

PHYSIOLOGICAL EFFECTS OF IAPP

There has been considerable interest in possible hormonal roles of IAPP (Table 1). The C-terminal amidation of IAPP suggests that the peptide has endocrine activity and its co-release with insulin from pancreatic B cells has implicated IAPP in glucose metabolism. In addition, the homologies of IAPP with calcitonin and CGRP suggest that IAPP could have a hormonal role in calcium metabolism. However, even after extensive *in vivo* and *in vitro* physiological studies, the exact role (or roles) of IAPP remains obscure.

Table 1 Roles of IAPP

Intrapancreatic
Formation of islet amyloid
Inhibition of insulin secretion
Extrapancreatic
Inhibition of insulin-stimulated glycogen synthesis in skeletal muscle
Promotion of lactate formation from skeletal muscle
Vasodilation
Inhibition of bone resorption
Suppression of food intake

Actions of IAPP on Glucose Metabolism

High concentrations of IAPP (10–100 nmol/l) have been shown to reduce insulin-stimulated uptake of glucose and incorporation of glucose into glycogen, and to activate glycogen phosphorylase in human and rat skeletal muscle strips *in vitro* [76, 81]. It was therefore proposed that IAPP modulates insulin resistance and, as such, would be a significant factor in the decreased insulin sensitivity in type 2 diabetes [82, 83, 84, 85]. However, studies with exogenous synthetic IAPP infusions *in vivo* in man and laboratory animals have produced results which do not support this hypothesis. IAPP in concentrations equivalent to those measured in the circulation in man (5–50 pmol/l) had no effect on glucose disposal in some experiments *in vivo* on rats or dogs [82, 83, 86, 87] and concentrations in the circulation as high as 1500 pmol/l had no effect on glucose disposal in man [88].

An additional hypothesis states that IAPP promotes lactate production by skeletal muscle which is used as a fuel for hepatic glycogen formation and increased glucose output (the Cori cycle) [89]. Although there is some preliminary evidence for increased lactate production in response to IAPP [89, 90, 91], the role of IAPP, and the relevance of this complex cascade to diabetes, has still to be demonstrated. Furthermore, observations in transgenic mice do not support a major role for IAPP in insulin resistance: elevated expression and high circulating concentrations of IAPP (2–15 times higher than controls) in transgenic mice expressing the gene for rat IAPP (identical to mouse IAPP) under transcriptional control of an insulin gene promoter, does not lead to hyperinsulinaemia, hyperglycaemia, elevated lactate concentrations or obesity [92, 93, 94].

Structural homology of IAPP with CGRP has led to some difficulties in identifying specific receptors for IAPP. CGRP and IAPP have similar biological effects and both peptides appear to act via CGRP-binding sites in skeletal muscle, hepatic cells [95] and other tissues, possibly involving activation of adenylate cyclase [96]. Some of these effects are inhibited by $CGRP_{8-37}$ or $IAPP_{8-37}$ both of which have been proposed as IAPP receptor blocking agents [97, 98]. However, the hypothesis of a specific action of IAPP on carbohydrate metabolism in diabetes via well characterised IAPP receptors, while attractive, remains unproven.

IAPP and Insulin Secretion

IAPP in relatively high concentrations (0.03–10 µmol/l) has been shown to inhibit glucose-stimulated insulin secretion from isolated pancreatic islets and in perfused pancreas [99, 100, 101]. However, other reports indicate a lack of effect of IAPP on glucose-induced insulin or glucagon secretion [102, 103, 104] and there is no evidence for an inhibitory effect in man *in vivo* with plasma concentrations of IAPP up to 1500 pmol/l [88, 106]. The islet is supplied by CGRP-containing nerves and CGRP affects insulin and glucagon secretion under various physiological conditions in rats and mice [107, 108], pigs [109] and dogs [110]. No effects of IAPP on proinsulin biosynthesis can be demonstrated [111] and the mechanisms involved in the effects of IAPP on glucose-stimulated insulin secretion remain obscure. It is possible that the structurally homologous IAPP molecule is acting on CGRP receptors in the islet to modulate insulin secretion.

Other Effects of IAPP

IAPP, like CGRP, acts as a vasodilator [97, 112] although IAPP is far less potent. A possibility therefore exists that IAPP co-secreted with insulin, together with CGRP from nerves, could facilitate insulin delivery to the circulation by dilatation of vessels in the islets or pancreas.

Infusions of IAPP decrease plasma calcium concentrations suggesting an action of IAPP on calcium metabolism [113]. IAPP has been shown to affect bone resorption, although, compared to calcitonin, it is 10–100 times less potent in this respect [113, 114]. In addition, effects of IAPP on the central nervous system causing anorexia have been reported [115]. It is likely that these actions of IAPP are mediated via calcitonin or CGRP receptors and reflect some evolutionary aspects of IAPP.

CONCLUSIONS

IAPP, a Role in Pathology or Therapy?

Islet amyloid polypeptide (IAPP) polymerises to form insoluble amyloid fibrils by as yet unknown mechanisms in the islets of type 2 diabetic patients.

Progressive accumulation of the amyloid deposits is likely to contribute to the deterioration of islet function during the course of the disease. Although IAPP is co-secreted with insulin its effects as a hormone are unclear. Studies *in vitro* have indicated that IAPP (amylin) has a role in glucose metabolism. Suggestions have been made that IAPP-like peptides could be used for the treatment of diabetes: in type 1 diabetes to reduce insulin-induced hypoglycaemia, and in type 2 diabetes to reduce insulin resistance, obesity and hyperglycaemia. However, directions for future research should include identification of therapeutic measures to reduce or prevent the formation of islet amyloid and thus minimise deterioration of islet function in type 2 diabetes.

Acknowledgements

We would like to thank Drs Barbara Hansen and Noni Bodkin for providing tissue from diabetic monkeys, Sophie Chargé for technical assistance and Dr John Morris for his interest and support. We are grateful to Toria Summers for her assistance in preparation of the manuscript and to the British Diabetic Association, the Oxford Medical Research Committee and Mallinkrodt Medical Inc. for financial support. Eelco de Koning is a Medical Research Council Training Fellow.

REFERENCES

1. Westermark P, Wernstedt C, Wilander E, Hayden DW, O'Brien TD, Johnson KH. Amyloid fibrils in human insulinoma and islets of Langerhans of the diabetic cat are derived from a neuropeptide-like protein also present in normal islet cells. Proc Natl Acad Sci USA 1987; 84: 3881–5.
2. Clark A, Cooper GJS, Lewis CE, Morris JF, Willis AC, Reid KBM, Turner RC. Islet amyloid formed from diabetes-associated peptide may be pathogenic in type 2 diabetes. Lancet 1987; ii: 231–4.
3. Cooper GJS, Willis AC, Clark A, Turner RC, Sim RB, Reid KBM. Purification and characterisation of a peptide from amyloid-rich pancreases of type 2 diabetic patients. Proc Natl Acad Sci USA 1987; 84: 8628–32.
4. Clark A, Edwards CA, Ostle LR, Sutton R, Rothbard JB, Morris JF, Turner RC. Localisation of islet amyloid peptide in lipofuscin bodies and secretory granules of human β-cells and in islets of type 2 diabetic subjects. Cell Tissue Res 1989; 257: 179–85.
5. Lukinius A, Wilander E, Westermark GT, Engström U, Westermark P. Co-localisation of islet amyloid polypeptide and insulin in the β-cell secretory granules of the human pancreatic islets. Diabetologia 1989; 32: 240–4.
6. Kahn SE, d'Alessio DA, Schwartz MW, Fujimoto WY, Ensinck JW, Taborsky GJ, Porte D. Evidence of co-secretion of islet amyloid polypeptide and insulin by β-cells. Diabetes 1990; 39: 634–8.

7. Sanke T, Bell GI, Sample C, Rubenstein AH, Steiner DF. An islet amyloid peptide is derived from an 89 amino acid precursor by proteolytic processing. J Biol Chem 1988; 263: 17243-6.

8. Nishi M, Chau SJ, Nagamatsu S, Bell GI, Steiner DF. Conservation of the sequence of islet amyloid polypeptide in five mammals is consistent with its putative role as an islet hormone. Proc Natl Acad Sci USA 1989; 86: 5738-42.

9. Ohagi S, Nishi M, Bell GI, Ensinck JW, Steiner DF. Sequences of islet amyloid polypeptide precursors of an old world monkey, the pig-tailed macaque *Macaca nemestrina* and the dog *Canis familiaris*. Diabetologia 1991; 34: 555-8.

10. Nishi M, Bell GI, Steiner DF. Sequence of a cDNA encoding Syrian hamster islet amyloid polypeptide precursor. Nucleic Acids Res 1990; 18: 6726.

11. Johnson KH, Wernstedt C, O'Brien TD, Westermark P. Amyloid in the pancreatic islets of the cougar *Felis concolor* is derived from islet amyloid polypeptide IAPP. Comp Biochem Physiol B 1991; 98: 115-19.

12. Leffert JD, Newgard CB, Okamoto H, Milburn JL, Luskey KL. Rat amylin: cloning and tissue-specific expression in pancreatic islets. Proc Natl Acad Sci USA 1989; 86: 3127-30.

13. Betzholtz C, Christmanson L, Engström U, Rorsman F, Jordan K, O'Brien TD et al. Structure of cat islet amyloid polypeptide and identification of amino acid residues of potential significance for islet amyloid formation. Diabetes 1990; 39: 118-22.

14. Jordan K, Murtaugh MP, O'Brien TD, Westermark P, Betsholtz C, Johnson KH. Canine IAPP cDNA sequence provides important clues regarding diabetogenesis and amyloidogenesis in type 2 diabetes. Biochem Biophys Res Commun 1990; 169: 502-8.

15. Clark A. Islet amyloid: an enigma of type 2 diabetes. Diabet Metab Rev 1992; 8: 117-32.

16. Christmanson L, Betzholtz C, Leckström A, Engström U, Cortie C, Johnson KH et al. Islet amyloid polypeptide in the rabbit and European hare: studies on its relationship to amyloidogenesis. Diabetologia 1993; 36: 183-8.

17. Nishi M, Steiner DF. Cloning of complementary DNAs encoding islet amyloid polypeptide insulin and glucagon precursors from a New World rodent, the degu, *Octodon degus*. Mol Endocrinol 1990; 4: 1192-8.

18. Mosselman S, Höppener JWM, Zandberg J, van Mansfield ADM, Geurts van Kessel AHM, Lips CJM, Jansz HS. Islet amyloid polypeptide IAPP: identification and chromosomal localization of the human gene. FEBS Lett 1988; 239: 227-32.

19. van Mansfield ADM, Mosselman S, Höppener JWM, Zandberg J, van Teefflen NAAM, Baas PD et al. Islet amyloid polypeptide: structure and upstream sequences of the IAPP genes in rat and man. Biochem Biophys Acta 1990; 1087: 235-40.

20. Höppener JWM, Oosterwijk C, Visser-Vernooy HJ, Lips CJM, Jansz HS. Characterisation of the human islet amyloid polypeptide/amylin gene transcripts: identification of a new polyadenylation site. Biochem Biophys Res Commun 1992; 189: 1569-77.

21. Mosselman S, Höppener JWM, de Wit L, Soeller W, Lips CJM, Jansz HS. IAPP/amylin gene transcriptional control region: evidence for negative regulation. FEBS Lett 1990; 271: 33-6.

22. German MS, Moss LG, Wang J, Rutter WJ. The insulin and islet amyloid polypeptide genes contain similar cell-specific promoter elements that bind identical β-cell nuclear complexes. Molec Cell Biol 1992; 12: 1777-88.

23. Lehto M, Eriksson J, Nakasato M. Could a mutation in the amylin gene promoter region explain hyperamylinaemia in individuals predisposed to NIDDM? Diabetes 1992; 41: 92A.

24. Nagamatsu S, Nishi M, Steiner DF. Biosynthesis of islet amyloid polypeptide. J Biol Chem 1991; 296: 13737-41.

25. Guest PC, Hutton JC. Biosynthesis of insulin secretory granule proteins. In Flatt PR (ed) Nutrient regulation of insulin secretion. London: Portland Press, 1992; pp 59-82.

26. Clark A, Lloyd J, Novials A, Hutton JC, Morris JF. Localisation of islet amyloid polypeptide and its carboxy-terminal flanking peptide in islets of diabetic man and monkey. Diabetologia 1991; 34: 449-51.

27. Clark A, de Koning EJP, Baker CA, Chargé S, Morris JF. Localisation of N-terminal pro-islet amyloid polypeptide in β cells of man and transgenic mice. Diabetologia 1993; 36: A136.

28. Porte D, Kahn SE Hyperproinsulinaemia and amyloid in NIDDM: clues to etiology of islet β-cell dysfunction. Diabetes 1989; 38: 1333-6.

29. Palsdottir A, Abrahamson M, Thorsteinsson L, Arnason A, Olafsson I, Grubb A, Jensson O. Mutation in cystatin C gene causes hereditary brain haemorrhage. Lancet 1988; ii: 603-4.

30. Pras M, Prelli F, Franklin EC, Frangione B. Primary structure of an amyloid pre-albumin variant in familial polyneuropathy of Jewish origin. Proc Natl Acad Sci USA 1983; 30: 539-42.

31. Nishi M, Bell GI, Steiner DF. Islet amyloid polypeptide (amylin): no evidence of an abnormal precursor sequence in 25 Type 2 (non-insulin dependent) diabetic patients. Diabetologia 1990; 33: 628-30.

32. Cook JT, Patel PP, Clark A, Höppener JW, Lips CJ, Mosselman S et al. Non-linkage of the islet amyloid polypeptide gene with type 2 non-insulin dependent diabetes mellitus. Diabetologia 1991; 34: 103-8.

33. Westermark P, Engström U, Johnson KH, Westermark GT, Betzholtz C. Islet amyloid polypeptide: pinpointing amino acid residues linked to amyloid fibril formation. Proc Natl Acad Sci USA 1990; 87: 5036-40.

34. Westermark P, Johnson KH, Engström U, Westermark GT, Betzholtz C. Islet amyloid polypeptide: synthetic peptides for study of the pathogenesis of islet amyloid. In Natvig JB, Førre Ø, Husby G et al (eds) Amyloid and amyloidosis. Dordrecht: Kluwer, 1991; pp 449-52.

35. Kirschner DA, Inouye H, Duffy LK, Sinclair A, Lind M, Selkoe DJ. Synthetic peptide homologous to beta protein from Alzheimer's disease forms amyloid-like fibrils *in vitro*. Proc Natl Acad Sci USA 1987; 84: 6953-7.

36. Howard CF. Longitudinal studies on the development of diabetes in individual *Macaca nigra*. Diabetologia 1986; 29: 301-6.

37. de Koning EJP, Bodkin NL, Hansen BC, Clark A. Diabetes mellitus in *Macaca mulatta* monkeys is characterised by islet amyloidosis and reduction in β-cell population. Diabetologia 1993; 36: 378-84.

38. O'Brien TD, Westermark P, Johnson KH. Islet amyloid polypeptide and calcitonin gene-related peptide immunoreactivity in amyloid and tumour cells of canine pancreatic endocrine tumours. Vet Pathol 1990; 27: 194–8.

39. Clark A, de Koning EJP, Morris JF. Formation of islet amyloid from islet amyloid polypeptide. Biochem Soc Trans 1993; 21: 169–73.

40. Borg LAH, Schnell AH. Lysosomes and pancreatic islet function: intracellular insulin degradation and lysosomal transformations. Diabet Res 1986; 3: 277–85.

41. In't Veld PA, Zang F, Madsen OD, Klöppel G. Islet amyloid polypeptide immunoreactivity in the human fetal pancreas. Diabetologia 1992; 35: 272–6.

42. de Krijger RR, Kranenburg G, Stevens M, Rahier JRD, Bruining GJ. The presence of islet amyloid polypeptide during the development of the human fetal pancreas. Diabetologia 1991; 34: A43.

43. Madsen OD, Nielsen JH, Michelsen B, Westermark P, Betsholtz C, Nishi M, Steiner DF. Islet amyloid polypeptide and insulin expression are controlled differently in primary and transformed islet cells. Mol Endocrinol 1991; 5: 143–8.

44. De Vroede M, Foriers A, Van de Winkel M, Madsen O, Pipeleers D. Presence of islet amyloid polypeptide in rat islet B and D cells determines parallelism and dissociation between rat pancreatic islet amyloid polypeptide and insulin content. Biochem Biophys Res Commun 1992; 182: 886–93.

45. Ferrier GJM, Pierson AM, Jones PM, Bloom SR, Girgis SI, Legon S. Expression of the rat amylin IAPP/DAP gene. Mol Endocrinol 1989; 3: R1–4.

46. Toshimori H, Navita R, Nakazato M, Asai J, Mitsukawa T, Kangawa K, Matsuo H, Matsukura S. Islet amyloid polypeptide (IAPP) in the gastrointestinal tract in pancreas of man and rat. Cell Tissue Res 1990; 262: 401–6.

47. Alam T, Chen L, Ogawa A, Leffert J, Unger RH, Luskey KL. Co-ordinate regulation of amylin and insulin expression in response to hypoglycaemia and fasting. Diabetes 1992; 41: 508–14.

48. Bretherton-Watt D, Ghatei MA, Legon S, Jamal H, Suda K, Bloom SR. Depletion of islet amyloid polypeptide in the spontaneously diabetic (BB) Wistar rat. J Mol Endocrinol 1991; 6: 3–7.

49. Kanatsuka A, Makino H, Ohsawa H, Tokuyama Y, Yamaguchi T, Yoshuda S, Adachi M. Secretion of islet amyloid polypeptide in response to glucose. FEBS Lett 1989; 259: 199–201.

50. Ogawa A, Harris V, McCorkle SK, Unger RH, Luskey KL. Amylin secretion from the rat pancreas and its selective loss after streptozotocin treatment. J Clin Invest 1989; 85: 973–8.

51. Inoue K, Hisatomi A, Umeda F, Nawata H. Release of amylin from perfused rat pancreas in response to glucose, arginine, beta hydroxybutyrate and gliclazide. Diabetes 1991; 40: 1005–9.

52. Moore CX, Cooper GJS. Co-secretion of amylin and insulin from cultured islet β cells: modulation by nutrient secretagogues, islet hormones and hypoglycaemic agents. Biochem Biophys Res Commun 1991; 179: 1–9.

53. O'Brien TD, Westermark P, Johnson KH. Islet amyloid polypeptide and insulin secretion from isolated perfused pancreas of fed, fasted, glucose-treated and dexamethazone-treated rats. Diabetes 1991; 40: 1701–6.

54. Jamal H, Bretherton-Watt D, Suda K, Ghatei MA, Bloom SR. Islet amyloid polypeptide-like immunoreactivity (amylin) in rats treated with dexamethasone and streptozotocin. J Endocrinol 1990; 126: 425–9.

55. Stridsberg M, Sandler S, Wilander E. Cosecretion of islet amyloid polypeptide (IAPP) and insulin from isolated rat pancreatic islets following stimulation or inhibition of β cell function. Regul Peptid 1993; 45: 363–70.

56. Gedulin B, Cooper GJS, Young AA. Amylin secretion from the perfused pancreas: dissociation from insulin and abnormal elevation in insulin-resistant diabetic rats. Biochem Biophys Res Commun 1991; 180: 782–9.

57. Novials A, Sarri Y, Casamitjana R, Rivera F, Gomis R. Regulation of islet amyloid polypeptide in human pancreatic islets. Diabetes 1993; 42: 1514–19.

58. Nakazato M, Miyazato M, Asai J, Mitsukawa T, Kangawa K, Matsuo H, Matsukura S. Islet amyloid polypeptide, a novel pancreatic peptide, is a circulating hormone secreted under glucose stimulation. Biochem Biophys Res Commun 1990; 169: 713–18.

59. Mitsukawa T, Takemura J, Asai J, Nakazato M, Nagawa K, Matsuo H, Mutsukura S. Islet amyloid polypeptide response to glucose, insulin and somatostatin analogue administration. Diabetes 1990; 39: 639–42.

60. Butler PC, Chou J, Carter WB, Wang Y-N, Bu B-H, Chang D, Chang J-K, Rizza RA. Effects of meal ingestion on plasma amylin concentration in NIDDM and non-diabetic humans. Diabetes 1990; 39: 752–6.

61. van Jaarsveld BC, Hackeng WHL, Lips CJM, Erkelens DW. Plasma concentrations of islet amyloid polypeptide after glucagon administration in type 2 diabetic patients and non-diabetic subjects. Diabet Med 1993; 10: 327–30.

62. Sanke T, Hanabusa T, Nakamo Y, Oki C, Okai K, Nishimura S, Kondo M, Nanjo K. Plasma islet amyloid polypeptide (amylin) levels and their responses to oral glucose in type 2 (non-insulin dependent) diabetic patients. Diabetologia 1991; 34: 129–32.

63. Ludvik B, Lell B, Hartter E, Schnack C, Prager R. Decrease of stimulated amylin release precedes impairment of insulin secretion in type 2 diabetes. Diabetes 1991; 40: 1615–19.

64. Hartter E, Svoboda T, Ludvik B, Schuller M, Lell B, Kuenburg E, Brunnbauer M, Woloszczuk W, Prager R. Basal and stimulated plasma levels of pancreatic amylin indicate its co-secretion with insulin in humans. Diabetologia 1991; 34: 52–4.

65. Ludvik B, Berzlanovich A, Hartter E, Lell B, Prager R, Graf H. Increased amylin levels in patients on chronic haemodialysis. Nephrol Dial Transplant 1990; 8: 694–5.

66. Watschinger B, Hartter E, Traindt O, Pohanka E, Pidlich J, Kovarik J. Increased levels of plasma amylin in advanced renal failure. Clin Nephrol 1992; 37: 131–4.

67. Nakazato M, Asai J, Kangawa K, Matsukura S, Matsuo H. Establishment of radioimmunoassay for human islet amyloid polypeptide and its tissue content and plasma concentration. Biochem Biophys Res Commun 1989; 164: 394–9.

68. Johnson KH, O'Brien TD, Betsholtz C, Westermark P. Islet amyloid, islet amyloid polypeptide and diabetes mellitus. New Engl J Med 1989; 321: 513–18.

69. O'Brien TD, Hayden DW, Johnson KH, Fletcher TF. Immunohistochemical morphometry of pancreatic endocrine cells in diabetic normoglycaemic glucose-intolerant and normal cats. J Comp Pathol 1986; 96: 357–69.

70. Johnson KH, O'Brien TD, Jordan K, Westermark P. Impaired glucose tolerance is associated with increased islet amyloid polypeptide (IAPP) immunoreactivity in pancreatic β cells. Am J Pathol 1989; 135: 245–50.

71. McCulloch DR, Koerker DJ, Kahn SE, Bonner-Weir S, Palmer JP. Correlations of in vivo β cell function tests with β cell mass and pancreatic insulin content in streptozotocin-administered baboons. Diabetes 1991; 40: 673–9.

72. Clark A, Wells CA, Buley ID, Cruickshank JK, Vanhegan RI, Matthews DR, et al. Islet amyloid, increased A cells, reduced β cells and exocrine fibrosis: quantitative changes in the pancreas in type 2 diabetes. Diabet Res 1988; 9: 151–60.

73. Schneider HM, Storkel S, Will W. Das Amyloid der Langerhansschen Inseln und seine Beziehung zum Diabetes Mellitus. Dtsch Med Wschr 1980; 105: 1143–7.

74. Clark A, Morris JF, Scott LA, McLay A, Foulis AK, Bodkin NL, Hansen BC. Intracellular formation of amyloid fibrils of human insulinoma and pre-diabetic monkey islets. In Natvig JB, Førre Ø, Husby G et al (eds) Amyloid and amyloidosis. Dordrecht: Kluwer, 1991: pp 453–6.

75. Lansbury PT. The structural basis for pancreatic amyloid formation. In Kisilevsky R, Benson MD, Frangione B, Gauldie S, Muckle TJ, Young ID (eds) Amyloid and amyloidosis: proceedings of VII International Symposium on Amyloidosis. New York: Parthenon, 1994.

76. Cooper GJS, Leighton B, Dimitriadis GD, Parry-Billings M, Kowalchuk JM, Howland K et al. Amylin found in amyloid deposits in human type 2 diabetes mellitus may be a hormone that regulates glycogen metabolism in skeletal muscle. Proc Natl Acad Sci USA 1988; 85: 7763–6.

77. Leighton B, Cooper GJS. Pancreatic amylin and calcitonin gene-related peptide cause resistance to insulin in skeletal muscle in vitro. Nature 1988; 335: 632.

78. Leighton B, Foot E. The effects of amylin on carbohydrate metabolism in skeletal muscle in vitro and in vivo. Biochem J 1990; 269: 19–23.

79. Young DA, Deems RO, Deacon RW, McIntosh RH, Foley JE. Effects of amylin on glucose metabolism and glycogenolysis in vivo and in vitro. Amer J Physiol 1990; 259: E457–61.

80. Zierath JR, Galuska D, Engström A, Johnson KH, Betzholtz C, Westermark P, Wallberg-Henriksson H. Human islet amyloid polypeptide at pharmacological levels inhibits insulin and phorbol-ester-stimulated glucose transport in in vitro incubated human muscle strips. Diabetologia 1992; 35: 26–31.

81. Young AA, Mott DM, Stone K, Cooper GJS. Amylin activates glycogen phosphorylase in the isolated soleus muscle of the rat. FEBS Lett 1991; 281: 149–51.

82. Frontoni S, Choi SB, Banduch D, Rossetti L. In vivo insulin resistance induced by amylin primarily through inhibition of insulin-stimulated glycogen synthesis in skeletal muscle. Diabetes 1991; 40: 568–73.

83. Koopmans SJ, van Mansfeld AD, Jansz HS, Krans HM, Radder JK, Frolich M, de Boer SF, Kreutter DK, Andrews GC, Maassen JA. Amylin induced in vivo insulin resistance in conscious rats: the liver is more sensitive to amylin than peripheral tissues. Diabetologia 1991; 34: 218–24.

84. Molina JM, Cooper GJS, Leighton B, Olefsky JM. Induction of insulin resistance in vivo by amylin and calcitonin gene-related peptide. Diabetes 1990; 39: 260–65.

85. Sowa R, Sanke T, Hrayama J, Tabata H, Furuta H, Nishimura S, Nanjo K. Islet amyloid polypeptide amide causes peripheral insulin resistance in vivo in dogs. Diabetologia 1990; 33: 118–20.

86. Tedstone AE, Nezzer T, Hughes SJ, Clark A, Matthews DR. The effect of islet amyloid polypeptide (amylin) and calcitonin-gene-related peptide on glucose removal in the anaesthetised rat and on insulin secretion from rat pancreatic islets in vitro. Biosci Rep 1990; 10: 339–45.

87. Kassir AA, Upadhyay AK, Lim TJ, Moossa AR, Olefsky JM. Lack of effect of islet amyloid polypeptide in causing insulin resistance in conscious dogs during euglycemic clamp studies. Diabetes 1991; 40: 998–1004.

88. Bretherton-Watt D, Gilbey SG, Ghatei MA, Beacham J, Machae AD and Bloom SR. Very high concentrations of islet amyloid polypeptide are necessary to alter the insulin response to intravenous glucose in man. J Clin Endocrinol 1992; 74: 1032–5.

89. Young AA, Crocker LB, Wolfe-Lopez D, Cooper GJS. Daily amylin replacement reverses hepatic glycogen depletion in insulin-treated streptozotocin diabetic rats. FEBS Lett 1991; 287: 203–5.

90. Young AA, Wang M-W, Cooper GJS. Amylin injection causes elevated plasma lactate and glucose in the rat. FEBS Lett 1991; 291: 101–4.

91. Deems RO, Cardinaux F, Deacon RW, Young DA. Amylin or CGRP (8–37) fragments reverse amylin-induced inhibition of ^{14}C-glycogen accumulation. Biochem Biophys Res Commun 1991; 181: 116–20.

92. de Koning EJP, Höppener JWM, Oosterwijk C, Verbeek SJ, Visser JH, Janz HS et al. Localisation of islet amyloid polypeptide (IAPP) in pancreatic islets of transgenic mice expressing the human or rat IAPP gene. Biochem Soc Trans 1992; 21: 26S.

93. Fox N, Schrementi J, Nishi M, Ohagi S, Chan SJ, Heisserman JA et al. Human islet amyloid polypeptide transgenic mice as a model of non-insulin dependent diabetes mellitus (NIDDM). FEBS Lett 1993; 323: 40–44.

94. Höppener JWM, Verbeek JS, de Koning EJP, Oosterwijk C, van Hulst KL, Visser-Vernooy HS et al. Chronic overproduction of islet amyloid polypeptide/amylin in transgenic mice: lysosomal localisation of human islet amyloid polypeptide and lack of marked hyperglycaemia or hyperinsulinaemia. Diabetologia 1993; 36: 1258–65.

95. Chantry A, Leighton B, Day AJ. Cross-reactivity of amylin with calcitonin gene-related peptide binding sites in rat liver and skeletal muscle membranes. Biochem J 1991; 277: 139–43.

96. Morishita T, Yamaguchi A, Fujita T, Chiba T. Activation of adenylate cyclase by islet amyloid polypeptide with COOH-terminal amide via calcitonin gene-related peptide receptors on rat liver plasma membranes. Diabetes 1990; 39: 875-7.

97. Gardiner SM, Compton AM, Kemp PA, Bennett T, Bose C, Foulkes R, Hughes B. Antagonistic effect of human alpha-calcitonin gene-related peptide (8-37) on regional hemodynamic actions of rat islet amyloid polypeptide in conscious Long-Evans rats. Diabetes 1991; 40: 948-51.

98. Wang ZL, Bennet WM, Ghatei MA, Byfield PGH, Smith DM, Bloom SR. Influence of islet amyloid polypeptide and the 8-37 fragment of islet amyloid polypeptide on insulin release from perifused rat islets. Diabetes 1993; 42: 330-35.

99. Ohsawa H, Kanatsuka A, Yamaguchi T, Makino H, Yoshida S. Islet amyloid polypeptide inhibits glucose-stimulated insulin secretion from isolated rat pancreatic islets. Biochem Biophys Res Commun 1989; 160: 961-7.

100. Silvestre RA, Peiro E, Degano P, Miralles P, Marco J. Inhibitory effect of rat amylin on the insulin responses to glucose and arginine in the perfused rat pancreas. Regul Peptid 1990; 31: 23-31.

101. Fehmann H-C, Weber V, Goke R, Goke B, Eissele R, Arnold R. Islet amyloid polypeptide (IAPP; amylin) influences the endocrine but not the exocrine rat pancreas. Biochem Biophys Res Commun 1990; 167: 1102-8.

102. O'Brien TD, Westermark P, Johnson KH. Islet amyloid polypeptide (IAPP) does not inhibit glucose-stimulated insulin secretion from isolated perfused rat pancreas. Biochem Biophys Res Commun 1990; 170: 1223-8.

103. Ar'Rajab A, Ahrén B. Effects of amidated rat islet amyloid polypeptide on glucose stimulated insulin secretion *in vivo* and *in vitro* in rats. Eur J Pharmacol 1991; 192: 443-5.

104. Broderick C, Brooke GS, diMarchi RD, Gold G. Human and rat amylin have no effects on insulin secretion in isolated rat pancreatic islets. Biochem Biophys Res Commun 1991; 177: 932-8.

105. Bretherton-Watt D, Gilbey SG, Ghatei MA, Beacham J, Bloom SR. Failure to establish islet amyloid polypeptide (amylin) as a circulating beta cell inhibiting hormone in man. Diabetologia 1990; 38: 115-17.

106. Wilding JPH, Khandan-Nia N, Gilbey SG, Bennet WM, Beacham J, Ghatei MA, Bloom SR. Amylin does not affect insulin sensitivity in humans. Diabetologia 1993; 36 (suppl. 1): A135.

107. Pettersson M, Ahrén B, Bottcher G, Sundler F. Calcitonin-gene-related peptide: occurrence in pancreatic islets in the mouse and the rat and inhibition of insulin secretion in the mouse. Endocrinology 1986; 119: 865-9.

108. Pettersson M, Lundquist I, Ahrén B. Neuropeptide Y and calcitonin gene-related peptide: effects on glucagon and insulin secretion in the mouse. Endocr Res 1987; 13: 407-17.

109. Ahrén B, Martinsson H, Nobin A. Effects of calcitonin-gene related peptide (CGRP) on islet hormone secretion in the pig. Diabetologia 1987; 30: 354-9.

110. Hermanson K, Ahrén B. Dual effects of calcitonin gene-related peptide on insulin secretion in the perfused dog pancreas. Regul Peptid 1990; 27: 149-57.

111. Nagamatsu S, Carroll J, Grodsky EM, Steiner DF. Lack of islet amyloid polypeptide regulation of insulin biosynthesis or secretion in normal rat islets. Diabetes 1990; 39: 871-4.

112. Brain SD, Williams TJ, Tippins JR, Morris HR, MacIntyre I. Calcitonin gene-related peptide is a potent vasodilator. Nature 1990; 313: 54-6.

113. Datta HK, Zaidi M, Wimalawansa SI, Ghatei MA, Beacham JL, Bloom SR, MacIntyre I. *In vivo* and *in vitro* effects of amylin and amylin-amide on calcium metabolism in the rabbit. Biochem Biophys Res Commun 1989; 162: 876-81.

114. Zaidi M, Datta HK, Bevis PJ, Wimalawansa SJ, MacIntyre I. Amylin amide: a new bone conserving peptide from the pancreas. Exp Physiol 1990; 75: 529-36.

115. Balasubramaniam A, Renugopalakrishnan V, Stein M, Fischer JE, Chance WT. Syntheses, structures and anorectic effects of human and rat amylin. Peptides 1991; 12: 919-24.

20

IGF-I, IGF-II, IGF-binding Proteins and Diabetes

Jan Frystyk and Hans Ørskov

Institute of Experimental Clinical Research, University Hospital, Aarhus, Denmark

INTRODUCTION

The term 'growth factor' is generally used to define a substance inducing cellular proliferation and/or differentiation, and embraces peptides among which the insulin-like growth factors (IGFs) constitute a major subclass [1]. The ubiquitous IGFs found in tissues and the circulation exert their effects through endocrine, paracrine and autocrine mechanisms [2]. Their biological actions were traditionally divided into metabolic insulin-like effects and promotion of cellular growth and differentiation. These can also be viewed in terms of time-scale: the metabolic response as short-term substrate regulation and the mitogenic response as long-term substrate regulation [3].

An association between diabetes mellitus and growth-promoting hormones was first recognized in 1937, when it was shown that anterior pituitary extracts precipitated diabetes in dogs [4]. Later, in 1950, it was shown that dogs given daily injections of purified growth hormone (GH) became permanently diabetic [5]. In 1969–70 further studies [6, 7] extended the evidence on the role of GH in diabetes by demonstrating that diabetic patients were GH-hypersecretory in a manner that was inversely related to metabolic control. Based on these and other findings, Lundbæk et al in 1970 put forward the as yet unproven hypothesis that the abnormalities in GH secretion were involved in the pathogenesis of diabetic angiopathy [8]. By this time hypophysectomy had already been used for treatment of proliferative retinopathy

[9]. Though this was the first proven efficacious therapy [10], it carried serious side-effects and was therefore abandoned with the appearance of argon-laser photocoagulation [11]. It is noteworthy that a follow-up study in 1987 including 100 surviving diabetic patients, who received pituitary [90]yttrium implantation in 1965, gave compelling evidence for protection against development of diabetic retinopathy [12].

The discovery of the insulin-like growth factors was based originally on three separate biological effects, which decided the early terminology: (a) the non-suppressible insulin-like activity of serum (NSILA) determined after addition of anti-insulin antiserum [13]; (b) the sulphation factor (SF) stimulating sulphate incorporation into cartilage [14]; and finally (c) the multiplication-stimulating activity (MSA), inducing mitogenic stimulation of cultured fibroblasts [15]. The term somatomedin was introduced when it became apparent that the observed biological effects, being partly under somatotropin (GH) regulation, were different expressions of the same peptides [16, 17]. Later, following molecular purification and sequencing, it became evident that the somatomedins consisted of GH-dependent as well as GH-independent peptides. Because of the pronounced structural homology with proinsulin and insulin [18, 19], and the mitogenic potential and the insulin-like effects in adipocytes and muscle tissue, they were re-named insulin-like growth factor I (IGF-I; formerly SF or Somatomedin C)

International Textbook of Diabetes Mellitus, Second Edition. Edited by K.G.M.M. Alberti, P. Zimmet, R.A. DeFronzo, and H. Keen (Honorary)
© 1997 John Wiley & Sons Ltd

and insulin-like growth factor II (IGF-II; formerly MSA) [20].

The first study of growth factors in diabetic patients was reported in 1969: the GH-dependent SF (IGF-I) was found to be subnormal in diabetic serum and to correlate negatively with fasting blood glucose [21]. Since then a multitude of clinical and experimental studies have focused on the regulation of circulating IGFs in diabetes mellitus and their possible pathogenic role in the metabolic derangement and, more recently, in the development of diabetic retinopathy and nephropathy.

This chapter will focus on current information on basic aspects of the IGFs, their physiological and pathophysiological roles with special reference to diabetes mellitus, the IGF-binding proteins (IGFBPs), and recent attempts to use recombinant IGF-I in the treatment of diabetes.

THE STRUCTURE, RECEPTORS AND BASIC MECHANISM OF ACTION OF IGFs

Molecular Structure of IGF-I and IGF-II

The amino acid sequence of the major form of each human IGF was determined in 1978, revealing IGF-I to consist of 70 amino acids (molecular weight (M_r) 7649 Da) and IGF-II of 67 amino acids (M_r 7471 Da), with a 65% homology between the peptides. The similarities with proinsulin/insulin were striking, as both growth factors, although single-stranded, contained three intrachain disulphide bridges and furthermore, the peptide chain could be divided into domains A and B (similar to insulin), C (analogous to C-peptide of proinsulin, but not cleaved away) and D (not present in insulin) [22–24]. Immunoactive IGF has been identified in practically all species studied, including non-mammalian and insect species, and the structure seems to have been conserved through evolution, since many different species produce highly similar IGF-peptides [18]. Human, porcine, bovine, ovine, rat and mouse IGF-I and IGF-II all consist of 70 and 67 amino acid residues, and the primary structure is maintained almost unchanged, human, porcine and bovine IGF-I being identical while rat and mouse IGF-I differ only in 3–4 amino acids. In IGF-II the divergence is restricted to 1–6 amino acids depending on species [24].

In addition to the classical forms of IGF-I and IGF-II, several variants with effectively identical molecular weights have been described: at least six different somatomedin-like peptides (three acidic peptides related to IGF-I and three basic peptides related to IGF-II) have been isolated from human plasma, all equally potent in a porcine costal cartilage *in vitro* assay [25].

These peptides are probably products of diverse post-translational processing of prepro- and pro-IGFs, since IGF-I and IGF-II are both single-gene products: in man the IGF-I gene is located on the long arm of chromosome 12, while the IGF-II gene is on the short arm of chromosome 11 in continuity with the insulin gene [26–28]. The possibility of allelic variation seems unlikely, since most IGF-forms are present in individual sera [29].

IGF variants of different length have also been characterized. Truncated IGF-I (also named *des*-[1–3]-IGF-I) lacking the amino-terminal tripeptide 'Gly-Pro-Glu' (GPE) was isolated from human fetal and adult brain tissue. This form had 1.4–5 times higher biological potency than 'normal' IGF-I in displacing ^{125}I-IGF-I from neuronal cell membranes, a finding probably connected to the reduced affinity of truncated IGF-I to low molecular weight IGF-binding proteins, leaving a higher proportion of IGF-I accessible for interaction with membrane-bound receptors. On the basis of these findings it was proposed that truncated IGF-I represents a paracrine/autocrine form of IGF-I [30, 31]. The proteolytic tripeptide GPE has itself been found to act as a potent stimulator of acetylcholine release [32].

Variants of human IGF-II include a shortened variant lacking the amino-terminal alanine residue, and several high molecular weight forms have been described in spinal fluid, brain tissue and serum [23, 33, 34]. Although the physiological role of this diversity remains unsolved, only negligible concentrations of these big pro-IGF-II forms are present in normal human serum (< 10% of total IGF-II), while under pathological circumstances some of the 'big' IGF-II (approximate M_r 15–25 kDa) constitutes up to 75% of total IGF-II immunoreactivity [35]. Big IGF-II is now regarded as being of pathogenetic importance in extrapancreatic (non-islet or non-B cell) tumour-induced hypoglycaemia (EPTH). Interest had already focused on the non-suppressible insulin-like activity (NSILA) in serum [36], supported by the findings of elevated IGF-II mRNA in tumours from some patients with symptomatic hypoglycaemia [37, 38]. However, when total immunoreactive IGF-II (irIGF-II) was measured, the concentration was reported as elevated or unchanged [39, 40]. Recently, after specific isolation of big IGF-II, a clearer picture emerged: in 25 out of 28 patients with EPTH, serum big IGF-II was elevated 1.5–8 times, while total irIGF-II was unchanged in all except two patients. Further, in four patients followed pre- and post-operatively, removal of the tumour caused big IGF-II concentrations to drop from 250 to 450% above normal to normal or below-normal values, with concomitant cessation of hypoglycaemic attacks [41].

The IGF Receptors

Hormones normally react via cell-bound receptors to elicit an intracellular response, and so do the IGFs and insulin. Three well characterized receptor complexes bind one or more of these peptides with high affinity. However, contrary to expectations based on the structural homology between the peptides, a similar conformation exists only between the insulin receptor and the IGF-I receptor. The distinctly different IGF-II receptor is identical to the cation-independent mannose-6-phosphate receptor, expressing a specific binding site for each ligand, and is therefore referred to as the IGF-II/mannose-6-phosphate receptor (IGF-II/Man-6-P) [42, 43]. Both the insulin receptor and the IGF-I receptor are heterotetrameric glycoproteins, composed of two α (M_r 115–135 kDa) and two β subunits (M_r 90 kDa): the α subunit contains the extracellular ligand binding site, while the β subunit holds a transmembrane and an intracellular tyrosine autophosphorylation (tyrosine kinase) domain. When IGF-I or insulin interacts with the receptor, cascades of phosphorylation and dephosphorylation events initiate the ligand-mediated effects. The IGF-II/Man-6-P receptor is structurally and functionally different from the IGF-I/insulin receptor, as it is composed of a mainly extracellularly located monomer of approximately 250 kDa without kinase activity [3, 44]. Two postreceptor signalling pathways are currently proposed: (a) the IGF-II/Man-6-P receptor contains a G-protein-associated sequence that may trigger the intracellular signal through G-protein-coupled signalling pathways; (b) IGF-II modulates the cellular uptake of lysosomal enzymes via the IGF-II/Man-6-P receptor [45, 46]. Finally, part of the receptor, apparently equal to the truncated major extracellular domain, has been demonstrated in sheep serum, where it serves as an IGF-II specific binding protein being maximal in fetal serum and declining steadily postnatally [47].

Ligand–Receptor Interaction

It is well known that supraphysiological concentrations of insulin and IGF induce mitogenic and insulin-like effects, respectively. These findings were interpreted as a result of the similar composition of IGF and insulin and the presence of an insulin receptor and an IGF receptor, each cross-reacting with lower affinity with the heterologous ligand: the metabolic effect was mediated through the insulin receptor, and the mitogenic action through the IGF receptor [48]. This theory was supported by studies using competitive binding and cross-linking experiments [49] and further confirmed using antireceptor antibodies [50]: naturally occurring Fab fragments directed against the insulin receptor almost abolished the insulin-binding, but not IGF binding to rat adipocytes (primarily expressing active insulin receptors), producing a thirty-fold rightward shift in the dose response for stimulation of glucose oxidation by both insulin and IGF. By contrast, in fibroblasts, insulin receptor blockade did not alter the dose response for stimulation of thymidine incorporation by either insulin or IGF. With the differentiation between IGF-I and IGF-II cell membrane receptors [49] and the appearance of the highly specific monoclonal IGF-I receptor-blocking antibody αIR-3 [51], this explanation was further extended: αIR-3 added to human fibroblast cultures strongly inhibited binding of ^{125}I-IGF-I, but not of ^{125}I-IGF-II. However, the antibody abolished both the IGF-I- and IGF-II-stimulated ^{3}H-thymidine incorporation, indicating that the mitogenic response was induced solely by the IGF-I receptor via ligand binding of either IGF-I or IGF-II [52]. This observation was in accordance with other experiments [53] and was further confirmed in various human cell lines [54, 55], thus questioning the importance and physiological relevance of the IGF-II peptide and IGF-II/Man-6-P receptor in growth promotion [56].

It now appears that insulin is capable of eliciting mitogenic responses via the insulin receptor even at low concentrations, and induces the same biological effect via the IGF-I receptor only at high concentrations [57, 58]. The opposite situation, in which low concentrations of IGF-I stimulate insulin-like effects via the IGF-I receptor, has emerged in studies using the monoclonal insulin receptor (MA-10) and αIR-3 antibodies [59]. These features are emphasized more directly in cells over-expressing either IGF-I or insulin receptors after transfection with the specific receptor cDNA sequence [60, 61].

As the interaction between IGF-II and the IGF-II/Man-6-P receptor is not a growth-promoting event, what is the 'purpose' of the receptor? Since the major part of the receptor targets lysosomal enzymes to lysosomes, and IGF-II interaction with the IGF-II/Man-6-P receptor inhibits enzyme binding, it is speculated that IGF-II might still influence cellular growth by altering enzymatic degradation [62]. Another study suggests that the receptor acts as a major degradation route for IGF-II: in cultured L6 myoblasts IGF-II is degraded after receptor interaction and internalization, actions strongly inhibited by the addition of receptor-blocking antibodies to the medium [54]. It is also possible that IGF-II 'only' acts as a regulator of the IGF-II/Man-6-P receptor, since in fibroblasts IGF-II is capable of upregulating the receptor through a redistribution from internal membranes to the cell surface [63].

In summary, in most cells the following relative binding affinities among the three ligands are: the *insulin receptor* binds insulin $\gg$ IGF-II > IGF-I; the *IGF-I receptor* binds IGF-I > IGF-II $\gg$ insulin and the *IGF-II/Man-6-P receptor* binds IGF-II > IGF-I (insulin does not bind) [3, 44].

INSULIN-LIKE GROWTH FACTOR
BINDING PROTEINS (IGFBPs)

While endocrine systems usually involve a typical hormone–target tissue relationship, this is not the case for IGFs: extracts of liver and other tissues contain only small amounts of IGF-activity during basal unstimulated conditions. This has been interpreted as a sign of *de novo synthesis* following stimulation, which is further supported by the interval seen before serum IGF-I levels increase after growth hormone administration [19]. However, these low tissue concentrations are in contrast to the high and relatively stable concentrations of IGF-I/IGF-II in the circulation, which may therefore be considered *the reservoir* for IGFs. It soon became apparent, however, that the plasma pool of IGFs was bound to several larger proteins: originally, using size exclusion gel chromatography, IGF activity presented in two fractions of approximately 150 kDa and 50 kDa, with almost no IGF being detected as free, unbound peptide [64, 65]. Because of major methodological problems, primarily those of preserving *in vivo* equilibria during *ex vivo* analyses, very few studies have attempted to calculate the distribution of IGFs between the three molecular fractions. One study estimated that the 150 kDa accounted for approximately 70–80% of all IGF (IGF-I and -II), while the 50 kDa fraction contained 20–30%, and only about 10% of IGF-I and less than 2% of IGF-II was 'free' [66]. The main role of these IGF-related binding proteins was considered to be the transport of IGFs, with the 150 kDa being the primary binding protein in the vascular compartment serving as an IGF-store reducing renal/hepatic clearance, and the 50 kDa fraction including transport proteins to the extravascular compartment determining the bioavailability of IGFs to the tissues [16]. It soon became clear, however, that the binding proteins possessed the 'intrinsic' ability to modulate the cellular response to IGFs. This opened up a complex world of new roles in the regulation, inhibition and, possibly, activation of IGFs.

Six different binding proteins (denoted IGFBP-1 to IGFBP-6) have now been discovered, all binding exclusively IGF-I and -II and, in contrast to the cell membrane receptors, without any cross-linking to insulin [3]. The liver is the major site for production of IGFBP-1 to -4 and the circulation is the main 'target organ'. IGFBP-5 and -6 appear to be synthesized locally in different tissues, although this has not been finally determined [67].

The 150 kDa complex consists of the IGFBP-3 acid-stable β-subunit (M_r 53 kDa, 264 amino acids), responsible for the high-affinity binding of either IGF-I or IGF-II, and the acid-labile α-subunit (ALS; M_r 85 kDa), which does not bind IGF and interacts with only moderate affinity with the binary IGFBP-3:IGF complex [18, 68, 69]. Since IGFBP-3 has very high affinity for IGF-I/-II, it is almost fully saturated, implying that the serum concentration of IGFBP-3 is usually equimolar to the combined molar concentrations of IGF-I and -II [70]. The circulating levels of IGFBP-3 do not vary diurnally and hence maintain constant serum levels of IGFs [71]. Furthermore, IGFBP-3 increases the half-life of serum IGF-I and -II when compared to unbound IGF (to approximately 16 hours vs. 10 minutes) [66], presumably as a result of reduced renal and hepatic clearance and of restricting the growth factor to the circulation [72]. The *in vivo* production of IGFBP-3 was initially believed to be growth hormone-dependent (hence the former designation 'the growth hormone-dependent IGF binding protein'), but is now considered to be regulated primarily by IGF-I increasing hepatic production directly. Formation of the 150 kDa complex is, however, only possible in the presence of GH [73]. This is in accordance with observations that the α-subunit has a strong correlation with growth hormone status [68]. *In vitro* IGFBP-3 is stimulated by various growth factors, including transforming growth factor β (TGF-β), platelet-derived growth factor (PDGF) and epidermal growth factor (EGF), and further by vasopressin and bombesin, whereas glucocorticoid reduces production [74, 75].

IGFBP-2 (289 amino acids) constitutes together with IGFBP-1 (264 amino acids) two of the components of the 50 kDa IGF complex. While IGFBP-3 and IGFBP-1 bind IGF-I and IGF-II with equal affinity, IGFBP-2 predominantly binds IGF-II, even though its affinity for both IGF forms is greater than that of IGFBP-1 [76, 77]. The half-life determined in normal rats was estimated as approximately $2-2\frac{1}{2}$ hours for IGFBP-1 and -2, being thus intermediate between those of IGFBP-3 and free IGF [78]. Insulin is apparently the most important physiological regulator of hepatic synthesis of IGFBP-1 [65, 79], and serum IGFBP-1 levels correlate inversely with circulating levels of insulin [80]. As a consequence, the IGFBP-1 concentration varies widely through the day [71, 81, 82]. Finally, it has recently been demonstrated that octreotide and lanreotide, two long-acting somatostatin analogues, and somatostatin itself independent of insulin, stimulate IGFBP-1 release [83–85]. Apart from transport, IGFBP-1 appears to have a distinct role in fetal growth and development: in maternal serum, levels of IGFBP-1 are markedly increased during pregnancy and reach their highest concentrations in amniotic fluid [86–88]. By contrast, the regulation of IGFBP-2 is far from understood. The influence of nutritional and hormonal status has recently been examined: in normal adults serum IGFBP-2 exhibited only moderate diurnal variation (less than twofold) and neither food intake nor glucose infusion changed IGFBP-2 levels, which are some five times higher than basal IGFBP-1 levels. In cord sera from normal term infants, mean IGFBP-2 was almost four times higher than in normal adults, while hypopituitary patients had twofold increased levels. By contrast, acromegalic patients showed no suppression of IGFBP-2, so apparently GH does not *per se* regulate IGFBP-2 [89].

The remaining three IGFBPs (IGFBP-4, -5 and -6) have only recently been identified, so are much less well described. IGFBP-4 is a 237 amino acid peptide with a molecular weight of approximately 24–25 kDa. Serum levels estimated using Western ligand blotting are reported to be relatively unchanging [67], and increasing evidence suggests that IGFBP-4 exerts its biological role through autocrine/paracrine mechanisms as an inhibitor of IGF bioactivity, most important perhaps in the regulation of bone cells: vitamin D is found to increase IGFBP-4 secretion *in vivo* and thereby decrease the actions of IGFs [90, 91]. Further, IGFBP-4 is found as the major IGFBP component in the connective tissue of perfused rat hearts [92]. IGFBP-5 is a 252 amino acid peptide (M_r 29 kDa) and, unlike the four IGFBPs already mentioned, is produced at highest levels in the kidney [93]. It binds IGF-II preferentially and appears to be associated with components of the extracellular matrix in cultured fibroblasts [94] and bone [95]. Interestingly, in cultured human osteoblasts IGFBP-5 has been shown to enhance mitogenic responses to IGF-I and IGF-II and to stimulate mitogenesis alone, without the presence of endogenous or exogenous IGF, via interaction with the cell membrane [96]. While no immunoassay exists for IGFBP-4 or -5, a radioimmunoassay (RIA) measuring IGFBP-6 (216 amino acids) has recently been developed [97]. The mean concentration in adult serum was 220 ± 110 µg/l; similar concentrations were found in umbilical serum and in amniotic fluid. In cerebrospinal fluid, where IGFBP-6 has been found to be the predominant IGF binding protein [98], the levels were slightly lower. Also, IGFBP-6 binds IGF-II with higher affinity than IGF-I.

In summary (Table 1), a number of different physiological functions have been suggested for the IGFBPs, but the exact role for each binding protein remains far from clear. It seems reasonable to assume that the binding proteins distribute IGFs to the different body compartments and are also able to modulate their action through diverse autocrine, paracrine and endocrine mechanisms. The dynamic insulin regulation of hepatic IGFBP-1 production and secretion could be an endocrine way of short-term regulating the access of IGFs to the fuel supplies, and hence cellular anabolism. Finally, the IGFBPs can be expected to prevent insulinomimetic IGF-induced hypoglycaemia by inhibiting

the interaction between IGF and the insulin receptor: this would explain how serum IGF present in thousandfold higher concentration than insulin, and having 5% insulin-like activity, still does not cause hypoglycaemia [18].

CIRCULATING LEVELS OF IGFs

It must be emphasized when referring to circulating levels of IGFs that these include unbound as well as IGFBP-bound peptides. Hence, two difficult and confounding aspects must be considered when evaluating 'total' IGF-I and IGF-II levels in serum. Firstly, the variable interaction in different immunoassays of the binding proteins which may induce spurious high or low values, means that the IGFBPs must be removed. Of the available methods acid gel chromatography is regarded as the gold standard, but is inordinately cumbersome in routine use, while micro-columns and acid–ethanol extraction are rapid and easy to use but less reliable, giving problems with residual IGFBPs and sometimes loss of antigen. Undoubtedly, most of the conflict in the results from different laboratories is due to inadequate methodology which also partly explains the confusion in the literature on IGFs and diabetes. The second aspect concerns the meaningfulness of the total serum IGF as a quantitative indicator of its impact on cells. By analogy with circulating thyroid hormones, it may be the free IGF-fraction which determines biological effects and feedback, but the situation is infinitely more complex for IGFs with small binding proteins, which diffuse through capillaries and are produced at the sites of action and at variable rates, and with IGFBP-1 concentration varying by a factor of ten during the day, probably inducing drastic changes in the level of free IGF-I. In contrast to what was successfully accomplished for free thyroid hormones, at the time of writing no methods exist for determining free IGF-I in circumstances mimicking the intravascular milieu.

The level of total circulating IGF, in contrast to many other hormones (including GH), exhibits no diurnal variation, but varies in an age-dependent manner. In man both IGF-I and -II are low in fetal plasma, rising from approximately 40 and 160 µg/l at mid-gestational age to 80 and 260 µg/l at term, respectively. Thereafter IGF-I increases slowly until the onset of puberty, when a maximum level (approximately 400 µg/l) occurs concomitantly with the pubertal growth surge; the IGF-I increase correlates better with Tanner pubertal stage than chronological age [99]. This rise in IGF-I is due to increased pituitary GH secretion and directly or indirectly to increased synthesis of sex steroids. After puberty IGF-I levels slowly decline and reach prepubertal

Table 1 IGFBPs—a summary

	Components	Regulation	Half-life (diurnal variation)	Ligand affinity	Biological effect
High molecular weight complex					
150 kDa; 75% of total IGF Ternary complexes	IGFBP-3 ALS	IGF-I ↑ /GH ↑ GH ↑	IGF within the ternary complex —16 hours (constant)	IGF-I = IGF-II	Circulating reservoir restricted to the circulation; stabilizing the concentration
Low molecular weight complex					Transport of IGFs to the extravascular compartment; modulators of IGF-bioactivity
	IGFBP-1	Insulin ↓ Somatostatin ↑	$2-2\frac{1}{2}$ hours (marked)	IGF-I = IGF-II	Inhibits IGF-bioactivity
	IGFBP-2	?	$2-2\frac{1}{2}$ hours (moderate)	IGF-II > IGF-I	?
50 kDa; 25% of total IGF Binary complexes	IGFBP-4	Vitamin D ↑	? (constant)	?	Inhibits IGF-bioactivity
	IGFBP-5	?	? (constant)	IGF-II > IGF-I	Intrinsic bioactivity
	IGFBP-6	?	? (constant)	IGF-II > IGF-I	Predominant IGFBP in CSF

Abbreviations: IGF = insulin-like growth factor; IGFBP = insulin-like growth factor binding protein; ALS = acid-labile subunit ($\sim \alpha$-subunit); ↑ = stimulation; ↓ = inhibition; CSF = cerebrospinal fluid; ? = unknown.

values at about 60 years of age [16, 100–103]. In contrast, IGF-II rises rapidly from low postnatal values to about 600 µg/l at the age of 1 year and then stays at this level independent of age [40, 104]. In addition to these different serum profiles of IGF-I and -II, their regulation also diverges. Even though production of IGFs is maintained in many tissues, probably reflecting paracrine/autocrine mechanisms, the liver, because of its mass, appears to contribute most to the plasma pool of IGF [19, 105]. The synthesis of IGF-I is mainly under strict growth hormone regulation, so that circulating serum levels generally reflect endogenous GH production [40], being significantly increased during GH excess (as in acromegaly) and reduced in GH deficiency. By contrast, serum IGF-II is much less influenced by GH, levels being unchanged in acromegaly but reduced in GH deficiency. The latter finding demonstrates that IGF-II is indirectly GH-dependent, probably through reduced production of IGFBP-3. The associations between IGF-I and GH are often referred to as the IGF-I/GH axis, and consist, in addition to the already mentioned GH stimulation of hepatic IGF-I production and release, of negative feed-back loops: IGF-I inhibits pituitary GH-release directly via a short loop and indirectly via a long loop by stimulating the inhibitory hypothalamic peptide somatostatin and inhibiting the stimulatory peptide GHRH (growth hormone releasing hormone) [106]. In many clinical situations, however, the nutritional condition is very important, since pronounced catabolism as seen in severe insulin dependent diabetes, kwashiorkor, chronic renal failure and critical illness involves a 'hepatic disconnection' between GH and IGF-I. The common feature of these conditions is low levels of IGF-I despite normal or elevated GH secretion, and it appears from data obtained in protein-restricted rats that the GH resistance occurs at a postreceptor level [107]. This hepatic GH insensitivity is abolished only when the catabolic situation is reversed, by refeeding or by insulin treatment [108–113]. Regulation involving IGF-I and -II seems also to take place: under circumstances with high serum levels of IGF-II (or IGF-II variants) such as during EPTH, the IGF-I concentration is reduced, possibly through IGF-II-mediated GH suppression [37]. In conditions of excess IGF-I, for instance after administration of recombinant IGF-I, the levels of IGF-II are reduced [114]. It is obvious that it may be through a competitive mechanism, a result of reduced binding of IGF-II to the IGFBPs and hence increased clearance. Finally, competent insulin secretory capacity is a prerequisite for adequate hepatic IGF-I release [115, 116].

In summary, serum levels of IGF-I are mainly regulated by: (a) growth hormone; (b) nutritional status;

and (c) insulin [117], without one being able to substitute for the other.

BIOLOGICAL EFFECTS OF IGF-I AND IGF-II

Despite the similarities in action and structure between IGF-I and insulin, the main *in vivo* action of insulin is metabolic, while IGF-I primarily regulates cellular growth and differentiation [3]. The closely intermingled receptor and postreceptor effects of IGF-I and insulin raise the question, how are the intracellular signals differentiated *in vivo?* Although this is largely unanswered, it must be emphasized that the abovementioned observations are based on *in vitro* experiments. Furthermore, while many effects of IGF-I are now well recognized and closely entwined with the actions of insulin, the effects and biological importance of IGF-II and the IGF-II/Man-6-P receptor remain speculative. Finally, the ubiquitous distribution of IGF receptors in a diversity of tissues complicates attempts to understand the biological effects of IGFs.

In Vitro Effects

The insulinomimetic effects of IGFs were studied in the classical insulin bioassay based on epididymal fat pads or adipocytes [118], and included enhanced cellular glucose uptake, glucose oxidation, glycogen synthesis, lipogenesis and antilipolysis [20]. The discovery of the 'anabolic' function of IGF-I was based on *in vitro* findings in isolated rat cartilage: serum from normal rats contained a substance that stimulated incorporation of sulphate (^{35}S) into cartilage, whereas serum from hypophysectomized animals had no stimulatory effect, but preceding growth hormone substitution to hypophysectomized rats reconstituted the ability to stimulate sulphate incorporation. These observations led to one of the cornerstones of IGF research, the somatomedin hypothesis: growth hormone itself does not lead directly to cellular growth, but rather to formation of a growth-enhancing serum substance originally termed the sulphation factor [119, 120].

Regarding the mitogenic actions, IGF-I was first found to be a potent stimulator of labelled thymidine incorporation into DNA of mesodermal origin (fibroblasts) [121] and later in cultures of chondrocytes, calvaria cells, premyoblasts and erythroid precursor cells [20]. In addition to the enhanced replication, the stimulated cells were also maintained in highly differentiated states, synthesizing their typical cellular products more efficiently in the presence of IGF-I. Thus IGF-I was found to stimulate alkaline phosphatase activity and type II collagen in osteoblasts, glycosaminoglycans in chondrocytes [122] and steroids in endocrine cells [123].

In brief, IGF-I (and to a lesser extent IGF-II via the IGF-I or insulin receptor) acts as a strong anabolic substance, increasing cellular fuel deposits and stimulating both intracellular and extracellular cell activities.

In Vivo Effects

With the appearance of purified and recombinant IGF-I, sufficient amounts of peptide became available to initiate *in vivo* studies, which clearly showed that the *in vitro* actions could once again be divided into short-term insulin-like and long-term growth-promoting effects, depending on the amount of IGF-I administered. In studies using bolus injections, acute hypoglycaemia was induced in the rat [124], dog [125] and man [126]. The latter study demonstrated that on a molar basis, IGF-I (100 µg/kg) was only 6% as potent as insulin in the induction of hypoglycaemia and approximately half as effective in reducing serum levels of free fatty acids. By contrast, levels of epinephrine, norepinephrine, growth hormone, glucagon and cortisol were reported to respond similarly to both agents. The concentration of free IGF-I was estimated to constitute 80% of total serum IGF-I in these experiments, leading to the assumption that all IGFBPs were saturated, drastically increasing the amount of bioavailable peptide to act with the cell membrane receptors. Lipogenesis and hypoglycaemia did not, however, occur when IGF-I (20 µg/kg) was administered in a continuous fashion, and furthermore, fasting insulin and blood glucose levels stayed within normal range [114].

With regard to growth and differentiation, an early study [127] demonstrated that continuous infusion of purified IGF-I dose-dependently stimulated weight gain and longitudinal growth in hypophysectomized rats, indistinguishable from effects induced by growth hormone administration. This was in excellent accordance with the general idea that GH stimulated hepatic synthesis of IGF-I, which via the circulation reached the organs [40, 128]. It is now clear, however, that GH is capable of inducing local production of IGF-I and IGF-BPs in chondrocytes and osteoblasts [129–131], making it difficult to distinguish *in vivo* between endocrine (hepatic) and autocrine/paracrine (local) IGF-I mediated actions. Furthermore, it now appears that some anabolic effects are mediated through additive and different mechanisms.

Two recent studies using recombinant human peptides examined the anabolic effects of either GH, or IGF-I, or the combination in hypocaloric normal volunteers: subcutaneous IGF-I infusion was as effective as GH in reducing nitrogen wasting, but caused hypoglycaemia, whereas the combination was substantially

more anabolic and eliminated the IGF-I induced hypoglycaemia [132, 133]. Some differences in 'potency' are found in the response of certain organs to administration of IGF-I or GH in hypophysectomized rats. The kidney, spleen and thymus are extremely responsive to growth-promoting peptides, and the IGF-I-induced organ growth exceeded that of GH [134]. These results are in accordance with findings in hypophysectomized neonatal rats, which at the age of 10 days were given either IGF-I alone or IGF-I + GH, or IGF-I + thyroxine (T_4): IGF-I alone restored serum levels and resulted in some organ growth (kidney, spleen and lung), but did not increase body weight, which was significantly increased by GH. Both peptides stimulated skeletal growth by 17%, whereas T_4 treatment resulted in a 50% increase without changing serum IGF-I [135]. Although these experiments may have used insufficient dosages, the authors suggested that in the neonatal rat, GH and T_4 regulate body weight and skeletal growth via endocrine mechanisms, while IGF-I primarily induces organ growth through autocrine/paracrine actions. These somehow contrasting results may be due to changing roles of IGF-I during development; from a primarily autocrine/paracrine mechanism during the neonatal period and early childhood to a more endocrine mechanism during puberty and adolescence. This is of course speculative, but might explain why in man, during early childhood when somatic growth is at its highest, the circulating levels of IGF-I are quite low, first increasing at the onset of puberty.

Although it is the consensus that cellular effects of IGF-II are primarily mediated through the IGF-I receptor, more specific IGF-II actions have been proposed. In rats the IGF-II/Man-6-P receptor is present throughout the gut, and the levels of receptors were found to increase twofold after 50% resection of the small intestine [136, 137]. Another study investigating post-ischaemic regeneration in rat skeletal muscles found that IGF-II was increased both at mRNA and peptide levels [138]. These findings suggest that IGF-II might play a role in cellular regenerative processes. Finally, normal and high-molecular IGF-II forms have been found in most areas in the human brain, without concomitant presence of IGF-I, supporting the concept that IGF-II is more a neuronal growth factor than a somatic growth factor [139].

REGULATION OF GH, IGFs AND IGFBPs IN DIABETES

Changes in the IGF-I/GH Axis

In man GH is secreted episodically from the pituitary gland, the bulk of GH being released at the onset of slow-wave sleep, with less conspicuous daytime spikes stimulated by the postprandial decline in blood glucose [140, 141]. In healthy volunteers, 24-hour serum GH profiles were accounted for by an average of 12 discrete GH secretory volleys, each consisting of four distinct bursts. Between these 'pulse-within-pulse' episodes, calculated GH secretory rates fell asymptotically to zero [142]. In the fasted state (5 days), the GH pulse frequency, 24-h integrated GH concentration and maximal pulse amplitude were significantly increased, with a concomitant decrease in serum IGF-I levels [143]. Similar changes are observed in insulin dependent diabetes mellitus (IDDM) and non-insulin dependent diabetes mellitus (NIDDM), especially during poor control [7, 144, 145]. In 48 adult IDDM patients, mean 24-h serum GH levels were elevated by up to 3.5 times, due to increased GH secretory pulse frequency (50%) and pulse amplitude and inter-pulse baseline levels, when compared to healthy controls [146]. Furthermore, this GH excess was related to metabolic control at the time: a modest rise in GH was observed in diabetic patients with clinically good control [144, 145], while normoglycaemia, obtained during intensified insulin therapy, tends to normalize GH [147, 148]. Moreover, inappropriate or exaggerated GH responses to a whole range of stimuli have been reported: to glucose, sleep, exercise, arginine, clonidine and GHRH [149]. In summary, there is no doubt that non-obese diabetic patients in general are exposed to higher amounts of circulating GH; the diurnal GH production of moderately controlled IDDM patients can be estimated at about 1.0 mg in comparison to 0.5 mg in non-diabetic subjects [150].

While the metabolically related GH hypersecretion in diabetic patients is generally accepted, the results of different studies on circulating levels of IGF-I are remarkably conflicting. The original study, describing the *bioactivity* of sulphation factors in serum from adult diabetic patients (IDDM and NIDDM), found decreased levels, correlating inversely with blood glucose concentration [21]. Two later studies, measuring *immunoreactive* IGF-I in adult IDDM patients [151] and in diabetic children [152], confirmed this observation, both demonstrating low levels of circulating IGF-I and an inverse correlation to glycosylated haemoglobin (HbA$_{1c}$). In another study, similar and significant reductions were found in adult NIDDM and IDDM patients, but IGF-I and HbA$_{1c}$ correlated only in the youngest IDDM patients [153]. Opposite findings were demonstrated in adult IDDM patients measuring both increased immunoreactive IGF-I levels [154] and enhanced IGF bioactivity [155, 156]. Finally, some studies have shown IGF-I levels to be identical in diabetic and control subjects [157, 158].

The same picture of conflicting results emerges in insulin-dependent diabetic children: normal serum IGF-I immunoreactivity was found in young adolescents and children less than 10 years of age, but a subgroup of the prepubertal children had low levels and responded to improved glycaemic control by increased serum IGF-I and entered puberty during therapy [159]. Low prepubertal IGF-I levels, being normalized during puberty, were in agreement with some studies [160], but differed from others [161], finding IGF-I levels in children less than 5 years old significantly reduced, while children between 5 and 18 years of age had normal values. Finally, comparing the pregnancy-induced rise in serum IGF-I in IDDM and healthy subjects, the normal increment was markedly reduced in the former group (50%), whereas cord blood from infants of diabetic mothers (independent of metabolic control) contained 100% more IGF-I than that from infants of healthy mothers. By contrast, no significant changes regarding IGF-II were obtained [162].

The reasons for these discrepancies are probably both *methodological* (assays with different IGF-I specificity and IGF-II cross-reaction, different extraction procedures performed to eliminate IGFBP interference) and *clinical* (matching of controls in terms of age, sex, weight, metabolic control, duration of diabetes, kidney and cardiovascular function, and insulin therapy regimen). However, when the GH hypersecretion is taken into account, the levels of serum IGF-I are relatively decreased, pointing to an imbalance in the IGF-I/GH axis, probably at hepatic level.

Of the few studies of circulating IGF-II and diabetes, one reported unchanged levels [157], another increased levels [163], but both agreed that IGF-II levels are independent of glycaemic control. The fact that IGF-I and IGF-II share the same IGF-binding proteins, makes it probable that changes affecting one growth factor also influence the other.

Changes in IGF-binding Proteins (IGFBPs)

As regards acute metabolic changes, IGFBP-1 is by far the most interesting binding protein, being regulated in an inverse manner by insulin. Without considering the presence of diabetic complications, IGFBP-1 levels are in general found to be elevated in insulin-dependent diabetic subjects [164, 165]. This might be a result of altered systemic and local somatostatin levels in IDDM patients [166, 167], since somatostatin analogues are shown to have a specific stimulatory effect on hepatic IGFBP-1 production independent of insulin [83, 85]. Alternatively, subnormal portal insulin levels and hence increased hepatic IGFBP-1 production could explain the raised serum IGFBP-1 levels, despite increased peripheral insulin concentrations. A recent study examined an 11-hour profile of IGFBP-1 levels in IDDM patients with or without diabetic neuropathy. Both groups had identical IGF-I levels and peripheral hyperinsulinaemia, but the neuropathic group had significantly raised IGFBP-1 levels when compared to non-neuropathic diabetic patients [80]. In NIDDM patients results are more conflicting. One study reported *mean* IGFBP-1 concentrations to be raised twofold in NIDDM patients, but fourfold in IDDM patients, although both groups showed similar relative decreases during acute hyperinsulinaemia [164]. Another study found decreased IGFBP-1 [168].

It is difficult to interpret the increased levels of IGFBP-1 in diabetes. One could speculate that in non-diabetic subjects, the binding protein functions as a short-term metabolic counter-regulator, increasing the amount of unbound IGF-I and hence IGF-I bioactivity in the case of excess fuel supplies, so that it is acting indirectly with insulin. During (poorly controlled) diabetes, on the other hand, the increased levels of IGFBP-1 might down-regulate the IGF-I induced cellular anabolism in accordance with the decreased access of metabolites. By contrast, studies in rats have demonstrated that IGFBP-1 injections caused a rise in plasma glucose [169], suggesting that elevated IGFBP-1 levels should be regarded as an adverse effect: poor metabolic control and decreased levels of bioactive IGF-I (qua increased IGFBP-1 levels) contribute to elevated GH secretion and increased insulin resistance.

Data regarding the other binding proteins are sparse. IGFBP-3 is reported to be slightly decreased, and the normal pubertal rise seems to be absent [67], in accordance with some but not all of the mentioned studies of reduced IGF-I levels in diabetic subjects. The other binding proteins have not yet been examined in human diabetes.

DIABETIC ANGIOPATHY

Traditionally, diabetic angiopathy is divided into *macroangiopathy*, most commonly affecting large muscular arteries, and *microangiopathy*, affecting arterioles and capillaries, especially important in the kidney and the retina. Since diabetic macroangiopathy comprises the same *clinical* manifestations as atherosclerosis, the phenomena have been considered to be identical [170]. Today, however, accumulating evidence supports the concept that diabetic macroangiopathy has certain characteristics in addition to those of atherosclerosis.

Diabetes Mellitus and Atherosclerosis

Atherosclerotic heart and vessel disease evolves in some ways differently from normal in the diabetic population. The male:female ratio is 1:1 instead of about 3:1, and it develops earlier in life and at an accelerated rate. This has been ascribed to the participation of a more specific diabetic macroangiopathy, but may also be partly due to a higher incidence of recognized risk factors in diabetes.

Peripheral hyperinsulinaemia is a predominant finding in diabetes [171]. Since increased insulin levels may accelerate development of cardiovascular disease, interest has focused on a possible role of peripheral hyperinsulinaemia or perhaps rather insulin resistance. In addition, since migration and proliferation of vascular smooth muscle cells into the intima occur in the early phases of atherosclerosis [172], IGF-I may be involved in the initial transformations. IGF-I is a known stimulator of DNA synthesis and proliferation of cultured vascular smooth muscle cells from various species, including man. Furthermore, these cells contain abundant IGF-I receptors, in contrast to the expression of insulin receptors, which is low or absent. Finally, the affinity of insulin for the IGF-I receptor and the ability to stimulate DNA synthesis is approximately 100–1000 times lower than for IGF-I, and antibody-induced IGF-I receptor blockade abolishes the effects of both IGF-I and insulin. This strongly suggests that growth of vascular smooth muscle cells is mediated via the IGF-I receptor [172–176]. Insulin is, however, able to modulate the cellular response to IGF-I: in the untreated insulinopenic diabetic rat, the content of IGF-I mRNA in the aorta is decreased, whereas elevated levels of IGF-I receptor mRNA are observed. Insulin treatment acutely down-regulates the levels of IGF-I receptor mRNA, and normalizes IGF-I mRNA in four days [177, 178]. *In vivo*, endothelial damage, induced by balloon catheterization of blood vessels, stimulates vascular smooth muscle proliferation [179, 180]. In hypophysectomized rats the proliferative response was markedly delayed, and in diabetic rats the maximal DNA synthesis was reduced, when compared to normal control animals [181, 182]. Since diabetic rats, *in contrast to humans, have low levels of circulating GH*, both conditions are characterized by reduced levels of GH and IGF-I. In the latter study, continuous IGF-I infusion to a group of diabetic rats restored DNA synthesis to the same extent as insulin treatment, but without affecting blood glucose levels. Finally, when non-diabetic rabbit aorta is balloon catheterized, three–fourfold elevated levels of extractable tissue IGF-I are demonstrated two and four days after vessel injury. Treatment with lanreotide, a somatostatin analogue, maintains the IGF-I content of the aorta at control levels [227] and has recently been shown to reduce myomedial proliferation postoperatively in rabbits [183].

In summary, increasing evidence supports the concept that IGF-I is directly involved in the growth regulation of vascular smooth muscle cells, whereas the role of insulin is more indirect, possibly via improved metabolic control.

Diabetic Macroangiopathy

The concept that macroangiopathy is different from atherosclerosis in non-diabetic subjects is supported by biochemical and morphological characteristics: (a) large amounts of periodic acid–Schiff (PAS)-positive, but glycosaminoglycan-poor, material are present in coronary arteries; (b) increased levels of collagen type IV and V are found in the aorta, together with; (c) an elevated amount of arterial basement membrane material. These features, also seen in diabetic microangiopathy, were demonstrated with and without evidence of atherosclerotic plaques and often unrelated to intimal lesions [184].

In vitro, GH increased the cellular growth of, and basement membrane material accumulation of, cultured arterial smooth muscle cells, and so did serum from IDDM and NIDDM subjects. In addition, GH antibodies added to the diabetic serum reduced the growth-promoting effects more than in non-diabetic serum [185–187]. This points to a direct or indirect effect of GH, and indicates that increased levels of circulating GH are of pathogenetic importance in diabetic macroangiopathy. A direct role for IGF-I has yet to be determined.

Diabetic Retinopathy

After the GH hypothesis was put forward in 1970, clinical trials and follow-up studies confirmed that hypophysectomy (surgical or by radiation) was an effective treatment, maintaining visual acuity and reducing blindness [10, 12]. There is evidence that it is the specific removal of GH which causes an improvement in diabetic retinopathy: (a) hypophysectomized patients received therapy with thyroxine, and adrenal and sex steroids, without any progression of their retinopathy [188]; (b) a positive correlation was found between the degree of GH deficiency following pituitary ablation and the beneficial effect on retinopathy [189]; (c) pituitary-intact diabetic patients with proliferative retinopathy had higher levels of GH than diabetic patients without retinopathy [190–193]. This evidence does not, however, prove a definite causal relation between GH and proliferative retinopathy.

The appearance of the IGF-I immunoassays gave new opportunities to investigate the connection between GH and retinopathy but, as already mentioned, contrasting results emerged. Most studies have been unable to differentiate between serum levels of IGF-I in diabetic patients with and without retinopathy [151, 157,

194, 195]. One study demonstrated acromegalic levels of circulating IGF-I in seven IDDM patients with 'accelerated' proliferative retinopathy [154], but suffered from sparsity of clinical data regarding the possible influence of nephropathy. Another group investigated NIDDM patients and reported elevated levels of IGF-I in patients with retinopathy, when compared to normal age-matched controls. However, the normal control levels were only about 40% of what should be expected, and furthermore, when the patients were subdivided according to the stage of retinopathy, the subgroups had identical IGF-I concentrations [196]. An explanation for these contrasting findings might be that increased serum IGF-I in patients with retinopathy is a transient phenomenon, as seen in kidney tissue during experimental diabetes [197].

A two-year follow-up study of diabetic patients contained one group with mild background retinopathy, and one with severe background or preproliferative retinopathy. Serum IGF-I levels were identical in the two groups throughout, as were the levels when compared to healthy controls. However, in eight patients from the second group, the disease progressed to proliferative retinopathy and at the time of the first neovascularization, serum IGF-I levels were significantly increased (271 ± 94 µg/l (mean $\pm$ SD) versus 196 ± 58 µg/l), but returned to previous values after four months. The authors concluded that despite the transient increase, the rise was not sufficiently great or early enough to be of clinical value as a predictor of retinal neovascularization [198]. However, some studies have demonstrated that acceleration of retinopathy sets in during the first year of intensified insulin treatment [199–201], when circulating IGF-I would also be expected to rise [202].

Few studies have examined IGF-I changes within the eye: increased levels of vitreous IGF-I were found in diabetic patients when compared to non-diabetic subjects undergoing vitrectomy for various reasons; the vitreous samples were considered to be without major blood contamination since only the 50 kDa IGFBPs were present [203].

Attempts to use long-acting somatostatin analogues in suppressing GH (and IGF-I) levels have suffered from side-effects or an incomplete suppression of GH, making it difficult to interpret the results [204, 205].

In summary, the GH hypothesis is still unanswered, and the IGF-I estimations have neither validated nor disproved it. It must again be emphasized that measurements of *total* IGF-I levels may be misleading, as the actions of IGF-I are modulated by the presence of IGFBPs. Further elucidation awaits the development of reliable methods for analysis of *free* IGF-I in plasma.

Diabetic Nephropathy

Diabetic nephropathy is caused primarily by advanced glomerulopathy, the renal expression of diabetic micro-angiopathy, and much interest has focused on diabetic glomerulosclerosis, since it is a major cause of end-stage renal failure (ESRF). The development of overt nephropathy is, however, a final step in a series of changes starting with renal enlargement and hyperfiltration (elevated RPF (renal plasma flow) and GFR (glomerular filtration rate)), and ending with sclerotic kidneys deprived of any renal function [206-208]. Since the initial renal changes occur in the early phase of diabetes, and may initiate and/or lead to progression to diabetic ESRF, several groups have studied possible means of intervention by investigating the initial renal enlargement, the mechanisms provoking this and the possible role in the development of diabetic ESRF [206, 209].

Regarding the dynamic aspects, GH and IGF-I have pronounced effects on renal function. However, whereas IGF-I infusion lasting only 20 minutes is capable of inducing acute changes in terms of increased RPF and GFR, the effects of GH are not seen until after approximately 24 hours, suggesting that they may be mediated through the increased IGF-I levels following GH injection [210-213]. The observed increase in RPF and GFR is a result of decreased renal vascular resistance, the effect of IGF-I being dose-dependent [214].

The kidney is a very active site for IGF-I synthesis, especially in the collecting ducts, but also in glomeruli. Furthermore, the expression of IGF-I receptors is abundant throughout the various renal cell lines [215]. The first evidence for a possible role of IGF-I in initial diabetic hypertrophy was the demonstration that renal tissue IGF-I accumulation was maximal 24-48 hours after induction of diabetes in streptozotocin (STZ)-treated rats, and returned to basal levels after 4 days. This transient IGF-I accumulation thus preceded the first demonstrable increase in kidney RNA, protein, function and size. Furthermore, both renal IGF-I tissue accumulation and the following hypertrophy were abolished during insulin treatment or administration of octreotide, the latter without affecting blood glucose levels [216-218]. Finally, the IGF-I increase was positively correlated to the prevailing blood glucose level [219]. The origin of the increased IGF-I content is unknown: (a) kidney IGF-I mRNA remained unchanged during the first four days of STZ-diabetes [217]; (b) in competitive binding experiments, the IGF-I receptor number and affinity were unaltered during the first seven days of diabetes [220]. Although these studies do not exclude changes in restricted localizations of IGF-I mRNA and receptors, undetectable with the chosen study design, it appears that IGF-I is accumulated through other mechanisms. One possible explanation is that (STZ-) diabetes induces decreased intracellular degradation of IGF-I.

To study a possible effect of long-term depression of renal growth, octreotide was injected (200 µg daily) to STZ-diabetic rats for six months [209]. Monthly measurements of urinary albumin excretion (UAE) revealed that UAE stayed at the control level throughout the study in octreotide-diabetic rats, in contrast to a pronounced increase in untreated diabetic rats. Furthermore, kidney weight increase and serum IGF-I were significantly reduced, all without changes in metabolic control, indicating a direct effect of the somatostatin analogue. In rats with diabetes of 15 weeks' duration, 3 weeks of octreotide treatment reversed renal size and proteinuria towards normal, and similar findings have been demonstrated in human insulin dependent diabetes [221-223]. These observations obviously do not prove a causal relation between diabetic kidney disease and initial renal hypertrophy, but they strongly support the suggestion that involvement of growth-promoting peptides, such as GH and IGF-I, is of pathogenetic importance. One study has investigated this in transgenic mice expressing either GH or IGF-I: IGF-I over-expressing mice developed modest glomerular hypertrophy but no glomerulosclerosis, which was a characteristic finding in GH over-expressing mice; the authors concluded that GH was more important than IGF-I in the development of ESRF [224]. An indication that GH is necessary for development of diabetic kidney hypertrophy was found in a recent study in diabetic rats with genetic GH deficiency. GH-deficient diabetic rats had significantly less kidney growth and increase in glomerular volume than intact or GH-treated GH-deficient diabetic animals [218].

In summary, several animal studies support the concept that growth hormone and IGF-I have important roles in diabetic nephropathy, in the initial hypertrophy and hyperfunction as well as at an intermediate stage, when increased urinary albumin excretion sets in. Strict causal relations and their significance in the later progression to overt diabetic kidney disease remain, however, to be determined.

THERAPEUTIC APPLICATIONS OF IGF-I IN DIABETES

Two major areas for a possible therapeutic use of IGF-I have been investigated: first, as an anabolic agent reversing the catabolic effects of the insulin deficiency in IDDM, and second, to improve the metabolic derangement in diseases characterized by relative insulin resistance. In poorly controlled IDDM patients and STZ-diabetic rats, the insulin deficiency causes a significant growth arrest. In STZ-rats this reverted toward normal with daily injections of IGF-I, without changes in glycaemia or glucosuria [117]. In NIDDM patients, characterized by obesity, insulin resistance, peripheral hyperinsulinaemia and hypertriglyceridaemia, two daily injections of IGF-I (120 µg/kg) normalized fasting and postprandial plasma glucose levels, and suppressed fasting insulin and C-peptide concentrations. Furthermore, triglyceride levels were improved [225]. Finally, attempts to use IGF-I in type A insulin resistance have been initiated [226]. Fasting plasma glucose and glucose tolerance improved, but the results are still preliminary. Since therapeutic use of IGF-I is still quite new, the long-term adverse effects are still unknown; speculations concern atherosclerosis, the possible induction of cancers and finally the role of IGF-I in diabetic angiopathy.

REFERENCES

1. Flyvbjerg A. Growth factors and diabetic complications. Diabet Med 1990; 7: 387–99.
2. Holly JMP, Wass JA. Insulin-like growth factors; autocrine, paracrine or endocrine? New perspectives of the somatomedin hypothesis in the light of recent developments. J Endocrinol 1989; 122: 611–18.
3. Humbel RE. Insulin-like growth factors I and II. Eur J Biochem 1990; 190: 445–62.
4. Young FG. Permanent diabetes produced by pituitary (anterior lobe) injections. Lancet 1937; ii: 372–4.
5. Campbell J, Davidson IWF, Lei HP. The production of permanent diabetes by highly purified growth hormone. Endocrinology 1950; 46: 588–90.
6. Yde H. Abnormal growth hormone response to ingestion of glucose in juvenile diabetics. Acta Med Scand 1969; 186: 499–504.
7. Hansen AaP, Johansen K. Diurnal pattern of blood glucose, serum FFA, insulin, glucagon, and growth hormone in normals and juvenile diabetics. Diabetologia 1970; 6: 27–33.
8. Lundbæk K, Christensen NJ, Jensen VA et al. Diabetes, diabetic angiopathy and growth hormone (hypothesis). Lancet 1970; ii: 131–3.
9. Luft R, Olivecrona H. Hypophysectomy in man: further experience in severe diabetes mellitus. Br Med J 1955; ii: 752–6.
10. Lundbæk K, Malmros R, Andersen HC. Proceedings of the Sixth Congress of the International Diabetes Federation, Amsterdam: Excerpta Medica, 1969; pp 127–39.
11. Flyvbjerg A, Ørskov H, Alberti KGMM. Introduction. In Flyvbjerg A, Ørskov H, Alberti KGMM (eds) Growth hormone and insulin-like growth factor I in human and experimental diabetes. Chichester: Wiley 1993; pp x–xii.
12. Sharp PS, Fallon TJ, Brazier J, Sandler LM, Joplin GF, Kohner EM. Long-term follow-up of patients who underwent yttrium-90 pituitary implantation for treatment of proliferative diabetic retinopathy. Diabetologia 1987; 30: 199–207.
13. Froesch ER, Burgi H, Ramseier EB, Bally P, Labhart A. Antibody-suppressible and non-suppressible

14. Salmon WDJ, Daughaday WH. A hormonally controlled serum factor which stimulates sulphate incorporation by cartilage *in vivo*. J Lab Clin Med 1957; 49: 825–36.
15. Pierson RWJ, Temin HE. The partial purification from calf serum of a fraction with multiplication-stimulating activity for chicken fibroblasts in the cell culture and with non-suppressible insulin-like activity. J Cell Physiol 1972; 79: 319–30.
16. Hall K, Tally M. The somatomedin-insulin-like growth factors. J Intern Med 1989; 225: 47–54.
17. Froesch ER, Schmid C, Schwander J, Zapf J. Actions of insulin-like growth factors. Ann Rev Physiol 1985; 47: 443–67.
18. Rutanen EM, Pekonen F. Insulin-like growth factors and their binding proteins. Acta Endocrinol (Copenh) 1990; 123: 7–13.
19. Underwood LE, D'Ercole AJ, Clemmons DR, Van Wyk JJ. Paracrine functions of somatomedins. Clin Endocrinol Metab 1986; 15: 59–77.
20. Froesch ER, Zapf J. Insulin-like growth factors and insulin: comparative aspects. Diabetologia 1985; 28: 485–93.
21. Yde H. The growth hormone dependent sulphation factor in serum from patients with various types of diabetes. Acta Med Scand 1969; 186: 293–7.
22. Rinderknecht E, Humbel RE. The amino acid sequence of human insulin-like growth factor I and its structural homology with proinsulin. J Biol Chem 1978; 253: 2769–76.
23. Rinderknecht E, Humbel RE. Primary structure of human insulin-like growth factor II. FEBS Lett 1978; 89: 283–6.
24. Daughaday WH, Rotwein P. Insulin-like growth factors I and II. Peptide, messenger ribonucleic acid and gene structures, serum, and tissue concentrations. Endocrin Rev 1989; 10: 68–91.
25. Blum WF, Ranke MB, Bierich JR. Isolation and partial characterization of six somatomedin-like peptides from human plasma Cohn fraction IV. Acta Endocrinol (Copenh) 1986; 111: 271–84.
26. Bell GI, Gerhard DS, Fong NM, Sanchez Pescador R, Rall LB. Isolation of the human insulin-like growth factor genes: insulin-like growth factor II and insulin genes are contiguous. Proc Natl Acad Sci USA 1985; 82: 6450–54.
27. Tricoli JV, Rall LB, Scott J, Bell GI, Shows TB. Localization of insulin-like growth factor genes to human chromosomes 11 and 12. Nature 1984; 310: 784–6.
28. Brissenden JE, Ullrich A, Francke U. Human chromosomal mapping of genes for insulin-like growth factors I and II and epidermal growth factor. Nature 1984; 310: 781–4.
29. Blum WF, Ranke MB, Lechner B, Bierich JR. The polymorphic pattern of somatomedins during human development. Acta Endocrinol (Copenh) 1987; 116: 445–51.
30. Carlsson Skwirut C, Lake M, Hartmanis M, Hall K, Sara VR. A comparison of the biological activity of the recombinant intact and truncated insulin-like growth factor 1 (IGF-1). Biochim Biophys Acta 1989; 1011: 192–7.
31. Adashi EY, Resnick CE, Ricciarelli E, Hurwitz A, Kokia E, Tedeschi C, et al. Granulosa cell-derived

insulin-like growth factor (IGF) binding proteins are inhibitory to IGF-I hormonal action. Evidence derived from the use of a truncated IGF-I analogue. J Clin Invest 1992; 90: 1593–9.

32. Sara VR, Carlsson Skwirut C, Bergman T, Jornvall H, Roberts PJ, Crawford M, et al. Identification of Gly-Pro-Glu (GPE), the aminoterminal tripeptide of insulin-like growth factor 1 which is truncated in brain, as a novel neuroactive peptide. Biochem Biophys Res Commun 1989; 165: 766–71.

33. Haselbacher G, Humbel R. Evidence for two species of insulin-like growth factor II (IGF-II and 'big' IGF-II) in human spinal fluid. Endocrinology 1982; 110: 1822–4.

34. Haselbacher G, Schwab ME, Pasi A, Humbel R. Insulin-like growth factor II (IGF-II) in human brain: regional distribution of IGF-II and higher molecular mass forms. Proc Natl Acad Sci USA 1985; 82: 2153–7.

35. Daughaday WH, Emanuele MA, Brooks MH, Barbato AL, Kapadia M, Rotwein P. Synthesis and secretion of insulin-like growth factor II by a leiomyosarcoma with associated hypoglycemia. New Engl J Med 1988; 319: 1434–40.

36. Kahn CR. The riddle of tumour hypoglycaemia revisited. Clin Endocrinol Metab 1980; 9: 335–60.

37. Ron D, Powers AC, Pandian MR, Godine JE, Axelrod L. Increased insulin-like growth factor II production and consequent suppression of growth hormone secretion: a dual mechanism for tumor-induced hypoglycemia. J Clin Endocrinol Metab 1989; 68: 701–6.

38. Lowe WLJ, Roberts CT, LeRoith D, Rojeski MT, Merimee TJ, Fui Teng S, et al. Insulin-like growth factor-II in non-islet cell tumors associated with hypoglycemia: increased levels of messenger ribonucleic acid. J Clin Endocrinol Metab 1989; 69: 1153–9.

39. Daughaday WH, Trivedi B, Kapadia M. Measurement of insulin-like growth factor II by a specific radioreceptor assay in serum of normal individuals, patients with abnormal growth hormone secretion, and patients with tumor-associated hypoglycaemia. J Clin Endocrinol Metab 1981; 53: 289–94.

40. Zapf J, Walter H, Froesch ER. Radioimmunological determination of insulin-like growth factors I and II in normal subjects and in patients with growth disorders and extrapancreatic tumor hypoglycemia. J Clin Invest 1981; 68: 1321–30.

41. Zapf J, Futo E, Peter M, Froesch ER. Can 'big' insulin-like growth factor II in serum of tumor patients account for the development of extrapancreatic tumor hypoglycemia? J Clin Invest 1992; 90: 2574–84.

42. Czech MP, Lewis RE, Corvera S. Multifunctional glycoprotein receptors for insulin and the insulin-like growth factors. Ciba Foundation Symposium No. 145. Chichester: Wiley, 1989; pp 27–41.

43. Tong PY, Tollefsen SE, Kornfeld S. The cation-independent mannose 6-phosphate receptor binds insulin-like growth factor II. J Biol Chem 1988; 263: 2585–8.

44. Gammeltoft S, Christiansen J, Nielsen FC, Verland S. Insulin-like growth factor II: complexity of biosynthesis and receptor binding. Adv Exp Med Biol 1991; 293: 31–44.

45. Funk B, Kessler U, Eisenmenger W, Hansmann A, Kolb H, Kiess W. Expression of the insulin-like growth factor II/mannose-6-phosphate receptor in multiple human tissues during fetal life and early infancy. J Clin Endocrinol Metab 1992; 75: 424–31.

46. Nishimoto I, Murayama Y, Katada T, Ui M, Ogata E. Possible direct linkage of insulin-like growth factor-II receptor with guanine nucleotide-binding proteins. J Biol Chem 1989; 264: 14029–38.

47. Gelato MC, Rutherford C, Stark RI, Daniel SS. The insulin-like growth factor II/mannose-6-phosphate receptor is present in fetal and maternal sheep serum. Endocrinology 1989; 124: 2935–43.

48. Megyesi K, Kahn CR, Roth J, Froesch ER, Humbel R, Zapf J, Neville DM Jr. Insulin and non-suppressible insulin-like activity (NSILA-s): evidence for separate plasma membrane receptors. Biochem Biophys Res Commun 1974; 57: 307–15.

49. Rechler MM, Nissley SP. The nature and regulation of the receptors for insulin-like growth factors. Ann Rev Physiol 1985; 47: 425–42.

50. King GL, Kahn CR, Rechler MM, Nissley SP. Direct demonstration of separate receptors for growth and metabolic activities of insulin and multiplication-stimulating activity (an insulin-like growth factor) using antibodies to the insulin receptor. J Clin Invest 1980; 66: 130–40.

51. Kull FCJ, Jacobs S, Su YF, Svoboda ME, Van Wyk JJ, Cuatrecasas P. Monoclonal antibodies to receptors for insulin and somatomedin-C. J Biol Chem 1983; 258: 6561–6.

52. Conover CA, Misra P, Hintz RL, Rosenfeld RG. Effect of an anti-insulin-like growth factor I receptor antibody on insulin-like growth factor II stimulation of DNA synthesis in human fibroblasts. Biochem Biophys Res Commun 1986; 139: 501–8.

53. Furlanetto RW, DiCarlo JN, Wisehart C. The type II insulin-like growth factor receptor does not mediate deoxyribonucleic acid synthesis in human fibroblasts. J Clin Endocrinol Metab 1987; 64: 1142–9.

54. Kiess W, Haskell JF, Lee L, Greenstein LA, Miller BE, Aarons AL, Rechler MM, Nissley SP. An antibody that blocks insulin-like growth factor (IGF) binding to the type II IGF receptor is neither an agonist nor an inhibitor of IGF-stimulated biologic responses in L6 myoblasts. J Biol Chem 1987; 262: 12745–51.

55. Mottola C, Czech MP. The type II insulin-like growth factor receptor does not mediate increased DNA synthesis in H-35 hepatoma cells. J Biol Chem 1984; 259: 12705–13.

56. Oka Y, Czech MP. The type II insulin-like growth factor receptor is internalized and recycles in the absence of ligand. J Biol Chem 1986; 261: 9090–93.

57. Chaiken RL, Moses AC, Usher P, Flier JS. Insulin stimulation of aminoisobutyric acid transport in human skin fibroblasts is mediated through both insulin and type I insulin-like growth factor receptors. J Clin Endocrinol Metab 1986; 63: 1181–5.

58. Flier JS, Usher P, Moses AC. Monoclonal antibody to the type I insulin-like growth factor (IGF-I) receptor blocks IGF-I receptor-mediated DNA synthesis: clarification of the mitogenic mechanisms of IGF-I and insulin in human skin fibroblasts. Proc Natl Acad Sci USA 1986; 83: 664–8.

59. Verspohl EJ, Maddux BA, Goldfine ID. Insulin and insulin-like growth factor I regulate the same biological functions in HEP-G2 cells via their own specific receptors. J Clin Endocrinol Metab 1988; 67: 169–74.

60. Hofmann C, Goldfine ID, Whittaker J. The metabolic and mitogenic effects of both insulin and insulin-like growth factor are enhanced by transfection of insulin receptors into NIH3T3 fibroblasts. J Biol Chem 1989; 264: 8606–11.

61. Steele Perkins G, Turner J, Edman JC, Hari J, Pierce SB, Stover C, Rutter WJ, Roth RA. Expression and characterization of a functional human insulin-like growth factor I receptor. J Biol Chem 1988; 263: 11486–92.

62. Kiess W, Kessler U, Schmitt S, Funk B. Growth hormone and insulin-like growth factor I: basic aspects. In Flyvbjerg A, Ørskov H, Alberti KGMM (eds) Growth hormone and insulin-like growth factor I in human and experimental diabetes. Chichester: Wiley 1993; pp 1–21.

63. Braulke T, Tippmer S, Chao HJ, von Figura K. Insulin-like growth factors I and II stimulate endocytosis but do not affect sorting of lysosomal enzymes in human fibroblasts. J Biol Chem 1990; 265: 6650–55.

64. Zapf J, Waldvogel M, Froesch ER. Binding of non-suppressible insulin-like activity to human serum: evidence for a carrier protein. Arch Biochem Biophys 1975; 168: 638–45.

65. Hintz RL, Liu F. Demonstration of specific plasma binding sites for somatomedin. J Clin Endocrinol Metab 1977; 45: 988–95.

66. Guler HP, Zapf J, Schmid C, Froesch ER. Insulin-like growth factors I and II in healthy man. Estimations of half-lives and production rates. Acta Endocrinol (Copenh) 1989; 121: 753–8.

67. Holly JMP. Insulin-like growth factor binding proteins in diabetic and non-diabetic states. In: Flyvbjerg A, Ørskov H, Alberti KGMM (eds) Growth hormone and insulin-like growth factor I in human and experimental diabetes. Chichester: Wiley, 1993: pp 47–76.

68. Baxter RC. Circulating levels and molecular distribution of the acid-labile (alpha) subunit of the high molecular weight insulin-like growth factor-binding protein complex. J Clin Endocrinol Metab 1990; 70: 1347–53.

69. Baxter RC. Glycosaminoglycans inhibit formation of the 140 kDa insulin-like growth factor-binding protein complex. Biochem J 1990; 271: 773–7.

70. Ranke MB, Blum WF, Bierich JR. Clinical relevance of serum measurements of insulin-like growth factors and somatomedin binding proteins. Acta Paediatr Scand Suppl. 1988; 347: 114–26.

71. Baxter RC, Cowell CT. Diurnal rhythm of growth hormone-independent binding protein for insulin-like growth factors in human plasma. J Clin Endocrinol Metab 1987; 65: 432–40.

72. Binoux M, Hossenlopp P. Insulin-like growth factor (IGF) and IGF-binding proteins: comparison of human serum and lymph. J Clin Endocrinol Metab 1988; 67: 509–14.

73. Zapf J, Hauri C, Waldvogel M, Futo E, Hasler H, Binz K, et al. Recombinant human insulin-like growth factor I induces its own specific carrier protein in hypophysectomized and diabetic rats. Proc Natl Acad Sci USA 1989; 86: 3813–17.

74. Martin JL, Baxter RC. Transforming growth factor-beta stimulates production of insulin-like growth factor-binding protein-3 by human skin fibroblasts. Endocrinology 1991; 128: 1425–33.

75. Corps AN, Brown KD. Mitogens regulate the production of insulin-like growth factor-binding protein by Swiss 3T3 cells. Endocrinology 1991; 128: 1057–64.

76. Bourner MJ, Busby WHJ, Siegel NR, Krivi GG, McCusker RH, Clemmons DR. Cloning and sequence determination of bovine insulin-like growth factor binding protein-2 (IGFBP-2): comparison of its structural and functional properties with IGFBP-1. J Cell Biochem 1992; 48: 215–26.

77. Oh Y, Muller HL, Lee DY, Fielder PJ, Rosenfeld RG. Characterization of the affinities of insulin-like growth factor (IGF)-binding proteins 1–4 for IGF-I, IGF-II, IGF-I/insulin hybrid, and IGF-I analogs. Endocrinology 1993; 132: 1337–44.

78. Young SC, Miles MV, Clemmons DR. Determination of the pharmacokinetic profiles of insulin-like growth factor binding proteins-1 and -2 in rats. Endocrinology 1992; 131: 1867–73.

79. Conover CA, Lee PD. Insulin regulation of insulin-like growth factor-binding protein production in cultured HepG2 cells. J Clin Endocrinol Metab 1990; 70: 1062–7.

80. Crosby SR, Tsigos C, Anderton CD, Gordon C, Young RJ, White A. Elevated plasma insulin-like growth factor binding protein-1 levels in type 1 (insulin-dependent) diabetic patients with peripheral neuropathy. Diabetologia 1992; 35: 868–72.

81. Lewitt MS, Baxter RC. Inhibitors of glucose uptake stimulate the production of insulin-like growth factor-binding protein (IGFBP-1) by human fetal liver. Endocrinology 1990; 126: 1527–33.

82. Rutanen EM, Seppala M, Pietila R, Bohn H. Placental protein 12 (PP12): factors affecting levels in late pregnancy. Placenta 1984; 5: 243–8.

83. Wolthers T, Grøfte T, Flyvbjerg A, Frystyk J, Vilstrup H, Ørskov H, Foegh M. Dose-dependent stimulation of insulin-like growth factor binding protein-1 by Lanreotide, a somatostatin analogue. J Clin Endocrinol Metab 1994; 78: 141–4.

84. Ørskov H, Wolthers T, Grøfte T, Flyvbjerg A, Vilstrup H, Hamberg O. Somatostatin stimulated IGFBP-1 release is abolished by hyperinsulinaemia. J Clin Endocrinol Metab 1994; 78: 138–40.

85. Ezzat S, Ren SG, Braunstein GD, Melmed S. Octreotide stimulates insulin-like growth factor-binding protein-1: a potential pituitary-independent mechanism for drug action. J Clin Endocrinol Metab 1992; 75: 1459–63.

86. Hall K, Hansson U, Lundin G, Luthman M, Persson B, Povoa G, Stangenberg M, Ofverholm U. Serum levels of somatomedins and somatomedin-binding protein in pregnant women with type I or gestational diabetes and their infants. J Clin Endocrinol Metab 1986; 63: 1300–306.

87. Drop SL, Kortleve DJ, Guyda HJ, Posner BI. Immunoassay of a somatomedin-binding protein from human amniotic fluid: levels in fetal, neonatal, and adult sera. J Clin Endocrinol Metab 1984; 59: 908–15.

88. Drop SL, Kortleve DJ, Guyda HJ. Isolation of a somatomedin-binding protein from preterm amniotic fluid. Development of a radioimmunoassay. J Clin Endocrinol Metab 1984; 59: 899–907.

89. Clemmons DR, Snyder DK, Busby WHJ. Variables controlling the secretion of insulin-like growth factor binding protein-2 in normal human subjects. J Clin Endocrinol Metab 1991; 73: 727–33.

90. Latour D, Mohan S, Linkhart TA, Baylink DJ, Strong DD. Inhibitory insulin-like growth factor-binding protein: cloning, complete sequence, and physiological regulation. Mol Endocrinol 1990; 4: 1806–14.

91. Scharla SH, Strong DD, Mohan S, Baylink DJ, Linkhart TA. 1,25-Dihydroxyvitamin D3 differentially regulates the production of insulin-like growth factor I (IGF-I) and IGF-binding protein-4 in mouse osteoblasts. Endocrinology 1991; 129: 3139–46.

92. Boes M, Booth BA, Sandra A, Dake BL, Bergold A, Bar RS. Insulin-like growth factor binding protein (IGFBP)-4 accounts for the connective tissue distribution of endothelial cell IGFBPs perfused through the isolated heart. Endocrinology 1992; 131: 327–30.

93. Shimasaki S, Shimonaka M, Zhang HP, Ling N. Identification of five different insulin-like growth factor binding proteins (IGFBPs) from adult rat serum and molecular cloning of a novel IGFBP-5 in rat and human. J Biol Chem 1991; 266: 10646–53.

94. Clemmons DR, Camacho Hubner C, Jones JI, McCusker RH, Busby WH. Modern concepts of insulin-like growth factors. New York: Elsevier, 1991: pp 475–86.

95. Bautista CM, Baylink DJ, Mohan S. Isolation of a novel insulin-like growth factor (IGF) binding protein from human bone: a potential candidate for fixing IGF-II in human bone. Biochem Biophys Res Commun 1991; 176: 756–63.

96. Andress DL, Birnbaum RS. Human osteoblast-derived insulin-like growth factor (IGF) binding protein-5 stimulates osteoblast mitogenesis and potentiates IGF action. J Biol Chem 1992; 267: 22467–72.

97. Baxter RC, Saunders H. Radioimmunoassay of insulin-like growth factor-binding protein-6 in human serum and other body fluids. J Endocrinol 1992; 134: 133–9.

98. Roghani M, Lassarre C, Zapf J, Povoa G, Binoux M. Two insulin-like growth factor (IGF)-binding proteins are responsible for the selective affinity for IGF-II of cerebrospinal fluid binding proteins. J Clin Endocrinol Metab 1991; 73: 658–66.

99. Luna AM, Wilson DM, Wibbelsman CJ, Brown RC, Nagashima RJ, Hintz RL, Rosenfeld RG. Somatomedins in adolescence: a cross-sectional study of the effect of puberty on plasma insulin-like growth factor I and II levels. J Clin Endocrinol Metab 1983; 57: 268–71.

100. Parker MW, Johanson AJ, Rogol AD, Kaiser DL, Blizzard RM. Effect of testosterone on somatomedin-C concentrations in prepubertal boys. J Clin Endocrinol Metab 1984; 58: 87–90.

101. Harris DA, Van Vliet G, Egli CA, Grumbach MM, Kaplan SL, Styne DM, Vainsel M. Somatomedin-C in normal puberty and in true precocious puberty before and after treatment with a potent luteinizing hormone-releasing hormone agonist. J Clin Endocrinol Metab 1985; 61: 152–9.

102. Hall K, Enberg G, Ritzen M, Fryklund L, Takano K. Somatomedin A levels in serum from healthy children and from children with growth hormone deficiency or delayed puberty. Acta Endocrinol (Copenh) 1980; 94: 155–65.

103. Juul A, Bang P, Hertel NT, Main K, Dalgaard P, Jørgensen K et al. Serum insulin-like growth factor-I in 1030 healthy children, adolescents and adults: relation to age, sex, stage of puberty, testicular size and body mass index. J Clin Endocrinol Metab 1994; 78: 744–52.

104. Enberg G, Hall K. Immunoreactive IGF-II in serum of healthy subjects and patients with growth hormone disturbances and uraemia. Acta Endocrinol (Copenh) 1984; 107: 164–70.

105. D'Ercole AJ, Stiles AD, Underwood LE. Tissue concentrations of somatomedin C: further evidence for multiple sites of synthesis and paracrine or autocrine mechanisms of action. Proc Natl Acad Sci USA 1984; 81: 935–9.

106. Marshall SM, Alberti KGMM. Alterations in the growth hormone/insulin-like growth factor I axis in human and experimental diabetes: differences and similarities. In: Flyvbjerg A, Ørskov H, Alberti KGMM (eds) Growth hormone and insulin-like growth factor I in human and experimental diabetes. Chichester: Wiley, 1993: pp 23–46.

107. Fliesen T, Maiter D, Gerard G, Underwood LE, Maes M, Ketelslegers JM. Reduction of serum insulin-like growth factor-I by dietary protein restriction is age dependent. Pediatr Res 1989; 26: 415–19.

108. Amiel SA, Sherwin RS, Hintz RL, Gertner JM, Press CM, Tamborlane WV. Effect of diabetes and its control on insulin-like growth factors in the young subject with type I diabetes. Diabetes 1984; 33: 1175–9.

109. Rieu M, Binoux M. Serum levels of insulin-like growth factor (IGF) and IGF binding protein in insulin-dependent diabetics during an episode of severe metabolic decompensation and the recovery phase. J Clin Endocrinol Metab 1985; 60: 781–5.

110. Rappaport R. New aspects of growth: its neuro-endo-paracrine regulation. Triangle 1989; 28: 57–67.

111. Ross R, Miell J, Freeman E, Jones J, Matthews D, Preece M, Buchanan C. Critically ill patients have high basal growth hormone levels with attenuated oscillatory activity associated with low levels of insulin-like growth factor-I. Clin Endocrinol (Oxf) 1991; 35: 47–54.

112. Mehls O, Blum WF, Schaefer F, Tönshoff B, Scharer K. Growth failure in renal disease. Baillières Clin Endocrinol Metab 1992; 6: 665–85.

113. Phillips LS, Unterman TG. Somatomedin activity in disorders of nutrition and metabolism. Clin Endocrinol Metab 1984; 13: 145–89.

114. Guler HP, Schmid C, Zapf J, Froesch ER. Effects of recombinant insulin-like growth factor I on insulin secretion and renal function in normal human subjects. Proc Natl Acad Sci USA 1989; 86: 2868–72.

115. Daughaday WH, Phillips LS, Mueller MS. The effects of insulin and growth hormone on the release of somatomedin by the isolated rat liver. Endocrinology 1976; 98: 1214–19.

116. Böni Schnetzler M, Binz K, Mary JL, Schmid C, Schwander J, Froesch ER. Regulation of hepatic expression of IGF I and fetal IGF binding protein mRNA in streptozotocin-diabetic rats. FEBS Lett 1989; 251: 253–6.

117. Froesch ER, Guler HP, Schmid C, Binz K, Zapf J. Therapeutic potential of insulin-like growth factor I. TEM 1990; 1: 254–60.

118. Froesch ER, Burgi H, Ramseier EB, Bally P, Labhart A. Antibody-suppressible and non-suppressible

insulin-like activities in human serum and their physiologic significance: an insulin assay with adipose tissue of increased precision and specificity. J Clin Invest 1963; 42: 1816–34.

119. Daughaday WH, Hall K, Raben MS, Salmon WDJ, van den Brande JL, Van Wyk JJ. Somatomedin: proposed designation for sulphation factor. Nature 1972; 235: 107.

120. Salmon WDJ, Daughaday WH. Sulfation factor, a serum component mediating the actions of growth hormone in stimulating incorporation of sulfate into cartilage. J Clin Invest 1956; 35: 733.

121. Morell B, Froesch ER. Fibroblasts as an experimental tool in metabolic and hormone studies. II. Effects of insulin and non-suppressible insulin-like activity (NSILA-S) on fibroblasts in culture. Eur J Clin Invest 1973; 3: 119–23.

122. Vetter U, Zapf J, Heit W, Helbing G, Heinze E, Froesch ER, Teller WM. Human fetal and adult chondrocytes. Effect of insulin-like growth factors I and II, insulin, and growth hormone on clonal growth. J Clin Invest 1986; 77: 1903–8.

123. Veldhuis JD, Furlanetto RW. Trophic actions of human somatomedin C/insulin-like growth factor I on ovarian cells: *in vitro* studies with swine granulosa cells. Endocrinology 1985; 116: 1235–42.

124. Zapf J, Hauri C, Waldvogel M, Froesch ER. Acute metabolic effects and half-lives of intravenously administered insulin-like growth factors I and II in normal and hypophysectomized rats. J Clin Invest 1986; 77: 1768–75.

125. Guler HP, Binz K, Eigenmann E, Jaggi S, Zimmermann D, Zapf J, Froesch ER. Small stature and insulin-like growth factors: prolonged treatment of mini-poodles with recombinant human insulin-like growth factor I. Acta Endocrinol (Copenh) 1989; 121: 456–64.

126. Guler HP, Zapf J, Froesch ER. Short-term metabolic effects of recombinant human insulin-like growth factor I in healthy adults. New Engl J Med 1987; 317: 137–40.

127. Schoenle E, Zapf J, Humbel RE, Froesch ER. Insulin-like growth factor I stimulates growth in hypophysectomized rats. Nature 1982; 296: 252–3.

128. Schwander JC, Hauri C, Zapf J, Froesch ER. Synthesis and secretion of insulin-like growth factor and its binding protein by the perfused rat liver: dependence on growth hormone status. Endocrinology 1983; 113: 297–305.

129. Nilsson A, Isgaard J, Lindahl A, Dahlstrom A, Skottner A, Isaksson OG. Regulation by growth hormone of number of chondrocytes containing IGF-I in rat growth plate. Science 1986; 233: 571–4.

130. Ernst M, Froesch ER. Growth hormone dependent stimulation of osteoblast-like cells in serum-free cultures via local synthesis of insulin-like growth factor I. Biochem Biophys Res Commun 1988; 151: 142–7.

131. Schmid C, Schläpfer I, Futo E, Waldvogel M, Schwander J, Zapf J, Froesch ER. Triiodothyronine (T_3) stimulates insulin-like growth factor-I (IGF-I) and IGF-binding protein (IGFBP)-2 production by rat osteoblasts *in vitro*. Acta Endocrinol (Copenh) 1992; 126: 467–73.

132. Clemmons DR, Smith Banks A, Underwood LE. Reversal of diet-induced catabolism by infusion of recombinant insulin-like growth factor-I in humans. J Clin Endocrinol Metab 1992; 75: 234–8.

133. Kupfer SR, Underwood LE, Baxter RC, Clemmons DR. Enhancement of the anabolic effects of growth hormone and insulin-like growth factor I by use of both agents simultaneously. J Clin Invest 1993; 91: 391–6.

134. Guler HP, Zapf J, Scheiwiller E, Froesch ER. Recombinant human insulin-like growth factor I stimulates growth and has distinct effects on organ size in hypophysectomized rats. Proc Natl Acad Sci USA 1988; 85: 4889–93.

135. Glasscock GF, Hein AN, Miller JA, Hintz RL, Rosenfeld RG. Effects of continuous infusion of insulin-like growth factor I and II, alone and in combination with thyroxine or growth hormone, on the neonatal hypophysectomized rat. Endocrinology 1992; 130: 203–10.

136. Heinz Erian P, Kessler U, Funk B, Gais P, Kiess W. Identification and *in situ* localization of the insulin-like growth factor-II/mannose-6-phosphate (IGF-II/M6P) receptor in the rat gastrointestinal tract: comparison with the IGF-I receptor. Endocrinology 1991; 129: 1769–78.

137. Grey V, Rouyer Fessard C, Gammeltoft S, Bourque M, Morin C, Laburthe M. Insulin-like growth factor II/mannose-6-phosphate receptors are transiently increased in the rat distal intestinal epithelium after resection. Mol Cell Endocrinol 1991; 75: 221–7.

138. Levinovitz A, Jennische E, Oldfors A, Edwall D, Norstedt G. Activation of insulin-like growth factor II expression during skeletal muscle regeneration in the rat: correlation with myotube formation. Mol Endocrinol 1992; 6: 1227–34.

139. Haselbacher GK, Schwab ME, Pasi A, Humbel RE. Insulin-like growth factor II (IGF II) in human brain: regional distribution of IGF II and of higher molecular mass forms. Proc Natl Acad Sci USA 1985; 82: 2153–7.

140. Takashahi Y, Kipnis DM, Daughaday WH. Growth hormone secretion during sleep. J Clin Invest 1968; 47: 2079–90.

141. Parker DC, Sassin JF, Mace JW, Gotlin RW, Rossman LG. Human growth hormone release during sleep: electroencephalographic correlation. J Clin Endocrinol Metab 1969; 29: 871–4.

142. Hartman ML, Faria AC, Vance ML, Johnson ML, Thorner MO, Veldhuis JD. Temporal structure of *in vivo* growth hormone secretory events in humans. Am J Physiol 1991; 260: E101–10.

143. Ho KY, Veldhuis JD, Johnson ML, Furlanetto R, Evans WS, Alberti KG, Thorner MO. Fasting enhances growth hormone secretion and amplifies the complex rhythms of growth hormone secretion in man. J Clin Invest 1988; 81: 968–75.

144. Johansen K, Hansen AaP. Diurnal serum growth hormone levels in poorly and well controlled juvenile diabetics. Diabetes 1971; 20: 239–45.

145. Vigneri R, Squatrito S, Pezzino V, Filetti S, Branca S, Polosa P. Growth hormone levels in diabetes: correlation with the clinical control of the disease. Diabetes 1976; 25: 167–72.

146. Asplin CM, Faria AC, Carlsen EC, Vaccaro VA, Barr RE, Iranmanesh A et al. Alterations in the pulsatile mode of growth hormone release in men and women with insulin-dependent diabetes mellitus. J Clin Endocrinol Metab 1989; 69: 239–45.

147. Tamborlane WV, Hintz RL, Bergman M, Genel M, Felig P, Sherwin RS. Insulin infusion pump treatment of diabetes. New Engl J Med 1981; 305: 303–5.

148. Press M, Tamborlane WV, Sherwin RS. Importance of raised growth hormone levels in mediating the metabolic derangements of diabetes. New Engl J Med 1984; 310: 810–14.

149. Flyvbjerg A, Frystyk J, Sillesen IB, Ørskov H. Growth hormone and insulin-like growth factor I in experimental and human diabetes. In: Alberti KGMM, Krall LP (eds) Diabetes annual/6. Amsterdam: Elsevier 1991: pp. 562–90.

150. Møller N. The Role of Growth Hormone in the Regulation of Human Fuel Metabolism. In Flyvbjerg A, Ørskov H, Alberti KGMM (eds) Growth hormone and insulin-like growth factor I in human and experimental diabetes. Chichester: Wiley, 1993: pp. 77–108.

151. Dills DG, Moss SE, Klein R, Klein BE, Davis M. Is insulin-like growth factor I associated with diabetic retinopathy? Diabetes 1990; 39: 191–5.

152. Tamborlane WV, Sherwin RS, Koivisto V, Hendler R, Genel M, Felig P. Normalization of the growth hormone and catecholamine response to exercise in juvenile onset diabetic subjects treated with a portable insulin pump. Diabetes 1979; 28: 785–8.

153. Tan K, Baxter RC. Serum insulin-like growth factor I levels in adult diabetic patients: the effect of age. J Clin Endocrinol Metab 1986; 63: 651–5.

154. Merimee TJ, Zapf J, Froesch ER. Insulin-like growth factors. Studies in diabetics with and without retinopathy. New Engl J Med 1983; 309: 527–30.

155. Cohen MP, Jasti K, Rye L. Somatomedin in insulin-dependent diabetes mellitus. J Clin Endocrinol Metab 1977; 45: 236–9.

156. Ashton IK, Dornan TL, Pocock AE, Turner RC, Bron AT. Plasma somatomedin activity and diabetic retinopathy. J Endocrinol 1983; 19: 105–10.

157. Lamberton RP, Goodman AD, Kassoff A, Rubin CL, Treble DH, Saba TM et al. Von Willebrand factor (VIII R:Ag), fibronectin, and insulin-like growth factors I and II in diabetic retinopathy and nephropathy. Diabetes 1984; 33: 125–9.

158. Horner JM, Kemp SF, Hintz RL. Growth hormone and somatomedin in insulin-dependent diabetes mellitus. J Clin Endocrinol Metab 1981; 53: 1148–53.

159. Merimee TJ, Gardner DF, Zapf J, Froesch ER. Effect of glycemic control on serum insulin-like growth factors in diabetes mellitus. Diabetes 1984; 33: 790–93.

160. Salardi S, Cacciari E, Ballardini D, Righetti F, Capelli M, Cicognani A et al. Relationships between growth factors (somatomedin-C and growth hormone) and body development, metabolic control, and retinal changes in children and adolescents with IDDM. Diabetes 1986; 35: 832–6.

161. Blethen SL, Sargeant DT, Whitlow MG, Santiago JV. Effect of pubertal stage and recent blood glucose control on plasma somatomedin C in children with insulin-dependent diabetes mellitus. Diabetes 1981; 30: 868–72.

162. Bhaumick B, Danilkewich AD, Bala RM. Insulin-like growth factors (IGF) I and II in diabetic pregnancy: suppression of normal pregnancy-induced rise of IGF-I. Diabetologia 1986; 29: 792–7.

163. Hall K, Johansson BL, Povoa G, Thalme B. Serum levels of insulin-like growth factor (IGF) I, II and IGF binding protein in diabetic adolescents treated with continuous subcutaneous insulin infusion. J Intern Med 1989; 225: 273–8.

164. Suikkari AM, Koivisto VA, Rutanen EM, Yki Jarvinen H, Karonen SL, Seppala M. Insulin regulates the serum levels of low molecular weight insulin-like growth factor-binding protein. J Clin Endocrinol Metab 1988; 66: 266–72.

165. Holly JMP, Biddlecombe RA, Dunger DB, Edge JA, Amiel SA, Howell R et al. Circadian variation of GH-independent IGF-binding protein in diabetes mellitus and its relationship to insulin: a new role for insulin? Clin Endocrinol 1988; 29: 667–75.

166. Gutniak M, Grill V, Wiechel KL, Efendic S. Basal and meal-induced somatostatin-like immunoreactivity in healthy subjects and in IDDM and totally pancreatectomised patients: effects of acute blood glucose normalisation. Diabetes 1987; 36: 802–7.

167. Segers O, De Vroede M, Michotte Y, Somers G. Basal and tolbutamide-induced plasma somatostatin in healthy subjects and in patients with diabetes and impaired glucose tolerance. Diabet Med 1989; 6: 232–8.

168. Brismar K, Gutniak M, Povoa G, Werner S, Hall K. Insulin regulates the 35 kDa IGF binding protein in patients with diabetes mellitus. J Endocrinol Invest 1988; 11: 599–602.

169. Lewitt MS, Denyer GS, Cooney GJ, Baxter RC. Insulin-like growth factor-binding protein-1 modulates blood glucose levels. Endocrinology 1991; 129: 2254–6.

170. Foulis AK. The pancreas. In Anderson JR (ed.) Muir's textbook of pathology, 12th edn. London: Edward Arnold, 1985; pp. 20.55–20.66.

171. DeFronzo RA, Ferrannini E. Insulin resistance. A multifaceted syndrome responsible for NIDDM, obesity, hypertension, dyslipidemia, and atherosclerotic cardiovascular disease. Diabetes Care 1991; 14: 173–94.

172. Bornfeldt KE, Arnqvist HJ. Actions of insulin-like growth factor I and insulin in vascular smooth muscle: receptor interaction and growth promoting effects. In Flyvbjerg A, Ørskov H, Alberti KGMM (eds) Growth hormone and insulin-like growth factor I in human and experimental diabetes. Chichester: Wiley 1993: pp 159–92.

173. King GL, Goodman AD, Buzney S, Moses A, Kahn CR. Receptors and growth-promoting effects of insulin and insulinlike growth factors on cells from bovine retinal capillaries and aorta. J Clin Invest 1985; 75: 1028–36.

174. Bornfeldt KE, Gidlof RA, Wasteson A, Lake M, Skottner A, Arnqvist HJ. Binding and biological effects of insulin, insulin analogues and insulin-like growth factors in rat aortic smooth muscle cells. Comparison of maximal growth promoting activities. Diabetologia 1991; 34: 307–13.

175. Lee PD, Hintz RL, Rosenfeld RG, Benitz WE. Presence of insulinlike growth factor receptors and lack of insulin receptors on fetal bovine smooth muscle cells. In Vitro Cell Dev Biol 1988; 24: 921–6.

176. Banskota NK, Taub R, Zellner K, Olsen P, King GL. Characterization of induction of proto-oncogene c-myc and cellular growth in human vascular smooth muscle cells by insulin and IGF-I. Diabetes 1989; 38: 123–9.

177. Bornfeldt KE, Skottner A, Arnqvist HJ. *In vivo* regulation of messenger RNA encoding insulin-like

growth factor-I (IGF-I) and its receptor by diabetes, insulin and IGF-I in rat muscle. J Endocrinol 1992; 135: 203–11.

178. Murphy LJ, Ghahary A, Chakrabarti S. Insulin regulation of IGF-I expression in rat aorta. Diabetes 1990; 39: 657–62.

179. Goldberg ID, Stemerman MB, Schnipper LE, Ransil BJ, Crooks GW, Fuhro RL. Vascular smooth muscle cell kinetics: a new assay for studying patterns of cellular proliferation *in vivo*. Science 1979; 205: 920–22.

180. Capron L, Jarnet J, Kazandjian S, Housset E. Growth-promoting effects of diabetes and insulin on arteries. Diabetes 1986; 35: 973–8.

181. Tiell ML, Stemerman MB, Spaet TH. The influence of the pituitary on arterial intimal proliferation in the rat. Circ Res 1978; 42: 644–9.

182. Bornfeldt KE, Arnqvist HJ, Capron L. *In vivo* proliferation of rat vascular smooth muscle in relation to diabetes mellitus insulin-like growth factor I and insulin. Diabetologia 1992; 35: 104–8.

183. Conte J, Foegh M, Calcagno D, Wallace R, Ramwell P. Peptide inhibition of proliferation following angioplasty in rabbits. Transpl Proc 1989; 21: 3686–8.

184. Heickendorff L, Thøgersen V, Ledet T. Diabetic macroangiopathy: possible roles of growth hormone and insulin-like growth factor I. In Flyvbjerg A, Ørskov H, Alberti KGMM (eds) Growth hormone and insulin-like growth factor I in human and experimental diabetes. Chichester: Wiley, 1993: pp 193–201.

185. Ledet T. Growth hormone antiserum suppresses the growth effect of diabetic serum: studies on rabbit aortic medial cell cultures. Diabetes 1976; 25: 1011–18.

186. Rasmussen LM, Ledet T. Serum from diabetic patients enhances the synthesis of arterial basement membrane-like material studied on rabbit aortic myomedial cell culture. Acta Pathol Microbiol Scand 1988; 96: 77–83.

187. Ledet T, Heickendorff L. Growth hormone effect on accumulation of arterial basement-like material studied on rabbit aortic myomedial cell cultures. Diabetologia 1985; 28: 922–7.

188. Sharp PS. Diabetic retinopathy: an analysis of the possible pathogenic roles of growth hormone and insulin-like growth factor I. In Flyvbjerg A, Ørskov H, Alberti KGMM (eds) Growth hormone and insulin-like growth factor I in human and experimental diabetes. Chichester: Wiley, 1993: pp 203–28.

189. Wright AD, Kohner EM, Oakley NW, Hartog M, Joplin GF, Fraser TR. Serum growth hormone and the responses of diabetic retinopathy to pituitary ablation. Br Med J 1969; ii: 346–8.

190. Powell EDU, Frantz AG, Rabkin MT, Field RA. Growth hormone in relation to diabetic retinopathy. New Engl J Med 1966; 275: 922–5.

191. Blickle JF, Schlienger JT, DeLaharpe F, Stephan F. Growth hormone response to thyrotropin releasing hormone in insulin dependent diabetics with or without severe microvascular lesions. Diabèt Métab 1982; 8: 197–201.

192. Sharp PS, Foley K, Vitelli F, Maneschi F, Kohner EM. Growth hormone response to hyperinsulinaemia in insulin dependent diabetics with and without retinopathy. Diabet Med 1984; 1: 55–8.

193. Kaneko K, Komine S, Maeda T, Ohta M, Tsushima T, Shizume K. Growth hormone responses to growth-hormone-releasing hormone and thyrotropin-releasing hormone in diabetic patients with and without retinopathy. Diabetes 1985; 34: 710–13.

194. Nardelli GM, Guastamacchia E, Di Paolo S, Balice A, Rosco M, Santoro G et al. Somatomedin-C (SM-C). Study in diabetic patients with and without retinopathy. Acta Diabetol Lat 1989; 26: 217–24.

195. Hyer SL, Sharp PS, Brooks RA, Burrin JM, Kohner EM. Serum IGF-1 concentration in diabetic retinopathy. Diabet Med 1988; 5: 356–60.

196. Sato K, Ikeda T, Miki T, Nishizawa Y, Morii H. Somatomedin-C and diabetic retinopathy. Jpn J Ophthalmol 1988; 32: 219–22.

197. Flyvbjerg A, Frystyk J, Thorlacius-Ussing O, Ørskov H. Somatostatin analogue administration prevents increase in kidney somatomedin C and initial renal growth in diabetic and uni-nephrectomized rats. Diabetologia 1989; 32: 261–5.

198. Hyer SL, Sharp PS, Brooks RA, Burrin JM, Kohner EM. A two-year follow-up study of serum insulin-like growth factor I in diabetics with retinopathy. Metabolism 1989; 38: 586–9.

199. Lauritzen T, Frost-Larsen K, Larsen HW, Deckert T. Two years experience with continuous subcutaneous insulin infusion in relation to retinopathy and nephropathy. Diabetes 1985; 34 (suppl. 3): 74–9.

200. Hanssen K, Dahl-Jørgensen K, Lauritzen T. Diabetic control and microvascular complications: the near normoglycaemic experience. Diabetologia 1986; 29: 677–84.

201. The Kroc Collaborative Study Group. Blood glucose control and the evolution of diabetic retinopathy and albuminuria. A preliminary multicenter trial. New Engl J Med 1984; 311: 365–72.

202. Hyer SL, Sharp PS, Sleightholm M, Burrin JM, Kohner EM. Progression of diabetic retinopathy and changes in serum insulin-like growth factor I (IGF I) during continuous subcutaneous insulin infusion (CSII). Horm Metab Res 1989; 21: 18–22.

203. Grant M, Russell B, Fitzgerald C, Merimee TJ. Insulin-like growth factors in vitreous. Studies in control and diabetic subjects with neovascularization. Diabetes 1986; 35: 416–20.

204. Hyer SL, Sharp PS, Brooks RA, Burrin JM, Kohner EM. Continuous subcutaneous octreotide infusion markedly suppresses IGF-I levels whilst only partially suppressing GH secretion in diabetics with retinopathy. Acta Endocrinol (Copenh) 1989; 120: 187–94.

205. Kirkegaard C, Nørgaard K, Snorgaard O, Bek T, Larsen M, Lund Andersen H. Effect of one-year continuous subcutaneous infusion of a somatostatin analogue, octreotide, on early retinopathy, metabolic control and thyroid function in type I (insulin-dependent) diabetes mellitus. Acta Endocrinol (Copenh) 1990; 122: 766–72.

206. Østerby R. Glomerular structural changes in type I (insulin dependent) diabetes mellitus: causes, consequences, and prevention. Diabetologia 1992; 35: 803–12.

207. Steffes MW, Østerby R, Chavers B, Mauer SM. Mesangial expansion as a central mechanism for loss of kidney function in diabetic patients. Diabetes 1989; 38: 1077–81.

208. Mogensen CE, Andersen MJF. Increased kidney size and glomerular filtration rate in early juvenile diabetes. Diabetes 1973; 22: 706-12.

209. Flyvbjerg A, Marshall SM, Frystyk J, Hansen KW, Harris AG, Ørskov H. Octreotide administration in diabetic rats: effects on renal hypertrophy and urinary albumin excretion. Kidney Int 1992; 41: 805-12.

210. Christiansen JS, Gammelgaard J, Ørskov H, Anderson A, Temler S, Parving HH. Kidney function and size in normal subjects before and during growth hormone administration for one week. Eur J Clin Invest 1981; 11: 487-90.

211. Parving HH, Noer I, Mogensen CE, Svendsen P. Kidney function in normal man during short-term growth hormone infusion. Acta Endocrinol (Copenh) 1978; 89: 796-800.

212. Hirschberg R, Kopple JD. Evidence that insulin-like growth factor I increases renal plasma flow and glomerular filtration rate in fasted rats. J Clin Invest 1989; 83: 326-30.

213. Hirschberg R, Kopple JD, Blantz RC, Tucker BJ. Effects of recombinant human insulin-like growth factor I on glomerular dynamics in the rat. J Clin Invest 1991; 87: 1200-206.

214. Haylor J, Singh I, El Nahas AM. Nitric oxide synthesis inhibitor prevents vasodilation by insulin-like growth factor I. Kidney Int 1991; 39: 333-5.

215. Hirschberg R, Kopple JD. The effects of growth hormone and insulin-like growth factor I on renal glomerular and tubular function. In Flyvbjerg A, Ørskov H, Alberti KGMM (eds) Growth hormone and insulin-like growth factor I in human and experimental diabetes. Chichester: Wiley 1993: pp 229-54.

216. Flyvbjerg A, Thorlacius-Ussing O, Naeraa R, Ingerslev J, Ørskov H. Kidney tissue somatomedin C and initial renal growth in diabetic and uni-nephrectomized rats. Diabetologia 1988; 31: 310-14.

217. Flyvbjerg A, Bornfeldt KE, Marshall SM, Arnqvist HJ, Ørskov H. Kidney IGF-I mRNA in initial renal hypertrophy in experimental diabetes in rats. Diabetologia 1990; 33: 334-8.

218. Flyvbjerg A, Frystyk J, Østerby R, Ørskov H. Kidney IGF-I and renal hypertrophy in GH-deficient diabetic dwarf rats. Am J Physiol 1992; 262: E956-62.

219. Flyvbjerg A, Ørskov H. Kidney tissue insulin-like growth factor I and initial renal growth in diabetic rats: relation to severity of diabetes. Acta Endocrinol (Copenh) 1990; 122: 374-8.

220. Marshall SM, Flyvbjerg A, Frystyk J, Korsgaard L, Ørskov H. Renal insulin-like growth factor I and growth hormone receptor binding in experimental diabetes and after unilateral nephrectomy in the rat. Diabetologia 1991; 34: 632-9.

221. Igarashi K, Nakazawa A, Tani N, Yamazaki M, Ito S, Shibata A. Effect of a somatostatin analogue (SMS 201-995) on renal function and excretion in diabetic rats. J Diabet Complications 1991; 5: 181-3.

222. Chateauneuf C, Babin T, Ducasse MCR, Harris AG. Preliminary results as regards the evolution of microalbuminuria in diabetic patients treated with Sandostatin. Diabete Metab 1989; 15: A18 (abstr).

223. Serri O, Beauregard H, Brazeau P, Abribat T, Lambert J, Harris A, Vachon L. Somatostatin analogue, octreotide, reduces increased glomerular filtration rate and kidney size in insulin-dependent diabetes. JAMA 1991; 265: 888-92.

224. Doi T, Striker LJ, Quaife C, Conti FG, Palmiter R, Behringer R et al. Progressive glomerulosclerosis develops in transgenic mice chronically expressing growth hormone and growth hormone releasing factor but not in those expressing insulin-like growth factor-1. Am J Pathol 1988; 131: 398-403.

225. Holzmann P, Zenobi PD, Riesen W, Froesch ER. Recombinant human insulin-like growth factor-I (rhIGF-I) improves lipid profile in type 2 diabetes mellitus. Diabetologia 1991; 34 (suppl. 2): A194.

226. Schoenle EJ, Zenobi PD, Torresani T, Werder EA, Zachmann M, Froesch ER. Recombinant human insulin-like growth factor I (rhIGF I) reduces hyperglycaemia in patients with extreme insulin resistance. Diabetologia 1991; 34: 675-9.

227. Howell M, Ørskov H, Frystyk J, Flyvbjerg A, Grønbæk H, Foegh M. Lanreotide, a somatostatin analogue, reduces insulin-like growth factor I accumulation in proliferating aortic tissue in rabbits in vivo. A preliminary study. Eur J Endocrinol 1994; 130: 422-5.

21

Insulin Receptors and Insulin Signaling in Normal and Disease States

C. Ronald Kahn

Elliott P. Joslin Research Laboratory, Joslin Diabetes Center, and Department of Medicine, Harvard Medical School, Boston, MA, USA

The pathophysiology of diabetes mellitus in all of its forms is ultimately due to a deficiency in insulin signaling. In type 1 diabetes, this is a result of deficiency in insulin itself, whereas in type 2 and most secondary forms of diabetes, the primary defect is resistance to insulin action at the target cell level. Thus, any understanding of diabetes requires an understanding of the mechanisms of insulin action and the effects of insulin in the cell.

Insulin action at the cellular level can be viewed as existing in three levels (Figure 1). Level 1 is the initiation of insulin action and depends upon insulin binding to and stimulating its receptor tyrosine kinase, which results in tyrosine phosphorylation of the receptor and intracellular substrates. Level 2 actions are the intermediate signals in the insulin action cascade and involve a number of serine kinases, such as MAP and S6 kinases, as well as lipid kinases, such as phosphatidylinositol (PI) 3-kinase. At level 3 are the final biological effectors of insulin signaling. These are the enzymes and transporters required for insulin's effects on glucose, lipid and protein metabolism. This chapter will focus on the early and intermediate components of the insulin signaling cascade, and their alterations in different physiological and pathological states.

THE INSULIN RECEPTOR

Insulin regulates numerous diverse metabolic processes through binding to high-affinity cell surface receptors [1–4]. The receptor can be found in classical target tissues, where it plays an essential role in determining the metabolic responses to insulin stimulation, as well as in tissues such as brain, red blood cells and gonads, which are not traditionally viewed as insulin-sensitive. Likewise, the postreceptor machinery of insulin signaling, including substrates of the receptor and other signaling intermediates, is present in most cells. Thus, there are probably many important insulin actions in both classical and non-classical target tissues which are yet to be determined.

Structure and Function

The receptor is a transmembrane glycoprotein complex with a molecular weight of about 460 kDa [5]. The basic structural characteristics of the receptor, as well as its binding properties, are highly conserved through evolution in organisms as distant as humans and *Drosophila* [6, 7], supporting the concept of an essential role of the insulin receptor signaling system in development and metabolic control. In all vertebrate species, the receptor complex consists of two 135 kDa α-subunits and two 95 kDa β-subunits (Figure 2). Both α- and β-subunits are derived from a single chain proreceptor encoded by a single gene. In humans the insulin receptor gene is located on the short arm of chromosome 19 [8–12]. In the mature receptor, the α- and β-subunits are linked by disulfide bonds to form a tetramer with a $\beta - \alpha - \alpha - \beta$ structure [5,

International Textbook of Diabetes Mellitus, Second Edition. Edited by K.G.M.M. Alberti, P. Zimmet, R.A. DeFronzo, and H. Keen (Honorary)
© 1997 John Wiley & Sons Ltd

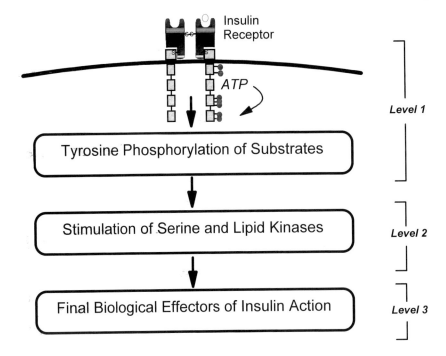

Figure 1   Three levels of insulin action

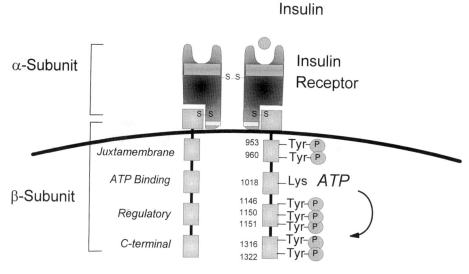

Figure 2   Insulin receptor structure. The insulin receptor consists of an α-subunit which is entirely extracellular and a β-subunit with an extracellular domain, a transmembrane domain and a large intracellular domain. Following insulin binding to the α-subunit, the tyrosine kinase activity of the β-subunit is activated, resulting in autophosphorylation of the receptor on at least six sites. Together with the kinase domain, these define the four subdomains of the intracellular portion of the β-subunit: the juxtamembrane region which contains tyrosine phosphorylation site 960, the regulatory region which contains three tyrosine sites of phosphorylation, and the C-terminal receptor domain which contains two tyrosine phosphorylation sites

13]. The α-subunit is entirely extracellular [5, 13], whereas the β-subunit is a transmembrane protein with a short extracellular domain, a single membrane-spanning region of about 23 amino acids, and an intracellular domain. Both subunits are glycoproteins with complex O- and N-linked carbohydrate side-chains [14, 15]. Removal of these carbohydrate residues by

glycosidase treatment results in a decrease in insulin binding suggesting that the carbohydrate residues provide some tertiary structural features required for full binding activity [16]. Based on biosynthetic labeling, the insulin receptor also appears to contain covalently bound fatty acid side chains [17]; the exact location and functional significance of this modification, however, is not clear. Differences in receptor subunit size and recognition by monoclonal antibodies have been noted in both human tissues [18] and rat tissues [19] suggesting that there is some micro-heterogeneity of receptor structure in different tissues. This is in part due to alternative splicing of exon 11 in the α-subunit which results in two forms of this subunit which differ by 12 amino acids near the C-terminus [20–22]. The α-subunits of insulin receptors in brain are also of lower molecular weight than those in other tissues due to altered glycosylation of the receptor in this tissue [23–25].

Insulin Binding Properties

Recognition of the insulin molecule by its receptor is a complex molecular event and is essential for signal transmission. This involves an interaction between a three-dimensional surface on the insulin molecule (composed of portions of the A and B chains of insulin) with the N-terminal half of the α-subunit of the receptor which contains the primary hormone binding region [1, 26, 27]. Recent data suggest that there is a secondary interaction between a domain on the opposite side of the insulin molecule and the second α-subunit in the receptor heterotetramer [28]. This bivalent binding of insulin to the receptor creates a high affinity interaction and 'cross-links' the receptor α-subunits, possibly contributing to the conformational change required for signaling [29, 30]. There is an almost perfect correlation between receptor-binding affinity and biological effect among over 200 analogues of insulin studied [1, 26, 28, 31], indicating that the structural requirements for insulin binding include all the features necessary for insulin's biological action.

The kinetics of insulin binding to its receptor are complex. Scatchard plots of binding data designed to estimate receptor number and affinity are not linear [32]. Two models of the insulin–receptor interaction have been suggested to explain this non-linear behavior. One model proposes that the binding of insulin leads to negative cooperativity, i.e. hormone binding causes a decrease in the affinity of the receptor for subsequent hormone molecules [33, 34]. The other model hypothesizes the existence of multiple binding sites, with either low or high affinity for the hormone [32, 35]. The fact that there is a single basic receptor structure and the recent evidence for a bivalent interaction between insulin and its receptor suggest that the cooperative model is the most appropriate, although the exon 11 polymorphism of the α-subunit does provide two structural forms of the receptor which have slightly different binding affinities for the hormone [22, 36–38]. Aggregation of insulin receptors on the cell surface is

induced by insulin binding, and this may play an additional role in cooperative binding effects, as well as in transmission of the hormone signal itself [39, 40].

The Insulin Receptor as a Tyrosine Kinase

One of the most important breakthroughs in understanding insulin action at the cellular level was the revelation that the insulin receptor is an enzyme of a class called receptor tyrosine protein kinases [41–43]. This class of receptor enzymes respond to ligand binding by catalyzing the transfer of phosphate groups from ATP to tyrosine residues of proteins (Figure 3A). In the case of the insulin receptor kinase, the tyrosine phosphorylation occurs on both the receptor itself (autophosphorylation) and on a range of intracellular substrates (Figure 3B). Although occasional studies have suggested other activities of the receptor, the tyrosine kinase activity of the insulin receptor appears to be essential for insulin signaling [44, 45]. The importance of kinases in insulin action cannot be overemphasized. Intermediate signaling involves protein kinases which can phosphorylate serine and threonine residues in proteins and lipid kinases, e.g. PI 3-kinase (Figure 3A). Interestingly, some of the final classical biological effects of insulin, such as activation of glycogen synthase, depend on enzymes which reverse phosphorylation, i.e. phosphatases (Figure 3A).

Functionally, the two subunits of the insulin receptor perform the different functions required for transmission of the insulin signal to the cell interior [4, 42]. Thus, the α-subunit binds insulin with high affinity and specificity. Although the exact binding site has not been mapped, it appears that this interaction involves several domains of the α-subunit, with the primary binding domain in the N-terminal one-third of the receptor. The function of the α-subunit in the unoccupied state is to repress the tyrosine kinase activity intrinsic to the β-subunit. Thus, removal or modification of the α-subunit leads to constitutive activation of the receptor [46, 47]. Binding of insulin leads to a propagated conformational change in the receptor which mimics the removal of the subunit and also leads to stimulation of the kinase activity of the β-subunit [48, 49].

Once activated, the β-subunit acts as the signal transducer through its tyrosine kinase activity. The β-subunit autophosphorylates itself on at least six tyrosine sites [50–52], as well as phosphorylating intracellular substrate proteins [53, 54]. Three of the six autophosphorylation sites identified in the β-subunit are at tyrosines 1146, 1150 and 1151 (or residues 1158, 1162 and 1163 in the +exon 11 form). These are considered to form a regulatory domain of the receptor, because once these tyrosines are phosphorylated, the activity of the receptor towards exogenous substrates is enhanced

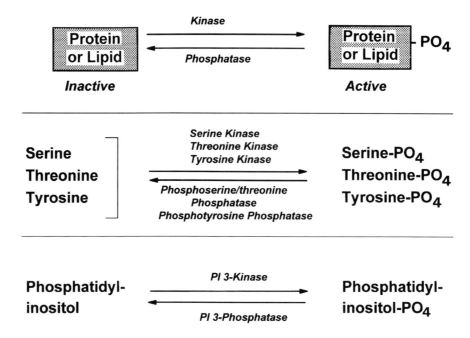

Figure 3A Kinases and phosphatases as signal transducers. Cells contain enzymes with both protein kinase and lipid kinase activity. These kinases can phosphorylate various amino acids (serine, threonine or tyrosine) or specific lipids (phosphatidylinositol) at highly specific sites. In most cases, this results in an activation or increased activity of the protein or lipid in some biological system. Phosphatases of specific types are present in the cell which can dephosphorylate these phosphorylated moieties and reverse the activation. In a few cases, such as glycogen synthase, dephosphorylation results in activation of the enzyme

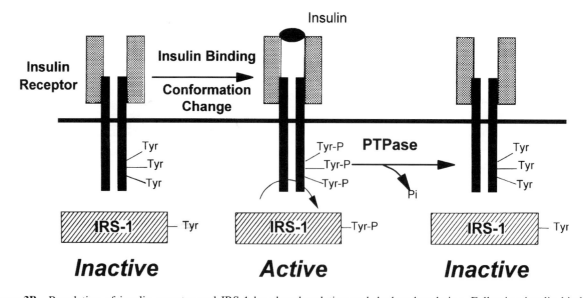

Figure 3B Regulation of insulin receptor and IRS-1 by phosphorylation and dephosphorylation. Following insulin binding, the insulin receptor undergoes autophosphorylation on tryosine residues which results in activation toward exogenous substrates such as IRS-1. When insulin dissociates from the receptor or is degraded, there is a loss of kinase activation, and intracellular protein tyrosine phosphatases (PTPases) dephosphorylate both the receptor and its substrates, leading to inactivation of the system

[50, 51, 55] (Figure 3B). Mutations that affect either the kinase activity of the receptor or its ability to undergo autophosphorylation in the regulatory region result in a loss of insulin action [44, 45, 56].

In addition to the phosphorylation sites in the regulatory region, there are three additional sites of autophosphorylation. These include tyrosine 960 (residue 972 in the +exon 11 receptor) in the juxtamembrane region of the receptor which is critical for interaction with most intracellular substrates of the receptor and is also important for insulin-stimulated receptor internalization [57–61]. The remaining two sites of phosphorylation are in the carboxy terminal region at tyrosines 1316 and 1322 (residues 1328 and 1334 in the +exon 11 receptor). The functional importance of the latter region remains debated, but it has been suggested that it is involved in growth-regulating pathways [62].

INSULIN RECEPTOR SUBSTRATES

Following activation, the insulin receptor tyrosine kinase can stimulate transfer of phosphate groups to tyrosine residues on intracellular substrate proteins. The first identified and best characterized substrate of the receptor was simply named insulin receptor substrate-1 (IRS-1) [63–68]. IRS-1 is a cytoplasmic protein of molecular weight 131 kDa. On SDS gels it has an apparent molecular weight of ~185 kDa, and was therefore originally termed pp185. IRS-1 is also a substrate for IGF-I receptors which are highly homologous to the insulin receptor, as well as for tyrosine kinases that are stimulated by several cytokine receptors, including the interleukin-4 and growth hormone receptors [69–74]. The primary sequence of IRS-1 is highly conserved among mammals. In man, the gene is located on chromosome 2q

36–37 [75]. Like the insulin and IGF-I receptors, IRS-1 has a wide tissue distribution and appears to be regulated during development and different physiological states [76–79].

Structurally, IRS-1 can be viewed as having two types of functional domains (Figure 4). In the N-terminal third of the molecule are two domains which are involved in interaction with the insulin receptor; they have been termed the PH (pleckstrin homology) and PTB (phosphotyrosine binding) domains [80, 81]. Scattered throughout the rest of the molecule are 22 potential tyrosine phosphorylation sites, at least seven or eight of which undergo rapid tyrosine phosphorylation following insulin stimulation [64]. This phosphorylation of IRS-1 provides the next step of insulin signaling by allowing IRS-1 to serve as an intracellular ligand and bind to other intracellular proteins involved in signal transduction via non-covalent interactions [4, 42, 82–84]. These interactions occur between the phosphorylated motifs of IRS-1 and specific domains on these other proteins, termed src homology-2 (SH2) domains [85] (Figure 5). IRS-1 binds to at least six different SH2 domain proteins, and this results in a rapid divergence of signal transduction to many pathways (Figures 4 and 6). Some of the SH2 domain proteins that bind to IRS-1 are enzymes, such as phosphatidylinositol 3-kinase (PI 3-kinase) [82, 86, 87] and the phosphotyrosine phosphatase SHPTP2 (also called Syp) [83, 88]. Binding of IRS-1 to these

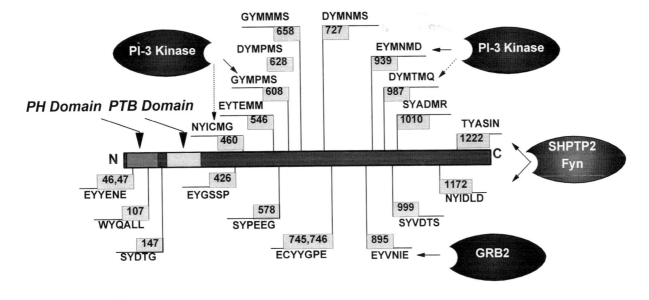

Figure 4 IRS-1 structure. In humans and rodents, IRS-1 is a molecule of about 1250 amino acids. Near the amino terminus (shown at the left) there are two domains involved in high affinity recognition by the insulin receptor. These are termed the pleckstrin homology (PH) and phosphotyrosine binding (PTB) domains. Scattered throughout the length of the molecule are 22 potential tyrosine phosphorylation sites. Several of these have been shown to bind specific SH2 domain proteins following phosphorylation. Some of the phosphorylation sites and their SH2 partners are indicated. These partners include the enzyme PI 3-kinase, the phosphotyrosine phosphatase SHPTP2 and the adaptor protein GRB2

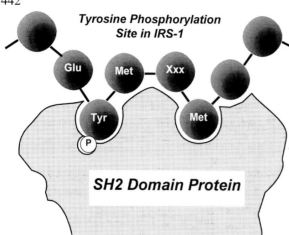

Figure 5 Binding of an SH2 domain protein to IRS-1 YMXM motif. Following phosphorylation, tyrosine residues in specific motifs bind to downstream proteins via recognition domains, termed SH2 (src homology 2) domains. These recognize the phosphotyrosine in the context of a few adjacent amino acids. The recognition site for the SH2 domain of PI 3-kinase has the sequence tyrosine–methionine–any amino acid–methionine (Tyr–Met–Xxx–Met)

SH2 proteins results in rapid stimulation of their enzymatic activity [82, 83, 87, 89]. Other SH2 proteins which bind to IRS-1 have no intrinsic enzymatic activity, but serve as adaptor proteins between IRS-1 and other signaling systems. The best characterized of these is the molecule GRB2 which links IRS-1 to the Ras pathway [90, 91]. Exactly how each of these intermediate signaling pathways leads to insulin action remains unknown, but most evidence suggests that PI 3-kinase is the major link between IRS-1 and the metabolic effects of insulin, while GRB2 may be the major link to growth stimulation [4].

PI 3-kinase consists of two subunits, a regulatory subunit of molecular weight 85 000 (p85) and a catalytic subunit with a molecular weight of 110 000 (p110). The p85 subunit contains two SH2 domains that allow this protein to associate with tyrosine phosphorylation motifs in IRS-1 which have the sequence YMXM or YVXM (Y = tyrosine, V = valine, M = methionine, X = any amino acid) (an example is shown

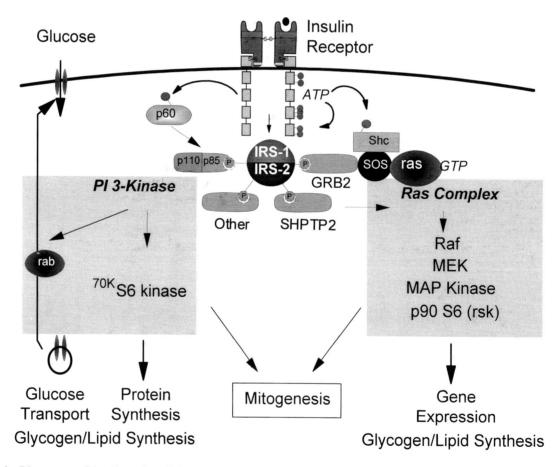

Figure 6 Divergence of insulin action. IRS-1 phosphorylation results in a divergence of the insulin action signal. The two major limbs are the result of stimulation of PI 3-kinase activity and the stimulation of Ras activity. The PI 3-kinase activity has been shown to be upstream of p70 S6 kinase and insulin stimulated glucose transporter translocation. The Ras pathway is upstream of a series of serine/threonine kinases called Raf, MEK, MAP, and p90 S6 kinase (rsk). The latter appear to be important in phosphorylation of various transcription factors and the growth-promoting actions of insulin. Insulin-stimulated mitogenesis depends on reconvergence of these divergent pathways

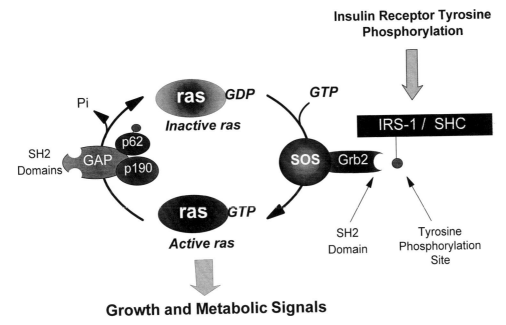

Figure 7 Ras pathway and its stimulation by insulin. Following insulin stimulation, Ras is converted from the GDP-bound form to the GTP-bound form by the presence of a guanine nucleotide exchange factor called SOS (son of sevenless). When insulin signaling is reversed, Ras GTP is reconverted to Ras GDP in the presence of a GTPase activating protein (GAP). The activated form of Ras, i.e. the GTP-bound form, is responsible for activation of the Raf–MAP kinase cascade

in Figure 5). The SH2 domains of PI 3-kinase appear to bind preferentially to the IRS-1 sequence around tyrosines 460, 608, 939 and 987 [53, 84]. This interaction results in a stimulation of PI 3-kinase activity [82, 86, 87], which in turn can catalyze the phosphorylation of phosphatidylinositol (PI), PI-4P and PI-4,5P_2 to PI-3P, PI-3,4P_2 and PI-3,4,5P_3, respectively. PI 3-kinase also has a tightly associated serine kinase activity, the function of which is poorly understood [92]. Although the exact mechanisms remain unknown, activation of PI 3-kinase appears to be a critical upstream step for insulin stimulation of Glut4 glucose transporter translocation and glucose uptake, as well as stimulation of some enzymes involved in protein synthesis, such as pp70 S6 kinase (Figure 6).

As noted above, IRS-1 also binds to GRB2 which links insulin to the Ras pathway. Ras (p21^{ras}) is an important protein involved in regulation of cell growth and metabolism. Ras cycles between an active GTP-bound form and an inactive GDP-bound form. Insulin shifts the equilibrium of Ras binding from GDP-bound toward GTP-bound (Figure 7). This regulation is mediated by a guanine nucleotide exchange factor termed SOS which promotes the exchange of GTP for GDP. In cells, SOS is complexed with the adaptor protein GRB2. Thus, after insulin stimulation, GRB2 binds to IRS-1 at phosphorylated tyrosine 895 via its SH2 domain [90, 93–97]. This activates the GDP/GTP exchange factor SOS in the GRB2/SOS complex, which in turn stimulates the GTP loading

of Ras [98–100]. Activation of Ras then results in stimulation of a cascade of serine/threonine phosphorylation involving Raf-1 kinase, MAP kinase kinase (also termed MEK), MAP kinase and p90 S6 kinase (also called rsk) (Figure 6) [4, 101, 102]. The p90 S6 kinase (rsk) then phosphorylates and activates several transcription factors which regulate gene expression. Phosphorylation by rsk also activates protein phosphatase-1 (PPG-1) which can dephosphorylate and activate three enzymes in the glycogen synthetic pathway: glycogen synthetase, phosphorylase kinase and glycogen phosphorylase [101]. Thus, one can envisage an 11-step process in which Ras forms the critical link between the insulin receptor and glycogen synthesis (Figure 8). However, recent data suggest that PI 3-kinase is probably more important than Ras as an upstream regulator of glycogen synthesis [103]. Thus, although the Ras–MAP–rsk pathway may play a role in the metabolic actions of insulin, this pathway is probably most important in control of transcription factor activity and mitogenesis [102, 104, 105].

ALTERNATIVE PATHWAYS IN INSULIN SIGNALING

Recent data suggest that there are several alternative pathways of insulin signaling. Mice in which the IRS-1 gene has been disrupted are clearly resistant to both IGF-I and insulin, and exhibit both growth retardation and impaired glucose tolerance [106, 107]. However,

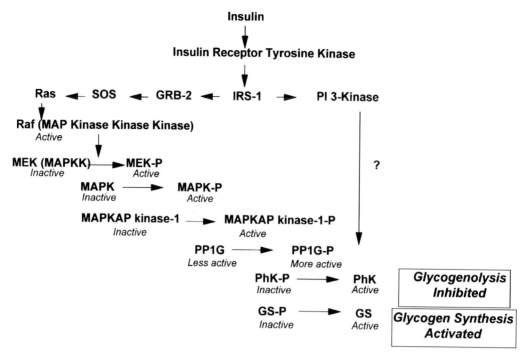

Figure 8 Presumed pathways of insulin stimulation of glycogen metabolism. Following insulin receptor and IRS-1 phosphorylation, it is possible to envision an 11-step sequential pathway resulting in stimulation of glycogen metabolism. This utilizes a cascade of kinases activated by the Ras pathway. Recent studies, however, also indicate that PI 3-kinase activation may contribute to stimulation of glycogen metabolism. Exactly where this has its effect in the cascade is at present unknown. MAPKAP kinase-1 is also referred to as p90 S6 kinase or rsk

there is residual IRS-1 independent signaling. Thus, at high concentrations insulin and IGF-I have some effect in lowering the blood glucose, and glucose uptake in isolated adipocytes shows about 50% of normal stimulation by insulin. This insulin stimulation is due to the presence of an alternative substrate of the insulin receptor termed IRS-2 [108].

IRS-2 is distinct from IRS-1, has a slightly higher molecular weight and is derived from a separate gene [109]. However, cloning and sequence analysis of this protein reveals many similarities to IRS-1, including highly homologous PH and PTB domains and many tyrosine phosphorylation sites with similar sequences. Like IRS-1, IRS-2 also participates in IGF-I and cytokine signaling and is widely distributed in tissues. Thus, following insulin stimulation, both IRS-1 and IRS-2 become tyrosine-phosphorylated on multiple sites and bind to and activate multiple SH2 domain proteins including PI 3-kinase, SHPTP2 and GRB-2-SOS (Figure 6).

The insulin receptor is also linked to PI 3-kinase and Ras by at least two lower molecular weight substrates (Figure 6). One involves the protein Shc which is phosphorylated in response to insulin stimulation and forms a complex with GRB2/SOS, leading to an increase of Ras activity [110]. This can occur in the absence of IRS-1 or IRS-2 phosphorylation, but has a slower time-course and may therefore play a lesser

role in normal insulin signaling. Shc does not, however, couple insulin to PI 3-kinase. On the other hand, insulin stimulates the phosphorylation of a protein or proteins of 55–60 kDa (p55 and p60) which appear to provide additional links to the PI 3-kinase pathway of signaling without affecting Ras activation [111, 112].

THE FINAL EFFECTORS OF INSULIN ACTION

An important frontier of current investigation is exactly how the intermediate signals generated by insulin lead to the final biological effects of the hormone. The major effect of insulin on glucose uptake in muscle and fat depends on the ability of insulin to stimulate a translocation of intracellular vesicles containing the insulin-sensitive Glut4 glucose transporter to the plasma membrane, where they fuse with the membrane and are active in promoting glucose uptake in the cells. This depends on activation of PI 3-kinase, specific intracellular GTP-binding proteins of the Rab family, and the presence of proteins involved in vesicular docking on both the Glut4 containing vesicle and the plasma membrane [113–116]. However, how PI 3-kinase activation promotes this translocation is unknown. Likewise, the specific mechanisms by which insulin stimulates protein synthesis and gene transcription remain unclear, although it is known that these processes are dependent on activation of the two major forms of S6 kinase, p70 S6 kinase and p90 rsk. Since these two enzymes are downstream of the two major limbs of the divergent signaling pathway, PI 3-kinase and Ras, these processes are clearly dependent on several different signaling intermediates.

LIFE CYCLE OF THE INSULIN RECEPTOR

The Insulin Receptor Gene and its Regulation

In humans, the insulin receptor gene is located on the short arm of chromosome 19 near the gene for the low-density lipoprotein receptor [11, 117]. The insulin receptor gene spans over 150 kilobases and consists of 22 exons separated by long introns [117, 118]. One alternative splicing site exists in the region surrounding exon 11; this results in two distinct mRNA species that encode different α-subunits differing by 12 amino acids at the carboxy terminus. As noted above, this alternative splicing may play a role in microheterogeneity of the receptor, subtle differences in insulin binding and differences in internalization [20, 38, 119]. While the ratio of +exon 11 to −exon 11 receptor (sometimes called the A and B forms of the receptor) varies, both receptor forms are found in most tissues [21, 22].

Although insulin receptors are expressed on virtually all mammalian tissues, the concentration of receptors varies from as few as 40 per cell on circulating erythrocytes to more than 200 000 per adipocyte or hepatocyte. Expression of the insulin receptor gene is regulated by both the metabolic status of the cell and the state of differentiation [120, 121]. For example, differentiation of fibroblasts into adipocytes and of myoblasts into myocytes leads to an increase in insulin receptor mRNA levels and increased receptor expression. The 5' upstream regulatory region of the receptor gene is rich in GC residues and has other structural features characteristic of 'house-keeping' promoters [117, 122, 123]. These promoters typically control the transcription of genes whose products are required by most cells for normal homeostasis and growth [124].

A number of elements involved in the control of basal levels of receptor expression have been defined by mutagenesis and gel shift studies [120, 122, 123, 125]. Glucocorticoids have been shown to stimulate insulin receptor gene transcription, with no apparent effect on mRNA half-life [126]. However, a sequence characteristic of the glucocorticoid element (GRE) has not yet been located in the receptor gene or its promoter. Besides the glucocorticoid effect, steady-state insulin receptor mRNA content is markedly stimulated by differentiation of pre-adipocyte cells into the

adipocyte phenotype, as well as during activation of peripheral lymphocytes [127]. Insulin itself does not appear to have a significant effect in the regulation of its receptor gene [128], although it dramatically shortens protein half-life.

Transcription of the insulin receptor gene produces multiple large mRNA species that vary in size and abundance among various tissues [129]. The four major human mRNA species range from 5.7 to 9.5 kb, all larger than the 4.2 kb required for the coding sequence. The bulk of the untranslated mRNA lies at the 3' end of the insulin receptor transcripts, and its function is not currently understood. The multiple mRNA species are regulated similarly with differentiation and also similarly regulated when glucocorticoids act to induce transcription of the receptor gene [129, 130]. The stability of insulin receptor mRNA varies significantly in different cell types, and may play a greater role in determining receptor abundance than changes in receptor gene transcription.

Insulin Receptor Biosynthesis and Processing

Both biosynthetic labeling studies and analysis of the gene structure have indicated that both subunits of the receptor are derived from a single precursor or proreceptor. The initial product of insulin receptor mRNA translation is a polypeptide of approximately 160 kDa on SDS gels [8, 10, 131]. This 'preprocursor' has a signal peptide which, when cleaved, leaves a single-chain proreceptor with the α-subunit sequence at the NH$_2$ terminus and the β-subunit sequence at the COOH portion (Figure 9). The subunit polypeptides are separated by a proteolytic cleavage site of four basic residues [8] that are required for processing [132]. Thus, the biosynthesis of the insulin receptor resembles in some ways that of the insulin molecule itself, which also contains two chains that are synthesized as a single chain precursor. The receptor precursor is co-translationally glycosylated to give a 190–210 kDa proreceptor [12, 131, 133, 134]. These proreceptors possess insulin binding and hormone-activated tyrosine kinase activity prior to cleavage into α- and β-subunits, although the level of activity is lower than that in the mature receptor [135, 136]. Additional steps in proreceptor maturation involve oligomerization [137], terminal glycosylation [12, 133, 134], fatty acid acylation [17], subunit cleavage [12, 138] and insertion of the mature $\alpha_2\beta_2$ holoreceptor into the plasma membrane [139]. The entire process of insulin receptor biosynthesis requires about 1.5–3 hours. The various processes involved in insulin receptor biosynthesis are important for determining the ultimate number of cell surface receptors. However, control of these biosynthetic events and the exact enzymes involved have not

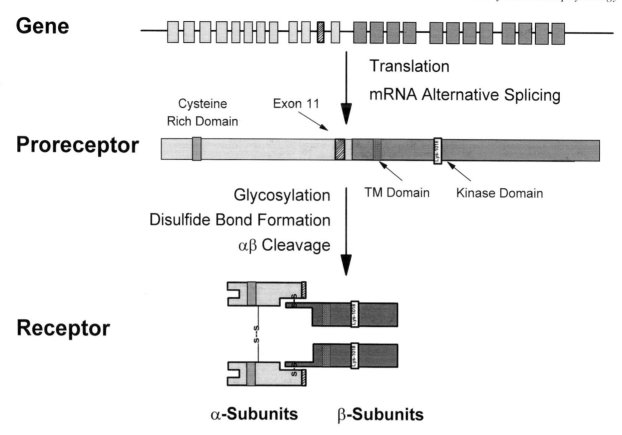

Figure 9 Insulin receptor biosynthesis. The insulin receptor gene is on the short arm of chromosome 19 and comprises 22 exons (shown by the boxes). These result in the formation of several mRNA species which undergo alternative splicing and translation to form the proreceptor. The proreceptor contains a linear sequence including both α- and β-subunits of the receptor separated by a four-amino-acid proteolytic processing site. The proreceptor then undergoes glycosylation, membrane insertion, and cleavage to α- and β-subunits to form the mature receptor

been well characterized. One patient has been described with a mutation in the processing site of the proreceptor; this individual presents the phenotype of insulin resistant diabetes [132].

Recycling and Down-regulation of the Insulin Receptor

Like all membrane proteins, the insulin receptor is highly dynamic and is in a constant state of turnover. The complete life-cycle of the receptor involves steps of biosynthesis, degradation, internalization and recycling [140–145]. The mature receptors on the cell surface are degraded and replaced with a half-life of about 7–12 hours [12, 138]. This involves two forms of receptor internalization—one which is constitutive and the other which is stimulated by ligand binding [61]. Although some insulin receptors recycle spontaneously, most receptors are internalized by a process of ligand-mediated endocytosis whereby insulin binding leads to internalization of the hormone–receptor complexes [141, 142]. Thus, when cells are incubated *in vitro* in medium containing insulin, the concentration

of receptors on the surface is acutely reduced in a time-dependent and temperature-dependent fashion [146–148]. This process has been studied in many cell types and is known as 'down-regulation'. Other ligands which bind to the receptor, such as anti-insulin receptor antibodies, can mimic this effect [149, 150]. Insulin has been shown to accelerate receptor degradation by reducing the half-life from 12 hours to about 2–3 hours [151]. Often, internalized receptors escape degradation and may make several cycles back to the membrane before being degraded [152]. Insulin receptors may also shuttle from one side of a cell to another and back in a process known as transcytosis [153]. This process occurs in endothelial cells and is believed to participate in the transport of insulin from the intravascular space to its site of action at the target cell.

The effect of insulin to regulate receptor turnover, or down-regulation, is important physiologically and is also apparent in cells and tissues isolated from patients and animals with a variety of diseases. In almost all situations, the number of cell surface insulin receptors correlates inversely with the level of insulin to which the cells have been exposed [146]. The phenomenon of down-regulation plays a central part in the regulation of plasma membrane insulin receptor number and in the pathogenesis of several states of insulin resistance, including obesity and type 2 diabetes [154].

REGULATION OF INSULIN RECEPTORS AND INSULIN SIGNALING IN PHYSIOLOGICAL STATES

Insulin receptors are central to insulin action, and thus defects in the receptor or post-receptor signaling contribute to the metabolic consequences of insulin resistance. Insulin resistance exists whenever normal concentrations of insulin produce a less than normal biological response [155]. In most disorders, this is accompanied by a compensatory increase in insulin secretion. When endogenous secretion does not completely compensate for the resistance, impaired glucose tolerance or diabetes results. Alterations in insulin receptor function and insulin action occur in both normal physiology and disease states. Many of the physiological regulators of signaling also play a role in pathological disorders.

Effects of Diet

Both the quantity and quality of calorie intake affect insulin binding and insulin action at a molecular level. In normal individuals on an *ad lib* diet, there is a diurnal variation in insulin binding to circulating monocytes [156]. This variation is apparently related to dietary intake and is abolished by total fasting. This circadian variation in insulin binding appears to be due to fluctuations in receptor binding affinity rather than changes in receptor concentration. An oral glucose load following a fast has also been shown to cause an acute increase in insulin binding affinity on circulating monocytes [157]. The mechanisms involved in these changes in affinity are unknown.

Dietary effects on the insulin receptor tyrosine kinase have also been observed in rodents and animal models of disease. In rats, fasting is associated with an increase in receptor number in liver (up-regulation), but a decrease in kinase activity and in the rate of substrate phosphorylation [158]. Conversely, autophosphorylation is increased in rats fed a high-carbohydrate diet [159]. Since fasting is known to cause insulin resistance and carbohydrate feeding enhances glucose action, these results support the physiological role of receptor autophosphorylation and substrate phosphorylation in insulin action. The dissociation between binding and kinase function in fasting suggests an uncoupling of the normal interaction between the α- and β-subunits. The exact mechanism of this uncoupling

is unknown. Fasting also leads to an increase in IRS-1 and IRS-2 in liver [77]. Thus, despite decreased receptor kinase activity, total IRS phosphorylation is increased. These results suggest that the insulin resistance observed in fasted rats may have an important post-receptor component, beyond or at the level of PI 3-kinase activation.

Exercise

Exercise enhances insulin sensitivity and glucose disposal in normal physiology [160]. This is associated with increased insulin binding to muscle [161], adipocytes [162, 163], monocytes [164, 165] and erythrocytes [166]. A study in rat muscle demonstrated a doubling of insulin receptor content within 4 weeks of exercise training, which was associated with little change in receptor autophosphorylation or tyrosine kinase activity [167]. Although chronic training will also increase receptor number in animals, in humans the major effect of exercise training is an increase in Glut4 glucose transporters in muscle [168, 169]. Acute exercise can also stimulate Glut4 translocation without activating the insulin receptor or PI 3-kinase [170]. Thus, exercise increases insulin sensitivity and mimics insulin action mainly at post-receptor levels.

Hormonal Regulation

Effects of Insulin

In most insulin resistant states elevated insulin levels result in down-regulation of the receptor, by increasing receptor internalization and degradation. Increased insulin levels also appear to decrease the receptor kinase activity, perhaps via altered serine/threonine phosphorylation of the receptor [171]. Several studies have shown that stimulation of serine kinases, including protein kinase A and protein kinase C, can result in serine phosphorylation of the insulin receptor. In contrast to tyrosine phosphorylation, which stimulates receptor kinase activity, serine and threonine phosphorylation produce significant decreases in receptor kinase activity [172, 173]. Thus, decreased receptor number and activity lead to decreased sensitivity of target tissues to insulin action.

In animal models, the higher the basal level of insulin, the greater the decrease in the number of insulin receptors [174, 175] (Figure 10). This has also been shown in patients with insulinoma [176]. Diet or weight loss reduces insulin levels and normalizes the receptor defect [177, 178]. Conversely, in insulin-deficient animal models and in patients with type 1 diabetes, an increase in insulin receptor number is seen (see below). These changes in receptor concentration and insulin sensitivity may occur within hours and

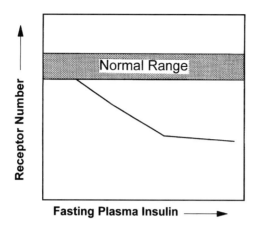

Figure 10 Schematic representation of relationship between insulin levels and insulin receptor levels. Both in intact animals, including humans, and in cultured cells there is an inverse relationship between the ambient insulin level and the level of the insulin receptors expressed. This is due to a stimulation by insulin of receptor internalization and degradation. This contributes to the 'down-regulation' of insulin receptor number and to the desensitization of insulin signaling in various hyperinsulinemic states

certainly within a day. Isolated cells incubated with insulin demonstrate a time-dependent loss of insulin receptors that reach a new steady state in 4–16 hours [146, 179, 180].

Prolonged exposure of cells to insulin leads to desensitization and reduced insulin-stimulated receptor autophosphorylation [181]. There is a normal level of autophosphorylation in relation to insulin bound, indicating that the decreased receptor phosphorylation in desensitized cells is due to the decrease in receptor number from down-regulation. Similar findings have been observed in adipocytes treated with insulin *in vitro* [171]. Chronic insulin treatment also causes a decrease in IRS-1 protein, secondary to increased IRS-1 protein degradation [182, 183]. Thus, the first two proteins in the signaling cascade are both down-regulated by hyperinsulinemia.

Other Hormones

Several hormones that act physiologically to counter the effects of insulin have distinct action on the abundance and function of insulin receptors. The insulin resistance induced by growth hormone excess in acromegaly is associated with a decrease in receptor number [184] and an increase in the affinity of the receptor [185]. Taken together with the recent finding that growth hormone signaling may also involve IRS-1 and IRS-2 [73, 74], the defects in insulin action in acromegaly and high growth hormone states are likely to involve post-receptor, as well as receptor sites in the signaling pathway.

Beta-adrenergic agents, such as isoproterenol, will cause a 50% reduction in apparent insulin binding affinity with no change in receptor number when incubated *in vitro* with adipocytes [186]. This effect is mimicked by cyclic AMP analogues and agents, such as methylxanthine, which elevate cellular cAMP levels. Compounds with α-adrenergic properties do not elicit these effects. Similarly, tumor-promoting phorbol diesters decrease the apparent affinity of insulin receptors in IM-9 lymphocytes [187]. The common denominator of all these agents is that they activate cellular serine/threonine kinases: cAMP acts on the cAMP-dependent protein kinase, and phorbol esters stimulate the calcium-dependent and phospholipid-dependent protein kinase, protein kinase C. Both of these kinases can phosphorylate the insulin receptor on serine/threonine residues, and this serine phosphorylation attenuates insulin receptor tyrosine kinase activity and insulin action [172, 173, 188–190]. In intact cells and tissues, insulin also stimulates increase in serine phosphorylation of the insulin receptor, but this occurs more slowly than the rapid increase in tyrosine phosphorylation [191]. This has led to the speculation that one of the insulin-stimulated serine/threonine kinases may act on the insulin receptor to slowly turn off or modulate insulin signaling action [192].

It is well known that when present in excess, glucocorticoids can produce a form of insulin-resistant diabetes and glucose intolerance. Studies *in vitro* have shown that the insulin receptor of various cell types responds in different ways to the presence of glucocorticoids. In many cell types, including hepatocytes, fibroblasts, monocytes and cultured lymphocytes, glucocorticoids stimulate insulin receptor binding due to increased receptor synthesis and increased cell surface receptor number [193–196]. This effect is due to enhanced transcription of the insulin receptor gene with a resultant increase in the steady-state level of receptor mRNA species [126, 130]. In contrast, there is no effect of glucocorticoids on receptor number or affinity in adipocytes [197], and glucocorticoids decrease insulin binding affinity in 3T3-L1 cells [198]. Some of these discrepancies are likely to be due to variations in experimental technique, but they may also reflect tissue differences in the response to glucocorticoids, either because of differences in the pathways of steroid hormone action or because of different mechanisms of insulin receptor regulation in different cell types. In adipocytes, glucocorticoid-induced insulin resistance appears to be primarily due to effects on post-receptor pathways [197, 199].

The effects of glucocorticoids on insulin receptor tyrosine kinase activity and substrate phosphorylation have been studied in only a few instances. Treatment of rats with dexamethasone produced an approximately

35% increase in insulin receptor phosphorylation in hepatocytes [200] and a smaller increase in receptor phosphorylation activity in adipocytes and muscle [79, 201]. In fasted animals, dexamethasone treatment decreases receptor phosphorylation by 25–50% [200]. IRS-1 and insulin-stimulated PI 3-kinase are similarly reduced in liver, but changes in muscle are less dramatic. In adrenal insufficiency, increase in insulin binding affinity to rat liver plasma membranes [202] and to circulating erythrocytes in patients [203] have been described. When cultured hepatoma cells are exposed to dexamethasone, there is an increase in insulin receptor number and IRS-1 phosphorylation [196, 204]. These studies provide further evidence for heterogeneity in the effect of glucocorticoids on the function of the insulin receptor kinase and the early post-receptor signaling cascade. These findings also suggest that an increase in insulin receptor binding may be at least partly responsible for the increase in insulin sensitivity in adrenal insufficiency [203].

REGULATION OF INSULIN RECEPTOR AND INSULIN ACTION IN PATHOLOGIC STATES

Obesity

In Westernized countries, obesity, with or without the presence of hyperglycemia, is almost certainly the most common state of insulin resistance. Obesity is typically associated with elevated fasting plasma insulin levels which correlate directly with the level of resistance and inversely with receptor number on circulating monocytes, adipocytes, skeletal muscle and liver [205–207] (Figure 10). This represents the effect of high circulating insulin to down-regulate insulin receptors in a number of tissues. Lowering of insulin levels by diet [178, 208], streptozotocin treatment [209] or diazoxide therapy [210] normalizes receptor number, even though the degree of obesity may not be significantly changed. Thus far no alterations in the insulin receptor gene or any of the genes encoding proteins in the insulin signal cascade have been shown to be abnormal in obesity when studied in the context of diabetes [211, 212], although there appears to be an interaction between obesity and the common polymorphisms in IRS-1 [213] (see below). Thus the defects are acquired because of either regulation of insulin signaling proteins or the presence of inhibitors of insulin action.

In humans several sites of insulin resistance have been identified in obesity. Insulin action on muscle metabolism is impaired, as demonstrated by decreased glycogen synthesis rate and decreased glucose uptake and phosphorylation in response to insulin [214, 215]. In adipocytes isolated from non-diabetic, non-obese

and obese subjects the ability of insulin to stimulate uptake of 3-*O*-methylglucose is also impaired [216]. However, activity of the insulin receptor kinase from liver biopsy specimens is only slightly impaired [217], and inhibition of glycogenolysis is near normal. Skeletal muscle Glut4 expression is normal in obesity [218, 219], but is decreased in fat tissue [220, 221]. Both tissues exhibit decreased glucose uptake, however, suggesting that defects in insulin-stimulated translocation must be present.

In addition to down-regulation of receptors secondary to the hyperinsulinemia, the obese state is characterized by post-binding defects in insulin action which can be demonstrated in euglycemic clamp and other studies [222, 223]. The greater the degree of insulin resistance and hyperinsulinemia, the greater the post-receptor defect. This defect can be correlated with an elevation in circulating plasma free fatty acids which is thought to contribute to this post-receptor defect. Recent studies indicate that genetic background may also modify the insulin resistance of obesity. For example, subjects who are offspring of type 2 diabetic patients become more insulin resistant with increasing weight than obese subjects without a positive family history [224].

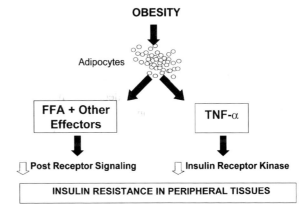

Figure 11 Possible role of TNF-α in insulin resistance. Studies have revealed that adipose tissues produce TNF-α in increased amounts in humans and rodents with obesity. This TNF-α can act on peripheral tissues such as fat, muscle and liver to induce insulin resistance by desensitization of the insulin signal at the level of the insulin receptor kinase activity. Increased fat mass also results in an increased concentration of circulating free fatty acid (FFA) levels. This contributes to the insulin resistant state at the post-receptor level

An important new potential mechanism of insulin resistance in obesity has been the observation that fat tissue itself may produce and secrete hormones or cytokines that affect metabolism and/or insulin sensitivity. The best studied of these cytokines is tumor necrosis factor-alpha (TNF-α) which is produced by fat and may act as an inhibitor of insulin action on fat, muscle and other tissues (Figure 11) [225]. This effect of TNF-α appears to involve an increase in serine phosphorylation of IRS-1 and an inhibition of insulin receptor kinase activity [226]. The major effect of TNF-α may be as a paracrine factor, since circulating levels of TNF-α are not increased in obesity. The importance of this mechanism in humans with obesity, however, is as yet unclear. Although neutralization of TNF-α significantly increases insulin sensitivity in obese rats [227, 228], two small studies performed in humans with obesity and type 2 diabetes failed to find any beneficial effect of anti-TNF treatments [229, 230]. Adipose tissue also produces the hormone leptin, which acts at the level of the brain to alter feeding behavior [231–233]. Whether leptin can also act on peripheral tissues to modulate insulin sensitivity has not yet been determined.

Type 2 Diabetes

The pathogenesis of type 2 (non-insulin dependent) diabetes mellitus is complex and involves defects in both insulin secretion from islet B cells and insulin action on target tissues [234–236]. These defects result from an interplay of genetic and environmental effects. The specific genes that confer the risk for development of diabetes are still unknown. Acquired defects, due to obesity and metabolic abnormalities, such as mild hyperglycemia, also play important roles in progression from normal glucose tolerance to diabetes [237].

A major component of insulin resistance appears to be genetically determined. Long-term studies involving children of type 2 diabetic parents or ethnic groups with high prevalence of diabetes, such as Pima Indians, reveal that low insulin sensitivity precedes and predicts type 2 diabetes [224, 238–242]. Studies of these high risk individuals also reveal that low insulin sensitivity tends to cluster in families [243]. In addition, individuals with this genetic predisposition to insulin resistance and type 2 diabetes have an even greater level of obesity-induced insulin resistance than do individuals from non-diabetic families [155]. However, at least two pathological defects are required for the development of type 2 diabetes—a decreased ability of insulin to act on peripheral tissues [155, 223, 235, 244, 245] and an inability of the islet B cells to compensate for this insulin resistance by increasing insulin secretion [234, 246–248]. Thus, despite the presence of insulin resistance, euglycemia can be maintained as long as insulin secretion is normal or increased. This pre-diabetic period may last for decades [238, 241, 249, 250].

Sites of Insulin Resistance in Type 2 Diabetes

There are multiple potential sites of insulin resistance in type 2 diabetes including the insulin receptor, IRS-1, SH2 domain proteins, glucose transporters, and the many cellular enzymes involved in glucose metabolism. People with insulin resistance have decreased insulin-stimulated glycogen synthesis and decreased glucose-6-phosphate formation (a measure of glucose transport) even prior to the development of type 2 diabetes [214, 242] (Figure 12). Animal studies, particularly in ob/ob mice, reveal defects in insulin receptor phosphorylation, IRS-1 phosphorylation and a decrease in insulin-stimulated PI 3-kinase activity. Decreases in insulin receptor kinase activity have also been observed in type 2 diabetic patients [206, 217, 251–257]. These defects appear to be acquired, since insulin receptors are structurally normal and kinase activity improves with weight reduction [258]. Glut4 glucose transporters are also normal in patients with type 2 diabetes [218, 259], although there is clearly a decrease in insulin-stimulated glucose uptake, due in large part to a defect in transporter translocation [220, 260]. Cells taken from type 2 diabetic individuals and put in culture have normal or near-normal insulin signaling, suggesting that most of these alterations are acquired [261, 262].

Scanning of candidate genes for type 2 diabetes, and linkage analysis, have failed to reveal a single cause of the genetically determined insulin resistance [263, 264]. Although defects in the insulin receptor and Glut4 transporter are rare in type 2 diabetes, differences in the ratio of expression of the two alternatively spliced forms of insulin receptor have been reported in some studies of type 2 diabetic patients [22], but not confirmed in others [21]. The significance of these, therefore, remains unclear.

Sequence polymorphisms in intracellular components of the insulin action cascade appear to be more common than those in the receptor. This is especially true for IRS-1, which shows single amino acid changes in about 5% of normal populations and between 10 and 15% of type 2 diabetic populations [265, 266] (Figure 13). Although these polymorphisms do not directly affect the tyrosine phosphorylation of IRS-1 by the insulin receptor, they do appear to reduce signaling in cultured cell models [267] and *in vivo* in patients studied by the euglycemic clamp [268].

Possible Inhibitors of Insulin Action

Four potential inhibitors of insulin action may also play a role in the insulin resistance of type 2 diabetes (Figure 14). One of these, TNF-α, has been discussed above in the section on obesity. Two others, αHS glycoprotein [269] and a protein designated PC-1 [270],

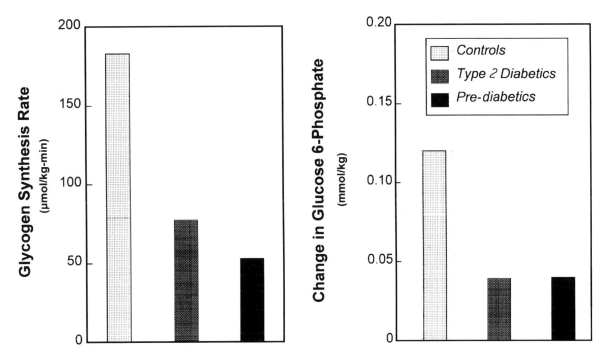

Figure 12 Altered insulin action in pre-type 2 diabetes demonstrated by NMR, which makes it possible to study muscle glucose transport and phosphorylation, as well as glycogen synthesis, in intact human beings. Studies by Rothman et al [242] have demonstrated decreased muscle glucose transport/phosphorylation, as well as decreased glycogen synthesis, in individuals with type 2 diabetes and in relatives at high risk for development of the disease, i.e. pre-type 2 diabetes

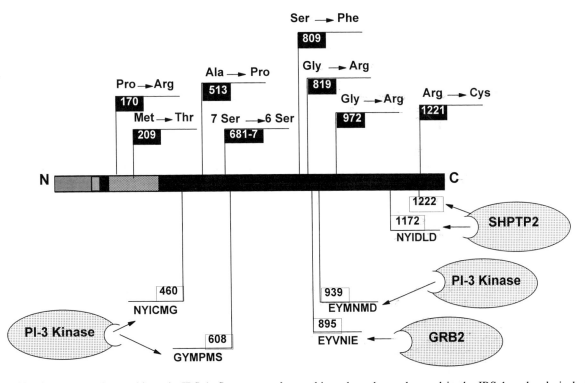

Figure 13 Sequence polymorphisms in IRS-1. Sequence polymorphisms have been observed in the IRS-1 molecule in both normal individuals and in individuals with type 2 diabetes. At least eight different polymorphisms have been identified, and these are shown schematically above the IRS-1 molecule as raised flags. The most common polymorphism occurs at amino acid 972 (sometimes called 971 due to the polymorphisms in sequence numbering). Some polymorphisms have only been observed in diabetic individuals. Taken together, there is about a two- to threefold increase in frequency of these polymorphisms in patients with type 2 diabetes as compared to non-diabetic populations

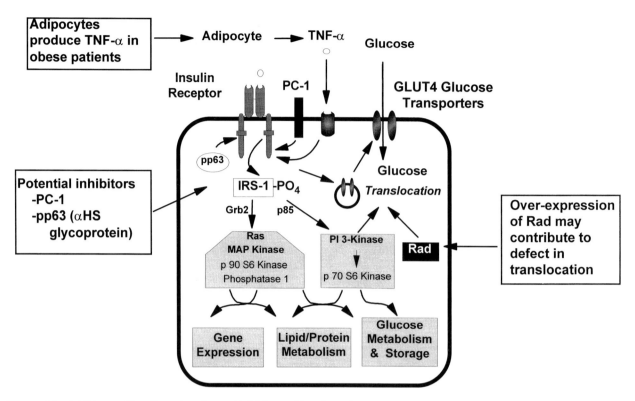

Figure 14 Inhibitors of insulin action. Several inhibitors of insulin action at both the receptor and post-receptor level have been described in a variety of disease states. These are illustrated schematically on a model of insulin action. They are described in more detail in the text

also act as inhibitors of tyrosine kinase activity of the insulin receptor. αHS glycoprotein is produced by the liver and released into the circulation, whereas PC-1 is a high molecular weight membrane glycoprotein which must interact with the receptor in the cell. Cells overexpressing PC-1 show decreased insulin-induced autophosphorylation of the insulin receptor β-subunit and decreased insulin receptor mediated phosphorylation of IRS-1. PC-1 appears to be the same as liver nucleoside pyrophosphatase and is found in other cells including placenta, kidney, brain, skeletal muscle and fat.

The fourth potential inhibitor of insulin action in type 2 diabetes is a novel Ras-related protein termed Rad. Rad is a 35 kDa protein with GTP-binding and GTPase activities [271]. It appears to be over-expressed in skeletal muscle of some people with type 2 diabetes. Although the exact function of Rad is unknown, overexpression appears to result in insulin resistance by inhibition of insulin-stimulated glucose uptake [272]. The full functions of PC-1, αHS glycoprotein, TNF-α and Rad on carbohydrate metabolism are as yet undefined, but each of these has become a potential therapeutic target for improving insulin resistance in type 2 diabetes.

Effects of Treatment in Type 2 Diabetes

Conventional treatment of type 2 diabetes may involve dietary restriction and exercise, or a combination of diet and/or exercise with oral hypoglycemic agents. Dietary restriction and weight loss lead to improved insulin sensitivity and a normalization or improvement in the binding of insulin to its receptor on various cells [273–275]. Insulin receptor kinase activity in adipocytes from obese diabetic patients reverts toward normal after weight reduction [276]. Weight loss also produces an improvement in glucose disposal rate in the non-diabetic controls without a change in receptor kinase activity, suggesting that the improvement in insulin sensitivity lies at a post-receptor site. Exercise training improves insulin sensitivity associated with an increase in Glut4 transporters in muscle [168, 169]. Clearly more studies are needed in this area to define these important mechanisms of regulation.

Although early studies suggested an effect of sulfonylureas to increase insulin receptor binding in patients with type 2 diabetes [277–279], this effect has been inconsistent. It seems likely that the major therapeutic effect of sulfonylureas in type 2 diabetes derives from their insulinotropic effects on the islet B cell which possesses receptors for these drugs [280]. Possible extra-pancreatic effects and early studies showing effects of these agents on hepatic glucose production did not take into account the significant insulin resistance caused by chronic hyperglycemia, and the possibility that sulfonylureas may improve insulin action by this indirect route [280]. The mechanism of action of biguanides, such as metformin, remains debated, but is unlikely to involve the insulin receptor or early insulin signaling. Biguanides do not have a hypoglycemic effect in normal subjects [281]. Metformin has been shown to reduce absorption of glucose from the gastrointestinal tract due to inhibition of glucose uptake at the mucosal surface [282], and to increase insulin-stimulated glucose uptake at the periphery, perhaps by stimulating the Glut4 glucose transporter [283].

Recently, a new class of agents for type 2 diabetes has been introduced in clinical trials which act primarily to improve insulin sensitivity [284]. These agents belong to the chemical family of thiazolidinediones, also called ciglitazones. Thiazolidinediones improve insulin sensitivity by acting at post-receptor levels. These agents bind to a nuclear receptor called PPAR-γ and increase the transcription of a number of genes, including the genes for glucose transporters [285, 286]. Some studies have also suggested an effect of ciglitazones to increase insulin-stimulated PI 3-kinase activity [287], but others have not observed this effect.

Experimentally, vanadium salts such as sodium vanadate and vanadyl sulfate have been shown to improve insulin sensitivity when given orally to both humans and rodents with type 2 diabetes [288–291]. Vanadium salts can be shown to mimic insulin action [292] and act as potent inhibitors of phosphotyrosine phosphatases (the enzymes which reverse insulin action) *in vitro* [293]. Whether the latter is their primary mechanism *in vivo*, however, is unclear. Since insulin resistance is such an important component of type 2 diabetes, identifying the sites of action of both the vanadium salts and thiazolidinediones may provide important clues for further pharmaceutical development.

Type 1 Diabetes Mellitus

Although type 1 diabetes (IDDM) is primarily a disease of insulin deficiency, insulin resistance is also a feature, both at initial presentation of the disease and during periods of poor control [294, 295]. This insensitivity and its normalization following insulin therapy are thought to be due to post-insulin binding defects. In newly diagnosed patients with type 1 diabetes, normal insulin-binding to adipocytes, monocytes and erythrocytes has been found, despite significantly

impaired insulin action *in vitro* [296]. Conventionally treated type 1 diabetic patients may develop impaired insulin binding to adipocytes [297, 298], associated with reduced sensitivity to the effects of insulin on glucose transport and lipolysis, suggesting both receptor and post-receptor alterations [297]. In contrast, patients treated with continuous subcutaneous insulin infusion have unaltered adipocyte insulin binding, suggesting that in the conventionally treated patients the adipocytes were subjected to higher degrees of hyperinsulinemia and consequent receptor down-regulation [299]. Dietary regimen has also been shown to affect cellular insulin binding in type 1 diabetes. Thus, patients fed high-carbohydrate and low-fat diets had significant elevations of monocyte insulin binding associated with an improvement of insulin-mediated glucose metabolism [300].

In animal models of hypoinsulinemic type 1 diabetes, effects have been observed at the level of insulin binding to target tissues, as well as in the receptor kinase activity. Increased insulin binding has been observed in adipocytes [301, 302], liver membranes [303] and skeletal muscle [304] from rats with insulin-deficient diabetes, due to increased receptor affinity [305] and/or increased receptor number [306]. The increased receptor binding apparently does not generate normal transmembrane signals, since insulin receptor kinase activity and insulin's effects on glucose transport and metabolism are usually somewhat blunted. The mechanism of this decrease in kinase activity is unknown, but may involve serine phosphorylation of the receptor [307].

Acidosis in type 1 diabetes has a profound effect on insulin receptor function because of the marked sensitivity of insulin binding to ambient pH [308, 309]. Experimental evidence has been presented that 3-hydroxybutyrate may have a beneficial effect for insulin binding in ketoacidosis, because it increases binding at low pH levels [310, 311] and potentiates the metabolic effect of insulin promoting glucose transport into adipocytes [312]. The complex milieu in ketoacidosis has potential effects that may modulate the function of the insulin receptor, as well as insulin action at post-receptor sites.

To address the paradox between increased binding and defective insulin action in type 1 diabetes, several studies have focused on the receptor kinase activity in this state. Early studies showed variable levels of insulin-receptor tyrosine kinase activity in type 1 diabetic animals [313–315]. Okamoto et al [316] studied hepatocytes from two hypoinsulinemic rat models (streptozotocin diabetes and the BB rat), and found that the diminished insulin receptor autophosphorylation and receptor tyrosine kinase activity in the diabetic state could be partially normalized by insulin treatment.

Other studies have confirmed a reduction in receptor kinase activity in streptozotocin diabetes which does not improve with a short (24 hours) fast which normalizes blood glucose levels [317]. An altered electrophoretic mobility of receptor β-subunits has been demonstrated in insulin receptors with defective kinase activity that were extracted from skeletal muscles of diabetic rats, suggesting an increase in serine phosphorylation or glycosylation [306]. This difference in receptor structure is apparently due, at least in part, to alterations in the sialic acid content of the receptor and is reversed by insulin treatment of diabetic rats for 60 hours. Although the precise cause of insulin resistance in these models is not yet clear, reduced receptor kinase activity and altered receptor carbohydrate structure may certainly have a pathophysiologic role.

Hypertension

The association of insulin resistance and hypertension has been recognized for over 30 years [245, 318–321], but the mechanism of insulin resistance in hypertension is unknown. Recent studies have shown that angiotensin II may partially mimic early insulin action by stimulating IRS-1 and IRS-2 phosphorylation. Somewhat surprisingly, however, this is associated with a decrease, rather than an increase, in PI 3-kinase activity [322].

It has also been suggested that insulin resistance leads to hypertension, rather than vice versa. Insulin has an antinatriuretic effect on both the proximal and distal nephron [323]. Another potential mechanism by which insulin may raise blood pressure is by its ability to affect activity of the sympathetic nervous system [324, 325]. Finally, the Na^+–K^+ exchanger has been implicated in the association between insulin resistance and hypertension. Insulin stimulates the activity of this exchanger in skeletal muscle and in adipocytes. Increased insulin levels result in an intracellular accumulation of Na^+ and an increase in cellular pH, and hence both enhanced reactivity of vascular smooth muscle to pressor effects, as well as increased protein synthesis and cellular proliferation [320].

GENETIC DISORDERS AFFECTING THE INSULIN RECEPTOR

Mutations of the insulin receptor are usually associated with severe insulin resistance and a collection of diverse clinical features including acanthosis nigricans, ovarian hyperandrogenism and impaired glucose tolerance or diabetes. To date, over 50 mutations of the receptor have been described (Figure 15). These can be classified into five categories, biochemically based on whether the mutation prevents receptor synthesis,

intracellular transport and post-translational processing, leads to defects in insulin binding, impairs tyrosine kinase activity, or accelerates receptor degradation [326]. The phenotypes associated with these mutations are remarkably broad and include leprechaunism, the Rabson–Mendenhall syndrome, the type A syndrome of insulin resistance, pseudoacromegaly, lipodystrophy and hyperandrogenism, and even mild NIDDM (Table 1). It is likely that different mutations alter distinct signals and that correlations of molecular structure and phenotype will require a much more thorough understanding of the effects of the mutations on the downstream events that mediate signaling.

Table 1 Genetic syndromes of insulin resistance

Insulin receptor mutations
Homozygous or compound heterozygous defects
    Leprechaunism
    Rabson–Mendenhall syndrome
Heterozygous defects
    Type A syndrome of insulin resistance
Post-receptor mutations at unknown sites
    Lipoatrophic diabetes
    Pseudoacromegaly syndrome

Type A Syndrome

The type A syndrome of insulin resistance was initially described in 1976 and is typically recognized in thin females between the ages of 8 and 30 years, with marked glucose intolerance, severe target cell insulin resistance, acanthosis nigricans and hyperandrogenism [327]. Since it was first recognized by its association with the skin lesion acanthosis nigricans, it was initially called the type A syndrome of insulin resistance and acanthosis nigricans. Although the syndrome has been described in both males and females, it is more easily recognized in females due to the associated hyperandrogenism. Usually these girls and young women appear normal until puberty, when they develop hirsutism, masculinization, oligomenorrhea or amenorrhea and acne, although careful history may disclose some early findings even in the first year of life. The insulin resistance is usually severe, and when treated these patients can require up to 50 000 U of insulin per day. Fasting insulin levels may be normal or above 600 µU/ml (400 pmol/l) [328]. Glucose tolerance may be normal, slightly impaired, or frankly diabetic. Patients in the same family with the same mutation have varying degrees of disease presentation. What accounts for this difference in clinical severity is not clear.

Almost all patients with the type A syndrome are heterozygous for mutations in the insulin receptor. Since the first report of an insulin receptor mutation in

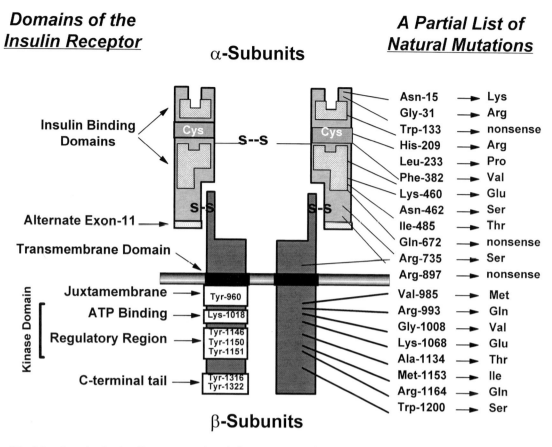

Figure 15 Mutations in the insulin receptor, in relation to structural domains. Mutations in the insulin receptor may occur in heterozygous, homozygous or compound heterozygous forms, and have been described in various residues throughout the α-subunit and the β-subunit. Some of these are depicted here schematically on the backbone of the insulin receptor's functional domains

a type A patient [329], there have been numerous additional reports of receptor mutations involving both the α- and β-subunits of the receptor [326, 330]. However, studies of some patients with typical clinical features of the type A syndrome have yielded no identifiable coding sequence mutation in the receptor. Potential defects in these patients might include mutations leading to decreased receptor expression or mutations in the post-receptor signaling cascade. In some studies, production of factors inhibiting insulin action, including PC-1, have also been reported [331–333].

Insulin Resistance and Pseudoacromegaly

One rare variant of the type A syndrome is found in patients with severe insulin resistance who also present with clinical features suggesting acromegaly. Unlike true acromegaly, however, these patients have no evidence of high growth hormone or IGF-I levels. There may also be significant obesity. In one extensively studied patient, the number and affinity of the insulin receptors was normal, and kinase activity was unimpaired [334]. However, studies of insulin action in cultured fibroblasts revealed a selective defect in insulin signaling. Thus, insulin could stimulate amino acid uptake and thymidine incorporation normally, but could not stimulate glucose uptake. Similar effects were noted *in vivo* during a euglycemic clamp, i.e. insulin failed to promote glucose disposal, but was able to suppress muscle proteolysis [334]. While the molecular basis of this patient's insulin resistance is unknown, it is likely that the patient has a mutation affecting function or expression of a protein required for coupling of the receptor to glucose transport.

Leprechaunism

Leprechaunism is a rare congenital syndrome characterized by elfin-like facies, decreased subcutaneous adipose tissue, hirsutism, acanthosis nigricans and growth retardation, failure to thrive and early death [335]. Metabolic abnormalities include severe insulin resistance with hyperinsulinemia and postprandial hyperglycemia. Paradoxically, fasting hypoglycemia is also common, presumably due to poor substrate availability for gluconeogenesis. The incidence of this disease has been estimated at approximately 1 per 4 000 000 live births.

At the cellular level a number of studies of skin fibroblasts or transformed lymphocytes demonstrated reduced receptor affinity and/or number [336–338]. The failure of anti-receptor antibodies to bind to insulin receptors of at least one patient (Ark-1) with this syndrome implicated a genetic defect [339]. Increased rates of receptor degradation have also been described in leprechaun patients [340]. In fact, in most cases leprechaunism appears to be due to mutations in both alleles of the insulin receptor. This was first recognized in 1988 in a patient who was a compound heterozygote in whom one allele of the receptor had a premature chain termination codon at 672 and the other allele had a mutation at Glu^{460}. The latter led to a decrease in the number of insulin receptors on monocytes *in vivo* and a decreased sensitivity of insulin binding to changes in temperature and pH [341]. A second patient designated Minn-1 also had two mutations in the receptor. The paternal allele contained a nonsense mutation at codon 897 which led to a truncated mRNA, while the allele from the mother (which was marked by a silent polymorphism at codon Asp^{234}) was underexpressed to a level representing only 10% of normal, suggesting an as yet unrecognized *cis*-acting mutation. Subsequently several other mutations in different sites on the insulin receptor, including homozygous mutations, have been found in patients with the leprechaun phenotype [338, 342, 343]. Some patients with this syndrome have also been defined who have no functional insulin receptor genes [334].

Rabson–Mendenhall Syndrome

Rabson–Mendenhall syndrome is another rare congenital syndrome characterized by insulin resistance, acanthosis nigricans and growth retardation. In addition, these patients have developmental abnormalities of bones and teeth, polycystic ovarian disease, genitomegaly, and pineal gland hyperplasia. Like patients with leprechaunism, these individuals when studied have been positive for mutations in both insulin receptor alleles [338, 345]. Again, why the phenotype is distinct from other patients with receptor mutations is unclear.

Lipodystrophy and Lipoatrophic Diabetes

These disorders encompass a heterogeneous group of rare syndromes characterized by insulin-resistant diabetes mellitus and a complete or partial absence of subcutaneous adipose tissue [346]. Other clinical features include severe insulin resistance and hyperinsulinemia, elevated metabolic rate, acanthosis nigricans, hyperlipidemia, hepatic disease and accelerated atherosclerosis. Thus, there is an overall likeness between this syndrome and both the type A syndrome and leprechaunism, the major difference being the lipodystrophy.

Generalized lipodystrophy (lipoatrophy) was first described in 1854 in two children with total absence of subcutaneous fat, impaired glucose tolerance and hepatomegaly, and has now been described in over 200 patients [347, 348]. In some families, the inheritance appears to be autosomal recessive, and there is consanguinity among parents. The associated phenotype is varied. Accelerated early growth with early epiphyseal closure and reduced final height has been reported. However, some patients have features of gigantism, and may resemble the pseudoacromegaly phenotype. Hepatic involvement is a poor prognostic sign, especially if it occurs early and progresses to cirrhosis. Total lipodystrophy may also be acquired, sometimes after an antecedent infection. The clinical features are otherwise similar to the congenital disorder. Accelerated atherosclerosis often occurs in these patients due to hyperlipidemia, and may result in premature cardiovascular death.

The pathophysiology of the syndrome is poorly understood. Glucose production is increased and cannot be suppressed by insulin. Similarly, levels of nonesterified fatty acids, glycerol and ketone bodies are elevated and do not respond to insulin infusion. It is possible that insulin cannot regulate lipolysis and that as a result the high levels of non-esterified fatty acids and glycerol promote gluconeogenesis in the liver [349]. In at least one study of fat from patients with acquired lipodystrophy, changes suggestive of adipose cell destruction were noted [350].

The role of the insulin receptor in lipoatrophy remains controversial. Impairment of insulin binding to circulating monocytes has been reported [351, 352]. In one study reduced receptor expression and altered receptor affinity was demonstrated using patient-derived fibroblasts and EBV-transformed lymphocytes, but different affected family members showed different alterations [353]. To date no mutation in the insulin receptor has been described, despite the similarity of features of this syndrome to the type A syndrome and leprechaunism [343, 354].

Lipodystrophy may also be partial and distributed in an uneven manner, such that certain areas exhibit lipoatrophy while others have normal fat or even hypertrophy. A familial form of lipodystrophy is face-sparing lipodystrophy. The pattern of inheritance suggests that this form is X-linked. Loss of adipose tissue begins in childhood or adolescence. Facial fat and truncal fat may be spared. Hyperlipidemia is not as severe as in generalized lipodystrophy, but many patients have hypertension. Biopsy of the affected area reveals small adipocytes. One postulated mechanism of this variant of lipodystrophy is that there is a regional increase in sympathetic nervous activity which leads to accelerated lipolysis [355]. One patient with this form of lipodystrophy has also been shown to be homozygous for a mutation in the insulin receptor gene (Ile^{485} to Thr); however, the functional significance of this mutation is unclear.

REFERENCES

1. Freychet P, Roth J, Neville DM Jr. Insulin receptors in the liver: specific binding of [^{125}I] insulin to the plasma membrane and its relation to insulin bioactivity. Proc Natl Acad Sci USA 1971; 68: 1833–7.
2. Cuatrecasas P. Affinity chromatography and purification of the insulin receptor of liver cell membranes. Proc Natl Acad Sci USA 1972; 69: 1277–81.
3. Rosen OM. After insulin binds. Science 1987; 237: 1452–8.
4. Cheatham B, Kahn CR. Insulin action and the insulin signaling network. Endocr Rev 1995; 16: 117–42.
5. Massague J, Pilch PF, Czech MP. Electrophoretic resolution of three major insulin receptor structures with unique subunit stoichiometries. Proc Natl Acad Sci USA 1982; 77: 7137–41.
6. Petruzzelli L, Herrera R, Arenas Garcia R, Fernandez R, Birnbaum MJ, Rosen OM. Isolation of a *Drosophila* genomic sequence homologous to the kinase domain of the human insulin receptor and detection of the phosphorylated *Drosophila* receptor with an anti-peptide antibody. Proc Natl Acad Sci USA 1986; 83: 4710–14.
7. Muggeo M, Ginsberg BH, Roth J, Neville DM Jr, DeMeyts P, Kahn CR. The insulin receptor in vertebrates is functionally more conserved during evolution than insulin itself. Endocrinology 1979; 104: 1393–1402.
8. Ullrich A, Bell JR, Chen EY et al. Human insulin receptor and its relationship to the tyrosine kinase family of oncogenes. Nature 1985; 313: 756–61.
9. Seino S, Seino M, Bell GI. Human insulin-receptor gene. Diabetes 1990; 39: 129–33.
10. Ebina Y, Edery M, Ellis L et al. Expression of a functional human insulin receptor from a cloned cDNA in Chinese hamster ovary cells. Proc Natl Acad Sci USA 1985; 82: 8014–18.
11. Yang Feng TL, Francke U, Ullrich A. Gene for human insulin receptor: localization to site on chromosome 19 involved in pre-B-cell leukemia. Science 1985; 228: 728–31.
12. Hedo JA, Kahn CR, Hayoshi M, Yamada KM, Kasuga M. Biosynthesis and glycosylation of the insulin receptor. Evidence for a single polypeptide precursor of the two major subunits. J Biol Chem 1983; 258: 10020–26.
13. Kasuga M, Hedo JA, Yamada KM, Kahn CR. The structure of the insulin receptor and its subunits: evidence for multiple non-reduced forms and a 210K possible proreceptor. J Biol Chem 1982; 257: 10392–9.
14. Hedo JA, Kasuga M, Van Obberghen E, Roth J, Kahn CR. Direct demonstration of glycosylation of insulin receptor subunits by biosynthetic and external

15. labeling: evidence for heterogeneity. Proc Natl Acad Sci USA 1981; 78: 4791–5.
15. Herzberg VL, Grigorescu F, Edge ASB, Spiro RG, Kahn CR. Characterization of insulin receptor carbohydrate by comparison of chemical and enzymatic deglycosylation. Biochem Biophys Res Commun 1985; 129: 789–96.
16. Capeau J, Picard J. The influence of glycosidases and lectins on insulin binding to Zajdela hepatoma cells. Growth Regul 1980; 118: 25–30.
17. Hedo JA, Collier E, Watkinson A. Myristyl and palmityl acylation of the insulin receptor. J Biol Chem 1987; 262: 954–7.
18. Caro JF, Raju SM, Sinha MK, Goldfine ID, Dohm GL. Heterogeneity of human liver, muscle and adipose tissue insulin receptor. Biochem Biophys Res Commun 1988; 151: 123–9.
19. Burant CF, Treutelaar MK, Block NE, Buse MG. Structural differences between liver- and muscle-derived insulin receptors in rats. J Biol Chem 1986; 261: 14361–4.
20. Seino S, Bell GI. Alternative splicing of human insulin receptor messenger RNA. Biochem Biophys Res Commun 1989; 159: 312–16.
21. Moller DE, Yokota A, Caro JF, Flier JS. Tissue-specific expression of two alternatively spliced insulin receptor mRNAs in man. Mol Endocrinol 1989; 3: 1263–9.
22. Kellerer M, Sesti G, Seffer E, Ullrich A, Haring HU. Altered pattern of insulin receptor isotypes in skeletal muscle membranes of NIDDM patients. Diabetologia 1993; 36: 628–32.
23. Heidenreich KA, Zahniser NR, Berhanu P, Brandenburg D, Olefsky JM. Structural differences between insulin receptors in the brain and peripheral tissues. J Biol Chem 1983; 258: 8527–30.
24. Lowe WL Jr, Boyd FT Jr, Clarke DW, Raizada MK, Hart C, LeRoith D. Development of brain insulin receptors: structural and functional studies of insulin receptors from whole brain and primary cell cultures. Endocrinology 1986; 119: 25–35.
25. Roth RA, Morgan DO, Beaudoin J, Sara V. Purification and characterization of the human brain insulin receptor. J Biol Chem 1986; 261: 3753–7.
26. Pullen RA, Lindsay DG, Wood SP et al. Receptor-binding region of insulin. Nature 1976; 259: 369–73.
27. Jacobs S, Shechter Y, Bissell K, Cuatrecasas P. Purification and properties of insulin receptors from rat liver membranes. Biochem Biophys Res Commun 1977; 77: 981–8.
28. Schaffer L. A model for insulin binding to the insulin receptor. Eur J Biochem 1994; 221: 1127–32.
29. DeMeyts P, Gu JL, Shymko RM, Kaplan BE, Bell GI, Whittaker J. Identification of a ligand-binding region of the human insulin receptor encoded by the second exon of the gene. Mol Endocrinol 1990; 4: 409–16.
30. Kjeldsen T, Andersen AS, Wiberg FC et al. The ligand specificities of the insulin receptor and the insulin-like growth factor I receptor reside in different regions of a common binding site. Proc Natl Acad Sci USA 1991; 88: 4404–8.
31. Anderson OP, Gliemann J, Gammeltoft S. Receptor binding and biological effect of insulin in human adipocytes. Diabetologia 1977; 13: 589–93.
32. Kahn CR, Freychet P, Neville DM Jr, Roth J. Quantitative aspects of the insulin–receptor interaction in

liver plasma membranes. J Biol Chem 1984; 249: 2249–57.

33. DeMeyts P, Bianco AR, Roth J. Site–site interactions among insulin receptors: characterization of the negative cooperativity. J Biol Chem 1976; 251: 1877–88.

34. DeMeyts P. The structural basis of insulin and insulin-like growth factor-1 receptor binding and negative cooperativity, and its relevance to mitogenic versus metabolic signaling. Diabetologia 1995; 37 (suppl. 2): s135–48.

35. Pollet RJ, Kempner ES, Standaert ML, Haase BA. Structure of the insulin receptor of cultured human lymphoblastoid cells IM-9: evidence suggesting that two subunits are required for insulin binding. J Biol Chem 1982; 257: 894–8.

36. Mosthaf L, Grako KA, Dull TJ, Coussens L, Ullrich A, McClain DA. Functionally distinct insulin receptors generated by tissue-specific alternative splicing. EMBO J 1990; 9: 2409–13.

37. Goldstein BJ, Dudley AL. The rat insulin receptor: Primary structure and conservation of tissue-specific alternative messenger RNA splicing. Mol Endocrinol 1990; 4: 235–44.

38. Yamaguchi Y, Flier JS, Yokota A, Benecke H, Backer JM, Moller DE. Functional properties of two naturally occurring isoforms of the human insulin receptor in Chinese hamster ovary cells. Endocrinology 1991; 129: 2058–66.

39. Kahn CR, Baird KL, Jarett DB, Flier JS. Direct demonstration that receptor cross-linking or aggregation is important in insulin action. Proc Natl Acad Sci USA 1976; 75: 4209–13.

40. Schlessinger J, Van Obberghen E, Kahn CR. Insulin and antibodies against insulin receptor cap on the membrane of cultured human lymphocytes. Nature 1980; 286: 729–31.

41. Kasuga M, Karlsson FA, Kahn CR. Insulin stimulates the phosphorylation of the 95 000-Dalton subunit of its own receptor. Science 1982; 215: 185–7.

42. White MF, Kahn CR. The insulin signaling system. J Biol Chem 1994; 269: 1–4.

43. Ullrich A, Schlessinger J. Signal transduction by receptors with tyrosine kinase activity. Cell 1990; 61: 203–12.

44. Chou CK, Dull TJ, Russell DS et al. Human insulin receptors mutated at the ATP-binding site lack protein tyrosine kinase activity and fail to mediate postreceptor effects of insulin. J Biol Chem 1987; 262: 1842–7.

45. Ebina Y, Araki E, Taira M et al. Replacement of lysine residue 1030 in the putative ATP-binding region of the insulin receptor abolishes insulin- and antibody-stimulated glucose uptake and receptor kinase activity. Proc Natl Acad Sci USA 1987; 84: 704–8.

46. Ellis L, Morgan DO, Clauser E, Roth RA, Rutter WJ. A membrane-anchored cytoplasmic domain of the human insulin receptor mediates a constitutively elevated insulin-independent uptake of 2-deoxyglucose. Mol Endocrinol 1987; 1: 15–24.

47. Shoelson SE, White MF, Kahn CR. Tryptic activation of the insulin receptor. J Biol Chem 1988; 263: 4852–60.

48. Perlman R, Bottaro DG, White MF, Kahn CR. Conformational changes in the α- and β-subunits of the insulin receptor identified by anti-peptide antibodies. J Biol Chem 1989; 264: 8946–50.

49. Baron V, Kaliman P, Gautier N, Van Obberghen E. The insulin receptor activation process involves localized conformational changes. J Biol Chem 1992; 267: 23290–94.

50. White MF, Takayama S, Kahn CR. Differences in the sites of phosphorylation of the insulin receptor *in vivo* and *in vitro*. J Biol Chem 1985; 260: 9470–78.

51. White MF, Shoelson SE, Keutmann H, Kahn CR. A cascade of tyrosine autophosphorylation in the β-subunit activates the insulin receptor. J Biol Chem 1988; 263: 2969–80.

52. Tornqvist HE, Pierce MW, Frackelton AR Jr, Nemenoff RA, Avruch J. Identification of insulin receptor tyrosine residues autophosphorylated *in vitro*. J Biol Chem 1987; 262: 10212–19.

53. Sun XJ, Crimmins DL, Myers MG Jr, Miralpeix M, White MF. Pleiotropic insulin signals are engaged by multisite phosphorylation of IRS-1. Mol Cell Biol 1993; 13: 7418–28.

54. Akiyama T, Kadowaki T, Nishida E et al. Substrate specificities of tyrosine-specific protein kinases toward cytoskeletal proteins *in vitro*. J Biol Chem 1986; 261: 14797–803.

55. Murakami MS, Rosen OM. The role of insulin receptor autophosphorylation in signal transduction. J Biol Chem 1991; 266: 22653–60.

56. Wilden PA, Siddle K, Haring E, Backer JM, White MF, Kahn CR. The role of insulin receptor kinase domain autophosphorylation in receptor-mediated activities. J Biol Chem 1992; 267: 13719–27.

57. Feener EP, Backer JM, King GL et al. Insulin stimulates serine and tyrosine phosphorylation in the juxtamembrane region of the insulin receptor. J Biol Chem 1993; 268: 11256–64.

58. White MF, Livingston JN, Backer JM et al. Mutation of the insulin receptor at tyrosine 960 inhibits signal transmission but does not affect its tyrosine kinase activity. Cell 1988; 54: 641–9.

59. Kaburagi Y, Momomura K, Yamamoto-Honda R et al. Site-directed mutagenesis of the juxtamembrane domain of the human insulin receptor. J Biol Chem 1993; 268: 16610–22.

60. Backer JM, Schroeder GG, Kahn CR et al. Insulin stimulation of phosphatidylinositol 3-kinase activity maps to insulin receptor regions required for endogenous substrate phosphorylation. J Biol Chem 1992; 267: 1367–74.

61. Carpentier JL, Paccaud JP, Backer JM, Gilbert A, Orci L, Kahn CR. Two steps of insulin receptor internalization depend on different domains of the beta subunit. J Cell Biol 1993; 122: 1243–52.

62. Pang L, Milarski KL, Ohmichi M, Takata Y, Olefsky JM, Saltiel AR. Mutation of the two carboxyl-terminal tyrosines in the insulin receptor results in enhanced activation of mitogen-activated protein kinase. J Biol Chem 1994; 269: 10604–8.

63. White MF, Maron R, Kahn CR. Insulin rapidly stimulates tyrosine phosphorylation of a Mr 185 000 protein in intact cells. Nature 1985; 318: 183–6.

64. Sun XJ, Rothenberg PL, Kahn CR et al. The structure of the insulin receptor substrate IRS-1 defines a unique signal transduction protein. Nature 1991; 352: 73–7.

65. Keller SR, Kitagawa K, Aebersold RH, Lienhard GE, Garner CW. Isolation and characterization of the

160 000-Da phosphotyrosyl protein, a putative participant in insulin signaling. J Biol Chem 1991; 266: 12817–20.

66. White MF, Stegmann EW, Dull TJ, Ullrich A, Kahn CR. Characterization of an endogenous substrate of the insulin receptor in cultured cells. J Biol Chem 1987; 262: 9769–77.

67. Nishiyama M, Wands JR. Cloning and increased expression of an insulin receptor substrate-1-like gene in human hepatocellular carcinoma. Biochem Biophys Res Commun 1992; 183: 280–85.

68. Araki E, Haag BL III, Kahn CR. Cloning of the mouse insulin receptor substrate-1 (IRS-1) gene and complete sequence of mouse IRS-1. Biochim Biophys Acta 1994; 1221: 353–6.

69. Condorelli G, Formisano P, Villone G, Smith RJ, Beguinot F. Insulin and insulin-like growth factor I (IGF I) stimulate phosphorylation of a M$_r$ 175 000 cytoskeleton-associated protein in intact FRTL cells. J Biol Chem 1989; 264: 12633–8.

70. Shemer J, Adamo M, Wilson GL, Heffez D, Zick Y, LeRoith D. Insulin and insulin-like growth factor-I stimulate a common endogenous phosphoprotein substrate (pp185) in intact neuroblastoma cells. J Biol Chem 1987; 262: 15476–82.

71. Wang LM, Myers MG Jr, Sun XJ, Aaronson SA, White MF, Pierce JH. IRS-1: Essential for insulin and IL-4-stimulated mitogenesis in hematopoietic cells. Science 1993; 261: 1591–4.

72. Myers MG Jr, Sun XJ, Cheatham B et al. IRS-1 is a common element in insulin and insulin-like growth factor-I signaling to the phosphatidylinositol 3′-kinase. Endocrinology 1993; 132(4): 1421–30.

73. Souza SC, Frick GP, Yip R, Lobo RB, Tai L-R, Goodman HM. Growth hormone stimulates tyrosine phosphorylation of insulin receptor substrate-1. J Biol Chem 1994; 269: 30085–8.

74. Argetsinger LS, Hsu GW, Myers MG Jr, Billestrup N, White MF, Carter-Su C. Growth hormone, interferon-gamma, and leukemia inhibitory factor promoted tyrosyl phosphorylation of insulin receptor substrate-1. J Biol Chem 1995; 270: 14685–92.

75. Araki E, Sun XJ, Haag BL III et al. Human skeletal muscle insulin receptor substrate-1: characterization of the cDNA, gene and chromosomal localization. Diabetes 1993; 42: 1041–54.

76. Rice KM, Lienhard GE, Garner CW. Regulation of the expression of pp 160, a putative insulin receptor signal protein, by insulin, dexamethasone, and 1-methyl-3-isobutylxanthine in 3T3-L1 adipocytes. J Biol Chem 1992; 267: 10163–7.

77. Saad MJA, Araki E, Miralpeix M, Rothenberg PL, White MF, Kahn CR. Regulation of insulin receptor substrate 1 in liver and muscle of animal models of insulin resistance. J Clin Invest 1992; 90: 1839–49.

78. Saad MJA, Folli F, Kahn JA, Kahn CR. Modulation of insulin receptor, insulin receptor substrate-1, and phosphatidylinositol 3-kinase in liver and muscle of dexamethasone-treated rats. J Clin Invest 1993; 92: 2065–72.

79. Giorgino F, Almahfouz A, Goodyear LJ, Smith RJ. Glucocorticoid regulation of insulin receptor and substrate IRS-1 tyrosine phosphorylation in rat skeletal muscle *in vivo*. J Clin Invest 1993; 91: 2020–30.

80. Myers MG Jr, Grammer TC, Brooks J et al. The pleckstrin homology domain in IRS-1 sensitizes insulin signaling. J Biol Chem 1995; 270: 11715–18.

81. Eck MJ, Dhe-Paganon S, Trub T, Nolte RT, Shoelson SE. Structure of the IRS-1 PTB domain bound to the juxtamembrane region of the insulin receptor. Cell 1996; 85: 695–705.

82. Backer JM, Myers MG Jr, Shoelson SE et al. Phosphatidylinositol 3′-kinase is activated by association with IRS-1 during insulin stimulation. EMBO J 1992; 11: 3469–79.

83. Sugimoto S, Wandless TJ, Shoelson SE, Neel BG, Walsh CT. Activation of the SH2-containing protein tyrosine phosphatase, SH-PTP2, by phosphotyrosine-containing peptides derived from insulin receptor substrate-1. J Biol Chem 1994; 269: 13614–22.

84. Songyang Z, Shoelson SE, Chaudhuri M et al. SH2 domains recognize specific phosphopeptide sequences. Cell 1993; 72: 767–78.

85. Koch CA, Anderson DJ, Moran MF, Ellis CA, Pawson T. SH2 and SH3 domains: elements that control interactions of cytoplasmic signaling proteins. Science 1991; 252: 668–74.

86. Ruderman N, Kapeller R, White MF, Cantley LC. Activation of phosphatidylinositol-3-kinase by insulin. Proc Natl Acad Sci USA 1990; 87: 1411–15.

87. Folli F, Saad MJA, Backer JM, Kahn CR. Insulin stimulation of phosphatidylinositol 3-kinase activity and association with IRS-1 in liver and muscle of the intact rat. J Biol Chem 1992; 267: 22171–7.

88. Xiao S, Roses DW, Sasaoka T et al. Syp (SH-PTP2) is a positive mediator of growth factor-stimulated mitogenic signal transduction. J Biol Chem 1994; 269: 21244–8.

89. Myers MG Jr, Backer JM, Sun XJ et al. IRS-1 activates the phosphatidylinositol 3′-kinase by associating with the src homology 2 domains of p85. Proc Natl Acad Sci USA 1992; 89: 10350–54.

90. Skolnik EY, Lee CH, Batzer AG et al. The SH2/SH3 domain-containing protein GRB2 interacts with tyrosine-phosphorylated IRS-1 and Shc: implications for insulin control of ras signalling. EMBO J 1993; 12: 1929–36.

91. Myers MG Jr, Wang LM, Sun XJ et al. The role of IRS-1/GRB2 complexes in insulin signaling. Mol Cell Biol 1994; 14: 3577–87.

92. Carpenter CL, Auger KR, Duckworth BC, Hou WM, Schaffhausen B, Cantley LC. A tightly associated serine/threonine protein kinase regulates phosphoinositide 3-kinase activity. Mol Cell Biol 1993; 13: 1657–65.

93. Lowenstein EJ, Daly RJ, Batzer AG et al. The SH2 and SH3 domain-containing protein GRB2 links receptor tyrosine kinases to ras signaling. Cell 1992; 70: 431–42.

94. Baltensperger K, Kozma LM, Cherniack AD et al. Binding of the Ras activator son of sevenless to insulin receptor substrate-1 signaling complexes. Science 1993; 260: 1950–2.

95. Skolnik EY, Batzer AG, Li N et al. The function of GRB2 in linking the insulin receptor to ras signaling pathways. Science 1993; 260: 1953–5.

96. Waters SB, Yamauchi K, Pessin JE. Insulin-stimulated disassociation of the SOS-Grb2 complex. Mol Cell Biol 1995; 15: 2791–9.

97. Holgado-Madruga M, Emlet DR, Moscatello DK, Godwin AK, Wong AJ. A Grb2-associated docking protein in EGF- and insulin-receptor signalling. Nature 1996; 379: 560–63.

98. Li N, Batzer AG, Daly RJ, Yajnik V, Skolnik E, Chardin P et al. Guanine-nucleotide-releasing factor mSos1 binds to Grb2 and links receptor tyrosine kinases to ras signalling. Nature 1993; 363: 85–8.

99. Buday L, Downward J. Epidermal growth factor regulates p21^ras through the formation of a complex of receptor, Grb2 adapter protein, and Sos nucleotide exchange factor. Cell 1993; 73: 611–20.

100. Egan SE, Giddings BW, Brooks MW, Buday L, Sizeland AM, Weinberg RA. Association of Sos ras exchange protein with Grb2 is implicated in tyrosine kinase signal transduction and transformation. Nature 1993; 363: 45–51.

101. Dent P, Lavoinne A, Nakielny S, Caudwell FB, Watt P, Cohen P. The molecular mechanisms by which insulin stimulates glycogen synthesis in mammalian skeletal muscle. Nature 1990; 348: 302–7.

102. Crews CM, Erikson RL. Extracellular signals and reversible protein phosphorylation: what to Mek of it all. Cell 1993; 74: 215–17.

103. Shepherd PR, Nave BT, Siddle K. Insulin stimulation of glycogen synthesis and glycogen synthase activity is blocked by wortmannin and rapamycin in 3T3-L1 adipocytes: evidence for the involvement of phosphoinositide 3-kinase and p70 ribosomal protein-S6 kinase. Biochem J 1995; 305: 25–8.

104. Schlessinger J. How receptor tyrosine kinases activate Ras. Trends Biochem Sci 1993; 18: 273–5.

105. Nakajima T, Fukamizu A, Takahashi J et al. The signal-dependent coactivator CBP is a nuclear target for pp 90$_{RSK}$. Cell 1996; 86: 465–74.

106. Araki E, Lipes MA, Patti ME et al. Alternative pathway of insulin signalling in mice with targeted disruption of the IRS-1 gene. Nature 1994; 372: 186–90.

107. Yamauchi T, Tobe K, Tamemoto H et al. Insulin signalling and insulin actions in the muscles and livers of insulin-resistant, insulin receptor substrate 1-deficient mice. Mol Cell Biol 1996; 16: 3074–84.

108. Patti ME, Sun XJ, Bruning JC et al. 4PS/IRS-2 is the alternative substrate of the insulin receptor in IRS-1 deficient mice. J Biol Chem 1995; 270: 24670–3.

109. Sun XJ, Wang LM, Zhang Y et al. Role of IRS-2 in insulin and cytokine signalling. Nature 1995; 377: 173–7.

110. Pellici G, Lanfrancone L, Grignani F et al. A novel transforming protein (SHC) with an SH2 domain is implicated in mitogenic signal transduction. Cell 1992; 70: 93–104.

111. Hosomi Y, Shii K, Ogawa W et al. Characterization of a 60-kiloDalton substrate of the insulin receptor kinase. J Biol Chem 1994; 269: 11498–502.

112. Pons S, Asano T, Glasheen EM et al. The structure and function of p55^PIK reveals a new regulatory subunit for the phosphatidylinositol-3 kinase. Mol Cell Biol 1995; 15: 4453–65.

113. Mastick CC, Aebersold RH, Lienhard GE. Characterization of a major protein in GLUT4 vesicles. J Biol Chem 1994; 269 (8): 6089–92.

114. Cheatham B, Vlahos CJ, Cheatham L et al. Phosphatidylinositol 3-kinase activation is required for insulin stimulation of pp 70 S6 kinase DNA synthesis and glucose transporter translocation. Mol Cell Biol 1994; 14: 4902–11.

115. Cormont M, Tanti JF, Zahraoui A, Vanobberghen E, Tavitian A, Le Marchand-Brustel Y. Insulin and okadaic acid induce Rab4 redistribution in adipocytes. J Biol Chem 1993; 268: 19491–7.

116. Volchuk A, Sargeant R, Sumitani S, Liu Z, He L, Klip A. Cellulbrevin is a resident protein of insulin-sensitive GLUT4 glucose transporter vesicles in 3T3-L1 adipocytes. J Biol Chem 1995; 270: 8233–40.

117. Seino S, Seino M, Nishi S, Bell GI. Structure of the human insulin receptor gene and characterization of its promoter. Proc Natl Acad Sci USA 1989; 86: 114–18.

118. Muller-Wieland D, Taub RA, Tewari DS, Kriauciunas KM, Reddy SSK, Kahn CR. The insulin receptor gene and its expression in patients with insulin resistance. Diabetes 1989; 38: 31–8.

119. Yamaguchi Y, Flier JS, Benecke H, Ransil BJ, Moller DE. Ligand-binding properties of the two isoforms of the human insulin receptor. Endocrinology 1993; 132: 1132–8.

120. Mamula PW, McDonald AR, Brunetti A et al. Regulating insulin-receptor-gene expression by differentiation and hormones. Diabetes Care 1990; 13: 288–301.

121. Rubin CS, Lai E, Rosen OM. Acquisition of increased hormone sensitivity during *in vitro* adipocyte development. J Biol Chem 1977; 252: 3554–7.

122. Araki E, Shimada F, Uzawa A, Mori M, Ebina Y. Characterization of the promoter region of the human insulin receptor gene. J Biol Chem 1987; 262: 16186–91.

123. Mamula PW, Wong KY, Maddux BA, McDonald AR, Goldfine ID. Sequence and analysis of promoter region of human insulin-receptor gene. Diabetes 1988; 37: 1241–6.

124. Dynan WS. Promoters for housekeeping genes. Trends in Genetics 1986; 2: 196–7.

125. Sibley E, Kastelic T, Kelly TJ Jr, Lane MD. Characterization of the mouse insulin receptor gene promoter. Proc Natl Acad Sci USA 1989; 86: 9732–6.

126. McDonald AR, Goldfine IG. Glucocorticoid regulation of insulin receptor gene transcription in IM-9 cultured lymphocytes. J Clin Invest 1988; 81: 499–504.

127. Reed JC, Alpers JD, Nowell PC, Hoover RG. Sequential expression of protoncogenes during lectin-stimulated mitogenesis of normal human lymphocytes. Proc Natl Acad Sci USA 1986; 83: 3982–6.

128. Maassen JA, Krans HMJ, Moller W. The effect of insulin, serum and dexamethasone on mRNA levels for the insulin receptor in the human lymphocytes. J Clin Invest 1987; 930: 72–8.

129. Goldstein BJ, Muller-Wieland D, Kahn CR. Variation in insulin receptor mRNA expression in human and rodent tissues. Mol Endocrinol 1987; 1(11): 759–66.

130. McDonald AR, Maddux BA, Okabayashi Y et al. Regulation of insulin-receptor mRNA levels by glucocorticoids. Diabetes 1987; 36: 779–81.

131. Goldstein BJ, Kahn CR. Initial processing of the insulin receptor precursor *in vivo* and *in vitro*. J Biol Chem 1988; 263: 12809–812.

132. Yoshimasa Y, Seino S, Whittaker J et al. Insulin-resistant diabetes due to a point mutation that prevents insulin proreceptor processing. Science 1988; 240: 784–7.

133. Ronnet GV, Knutson VP, Kohanski RA, Simpson TL, Lane MD. Role of glycosylation in the processing of newly translated insulin proreceptor in 3T3-L1 adipocytes. J Biol Chem 1983; 259: 4566–75.

134. Forsayeth JR, Maddux BA, Goldfine ID. Biosynthesis and processing of the human insulin receptor. Diabetes 1986; 35: 837–46.

135. Rees-Jones R, Hedo HA, Zick Y, Roth J. Insulin-stimulated phosphorylation of the insulin receptor precursor. Biochem Biophys Res Commun 1983; 116: 417–22.

136. Blackshear PJ, Nemenoff RA, Avruch J. Insulin binds to and promotes the phosphorylation of a M_r 210 000 component of its receptor in detergent extracts of rat liver microsomes. Growth Regul 1983; 158: 243–6.

137. Olson TS, Bamberger MJ, Lane MD. Post-translational changes in tertiary and quaternary structure of the insulin proreceptor. Correlation with acquisition of function. J Biol Chem 1988; 263: 7342–51.

138. Deutsch PJ, Wan CF, Rosen OM, Rubin CS. Latent insulin receptors and possible receptor precursors in 3T3-L1 adipocytes. Proc Natl Acad Sci USA 1983; 80: 133–6.

139. Hedo JA, Gorden P. Biosynthesis of the insulin receptor. Horm Metab Res 1985; 17: 487–90.

140. Goldfine ID, Jones AL, Hradek GT, Wong KY, Mooney JS. Entry of insulin into cultured lymphocytes: electron microscopic autoradiographic analysis. Science 1979; 202: 760–63.

141. Carpentier JL, Gorden P, Freychet P, LeCam A, Orci L. Relationship of binding to internalization of ^{125}I-insulin in isolated rat hepatocytes. Diabetologia 1979; 17: 379–84.

142. Posner BI, Bergeron JJM, Josefsberg Z et al. Polypeptide hormones: intracellular receptors and internalization. Recent Prog Horm Res 1981; 37: 539–78.

143. Fehlmann M, Carpentier JL, Obberghen EV et al. Internalized insulin receptors are recycled to the cell surface in rat hepatocytes. Proc Natl Acad Sci USA 1982; 79: 5921–5.

144. Huecksteadt T, Olefsky JM, Brandenberg D, Heidenreich KA. Recycling of photoaffinity-labeled insulin receptors in rat adipocytes. Dissociation of insulin-receptor complexes is not required for receptor recycling. J Biol Chem 1986; 261: 8655–9.

145. Hedo JA, Simpson IA. Internalization of insulin receptors in the isolated rat adipose cell. J Biol Chem 1984; 259: 11083–9.

146. Gavin JR III, Roth J, Neville DM Jr, DeMeyts P, Buell DN. Insulin-dependent regulation of insulin-receptor concentration. Proc Natl Acad Sci USA 1974; 71: 84–8.

147. Simpson IA, Hedo JA, Cushman SW. Insulin-induced internalization of the insulin receptor in the isolated rat adipose cell: detection of both major receptor subunits following their biosynthetic labeling in culture. Diabetes 1984; 33: 13–18.

148. Knutson VP, Ronnett GV, Lane MD. Rapid reversible internalization of cell surface insulin receptors. Correlation with insulin-induced down-regulation. J Biol Chem 1983; 258: 12139–42.

149. Roth RA, Maddux BA, Cassell DJ, Goldfine ID. Regulation of the insulin receptor by a monoclonal anti-receptor antibody. J Biol Chem 1983; 258: 12094–7.

150. Taylor SI, Marcus-Samuels B. Anti-receptor antibodies mimic the effect of insulin to down-regulate insulin receptors in cultured human lymphoblastoid (IM-9) cells. J Clin Endocrinol Metab 1984; 58: 182–6.

151. Kasuga M, Kahn CR, Hedo JA, Van Obberghen E, Yamada KM. Insulin-induced receptor loss in cultured human lymphocytes is due to accelerated receptor degradation. Proc Natl Acad Sci USA 1981; 78: 6917–21.

152. Marshall S, Olefsky JM. Separate intracellular pathways for insulin receptor recycling and insulin degradation in isolated rat adipocytes. J Cell Physiol 1983; 117: 195–203.

153. King GL, Johnson SM. Receptor mediated transport of insulin across endothelial cells. Science 1985; 219: 865–9.

154. Flier JS. Insulin receptors and insulin resistance. Ann Rev Med 1983; 34: 145–60.

155. Kahn CR. Insulin resistance, insulin insensitivity, and insulin unresponsiveness: a necessary distinction. Metabolism 1978; 27: 1893–1902.

156. Beck-Nielsen H, Pedersen O. Diurnal variation in insulin binding to human monocytes. J Clin Endocrinol Metab 1978; 47: 385–90.

157. Muggeo M, Bar RS, Roth J. Changes in affinity of insulin receptors following oral glucose in normal adults. J Clin Endocrinol Metab 1977; 44: 1206–9.

158. Friedenberg GR, Klein HH, Cordera R, Olefsky JM. Insulin receptor kinase activity in rat liver. Regulation by fasting and high carbohydrate feeding. J Biol Chem 1985; 260: 12444–53.

159. Olefsky JM, Saekow M. The effects of dietary carbohydrate content on insulin binding and glucose metabolism by isolated rat adipocytes. Endocrinology 1978; 103: 2252–63.

160. Rosenthal M, Haskell WL, Solomon R, Widstrom A, Reaven GM. Demonstration of a relationship between level of physical training and insulin-stimulated glucose utilization in normal humans. Diabetes 1983; 32: 408–11.

161. Tan MH, Bonen A. Physical training enhances insulin binding and glucose uptake by skeletal muscle. Clin Invest Med 1982; 5: 39B.

162. Vinten J, Galbo H. Effect of physical training on transport and metabolism of glucose in adipocytes. Am J Physiol 1983; 244: E129–34.

163. Craig BW, Hammons GT, Garthwaite SM, Jarett J, Holloszy JO. Adaptation of fat cells to exercise: response of glucose uptake and oxidation to insulin. J Appl Physiol 1981; 51: 1500–1506.

164. Koivisto VA, Soman V, Conrad P, Hendler R, Nadel E, Felig P. Insulin binding to monocytes in trained athletes. J Clin Invest 1979; 64: 1011–15.

165. LeBlanc J, Nadeau A, Boulay M, Rousseau-Migneron S. Effects of physical training and adiposity on glucose metabolism and ^{125}I-insulin binding. J Appl Physiol 1979; 46: 235–9.

166. Burstein R, Polychronakos C, Toews J, MacDougall JD, Guyda HJ, Posner BI. Acute reversal of the enhanced insulin action in trained athletes. Association with insulin receptor changes. Diabetes 1985; 34: 756–60.

167. Dohm GL, Sinha MK, Caro JF. Insulin receptor binding and protein kinase activity in muscles of trained rats. Am J Physiol 1987; 252: E170–75.

168. Hughes VA, Fiatarone MD, Fielding RA et al. Exercise increases muscle GLUT-4 levels and insulin action in subjects with impaired glucose tolerance. Am J Physiol 1993; 264: E855–62.

169. Dela F, Plough T, Handberg A et al. Physical training increases muscle GLUT4 proteins and mRNA in patients with NIDDM. Diabetes 1994; 43: 862–5.

170. Goodyear LJ, Giorgino F, Balon TW, Condorelli G, Smith RJ. Effects of contractile activity on tyrosine phosphoproteins and phosphatidylinositol 3-kinase activity in rat skeletal muscle. Am J Physiol 1995; 268: E987–95.

171. Arsenis G, Livingston JN. Alterations in the tyrosine kinase activity of the insulin receptor produced by *in vitro* hyperinsulinemia. J Biol Chem 1986; 261: 147–53.

172. Takayama S, White MF, Kahn CR. Phorbol ester-induced serine phosphorylation of the insulin receptor decreases its tyrosine kinase activity. J Biol Chem 1988; 263: 3440–47.

173. Roth RA, Beaudoin J. Phosphorylation of purified insulin receptor by cAMP kinase. Diabetes 1987; 36: 123–6.

174. Kahn CR. Role of insulin receptors in insulin resistant states. Metabolism 1980; 29: 455–67.

175. Kobayashi M, Olefsky JM. Effect of experimental hyperinsulinemia on insulin binding and glucose transport in isolated rat adipocytes. Am J Physiol 1978; 235: E53–62.

176. Bar RS, Gorden P, Roth J et al. Insulin receptors in patients with insulinomas. J Clin Endocrinol Metab 1977; 44: 1210–13.

177. Archer JA, Gorden P, Gavin JR III et al. Insulin receptors in human circulating lymphocytes: application to the study of insulin resistance in man. J Clin Endocrinol Metab 1973; 36: 627–37.

178. Bar RS, Gorden P, Roth J, Kahn CR, DeMeyts P. Fluctuations in the affinity and concentration of insulin receptors on circulating monocytes of obese patients: effects of starvation, refeeding and dieting. J Clin Invest 1976; 58: 1123–35.

179. Blackard WG, Guzelian PS, Small ME. Down regulation of insulin receptors in primary cultures of adult rat hepatocytes in monolayer. Endocrinology 1978; 103: 548–53.

180. Livingston JM, Purvis BJ, Lockwood DH. Insulin-induced changes in insulin binding and insulin-sensitivity of adipocytes. Metabolism 1978; 27 (suppl. 2): 2009–14.

181. Kahn CR, Crettaz M, Grigorescu F, Takayama S, Ganda OP, Flier JS. The role of insulin receptor kinase activity in insulin action: implications from insulin-resistant states. In Labrie F, Proulx L (eds) Endocrinology. New York: Elsevier, 1984; 249–56.

182. Saad MJA, Folli F, Araki E, Hashimoto N, Csermely P, Kahn CR. Regulation of insulin receptor, insulin receptor substrate-1, and phosphatidylinositol 3-kinase in 3T3-F442A adipocytes. Effects of differentiation, insulin and dexamethasone. Mol Endocrinol 1994; 8: 545–57.

183. Ruan Y, Chen C, Cao Y, Garofalo RS. The *Drosophila* insulin receptor contains a novel carboxyl-terminal extension likely to play an important role in signal transduction. J Biol Chem 1995; 270: 4236–43.

184. Beck P, Schalch DS, Parker ML et al. Correlative studies of growth hormone and insulin plasma concentrations with metabolic abnormalities in acromegaly. J Lab Clin Med 1965; 66: 366–7.

185. Muggeo M, Bar RS, Roth J, Kahn CR, Gorden P. The insulin resistance of acromegaly: evidence for two alterations in the insulin receptor on circulating monocytes. J Clin Endocrinol Metab 1979; 48: 17–25.

186. Pessin JE, Gitomer W, Oka Y, Oppenheimer CL, Czech MP. β-Adrenergic regulation of insulin and epidermal growth factor receptors in rat adipocytes. J Biol Chem 1983; 258: 7386–94.

187. Grunberger G, Gorden P. Affinity alteration of insulin receptor induced by a phorbol ester. Am J Physiol 1982; 243: E319–24.

188. Jacobs S, Cuatrecasas P. Phosphorylation of receptors from insulin and insulin-like growth factor I. Effects of hormones and phorbol esters. J Biol Chem 1984; 261: 934–9.

189. Stadtmauer L, Rosen OM. Increasing the cAMP content of IM-9 cells alters the phosphorylation state and protein kinase activity of the insulin receptor. J Biol Chem 1986; 261: 3402–7.

190. Takayama S, White MF, Lauris V, Kahn CR. Phorbol esters modulate insulin receptor phosphorylation and insulin action in hepatoma cells. Proc Natl Acad Sci USA 1984; 81: 7797–801.

191. Kasuga M, Zick Y, Blithe DL, Karlsson FA, Haring HU, Kahn CR. Insulin stimulation of phosphorylation of the β-subunit of the insulin receptor: formation of both phosphoserine and phosphotyrosine. J Biol Chem 1982; 257: 9891–4.

192. Czech MP, Klarlund JK, Yagaloff KA, Bradford AP. Lewis RE. Insulin receptor signaling. Activation of multiple serine kinases. J Biol Chem 1988; 263: 11017–20.

193. Rouiller DG, McElduff A, Hedo JA, Gorden P. Induction of the insulin proreceptor by hydrocortisone in cultured lymphocytes (IM-9 line). J Clin Invest 1985; 76: 645–9.

194. Knutson VP, Ronnet GV, Lane MD. Control of insulin receptor level in 3T3 cells: effect of insulin-induced down-regulation on the rate of receptor inactivation. Proc Natl Acad Sci USA 1982; 79: 2822–6.

195. Robert A, Grunberger G, Carpentier JL, Dayer JM, Orci L, Gorden P. The insulin receptor of a human monocyte-like cell line: characterization and function. Endocrinology 1984; 114: 247–53.

196. Salhanick AI, Krupp MN, Amatruda JM. Dexamethasone stimulates insulin receptor synthesis in cultured rat hepatocytes. J Biol Chem 1983; 258: 14130–5.

197. Malchoff DM, Maloff BL, Livingston JN, Lockwood DH. Influence of dexamethasone on insulin action: inhibition of basal and insulin-stimulated hexose transport is dependent on length of exposure *in vitro*. Endocrinology 1982; 110: 2081–7.

198. Grunfeld C, Baird KL, Van Obberghen E, Kahn CR. Glucocorticoid-induced insulin resistance *in vitro*: evidence for both receptor and post-receptor defects. Endocrinology 1981; 109: 1723–30.

199. Olefsky JM. Effect of dexamethasone on insulin binding, glucose transport and glucose oxidation of isolated rat adipocytes. J Clin Invest 1975; 56: 1499–1508.

200. Karasik A, Kahn CR. Dexamethasone-induced changes in phosphorylation of the insulin and epidermal growth factor receptors and their substrates in intact rat hepatocytes. Endocrinology 1988; 123: 2214–22.

201. Truglia JA, Hayes GR, Lockwood DH. Intact adipocyte insulin-receptor phosphorylation and *in vitro* tyrosine kinase activity in animal models of insulin resistance. Diabetes 1988; 37: 147–53.

202. Kahn CR, Goldfine ID, Neville DM Jr, DeMeyts P. Alterations in insulin binding induced by changes

in vivo in the level of glucocorticoids and growth hormone. Endocrinology 1978; 103: 1054-66.

203. Takeda N, Yasuda K, Kitabchi AE, Horiya T, Jallepalli P, Miura K. Increased insulin binding of erythrocytes and insulin sensitivity in adrenal insufficiency. Metabolism 1987; 36: 1003-66.

204. Saad MJA, Folli F, Kahn CR. Insulin and dexamethasone regulate insulin receptors, insulin receptor substrate-1, and phosphatidylinositol 3-kinase in Fao hepatoma cells. Endocrinology 1995; 136: 1579-88.

205. Bar RS, Harrison LC, Muggeo M et al. Regulation of insulin receptors in normal and abnormal physiology in humans. Adv Int Med 1978; 24: 23-52.

206. Maegawa H, Shigeta Y, Egawa K, Kobayashi M. Impaired autophosphorylation of insulin receptors from abdominal skeletal muscles in non-obese subjects with NIDDM. Diabetes 1991; 40: 815-19.

207. Sinha MK, Pories WJ, Flickinger EG, Meelheim D, Caro JF. Insulin-receptor kinase activity of adipose tissue from morbidly obese humans with and without NIDDM. Diabetes 1987; 36: 620-25.

208. Archer JA, Gorden P, Roth J. Defect in insulin binding to receptors in obese man. Amelioration with caloric restriction. J Clin Invest 1975; 55: 166-74.

209. Olefsky JM, Bacon VC, Baur S. Insulin receptors of skeletal muscle: specific insulin binding sites and demonstration of decreased numbers of sites in obese rats. Metabolism 1976; 25: 179-91.

210. Wigand JP, Blackard WG. Down-regulation of insulin receptors in obese man. Diabetes 1979; 28: 287-91.

211. Moller DE, Yokota A, Flier JS. Normal insulin receptor cDNA sequence in Pima Indians with NIDDM. Diabetes 1989; 38: 1496-1500.

212. Cama A, Patterson AP, Kadowaki T et al. The amino acid sequence of the insulin receptor is normal in an insulin resistant Pima Indian. J Clin Endocrinol Metab 1990; 70: 1155-61.

213. Clausen JO, Hansen T, Bjorbaek et al. Insulin resistance: interactions between obesity and a common variant of insulin receptor substrate-1. Lancet 1995; 346: 397-402.

214. Rothman DL, Shulman RG, Shulman GI. ^{31}P nuclear magnetic resonance measurements of muscle glucose-6-phosphate. Evidence for reduced insulin-dependent muscle glucose transport or phosphorylation activity in non-insulin dependent diabetes mellitus. J Clin Invest 1992; 89: 1069-75.

215. Bonadonna RC, Del Prato S, Bonora E, Saccomani MP, Gulli G, Natali A et al. Roles of glucose transport and glucose phosphorylation in muscle insulin resistance of NIDDM. Diabetes 1996; 45: 915-25.

216. Ciaraldi TP, Kolterman OG, Olefsky JM. Mechanism of the postreceptor defect in insulin action in human obesity. J Clin Invest 1981; 68: 875-80.

217. Caro JF, Ittoop O, Pories WJ et al. Studies on the mechanism of insulin resistance in the liver from humans with non-insulin-dependent diabetes. J Clin Invest 1986; 78: 249-58.

218. Garvey WT, Maianu L, Hancock JA, Golichowski AM, Baron AD. Gene expression of GLUT4 in skeletal muscle from insulin-resistant patients with obesity, IGT, GDM, and NIDDM. Diabetes 1992; 41: 715-22.

219. Friedman JE, Dohm GL, Leggett-Frazier N et al. Restoration of insulin responsiveness in skeletal muscle of morbidly obese patients after weight loss. Effect on muscle glucose transport and glucose transporter GLUT4. J Clin Invest 1992; 89: 701-5.

220. Kahn BB. Alterations in glucose transporter expression and function in diabetes: mechanisms for insulin resistance. J Cell Biochem 1992; 48: 122-8.

221. Garvey WT, Maianu L, Huecksteadt TP, Birnbaum MJ, Molina JM, Ciaraldi TP. Pretranslational suppression of a glucose transporter protein causes insulin resistance in adipocytes from patients with non-insulin-dependent diabetes mellitus and obesity. J Clin Invest 1991; 87: 1072-81.

222. Olefsky JM, Reaven GM. Insulin binding in diabetes: relationships with plasma insulin levels and insulin sensitivity. Diabetes 1977; 26: 680-88.

223. Kolterman OG, Gray RS, Griffin J et al. Receptor and postreceptor defects contribute to the insulin resistance in non-insulin-dependent diabetes mellitus. J Clin Invest 1981; 68: 957-69.

224. Warram JH, Martin BC, Krolewski AS, Soeldner JS, Kahn CR. Slow glucose removal rate and hyperinsulinemia are predictors of the risk of type II diabetes in offspring of diabetic parents. Ann Intern Med 1990; 113: 909-15.

225. Hotamisligil GS, Shargill NS, Spiegelman BM. Adipose expression of tumor necrosis factor-α: direct role in obesity-linked insulin resistance. Science 1993; 259: 87-91.

226. Sims RE, Rushford FE, Huston DP, Cunningham GR. Successful immunosuppressive therapy in a patient with autoantibodies to insulin receptors and immune complex glomerulonephritis. South Med J 1987; 80: 903-6.

227. Hotamisligil GS, Budavari A, Murray D, Spiegelman BM. Reduced tyrosine kinase activity of the insulin receptor in obesity-diabetes. Central role of tumor necrosis factor-alpha. J Clin Invest 1994; 94: 1543-9.

228. Hofmann CA, Lorenz K, Braithwaite SS et al. Altered gene expression for tumor necrosis factor-alpha and its receptors during drug and dietary modulation of insulin resistance. Endocrinology 1994; 134: 264-70.

229. Ofei F, Hurel S, Newkirk J, Sopwith M, Taylor R. Effects of an engineered human anti-TNF-α antibody (CDP571) on insulin sensitivity and glycemic control in patients with NIDDM. Diabetes 1996; 45: 881-5.

230. Scheen AJ, Castillo MJ, Paquot N, Lefebvre PJ. No effect of neutralization of TNF-α on insulin-mediated glucose disposal in obese insulin resistant subjects. Diabetologia 1996; 39 (suppl. 1): A153 (abstr).

231. Zhang Y, Proenca R, Maffei M, Barone M, Leopold L, Friedman JM. Positional cloning of the mouse obese gene and its human homologue. Nature 1994; 372: 425-32.

232. Rohner-Jeanrenaud F, Jeanrenaud B. Obesity, leptin and the brain. New Engl J Med 1996; 334: 324-5.

233. Ahima RS, Prabakaran D, Mantzoros CS et al. Role of leptin in the neuroendocrine response to fasting. Nature 1996; 382: 250-52.

234. Porte DJ. Banting lecture 1990. Beta-cells in type II diabetes mellitus. Diabetes 1991; 40: 166-80.

235. DeFronzo RA, Bonadonna RC, Ferrannini E. Pathogenesis of NIDDM: a balanced overview. Diabetes Care 1992; 15: 318-68.

236. Kahn CR. Insulin action, diabetogenes, and the cause of type II diabetes (Banting Lecture). Diabetes 1994; 43: 1066-84.

237. Rossetti L, Giaccari A, DeFronzo RA. Glucose toxicity. Diabetes Care 1990; 13: 610–30.

238. Martin BC, Warram JH, Krolewski AS, Bergman RN, Soeldner JS, Kahn CR. Role of glucose and insulin resistance in development of type II diabetes mellitus: results of a 25-year follow-up study. Lancet 1992; 340: 925–9.

239. Lillioja S, Mott DM, Howard BV et al. Impaired glucose tolerance as a disorder of insulin action: longitudinal and cross-sectional studies in Pima Indians. New Engl J Med 1988; 318: 1217–25.

240. Bogardus C, Lillioja S, Nyomba BL et al. Distribution of in vivo insulin action in Pima Indians as mixture of three normal distributions. Diabetes 1989; 38: 1423–32.

241. Gulli G, Ferrannini E, Stern M, Haffner SM, DeFronzo RA. The metabolic profile of NIDDM is fully established in glucose-tolerant offspring of two Mexican-American NIDDM parents. Diabetes 1992; 41: 1575–86.

242. Rothman DL, Magnusson I, Cline G et al. Decreased muscle glucose transport/phosphorylation is an early defect in the pathogenesis of non-insulin-dependent diabetes mellitus. Proc Natl Acad Sci USA 1995; 92: 983–7.

243. Martin BC, Warram JH, Rosner B, Rich SS, Soeldner JS, Krolewski AS. Familial clustering of insulin sensitivity. Diabetes 1992; 41: 850–54.

244. Olefsky JM. Insulin resistance and insulin action: an in vitro and in vivo perspective. Diabetes 1981; 30: 148–62.

245. Reaven GM. Role of insulin resistance in human disease. Diabetes 1988; 37: 1595–1607.

246. Leahy JL, Bonner-Weir S, Weir G. β-Cell dysfunction induced by chronic hyperglycemia—current ideas on mechanism of impaired glucose-induced insulin secretion. Diabetes Care 1992; 15: 442–5.

247. Turner R, Hattersley A, Cook J. Type II diabetes: search for primary defects. Ann Med 1992; ·24: 511–16.

248. Orci L, Unger RH, Ravazzola M et al. Reduced beta-cell glucose transporter in new onset diabetic BB rats. J Clin Invest 1990; 86: 1615–22.

249. Lillioja S, Nyomba BL, Saad MF et al. Exaggerated early insulin release and insulin resistance in a diabetes-prone population: a metabolic comparison of Pima Indians and Caucasians. J Clin Endocrinol Metab 1991; 73(4): 866–76.

250. Zimmet P, Dowse G, Finch CE, Serjeantson S, King H. The epidemiology and natural history of NIDDM—lessons from the South Pacific. Diabetes Metab Rev 1990; 6: 91–124.

251. Arner P, Engfeldt P, Skarfors E, Lithell H, Bolinder J. Insulin receptor binding and metabolic effects of insulin in human subcutaneous adipose tissue in untreated non-insulin dependent diabetes mellitus. Ups J Med Sci 1987; 92: 47–58.

252. Caro JF, Sinha MK, Raju SM et al. Insulin receptor kinase in human skeletal muscle from obese subjects with and without non-insulin-dependent diabetes. J Clin Invest 1987; 79: 1330–37.

253. Arner P, Einarsson K, Ewerth S, Livingston J. Studies of the human liver insulin receptor in non-insulin-dependent diabetes mellitus. J Clin Invest 1986; 77: 1716–18.

254. Takayama S, Kahn CR, Kubo K, Foley JE. Alterations in insulin receptor autophosphorylation in insulin resistance: correlation with altered sensitivity to glucose transport and anti-lipolysis to insulin. J Clin Endocrinol Metab 1988; 66: 992–9.

255. Obermaier-Kusser B, White MF, Pongratz DE et al. A defective intramolecular autoactivation cascade may cause the reduced kinase activity of the skeletal muscle insulin receptor from patients with non-insulin-dependent diabetes mellitus. J Biol Chem 1989; 264: 9497–504.

256. Thies RS, Molina JM, Ciaraldi TP, Freidenberg GR, Olefsky JM. Insulin-receptor autophosphorylation and endogenous substrate phosphorylation in human adipocytes from control, obese, and NIDDM subjects. Diabetes 1990; 39: 250–59.

257. Arner P, Pollare T, Lithell H, Livingston JN. Defective insulin receptor tyrosine kinase in human skeletal muscle in obesity and type II (non-insulin-dependent) diabetes mellitus. Diabetologia 1987; 30: 437–40.

258. Freidenberg GR, Reichart D, Olefsky JM, Henry RR. Reversibility of defective adipocyte insulin receptor kinase activity in non-insulin-dependent diabetes mellitus. Effect of weight loss. J Clin Invest 1988; 82: 1398–1406.

259. Choi WH, O'Rahilly S, Buse JB et al. Molecular scanning of insulin-responsive glucose transporter (GLUT4) gene in NIDDM subjects. Diabetes 1991; 40: 1712–18.

260. King PA, Horton ED, Hirschman MF, Horton ES. Insulin resistance in obese Zucker rat (fa/fa) skeletal muscle is associated with a failure of glucose transporter translocation. J Clin Invest 1992; 90: 1568–75.

261. Wells AM, Sutcliffe IC, Johnson AB, Taylor R. Abnormal activation of glycogen synthesis in fibroblasts from NIDDM subjects. Evidence for an abnormality specific to glucose metabolism. Diabetes 1993; 42: 583–9.

262. Prince MJ, Tsai P, Olefsky JM. Insulin binding, internalization and insulin receptor regulation in fibroblasts from type II (non-insulin-dependent) diabetic subjects. Diabetes 1981; 30: 596–600.

263. Elbein SC, Chiu KC, Hoffman MD, Mayorga RA, Bragg KL, Leppert MF. Linkage analysis of 19 candidate regions for insulin resistance in familial NIDDM. Diabetes 1995; 44: 1259–65.

264. Biorbaek C, Echwald SM, Hubricht P et al. Genetic variants in promoters and coding regions of the muscle-glycogen synthase and the insulin-responsive GLUT4 genes in NIDDM. Diabetes 1994; 43: 976–83.

265. Almind K, Biorbaek C, Vestergaard H, Hansen T, Echwald SM, Pedersen O. Amino acid polymorphisms of insulin receptor substrate-1 in non-insulin-dependent diabetes mellitus. Lancet 1993; 342: 828–32.

266. Hager J, Zouali H, Velho G, Froguel P. Insulin receptor substrate (IRS-1) gene polymorphism in French NIDDM families. Lancet 1993; 342: 1430.

267. Almind K, Inoue G, Pedersen O, Kahn CR. A common amino acid polymorphism in insulin receptor substrate-1 causes impaired insulin signaling. Evidence from transfection studies. J Clin Invest 1996; 97: 2569–75.

268. Ura S, Araki E, Kishikawa H et al. Molecular scanning of the IRS-1 gene in Japanese patients with non-insulin-dependent diabetes mellitus: identification of five novel mutations in IRS-1 gene. Diabetologia 1996; 39: 600–608.

269. Srinivas PR, Wagner AS, Reddy LV et al. Serum alpha 2 HS-glycoprotein is an inhibitor of the human insulin receptor at the tyrosine kinase level. Mol Endocrinol 1993; 7: 1445–55.

270. Maddux BA, Sbraccia P, Kumakura S et al. Membrane glycoprotein PC-1 in the insulin resistance of non-insulin dependent diabetes mellitus. Nature 1995; 373: 448–51.

271. Reynet C, Kahn CR. Rad: a member of the ras family overexpressed in muscle of type II diabetic humans. Science 1993; 262: 1441–4.

272. Moyers JS, Bilan PJ, Reynet C, Kahn CR. Overexpression of Rad inhibits glucose uptake in cultured muscle and fat cells. J Biol Chem 1996; 271: 23111–16.

273. Beck-Nielsen H, Pedersen O, Sovensen NS. Effects of dietary changes on cellular insulin binding and *in vivo* insulin sensitivity. Metabolism 1980; 29: 482–7.

274. Pedersen O, Hjollund E, Sovensen NS. Insulin receptor binding and insulin action in human fat cells: effects of obesity and fasting. Metabolism 1982; 31: 884–95.

275. Cech JM, Freeman RB Jr, Caro JF, Amatruda JM. Insulin action and binding in isolated hepatocytes from fasted streptozotozin-diabetic, and older, spontaneously obese rats. Biochem J 1980; 188: 839–45.

276. Friedenberg GR, Reichard D, Olefsky JM, Henry RR. Reversibility of defective adipocyte insulin receptor kinase activity in non-insulin-dependent diabetes mellitus. Effect of weight loss. J Clin Invest 1988; 82: 1398–1406.

277. Olefsky JM, Reaven GM. Effects of sulfonylurea therapy on insulin binding to mononuclear leukocytes of diabetic patients. Am J Med 1976; 60: 89–95.

278. Beck-Nielsen H, Pedersen O, Lindskov HO. Increased insulin sensitivity and cellular insulin binding in obese diabetics following treatment with glibenclamide. Acta Endocrinol 1979; 90: 451–62.

279. Grunberger G, Ryan J, Gorden P. Sulfonylureas do not affect insulin binding or glycemic control in insulin-dependent diabetics. Diabetes 1982; 31: 890–96.

280. Groop LC, Luzi L, Melander A et al. Different effects of glyburide and glipizide on insulin secretion and hepatic glucose production in normal and NIDDM subjects. Diabetes 1987; 36: 1320–28.

281. Bailey CJ. Metformin revisited: its actions and indications for use. Diabet Med 1988; 5: 315–20.

282. Caspary WF, Creutzfeldt W. Analysis of the inhibitory effect of biguanides on glucose absorption: inhibition of sugar transport. Diabetologia 1971; 7: 379–82.

283. Klip A, Leiter LA. Cellular mechanisms of action of metformin. Diabetes Care 1990; 13: 696–704.

284. Nolan JJ, Ludvik B, Beerdsen P, Joyce M, Olefsky J. Improvement in glucose tolerance and insulin resistance in obese subjects treated with troglitazone. New Engl J Med 1994; 331: 1188–93.

285. Lehmann JM, Moore LB, Smith-Oliver TA, Wilkison WO, Willson TM, Kliewer SA. An antidiabetic thiazolidinedione is a high affinity ligand for peroxisome proliferator-activated receptor gamma. J Biol Chem 1995; 270: 12953–6.

286. Forman BM, Tontonoz P, Chen J, Brun RP, Spiegelman BM, Evans RM. 15-deoxy-delta^{12,14}-prostaglandin J$_2$ is a ligand for the adipocyte determination factor PPAR gamma. Cell 1995; 83: 803–12.

287. Zhang B, Szalkowski D, Diaz E, Hayes NS, Smith R, Berger J. Potentiation of insulin stimulation of phosphatidylinositol 3-kinase by thiazolidinedione-derived antidiabetic agents in Chinese hamster ovary cells expressing human insulin receptors and L6 myotubes. J Biol Chem 1994; 269: 25735–41.

288. Ramanadham S, Mongold JJ, Brownsey RW, Cros GH, McNeill JH. Oral vanadyl sulfate in treatment of diabetes mellitus in rats. Am J Physiol 1989; 257: H904–11.

289. Cohen N, Halberstam M, Shlimovich P, Chang CJ, Shamoon H, Rossetti L. Oral vanadyl sulfate improves hepatic and peripheral insulin sensitivity in patients with non-insulin-dependent diabetes mellitus. J Clin Invest 1995; 95: 2501–9.

290. Meyerovitch J, Farfel Z, Sack J, Shechter Y. Oral administration of vanadate normalizes blood glucose levels in streptozotocin-treated rats. Characterization and mode of action. J Biol Chem 1987; 262: 6658–62.

291. Goldfine AB, Simonson DC, Folli F, Patti ME, Kahn CR. Metabolic effects of sodium metavanadate in humans with insulin-dependent and non-insulin-dependent diabetes mellitus—*in vivo* and *in vitro* studies. J Clin Endocrinol Metab 1995; 80: 3311–20.

292. Scimeca JC, Ballotti R, Filloux C, Van Obberghen E. Insulin and orthovanadate stimulate multiple phosphotyrosine-containing serine kinases. Mol Cell Biochem 1992; 109: 139–47.

293. Fantus IG, Ahmad F, Deragon G. Vanadate augments insulin-stimulated insulin receptor kinase activity and prolongs insulin action in rat adipocytes. Evidence for transduction of amplitude of signaling into duration of response. Diabetes 1994; 43: 375–83.

294. Pedersen O, Beck-Nielsen H. Insulin-resistance and insulin-dependent diabetes mellitus. Diabetes Care 1987; 10: 516–23.

295. Kruszynska YT, Home PD. Insulin insensitivity in type 1 diabetes. Diabet Med 1987; 4: 414–22.

296. Hjollund E, Pedersen O, Richelsen B, Beck-Nielsen H, Sorensen NS. Glucose transport and metabolism in adipocytes from newly diagnosed untreated insulin-dependent diabetics. Severely impaired basal and postinsulin binding activities. J Clin Invest 1985; 76: 2091–6.

297. Pedersen O, Hjollund E. Insulin receptor binding to fat and blood cells and insulin action in fat cells from insulin-dependent diabetics. Diabetes 1982; 31: 706–15.

298. Pedersen O, Beck-Nielsen H, Heding L. Insulin receptors on monocytes from patients with ketosis-prone diabetes mellitus. Diabetes 1978; 27: 1098–1104.

299. Pedersen O, Hjllund E, Beck-Nielsen H, Richelsen B, Srensen NS. Continuous subcutaneous insulin infusion fails to correct impaired basal glucose metabolism and impaired insulin sensitivity of adipocytes from patients with type 1 (insulin-dependent) diabetes. Diabetes Res 1986; 3: 17–23.

300. Pedersen O, Hjollund E, Lindskov HO, Helms P, Sorensen NS, Ditzel J. Increased insulin receptor binding to monocytes from insulin-dependent diabetic patients after a low-fat, high starch, high fiber diet. Diabetes Care 1982; 5: 284–91.

301. Kasuga M, Akanuma Y, Iwamoto Y, Kosaka K. Insulin binding and glucose metabolism in adipocytes of streptozotocin-diabetic rats. Am J Physiol 1978; 235: E175–82.

302. Kobayashi M, Olefsky JM. Effects of streptozotocin-induced diabetes on insulin binding, glucose transport, and intracellular glucose metabolism in isolated rat adipocytes. Diabetes 1979; 28: 87–95.

303. Davidson MB, Kaplan SA. Increased insulin binding by hepatic plasma membranes from diabetic rats. J Clin Invest 1977; 59: 22–30.

304. Le Marchand-Brustel Y, Freychet P. Effect of fasting and streptozotocin diabetes on insulin binding and action in the isolated mouse soleus muscle. J Clin Invest 1979; 64: 1505–15.

305. Okamoto M, Kuzuga H, Imura H. Increased affinity of insulin receptors on hepatocytes from streptozotocin-induced diabetic rats. Endocrinology 1984; 31: 235–43.

306. Burant CF, Treutelaar MK, Buse MG. Diabetes-induced functional and structural changes in insulin receptors from rat skeletal muscle. J Clin Invest 1986; 77: 260–70.

307. Freidenberg GR, Henry RR, Klein HH, Reichart DR, Olefsky JM. Decreased kinase activity of insulin receptors from adipocytes of non-insulin dependent diabetic subjects. J Clin Invest 1987; 79: 240–50.

308. Whittaker J, Cuthbert C, Hammond VA, Alberti KGMM. Impaired insulin binding to isolated adipocytes in experimental diabetic ketoacidosis. Diabetologia 1981; 21: 563–8.

309. Pedersen O, Gliemann J. Hexose transport in human adipocytes: factors influencing the response to insulin and kinetics of methylglucose and glucose transport. Diabetologia 1981; 20: 630–35.

310. Merimee TJ, Pulkkinen AJ, Lotton S. Increased insulin binding by lymphocyte receptors induced by betahydroxybutyrate. J Clin Endocrinol Metab 1976; 43: 1190–92.

311. Hidaka H, Howard BV, Ishibashi F, Kosmakos FC. Effect of pH and 3-hyroxybutyrate on insulin binding and action in cultured human fibroblasts. Diabetes 1981; 30: 402–6.

312. Green A, Bustillos DP, Misbin RI. β-Hydroxybutyrate increases the insulin sensitivity of adipocyte glucose transport at a postreceptor level. Diabetes 1984; 33: 1045–50.

313. Blackshear PJ, Nemenoff RA, Avruch J. Characteristics of insulin and epidermal growth factor stimulation of receptor autophosphorylation in detergent extracts of rat liver and transplantable rat hepatomas. Endocrinology 1984; 114: 141–52.

314. Kadowaki T, Kasuga M, Akanuma Y, Ezaki O, Takaku F. Decreased autophosphorylation of the insulin receptor-kinase in streptozotocin-diabetic rats. J Biol Chem 1984; 259: 14208–16.

315. Amatruda JM, Roncone AM. Normal hepatic insulin receptor autophosphorylation in non-ketotic diabetes mellitus. Biochem Biophys Res Commun 1985; 129: 163–70.

316. Okamoto M, White MF, Maron R, Kahn CR. Autophosphorylation and kinase activity of insulin receptor in diabetic rats. Am J Physiol 1986; 251: E542–50.

317. Gherzi R, Andraghetti G, Ferrannini E, Cordera R. Insulin receptor autophosphorylation and kinase activity in streptozotocin diabetic rats. Effect of a short fast. Biochem Biophys Res Commun 1986; 140: 850–56.

318. Ferrannini E, Buzzigoli G, Bonadonna R et al. Insulin resistance in essential hypertension. New Engl J Med 1987; 317: 350–57.

319. Krotkiewski M, Mandroukas K, Sjostrom L, Sullivan L, Wetterqvist H, Bjorntorp P. Effect of long-term physical training on body fat, metabolism and blood pressure in obesity. Metabolism 1979; 28: 650–58.

320. DeFronzo RA, Ferrannini E. Insulin resistance. A multifaceted syndrome responsible for NIDDM, obesity, hypertension, dyslipidemia, and atherosclerotic cardiovascular disease. Diabetes Care 1991; 14 (3): 173–94.

321. Lithell H. Effect of antihypertensive drugs on insulin, glucose and lipid metabolism. Diabetes Care 1991; 14: 203–9.

322. Velloso LA, Folli F, Sun XJ, White MF, Saad MJA, Kahn CR. Cross-talk between the insulin and angiotensin signaling system. Proc Natl Acad Sci USA 1996; 93: 12490–5.

323. DeFronzo RA, Goldberg M, Agus ZS. The effects of glucose and insulin on renal electrolyte transport. J Clin Invest 1976; 58: 83–90.

324. Young JB, Cohen WR, Rappaport EB, Landsberg L. High plasma norepinephrine concentrations at birth in infants of diabetic mothers. Diabetes 1979; 28: 697–9.

325. Liang CM, Doherty JU, Faillace R et al. Insulin infusion in conscious dogs: effects on systemic and coronary hemodynamics, regional blood flows and plasma catecholamines. J Clin Invest 1982; 69: 1321–36.

326. Taylor SI, Moller DE. Mutations of the insulin receptor gene. In Moller DE (ed.) Insulin resistance. Chichester: Wiley, 1993; pp 83–121.

327. Kahn CR, Flier JS, Bar RS et al. The syndromes of insulin resistance and acanthosis nigricans: insulin receptor disorders in man. New Engl J Med 1976; 294: 739–45.

328. Bar RS, Muggeo M, Roth J, Kahn CR, Havrankova J, Imperato-McGinley J. Insulin resistance, acanthosis nigricans and normal insulin receptors in a young woman: evidence for a post-receptor defect. J Clin Endocrinol Metab 1978; 47: 620–25.

329. Moller DE, Flier JS. Detection of an alteration in the insulin-receptor gene in a patient with insulin resistance, acanthosis nigricans, and the polycystic ovary syndrome (type A insulin resistance). New Engl J Med 1988; 319: 1526–9.

330. Flier JS. Lilly Lecture. Syndromes of insulin resistance: from patient to gene and back again. Diabetes 1992; 41: 1207–19.

331. Harrison LC, Dean B, Peluso I, Clark S, Ward G. Insulin resistance, acanthosis nigricans, and polycystic ovaries have been associated with a circulating inhibitor of postbinding insulin action. J Clin Endocrinol Metab 1985; 60: 1047–52.

332. Misbin RI, Green A, Alvarez IM, Almira EC, Dohm GL, Caro JF. Inhibition of insulin-stimulated glucose transport by factor extracted from serum of insulin-resistant patient. Diabetes 1988; 37: 1217–25.

333. Sbraccia P, Goodman PA, Maddux BA et al. Production of inhibitor of insulin-receptor tyrosine kinase in fibroblasts from patient with insulin resistance and NIDDM. Diabetes 1991; 40: 295–9.

334. Flier JS, Moller DE, Moses AC et al. Insulin-mediated pseudoacromegaly: clinical and biochemical characterization of a syndrome of selective insulin resistance. J Clin Endocrinol Metab 1993; 76: 1533–41.

335. Donahue WL, Uchida I. Leprechaunism: euphemism for a rare familial disorder. J Pediatr 1954; 45: 505–19.

336. Kobayashi M, Olefsky JM, Elders J et al. Insulin resistance due to a defect distal to the insulin receptor: demonstration in a patient with leprechaunism. Proc Natl Acad Sci USA 1978; 75: 3469–73.

337. Schilling EE, Rechler MM, Grunfeld C, Rosenberg AM. Primary defect of insulin receptors in skin fibroblasts cultured from an infant with leprechaunism and insulin resistance. Proc Natl Acad Sci USA 1979; 76: 5877–81.

338. Taylor SI. Lilly Lecture: Molecular mechanisms of insulin resistance—Lessons from patients with mutations in the insulin receptor gene. Diabetes 1992; 41: 1473–90.

339. Cama A, Marcus-Samuels B, Taylor SI. Immunological abnormalities in insulin receptors on cultured EBV-transformed lymphocytes from insulin-resistant patient with leprechaunism. Diabetes 1988; 37: 982–8.

340. McElduff A, Hedo JA, Taylor SI, Roth J, Gorden P. Insulin receptor degradation is accelerated in cultured lymphocytes from patients with genetic syndromes of extreme insulin resistance. J Clin Invest 1984; 74: 1366–74.

341. Taylor SI, Roth J, Blizzard RM, Elders MJ. Qualitative abnormalities in insulin binding in a patient with extreme insulin resistance: decreased sensitivity to alterations in temperature and pH. Proc Natl Acad Sci USA 1981; 78: 7157–61.

342. Van der Vorm ER, Lindhout D, Wit JM, Odink RJ, Krans HM, Maassen JA. Molecular heterogeneity of congenital forms of insulin resistance [in Dutch]. Nederlands Tijdschrift Voor Geneeskunde 1991; 135: 1165–70.

343. Moller DE, O'Rahilly S. Syndromes of severe insulin resistance: clinical and pathophysiological features. In Moller DE (ed.) Insulin resistance. Chichester: Wiley, 1993; pp 49–81.

344. Hone J, Accili D, Psiachou H et al. Homozygosity for a null allele of the insulin receptor gene in a patient with leprechaunism. Hum Mutat 1995; 6: 17–22.

345. Moncada VY, Hedo JA, Serrano Rios M, Taylor SI. Insulin-receptor biosynthesis in cultured lymphocytes from an insulin-resistant patient (Rabson–Mendenhall syndrome). Evidence for defect before insertion of receptor into plasma membrane. Diabetes 1986; 35: 802–7.

346. Senior B, Gellis SS. The syndromes of total lipodystrophy and of partial lipodystrophy. Pediatrics 1964; 330: 593–612.

347. Seip M. Lipodystrophy and gigantism with associated endocrine manifestations: a new diencephalic syndrome? Acta Paediatr 1995; 48: 555–74.

348. Seip M. Generalized lipodystrophy. Ergeb Inn Med Kinderheilkd 1871; XXXI: 59–69.

349. Beylot M, Sautot G, Laville M, Cohen R. Metabolic studies on lipatrophic diabetes: mechanism of hyperglycemia and evidence of resistance to insulin of lipid metabolism. Diabète Métab 1988; 14: 20–24.

350. Kobberling J. Genetic syndromes associated with lipoatrophic diabetes. In Creutzfeldt W, Kobberling J, Neel JV (eds) The genetics of diabetes mellitus. New York: Springer-Verlag, 1976; pp 147–54.

351. Oseid S, Beck-Nielsen H, Pedersen O et al. Decreased binding of insulin to its receptor in patients with congenital generalized lipodystrophy. New Engl J Med 1977; 296: 245–8.

352. Wachslicht-Rodbard H, Muggeo M, Kahn CR et al. Heterogeneity of the insulin-receptor interaction in lipoatrophic diabetes. Evidence for heterogeneous postbinding defects. Diabetes 1988; 37: 421–8.

353. Kriaauciunas KM, Kahn CR, Muller-Wieland D, Reddy SSK, Taub R. Altered expression and function of the insulin receptor in a family with lipoatrophic diabetes. J Clin Endocrinol Metab 1988; 67: 1284–93.

354. Desbois-Mouthon C, Magre J, Amselem S et al. Lipoatrophic diabetes: genetic exclusion of the insulin receptor gene. J Clin Endocrinol Metab 1995; 80: 314–19.

355. Davidson MB, Young RT. Metabolic studies in familial partial lipodystrophy of the lower trunk and extremities. Diabetologia 1975; 11: 561–8.

22

Molecular Basis of Insulin Actions on Intracellular Metabolism

Richard M. Denton and Jeremy M. Tavaré

Department of Biochemistry, University of Bristol, UK

The initial event in the action of insulin is its binding to—and activation of—a specific receptor protein in the plasma membrane of target tissues, the most important of which are liver, fat and muscle. The subsequent intracellular signals emanating from the insulin receptor remain rather elusive and poorly understood despite a great deal of progress in recent years towards their identification.

The effects of insulin range over a wide time-scale, from the acute (for example the regulation of many enzymes in carbohydrate and fat metabolism by reversible phosphorylation) which occur within minutes, to the long-term (including the regulation of DNA transcription and translation), often taking a matter of several hours or longer. Any plausible explanation as to the nature of the intracellular signals for insulin action must, therefore, take into account not only a diverse array of responses but also their widely differing time-courses. Furthermore, there is a considerable degree of amplification involved between the binding of insulin to as few as 2000 insulin receptors on the plasma membrane of each fat or other cell, and the resulting regulation of the activity of many millions of target enzymes and other molecules within the cell, such as glucose transporters, glycogen synthase and acetyl-CoA carboxylase.

A good deal is known about the general effects of insulin on carbohydrate and lipid metabolism (see Tables 1 and 3). Their combined effect is to increase the net uptake of glucose from the blood and increase its conversion to storage products such as glycogen and fat. At the same time, insulin inhibits the breakdown of triacylglycerol and glycogen and, under appropriate conditions, fatty acid oxidation, ketone body formation and gluconeogenesis in the liver. The effects of insulin on DNA synthesis and transcription and on protein synthesis are perhaps less well understood than its effects on carbohydrate and lipid metabolism. In this chapter we cover each of these aspects in turn and then consider some of the more promising mechanisms that have been proposed recently to be involved in bringing about the effects of this hormone. Many aspects of insulin action have also been considered in a number of recent reviews [1–6].

EFFECTS OF INSULIN ON CARBOHYDRATE METABOLISM

Figure 1 and Table 1 summarize the principal effects of insulin on carbohydrate metabolism, which occur within minutes after the exposure of liver, muscle or adipose tissue to insulin. There are, in addition, longer-term effects involving changes in gene expression and, possibly, translation rates, which result in alterations in the concentration of specific enzymes in tissues. Examples of such effects include the induction of the NADP-linked dehydrogenases of the pentose cycle and liver L-type pyruvate kinase and glucokinase, together with the repression of liver phospho-enol-pyruvate carboxykinase (see later).

International Textbook of Diabetes Mellitus, Second Edition. Edited by K.G.M.M. Alberti, P. Zimmet, R.A. DeFronzo, and H. Keen (Honorary)
© 1997 John Wiley & Sons Ltd

Table 1 Principal acute effects of insulin on carbohydrate metabolism. The changes listed under 'mechanisms involved' are not necessarily complete. Step numbers are those indicated in Figure 1

Process	Effect	Tissue*	Mechanisms involved
Glucose transport	Increase	F, M	Translocation of glucose transporters (step 1)
Glycogen synthesis	Increase	L, F, M	Dephosphorylation of glycogen synthase (step 2)
Glycogen breakdown	Decrease†	L, F, M	Dephosphorylation of phosphorylase kinase and hence phosphorylase (step 3)
Glycolysis	Increase†	L	Dephosphorylation of pyruvate kinase (step 6) and
Gluconeogenesis	Decrease†	L	fructose 2,6-bisphosphate kinase
Pyruvate → acetyl-CoA	Increase	(L), F	Dephosphorylation of pyruvate dehydrogenase (step 7)

*Abbreviations: F, white and brown adipose tissue; M, muscle; L, liver.
†These effects are not usually apparent unless tissue cAMP levels are increased by the presence of another hormone.
For further details, including specific references, see reference 1.

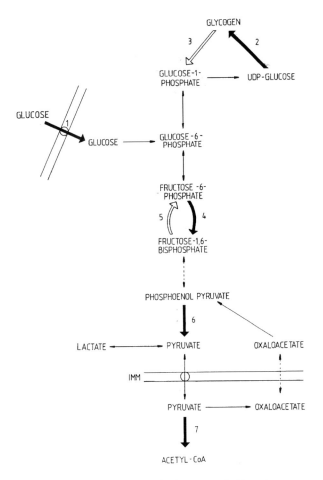

Figure 1 Outline of carbohydrate metabolism in mammalian tissues emphasizing the main sites of acute regulation by insulin. Numbered steps indicated by solid arrows are stimulated whereas those by open arrows are inhibited in appropriate tissues. Enzymes catalysing these steps are: (1) glucose transporter; (2) glycogen synthase; (3) phosphorylase; (4) phosphofructokinase (PFK); (5) fructose 1,6-bisphosphatase; (6) pyruvate kinase (liver isoenzyme); (7) pyruvate dehydrogenase. Note: regulation of steps 4 and 5, at least in liver, probably occurs mainly through changes in fructose 2,6-bisphosphate as a result of alterations in the activity of fructose 2,6-bisphosphate kinase. Regulation of phosphorylase is brought about through changes in the activity of phosphorylase kinase. IMM, inner mitochondrial membrane

In this section we summarize first the recent progress in our understanding of the action of insulin on glucose transport, and in particular the extent to which it may be explained by the translocation of glucose transporters to the plasma membrane from an intracellular location. We then consider the means whereby insulin may alter the activity of intracellular proteins, with particular emphasis on glycogen synthase and pyruvate dehydrogenase. The action of insulin on these two enzymes is of special interest because their dephosphorylation and activation is most easily observed under basal conditions (i.e. in the absence of other hormones) when there are typically no detectable changes in cAMP levels and dephosphorylation occurs at sites that are probably not phosphorylated by cAMP-dependent protein kinase. By contrast, the dephosphorylation of the other proteins can be explained, at least in part, by a decrease in the activity of cAMP-dependent protein kinase secondary to a lowering of the concentration of cAMP. Such effects of insulin are usually only evident when cell cAMP concentrations are first elevated by other hormones such as glucagon or β-adrenergic agonists. Examples in carbohydrate metabolism include phosphorylase kinase (and hence phosphorylase), pyruvate kinase and fructose 2,6-bisphosphate kinase. The mechanisms whereby insulin lowers intracellular cAMP under such conditions are of considerable relevance to an understanding of insulin actions in general and are discussed later in this chapter.

Glucose Transport

The entry of glucose into most mammalian cells is mediated by an integral membrane transport protein through a facilitated diffusion mechanism. However, in only two mammalian tissues—muscle and adipose tissue—is glucose uptake acutely regulated by insulin. Most studies have been carried out using isolated fat cells prepared by collagenase digestion of adipose tissue, as these cells have proved more amenable to the detailed study of the mechanisms involved.

The elegant independent studies of Kono and Cushman and their respective co-workers have revealed that the binding of insulin to its receptor results in the rapid translocation of glucose transporter proteins from an apparently intracellular membrane location to the plasma membrane [7, 8]. Early studies involved the use of either the binding of cytochalasin B (a specific inhibitor of glucose transport) to glucose transporters in subcellular membrane fractions or the reconstitution of glucose transport activity derived from similar subcellular membrane fractions into artificial liposomes. This has been substantiated by the use of photochemical crosslinking of glucose transporters with [^{3}H]cytochalasin B or glucose analogues and the use of specific antisera for Western blotting and immunocytochemistry [9, 10, 107, 108]. The use of such antisera has also allowed the isolation and sequencing of the genes coding for the facilitative glucose transporters in mammalian tissues [11, 12]. There are at least six isoforms (Glut1–6) with distinct tissue distributions. In muscle and adipose tissue, the major isoform is Glut4 with a lesser amount of Glut1. In these tissues, insulin appears to be able to initiate the translocation of both isoforms [11–13]. The bulk of the insulin-mediated increase in transport, however, is due to translocation of the Glut4 isoform caused by an increase in externalization rather than internalization of the transporter [128].

In unstimulated fat cells, it appears that less than 5% of the total cellular complement of glucose transporters reside in the plasma membrane. Addition of insulin to cells markedly increases this number, with a concomitant decrease in the number of glucose transporters associated with the intracellular membrane compartment. This translocation event is energy-dependent, protein synthesis-independent, and occurs with a half-time of 2–3 min (Table 2). It explains earlier observations that under most conditions insulin increased the maximal rate of glucose transport into fat cells without having a major effect on the K_m [14]. Evidence for translocation has also been obtained in rat heart and diaphragm muscle [14]. However, translocation does not appear to account fully for the overall increase in glucose transport in fat cells, as the increase in plasma membrane-associated transporters is considerably less than the increase in glucose transport [14, 15].

Phorbol esters mimic the effects of insulin on translocation of glucose transporters to the plasma membrane of both rat fat cells and Swiss mouse 3T3-L1 cells [16]. However, although phorbol esters cause a translocation of equivalent magnitude even to that seen with insulin, they have a considerably smaller overall effect on glucose transport compared with insulin [16]. This strongly suggests that insulin (but not phorbol esters) is capable of inducing an increase in the inherent activity of glucose transporters once they are inserted into the plasma membrane. Such an increased activity might explain recent reports of decreases in K_m of the transporter for glucose [17], and that insulin, in the presence of cycloheximide, is capable of bringing about near-maximal stimulation of glucose transporters without increasing the number of transporters present in the plasma membrane [18].

An increase in the activity of glucose transporters once inserted in the plasma membrane could be brought about through their covalent modification by phosphorylation. However, so far no evidence has been found for any changes in phosphorylation of glucose transporters following exposure of cells to insulin [19]. However, okadaic acid, which is a potent and specific inhibitor of protein phosphatases 1 and 2A, stimulates glucose transport into both fat and muscle cells [109, 110], suggesting that some component of the system is regulated by reversible phosphorylation.

Insulin also promotes the translocation of insulin-like growth factor II (IGF-II) receptors and transferrin receptors to the plasma membrane from an intracellular membrane compartment with similar characteristics to that which contains the insulin-sensitive pool of glucose transporters [20, 21]. The time-courses and extents of the translocations of glucose transporters, IGF-II receptors and transferrin receptors are also broadly similar (Table 2). By contrast, insulin promotes the translocation of occupied insulin receptors from the plasma membrane to an 'endocytic' subcellular membrane compartment. The half-maximal response of this internalization closely parallels that of the binding of

Table 2 Effects of insulin on the distribution of fat-cell membrane proteins. The table indicates the approximate time-courses and half-maximal responses to insulin of the listed proteins. Class I represents proteins that move out of the plasma membrane to an intracellular membrane fraction in response to insulin. Class II proteins move in the opposite direction

Class	Protein	Time-course of response		ED_{50} for insulin
		$t_{1/2}$	Steady state	
I	Insulin receptor	2–3 min	5–10 min	3 nmol/l
II	Glucose transporter	2–3 min	10 min	0.1 nmol/l
	IGF-II receptor	1 min	10 min	0.1 nmol/l
	Transferrin receptor	<2 min	2 min	1 nmol/l

insulin to its receptor [22]. However, the response to insulin of the translocation of glucose transporters and IGF-II receptors is shifted an order of magnitude to the left of insulin binding (Table 2), suggesting that the mechanisms involved differ. There are also large differences in the numbers involved. It can be calculated that the binding of insulin to about 2000 receptors per fat cell is sufficient to cause the translocation of more than one million glucose transporters.

Major questions remain to be answered regarding the relationships between all these translocation events in both spatial and mechanistic terms. Some progress has been made with identifying some of the other components of the Glut4-rich intracellular vesicles [12, 129].

Glycogen Synthase

Insulin activates rabbit muscle glycogen synthase through stimulating its dephosphorylation on specific serine residues termed 3a, b, c (or C30, C34, C38) and, perhaps, C42 plus N7 [3, 4, 23–26] and it is in this tissue that the enzyme has been most extensively studied. Insulin has also been shown to activate glycogen synthase through an apparently similar dephosphorylation mechanism in both rat adipocytes [3, 24] and rat diaphragm [3, 25].

Glycogen synthase can be phosphorylated on nine serines by at least seven distinct protein kinases. In the resting state, the enzyme contains about 3 moles of phosphate per mole of enzyme shared between the various phosphorylation sites. Agents such as adrenaline and glucagon, which promote increases in cAMP concentrations, inhibit glycogen synthase activity through increasing the phosphorylation state of sites 3a, b, c, together with two further sites (1a, b).

Sites 3a, b, c are phosphorylated by a cAMP- and Ca^{2+}-independent protein kinase known as GSK-3 and dephosphorylated mainly by protein phosphatase 1. It can be argued, therefore, that insulin could act through inhibition of GSK-3, activation of protein phosphatase 1 or a combination of these events [4, 24]. Present evidence, largely from the laboratory of Philip Cohen, suggests that both mechanisms may operate [4, 27–31].

Glycogen particles from skeletal muscle contain phosphatase-1 which is composed of a catalytic subunit complexed with a glycogen binding (G) subunit. Phosphorylation of the G-subunit on a particular site (site 1) increases the ability of the phosphatase to act on glycogen synthase and hence activate the enzyme [4, 27, 112]. The extent of phosphorylation of this site in rabbit skeletal muscle has been shown to be increased following administration of insulin to the animals and further studies have shown that the site can be phosphorylated by an insulin-activated kinase known as p90^{rsk} (or

MAPKAPK-1). In turn this kinase can be activated by another insulin-activated kinase called MAP-kinase, as first demonstrated by Sturgill et al (reviewed in [84]).

In earlier studies, no evidence was obtained of any inhibition of GSK-3 in skeletal muscle following administration of insulin to rabbits [4, 27]. However, in more recent studies, Welsh and Proud [130] showed that insulin decreased the activity of GSK-3 in CHO cells and subsequently decreases have also been observed in a rat skeletal muscle cell line L6 and in the skeletal muscle of insulin-treated rabbits [30]. The effects of insulin are reversed by treatment of partially purified GSK-3 with protein phosphatase 2A [130], suggesting that the decrease in activity involves changes in phosphorylation of GSK-3. A search for the kinase involved has indicated that it is likely to be p90^{rsk} [31, 111].

Activation of MAP-kinase and hence p90^{rsk} may therefore result in the dephosphorylation of glycogen synthase through activation of phosphatase-1 and/or inhibition of GSK-3. This is summarized in Figure 5 and will be discussed later together with the role of the other insulin-activated protein kinases.

An alternative view is that of Larner and colleagues who have argued that insulin acts through low molecular weight mediators released at the plasma membrane, which not only stimulate phosphatase activity but may also inhibit cAMP-dependent protein kinase activity [131]. Similar substances may also be involved in the regulation of pyruvate dehydrogenase, cAMP phosphodiesterase and other intracellular effects of insulin and are discussed further in the following section.

Pyruvate Dehydrogenase

Once pyruvate is converted to acetyl-CoA by this exclusively intramitochondrial enzyme complex, there is no means in mammals whereby the acetyl-CoA can be used for the resynthesis of glucose. The enzyme must, therefore, be under exact control and, in particular, during starvation the enzyme must be greatly inhibited to conserve the restricted reserves of carbohydrate. Regulation of the enzyme is achieved in part by end-product inhibition by acetyl-CoA and NADH and in part by reversible phosphorylation [32, 33]. The phosphorylated form of the enzyme is essentially inactive [32, 33].

Exposure to insulin of tissues such as adipose tissue and mammary gland results in the rapid activation of pyruvate dehydrogenase where the complex has an essentially biosynthetic role (since much of the acetyl-CoA formed is used for the synthesis of fatty acids). Such short-term effects are not found in muscle and CNS, where pyruvate dehydrogenase has essentially a catabolic role as the acetyl-CoA formed is mainly oxidized via the citrate cycle to CO_2. Most studies have been concerned with the means whereby insulin causes a twofold to threefold increase in activity in rat epididymal fat cells [34]. The increase in activity persists during the preparation and subsequent incubation of intact mitochondria and this property has greatly facilitated investigations into the mechanism involved. In particular, it has allowed good evidence to be obtained that the effect of insulin is brought about by the activation of pyruvate dehydrogenase phosphatase rather than inhibition of the kinase. However, no changes in phosphatase activity are detectable in extracts of mitochondria from insulin-treated tissue. This suggests that insulin may cause a change in the concentration of some effector of the phosphatase within mitochondria which then dissociates from the phosphatase during the preparation of extracts [34].

The activity of the phosphatase is known to be regulated by Ca^{2+}, Mg^{2+} and possibly changes in the $NADH : NAD^+$ ratio, but there is considerable evidence that insulin does not alter the activity of the phosphatase through changes in these particular regulators [34, 35]. For example, the effect of insulin still persists within mitochondria made permeable to Mg^{2+} or Ca^{2+} by incubation with A23187, or to all substances up to a molecular weight of 1000–2000 by treatment with toluene. Further studies of the persistent effect of insulin in these permeabilized mitochondria have shown that insulin causes an increase in the sensitivity of pyruvate dehydrogenase phosphatase to Mg^{2+} with little effect apparent on the maximum velocity [34].

Spermine has a similar effect on purified preparations of pyruvate dehydrogenase phosphatase. However, it is unlikely that insulin acts by increasing the concentration of spermine in the appropriate cell compartments because the cell content of spermine would appear to be too high to have a conventional second messenger role and insulin appears to have little or no short-term effect on the amount of spermine in mitochondria [35].

The simplest explanation of these observations on pyruvate dehydrogenase would appear to be that insulin causes a change in the concentration of a spermine-like compound in mitochondria. However, the persistence of the activation in toluene-permeabilized mitochondria suggests that the compound is probably not small. An attractive explanation would be that insulin may promote some change in the interactions between the pyruvate dehydrogenase system and the inner mitochondrial membrane [34, 35]. However, such an explanation is not easily reconciled with the proposal of Jarett [36] that the activation of pyruvate dehydrogenase by insulin involves a low molecular weight mediator apparently similar to that proposed by Larner

to be involved in the activation of glycogen synthase. This putative mediator was first proposed following the demonstration that addition of insulin to fat cell plasma membranes resulted in formation of a low molecular weight factor that was capable of increasing pyruvate dehydrogenase activity when added to fat cell mitochondria. The mediator appears to act by stimulating the phosphatase but characterization has been difficult. One reason for this may be the assay systems used, which would appear to be far from optimal (see reference 34).

So far we have been concerned with the mechanism whereby insulin activates pyruvate dehydrogenase activities within a few minutes. This effect of insulin appears to be restricted to tissues that carry out fatty acid synthesis and is exerted through a stimulation of the phosphatase. Insulin also has important long-term effects on the pyruvate dehydrogenase system, exerted through changes in the activity of the kinase, and these have been extensively studied by Randle, Kerbey and colleagues [37–40]. Starvation or experimental diabetes decreases the proportion of the active, non-phosphorylated form of the complex to very low levels in heart and most other tissues. These effects are of great importance in effectively blocking carbohydrate oxidation. They can be reversed over 1–2 days *in vivo* by glucose refeeding or insulin treatment, respectively. It is now clear that long-term insulin deficiency results in a substantial increase in the activity of pyruvate dehydrogenase kinase [37–40]. Studies involving culture of rat hepatocytes or cardiac myocytes have shown that the increase in kinase activity may involve a combination of an increase in cell cyclic AMP and in fatty acid oxidation. The detailed mechanisms involved are still unclear but the result is an increase in the specific activity of the kinase rather than changes in the amount [37, 38].

EFFECTS OF INSULIN ON LIPID METABOLISM

Probing the molecular basis of insulin action on lipid metabolism has been dogged to some extent by the practical problems confronting the researcher in this area. In contrast to carbohydrate metabolism, which generally involves the interconversion of water-soluble intermediates by enzymes that are probably free in the cell cytoplasm or within the mitochondrial matrix, lipid metabolism involves hydrophobic intermediates and many membrane-bound enzymes which are often very difficult to study *in vitro*.

The major acute effects of the hormone are summarized in Table 3. The overall effect is undoubtedly to increase fatty acid synthesis and the storage of fatty acids as triacylglycerol, especially in adipose tissue. In

Table 3 Principal acute effects of insulin on lipid metabolism

Process	Effect	Tissue	Mechanisms involved
Fatty acid synthesis	Increase	F, L, MT	Activation and increased phosphorylation of acetyl-CoA carboxylase (step 8)
Fatty acid oxidation	Decrease	L, (F)	Inhibition of carnitine acyltransferase (steps 12 and 13)
Triacylglycerol synthesis	Increase	F, (L, M)	Stimulation of esterification of glycerol phosphate (step 16)
Triacylglycerol breakdown*	Decrease	F	Dephosphorylation of triacylglycerol lipase (step 19)
Cholesterol synthesis	Increase	L, (F)	Activation and dephosphorylation of HMG-CoA reductase
Cholesterol ester breakdown	Decrease (?)	(L, F)	Dephosphorylation of cholesterol esterase (?)
Phospholipid metabolism	Various	(all)	See text

The changes listed under 'mechanisms involved' are not necessarily complete.
Step numbers are those indicated in Figures 2 and 3.
F, white and brown adipose tissue; M, muscle; L, liver; MT, mammary tissue.
*This effect is not usually apparent unless tissue cAMP levels are increased by the presence of another hormone.

addition, the hormone may also promote cholesterol synthesis and cholesterol ester storage and have some important effects on phospholipid metabolism. Insulin undoubtedly has longer-term effects involving changes in gene expression which result in alterations in the concentration of specific enzymes involved. The best established is the parallel induction of the enzymes that bring about fatty acid synthesis, namely ATP-citrate lyase, acetyl-CoA carboxylase and fatty acid synthase.

Fatty Acid Synthesis

In mammals, the principal sites of fatty acid synthesis are white and brown adipose tissue, liver and lactating mammary gland. Insulin stimulates fatty acid synthesis in all four tissues within a few minutes but the greatest proportional effects are observed in the adipose tissue of rats and mice fed a high-carbohydrate diet. In contrast, hormones that increase cellular cAMP levels, such as β-adrenergic agonists and glucagon, cause a marked decrease in fatty acid synthesis in adipose tissue and liver in particular [41, 42]. All these changes in fatty acid synthesis appear to be brought about largely through changes in the activity of acetyl-CoA carboxylase, although alterations in rates of glucose transport and pyruvate dehydrogenase may also be important as these determine the rate of supply of acetyl-CoA (Figure 2).

Acetyl-CoA Carboxylase

It is well established that exposure of rat epididymal fat cells to insulin leads to a twofold to threefold increase in enzyme activity, and that this increase is associated both with a greater proportion of the enzyme occurring in its more active polymerized form and with increased phosphorylation of the enzyme [41–43]. This phosphorylation probably occurs on at least two different sites on the enzyme. One site (referred to as the I-site) was first identified by Brownsey and Denton [44] and exhibits a threefold to fivefold increase in

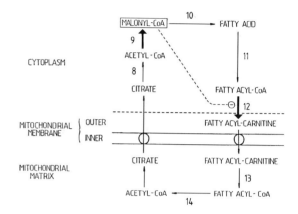

Figure 2 Compartmentation and interrelationships between the pathways of fatty acid synthesis and fatty acid oxidation. The major enzymes involved are: (8) ATP-citrate lyase; (9) acetyl-CoA carboxylase; (10) fatty acid synthase; (11) fatty acyl-CoA synthetase; (12) carnitine palmitoyl transferase I; (13) carnitine palmitoyl transferase II. Step 14 represents β-oxidation

phosphorylation with insulin. It has been demonstrated that after purification from extracts of insulin-treated tissue a greater proportion of the enzyme was present in an active polymerized form, which exhibited a high degree of phosphorylation within the tryptic peptide containing the I-site [41, 43]. The other site, which exhibits a smaller increase in phosphorylation, has been sequenced and contains a serine residue which is also phosphorylated by purified casein kinase 2 *in vitro* [42, 45]. These sites of phosphorylation are quite distinct from the sites phosphorylated by cAMP-dependent protein kinase (and other kinases) which result in inhibition of enzyme activity [42, 45]. What is a matter of some debate is whether the undoubted increases in phosphorylation of acetyl-CoA carboxylase promoted by insulin lead directly to its increased activity. The activity of casein kinase 2 has been shown to be increased by insulin in fat cells [113] but phosphorylation of the enzyme by casein kinase 2 does not appear to alter the activity of the enzyme [42]. On the other hand, another insulin-activated acetyl-CoA carboxylase kinase has been separated from rat epididymal adipose tissue which appears to phosphorylate the enzyme within the I-peptide with a concomitant increase in activity [46, 47].

ATP-Citrate Lyase

ATP-citrate lyase, which catalyses the step immediately preceding that catalysed by acetyl-CoA carboxylase in fatty acid synthesis, also exhibits marked increases in phosphorylation following exposure of fat and other cells to insulin. The role of this phosphorylation is an enigma. Hormones that increase the cell content of cyclic AMP, such as glucagon and β-adrenergic agonists, cause comparable increases in phosphorylation of the enzyme on precisely the same serine but have the opposite effect to insulin on fatty acid synthesis [48]. No regulatory role for this phosphorylation has been found, beyond a small change in ATP affinity [49] and a possible subcellular redistribution [50].

Increases and decreases in ATP-citrate lyase kinase activity are evident in the supernatant fractions of fat cells previously exposed to insulin [46, 132]. The activated kinase has not been well characterized but it phosphorylates the major site phosphorylated in fat cells exposed to insulin. The inhibited kinase phosphorylates a different site and has turned out to be GSK-3 [132]. The physiological role of the phosphorylation of ATP-citrate lyase by either kinase is a mystery.

Fatty Acid Oxidation

Effects of insulin on the oxidation of fatty acids have not been extensively studied. Inhibition of fatty acid oxidation is evident in noradrenaline-stimulated brown fat cells. In the liver, insulin can reverse the increases observed both with glucagon and with starvation or experimental diabetes [51]. These increases are thought to be due, at least in part, to changes in the activity of carnitine palmitoyl transferase I (CPT-I; see Figure 2). This enzyme is located on the outer membrane of mitochondria and represents the first step in the system that allows the transfer of long-chain acyl groups into mitochondria for β-oxidation. Important determinants of its activity are probably the concentration of its substrate (long-chain fatty acyl-CoA esters) and of malonyl-CoA which, via binding to an apparently distinct regulatory binding site, is a potent inhibitor. Effects of insulin are likely to involve a combination of a lowering in fatty acyl-CoA esters secondary to a diminished supply of fatty acids (e.g. from lipolysis) as well as an increase in the concentration of malonyl-CoA. The concentration of malonyl-CoA changes broadly in parallel with rates of fatty acid synthesis and hence any increase in the

rate of fatty acid synthesis caused by insulin is likely to be associated with an increase in malonyl-CoA and hence inhibition of CPT-I [51].

It is now becoming increasingly evident that further mechanisms of control of CPT-I probably occur. In particular, fasting and experimental diabetes result in a marked increase in sensitivity to malonyl-CoA and this may be reversed by insulin in less than 2 hours [52]. The mechanisms underlying these changes in sensitivity have not been established. They may involve rapid changes in protein synthesis, but it seems more likely that some covalent modification of existing CPT-I and/or its malonyl-CoA binding regulatory subunit is involved.

Triacylglycerol Synthesis and Breakdown

The promotion of triacylglycerol storage in fat and to a lesser extent in liver cells is one of the most important of the actions of insulin. The hormone has effects on both the synthetic (esterification) and breakdown (lipolysis) pathways.

Triacylglycerol Synthesis

The pathway of triacylglycerol synthesis is given in Figure 3. All the enzymes involved are associated to varying extents with intracellular membranes, including the endoplasmic reticulum and the outer mitochondrial membrane. Considerable difficulties have been encountered in the assay, purification and characterization of the enzymes; hence, knowledge of the mechanisms involved in their short-term regulation by insulin and other hormones is very incomplete. Insulin stimulates the rate of glycerol phosphate esterification in fat cells by up to tenfold within minutes, whereas the effect on liver, at least with *in vitro* preparations, is rather modest and certainly less than twofold. These stimulated rates may be due in part to increase

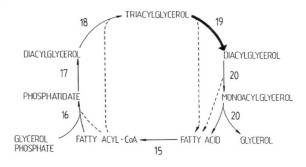

Figure 3 Pathways of triacylglycerol synthesis (esterification) and breakdown (lipolysis). The major enzymes involved are: (15) fatty acyl-CoA synthetase; (16) glycerol 3-phosphate acyltransferase; (17) phosphatidate phosphohydrolase; (18) diacyglycerol acyltransferase; (19) triacylglycerol lipase; (20) monoacylglycerol lipase

in glycerol phosphate concentration [53], but this is unlikely to be the entire explanation. For example, insulin causes a twofold to threefold increase in triacylglycerol synthesis without affecting glycerol phosphate levels in rat epididymal adipose tissue incubated with adrenaline [53].

There appears to be little evidence of any change in the activity of any enzymes in this pathway induced by insulin in the absence of other hormones, although under these conditions insulin causes substantial increases in esterification, especially in fat cells. However, in fat cells noradrenaline can cause marked reductions in the activity of fatty acyl-CoA synthetase, glycerol phosphate acyltransferase and phosphatidate phosphohydrolase, and these are reversed rapidly by insulin [54]. The activities of these same enzymes are also diminished in streptozotocin-induced diabetes, but insulin is only able to reverse these effects after 2 hours [54].

The mechanisms involved in these effects of insulin are poorly understood. It appears unlikely that glycerol phosphate acyltransferase is regulated by reversible phosphorylation.

Lipolysis

The short-term regulation of lipolysis, at least in adipose tissue, is better understood than that of esterification, but a number of important problems still remain. The rate-limiting step is the first reaction catalysed by triacylglycerol lipase (TG-lipase; see Figure 3), and regulation of this enzyme is the major means whereby lipolysis is controlled by insulin and other hormones. The release of fatty acids from fat cells appears to involve a specific plasma membrane carrier system which may also be a site of potential hormonal control.

Insulin has little effect on basal rates of lipolysis from fat cells but reverses the stimulation caused by counter-regulatory hormones such as adrenaline, ACTH and glucagon, which increase the cellular content of cAMP. The counter-regulatory hormones appear to lead to the activation of this enzyme through its phosphorylation (probably on a single serine) by cAMP-dependent protein kinase [55]. In general, increases in phosphorylation within intact cells correlate well with increases in lipolysis. The effect of insulin is to reverse this increased phosphorylation of the enzyme and hence to diminish the rate of lipolysis [55]. Under many conditions, the insulin-stimulated decreases in lipolysis correlate well with decreases in activity of cAMP-dependent protein kinase [55] and hence are presumably brought about by decreases in cAMP concentrations (see later discussion). However, there are conditions where the inhibition of lipolysis by insulin cannot be fully explained in terms of the

effects of the hormone on cAMP concentrations. For example, an extensive and careful study showed that in more highly stimulated cells the effect of insulin on lipolysis was substantially greater than that appropriate for the inhibition of cAMP-dependent protein kinase activity [56]. One explanation of these observations is that insulin may also be increasing protein phosphatase activity, so enhancing the dephosphorylation of TG-lipase. Direct evidence for such a stimulation is lacking, but it could also explain the dephosphorylation of other key enzymes such as phosphorylase kinase, pyruvate kinase and glycogen synthase, as discussed earlier in this chapter.

Metabolism of Other Lipids

Cholesterol Metabolism

The effects of insulin on cholesterol synthesis and its storage in cells as cholesterol esters have not been extensively studied, but a number of interesting analogies can be made with the effects of insulin on fatty acid synthesis and triacylglycerol storage [133].

Insulin stimulates cholesterol synthesis, at least in rat liver, and this effect is reversed by glucagon. There is a marked diurnal cycle of changes in rates of both cholesterol and fatty acid synthesis in the livers of fed rats and it seems likely that these parallel changes are the result of changes in the insulin:glucagon ratio. Regulation of cholesterol synthesis appears to be exerted mainly by hydroxymethylglutaryl-CoA reductase (HMG-CoA reductase). It is well established both *in vitro* and *in vivo* that insulin results in activation of the enzyme, probably through dephosphorylation, and that this is reversed by glucagon [57].

There is mounting evidence that cholesterol esterase, the enzyme that controls the breakdown of cholesterol ester, is very similar (if not identical) to TG-lipase [58]. Certainly, like TG-lipase, the enzyme is phosphorylated and activated by cAMP-dependent protein kinase [55] and hence, under appropriate conditions, it is to be expected that exposure of tissues to insulin will lead to decreases in rates of cholesterol ester breakdown.

Phosphoinositol Metabolism

Phosphatidic acid is an intermediate in the synthesis of both storage triacylglycerol and phospholipids (Figure 4). Phosphatidylcholine, phosphatidylethanolamine and phosphatidylserine are important structural components of biological membranes. The polyphosphoinositides (PI, PIP and PIP$_2$; see legend to Figure 4 for definition of abbreviations) are also crucial precursors of the inositol phosphates (IP, IP$_2$ and IP$_3$) and diacylglycerol, which are, in turn, involved as second

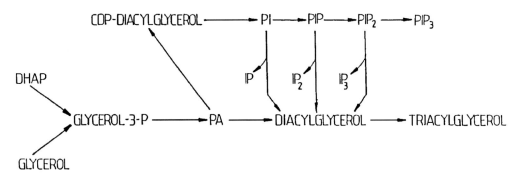

Figure 4 Relationship between the pathways of phospholipid and triacylglycerol synthesis. Abbreviations: phosphatidylinositol, PI; phosphatidylinositol phosphate, PIP; phosphatidylinositol bisphosphate, PIP$_2$; phosphatidylinositol triphosphate, PIP$_3$ inositol phosphate, IP; inositol bisphosphate, IP$_2$; inositol trisphosphate, IP$_3$; dihydroxyacetone phosphate, DHAP; phosphatidic acid, PA

messengers in the actions of several hormones. The hydrolysis of PIP$_2$ by a phospholipase C yields two products, inositol trisphosphate (IP$_3$) and diacylglycerol (DAG) [59]. IP$_3$ is now known to promote a rise in cytosolic Ca^{2+} by mediating Ca^{2+} release from intracellular stores. DAG is an activator of protein kinase C and is thus thought to have a pivotal role in the action of several hormones, growth factors and phorbol esters through regulation of protein phosphorylation. Increasing attention, therefore, has been focused in recent years on the role of phospholipids in insulin action (see reference 60).

Insulin appears to increase the synthesis *de novo* of phosphatidic acid, phosphatidylethanolamine, PI, PIP, PIP$_2$ and PIP$_3$, at least in some cells.

There are conflicting reports as to the effect of insulin on the breakdown of PIP$_2$ (or of the other polyphosphoinositides) and thus rises in IP$_3$ levels (or of the other inositol phosphates) [61]. However, although small transient elevations in IP, IP$_2$ and IP$_3$ levels in rat epididymal fat pads and insulin-stimulated phospholipase C activity have been reported, the great body of evidence suggests that insulin does not cause any general increase in cytosolic Ca^{2+} levels. It remains possible that insulin-stimulated rises in PI, PIP and PIP$_2$ levels are simply a reflection of increased phosphatidic acid synthesis.

What is much more certain is that insulin activates phosphatidylinositol 3-kinase (PtdIns 3-kinase), as do many growth factors, and that this could be a central element in the insulin signalling system [114]. The mechanism of this action is discussed in a later section.

EFFECTS OF INSULIN ON TRANSCRIPTION AND TRANSLATION

Insulin increases the overall rate of protein synthesis in many tissues. This effect appears to be mainly exerted through increases in the initiation phase of translation of mRNA by ribosomes. However, as well as this general effect, insulin also regulates the synthesis of many individual proteins. We have already given a number of examples of such enzymes in carbohydrate and lipid metabolism. These longer-term effects of insulin arise mainly from alterations in the level of the mRNA itself due to changes in the rate of transcription of the corresponding gene.

Transcription

The advances in molecular cloning techniques made during the late 1970s and early 1980s have led to the isolation of an ever-increasing number of genes. This in turn has provided the necessary methodology to examine the molecular mechanisms underlying transcriptional control.

Insulin can both increase and decrease the levels of specific mRNAs for a considerable number of enzymes and secretory proteins, and proteins involved in reproduction (Table 4). Many examples of this phenomenon have come from rat liver, but studies have recently turned to the use of cells in tissue culture where long-term experiments can be performed and the molecular mechanisms underlying transcription can be more easily examined [65] (see also Chapter 23).

In many cases *in vivo*, insulin has been shown to reverse the effects of experimental diabetes; however, insulin is capable of having a direct effect on mRNA levels in tissues from normal animals, either alone or when added with a permissive factor such as dexamethasone (see Table 4). The effects of insulin in many of these systems appear to occur directly through the insulin rather than through the insulin-like growth factor I receptor. In some cases, such as fatty acid synthase, acetyl-CoA carboxylase and liver pyruvate kinase the effect of insulin appears to be secondary to the stimulation of glucose metabolism. In other cases, such as glucokinase, phosphoenolpyruvate carboxykinase and c-fos induction, the effect

Table 4 Insulin-induced changes in specific mRNA levels

Change	Tissue	Specific mRNAs
Increase	Liver	Glucokinase, glucose-6-phosphate dehydrogenase, pyruvate kinase, fatty acid synthase*, malic enzyme*, tyrosine aminotransferase, $\alpha2\mu$-globulin, p33, albumin†, c-fos, c-myc, acetyl-CoA carboxylase
	Fat	Glyceraldehyde-3-phosphate dehydrogenase, glycerol-3-phosphate dehydrogenase, pyruvate carboxylase*, c-fos
	Mammary gland	Casein*
	Pancreas	Amylase
	Chick oviduct	Ovalbumin*
Decrease	Liver	Phospho-enol-pyruvate carboxykinase, carbamoyl phosphate synthetase*

*Indicates that insulin only has an effect in the presence of a 'permissive' factor.
†Decreases have also been demonstrated.

of insulin is glucose-independent and thus more direct [65, 69].

The time-courses of the effects of insulin vary considerably. For example, insulin causes a transient increase in c-fos mRNA levels with levels peaking at 15 min and returning to basal after 60 min [62]. Tyrosine aminotransferase mRNA levels also peaked at 15 min but remained elevated at 5 hours [63]. In contrast, the effect of insulin can often take several hours to become apparent [64].

The changes in mRNA levels for phosphoenol-pyruvate carboxykinase [66], tyrosine amino-transferase [63], albumin [64], c-fos [67] and glucokinase [68] appear to be brought about through changes in the rate of gene transcription. This has been shown through the use of the transcript elongation assay, in which nuclei isolated from control or insulin-treated tissues are incubated with radiolabelled nucleotides and the level of incorporation into specific mRNAs is assessed by hybridization with a complementary DNA probe.

Clearly, an important goal is the identification of the factors involved in the binding to the response elements which are often located upstream of the initiation site and regulate gene transcription. Some progress has been made in characterizing both the nucleotide sequences involved and the protein transcription factors which bind to the sequences [69]. In general, little is known about the mechanisms which regulate the transcription factors but it seems likely that changes in phosphorylation will prove to be important. This is now only well established for two transcription factors (p62[TCF]/Elk-1 and c-Jun) which interact with the 'serum-response element' (SRE) and the 'TPA-response element' (TRE) respectively. These elements are found in the promoters of a number of different genes mainly associated with growth; both are present in the promoter for the c-fos gene [70, 71]. The activities of the two transcription factors involved are altered following phosphorylation by a number of different protein kinases. In particular, phosphorylation by MAP-kinase increases the transcriptional activity of both factors and this may be the mechanism whereby

insulin (and growth factors) cause the rapid induction of c-fos. It needs to be emphasized that the long-term effects of insulin on the various metabolic enzymes listed in Table 4 do not appear to involve these particular transcription factors as the promoter regions for the relevant genes do not contain TRE or SRE.

Translation

Increases in protein synthesis in tissues and cells exposed to insulin (or growth factors) are associated with rapid increases in the proportion of ribosomes bound to mRNA to form active polysomes. This indicates that the major effect of insulin and growth factors is exerted at the initiation stage of translation. However, a single site of action is unlikely as these hormones not only cause a general increase in mRNA translation but also cause selective increases in the translation of particular mRNAs—especially those encoding growth-related proteins [72]. In the last few years evidence has been obtained that three different sites may be involved and these will be discussed in turn.

It has been known for more than 10 years that there is a substantial increase in the phosphorylation of the S6 protein (which is a component of the small 40S subunit of ribosomes) under conditions of increased protein synthesis including stimulation by insulin. It has proved difficult to establish how S6 phosphorylation might influence mRNA translation, but recent evidence indicates that phosphorylation of S6 may allow the binding and selective translation of a family of mRNAs which are characterized by having a polypyrimidine tract close to their 5' cap [73]. Many mRNAs with polypyrimidine tracts encode for ribosomal proteins and thus this in turn may result in a general increase in protein synthesis. Two types of kinases have been implicated in bringing about the increased phosphorylation of S6. These kinases are p70[S6k] and p90[rsk]. Both readily phosphorylate S6 *in vitro* and both are activated by insulin and growth factors [74]. Considerable evidence now indicates that the increased phosphorylation of S6 in intact cells

(a)

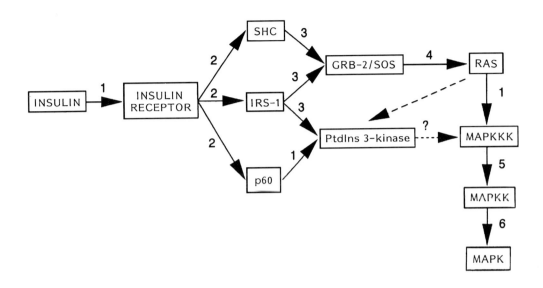

(b)

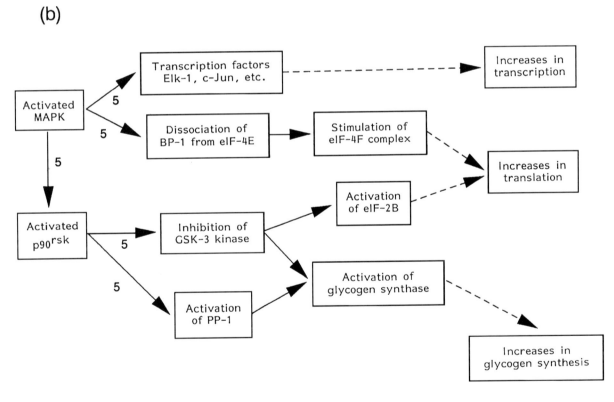

Figure 5 (a) Possible links between the insulin receptor and the activation of MAP kinase. (b) Possible links between activated MAP-kinase and transcription, translation and the regulation of glycogen synthesis. Interactions are: 1, binding; 2, tyrosine phosphorylation; 3, binding through SH2 domains; 4, guanine nucleotide exchange (on Ras); 5, serine/threonine phosphorylation; 6, threonine/tyrosine phosphorylation

treated with insulin is largely if not exclusively brought about by p70^{S6k} rather than p90^{rsk} [72]. As mentioned in a previous section the role of p90^{rsk} may be largely in the regulation of glycogen synthase. The activation of p70^{S6k} by insulin is known to be brought about by phosphorylation but the kinase involved has not been identified and is not MAP-kinase. On the other hand, MAP-kinase is implicated in the other two regulatory mechanisms through which insulin might activate protein synthesis.

Initiation of protein synthesis requires the binding of Met-tRNA to the ribosome and this in turn involves eIF-2GTP. In the subsequent formation of the 80S initiation complex, eIF-2GDP is released which cannot bind Met-tRNA and therefore GDP on eIF-2 must be exchanged for GTP before Met-tRNA binding can again occur [72]. This exchange is catalysed by eIF-2B. Recently, it has been shown that insulin and growth factors can enhance the activity of eIF-2B and a possible mechanism is through a decrease in the phosphorylation of this translation factor caused by the inhibition of GSK-3 [75]. As mentioned earlier in the context of the regulation of glycogen synthase, insulin and growth factors bring about the inhibition of GSK-3, probably through its phosphorylation by p90^{rsk}, which in turn is activated by phosphorylation by MAP-kinase. The possible links involved are illustrated in Figure 5.

Cytosolic mRNAs in eukaryotic cells are 'capped' at the extreme 5′-end with 7-methyl guanosine. This cap structure is bound by eIF-4E which is part of a complex of initiation factors termed eIF-4F. The binding of this complex to the mRNA is thought to be involved in the mRNA scanning process which aligns the 40S ribosomal subunit with the initiation codon [76]. The cap-binding and scanning processes provide the potential for general control of the translation of all mRNAs as well as control of the translation of specific mRNAs [76]. A protein termed eIF-4E BP-1 has been identified, initially on the basis of its ability to bind eIF-4E [134]. This protein had been recognized earlier as a target for insulin-stimulated phosphorylation [135–137]. It has now become evident that binding of this protein to eIF-4E inhibits translation of capped mRNA and that its phosphorylation in insulin stimulated cells is associated with decreased binding to eIF-4E. The stimulation of translation by insulin may thus involve, in part, the release of eIF-4E from inhibition by BP-1. This protein has been shown to be phosphorylated *in vitro* by MAP-kinase [138] and this may result in the dissociation of BP-1 from eIF-4E and hence enhanced eIF-4F activity and increased mRNA translation (Figure 5).

MECHANISMS INVOLVED IN INSULIN ACTION

A full understanding of the molecular mechanisms by which insulin brings about the wide diversity of metabolic effects described in the first part of this chapter is one of the most important challenges in endocrinology. Most of the effects are observed within minutes. However, those involving changes in transcription and to some extent translation can take hours, if not days, before the long-term alterations in the concentration of specific proteins become fully established. Many of the effects of insulin are accompanied by changes in the phosphorylation state of serines and threonines on specific proteins. Examples of both increases and decreases in protein phosphorylation are listed in Table 5.

Table 5 Examples of proteins exhibiting changes in serine/threonine phosphorylation in intact cells exposed to insulin

Change in phosphorylation	Protein	Cell compartment	Tissue type
Increases	Acetyl-CoA carboxylase	Cytoplasm	F, L
	ATP-citrate lyase	Cytoplasm	F, L
	Insulin receptor	Plasma membrane	F, L
	cAMP-phosphodiesterase	Membrane-bound	F, L
	S6-ribosomal protein	Microsomes	F, L
	eIF-4E BP-1	Cytoplasm/ribosomes	F, L, M
Decreases	Glycogen synthase	Glycogen particles	F, L, M
	Phosphorylase*	Glycogen particles	F, L, M
	Phosphorylase kinase*	Glycogen particles	F, L, M
	Pyruvate kinase	Cytoplasm	L
	HMG-CoA reductase*	Microsomes	L
	Phenylalanine hydroxylase†	Cytoplasm	L
	Triglyceride lipase†	Triacylglycerol complex	F
	Pyruvate dehydrogenase	Mitochondria	F, L
	Inhibitor I†	Cytoplasm	F, L

Abbreviations: F, fat; L, liver; M, muscle
*Inferred from changes in activity.
†Indicates that the insulin effect is only apparent if cellular cAMP levels are previously elevated by another hormone.

Originally, it appeared that a common feature of the intracellular effects of insulin might be the dephosphorylation of regulatory enzymes in metabolism, such as glycogen synthase, pyruvate dehydrogenase, phosphorylase kinase and triglyceride lipase. As already discussed, in some cases, notably glycogen synthase and pyruvate dehydrogenase, insulin causes changes in dephosphorylation in the absence of changes in cAMP. In other cases, however, insulin can only promote dephosphorylation once cAMP levels and hence cAMP-dependent protein kinase activity have been previously elevated by other hormones, such as glucagon or β-adrenergic agonists (Table 5) [1]. It has been proposed that small molecular weight 'mediators' may be produced at the cell membrane following the binding of insulin to the cell surface receptors and that these 'mediators' may be responsible for the intracellular effects of insulin through their effects on protein phosphatase or cAMP phosphodiesterase activities [77, 78, 120]. The characterization of the putative mediators has proved difficult but it has been proposed that they may be phosphoinositol glycans released from plasma membrane-associated glycolipids by the action of a specific insulin-activated phospholipase C [78, 79]. Partially purified preparations of the phosphoinositol glycans have been reported to stimulate cAMP phosphodiesterase and pyruvate dehydrogenase phosphatase in subcellular fractions and to elicit a number of insulin-like actions including the stimulation of fat synthases and inhibition of lipolysis when added to intact cells [77–81]. However, to date it has not proved possible to define the structure of the putative mediators and there is considerable doubt about the extent to which such compounds play a role in the insulin signalling system [34]. It also seems likely that the glycolipid precursors will be orientated so that the proposed mediators would be released on the outside of cells although their effects would have to be exerted on intracellular targets [82].

In the last 10–15 years, the number of proteins found which exhibit increased phosphorylation on serine/threonine residues following exposure of cells to insulin has been growing rapidly. Important examples we have mentioned already are acetyl-CoA carboxylase, ATP-citrate lyase, ribosomal protein S6 and cAMP-phosphodiesterase (Table 5). Moreover, a number of different serine/threonine protein kinases have been found to be activated following exposure to insulin. Many of these kinases have also been mentioned in earlier sections, such as MAP kinases, casein kinase 2, p70^{S6k} and p90^{rsk}. A fuller list is given in Table 6. There is now substantial evidence that these kinases play important roles in the insulin signalling system and we discuss this further in the penultimate section of this chapter.

If MAP kinase and the other insulin activated kinases are a central component of the insulin signalling system, the obvious question arises as to how they could give rise to the decreases in protein phosphorylation which are certainly important in the metabolic effects of insulin. Three mechanisms can be envisaged [83]. These are that a primary activation of protein kinases can result in: (a) inhibition of a protein kinase; (b) activation of a protein phosphatase; (c) activation of cAMP phosphodiesterase. It is now becoming evident that all three mechanisms may play a role. Examples of mechanisms (a) and (b) have been suggested to be important in the regulation of glycogen synthase and protein synthesis (Figure 5). In the case of mechanism (c), it is well established that insulin activates a membrane-bound cAMP phosphodiesterase in fat and liver, which can result in a decrease in activity of cAMP-dependent protein kinase and hence decreases in the phosphorylation of triglyceride lipase, phosphorylase kinase and other proteins [84]. The activation of the phosphodiesterase is probably caused by an increase in phosphorylation, and evidence for an insulin-activated kinase which phosphorylates

Table 6 Examples of insulin-induced increases in serine- and threonine-specific protein kinase activities

Kinase	Alternative name (specific examples)	Substrates*
MAP kinase kinase kinase	MAPKKK (Raf-1, c-Mos)	MAP kinase kinase
MAP kinase kinase†	MAPKK, MEK (MAPKK-1, MAPKK-2)	MAP kinase
MAP kinase	MAPK (Erk-1, Erk-2)	Many (see Figure 5)
p90^{rsk}	p90 ribosomal S6 kinase, MAPKAPK-1,	PP-1 G-subunit/GSK-3
p70^{rsk}	p70/p85 S6 kinase	Ribosomal protein S6
Casein kinase 2	–	Many
Protein kinase C	–	Many
Insulin receptor kinase	IRSK	β-subunit of insulin receptor
ATP-citrate lyase kinase	–	ATP-citrate lyase
Acetyl-CoA carboxylase kinase	–	Acetyl-CoA carboxylase
cAMP phosphodiesterase kinase	–	cAMP-phosphodiesterase

*Most likely intracellular substrates are given. †This kinase phosphorylates MAP kinases at both threonine and tyrosine; all the other kinases appear to be specific for serines and threonines.

the appropriate phosphodiesterase has been obtained [84–86].

In the remainder of this chapter, we discuss first early events which follow directly from the activation of the tyrosine kinase activity of the insulin receptor, then the likely links between these events and the activated serine/threonine protein kinases, and finally summarize the possible roles of these kinases in the metabolic effects of insulin.

Insulin Receptor Tyrosine Kinase Activity and Early Events in the Insulin Signalling System

Without doubt the first event after the binding of insulin to the α subunit of its receptor is the activation of a protein kinase activity intrinsic to the receptor β subunit, which specifically phosphorylates tyrosine residues on both the β subunit itself and exogenous substrates. This aspect of insulin action is dealt with in more detail elsewhere in this book (see Chapter 21), but a number of important points are pertinent here.

The integrity of the protein tyrosine kinase activity of the insulin receptor appears to be essential for the effects of insulin [87, 88]. Furthermore, the activity of the tyrosine kinase may be decreased in insulin resistance and experimental diabetes [5, 89]. Activation of the tyrosine kinase of the intrinsic kinase domain of the insulin receptor results in autophosphorylation on at least five tyrosines within the intracellular part of the β-subunits [88]. Three of these sites are clustered together within the kinase domain and their phosphorylation is necessary for activation of the kinase towards other substrates [88, 90, 91]. A number of endogenous substrates which are likely to be involved in insulin signal transduction have been characterized. The most prominent and widespread is IRS-1 (insulin receptor substrate-1) [5, 92, 93]. The activated insulin receptor phosphorylates IRS-1 on several different tyrosines, forming binding sites for other proteins which contain SH2 domains (src homology 2 domain—a region of a protein which binds to specific domains on other proteins which contain phosphorylated tyrosine). These proteins include GRB-2 and phosphatidylinositol 3-kinase (PtdIns3-kinase) which are certainly central to the actions of insulin (Figure 5a) [5, 92, 93].

GRB-2 is a small adaptor protein which is strongly associated (through SH3 domains) to SOS ('son-of-sevenless'—a guanine nucleotide exchange factor which promotes the exchange of GTP for GDP on Ras, yielding activated Ras-GTP) [94]. Binding of GRB-2 to a specific phosphotyrosine-containing domain of IRS-1 probably brings SOS into conjunction with Ras which is located on the inner face of the plasma membrane.

The end result is an observed increase in the amount of Ras-GTP, and there is mounting evidence that this is important in bringing about a number of the effects of insulin, including a cascade of activated kinases leading to activated MAP kinase (see next section and Figure 5a) [93–96].

Binding of PtdIns3-kinase to IRS-1 results in the activation of the enzyme and one result is an increase in the product phosphatidylinositol (3,4,5) trisphosphate [96, 114]. Wortmannin, which is a potent and apparently specific inhibitor of the enzyme, blocks many of the effects of insulin, including the stimulation of glucose transport, glycogen synthase, phosphodiesterase and acetyl-CoA carboxylase [30, 86, 97, 98]. The stimulation of pyruvate dehydrogenase is one of the few metabolic effects of insulin which is not blocked by wortmannin [98]. It has been suggested that phosphatidylinositol (3,4,5) trisphosphate may activate a protein kinase such as protein kinase C zeta [99], and evidence has been obtained that PtdIns3-kinase itself is a protein kinase able to phosphorylate one of its subunits as well as IRS-1 [100].

IRS-1 is not absolutely necessary for the actions of insulin, since the hormone clearly acts in transgenic mice which lack IRS-1 [101]. However, these animals do show impaired intrauterine growth with evidence of some impaired glucose tolerance and insulin resistance. Alternative signalling pathways may include: (a) Shc, which, like IRS-1 can bind to GRB-2 and through SOS activate Ras [102]; (b), 60 kDa proteins which interact with PtdIns3-kinase [103]; (c), a protein tentatively called 'IRS-2' [101]. All these proteins are phosphorylated on tyrosines by the activated insulin receptor. A further complicating twist is that activated Ras can itself interact directly with the catalytic subunit of PtdIns3-kinase causing its stimulation [104]. Altogether there appears to be a web of pathways between the receptor on the one hand, and Ras and/or PtdIns3-kinase on the other.

Insulin Action Involves Cascades of Protein Kinases

Table 6 gives examples of serine/threonine specific protein kinases which are activated by insulin. In the case of MAP kinase (which may play a key role in insulin action) activation can be linked via a cascade of kinases initiated by the activation of Ras. We discuss this cascade system first, then a second cascade which involves p70^{S6k} and finally some of the other insulin-activated kinases which are not so well characterized.

MAP Kinase Cascade

A number of different isoforms of MAP kinases are found in mammalian cells [105]. Two members of the

MAP kinase family called Erk-1 and Erk-2 are very similar to each other, expressed in virtually all cells and activated by both insulin and many growth factors such as epidermal growth factor. The other members of the family do not appear to be activated by insulin and for the sake of simplicity MAP kinase in this chapter refers to Erk-1 plus Erk-2. The enzymes are essentially inactive when not phosphorylated; activation requires the phosphorylation of both threonine and tyrosine residues in the sequence—TEY—and is brought about by the dual-specificity MAP kinase kinase, MAPKK-1 and MAPKK-2 [106]. The MAP kinase kinases are in turn activated by phosphorylation on serine and threonine residues by MAP kinase kinase kinases (MAPKKK). These include Raf-1, c-mos and probably others. Raf-1 has been shown to be activated by insulin [30, 140]. Ras-GTP but not Ras-GDP has been shown to bind to Raf-1, but simple association of Raf-1 with Ras-GTP does not cause activation of Raf-1. Rather it seems likely that this binding may bring Raf-1 into juxtaposition with other components of a signalling complex associated with the plasma membrane [139]. One such component might be PtdIns3-kinase. Inhibition of PtdIns3-kinase activity by wortmannin blocks the activation of MAP kinase by insulin (Figure 5a) [30, 140].

The array of potential substrates for the MAP kinases is very extensive [6]. They include upstream components of the insulin signalling pathway to MAP kinase such as SOS and MAPKK-1, and this may be part of a complicated feedback inhibition system. Other major substrates of MAP kinases we have mentioned earlier in this chapter include transcription factors (such as c-Jun and Elk-1), p90^{rsk} and eIF-4E. As summarized in Figure 5b, and the relevant earlier sections, these phosphorylations may be important in the regulation of gene transcription, glycogen synthase activity and mRNA translation. Certainly the phosphorylations are known to occur in insulin-treated cells.

A difficulty arises with the possible role of MAP kinase in the regulation of glycogen synthase. In fat and liver cells, EGF also activates MAP kinase and, indeed, activates it to a greater extent than insulin, yet does not activate glycogen synthase [115, 116]. This would appear to suggest that an increase in MAP kinase is not sufficient to cause an increase in glycogen synthase activity and may even indicate that MAP kinase activation is not involved at all, at least in these two tissues. Alternatively, EGF may have an additional effect within the cells which may over-ride the effects of the activation of MAP kinase; EGF, but not insulin, activates phospholipase C gamma, which results in increases in cell calcium and protein kinase C activity and hence may cause compensating increases in phosphorylation of glycogen synthase.

p70^{S6k}/p85^{S6k} Cascade

This was one of the first protein kinases to be shown to be activated in cells exposed to insulin, and its major substrate appears to be the ribosomal protein S6. It occurs in cells as two alternative splice products of approximate molecular weights 70 and 85 kDa. Insulin and growth factors cause its activation through increasing the phosphorylation of the kinase on serine and threonine residues [117, 118]. This points to the involvement of another kinase kinase immediately upstream. The identity of this kinase is unknown but it appears to be involved in a signalling pathway from tyrosine kinase receptors which involves PtdIns3-kinase, as it is inhibited by wortmannin but apparently not Ras [119, 120]. The signalling pathway also contains the target of rapamycin (TOR). Rapamycin inhibits the activation of p70^{S6k}/p85^{S6k} and another component which is involved in the increased phosphorylation of S6 protein in cells exposed to insulin and growth factors. In contrast TOR is not part of the MAP kinase cascade as rapamycin is without effect on the activation of MAP kinase.

Other Insulin-activated Protein Kinases

Insulin-activated kinases which act on ATP-citrate lyase, acetyl-CoA carboxylase and cAMP phosphodiesterase have been discussed in earlier sections of this chapter. They appear to be fairly specific for their substrates but the molecular basis of their activation has not been established. The activation by insulin of casein kinase 2 has been shown in fat cells [121]. This enzyme has a number of potentially physiologically important substrates including IRS-1, acetyl-CoA carboxylase and eIF-4E, but direct evidence that it plays an important role in insulin signalling has yet to be obtained. The molecular basis of its activation is also a mystery—there is no evidence that it is activated by phosphorylation by any other kinases [122].

CONCLUSION

The links indicated in Figure 5a, b represent a plausible signalling system between the insulin receptor and three of the main effects of insulin—namely the activation of the transcription of some genes, mRNA translation and glycogen synthase. However, it must be emphasized that many of the effects of insulin are not explained by this system. These include the long-term effects of insulin on the transcription of genes encoding a number of important metabolic enzymes such as phosphoenolpyruvate carboxykinase and glucokinase, as well as the short-term effects of the hormone on glucose transport, pyruvate dehydrogenase, acetyl-CoA carboxylase and cAMP phosphodiesterase. The over-all signalling system for insulin has to be such that insulin brings about a whole range of different effects on the metabolism of fat, muscle, liver and other target cells. Some of these are markedly different from those of growth factors such as epidermal growth factor which also act via a tyrosine kinase receptor and activate the MAP kinase cascade. It seems likely that the MAP kinase cascade is, at least, involved in the growth-related effects of insulin such as c-fos induction and mRNA translation, since insulin and growth factors have similar effects on these processes.

There is mounting evidence that insulin acts through a number of different signalling pathways—some of which are not employed by growth factors. Some evidence in favour of a divergence between the mitogenic and metabolic effects of insulin comes from studies on a naturally occurring mutation of the insulin receptor tyrosine kinase domain (W1200S), which greatly decreases the ability of the receptor to stimulate mitogenesis but has no effect on insulin-stimulated glucose uptake and glycogen synthesis [123]. Consistent with this view, deletions of the C-terminus of the insulin receptor β-subunit promote a parallel enhancement of insulin-stimulated MAP kinase activity and the mitogenic effect of the hormone [124–126]. There may be at least three signalling pathways involved in insulin action in addition to that involving MAP kinase. One, as described above, leads to the activation of p70^{S6k} resulting in the phosphorylation of the ribosomal protein S6; this pathway is inhibitable by rapamycin and is apparently independent of Ras. A further potential pathway, which is inhibitable by wortmannin but is probably independent of MAP kinase, leads to increased glucose transport via Glut4 translocation [97, 127] and increased acetyl-CoA carboxylase activity. Finally, there is the pathway leading to the activation of pyruvate dehydrogenase, which is apparently insensitive to both wortmannin and rapamycin [98].

REFERENCES

1. Denton RM. Early events in insulin actions. Adv Cyclic Nucleotide Prot Phos Res 1986; 20: 293–341.
2. Zick Y. The insulin receptor—structure and function. Crit Rev Biochem Mol Biol 1989; 24: 217–69.
3. Lawrence JC. Signal transduction and protein phosphorylation in the regulation of cellular metabolism by insulin. Ann Rev Physiol 1992; 54: 177–93.
4. Cohen P, Campbell DG, Dent P et al. Dissection of the protein kinase cascades involved in insulin and nerve growth factor action. Biochem Soc Trans 1992; 20: 671–4.
5. Kahn CR. Insulin action, diabetogenes, and the cause of type 2 diabetes. Diabetes 1994; 43: 1066–84.
6. Denton RM, Tavaré JM. Does mitogen-activated protein kinase have a role in insulin action? The case for and against. Eur J Biochem 1995; 227: 597–611.
7. Cushman SW, Wardzala LJ. Potential mechanism of insulin action on glucose transport in the isolated rat adipose cell: apparent translocation of intracellular transport systems to the plasma membrane. J Biol Chem 1980; 255: 4758–62.
8. Suski K, Kono T. Evidence that insulin causes translocation of glucose transport activity to the plasma membrane from an intracellular storage site. Proc Natl Acad Sci USA 1980; 77: 2542–5.
9. Oka Y, Czech MP. Photoaffinity labelling of insulin-sensitive hexose transporters in intact rat adipocytes. Direct evidence that latent transporters become exposed to the extracellular space in reponse to insulin. J Biol Chem 1984; 259: 8125–33.
10. Blak J, Gibbs EM, Lienhard GE, Slot JW, Geuve HJ. Insulin-induced translocation of glucose transporters from post-golgi compartments to the plasma membrane of 3T3-LI adipocytes. J Cell Biol 1988; 106: 69–76.
11. Bell GI, Kayano T, Buse JB et al. Molecular biology of mammalian glucose transporters. Diabetes Care 1990; 13: 198–208.
12. Gould GW, Holman GD. The glucose transporter family—structure, function and tissue-specific expression. Biochem J 1993; 295: 329–41.
13. Calderhead DM, Kitagawa K, Tanner LI et al. Insulin regulation of the 2 glucose transporters in 3T3-L1 adipocytes. J Biol Chem 1990; 265: 13800–8.
14. Simpson IA, Cushman SW. Hormonal regulation of mammalian glucose transport. Ann Rev Biochem 1986; 55: 1059–89.
15. Calderhead DM, Lienhard GE. Labelling of glucose transport at the cell surface in 3T3-L1 adipocytes. J Biol Chem 1988; 263: 12171–4.
16. Muhlbacher C, Karnieli E, Schaff P. Obermaier B, Mushack J, Rattenhuber E, Häring HV. Phorbol esters imitate in rat fat cells the full effect of insulin on glucose-carrier translocation, but not on 3-O-methylglucose transport activity. Biochem J 1988; 249: 865–70.
17. Whitesell RR, Abumrad NA. Increased affinity predominates in insulin stimulation of glucose transport in the adipocyte. J Biol Chem 1985; 260: 2894–9.
18. Baly DL, Horuk R. Dissociation of insulin-stimulated glucose transport from the translocation of glucose carriers in rat adipose cells. J Biol Chem 1987; 262: 21–4.
19. Piper RC, James DE, Slot JW et al. Glut4 phosphorylation and inhibition of glucose transport by dibutyryl cAMP. J Biol Chem 1993; 268: 16557–63.
20. Oka Y, Mottola C, Oppenheimer CL, Czech MP. Insulin activates the appearance of insulin-like growth-factor II receptors on the adipocyte cell surface. Proc Natl Acad Sci USA 1984; 81: 4028–32.
21. Davis RJ, Corvera S, Czech MP. Insulin stimulates cellular iron uptake and causes the redistribution of intracellular transferrin receptors to the plasma membrane. J Biol Chem 1986; 261: 8708–11.
22. Sonne O, Simpson IA. Internalisation of insulin and its receptor in the isolated rat adipose cell. Time-course and insulin concentration dependency. Biochim Biophys Acta 1984; 804: 404–13.
23. Cohen P. Role of multisite phosphorylation in the hormonal control of glycogen synthase from mammalian muscle. In Krebs EG, Boyer PD (eds) The enzymes, vol. 18. Orlando: Academic Press, 1986: pp 462–99.

24. Lawrence JC, James C. Activation of glycogen synthase by insulin in rat adipocytes. Evidence of hormonal stimulation of multisite dephosphorylation by glucose transport-dependent and -independent pathways. J Biol Chem 1984; 259: 7975–82.

25. Lawrence JC Jr, Hiken JF, Depaoli-Roach AA et al. Hormonal control of glycogen synthase in rat hemidiaphragms. J Biol Chem 1983; 258: 10710–19.

26. Poulter L, Ang SG, Gibson BW et al. Analysis of the in vivo phosphorylation sites of rabbit skeletal muscle glycogen synthase by fast atom bombardment mass spectrometry. Eur J Biochem 1988; 175: 497–510.

27. Cohen P. Dissection of the protein phosphorylation cascades involved in insulin and growth factor action. Biochem Soc Trans 1993; 21: 555–67.

28. Sutherland C, Campbell DG, Cohen P. Identification of insulin-stimulated protein kinase-1 as the rabbit equivalent of rsk(mo)-2—identification of 2 threonines phosphorylated during activation by mitogen-activated protein kinase. Eur J Biochem 1993; 212: 581–8.

29. Hubbard MJ, Cohen P. On target with a new mechanism for the regulation of protein phosphorylation. TIBS 1993; 18: 172–7.

30. Cross DAE, Alessi DR, Vanderheede JR et al. The inhibition of glycogen synthase kinase-3 by insulin or insulin-like growth factor 1 in the rat skeletal muscle cell line L6 is blocked by wortmannin but not by rapamycin. Biochem J 1994; 303: 21–6.

31. Sutherland C, Cohen P. The alpha-isoform of glycogen synthase kinase-3 from rabbit skeletal muscle is inactivated by p70 S6 kinase or Map kinase-activated protein kinase-1 in vitro. FEBS Lett 1994; 338: 37–42.

32. Denton RM, Halestrap AP. Regulation of pyruvate metabolism in mammalian tissues. Essays Biochem 1979; 15: 37–77.

33. Behal RH, Buxton DB, Robertson JG. Regulation of the pyruvate dehydrogenase multienzyme complex. Ann Rev Nutr 1993; 13: 497–520.

34. Denton RM, Midgley PJW, Rutter GA, Thomas AP, McCormack JG. Studies into the mechanism whereby insulin activates pyruvate dehydrogenase in adipose tissue. Ann NY Acad Sci 1989; 573: 285–96.

35. Rutter GA, Diggle TA, Denton RM. Regulation of pyruvate dehydrogenase by insulin and polyamines within electropermeabilized fat-cells and isolated mitochondria. Biochem J 1992; 285: 435–9.

36. Gottschalk WK, Jarett L. The insulinomimetic effects of the polar head group of an insulin-sensitive glycophospholipid on pyruvate dehydrogenase in both subcellular and whole cell assays. Arch Biochem Biophys 1988; 261: 175–85.

37. Mistry SC, Priestman DA, Kerbey AL. Evidence that rat liver pyruvate dehydrogenase kinase activator protein is a pyruvate dehydrogenase kinase. Biochem J 1991; 275: 775–9.

38. Priestman DA, Mistry SC, Halsall A et al. Role of protein synthesis and of fatty acid metabolism in the longer-term regulation of pyruvate dehydrogenase. Biochem J 1994; 300: 659–64.

39. Randle PJ. Fuel selection in animals. Biochem Soc Trans 1986; 14: 799–806.

40. Marchington DR, Kerbey AL, Randle PJ. Longer-term regulation of pyruvate dehydrogenase kinase in cultured rat cardiac myocytes. Biochem J 1990; 267: 245–7.

41. Brownsey RW, Denton RM. Acetyl-CoA carboxylase. In Krebs EG, Boyer PD (eds) The enzymes, vol. 18. New York: Academic Press, 1987; pp 123–46.

42. Hardie DG. Regulation of fatty acid synthesis via phosphorylation of acetyl-CoA carboxylase. Prog Lipid Res 1989; 28: 117–46.

43. Borthwick AC, Edgell NJ, Denton RM. Use of rapid gel-permeation chromatography to explore the inter-relationships between polymerisation and activity of acetyl-CoA carboxylase. Effects of insulin and phosphorylation by cyclic-AMP dependent protein kinase. Biochem J 1987; 241: 773–82.

44. Brownsey RW, Denton RM. Evidence that insulin activates acetyl-CoA carboxylase by increased phosphorylation of a specific site. Biochem J 1982; 202: 77–86.

45. Haystead TAJ, Campbell DG. Hardie DG. Analysis of sites phosphorylated on acetyl-CoA carboxylase in response to insulin in isolated adipocytes. Comparison with sites phosphorylated by casein kinase-2 and the calmodulin-dependent multiprotein kinase. Eur J Biochem 1988; 175: 347–54.

46. Brownsey RW, Edgell NJ, Hopkirk TJ, Denton RM. Studies on insulin-stimulated phosphorylation of acetyl-CoA carboxylase, ATP-citrate lyase and other proteins in rat epididymal adipose tissue. Evidence for activation of a cyclic AMP independent protein kinase. Biochem J 1984; 218: 733–43.

47. Borthwick AC, Edgell NJ, Denton RM. Protein-serine kinase from rat epididymal adipose tissue which phosphorylates and activates acetyl-CoA carboxylase: possible role in insulin action. Biochem J 1990; 270: 795–801.

48. Pierce MW, Palmer JL, Keutmann HT et al. The insulin-directed phosphorylation site on ATP-citrate lyase. J Biol Chem 1982; 257: 10681–6.

49. Houston B, Nimmo HG. Effects of phosphorylation on the kinetic properties of rat liver ATP-citrate lyase. Biochim Biophys Acta 1985; 844: 233–9.

50. Stralfors P. Isoproterenol and insulin control the cellular localization of ATP-citrate lyase through its phosphorylation in adipocytes. J Biol Chem 1987; 262: 11486–9.

51. McGarry JD, Foster DW. Regulation of hepatic fatty acid oxidation and ketone body production. Ann Rev Biochem 1980; 49: 395–440.

52. Cook GA, Gamble MS. Regulation of carnitine palmitoyl transferase by insulin results in decreased activity and decreased apparent K_i values for malonyl-CoA. J Biol Chem 1987; 262: 2050–55.

53. Denton RM, Halperin ML. The control of fatty acid and triglyceride synthesis in rat epididymal adipose tissue. Biochem J 1968; 110: 27–38.

54. Saggerson ED, Carpenter CA. Effects of streptozotocin-diabetes and insulin administration in vivo or in vitro on the activities of five enzymes in the adipose tissue triacylglycerol-synthesis pathway. Biochem J 1987; 243: 289–92.

55. Stralfors P, Olsson H, Belfrage P. Hormone sensitive lipase. In Boyer PD, Krebs EG (eds) The enzymes, vol 18B. New York: Academic Press, 1985: pp 147–79.

56. Londos C, Honnor RC, Dhillon GS. cAMP-dependent protein kinase and lipolysis in rat adipocytes. III. Multiple modes of insulin regulation of lipolysis and regulation of insulin responses by adenylate cyclase regulators. J Biol Chem 1985; 260: 15139–45.

57. Gibson DM, Parker RA. Hydroxymethyl-glutaryl CoA reductase. In Boyer PD, Krebs EG (eds) The enzymes, vol 18B New York: Academic Press, 1985: pp 180–215.

58. Cook KG, Yeaman, SJ, Stralfors P et al. Direct evidence that cholesterol ester hydrolase from adrenal cortex is the same enzyme as hormone sensitive lipase from adipose tissue. Eur J Biochem 1982; 125: 245–9.

59. Downes P, Michell RH. Inositol phospholipid breakdown as a receptor controlled generator of second messengers. In Cohen P, Houslay M (eds) Molecular mechanisms of transmembrane signalling, vol 4. Amsterdam: Elsevier, 1986: pp 3–56.

60. Farese RV, Konda TS, Davis JS et al. Insulin rapidly increases diacylglycerol by activating de novo phosphatidic acid synthesis. Science 1987; 236: 586–9.

61. Pennington SR, Martin BR. Insulin stimulated phosphoinositide metabolism in isolated fat cells. J Biol Chem 1985; 260: 11039–45.

62. Stumpo DJ, Blackshear PJ. Insulin and growth factor effects on *c-fos* expression in normal and protein kinase C-deficient 3T3-L1 fibroblasts and adipocytes. Proc Natl Acad Sci USA 1986; 83: 9453–7.

63. Crettaz M, Muller-Wieland D, Kahn CR. Transcriptional and post-transcriptional regulation of tyrosine aminotransferase by insulin in rat hepatoma cells. Biochemistry 1988; 27: 495–500.

64. Straus DS, Takemato CD. Insulin negatively regulates albumin mRNA at the transcriptional and post-transcriptional level in rat hepatoma cells. J Biol Chem 1987; 262: 1955–60.

65. O'Brien RM, Granner DK. Regulation of gene expression by insulin. Biochem J 1991; 278: 609–19.

66. Sasaki K, Cripe TP, Koch SR, Andreone TL, Peterson DD, Beale EG, Granner DK. Multihormonal regulation of phosphoenol pyruvate carboxylase gene transcription. J Biol Chem 1984; 259: 15242–51.

67. Stumpo DJ, Stewart TN, Gilman MZ, Blackshear PJ. Identification of *c-fos* sequences involved in induction by insulin and phorbol esters. J Biol Chem 1988; 263: 1611–14.

68. Iynedjian PB, Gjinovci A, Renold AE. Stimulation by insulin of glucokinase gene transcription in liver of diabetic rats. J Biol Chem 1988; 263: 740–4.

69. Lemaigre FP, Rousseau GG. Transcriptional control of genes that regulate glycolysis and gluconeogenesis in adult liver. Biochem J 1994; 303: 1–14.

70. Karim M. Signal transduction from the cell surface to the nucleus through phosphorylation of transcription factors. Curr Opinions Cell Biol 1994; 6: 415–24.

71. Woodgett JR, Pulverer BJ, Nikolalaki E, Plyte S, Hughes K, Franklin CC et al. Regulation of jun/ap-1 oncoproteins by protein phosphorylation. Adv Second Messenger Prot Phos Res 1993; 8: 261–9.

72. Redpath NT, Proud CG. Molecular mechanisms in the control of translation by hormones and growth factors. Biochim Biophys Acta 1994; 1220: 147–62.

73. Jefferies HBJ, Reinhard C, Kozma SC, Thomas G. Rapamycin selectively represses translation of the 'polypyrimidine tract' mRNA family. Proc Natl Acad Sci USA 1994; 91: 4441–5.

74. Kozma SC, Thomas G. Serine/threonine kinases in the propagation of the early mitogenic response. Rev Physiol Biochem Pharmacol 1993; 119: 123–55.

75. Welsh GI, Proud CG. Glycogen synthase kinase-3 is rapidly inactivated in response to insulin and phosphorylates eukaryotic initiation factor eIF-2B. Biochem J 1993; 294: 625–9.

76. Sonenberg N. Translation factors as effectors of cell growth and tumorigenesis. Current Opinion Cell Biology 1993; 5: 955–60.

77. Larner J. Insulin signalling mechanisms. Lessons from the old testament of glycogen metabolism and the new testament of molecular biology. Diabetes 1988; 37: 262–75.

78. Saltiel AR, Cuatrecasas P. In search of a second messenger for insulin. Amer J Physiol 1988; 255: C1–10.

79. Saltiel AR, Fox JA, Sherline P, Cuatrecasas P. Insulin stimulated hydrolysis of a novel glycolipid generates modulators of cAMP phosphodiesterase. Science 1986; 233: 967–72.

80. Villalba M, Kelly KL, Mato JM. Inhibition of cyclic AMP-dependent protein kinase by the polar head group of an insulin sensitive glycophospholipid. Biochim Biophys Acta 1988; 968: 69–76.

81. Gottschalk WK, Jarett L. The insulinomimetic effects of the polar head group of an insulin sensitive glycophospholipid on pyruvate dehydrogenase in both subcellular and whole cell assays. Arch Biochem Biophys 1988; 261: 175–85.

82. Alvarez JF, Varela I, Ruiz-Albusac JM, Mato JM. Localization of the insulin-sensitive phosphatidylinositol glycan at the outer surface of the cell membrane. Biochem Biophys Res Commun 1988; 152: 1455–62.

83. Denton RM, Tavaré JM, Borthwick A et al. Insulin-activated protein kinases in fat and other cells. Biochem Soc Trans 1992; 20: 659–64.

84. Makino H, Manganiello VC, Kono T. Roles of ATP in insulin action. Ann Rev Physiol 1994; 56: 273–95.

85. Degerman E, Smith CJ, Tornqvist H et al. Evidence that insulin and isoprenaline activate the cGMP-inhibited low-km cAMP phosphodiesterase in rat fat cells by phosphorylation. Proc Nat Acad Sci USA 1990; 87: 533–7.

86. Rahn T, Ridderstrale M, Tornqvist H et al. Essential role of phosphatidylinositol 3-kinase in insulin-induced activation and phosphorylation of the cGMP-inhibited cAMP phosphodiesterase in rat adipocytes. Studies using the selective inhibitor wortmannin. FEBS Lett 1994; 350: 314–18.

87. Rosen OM. After insulin binds. Science 1987; 237: 1452–8.

88. Tavaré JM, Siddle K. Mutational analysis of insulin receptor function—consensus and controversy. Biochim Biophys Acta 1993; 1178: 21–39.

89. Saad MJA, Araki E, Miralpeix M et al. Regulation of insulin receptor substrate-1 in liver and muscle of animal models of insulin resistance. J Clin Invest 1992; 90: 1839–49.

90. Tavaré JM, OBrien RM, Siddle K, Denton RM. Analysis of insulin receptor phosphorylation sites in intact cells by two-dimensional phosphopeptide mapping. Biochem J 1988; 253: 783–8.

91. White MF, Shoelson SE, Keutmann H, Kahn CR. A cascade of tyrosine autophosphorylation in the β-subunit activates the phosphotransferase of the insulin receptor. J Biol Chem 1988; 263: 2669–80.

92. Sun XJ, Rothenberg P, Kahn CR et al. Structure of the insulin receptor substrate IRS-1 defines a unique signal transduction protein. Nature 1991; 352: 73–7.

93. White MF, Kahn CR. The insulin signaling system. J Biol Chem 1994; 269: 1–4.

94. McCormick F. Signal transduction—how receptors turn Ras on. Nature 1993; 363: 15–16.
95. Skolnik EY, Batzer A, Li N et al. The function of GRB2 in linking the insulin receptor to Ras signaling pathways. Science 1993; 260: 1953–5.
96. Myers MG, Sun XJ, White MF. The IRS-1 signaling system. TIBS 1994; 19: 289–93.
97. Clarke JF, Young PW, Yonezawa K et al. Inhibition of the translocation of Glut1 and Glut4 in 3T3-L1 cells by the phosphatidylinositol 3-kinase inhibitor, wortmannin. Biochem J 1994; 300: 631–5.
98. Moule SK, Edgell NJ, Welsh GI, Diggle TA, Foulstone EJ, Heesom KJ, Proud CG, Denton RM. Multiple signalling pathways involved in the stimulation of fatty acid and glycogen synthesis by insulin in rat epididymal fat cells. Biochem Soc Trans 1995; 311: 595–601.
99. Nakaniski H, Brewer KA, Exton JH. Activation of the zeta-isozyme of protein kinase C by phosphatidylinositol 3,4,5-triphosphate. J Biol Chem 1993; 268: 13–16.
100. Lam K, Carpenter CL, Ruderman NB, Friel JC, Kelly KL. The phosphatidylinositol 3-kinase serine kinase phosphorylates IRS-1—stimulation by insulin and inhibition by wortmannin. J Biol Chem 1994; 269: 20648–52.
101. Araki E, Lipes MA, Patti M, Bruning JC, Haag B, Johnson RS et al. Alternative pathway of insulin signalling in mice with targeted disruption of the IRS-1 gene. Nature 1994; 372: 186–90 (erratum p. 710).
102. Sasaoka T, Rose DW, Jhun BH et al. Evidence for a functional role of Shc proteins in mitogenic signaling induced by insulin, insulin-like growth factor-1, and epidermal growth factor. J Biol Chem 1994; 269: 13689–94.
103. Hosomi Y, Shii K, Ogawa W et al. Characterization of a 60-kilodalton substrate of the insulin receptor kinase. J Biol Chem 1994; 269: 11498–502.
104. Rodriguez-Viciana P, Warne PH, Dhand R et al. Phosphatidylinositol-3-OH kinase as a direct target of Ras. Nature 1994; 370; 527–32.
105. Blumer KJ, Johnson GL. Diversity in function and regulation of MAP kinase pathways. TIBS 1994; 19: 236–40.
106. Zheng CF, Guan KL. Properties of MEKs, the kinases that phosphorylate and activate the extracellular signal-regulated kinases. J Biol Chem 1993; 268: 23933–9.
107. Clark AE, Holman GD. Exofacial photolabelling of the human erythrocyte glucose transporter with an azitrifluoroethylbenzoyl-substituted bismannose. Biochem J 1990; 269: 615–22.
108. Holman GD, Kozka IJ, Clark AE et al. Cell surface labelling of glucose transporter isoform glut-4 by bis-mannose photolabel: correlation with stimulation of glucose transport in rat adipose cells by insulin and phorbol ester. J Biol Chem 1990; 265: 18172–9.
109. Haystead TAJ, Sim AYR, Carling D et al. Effects of the tumour promotor okadaic acid on intracellular protein phosphorylation and metabolism. Nature 1989; 337: 78–81.
110. Tanti JF, Gremeaux T, Van-Obberghen E, Le Marchand-Brustel Y. Effects of okadaic acid, an inhibitor of protein phosphatases-I and phosphatases-2A, on glucose transport and metabolism in skeletal muscle. J Biol Chem 1991; 266: 2099–103.
111. Welsh GI, Foulstone EJ, Young SW, Tavaré JM, Proud CG. Wortmannin inhibits the effects of insulin and serum on the activities of glycogen synthase kinase-3 and mitogen-activated protein kinase. Biochem J 1994; 303: 15–20.
112. Dent P, Lavoinne A, Nakielny S et al. The molecular mechanism by which insulin stimulates glycogen synthesis in mammalian skeletal muscle. Nature 1990; 348: 302–8.
113. Diggle TA, Schmitz-Peiffer C, Borthwick AC et al. Evidence that insulin activates casein kinase 2 in rat epididymal fat cells and that this may result in the increased phosphorylation of an acid-soluble 22 kDa protein. 1991; 279: 545–51.
114. Fry MJ. Structure, regulation and function of phosphoinositide 3-kinases. Biochim Biophys Acta 1994; 1226: 237–68.
115. Lin T, Lawrence JC. Activation of ribosomal protein S6 kinases does not increase glycogen synthesis or glucose transport in rat adipocytes. J Biol Chem 1994; 269: 21255–61.
116. Peak M, Yeaman SJ, Agius L. Epidermal growth factor and insulin stimulate MAP kinase activity in cultured hepatocytes. Biochem Soc Trans 1993; 21: 494S.
117. Ballou LM, Luther H, Thomas G. MAP2 kinase and 70K-S6 kinase lie on distinct signalling pathways. Nature 1991; 349: 348–50.
118. Kyriakis JM, Avruch J. Insulin, epidermal growth factor and fibroblast growth factor elicit distinct patterns of protein tyrosine phosphorylation in Bc3H1 cells. Biochim Biophys Acta 1990; 1054: 73–82.
119. Chung JK, Grammer TC, Lemon KP et al. PDGF- and insulin-dependent pp70(S6k) activation mediated by phosphatidylinositol-3-OH kinase. Nature 1994; 370: 71–5.
120. Ming X, Burgering BMTh, Wennstrom S et al. Activation of p70/p85 S6 kinase by a pathway independent of p21ras. Nature 1994; 371: 426–9.
121. Diggle TA, Schmitz-Peiffer C, Borthwick AC, Welsh GI, Denton RM. Evidence that insulin activates casein kinase-2 in rat epididymal fat-cells and that this may result in the increased phosphorylation of an acid-soluble 22 kDa protein. Biochem J 1991; 279: 545–51.
122. Pinna LA. Casein kinase-2—an eminence-grise in cellular regulation. Biochim Biophys Acta 1990; 1054: 267–84.
123. Moller DE, Benecke H, Flier JS. Biologic activities of naturally occurring human insulin receptor mutations—evidence that metabolic effects of insulin can be mediated by a kinase-deficient insulin receptor mutant. J Biol Chem 1991; 266: 10995–11001.
124. Thies RS, Ullrich A, McClain DA. Augmented mitogenesis and impaired metabolic signalling mediated by a truncated insulin receptor. J Biol Chem 1988; 24: 12820–25.
125. Dickens M, Chin JE, Roth RA et al. Characterization of insulin-stimulated protein serine/threonine kinases in CHO cells expressing human insulin receptors with point and deletion mutations. Biochem J 1992; 287: 201–9.
126. Pang L, Milarki KL, Ohmichi M et al. Mutation of the 2 carboxyl-terminal tyrosines in the insulin receptor results in enhanced activation of mitogen-activated protein kinase. J Biol Chem 1994; 269: 10604–8.

127. Fingar DC, Birnbaum MJ. Characterization of the mitogen-activated protein kinase 90-kilodalton ribosomal protein Sb kinase signaling pathway in 3T3-L1 adipocytes and its role in insulin-stimulated glucose transport. Endocrinology 1994; 134: 728–35.

128. Yang J, Holman GD. Comparison of Glut4 and Glut1 subcellular trafficking in basal and insulin-stimulated 3T3-L1 cells. J Biol Chem 1993; 268: 4600–603.

129. Kandror K, Pilch PF. Identification and isolation of glycoproteins that translocate to the cell surface from Glut4-enriched vesicles in an insulin-dependent fashion. J Biol Chem 1994; 269: 138–42.

130. Welsh GI, Proud CG. Glycogen synthase kinase-3 is rapidly inactivated in response to insulin and phosphorylates eukaryotic initiation factor eIF-2B. Biochem J 1993; 294: 625–9.

131. Larner J. Insulin signalling mechanisms. Lessons from the Old Testament of glycogen metabolism and the New Testament of molecular biology. Diabetes 1988; 37: 262–75.

132. Hughes K, Ramakrishna S, Benjamin WB et al. Identification of multifunctional ATP-citrate lyase kinase as the alpha-isoform of glycogen synthase kinase-3. Biochem J 1992; 288: 309–14.

133. Hardie DG. Regulation of fatty acid and cholesterol metabolism by the AMP-activated protein kinase. Biochim Biophys Acta 1992; 1123: 231–8.

134. Pause A, Belsham GJ, Donzé O, Lin T, Lawrence JC, Sonenberg N. Insulin-dependent stimulation of protein synthesis via phosphorylation of a regulator of 5'-cap function. Nature 1994; 371: 762–7.

135. Belsham G, Brownsey RW, Hughes WH, Denton RM. Anti-insulin receptor antibodies mimic the effects of insulin on the activities of pyruvate dehydrogenase and acetyl-CoA carboxylase and on specific protein phosphorylation in rat epididymal fat cells. Diabetologia 1980; 18: 307–12.

136. Hu CB, Pang SH, Kong XM. Molecular cloning and tissue distribution of Phas-I, an intracellular target for insulin and growth factors. Proc Natl Acad Sci USA 1994; 91: 3730–34.

137. Diggle TA, Bloomberg GB, Denton RM. Further characterisation of the acid soluble phosphoprotein (SDS/PAGE apparent molecular weight of 22 kDa) in rat fat cells by peptide sequencing and immuno-analysis. Effects of insulin and isoproterenol. Biochem J 1995; 306: 135–9.

138. Haystead TAJ, Haystead CMM, Hu C, Lin T, Lawrence JC Jr. Phosphorylation of PHAS-I by mitogen-activated protein (MAP) kinase. Identification of a site phosphorylated by MAP kinase in vitro and in response to insulin in rat adipocytes. J Biol Chem 1994; 269: 23185–91.

139. Leevers SJ, Paterson HF, Marshall CJ. Requirement for Ras in Raf activation is overcome by targeting Raf to the plasma membrane. Nature 1994; 369: 411–14.

140. Porras A, Muszynski K, Rapp UR, Santos E. Dissociation between activation of Raf-1Kinase and the 42-kDa mitogen-activated protein kinase/90-kDa S6 kinase (Mapk/Rsk) cascade in the insulin/Ras pathway of adipocytic differentiation of 3T3 L1 cells. J Biol Chem 1994; 269: 12741–8.

23

The Regulation of Gene Transcription by Insulin and the Search for Diabetogenes

Calum Sutherland, Richard M. O'Brien and Daryl K. Granner

Department of Molecular Physiology and Biophysics, Vanderbilt University Medical School, Nashville, Tennessee, USA

INTRODUCTION

Diabetes Mellitus

The inability to produce functional insulin molecules results in insulin-dependent diabetes mellitus (IDDM), a disorder that can be treated by daily injections of the hormone. In contrast, patients with fully developed non-insulin dependent diabetes mellitus (NIDDM) exhibit alterations in insulin secretion from the pancreas, and also have a reduced ability. to respond to the hormone (insulin resistance) [1, 2]. It remains controversial as to whether abnormalities in insulin secretion or insulin resistance constitute the primary lesion leading to the development of NIDDM in humans, although epidemiological studies suggest that either is possible (for review, see [3]). Many NIDDM patients exhibit increased insulin secretion early in the development of the disorder. This may constitute a secondary response to the hyperglycemia that results from the emergence of insulin resistance. However, by the time NIDDM is fully developed there is almost always a reduction in glucose-stimulated secretion of insulin from the pancreatic islet B-cells [3]. What is clear is that this disease contains a genetic component(s), since offspring of two diabetic parents have a manifold greater risk of developing the disorder compared with offspring of healthy individuals [4, 5]. In addition, distinct genetic populations have an increased risk of developing NIDDM (e.g. Pima Indians [6]). This disorder can take 40–60 years to develop fully, and can be classified by a series of well defined stages (for review, see [2]), possibly suggesting that it does not occur due to the loss of an individual gene product or activity. A more complicated multi-component syndrome may explain the gradual progression of the disease, with environmental factors (e.g. nutrition, exercise, etc.) as well as genetic factors having a role. This may also explain the variations observed in the diabetic phenotype.

The question arises as to how a treatment for such a complex disorder can be developed. Initially, the cause(s) of insulin resistance must be determined, a process that will require a better understanding of the molecular mechanisms engaged by insulin to bring about its various metabolic functions.

Insulin Action

Insulin is secreted from the pancreatic B-cells in response to increased levels of plasma glucose and amino acids (i.e. postprandially). The hormone elicits a variety of metabolic changes in many mammalian tissues, primarily adipose tissue, liver and muscle [7]. These include increased glucose transport and increased glycogen, fatty acid and protein synthesis along with decreased protein, lipid and glycogen breakdown and reduced glucose biosynthesis (gluconeogenesis). The result is a general increase in

International Textbook of Diabetes Mellitus, Second Edition. Edited by K.G.M.M. Alberti, P. Zimmet, R.A. DeFronzo, and H. Keen (Honorary)
© 1997 John Wiley & Sons Ltd

anabolism and, in certain circumstances, growth of responsive tissues.

One of the most important actions of insulin is to maintain glucose homeostasis [2]. It is a breakdown in glucose homeostasis that manifests itself as NIDDM (due to alterations in insulin secretion and development of insulin resistance primarily in the liver, adipose tissue and muscle).

Insulin Resistance

Several potential mechanisms have been postulated to explain the cause of insulin resistance (for review see [8]) but none can adequately account for the cause of insulin resistance in the majority of patients (see Chapter 21). In order to identify potential therapeutic targets for this syndrome, the molecular mechanisms that underlie insulin signaling must first be elucidated. Alterations in the activity of a multitude of proteins occur within minutes of insulin administration to liver, muscle and adipose tissue [9, 10]. Similarly, by regulating their rate of production, insulin can affect the concentration of over 100 proteins (Table 1: for review, see [11]). The loss of the appropriate regulation of the expression of specific gene(s) by insulin could cause or contribute to resistance to this hormone.

REGULATION OF GENE EXPRESSION BY INSULIN

Gene Expression and NIDDM

The level of activity of a given metabolic process can be influenced by an alteration of the amount as well as the inherent activity of specific protein(s). Insulin affects the expression of over 100 genes (for complete list, see [11, 12]), and there is little doubt that this number will continue to rise. These genes have been identified using a variety of approaches, such as subtraction screening of cDNA libraries generated from patients with NIDDM [13] as well as carbohydrate-fed animals (such feeding leads to elevated insulin secretion) [14] and insulin-treated cell lines [15, 16]. In addition, two-dimensional gel electrophoresis has been used to show that the concentration of a number of other, as yet undefined, proteins changes in insulin-treated cells [17, 18]. It is possible that the loss of the regulation of one or more of these genes by insulin is responsible for insulin resistance. However, it is also possible that partial loss of the regulation of several genes would have a similar effect. In addition, it is feasible that an increase or decrease in basal expression of one or more genes (not necessarily an insulin-regulated gene) could participate in the generation of NIDDM. It is clearly important to understand the molecular mechanisms by

Table 1 Representative genes affected by insulin (from a list of >100 [11, 12])

Protein	Cell type studied
Pyruvate kinase (+)	Hepatocytes
GAPDH (+)	Hepatocytes/adipocytes
Gene 33 (+)	Hepatocytes
PEPCK (−)	Hepatocytes
MTP (−)	Hepatocytes
Tyrosine aminotransferase (−)	Hepatocytes
IGFBP-1 (−)	Hepatocytes
Glucagon (−)	Pancreatic islet A-cells
Neuropeptide Y (−)	Brain
Fatty acid synthetase (+)	Adipocytes/hepatocytes
Acetyl-CoA carboxylase (+)	Adipocytes
Hexokinase-II (+)	Myocytes
Thyrotropin (TSH) receptor (+)	Thyroid
Thyroglobulin (+)	Thyroid
Prolactin (+)	Pituitary
c-fos (+)	Multiple
c-jun (+)	Multiple
p21Ras (+)	Multiple
δ1-Crystallin (+)	Lens epithelium
Casein (+)	Mammary gland

Stimulation (+) or inhibition (−) of transcription by insulin is indicated in parentheses. Abbreviations: GAPDH, glyceraldehyde-3-phosphate dehydrogenase; PEPCK, phosphoenolpyruvate carboxykinase; MTP, microsomal triglyceride transfer protein, large subunit; IGFBP-1, insulin-like growth factor binding protein 1

which insulin regulates gene expression, as defects in the regulatory machinery of gene expression, as well as the transcriptional machinery, may well contribute as a primary cause of NIDDM.

Although a large number of genes appear to be regulated by insulin, only a subset of these have, to date, been demonstrated to be directly regulated at the transcriptional level by this hormone (see below). Many of the studies mentioned above do not discriminate between direct and indirect regulation of gene transcription by insulin. Thus, the effects of insulin on gene transcription may be due to an effect on the expression or action of another hormone. In addition, the potential role of insulin-stimulated changes in glucose concentration in the regulation of gene expression must be considered. The remainder of this chapter reviews the mechanisms identified to date by which insulin has been shown to regulate gene transcription directly. We also discuss the relevance of this regulation to NIDDM.

Identification of Insulin Response Sequences

In order to confer regulation by insulin, a given gene promoter must contain a specific sequence(s) of DNA.

The binding of a specific protein to this sequence is required for reception of the ultimate insulin 'signal'. It is widely accepted that extracellular signals regulate gene transcription through such a *cis/trans* mechanism. The specific DNA sequence within the promoter is designated a *cis*-acting element, and the protein that interacts with this element is termed a *trans*-acting factor; it is this factor that receives the given signal. These two elements together transmit the signal to the basal promoter apparatus (Figure 1).

In several cases a DNA sequence has been designated an insulin response sequence when mutation of the sequence reduced the ability of a given promoter to confer a specific response to insulin. However, this interpretation can be complex and is easier to demonstrate if such mutations do not affect the regulation of gene expression by another hormone or the basal activity of the promoter. Additional evidence that the sequence does function as an insulin response sequence comes from a demonstration that the sequence confers insulin responsiveness when fused to a heterologous promoter. These criteria have been met for several sequences within the promoters of a number of the genes identified to date that are known to be regulated by insulin. Some of the genes that have met at least one of the above criteria are discussed in this chapter.

Insulin Response Sequences

Interestingly, no general consensus sequence has been found for an insulin response sequence, and no insulin-specific *trans*-acting factor has yet been identified, although several promoter elements that confer insulin responsiveness have been examined in detail.

The Serum Response Element (SRE)

The serum response element (SRE) is found in the promoter of a number of insulin-regulated genes [19, 20]. A potential signaling pathway by which insulin could regulate transcription through the SRE is described below, in the section on insulin signaling.

c-fos The best studied SRE lies within the promoter of the c-fos gene (for review see [19, 21]). c-fos is a component of the activator protein-1 (AP-1) transcription factor complex and its actions are discussed more fully below. Insulin increases the transcription of the c-fos gene in NIH 3T3 cells, in CHO cells that overexpress the insulin receptor [22], and in H4IIE cells [23]. Experiments that utilized promoter–reporter fusion genes located an insulin response sequence between residues −320 and −298 of the c-fos promoter [24, 25]. This DNA segment contains the c-fos SRE (Figure 2), and when this SRE was fused to a reporter

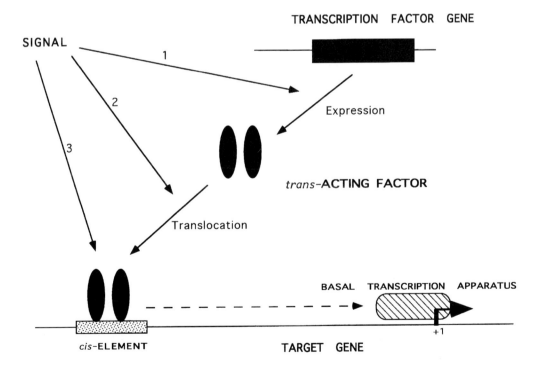

Figure 1 Schematic diagram of the *cis/trans* model for the regulation of gene transcription. The model predicts several potential regulatory mechanisms; e.g. at the level of expression of the transcription factor (1), the transport of the factor to the nucleus (2) and the binding and transactivation capability of the transcription factor (3). Protein phosphorylation and protein–protein interactions are the best described mechanisms of regulation to date (see text)

Gene promoter	Serum response element
c-fos (-299)	5'-TTACAC**AGGA**TGT<u>CCATATTAGG</u>ACATCT
Glut-1 (-2700)	<u>5'-CCTTTAAAGG</u>

Gene promoter	Activator protein-1 motif
Collagenase (-60)	5'-TAAAGCA<u>TGAGTCA</u>GACACC

Figure 2 Serum response element (SRE) and activator protein-1 (AP-1) sequences located in the promoters of insulin-regulated genes. The numbers in parentheses refer to the position of the 3'-nucleotide relative to the transcription start site

gene it conferred a fourfold stimulation upon insulin treatment. The SRE is known to bind a number of proteins, including the serum response factor (p67^{SRF}), NFIL6, Phox 1 and DBF (for review, see [19]). The c-fos SRE consists of a p67^{SRF} binding element that is located 3' to an Ets binding element (CAGGAT). This Ets binding element increases the responsiveness of the c-fos p67^{SRF} binding element to insulin from 4- to 13-fold when the elements are linked in series to a heterologous promoter [24]. However, it should be noted that these experiments compared a single copy of the p67^{SRF} binding element with two copies of an Ets-p67^{SRF} binding element linked in series [24]. Insulin does stimulate the binding of protein(s) to the Ets domain [26], and a protein, termed ternary complex factor (p62^{TCF}), is known to bind to the c-fos Ets sequence *in vitro*, but only in combination with p67^{SRF} [19]. The protein p62^{TCF} is phosphorylated *in vitro* by the p42/p44 MAP kinase(s), enzymes that are stimulated by insulin in several cell types, including hepatoma cells [27]. This phosphorylation leads to a stimulation of DNA binding *in vitro* [28], or an increase in the transactivation potential of p62^{TCF} [29]. In addition, an inhibitor of insulin-stimulated MAP kinase activity blocked induction of c-fos transcription by insulin [30], which suggests that this phosphorylation cascade is required for regulation of c-fos transcription by insulin.

Glut-1 This gene encodes a protein that is involved in the transport of glucose across the cell membranes of most tissues [31]. In 3T3 F442A adipocytes and L6 myocytes insulin stimulates the transcription of Glut-1 five- and threefold respectively, although this effect appears to require insulin levels generally considered to be higher than physiologic [32]. By contrast, insulin does not stimulate Glut-1 gene expression in adipocytes isolated from streptozotocin-induced diabetic rats, although it does result in decreased

expression of the Glut-4 transporter [33]. The Glut-1 gene contains two enhancer elements that are required for responsiveness to serum, growth factor and oncogenes and to insulin [34, 35]. Enhancer-1 (located 2.7 kilobases upstream of the cap site) contains an SRE that is required for the response to insulin [35].

Other examples An SRE within the promoter of the β-actin gene also mediates a positive insulin response [36], and a number of other genes that contain SREs within their promoters are also positively regulated by insulin (e.g. egr-1, c-jun, Jun B and Jun D), although the role of the SREs with respect to insulin responsiveness in these cases has not been determined [17, 37].

The TPA Response Element (TRE)/AP-1

The DNA sequence (TGAGTCA) mediates a transcriptional response to the phorbol ester, 12-*O*-tetradecanoyl phorbol 13-acetate (TPA; thus the TPA response element, TRE) [38, 39]. It is now more generally referred to as the activator protein-1 (AP-1) motif, although recent evidence suggests that negative as well as positive effects on transcription are mediated through this element (for review, see [39]). The AP-1 motif mediates the transcriptional stimulation by insulin of the collagenase gene [40], and is found in other insulin-responsive genes, such as c-jun, α2-microglobulin, PEPCK (phosphoenolpyruvate carboxykinase) and albumin, although the role of this element in the regulation of these genes by insulin remains unclear [41–43]. The sequence can elicit a positive insulin response when multimerized and linked to a heterologous promoter [44]. Members of the jun and fos family of transcription factors bind this element as a variety of homo- and hetero-dimers (for review, see [39]), and the configuration of partners can determine the type (positive or negative) and magnitude of the effect on transcription. Interestingly, insulin can modulate transcription through the AP-1 motif by regulating the levels of c-fos and c-jun proteins, and also by modulating the phosphorylation state of these transcription factors (for review see [21, 45, 46]).

The T(G/A) TTT-like Motif (Figure 3)

Phosphoenolpyruvate carboxykinase (PEPCK) The PEPCK gene has been studied extensively due to its importance as the gene encoding the rate-limiting enzyme in hepatic gluconeogenesis. Glucagon (via the second messenger cAMP), and glucocorticoids stimulate the transcription of the PEPCK gene, whereas insulin and phorbol esters inhibit, in a dominant fashion, these stimulatory effects [12, 47, 48]. Many of the positive *cis*-acting elements within the PEPCK promoter have been identified through the analysis of a

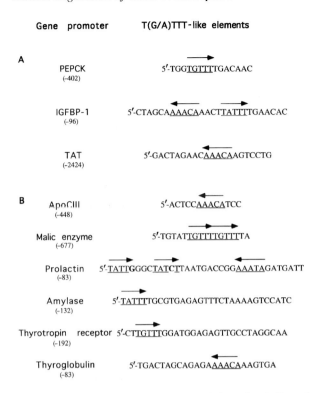

Gene promoter **T(G/A)TTT-like elements**

A

PEPCK
(-402)
5'-TGGTGTTTTGACAAC

IGFBP-1
(-96)
5'-CTAGCAAAACAAACTTATTTTGAACAC

TAT
(-2424)
5'-GACTAGAACAAACAAGTCCTG

B

ApoCIII
(-448)
5'-ACTCCAAACATCC

Malic enzyme
(-677)
5'-TGTATTGTTTTGTTTTA

Prolactin
(-83)
5'-TATTGGGCTATCTTAATGACCGGAAATAGATGATT

Amylase
(-132)
5'-TATTTTGCGTGAGAGTTTCTAAAAGTCCATC

Thyrotropin receptor
(-192)
5'-CTTGTTTGGATGGAGAGTTGCCTAGGCAA

Thyroglobulin
(-83)
5'-TGACTAGCAGAGAAAACAAAGTGA

Figure 3 T(G/A)TTT-like sequences (orientation indicated by arrows) located in the promoters of insulin-regulated genes. The numbers in parentheses refer to the position of the 3'-nucleotide relative to the transcription start site. A, Sequences that have been proven to confer a functional insulin response; B, Sequences that have not yet been shown to confer insulin regulation

variety of PEPCK–CAT fusion genes in transient transfection experiments (Figure 4; [11]). The stimulatory action of glucocorticoids is mediated by a complex glucocorticoid response unit (GRU) ([49]; D. Scott, personal communication) that consists of three accessory factor binding sites (AF1, from −455 to −431; AF2, from −420 to −403; AF3, from −337 to −312) and two glucocorticoid receptor binding sites (GR1 and GR2, from −395 to −349). The accessory factor

binding sites alone do not mediate a response to glucocorticoids. However, if any one of these elements is mutated within the context of the PEPCK promoter, approximately 60% of the ability to respond to glucocorticoids is lost. Similarly, when two out of three of the elements are mutated the promoter is almost unresponsive to glucocorticoids. Thus, GR1 and GR2 are inert by themselves, at least in the context of the PEPCK promoter ([49]; D. Scott, personal communication). In addition, at least four cis-acting elements (designated CRE, P3[I], P3[II] and P4) are required for cAMP-stimulated PEPCK gene transcription [48, 50]. Together these elements form a cAMP response unit. Interestingly, CRE is also required for the full glucocorticoid response and thus also forms part of the complex GRU [51, 52].

The identification of multiple elements required for the dominant negative effect of insulin was achieved using both transient and stable transfection techniques [11]. At least one such insulin response sequence resides in the region between −271 and +69, but its exact location remains to be determined. Another, the distal insulin response sequence, located between −413 and −407, has been well characterized [53]. This sequence is located within the AF2 binding region, and mediates both an insulin and a phorbol ester inhibitory signal in the PEPCK promoter [47], although insulin treatment does not alter DNA footprints over this region [54]. This distal sequence has the core sequence T(G/A)TTTG, and confers insulin responsiveness when fused to a reporter gene; the same response is seen whether the second residue of the sequence is a guanosine or an adenosine (R. O'Brien, in preparation). A number of proteins, including C/EBPα and -γ, and HNF3α and -β bind, in vitro, to oligonucleotides that contain this sequence ([53, 55]; R. O'Brien, in preparation). However, since there is no correlation between the binding of any of these proteins and insulin-regulated transcription via this element, it remains unclear which, if any, of these DNA binding

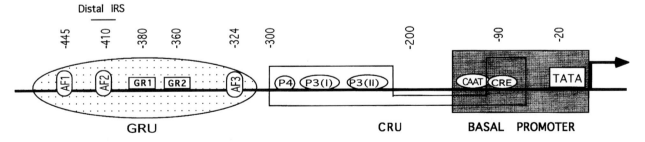

Figure 4 Schematic diagram of the PEPCK promoter, detailing the major elements involved in the transcriptional responses to cAMP, glucocorticoids and insulin. The numbers identify nucleotide positions relative to the transcription initiation site. In the GRU the distances in nucleotides from the transcription initiation site are measured to the center of each element. IRS, insulin response sequence; AF, accessory factor; GR, glucocorticoid receptor binding site; GRU, glucocorticoid response unit; CRE, cAMP response element; CRU, cAMP response unit

proteins actually mediates the action of insulin on PEPCK gene transcription *in vivo*.

Insulin-like growth factor binding protein-1 (IGFBP-1) IGFBP-1 binds the hormones IGF-I and IGF-II, but does not bind insulin (for review see [56]). IGFBP-1 inhibits IGF action in many systems, although it has been shown to potentiate the mitogenic effects of IGF-I under certain circumstances [57]. Insulin inhibits transcription of the IGFBP-1 gene in human HepG2 [58] and rat H4IIE hepatoma [59] cells. This effect, like the action of insulin on PEPCK gene transcription, is dominant over the cAMP and glucocorticoid-stimulated transcription of the gene [59–61]. The human IGFBP-1 gene promoter contains an insulin response sequence located between residues −120 and −96 that was identified by fusion gene experiments [62]. This contains two T(G/A)TTTTG motifs arranged as an inverted palindrome (Figure 3), and matches the distal insulin response sequence of the PEPCK promoter (see above). In addition, the IGFBP-1 insulin response sequence overlaps with another sequence identified as an accessory element required for full glucocorticoid responsiveness of the IGFBP-1 promoter [63]. This sequence, like that in the AF2 region of the PEPCK promoter, binds HNF3 [53, 64]. Thus a model has been proposed in which T(G/A)TTTTG binds a repressor (that functions upon insulin treatment) that 'interferes' with HNF3 action and thus blocks glucocorticoid-stimulated PEPCK and IGFBP-1 gene transcription [53].

Tyrosine aminotransferase (TAT) The TAT gene represents another example of a gene whose expression is stimulated by both cAMP and glucocorticoids, and inhibited, in a dominant fashion, by insulin [65, 66]. In addition the TAT gene promoter contains a T(G/A)TTT motif (Figure 3) that is located in an enhancer element located about −2.5 kilobases upstream from the transcription start site [66]. Insulin response sequences have been located both at the −2.5 kbp enhancer and at a −3.6 kbp enhancer element [67]. The −3.6 kbp element is required for the action of cAMP, whereas the 2.5 kbp element (and potentially a 5.4 kbp element [65]) is required for the action of glucocorticoids on TAT gene expression. The TAT gene promoter also contains a number of accessory factor binding sites that are required for full responsiveness to these hormones [66, 68], so this gene also serves as a model for complex hormone response domains [69]. As with the PEPCK and IGFBP-1 genes, the T(G/A)TTT motif in the 2.5 kbp enhancer overlaps with a sequence that binds HNF3 [66]. Thus, antagonism of HNF3 function may be involved in the regulation of TAT gene transcription by insulin. A number of other genes whose products are involved in amino acid and cholesterol metabolism are positively

regulated by glucocorticoids and negatively regulated by insulin [11], but a role for a T(G/A)TTT-like motif within the relevant promoters has not yet been demonstrated.

Apolipoprotein CIII (apo-CIII) The apolipoprotein apo-CIII is one of the major constituents of chylomicrons and VLDL, the lipoproteins that transport triglycerides, cholesterol esters and phospholipids from the intestine to the liver. Over-expression of apo-CIII in transgenic mice results in hypertriglyceridemia (HTG) [70], a disorder closely associated with the development of atherosclerosis and coronary heart disease. Interestingly, hepatic apo-CIII gene expression is increased in streptozotocin-treated animals, an effect that is reversed by insulin administration [71]. Apo-CIII–luciferase fusion gene expression in transfected Hep G2 cells is potently inhibited by insulin, and additional experiments suggest that an insulin response sequence is located between residues −854 and +22 [71]. Five polymorphisms are present in the human apo-CIII gene promoter, and the less common allele of each is associated with severe hypertriglyceridemia [72]. Two of these polymorphisms map to a region that contains an inverted T(G/A)TTT motif (between −461 and −453, Figure 3) [72]. This region confers an inhibitory action of insulin in the context of a minimal apo-CIII promoter (T. Leff, personal communication), but the two mutations that abolish insulin responsiveness, and result in severe hypertriglyceridemia in humans, lie outside the T(G/A)TTT motif and one of these actually results in a sequence that more closely resembles the PEPCK distal insulin response sequence. Thus, additional studies are required to address fully the role of this element in the regulation of apo-CIII gene expression by insulin.

Malic enzyme In contrast to the three examples cited above, malic enzyme gene transcription is stimulated by insulin [73, 74]. This effect is blocked by cycloheximide [73]. The promoter of the malic enzyme gene contains a T(G/A)TTT-like motif located between residues −692 and −683 relative to the transcription start site, and protein binding to this region is inhibited by insulin treatment [74]. This promoter also contains an element similar to the insulin response sequence found in the GAPDH gene promoter (see below). This latter sequence is located between residues −170 and −161 of the malic enzyme promoter, and in contrast to the T(G/A)TTT-like motif, protein binding to this element is stimulated by insulin [74]. Interestingly, this sequence functions as a positive element in the context of the GAPDH promoter. However, it is not yet known whether either of these elements actually functions as an insulin response sequence within the malic enzyme gene promoter.

Aspartate aminotransferase (AAT) and amylase
The promoters of cytosolic aspartate aminotransferase (AAT) and amylase genes both contain the T(G/A)TTT-like motif [75–77]. However, although AAT gene transcription is stimulated by glucocorticoids and cAMP and inhibited by insulin, this motif apparently does not function as an insulin response sequence. Similarly, this sequence in the amylase promoter appears to confer no function with regard to insulin-regulated gene transcription. Indeed, a distinct insulin response sequence has been identified elsewhere in the promoter (see below).

Prolactin Insulin stimulates transcription of the prolactin gene [78–80] and, in combination with thyroid hormone, provides a response that is five- to tenfold greater than that afforded by either hormone alone [81]. The prolactin insulin response sequence is located between residues −97 and −87 [79, 80], and insulin stimulates the binding of a protein to this region. The prolactin insulin response sequence functions as an insulin response sequence in a heterologous context [79] and this element contains a region homologous to an inverted T(G/A)TTT motif (Figure 3) but also contains a region that is similar to the Ets binding domain (CAGGAT) that is located within the c-fos promoter (see above). Most recently, Jacob et al have demonstrated that the Ets binding element is required for insulin responsiveness of the prolactin, somatostatin and thymidine kinase promoters [82], which suggests that, in the prolactin promoter, the Ets binding element is indeed an insulin response sequence.

Other examples Several other genes that are responsive to insulin contain the T(G/A)TTT-like motif in their promoters, and more examples will no doubt be identified. The thyroglobulin promoter contains this motif (Figure 3), although it appears to be only one of three elements (which bind three distinct factors) required for insulin responsiveness (stimulation), while a protein that binds this region is a thyroid cell specific factor (TTF-2) [83]. The binding of TTF-2 to this T(G/A)TTT-like element is dependent upon insulin treatment [83]. In distinct contrast to PEPCK, the insulin effect is blocked by cycloheximide [83]. Transcription of the thyrotropin receptor gene is stimulated by insulin [84, 85], an effect that, in part, requires a thyroid transcription factor-1 binding site (−189 to −175) [85]. Adjacent to this site lies a region (−220 to −192; Figure 3) that, when fused to a CAT reporter gene, confers insulin responsiveness in FRTL-5 cells [85]. However, the endogenous gene requires both this novel insulin response sequence and the TTF-1 binding site for insulin responsiveness, and although the promoter of this gene contains a T(G/A)TTT-like element, mutation of this sequence does not affect the stimulation of gene transcription elicited by insulin [85].

The CCCGCCT-like Element

The sequence CCCGCCT was first demonstrated to act as an insulin response sequence within the context of the GAPDH promoter [86]. Homologous sequences have since been identified in a number of insulin-regulated gene promoters. Interestingly, this sequence is very similar to the Sp-1 binding site; however, only one of the insulin-regulated genes described below (δ1-crystallin) appears to utilize this transcription factor to mediate the action of insulin.

GAPDH The product of the GAPDH gene catalyzes a rate-limiting glycolytic step in adipocytes [87]. Transcription of GAPDH is increased in the genetically obese Zucker rat [88] while in a fasted, high-carbohydrate/low fat re-fed rat, the expression of GAPDH is increased 8- to 20-fold [86]. Expression of GAPDH is increased three- and tenfold respectively by insulin in hepatoma and adipocyte cell lines [86]. By utilizing GAPDH–CAT fusion genes, two insulin response sequences were identified within this promoter, one located between −488 and −409 and another between −308 and −269, relative to the transcription start site. These were termed IRE-A and IRE-B, respectively (Figure 5; [86]). Interestingly, two IRE-A binding proteins, designated IRE-A binding protein (IRE-ABP) [89] and insulin response protein (IRP-A) [86], have been identified. Insulin treatment increases the binding of IRP-A to the IRE-A, and IRP-A binding to the IRE-A is also increased in the fasted/re-fed rat [86]. In the same animals, a nutritional switch from fasted to re-fed induced the expression of IRE-ABP. IRE-ABP contains an HMG box domain that is 67% identical to that of the testis determining factor, SRY [90]. The sequence of the GAPDH-IRE-A is found in a number of other insulin-regulated gene promoters. However, as yet it is unclear as to how IRE-ABP and IRP-A interact to mediate the regulation of GAPDH transcription by insulin, although it is interesting to note that insulin alters the phosphorylation state of both of these proteins [91, 92].

Glucagon The actions of this hormone are frequently antagonistic to the actions of insulin, and the transcription of the glucagon gene is inhibited by insulin [93]. Interestingly, an insulin response sequence with homology to the GAPDH IRE-A (Figure 5), located between residues −274 and −234 of the glucagon promoter, confers insulin responsiveness to a heterologous promoter [94]. This suggests that, depending on context, this element may confer a positive or a negative insulin signal. It is worth noting, however, that in contrast

Gene promoter	CCCGCCT-like elements

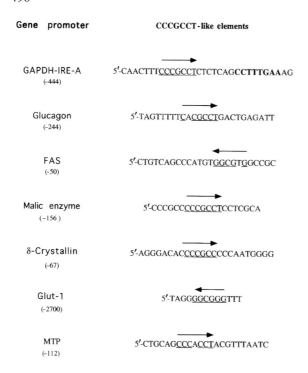

GAPDH-IRE-A
(-444)
5'-CAACTTT<u>CCCGCCT</u>CTCTCAGC**CTTTGAAA**G

Glucagon
(-244)
5'-TAGTTTTTC<u>AC</u>G<u>CCT</u>GACTGAGATT

FAS
(-50)
5'-CTGTCAGCCCATGT<u>GGC</u>G<u>T</u>GGCCGC

Malic enzyme
(-156)
5'-CCCGCC<u>CCCGCCT</u>CCTCGCA

δ-Crystallin
(-67)
5'-AGGGACAC<u>CCCGCC</u>CCCAATGGGG

Glut-1
(-2700)
5'-TAGG<u>GGCGGG</u>TTT

MTP
(-112)
5'-CTGCAG<u>CCCACCT</u>ACGTTTAATC

Figure 5 CCCGCCT-like sequences located in the promoters of insulin-regulated genes. The numbers in parentheses refer to the position of the 3'-residue relative to the transcription start site. GAPDH, glyceraldehyde-3-phosphate dehydrogenase; IRE, insulin response element; FAS, fatty acid synthetase; MTP, microsomal triglyceride transfer protein

to the GAPDH promoter, the transcription factors that bind this insulin response sequence in the glucagon promoter are islet cell-specific [95], and insulin does not affect protein binding to the glucagon insulin response sequence [94]. Thus, the glucagon insulin response sequence, although it shares sequence homology with the GAPDH IRE-A, appears to be functionally distinct from that in the GAPDH promoter.

δ1-Crystallin The δ1-crystallin gene product functions as a structural protein in the lens. Expression of the gene is stimulated by insulin and also by IGF-I, and an insulin response sequence has been located between residues −120 and −43 [96]. Within this region there exists the sequence CCCGCC<u>C</u> (the difference from the GAPDH-IRE-A is underlined). Interestingly, IGF-I stimulates protein binding to the region between −120 and +23, but in contrast to the GAPDH IRE-A, this binding was prevented by oligonucleotides that contain an Sp-1 binding element [96]. Thus, as with the glucagon insulin response sequence, the regulation of this insulin response sequence appears to be functionally distinct from that in the GAPDH promoter.

Fatty acid synthetase (FAS) Transcription of the gene that encodes the key lipogenic enzyme, FAS [97],

is increased by insulin [14, 88, 98]. The stimulation of FAS gene transcription by insulin can be blocked by cAMP, or by cycloheximide [14]. However, an insulin response sequence with some homology to the GAPDH IRE-A has been located between residues −68 and −52 ([99]; Figure 5). This sequence confers insulin responsiveness to a heterologous promoter. While nuclear factors have been identified that bind this sequence *in vitro*, there appears to be no effect of insulin on binding [99]. This is in contrast to the effect insulin has on the binding of proteins to the GAPDH promoter (see above). Therefore, this insulin response sequence, like those of glucagon and δ1-crystallin, exhibits a regulatory mechanism which is different from that of the GAPDH IRE-A.

Malic enzyme and Glut-1 As discussed earlier, malic enzyme and Glut-1 contain sequences homologous to the T(G/A)TTT and SRE motifs, respectively, within their promoters. However, both promoters also contain sequences homologous to the GAPDH IRE-A (Figure 5). Insulin stimulates the expression of malic enzyme and also increases protein binding to the CCCGCCT-like element in the malic enzyme promoter [74]. Which element (T(G/A)TTT or CCCGCCT), if either, is involved in the response of this promoter to insulin is not yet clear. The Glut-1 gene requires an SRE for the observed insulin responsiveness, but evidence to date suggests that the CCCGCCT-like element (located within the −2.7 kbp enhancer [35]) is not important.

Microsomal triglyceride transfer protein (MTP), large subunit MTP plays a key role in the production of lipoproteins, chylomicrons and VLDL. It exists as a heterodimer complex of 58 kDa and 88 kDa subunits. The smaller subunit has protein disulphide isomerase activity and the larger subunit has an unknown function, but mutations in the gene encoding the latter have been linked to the lipid disorder, abetalipoproteinemia [100]. Transcription of the endogenous small subunit is inhibited by insulin [101], but hormonal regulation of the large subunit *in vivo* has not been reported as yet. In fusion gene experiments, however, insulin inhibits the transcription of the large subunit promoter ligated to luciferase, and the region from −124 to −112 contains an insulin response sequence [102]. Within this region there is a sequence homologous to the GAPDH IRE-A (CCC<u>A</u>CCT, Figure 5), but the role of this sequence in the regulation of this promoter by insulin has not been studied in detail. In addition, the response of this fusion gene to insulin requires higher concentrations of the hormone than most genes reported thus far [102], so IGF-I receptors may actually mediate the insulin response.

Miscellaneous

Several other unique sequences required for insulin responsiveness have been reported (see [11, 12]). A novel insulin response sequence has been located within the promoter of one of the amylase genes (Amy 2.2) [77, 103]. The region from −167 to −138 of this gene promoter is sufficient to confer insulin stimulation when linked to a heterologous promoter and when expressed in transgenic animals [104]. Although a T(G/A)TTT-like sequence is present in this region of the Amy 2.2 promoter (Figure 3), it does not lie within the core insulin response sequence that has recently been more accurately located between residues −145 and −136 [77].

Expression of the acute phase protein, α_1-acid glycoprotein (AGP) in hepatoma cells, is stimulated by IL-1 and IL-6, and these effects are blocked by insulin [105, 106]. Surprisingly, a subclone of the same hepatoma cell line exhibits insulin-stimulated AGP gene transcription. The molecular differences between these clones are unknown [107]. Using this subclone, an insulin response sequence has been found that overlaps the IL-1 response element and represents a binding site for the transcription factor C/EBPβ [107, 108]. Campos et al proposed that insulin regulates AGP gene transcription indirectly, through stimulation of the synthesis of C/EBPβ in the AGP promoter. The only other element described above that resembles a binding site for C/EBPβ is the SRE, but there is no evidence that a C/EBPβ/SRE complex has a role in the regulation of gene transcription by insulin.

The classification system employed in this chapter is an attempt to group homologous sequences from insulin-regulated gene promoters, in the hope of identifying common patterns of regulatory mechanisms. However, the evidence presented would argue that these sequences are not general consensus elements but that a particular sequence may confer insulin regulation within a certain context (e.g. the T(G/A)TTTT motif within the PEPCK, TAT and IGFBP-1 genes mediates an inhibitory response to glucocorticoid stimulation).

INSULIN SIGNALING AND GENE EXPRESSION

The signaling pathways involved in the regulation of gene transcription by insulin have only recently begun to be mapped [46, 109–112]. The insulin receptor is linked to the c-fos promoter via a cascade of proteins including adaptor proteins, GTPases and protein kinases, that constitute the 'Ras/MAP kinase' cascade (for review, see [19]). This signaling pathway results in the phosphorylation of p62[TCF] (the protein that binds to the Ets domain of the c-fos promoter just proximal to the p67[SRF] binding site), with a resultant increase in the ability of this protein to bind to and/or transactivate the c-fos gene. Other pathways almost certainly exist and probably synergize with the 'Ras/MAP kinase' pathway in the regulation of c-fos gene transcription [19]. A second insulin signaling pathway involves the enzyme phosphatidylinositol 3-kinase (PI 3-kinase). This enzyme generates putative 'second messenger' phosphorylated inositol lipids [113], and is required for the insulin regulation of transcription of the genes for PEPCK [114] and hexokinase II (HKII) (H Osawa and DK Granner, in preparation). Interestingly, in contrast to the c-fos gene, the Ras/MAP kinase pathway is not required for the action of insulin on the PEPCK [27] or HKII (H Osawa and DK Granner, in preparation) promoter. In addition, the activation of the protein kinase p70[S6K] by insulin is not required for the inhibition of PEPCK transcription by insulin in hepatoma cells [114], but is required for the positive regulation of HKII transcription by the same hormone in L6 myocytes (H Osawa and DK Granner, in preparation). Therefore, insulin utilizes distinct signaling pathways for the regulation of transcription of distinct genes. Much work remains to be done in this area, but the identification of the insulin response sequence(s) is the first step in linking the insulin-responsive genes to the insulin receptor. Only by identifying the insulin response sequence(s) can the associated *trans*-acting factors be characterized and the mechanism by which they receive the insulin 'signal' be determined.

THE SEARCH FOR GENETIC DETERMINANTS OF NIDDM

Since it remains unclear whether a defect in insulin secretion or insulin action is responsible for the primary defect that leads to the development of NIDDM in humans, any molecule required for either process constitutes a potential 'diabetogene'. Researchers have attempted to determine whether the activities of specific enzymes involved in the metabolic processes known to be defective in patients with NIDDM are indeed altered. In insulin resistance there is an increase in hepatic glucose production and a reduction in peripheral glucose uptake. Thus the question arises as to whether the activities of the enzymes required for gluconeogenesis (e.g. PEPCK) are also increased. Similarly, a reduction of peripheral glucose uptake could result if there is a reduced activity of hexokinase II, the enzyme that maintains the inward glucose gradient in muscle and adipose tissue, or if there is reduced expression of the facilitative glucose transporters in these tissues. In addition, the reduced insulin secretion observed in patients with NIDDM could be due to loss of expression or decreased activity of the glucose sensor in the pancreatic islet B-cells. Much research has focused on the activities and expression of these proteins in diabetic patients and in animal models of this disease. The general findings are discussed below.

Glut-2

In two different rat models of NIDDM there is a reduction of the amount of the Glut-2 glucose transporter in the pancreatic islet B-cells [115, 116], and expression of antisense RNA to the Glut-2 gene in the pancreases of transgenic mice produces a diabetic phenotype [117]. Unfortunately, kinetic data on glucose transport in the islet B-cells suggest that Glut-2 defects cannot be the primary B-cell defect [2, 31]. Firstly, glucose transport is not normally limiting in B-cells [118]. Secondly, in B-cells isolated from streptozotocin-administered or partially pancreatectomized rats the complete loss of glucose-induced insulin secretion is seen with only a partial reduction in Glut-2 and glucose transport [119, 120].

Glucokinase

Hexokinase IV, generally termed glucokinase, is the major hexokinase isoform in liver and islet B-cells. Although both these tissues express the same isoform of hexokinase, its expression is differentially regulated due to the existence of alternative, tissue-specific promoters [121]. In the liver, expression of glucokinase is stimulated by insulin (at the transcriptional level) [122, 123] and unaffected by glucose [124]. By contrast, glucose regulates glucokinase expression in the pancreatic B-cell [125, 126]. Many of the individuals suffering from the rare form of NIDDM, MODY, contain glucokinase gene mutations that result in reduced activity of glucokinase (for review, see [126]). However, these mutations are only found in MODY 2 patients, and not in MODY 1 or 3 [127] (see also Chapter 3).

PEPCK

Transgenic animals that overexpress PEPCK exhibit a diabetic-like phenotype [128, 129], while in H4IIE cells replacement of the PEPCK promoter with a non-insulin responsive viral promoter resulted in increased gluconeogenesis and therefore a higher rate of hepatic glucose production [129]. No mutations were located in the PEPCK promoter of a sample of patients with NIDDM [130], so a mutation of the insulin response sequence in the PEPCK gene promoter does not contribute to the NIDDM phenotype in the group studied. Loss of insulin repression of PEPCK does occur in at least one animal model, the obese hyperglycemic Wistar rat. These animals have reduced regulation of

PEPCK gene expression by insulin (and also glucokinase expression) [131]. However, this may result from a defect other than loss of a functional insulin response sequence, such as a defect in insulin signaling (see below).

Hexokinase II

As with PEPCK, the expression of HKII in animal models of NIDDM is altered [132]. No mutations in the coding region of this gene were found in recent studies of patients with NIDDM [133–135]. Studies to determine whether mutations exist in the HKII gene promoter in patients with NIDDM are ongoing.

Molecules Involved in Insulin Signal Transduction

The signaling molecules that mediate the connection between the insulin receptor at the cell surface and the various catalytic activities influenced by insulin also constitute candidate 'diabetogenes'. Insulin employs a series of 'molecular highways' in order to link the insulin receptor to the promoters of insulin responsive genes. Two general approaches have been employed to determine the molecular paths utilized by insulin. Researchers have studied the substrates of the insulin receptor tyrosine kinase and have attempted to map the signals that are initiated as a consequence of the binding of insulin to its receptor. Alternatively, well characterized actions of insulin (e.g. the stimulation of glycogen synthesis) are used as 'end points' of a pathway, and the regulatory mechanisms that mediate the action of insulin at these specific 'end points' are studied so that researchers can subsequently 'walk' back up the signaling pathway and eventually arrive back at the insulin receptor. These approaches have already identified several insulin signaling molecules, and the role of some of these molecules in NIDDM has been investigated. Each gene that encodes a specific mediator of such a pathway represents a potential 'diabetogene'. There are reports of defects in insulin receptor gene expression in patients with extreme insulin resistance (e.g. leprechaunism), but a similar defect is uncommon in patients with NIDDM [136]. The insulin-stimulated activity of a key signaling molecule, PI 3-kinase, that is required for insulin regulation of PEPCK [27, 114] and HKII (H Osawa and DK Granner, in preparation) gene expression, is reduced in skeletal muscle of insulin-resistant obese subjects [137]. Of course, the effect may simply be due to the reduction in insulin responsiveness of the insulin receptor tyrosine kinase that is also observed in these patients. There have been no studies as yet to determine whether patients with NIDDM contain mutations in any of the genes that encode the subunits of PI 3-kinase. In Pima Indians, a population with an abnormally high incidence of NIDDM, the activity of an insulin-stimulated protein kinase, $p70^{S6K}$, is reduced [138]. This protein kinase may be involved in the regulation of protein synthesis by insulin [139, 140].

A second insulin-stimulated ribosomal S6 protein kinase, $p90^{rsk}$, lies on a distinct insulin signaling pathway to the $p70^{S6K}$ [141] and has been implicated in the regulation of glycogen synthesis by insulin [141–143]. Also implicated in this pathway is the type 1 protein phosphatase (PP1) [144]. Since the regulation of glycogen synthase activity by insulin is impaired in insulin resistance [145], Bjorbaek et al examined the coding region of $p90^{rsk}$ and the three isoforms of PP1 (α, β and γ), that are expressed in the muscle of a number of NIDDM patients [146]. No mutations associated with NIDDM were identified, and no differences were found in the mRNA levels of any of these signaling molecules between normal and NIDDM subjects [146]. Since there was a clear reduction in the specific activity of glycogen synthase in the NIDDM patients examined, the authors suggest that the defect must lie in the insulin signaling pathway upstream of PP1 and $p90^{rsk}$ [146].

Antagonists of Insulin Action

Abnormal expression of molecules that antagonize one or more of these insulin-signaling pathways could result in the phenomenon of insulin resistance. The gene 'Ras associated with diabetes' (Rad), was identified by a subtraction cloning technique [8, 13]. Rad, a member of the Ras superfamily of GTPases, is expressed in muscle and adipose tissue but not liver, and is excessively expressed in persons with NIDDM [13]. It has been proposed to act as an antagonist of insulin action, potentially by blocking glucose transporter translocation [13]. Tumor necrosis factor-α (TNF-α) also suppresses insulin action (at least in adipocytes and myocytes), probably by reducing insulin receptor tyrosine kinase activity [147, 148]. TNF-α levels are increased in animal models of obesity and diabetes [149]. A membrane glycoprotein, PC-1, is also expressed at high levels in some NIDDM patients. This protein apparently antagonizes insulin action by blocking the insulin receptor tyrosine kinase [150, 151]. However, this molecule does not appear to be present in liver, one of the major sites of insulin resistance. A third endogenous inhibitor of the insulin receptor tyrosine kinase is the plasma protein, pp63 [152], but there is no evidence that its levels are altered in NIDDM. However, only the phosphorylated form of pp63 inhibits the receptor tyrosine kinase [152], and therefore the level of phosphorylated pp63 is more relevant than absolute measurements of the protein.

Thus, there are a number of candidates that may act as antagonists of insulin signal transduction and may, if abnormally expressed or regulated, lead to an insulin-resistant state.

SUMMARY

With the continuing characterization of insulin response sequences it becomes increasingly evident that no single overall consensus sequence for such an element exists within the numerous gene promoters regulated by insulin. In addition, no consensus sequences exist for positively or negatively regulated genes, or for genes involved in similar biologic processes (e.g. membrane proteins, enzymes of metabolism, hormones). In addition, in contrast to agents such as glucocorticoids, estrogen and retinoic acid, no single transcription factor specifically involved in insulin signaling has yet been unequivocally identified. Interestingly, a relatively short and simple motif (T(G/A)TTT) is found in the promoters of several genes that respond to insulin (Figure 3). However, the mechanism by which insulin signals to this motif appears to be distinct for many of these genes, the exception being the PEPCK, IGFBP-1 and TAT genes. This group of hepatic, insulin-regulated genes shares the ability to bind the glucocorticoid accessory factor, HNF3, at or very close to their T(G/A)TTT-motif. Although this protein does not appear to mediate the response of the PEPCK promoter to insulin directly, it is possible that its role as an accessory factor may be compromised by the actual insulin response factor. In contrast, the genes that contain a CCCGCCT motif within their insulin response sequences (Figure 5) do not appear to share a common regulatory mechanism. Thus, it would appear that insulin utilizes a number of distinct sequences, and several distinct mechanisms in order to regulate gene transcription, and the task of identifying an insulin response sequence in each insulin-regulated gene promoter will therefore be complex.

Acknowledgments

This work was supported by NIH grants DK35107, DK20593 (the Vanderbilt Diabetes Research and Training Center) and DK46867. CS is a recipient of an American Diabetes Association Mentor-based Fellowship (DKG).

REFERENCES

1. DeFronzo RA. The triumvirate: β-cell, muscle, liver. A collusion responsible for NIDDM. Diabetes 1988; 37: 667–87.

2. Granner DK, O'Brien RM. Molecular physiology and genetics of NIDDM. Diabetes Care 1992; 15: 369–95.

3. DeFronzo RA, Bonadonna RC, Ferrannini E. Pathogenesis of NIDDM. Diabetes Care 1992; 15: 318–68.

4. Warram JH, Martin BC, Krolewski AS, Soeldner JS, Kahn CR. Slow glucose removal rate and hyperinsulinemia precede the development of type 2 diabetes in the offspring of diabetic parents. Ann Intern Med 1990; 113: 909–15.

5. Martin BD, Warram JH, Krolewski AS, Bergman RN, Soeldner JS, Kahn CR. Role of glucose and insulin resistance in development of type 2 diabetes mellitus: results of a 25-year follow-up study. Lancet 1992; 340: 925–9.

6. Lillioja S, Mott DM, Howard BV, Bennett PH, Yki-Jarvinen H, Freymond BL et al. Impaired glucose tolerance as a disorder of insulin action: longitudinal and cross-sectional studies in Pima Indians. New Engl J Med 1988; 318: 1217–25.

7. Denton RM. Early events in insulin actions. Adv Cycl Nucl Prot Phos Res 1986; 20: 293–341.

8. Kahn CR. Insulin action, diabetogenes and the cause of type 2 diabetes. Diabetes 1994; 43: 1066–84.

9. Myers MG, Grammer TC, Wang L-M, Sun XJ, Pierce JH, Blenis J, White MF. IRS-1 mediates PI 3-kinase and p70^{s6k} signaling during insulin, IGF-1 and IL-4 stimulation. J Biol Chem 1994; 269: 28783–9.

10. White MF, Kahn CR. The insulin signalling system. J Biol Chem 1994; 269: 1–4.

11. O'Brien RM, Granner DK. Regulation of PEPCK gene expression by insulin. Physiol Rev 1996; 76: 1–53.

12. O'Brien RM, Granner DK. Regulation of gene expression by insulin. Biochem J 1991; 278: 609–19.

13. Reynet C, Kahn CR. Rad: a member of the Ras family overexpressed in muscle of type 2 diabetic humans. Science 1993; 262: 1441–4.

14. Paulauskis JD, Sul HS. Cloning and expression of mouse fatty acid synthase and other specific mRNAs. J Biol Chem 1988; 263: 7049–54.

15. Levenson RM, Nairn AC, Blackshear PJ. Insulin rapidly induces the biosynthesis of elongation factor 2. J Biol Chem 1989; 264: 11904–11.

16. Shanker R, Neeley WE, Dillmann WH. Rapid effects of insulin on *in vitro* translational activity of specific mRNA in diabetic rat heart. Am J Physiol 1986; 250: E558–63.

17. Mohn KL, Laz TM, Melby AE, Taub R. Immediate-early gene expression differs between regenerating liver, insulin-stimulated H-35 cells, and mitogen-stimulated Balb/c 3T3 cells. J Biol Chem 1990; 265: 21914–21.

18. Mohn KL, Laz TM, Hsu J-C, Melby AE, Bravo R, Taub R. The immediate–early growth response in regenerating liver and insulin-stimulated H-35 cells: comparison with serum-stimulated 3T3 cells and identification of 41 novel immediate–early genes. Mol Cell Biol 1991; 11: 381–90.

19. Treisman R. The serum response element. TIBS 1992; 17: 423–6.

20. Whitmarsh AJ, Shore P, Sharrocks AD, Davis RJ. Integration of MAP kinase signal transduction pathways at the serum response element. Science 1995; 269: 403–6.

21. Karin M, Hunter T. Transcriptional control by protein phosphorylation: signal transmission from the cell surface to the nucleus. Current Biology 1995; 5: 747–57.

22. Medema RH, Wubbolts R, Bos JL. Two dominant inhibitory mutants of p21ras interfere with insulin-induced gene expression. Mol Cell Biol 1991; 11: 5963–7.

23. Messina JL, Standaert ML, Ishizuka T, Weinstock RS, Farese RV. Role of PKC in insulin regulation of c-fos transcription. J Biol Chem 1992; 267: 9223–8.

24. Yamauchi K, Holt K, Pessin J. PI 3-kinase functions upstream of ras and raf in mediating insulin stimulation of c-fos transcription. J Biol Chem 1993; 268: 14597–600.

25. Buchou T, Gaben A-M, Phan-Dhin-Tuy F, Mester J. Insulin/IGF1 induce actin transcription in mouse fibroblasts expressing constitutively myc gene. Mol Cell Endocrin 1991; 75: 181–7.

26. Thompson MJ, Roe MW, Malik RK, Blackshear PJ. Insulin and other growth factors induce binding of the ternary complex and a novel protein complex to the c-fos serum response element. J Biol Chem 1994; 269: 8679–82.

27. Gabbay RA, Sutherland C, Gnudi L, Kahn BB, O'Brien RM, Granner DK, Flier JS. Insulin regulation of PEPCK gene expression does not require activation of the Ras/MAP kinase signaling pathway. J Biol Chem 1996; 271: 1890–7.

28. Gille H, Sharrocks A, Shaw P. Phosphorylation of p62TCF by MAP kinase stimulates ternary complex formation at the c-fos promoter. Nature 1992; 358: 414–17.

29. Marais R, Wynne J, Treisman R. The SRF accessory protein ELK-1 contains a growth factor regulated transcription domain. Cell 1993; 73: 381–93.

30. Lazar DF, Wiese RJ, Brady MJ, Mastick CC, Waters SB, Yamauchi K et al. MAP kinase kinase inhibition does not block the stimulation of glucose utilization by insulin. J Biol Chem 1995; 270: 20801–7.

31. Mueckler M. Facilitative glucose transporters. Eur J Biochem 1994; 219: 713–25.

32. Garcia de Herreros A, Birnbaum MJ. The regulation of glucose transporter gene expression in 3T3 adipocytes. J Biol Chem 1989; 264: 9885–90.

33. Kahn BB, Schulman GI, DeFronzo RA, Cushman SW, Rossetti L. Normalization of blood glucose in diabetic rats with phlorizin treatment reverses insulin-resistant glucose transport in adipose cells without restoring glucose transporter gene expression. J Clin Invest 1991; 87: 561–70.

34. Murakami T, Nishiyama T, Shirotani T, Shinohara Y, Kan M, Ishii K et al. Identification of two enhancer elements in the gene encoding the type 1 glucose transporter from the mouse which are responsive to serum, growth factor, and oncogenes. J Biol Chem 1992; 267: 9300–6.

35. Todaka M, Nishiyama T, Murakami T, Saito S, Ito K, Kanai F et al. The role of insulin in activation of two enhancers in the mouse Glut-1 gene. J Biol Chem 1994; 269: 29265–70.

36. Onyia JE, Halladay DL, Messina JL. One of the three CCArGG box/SREs of the β-actin gene is an insulin response element. Endocrinology 1995; 136: 306–15.

37. Metz R, Ziff E. cAMP stimulates the C/EBP-related transcription factor rNFIL-6 to translocate to the nucleus and induce c-fos transcription. Genes Develop 1991; 5: 1754–66.

38. Angel P, Imagawa M, Chiu R, Stein B, Imbra RJ, Rahmsdorf HJ et al. Phorbol ester-inducible genes contain a common *cis* element recognized by a TPA-modulated *trans*-acting factor. Cell 1987; 49: 729–39.

39. Angel P, Karin M. The role of jun, fos and the AP-1 complex in cell proliferation and transformation. Biochim Biophys Acta 1991; 1072: 129–57.

40. Rutter GA, White MRH, Tavare JM. Involvement of MAP kinase in insulin signaling revealed by non-invasive imaging of luciferase gene expression in single living cells. Curr Biol 1995; 5: 890–9.

41. van Dijck P, Schoonjans K, Sassone-Corsi P, Auwerx J, Verhoeven G. A fos-jun element in the first intron of an α-globulin gene. Mol Cell Biochem 1993; 125: 127–36.

42. Straus DS, Takemoto CD. Insulin negatively regulates albumin mRNA at the transcriptional and post-transcriptional level in rat hepatoma cells. J Biol Chem 1987; 262: 1955–60.

43. Mira E, Castano JG. Insulin short-term control of rat liver α$_2$-microglobulin gene transcription. J Biol Chem 1989; 264: 18209–12.

44. Kim S-J, Kahn CR. Insulin stimulates phosphorylation of c-jun, c-fos, and fos-related proteins in cultured adipocytes. J Biol Chem 1994; 269: 11887–92.

45. Davis RJ. MAPKs: new JNK expands the group. TIBS 1994; 19: 470–3.

46. Karin M. Signal transduction from the cell surface to the nucleus through the phosphorylation of transcription factors. Curr Opin Cell Biol 1994; 6: 415–24.

47. O'Brien RM, Bonovich MT, Forest CD, Granner DK. Signal transduction convergence: phorbol esters and insulin inhibit PEPCK gene transcription through the same 10-base-pair sequence. Proc Natl Acad Sci 1991; 88: 6580–4.

48. Hanson RW, Patel YM. PEPCK: the gene and the enzyme. Adv Enzymol 1994; 69: 203–81.

49. Imai E, Stromstedt P-E, Quinn PG, Carlstedt-Duke J, Gustafsson J-A, Granner DK. Characterization of a complex glucocorticoid response unit in the PEPCK gene. Mol Cell Biol 1990; 10: 4712–19.

50. Liu J, Park EA, Gurney AL, Roesler WJ, Hanson RW. cAMP induction of PEPCK gene transcription is mediated by multiple promoter elements. J Biol Chem 1991; 266: 19095–102.

51. Imai E, Miner JN, Mitchell JA, Yamamoto KR, Granner DK. Glucocorticoid receptor–cAMP response element-binding protein interaction and the response of the PEPCK gene to glucocorticoids. J Biol Chem 1993; 268: 5353–6.

52. Angrand P-O, Coffinier C, Weiss MC. Response of the PEPCK gene to glucocorticoids depends on the integrity of the cAMP pathway. Cell Growth Diff 1994; 5: 957–66.

53. O'Brien RM, Noisin EL, Suwanichkul A, Yamasaki T, Lucas PL, Wang J-C et al. HNF3 and hormone-regulated expression of the PEPCK and insulin-like growth factor-binding protein 1 genes. Mol Cell Biol 1995; 15: 1747–58.

54. Faber S, O'Brien RM, Imai E, Granner DK, Chalkley R. Dynamic aspects of DNA/protein interactions in the transcriptional initiation complex and the hormone-responsive domains of the PEPCK promoter *in vivo*. J Biol Chem 1993; 268: 24976–85.

55. O'Brien RM, Lucas PL, Yamasaki T, Noisin EL, Granner DK. Potential convergence of insulin and cAMP signal transduction systems at the PEPCK gene promoter through C/EBP. J Biol Chem 1994; 269: 30419–28.

56. Rechler MM. Insulin like growth factor binding proteins. Vitamins Horm 1993; 47: 1–114.

57. Elgin RG, Busby WH, Clemmons DR. An insulin-like growth factor binding protein enhances the biologic response to IGF-1. Proc Natl Acad Sci 1987; 84: 3254–8.

58. Powell DR, Suwanichkul A, Cubbage ML, DePaolis LA, Snuggs MB, Lee PDK. Insulin inhibits transcription of the human gene for IGFBP-1. J Biol Chem 1991; 266: 18868–76.

59. Orlowski CC, Ooi GT, Brown DR, Yang YW-H, Tseng LY-H, Rechler MM. Insulin rapidly inhibits IGFBP-1 gene expression in H4-II-E rat hepatoma cells. Mol Endocrinol 1991; 5: 1180–7.

60. Suh D-S, Ooi GT, Rechler MM. Identification of *cis*-elements mediating the stimulation of rat IGFBP-1 promoter activity by dexamethasone, cAMP and phorbol esters and inhibition by insulin. Mol Endocrinol 1994; 8: 794–805.

61. Unterman TG, Oehler DT, Murphy LJ, Lacson RG. Multihormonal regulation of IGFBP-1 in rat H4IIE hepatoma cells: the dominant role of insulin. Endocrinology 1991; 128: 2693–701.

62. Suwanichkul A, Morris SL, Powell DR. Identification of an IRE in the promoter of the human gene for IGFBP-1. J Biol Chem 1993; 268: 17063–8.

63. Suwanichkul A, Allander SV, Morris SL, Powell DR. Glucocorticoids and insulin regulate expression of the human gene for IGFBP-1 through proximal promoter elements. J Biol Chem 1994; 269: 30835–41.

64. Unterman TG, Fareeduddin A, Harris MA, Goswami RG, Porcella A, Costa RH, Lacson RG. HNF3 binds to the insulin response sequence in the IGFBP-1 promoter and enhances promoter function. Biochem Biophys Res Comm 1994; 203: 1835–41.

65. Grange T, Roux J, Rigaud G, Pictet R. Cell-type specific activity of two glucocorticoid responsive units of the rat TAT gene is associated with multiple binding sites for C/EBP and a novel liver-specific nuclear factor. Nucl Acids Res 1991; 19: 131–9.

66. Nitsch D, Boshart M, Schutz G. Activation of the tyrosine aminotransferase gene is dependent on synergy between liver-specific and hormone-responsive elements. Proc Natl Acad Sci 1993; 90: 5479–83.

67. Ganss R, Weih F, Schutz G. The cAMP and the glucocorticoid dependent enhancers are targets for insulin repression of tyrosine aminotransferase gene transcription. Mol Endocrinol 1994; 8: 895–903.

68. Granner DK, O'Brien RM. Regulation of transcription by insulin. In Cohen P, Foulkes JG (eds) The hormonal regulation of gene transcription. Amsterdam: Elsevier, 1991; 309–32.

69. Lucas PC, Granner DK. Hormone response domains in gene transcription. Annu Rev Biochem 1992; 61: 1131–73.

70. Ito Y, Azrolan N, O'Connell A, Walsh A, Breslow JL. Hypertriglyceridemia as a result of human apo-CIII gene expression in transgenic mice. Science 1990; 249: 790–3.

71. Chen M, Breslow JL, Li W, Leff T. Transcriptional regulation of the apo-CIII gene by insulin in diabetic mice: correlation with changes in plasma triglyceride levels. J Lipid Res 1994; 35: 1918–24.

72. Dammerman M, Sandkuul LA, Halaas JL, Chung W, Breslow JL. An apolipoprotein-CIII haplotype protective against HTG is specified by promoter and 3′ untranslated region polymorphisms. Proc Natl Acad Sci 1993; 90: 4562–6.

73. Katsurada A, Iritani N, Fukada H, Matsumura Y, Noguchi T, Tanaka T. Effects of insulin and fructose on transcriptional and post-transcriptional regulation of malic enzyme synthesis in diabetic rat liver. Biochim Biophys Acta 1989; 1004: 103–7.

74. Garcia-Jimenez C, Benito B, Jolin T, Santisteban P. Insulin regulation of malic enzyme gene expression in rat liver: evidence for nuclear proteins that bind to two putative insulin response elements. Mol Endocrinol 1994; 8: 1361–9.

75. Barouki R, Pave-Preux M, Bousquet-Lemercier B, Pol S, Bouguet J, Hanoune J. Regulation of cytosolic aspartate aminotransferase mRNAs in the Fao rat hepatoma cell line by dexamethasone, insulin and cAMP. Eur J Biochem 1989; 186: 79–85.

76. Aggerbeck M, Garletti M, Feilleux-Duche S, Veyssier C, Daheshia M, Hanoune J, Barouki R. Regulation of the cytosolic aspartate aminotransferase housekeeping gene promoter by glucocorticoids, cAMP, and insulin. Biochemistry 1993; 32: 9065–72.

77. Johnson TM, Rosenberg MP, Meisler MH. An insulin-responsive element in the pancreatic enhancer of the amylase gene. J Biol Chem 1993; 268: 464–8.

78. Stanley FM. An element in the prolactin promoter mediates the stimulatory effect of insulin on transcription of the prolactin gene. J Biol Chem 1992; 267: 16719–26.

79. Jacob KK, Stanley FM. The insulin and cAMP response elements of the prolactin gene are overlapping sequences. J Biol Chem 1994; 269: 25515–20.

80. Jacob KK, Stanley FM. Insulin and cAMP increase prolactin gene expression through different response pathways. Mol Cell Endocrinol 1995; 109: 175–81.

81. Stanley F. Stimulation of prolactin gene expression by insulin. J Biol Chem 1988; 263: 13444–8.

82. Jacob KK, Ouyang L, Stanley FM. A consensus insulin response element is activated by an ETS-related transcription factor. J Biol Chem 1995; 270: 27773–9.

83. Santisteban P, Acebron A, Polycarpou-Schwarz M, Di Lauro R. Insulin and IGFBP-1 regulate a thyroid-specific nuclear protein that binds to the thyroglobulin promoter. Mol Endocrinol 1992; 6: 1310–17.

84. Saji M, Akamizu T, Sanchez M, Obici S, Avvedimento E, Gottesman ME, Kohn LD. Regulation of thyrotropin receptor gene expression in rat FRTL-5 thyroid cells. Endocrinology 1992; 130: 520–33.

85. Shimura Y, Shimura H, Ohmori M, Ikuyama S, Kohn LD. Identification of a novel insulin-responsive element in the rat thyrotropin receptor promoter. J Biol Chem 1994; 269: 31908–14.

86. Nasrin N, Ercolani L, Denaro M, Kong X-F, Kang I, Alexander M. An insulin response element in the GAPDH gene binds a nuclear protein induced by insulin in cultured cells and by nutritional manipulations *in vivo*. Proc Natl Acad Sci 1990; 87: 5273–7.

87. Dugail I, Quignard-Boulange A, Bazin R, Le Liepvre X, Lavau M. Adipose-tissue specific increase in GAPDH activity and mRNA amounts in suckling pre-obese Zucker rats. Biochem J 1988; 254: 483–7.

88. Rolland V, Dugail I, Le Liepvre X, Lavau M. Evidence of increased GAPDH and fatty acid synthase promoter activities in transiently transfected adipocytes from genetically obese rats. J Biol Chem 1995; 270: 1102–6.

89. Nasrin N, Buggs C, Kong X-F, Carnazza J, Goebl M, Alexander-Bridges M. DNA-binding properties of the product of the testis-determining gene and a related protein. Nature 1991; 354: 317–20.

90. Alexander-Bridges M, Ercolani L, Kong XF, Nasrin N. Identification of a core motif that is recognized by three members of the HMG class of transcriptional regulators: IRE-ABP, SRY, and TCF-1α. J Cell Biochem 1992; 48: 129–35.

91. Alexander-Bridges M, Buggs C, Giere L, Denaro M, Kahn B, White M et al. Models of insulin action on metabolic and growth responses. Mol Cell Biochem 1992; 109: 99–105.

92. Alexander-Bridges M, Mukhopadhyay NK, Jhala U, Denaro M, Kong X-F, Avruch J, Maller J. Growth factor-activated kinases phosphorylate IRE-ABP. Biochem Soc Trans 1992; 20: 691–3.

93. Philippe J. Glucagon gene transcription is negatively regulated by insulin in a hamster islet cell line. J Clin Invest 1989; 84: 672–7.

94. Philippe J. Insulin regulation of the glucagon gene is mediated by an insulin-responsive DNA element. Proc Natl Acad Sci 1991; 88: 7224–7.

95. Philippe J, Morel C, Cordier-Bussat M. Islet-specific proteins interact with the insulin response element of the glucagon gene. J Biol Chem 1995; 270: 3039–45.

96. Alemany J, Borras T, DePablo F. Transcriptional stimulation of the δ_1-crystallin gene by IGF-1 and insulin requires DNA *cis* elements in chicken. Proc Natl Acad Sci 1990; 87: 3353–7.

97. Wakil SJ, Stoops JK, Joshi VC. Fatty acid synthesis and its regulation. Annu Rev Biochem 1983; 52: 537–79.

98. Paulauskis JD, Sul HS. Hormonal regulation of mouse fatty acid synthase gene transcription in liver. J Biol Chem 1989; 264: 574–7.

99. Moustaid N, Beyer RS, Sul HS. Identification of an insulin response element in the fatty acid synthase promoter. J Biol Chem 1994; 269: 5629–34.

100. Sharp D, Blinderman L, Combs KA, Kienzle B, Ricci B, Wager-Smith K et al. Cloning and gene defects in microsomal triglyceride transfer protein associated with abetalipoproteinaemia. Nature 1993; 365: 65–9.

101. Nieto A, Mira E, Castano JG. Transcriptional regulation of rat liver protein disulphide-isomerase gene by insulin and in diabetes. Biochem J 1990; 267: 317–23.

102. Hagan DL, Kienzle B, Jamil H, Hariharan N. Transcriptional regulation of human and hamster microsomal triglyceride transfer protein genes. J Biol Chem 1994; 269: 28737–44.

103. Keller SA, Rosenberg MP, Johnson TM, Howard G, Meisler MH. Regulation of amylase gene expression in diabetic mice is mediated by a *cis*-acting upstream element close to the pancreas-specific enhancer. Gen Dev 1990; 4: 1316–21.

104. Schmid RM, Meisler MH. Dietary regulation of pancreatic amylase in transgenic mice mediated by a 126-base pair DNA fragment. Am J Physiol 1992; 262: G971–6.

105. Thompson D, Harrison SP, Evans SW, Whicher JT. Insulin modulation of acute phase protein production

in a human hepatoma cell line. Cytokine 1991; 3: 619–26.

106. Campos SP, Baumann H. Insulin is a prominent modulator of the cytokine-stimulated expression of acute-phase plasma protein genes. Mol Cell Biol 1992; 12: 1789–97.

107. Campos SP, Wang Y, Koj A, Baumann H. Insulin cooperates with IL-1 in regulating expression of α_1-acid glycoprotein gene in rat hepatoma cells. Cytokine 1994; 6: 485–92.

108. Baumann H, Jahreis GP, Morella KK, Won K-A, Pruitt SC, Jones VE. Transcriptional regulation through cytokine and glucocorticoid response elements of rst acute phase plasma protein genes by C/EBP and Jun-B. J Biol Chem 1991; 266: 20390–9.

109. Shiran R, Aronheim A, Rosen A, Park CW, Leshkowitz D, Walker MD. Positive and negative regulation of insulin gene transcription. Biochem Soc Trans 1993; 21: 150–4.

110. Denton RM, Tavare JM. Does mitogen-activated-protein kinase have a role in insulin action? The cases for and against. Eur J Biochem 1995; 227: 597–611.

111. Cheatham B, Kahn CR. Insulin action and the insulin signaling network. Endocr Rev 1995; 16: 117–47.

112. Hill CS, Treisman R. Transcriptional regulation by extracellular signals: mechanisms and specificity. Cell 1995; 80: 199–211.

113. Auger KR, Serunian LA, Soltoff SP, Libby P, Cantley LC. PDGF-dependent tyrosine phosphorylation stimulates production of novel polyphosphoinositides in intact cells. Cell 1989; 57: 167–75.

114. Sutherland C, O'Brien RM, Granner DK. Phosphatidylinositol 3-kinase, but not p70/p85 ribosomal S6 protein kinase, is required for the regulation of phosphoenolpyruvate carboxykinase gene expression by insulin. J Biol Chem 1995; 270: 15501–6.

115. Johnson JH, Ogawa A, Chen L, Orci L, Newgard CB, Alam T, Unger RH. Underexpression of β-cell high Km glucose transporters in NIDDM. Science 1990; 250: 546–9.

116. Burcelin R, Eddouks M, Kande J, Assan R, Girard J. Evidence that Glut-2 mRNA and protein concentrations are decreased by hyperinsulinaemia and increased by hyperglycaemia in liver of diabetic rats. Biochem J 1992; 288: 675–9.

117. Valera A, Solanes G, Fernandez-Alvarez J, Pujol A, Ferrer J, Asins G et al. Expression of Glut-2 antisense RNA in β cells of transgenic mice leads to diabetes. J Biol Chem 1994; 269: 28543–6.

118. Meglasson MD, Matschinsky FM. Pancreatic islet glucose metabolism and regulation of insulin secretion. Diabet Metab Rev 1986; 2: 163–214.

119. Leahy JL. Natural history of β-cell dysfunction in NIDDM. Diabetes Care 1990; 13: 992–1010.

120. Collela RM, May JM, Bonner-Weir S, Leahy JL, Weir GC. Glucose utilization in islets of hyperglycemic rat models with impaired glucose-induced insulin secretion. Metabolism 1987; 36: 335–7.

121. Magnuson MA. Glucokinase gene structure. Diabetes 1990; 39: 523–7.

122. Magnuson MA, Andreone TL, Printz RL, Koch S, Granner DK. Rat glucokinase gene: structure and regulation by insulin. Proc Natl Acad Sci 1989; 86: 4838–42.

123. Iynedjian PB, Jotterand D, Nouspikel T, Asfari M, Pilot P-R. Transcriptional induction of the glucokinase gene by insulin in cultured liver cells and its repression by the glucagon-cAMP system. J Biol Chem 1989; 264: 21824–9.

124. Vaulont S, Kahn A. Transcriptional control of metabolic regulation genes by carbohydrates. FASEB J. 1994; 8: 28–35.

125. Bedoya FJ, Matschinsky FM, Shimizu T, O'Neil JJ, Appel MC. Differential regulation of glucokinase activity in pancreatic islets and liver of the rat. J Biol Chem 1986; 261: 10760–4.

126. Printz RL, Magnuson MA, Granner DK. Mammalian glucokinase. Annu Rev Nutr 1993; 13: 463–96.

127. Turner RC, Hattersley AT, Shaw JTE, Levy JC. Type 2 diabetes: clinical aspects of molecular biological studies. Diabetes 1995; 44: 1–10.

128. Valera A, Pujol A, Pelegrin M, Bosch F. Transgenic mice overexpressing PEPCK develop NIDDM. Proc Natl Acad Sci 1994; 91: 9151–4.

129. Rosella G, Zajac JD, Kaczmarczyk SJ, Andrikopoulos S, Proietto J. Impaired suppression of gluconeogenesis induced by overexpression of a non-insulin-responsive PEPCK gene. Mol Endocrinol 1993; 7: 1456–62.

130. Ludwig DS, Puig AV, O'Brien RM, Printz RL, Granner DK, Moller DF, Flier JS. Examination of the PEPCK promoter in patients with NIDDM. J Cell Endocrinol Metab 1996; 81: 503–6.

131. Noguchi T, Matsuda T, Tomari Y, Yamada K, Imai E, Wang Z et al. The regulation of gene expression by insulin is differentially impaired in the liver of the genetically obese-hyperglycemic Wistar fatty rat. FEBS Lett. 1993; 328: 145–8.

132. Braithwaite SS, Palazuk B, Colca JR, Edwards CW, Hofmann C. Reduced expression of HKII in insulin resistant diabetes. Diabetes 1995; 44: 43–8.

133. Vidal-Puig A, Printz RL, Stratton IM, Granner DK, Moller DE. Analysis of the HKII gene in subjects with insulin resistance and NIDDM and detection of a Gln 142: His substitution. Diabetes 1995; 44: 340–6.

134. Echwald SM, Bjorbaek C, Hansen T, Clausen JO, Vestergaard H, Zierath JR et al. Identification of four amino acid substitutions in hexokinase II and studies of relationships to NIDDM, glucose effectiveness, and insulin sensitivity. Diabetes 1995; 44: 347–53.

135. Vestergaard H, Bjorbaek C, Hansen T, Larsen FS, Granner DK, Pedersen O. Impaired activity and gene expression of hexokinase II in muscle from NIDDM patients. J Clin Invest 1996; 96: 2639–45.

136. Taylor SI, Accili D, Imai Y. Insulin resistance or insulin deficiency. Diabetes 1994; 43: 735–40.

137. Goodyear LJ, Giorgio F, Sherman LA, Carey J, Smith RJ, Dohm GL. Insulin receptor phosphorylation, IRS-1 phosphorylation, and PI 3-kinase activity are decreased in intact skeletal muscle strips from obese subjects. J Clin Invest 1995; 95: 2195–204.

138. Sommercorn J, Fields R, Raz I, Maeda R. Abnormal regulation of ribosomal S6 kinase by insulin in skeletal muscle of insulin-resistant humans. J Clin Invest 1993; 91: 509–13.

139. Terada N, Patel HR, Takase K, Kohno K, Nairn AC, Gelfand EW. Rapamycin selectively blocks translation of mRNAs encoding elongation factors and ribosomal proteins. Proc Natl Acad Sci 1994; 91: 11477–81.

140. Jefferies HBJ, Reinhard C, Kozma SC, Thomas G. Rapamycin selectively represses translation of the

polypyrimidine tract mRNA family. Proc Natl Acad Sci 1994; 91: 4441–5.

141. Cohen P, Campbell DG, Dent P, Gomez N, Lavoinne A, Nakielny S et al. Dissection of the protein kinase cascades involved in insulin and nerve growth factor action. Biochem Soc Trans 1992; 20: 671–4.

142. Sutherland C, Leighton IA, Cohen P. Inactivation of glycogen synthase kinase-3β by phosphorylation: new kinase connections in insulin and growth factor signalling. Biochem J 1993; 296: 15–19.

143. Sutherland C, Cohen P. The α-isoform of glycogen synthase kinase-3 from rabbit skeletal muscle is inactivated by p70 S6 kinase or MAP kinase-activated protein kinase-1 *in vitro*. FEBS Lett 1994; 338: 37–42.

144. Dent P, Lavoinne A, Nakielny S, Caudwell FB, Watt P, Cohen P. The molecular mechanism by which insulin stimulates glycogen synthesis in mammalian skeletal muscle. Nature 1990; 348: 302–8.

145. Freymond D, Bogardus C, Okubo M, Stone K, Mott D. Impaired insulin-stimulated muscle glycogen synthase activation *in vivo* in man is related to low fasting glycogen synthase phosphatase activity. J Clin Invest 1988; 82: 1503–9.

146. Bjorbaek C, Vik TA, Echwald SM, Yang PY, Vestergaard H, Wang JP et al. Cloning of a human insulin-stimulated protein kinase-1 (ISPK-1) gene and analysis of coding regions and mRNA levels of the ISPK-1

and the protein phosphatase-1 genes in muscle from NIDDM patients. Diabetes 1995; 44: 90–7.

147. Feinstein R, Kanety H, Papa MZ, Lunenfeld B, Karasik A. TNF-α suppresses insulin-induced tyrosine phosphorylation of insulin receptor and its substrates. J Biol Chem 1993; 268: 26055–8.

148. Hotamisligil GS, Murray DL, Choy LN, Spiegelman BM. Tumour necrosis factor α inhibits signaling from the insulin receptor. Proc Natl Acad Sci 1994; 91: 4854–8.

149. Hotamisligil GS, Shargill NS, Spiegelman BM. Adipose expression of TNF-α: direct role in obesity-linked insulin resistance. Science 1993; 259: 87–91.

150. Sbraccia P, Goodman PA, Maddux BA, Wong KY, Chen Y-DI, Reaven GM, Goldfine ID. Production of an inhibitor of insulin-receptor tyrosine kinase in fibroblasts from patients with insulin resistance and NIDDM. Diabetes 1991; 40: 295–9.

151. Maddux BA, Sbraccia P, Kumakura S, Sasson S, Youngren J, Fisher A et al. Membrane glycoprotein PC-1 and insulin resistance in non-insulin-dependent DM. Nature 1995; 373: 448–51.

152. Auberger P, Falquerho L, Contreres JO, Pages G, Le Cam G, Rossi B, Le Cam A. Characterisation of a natural inhibitor of the insulin receptor tyrosine kinase. Cell 1989; 59: 631–40.

24

Insulin Actions *In Vivo*: Glucose Metabolism

Ele Ferrannini*† and Ralph A. DeFronzo†

*Metabolism Unit of the CNR Institute of Clinical Physiology at the University of Pisa, Italy, and †Diabetes Division, Department of Medicine, University of Texas Health Science Center, San Antonio, Texas, USA

INTRODUCTION

Glucose

Glucose is widespread in living organisms, in which, with protein and fat, it completes the triad of the major metabolic fuels. To a much lesser extent than in plants, glucose also constitutes a building block for structural and enzymatic components of cells as well as the extracellular matrix. As a metabolic substrate, glucose is present in organisms essentially in its simple, monomeric form (α-D-glucopyranose), and as a branched polymer of α-glucose, namely glycogen. Disaccharides of glucose (lactose, maltose, and sucrose) are quantitatively less important.

Glucose is present in plasma water at a concentration that—in a healthy adult who has fasted overnight—ranges between 3.6 mmol/l and 5.8 mmol/l (65–105 mg/dl). A family of proteins residing in the plasma membrane (and in microsomal membranes) can specifically and reversibly bind glucose molecules, and transfer them across plasma cell membranes in both directions. Of such proteins, known as glucose transporters, there are five different species that have so far been identified and characterized [1]. They differ from one another both in tissue distribution and physiologic regulation, particularly in respect to sensitivity to insulin stimulation. More than one species of glucose transporter is usually expressed in a tissue. Present knowledge in this rapidly evolving field indicates that only one type of glucose transporter (termed Glut4) shows clear sensitivity to acute insulin stimulation *in vivo*, and it is this transporter that is abundantly expressed in the classic insulin-sensitive tissues (adipocyte, brown fat, skeletal, heart and smooth muscle). Variable dominance of the other four types of glucose transporters is found in tissues in which glucose metabolism does not respond to insulin acutely (erythrocyte, liver, kidney, brain, pancreatic B cells). Some basic features of glucose distribution and metabolism can be suitably interpreted on the basis of current information on glucose transport.

A non-insulin-regulatable transporter (GT1) effects facilitated glucose diffusion in red blood cells (RBCs). The abundance of this transporter in RBCs has the following physiological consequences. Firstly, glucose diffuses very rapidly across RBC membranes, with an estimated equilibration time of only 4 s (a total RBC mass of 25×10^9 cells with a mean diameter of 7 µm and a spherical shape occupies a surface area of approximately 4 m^2) [2]. The rate of glycolytic utilization of transported glucose by the erythrocyte mass is estimated to be 25 µmol/min, or about 6 µmol/min per m^2 of diffusion surface. As such a rate is about 17 000 times less than the rate of glucose transport in these cells, glucose concentration will, in general, be the same in plasma and erythrocyte water. Plasma proteins make up some 8% of plasma volume, while RBC proteins and ghost occupy about 38% of packed red

International Textbook of Diabetes Mellitus, Second Edition. Edited by K.G.M.M. Alberti, P. Zimmet, R.A. DeFronzo, and H. Keen (Honorary)
© 1997 John Wiley & Sons Ltd

cell volume (which, in turn, averages 40% of blood volume). Thus, 20% (i.e. $0.38 \times 0.4 + 0.08 \times 0.6 = 0.2$) of total blood volume is inaccessible to glucose. It follows that glucose concentration should be identical in plasma and RBC water under most circumstances, and that a *blood water* glucose concentration of 5.0 mmol/l translates into a *plasma* glucose concentration of 4.6 mmol/l and a *whole-blood* glucose concentration of 4.0 mmol/l, i.e. a 15% systematic difference between plasma and whole-blood glucose level under typical conditions of hematocrit, proteinemia, and erythrocyte volume.

Secondly, as both RBC and plasma convey glucose, the total amount of the sugar reaching any given organ is the product of arterial whole-blood glucose concentration times the total blood flow to that organ. Similarly, the total amount of glucose leaving a body region is the product of whole-blood glucose level in the venous effluent times the blood flow rate. Thus, under steady state conditions of blood flow (F), arterial glycemia (A) and organ metabolism, the net balance of glucose movements across a body region is given by the product of blood flow and the arterio-venous (A−V) whole-blood glucose concentration difference ($[A - V] \times F$, or Fick principle) (Figure 1) [3]. It is evident that the use of *plasma* flow rates and glucose concentrations systematically underestimates the net organ balance of glucose (and, for that matter, of any substance that travels in plasma as well as in erythrocytes, e.g. lactate, some amino acids, etc.). In fact, plasma flow is less than blood flow by an amount equal to the hematocrit (∼40%), while plasma glucose is higher than whole-blood glucose by only 15% ($0.6 \times 1.15 = 0.69$, i.e. a 31% underestimation).

NET BALANCE = INPUT − OUTPUT; U − R = F (A−V)

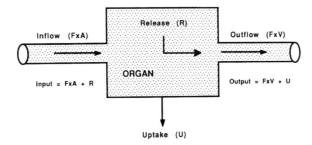

Figure 1 Scheme of an organ perfused by a blood flow (F) carrying a substrate that is both removed by irreversible metabolism and produced *de novo* by intraorgan synthesis. All equations shown are valid when blood flow, arterial substrate concentration and rates of intraorgan substrate metabolism are constant (Fick principle)

Two non-insulin-regulatable glucose transporters (Glut1 and Glut3) have been identified in the blood–brain barrier and placenta [1], where trans-endothelial glucose passage occurs via facilitated diffusion. This is the structural basis for the long-held notion that brain and placental glucose utilization are outwith insulin control, so that vital functions for the adult and fetal organism can be maintained in the face of variable metabolic conditions. In other tissues, the mechanism of extravascular glucose transfer is still undefined.

In general, diffusion of glucose from the intravascular compartment into the interstitial fluid space is known to be very rapid. Whether this is accomplished by facilitated diffusion mediated by specific cell transporters (as in the brain) or by simple diffusion through intercellular clefts of endothelial cells is still uncertain. A lower limit of glucose diffusion through endothelial membranes is represented by cellular glucose uptake (which does not include glucose back-diffusion into the intravascular compartment), and can be estimated by carrying out the following calculation. In healthy subjects under conditions of maximal stimulation (i.e. combined hyperinsulinemia and hyperglycemia), whole-body glucose uptake can reach 12 mmol/min which, for a total capillary surface of $700\ m^2$ available for diffusion (and considering a mean capillary surface of $19\,000\ \mu m^2$ [4]), corresponds to 0.3 pmol/min per capillary. Thus, about 200 billion glucose molecules must pass through each capillary surface each minute to travel cell-bound through the interstitial space. What kind of radial gradient (from the center of the capillary to the cell surface) is generated by the irreversible removal of glucose by cell metabolism *in vivo* is not known, but theoretically this gradient is a function of the rate of diffusion through the endothelium, the distance between the capillary and the cell, and the rate of net glucose transport through the cell membrane. Furthermore, the presence of active glucose uptake also creates a longitudinal glucose concentration gradient along the axis of the capillary, as the glucose supplied at the arterial end of the capillary tree is progressively lost to cells and subtracted from the venous return. The two gradients are obviously dependent on one another, and together determine, at any given rate of cellular glucose uptake, the concentration of glucose at the cell surface (Figure 2). Further complexity is added by the three-dimensional structure of tissues. Direct measurement of interstitial glucose concentrations has proven to be difficult, and has yielded conflicting results. Collection of subcutaneous filtrate, equilibration of perfusates through ultrafiltration membranes, and microdialysis-based methods have been employed. In one study in which these techniques were used simultaneously in the abdominal subcutaneous tissue of healthy volunteers, interstitial fluid glucose concentrations were found to be ~50% lower than venous blood glucose levels, both under fasting circumstances and in response to i.v. glucose-induced hyperglycemia [4]. Difficult as it may be to measure or calculate this 'bathing' concentration of glucose, it is this concentration that dictates the activity of cellular glucose transport together with the state of specific activation of the transporter.

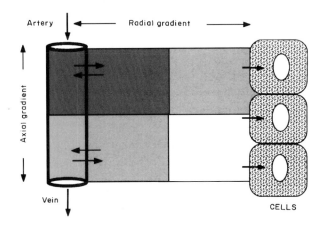

Figure 2 Schematic representation of substrate gradients in an idealized tissue. A capillary (human mean capillary length is 0.75–1.00 mm) receives the substrate from the arterial end (with a flow of $0.5 \times 10^{-6}\ \mu l^3$ per min at a linear velocity of 17 mm/min) and delivers it back to the circulation at the venous end. During its transit time along the capillary (3.5 s), the substrate permeates the capillary endothelial membrane by facilitated diffusion (through a surface that averages $19\,000\ \mu m^2$ per capillary), distributes radially into the tissue interstitium (in about 0.1 s), and is actively removed by cell metabolism. Because of the latter, there exists a dynamic steady state whereby a radial substrate gradient is compounded by an axial gradient along the capillary. Four degrees of shading represent in the scheme what must be a continuous distribution of interstitial gradients

In addition to hormonal stimulation and substrate mass action, cellular glucose uptake is influenced by changes in blood flow in at least two ways. First, an increase in blood supply to a given tissue unit will dissipate—at least in part—the longitudinal glucose gradient (along the axis of the capillary tree), thereby also flattening the radial gradient (capillary to cell surface) and raising the glucose concentration bathing the cell. Intuitively, this increase in the operating glucose level should by itself enhance glucose transport; the converse will happen if blood flow slows down. To quantify this phenomenon, it is pertinent to recall the laws that govern cellular uptake of permeable solutes. According to the Renkin–Crone model of capillary exchange and tissue metabolism [5, 6], the following general equation applies:

$$J_s = [S]_a \cdot F \cdot (1 - e^{-PS/F})$$

where J_s is the net flux of solute from blood into tissue, $[S]_a$ is the arterial blood solute concentration, F is the blood flow rate, and PS is the product of permeability of exchange surface to solute (P) and exchange surface area (S). Although such a model is only valid for uniformly perfused capillary networks, it can be applied to real (heterogeneous) systems to dissect out the relative role of blood flow and the PS product in regulating glucose uptake. Note that the PS product for glucose refers to the slower of the two exchange surfaces (namely, the capillary exchange surface and the cell membrane surface) that are interposed between the bloodstream and intracellular glucose disposal. Thus, as alluded to above, the glucose PS underestimates the actual unidirectional transfer of glucose across the capillary walls. For a given capillary surface, P is equivalent to net transmembrane glucose transport, and therefore is the target of hormonal influences. By combining the above equation (with $[S]_a = A$) with the Fick equation ($J_s = F \cdot (A - V)$), one can estimate PS from perfused forearm experiments, in which forearm blood flow and the A–V glucose gradient are directly measured, by using the following equation:

$$PS = -F \cdot \log_e (V/A)$$

As exemplified in Figure 3, in healthy subjects under conditions of physiological hyperinsulinemia at an arterial glycemia of 5 mmol/l, one measures a deep forearm venous glucose level of 4 mmol/l combined with a total forearm blood flow of 50 ml/min/kg of deep forearm tissues. The corresponding value (0.223) of

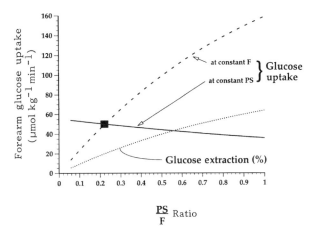

Figure 3 Forearm glucose uptake as a function of the PS/F ratio. The hatched square indicates the actual values of PS/F ratio (0.223) and forearm glucose uptake (50 μmol min^{-1}kg^{-1}) as measured in healthy volunteers during a euglycemic (5 mmol/l) hyperinsulinemic (~80 mU/l) clamp experiment. Forearm glucose uptake is then calculated over a 20-fold range of PS/F values, once by varying blood flow (at constant PS) and again by varying PS (at constant F). In the face of the same extraction ratio, glucose uptake changes little at constant PS and markedly at constant flow

the glucose PS/F ratio (corresponding to a PS of 11 ml/min/kg of tissue), is indicated by the hatched box in Figure 3. If the value of PS/F is allowed to vary over a 20-fold range of forearm blood flow (200 to 11 ml/min/kg) while holding PS constant, forearm glucose uptake declines sluggishly, by some 30% at most. Thus, blood flow has little effect on glucose uptake provided that the permeability–surface product is maintained.

Second, additional metabolic units may be recruited by vasodilation, i.e. through the opening-up of previously unperfused or hypoperfused capillary sectors. Capillaries display vasomotion under the control of feeding arterioles and precapillary sphincters. In response to exercise or hypoxia, the number of capillaries open at any moment and the integrated time that capillaries remain open increase. As a consequence, PS increases because of a larger capillary exchange surface. To the extent that a corresponding surface of cell membranes is exposed to perfusion (i.e. metabolic recruitment), glucose uptake will be stimulated. As shown in Figure 3, when the forearm PS/F is allowed to vary over the same range by changing PS while holding flow constant, forearm glucose uptake increases sharply with PS. In other words, changes in the PS product are much more important than blood flow changes in regulating glucose uptake. Of note is that the glucose extraction ratio (i.e. ER = (A − V)/A) across forearm tissues, which in Crone–Renkin terms is equal to:

$$ER = 1 - e^{-PS/F}$$

is the same regardless of whether the PS/F ratio changes as a result of changes in PS or F. Thus, although the extraction ratio is a measure of the specific ability of cells to extract glucose from the arterial influx, it does not discriminate between simple acceleration of blood flow through already perfused areas and true metabolic recruitment. If both the extraction ratio and the blood flow rate through metabolically active tissue are known, glucose (and other substrates) metabolism can be determined with good accuracy. The key condition is that the measured changes in blood flow do occur in the tissue that drains into the sampling vein.

With regard to flow-dependent metabolic recruitment, Baron and his co-workers have fostered the concept that insulin itself is a vasodilator in humans, and that this hemodynamic effect contributes to the metabolic actions of the hormone [7]. In these investigators' hands the response to systemic insulin administration—either with maintenance of euglycemia or with graded changes in plasma glucose from basal to high levels—comprises an increase in glucose uptake by leg tissues paralleled by a major (2–3-fold) increase in leg blood flow. The simultaneous infusion of somatostatin, to inhibit endogenous insulin release, abolishes the vasodilatory effect of hyperglycemia.

In obese or diabetic subjects with insulin resistance, insulin fails to cause vasodilation in the leg. In healthy, insulin-sensitive volunteers, insulin-mediated increments in leg blood flow correlate with both glucose utilization and blood pressure levels. These findings have been interpreted to indicate that insulin-induced vasodilation recruits metabolically responsive muscle tissue and, in this capacity, it is a mechanism, or pre-requisite, of insulin-mediated glucose uptake (or insulin sensitivity): resistance to insulin action on blood vessels contributes to metabolic insulin resistance.

This interpretation presents some difficulties. In other laboratories and with a different experimental model (e.g. the forearm), insulin-induced vasodilation has generally been modest (25–40%), particularly at physiological insulin levels. Differences in patient selection, experimental conditions, and techniques to measure blood flow (thermodilution, strain-gauge plethysmography, indicator dilution) possibly account for this discrepancy. More importantly, no direct evidence has been provided that the observed increase in limb blood flow involves recruitment of muscle tissue rather than increased blood velocity through already well-perfused regions. Finally, if the increase in blood flow was rate-limiting for insulin action on glucose metabolism, forcing vasodilation should overcome insulin resistance. However, in lean patients with essential hypertension, doubling forearm blood flow by a local intra-arterial adenosine infusion does not increase oxygen uptake (which should follow recruitment of metabolically active tissue) and fails to modify insulin-stimulated glucose uptake [8]. Thus, impaired insulin-induced vasodilation appears to be another manifestation (possibly, even a consequence) of insulin resistance rather than a causally related phenomenon.

Another form of non-insulin-regulatable glucose transporter (Glut2) is amply expressed in the plasma membrane of liver, kidney, intestinal cells, and pancreatic B cells. In liver and kidney, net glucose release occurs *in vivo*. Thus, in the only organs in the body in which the presence of glucose 6-phosphatase (G6Pase)—the enzyme catalyzing the formation of free intracellular glucose from glucose 6-phosphate (G6P)—makes glucose available to the circulation, the transporter is of a type that only responds to the concentration gradient between the internal and external side of the plasma membrane. This ensures that, when insulin is around to stimulate inward glucose transport in tissues with sensitive transporters, the liver can release glucose into the blood stream as long as sufficient G6P is derived from glycogenolysis or gluconeogenesis (or both) and sufficient G6Pase activity is there to accumulate free glucose on the inside of the plasma membrane. Under these conditions of reversed gradient, the presence of insulin-responsive glucose transport activity on hepatocyte cell membranes would enhance glucose *outflow*, thereby opposing the plasma glucose-lowering action of insulin. In contrast, the physiologic control of the direction and rate of glucose flux through the hepatocyte membrane is not on the transport step but on intracellular processes.

In summary, the differential distribution and acute insulin sensitivity of the various classes of glucose transporters appear to provide the skeleton for the functional characteristics of glucose distribution and exchange in the body. On the whole, free glucose is present in blood water, interstitial fluid and the intracellular water compartment of insulin-independent tissues (liver, brain, kidney, intestine, placenta) in total amounts which, in the overnight-fasted healthy adult, average 80 mmol (14 g or 1.2 mmol/kg of body weight), of which one-fifth is in the blood volume. Free glucose is found at concentrations that (a) are uniform in the intravascular water compartment; (b) decline across the interstitial space towards the cell; (c) fall precipitously within cells that consume glucose avidly (e.g. brain) or in which glucose transport is relatively slow in the basal state (e.g. muscle, adipose tissue); (d) are increased in the cytoplasm of cells that produce free glucose (mostly liver); and (e) gradually and continuously decrease in the vascular bed as arterial blood turns into capillary blood and then runs back towards the right heart as venous blood. The regional characteristics of tissue composition, blood flow rate, capillary density (i.e. the average distance between the capillary axis and the cell surface) and cellular glucose uptake concur to determine the A–V glucose gradient in any region of the body (Figure 2).

Glycogen

Glycogen is present in most cells, in cytoplasmic granules which encase the enzymes that regulate its metabolism. In normal humans, the largest part of glycogen stores is in liver and skeletal muscle. In the former, 3–4 g of glycogen are packed in each 100 g of parenchyma; in striated muscle, the concentration is much lower (0.7–1.0% weight by weight). As a consequence, a normal human liver (1.5 kg) contains some 60 g of glycogen, whereas muscle (28 kg) depots keep 250 g. Thus, approximately 25 times more glycosyl units are stored in intracellular depots as glycogen than are dissolved in body water as free glucose.

Glycogen metabolism is controlled by irreversible cascades of enzymatic reactions ultimately acting upon the proximal enzymes that catalyze glycogen synthesis (glycogen synthase) and degradation (glycogen phosphorylase). For the two symmetric pathways, reverse phosphorylation/dephosphorylation cycles convert inactive enzymes into their active counterparts

[9]. Both synthesis and breakdown of glycogen are regulated by multiple, complex mechanisms involving substrates as well as hormones [10]. In this chapter, we recall only those established notions of glycogen metabolism that are the key to understanding some aspects of glucose metabolism.

Points of Clinical Interest

(1) Plasma glucose concentration is on average 15% higher than the whole-blood glucose concentration under ordinary circumstances.

(2) Arterial glucose levels are higher than capillary glucose concentrations, which in turn are higher than venous levels. The extent of these differences depends on the circulatory region and on its rate of glucose utilization.

(3) Both plasma and erythrocytes carry glucose to and from consuming tissues.

(4) In brain, liver, kidney, intestine and placenta, glucose utilization is insulin independent; in adipose tissue, skeletal and heart muscle, glucose uptake depends on insulin.

(5) The whole-body reserves of carbohydrate are quite small.

GLUCOSE METABOLISM

Introduction

Any given concentration of glucose in plasma (and in the space in equilibrium with plasma) is the result of simultaneous release of glucose into the circulation and uptake of glucose from the blood stream into cells. Whenever plasma glucose concentration is stable, the concurrent rates of its release and overall uptake must be equal. Glucose turnover (TR) is this rate of constant flux through its system. Accepted terminology refers to stationary conditions of glucose concentrations and flux rate as the 'steady state', with the understanding that any physiological steady state is only an approximation of the true, ideal steady state. Furthermore, the 'glucose system' refers to the whole space or volume into which glucose is present as free glucose, regardless of how many compartments this system consists of, where they are physically located in the body, and how they are interconnected. Finally, the reference pool for glucose kinetics customarily is the plasma, for in most clinical or experimental circumstances the plasma is the only site accessible for sampling.

When the plasma glucose concentration changes over time, one rate of glucose flux (entry or removal) is being exceeded by the other. Under these non-steady state conditions, the glucose rates of entry and removal are called rate of appearance (R_a) and disappearance (R_d), respectively. The glucose system is strongly homeostatic with respect to glucose levels, in that the normal variations in human plasma glucose concentration throughout a day of life are confined within a surprisingly narrow range. This in itself implies that multiple mechanisms must contribute to controlling glycemia in a highly integrated fashion. It should also be recalled that glycosuria is called upon whenever glycemia exceeds the renal threshold, as if a safety measure had been set to cope with emergency when metabolic control fails. These considerations alone suggest that the body does not tolerate either hypoglycemia or hyperglycemia. For the former, the obligate dependence of brain function on the use of glucose as fuel has classically offered a rational explanation. For hyperglycemia, the evidence—and hence the concept—that high glucose levels, if not immediately life-threatening, are nonetheless intolerable to bodily functions, is more recent but no less compelling, and currently goes under the name of 'glucose toxicity' (see Chapter 32).

Methods

Under the conditions of an overnight fast the liver is the only organ that makes free glucose and pours it into the systemic circulation. In theory, therefore, placing catheters across the splanchnic bed (one into a hepatic vein and another one into any artery) and measuring splanchnic blood flow (e.g. by infusing a dye, such as indocyanine green, that is only cleared by the hepatocyte) would allow the measurement of glucose turnover as the product of A–V difference and blood flow (Figure 1). However, the liver and extrahepatic splanchnic tissues (gut, pancreas, spleen, etc.) also take up glucose; the application of the Fick principle will therefore estimate the net balance between glucose uptake and release in the splanchnic area, not the total rate of glucose turnover (Figure 1). One must therefore resort to glucose tracers, such as radioactive (e.g. ^{3}H-glucose or ^{14}C-glucose) or stable (e.g. ^{2}H-glucose or ^{13}C-glucose) isotopes of glucose. The use of the isotope dilution method to measure glucose turnover has become popular among clinical investigators because of its good feasibility, and has generated large amounts of information; it therefore warrants description here. The details of the tracer technique as applied to glucose turnover measurement can be found in several reviews and treatises [11–13]. In brief, the choice of a tracer is dictated essentially by cost (of the isotope and the experimental apparatus to measure it) and safety (in terms of radiation burden to the patient in the case of radioactive isotopes). The format of tracer administration (pulse injection or constant intravenous infusion)

can also be chosen on the basis of practical ease. Problems arise in the calculation and interpretation of the data, however. Under steady-state conditions applying to both tracee (i.e. glucose) and tracer, glucose turnover rate is simply given by the ratio of the tracer infusion rate (IR) to the equilibrium plasma glucose specific activity (SA = tracer/tracee concentration). Equilibrium is the time (usually 2 hours after starting the tracer infusion) when unchanging plasma tracer concentrations indicate that glucose specific activity has become uniform throughout its distribution space. This formula, IR/SA, is not based on any assumptions. On the other hand, in the non-steady state this approach cannot be used because either the tracer or tracee concentration (or both) change over the period of measurement. Unfortunately, in the patient with diabetes the glucose system is unsteady for most of the time, precisely because homeostasis has been lost. Using a steady-state means to probe an ever-changing state sounds like a violation of Heisenberg's principle of indetermination (one cannot precisely measure position and speed of a subatomic particle at the same time). Practicable ways around the problem do, however, exist. Their common rationale is provided by the theory [14] that proves that the degree and rate of change in glucose specific activity are the principal factors affecting non-steady state analysis of isotope data. The larger the swings in glucose specific activity the more uncertain is the estimation of actual rates of appearance and disappearance from plasma data. Intuitively, when a change occurs at the cellular level, the interposition of an undetermined number of compartments, each with its own kinetics of distribution and metabolism, blurs the image of that change which is reconstructed from a narrow window such as plasma. All the formal models that have been proposed to represent the glucose system become progressively weaker as plasma specific activity is allowed to fluctuate freely. Therefore, one of two strategies can be followed: either the tracer administration is repeated when the glucose system has reached a new, reasonably steady state, or the format of tracer infusion is adjusted empirically to follow plasma cold glucose changes. In both cases, the aim is to minimize the changes in specific activity, thereby meeting the conditions under which steady state equations can be used reliably. In reporting results of glucose turnover obtaining under non-steady state conditions, we shall have to make some selection of available data, and the reader will have to use some caution in accepting them at face value.

Glucose tracers also are useful in the study of regional metabolism in two respects. First, for organs in which glucose uptake and release occur simultaneously (typically, the liver) the A–V difference for the tracer offers a measure of absolute uptake (for the tracer is not produced by the organ), while absolute release can be calculated as the difference between net balance (as measured by the Fick principle) and uptake. In formula, if A^* and V^* and A and V are the arterial and venous tracer and tracee concentrations respectively, and F is the blood flow:

$$\text{absolute uptake rate (GU)} = (A^* - V^*)/A^* \times A \times F$$

$$\text{net balance (NB)} = (A - V) \times F$$

$$\text{absolute release rate (GP)} = NB - GU$$
$$= F \times A \times (V^*/A^* - V/A)$$

Second, as tracer glucose is metabolized its label will appear in one or more degradation products (P^*). For any product, the ratio of its labeled moiety to the specific activity of glucose (i.e. $P^* \times A/A^*$) is the amount of that product generated from glucose (in units of concentration). For example, measuring ^{14}C-lactate and ^{14}C-carbon dioxide during the infusion of ^{14}C-glucose makes it possible to estimate the amounts of glucose that were glycolyzed and completely oxidized, respectively. If, then, the kinetics of precursor and product are separately determined, all of these precursor–product relationships can be converted into fluxes of interconversion, regionally as well as at the whole body level.

An important concept in kinetics and physiology is that of glucose clearance. When referred to the plasma volume, glucose clearance is the volume of plasma that is completely cleared of glucose per unit time. Glucose clearance (CR) is related to glucose turnover rate as follows: $TR = CR \times G$ (where G is the glucose concentration in the same pool, plasma or blood, arterial or venous, in which the tracer concentration was determined). At the level of an organ that only consumes glucose—i.e. in which $U = F \times (A - V)$, Figure 1—glucose clearance is also given by U/A or $F \times (A - V)/A$. (The latter formula calculates *net* glucose clearance in organs in which there is simultaneous glucose uptake and release.) As the ratio $(A - V)/A$ is the extraction ratio (or fractional extraction) of glucose, the product $F \times (A - V)/A$ is the fraction of the flow to an organ that is totally cleared of glucose at any glucose concentration. Thus, the clearance rate is a measure of the efficiency of glucose removal regardless of glycemia; as such, it 'feels' the impact of specific stimuli (e.g. insulin) independently of the mass action of glucose. It is important in this context to bear in mind that the tracer method actually measures glucose clearance (as the ratio of the tracer infusion rate to the equilibrium plasma tracer concentration), and derives glucose turnover rate as the product of clearance and glycemia.

THE BASAL STATE

Glucose Production

By convention, the basal state is the metabolic condition prevailing in the morning after an overnight (10–14 hours) fast. This time marks the end of the longest period of fasting in ordinary life (for the rest of the day humans are in a more or less fed state); this time is also the most common point of clinical observation and physiological measurements.

The true value of basal endogenous glucose production is the one that would be reproducibly measured with the use of an irreversible glucose tracer, which loses its label at the earliest possible intracellular step without ever getting it reincorporated into a circulating tracer molecule [13]. Carbon isotopes systematically underestimate glucose turnover because of the efficient reincorporation of carbons (via 3-carbon fragments such as lactate) into new glucose in the liver (gluconeogenesis) (Figure 4). Obviously, gluconeogenesis can occur in other tissues (e.g. skeletal muscle [15]), but the absence of significant G6Pase activity in tissues other than the liver prevents labeled breakdown products from re-entering the circulation as glucose, where they would alter the estimation of glucose turnover. As for tritiated or deuterated isotopes, labels in positions 3, 4, 5 and 6 are lost at the triosephosphate step or further downstream in anaerobic glycolysis, while a label in position 2 is largely lost at the (phosphogluco)isomerase step (a near-equilibrium reaction) soon after phosphorylation [16] (Figure 4). In neither case does the detached label (essentially in equilibrium with the hydrogen of the body water pool) recycle back into a new glucose molecule to any detectable extent. Therefore, everywhere in the body the clearance of any species of tritiated or deuterated glucose reflects the first, irreversible step in intracellular glucose metabolism, i.e. phosphorylation (= hexokinase activity). In the liver, in contrast, hydrogen isotopes can retrace their way back to free glucose because phosphorylation is reversed by G6Pase. H-2 isotopes are an exception because they lose most of their label (75%) in one turn of the isomerase cycle; the latter being faster than the phosphorylation/dephosphorylation cycle, very little labeled hexose regurgitates back to the free glucose pool. For this reason, the closest estimate of 'true' glucose clearance is that provided by ^{3}H-2-glucose or ^{2}H-2-glucose, which reflects the activity of glucokinase for the forward reaction, and that of G6Pase for the reverse reaction (Figure 4).

It should be recalled that any free glucose molecule produced via the G6Pase reaction but reutilized before secretion into the central hepatic vein will not be detected by any tracer method precisely because it does not contribute to diluting the tracer. Glucose production

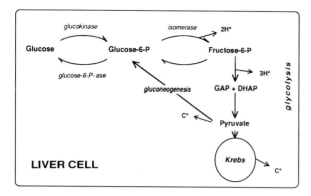

Figure 4 In liver cells, hydrogen labels in position 3 of the glucose molecule are almost exclusively lost at the triosephosphate step; they can therefore travel backwards through the phosphoglucoisomerase reaction to glucose 6-phosphate, and on to free glucose via glucose 6-phosphatase. In contrast, hydrogen labels in position 2 are largely lost in the isomerase reaction (by 75% for each complete cycle), and are therefore prevented from recycling to the free glucose pool. Carbon labels of glucose are lost to carbon dioxide following complete oxidation of glucose in the Krebs (TCA) cycle, but can also recycle to glucose *de novo* through 3-carbon precursors via gluconeogenesis

and reuptake can occur in the same cell; alternatively, since pericentral and periportal liver cells appear to be specialized metabolically (i.e. metabolic zonation [17]), intrahepatic exchange of free glucose may exist. Thus, biochemical free glucose production may be in excess of physiologic glucose secretion.

In the basal state, glucose output in healthy adults averages 840 µmol/min (or 12 µmol/min/kg of body weight). The scatter around this mean estimate is significant (20–30%), with an unknown contribution of genetic and environmental factors. Whether, and how much, fasting glucose output varies as a consequence of changes in dietary habits, caloric intake, physical fitness, etc. has not been investigated. Intrafamilial covariance of this physiological variable is also undetermined. Under standard nutritional conditions, the fasting liver depletes its glycogen stores at a rate of about 0.6 mmol/min or 11%/hour, such that glycogen depots would empty after about 10 hours. Since fasting can be prolonged well beyond 10 hours, obviously gluconeogenesis must progressively replace glycogenolysis as fast continues. Note that in animal species in which the basal rate of glucose turnover is higher than in humans (e.g. dogs, 20 µmol/min/kg; rats, 40 µmol/min/kg), the limited capacity of the liver to store glycogen confers an increasing role to gluconeogenesis for the maintenance of basal glycemia. This limitation on glycogen accumulation has an anatomical basis: overcrowding of cytoplasm with glycogen granules impairs cellular functions, leading to infiltration of nuclei, and, eventually, to cell death. Such is in

fact the sequence of events in several glycogen storage diseases associated with liver damage [18].

In the normal fasting state, gluconeogenesis is classically reputed to contribute to hepatic glucose release. The size of this contribution is, however, somewhat controversial [19]. Recent investigations employing a multiple tracer method estimated that gluconeogenesis is responsible for ~30% of basal hepatic glucose release, the remaining 64% being, by default, glycogenolysis [20]. Rothman and co-workers [21], by measuring ^{13}C-glycogen in human liver *in situ* with the use of ^{13}C nuclear magnetic resonance spectroscopy, reversed these estimates, and concluded that only 36% of fasting liver glucose output is supplied by glycogenolysis. In the latter study, however, the substrates for this *de novo* glucose synthesis were not identified. Circulating lactate, pyruvate, glycerol, alanine and other gluconeogenic amino acids are natural candidate precursors, and undoubtedly transfer their carbons to newly synthesized glucose molecules (as proven, for example, by the incorporation of labeled lactate into glucose, or the Cori cycle). However, trans-splanchnic catheterization in humans has shown that *net* uptake of circulating precursors is rather scanty in the basal state, accounting for only about 15–20% of endogenous glucose production [22]. The discrepancy (1–2 µmol/min/kg) between radioisotopic estimates of basal gluconeogenic rate [20] and accountable circulating precursors [22] suggests that the blood may not be the only route of gluconeogenic supply. Within the splanchnic area, the intestine returns 10–20% of its glucose uptake to the liver as alanine (0.5 µmol/min/kg) [23], thereby filling part of the gap. Intrahepatic lipolysis (i.e. glycerol), proteolysis, and glycolysis theoretically could guarantee ample provision of precursors as an alternative or in addition to those in the circulation. However, the liver can supply gluconeogenic amino acids only at the cost of breaking down liver tissue. It has been calculated that to produce glucose at a rate of 5.6 µmol/min/kg (i.e. 50% of fasting hepatic output) would require the consumption of all the protein in 40 g of liver tissue every hour [19]. Thus, both the amount and source of the gluconeogenic flux in fasting humans remain elusive.

In general, and with reference to the schemes in Figures 1 and 4, a complete description of a precursor–product pathway in any organ requires (1) measuring the rate of intraorgan conversion of the precursor into the product, for which the specific activity and flux rate of both are needed; and (2) measuring the net exchange of the precursor across the organ. For Cori cycle activity, for example, one must determine whole-body glucose and lactate kinetics with tracers, then measure the lactate label appearing in glucose, next determine the intrahepatic specific activity of the *immediate* precursor of new glucose (i.e. fructose 1,6-bisphosphate, triosephosphates or phosphoenolpyruvate), and finally the net hepatic balance of lactate. This painstaking sequence is imposed by the facts that (a) lactate carbons can be found in new glucose without there being net lactate incorporation into glucose (as the liver simultaneously produces and takes up lactate), and (b) lactate specific activity is progressively diluted as other gluconeogenic precursors enter the oxaloacetate pool (e.g. alanine) or the triosephosphate pool (e.g. glycerol). This discussion is also meant to exemplify the intricacies and experimental difficulties that are involved in furnishing answers even to basic physiologic questions in glucose metabolism.

The main control of basal hepatic glucose production is exerted by the sum of several neurohormonal and metabolic stimuli, some stimulatory, others inhibitory. Figure 5 sketches the control system as a simple balance between inhibition and stimulation. Both parasympathetic and sympathetic fibres supply the liver via the splanchnic nerves, allowing autonomic nervous modulation of both glucose production and uptake. An increase in parasympathetic impulses restrains glycogenolysis and enhances glycogen synthesis (at least in animals), while a strengthening of sympathetic outflow to the liver stimulates glucose output via potentiation of both glycogenolysis and gluconeogenesis [24]. In the human, the influence of the sympathetic nervous system on hepatic glucose metabolism can be demonstrated under conditions of acute stimulation, but the contribution of the autonomic nervous system to the maintenance of basal glucose production remains undetermined. ˙

HEPATIC GLUCOSE PRODUCTION

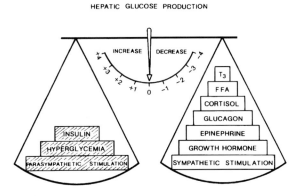

Figure 5 Inhibitory (on the left) and stimulatory (on the right) factors controlling hepatic glucose production

As for metabolic signals, hyperglycemia *per se* can effectively inhibit liver glucose output in normal humans. As shown in Figure 6, during constant hyperglycemia (maintained by a hyperglycemic clamp)

hepatic glucose production is significantly reduced in comparison with euglycemia, even when the endogenous insulin response to hyperglycemia is blocked by somatostatin. It is evident from Figure 6 that normally the two inhibitory signals, hyperglycemia and endogenous hyperinsulinemia, concur to shut off glucose production [25]. That hypoglycemia by itself may trigger an increase in hepatic glucose release is suggested by the fact that during insulin-induced hypoglycemia the rise in tracer-determined R_a of glucose occurs even when one or more counter-regulatory influences are paralyzed [26] and seems to precede in time any measurable increment in circulating anti-insulin hormones. Within the limits of reliability of current tracer methods, the evidence does suggest that glucose *per se* is a signal for liver cell glucose metabolism. This concept is, on the other hand, fully compatible with the idea that the net movement of glucose across the hepatocyte membrane is ultimately determined by the transmembrane gradient, which is the result of intracellular events (i.e. the balance between free glucose generation and disposal) and the extracellular glucose level.

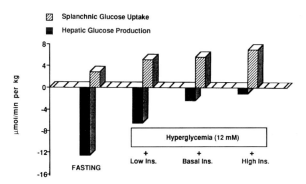

Figure 6 Splanchnic glucose uptake (crosshatched bars) and hepatic glucose production (solid bars) in healthy adults under four experimental conditions: (1) overnight fast; (2) hyperglycemia with somatostatin block of endogenous insulin release (low ins.); (3) hyperglycemia with somatostatin block but replacement of fasting insulin concentrations (basal ins.); and (4) hyperglycemia and unopposed endogenous insulin release (high ins.). Note that hyperglycemia *per se* inhibits glucose production, and that hyperglycemia synergizes insulin in suppressing liver glucose output. In contrast, hyperglycemia stimulates splanchnic glucose uptake to approximately the same extent whether an insulin response is present or not, i.e. mostly by mass action

Of other metabolic signals not very much is known, except that it is very difficult to demonstrate in humans a detectable augmentation of hepatic glucose production by infusing large quantities of glycerol, lactate or a mixture of amino acids, at least as long as there is physiological hyperinsulinemia to balance out such gluconeogenic push. Note that an increased provision of precursors may well lead to increased intrahepatic formation of G6P, but the eventual fate of this intermediate may be glycogen rather than free glucose if control of the rate-limiting step for free glucose production, namely G6Pase activity, is not simultaneously loosened. However, free fatty acids (FFAs) stand out as one substrate that may play an important part in setting the level of hepatic glucose production. Only odd-chain FFAs (i.e. propionate) can donate their carbon to oxaloacetate in the tricarboxylic acid cycle; most physiological FFAs, being even-chain, exchange their carbon moieties with tricarboxylic acid cycle intermediates but do not contribute to *de novo* glucose synthesis. Nevertheless, enriching the perfusion medium of isolated rat liver with oleate or palmitate induces an increase in new glucose formation from lactate or pyruvate [27–29]. Moreover, FFAs (or, rather, products of their oxidation such as citrate and acetyl-CoA) activate key enzymes of gluconeogenesis such as pyruvate carboxylase, phophoenol-pyruvate carboxykinase, and G6Pase [29]. In addition, raised FFA concentrations *in vivo* are accompanied by raised glycerol levels, both resulting from hydrolysis of triglycerides; therefore, accelerated lipolysis normally supplies both the stimulus (FFA) and the substrate (glycerol) for gluconeogenesis. Finally, the liver takes up FFAs avidly, and oxidizes them efficiently (as indicated by the low respiratory quotient of the organ) [30–32]. Thus, there are all the requisites to consider FFA oxidation in the liver as the energy-providing process that is coupled to energy-requiring gluconeogenesis. In isolated hepatocytes, FFAs in micromolar amounts have also been shown to inhibit glycogen synthase [33], which suggests that an additional interaction of this substrate with hepatic glucose metabolism may be at the level of glycogen metabolism. In healthy volunteers, short-term infusion of triglycerides (with heparin, to activate lipoprotein lipase) results in an increase in hepatic glucose output under conditions (hyperglycemia and somatostatin block of endogenous insulin response) mimicking the key features of diabetes [34]. A large part of this effect can be reproduced by infusing, under the same experimental circumstances, glycerol alone. On the other hand, when endogenous insulin is allowed to rise, or when exogenous insulin is administered, the stimulatory effect of triglyceride infusion or hepatic glucose release is easily overcome [34]. In summary, long-chain FFAs may regulate glucose production both by acting upon key enzymes of gluconeogenesis (through products of FFA oxidation) and by virtue of the substrate push of glycerol. In the normal subject this regulatory loop would appear to be operative particularly when insulin secretion is not stimulated, i.e. in the basal state.

Insulin and the classic counter-regulatory hormones—glucagon, cortisol, growth hormone (GH), catecholamines and triiodothyronine (T_3)—form one of the best-described agonist–antagonist regulatory systems (Figure 7). Insulin is a potent, specific and rapid-acting inhibitor of hepatic glucose production. It restricts both glycogenolysis and gluconeogenesis, although with different dose–response characteristics (gluconeogenesis being less sensitive [35]). Moreover, by restraining lipolysis and proteolysis, insulin also reduces the delivery of potential glucose precursors (glycerol, amino acids) to the liver. In its capacity as the inhibitory signal for glucose release, insulin is greatly favored by the anatomical connection between the pancreas and the liver. In fact, the pancreatic venous effluent being a tributary of the portal vein, secreted insulin reaches the liver at a concentration that in fasting humans is three to four times higher than the peripheral (arterial) concentration [36]. Such portosystemic gradient is maintained by a high rate of insulin degradation by hepatic tissues (with a fractional extraction of about 50%). Thus, a small secretory stimulus to the B cell will raise mostly portal insulin levels, thereby selectively acting upon glucose production rather than also enhancing peripheral glucose utilization. In addition to short-circuiting the general circulation, pancreatic insulin release is potentiated by several gastrointestinal hormones (e.g. cholecystokinin-pancreozymin, gastric inhibitory polypeptide). Therefore, anatomical and physiologic connections in the gut–liver–pancreas circle ensure that the primary station for the handling of foodstuff, the liver, is under close control by a nearby, well-informed unit, the B cell.

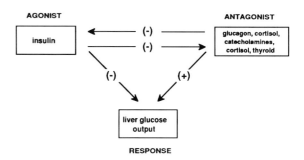

Figure 7 Insulin and the counterinsulin hormones make a complete regulatory system for hepatic glucose production

The role of insulin in regulating basal glucose production is best exemplified by the situation observed in type 1 diabetes: selective B cell failure is associated with a marked increase in fasting glucose production despite the inhibitory influence of hyperglycemia. Furthermore, in the natural history of type 1 diabetes, progressive exhaustion of B-cell function is marked by a gradual rise in hepatic glucose output, and insulin treatment of even extreme diabetic hyperglycemia essentially aims at cutting down glucose release.

The anti-insulin hormones all counter insulin action on the liver by facilitating both glycogenolysis and gluconeogenesis. They do so, however, with different dose–response kinetics and time-courses. Thus, glucagon and catecholamines act rapidly, while cortisol, GH and thyroid hormones (in that order) are involved in the long-range control of glucose release. Glucagon has been shown to play a major part in the tonic support of hepatic glucose release: in the dog, suppression of glucagon release with preservation of basal insulin secretion causes a fall of glucose production of over one-third [37]. The precise quantitative contribution of the other hormones of the counter-regulatory system to the maintenance of basal glucose output has not been assessed. What has become established, however, is the strongly synergistic pattern of interaction between the anti-insulin hormones, such that their cumulative effect is larger than the sum of the individual effects [38, 39]. This interaction may also be expressed at the level of the components of glucose production, glycogenolysis and gluconeogenesis, as well as at the level of peripheral tissues (as discussed later in this chapter). An added feature of this homeostatic complex is the dual negative feedback between agonist and antagonists (Figure 7). A cells and B cells 'talk' to each other in the islets of Langerhans via paracrine influences (some of which may possibly be mediated by somatostatin). For example, insulin infusion *in vivo* reduces circulating glucagon levels by 20–30% even when changes in glycemia are prevented. Another example is the direct modulation of B cell secretion by catecholamines, α-adrenergic stimulation (mostly α-2) depressing, and β-adrenergic stimulation exciting, B-cell secretory activity. Of note in this control system is that a host of hormones is required to balance the action of only one agonist, insulin; such redundance of the antagonistic set-up is typical of any system involved in a vital function. This fact must arise from the inhibitory nature of insulin's effect on the production of a fuel on which brain cell viability depends in an obligatory manner.

Points of Clinical Interest

(1) After a subject has fasted overnight, all the glucose entering the circulation (at a mean rate of 12 μmol/min/kg, or about 220 g/day) derives from liver glycogenolysis and gluconeogenesis, in estimated relative proportion of 70 to 30%.

(2) As fasting continues, glucose production becomes progressively more dependent on gluconeogenesis, and the kidneys may contribute to it. Consequently, substances interfering with gluconeogenesis (e.g. ethanol) may cause dangerous hypoglycemia in the fasting individual.

(3) Any given rate of glucose output is the net result of the inhibitory actions of insulin, hyperglycemia, parasympathetic nervous activity and substrate shortage on the one hand, and the stimulatory actions of counter-regulatory hormones, hypoglycemia, sympathetic nervous activity and gluconeogenic substrate load on the other. Among substrates, lipids may have an added regulatory value for glucose output.

(4) Inappropriate insulin can be life-threatening in the fasting state by shutting off endogenous glucose supply to the brain. Insulin counter-regulation therefore is entrusted to several hormones, providing both short-term and long-term control. The entire hormonal system is the best known in metabolism, and one of the best known in the whole of human physiology.

Glucose Disposal

In the basal state, whole-body glucose disposal equals hepatic glucose production (by definition). Data on the individual contribution of organs and tissues to total glucose uptake have been obtained in regional catheterization studies. In the case of the splanchnic area, in which glucose uptake and production both occur, such data have been derived from the combined use of glucose tracers and indwelling catheters, as diagrammatically shown in Figure 1. By collating the available information, the organ–circulation model of Figure 8 can be drawn, in which steady state inter-organ exchanges of blood and glucose, and regional glucose gradients, are calibrated at a rate of hepatic glucose release of 840 μmol/min. In this model, it is seen that roughly 70% of basal glucose disposal takes place in insulin-independent tissues (brain, liver, kidney, intestine, erythrocytes). It can also be appreciated that the fractional extraction of glucose (as defined earlier) is quite low everywhere in the body (ranging from 1.7% to 2.8%) except in the brain (9%). In particular, if it is assumed that skeletal muscle (40% of body weight) receives 16% of cardiac output and is responsible for one-quarter of overall glucose disposal (~245 μmol/min, Figure 8), then muscle glucose clearance averages 1.3 ml/min/kg of tissue. This value can be compared with those of other organs and tissues (Table 1) similarly obtained by dividing the organ glucose clearance by the estimated organ weight. In the rank of efficiency of glucose utilization in the basal state, resting muscle is last, being 10 times less active than the liver, and 50 times less avid than the brain. In

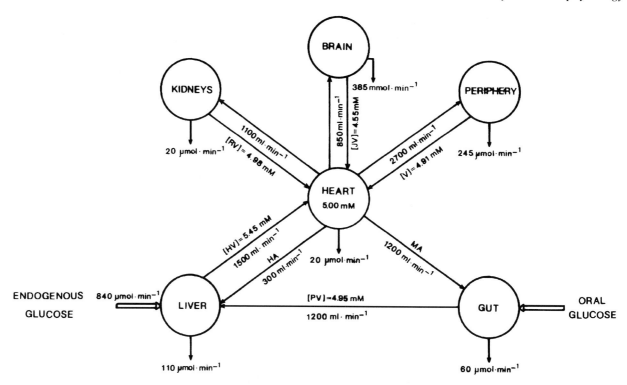

Figure 8 Organ–circulation model for glucose metabolism in the basal state. Average data for healthy adults (from various literature sources) are indicated. The arrow labeled 'oral glucose' indicates the site of dietary glucose entry in the postprandial state. 'Periphery' encompasses all tissues other than liver, gut, kidneys, brain, and heart; 'gut' includes organs (spleen, pancreas, etc.) draining their blood supply into the portal circulation. Abbreviations: PV, portal vein; MA, mesenteric arteries; HA, hepatic artery; HV, hepatic veins; RV, renal veins; JV, jugular veins; V, peripheral veins. Numbers are blood flow rates (ml/min) or glucose flux rates (μmol/min); blood glucose concentrations are given as mM

Table 1 Regional glucose disposal in the basal state

Organ	Weight (kg)	Blood flow (1/min)	Uptake (μmol/min)	Extraction (%)	Clearance* (ml/min per kg)
Brain	1.2	0.85	385	9.1	64
Liver	1.5	1.50	110	2.3	15
Kidneys	0.28	1.10	20	1.9	15
Heart	0.30	0.25	20	1.7	13
Gut	5.00	1.20	60	1.0	2.4
Muscle	28.00	1.05	245	3.5	1.3

*Organ clearance rate divided by organ weight.

tissues in which specific glucose clearance is already high (brain, liver, kidneys), the effect on glucose uptake of acutely raising plasma insulin levels above fasting values is small or absent, while in muscle glucose clearance can increase by a factor of 10 over the physiological range of insulin concentrations. The intermediate position of heart muscle in the list is solely accounted for by its working state. As mentioned earlier, these characteristics can now be seen as the physiologic equivalent of the type and abundance of specific glucose transporters with which the various tissues are endowed. They also narrow the concept of insulin-independent tissue: in the latter, if raising insulin does not accelerate glucose clearance, lowering insulin may

reduce the efficiency of glucose removal. In fact, even non-insulin-regulatable glucose transporters are subject to chronic regulation by insulin, as proven by the fact that animal models of insulin deficient diabetes are associated with a depletion of all types of glucose transporters. This prediction has recently been verified in humans for at least two insulin independent tissues: the liver and the brain. For the former, selective hypoinsulinemia (induced with somatostatin and glucagon replacement) lowers splanchnic glucose uptake below the basal value in healthy volunteers (Figure 6) [25]. For the latter, indirect calculations indicate that brain glucose clearance is reduced in type 2 diabetics with moderate fasting hyperglycemia [40].

The intracellular disposition of transported glucose can be studied by using glucose tracers, and then tracking down the appearance of the label in specific metabolic products, such as lactate (i.e. anaerobic glycolysis) or carbon dioxide (i.e. complete oxidation) (see earlier). It is self-evident that these techniques, even when correctly applied, provide estimates of the metabolic fate of *plasma* glucose, which is the labeled pool. If, for example, there should be direct oxidation of glycogen in muscle, the plasma glucose specific activity would miss it (because of the lack of G6Pase in this tissue). Total carbon dioxide production, however, would include the oxidized glycogen together with all the other oxidized substrates. In general, measuring the exchange of oxygen and carbon dioxide makes it possible to obtain estimates of net rates of substrate oxidation. The method, which goes under the name of indirect calorimetry, does depend on a number of assumptions and, consequently, suffers from limitations. Theoretical analysis has, however, at least set the boundaries of validity of indirect calorimetry [41], which has the formidable advantage over tracer methods of being easy to apply and fully non-invasive. Furthermore, indirect calorimetry also supplies a close estimate of the rate of energy expenditure, can be done at the bedside, and complements information obtained by tracer methods.

In the basal state and under ordinary nutritional circumstances, oxygen consumption averages 250 ml/min, while carbon dioxide production is 200 ml/min, i.e. a whole-body respiratory quotient of 0.8 (RQ = carbon dioxide production/oxygen consumption). Simple calculations (Table 2) thus estimate whole-body net carbohydrate oxidation at about 60% of total glucose uptake. As the brain uses 46% of glucose turnover (Table 1) and readily oxidizes the transported sugar, it follows that three-quarters (i.e. 46/60 = 77%) of basal glucose oxidation occurs in the brain. Little is left for other tissues, which preferentially derive their metabolic energy from the oxidation of fatty substrates and return most of the glucose to the liver after conversion into lactate (Cori cycle). Skeletal muscle, for example, has a respiratory quotient of 0.75 and relies on fat oxidation for the production of 80% of the energy it needs in the resting state [36]. Thus, the basal state is characterized by parsimonious usage of glucose as fuel, which

is selectively channeled to organs that cannot rely on alternative energy sources. Altogether over one-half of total energy production (5 kJ/min) is generated via oxidation of fat, of which there are plentiful (~500 MJ) and almost unlimited stores (e.g. morbid obesity). The role of insulin in maintaining this metabolic set-up is permissive rather than determinant. Through a loose brake on lipolysis, insulin lets FFA over-ride glucose in the competition between the two chief substrates, keeps glucose transport and metabolism in its own target tissues at a minimum, and restrains protein breakdown (which contributes only about 15% to energy metabolism). The part that counter-regulation plays in basal glucose uptake is less well defined, but probably is centered upon maintenance of lipolysis, since all the anti-insulin hormones are more or less potent lipolytic stimuli.

Glucose Cycles

After transport through the plasma membrane, glucose does not necessarily follow a straight path to its eventual fate—be it glycogen, pyruvate or pentoses—but may go around in what are known as 'futile cycles'. A metabolic futile cycle is one in which a precursor is converted into a product by a forward reaction, which is then reversed to resynthesize the precursor. In this way, no net product accumulates, but energy (ATP) is used. One example of a futile cycle, G6P to fructose 6-phosphate and back through the phosphoglucoisomerase reaction, has been previously discussed in relation to the possibility of measuring it (as the difference between the turnover rate as estimated by ^{2}H and ^{3}H isotopes of glucose). Another example is glucose to G6P via glucokinase and back via G6Pase. In general terms, whenever bidirectional flux through a metabolic pathway is simultaneously operative, there exists a cycle, regardless of the number of intermediate reactions and of whether one or more tissues are involved. In this sense, lipolysis in adipose tissue followed by partial re-esterification of FFA in the liver is a complete cycle. Another one is protein breakdown in skeletal muscle with reincorporation of amino acids into proteins in the liver. The derogatory connotation of futility has traditionally been reserved for those cycles that go on in the same cell. They are, however, anything

Table 2 Formulae of indirect calorimetry

Net carbohydrate oxidation (μmol/min)	$= 25.3 V_{CO_2} - 17.8 V_{O_2} - 16.0 N$
Net lipid oxidation (μmol/min)	$= 6.5 (V_{O_2} - V_{CO_2}) - 7.5 N$
Energy expenditure (kJ/min)	$= 0.0164 V_{O_2} + 0.0046 V_{CO_2} - 0.014 N$

V_{O_2} = oxygen consumption (in ml/min); V_{CO_2} = carbon dioxide production (in ml/min); N = urinary non-protein nitrogen excretion (in mg/min).

but futile. As elegantly discussed by Newsholme [9], a metabolic cycle with an internal loop is the best kinetic stratagem to keep the enzymes of a dormant pathway at a minimum of activity, and to ensure a sensitivity gain, for ready amplification of incoming signals. The ATP cost of these cycles is itself a means of increasing the efficiency of energy dissipation. The fact that the activity of these cycles is under hormonal control (e.g. catecholamines and thyroid hormones enhance the cycling rate) makes room for modulation; in this way, these cycles become components of facultative thermogenesis (see below).

Points of Clinical Interest

(1) Of fasting glucose uptake, 70% occurs in insulin-independent tissues, and two-thirds of the glucose is completely oxidized. Much of this distribution is due to the obligatory use of glucose as fuel by the brain.

(2) In insulin-independent tissues, raising insulin does not stimulate glucose metabolism, but insulin lack may decrease the efficiency of glucose utilization (glucose clearance).

(3) Fat is the preferred substrate of insulin-dependent tissues in the basal state.

(4) Over 50% of basal energy production relies on fat oxidation.

THE FED STATE

Introduction

The fed state is the absorptive period between meals. Carbohydrates are normally mixed with lipids and protein in the diet, of which they make up 40–60% of the caloric contents. Absorption of dietary carbohydrates is influenced by their chemical form (refined sugars or complex carbohydrates) and by other components of food. Furthermore, disposal of dietary carbohydrate is indirectly affected by fats and protein to the extent that these latter (a) compete with glucose as substrates, and (b) interfere with glucoregulatory hormones (both FFA and some amino acids are insulin secretagogues).

To circumvent the difficulties of study of glucose ingestion, the regulation of glucose homeostasis during the fed state has classically been investigated with the use of intravenous glucose, which can be administered in formats more suitable for formal analysis.

Methods (see also Chapter 28)

Glucose can be injected intravenously as a single bolus—0.33 or 0.5 g (1.8 or 2.8 mmol) per kg of body weight—and the decline in plasma glucose

concentration after the initial peak followed for 60–90 min (intravenous glucose tolerance test or IVGTT). As, between 10 and 60 min, glycemia decreases approximately as a single exponential function of time, a decay constant (k value) can be easily calculated, and taken to estimate tolerance to intravenous glucose (Figure 9). The IVGTT has several drawbacks. First, the time-course of glucose fall is a multiexponential function of time, so that the decay constant takes on different values according to which segment of the curve is used for analysis. Second, over the same time interval, different curves can have similar k values (as exemplified in Figure 9); for this reason, the area under the glycemic excursion is sometimes used instead of the k value. The area under the curve, on the other hand, is also influenced by the volume into which the injected glucose is distributed. Third, and most important, the shape of the glucose curve is heavily affected by the endogenous insulin response to the acute hyperglycemia caused by the intravenous bolus. Such response is highly irregular, and after an initial peak proceeds in two or three smaller spikes tightly synchronized with similar glycemic spikes [43]. In general, in the presence of an intact feedback loop between glucose and insulin, glucose tolerance is the integrated outcome of multiple changes in the glucose as well as the insulin system: distribution of the exogenous glucose, stimulation of peripheral glucose uptake by insulin and hyperglycemia, suppression of hepatic glucose output, and secretion, distribution, and degradation of insulin. It is therefore not surprising that the information provided by an IVGTT is somewhat ambiguous, and that the test itself is neither very sensitive nor well reproducible.

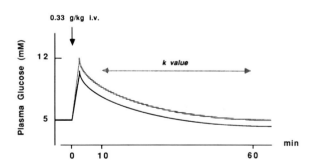

Figure 9 Schematic representation of the time-course of plasma glucose concentrations following the bolus injection of 0.33 g/kg of glucose in a healthy individual. The k value is the rate constant of glucose removal from the plasma between 10 and 60 min after injection (calculated after logarithmic transformation of plasma glucose values). The two curves shown have similar k values but different areas under the time–concentration curve

A modern version of the IVGTT is that which interprets the changes in glucose and peripheral insulin concentrations (measured at frequent intervals following the bolus) on the basis of a 'minimal' mathematical model of the glucose and insulin systems and their interactions [44]. The model generates a parameter reflecting the ability of hyperglycemia to stimulate insulin secretion, another parameter estimating the ability of insulin to stimulate glucose metabolism, and an index of the ability of glucose to promote its own disposal. Although attractive for its simplicity, the minimal model approach generally falls short of its ambitious goal, i.e. to describe all aspects of glucose tolerance with a minimum of data. In particular, the minimal model does not work when the endogenous insulin response is diminished, e.g. in diabetic patients. Several updates of the technique have been devised. Labeled (tritiated or deuterated) glucose can be co-injected with cold glucose; appropriate model analysis of the tracer data makes it possible to dissect out the effects of insulin on the liver and on peripheral tissues [45]. A secondary injection of exogenous insulin or tolbutamide has been used to circumvent the failure of the minimal model in case of insufficient endogenous insulin response [46]. The merits of the latter versions are at least controversial.

A simple way to estimate whole-body sensitivity to insulin is to inhibit endogenous insulin release with a constant infusion of somatostatin (at a rate of 0.3–0.5 mg/h) while simultaneously infusing glucose (at a rate of 1.35 mmol/min/m^2 of body surface area) and regular insulin (at a rate of 50 mU/min/m^2). With this technique (also known as the pancreatic suppression test) [46], steady hyperinsulinemia (of about 80 mU/l) is associated with a level of hyperglycemia that is inversely proportional to the ability of whole-body tissues to increment their glucose utilization in response to insulin. This test suffers from the fact that somatostatin inhibits the release of other glycoactive hormones (e.g. glucagon). With this limitation, however, it is simple and reliable enough for clinical use.

The glucose clamp technique has become the reference method in the study of glucose metabolism [47]. Figure 10 exemplifies the euglycemic, or insulin, version of the clamp technique. An exogenous infusion of regular insulin is started at time zero in a format comprising a prime followed by a constant infusion (usually at a rate of 1 mU/min/kg); such infusion quickly establishes a hyperinsulinemic plateau of about 60–70 mU/l. A few minutes after starting the insulin infusion, an infusion of glucose is begun, at a rate which is adjusted every 5–10 min on the basis of on-line plasma glucose measurements obtained with the same frequency. Over the second hour of a 2-hour experiment, euglycemia in the face of constant hyperinsulinemia is maintained by an approximately constant glucose infusion, which in a healthy adult ranges between 25 and 50 μmol/min/kg (a mean value is shown in the figure). Such a rate equals the overall rate of glucose uptake (also called *M*) in a subject in whom endogenous glucose production is nil. Relative insulin insensitivity or insulin resistance is a low *M* value at comparable levels of glycemia and insulinemia. The technique has the following advantages: (a) any preset combination of plasma glucose and insulin levels can be easily achieved; (b) the time-course of insulin action can be determined with a time resolution of about 10 min; (c) controlled hypoglycemia can be realized for study purposes; (d) other techniques, such as tracer glucose infusion and indirect calorimetry, can be readily combined with a clamp protocol; (e) the interference of other hormones or substances with insulin action can be quantitated by co-infusing them during a clamp study; and (f) although computerized algorithms are available to run a clamp, manual operation with a minimum of experience does just as well. The drawbacks of the euglycemic clamp are the need to draw frequent blood samples from an arterialized vein (e.g. a heated wrist or hand vein), and the cost of the equipment (glucose analyzer and precise infusion pumps).

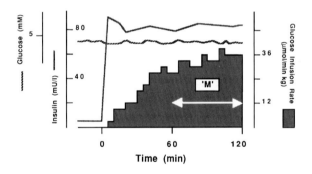

Figure 10 The euglycemic insulin clamp (see text for explanation)

The hyperglycemic version of the glucose clamp (schematized in Figure 11) consists of acutely raising plasma glucose to any desired level, and then clamping it at that level, by means of a primed glucose infusion followed by an adjustable infusion (as in the euglycemic version). The hyperglycemic step evokes an endogenous insulin response that typically is biphasic: an early output (presumably of preformed hormone) lasts 10–15 min, and is followed by a gradual, continuous rise in insulin levels, reflecting glucose-induced triggering and potentiation of B cell secretory activity. By analogy with the euglycemic counterpart, the hyperglycemic clamp provides an *M* value, which represents the combined effect of endogenous hyperinsulinemia and hyperglycemia on whole-body glucose disposal.

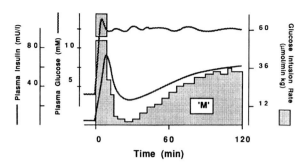

Figure 11 The hyperglycemic glucose clamp (see text for explanation)

Intravenous Glucose

Even when euglycemia is maintained—thereby avoiding the inhibitory effect of raised plasma glucose levels—insulin displays a potent suppressive action on hepatic glucose production, such that portal insulin concentrations of less than 100 mU/l abolish glucose entry into the circulation. Figure 12 shows a typical time-course for endogenous glucose production following an acute increase in plasma insulin to levels of 60–70 mU/l in a healthy subject. Dose–response curves relating calculated portal plasma insulin concentrations to suppression of glucose production (such as that in Figure 13) indicate a half-maximal effect at levels of about 30 mU/l, corresponding to increments in portal insulin in the range of only 5–10 mU/l. Note

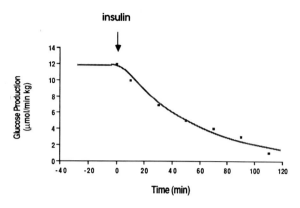

Figure 12 The time-course of hepatic glucose production at euglycemia in response to insulin infusion (plasma levels of ~80 mU/l) in a healthy adult as reconstructed by using a tritium-labeled glucose isotope and non-steady state analysis of the data (redrawn from reference 14)

that in its capacity of a glucose-producing organ the liver is insulin sensitive, while it is insulin independent as a glucose consumer. Hyperglycemia induced by intravenous glucose administration strongly synergizes this inhibitory action of insulin (see Figure 6): in normal adults, a rise in arterial plasma glucose levels of only about 2 mmol/l is sufficient to reduce glucose output promptly by over 80% [25].

Figure 13 also shows the dose–response curves of insulin-stimulated whole-body glucose disposal. The apparent maximum at euglycemia is in the

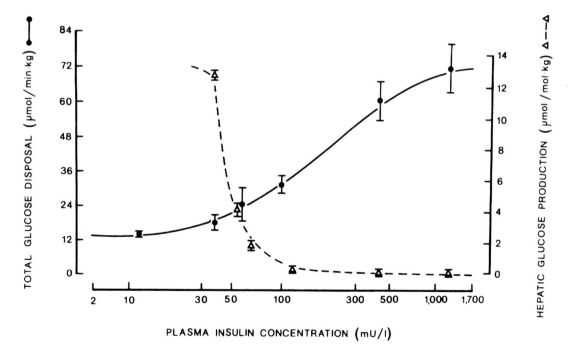

Figure 13 Dose–response curves for hepatic glucose production and whole-body glucose disposal in healthy subjects studied at five steady plasma insulin concentrations with euglycemia by the insulin clamp technique. The insulin concentrations shown are peripheral levels in the case of total glucose disposal, and portal levels in the case of hepatic glucose production. Note the logarithmic scale for insulin (from reference 25, with permission)

order of 60 μmol/min/kg in healthy adult subjects, whereas the half-maximum lies around 70–110 mU/l of peripheral (systemic) plasma insulin concentrations. A dose–response curve of similar shape is derived when progressively higher insulin doses are applied locally in forearm tissues, about 70% of which consists of skeletal muscle [48]. Extrapolating the latter data to total body muscle mass makes it possible to estimate that, with prevailing peripheral plasma insulin concentrations in the high physiological range (60–90 mU/l), 50–70% of a total glucose flux of 30–40 μmol/min/kg is disposed of in muscle tissue. Obviously, this percentage increases further at still higher insulin levels as the contribution of insulin-independent tissues declines.

The control of glucose production and utilization by insulin is dependent on both concentration and time. At any given hormone concentration, there is a finite time before the effect sets in and reaches its maximum. Such onset time is the sum of a circulatory delay (from arterial blood to cell surface, see Figure 1) and a cellular lag (intracellular diffusion and effector activation). Similarly, insulin's effect is present for some time (offset) after the circulating concentrations have returned to prestimulatory levels. Figure 14 shows the activation and deactivation times of insulin calculated at euglycemia over a wide range of plasma hormone levels (up to 1000 mU/l) [49]. With the reservations inherent in the analysis of non-steady state tracer data, these results provide evidence that activation and deactivation are inversely related to one another; thus, at higher insulin doses the effect is more rapid and takes longer to wane. Also of physiological interest is that the relationship between onset and offset time is

different for the liver (in terms of suppression of glucose release) and for peripheral tissue (as stimulation of glucose uptake): at any insulin dose, the liver is activated more rapidly and more persistently. The latter phenomenon may have to do with the shorter diffusion time of blood-borne substances into highly perfused organs (1 ml/min/g of tissue in the liver versus a corresponding value of 0.04 ml/min/g in resting skeletal muscle, Table 1).

The inter-individual variation of insulin-stimulated glucose disposal is large, covering a twofold span even in relatively homogeneous groups of healthy subjects. Adipose mass and degree of physical fitness are powerful determinants of insulin sensitivity, in that weight loss and regular aerobic training are associated with demonstrable gains in insulin sensitivity. On the other hand, age, gender, distribution of body fat, diet and menstrual phase are general physiological covariates of insulin sensitivity. Evidence obtained in Pima Indians [50] has proved that genetic factors are at work in the distribution of insulin sensitivity (estimated as the glucose disposal occurring at euglycemia with submaximal doses of insulin) in the population.

By combining indirect calorimetry with dose–response studies using the clamp technique, it has been possible to quantitate the two major components of whole-body glucose disposal, i.e. glucose oxidation and non-oxidative glucose disposal—the latter consisting of glycogen synthesis for the most part (>90%), the remainder being net lactate production. Figure 15 shows that the two daughter curves retain the sigmoidal shape of the mother curve but with distinctly different dose kinetics. Thus, glucose oxidation is more sensitive (lower apparent half-maximum) but saturates earlier (lower maximum) than glycogen synthesis; the latter behaves as a pathway with low sensitivity and high capacity. Whereas skeletal muscle has been identified as the predominant site of insulin-mediated net glycogen synthesis, the increment in carbohydrate oxidation that follows systemic insulin administration occurs in muscle as well as other tissues (possibly the liver) in an approximate ratio of 1 to 2. Insulin inhibits lipolysis and lipid utilization very effectively. As shown in Figure 16, plasma FFA concentrations decline steeply in response to small increments in circulating insulin levels at euglycemia; this is the result of a drastic reduction of the rate of FFA appearance into the circulation. The consequence of the reduced availability of FFA is a parallel reduction in both FFA oxidation and non-oxidative FFA disposal, i.e. re-esterification (Figure 17).

The inverse patterns of change of glucose disposal and oxidation on the one hand, and lipid utilization on the other, introduce the issue of substrate competition. Glucose and long-chain FFAs are the first and

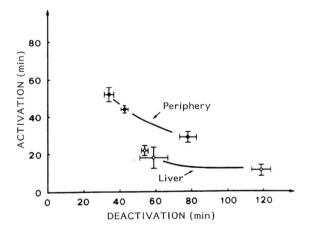

Figure 14 Relationship between activation and deactivation times for insulin stimulation of peripheral glucose uptake and inhibition of hepatic glucose production at three insulin infusion rates (15, 40, and 120 mU/min/m² of body surface area) (reconstructed from reference 49)

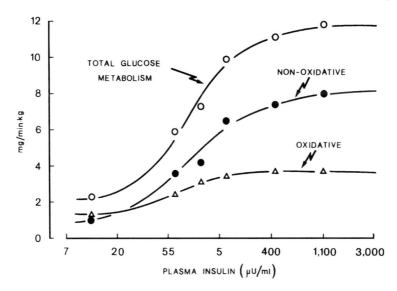

Figure 15 Dose-response curves for total glucose disposal and its components, oxidation and non-oxidative glucose uptake, in healthy subjects during euglycemic insulin clamps

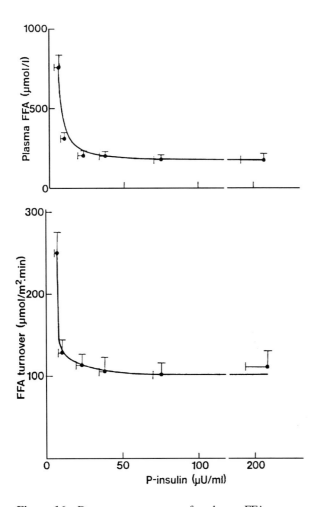

Figure 16 Dose-response curves for plasma FFA concentrations (top) and rates of FFA turnover (bottom), as estimated by ^{14}C-palmitate turnover, in healthy subjects during euglycemic insulin clamps

best-known example of substrates in mutual competition for use by insulin-dependent tissues as fuels. Physiologically, a rise in plasma glucose concentration increases the rate of glucose uptake into cells by mass action; the resulting increase in the generation of α-glycerolphosphate during anaerobic glycolysis supplies the substrate for augmented re-esterification of tissue FFAs, thereby limiting their release into the blood stream. This effect is reinforced by the glucose-induced rise in insulin, which further reduces the supply of lipid substrates to the oxidative machinery. This glucose-on-FFA feedback is balanced by an FFA-on-glucose negative feedback. A rise in FFA availability enhances lipid oxidation, and restrains pyruvate oxidation (at the pyruvate dehydrogenase step) and glycolysis (at the phosphofructokinase step), causing a backward accumulation of glycolytic intermediates, of which G6P in particular has the potential of slowing down glucose transport by allosterically inhibiting phosphorylation (at the hexokinase step). This sequence of biochemical events, and the intracellular signals that trigger it (citrate, ATP and a high acetyl-CoA:CoA ratio) were elucidated by Randle and co-workers in an elegant series of experiments in rat hearts and diaphragms [51]. In the human, experimental elevations in FFA concentrations inhibit insulin-mediated glucose disposal [52] in a fashion that is both dose-dependent and time-dependent [53]. The insulin dose-response curves for glucose oxidation and glycogen synthesis are both shifted downwards during concomitant administration of an intravenous lipid load (Figure 18), supporting the idea that an excess of lipid supply may have inhibitory effects not only on glucose oxidation but also on glycogen synthase [33] or on glucose transport.

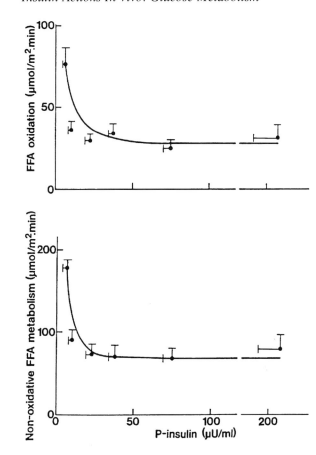

Figure 17 Dose-response curves for whole-body rates of FFA oxidation (top) and non-oxidative disposal (i.e. re-esterification, bottom) estimated from ^{14}C-carbon dioxide production during ^{14}C-palmitate infusion in healthy subjects during euglycemic insulin clamps

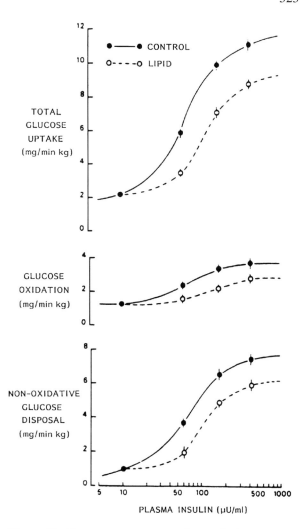

Figure 18 Dose-response curves for total glucose metabolism, glucose oxidation and non-oxidative glucose disposal (i.e. glycogen synthesis) in healthy subjects during euglycemic insulin clamps with (lipid) or without (control) a concomitant infusion of a triglyceride emulsion

The extent to which insulin action in target tissues is direct rather than mediated by shifts in substrate supply can be appreciated by comparing systemic with local insulin administration. When infused intra-arterially into the forearm, insulin does not alter the circulating substrate supply, in that neither FFA nor glucose levels change in the arterial blood recirculating to the forearm tissues. Under these conditions, insulin stimulates forearm glucose uptake and lactate release (Figure 19), but induces only minimal changes in the local respiratory quotient (0.76). This indicates that the forearm tissues continue to rely mostly on lipid oxidation for energy production, and that the vast majority of insulin-stimulated glucose uptake is channeled to glycogen [42]. In contrast, when comparable hyperinsulinemia is created by systemic insulin administration (with maintenance of euglycemia), the leg respiratory quotient increases from 0.74 to almost 1.00, i.e. glucose oxidation increases while lipid oxidation is markedly depressed [54]. Thus, the direct effects of insulin are to promote glucose transport, glycolysis and glycogen synthesis; the effect of the

hormone on glucose oxidation is mediated by a fall in lipid availability. The insulin–glucose system therefore offers a paradigm of coordinate actions at multiple levels within the cell (transport, enzymes of glycolysis, glycogen synthesis and pyruvate oxidation) as well as the whole-body level (suppression of glucose release, stimulation of glucose uptake, inhibition of lipolysis).

Amino acids, too, can enter a competition cycle with glucose, although somewhat less effectively than FFAs. Increased amino acid provision enhances glucose production under conditions of insulin deficiency or resistance, and limits glucose utilization in the insulinized state [55]. Furthermore, raising FFAs has a hypoaminoacidemic effect in humans [56]. In summary, each of the three major substrates, if present in excessive amounts (whether by endogenous production or exogenous administration), can lower the

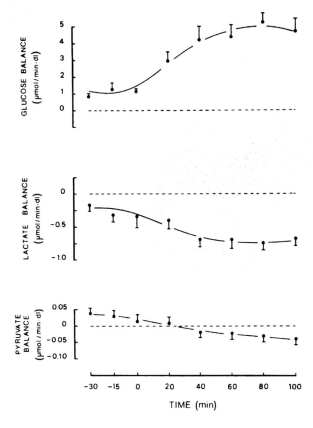

Figure 19 Net glucose, lactate and pyruvate balances across the human forearm of healthy volunteers in the fasting state (time −30 min to 0) and during 100 min of intra-arterial insulin infusion, raising local insulin concentrations to ~120 mU/l (from reference 42, with permission)

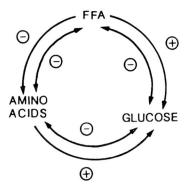

Figure 20 The glucose–FFA–amino acid cycle. Because glucose, FFA and amino acids are all insulin secretagogues, isolated increases of each of them will lower the circulating levels of the other two via hyperinsulinemia (inner ring of the scheme). By substrate competition (outer ring), an increased supply of either FFA or amino acids will spare glucose; in addition, FFAs have a hypoaminoacidemic effect of their own (see text for further explanation)

level of the other two by stimulating insulin release. In this capacity, glucose is obviously favored, being a much more potent secretagogue than fat or amino acids. In addition, multiple substrate effects (not mediated by changes in insulin release) participate in the regulation of the substrates themselves: high FFAs and amino acids raise glucose, high FFAs lower amino acids (Figure 20).

Intravenous glucose administration is thermogenic. Thus, during a standard euglycemic insulin clamp (such as that schematized in Figure 10), basal resting energy expenditure consistently increases by 6–10%. This effect, termed diet-induced thermogenesis (DIT), is also observed with fat and protein [57]. Part of the increase in energy production is evidently directed at meeting the cost of transporting and storing the excess nutrient. This obligatory component of DIT is even larger when the nutrients are ingested rather than infused, in keeping with the added expense of absorbing foodstuffs. The remaining component of DIT is called facultative; substrate cycling, in the form of interconversion or futile cycles, is believed to make up this component. The adrenergic system and thyroid

hormones effect short-term and long-term adjustments, respectively, of facultative DIT; dysregulation of these adjustments is reputed to have pathogenetic relevance for the development of obesity. With regard to this, it is important to note that obesity and type 2 diabetes, both states of insulin resistance, are characterized by a defective DIT, and that in both cases normalization of glucose utilization with extra insulin brings about a recovery of DIT [57]. It is therefore logical to suppose that an intact insulin action on carbohydrate oxidation is required for DIT. In support of this are the following observations in healthy volunteers: (a) if the same total glucose flux is realized by a combination of high insulin (80 mU/l) and euglycemia (5 mmol/l) or low insulin (20 mU/l) plus hyperglycemia (15 mmol/l), the intracellular routing of the transported glucose is different; with less insulin, glucose oxidation is significantly lower and the thermogenic effect of glucose is abolished [58]; (b) when insulin is infused locally into the forearm, muscle glucose oxidation is not stimulated, and no thermogenic effect is evident [42]. In contrast, systemic hyperinsulinemia increases both glucose oxidation and energy expenditure in leg tissues [54].

As discussed at the start of this chapter, whole-body glucose disposal may be influenced by hemodynamic responses. In particular, vasodilation can potentiate the effect of insulin on glucose uptake by exposing more sensitive tissue to hormone action; the converse can happen with vasoconstriction. Current evidence suggests that high rates of glucose uptake, whether maintained by hyperinsulinemia or a combination of hyperinsulinemia and hyperglycemia, may reduce peripheral vascular resistance; the attending vasodilation may contribute to overall glucose disposal by recruiting metabolically responsive tissue [59, 60].

Prolonged intravenous administration of insulin at a constant rate impairs insulin action *in vivo*, possibly through downregulation of insulin binding to its receptors [61]. Such an effect might be prevented by pulsatile, rather than constant, insulin infusion [62], the rationale being that basal endogenous insulin secretion oscillates cyclically [63].

Counter-regulatory hormones in general impede insulin-stimulated glucose metabolism. Both direct effects on glucose transport (or some intracellular step of glucose utilization) and indirect effects are implicated. The latter comprise an increased supply of competitive substrates (notably, FFA) via stimulation of lipolysis. The mechanisms and time-courses of action of the various member hormones of the counter-regulatory system are different. For example, the inhibition of insulin-mediated glucose disposal by epinephrine or cortisol is acute, whereas it takes prolonged hyperglucagonemia or a chronic, large excess of thyroid hormones to impair glucose metabolism (see references 64, 65 for reviews). Once again, the anti-insulin system operates in a synergistic, coordinated fashion to oppose insulin action on glucose uptake.

Oral Glucose

At any point in time, the glycemic response to exogenous glucose is the balance between the rate at which glucose appears in the systemic circulation (from oral as well as endogenous sources) and the rate at which glucose is disposed of. Oral glucose appearance in the peripheral circulation depends on: (a) the rate at which the gastric contents are passed on to the small intestine; (b) the rate of intestinal glucose absorption; (c) the extent of gut glucose utilization; (d) the degree of hepatic glucose trapping; and (e) the dynamics of glucose transfer through gut, liver and posthepatic circulation on to the right heart. The contribution of endogenous glucose to the glycemic response to feeding depends on the extent and rate of change of hepatic glucose release. Finally, glucose disposal depends on changes in the pattern of hormonal stimuli and substrate availability. Being a summation phenomenon, the response to oral glucose explores the whole of glucose tolerance, not the individual contribution of the various components.

The rate-limiting step in the transfer of ingested glucose from the stomach to the liver is the rate of gastric emptying. This depends on the volume, temperature and osmolarity of the glucose solution in a case in which glucose alone is ingested. Glucose absorption through the intestinal lining cells is rapid and efficient, the capacity of the whole small intestine being far in excess of ordinary needs. The presence

of sodium chloride in the glucose drink enhances glucose absorption, and potentiates the release of such gut hormones as gastric inhibitory polypeptide [66]. Glucose utilization by intestinal tissues is small when glucose is presented on the vascular side, i.e. when there is no oral glucose (Table 1); whether the presence of glucose at relatively high concentrations on the luminal side increases gut glucose metabolism is likely (in view of the increased energy needs for absorption) but undetermined in the human. The possibility also exists that systemic hyperglycemia and/or hyperinsulinemia may impede intestinal glucose absorption. Glucose uptake by the liver is stimulated by portal hyperglycemia (see below), but traversing the hepatic space is unlikely to introduce a significant delay in the systemic appearance of oral glucose. On the whole, the dynamics of oral glucose appearance are essentially dictated by gastric emptying, while intestinal transit, crossing of the mucosa to enter portal blood, and transhepatic passage together introduce only a small time delay. In other words, if neither gut nor liver tissues used glucose, the time-course of oral glucose appearance would only follow gastric emptying, with a time shift of a few minutes. For this reason, the absorption step is a major component of the shape of the glycemic response to glucose.

Figure 21 shows the pattern of appearance of ingested glucose in the systemic circulation in healthy individuals, as reconstructed by a double tracer technique [67]. Glucose arrival peaks within 30–45 min,

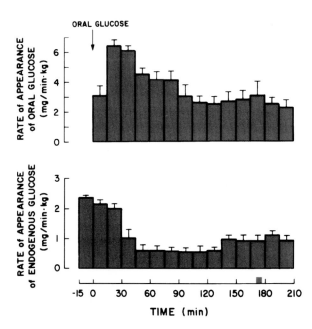

Figure 21 Rates of appearance of oral (top) and endogenous (bottom) glucose following the ingestion of a glucose load of 1 g/kg in healthy subjects (from reference 67, with permission)

declines slowly thereafter, and is still significantly above zero 210 min after glucose ingestion. A secondary rise in oral glucose appearance is sometimes seen between 2 and 3 hours after ingestion [67]. Figure 21 also shows the time-course of suppression of endogenous glucose release by oral glucose. A sustained nadir of 90 min is followed by a slow return towards fasting rates; hepatic glucose production is still significantly inhibited 210 min after the glucose challenge. Overall suppression of endogenous glucose production during 3–4 hours after ingestion averages 50%, surprisingly less than what would be expected on the basis of the combined portal hyperglycemia and hyperinsulinemia (see Figure 6). Relative to intravenous glucose/insulin administration, glucose ingestion evidently reinforces counter-regulatory influences (circulating catecholamines? adrenergic discharge?) which keep liver glucose outflow open.

In Figure 22 the observed arterial plasma glucose concentration is broken down into the component contributed by oral glucose appearance and that provided by hepatic glucose production. While the resemblance of oral R_a to the plasma glucose curve is evident (especially during the first 60–90 min), less appreciated is the fact that absorption is still incomplete 3–4 hours after ingestion. Figure 23 depicts the time-course of total glucose disposal (R_d) following oral glucose: with a lag of some 30 min, glucose uptake is stimulated by 50–110% throughout the period of observation. Hyperglycemia contributes more to whole-body glucose disposal during the first half of the test; thereafter, hyperinsulinemia predominates. Oral glucose elicits vasodilation of the splanchnic vascular bed; this, too, is a change that persists for at least 4 hours

[67]. Thus, both the metabolic and the hemodynamic perturbations induced by oral glucose extend beyond the time of return of plasma glucose to preingestion levels.

The tissue destination of absorbed glucose has been the subject of intense investigation. While the liver was classically reputed to be responsible for the eventual disposal of the majority of oral glucose [68], the weight of more recent evidence [69, 70] favors the view that peripheral tissues collect between one-half and two-thirds of glucose uptake, while the splanchnic tissues account for the remainder. Naturally, these approximate proportions vary according to the time period over which they are observed, as well as the nature of individual responses to glucose ingestion. A robust insulin secretory response directs more posthepatic glucose to the periphery, while a large increase in splanchnic blood flow increases the delivery of incoming sugar to the liver. In humans, for example, a glucose drink sipped over 3.5 hours rather than swallowed in one bolus generates the same overall glucose curve but a 50% smaller endogenous insulin response [71].

In animals the route of administration seems to influence the metabolic fate of glucose [72, 73], in that the portosystemic glucose gradient *per se* enhances liver glucose uptake independently of portal glycemia and total glucose delivery to the organ. In humans, however, good evidence for such a phenomenon is lacking. In fact, the available data (together with inevitable assumptions and approximations) rather suggest that the human liver takes up glucose in simple proportion to delivery (i.e. with a fixed efficiency) regardless of the route of administration [74].

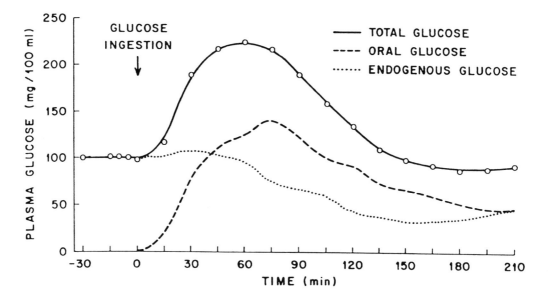

Figure 22 Separation of actual arterial plasma glucose concentration into its components contributed by endogenous and oral glucose (reconstructed by tracer analysis)

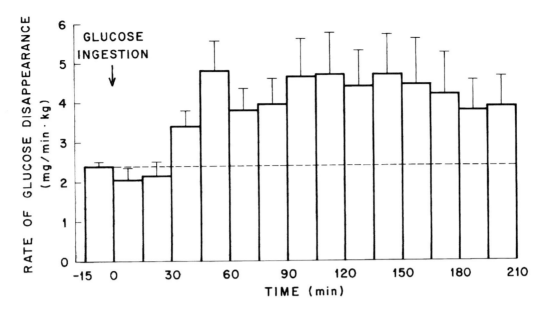

Figure 23 Total whole-body rates of glucose disappearance in healthy subjects following the ingestion of a glucose load of 1 g/kg (from reference 67, with permission)

Limited information is available on the intracellular fate of ingested glucose. While glucose oxidation in the brain continues unabated during the absorptive period, some 50% of the glucose taken up by peripheral tissues (muscle) is oxidized, the remainder being stored as muscle glycogen or as lactate in the lactate pool [70]. During absorption, there is an increase in lactate release by both the splanchnic area as a whole and the intestine [22, 23]. In the latter, it has been estimated that some 5% of the ingested load is converted into 3-carbon precursors of glucose (lactate, pyruvate and alanine) and passed on to the liver [23, 75]. The net release of lactate by the splanchnic area therefore suggests that the sum of hepatic lactate production and gut lactate formation exceeds hepatic lactate extraction. Liver glycogen formation during absorption of oral glucose certainly occurs both directly from glucose and indirectly via gluconeogenesis. The relative contribution of the direct versus indirect pathway to hepatic glycogen synthesis is somewhat uncertain due to methodological difficulties [76]. Current data [77] suggest that gluconeogenesis participates in liver glycogen repletion to a much lesser extent in humans than in rats [78, 79].

Points of Clinical Interest

(1) The liver (hepatic glucose production) is three times more sensitive to the inhibitory action of insulin than peripheral tissues (glucose uptake) are sensitive to the stimulatory action of the hormone.

(2) Insulin action on glucose metabolism is both direct (enhancement of glucose transport, glycolytic breakdown and incorporation into glycogen) and indirect (inhibition of lipolysis, lipid oxidation and protein degradation).

(3) In insulin-sensitive tissues, the three major substrates (glucose, FFAs, amino acids) are in competition with one another.

(4) The counter-regulatory hormones oppose both the direct and the indirect actions of insulin on glucose disposal.

(5) Stimulation of glucose uptake by insulin increases energy production (diet-induced thermogenesis).

(6) The shape of the oral glucose tolerance curve is dominated by absorption processes, especially early after ingestion. Later on, insulin action prevails.

(7) Insulin controls oral glucose tolerance by suppressing endogenous glucose production and promoting glucose uptake into muscle. Hyperglycemia enhances liver splanchnic glucose uptake.

REFERENCES

1. Kahn BB, Flier JS. Regulation of glucose-transporter gene expression *in vitro* and *in vivo*. Diabetes Care 1990; 13: 548–64.
2. Jacquez JA. Red blood cell as glucose carrier: significance for placental and cerebral glucose transfer. Am J Physiol 1984; 246: R289–98.
3. Zierler KL. Theory of the use of arteriovenous concentration differences for measuring metabolism in

steady and non-steady states. J Clin Invest 1961; 40: 2111-25.

4. Schmidt FJ, Sluiter WJ, Schoonen AJM. Glucose concentration in subcutaneous extracellular space. Diabetes Care 1993; 16: 695-700.

5. Crone C, Levitt DG. Capillary permeability to small solutes. In Handbook of physiology—the cardiovascular system IV. Bethesda, MD: American Physiological Society, 1984: pp 411-66.

6. Renkin E. Control of microcirculation and blood tissue exchange. In Handbook of physiology. The cardiovascular system. Microcirculation, sect. 4, vol. 4. Bethesda, MD: American Physiological Society, 1984; pp 627-87.

7. Baron AD. Cardiovascular actions of insulin in humans. Implications for insulin sensitivity and vascular tone. In Ferrannini E (ed.) Insulin resistance and disease. Baillière's clinical endocrinology and metabolism, vol. 7(4). London: WB Saunders, 1993: pp 961-88.

8. Natali A, Bonadonna R, Santoro D, Quiñones Galvan A, Baldi S, Frascerra S et al. Insulin resistance and vasodilation in essential hypertension. Studies with adenosine. J Clin Invest 1994; 94: 1570-6.

9. Newsholme EA, Leech AR. Biochemistry for the medical sciences. Chichester: John Wiley, 1983: pp 308-10.

10. Hers HG. The control of glycogen metabolism in the liver. Ann Rev Biochem 1976; 45: 167-89.

11. Shipley RA, Clark RE. Tracer methods for in vivo kinetics. New York: Academic Press, 1972.

12. Wolfe RR. Tracers in metabolic research. Radio-isotope and stable isotope/mass spectrometry methods. New York: Alan R. Liss, 1984.

13. Ferrannini E, Del Prato S, DeFronzo RA. Glucose kinetics: tracer methods. In Clarke WL, Larner J, Pohl SL (eds) Methods in diabetes research, vol. II: Clinical methods. New York: John Wiley, 1986: pp 107-42.

14. Cobelli C, Mari A, Ferrannini E. The non-steady state problem: error analysis of Steele's model and developments for glucose kinetics. Am J Physiol 1987; 252: E679-87.

15. Bonen A, McDermott JC, Tan MH. Glycogenesis and glyconeogenesis in skeletal muscle: effects of pH and hormones. Am J Physiol 1990; 258: E693-700.

16. Katz J, Golden S, Dunn A, Chenoweth M. Estimation of glucose turnover in rats *in vivo* with tritium labeled glucoses. Hoppe-Seyler's Z Physiol Chem 1976; 357: 1387-94.

17. Jungerman K. Metabolic zonation of liver parenchyma: significance for the regulation of glycogen metabolism, gluconeogenesis and glycolysis. Diabetes Metab Rev 1987; 3: 260-93.

18. Hers H-G, Van Hoof F, de Barsy T. Glycogen storage diseases. In Scriver CR, Beaudet AL, Sly NS, Valle D (eds) The metabolic basis of inherited disease. New York: McGraw-Hill, 1989: pp 425-52.

19. Barrett EJ, Liu Z. Hepatic glucose metabolism and insulin resistance in NIDDM. In Ferrannini E (ed) Insulin resistance and disease. Baillière's clinical endocrinology and metabolism, vol. 7(4). London: WB Saunders, 1993: pp 875-902.

20. Consoli A, Kennedy FP, Miles J, Gerich JE. Determination of Krebs cycle metabolic carbon exchange *in vivo* and its use to estimate individual contributions of gluconeogenesis and glycogenolysis to overall glucose output in man. J Clin Invest 1987; 80: 1303-10.

21. Rothman DL, Magnusson I, Katz LD, Shulman RG, Shulman GI. Quantitation of hepatic glycogenolysis and gluconeogenesis in fasting human with ^{13}C NMR. Science 1991; 254: 573-6.

22. Felig P, Sherwin RS. Carbohydrate homeostasis, liver and diabetes. Prog Liver Dis 1976; 5: 169-71.

23. Bjorkman O, Eriksson LS, Nyberg B, Wahren J. Gut exchange of glucose and lactate in basal state and after oral glucose ingestion in postoperative patients. Diabetes 1990; 39: 747-51.

24. Shimazu T. Neuronal regulation of hepatic glucose metabolism in mammals. Diabetes Metab Rev 1987; 3: 185-206.

25. DeFronzo RA, Ferrannini E, Hendler R, Felig P, Wahren J. Regulation of splanchnic and peripheral glucose uptake by insulin and hyperglycemia in man. Diabetes 1983; 32: 35-45.

26. Gerich JE, Campbell PJ. Overview of counter-regulation and its abnormalities in diabetes mellitus and other conditions. Diabetes Metab Rev 1988; 4: 93-112.

27. Struck E, Ashmore J, Wieland O. Effects of glucagon and long-chain fatty acids on glucose production by isolated perfused rat liver. Adv Enzyme Regul 1966; 4: 219-24.

28. Williamson JR, Kreisberg RA, Felts PW. Mechanism for the stimulation of gluconeogenesis by fatty acids in perfused rat liver. Proc Natl Acad Sci USA 1966; 56: 247-54.

29. Friedman B, Goodman EH Jr, Weinhouse S. Effects of insulin and fatty acids on gluconeogenesis in the rat. J Biol Chem 1967; 242: 3620-7.

30. Havel RJ, Kane JP, Balasse EO, Segel N, Basso LV. Splanchnic metabolism of free fatty acids and production of triglycerides of very low density lipoproteins in normotriglyceridemic and hypertriglyceridemic humans. J Clin Invest 1970; 49: 2017-35.

31. Basso LV, Havel RJ. Hepatic metabolism of free fatty acids in normal and diabetic dogs. J Clin Invest 1970; 49: 537-47.

32. Wahren J, Hagenfeldt L, Felig P. Splanchnic and leg exchange of glucose, amino acids, and free fatty acids during exercise in diabetes mellitus. J Clin Invest 1975; 55: 1303-14.

33. Wititsuwannakul D, Kim K. Mechanism of palmityl coenzyme A inhibition of liver glycogen synthase. J Biol Chem 1977; 252: 7812-17.

34. Ferrannini E, Barrett EJ, Bevilacqua S, DeFronzo RA. Effect of fatty acids on glucose production and utilization in man. J Clin Invest 1983; 72: 1737-47.

35. Chiasson JL, Liljenquist JE, Finger FE, Lacy WW. Differential sensitivity of glycogenolysis and gluconeogenesis to insulin infusion in the dog. Diabetes 1976; 25: 283-91.

36. Ferrannini E, Cobelli C. The kinetics of insulin in man. II. Role of the liver. Diabetes Metab Rev 1987; 3: 365-97.

37. DeFronzo RA, Ferrannini E. Regulation of hepatic glucose metabolism in humans. Diabetes Metab Rev 1987; 3: 415-59.

38. Eigler NL, Sacca L, Sherwin RS. Synergistic interactions of physiologic increments of glucagon, epinephrine, and cortisol in the dog. A model for stress-induced hyperglycemia. J Clin Invest 1979; 63: 114-23.

39. Gerich J, Cryer P, Rizza R. Hormonal mechanisms in acute glucose counter-regulation: the relative roles

of glucagon, epinephrine, norepinephrine, growth hormone and cortisol. Metabolism 1980; 29: 1164–75.

40. Gerich JE, Mitrakou A, Kelley D et al. Contribution of impaired muscle glucose clearance to reduced postabsorptive systemic glucose clearance in NIDDM. Diabetes 1990; 39: 211–16.

41. Ferrannini E. The theoretical bases of indirect calorimetry: a review. Metabolism 1988; 37: 287–301.

42. Natali A, Buzzigoli G, Taddei S, Santoro D, Cerri M, Pedrinelli R, Ferrannini E. Effects of insulin on hemodynamics and metabolism in human forearm. Diabetes 1990; 39: 490–500.

43. Ferrannini E, Pilo A. Pattern of insulin delivery after intravenous glucose injection, and its relation to plasma glucose disappearance. J Clin Invest 1979; 64: 243–54.

44. Bergman RN, Ider YZ, Bowden CR, Cobelli C. Quantitative estimation of insulin sensitivity. Am J Physiol 1979; 236: E667–77.

45. Cobelli C, Pacini G, Toffolo G, Sacca L. Estimation of insulin sensitivity and glucose clearance from minimal model: new insights from labeled IVGTT. Am J Physiol 1986; 253: E551–64.

46. Bergman RN, Finegood DT, Ader M. Assessment of insulin sensitivity *in vivo*. Endocr Rev 1985; 6: 45–86.

47. DeFronzo RA, Tobin J, Andres R. Glucose clamp technique: a method for quantifying insulin secretion and insulin resistance. Am J Physiol 1979; 237: E214–23.

48. Yki-Jarvinen H, Young AA, Lamkin C, Foley J. Kinetics of glucose disposal in whole body and across the forearm in man. J Clin Invest 1987; 79: 1713–19.

49. Prager R, Wallace P, Olefsky JM. *In vivo* kinetics of insulin action on peripheral glucose disposal and hepatic output in normal and obese subjects. J Clin Invest 1986; 78: 472–81.

50. Lillioja S, Mott DM, Zawadzki JK et al. *In vivo* insulin action is familial characteristic in non-diabetic Pima Indians. Diabetes 1987; 36: 1329–35.

51. Randle PJ, Newsholme EA, Garland PB. Regulation of glucose uptake by muscle. Effects of fatty acids, ketone bodies, and pyruvate, and of alloxan diabetes and starvation, on the uptake and metabolic fate of glucose in rat heart and diaphragm muscles. Biochem J 1964; 93: 652–65.

52. Thiebaud D, Jacot E, DeFronzo RA, Maeder E, Jéquier E, Felber JP. The effect of graded doses of insulin on total glucose uptake, glucose oxidation, and glucose storage in man. Diabetes 1982; 31: 957–63.

53. Bonadonna RC, Zych K, Boni C, Ferrannini E, DeFronzo RA. Time dependence of the interaction between glucose and lipid in man. Am J Physiol 1989; 257: E49–57.

54. Kelley DE, Reilly JP, Veneman T, Mandarino LJ. Effects of insulin on skeletal muscle glucose storage, oxidation, and glycolysis in humans. Am J Physiol 1990; 258: E923–9.

55. Ferrannini E, Bevilacqua S, Lanzone L et al. Metabolic interactions of amino acids and glucose in healthy humans. Diab Nutr Metab 1988; 3: 175–86.

56. Ferrannini E, Barrett EJ, Bevilacqua S, Jacob R, Walesky M, Sherwin RS, DeFronzo RA. Effect of free fatty acids on blood amino acid levels in humans. Am J Physiol 1986; 250: E686–94.

57. Jequier E, Schutz Y. Energy expenditure in obesity and diabetes. Diabetes Metab Rev 1988; 4: 583–94.

58. Ferrannini E, Locatelli L, Jéquier E, Felber JP. Differential effects of insulin and hyperglycemia on intracellular glucose disposition in man. Metabolism 1989; 38: 459–67.

59. Edelman SV, Laakso M, Wallace P, Brechtel G, Olefsky JM, Baron AD. Kinetics of insulin-mediated and non-insulin-mediated glucose uptake in humans. Diabetes 1990; 39: 955–64.

60. Laakso M, Edelman SV, Brechtel G, Baron AD. Decreased effect of insulin to stimulate skeletal muscle blood flow in obese man. A novel mechanism for insulin resistance. J Clin Invest 1990; 85: 1844–52.

61. Rizza RA, Mandarino LJ, Genest J, Baker BA, Gerich JE. Production of insulin resistance by hyperinsulinaemia in man. Diabetologia 1985; 28: 70 5.

62. Ward GM, Walters J, Aitken PM, Best JD, Alford FP. Effects of prolonged pulsatile hyperinsulinemia in humans: enhancement of insulin sensitivity. Diabetes 1990; 39: 501–7.

63. Lang DA, Matthews DR, Peto J, Turner RC. Cyclic oscillations of basal plasma glucose and insulin concentrations in human beings. N Engl J Med 1979; 301: 1023–7.

64. Gerich JE, Rizza R, Haymond M, Cryer P. Hormonal mechanisms in acute glucose counter-regulation: the relative roles of glucagon, epinephrine, norepinephrine, growth hormone and cortisol. Metabolism 1981; 29 (suppl. 2): 1164–75.

65. Bratusch-Marrain PR. Insulin-counteracting hormones: their impact on glucose metabolism. Diabetologia 1983; 24: 74–9.

66. Ferrannini E, Barrett E, Bevilacqua S, Dupre J, DeFronzo RA. Sodium elevates the plasma glucose response to glucose ingestion in man. J Clin Endocrinol Metab 1982; 54: 455–8.

67. Pilo A, Ferrannini E, Biörkman O, Wahren J, Reichard GA, Felig P, DeFronzo RA. Analysis of glucose production and disappearance rates following an oral glucose load in normal subjects: a double tracer approach. In Cobelli C, Bergman RN (eds) Carbohydrate metabolism. New York: Wiley, 1981: pp 221–38.

68. Felig P, Wahren J, Hendler R. Influence of maturity-onset diabetes on splanchnic balance after oral glucose ingestion. Diabetes 1978; 27: 121–6.

69. Ferrannini E, Bjorkman O, Reichard GA, Pilo A, Olsson M, Wahren J, DeFronzo RA. The disposal of an oral glucose load in healthy subjects. A quantitative study. Diabetes 1985; 34: 580–8.

70. Kelley D, Mitrakou A, Marsh H et al. Skeletal muscle glycolysis, oxidation, and storage of an oral glucose load. J Clin Invest 1988; 81: 1563–71.

71. Jenkins DJA, Wolever TMS, Ocana AM et al. Metabolic effects of reducing rate of glucose ingestion by single bolus versus continuous sipping. Diabetes 1990; 39: 775–81.

72. Ishida T, Chap Z, Chen J, Lewis R, Hartley C, Entman M, Field J. Differential effects of oral, peripheral intravenous, and intraportal glucose on hepatic glucose uptake and insulin and glucagon extraction in conscious dogs. J Clin Invest 1983; 72: 590–601.

73. Adkins BA, Myers SR, Hendrick GK, Williams PE, Stevenson RW, Cherrington AD. Importance of route of intravenous glucose delivery on hepatic glucose balance in the conscious dog. J Clin Invest 1987; 79: 557–65.

74. Ferrannini E, Katz LD, Glickman MG, DeFronzo RA. Influence of combined intravenous and oral glucose administration on splanchnic glucose uptake in man. Clin Physiol 1990; 10: 527–38.

75. Abumrad NN, Cherrington AD, Williams PE, Lacy WW, Rabin D. Absorption and disposition of a glucose load in the conscious dog. Am J Physiol 1982; 242: E398–406.

76. Radziuk J. Mathematical basis for the measurement of the rates of glucose appearance and synthesis *in vivo*. In Clarke WL, Larner J, Pohl SL (eds) Methods in diabetes research. Vol. II: Clinical methods. New York: John Wiley, 1986: pp 143–64.

77. Radziuk J. Carbon transfer in the measurement of glycogen synthesis from precursors during absorption of an ingested glucose load. Fed Proc 1982; 41: 88–90.

78. Newgard CB, Hirsch LJ, Foster DW, McGarry JD. Studies on the mechanism by which exogenous glucose is converted into liver glycogen in the rat. J Biol Chem 1983; 258: 8046–52.

79. Shulman GI, Rothman DL, Smith D, Johnson CM, Blair JB, Shulman RG, DeFronzo RA. Mechanism of liver glycogen repletion *in vivo* by nuclear magnetic resonance spectroscopy. J Clin Invest 1985; 76: 1229–36.

25

Insulin Actions *In Vivo*: Insulin and Lipoprotein Metabolism

Barbara V. Howard

Medlantic Research Institute, Washington, D.C., USA

INTRODUCTION

The insulin resistance syndrome [1], also referred to as 'syndrome X' [2] or 'The Deadly Quartet' [3] has been defined as the presence of increased insulin concentrations in association with other disorders, including central obesity, hyperglycemia, hypertension, dyslipidemia and sometimes hyperuricemia and renal dysfunction (see also Chapter 12). This syndrome has particular significance because it has been shown to be an antecedent of both non-insulin dependent diabetes mellitus (NIDDM) and atherosclerosis [1–3]. The aim of this chapter is to concentrate on the dyslipidemia (high VLDL, low HDL and altered LDL composition) that accompanies the disorder and the possible relationships between lipoprotein metabolism, insulin concentrations and insulin resistance.

POPULATION STUDIES ESTABLISHING THE RELATIONSHIP BETWEEN INSULIN AND LIPOPROTEIN CONCENTRATIONS

A possible relationship between insulin and plasma lipids was suggested as early as the 1960s, soon after the techniques to measure plasma insulin became available. Patients who had elevated VLDL-triglycerides, either type IV or V hyperlipidemia, were found to have higher insulin concentration after an oral glucose tolerance test [4], and Reaven et al described a significant relationship between plasma insulin concentrations and triglyceride increases in response to a high carbohydrate diet [5]. Relationships between insulin and triglyceride levels over a wide range of plasma triglycerides were then further described by Brunzell et al [6]. Although the relationships between insulin and plasma lipids were initially observed in metabolic ward studies focusing on individuals with triglyceride disorders, a consistent relationship between insulin and plasma lipids has subsequently been established in population-based studies in both men and women in diverse ethnic groups. In the first study, insulin and triglyceride concentrations were measured in a group of 323 non-diabetic first-degree relatives of insulin-dependent diabetic patients, and significant positive correlations were shown between triglycerides and fasting insulin or the 3-hour area under the insulin curve during an oral glucose tolerance test, and an inverse correlation between these variables and HDL-cholesterol [7]. Howard et al examined relationships between plasma insulin, plasma lipids, and lipoprotein concentrations in 1391 Pima Indians [8]. Significant positive correlations between insulin and total or VLDL-triglycerides were observed in non-diabetic men and women, and negative correlations with HDL-cholesterol in a multivariate analysis adjusted for age, body mass index (BMI), smoking and alcohol consumption.

Subsequent population-based studies have almost universally confirmed the relationship between insulin, triglycerides and HDL-cholesterol. In the Paris Prospective Study, entrance data on 2144 healthy, middle-aged men showed significant positive relations between insulin and triglycerides and a negative correlation between insulin and HDL-cholesterol, after adjustment for BMI, plasma glucose, age, alcohol consumption and cigarette smoking [9]. In a county-wide study in Pennsylvania, HDL-cholesterol and insulin were negatively associated in young adult men in a multiple regression adjusted for BMI [10]. This study found that insulin was independently associated with HDL-cholesterol, even when triglycerides were included in the regression model.

The relations between insulin, triglycerides and HDL-cholesterol were shown in Hispanics in the San Antonio Heart Study, which examined a population-based sample of Mexican Americans and non-Hispanic Whites of varying socioeconomic status [11]. Insulin was positively correlated with triglycerides and negatively with HDL-cholesterol in both men and women in a multivariate analysis controlled for BMI and body fat distribution. The relationships between insulin and triglycerides and HDL-cholesterol were also reported in a second group of Hispanics in the San Luis Valley Diabetes Study, which reported positive relationships between plasma insulin and triglycerides and a negative relationship between insulin and HDL-cholesterol [12]. Elevated triglyceride levels and low HDL-cholesterol were shown to be associated with plasma insulin in a study of Asians (Indians, Pakistanis and Bangladeshis) living in the UK [13]. In the Israel Study of glucose tolerance, obesity, and hypertension (Israel GOH Study), a constellation of dyslipidemia, including elevations in VLDL-triglycerides and LDL-cholesterol and decreases in HDL-cholesterol were shown in hyperinsulinemic individuals in the population-based cohort [14]. A study in Central Italy examined 607 factory workers who were normotensive, non-obese and without a family history of diabetes [15]. When they were divided into hyperinsulinemic and normoinsulinemic groups, those with hyperinsulinemia had higher triglycerides and lower HDL-cholesterol, even after adjusting for glucose tolerance, alcohol consumption, smoking and physical activity.

The CARDIA Study examined insulin and lipids in both Black and White young adults in the USA [16]. Positive relationships of insulin with triglycerides and negative relationships with HDL were found among both Blacks and Whites and they persisted after adjustment for BMI, age and gender. The French Telecom Study also compared characteristics of the insulin resistance syndrome in Caribbeans and Europids [17]. Higher insulin concentrations in the Caribbean group were associated with higher levels of triglyceride after adjustment for age and BMI. Associations between insulin and plasma lipids have been observed in Orientals in a study of Japanese Americans [18]. Significant positive relations between triglycerides and plasma insulin, and inverse relationships with HDL-cholesterol were confirmed. Finally, data derived from the Pima Indians have recently been extended to American Indians from 12 other tribes who participated in the Strong Heart Study [19]. Examinations of relationships between plasma insulin and lipoprotein variables showed significant positive correlations between insulin and total and VLDL-triglycerides and a negative correlation between insulin and HDL-cholesterol. These relationships were significant after adjustment for age, BMI, waist:hip ratio and plasma glucose.

Taken as a whole, the population-based studies have universally and consistently found positive associations between insulin and plasma total or VLDL-triglycerides and negative associations between insulin and HDL-cholesterol. These have remained significant when adjusted for covariates such as obesity and age. They appear to be consistent in both genders and among various populations, with convincing data available in Whites, Blacks, Hispanics, Asians, Indians, Orientals and American Indians.

RELATIONSHIPS BETWEEN INSULIN RESISTANCE AND PLASMA LIPOPROTEINS (Table 1)

The direct assessment of insulin sensitivity requires complex metabolic techniques which are generally not applicable to large population-based studies. Thus, in the large-scale studies reviewed in the above section plasma insulin was taken as an index of insulin sensitivity. The validity of plasma insulin concentrations as a marker for insulin sensitivity has not been thoroughly evaluated, but correlation coefficients between fasting insulin concentrations and insulin-mediated glucose disposal as measured by the euglycemic clamp technique can be as high as 0.74 [20]. The tightness of the correlation may in part be influenced by the precision of the insulin assay itself.

Table 1 Dyslipidemia in the insulin resistance syndrome

- Higher triglycerides (TG)
- Higher VLDL-TG
- Lower HDL-cholesterol
- Small dense LDL
- Higher apo B
- Lower apo A1

Several studies have directly examined the relationships between plasma lipoproteins and insulin action. This was first accomplished by Bernstein et al, who reported impaired insulin response in individuals with hypertriglyceridemia [21]. Relationships between plasma lipoprotein concentrations and insulin action as measured by the euglycemic clamp technique were first reported by Abbott et al in a study of 141 non-diabetic Southwestern American Indians [22]. Indices of total insulin-mediated glucose disposal, glucose storage and glucose oxidation were all significantly inversely correlated with total and VLDL-triglyceride concentrations, and HDL-cholesterol was positively related to these indices. The relationships between insulin action and lipoprotein concentrations were independent of obesity and fasting insulin, and the relationships of triglycerides and HDL-cholesterol with insulin action were independent of each other. The relationships between *in vivo* insulin action as measured by the euglycemic clamp and lipoproteins was also reported in non-diabetic young White men by Garg et al [23], and the relationships between insulin resistance and lipoproteins were extended to individuals who had varying degrees of glucose intolerance by Laakso et al [24]. The latter found that in groups with normal glucose tolerance, impaired glucose tolerance and NIDDM, lower concentrations of HDL-cholesterol and higher total and VLDL-triglycerides were found in those who were more insulin-resistant.

These associations were independent of fasting, insulin, age, obesity, waist:hip ratio, 2-hour glucose and fatty acid concentrations, and HDL-cholesterol and VLDL-triglycerides were independently associated with insulin action. Most recently, relationships between serum lipoproteins and measures of glucose metabolism were reported in men over a wide range of age and BMI. Godsland et al [25], using the frequently sampled intravenous glucose tolerance test (FSIGT) as a measure of insulin action and insulin secretion, showed significant positive associations with triglycerides which were independent of age, BMI and body fat distribution. Hepatic insulin throughput, a measure inversely related to hepatic insulin uptake, was independently associated with HDL$_2$-cholesterol.

INSULIN RESISTANCE AND SMALL DENSE LDL

A description of the dyslipidemia that occurs in the insulin resistance syndrome in the population studies was limited to elevated total or VLDL-triglycerides and lower HDL-cholesterol. More recent detailed studies have suggested that an additional component of the dyslipidemia is altered LDL composition. LDL particles occur over a range of size and density. The presence of small dense LDL has been shown in multiple studies to be correlated with coronary heart disease [26–28], and Austin et al have shown that most

individuals can be segregated into two LDL subclass patterns, A and B, and that this pattern is determined by a major dominant gene [27]. Many of the studies describing small dense LDL showed them to be associated with metabolic components of the insulin resistance syndrome, specifically, high triglycerides and low HDL-cholesterol. Barakat et al had originally described a relationship between hyperinsulinemia and LDL structure and composition [29], and Reaven et al have reported that LDL size is negatively associated with plasma insulin concentrations and insulin action, and that insulin-resistant individuals tend to have a higher proportion of LDL subclass pattern B [30]. Selby et al demonstrated that LDL size and the B subclass pattern were associated with a cluster of risk factors defining the insulin resistance syndrome [31]. The association between LDL size and subclass patterns and plasma insulin has also been demonstrated in a population-based sample of Mexican Americans and non-Hispanic Whites [32], and the association of LDL size and pattern with a clustering of risk factors of the insulin resistance syndrome was confirmed in both ethnic groups. In these latter three studies, the association of the occurrence of small dense LDL with insulin has been shown to be independent of plasma triglycerides and HDL-cholesterol.

Thus, the dyslipidemia in individuals with insulin resistance appears to include LDL, depleted in core cholesterol ester and relatively enriched in apo B, with a smaller diameter, a lower flotation constant (Sf) and a higher average density. This abnormality, coupled with the elevated triglycerides and low HDL-cholesterol, brings to a total of three the facets of dyslipidemia that may accelerate the atherosclerotic process in insulin-resistant individuals.

MECHANISMS EXPLAINING THE ASSOCIATION BETWEEN INSULIN RESISTANCE AND LIPOPROTEIN METABOLISM

VLDL-triglycerides (Table 2)

Many reports of the association between total or VLDL-triglycerides, and insulin have suggested that the relationship might be explained by the direct stimulation of VLDL production by insulin. Observations of individuals with insulin dependent diabetes have indicated that insulin is required for hepatic production of VLDL as well as for most other hepatic proteins [33], and in studies of diabetic animals insulin has a stimulatory effect on hepatic lipogenesis [34, 35]. An insulin receptor-mediated pathway for short-term insulin regulation of apo B metabolism in rat liver has also been shown. Hyperinsulinism was associated with increased lipoprotein production in rat liver, and thus it has been hypothesized that hyperinsulinemia may stimulate apo B mRNA levels [36]. On the other hand, several lines of evidence suggest that the association between insulin and VLDL is not the result of a direct stimulatory effect of elevated insulin concentrations on VLDL production. Examination of a large cohort of patients with insulinomas indicated no abnormalities in lipoproteins compared to individuals matched by age, gender and race [37]. Intensive insulin therapy in persons with diabetes almost always decreases plasma triglyceride, because higher insulin concentrations lower glucose and free fatty acids (FFA), the precursors of VLDL-triglyceride [38]. Furthermore, insulin is a stimulator of lipoprotein lipase (LPL) activity [40]; thus, hyper-insulinemia would be expected to facilitate VLDL clearance, and lower concentrations of VLDL. Steiner and co-workers have recently examined the effect of short-term hyperinsulinemia on the production of both VLDL-triglyceride and apo B [41]. Hyperinsulinemia was found to inhibit VLDL-triglyceride production and VLDL apo B production, and plasma triglyceride and VLDL particle size decreased.

While hyperinsulinemia *per se* may not be the major determinant of the elevated VLDL in insulin-resistant subjects, the insulin-resistant state itself might induce elevated VLDL. Insulin resistance is strongly associated with central obesity [42, 43]. Individuals with central obesity have increased free fatty acids and increased fatty acid flux through the splanchnic area, since abdominal fat cells are more resistant to insulin suppression of lipolysis than fat cells from other depots [44]. Fatty acids have been shown to increase triglyceride synthesis and apo B secretion by hepatocytes *in vitro*. In addition, the tendency toward hyperglycemia in insulin-resistant subjects provides additional substrate to stimulate hepatic VLDL production. The scenario of increased fatty acid and glucose flux in insulin-resistant individuals is supported by data from individuals with hypertriglyceridemia, showing that insulin's antilipolytic effect appears to be blunted and accompanied by increases of free fatty acids [45].

Table 2 Possible mechanisms for elevations in VLDL

- Elevated FFA and glucose flux to liver
- VLDL-TG production increased
- VLDL apo B increased
- LPL activity lower

A major effect of insulin *in vivo* is to increase the metabolism of VLDL-triglycerides by its activation of LPL [46]. Insulin enhances the rate of synthesis of this enzyme, via increases in LPL mRNA [47, 48]. Stability of the LPL mRNA and the newly

formed enzyme are also enhanced by insulin [48], and insulin stimulates the release of LPL from the cell [49]. LPL activity in skeletal muscle of insulin-resistant subjects has been shown to be lower [50]. This suggests that in insulin-resistant subjects, regulation of LPL by insulin might be defective. If this is the case, then clearance of VLDL-triglycerides would be impaired, causing VLDL elevation. It has been demonstrated in insulin-resistant persons with NIDDM that there is in fact an impaired insulin suppression of plasma free fatty acid concentrations [51]. This was demonstrated using small increments in plasma insulin during hyperglycemic clamp studies, levels much lower than those necessary to demonstrate a defect in insulin-stimulated glucose uptake. Obesity and a low level of physical fitness, traits both associated with insulin resistance, have also been shown to be related to a reduced ability of insulin to suppress plasma free fatty acids [52].

HDL (Table 3)

The complexity of the mechanisms controlling HDL metabolism and the lack of understanding of many of the key mechanisms regulating HDL impedes the examination of possible associations between insulin resistance and HDL. Most studies of lipoproteins have shown an inverse relationship between VLDL-triglycerides and HDL-cholesterol. Factors that interfere with VLDL metabolism, such as impaired lipolysis, would result in lowered HDL-cholesterol because the HDL compartment is augmented during the lipolytic process by transfer of material (apoproteins and cholesterol ester) from triglyceride-rich lipoproteins [53]. Thus the lower HDL in hyperinsulinemic or insulin-resistant individuals could be related to their elevated VLDL. However, both population-based studies and those relating lipoproteins to euglycemic clamp measurements have demonstrated that the relationship between HDL-cholesterol and insulin/insulin action is independent of VLDL-triglyceride concentrations. Thus, a more direct connection may exist between insulin resistance and HDL metabolism. As with VLDL, elevated insulin concentration *per se* may not directly influence HDL. Data on insulin-treated subjects with insulin dependent diabetes mellitus and some studies of insulin therapy of non-insulin-therapy-dependent diabetes mellitus show that introduction of insulin therapy leads to higher HDL-cholesterol concentrations [54]. *In vitro* studies in hepatocytes showed no evidence of insulin action on apo A1 secretion [39]. Therefore, there may be direct relationships between insulin resistance and HDL metabolism. Hepatic lipase (HL) activity has been shown to be increased in insulin resistance states [55]. Since it is active in the clearance of HDL, elevated HL might contribute to reduced HDL in insulin resistance. Another possible site of control might be in the production of apo A1 or hepatic secretion of nascent HDL. The alterations in hepatic function in the insulin-resistant individual might inhibit either or both of these processes. Godsland et al have recently demonstrated a close relationship between hepatic insulin extraction and HDL_2 concentrations that is independent of triglyceride metabolism [25]. This would imply that insulin in the liver does have a direct effect on HDL concentrations in the plasma. Cholesterol ester transfer protein (CETP) and lecithin-cholesterol acyl transferase (LCAT) are both enzymes which play major roles in the regulation of HDL. If either of these were altered in the insulin-resistant state they could explain changes in HDL-cholesterol. Finally, when there are higher plasma triglyceride concentrations, there is a greater rate of exchange between triglycerides in triglyceride-rich lipoproteins and in HDL, with HDL being depleted of cholesterol. This has been one of the mechanisms invoked to explain the negative association between HDL and triglyceride concentrations and this may also contribute to the lower HDL-cholesterol in insulin-resistant individuals [56]. Thus, there are several possibilities for altered HDL metabolism in insulin resistance and it is not certain which or which combination of these parameters is affected by the insulin-resistant state and is operative in causing the lower HDL-cholesterol concentrations.

Table 3 Possible mechanisms for decreases in HDL

- Impaired lipolysis of TG-rich lipoproteins
- Increased hepatic triglyceride lipase (HTGL)
- Decreased hepatic production

LDL (Table 4)

In considering possible associations between insulin and LDL metabolism, there is only contradictory evidence for the possibility that elevated insulin concentrations might cause increases in LDL-cholesterol concentrations. LDL receptor activity in skin fibroblasts is stimulated by the addition of insulin to the medium [57]. Also, insulin causes accelerated disappearance of ^{125}I-labeled LDL from plasma [58]. Thus, insulin *in vivo* probably stimulates LDL receptor activity and thus would be expected to lower LDL. Although LDL-cholesterol concentrations do not appear to be significantly elevated in most studies of individuals with the insulin resistance syndrome, they appear to have small dense LDL. These might result from some of the alterations in VLDL metabolism discussed above, since almost all studies have demonstrated a tight (inverse)

association between VLDL-triglyceride concentrations and LDL size. The metabolic mechanisms controlling the size of LDL are not well understood. One possibility is that if there is impaired lipase activity in insulin-resistant subjects, persistence of VLDL remnants may result in smaller LDL particles. There is some evidence from animal studies that in fact, smaller VLDL are converted to small LDL [59], and Packard et al showed that therapy with simvastatin lowered the synthesis of large VLDL and also resulted in more dense LDL [60]. High levels of plasma triglyceride-rich lipoproteins may serve as acceptors for cholesterol esters and other constituents from LDL in exchange for triglyceride, mediated by lipid transfer proteins [56]. The triglycerides in the LDL particles can then be removed by the action of lipoprotein lipase, thus resulting in lipid-poor, protein-rich, dense LDL particles.

Table 4 Possible mechanisms for small dense LDL

- Impaired lipolysis
- Depletion of core cholesterol ester (CE) because of elevated VLDL-TG
- Larger VLDL→LDL

CAN ELEVATED VLDL (OR OTHER DYSLIPIDEMIA) INFLUENCE INSULIN ACTION ?

The possibility that abnormal lipid or lipoprotein concentrations can impair insulin action must be considered. This is suggested by *in vitro* observations that incubation with βVLDL results in resistance to the action of insulin in cultured cells [61]. Studies have also shown that VLDL *in vitro* is able to regulate insulin receptors on monocytes [62]. Finally, *in vivo* infusion of Intralipid results in significant reductions in total body glucose uptake through inhibition of both glucose storage and glucose oxidation [63, 64]; however, it might have been the free fatty acids in the infusion mixture in these studies that caused the impairment of insulin action. There is some evidence that insulin resistance precedes the development of lipid abnormalities. Haffner et al have demonstrated in an 8-year prospective study that baseline insulin concentrations predict the future development of both hypertriglyceridemia and low HDL-cholesterol, and these changes in lipids were independent of weight gain [65]. On the other hand, Schumacher et al have reported that normoglycemic members of NIDDM families have increased prevalence of dyslipidemia [66], and Sane and Taskinen have shown that baseline concentrations of triglycerides are an independent predictor of impaired glucose tolerance (IGT) and NIDDM in families with hypertriglyceridemia [67]. Thus, while it remains most likely that dyslipidemia is caused by the fundamental metabolic defect which causes insulin resistance, it is also possible that there may be a self-augmenting process where the hypertriglyceridemia exacerbates the insulin resistance.

POSSIBLE ROLES OF SEX HORMONES IN THE ETIOLOGY OF DYSLIPIDEMIA

The central obesity that accompanies insulin resistance has been shown to be accompanied by multiple metabolic and endocrine derangements [68]. Kissebah et al have shown that upper body obesity is associated with increased free testosterone and decreased sex hormone binding globulin (SHBG) [69] and several studies have shown relationships between higher glucose and insulin concentrations, higher free testosterone, and decreased SHBG [69, 70]. Studies in which testosterone is administered show an absolute fall in HDL-cholesterol [71, 72]. High levels of free testosterone and low SHBG have been associated in several studies with higher triglycerides and lower HDL [73, 74]. Finally, women with polycystic ovarian disease who have higher levels of free testosterone have higher triglycerides and low HDL concentrations [75]. On the other hand, estrogen has been shown to raise HDL-cholesterol and lower

plasma LDL-cholesterol [76, 77]. Thus, it may be that in insulin-resistant individuals, particularly women, altered hormones or SHBG may contribute to the dyslipidemia.

POSSIBLE INVOLVEMENT OF THE SYMPATHETIC NERVOUS SYSTEM IN THE DYSLIPIDEMIA ASSOCIATED WITH INSULIN RESISTANCE

Hyperinsulinemia appears to stimulate the sympathetic nervous system independently of its effects on blood glucose. Plasma concentrations of norepinephrine increase in diabetic patients receiving insulin [78], and studies using the euglycemic clamp technique have shown that insulin infusion produces a dose-dependent increase in norepinephrine and activation of muscle sympathetic nerves [79]. These effects appear to be centrally mediated [80]. Norepinephrine in turn plays a role in the regulation of plasma free fatty acids. It stimulates lipolysis, antagonizes the effect of insulin on adipocytes, and thereby increases plasma free fatty acids [81]. Since fatty acids are the major substrates for VLDL-triglyceride synthesis, increases in sympathetic nervous system activity could then lead to increases in plasma triglyceride concentrations and possibly other aspects of the dyslipidemia associated with insulin.

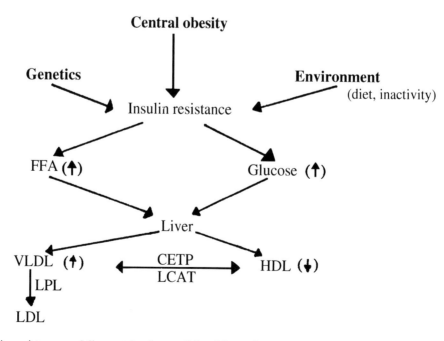

Figure 1 Insulin resistance and lipoprotein abnormalities. Most of the putative causes of insulin resistance including diet, central obesity and physical inactivity result in increased flux of glucose and fatty acids to the liver. This increased availability of substrate can induce increased production of VLDL and may concomitantly inhibit HDL or apo A1 production. Impaired lipoprotein lipase (LPL) may slow VLDL clearance and thus indirectly influence the flux of material to the HDL compartment. Further effects of insulin resistance might include inhibition of cholesterol ester-transfer protein (CETP) or lecithin cholesterol acyl transferase (LCAT). Alterations within the lipolytic cascade might result in more dense or altered LDL particles

CONCLUSIONS (Figure 1)

Although it is controversial whether alterations such as hypertension, atherosclerosis or renal disease always appear with the insulin resistance syndrome, the dyslipidemia does appear to be an integral part of the insulin resistance syndrome and is associated with hyperinsulinemia in individuals over a wide range of age and ethnic groups. This dyslipidemia appears to be manifested as an elevation in VLDL-triglycerides, a decrease in HDL-cholesterol, and the presence of small dense LDL particles. All three of these changes are known to be associated with atherogenesis. Most of the metabolic data to date indicate that the cause of the alterations in lipoproteins in insulin resistance is not elevation of insulin concentrations *per se*, but more fundamental effects of the insulin-resistant state itself on lipoprotein metabolism. Thus, fundamental aspects of insulin-resistant muscle, adipose tissue and/or liver must cause the defective lipoprotein metabolism. A plausible unifying hypothesis for the dyslipidemia associated with insulin resistance starts with an increase in free fatty acid flux that probably results from the central adiposity that occurs in insulin-resistant subjects. The insulin-resistant liver, presented with increased flux of fatty acids and also elevated levels of glucose, probably over-produces VLDL and somehow, by less understood mechanisms, either produces less HDL or accelerates its clearance. Small dense LDL then result either from the impaired metabolism of VLDL (insulin-resistant LPL) or through the lipoprotein transfer process whereby triglycerides are exchanged for cholesterol in the LDL core. Much further work is needed to understand the mechanisms that control VLDL, LDL and HDL metabolism and how they are altered in the insulin-resistance state. This knowledge will undoubtedly contribute to the understanding of the etiology of the insulin resistant syndrome and suggest possible strategies for the prevention of the associated atherosclerosis.

REFERENCES

1. DeFronzo RA, Ferrannini E. Insulin resistance: a multifaceted syndrome responsible for NIDDM, obesity, hypertension, dyslipidemia, and atherosclerotic cardiovascular disease. Diabetes Care 1991; 14: 173–94.
2. Reaven GM. Role of insulin resistance in human disease. Diabetes 1988; 37: 1595–607.
3. Kaplan NM. The deadly quartet. Arch Intern Med 1989; 149: 1514–20.
4. Glueck CJ, Levy RI, Frederickson DS. Immunoreactive insulin, glucose tolerance, and carbohydrate inducibility in Types II, III, IV, and V hyperlipoproteinemia. Diabetes 1969; 18: 739–47.
5. Reaven GM, Lerner RL, Stern MP, Farquhar JW. Role of insulin in endogenous hypertriglyceridemia. J Clin Invest 1967; 46: 1756–67.
6. Brunzell JO, Chait A, Bierman EL. Pathophysiology of lipoprotein transport. Metabolism 1978; 27: 1109–27.
7. Orchard TJ, Becker DJ, Bates M, Kuller LH, Drash AL. Plasma insulin and lipoprotein concentrations: an atherogenic association? Am J Epidemiol 1983; 118: 326–37.
8. Howard BV, Knowler WC, Vasquez B, Kennedy AL, Pettitt DJ, Bennett PH. Plasma and lipoprotein cholesterol and triglyceride in the Pima Indian population. Arteriosclerosis 1984; 4: 462–71.
9. Cambien FJ, Warnet M, Eschwege E, Jacqueson A, Richard JL, Rosselin G. Body mass, blood pressure, glucose, and lipids, does plasma insulin explain their relationships? Arteriosclerosis 1987; 7: 197–202.
10. Donahue RP, Orchard TJ, Becker DJ, Kuller LH, Drash AL. Sex differences in the coronary heart disease risk profile: a possible role for insulin. Am J Epidemiol 1987; 125: 650–7.
11. Haffner SM, Fing D, Hazuda HP, Pugh JA, Patterson JK. Hyperinsulinemia, upper body adiposity, and cardiovascular risk factors in non-diabetics. Metabolism 1988; 37: 338–45.
12. Burchfiel CM, Hamman RF, Marshall JA, Baxter JH, Kahn LB, Amirant JJ. Cardiovascular risk factors and impaired glucose tolerance: the San Luis Valley diabetes study. Am J Epidemiol 1990; 131: 57–70.
13. McKeigue PM, Miller GJ, Marmot MG. Coronary heart disease in South Asians overseas: a review. J Clin Epidemiol 1989; 42: 597–609.
14. Modan M, Halkin H, Lusky A, Segal P, Fuchs A, Chetrit A. Hyperinsulinemia is characterized by jointly disturbed plasma VLDL, LDL, and HDL levels. Arteriosclerosis 1988; 8: 227–36.
15. Zavaroni I, Dall'Aglio E, Alpi O, Bruschi F, Bonora E, Pezzarossa A, Butturini U. Evidence for an independent relationship between plasma insulin and concentration of high density lipoprotein cholesterol and triglyceride. Atherosclerosis 1985; 55: 259–66.
16. Manolio TA, Savage PJ, Burke GL, Liu K, Wagneknecht LE, Sidney S et al. Association of fasting insulin with blood pressure and lipids in young adults. Arteriosclerosis 1990; 10: 430–6.
17. Fontbonne A, Papoz L, Eschwege E, Roger M, Saint-Paul M, Simon D. Features of insulin-resistance syndrome in men from French Caribbean Islands. Diabetes 1992; 41: 1385–9.
18. Fujimoto WY. Diabetes in Asian and Pacific Islander Americans. Diabetes in America (2nd edn), NIH publication no. 95-1468 1995; pp 661–81.
19. Howard BV, Welty TK, Fabsitz RR, Cowan LD, Oopik A, Le NA et al. Risk factors for coronary heart disease in diabetic and non-diabetic Native Americans. Diabetes 1992; 41 (suppl 2): 4–11.
20. Bennett PH, Bogardus C, Knowler WC, Lillioja S. Recent epidemiological contributions to the pathogenesis and etiology of non-insulin dependent diabetes. J Med Assn Thailand 1987; 70(2): 5–10.
21. Bernstein RM, Davis BM, Olefsky JM, Reaven GM. Hepatic insulin responsiveness in patients with endogenous hypertriglyceridemia. Diabetologia 1978; 14: 249–53.
22. Abbott WGH, Lillioja S, Young AA, Zawadzki JK, Yki-Jarvinen H, Christin L, Howard BV. Relationships

between plasma lipoprotein concentrations and insulin action in an obese hyperinsulinemic population. Diabetes 1987; 36: 897–904.

23. Garg AJ, Helderman H, Koffler M, Ayuso R, Rosenstock J, Raskin P. Relationship between lipoprotein levels and *in vivo* insulin action in normal young white men. Metabolism 1988; 37: 982–7.

24. Laakso M, Sarlund H, Mykkanen L. Insulin resistance is associated with lipid and lipoprotein abnormalities in subjects with varying degrees of glucose tolerance. Arteriosclerosis 1990; 10: 223–31.

25. Godsland IF, Crook D, Walton C, Wynn V, Oliver MF. Influence of insulin resistance, secretion, and clearance on serum cholesterol, triglycerides, lipoprotein cholesterol, and blood pressure in healthy men. Arterioscler Thromb 1992; 12: 1030–5.

26. Crouse JR, Parks JS, Schey HM, Kahl FT. Studies of low density lipoprotein molecular weight in human beings with coronary artery disease. J Lipid Res 1985; 26: 566–74.

27. Austin MA, Breslow JL, Hennekens CH, Buring JE, Willett WC, Krauss RM. Low density lipoprotein subclass patterns and risk of myocardial infarction. JAMA 1988; 260: 1917–21.

28. Campos H, Genest JJ, Blijlevens E, McNamara JR, Jenner JL, Ordovas JM et al. Low density lipoprotein particle size and coronary artery disease. Arteriosclerosis 1992; 12: 187–95.

29. Barakat HA, Carpenter JW, McLendon VD, Khazanie P, Leggett N, Heath J, Marks R. Influence of obesity, impaired glucose tolerance and NIDDM on LDL structure and composition. Diabetes 1990; 39: 1527–33.

30. Reaven GM, Chen YDI, Jeppesen J, Mabeux P, Krauss RM. Insulin resistance and hyperinsulinemia in individuals with small dense low density lipoprotein particles. J Clin Invest 1993; 92: 141–6.

31. Selby JV, Austin MA, Newman B, Zhang D, Queensberry CP, Mayer EJ, Krauss RM. LDL subclass pattern and the insulin resistance syndrome in women. Circulation 1993; 88: 381–7.

32. Haffner SM, Mykkanen L, Valdez RA, Paidi M, Stern MP, Howard BV. LDL size and subclass pattern in a biethnic population. Arterioscler Thromb 1993; 13: 1623–30.

33. Owen OE, Block BSB, Patel M, Boden G, McDonough M, Kreulen T et al. Human splanchnic metabolism during diabetic ketoacidosis. Metabolism 1977; 26: 381–98.

34. Hollenberg CH. Effect of nutrition on activity and release of lipase from rat adipose tissue. Am J Physiol 1959; 197: 667–73.

35. Reaven EP, Reaven GM. Mechanisms for development of diabetic hypertriglyceridemia in streptozotocin treated rats: effect of diet and duration of insulin deficiency. J Clin Invest 1974; 54: 167–78.

36. Kissebah AH. Insulin actions *in vivo*: insulin and lipoprotein metabolism. In Alberti KGMM, DeFronzo RA, Keen H, Zimmet P (eds) International Textbook of Diabetes Mellitus, 1st edn. Chichester: Wiley, 1992: pp 439–58.

37. O'Brien T, Young WF, Palumbo PJ, O'Brien PC, Service FJ. Hypertension and dyslipidemia in patients with insulinoma. Mayo Clin Proc 1993; 68: 141–6.

38. Howard BV. Lipoprotein metabolism in diabetes mellitus. J Lipid Res 1987; 28: 613–28.

39. Sparks CE, Sparks JD, Bolognino M, Salhanick A, Strumph PS, Amatrude JM. Insulin effects on apolipoprotein synthesis and secretion by primary cultures of rat hepatocytes. Metabolism 1986; 35: 1128–36.

40. Eckel RH. Lipoprotein lipase and diabetes mellitus. In Draznin B, Eckel RH (eds) Diabetes and atherosclerosis. Molecular basis and clinical aspects. New York: Elsevier, 1993; pp 77–102.

41. Lewis GF, Uffelman KD, Szeto LW, Steiner G. Effects of acute hyperinsulinemia on VLDL triglyceride and VLDL apoB production in normal weight and obese individuals. Diabetes 1993; 42: 833–42.

42. Peiris AN, Aiman EJ, Drucker WD, Kissebah AH. The relative contributions of hepatic and peripheral tissue to insulin resistance in hyperandrogenic women. J Clin Endocrinol Metab 1989; 68: 715–20.

43. Fujioka S, Matsuzawa Y, Tokunage K, Tarui S. Contribution of intra-abdominal fat accumulation to the impairment of glucose and lipid metabolism in human obesity. Metabolism 1987; 36: 54–9.

44. Anderson AJ, Sobocinski KA, Freedman DS, Barboriak JJ, Rimm AA, Gruchow HW. Body fat distribution, plasma lipids, and lipoproteins. Arteriosclerosis 1988; 8: 88–94.

45. Yki-Jarvinen H, Taskinen MR. Interrelationships among insulin's antilipolytic and glucoregulatory effects and plasma triglycerides in non-diabetic and diabetic patients with endogenous hypertriglyceridemia. Diabetes 1988; 37: 1271–8.

46. Bagdade JD, Porte D Jr, Bierman EL. Acute insulin withdrawal and the regulation of plasma triglyceride removal in diabetic subjects. Diabetes 1968; 17: 127–32.

47. Ong JM, Kirchgessner TG, Schotz MC, Kern PA. Insulin increases the synthetic rate and mRNA level of lipoprotein lipase in isolated rat adipocytes. J Biol Chem 1988; 263: 12933–8.

48. Raynolds MV, Awald PD, Gordon DF et al. Lipoprotein lipase gene expression in rat adipocytes is regulated by isoproterenol and insulin through different mechanisms. Mol Endocrin 1990; 4: 1416–22.

49. Eckel RH, Fujimoto WY, Brunzell JD. Insulin regulation of lipoprotein lipase in cultured 3T3-L1 cells. Biochem Biophys Res Commun 1978; 84: 1069–75.

50. Pollare T, Vessby B, Lithell H. Lipoprotein lipase activity in skeletal muscle is related to insulin sensitivity. Arterioscler Thromb 1991; 11: 1192–1203.

51. Chen YDI, Golay A, Swislocki ALM et al. Resistance to insulin suppression of plasma free fatty acid concentrations and insulin stimulation of glucose uptake in non-insulin dependent diabetes mellitus. J Clin Endocrinol Metab 1987; 64: 17–21.

52. Coon PJ, Rogus EM, Goldberg AP. Time course of plasma free fatty acid concentration in response to insulin: effect of obesity and physical fitness. Metabolism 1992; 41: 711–16.

53. Eisenberg S. High density lipoprotein metabolism. J Lipid Res 1984; 25: 1017–58.

54. Howard BV, Howard WJ. Dyslipidemia in non-insulin diabetes mellitus. Endocr Rev 1994; 15: 263–74.

55. Taskinen MR. Insulin resistance and lipoprotein metabolism. Curr Opin Lipidol 1995; 6: 153–60.

56. Deckelbaum RJ, Granot E, Oschry Y, Rose L, Eisenberg S. Plasma triglyceride determines structure-composition in low and high density lipoproteins. Arteriosclerosis 1984; 4: 225–31.

57. Chait A, Bierman EL, Albers JL. Low-density lipoprotein receptor activity in cultured human skin fibroblasts. J Clin Invest 1979; 64: 1309–19.

58. Mazzone T, Foster D, Chait A. *In vivo* stimulation of low-density lipoprotein degradation by insulin. Diabetes 1984; 33: 333–8.

59. Shames DM, Yamada N, Havel RJ. Metabolism of apoB-100 in lipoproteins separated by density gradient ultracentrifugation in normal and Watanabe heritable hyperlipidemic rabbits. J Lipid Res 1990; 31: 753–62.

60. Gaw A, Packard CJ, Murray EF, Lindsay GM, Griffin BA, Caslake MJ et al. Effects of simvastatin on apoB metabolism and LDL subfraction distribution. Arterioscler Thromb 1993; 13: 170–89.

61. Berliner A, Frank HJL, Karasic D, Capdeville M. Lipoprotein-induced insulin resistance in aortic endothelium. Diabetes 1984; 33: 1039–44.

62. Bieger WP, Michel G, Barwich D, Biehl K, Wirth A. Diminished insulin receptors on monocytes and erythrocytes in hypertriglyceridemia. Metabolism 1984; 33: 982–7.

63. Bevilacqua S, Bonadonna R, Buzzigoli G, Boni C, Ciociaro D, Maccari F et al. Acute elevation of free fatty acid levels leads to hepatic insulin resistance in obese subjects. Metabolism 1987; 36: 502–6.

64. Thierbaud D, DeFronzo RA, Jacot E, Golay A, Acheson K, Maeder E, Felber JP. Effect of long chain triglyceride infusion on glucose metabolism in man. Metabolism 1982; 31: 1128–36.

65. Haffner SM, Valdez RA, Hazuda HP, Mitchell BD, Stern MP. Prospective analysis of the insulin resistance syndrome (syndrome X). Diabetes 1992; 41: 15–22.

66. Schumacher MC, Maxwell TM, Wu LL, Hunt SC, Williams RR, Elbein SC. Dyslipidemias among normoglycemic members of familial NIDDM pedigrees. Diabetes Care 1992; 15: 1285–9.

67. Sane T, Taskinen MR. Does familial hypertriglyceridemia predispose to non-insulin dependent diabetes? Diabetes Care 1993; 16: 1494–1501.

68. Krotkiewski M, Björntorp P, Sjöström L et al. Impact of obesity on metabolism in men and women. Importance of regional adipose tissue distribution. J Clin Invest 1983; 72: 1150–62.

69. Evans DJ, Hoffmann RG, Kalkhoff RK et al. Relationship of androgenic activity to body fat topography, fat cell morphology, and metabolic aberrations in premenopausal women. J Clin Endocrinol Metab 1983; 57: 304–310.

70. Haffner SM, Katz MS, Stern MP. The relationship of sex hormones to hyperinsulinemia. Metabolism 1988; 37: 681–8.

71. Friedl KE, Jones RE, Hannan CJ, Plymate SR. The administration of pharmacological doses of testosterone or 10-nortestosterone to normal men is not associated with increased insulin secretion or impaired glucose tolerance. J Clin Endocrinol Metab 1989; 62: 971–5.

72. Friedl KE, Hannan CJ, Jones RE, Plymate SR. High-density lipoprotein cholesterol is not decreased if an aromatizable androgen is administered. Metabolism 1990; 39: 69–74.

73. Soler JT, Folsom AR, Kaye SA, Prineas RJ. Associations of abdominal adiposity, fasting insulin, sex hormone binding globulin, and estrone with lipids and lipoproteins in post-menopausal women. Atherosclerosis 1989; 79: 21–7.

74. Haffner SM, Dunn JF, Katz MS. Relationship of sex hormone-binding globulin to lipid, lipoprotein, glucose, and insulin concentrations in post-menopausal women. Metabolism 1992; 41: 278–84.

75. Wild RA, Applebaum-Bowden D, Demers LM, Bartholemew M, Landis JR, Hazzard WR et al. Lipoprotein lipids in women with androgen excess: independent associations with increased insulin and androgen. Clin Chem 1990; 36: 283–9.

76. Matthews KA, Meilahn E, Kuller LH et al. Menopause and risk factors for coronary heart disease. N Engl J Med 1989; 321: 641–6.

77. Wahl PW, Walden CE, Knopp RH et al. Lipid and lipoprotein triglyceride and cholesterol interrelationships: effects of sex, hormone use, and hyperlipidemia. Metabolism 1984; 33: 502–8.

78. Christensen NJ, Gundersen HJG, Hegedus L et al. Acute effects of insulin on plasma noradrenaline and the cardiovascular system. Metabolism 1980; 29: 1138–45.

79. Rowe JW, Young JB, Minaker KL et al. Effect of insulin and glucose infusions on sympathetic nervous system activity in normal man. Diabetes 1981; 30: 219–25.

80. Anderson EA, Balon TW, Hoffman RP et al. Insulin increases sympathetic activity but not blood pressure in borderline hypertensive humans. Hypertension 1992; 19: 621–7.

81. Howard BV, Schneiderman N, Falkner B. Haffner SM, Laws A. Insulin, health behaviors, and lipid metabolism. Metabolism 1993; 42: 25–35.

26

Insulin Actions *In Vivo*: Role in the Regulation of Ketone Body Metabolism

M. Walker and K.G.M.M. Alberti

Department of Medicine, University of Newcastle upon Tyne, UK

The ketone bodies, acetoacetate and 3-hydroxy-butyrate, are important substrates for oxidation for the majority of tissues during catabolic states, for example starvation, and serve to limit the utilisation of glucose under these conditions. Following an overnight fast, the total ketone body levels in the normal human are around 0.1–0.4 mmol/l with a comparatively high rate of ketogenesis of 0.2–0.4 mmol/min [1]. Fasting for 5 days is accompanied by an increase in the rate of ketogenesis to 1.5–2.5 mmol/min; because of limited peripheral ketone body clearance, this is associated with a much greater increase in the total ketone body levels to around 7–10 mmol/l, tending to remain at this level with more prolonged fasting [1].

Insulin is the principal anabolic hormone, and during the fed state the emphasis is on fuel storage rather than utilisation. Ketogenesis is suppressed by a decrease in the supply of substrate, non-esterified fatty acids (NEFA), and by a direct effect of insulin at the liver. Conversely, during catabolic states insulin levels fall or remain unchanged while the secretion of glucagon, cortisol, growth hormone, adrenaline and noradrenaline are relatively or absolutely increased; the restraining influence of insulin is overcome and ketogenesis is stimulated as part of the general process of fuel mobilisation.

Insulin has a central role in the regulation of ketogenesis, and this is exemplified in insulin dependent diabetes mellitus (IDDM) when absolute insulin deficiency can lead to unrestrained ketogenesis and life-threatening ketoacidosis. In this chapter, a brief synopsis of ketone body metabolism is provided before the regulatory role of insulin is considered. More specific details of ketone body metabolism are available in other reviews [1–6].

OVERVIEW OF KETONE BODY METABOLISM

Although there is evidence that ketogenesis can occur in the extrahepatic tissues [7, 38], the liver remains the primary source of ketone bodies in humans. The hormonal regulation of ketone body metabolism is mediated at the liver, adipose tissue and other extrahepatic tissues; the individual effects of the relevant hormones are summarised in Table 1.

Regulation at Adipose Tissue

Long-chain NEFA are the major substrate for ketogenesis at the liver, and, as a consequence, the rate of supply of NEFA is a critical regulator of the rate of ketogenesis. In turn, the supply of NEFA from adipose tissue is determined by the relative rates of lipolysis and re-esterification, and both pathways are under direct hormonal control. These pathways are shown schematically in Figure 1.

Adipose tissue triacylglycerol is hydrolysed to glycerol and fatty acids by two enzymes, hormone-sensitive lipase (HSL) and monoacylglycerol lipase [8]. The removal of the first fatty acid to leave diacylglycerol is

International Textbook of Diabetes Mellitus, Second Edition. Edited by K.G.M.M. Alberti, P. Zimmet, R.A. DeFronzo, and H. Keen (Honorary)

Table 1 Summary of the hormonal regulation of ketone body metabolism

Hormone	Effect	Proposed mechanisms of action
Insulin	Inhibition of lipolysis	Decreases cAMP levels and HSL activity
	Inhibition of hepatic ketogenesis	Increases malonyl-CoA levels, and CPT-I affinity for this inhibitor
		Decreases affinity of CPT-I for fatty acyl-CoA
	Stimulation of ketone body clearance	Mechanism unknown
Glucagon	Stimulation of lipolysis	Increases cAMP levels and HSL activity
	Stimulation of hepatic ketogenesis	Decreases malonyl-CoA levels
Catecholamines	Stimulation of lipolysis	Increase cAMP levels and HSL activity
	Stimulation of hepatic ketogenesis	Mechanism unknown
Growth hormone	Stimulation of lipolysis	Slow mechanism, possibly by stimulation of protein synthesis
Cortisol	Stimulation of lipolysis	Promotes lipolytic action of other catabolic hormones
Thyroxine	Stimulation of lipolysis	Direct effect, and promotes lipolytic action of catecholamines
	Stimulation of ketone body clearance	Mechanism unknown
	? Stimulation of hepatic ketogenesis	Mechanism unknown

HSL, hormone-sensitive lipase: CPT-I, carnitine palmitoyltransferase I.

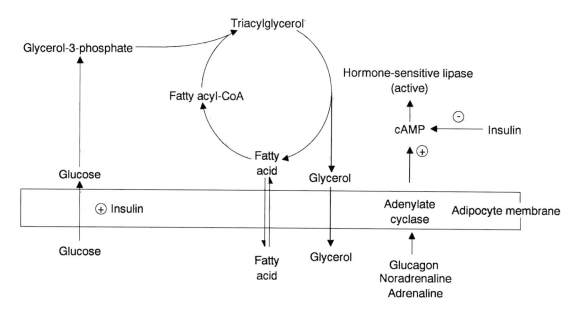

Figure 1 The hormonal regulation of adipose tissue lipolysis and re-esterification

specifically catalysed by HSL and is the rate-limiting step. In this context, it is appropriate that the hormonal regulation of lipolysis is mediated through HSL. The glycerol is not significantly metabolised in adipose tissue, and is released and transported to the liver, where it enters the pathway of gluconeogenesis or is oxidised. The NEFA are either released or immediately re-esterified. This latter pathway requires the availability of glycerol 3-phosphate which is synthesised *de novo* from glucose within the adipocyte.

It has been demonstrated *in vitro* that the catecholamines and glucagon stimulate lipolysis by increasing the intracellular levels of cAMP through the activation of adenylate cyclase [2]. Growth hormone stimulates lipolysis by a slower, alternative pathway, while cortisol exerts a permissive effect on the stimulatory action of these catabolic hormones [2]. The effect of these hormones *in vivo* is considered later, but it is pertinent to point out that, with the exception of the catecholamines, the infusion of these hormones into the normal human does not produce a significant increase in plasma NEFA levels.

Insulin inhibits the release of NEFA from the adipocyte by both inhibiting lipolysis and stimulating re-esterification. The antilipolytic action would appear to be mediated in part by a decrease in the intracellular cAMP levels following the activation of a cAMP phosphodiesterase [8]; the increase in re-esterification is thought to be promoted by an increase in glucose uptake into the adipocyte leading to the formation of glycerol 3-phosphate [2].

Other factors influence the rate of NEFA release from adipose tissue. Both lactate [9] and ketone bodies *per se* [1, 10] appear to have a direct antilipolytic effect, while recent evidence suggests that hyperglycaemia at basal insulin levels does not exert an independent effect on the rate of lipolysis [11].

Regulation at the Liver

Although the hepatic uptake of NEFA is concentration dependent [12], the rate of ketogenesis is not determined by the rate of substrate supply and points to a second intrahepatic site for the regulation of ketogenesis. This was demonstrated by McGarry et al [13] using the isolated perfused rat liver. Rats were fasted for progressive intervals, and then the livers were perfused with the same concentration of oleic acid. Despite constant oleic acid levels, the rate of ketogenesis was found to be low for the first 6 hours of fasting but then increased rapidly between 6 and 9 hours before remaining steady. McGarry et al concluded that a change in intrahepatic metabolism with fasting had led to the stimulation of ketogenesis. However, intrahepatic NEFA are not committed to ketogenesis and the possible routes of metabolism are shown in Figure 2. Following conversion to their coenzyme A (CoA) derivatives, they can either re-enter a storage phase with re-esterification to triacylglycerol or they can cross into the mitochondria to undergo β-oxidation to acetyl-CoA. This in turn can be completely oxidised in the tricarboxylic acid cycle or can enter the pathway for ketone body synthesis. Such a complex system of pathways requires careful regulation.

Initially, it was thought that the pathway of re-esterification was the site of regulation, so that diminished re-esterification allowed an increase in ketogenesis. However, this was shown to be incorrect as specific inhibitors of fatty acid oxidation led to a resumption of re-esterification [13, 14]. Attention then turned to the transport of fatty acyl-CoA derivatives across the mitochondrial membranes as a potential site for the regulation of ketogenesis. The inner mitochondrial membrane is permeable to medium-chain (but not long-chain) fatty acyl-CoA derivatives. Therefore, the movement of long-chain fatty acyl-CoA into the mitochondrion

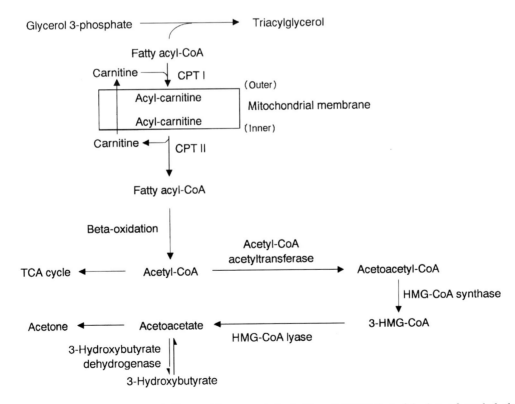

Figure 2 The pathways of fatty acid metabolism and ketogenesis in the liver (3-HMG-CoA, 3-hydroxy-3-methyl-glutaryl-CoA; CPT, carnitine palmitoyltransferase; TCA cycle, tricarboxylic acid cycle)

requires a specific transport system, which is called the carnitine shuttle. The importance of this shuttle in the regulation of long-chain fatty acyl-CoA oxidation was first demonstrated by McGarry and colleagues [15]. They showed that the rate of medium-chain fatty acid oxidation was the same in the livers from fed and fasted animals, whereas the oxidation of long-chain fatty acids was increased sixfold with fasting. The carnitine shuttle comprises two enzymes, carnitine palmitoyltransferases I and II (CPT-I and II, respectively), as shown in Figure 2. The CPT-I protein is located on the inner aspect of the outer mitochondrial membrane, and requires the structural integrity of the membrane for its function in the formation of fatty acyl carnitine [16]. The structure of CPT-I differs between tissues, and it includes the binding sites of the inhibitors of the carnitine shuttle [16]. Conversely, the activity of CPT-II is not strictly regulated and the structure of the enzyme is conserved across different tissue types. It is located on the inner mitochondrial membrane and catalyses the conversion of fatty acyl carnitine back to fatty acyl-CoA.

It has been shown that malonyl-CoA, an intermediate in the synthesis of long-chain fatty acids, is a potent inhibitor of CPT-I activity [3, 6]. This provides a possible explanation for the regulation of hepatic fuel metabolism. In the fed state, the rate of glycolysis will be high, leading to the production of malonyl-CoA and long-chain fatty acid synthesis. The high levels of malonyl-CoA will inhibit CPT-I activity so that the newly synthesised fatty acid is not immediately oxidised but is esterified to triacylglycerol. Conversely, in the fasting state the rate of glycolysis will be low, with decreased levels of malonyl-CoA and no significant lipid synthesis. The activity of CPT-I will increase, which will favour the oxidation of the incoming fatty acids with the potential for ketogenesis. The activity of CPT-I would also appear to be under direct hormonal regulation, which is considered below.

Within the mitochondrion the long-chain fatty acids undergo β-oxidation with the formation of acetyl-CoA. As shown in Figure 2, this can either enter the tricarboxylic acid (TCA) cycle or the pathway for the formation of acetoacetate. The proportion of acetoacetate converted to 3-hydroxybutyrate is dependent upon the redox state within the mitochondrion [2]. Acetone is formed by the decarboxylation of acetoacetate, which is not dependent upon the assistance of enzyme catalysis [17]. Although the two pathways of acetyl-CoA metabolism provide a further potential regulatory site for the control of ketogenesis, there is no experimental evidence to suggest that it is of physiological significance [2]; the principal site for the regulation of hepatic ketogenesis, therefore, remains the carnitine shuttle at

the partition of the pathways of fatty acid oxidation and esterification.

Extrahepatic Ketone Body Utilisation and Synthesis

The ketone bodies synthesised at the liver are released into the circulation to be taken up and utilised by the extrahepatic tissues. The 3-hydroxybutyrate is first converted to acetoacetate by 3-hydroxybutyrate dehydrogenase, which requires the cofactor NAD. If this is in limited supply, the 3-hydroxybutyrate may not be immediately utilised and is free to re-enter the tissue circulation. The acetoacetate is converted to acetyl-CoA by the following reactions [2]:

$$\text{acetoacetate} + \text{succinyl-CoA}$$
$$\xrightarrow{\text{3-oxoacid CoA transferase}} \begin{array}{l} \text{acetoacetyl-CoA} \\ + \text{ succinate} \end{array} \quad (1)$$
$$\text{acetoacetyl-CoA} + \text{CoA} \xrightarrow{\text{thiolase}} 2 \text{ acetyl-CoA} \quad (2)$$

Both enzymes involved in the peripheral utilisation of ketone bodies are located within the mitochondrion, and the acetyl-CoA is available for complete oxidation within the TCA cycle. The absence of 3-oxoacid CoA transferase in the liver ensures that the synthesised ketone bodies are not immediately utilised and are available for export to the extrahepatic tissues. Extrahepatic utilisation represents a third site for the regulation of ketone body metabolism. Hyperketonaemia *per se* has been shown to exert a powerful inhibitory effect on peripheral utilisation [18, 19], although there appears to be only a limited hormonal influence on this process.

There is evidence to suggest that the extrahepatic tissues also possess the capacity for ketogenesis. As the enzyme 3-hydroxy-3-methylglutaryl-CoA (HMG-CoA) synthase is virtually absent from the extrahepatic tissues, this would not involve the same pathway as that used by the liver [7]. Alternatively, it has been proposed that excess acetyl-CoA might be diverted away from the TCA cycle and participate in ketone body formation through the reversal of the reactions (equations 1 and 2) normally involved in ketone body utilisation [7]. The release of unlabelled ketone bodies following futile cycling of the infused labelled ketone bodies (pseudoketogenesis) was thought to provide an explanation for this apparent ketogenesis [20]. However, recent work would suggest that pseudoketogenesis makes an insignificant contribution to the appearance of ketone bodies across the human forearm [38].

THE ROLE OF INSULIN IN KETONE BODY METABOLISM

Insulin has a central role in the control of ketone body metabolism, and appears to act at all three sites of regulation.

Regulation at Adipose Tissue

The greatest effect of insulin is probably mediated through the regulation of the supply of NEFA from adipose tissue, and it is well established that this is exquisitely sensitive to the inhibitory effect of insulin [21–23]. It has been shown that fasting insulin levels continue to regulate the supply of NEFA from adipose tissue; the infusion of somatostatin produced a decrease in mean fasting insulin levels from 14 mU/l to 5 mU/l, and this was accompanied by a significant rise in the plasma NEFA concentration [21]. This sensitivity has been reaffirmed [22, 23], and it has been calculated that the half-maximal suppression of adipose tissue lipolysis is achieved at a plasma free insulin concentration of around 2 mU/l in normal humans [23]. Interestingly, patients with poorly controlled IDDM display a degree of insensitivity to the antilipolytic action of insulin [23], which would promote the release of NEFA and exacerbate the tendency to ketogenesis under conditions of absolute insulin deficiency.

Regulation at the Liver

There is increasing evidence to suggest that insulin inhibits hepatic ketogenesis directly. It has been shown that anti-insulin serum increases ketogenesis in the isolated perfused rat liver [24], while insulin and proinsulin inhibit ketogenesis directly in rat hepatocyte monolayer preparations [25]. The direct effect of insulin on hepatic ketogenesis has been investigated in normal humans [26, 27, 40]. In these studies, the effect of insulin at the liver, independent of its effect on substrate supply, was examined by the infusion of triacylglycerol to maintain constant plasma NEFA levels. At low insulin levels, insulin did not have an independent effect on ketogenesis [26, 40]. Conversely, when insulin levels were raised from basal levels into the high physiological range, there was a significant decrease in the rate of ketogenesis [27]. These observations can be brought together into a possible system for the control of ketogenesis. During the fasting state the major effect of insulin is through the regulation of NEFA supply with little or no effect at the liver. During feeding, however, there will still be a supply of NEFA to the liver from the gut and from *de novo* lipogenesis; to prevent persistent and unnecessary ketogenesis, therefore, this will be suppressed directly by the postprandial levels of insulin.

The mechanism by which insulin inhibits hepatic ketogenesis has not been fully elucidated. It is possible that insulin has a direct effect on CPT-I. Support for this comes from a study by Gamble and Cook who showed that the affinity of CPT-I for the inhibitor, malonyl-CoA, was decreased in streptozotocin-diabetic rats and that this was reversed with insulin treatment [28]. An alternative or, indeed, additional explanation is that insulin increases the concentration of malonyl-CoA through the stimulation of glycolysis [3, 6]. We have shown that insulin also decreases the affinity of CPT-I for the substrate, palmitoyl-CoA, and increases the concentration of glycerol 3-phosphate [25]. This might contribute to the inhibitory action of insulin by increasing intrahepatic esterification and diverting NEFA away from β-oxidation and ketogenesis.

Regulation at the Extrahepatic Tissues

Conflicting results have been produced by studies investigating the action of insulin on the peripheral utilisation of ketone bodies. As hyperketonaemia *per se* reduces ketone body clearance, it has been difficult to ascertain *in vivo* whether insulin improves peripheral utilisation directly, or indirectly by decreasing ketogenesis and lowering blood ketone body levels. Sherwin and colleagues showed that insulin increased the clearance of infused ketone bodies in normal and IDDM subjects [29]. Although ketogenesis was not directly measured in this study, it was presumed to be suppressed, and it was therefore concluded that insulin had a direct effect on ketone body clearance. Subsequently, 3-^{14}C labelled and unlabelled acetoacetate infusions have been administered to normal subjects in order to measure ketone body clearance and production under conditions of constant peripheral ketone body levels [18]. Hyperketonaemia alone had a significant inhibitory effect on ketogenesis and ketone body clearance, whereas the elevation of the serum insulin concentration to high physiological levels partially reversed the suppressive action of hyperketonaemia on peripheral utilisation. However, it is recognised that the use of a single tracer is not the most accurate method of assessing total ketone body turnover [4]. On balance, it would seem that insulin does have a small, direct stimulatory effect on ketone body clearance, although the mechanism remains to be determined.

INSULIN DEFICIENCY AND KETOACIDOSIS

The importance of the inhibitory effect of insulin on ketone body metabolism *in vivo* really becomes apparent only in the insulin-deficient state. This is reinforced by the observation that glucagon, cortisol and growth hormone infusions in normal subjects have no significant effect on circulating plasma NEFA and blood ketone body levels in the presence of insulin [30–32]. It is only when serum insulin levels are suppressed by the simultaneous administration of somatostatin that these catabolic hormones increase ketone body levels. Glucagon appears to have a direct effect on hepatic ketogenesis, whereas cortisol and growth hormone seem to act by increasing the supply of NEFA [2, 30–32]. Adrenaline and noradrenaline differ in that the infusion of these hormones in normal subjects leads to an increase in ketone body levels, even in the presence of basal insulin levels [4, 33]. As the increase in ketogenesis occurs at much lower plasma NEFA levels with noradrenaline than with adrenaline, it has been suggested that noradrenaline exerts a greater direct stimulatory effect on hepatic ketogenesis [4]. However, this suggestion must remain speculative without data for the rate of NEFA turnover and hepatic extraction. Not surprisingly, the ketogenic effects of adrenaline and noradrenaline are markedly enhanced when insulin levels are suppressed by the co-infusion of somatostatin [33], which underlines the great ketogenic capacity of these hormones when insulin deficiency develops in IDDM.

It would appear that the ketogenic potential is different between patients with IDDM and healthy control subjects [39]. Thus, at low insulin levels the ketogenic response to infused adrenaline was greater in the patients with IDDM and was independent of the supply of NEFA.

A number of studies have examined the metabolic changes in response to acute insulin withdrawal in patients with IDDM. Whereas there is no immediate change in cortisol and growth hormone levels, hyperglucagonaemia quickly develops and is associated with a progressive increase in ketone body concentrations [34, 35]. This emphasises the importance of combined hyperglucagonaemia and insulin deficiency in the initiation of ketoacidosis. Using both labelled acetoacetate and 3-hydroxybutyrate infusions, it has been shown that production of both ketone bodies is increased under these conditions, together with a selective defect of 3-hydroxybutyrate clearance which may be related to a change in the redox state at the periphery [36, 37].

From these studies it is easy to appreciate how insulin deficiency in IDDM will lead to escalating ketone body levels. The combination of an additional stress, for example infection or myocardial infarction, will lead to a surge of the catabolic hormones with a further stimulus to ketogenesis and the possibility of life-threatening ketoacidosis.

CONCLUSION

In conclusion, insulin acts at all three principal sites for the regulation of ketone body metabolism. The major effect appears to be through the regulation of NEFA supply, although it also inhibits hepatic ketogenesis and promotes peripheral ketone body clearance. The importance of insulin as a regulator of ketogenesis becomes apparent in the insulin-deficient state, when the ketogenic potential of the catabolic hormones can be fully realised.

REFERENCES

1. Balasse EO, Fery F. Ketone body production and disposal: effects of fasting, diabetes and exercise. Diabetes Metab Rev 1989; 5: 247–70.
2. Johnston DG, Alberti KGMM. Hormonal control of ketone body metabolism in the normal and diabetic state. Clin Endocrinol Metab 1982; 11: 329–61.
3. McGarry JD, Woeltje KF, Kuwajima M, Foster DW. Regulation of ketogenesis and the renaissance of carnitine palmitoyltransferase. Diabetes Metab Rev 1989; 5: 271–84.
4. Keller U, Lustenberger M, Muller-Brand J, Gerber PPG, Stauffacher W. Human ketone body production and utilization studied using tracer techniques: regulation by free fatty acids, insulin, catecholamines, and thyroid hormones. Diabetes Metab Rev 1989; 5: 285–98.
5. Nosadini R, Avagaro A. Ketone body metabolism in diabetes mellitus. In Alberti KGMM, Krall LP (eds) Diabetes annual 6. Amsterdam: Elsevier, 1991; pp 611–33.
6. Foster DW. Banting Lecture 1984. From glycogen to ketones—and back. Diabetes 1984; 33: 1188–99.
7. Nosadini R, Avogaro A, Sacca L et al. Ketone body metabolism in normal and diabetic skeletal muscle. Am J Physiol 1985; 249: E131–6.
8. Yeaman SJ. Hormone sensitive lipase—a multipurpose enzyme in lipid metabolism. Biochim Biophys Acta 1990; 1052: 128–32.
9. Björntorp P. The effect of lactic acid on adipose tissue metabolism in vitro. Acta Med Scand 1965; 178: 253–5.
10. Moller N, Jorgensen JOL, Moller J, Bak JF, Porksen N, Alberti KGMM, Schmitz O. Substrate metabolism during modest hyperinsulinemia in response to isolated hyperketonemia in insulin-dependent diabetic subjects. Metabolism 1990; 12: 1309–13.
11. Caruso M, Divertie GD, Jensen MD, Miles JM. Lack of effect of hyperglycemia on lipolysis in humans. Am J Physiol 1990; 259: E542–7.
12. Woodside WF, Heimberg M. Hepatic metabolism of free fatty acids in experimental diabetes. Israeli J Med Sci 1972; 8: 309–16.
13. McGarry JD, Meier JM, Foster DW. The effects of starvation and refeeding on carbohydrate and lipid metabolism in vivo and in the perfused rat liver. The relationship between fatty acid oxidation and esterification in the regulation of ketogenesis. J Biol Chem 1973; 248: 270–8.
14. Williamson JR, Scholz R, Browning ET. Control mechanisms of gluconeogenesis and ketogenesis. Interaction between fatty acid oxidation and the citric acid cycle in perfused rat liver. J Biol Chem 1969; 244: 4617–27.
15. McGarry JD, Foster DW. The regulation of ketogenesis from octanoic acid: the role of the tricarboxylic acid

cycle and fatty acid synthesis. J Biol Chem 1971; 246: 1149–59.

16. Woeltje KF, Esser V, Weis BC et al. Inter-tissue and inter-species characteristics of the mitochondrial carnitine palmitoyltransferase enzyme system. J Biol Chem 1990; 265: 10714–19.

17. Walker M, Marshall SM, Alberti KGMM. Clinical aspects of diabetic ketoacidosis. Diabetes Metab Rev 1989; 5: 651–63.

18. Keller U, Lustenberger M, Stauffacher W. Effect of insulin on ketone body clearance studied by a ketone body 'clamp' technique in normal man. Diabetologia 1988; 31: 24–9.

19. Fery F, Balasse EO. Ketone body production and disposal in diabetic ketosis. A comparison with fasting ketosis. Diabetes 1985; 34: 326–32.

20. Des Rosiers C, Montgomery JA, Garneau M et al. Pseudoketogenesis in hepatectomized dogs. Am J Physiol 1990; 258: E519–28.

21. Swislocki ALM, Chen YDI, Golay A, Chang MO, Reaven GM. Insulin suppression of plasma free fatty acid concentration in normal individuals and patients with type 2 (non-insulin dependent) diabetes. Diabetologia 1987; 30: 622–6.

22. Jensen MD, Caruso M, Heiling V, Miles J. Insulin regulation of lipolysis in non-diabetic and IDDM subjects. Diabetes 1989; 38: 1595–1601.

23. Bonadonna RC, Groop LC, Zych K, Shank M, DeFronzo RA. Dose-dependent effect of insulin on plasma free fatty acid turnover and oxidation in humans. Am J Physiol 1990; 259: E736–50.

24. McGarry JD, Wright PH, Foster DW. Hormonal control of ketogenesis. Rapid activation of hepatic ketogenic capacity in fed rats by anti-insulin serum and glucagon. J Clin Invest 1975; 55: 1202–9.

25. Agius L, Chowdhury MH, Davis SN, Alberti KGMM. Regulation of ketogenesis, gluconeogenesis and glycogen synthesis by insulin and proinsulin in rat hepatocyte monolayer cultures. Diabetes 1986; 35: 1286–93.

26. Miles JM, Haymond MW, Nissen SL, Gerich JE. Effects of free fatty acid availability, glucagon excess and insulin deficiency on ketone body production in post-absorptive man. J Clin Invest 1983; 71: 1554–61.

27. Keller U, Gerber PP, Stauffacher W. Fatty acid independent inhibition of hepatic ketone body production by insulin in humans. Am J Physiol 1988; 254: E694–9.

28. Gamble SM, Cook GA. Alteration of the apparent K_i of carnitine palmitoyl transferase for malonyl-CoA by the diabetic state and reversed by insulin. J Biol Chem 1985; 260: 9516–19.

29. Sherwin RS, Hendler RG, Felig P. Effect of diabetes mellitus and insulin on the turnover and metabolic response to ketones in man. Diabetes 1976; 25: 776–84.

30. Gill A, Johnston DG, Orskov H, Batsone GF, Alberti KGMM. Metabolic interactions of glucagon and cortisol in normal and insulin-deficient man. Metabolism 1982; 31: 305–11.

31. Johnston DG, Gill A, Orskov H, Batsone GF, Alberti KGMM. Metabolic effects of cortisol in normal and insulin-deficient man. Metabolism 1982; 31: 312–17.

32. Metcalfe P, Johnston DG, Nosadini R, Orskov H, Alberti KGMM. Metabolic effects of acute and chronic growth hormone excess in normal and insulin-deficient man. Diabetologia 1981; 20: 123–8.

33. Pernet A, Walker M, Gill GV, Orskov H, Alberti KGMM, Johnston DG. Metabolic effects of adrenaline and noradrenaline in man: studies with somatostatin. Diabète Métab 1984; 10: 98–105.

34. Alberti KGMM, Christensen NJ, Iverson J, Orskov H. Role of glucagon and other hormones in development of diabetic ketoacidosis. Lancet 1975; i: 1307–11.

35. Miles JM, Rizza RA, Haymond MW, Gerich JE. Effect of acute insulin deficiency on glucose and ketone body turnover in man. Evidence for the primary overproduction of glucose and ketone bodies in the genesis of diabetic ketoacidosis. Diabetes 1980; 29: 926–30.

36. Hall SEH, Wastney ME, Bolton TM, Braaten JT, Berman M. Ketone body kinetics in humans; the effect of insulin-dependent diabetes, obesity and starvation. J Lipid Res 1984; 25: 1184–94.

37. Nosadini R, Avogaro A, Trevisan R et al. Acetoacetate and 3-hydroxybutyrate kinetics in obese and insulin-dependent diabetic humans. Am J Physiol 1985; 248: R611–20.

38. Avogaro A, Doria A, Gnudi L et al. Forearm ketone body metabolism in normal and in insulin-dependent diabetic patients. Am J Physiol 1992; 263: E261–7.

39. Avogaro A, Valerio A, Gnudi L et al. The effects of different plasma insulin concentrations on lipolytic and ketogenic responses to epinephrine in normal and type 1 (insulin-dependent) diabetic humans. Diabetologia 1992; 35: 129–38.

40. Beylot M, Picard S, Chambrier C et al. Effect of physiological concentrations of insulin and glycagon on the relationship between non-esterified fatty acids availability and ketone body production in humans. Metabolism 1991; 40: 1138–46.

27

Insulin Actions *In Vivo*: Protein Metabolism

Ralph A. DeFronzo* and **William S. Stirewalt†**

Diabetes Division, University of Texas Health Science Center, San Antonio, TX, and
†*Departments of Obstetrics and Gynecology, and Molecular Physiology and Biophysics, University of Vermont,*
Burlington, VT, USA

The net protein balance, whether viewed at the whole body or organ level, represents the sum of two simultaneously ongoing processes: protein synthesis and protein degradation. It is well established that insulin promotes a protein anabolic state, whereas insulin deficiency and diabetes mellitus are characterized by protein catabolism, negative nitrogen balance, and muscle wasting [1–3]. Children with insulin-dependent diabetes mellitus fail to grow normally [4, 5], and when treated with insulin, demonstrate accelerated or 'catch-up' growth [6, 7]. These simple clinical observations underscore the important role of insulin in the regulation of protein metabolism.

In order for insulin to work it must first bind to specific receptors which are present on all insulin target tissues [8]. Following this initial step, insulin receptor tyrosine kinase is activated and serves as an obligatory initial step in the intracellular signaling process that promotes the many and varied actions of the hormone [9, 10, 11]. Following the activation of receptor tyrosine kinase, amino acid flux into the cell is enhanced [12, 13], ensuring an adequate supply of substrate for protein synthesis. Moreover, amino acids themselves are potent insulin secretagogues [14] and also augment protein synthesis directly [15, 16]. Thus, following the ingestion of a mixed meal the concomitant presence of hyperaminoacidemia and hyperinsulinemia conspire to augment protein anabolism. Over the last decade convincing evidence has accumulated to indicate that insulin stimulates the synthesis of protein by modulating the rate of both transcription and translation. Transcription is a complex sequence which involves transfer of the genetic code from DNA in the nucleus to messenger RNA (mRNA) [17]. The mRNA is then exported from the nucleus through nuclear pores into the cytoplasm, where the information contained in the mRNA is translated into specific proteins (translation). Not all tissues respond in the same way to insulin. In some tissues insulin augments protein synthesis by increasing the efficiency and/or capacity of the steps involved in translation [18–22], while in others it acts directly on genes, stimulating or inhibiting their rate of transcription [17, 23–28]. Lastly, insulin can promote net protein anabolism by suppressing the rate of protein degradation [29–32]. In the subsequent sections we will detail the basic cellular mechanisms involved in the regulation of protein synthesis and protein degradation and then review what is known about the effect of insulin and diabetes mellitus on these intracellular regulatory steps (Table 1).

Table 1 Potential steps involved in the regulation of protein metabolism by insulin

Insulin receptor signaling mechanism
Amino acid transport
Stimulation of protein synthesis
Gene transcription
Translation of mRNA
Initiation
Elongation
Termination
Inhibition of protein degradation

PROTEIN SYNTHESIS: NORMAL REGULATION

The Gene: DNA

The genetic code for the synthesis of all proteins resides within the nucleotide sequence of the double-stranded, helical molecules of DNA [17]. Each nucleotide has three components (Figure 1): (a) phosphoric acid, (b) a sugar, deoxyribose, (c) a nitrogenous base. There are four bases: two purines, adenine and guanine, and two pyrimidines, thymine and cytosine. The nucleotides are linked together in such a way that deoxyribose and phosphoric acid alternate with each other in the two separate DNA strands, which are held together by hydrogen bonding between the purine and pyrimidine bases (Figure 2). The purine base adenine (A) always binds with the pyrimidine base thymine (T) while the purine, guanine (G), always binds with the pyrimidine, cytosine (C).

Each amino acid is specified by a distinct codon, which is defined by three successive base triplets. However, many amino acids are specified by more than one codon. By convention the code is specified in terms of the nucleotides in RNA, where uracil (U) replaces

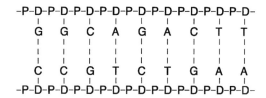

Figure 2 Arrangement of nucleotides in deoxyribonucleic acid (DNA). Deoxyribose (D) and phosphoric acid (P) alternate with each other in forming the backbone. The complementary bases (adenine and thymine; guanine and cytosine) are loosely bound to each other by hydrogen bonding

thymine (see below). Of the 64 possible base combinations, 61 are used to code for a specific amino acid, while three (UAG, UGA, UAA) are stop codons which serve to terminate translation of polypeptide synthesis and define the completion of the coded protein. All proteins start at the amino end with one amino acid, methionine, whose codon is AUG (see subsequent discussion on protein chain initiation). For an average size protein of 400 amino acids, a portion of DNA comprising 1200 nucleotide pairs is required, since each codon consists of three nucleotides. Since this is much smaller than the number of base pairs in the smallest

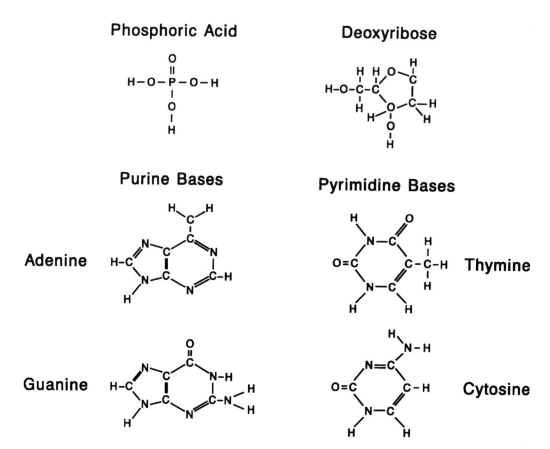

Figure 1 Deoxyribonucleic acid (DNA) comprises three building blocks: phosphoric acid, deoxyribose and four nitrogenous bases. There are two purine bases (adenine and guanine) and two pyrimidine bases (thymine and cytosine). One molecule of deoxyribose, one molecule of phosphoric acid, and one of the four bases combine to form a nucleotide

DNA molecule, it is obvious that most DNA molecules contain many genes.

Transcription: DNA to RNA

The synthesis of proteins involves the transfer of the encoded information in DNA in the cell nucleus to single stranded messenger RNA (mRNA) molecules in a process called DNA transcription. The chemical structure of the messenger RNA is similar to that of DNA with two exceptions: (a) the sugar ribose replaces deoxyribose and (b) the pyrimidine base uracil replaces thymidine. The synthesis of mRNA requires that the double-stranded DNA helix first unravel. One of the strands then serves as a template for the synthesis of a linear sequence of ribonucleotides complementary to the sequence information in DNA. The codons in the mRNA define the amino acid sequence of the protein by serving as a template during the process of protein synthesis (translation) which takes place in the cytoplasm of the cell.

The synthesis of most mRNAs is controlled by a complex protein binding system which is located at the start or promoter site, i.e. the 5′ end, of the DNA molecule immediately prior to the gene that is being transcribed (Figure 3). This binding system has been referred to as the *cis/trans* model [33, 34]. Regions of DNA that bind proteins are called *cis* elements, while the proteins that bind to the *cis* elements are called *trans* factors. A *trans* factor is synthesized by a transcription unit that is not associated with the DNA sequence being regulated. One potential site for the regulation of protein synthesis by insulin resides in the formation of specific *trans* factors which regulate the synthesis of specific mRNAs.

Assembly of the mRNA molecule is under the control of the enzyme RNA polymerase II [35]. This enzyme contains the appropriate complementary

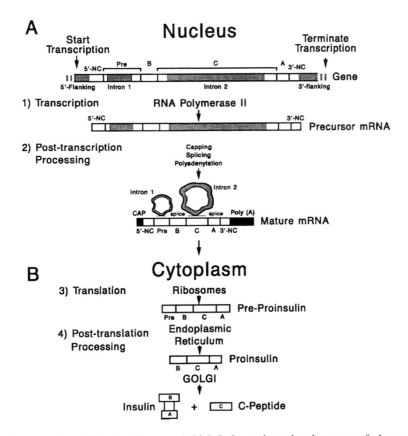

Figure 3 Steps in the expression of the insulin gene (which is located on the short arm of chromosome 11). (A) Nuclear events include transcription (step 1) and post-transcriptional processing (step 2). Arrow indicates transcription of gene to mRNA when RNA polymerase II binds 5′-flanking region of gene and proceeds in the direction from 5′ to 3′. Primary transcript or precursor mRNA is colinear with gene. Post-transcriptional processing involves capping of 5′ end of mRNA with 7-methylguanosine, splicing out of 2 introns, and polyadenylation on the 3′ end. (B) Cytoplasmic events include translation (step 3) and post-translational (step 4) processing. Mature proinsulin mRNA exits the nucleus and is bound by ribosomes. Translation of messenger RNA occurs in 5′ to 3′ direction and preproinsulin peptide, synthesized from NH$_2$-terminal to COOH-terminal, is immediately sequestered into membranous vesicles of the endoplasmic reticulum. Processing involves cleavage of pre-portion of the peptide during translation. Post-translational conversion of proinsulin to insulin and C-peptide occurs within the Golgi apparatus. From reference 425, with permission

structure that recognizes and binds to a specific nucleotide sequence in the promoter region of the DNA strand located upstream of the transcribed nucleotide sequence of the gene. The binding of a specific *trans* factor to the promoter region can enhance (or inhibit) the attachment of RNA polymerase. After the RNA polymerase has attached to the promoter, it causes the two complementary DNA strands to unwind and moves along one of the strands of DNA directing the assembly of the complementary linear sequence of RNA nucleotides. When the RNA polymerase reaches the end of the gene, it encounters a chain-terminating sequence of DNA nucleotides which cause the polymerase to break away from the DNA strand. The newly formed messenger RNA subsequently breaks away from the DNA template and is released into the nucleoplasm.

For most genes the nucleotide sequence contained in the nuclear DNA is significantly different from that in the mature messenger RNA which participates in the synthesis of protein [17, 36, 37]. The DNA segments which actually encode the messenger RNA are called exons and these exons are interrupted by non-coding sequences called introns. Within the nucleus the entire DNA sequence, including both exons and introns, is copied during the process of transcription to produce a primary RNA transcript. This transcript then undergoes a complex editing process in which the introns are cleared out and the exons are spliced

back together. After this splicing process has been completed, the mature messenger RNA, which now contains an uninterrupted linear sequence of codons, is exported from the nucleus to the cytoplasm [38].

Translation: RNA to Protein

The actual process by which proteins are synthesized is extremely complex [17, 19, 20, 39, 40] and involves three separate types of RNA: messenger RNAs (mRNA) which carry the genetic code, transfer RNAs (tRNA) which function as donors of amino acids during the process of protein synthesis, and ribosomal RNAs (rRNA), which are major components of the ribosome, the structure upon which proteins are synthesized (Figure 4).

There is a specific transfer RNA for each amino acid. At the 3' end of the tRNA is an adenylic acid molecule to which the designated amino acid is attached by enzymes specific for each amino acid (aminoacyl-synthetases). Each tRNA possesses within its linear structure a specific triplet of nucleotide bases, called an anticodon, which recognizes a specific codon in the messenger RNA and appropriately aligns the amino acid for incorporation into the newly forming protein. The tRNA is small in comparison to the mRNA and contains only 80 nucleotides which are folded into a cloverleaf structure (Figure 4). The anticodon is located close to the middle of the tRNA at the bottom

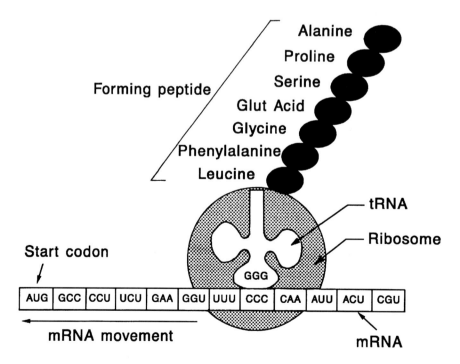

Figure 4 Mechanism of protein synthesis. Messenger RNA (mRNA) binds to a ribosome and initiates the process of translation. Transfer RNAs (tRNA) act as carriers to transport a specific amino acid to the mRNA-ribosome complex and to guide its insertion into the newly forming peptide chain. See text for a more detailed discussion

of the clover leaf and its triplet of nucleotides combines loosely through hydrogen bonding with the codon bases of the mRNA to establish the designated amino acid sequence.

Ribosomal RNA comprises about 60% of the ribosome, and protein constitutes the remainder. Each ribosome (80S) is made up of one small (40S) and one large subunit (60S). The small subunit contains a messenger RNA binding site while the large subunit contains the enzymatic activity that promotes peptide linkages between successive amino acids. Transfer RNA spans these two sites in the 80S ribosome during the synthesis of protein. Protein synthesis is initiated by the binding of mRNA to the ribosome at a site which appropriately positions the AUG start codon [41–44] (Figure 4). Subsequently the amino acid sequence code contained in mRNA is translated by the linear movement of mRNA relative to the ribosome. A single mRNA usually has several ribosomes attached and in the process of translating. This complex of ribosomes is referred to as a polysome.

In eukaryotic cells protein synthesis is an extremely complex process which involves a number of discrete metabolic steps. For simplicity of discussion, the process of translation has been separated into three phases: (a) *initiation*; (b) *elongation*; and (c) *termination*.

Initiation of Translation

The steps involved in the initiation of peptide chain formation are shown in Figure 5. Although there are 64 potential triplets which encode 20 different amino acids, only codon AUG recognizes methionyl-tRNA (met-tRNA) and serves as the initiator of translation [19, 20]. The initiation of translation is complex and involves a number of eukaryotic initiation factors (eIF) which promote the binding of the initiator methionyl-tRNA to messenger RNA to form a translationally competent ribosome (Figure 5). Many of these initiation factors have been purified and their structure elucidated [19, 45, 46]. The most extensive isolation of these initiation factors has been carried out in reticulocyte preparations, but a similar sequence has been described in a number of other cell types, including mammalian fat cells, liver and muscle [47]. In the first step of the initiation process a ternary

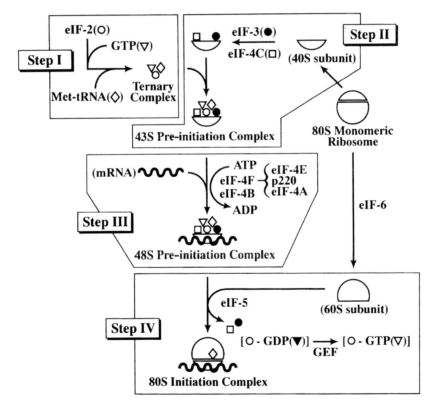

Figure 5 Initiation of protein synthesis. The first step (I) in the initiation of protein synthesis results in the formation of a ternary complex between eIF-2, GTP and Met-tRNA. In step II the ternary complex then binds to a 40S ribosomal subunit that is complexed with eIF-3 and eIF-4C to form a 43S preinitiation complex. The binding of an mRNA molecule to the 43S preinitiation complex (step III) involves initiation factors, the protein p220, and the hydrolysis of ATP. In the last step (IV) eIF-5 promotes the release of the initiation factors bound to the 40S ribosomal subunit, which allows the 60S ribosomal subunit to join with the 40S ribosomal subunit and form an 80S initiation complex. See text for a more detailed discussion. Redrawn from reference 18, with permission

complex is formed by the binding of eIF-2 and guanidine triphosphate (GTP) with met-tRNA. In step two the ternary complex binds to the 40S ribosomal subunit to form the 43S pre-initiation complex. The 40S ribosomal subunit is derived from an 80S monomeric ribosomal precursor and binds to the initiation factors eIF-3 and eIF-4C. Although met-tRNA can bind to the 40S subunit in the absence of eIF-3 and eIF-4C, the reaction is markedly accelerated by these initiation factors [48, 49]. The interactions between the initiation factors and the other components of the translational process are highly specific [50, 51]. Thus, eIF-2 binds to the 40S ribosomal subunit and met-tRNA, but does not react with any other aminoacyl-tRNA or the 80S ribosome. The significance of this is readily apparent when one remembers that only met-tRNA can initiate translation. The initiation factor eIF-2 is believed to be a site at which hormones, including insulin, can regulate protein synthesis [44, 46, 52]. The α subunit of eIF-2 is phosphorylated by a kinase called eIF-2α kinase and contains a GDP binding site [50], while the β subunit is phosphorylated by casein kinase II [51]. The δ subunit can be phosphorylated by either kinase and binds met-tRNA and mRNA [50]. Since guanine nucleotides and phosphorylation-dephosphorylation reactions have been implicated as intracellular elements involved in insulin action [11], binding of the ternary complex (which contains eIF-2) to the 40S ribosomal subunit represents an early step at which insulin could potentially regulate protein synthesis [44, 45, 53, 54, 55].

Step three in the initiation process involves the binding of the 43S pre-initiation complex to mRNA, leading to the formation of the 48S pre-initiation complex (Figure 5). This step involves several initiation factors and the hydrolysis of ATP. Initiation factors eIF-4E and eIF-4A and the protein p220 together form a complex (called eIF-4F) and, in conjunction with eIF-4B, bind to the 'cap' structure at the 5' end of mRNA upstream of the initiating AUG codon [45, 56]. The cap structure (m7GpppN, where N is any nucleotide and m is a methyl group) is common to all eukaryotic mRNAs. These interactions result in the unwinding of the mRNA 5' secondary structure and facilitate the attachment of the 43S preinitiation complex to mRNA to form the 48S pre-initiation complex. Recent evidence suggests that the modulation of the availability of eIF-4E to participate in this important step is a major mechanism by which insulin stimulates protein synthesis at the level of initiation [57, 58] (and see subsequent discussion; regulation of peptide chain initiation).

In step four of initiation the 48S pre-initiation complex is bound to the large 60S ribosomal subunit to form the final 80S initiation complex [59] (Figure 5).

This step is catalyzed by another initiation factor, eIF-5, which promotes the release of bound factors from the 48S pre-initiation complex in association with the hydrolysis of GTP to GDP. The GDP is released in complex with eIF-2. Before the eIF-2 can bind to another met-tRNA and participate in another round of protein chain initiation, the eIF-2-GDP complex must be converted to eIF-2-GTP, a reaction which is catalyzed by the guanine nucleotide exchange factor (GEF). Phosphorylation/dephosphorylation of GEF may also play an important role in the regulation of polypeptide chain initiation [60] and insulin has been shown to regulate GEF activity, providing another control mechanism via which the hormone can modulate protein synthesis [60–62]. Once formed, the 80S ribosome complex with its attached mRNA and start met-tRNA is ready to initiate peptide chain elongation.

Peptide Chain Elongation

The met-tRNA of the 80S ribosome is bound to a specific ribosomal site, referred to as the donor site, and its anticodon is base-paired at that site with the initiation codon AUG in the mRNA. The site immediately adjacent to the donor site is referred to as the acceptor site and initially is unoccupied. The appropriate aminoacyl-tRNA, dictated by the codon, then binds to the acceptor site via a reaction that is catalyzed by the hydrolysis of GTP and requires a specific elongation factor, eEF-1 [63]. After the incoming aminoacyl-tRNA has bound to the ribosome at the acceptor site, a peptidyl transferase (a component of the 60S ribosomal unit) catalyzes the peptide linkage of the amino group of the aminoacyl-tRNA to the start amino acid, methionine. Following the creation of this peptide bond, a translocation step ensues, the deacylated tRNA is released from the ribosome, and the mRNA and ribosome shift relative to each other by one codon (i.e. three bases). This shift is catalyzed by another elongation factor, eEF-2, and requires the hydrolysis of GTP. Repeated cycles of this process lead to peptide chain elongation and the formation of the mature protein [64].

Peptide Chain Termination

Elongation of the peptide chain continues until one of three termination codons (UAA, UAG, UGA) occupies the acceptor site. At this point the termination factor, RF (release factor), binds to the acceptor site and, with the hydrolysis of GTP, catalyzes the release of the completed peptide chain from the ribosome. There is little information to suggest that the process of termination is regulated *in vivo*.

PROTEIN DEGRADATION: NORMAL REGULATION

Knowledge about the specific pathways of protein degradation has lagged behind elucidation of the steps involved in protein synthesis. In recent years, however, a clearer picture of the pathways involved in protein degradation has begun to emerge [29, 31, 32, 65–70]. Multiple pathways for the degradation of protein have been identified in mammalian tissues (Table 2). The relative importance of these pathways varies from tissue to tissue and the physiological factors which regulate their activity are quite distinct.

Table 2 Pathways of protein degradation in mammalian tissues

- Lysosomal pathway
- Calcium-dependent proteases
- ATP-dependent proteolysis

In the post-absorptive state and following prolonged fasting, intracellular protein stores represent the major source of amino acids for metabolic needs. Unlike glycogen, which represents a specific storage molecule, proteins are integral parts of the normal cellular constituents. Therefore, it is not surprising that protein breakdown is finely regulated by hormones, amino acids and other factors. Certain organs, including liver, kidney and intestine, display a rapid rate of protein turnover, whereas other tissues, primarily muscle, have a slower rate of protein turnover [29–32, 71, 72]. During the first 24–48 hours of fasting, liver protein is rapidly depleted whereas skeletal muscle protein content changes little [29, 71–74]. After 48 hours, skeletal muscle protein breakdown accelerates to generate amino acids for gluconeogenesis [75, 76]. This switch from protein anabolism to protein catabolism is primarily regulated by a decline in plasma insulin concentration [75, 76]. In addition to providing amino acids during food deprivation, increase in the rate of proteolysis in muscle is a major contributing factor in the atrophy of muscle in prolonged disease and after denervation [68]. Degradation of specific proteins also plays an important role in modulating rapid changes in the concentration of short-lived regulatory proteins and rate-limiting enzymes and mediating the rapid removal of abnormal proteins whose presence might compromise cell function [77, 78]. The cellular mechanisms that have evolved to meet the individual requirements of specific tissues to modulate proteolysis are poorly understood. However, recent evidence suggests that ATP-dependent non-lysosomal pathways play a dominant role in skeletal muscle proteolysis in both the normal turnover of proteins and the adaptive changes that occur in response to starvation and muscle disuse

[65, 67, 69], while lysosomal proteolysis is the dominant pathway regulated in liver cells in response to insulin deficiency and starvation [79].

ATP-dependent Proteolysis

In most cells, including skeletal muscle, ATP depletion leads to a marked reduction in the rate of protein degradation [80]. Depletion of ATP with dinitrophenol to inhibit oxidative phosphorylation leads to a generalized decline in proteolysis, including degradation of myofibrillar components, which decreases by 50–70% [31, 81–83]. The best characterized of these systems is the ATP-dependent ubiquitin proteolytic pathway [65, 68, 69, 82, 85–89]. In the first part of the pathway, protein to be degraded is covalently attached to multiple ubiquitin molecules. This tags the protein for subsequent hydrolysis by a large cytoplasmic enzyme complex called the 26S proteasome (the ubiquitin-conjugate-degrading enzyme) during which ubiquitin is released and re-utilized. Both the polyubiquitination and hydrolysis steps require hydrolysis of ATP. The 26S proteasome is composed of a 19S complex of proteins which contains ATPases and a binding site for ubiquitin chains [89, 90], and a 20S cylindrical structure with internal hydrolytic sites which serves as the proteolytic core [47, 91, 92]. Recent X-ray crystallographic analysis of the 20S proteasome subunit from a thermophilic organism has defined its cylindrical structure as being composed of four stacked rings, each composed of seven subunits. The dimensions of the open ends and inner chambers suggest that only unfolded protein has access to the hydrolytic chamber [47]. Given the property of the 19S subunit to bind ubiquitin-conjugated proteins, it is reasoned that protein access to the interior of the proteolytic 20S subunit is regulated by the 19S complex. It has been suggested, based on the selective inhibition of lysosomal and calcium-activated proteolysis, that the ATP-dependent ubiquitin proteolytic pathway is responsible for the majority of protein turnover in eukaryotic cells [31, 84]. This conclusion is supported by the finding that the degradation rates of both long-lived and short-lived proteins in lymphoblasts are inhibited by over 80% by inhibitors shown to be selective for proteasomal proteolytic activity [67]. Significantly, the ATP-requiring non-lysosomal degradative system is activated in muscle following starvation and denervation atrophy [68, 93]. Under these same conditions the levels of polyubiquitin, polyubiquitin mRNA and mRNA for several proteasome subunits are elevated substantially [68]. The recent characterization of a selective inhibitor (lactacystin) of 20S proteasome proteolytic activity in intact cells [94] should prove to be a valuable tool in the continuing assessment of the importance of this pathway in protein degradation under the influence of a variety of physiological variables.

Lysosomal Pathway

The lysosome represents the most extensively investigated protein degradative pathway in mammalian cells [29–32, 66]. These organelles contain a variety of acid proteases and other acid hydrolases which rapidly degrade proteins. The lysosome is a major site of breakdown of glycoproteins, membrane proteins and peptide hormones, including the insulin receptor and insulin [95]. In addition, the lysosome is capable of degrading many soluble proteins under poor nutritional conditions, especially hypoinsulinemia and amino acid deficiency [29–32]. This system has been best characterized in liver [29, 32, 66, 79, 96–102] but has also been shown to be present in other cells including muscle [103–105] and cultured fibroblasts [106–108]. Omission of amino acids or insulin from the liver perfusate leads to the formation of early autophagic vacuoles which subsequently fuse with type R secondary lysosomes, thereby acquiring the full complement of acid hydrolases needed for the complete digestion of sequestered cytoplasm [29, 109–111]. The sequestration of cytosolic proteins by the lysosome has been explained by several mechanisms including transmembrane flow of protein molecules, invagination of lysosomal membrane, and formation of single-walled vesicles followed by lysosomal fusion [29]. In the perfused liver preparation the volume of hepatocyte cytoplasm sequestered by these autophagocytic lysosomes correlates closely with the rate of protein degradation [29, 98, 112] (Figure 6). Deficiency of insulin and amino acids are the most powerful initiators of this autophagic protein degradation response in liver and the addition of insulin and amino acids to the perfusion medium promptly suppresses the accelerated rate of proteolysis [29, 32, 96, 97, 99, 111]. Accelerated protein degradation via macroautophagic lysosomes has also been demonstrated in skeletal muscle [103, 104, 113, 114], heart [96, 103, 115] and cultured cells [106, 108, 116] following deprivation of insulin and amino acids.

It has been suggested that the lysosome has a role in the accelerated proteolysis associated with insulin and amino acid deficiency in muscle and liver, based on studies employing inhibitors of lysosomal function [96, 104, 105, 107, 108, 117, 118, 119]. Agents which raise intralysosomal pH (i.e. weak bases such as methylamine and chloroquine) or inhibit lysosomal proteases (i.e. leupeptin or E64 which inhibit cathepins) suppress overall cellular proteolysis in liver. Similarly, when muscles are maintained under optimal conditions with proper tension and presence of insulin and amino acids,

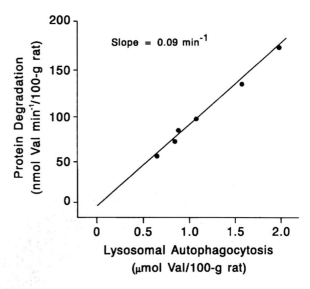

Figure 6   Direct relationship between the rate of lysosomal autophagocytosis of protein and rate of protein degradation in livers of fed, 24 hour starved and 48 hour starved rats. From reference 32, with permission

proteolysis is not enhanced and inhibitors of lysosomal function have little effect [31, 104, 105, 120]. Conversely, if muscles are incubated in the absence of insulin and amino acids or if appropriate tension is not maintained, proteolysis is markedly enhanced and this accelerated rate of protein breakdown can be returned to baseline values by inhibiting lysosomal activity. Until recently, it was believed that the lysosomal pathway represented a non-specific mechanism that was activated under non-physiological conditions, i.e. starvation, insulin deficiency or stress. However, recent studies by Dice et al have indicated that certain cytosolic proteins, when microinjected into cultured cells, are specifically targeted for autophagy by lysosomes by the presence of designated amino acid sequences [66, 106, 121, 122]. This indicates the existence of a specific intracellular recognition process.

Despite the impressive body of data reviewed above, the lysosome has not received universal acceptance as the primary regulatory mechanism for proteolysis under all conditions. In liver, in response to insulin deficiency and nutrient deprivation, there is agreement that autophagic lysosomal degradation represents the predominant pathway for protein catabolism. However, under basal conditions and especially in muscle, pathways other than the lysosome appear to be involved in protein degradation. First, morphological studies have failed to demonstrate active lysosomal sequestration [29, 31, 32] and, second, inhibition of lysosomal proteolysis with weak bases and protease inhibitors does not uniformly suppress basal protein turnover [31, 104, 105, 108, 120, 123, 124].

Calcium-dependent Proteases

Muscle tissue contains significant amounts of calcium-dependent proteases, calpins I and II, which are active at neutral pH [30, 31, 125, 126]. These proteases can be activated by maneuvers that increase intracellular calcium, including calcium ionophores, depolarization and muscle contraction [127, 128]. Although it is clear that this calcium-dependent protease system does not participate in the normal turnover of myofibrillar proteins, i.e. actin and myosin, it appears to play an important role following muscle injury [104, 105, 124, 129]. A commonly proposed function of these calcium-dependent neutral peptidases is the disassembly of myofibrils, starting with the removal of Z-discs and the subsequent release of actin and myosin, which are then degraded by other proteolytic systems [30].

PROTEIN TURNOVER: EFFECTS OF INSULIN AND DIABETES MELLITUS

Protein Synthesis

In diabetic animals protein synthesis is markedly impaired in skeletal muscle, heart and liver and can be restored to normal with insulin therapy [19, 21–23, 130]. In contrast, protein synthesis is enhanced in kidney and gut tissue of diabetic rats [131–133]. This apparent paradox is explained as follows. Since both the kidney and the gastrointestinal tissue are insulin insensitive, insulin deficiency does not alter their rate of protein synthesis. In insulin sensitive tissues, such as muscle and liver, insulin lack is associated with a decreased rate of protein synthesis and an accelerated rate of protein degradation and this leads to an increase in the plasma amino acid concentration. The resultant hyperaminoacidemia in turn provides a potent stimulus for protein synthesis in kidney and gut [133–139].

In skeletal muscle and heart of diabetic animals, protein synthesis has been shown to be reduced, both *in vivo* and *in vitro*. This observation has been consistently observed in all species studied, is independent of the means via which diabetes is induced, and can be demonstrated both *in vivo* and *in vitro* [21, 130, 140–153]. Moreover, insulin replacement returns protein synthetic rates to values which are similar to those observed in controls. It is important to note, however, that insulin never has been shown to increase the rates of protein synthesis to levels above those in non-diabetic control animals. Protein synthesis in livers from diabetic animals has also been shown to be reduced and is returned to normal with insulin therapy [133, 140, 154–162]. Although insulin deficiency is uniformly associated with impaired protein synthesis in skeletal muscle, heart and liver, the time-course of

development of the defect varies considerably in these three tissues, and striking differences exist amongst different muscle types [18, 22, 141, 147, 148]. Muscles are composed of three major fiber types: fast-twitch red (high glycolytic and high oxidative rates), fast-twitch white (high glycolytic and low oxidative rates), and slow-twitch red (low glycolytic and high oxidative rates). In diabetic rats (Figure 7) protein synthesis is reduced in all muscle fiber types but the most dramatic decreases (40–50%) are observed in mixed fast-twitch muscles (tibialis anterior and gastrocnemius) with the least inhibition (20%) in slow-twitch red fibers (soleus) [148]. Insulin replacement returns the diminished rates of protein synthesis to normal in mixed fast-twitch fibers (tibialis anterior and gastrocnemius) but is without effect in slow-twitch red fibers (soleus) [148] (Figure 8).

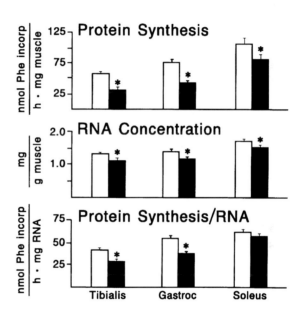

Figure 7 Rates of protein synthesis, RNA concentration and protein synthesis per RNA in skeletal muscle of control (open bars) and diabetic (solid bars) rats. Muscle samples were taken from rat hemicorpus perfused for 50 minutes. Perfusions were carried out 2 days after intravenous injection of saline (control) or 60 mg/kg of body weight alloxan (diabetic). Tibialis anterior (tibialis), whole gastrocnemius (gastroc), and soleus muscles were sampled and analyzed for the incorporation of [U-14C]phenylalanine into protein and for RNA concentration. Redrawn from reference 18, with permission

In a variety of isolated muscle preparations, as well as in the isolated perfused hemicorpus, heart and liver, insulin also has been shown to stimulate protein synthesis in normal animals [18–21, 163–172]. However, in all of these preparations the animals were fasted prior to study and/or important growth factors (i.e. serum, amino acids, insulin) were deleted from the

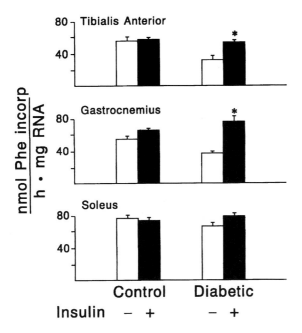

Figure 8 Acute effect of insulin on rates of protein synthesis relative to RNA concentration in perfused skeletal muscle of control (open bars) and diabetic (solid bars) rats. Protein synthesis values are expressed relative to RNA concentration for each muscle sample from experiments with (+) or without (−) addition of insulin to perfusion medium; *p < 0.01 vs. no insulin (−). Redrawn from reference 18, with permission

incubation medium or perfusate in order to put the muscle/liver into a catabolic state. Under these conditions insulin augments protein synthesis. However, the rates of protein synthesis returned to—but not above—those observed in control animals. In contrast to the diabetic and fasted state, a stimulatory effect of insulin on protein synthesis in muscle of fed, healthy animals has been difficult to demonstrate [103, 141, 172–179]. These results suggest that the major stimulatory effect of insulin on protein synthesis is seen within the range of plasma insulin concentrations from zero to basal (i.e. 0–10 µU/ml) and that increasing the plasma insulin concentration above basal levels (i.e. >10 µU/ml) has little, if any, effect in enhancing protein synthesis. By contrast, a decrease in the plasma insulin concentration below baseline leads to a dramatic decline in the rate of protein synthesis (see subsequent discussion on the effects of insulin *in vivo* in man).

Protein Degradation

As discussed in the preceding section, the stimulatory effects of insulin on protein synthesis are difficult to demonstrate in normal animals which have not been fasted prior to study. Nonetheless, the ability of insulin to promote positive nitrogen balance and to augment growth is well established. This implicates an anabolic effect of insulin mediated by an inhibition of protein

degradation. Experimentally induced diabetes is associated with a marked acceleration of proteolysis and this can be inhibited by insulin replacement [29–32, 103, 146, 147, 169, 180, 181]. Similarly, hypoinsulinemia induced by fasting causes an accelerated rate of protein breakdown which can be reversed by feeding [29–32, 75, 76, 115, 120, 136, 137, 164, 182–185]. The enhanced rate of protein degradation observed with insulin deficiency has been observed both *in vivo* and *in vitro* and in essentially all tissue preparations that have been studied, including skeletal [31, 103, 136, 147, 148, 169, 181] and cardiac [21, 103, 147, 149, 186, 187] muscle, liver [29, 32, 101, 112, 113], kidney [188], and adipose tissue [189]. Omission of insulin from the perfusion or incubation medium also leads to an accelerated rate of protein degradation in liver, skeletal muscle and heart [21, 29, 31, 96, 104, 107, 136, 169]. An important difference between the anabolic effects of insulin on protein degradation and protein synthesis relates to the ability of physiological increments in the hormone to suppress proteolysis to rates below those that are observed in the basal state. This is in contrast to the inability of insulin to enhance protein synthesis to values greater than observed in the postabsorptive state in animal models [103, 141, 173–180].

EFFECT OF AMINO ACIDS ON PROTEIN METABOLISM

Amino acids play an important role in the regulation of both protein synthesis and protein degradation, and recent studies suggest that the plasma amino acid concentration is an important regulator of protein synthesis *in vivo* [15, 190]. In fact, as reviewed in the preceding section, it has been difficult to demonstrate a stimulatory effect of insulin on protein synthesis [15].

The importance of amino acids *per se* in regulating protein metabolism was originally appreciated from studies conducted with isolated muscle preparations. These preparations are highly catabolic, with rates of protein degradation exceeding rates of protein synthesis [31, 136, 191, 192]. When isolated muscles are incubated in the presence of all 20 amino acids, protein synthesis is enhanced, proteolysis is markedly inhibited, and positive protein balance is achieved. Starvation is a potent stimulus which activates the protein degradative system, and when skeletal muscle and heart from fasted animals are perfused *in vitro,* accelerated rates of proteolysis are evident [31, 120, 152, 172, 182]. Addition of insulin to the perfusion medium inhibits the breakdown of many cytosolic proteins, but has little measurable effect on myofibrillar proteins, as estimated from the release of 3-methyl histidine [31, 105]. Refeeding with carbohydrate, which stimulates insulin secretion, does not suppress the elevated rate of myofibrillar protein breakdown [193], whereas refeeding with a balanced diet containing both protein and carbohydrate decreases myofibrillar proteolysis [152, 182, 193].

In addition to their inhibitory action on protein breakdown, amino acids have been demonstrated to augment protein synthesis in both incubated and perfused muscles [136–138, 192, 194]. Infusion of amino acids has been suggested to enhance the sensitivity of muscle protein synthesis to insulin *in vivo* in rats [135, 195], but this issue is somewhat controversial since infusing amino acids, while maintaining basal insulinemia, has been shown to be as effective as combined hyperinsulinemia plus hyperaminoacidemia in stimulating protein synthesis in man [15]. In skeletal muscle the non-essential amino acids appear to have little, if any, effect on protein synthesis [31, 135]. Methionine, which occupies a unique position as the initiator of protein synthesis, also has no effect on protein synthesis [13]. Of the essential amino acids, the branched chain amino acids appear to play the predominant role [18, 31, 135–139] and a specific role for leucine has been proposed [135, 138, 196]. Amino acids exert their anabolic effect by stimulating peptide chain initiation [18, 196]. The mechanism by which the amino acids do so is unknown.

Amino acids also have been shown to exert protein anabolic effects on the liver [29, 32]. Omission of amino acids from the perfused rat liver markedly accelerates protein degradation and leads to the formation of autophagic vacuoles [97, 111]. Although the number of amino acids which directly inhibit hepatic proteolysis is small [185, 197–199], it is considerably greater than in muscle where the branched chain amino acids predominate [135–139, 196]. In the perfused rat liver, leucine, tyrosine, phenylalanine, glutamine, proline, histidine, tryptophan and methionine are effective and collectively can mimic the inhibition observed with all 20 plasma amino acids [185]. It is of interest, however, that leucine is the most effective inhibitor in the perfused liver, while valine and isoleucine are without effect [185].

DIABETES MELLITUS, INSULIN, AND PROTEIN METABOLISM IN MAN

Methodological Considerations

Until recently the gold standard for measuring whole body protein metabolism in man has been the nitrogen balance technique [200, 201]. Although this approach has provided much knowledge about the regulation of protein metabolism in health and disease, it is now recognized to have serious shortcomings [200–202] (Table 3). First, it is tedious and time-consuming, and provides only a static measure of protein turnover. Moreover, it cannot provide any information about acute changes in protein turnover, as would occur following the ingestion/infusion of amino acids and/or insulin. Second, it cannot provide any insight into the basic biochemical mechanisms, i.e. alterations in protein synthesis vs. protein degradation, via which 'balance' is achieved. Neither can it provide any information about the specific contribution of individual organs, e.g. muscle vs. liver, to the maintenance of (or changes in) nitrogen balance. Third, the nitrogen balance technique uniformly yields positive numbers for nitrogen balance in adults in whom no net growth is occurring. The explanation of this physiological impossibility remains uncertain but at least two sources of error have been identified: nitrogen losses may be underestimated (incomplete urine/stool collections; unmeasured losses from sweat, skin, and blood; gaseous nitrogen loss), while nitrogen intake may be overestimated (food sticking to plates, pots, etc.). Since the net balance represents the very small difference between two very large values, i.e. nitrogen intake vs. nitrogen loss, even small errors can produce large errors in the overall balance. Moreover, these errors are not

Table 3 Interpretative problems and errors associated with the nitrogen balance technique

Tedious and time-consuming
Provides only a static measure of protein turnover
Provides no information about biochemical mechanisms, i.e. protein synthesis vs. protein degradation,
    responsible for changes in nitrogen balance
Provides no information about protein metabolism by specific organs
Non-growing adults, who by definition must be in neutral protein balance, display positive nitrogen balance, perhaps because:
    Nitrogen losses are underestimated
    Nitrogen intake is overestimated
    Errors in cumulative balance resulting from nitrogen losses and intake are propagated
    Other unrecognized error
Choice of the 'balance' point affects amino acid requirements
Non-steady state conditions induce major errors:
    Delay time for system to react and re-establish nitrogen balance
    Ability to achieve nitrogen equilibrium is dependent upon the distance from the 'balance' point
Energy intake has an independent effect on nitrogen balance
Nitrogen balance does not reflect overall nutritional status or adequacy of organ protein metabolism

random and summate with time when calculating the cumulative balance. Fourth, one also must be careful in choosing the so-called 'balance' point [203], since significant differences in amino acid requirements exist and are dependent upon the value chosen for daily unmeasured nitrogen loss. Fifth, the nitrogen balance technique cannot take into account either the delay or non-linearity of body protein dynamics following a change in nitrogen balance. When protein intake is altered, there is a considerable delay in the time required for the re-establishment of nitrogen balance. Moreover, the efficiency of nitrogen retention/loss is very much influenced by the individual's distance from his balance point and whether the change represents an increase or decrease in daily protein intake [204, 205]. Sixth, an alteration in dietary energy intake exerts a major influence on nitrogen balance in subjects ingesting similar dietary protein intakes [206]. Lastly, total body nitrogen equilibrium cannot be equated with nutritional status or adequacy of organ protein metabolism because it does not reflect changes in the quality, magnitude or distribution of tissue protein metabolism [207, 208]. This is best appreciated by the following example. Two groups of subjects are placed on a low protein diet and both come into nitrogen balance after 4 weeks. However, in the first group the achievement of nitrogen balance is accomplished primarily by a reduction in amino acid oxidation, with little change in protein synthesis; this obviously is a very adaptive change. In the second group nitrogen balance is accomplished primarily via a reduction in protein synthesis, with little reduction in amino acid oxidation; this represents a maladaptive response and the net flux of amino acids into protein is clearly reduced compared to the first group. Nonetheless, the nitrogen balance technique depicts both groups as being 'in balance'.

Because of the many problems associated with the nitrogen balance technique, tracers have been widely employed to investigate protein turnover in man. This approach has its own interpretative problems and assumptions (for a more in-depth discussion of these considerations, see references [202, 209]). A number of amino acids have been utilized to provide an index of the rates of protein degradation and protein synthesis. If an essential amino acid is chosen and the study is carried out in the postabsorptive state, the only source of the amino acid is from body protein stores. Consequently, the rate of amino acid appearance provides a measure of proteolysis. Moreover, if one chooses an essential amino acid, e.g. phenylalanine, whose only metabolic fate is incorporation into protein, its rate of disappearance from plasma provides a measure of protein synthesis, while its rate of appearance provides a measure of proteolysis [210, 211]. Moreover, by catheterizing a deep vein draining

the forearm/leg or the hepatic vein, one can derive a measure of muscle or liver protein metabolism, respectively [212–214]. Leucine, another amino acid which has been widely employed to study protein metabolism, has two metabolic fates: incorporation into protein and oxidation to carbon dioxide. Since the latter can be easily quantitated by indirect calorimetry [15], the rate of non-oxidative leucine disposal (i.e. total body leucine disappearance minus leucine oxidation) provides an index of protein synthesis [15, 215, 216]. As can be seen in Figure 9, all the essential amino acids yield rates of appearance which are directly proportional to their concentration in muscle. This observation supports the hypothesis that the plasma amino acid appearance rate in the postabsorptive state provides an accurate index of the rate of whole body proteolysis, since protein stores represent the only source of essential amino acids. The three amino acids (glutamine, alanine, glycine) that are responsible for the majority of interorgan nitrogen exchange yield plasma appearance rates which are much higher than those obtained with the essential amino acids. This indicates that much of their appearance in plasma is derived from *de novo* synthesis. Consequently, these amino acids cannot be used to provide quantitative estimates of protein synthesis *in vivo*.

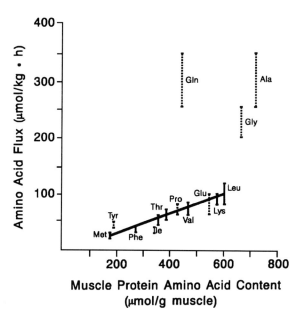

Figure 9 Relationship between the rate of protein synthesis measured with specific amino acids and their concentration in muscle. All of the essential amino acids (solid lines) yield rates which are proportional to their concentrations in muscle. The brackets represent the range. From reference 202, with permission

The use of tracers to evaluate rates of protein synthesis and proteolysis is associated with two major problems. First, the measured values represent rates of whole body protein turnover and thus reflect the composite of multiple tissues. This problem can be circumvented by combining the tracer technique with regional catheterization of the artery and vein draining the particular organ to be studied. As discussed previously, this technique, reviewed by Barrett and Gelfand [214], provides a powerful tool for the evaluation of protein metabolism *in vivo* and, when combined with measurement of whole body protein turnover, yields an integrated picture of protein metabolism in man. A second and more difficult problem with tracer kinetic studies centers on measurement of the specific activity of the precursor for protein synthesis. This concern applies to all amino acids, since the tracer is infused into the plasma compartment which also represents the sampled compartment for the determination of amino acid specific activity. However, the immediate precursor for protein synthesis is the amino acid acyl-tRNA and its measurement is both difficult and requires tissue biopsy [217]. For leucine this problem can be partly circumvented by measuring the plasma α-ketoisocaproate (KIC) specific activity in plasma [218]. KIC is generated from the transamination of leucine within the cell and it is in rapid equilibration with the extracellular compartment. Consequently, determination of the plasma KIC specific activity provides a good index of the intracellular free leucine concentration after dilution by unlabeled leucine which arises from proteolysis. *In vitro* studies have shown that the intracellular free leucine specific activity agrees well with the leucine tRNA specific activity in most tissues, including muscle [219, 220]. Other investigators have employed a radiolabeled 'flooding' technique in which a labeled amino acid, usually phenylalanine, is given with a large bolus of unlabeled amino acid to examine muscle protein metabolism [221]. The theory behind this methodology has been discussed previously [222].

Effects of Insulin and Amino Acids

The most comprehensive study of the effect of insulin and amino acids on protein metabolism in man has been provided by Castellino et al [15]. Subjects were studied on four occasions to produce all of the various combinations of changes in plasma insulin (while maintaining euglycemia) and amino acid concentrations (Table 4). ^{14}C-leucine was employed with indirect calorimetry to quantitate rates of endogenous leucine flux (proteolysis), non-oxidative leucine disposal (protein synthesis), and leucine oxidation. When insulin alone was infused (Study I), proteolysis (endogenous leucine flux) declined by almost 50% (Figure 10) and this was associated with a parallel decline in intracellular

Table 4 Summary of the plasma insulin and amino acid concentrations during studies designed to quantify rates of protein synthesis (see Figure 11) and protein degradation (see Figure 10)

	Plasma insulin	Plasma amino acid
Study I	↑	↓
Study II	↑	Basal
Study III	↑	↑
Study IV	Basal	↑

[223–225] and plasma [15] amino acid concentrations. Not surprisingly (see earlier discussion), the fall in intracellular amino acid levels was associated with a

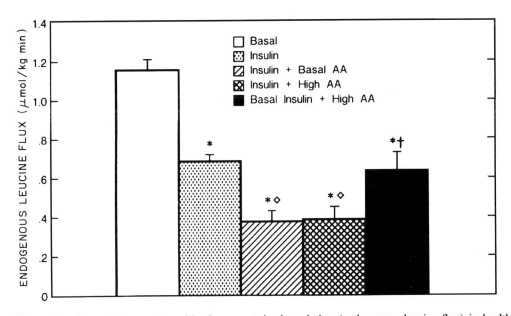

Figure 10   Effect of insulin and hyperaminoacidemia on protein degradation (endogenous leucine flux) in healthy subjects. See study design in Table 4. From reference 15, with permission

decrease in protein synthesis (non-oxidative leucine disposal) (Figure 11) despite the presence of hyperinsulinemia (about 75 µU/ml). This decrease in whole body and muscle protein synthesis following insulin infusion has been confirmed by many investigators [212, 215, 216, 226–228]. When insulin was infused with a balanced amino acid solution to clamp the plasma amino acid concentrations constant at their basal levels (Study II), a greater inhibition of proteolysis (compared to insulin alone; Study I) occurred (Figure 10), but no stimulation of protein synthesis (non-oxidative leucine disposal) was observed (Figure 11). These results are entirely consistent with *in vivo* and *in vitro* studies in animals (see earlier discussion) and indicate that an increment in plasma insulin concentration above baseline does not acutely stimulate protein synthesis. Rather, the stimulatory effect of insulin is already maximally manifest with basal levels of the hormone (10–15 µU/ml). It is important to recognize, however, that a decrease in plasma insulin concentration below basal levels is associated with a decline in protein formation in isolated tissues [18–21, 140–153, 163–171].

When insulin was infused with a balanced amino acid infusion designed to increase the plasma amino acid concentrations 1.5–2-fold above baseline (Study III), protein synthesis increased to a value that was 50% greater than in the postabsorptive state (Figure 11). It is noteworthy that when the plasma amino acid concentration was raised while the basal plasma insulin concentration was kept constant (Study IV), the stimulation of protein synthesis was as great as that observed with combined hyperinsulinemic hyperaminoacidemia (Figure 11). These results indicate that hyperaminoacidemia, not hyperinsulinemia, is the major stimulator of protein synthesis in man, a conclusion consistent with results obtained in animals [18, 21, 31, 135–138, 192–196] and in other studies in man [224, 228, 229, 230]. It also is noteworthy that hyperaminoacidemia alone (Study IV) was a powerful inhibitor of proteolysis (Figure 10), an observation again consistent with animal studies [29–32, 97, 111, 120, 136, 137, 152, 182, 191, 193]. Similar results have been reported by others [228, 229, 230–233] and these findings are summarized in Table 5. From the clinical standpoint it should be emphasized that during the ingestion of a typical mixed meal, the plasma amino concentration rises and insulin secretion is stimulated. Such conditions would favor, simultaneously, the stimulation of protein synthesis and the inhibition

Table 5 Summary of the effects of insulin and amino acids on protein synthesis (non-oxidative leucine disposal), protein degradation (endogenous leucine flux) and leucine oxidation. Based on the results presented in references 15, 223 and 232 (see experimental design in Table 4 and results presented in Figures 10 and 11). The number of arrows is commensurate with the magnitude of the effect

	Protein synthesis	Proteolysis	Leucine oxidation
Insulin	0	↓↓	↑
Amino acids	↑↑	↓↓	↑↑
Insulin + amino acids	↑↑	↓↓↓	↑↑↑

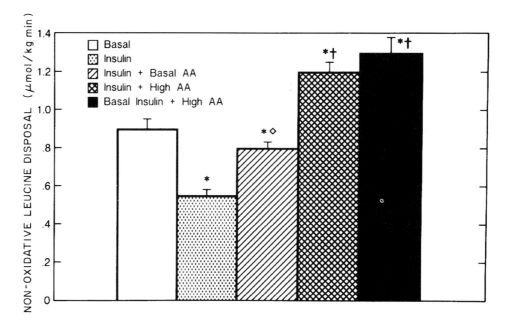

Figure 11 Effect of insulin and hyperaminoacidemia on protein synthesis (non-oxidative leucine disposal) in healthy subjects. See study design in Table 4. From reference 15, with permission

of proteolysis, thereby maximally enhancing protein anabolism. Indeed, this scenario has been documented in man by a number of investigators [190, 210, 234]. The dose–response curve relating the plasma insulin concentration to whole body [235, 236] and muscle [212] proteolysis is quite steep within the physiological range of plasma insulin levels, with maximum suppression being observed with a plasma insulin concentration of approximately 50–60 µU/ml (Figure 12).

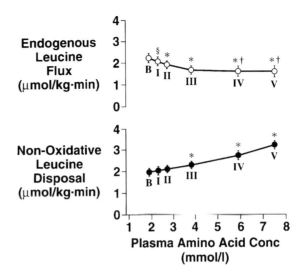

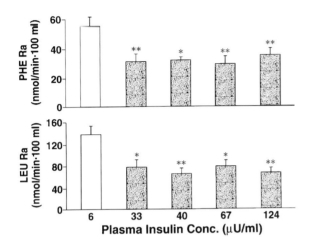

Figure 12 Effect of progressively increasing insulin infusion rates (0, 0.01, 0.02, 0.035, and 0.05 mU/kg/min) on forearm skeletal muscle proteolysis, as determined independently from the rates of appearance (Ra) of phenylalanine (PHE) (top) and leucine (LEU) (bottom). The steady-state plasma insulin concentration achieved at each insulin infusion rate is shown at the bottom of each bar. $^*p < 0.05$; $^{**}p < 0.01$. From reference 212, with permission

Figure 13 Relationship between the plasma amino concentration and proteolysis (endogenous leucine flux) and protein synthesis (non-oxidative leucine disposal) in healthy subjects. A balanced amino acid infusion was given at five different rates (I–V) to create plasma amino acid concentrations spanning the physiologic and pharmacologic range. B = basal plasma amino acid concentration. $^*p < 0.01$ vs. basal; $\dagger p = $ NS vs. study III; $\S p < 0.05$ vs. basal. From reference 237, with permission

Only one study has examined the dose–response curve relating the increment in plasma amino acid concentration to the stimulation of protein synthesis. In this study Giordano et al [237] infused a balanced amino acid solution at five different rates to increase the total plasma amino acid concentration by 21%, 42%, 103%, 211% and 296%, respectively (Figure 13). Maximal suppression of proteolysis (endogenous leucine flux) was observed with increments (21–103%) in plasma amino acid concentrations within the physiological range. Further increments (>103%) in plasma amino acid levels failed to inhibit proteolysis any further but were associated with a progressive, dose-related increase in protein synthesis (non-oxidative leucine disposal).

Barrett and colleagues [212, 214, 228, 238] as well as others [211, 213, 215, 229], have employed forearm catheterization in combination with ³H-phenylalanine/¹⁴C-leucine infusion to quantitate rates of forearm muscle and whole body protein synthesis and proteolysis. Phenylalanine is an especially good

tracer since its only metabolic fate is uptake into protein and its only source is from breakdown of body protein stores [214]. Moreover, since muscle protein turns over slowly, recycling of labeled phenylalanine is trivial [214]. In response to insulin (while maintaining euglycemia) Gelfand and Barrett demonstrated reversal of the net forearm muscle balance of phenylalanine from a net output to a net uptake (Figure 14). This was entirely due to an inhibition of proteolysis; forearm muscle protein synthesis was not stimulated by insulin (Figure 14). Identical results were observed for leucine both at the forearm (Figure 14) and whole body level [212, 213, 216, 228, 229, 239]. These findings are internally consistent and demonstrate that at the tissue level an increment in insulin above baseline does not stimulate muscle protein synthesis. The necessity of hyperaminoacidemia in order to observe a stimulation of muscle and liver protein synthesis has been documented by a number of investigators [15, 228–233, 240]. In the study by Gelfand et al [240] amino acids were infused to double the plasma amino acid concentration without significantly increasing circulating plasma insulin levels; liver and muscle amino acid kinetics were assessed by combined liver/leg catheterization and ¹⁴C-leucine. Whole body leucine disposal (an index of protein synthesis) rose significantly while leucine release (an index of proteolysis) declined (Figure 15). The increase in whole body leucine disposal following

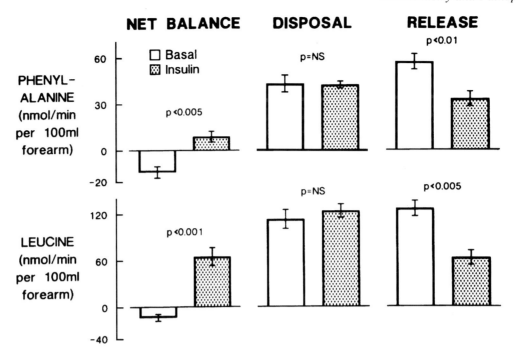

Figure 14 Effect of insulin on forearm muscle rates of phenylalanine and leucine disposal (protein synthesis) and release (proteolysis) in healthy subjects. From reference 214, with permission

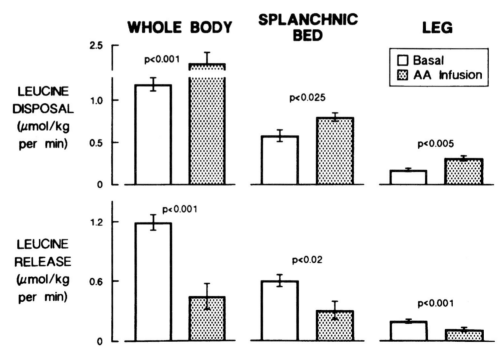

Figure 15 Effect of hyperaminoacidemia on rates of whole body, leg muscle, and splanchnic leucine disposal (an index of protein synthesis) and leucine appearance (an index of proteolysis) in normal subjects receiving a balanced infusion of amino acids. From reference 240, with permission

amino acid infusion was accounted for almost equally by increased splanchnic (liver) and leg (muscle) leucine disposal. Inhibition of proteolysis by hepatic and muscle tissues also contributed to the decline in whole body protein degradation following amino acid infusion

(Figure 15). Similar results have been reported by Bennet et al [241].

It should be emphasized that the use of radiolabeled tracers to quantitate rates of whole body, limb or liver protein synthesis and degradation reflects the composite turnover rate of a large number of proteins, each with different synthetic and degradative rates. Thus, a stimulatory effect of insulin on protein synthesis could be obscured by an inhibitory action on some proteins. This concept is supported by *in vitro* studies which demonstrate differential regulation of specific mRNAs by insulin [242–244]. Consistent with this, De Feo et al [245] have demonstrated that insulin withdrawal in IDDM patients has a differential effect on albumin and fibrinogen synthesis. In follow-up studies, these same investigators [226] showed that insulin infusion in healthy subjects had very different effects on the fractional synthetic rates of four hepatic proteins (Figure 16).

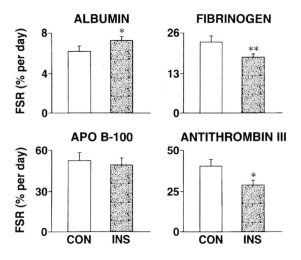

Figure 16 Fractional synthetic rate (FSR) of albumin, fibrinogen, apo B-100, and antithrombin III during saline (CONtrol study) and INSulin (0.4 mU/kg.min) infusion in healthy young subjects. *$p = 0.015$ for albumin; *$p = 0.007$ for antithrombin II; **$p = 0.05$. From reference 226, with permission

Recently, considerable attention has focused on insulin-like growth factor-I (IGF-I) because of its similarity to insulin with respect to glucose metabolism and its potential role in the treatment of diabetic patients [246] (see Chapter 20). Using radiolabeled leucine, Giordano et al [227] compared doses of insulin and IGF-I that caused similar declines in plasma concentrations of branched-chain amino acids. Qualitatively, the effects of IGF-I and insulin on protein metabolism were similar (Figure 17), but quantitatively IGF-I was 14-fold less potent than insulin. Similar findings have been reported by others [216, 247]. In these studies IGF-I inhibited proteolysis, leading to a generalized decline in most plasma amino acid concentrations. The resultant hypoaminoacidemia most likely accounted for the reduction in protein synthesis observed in these studies. To circumvent the confounding variable

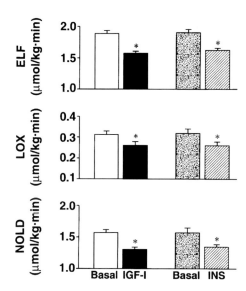

Figure 17 Endogenous leucine flux (ELF) (proteolysis), leucine oxidation (LOX), and non-oxidative leucine disposal (NOLD) (protein synthesis) in the basal state and during insulin-like growth factor-I (IGF-I) and insulin (INS) infusion. *$p < 0.01$ vs. basal. From reference 227, with permission

of hypoaminoacidemia, Fryburg [248] infused IGF-I locally into the forearm and documented a direct stimulatory effect on protein synthesis. In a follow-up study, Fryburg et al [228] demonstrated that IGF-I plus hyperaminoacidemia increased protein synthesis above that with either IGF-I alone or hyperaminoacidemia alone. In marked contrast, insulin, even in the presence of hyperaminoacidemia, was not capable of stimulating protein synthesis above that observed with hyperaminoacidemia alone (Figure 18). Russell-Jones et al [249] have also shown that IGF-I directly enhances protein synthesis under conditions of adequate substrate supply.

In summary, the results of both *in vivo* and *in vitro* studies in animals, as well as *in vivo* studies in man, are in agreement and indicate that the primary action of insulin on protein metabolism is the inhibition of proteolysis. Hyperaminoacidemia has two effects: stimulation of protein synthesis and inhibition of protein degradation.

Insulin-dependent Diabetes Mellitus (IDDM)

It is well recognized that children with poorly controlled insulin-dependent diabetes mellitus fail to grow normally [1–3] and, following the institution of tight glycemic control with insulin treatment, they demonstrate 'catch-up' growth [6, 7] (Figure 19). As originally shown by Atchley et al [1] and others [2, 3], insulin deficiency is associated with negative nitrogen balance, muscle wasting and protein catabolism.

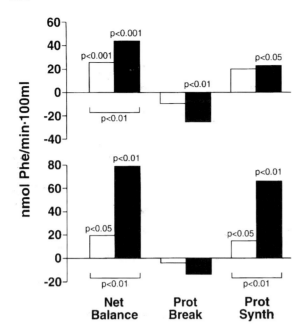

Figure 18 Comparisons of the changes in phenylalanine balance, and protein breakdown and synthesis due to amino acids alone (open bars) or insulin + amino acids (solid bars) in top panel, and amino acids alone (open bars) or insulin-like growth factor I + amino acids (solid bars) in lower panel. Significant changes from baseline for each variable are shown above each bar. Comparisons between amino acids and insulin + amino acids or IGF-I + amino acids are shown below a pair of bars. From reference 228, with permission

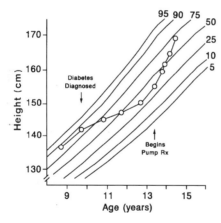

Figure 19 'Catch-up growth' in a poorly controlled IDDM patient following the institution of insulin therapy. Percentiles for growth curves of normal children are indicated. From reference 6, with permission

A number of investigators, using radioisotopic turnover techniques, have examined the effect of insulin deficiency on whole body [250–258] and regional [258–260] protein metabolism in IDDM. The results have been somewhat surprising, although amazingly consistent, and are typified by the findings of Luzi et al [250] (Figures 20 and 21). In IDDM

patients in poor control the whole body rate of protein degradation (endogenous leucine flux) in the postabsorptive state was significantly increased compared to controls and was returned to normal following 1–2 months of an intensified insulin regimen (Figure 21). These observations are consistent with a large number of *in vitro* and *in vivo* animal studies, which have shown that insulin is a powerful inhibitor of proteolysis (see above). Surprisingly, however, the rate of protein synthesis (non-oxidative leucine disposal) in the postabsorptive state was significantly increased in poorly controlled IDDM patients and returned to normal with intensified insulin treatment (Figure 20). Similar results have been reported by all other investigators [251–258]. These somewhat paradoxical observations are explained as follows (Figure 22). In the presence of insulin deficiency, proteolysis is enhanced and a brief period of negative protein balance ensues. The accelerated rate of protein degradation leads to a generalized increase in the plasma (and presumably intracellular) amino acid concentrations [261]. The resultant hyperaminoacidemia in turn stimulates protein synthesis [15, 232, 233], thereby returning the net balance of amino acids into and out of protein to values which are close to those observed in control subjects (Figure 23). This increase in protein synthesis can be viewed as a compensatory response that prevents excessive protein wasting during periods of insulin deficiency. Recently, the tissues responsible for enhanced protein synthesis in response to hyperaminoacidemia have been examined using the organ balance technique. Studies by Pacy et al [259] suggest that enhanced skeletal muscle protein synthesis accounts for only a small fraction (15–25%) of the increase in total body protein synthesis. In diabetic rats hyperaminoacidemia has been shown to be associated with an increased rate of gut protein synthesis [133], and this has been confirmed by Nair et al [213]. Using radiolabeled leucine and radiolabeled phenylalanine in combination with splanchnic and leg catheterization, they demonstrated that in insulin-withdrawn IDDM patients both the splanchnic (liver plus gut) and muscle tissues contributed to the accelerated rate of whole body proteolysis. In contrast, splanchnic tissues accounted for approximately 80–90% of the increase in whole body protein synthesis in these insulinopenic IDDM patients. Since amino acids are potent stimulators of muscle protein synthesis [228, 229], these observations imply that muscle tissue in IDDM patients must be resistant to the stimulatory effect of hyperaminoacidemia on protein synthesis. Insulin therapy corrected the disturbances in splanchnic/muscle proteolysis and splanchnic protein synthesis without any effect on muscle protein synthesis.

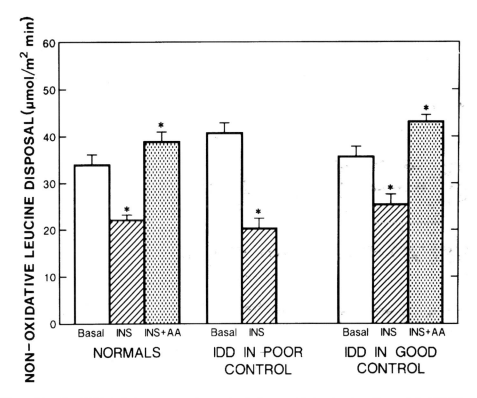

Figure 20 Effect of insulin (INS) infusion on protein synthesis (non-oxidative leucine disposal) in IDDM patients (IDD) in poor control and after 1–2 months of tightened glycemic control with insulin (good control). The effect of infusing insulin together with amino acids (INS + AA) is also shown for the good control group as compared with non-diabetic controls. $^*p < 0.01$ vs. basal. From reference 250, with permission

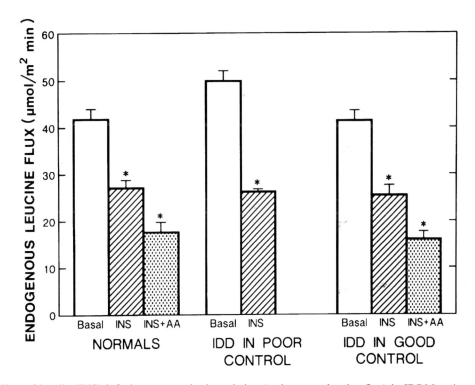

Figure 21 Effect of insulin (INS) infusion on protein degradation (endogenous leucine flux) in IDDM patients (IDD) in poor control and after 1–2 months of tightened glycemic control with insulin (good control). The effect of infusing insulin together with amino acids (INS + AA) is also shown for the good control group as compared with non-diabetic controls. $^*p < 0.01$ vs. basal. From reference 250, with permission

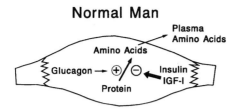

Normal Man

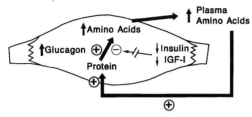

Insulin Dependent Diabetes Mellitus

Figure 22 Effect of insulin deficiency on protein metabolism in normal (upper) and IDDM (lower) subjects. Insulin deficiency leads to an accelerated rate of proteolysis and an increase in the plasma amino acid concentration. The resultant hyperaminoacidemia in turn stimulates protein synthesis and the net amino acid flux into and out of protein remains close to normal. In the presence of insulin deficiency plasma glucagon levels rise and insulin-like growth factor I (IGF-I) declines, promoting a more protein catabolic state

When insulin (insulin clamp technique) is infused acutely in poorly controlled IDDM patients [250],

proteolysis (endogenous leucine flux) is promptly inhibited to values observed in healthy subjects receiving an identical insulin infusion (Figure 21). Since the basal rate of proteolysis in IDDM individuals was significantly greater than in controls, it follows that the absolute decline in protein degradation in poorly controlled diabetic patients was actually greater than in control subjects. These results indicate that there is no resistance to the ability of insulin to inhibit proteolysis in IDDM, even though the insulin-mediated rate of glucose uptake measured simultaneously in the same subjects was reduced by more than 50% [250]. These results demonstrate a clear-cut disassociation between the effects of insulin on glucose and protein metabolism. Protein synthesis, which was elevated in poorly controlled IDDM subjects in the basal state, declined significantly in response to acute insulin infusion. This paradoxical result is explained by the reduction in elevated plasma amino acid concentration that occurs secondary to the inhibition of proteolysis by insulin. Although protein synthesis fell, the net flux of leucine into protein actually improved because the rate of proteolysis declined more than the decrease in protein formation. It is noteworthy that, similar to the situation in control subjects, insulin was not capable of promoting a *net positive* protein balance (Figure 23).

Although insulin deficiency clearly plays a major role in the elevated rates of proteolysis in poorly

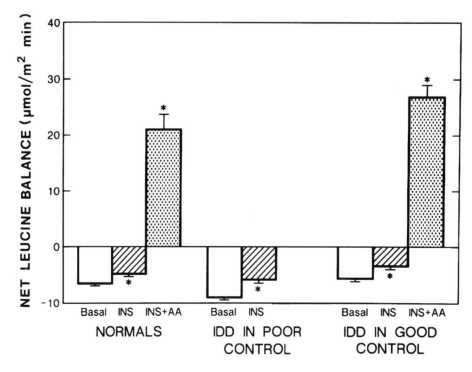

Figure 23 Effect of insulin (INS) infusion on net balance of leucine (into and out of protein) in IDDM patients (IDD) in poor control and after 1–2 months of tightened glycemic control with insulin (good control). The effect of infusing insulin together with amino acids (INS + AA) is also shown for the good control group as compared with non-diabetic controls. *$p < 0.01$ vs. basal. From reference 250, with permission

controlled IDDM patients, it is not the only factor. Insulin deficiency is associated with hyperglucagonemia and low circulating IGF-I levels. Recent studies have shown that glucagon is protein catabolic in man [262] and that IGF-I promotes protein anabolism [263]. Hyperglycemia *per se* has no effect on either proteolysis or protein synthesis [250].

In man amino acids are the primary regulator of protein synthesis [15]. Two groups have examined the effect of hyperaminoacidemia on protein synthesis in IDDM patients [250, 260]. In well controlled IDDM patients the ability of amino acids to promote whole body protein synthesis and to inhibit proteolysis was normal [250]. Somewhat different results were reported by Bennet et al [260], who found that the ability of combined amino acid/insulin infusion to augment whole body leg muscle protein synthesis was diminished in IDDM individuals. However, these later studies are difficult to compare, since the IDDM patients examined by Bennet et al [260] were in poor metabolic control, whereas those of Luzi et al [250] were well controlled. Moreover, Bennet et al [260] infused amino acids during the 3-hour 'basal' period, so a true baseline was never obtained. It is likely that this amino acid infusion altered the postabsorptive rate of protein turnover and made it appear that the IDDM subjects were resistant to combined insulin/amino acid infusion. In a recent study by Biolo et al [210], ingestion of a mixed meal (containing 18% of the calories in the form of crystalline amino acids) by insulin-deprived IDDM patients caused a marked suppression of whole body proteolysis, indicating a direct suppressive effect of hyperaminoacidemia on protein breakdown. Protein synthesis was not quantified in this study.

In summary, in well-controlled IDDM subjects basal protein turnover is normal, the ability of insulin to inhibit proteolysis is not impaired, and the stimulatory effect of amino acids on protein synthesis is intact. In poorly controlled IDDM individuals basal rates of proteolysis and protein synthesis are both augmented and the net flux of amino acids into protein is maintained close to normal. The ability of insulin to inhibit proteolysis is normal or even increased in poorly controlled IDDM subjects; the ability of amino acids to augment protein synthesis most likely is normal, although this area is deserving of further investigation. It should be noted, however, that this is a difficult issue to address since plasma amino acid levels are already markedly increased in the postabsorptive state in the presence of insulin deficiency, and this hyperaminoacidemia is associated with an enhanced rate of basal protein synthesis. At present the dose–response relationship between the plasma amino acid concentration and protein synthetic rate has not been defined. If the generalized increase in basal plasma amino acid

concentration has maximally or near maximally stimulated protein synthesis in IDDM, any further hyperaminoacidemia obviously would be expected to have a blunted effect.

Non-insulin Dependent Diabetes Mellitus

Protein metabolism in non-insulin dependent diabetes mellitus (NIDDM) has received much less attention compared to insulin dependent diabetes mellitus. This is somewhat surprising since insulin resistance, at the level of both muscle and liver, is well established as the hallmark of NIDDM [264] (see Chapter 31). Five groups have examined whole body protein turnover in poorly controlled NIDDM individuals [211, 265–268]. In the postabsorptive state the plasma amino acid concentrations have uniformly been reported to be normal. In three of the five published studies the rates of whole body protein synthesis and degradation in the postabsorptive state were identical to those of healthy control subjects [265–267], while in two studies they were slightly elevated [211, 268]. This is in contrast to poorly-controlled IDDM subjects [250–260], who have markedly accelerated rates of both protein synthesis and proteolysis and elevated plasma amino acid levels. These seemingly discrepant findings are explained by the different fasting plasma insulin levels in the two poorly-controlled groups: decreased in IDDM and elevated in NIDDM (Table 6). Since even small increments in plasma insulin concentration above baseline are capable of inhibiting proteolysis in normal individuals [212, 235, 236], the presence of a normal basal rate of protein degradation in the face of fasting hyperinsulinemia suggests that proteolysis is resistant to the action of insulin in NIDDM. However, when the plasma insulin concentration is raised above baseline in NIDDM patients, a normal suppression of whole body proteolysis is observed [211, 265] (Figure 24). Similarly, the ability of amino acids to augment protein synthesis and inhibit proteolysis is perfectly normal in NIDDM [265] (Figures 24 and 25).

Obesity

Obese subjects are characterized by severe insulin resistance with regard to glucose and lipid metabolism. Surprisingly, few studies have examined the effect of insulin on protein metabolism in non-diabetic obese subjects. Some [269–271] but not all [272, 273] studies have demonstrated that the decline in plasma amino acid concentration in response to carbohydrate ingestion or insulin infusion is blunted in obese subjects. In the postabsorptive state, the rate of protein breakdown has been shown to be either normal [274, 275] or increased [272, 276]. However, in the presence

Table 6 Protein synthesis and proteolysis in IDDM and NIDDM subjects during the basal state and in response to amino acid and insulin infusion

	Basal				Response to insulin infusion		Response to amino acid infusion	
	Plasma insulin conc.	Plasma amino acid conc.	Protein synthesis	Proteolysis	Protein synthesis	Proteolysis	Protein synthesis	Proteolysis
IDDM—poor control	↓	↑	↑	↑	↓*	↓	?	↓
IDDM—good control	N-↑	N	N	N	↓*	↓	↑	↓
NIDDM—poor control	↑	N	N	N	↓*	↓	↑	↓

* Protein synthesis declines secondary to the inhibition of proteolysis and the decrease in plasma/intracellular amino acid concentrations.
? Indicates inadequate data available.

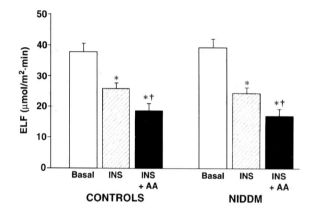

Figure 24 Endogenous leucine flux (ELF) (proteolysis) in the basal state (open bars), during insulin infusion (INS) (cross-hatched bars) and during insulin plus amino acid (AA) infusion (solid bars) in control subjects (left) and non-insulin dependent diabetic patients (NIDDM) (right). *$p < 0.01$ vs. basal; †$p < 0.01$ vs. insulin alone. From reference 265, with permission

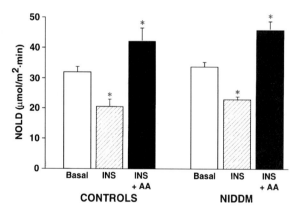

Figure 25 Non-oxidative leucine disposal (NOLD) (protein synthesis) in the basal state (open bars), during insulin infusion (INS) (cross-hatched bars), and during insulin plus amino acid (AA) infusion (solid bars) in control subjects (left) and non-insulin dependent diabetic patients (NIDDM) (right). *$p < 0.01$ vs. basal. From reference 265, with permission

of fasting hyperinsulinemia (which should suppress proteolysis) even a normal rate of protein breakdown

is abnormal. Thus, all four of these studies indicate the presence of insulin resistance with regard to the hormone's suppressive effect on protein breakdown. Two studies have shown that the ability of insulin to inhibit protein degradation in obese individuals is normal [272, 277], while two studies have shown it to be impaired [274, 275]. These apparently conflicting results are most likely explained by the different steady-state plasma insulin concentrations used by different investigators. Luzi et al [275] examined the effects of a low physiological (10 mU/m² min) and high physiological (40 mU/m² min) insulin infusion rate on rates of proteolysis and protein synthesis. In response to low physiological levels of hyperinsulinemia, suppression of proteolysis was impaired in obese subjects; however, the insulin resistance could be overcome at high physiological insulin levels. No abnormality in protein synthesis in response to insulin was observed at either the low or higher insulin levels in this study [275]. The ability of hyperaminoacidemia to stimulate protein synthesis and impair proteolysis was normal in obese subjects.

CELLULAR REGULATION OF PROTEIN METABOLISM BY INSULIN AND DIABETES MELLITUS

Insulin Receptor—Signal Transduction

In order for insulin to exert its many and varied biological effects, it must first bind to specific receptors which are present on the cell surface of all insulin target tissues [8] (Figure 26). Any maneuver which decreases the number of insulin receptors or alters their structure/function will result in a defect in insulin action and impair the hormone's ability to exert its anabolic effects on protein metabolism [8, 10, 11, 278, 279]. The insulin receptor itself is a tetrameric glycoprotein which is comprised of two α-subunits and two β-subunits, linked by sulfhydryl bonds. The α-subunit faces the outside of the cell and is anchored into the cell membrane, while the β-subunit contains a tyrosine kinase domain. When insulin is bound to its receptor, the tyrosine kinase is activated by a process involving receptor autophosphorylation of tyrosine residues at positions 1146, 1150 and 1151 of the β-subunit [280–282]. The activation of the receptor tyrosine kinase is mandatory for insulin to exert most, if not all, of its many biological effects [8, 11, 278–284]. Mutations or deletions of 1, 2 or 3 tyrosine residues in this regulatory region of the receptor progressively reduce tyrosine kinase activity, with a parallel loss of the biological effectiveness of insulin [11, 285]. The insulin receptor is also phosphorylated on serine and threonine sites, and the alteration of the state of phosphorylation of these sites by other intracellular regulators may modify insulin-stimulated receptor tyrosine kinase activity [11, 284].

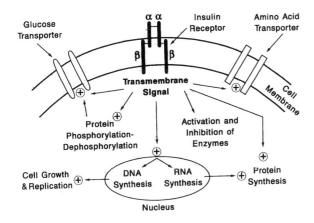

Figure 26 Schematic representation of insulin action on membrane, cytoplasmic and nuclear events involved in cell growth and metabolism. See text for a more detailed discussion

Once activated, insulin receptor tyrosine kinase initiates a chain of events mediated by intercommunicating proteins which sequentially pass signaling information to various downstream targets. While the precise molecular events linking the activated insulin receptor kinase to all of the hormone's target responses remain elusive, rapid advances in the past several years have contributed substantially to our understanding of several key features of the signal transduction pathway mediating the anabolic effects of the hormone. Among the advances has been the identification of specific intracellular protein substrates for the ligand-activated receptor tyrosine kinase. The first of these to be described was a large phosphotyrosine-containing protein (Mr170K) called insulin receptor substrate-1 (IRS-1) [286]. To propagate the signal, IRS-1 binds several different cytoplasmic signaling proteins containing Src homology 2 domains (SH2 proteins) to sites defined by the amino acid sequence motif around the phosphotyrosine residues [287, 288]. Included among

the several identified SH2 proteins is phosphatidylinositol (PI) 3'-kinase, which is activated upon binding to IRS-1 and is probably involved in the translocation of glucose receptors [289–291]. Another important SH2 protein bound to tyrosine phosphorylated IRS-1 is growth factor receptor bound protein 2 (Grb2) [292, 293] which has been linked to activation of p21 ras and the mitogen-activated protein (MAP) kinase cascade [11, 294]. Accordingly, IRS-1 appears to function as a docking protein by binding to several SH2 proteins which function as early components in different insulin signaling pathways [295]. However, the central importance of IRS 1 may not be unique, as evidenced by the recognition of the involvement of other insulin receptor tyrosine kinase substrates which also contain SH2 binding domains, including Shc [296–299] and IRS-2 [300]. Despite current uncertainty as to the relative importance of IRS-1, Shc and IRS-2 in mediating the activation of PI 3-kinase, Grb2 and other SH2 proteins, the basic nature of the linkage between the insulin receptor and early downstream events appears established.

The membrane-associated protein, p21 ras, is a key molecule in the mitogenic signaling pathway initiated by insulin [301, 302]. p21 ras is activated when it is converted from a GDP- to GTP-bound form by its association with the guanine nucleotide releasing factor (mSos). mSos is bound to Grb2 and is activated by the binding of Grb2 to a SH2 domain of IRS-1 (and/or Shc, IRS-2 as discussed above) following the binding of insulin to its receptor. The formation of p21 ras-GTP results in the activation of raf-1, a MAP kinase kinase kinase (MAPKKK). From here the signal is transmitted to the next kinase in the cascade, MEK (MAPKK) [303]. Activated MEK has a high degree of specificity for its downstream substrate, MAP kinase (MAPK or ERK), which is activated by phosphorylation of Tyr and Thr residues [294, 304]. One of the substrates for MAPK is PHAS-1, an eIF-4E binding protein which plays a critical role in the control of protein synthesis, as discussed below. In addition, MAPK phosphorylates a number of regulatory proteins, including factors in the nucleus which participate in the regulation of gene transcription [305].

The recent discovery of a linkage between the p21 ras/MAP kinase pathway activated by insulin and the regulation of the availability of the initiation factor, eIF-4E has contributed substantially to our understanding of the signal transduction pathway by which insulin effects the stimulation of protein synthesis [57, 58]. Under basal conditions, a portion of eIF-4E has been shown to be bound to non-phosphorylated PHAS-1 (phosphorylated heat- and acid-stable protein) and unavailable to participate in the initiation step. Upon phosphorylation of a serine residue (ser64) by MAP kinase, PHAS-1 dissociates from eIF-4E permitting it to function in protein chain initiation. While many details of this pathway need to be examined [306] including the modulation of PHAS-1 by other signal pathways [307], the definition of the elements of a complete pathway from receptor activation to a specific downstream effect has been a major advance in the field of growth factor research.

Insulin-induced phosphorylation of multiple serine residues of the ribosomal S6 protein is believed to play an important role in the stimulation of protein synthesis [308]. It should be noted, however, that phosphorylation of the S6 protein does not always correlate with the rate of protein synthesis [309–312]. Without a clear understanding of the functional consequences of the reversible phosphorylation of this protein, the importance of this insulin effect remains obscure.

Amino Acid Transport

All cells require amino acids for protein synthesis and this requirement is met by a combination of *de novo* synthesis of some amino acids and amino acid transport into the cell for others. For the neutral amino acids there are three main transport systems, called systems A, ASC and L. These systems differ in their Na$^+$ dependency, pH sensitivity, *trans*-inhibition/stimulation and amino acid specificity [12, 13] (Table 7).

System A recognizes a broad spectrum of amino acids, including those with short, polar and linear side-chains. This system is sodium dependent, displays reduced activity in response to low pH, and is inhibited by an increase in intracellular amino acid concentration, a kinetic phenomenon referred to as *trans*-inhibition. Methylaminoisobutyric acid is the model non-metabolizable amino acid that has been employed to trace the activity of this system. System A is subject to regulation by amino acid availability and hormones, especially insulin. The transport characteristics of systems ASC and L are shown in Table 7.

System ASC transports alanine, serine, cysteine, threonine and homologous amino acids up to five carbons. Aminoisobutyric acid is transported in shared fashion by systems ASC and L. System L transports the branched chain amino acids and phenylalanine, and its model non-metabolizable amino acid is aminobicyclo-heptane dicarboxylic acid. Cycloleucine, a non-metabolizable amino acid, is transported by both systems L and A. It is important to note that many amino acids are transported by more than one system.

Insulin has long been known to exert a powerful effect on amino acid transport in a variety of tissues including skeletal [313–315] and cardiac [316, 317] muscle, adipocytes [318], and liver [319, 320]. Insulin regulates predominantly or entirely those amino acids which are transported by system A [320–323]. The hormone acts by impairing the inactivation of the amino acid transport proteins and by increasing the rate of synthesis of these proteins at a post-transcriptional site [322, 324]. The stimulatory effect of insulin on amino acid transport requires binding of the hormone to its cell surface receptor [320] and is reduced in proportion to the decrease in insulin receptor number [325–327].

Since insulin has been shown to enhance amino acid transport, this step represents a potential regulatory role for the hormone on protein synthesis. If this were the rate-limiting step for protein synthesis, one would expect an increase in the intracellular free amino acid concentration in response to insulin. On the contrary, hyperinsulinemia has uniformly been associated with a generalized decline in intracellular amino acid levels [103, 169, 223, 328]. This observation indicates that steps distal to amino acid transport are rate-limiting for protein synthesis and that the decrease in cell amino acid concentration results from a primary stimulation of protein synthesis.

Regulation of Gene Transcription

The ability of insulin to augment the synthesis of specific mRNAs and proteins is well established and

Table 7 Summary of the characteristics of the three neutral amino acid transport systems

	System		
	A	ASC	L
Preferred substrate	Ala, Pro, Ser, Gly, Met	Ala, Ser, Cys, Thr	Leu, Ile, Val, Met, Phe
Model non-metabolizable amino acid probe	Methylaminoisobutyric acid	Unknown	Amino-bicyclo-heptane dicarboxylic acid
Na$^+$ dependent	Yes	Yes	No
pH sensitive	Yes (low pH inhibits)	Yes (low pH stimulates)	Yes
Substrate regulation	Trans-inhibition	Trans-stimulation	Trans-stimulation
Insulin sensitive	Yes	No	No

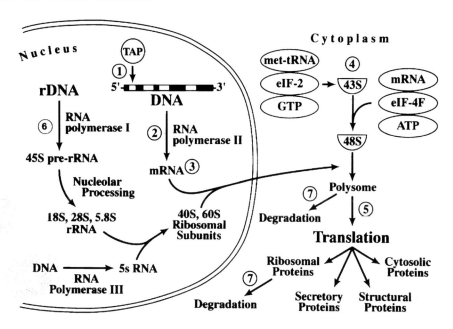

Figure 27 Schematic representation of cellular mechanisms involved in the stimulation of protein synthesis. The circled numbers represent steps where insulin has been shown to work. See text for a more detailed discussion

the list is rapidly growing [23–26, 329–331]. As described in the beginning of this chapter, synthesis of mRNAs is under the control of RNA polymerase II (Figure 27). The transcription process is initiated by the interaction of a *trans*-acting protein with the *cis*-acting DNA element, also referred to as the hormone response element (HRE). The hormone response element(s) for a number of hormones have been identified, including steroid hormones, cyclic AMP, thyroid hormones, and others [24, 25, 33, 34, 332, 333]. Although insulin has been shown to gain access to the nucleus [334–337], at present there is no evidence that insulin *per se* binds directly to any specific DNA sequence. Most [333], but not all authorities [338] believe that the transcriptional effects of insulin are regulated by the induction of other nuclear proteins which interact with a specific *cis*-acting DNA sequence, i.e. the hormone response element (Figure 27, step 1). The insulin responsive promoter DNA regions have been identified for several insulin-regulated genes: phosphoenolpyruvate carboxykinase [25]; glucokinase [26]; glyceraldehyde-3-phosphate dehydrogenase [339]; amylase [340]; the proto-oncogenes c-fos [341] and egr-1 [342]. An important goal of future investigation will be to isolate the insulin-response nuclear proteins that directly mediate the transcriptional effects of insulin. Two approaches have been employed to identify such regulatory proteins: biochemical isolation of nuclear proteins based upon their high affinity for specific DNA sequences [343] and screening of expression libraries with oligonucleotide probes containing the particular binding sequence in question [344]. Insulin could alter

transcription by: increasing (or decreasing) the amount of nuclear binding protein available for interacting with the hormone response element; covalently modifying the nuclear binding protein, thereby altering its interaction with the hormone response element; or producing a nuclear binding protein which interacts with the *trans*-acting protein, leading to an alteration in its configuration [333]. The transduction pathways by which insulin effects transcriptional regulation have not been defined. The regulation of PEPCK gene expression by insulin appears to require the participation of PI-3-kinase [345]. However, it is unlikely that there is a single pathway mediating the effects of insulin on transcription, since it has been demonstrated that the insulin stimulation of c-fos and egr-1 mRNA expression probably involves different transduction pathways [331].

Insulin also can alter gene transcription via mechanisms that do not involve the synthesis of *trans*-acting nuclear binding proteins. This has been most conclusively demonstrated for transcription of the gene for phosphoenolpyruvate carboxykinase (PEPCK), the rate-limiting enzyme for gluconeogenesis [25]. When nuclei from hepatocytes are incubated with insulin, the mRNA for PEPCK decreases rapidly and this inhibitory action of the hormone is not impaired if protein synthesis is blocked with cycloheximide or puromycin [25]. There are three general processes involved in the transcription of a gene: initiation, elongation and termination. In addition, transcription can be regulated by attenuation, a process in which the mRNA transcript is blocked by a specific base sequence in the gene.

Conversely, relief of attenuation can stimulate transcription. With respect to the PEPCK gene, Granner and colleagues [25, 346] have shown that the major effect of insulin on PEPCK gene transcription centers on inhibition of the RNA polymerase II complex initiation (Figure 27, step 2). Of note, dexamethasone and cyclic AMP, which stimulate the synthesis of PEPCK, increase RNA polymerase II initiation. Insulin also has been shown to retard elongation of the PEPCK transcript but this effect was minor compared to its inhibitory effect on transcript initiation. No effect of insulin on transcript attenuation or termination could be demonstrated [25, 346]. Proteins whose transcription is positively regulated by insulin include glucokinase, pyruvate kinase, glyceraldehyde-phosphate dehydrogenase and amylase [26, 333, 339, 340], although the precise mechanism whereby transcription is enhanced is less well delineated for these proteins than for PEPCK.

Insulin also regulates the transcription of secretory proteins, such as albumin. Following the induction of diabetes in rats, the rate of hepatic albumin synthesis falls dramatically and this decline is paralleled by a reduction in albumin mRNA [18, 329, 330] (Figure 28). Although total hepatic protein synthesis also declined, the fall in albumin synthesis was proportionally greater, indicating a selective effect of insulin on this specific protein. The decrease in albumin synthesis and mRNA was reversed following treatment with insulin (Figure 28). Identical changes in albumin synthetic rates and mRNA levels have been demonstrated following insulin withdrawal in the BB rat [347]. A similar result has been observed in studies of cultures of hepatocytes [348]. The nuclei of hepatocytes cultured in the absence of insulin demonstrate a progressive decline in albumin gene transcription and this is associated with a decrease in albumin mRNA

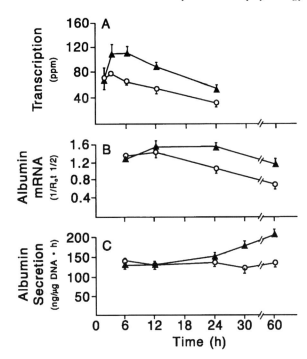

Figure 29 Albumin gene transcription (upper panel), albumin mRNA levels (middle panel) and albumin secretion (bottom panel) in hepatic nuclei of rats incubated in the presence (solid triangles) and absence (open circles) of insulin. From reference 18, with permission

and albumin secretion rate [349] (Figure 29). When insulin is added to the hepatocytes, albumin gene transcription is enhanced and this is associated, after a 12-hour delay, with an increase in albumin mRNA and albumin synthesis (Figure 29). The increased rate of albumin gene transcription displays a dose-dependent response to the insulin concentration.

In summary, it is clear that for many proteins insulin is capable of regulating their synthesis by altering

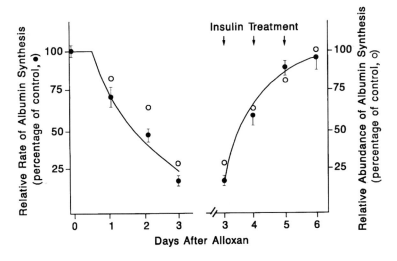

Figure 28 Effect of diabetes mellitus (left panel) and insulin treatment (right panel) on hepatic albumin synthesis (solid circles) and albumin mRNA (open circles) in rats. From reference 18, with permission

the transcription process. This regulation is brought about by an alteration in the amount or structural configuration of a *trans*-acting protein which interacts with the hormone (insulin) response element of the gene (see also Chapter 23).

Non-transcriptional Regulation of mRNA Levels

The level of mRNA (Figure 27, step 3) within the cytoplasm can be influenced by alterations in a number of steps (Table 8), not just by direct effects on transcription.

Table 8 Regulation of cytoplasmic mRNA level

Alteration in gene transcription
Altered processing of mRNA within the nucleus, i.e. splicing
Change in the stability of nuclear mRNA
Altered transport of mRNA out of the nucleus
Change in the degradation rate of mRNA in the cytoplasm

Jefferson and colleagues have demonstrated that the diabetes/insulin-induced changes in albumin mRNA levels are not due to increased/decreased degradation of mRNA or to an altered nuclear processing of the mRNA [18, 347, 349]. However, for other proteins including L-pyruvate kinase [350], tubulin [351], and malic enzyme [352], diabetes and insulin have been shown to respectively decrease and increase protein synthesis by altering the stability of the mRNA, thereby altering its half-life.

Selective Translation of mRNA Transcripts

Stimulation of protein synthesis by insulin can be brought about by enhancing the efficiency of translation (e.g. increasing the rate of peptide chain initiation) and/or by enhancing the capacity of translation (increasing the number of ribosomes) (Figure 27, step 4). Each of these actions would be expected to lead to a generalized increase in the synthesis of all cell proteins. However, several reports have documented that insulin causes a transcription-independent increase in synthesis of specific cell proteins including fatty acid synthase [353], lipoprotein lipase [354], a number of pancreatic acinar proteins [355], human insulin-like growth factor II [356], and ribosomal protein [357]. In all instances [353–357] increased protein synthesis was observed without any increase in the mRNA for the protein. At present, the mechanism by which insulin brings about this preferential translation of specific mRNAs (Figure 27, step 3) is unknown. However, it is likely to involve specific translational control by protein/RNA interactions in the 5′-motifs of specific mRNAs upstream from the AUG start codon [358] as has been demonstrated for the translation of ornithine decarboxylase [359], ferritin [360] and ribosomal proteins [361]. The selective increase in translation of ribosomal protein mRNA into actively translating polysomes by insulin [357] is especially important, since this would be expected to lead to a generalized increase in the capacity for protein synthesis.

Regulation of Peptide Chain Initiation

The rate of protein synthesis is dependent upon both the efficiency and capacity of the steps involved in translation (Figure 27, step 4). The capacity of any given tissue to synthesize protein is dependent upon the number of ribosomes and can be assessed by measuring the amount of total RNA, since ribosomal RNA (rRNA) comprises the great majority of tissue RNA. The efficiency of protein synthesis is quantified by expressing the amount of protein synthesized per amount of total RNA. There is now a large amount of evidence that diabetes mellitus and insulin exert profound effects on both the efficiency and capacity of protein synthesis, and we review here first the effects on peptide chain initiation, then the changes in ribosomal number.

In skeletal and cardiac muscle from diabetic animals both the efficiency and capacity (see Figure 7) of protein synthesis are reduced [18, 103, 140, 141, 148, 153, 169, 362–364]. This is most evident in muscles containing mixed fast-twitch (high glycolytic rate) fibers and least evident in slow-twitch red fibers (low glycolytic rate) such as the soleus. Conversely, insulin enhances the efficiency of protein synthesis (Figure 27, step 4) in both cardiac and skeletal muscle [18, 103, 140, 141, 147, 148, 153, 169, 362–364] (see Figure 8), and this action of insulin is not blocked by inhibitors of RNA synthesis [18, 130, 363]. As discussed previously, translation of the genetic code contained in the mRNA involves three steps (peptide chain initiation, elongation and termination) and defects in these steps can be inferred from analysis of the relative amounts of ribosomal subunits, monomers and polysomes [130, 363]. In fast-twitch muscles from diabetic rats, or in muscles from non-diabetic animals incubated in the absence of insulin, the number of monomeric ribosomes increases, while the number of polysomes decreases [18, 130, 146–148, 169, 350, 364]. Similar observations have been made for polysome profiles of liver homogenates from acutely and chronically diabetic rats [365–370]. These observations indicate that both diabetes (i.e. insulin lack) and insulin control protein synthesis at the step of peptide chain initiation (Figure 27, step 4). Inhibition of protein synthesis in soleus and cardiac muscle appears to be less affected by diabetes mellitus, but after 48 hours a decrease in peptide chain initiation can be demonstrated even in these muscles [3, 18, 350].

An impairment in peptide chain initiation could result from one or more of a number of steps (see Figure 5). In order to examine whether binding of the ternary complex (met-tRNA/eIF-2/GTP) to the 40S ribosomal subunit is impaired, Kelly and Jefferson [44] perfused muscles of diabetic rats with [^{35}S]-methionine in the presence and absence of insulin. Diabetic muscles demonstrated a marked decrease in the amount of ternary complex bound to ribosomal subunits and this defect was reversed by insulin. Similar observations have been made by Harmon et al [53] and Jeffrey et al [364] in cell-free extracts of gastrocnemius muscle. In the latter study, addition of eIF-2 to the muscle extract of diabetic animals returned the binding of met-tRNA to 40S ribosomal subunits to normal, suggesting that eIF-2 is directly related to the defect in peptide chain initiation. It is noteworthy that labeling of 43S initiation complexes with [^{35}S]-methionine also is diminished in perfused rat livers [371] and cultured Ehrlich ascites-tumor cells [372] deprived of essential amino acids. These observations may explain the biochemical basis by which amino acids stimulate protein synthesis *in vivo* and why hyperaminoacidemia causes an inhibition of protein synthesis [15]. Perfusion of diabetic rat livers with high amino acid concentration also causes a reaggregation of ribosomes and a return of protein synthesis to normal.

A guanine exchange factor (GEF) is required to convert GDP to GTP and to release eIF-2 at the end of each round of peptide chain initiation [18]. A defect in GDP/GTP exchange would effectively tie up eIF-2 and render it inactive. This would explain why addition of eIF-2 to muscle extracts of diabetic animals restores peptide chain initiation and protein synthesis to normal [53]. In fast-twitch muscles (gastrocnemius and psoas) of diabetic rats, GEF activity was reduced and was restored to normal with insulin. The change in GEF activity paralleled the changes in protein synthetic rate [373]. In two slow-twitch muscles GEF activity was unchanged in diabetic animals. In these slow-twitch muscles protein synthesis was not impaired and insulin had no effect on GEF activity [373].

Several mechanisms could explain the decrease in GEF activity observed in diabetic rats. It has been shown that phosphorylation of the α-subunit of eIF-2 inhibits GEF activity by causing the formation of a very stable GEF-eIF-2 complex, thereby inhibiting GDP/GTP exchange [19]. However, neither Clemens et al [60, 61, 364] nor Kimball and Jefferson [18] observed any change in the phosphorylation state of the α-subunit of eIF-2 in diabetic animals or following insulin treatment. Recent studies have shown

that casein kinase II phosphorylates the Mr subunit of GEF [18], markedly increasing its activity. Since insulin activates casein kinase II [62], this establishes a potential mechanism by which insulin could regulate peptide chain initiation. However, this interesting hypothesis has yet to receive direct experimental validation.

Another step in peptide chain initiation shown to be controlled by insulin is the regulation of the availability of the initiation factor eIF-4E to participate in initiation as described earlier (see insulin receptor signal transduction). The relative importance of the modulation of eIF-2B vs. the modulation of eIF-4E in mediating the effects of insulin in different tissues and different physiological states has not been assessed. While it is clear that only one of the steps can be rate-limiting for protein synthesis at any one time in a cell, it is possible that different steps assume this role under catabolic vs. anabolic conditions. It has been suggested [374] that the binding of the initiator tRNA to the 43S ribosomal subunit (involving eIF-2B) may be a control point in the down-regulation of protein synthesis in response to metabolic stress [52], whereas the binding of mRNA to the pre-initiation complex involving eIF-4E may be rate-limiting in most other circumstances [40, 45, 374]. With the recent discovery of insulin-modulated PHAS-1 protein (eIF-4E binding protein) [18, 58], these issues are likely to be addressed in the near future.

Peptide Chain Elongation

The regulation of peptide chain elongation has received much less attention. Short-term (24–48 hours) insulin deficiency in skeletal muscle causes a disaggregation of polysomes and an increase in monomeric ribosomes, indicating a block in peptide chain initiation. These changes are reversed by insulin [130]. However, if the diabetic state is allowed to persist for 7–10 days without insulin therapy, diminution of the rate of peptide chain elongation in the heart and soleus muscle can be demonstrated [148, 153]. These results indicate that the acute effects of diabetes and insulin are exerted on peptide chain initiation, while the more chronic effects of diabetes involve decreases in both peptide chain elongation and initiation.

Regulation of Ribosomal Turnover

The capacity for protein synthesis is dependent on the total number of ribosomes and consequently on the total amount of ribosomal rRNA within the tissue (Figure 27, step 6). In diabetic animals, the amount of rRNA is decreased in muscle and liver tissue (see

Figure 7) and returns to normal following insulin treatment [18, 103, 140, 141, 147, 148, 153, 169, 362]. In mixed fast-twitch muscle of diabetic rats, a decreased efficiency of ribosomal protein synthesis precedes alterations in ribosomal number [147, 148] and is the primary factor contributing to the decreased rate of protein synthesis. By contrast, a decrease in ribosomal number is responsible for a substantial portion of the decrease in the protein synthetic rate in heart and slow-twitch red muscle [148, 153].

By following the incorporation of labeled amino acids into ribosomal core proteins, insulin has been shown to increase their synthesis in muscle and liver [140, 375, 376]. Conversely, diabetes is associated with a reduction in ribosomal protein synthesis in both skeletal and cardiac muscle and in liver [140, 141, 146–148] (Figure 27, step 6). In these studies insulin treatment rapidly reversed the defect in ribosomal protein synthesis. In all of these studies, however, the decrease in RNA content (ribosomes) was more than could be accounted for by the modest reduction in ribosomal protein synthesis. Instead, ribosomal degradation increased 5–10-fold and was primarily responsible for the precipitous fall in ribosome content (Figure 27, step 7).

Little information is available concerning the mechanism(s) via which insulin regulates ribosome synthesis. Eukaryotic ribosomes are made up of equimolar amounts of 70–80 ribosomal proteins and four rRNAs. Potential regulatory sites include transcription of rRNA and mRNA for ribosomal proteins, nucleolar processing of these transcripts, and cytoplasmic translation of mRNA for ribosomal proteins [361]. The genetic DNA which encodes the ribosomal proteins resides within the nucleolar chromatin and is transcribed by RNA polymerase I into a 45S pre-ribosomal RNA [377]. The pre-ribosomal RNA undergoes nuclear processing, including several cleavages, methylation and addition of ribosomal proteins [378, 379], before ending up as mature 40S and 60S ribosomal subunits. Hammond and Bowman [357], using mouse myoblasts, have identified several steps at which insulin influences ribosomal protein synthesis. First, the hormone augmented the translation of a number of preformed mRNAs that were not previously being translated. Second, insulin also enhanced the transcription of the rDNAs for these untranslated mRNAs, while at the same time enhancing the transcription of a number of other rDNAs (Figure 27, step 6). Both processes were maximally stimulated within 15 minutes. Insulin had no effect on mRNA stability [357]. Similar results have been reported by others in different cell types [380, 381]. Several recent studies have demonstrated that the ability of insulin to stimulate RNA synthesis in myoblasts is inhibited by cyclo-oxygenase inhibitors [382–384]. This suggests that an arachidonate metabolite is involved in the signal transduction mechanism via which insulin stimulates RNA synthesis.

Current knowledge concerning the mechanisms involved in ribosomal degradation is even sketchier than for ribosomal protein synthesis. As discussed earlier, ribosomal degradation is enhanced in diabetes and inhibited by insulin [140, 146] (Figure 27, step 7). Both lysosomal and non-lysosomal pathways of degradation are involved and their relative contributions differ under different physiological conditions. Ribosomes are known to turn over as a unit. Consistent with this, the half-lives of ribosomal proteins and rRNA are similar [385, 386]. Therefore, it has been suggested that the major route of ribosomal degradation is as a whole unit by macroautophagic lysosomes [385–387]. However, a discriminatory mechanism of ribosomal degradation also must exist to explain the results of Ashford and Pain [140, 146].

Proteolysis

Unlike the effects of insulin on protein synthesis, the basic cellular signaling mechanisms by which the hormone inhibits proteolysis have been poorly characterized. Insulin deficiency both *in vivo* and *in vitro* is associated with an activation of proteolysis in essentially all tissues, including skeletal and cardiac muscle, liver, gut tissue, kidney, adipocytes and fibroblasts [29–32, 71–76]. The stimulation of protein degradation correlates closely with enhanced lysosomal autophagic activity [29–32, 96–116]. In the myocyte, however, macroautophagic activity of lysosomes is limited to non-myofibrillar proteins [29–32, 114, 115, 388–390]. Unfortunately, the cellular mechanisms via which insulin deficiency leads to an activation of lysosomal degradative activity have not been elucidated. Since this system digests large volumes of cytoplasm, it is difficult to envision how it can degrade specific proteins, although recent evidence by Dice et al [66, 106, 121, 122] suggests that the lysosomal system can recognize specific amino acid sequences within proteins. The calcium-dependent protease system is activated by lack of tension and cell injury, and does not appear to be regulated by insulin. The ATP-dependent ubiquitin–proteasome proteolytic system is activated by denervation and starvation [31, 68, 69, 93]. The effect of insulin *per se* on this degradative pathway has not yet been examined. However, its activation by starvation, a metabolic state characterized by a decrease in circulating insulin levels, together with the indications that this system is the dominant pathway for normal turnover of proteins [65, 67], suggest that insulin may have an important role in regulating the activity of this proteolytic system.

INTERORGAN EXCHANGE OF AMINO ACIDS

In the postabsorptive state, muscle tissue of normal humans is in net negative nitrogen balance (Figure 30), demonstrating a net release of amino acids [261, 391–404]. Although most amino acids are released by muscle, alanine and glutamine predominate, accounting for more than 50% of total amino acid release [261, 391–404]. The glutamine is taken up by the kidney where its nitrogen groups are utilized for ammonia production, and by the gut where glutamine serves as an important energy-yielding fuel [395, 397, 398, 400–402, 405–407]. Recent studies suggest that hepatic glutamine uptake and conversion to plasma glucose also is a major fate of glutamine and that this pathway may be quantitatively as important as that involving alanine in gluconeogenesis [403, 404]. In turn both the kidney and the gut release small amounts of alanine which, together with the alanine released by muscle, is taken up by the liver and used in glucose production [261, 392, 395, 398, 399, 401, 402, 408, 409]. Since alanine and glutamine account for only 10% of the amino acid residues in muscle, their predominance in the outflow of amino acids has been explained on the basis of *de novo* synthesis in muscle. Felig et al [261] and Mallete et al [410] suggested that the carbon skeleton of alanine is derived from circulating glucose. Most *in vivo* and *in vitro* studies [261, 395, 411] have indicated that alanine is formed by the transamination of pyruvate, and Chang and Goldberg [412] have directly documented that

over 97% of the carbons of alanine and pyruvate released by rat muscle *in vitro* are derived from exogenous glucose and not from endogenous protein degradation. A similar conclusion has been reached from analyzing previously published data by Pozefsky et al [391] on the arteriovenous difference of α-amino nitrogen and glucose across human forearm in the postabsorptive state. The branched-chain amino acids (BCAA) (leucine, isoleucine, valine) provide the nitrogen for glutamate production and ultimately for the formation of alanine [261, 395, 412, 413]. Concerning the formation of glutamine in skeletal muscle, Chang and Goldberg [414] have shown that a major portion of the carbon chains are contributed by amino acids derived from protein breakdown.

Alanine and glutamine represent the primary amino acids taken up by the splanchnic bed [261, 392, 395, 397–402]. With respect to the relative contributions of hepatic vs. extrahepatic tissues to net splanchnic balances, the gut represents the primary site of glutamine uptake [400–402, 415] whereas the liver is the major splanchnic organ which extracts alanine [261, 395, 401, 402, 409, 416]. However, two recent studies [403, 404] suggest that a significant amount of glutamine is taken up by the liver and converted to glucose, and that glutamine may be as important as alanine in its quantitative contribution to gluconeogenesis. Studies in experimental animals have confirmed and extended these observations by demonstrating that alanine also is released by the gut and contributes up to 50% of the total hepatic alanine uptake under fasting

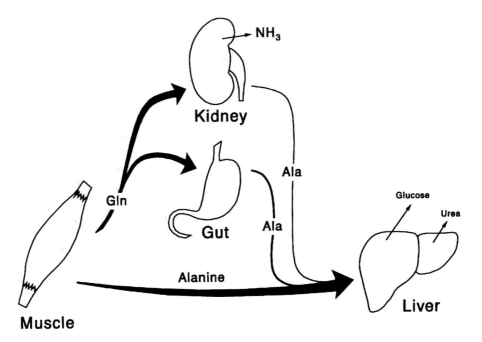

Figure 30   Normal physiology of the interorgan exchange of amino acids in the postabsorptive state in healthy subjects. See text for a more detailed discussion. Redrawn from reference 261, with permission

conditions (the remainder representing output from peripheral tissues).

Uptake of alanine by the liver is followed by its rapid conversion to glucose [410, 417, 418]. Alanine is thus not only a major vehicle for nitrogen release from muscle but is quantitatively the most important amino acid precursor for hepatic gluconeogenesis. On this basis, Felig et al [409] and Mallete et al [410] proposed the existence of a glucose–alanine cycle (Figure 30). According to this, alanine is synthesized in muscle by transamination of glucose-derived pyruvate and is then transported to the liver. Here its nitrogen moiety enters the urea cycle while its carbon skeleton is reconverted to glucose. Release of glucose into the blood and its return to muscle completes the cycle.

Protein Feeding in Normal Humans

Muscle tissue is in negative nitrogen balance in the postabsorptive state. Therefore, repletion of muscle nitrogen depends on a net uptake of amino acids in response to protein feeding. After the ingestion of a protein meal in normal man and animals, the pattern of amino acid rise does not parallel the relative amino acid concentrations in the protein meal [392, 402, 419]. The most marked increments, amounting to 200–300% of fasting values, are observed for the BCAA. In contrast, most other amino acids (such as alanine) show little or no change in plasma concentration after protein feeding. This peripheral amino acid profile following the ingestion of a protein meal (lean beef) is reflective of a selective escape of the BCAA from the splanchnic bed [392, 402]. Although leucine, isoleucine and valine constitute only 20% of the total amino acids in the beef meal, they constitute approximately 70% of the total amino acids entering the systemic circulation (Figure 31). By contrast, only a small and transient splanchnic escape is observed for most other amino acids, accounting for their smaller increments in the systemic circulation. In summary: (a) gut tissues quantitatively transfer the ingested amino acids to the portal blood; (b) the liver represents the major site of disposal of the gluconeogenic amino acids; (c) only the BCAA demonstrate a net release from the splanchnic tissues [392, 402].

Simultaneous with the net splanchnic release of amino acids following a protein meal, muscle exchange of most amino acids reverts from a basal net output to net uptake [392, 402] Complementing the pattern of splanchnic amino acid output, the BCAA are responsible for most of the amino acid uptake by muscle (Figure 32). They account for more than 50% of the total peripheral amino acid uptake in the first hour after protein ingestion and more than 80% during the third hour. It is likely that the high circulating and

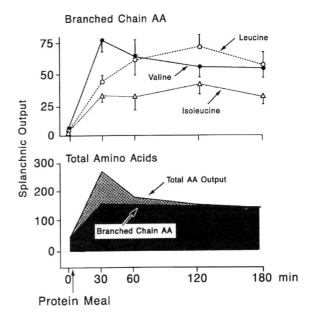

Figure 31 Splanchnic amino acid release (μmol/min) after the ingestion of a protein meal. Although branched-chain amino acids comprised only 20% of the total amino acids in the beef meal, they constituted almost 70% of the total amino acids entering the systemic circulation. From reference 392, with permission

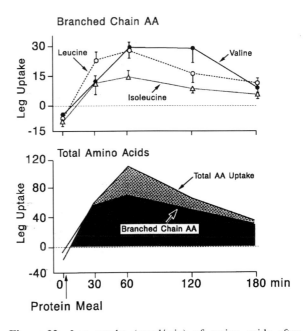

Figure 32 Leg uptake (μmol/min) of amino acids after protein ingestion. The branched chain amino acids account for 60–80% of the total uptake of amino acids by muscle. From reference 392, with permission

intracellular levels of BCAA have importance beyond the delivery of nitrogen, since studies by Buse and Reid have indicated that the BCAA, particularly leucine, may have a specific regulatory role in enhancing protein synthesis [138, 139]. The pattern of splanchnic and muscle amino acid uptake following intravenous amino acid infusion [398, 399, 401] is similar to that observed following protein ingestion [392, 402] (Figure 33).

The interorgan exchange of the BCAA after protein feeding can be summarized as follows (Figure 30). A nitrogen shuttle exists whereby the BCAA are responsible for nitrogen repletion in muscle tissue. The nitrogen thus delivered is released as alanine and glutamine in the fed as well as in the fasted condition. This occurs via transfer of the amino groups of the BCAA to α-ketoglutarate and eventually to alanine and glutamine. The liver removes about 30% of the BCAA and essentially 100% of the gluconeogenic amino acids contained in the protein meal.

Diabetes Mellitus: the Postabsorptive State

The diabetic patient who lacks insulin is in a state of negative nitrogen balance. This is not surprising since insulin deficiency is associated with a decrease in protein synthesis and a stimulation of proteolysis (see previous discussion). The interface between diabetes and protein metabolism also involves gluconeogenesis, since significant changes in the metabolism of alanine, the chief gluconeogenic amino acid precursor, are known to result from insulin lack [261, 393, 394, 420]. The arterial concentration of alanine (Figure 34, panel 1) is significantly reduced in IDDM patients compared with control subjects [261, 293, 294]. The decrease in circulating alanine levels cannot be accounted for by diminished muscle release of

alanine, since this is similar in diabetic and control subjects. Instead, a twofold increase in the splanchnic fractional extraction of alanine totally accounts for the decrease in arterial alanine concentration in diabetic subjects (Figure 34, panels 2 and 3). As a consequence of this increase in alanine uptake, gluconeogenesis can potentially account for over 40% of hepatic glucose production in diabetic patients, compared to 15–20% in normal humans [393, 420]. These findings are in keeping with the known inhibitory effect of insulin on alanine uptake and conversion to glucose by the liver [421, 422]. In the absence of this restraining effect (due either to insulin deficiency or insulin resistance), hepatic alanine uptake and gluconeogenesis are accelerated.

In addition to the decrease in fasting alanine levels, elevation of the three BCAA (valine, leucine, isoleucine) is characteristic of insulin dependent diabetes [261, 392, 393, 423]. The increase in arterial levels cannot be explained by increased BCAA release from muscle or liver. Instead, the elevated BCAA levels appear to result from a 30–40% decrease in their metabolic clearance rate, which can be reversed by physiological insulin replacement [424].

Diabetes Mellitus: Protein Feeding

In addition to the abnormalities in amino acid metabolism during the fasting state, repletion of muscle nitrogen after protein feeding is impaired in the insulin-dependent diabetic patient [392]. After the ingestion of a protein meal the rise in each of the three BCAA

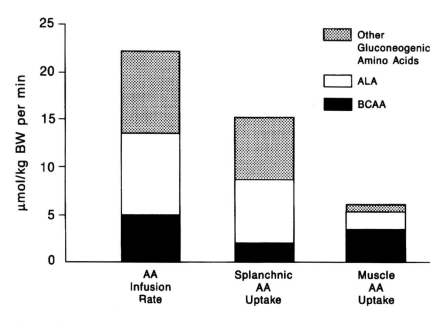

Figure 33 Splanchnic (middle bar) and leg muscle (right bar) uptake of infused amino acids (left bar) following intravenous infusion of a balanced amino acid solution. From both the qualitative and quantitative standpoints, the pattern of amino acid disposal was similar to that observed following ingestion of a protein meal. ALA, alanine; BCAA, branched chain amino acids. From reference 398, with permission

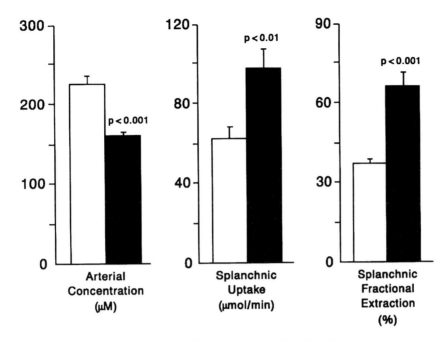

Figure 34 Alanine metabolism in insulin-dependent diabetic patients. The diminished circulating alanine levels are due to increased splanchnic extraction. Muscle release of alanine is similar in IDDM (solid bars) and control (open bars) subjects. From reference 393, with permission

is 30–50% greater in diabetic patients than in control subjects despite comparable rates of BCAA release from the splanchnic bed. The increase in arterial BCAA levels is due primarily to diminished uptake by muscle tissue [392]. In control subjects following protein ingestion, leg uptake of BCAA reverts from a small negative balance in the postabsorptive state to a markedly positive balance during the 3 hours after protein ingestion. By contrast, diabetic patients demonstrate a net uptake of BCAA only at 60 min. At 120 and 180 min after protein ingestion a net efflux of all three BCAA from muscle is observed. Since selective hepatic escape of BCAA and their preferential uptake by muscle represent an important mechanism of peripheral tissue (muscle) nitrogen repletion, the defect in muscle BCAA uptake in poorly controlled IDDM subjects partly explains the negative nitrogen balance, muscle wasting and growth failure in insulin deficient diabetic individuals [1–3].

REFERENCES

1. Atchley DW, Loeb RF, Richards DW Jr, Benedict EM, Driscoll ME. On diabetic acidosis: a detailed study of electrolyte balances following the withdrawal and reestablishment of insulin therapy. J Clin Invest 1933; 12: 297–326.
2. Walsh CH, Soler NG, James H et al. Studies in whole body potassium and whole body nitrogen in newly diagnosed diabetics. Q J Med 1976; 45: 295–301.
3. Best CH. Insulin. The Banting Memorial Lecture. Diabetes 1952; 1: 257–67.
4. Tattersall RB, Pyke DA. Growth in diabetic children: studies in identical twins. Lancet 1973; 2: 1105–9.
5. Guest CM. The Mauriac syndrome: dwarfism, hepatomegaly, and obesity with juvenile diabetes mellitus. Diabetes 1953; 2: 415–17.
6. Blethen SL, White NH, Santiago JV, Daughaday WH. Plasma somatomedins, endogenous insulin secretion, and growth in transient neonatal diabetes mellitus. J Clin Endocrinol Metab 1981; 52: 144–7.
7. Tamborlane WV, Hintz RL, Bergman M, Genel M, Felig P, Sherwin RS. Insulin-infusion-pump treatment of diabetes. Influence of improved metabolic control on plasma somatomedin levels. New Engl J Med 1981; 305: 303–7.
8. Olefsky JM. Perspectives in diabetes. The insulin receptor. A multifunctional protein. Diabetes 1990; 39: 1009–15.
9. Saltiel AR. Diverse signal pathways in the cellular actions of insulin. Am J Physiol 1996; 270: E375–85.
10. White MF, Kahn CR. The insulin signaling system. J Biol Chem 1994; 269: 1–4.
11. Cheatham B, Kahn CR. Insulin action and the insulin signaling network. Endocrine Rev 1995; 16: 117–42.
12. Guidotti GG, Borghetti AF, Gazzola GC. The regulation of amino acid transport in animal cells. Biochim Biophys Acta 1978; 515: 329–66.
13. Collarini EJ, Oxender DL. Mechanisms of transport of amino acids across membranes. Ann Rev Nutr 1987; 7: 75–90.
14. Palmer JP, Benson JW, Walter RM, Ensinck JW. Arginine-stimulated acute phase of insulin and glucagon secretion in diabetic subjects. J Clin Invest 1976; 58: 565–70.
15. Castellino P, Luzi L, Simonson DC, Haymond M, DeFronzo RA. Effect of insulin and plasma amino acid concentrations on leucine metabolism in man. Role of substrate availability on estimates of whole

body protein synthesis. J Clin Invest 1987; 80: 1784–93.

16. Li JB, Jefferson LS. Influence of amino acid availability on protein turnover in perfused skeletal muscle. Biochim Biophys Acta 1978; 544: 351–9.

17. Watson JD, Tooze J, Kurtz DT. Recombinant DNA. A short course. New York: W.H. Freeman, 1983.

18. Kimball SR, Jefferson LS. Cellular mechanisms involved in the action of insulin on protein synthesis. Diabetes Metab Rev 1988; 4: 773–87.

19. Pain VM. Initiation of protein synthesis in mammalian cells. Biochem J 1986; 235: 625–37.

20. Moldave K. Eukaryotic protein synthesis. Ann Rev Biochem 1985; 54: 1109–49.

21. Russo LA, Morgan HE. Control of protein synthesis and ribosome formation in rat heart. Diabetes Metab Rev 1989; 5: 31–47.

22. Kimball SR, Vary TC, Jefferson LS. Regulation of protein synthesis by insulin. Ann Rev Physiol 1994; 56: 321–48.

23. Meisler MH, Howard G. Effects of insulin on gene transcription. Ann Rev Physiol 1989; 51: 701–14.

24. Dillmann WH. Diabetes mellitus-induced changes in the concentration of specific mRNAs and proteins. Diabetes Metab Rev 1988; 4: 789–97.

25. O'Brien RM, Granner DK. PEPCK gene as model of inhibitory effects of insulin on gene transcription. Diabetes Care 1990; 13: 327–39.

26. Magnuson MA. Perspectives in diabetes. Glucokinase gene structure. Functional implications of molecular genetic studies. Diabetes 1990; 39: 523–7.

27. Johnson TM, Rosenberg MP, Meisler MH. An insulin-reponsive element in the pancreatic enhancer of the amylase gene. J Biol Chem 1993; 268: 464–8.

28. Philippe J. Insulin regulation of the glucagon gene is mediated by an insulin-responsive DNA element. Proc Natl Acad Sci USA 1991; 88: 7224–7.

29. Mortimore GE, Pösö AR. Intracellular protein catabolism and its control during nutrient deprivation and supply. Ann Rev Nutr 1987; 7: 539–64.

30. Pontremoli S, Melloni E. Extralysosomal protein degradation. Ann Rev Biochem 1986; 55: 455–81.

31. Kettelhut IC, Wing SS, Goldberg AL. Endocrine regulation of protein breakdown in skeletal muscle. Diabetes Metab Rev 1980; 4: 751–72.

32. Mortimore GE, Pösö AR, Lardeux BR. Mechanism and regulation of protein degradation in liver. Diabetes Metab Rev 1989; 5: 49–70.

33. Mitchell PJ, Tjian R. Transcriptional regulation in mammalian cells by sequence-specific DNA binding proteins. Science 1989; 245: 371–8.

34. Jones NC, Rigby PWJ, Ziff EB. Trans-acting protein factors and the regulation of eukaryotic transcription: lessons from studies on DNA tumor viruses. Genes Dev 1988; 2: 267–81.

35. Weiss SB. Enzymatic incorporation of ribonucleotide triphosphates into the interpolynucleotide linkages of ribonucleic acid. Proc Natl Acad Sci USA 1960; 46: 1020–30.

36. Chirgwin JM. Molecular biology for non-molecular biologists. Diabetes Care 1990; 13: 188–97.

37. Bell GI, Pictet RL, Rutter W, Cordell B, Tischer E, Goodman HM. Sequence of the human insulin gene. Nature 1980; 284: 26–32.

38. Csermely P, Schnaider T, Cheatham B, Olson MOJ, Kahn CR. Insulin induces the phosphorylation of nucleolin. A possible mechanism of insulin-induced RNA efflux from nuclei. J Biol Chem 1993; 268: 9747–52.

39. Merrick WC. Eukaryotic protein synthesis: an *in vitro* analysis. Biochimie 1994; 76: 822–30.

40. Kozak M. Determinants of translational fidelity and efficiency in vertebrate mRNAs. Biochimie 1994; 76: 815–21.

41. Goldfine ID, Purrello F, Vigneri R, Clawson GA. Insulin and the regulation of isolated nuclei and nuclear subfractions: potential relationships to mRNA metabolism. Diabetes Metab Rev 1985; 1: 119–38.

42. Schroer RA, Moldave K. Interaction of rat liver ribosomal subunits with homologous Met-tRNAs. Arch Biochem Biophys 1973; 154: 422–30.

43. Valenzuela DM, Chaudhuri A, Maitra U. Eukaryotic ribosomal subunit anti-association activity of calf liver is contained in a single polypeptide chain protein of $M_r = 25\,500$ (eukaryotic initiation factor 6). J Biol Chem 1982; 257: 7712–19.

44. Kelly FJ, Jefferson LS. Control of peptide-chain initiation in rat skeletal muscle. Development of methods for preparation of native ribosomal sub-units and analysis of the effect of insulin on formation of the 40S initiation complexes. J Biol Chem 1985; 260: 6677–83.

45. Rhoads RE, Joshi B, Minich WB. Participation of initiation factors in the recruitment of mRNA to ribosomes. Biochimie 1994; 76: 831–8.

46. Kimball SR, Jefferson LS. Mechanisms of translational control in liver and skeletal muscle. Biochimie 1994; 76: 729–36.

47. Lowe J, Stock D, Jap B, Zwicki P, Baumeister W, Huber R. Crystal structure of the 20S proteosome from the archaeon *T. acidophilum* at 3.4 A resolution. Science 1995; 268: 533–9.

48. Seal SN, Schmidt A, Marcus A. Fractionation and partial characterization of the protein synthesis system of wheat germ. J Biol Chem 1983; 258: 866–71.

49. Benne R, Hershey JWB. The mechanism of action of protein synthesis initiation factors from rabbit reticulocytes. J Biol Chem 1978; 253: 3078–87.

50. Barrieux A, Rosenfeld M. Characterization of GTP-dependent Met-tRNA$_f$ binding protein. J Biol Chem 1977; 252: 3843–7.

51. Tahara SM, Traugh JA, Sharp SB, Lundak TS, Safer B, Merrick WC. Effect of hemin on site-specific phosphorylation of eukaryotic initiation factor 2. Proc Natl Acad Sci USA 1978; 75: 789–93.

52. Pain VM. Translational control during amino acid starvation. Biochimie 1994; 76: 718–28.

53. Harmon CS, Proud CB, Pain VM. Effects of starvation, diabetes and acute insulin treatment on the regulation of polypeptide-chain initiation in rat skeletal muscle. Biochem J 1984; 223: 687–96.

54. Towle CA, Mankin HJ, Avruch J, Treadwell BV. Insulin promoted decrease in the phosphorylation of protein synthesis initiation factor eIF$_2$. Biochem Biophys Res Commun 1984; 121: 134–40.

55. Karinch AM, Kimball SR, Vary TC, Jefferson LS. Regulation of eukaryotic initiation factor 2B activity in muscle of diabetic rats. Am J Physiol 1993; 264: E101–8.

56. Sonenberg N. Regulation of translation and cell growth by eIF-4E. Biochimie 1994; 76: 839–46.

57. Pause A, Belsam GJ, Gingras AC et al. Insulin-dependent stimulation of protein synthesis by phosphorylation of a regulator of 5'-cap function. Nature 1994; 371: 762–7.

58. Lin TA, Kong X, Hayustead TA, Pause A, Belsham G, Sonenberg N. PHAS-1 as a link between mitogen-activated protein kinase and translation initiation. Science 1994; 266: 653–6.

59. Kozak M. How do eucaryotic ribosomes select initiation regions in messenger RNA? Cell 1978; 15: 1109–23.

60. Dholakia JN, Wahba AJ. Phosphorylation of the guanine nucleotide exchange factor from rabbit reticulocytes regulates its activity in polypeptide chain initiation. Proc Natl Acad Sci USA 1988; 85: 51 4.

61. Clemens MJ, Galpine AR, Austin SA et al. The role of phosphorylation of eIF-2α in translational regulation in non-erythroid cells. In Mathews MB (ed.) Current Communications in Molecular Biology. New York: Cold Spring Harbor Laboratory, 1986; pp 63–9.

62. Sommercorn J, Mulligan JA, Lozeman FJ, Krebs EG. Activation of casein kinase II in response to insulin and to epidermal growth factor. Proc Natl Acad Sci USA 1987; 84: 8834–8.

63. Nielson JBK, Plant PW, Haschemeyer AEV. Polypeptide elongation factor 1 and the control of elongation rate in rat liver *in vivo*. Nature 1976; 264: 804–6.

64. Moldave K, Harris J, Sabo W, Sadnik I. Protein synthesis and aging: studies with cell-free mammalian systems. Fed Proc 1979; 38: 1979–83.

65. Ciechanover A. The ubiquitin-proteasome proteolytic pathway. Cell 1994; 79: 13–21.

66. Terlecky SR, Dice JF. Polypeptide import and degradation by isolated lysosomes. J Biol Chem 1993; 268: 23490–5.

67. Rock KL, Gramm C, Rothstein L et al. Inhibitors of the proteosome block degradation of most cell proteins and the generation of peptides presented on MHC Class I molecules. Cell 1994; 78: 761–71.

68. Wing SS, Haas AL, Goldberg AL. Increase in ubiquitin–protein conjugates concomitant with the increase in proteolysis in rat skeletal muscle during starvation and atrophy denervation. Biochem J 1995; 307: 639–45.

69. Medina R, Wing SS, Goldberg AL. Increase in levels of polyubiquitin and proteosome mRNA in skeletal muscle during starvation and denervation atrophy. Biochem J 1995; 307: 631–7.

70. Millward DJ, Garlick PJ, James WP, Nnanyelugo DO, Ryatt JS. Relationship between protein synthesis and RNA content in skeletal muscle. Nature 1973; 241: 204–5.

71. Addis T, Poo LJ, Lew W. The quantities of protein lost by the various organs and tissues of the body during a fast. J Biol Chem 1936; 115: 111–18.

72. Mortimore GE, Hutson NJ, Surmacz CA. Quantitative correlation between proteolysis and macro- and microautophagy in mouse hepatocytes during starvation and refeeding. Proc Natl Acad Sci USA 1983; 80: 2179–83.

73. Millward DJ, Nnanyelugo DO, James WPT, Garlick PJ. Protein metabolism in skeletal muscle: the effect of feeding and fasting on muscle RNA, free amino acids, and plasma insulin concentrations. Br J Nutr 1974; 32: 127–42.

74. Millward DJ, Waterlow JC. Effect of nutrition on protein turnover in skeletal muscle. Fed Proc 1978; 37: 2283–9.

75. Felig P. Amino acid metabolism in man. Ann Rev Biochem 1975; 44: 933–55.

76. Cahill GF Jr. Starvation in man. New Engl J Med 1970; 282: 668–75.

77. Ciechanover A, Finley D, Varshavsky A. Ubiquitin dependence of selective protein degradation demonstrated in the mammalian cell cycle mutant ts85. Cell 1984; 37: 57–66.

78. Gropper R, Brandt R, Elias S et al. The ubiquitin-activated enzyme, E1, is required for stress-induced lysosomal degradation of cellular proteins. J Biol Chem 1991; 266: 3602–10.

79. Venerando R, Mioyyo G, Kadowski M, Siliprandi N, Mortimore GE. Multiphasic control of proteolysis by leucine and alanine in the isolated rat hepatocyte. Am J Physiol 1994; 266: C455–61.

80. Goldberg AL, St. John AC. Intracellular protein degradation in mammalian and bacterial cells. Part 2. Ann Rev Biochem 1976; 45: 747–803.

81. Bond JS, Butler PE. Intracellular proteases. Ann Rev Biochem 1987; 56: 333–64.

82. Fagan JM, Waxman L, Goldberg AL. Skeletal muscle and liver contain a soluble ATP + ubiquitin-dependent proteolytic system. Biochem J 1987; 243: 335–43.

83. Driscoll J, Goldberg AL. Skeletal muscle proteasome can degrade proteins in an ATP-dependent process that does not require ubiquitin. Proc Natl Acad Sci USA 1989; 86: 787–91.

84. Goldberg AL. The mechanism and functions of ATP-dependent proteases in bacterial and animal cells. Sem Cell Biol 1990; 1: 425–32.

85. Driscoll J, Goldberg AL. The proteasome (multicatalytic protease) is a component of the 1500-kDa proteolytic complex which degrades ubiquitin-conjugated proteins. J Biol Chem 1990; 265: 4789–92.

86. Ganoth D, Leshinsky E, Eytan E, Hershkov A. A multicomponent system that degrades proteins conjugated to ubiquitin. Resolution of factors and evidence for ATP-dependent complex formation. J Biol Chem 1989; 263: 12412–19.

87. Matthews W, Driscoll J, Tanaka K, Ichihara A, Goldberg AL. Involvement of the proteasome in various degradation processes in mammalian cells. Proc Natl Acad Sci USA 1989; 86: 2597–601.

88. Eytan E, Ganoth D, Armon T, Hershko A. ATP-dependent incorporation of 20S protease into the 26S complex that degrades proteins conjugated to ubiquitin. Proc Natl Acad Sci USA 1989; 86: 7751–5.

89. Rechsteiner M, Hoffman L, Dubiel W. The multicatalytic and 26S proteases. J Biol Chem 1993; 268: 6065–8.

90. DeMartino GN, Moomaw CR, Zagnitko OP et al. PA700—An ATP-dependent activator of the 20S proteasome, is an ATPase containing multiple members of a nucleotide-binding protein family. J Biol Chem 1994; 269: 20878–84.

91. Peters J. Proteasomes: protein degradation machines of the cell. Trends Biochem Sci 1994; 19: 377–82.

92. Seemiller E, Lupass A, Stock D, Lowe J, Huber R, Baumeister W. Proteasome from *Thermoplasma acidophilum*: a threonine protease. Science 1995; 268: 579–82.

93. Furano K, Goodman MN, Goldberg AL. Role of different proteolytic systems in the degradation of muscle proteins during denervation atrophy. J Biol Chem 1990; 265: 8550-7.

94. Fenteany G, Standaert RF, Lane WS, Choi S, Corey EJ, Schreiber SL. Inhibition of proteasome activities and subunit specific amino-terminal threonine modification by lactacystin. Science 1995; 268: 726-33.

95. Gorden P, Carpentier JL, Orci L. Insulin action at the cellular level: anatomical considerations. Diabetes Metab Rev 1985; 1: 99-117.

96. Ward WF, Chua BL, Li JB, Morgan HE, Mortimore GE. Inhibition of basal and deprivation-induced proteolysis by leupeptin and pepstatin in perfused rat liver and heart. Biochem Biophys Res Commun 1989; 87: 92-8.

97. Mortimore GE, Shworer CM. Induction of autophagy by amino acid deprivation in perfused rat liver. Nature 1977; 270: 174-6.

98. Mortimore GE, Ward WF. Internalization of cytoplasmic protein by hepatic lysosomes in basal and deprivation-induced proteolytic states. J Biol Chem 1981; 256: 7659-65.

99. Neely AN, Nelson PB, Mortimore GE. Osmotic alterations of the lysosomal system during rat liver perfusion: reversible suppression by insulin and amino acids. Biochim Biophys Acta 1974; 338: 458-72.

100. Mortimore GE, Lardeux BR, Wert JJ Jr, Adams CE. Adaptive regulation of basal autophagy and protein turnover in rat liver: effects of short-term starvation. J Biol Chem 1988; 263: 2506-12.

101. Mortimore GE, Mondon C. Inhibition by insulin of valine turnover in liver. J Biol Chem 1970; 245: 2375-83.

102. Blommaart EFC, Luiken JFP, Blommaart PJE, vanWoerkom GM, Meijer AJ. Phosphorylation of ribosomal protein S6 is inhibitory for autophagy in isolated rat hepatocytes. J Biol Sci 1995; 270: 2320-6.

103. Jefferson LS, Rannels DE, Munger BL, Morgan HE. Insulin in the regulation of protein turnover in heart and skeletal muscle. Fed Proc 1974; 33: 1098-104.

104. Furuno K, Goldberg AL. The activation of protein degradation in muscle by calcium or muscle injury does not involve a lysosomal mechanism. Biochem J 1986; 237: 859-64.

105. Furuno K, Goodman MN, Goldberg AL. Role of different proteolytic systems in the degradation of muscle proteins during denervation atrophy. J Biol Chem 1990; 265: 8550-7.

106. Chiang HL, Dice JF. Peptide sequences that target proteins for enhanced degradation during serum withdrawal. J Biol Chem 1988; 263: 6797-805.

107. Gronostajski R, Goldberg AL, Pardee AB. The role of increased proteolysis in the atrophy and arrest of proliferation in serum-deprived fibroblasts. J Cell Physiol 1984; 121: 189-98.

108. Amenta JS, Brocher SC. Mechanisms of protein turnover in cultured cells. Life Sci 1981; 28: 1195-1208.

109. Glaumann H, Ericsson JLE, Marzella L. Mechanisms of intralysosomal degradation with special reference to autophagocytosis and heterophagocytosis of cell organelles. Int Rev Cytol 1981; 73: 149-82.

110. Grinde B. Autophagy and lysosomal proteolysis in the liver. Experientia 1985; 41: 1089-95.

111. Schworer CM, Shiffer KA, Mortimore GE. Quantitative relationship between autophagy and proteolysis during graded amino acid deprivation in perfused rat liver. J Biol Chem 1981; 256: 7652-8.

112. Mortimore GE, Neely AN, Cox JR, Guinivan RA. Proteolysis in homogenates of perfused rat liver; responses to insulin, glucagon, and amino acids. Biochem Biophys Res Commun 1973; 54: 89-95.

113. Neely AN, Cox JR, Fortney JA, Schworer CM, Mortimore GE. Alterations of lysosomal size and density during rat liver perfusion: suppression by amino acids and insulin. J Biol Chem 1977; 252: 6948-54.

114. Li JB, Wassner SJ. Effects of food deprivation and refeeding on actomyosin degradation. Am J Physiol 1978; 246: E32-7.

115. Smith DM, Sugden PH. Contrasting response of protein degradation to starvation and insulin as measured by release of N^t-methylhistidine or phenylalanine from the perfused rat heart. Biochem J 1986; 237: 391-5.

116. Mitchener JS, Shelburne JD, Bradford WD, Hawkins HK. Cellular autophagocytosis induced by deprivation of serum and amino acids in HeLa cells. Am J Pathol 1976; 83: 485-98.

117. Neff NT, DeMartino GN, Goldberg AL. The effect of protease inhibitors and decreased temperature on the degradation of different classes of proteins in cultured hepatocytes. J Cell Physiol 1979; 101: 439-58.

118. Vandenburgh H, Kaufman S. Protein degradation in embryonic skeletal muscle. Effects of medium, cell type, inhibitors, and passive stretch. J Biol Chem 1980; 255: 5826-33.

119. Ward WF, Chua BL, Li JB, Morgan HE, Mortimore GE. Inhibition of basal and deprivation-induced proteolysis by leupeptin and pepstatin in perfused rat liver and heart. Biochem Biophys Res Commun 1979; 87: 92-8.

120. Lowell BB, Ruderman NB, Goodman NM. Evidence that lysosomes are not involved in the degradation of myofibrillar proteins in rat skeletal muscle. Biochem J 1986; 234: 237-40.

121. Dice JF, Backer JM, Miao P, Bourret L, McElligott MA. Regulation of catabolism of ribonuclease A microinjected into human fibroblasts. Intracellular protein catabolism. In Khairallah EA, Bond JS, Bird JWC (eds) New York: Alan R. Liss, 1985; pp 385-94.

122. Dice JF, Chiang H-L, Spencer EP, Backer JM. Regulation of catabolism of microinjected ribonuclease A. Identification of residues 7-11 as the essential pentapeptide. J Biol Chem 1986; 261: 6853-9.

123. Ord JM, Wakeland JR, Crie JS, Wildenthal K. Mechanisms of degradation of myofibrillar and non-myofibrillar protein in heart. Adv Myocardiol 1983; 4: 198-9.

124. Zeman RJ, Kameyama T, Matsumoto K, Bernstein P, Etlinger JD. Regulation of protein degradation in muscle by calcium. J Biol Chem 1985; 260: 13619-24.

125. Mellgren R. Calcium-dependent proteases: an enzyme system active at cellular membranes. FASEB J 1987; 1: 110-15.

126. Murachi T, Tanaka K, Hatanaka M, Murakami T. Intracellular Ca^{2+}-dependent protease (calpain) and its high molecular weight endogenous inhibition (calpastatin). Adv Enzyme Regul 1981; 19: 407-24.

127. Baracos VE, Greenberg RE, Goldberg AL. Influence of calcium and other divalent cations on protein turnover in rat skeletal muscle. Am J Physiol 1986; 250: E702-10.

128. Rodemann HP, Waxman L, Goldberg AL. The stimulation of protein degradation in muscle by Ca^{2+} is mediated by prostaglandin E2 and does not require the calcium-activated protease. J Biol Chem 1982; 257: 8716-23.

129. Sugden PH. The effects of calcium ions, ionophore A23187 and inhibition of energy metabolism on protein degradation in the rat diaphragm and epitrochlearis muscles *in vitro*. Biochem J 1980; 190: 593-603.

130. Stirewalt WS, Wool IG, Cavicchi P. The relation of RNA and protein synthesis to the sedimentation of muscle ribosomes: effects of diabetes and insulin. Proc Natl Acad Sci USA 1967; 57: 1885-92.

131. Pain VM, McNurlan MA, Albertse BC, Clemens MJ, Garlick PJ. Effect of streptozotocin diabetes on protein synthesis in the liver, kidney and intestinal mucosa of young rats. Proc Nutr Soc 1978; 37: 104A.

132. Ross R, Goldman JK. Effect of streptozotocin-induced diabetes on kidney weight and compensatory hypertrophy in the rat. Endocrinology 1971; 88: 1079-82.

133. McNurlan MA, Garlick PJ. Protein synthesis in liver and small intestine in protein deprivation and diabetes. Am J Physiol 1981; 241: E238-45.

134. Castellino P, Luzi L, Simonson DC, Haymond M, DeFronzo RA. Effect of insulin and plasma amino acid concentrations on leucine metabolism in man. Role of substrate availability on estimates of whole body protein synthesis. J Clin Invest 1987; 80: 1784-93.

135. Garlick PJ, Grant I. Amino acid infusion increases the sensitivity of muscle protein synthesis *in vivo* to insulin. Effect of branched-chain amino acids. Biochem J 1988; 254: 579-84.

136. Fulks RM, Li JB, Goldberg AL. Effects of insulin, glucose, and amino acids on protein turnover in rat diaphragm. J Biol Chem 1975; 250: 290-8.

137. Li JB, Higgins JE, Jefferson LS. Changes in protein turnover in skeletal muscle in response to fasting. Am J Physiol 1978; 236: E222-8.

138. Buse MG, Reid SS. Leucine. A possible regulator of protein turnover in muscle. J Clin Invest 1975; 56: 1250-61.

139. May ME, Buse MG. Effects of branched chain amino acids on protein turnover. Diabetes Metab Rev 1989; 5: 227-46.

140. Ashford AJ, Pain VM. Insulin stimulation of growth in diabetic rats. Stimulation and degradation of ribosomes and total tissue protein in skeletal muscle and heart. J Biol Chem 1986; 261: 4066-70.

141. Pain VM, Garlick PJ. Effect of streptozotocin diabetes and insulin treatment on the rate of protein synthesis in tissues of the rat *in vivo*. J Biol Chem 1974; 249: 4510-14.

142. Hay AM, Waterlow JC. The effect of alloxan diabetes on muscle and liver protein synthesis in the rat, measured by constant infusion of L-[^{14}C]lysine. J Physiol (Lond) 1967; 191: 111-12P.

143. Odedra BR, Shreedevi SD, Millward DJ. Muscle protein synthesis in the streptozotocin-diabetic rat. A possible role for corticosterone in the insensitivity to insulin infusions *in vivo*. Biochem J 1982; 202: 363-8.

144. Millward DJ, Garlick PJ, Nnanyelugo DO, Waterlow JC. The relative importance of muscle protein synthesis and breakdown in the regulation of muscle mass. Biochem J 1976; 156: 185-8.

145. Forker LL, Chaikoff IL, Entenman C, Tarver H. Formation of muscle protein in diabetic dogs studied with S^{35}-methionine. J Biol Chem 1951; 188: 37-48.

146. Ashford AJ, Pain VM. Effect of diabetes on the rates of synthesis and degradation of ribosomes in rat muscle and liver *in vivo*. J Biol Chem 1986; 261: 4059-65.

147. Pain VM, Albertse EC, Garlick PJ. Protein metabolism in skeletal muscle, diaphragm, and heart of diabetic rats. Am J Physiol 1983; 245: E604-10.

148. Flaim KE, Copenhaver ME, Jefferson LS. Effects of diabetes on protein synthesis in fast- and slow-twitch rat skeletal muscle. Am J Physiol (Endocrinol Metab 2) 1980; 239: E88-95.

149. Williams IH, Chua BHL, Sahms RH, Siehl D, Morgan HE. Effects of diabetes on protein turnover in cardiac muscle. Am J Physiol (Endocrinol Metab 2) 1980; 239: E178-85.

150. Gulve EA, Dice JF. Regulation of protein synthesis and degradation in L8 myotubes. Effects of serum insulin and insulin-like growth factors. Biochem J 1989; 260: 377-87.

151. Rannels DE, Hjalmarson AC, Morgan HE. Effects of noncarbohydrate substrates on protein synthesis in muscle. Am J Physiol 1974; 226: 528-39.

152. Smith DM, Fuller SJ, Sugden PH. The effects of lactate, acetate, glucose, insulin, starvation and alloxan-diabetes on protein synthesis in perfused rat hearts. Biochem J 1986; 236: 543-7.

153. Williams IH, Chua BHL, Sahms RH, Siehl D, Morgan HE. Effects of diabetes on protein turnover in cardiac muscle. Am J Physiol 1980; 239: E178-85.

154. Krahl ME. Incorporation of C^{14}-amino acids into glutathione and protein fractions of normal and diabetic rat tissues. J Biol Chem 1953; 200: 99-109.

155. Green M, Miller LL. Protein catabolism and protein synthesis in perfused livers of normal and alloxan-diabetic rats. J Biol Chem 1960; 235: 3202-8.

156. Penhos JC, Krahal ME. Stimulus of leucine incorporation into perfused liver protein by insulin. Am J Physiol 1963; 204: 140-2.

157. Peavy DE, Taylor JM, Jefferson LS. Correlation of albumin production rates and albumin mRNA levels in livers of normal, diabetic, and insulin-treated diabetic rats. Proc Natl Acad Sci USA 1978; 75: 5879-83.

158. Jefferson LS, Liao WSL, Peavy DE, Miller TB, Appel MC, Taylor JM. Diabetes-induced alterations in liver protein synthesis. Changes in the relative abundance of mRNAs for albumin and other plasma proteins. J Biol Chem 1983; 258: 1369-75.

159. Marsh JB. Effects of fasting and alloxan diabetes on albumin synthesis by perfused rat liver. Am J Physiol 1961; 201: 55-7.

160. Reaven EP, Peterson DT, Reaven GM. The effect of experimental diabetes mellitus and insulin replacement on hepatic ultrastructure and protein synthesis. J Clin Invest 1973; 52: 248-62.

161. Guzdek A, Sarnecka-Keller M, Dubin A. The activities of perfused livers of control and streptozotocin diabetic rats in the synthesis of some plasma proteins and peptides. Horm Metab Res 1979; 11: 107-11.

162. Berry EM, Ziv E, Bar-On H. Protein and glycoprotein synthesis and secretion by the diabetic liver. Diabetologia 1980; 19: 535-40.

163. Manchester KL, Young FG. The effect of insulin on incorporation of amino acids into protein of normal rat diaphragm *in vitro*. Biochem J 1958; 70: 353-8.

164. Preedy VR, Smith DM, Kearney NF, Sugden PH. Rates of protein turnover *in vivo* and *in vitro* in ventricular muscle of hearts from fed and starved rats. Biochem J 1984; 222: 395–400.

165. Morgan HE, Jefferson LS, Wolpert EB, Rannels DE. Regulation of protein synthesis in heart muscle. II. Effect of amino acid levels and insulin on ribosomal aggregation. J Biol Chem 1971; 246: 2163–70.

166. Jefferson LS, Koehler JO, Morgan HE. Effect of insulin on protein synthesis in skeletal muscle of an isolated perfused preparation of rat hemicorpus. Proc Natl Acad Sci USA 1972; 69: 816–20.

167. Stirewalt WS, Low RB, Slaiby JM. Insulin sensitivity and responsiveness of epitrochlearis and soleus muscles from fed and starved rats. Recognition of differential changes in insulin sensitivities of protein synthesis and glucose incorporation into glycogen. Biochem J 1985; 227: 355–62.

168. Hait G, Kypson J, Massih R. Amino acid incorporation into myocardium: effect of insulin, glucagon, and dibutyryl 3', 5'-AMP. Am J Physiol 1972; 222: 404–8.

169. Jefferson LS, Li JB, Rannels SR. Regulation by insulin of amino acid release and protein turnover in the perfused rat hemicorpus. J Biol Chem 1977; 252: 1476–83.

170. Ballard FJ, Francis GL. Effects of anabolic agents on protein breakdown in L6 myoblasts. Biochem J 1983; 210: 243–9.

171. Clark RL, Hansen RJ. Insulin stimulates synthesis of soluble proteins in isolated rat hepatocytes. Biochem J 1980; 190: 615–19.

172. Stirewalt WS, Low RB. Effects of insulin *in vitro* on protein turnover in rat epitrochlearis muscle. Biochem J 1983; 210: 323–30.

173. Garlick PJ, Fern M, Preedy VR. The effect of insulin infusion and food intake on muscle protein synthesis in postabsorptive rats. Biochem J 1983; 210: 669–76.

174. Oddy VH, Lindsay DB, Barker PJ, Northrop AJ. Effect of insulin on hind-limb and whole-body leucine and protein metabolism in fed and fasted lambs. Br J Nutr 1987; 58: 437–52.

175. Nissen S, Haymond MW. Changes in leucine kinetics during meal absorption: effects of dietary leucine availability. Am J Physiol 1986; 250: E695–701.

176. Mortimore GE, Mondon CE. Inhibition by insulin of valine turnover in liver. Evidence for a general control of proteolysis. J Biol Chem 1970; 245: 2375–83.

177. Baillie AGS, Garlick PJ. Responses of protein synthesis in different skeletal muscles to fasting and insulin in rats. Am J Physiol 1991; 260 (Endocrinol Metab 23): E891–6.

178. Frayn KN, Maycock PF. Regulation of protein metabolism by a physiological concentration of insulin in mouse soleus and EDL muscles. Biochem J 1979; 184: 323–30.

179. Palmer RM, Bain PA, Reeds RJ. The effect of insulin and intermittent mechanical stretching on rates of protein synthesis and degradation in isolated rabbit muscle. Biochem J 1985; 230: 117–23.

180. Dice JF, Walker CD, Byrne B, Cardiel A. General characteristics of protein degradation in diabetes and starvation. Proc Natl Acad Sci USA 1978; 75: 2093–7.

181. Gulve EA, Dice JF. Regulation of protein synthesis and degradation in L8 myotubes. Effects of serum, insulin and insulin-like growth factors. Biochem J 1989; 260: 377–87.

182. Li JB, Wassner SJ. Effects of food deprivation and refeeding on total protein and actomyosin degradation. Am J Physiol 1984; 246: E32–7.

183. Li JB, Goldberg AL. Effects of food deprivation on protein synthesis and degradation in rat skeletal muscles. Am J Physiol 1976; 231: 441–8.

184. Goodman MN, Larsen PR, Kaplan MM, Aoki TT, Young VR, Ruderman NB. Starvation in the rat. II. Effect of age and obesity on protein sparing and fuel metabolism. Am J Physiol 1980; 239: E277–86.

185. Pösö AR, Wert JJ Jr, Mortimore GE. Multi-functional control by amino acids of deprivation-induced proteolysis in liver: role of leucine. J Biol Chem 1982; 257: 12114–20.

186. Rannels DE, Kao R, Morgan HE. Effect of insulin on protein turnover in heart muscle. J Biol Chem 1975; 250: 1694–1701.

187. Sugden PH, Smith DM. The effects of glucose, acetate, lactate and insulin on protein degradation in the perfused rat heart. Biochem J 1982; 206: 467–72.

188. Pfeifer U, Warmuth-Metz M. Inhibition by insulin of cellular autophagy in proximal tubular cells of rat kidney. Am J Physiol 1983; 244: E109–14.

189. Tischler ME, Ost AH, Spina B, Cook PH, Coffman J. Regulation of protein turnover by glucose, insulin, and amino acids in adipose tissue. Am J Physiol 1984; 247: C228–33.

190. Nissen S, Haymond MW. Changes in leucine kinetics during meal absorption: effects of dietary leucine availability. Am J Physiol 1986; 250 (Endocrinol Metab 13): E695–701.

191. Baracos VE, Goldberg AL. Maintenance of normal length improves protein balance and energy status in isolated rat skeletal muscles. Am J Physiol 1986; 251: C588–96.

192. Li JB, Jefferson LS. Influence of amino acid availability on protein turnover in perfused skeletal muscle. Biochim Biophys Acta 1978; 544: 351–9.

193. Goodman MN, Gomez MDP. Decreased myofibrillar proteolysis after refeeding requires dietary proteins or amino acids. Am J Physiol 1987; 253: E53–8.

194. Lundholm K, Schersten T. Protein synthesis in human skeletal muscle tissue: influence of insulin and amino acids. Eur J Clin Invest 1977; 7: 531–6.

195. Preedy VR, Garlick PJ. The response of muscle protein synthesis to nutrient intake in postabsorptive rats: the role of insulin and amino acids. Biosci Rep 1986; 2: 177–83.

196. Buse MG, Atwell R, Mancusi V. *In vitro* effect of branched chain amino acids on the ribosomal cycle in muscles of fasted rats. Horm Metab Res 1979; 11: 289–92.

197. Woodside KH, Ward WF, Mortimore GE. Effects of glucagon on general protein degradation and synthesis in perfused rat liver. J Biol Chem 1974; 249: 5458–5463.

198. Hopgood MF, Clark MG, Ballard FJ. Inhibition of protein degradation in isolated rat hepatocytes. Biochem J 1977; 164: 399–407.

199. Seglen PO, Gordon PB. Amino acid control of autophagic sequestration and protein degradation in isolated rat hepatocytes. J Cell Biol 1984; 99: 435–44.

200. Munro HN. Historical perspective on protein requirements: Objectives for the future. In Blaxter KC and Waterlow JC (eds) Nutritional adaptation in man. London: John Libbey, 1985; pp 155–67.

201. Kopple JD. Uses and limitations of the balance technique. J Parent Ent Nut 1987; 11: 79S–85S.

202. Bier DM. Intrinsically difficult problems: the kinetics of body proteins and amino acids in man. Diabetes Metab Rev 1989; 5: 111–32.

203. Hegsted DM. Variation in requirements of nutrients amino acids. Fed Proc 1963; 22: 1424–9.

204. Hegsted DM. Balance studies. J Nutr 1976; 106: 307–11.

205. Young VR, Scrimshaw NS, Bier DM. Whole body protein and amino acid metabolism: relation to protein quality evaluation in human nutrition. J Agricult Food Chem 1981; 29: 440–7.

206. Garza C, Scrimshaw NS, Young VR. Human protein requirements: the effect of variations in energy intake within the maintenance range. Am J Clin Nutr 1976; 29: 280–7.

207. Young VR. 1987 McCollum award lecture. Kinetics of human amino acid metabolism: nutritional implications and some lessons. Am J Clin Nutr 1987; 46: 709–25.

208. Waterlow JC. What do we mean by adaptation? In Blaxter K, Waterlow JC (eds) Nutritional adaptation in man. London: John Libbey, 1985; pp 1–11.

209. Waterlow JC, Garlick PJ, Millward DJ. Protein turnover in mammalian tissues and in the whole body. New York: Elsevier/North Holland, 1978; p 804.

210. Biolo G, Inchiostro S, Tiengo A, Tessari P. Regulation of postprandial whole-body proteolysis in insulin-deprived IDDM. Diabetes 1995; 44: 203–9.

211. Denne SC, Brechtel G, Johnson A, Liechty EA, Baron AD. Skeletal muscle proteolysis is reduced in non-insulin-dependent diabetes mellitus and is unaltered by euglycemic hyperinsulinemia or intensive insulin therapy. J Clin Endocrinol Metab 1995; 80: 2371–7.

212. Louard RJ, Fryburg DA, Gelfand RA, Barrett EJ. Insulin sensitivity of protein and glucose metabolism in human forearm skeletal muscle. J Clin Invest 1992; 90: 2348–54.

213. Nair KS, Gord GC, Ekberg K, Fernqvist-Forbes E, Wahren J. Protein dynamics in whole body and in splanchnic and leg tissues in type I diabetic patients. J Clin Invest 1995; 95: 2926–37.

214. Barrett EJ, Gelfand RA. The *in vivo* study of cardiac and skeletal muscle protein turnover. Diabetes Metab Rev 1989; 5: 133–48.

215. Heslin MJ, Newman E, Wolf RF, Pisters PWT, Brennan MF. Effect of hyperinsulinemia on whole body and skeletal muscle leucine carbon kinetics in humans. Am J Physiol 1992; 262: E911–18.

216. Laager R, Ninnis R, Keller U. Comparison of the effects of recombinant human insulin-like growth factor-I and insulin on glucose and leucine kinetics in humans. J Clin Invest 1993; 92: 1903–9.

217. Rennie MJ, Ahmed A, Thompson GWA, Smith K, Bennet WM, Watt PW. Effects of insulin on amino acid transport and protein synthesis in skeletal muscle. In Nair KS (ed.) Protein metabolism in diabetes mellitus. London: Smith, Gordon, 1992: pp 173–80.

218. Schwenk WF, Beaufrere B, Haymond MW. Use of reciprocal pool specific activities to model leucine metabolism in humans. Am J Physiol 1985; 249 (Endocrinol Metab 12): E646–50.

219. McKee EE, Cheung JY, Rannels DE, Morgan HE. Measurement of the rate of protein synthesis and compartmentation of heart phenylalanine. J Biol Chem 1978; 253: 1030–40.

220. Watt PW, Stenhouse MG, Corbett ME, Rennie MJ. tRNA charging in pig muscle measured by [1-^{13}C]-leucine during fasting and infusion of amino acids. Clin Nutr 1989; 8 (suppl): 47.

221. McNurlan MA, Essen P, Thorell A et al. Response of protein synthesis in human skeletal muscle to insulin: an investigation with L-[^{2}H$_5$]phenylalanine. Am J Physiol 1994; 267: E102–8.

222. Garlick PJ, McNurlan MA, Preedy VR. A rapid and convenient technique for measuring the rate of protein synthesis in tissues by injection of ^{3}H-phenylalanine. Biochem J 1980; 192: 719–23.

223. Alvestrand A, DeFronzo RA, Smith D, Wahren J. Influence of hyperinsulinaemia on intracellular amino acid levels and amino acid exchange across splanchnic and leg tissues in uraemia. Clinical Science 1988; 74: 155–63.

224. Essen P, Heys SD, Garlick P, Wernerman J. The separate and combined effect of leucine and insulin on muscle free amino acids. Clin Physiol 1994; 14: 513–25.

225. Biolo G, Fleming RYD, Wolfe RR. Physiologic hyperinsulinemia stimulates protein synthesis and enhances transport of selected amino acids in human skeletal muscle. J Clin Invest 1995; 95: 811–19.

226. De Feo P, Volpi E, Lucidi P et al. Physiological increments in plasma insulin concentrations have selective and different effects on synthesis of hepatic proteins in normal humans. Diabetes 1993; 42: 995–1002.

227. Giordano M, Castellino P, DeFronzo RA. Comparison of the effects of human recombinant insulin-like growth factor I and insulin on plasma amino acid concentrations and leucine kinetics in humans. Diabetologia 1995; 38: 732–8.

228. Fryburg DA, John LA, Hill SA, Oliveras DM, Barrett EJ. Insulin and insulin-like growth factor-I enhance human skeletal muscle protein anabolism during hyperaminoacidemia by different mechanisms. J Clin Invest 1995; 96: 1722–9.

229. Newman E, Heslin MJ, Wolf RF, Pisters PWT, Brennan MF. The effect of systemic hyperinsulinemia with concomitant amino acid infusion on skeletal muscle protein turnover in the human forearm. Metabolism 1994; 43: 70–8.

230. Bennet WM, Connacher AA, Scrimgeour CM, Rennie MJ. The effect of amino acid infusion on leg protein turnover assessed by L-[^{15}N]phenylalanine and L-[1-^{13}C]leucine exchange. Eur J Clin Invest 1990; 20: 37–46.

231. Bennett WM, Connacher AA, Scrimgeour CM, Jung RT, Rennie MJ. Euglycemic hyperinsulinemia augments amino acid uptake by leg tissues during hyperaminoacidemia. Am J Physiol 1990; 259: E185–94.

232. Fukagawa NK, Minaker KL, Young VR, Matthews DE, Bier DM, Rowe JW. Leucine metabolism in aging humans: effect of insulin and substrate availability. Am J Physiol 1989; 256 (Endocrinol Metab 19): E288–94.

233. Tessari P, Inchiostro S, Biolo G et al. Differential effects of hyperinsulinemia and hyperaminoacidemia on leucine-carbon metabolism *in vivo*. Evidence for distinct mechanisms in regulation of net amino acid deposition. J Clin Invest 1987; 79: 1062–9.

234. Ferrando AA, Williams BD, Stuart CA, Lane HW, Wolfe RR. Oral branched-chain amino acids decrease

whole-body proteolysis. J Parent Ent Nutr 1995; 19: 47–54.

235. Fukagawa NK, Minaker KL, Rowe JW, Goodman MN, Matthews DE, Bier DM, Young VR. Insulin-mediated reduction of whole body protein breakdown. Dose–response effects on leucine metabolism in postabsorptive men. J Clin Invest 1985; 76: 2306–11.

236. Tessari P, Trevisan R, Inchiostro S et al. Dose-response curves of effects of insulin on leucine kinetics in humans. Am J Physiol 1986; 251 (Endocrinol Metab 14): E334–42.

237. Giordano M, Castellino P, DeFronzo RA. Differential responsiveness of protein synthesis and degradation to amino acid availability in humans. Diabetes 1996; 45: 393–9.

238. Fryburg DA, Louard RJ, Gerow KE, Gelfand RA, Barrett EJ. Growth hormone stimulates skeletal muscle protein synthesis and antagonizes insulin's antiproteolytic action in humans. Diabetes 1992; 41: 424–9.

239. Gelfand RA, Barrett EJ. Effect of physiologic hyperinsulinemia on skeletal muscle protein synthesis and breakdown in man. J Clin Invest 1987; 80: 1–6.

240. Gelfand RA, Glickman MG, Castellino P, Louard RJ, DeFronzo RA. Measurement of L-[14C]leucine kinetics in splanchnic and leg tissues in humans. Diabetes 1988; 37: 1365–72.

241. Bennet WM, Connacher AA, Scrimgeour CM, Jung RT, Rennie MJ. Euglycemic hyperinsulinemia augments amino acid uptake by human leg tissues during hyperaminoacidemia. Am J Physiol 1990; 259 (Endocrinol Metab 22): E185–94.

242. Flaim KE, Hutson SM, Lloyd CE, Taylor JM, Shiman R, Jefferson LS. Direct effect of insulin on albumin gene expression in primary cultures of rat hepatocytes. Am J Physiol 1985; 249: E447–53.

243. Granner DK, Andreone T, Sasake K, Beale E. Inhibition of transcription of the phosphoenolpyruvate carboxylase gene by insulin. Nature (Lond) 1983; 305: 549–51.

244. Dillmann WH. Diabetes mellitus-induced changes in the concentration of specific mRNAs and proteins. Diabetes Metab Rev 1988; 4: 789–97.

245. De Feo P, Gan Gaisano M, Haymond MW. Differential effects of insulin deficiency on albumin and fibrinogen synthesis in humans. J Clin Invest 1991; 88: 833–40.

246. Cusi K, DeFronzo RA. Treatment of NIDDM, IDDM, and other insulin-resistant states with IGF-I. Diabetes Rev 1995; 3: 206–36.

247. Turkalj I, Keller U, Ninnis R, Vosmeer S, Stauffacher W. Effect of increasing doses of recombinant human insulin-like growth factor-I on glucose, lipid, and leucine metabolism in man. J Clin Endocrinol Metab 1992; 75: 1186–91.

248. Fryburg DA. Insulin-like growth factor I exerts growth hormone- and insulin-like actions on human muscle protein metabolism. Am J Physiol 1994; 267: E331–6.

249. Russell-Jones DL, Umpleby AM, Hennessy TR et al. Use of a leucine clamp to demonstrate that IGF-I actively stimulates protein synthesis in normal humans. Am J Physiol 1994; 267: E591–8.

250. Luzi L, Castellino P, Simonson DC, Petrides AS, DeFronzo RA. Leucine metabolism in IDDM. Role of insulin and substrate availability. Diabetes 1990; 39: 38–48.

251. Umpleby AM, Boroujerdi MA, Brown PM, Carson ER, Sönksen PH. The effect of metabolic control on leucine metabolism in type 1 (insulin-dependent) diabetic patients. Diabetologia 1986; 29: 131–41.

252. Nair KS, Ford GC, Halliday D. Effect of intravenous insulin treatment on *in vivo* whole body leucine kinetics and oxygen consumption in insulin-deprived type 1 diabetic patients. Metabolism 1987; 36: 491–5.

253. Robert JJ, Beaufrere B, Koziet J et al. Whole body *de novo* amino acid synthesis in type 1 (insulin-dependent) diabetes studied with stable isotope-labeled leucine, alanine, and glycine. Diabetes 1985; 34: 67–73.

254. Tessari P, Nosadini R, Trevisan R et al. Defective suppression by insulin of leucine-carbon appearance and oxidation in type 1, insulin-dependent diabetes mellitus. Evidence for insulin resistance involving glucose and amino acid metabolism. J Clin Invest 1986; 77: 1797–1804.

255. Nair KS, Garrow JS, Ford C, Mahler RF, Halliday D. Effect of poor diabetic control and obesity on whole body protein metabolism in man. Diabetologia 1983; 25: 400–3.

256. Nair KS, Ford GC, Halliday D. Effect of intravenous insulin treatment on *in vivo* whole body leucine kinetics and oxygen consumption in insulin-deprived type 1 diabetic patients. Metabolism 1987; 36: 491–5.

257. Tessari P, Pehling G, Nissen SL et al. Regulation of whole-body leucine metabolism with insulin during mixed-meal absorption in normal and diabetic humans. Diabetes 1988; 37: 512–19.

258. Tessari P, Biolo G, Inchiostro S et al. Effects of insulin on whole body and forearm leucine and KIC metabolism in type 1 diabetes. Am J Physiol 1990; 259 (Endocrinol Metab 22): E96–103.

259. Pacy PJ, Nair KS, Ford C, Halliday D. Failure of insulin infusion to stimulate fractional muscle protein synthesis in type I diabetic patients. Anabolic effect of insulin and decreased proteolysis. Diabetes 1989; 38: 618–24.

260. Bennet WM, Connacher AA, Jung RT, Stehle P, Rennie MJ. Effects of insulin and amino acids on leg protein turnover in IDDM patients. Diabetes 1991; 40: 499–508.

261. Felig P. Amino acid metabolism in man. Ann Rev Biochem 1975; 44: 933–55.

262. Nair KS, Halliday D, Matthews DE, Welle SL. Hyperglucagonemia during insulin deficiency accelerates protein catabolism. Am J Physiol 1987; 253: E208–13.

263. Jacob R, Barrett E, Plewe G, Fagin K, Sherwin R. Acute effects of insulin-like growth factor I on glucose and amino acid metabolism in the awake fasted rat. J Clin Invest 1989; 83: 1717–23.

264. DeFronzo RA. Lilly Lecture 1987. The triumvirate: beta-cell, muscle, liver. A collusion responsible for NIDDM. Diabetes 1988; 37: 667–87.

265. Luzi L, Petrides AS, DeFronzo RA. Different sensitivity of glucose and amino acid metabolism to insulin in NIDDM. Diabetes 1993; 42: 1868–77.

266. Staten MA, Matthews DE, Bier DM. Leucine metabolism in type 2 diabetes mellitus. Diabetes 1986; 35: 1249–53.

267. Welle SL, Nair KE. Effect of insulin and glyburide treatment on protein metabolism in type 2 diabetes mellitus. Int J Obesity 1990; 16: 701–10.

268. Gougeon R, Pencharz PB, Marliss EB. Effect of NIDDM on the kinetics of whole-body protein metabolism. Diabetes 1994; 43: 318–28.

269. Caballero B, Finer N, Wurtman RJ. Plasma amino acids and insulin levels in obesity: response to carbohydrate intake and tryptophan supplements. Metab Clin Exp 1988; 37: 672–6.

270. Forlani G, Vannini G, Marchesini G, Zoli M, Ciavarella A, Pisi E. Insulin dependent metabolism of branched chain amino acids in obesity. Metab Clin Exp 1984; 33: 147–50.

271. Rice DE, Flakoll PJ, May MM, Hill JO, Abumrad NN. The opposing effects of insulin and hyperglycemia in modulating amino acid metabolism during a glucose tolerance test in lean and obese subjects. Metab Clin Exp 1994; 43: 211–16.

272. Pijl H, van Loon BJP, Toornvliet AC et al. Insulin-induced decline of plasma amino acid concentrations in obese subjects with and without non-insulin-dependent diabetes. Metab Clin Exp 1994; 43: 640–6.

273. Welle S, Statt M, Barnard R, Amatruda J. Differential effect of insulin on whole-body proteolysis and glucose metabolism in normal-weight, obese, and reduced-obese women. Metab Clin Exp 1994; 43: 441–5.

274. Jensen MD, Haymond MW. Protein metabolism in obesity: effects of body fat distribution and hyperinsulinemia on leucine turnover. Am J Clin Nutr 1991; 53: 172–6.

275. Luzi L, Castellino P, DeFronzo RA. Insulin and hyperaminoacidemia regulate by a different mechanism leucine turnover and oxidation in obesity. Am J Physiol 1996; 33: E273–81.

276. Welle S, Barnard RR, Statt M, Amatruda JM. Increased protein turnover in obese women. Metabolism 1992; 41: 1028–34.

277. Caballero B, Wurtman RJ. Differential effects of insulin resistance on leucine and glucose kinetics in obesity. Metab Clin Exp 1991; 40: 51–8.

278. Taylor SI, Kadowaki T, Kadowaki H, Accili D, Cama A, McKeon C. Mutations in insulin-receptor gene in insulin-resistant patients. Diabetes Care 1990; 13: 257–75.

279. McClain DA. Insulin action in cells expressing truncated or kinase-defective insulin receptors. Dissection of multiple hormone-signaling pathways. Diabetes Care 1990; 13: 302–16.

280. Wente SR, Rosen OM. Insulin-receptor approaches to studying protein kinase domain. Diabetes Care 1990; 13: 280–7.

281. Ellis LE, Clauser E, Morgan ME, Roth RA, Rutter WJ. Replacement of insulin receptor tyrosine residues 1162 and 1163 compromises insulin-stimulated kinase activity and uptake of 2-deoxyglucose. Cell 1986; 45: 721–32.

282. Taylor SI, Kadowaki T, Kadowaki H, Accili D, Cama A, McKeon C. Mutations in insulin-receptor gene in insulin-resistant patients. Diabetes Care 1990; 13: 257–75.

283. Chou CK, Dull TJ, Russell DS et al. Human insulin receptors mutated at the ATP-binding site lack protein tyrosine kinase activity and fail to mediate post-receptor effects of insulin. J Biol Chem 1987; 262: 1842–7.

284. Wilden PA, Kahn CR. The level of insulin receptor tyrosine kinase activity modulates the activities of phosphatidylinositol 3-kinase, microtubule-associated protein, and S6 kinases. Molecular Endocrinology 1994; 8: 558–67.

285. Wilden PA, Siddle K, Haring E, Backer JM, White MF, Kahn CR. The role of insulin receptor kinase domain autophosphorylation in receptor-mediated activities. Analysis with insulin and anti-receptor antibodies. J Biol Chem 1992; 267: 13719–27.

286. White MF, Maron R, Kahn CR. Insulin rapidly stimulates tyrosine phosphorylation of a Mr-185 000 protein in intact cells. Nature 1985; 318: 183–6.

287. Cantley LC, Auger KR, Carpenter C et al. Oncogenes and signal transduction. Cell 1991; 64: 281–302.

288. Koch CA, Anderson D, Moran MF, Ellis C, Pawson T. SH2 and SH3 domains: elements that control interactions of cytoplasmic signaling. Science 1991; 252: 668–74.

289. Okada T, Kawano Y, Sakakibara T, Hazeki O, Ui M. Essential role of phosphatidylinositol 3-kinase in insulin-induced glucose transport and antilipolysis in rat adipocytes. Studies with a selective inhibitor, wortmannin. J Biol Chem 1994; 269: 3568–73.

290. Hara K, Yonezawa K, Sakaue H et al. 1-phosphatidylinositol 3-kinase activity is required for insulin-stimulated glucose transport but not for Ras activation in CHO cells. Proc Natl Acad Sci USA 1994; 91: 7415–19.

291. Cheatham B, Vlahos CJ, Cheatham L, Wang L, Blenis J, Kahn CR. Phosphatidylinositol 3-kinase activation is required for insulin stimulation of pp70 S6 kinase, DNA synthesis, and glucose transporter translocation. Mol Cell Biol 1994; 14: 4902–11.

292. Downward J. The grb2/Sem-5 adaptor protein. FEBS Letters 1994; 338: 113–17.

293. Scolnick EY, Batzer A, Li N et al. The function of GRB2 in linking the insulin receptor to Ras signaling pathways. Science 1993; 260: 1953–5.

294. Seger R, Krebs EG. The MAPK signaling cascade. FASEB J 1995; 9: 726–35.

295. Sun XJ, Rothenberg P, Kahn CR et al. Structure of the insulin receptor substrate IRS-1 defines a unique signal transduction protein. Nature 1991; 352: 73–7.

296. Yamauchi K, Pessin JE. Insulin receptor substrate-1 (IRS1) and Shc compete for a limited pool of Grb2 in mediating insulin downstream signaling. J Biol Chem 1994; 269: 31107–14.

297. Ouwens DM, van der Zon GCM, Pronk GJ et al. A mutant insulin receptor induces formation of a Shc-growth factor receptor bound protein 2 (Grb2) complex and p21ras-GTP without detectable interaction of insulin receptor substrate 1 (IRS1) with Grb2. J Biol Chem 1994; 269: 33116–22.

298. Sasaoka T, Draznin B, Leitner JW, Langlois WJ, Olefsky JM. Shc is the predominant signaling molecule coupling insulin receptors to activation of guanine nucleotide releasing factor and p21ras-GTP formation. J Biol Chem 1994; 269: 10734–8.

299. Sasaoka T, Rose DW, Jhun BH, Saltiel AR, Draznin B, Olefsky JM. Evidence for a functional role of Shc proteins in mitogenic signaling induced by insulin, insulin-like growth factor-1, and epidermal growth factor. J Biol Chem 1994; 269: 13689–94.

300. Araki E, Lipes MA, Patti ME et al. Alternative pathway of insulin signalling in mice with targeted disruption of the IRS-1 gene. Nature 1994; 372: 186–90.

301. Boudewijn M, Burgering T, Bos JL. Regulation of Ras-mediated signalling: more than one way to skin a cat. TIBS 1995; 20: 18–22.

302. Langlois WJ, Sasaoka T, Saltiel AR, Olefsky JM. Negative feedback regulation and desensitization of

insulin- and epidermal growth factor-stimulated p21ras activation. J Biol Chem 1995; 270: 25320-3.

303. Sakaue M, Bowtell D, Kasuga M. A dominant-negative mutant of mSOS1 inhibits insulin-induced Ras activation and reveals Ras-dependent and Ras-independent insulin signaling pathways. Mol Cell Biol 1995; 15: 379-88.

304. Campbell JS, Seger R, Graves JD, Graves LM, Jensen AM, Krebs EG. The MAP kinase cascade. Rec Prog Horm Res 1995; 50: 131-59.

305. Edlar-Finkelman H, Seger R, Vandenheede JR, Krebs EG. Inactivation of glycogen synthase kinase-3 by epidermal growth factor is mediated by mitogen-activated protein kinase/p90 ribosomal protein S6 kinase signaling pathway in HIH/3T3 cells. J Biol Chem 1995; 270: 987-90.

306. Denton RM, Tavare JM. Does mitogen-activated-protein kinase have a role in insulin action? The cases for and against. Eur J Biochem 1995; 227: 597-611.

307. Haystead TA, Haystead CM, Hu C, Lin TA, Lawrence JC. Phosphorylation of PHAS-1 by mitogen-activated protein (MAP) kinase. Identification of a site phosphorylated by MAP kinase *in vitro* and in response to insulin in rat adipocytes. J Biol Chem 1994; 269: 23185-91.

308. Traugh JA, Pendergast AM. Regulation of protein synthesis by phosphorylation of ribosomal protein S6 and aminoacyl-tRNA synthetases. Prog Nucleic Acid Res Mol Biol 1986; 33: 195-230.

309. Gressner AM, Wool IG. The stimulation of the phosphorylation of ribosomal protein S6 by cycloheximide and puromycin. Biochem Biophys Res Commun 1974; 60: 1482-90.

310. Nielsen PJ, Manchester KL, Towbin H, Gordon J, Thomas G. The phosphorylation of ribosomal protein S6 in rat tissues following cycloheximide injection, in diabetes, and after denervation of diaphragm. A simple immunological determination of the extent of S6 phosphorylation on protein blots. J Biol Chem 1982; 257: 12316-21.

311. Gressner AM, Wool IG. Effect of experimental diabetes and insulin on phosphorylation of rat liver ribosomal protein S6. Nature 1976; 259: 148-50.

312. Proud CG. Protein phosphorylation in translational control. Curr Topics Cell Reg 1992; 32: 243-69.

313. Kipnis DM, Noall MW. Stimulation of amino acid transport by insulin in the isolated rat diaphragm. Biochim Biophys Acta 1958; 28: 226-7.

314. Akedo H, Christensen HN. Nature of insulin action on amino acid uptake by the isolated diaphragm. J Biol Chem 1962; 237: 118-22.

315. Wool IG, Castles JJ, Moyer AN. Regulation of amino acid accumulation in isolated rat diaphragm: effect of puromycin and insulin. Biochim Biophys Acta 1965; 107: 333-45.

316. Manchester KL, Wool IG. Insulin and incorporation of amino acids into protein of muscle. 2. Accumulation and incorporation studies with the perfused rat heart. Biochem J 1963; 89: 202-9.

317. Guidotti GG, Borghetti AF, Gaja G, Loreti L, Ragnotti G, Foá PP. Amino acid uptake in the developing chick embryo heart. The effect of insulin on alpha-aminoisobutyric acid accumulation. Biochem J 1968; 107: 565-74.

318. Touabi M, Jeanrenaud B. Alpha-aminoisobutyric acid uptake in isolated mouse fat cells. Biochim Biophys Acta 1969; 173: 128-40.

319. Schwartz A. Hormonal regulation of amino acid accumulation in human fetal liver explants. Effects of dibutyryl cyclic AMP, glucagon and insulin. Biochim Biophys Acta 1974; 362: 276-89.

320. Le Cam A, Freychet P. Effect of insulin on amino acid transport in isolated rat hepatocytes. Diabetologia 1978; 15: 117-23.

321. Riggs TR, McKirahan KJ. Action of insulin on transport of L-alanine into rat diaphragm *in vitro*. Evidence that the hormone affects only one neutral amino acid transport system. J Biol Chem 1973; 248: 6450-5.

322. Guidotti GG, Franchi-Gazzola R, Gazzola GC, Ronchi P. Regulation of amino acid transport in chick embryo heart cells. IV. Site and mechanism of insulin action. Biochim Biophys Acta 1974; 356: 219-30.

323. Elsas LJ, Wheeler FB, Danner DJ, DeHaan RL. Amino acid transport by aggregates of cultured chicken heart cells. J Biol Chem 1975; 250: 9381-90.

324. Elsas LJ, MacDonell RC Jr, Rosenberg LE. Influence of age on insulin stimulation of amino acid uptake in rat diaphragm. J Biol Chem 1971; 246: 6452-9.

325. Goldfine ID, Gardner JD, Neville DM Jr. Insulin action in isolated rat thymocytes. I. Binding of ^{125}I-insulin and stimulation of α-aminoisobutyric acid transport. J Biol Chem 1972; 247: 6919-26.

326. Goldfine ID. Binding of insulin to thymocytes from suckling and hypophysectomized rats: evidence for two mechanisms regulating insulin sensitivity. Endocrinology 1975; 97: 948-54.

327. Soll AH, Goldfine ID, Roth J, Kahn CR. Thymic lymphocytes in obese (ob-ob) mice. A mirror of the insulin receptor defect in liver and fat. J Biol Chem 1974; 249: 4127-31.

328. Bennet WM, Connacher AA, Smith K, Jung RT, Rennie MJ. Inability to stimulate skeletal muscle or whole body protein synthesis in type 1 (insulin-dependent) diabetic patients by insulin-plus-glucose during amino acid infusion: studies of incorporation and turnover of tracer L-[1-^{13}C]leucine. Diabetologia 1990; 33: 43-51.

329. Peavy DE, Taylor JM, Jefferson LS. Correlation of albumin production rates and albumin mRNA levels in livers of normal, diabetic, and insulin-treated diabetic rats. Proc Natl Acad Sci USA 1978; 75: 5879-83.

330. Peavy DE, Taylor JM, Jefferson LS. Time course of changes in albumin synthesis and mRNA in diabetic and insulin-treated diabetic rats. Am J Physiol 1985; 248: E656-63.

331. Jhun BH, Haruta T, Meinkoth JL et al. Signal transduction pathways leading to insulin-induced early gene expression. Biochemistry 1995; 34: 7996-8004.

332. Maniatis T, Goodbourn S, Fischer JA. Regulation of inducible and tissue-specific gene expression. Science 1987; 236: 1237-45.

333. Meisler MH, Howard G. Effects of insulin on gene transcription. Annu Rev Physiol 1989; 51: 701-14.

334. Goldfine ID. Interaction of insulin, polypeptide hormones and growth factors with intracellular membranes. Biochim Biophys Acta 1981; 650: 53-67.

335. Goldfine ID, Smith GJ. Binding of insulin to isolated nuclei. Proc Natl Acad Sci USA 1976; 73: 1427-31.

336. Peralta Soler A, Thompson KA, Smith RM, Jarett L. Immunological demonstration of the accumulation of insulin, but not insulin receptors, in nuclei of insulin-treated cells. Proc Natl Acad Sci USA 1989; 86: 6640-4.

337. Thompson KA, Peralta Soler A, Smith RM, Jarett L. Intranuclear localization of insulin in rat hepatoma cells: insulin/matrix association. Eur J Cell Biol 1989; 50: 442–6.

338. Miller DS. Stimulation of RNA and protein synthesis by intracellular insulin. Science 1988; 240: 506–9.

339. Alexander MC, Lomanto M, Nasrin N, Ramaika C. Insulin regulates glyceraldehyde-3-phosphate dehydrogenase (GAPDH) gene expression through *cis*-acting DNA sequences. Proc Natl Acad Sci USA 1988; 85: 5092–6.

340. Osborn LO, Rosenberg MP, Keller SA, Meisler M. Tissue-specific and insulin-dependent expression of a pancreatic amylase gene in transgenic mice. Mol Cell Biol 1987; 7: 326–34.

341. Stumpo DJ, Stewart TN, Gilman MZ, Blackshear PJ. Identification of c-*fos* sequences involved in induction by insulin and phorbol esters. J Biol Chem 1988; 263: 1611–14.

342. Stumpo DJ, Blackshear PJ. Cellular expression of mutant insulin receptors interferes with rapid transcriptional response to both insulin and insulin-like-growth factor 1. J. Biol Chem 1991; 266: 455–60.

343. Kadonaga JT, Tjian R. Affinity purification of sequence-specific DNA binding proteins. Proc Natl Acad Sci USA 1986; 83: 5889–93.

344. Singh H, LeBowitz JH, Baldwin AS, Sharp PA. Molecular cloning of an enhancer binding protein: isolation by screening of an expression library with a recognition site DNA. Cell 1988; 52: 415–23.

345. Sutherland C, O'Brien RM, Granner DK. Phosphatidylinositol 3-kinase, but not p70/p85 ribosomal S6 protein kinase, is required for the regulation of phosphoenolpyruvate carboxy kinase (PEPCK) gene expression by insulin. Dissociation of signaling pathways for insulin and phorbol ester regulation of PEPCK gene expression. J Biol Chem 1995; 270: 15501–6.

346. Sasaki K, Granner DK. Regulation of phosphoenolpyruvate carboxykinase gene transcription by insulin and cAMP: reciprocal actions on initiation and elongation. Proc Natl Acad Sci USA 1988; 85: 2954–8.

347. Jefferson LS, Liao WSL, Peavy DE, Miller TB, Appel MC, Taylor JM. Diabetes-induced alterations in liver protein synthesis. Changes in the relative abundance of mRNAs for albumin and other plasma proteins. J Biol Chem 1983; 258: 1369–75.

348. Kimball SR, Horetsky RL, Jefferson LS. Hormonal regulation of albumin gene expression in primary cultures of rat hepatocytes. Am J Physiol 1995; 268: E6–14.

349. Lloyd CE, Kalinyak JE, Hutson SM, Jefferson LS. Stimulation of albumin gene transcription by insulin in primary cultures of rat hepatocytes. Am J Physiol 1987; 252: C205–14.

350. Decaux J-F, Antoine B, Kahn A. Regulation of the expression of the L-type pyruvate kinase gene in adult rat hepatocytes in primary culture. J Biol Chem 1989; 264: 11584–90.

351. Fernyhough P, Mill JF, Roberts JL, Ishii DN. Stabilization of tubulin mRNAs by insulin and insulin-like growth factor I during neurite formation. Brain Res Mol Brain Res 1989; 6: 109–20.

352. Davis BB, Magge S, Mucenski CG, Drake RL. Insulin-mediated post-transcriptional regulation of hepatic malic enzyme and albumin mRNAs. Biochem Biophys Res Commun 1988; 154: 1081–7.

353. Wilson SB, Back DW, Morris SM Jr, Swierczynski J. Hormonal regulation of lipogenic enzymes in chick embryo hepatocytes in culture. Expression of the fatty acid synthetase gene is regulated at both translational and pretranslational steps. J Biol Chem 1986; 261: 15179–82.

354. Semenkovich CF, Wims M, Noe L, Etienne J, Chan L. Insulin regulation of lipoprotein lipase activity in 3T3-L1 adipocytes is mediated at post-transcriptional and post-translational levels. J Biol Chem 1989; 264: 9030–8.

355. Okabayashi Y, Moessner J, Logsdon CD, Goldfine ID, Williams JA. Insulin and other stimulants have non-parallel translational effects on protein synthesis. Diabetes 1987; 36: 1054–60.

356. Nielsen FC, Gammeltoft S, Christiansen J. Translational discrimination of mRNAs coding for human insulin-like growth factor II. J Biol Chem 1990; 265: 13431–4.

357. Hammond ML, Bowman LH. Insulin stimulates the translation of ribosomal proteins and the transcription of rDNA in mouse myoblasts. J Biol Chem 1988; 263: 17785–91.

358. Standart N, Jackson RJ. Regulation of translation by specific protein/mRNA interactions. Biochimie 1994; 76: 867–79.

359. Manzella JM, Rychlik W, Phoads RE, Hershey JWB, Blackshear PJ. Insulin induction of ornithine decarboxylase: importance of mRNA secondary structure and phosphorylation of eucaryotic initiation factors eIF-4B and eIF-4E. J Biol Chem 1991; 266: 2383–9.

360. Klausner RD, Rouault TA, Hartford JB. Regulating the fate of mRNA: the control of cellular iron metabolism. Cell 1993; 72: 19–28.

361. Levy S, Avni D, Hariharan N, Perry RP, Meyuhas O. Oligopyrimidine tract at the 5′ end of mammalian ribosomal protein mRNAs is required for their translational control. Proc Natl Acad Sci USA 1991; 88: 3319–23.

362. Rannels DE, Jefferson LS, Hjalmarson AC, Wolpert EB, Morgan HE. Maintenance of protein synthesis in hearts of diabetic animals. Biochem Biophy Res Comm 1970; 40: 1110–16.

363. Jefferson LS, Flaim KE, Morgan HE. Peptide-chain initiation in heart and skeletal muscle. In Atkinson DE, Fox CF (eds) Modulation of Protein Function. New York: Academic Press, 1979; pp 369–89.

364. Jeffrey IW, Kelly FJ, Duncan R, Hershey JWB, Pain VM. Effect of starvation and diabetes on the activity of the eukaryotic initiation factor eIF-2 in rat skeletal muscle. Biochimie 1990; 72: 751–7.

365. Peterson DT, Alfor EP, Reaven EP, Ueyama I, Reaven GM. Characteristics of membrane-bound and free hepatic ribosomes from insulin-deficient rats. I. Acute experimental diabetes mellitus. J Clin Invest 1973; 52: 3201–11.

366. Tragl KH, Reaven GM. Effect of insulin deficiency on hepatic ribosomal aggregation. Diabetes 1972; 21: 84–8.

367. Pilkis SJ, Korner A. Effect of diabetes and insulin treatment on protein synthetic activity of rat liver ribosomes. Biochim Biophys Acta 1971; 247: 597–608.

368. Wittman JS III, Lee K-L, Miller ON. Dietary and hormonal influences on rat liver polysome profiles; fat, glucose and insulin. Biochim Biophys Acta 1969; 174: 536–43.

369. Korner A. Alloxan diabetes and *in vitro* protein biosynthesis in rat liver microsomes and mitochondria. J Endocrinol 1960; 20: 256-65.

370. Pain VM. Protein synthesis in a postmitochondrial supernatant system from rat liver. An effect of diabetes at the level of peptide chain initiation. FEBS Lett 1973; 35: 169-71.

371. Flaim KE, Liao WSL, Peavy DE, Taylor JM, Jefferson LS. The role of amino acids in the regulation of protein synthesis in perfused rat liver. II. Effects of amino acid deficiency on peptide chain initiation, polysomal aggregation, and distribution of albumin mRNA. J Biol Chem 1982; 257: 2939-46.

372. Pain VM, Henshaw EC. Initiation of protein synthesis in Ehrlich ascites tumour cells. Evidence for physiological variation in the association of methionyl-$tRNA_f$ with native 40-S ribosomal subunits *in vivo* Eur J Biochem 1975; 57: 335-42.

373. Kimball SR, Jefferson LS. Effect of diabetes on guanine nucleotide exchange factor activity in skeletal muscle and heart. Biochem Biophys Res Commun 1988; 156: 706-11.

374. Morley SJ. Signal transduction mechanisms in the regulation of protein synthesis. Mol Biol Rep 1994; 19: 221-31.

375. Kurihara K, Wool IG. Effect of insulin on the synthesis of sarcoplasmic and ribosomal proteins of muscle. Nature 1968; 219: 721-4.

376. Raw I, Juliani MH, Rocha MC, Maia JCC. Effect of insulin on the synthesis of rat liver ribosomal and endoplasmic reticulum proteins. Braz J Med Biol Res 1985; 18: 421-6.

377. Long EO, Dawic IB. Repeated genes in eukaryotes. Ann Rev Biochem 1980; 49: 727-64.

378. Wolf SF, Schlessinger D. Nuclear metabolism of ribosomal RNA in growing, methionine-limited and methionine-treated HeLa cells. Biochemistry 1977; 16: 2783-91.

379. Greenberg H, Penman S. Methylation and processing of ribosomal RNA in HeLa cells. J Mol Biol 1966; 21: 527-35.

380. DePhilip RM, Rudert WA, Lieberman I. Preferential stimulation of ribosomal protein synthesis by insulin and in the absence of ribosomal and messenger ribonucleic acid formation. Biochemistry 1980; 19: 1662-9.

381. Ignotz GG, Hokari S, DePhilip RM, Tsukada K, Lieberman I. Biochemistry 1981; 20: 2550-8.

382. Palmer RM, Bain PA. Indomethacin inhibits the insulin-induced increases in RNA and protein synthesis in L6 skeletal muscle myoblasts. Prostaglandins 1989; 37: 193-6.

383. Palmer RM, Campbell GP, Whitelaw PF, Brown DS, Bain PA, Hesketh JE. The cyclo-oxygenase inhibitors indomethacin and ibuprofen inhibit the insulin-induced stimulation of ribosomal RNA synthesis in L6 myoblasts. Biochem J 1989; 262: 101-6.

384. Sameshima M, Liebhaber SA, Schlessinger D. Dual pathways for ribonucleic acid turnover in WI-38 but not in I-cell human diploid fibroblasts. Mol Cell Biol 1981; 1: 75-81.

385. Hirsch CA, Hiatt HH. Turnover of liver ribosomes in fed and in fasted rats. J Biol Chem 1966; 241: 5936-40.

386. Tsurugi K, Morita T, Ogata K. Mode of degradation of ribosomes in regenerating rat liver *in vivo*. Eur J Biochem 1974; 45: 119-26.

387. Lardeux BR, Mortimore GE. Amino acid and hormonal control of macromolecular turnover in perfused rat liver. Evidence for selective autophagy. J Biol Chem 1987; 262: 14514-19.

388. Bates PC, Millward DJ. Myofibrillar protein turnover. Biochem J 1983; 214: 587-92.

389. Pfeifer U, Strauss P. Autophagic vacuoles in heart muscle and liver. A comparative morphometric study including circadian variations in meal-fed rats. J Mol Cell Cardiol 1981; 13: 37-49.

390. Schiaffiano SS, Hanzilkova V. Studies on the effect of denervation in developing muscle. II. The lysosomal system. J Ultrastruct Res 1972; 39: 1-14.

391. Pozefsky T, Felig P, Tobin J, Soeldner JS, Cahill GF. Amino acid balance across the tissues of the forearm in postabsorptive man: effects of insulin at two dose levels. J Clin Invest 1969; 48: 2273-82.

392. Wahren J, Felig P, Hagenfeldt J. Effect of protein ingestion on splanchnic and leg metabolism in normal man and in patients with diabetes mellitus. J Clin Invest 1976; 57: 987-99.

393. Wahren J, Felig P, Cerasi E, Luft R. Splanchnic and peripheral glucose and amino acid metabolism in diabetes mellitus. J Clin Invest 1972; 51: 1870-8.

394. Chang TW, Goldberg AL. The metabolic fates of amino acids and the formation of glutamine in skeletal muscle. J Biol Chem 1978; 253: 3685-93.

395. Ruderman NB. Muscle amino acid metabolism and gluconeogenesis. Ann Rev Med 1975; 26: 245-58.

396. Elia M, Neale G, Lively G. Alanine and glutamine release from the human forearm: effects of glucose administration. Clinical Science 1985; 69: 123-33.

397. Marliss EB, Aoki TT, Pozefsky T, Most AS, Cahill GF. Muscle and splanchnic glutamine and glutamate metabolism in postabsorptive and starved man. J Clin Invest 1971; 50: 814-17.

398. Gelfand RA, Glickman MG, Jacob R, Sherwin RS, DeFronzo RA. Removal of infused amino acids by splanchnic and leg tissues in humans. Am J Physiol 1986; 250: E407-13.

399. Gelfand RA, Glickman MG, Castellino P, Louard RJ, DeFronzo RA. Measurement of L-[1-^{14}C]leucine kinetics in splanchnic and leg tissues in humans. Diabetes 1988; 37: 1365-72.

400. Felig P, Wahren J, Karl I, Cerasi E, Luft R, Kipnis DM. Glutamine and glutamate metabolism in normal and diabetic subjects. Diabetes 1973; 22: 573-6.

401. Ferrannini E, DeFronzo RA, Gusberg R. Splanchnic amino acid and glucose metabolism during amino acid infusion in dogs. Diabetes 1988; 37: 237-45.

402. Barrett EJ, Gusberg R, Ferrannini E et al. Amino acid and glucose metabolism in the postabsorptive state and following amino acid ingestion in the dog. Metabolism 1986; 35: 709-17.

403. Perriello G, Jorde R, Nurjhan N et al. Estimation of glucose-alanine-lactate-glutamine cycles in postabsorptive humans: role of skeletal muscle. Am J Physiol 1995; 269: E443-50.

404. Nurjhan N, Bucci A, Perriello G et al. Glutamine: a major gluconeogenic precursor and vehicle for interorgan carbon transport in man. J Clin Invest 1995; 95: 272-7.

405. Owen EE, Robinson RR. Amino acid extraction and ammonia metabolism by the human kidney during the prolonged administration of ammonium chloride. J Clin Invest 1963; 42: 263-76.

406. Addae SK, Lotspeich WD. Relation between glutamine utilization and production in metabolic acidosis. Am J Physiol 1968; 215: 269–77.

407. Windmueller HG, Spaeth AE. Identification of ketone bodies and glutamine as the major respiratory fuels *in vivo* for postabsorptive rat small intestine. J Biol Chem 1978; 253: 69–76.

408. Felig P, Owen OE, Wahren J, Cahill GF. Amino acid metabolism during prolonged starvation. J Clin Invest 1969; 48: 584–94.

409. Felig P, Pozefsky T, Marliss E, Cahill GF. Alanine: key role in gluconeogenesis. Science 1979; 167: 1003–4.

410. Mallete LE, Exton JH, Park CR. Control of gluconeogenesis from amino acids in the perfused rat liver. J Biol Chem 1969; 244: 5713–23.

411. Felig P, Wahren J, Sherwin R, Palaiologos G. Amino acid and protein metabolism in diabetes mellitus. Arch Intern Med 1977; 137: 507–13.

412. Chang TW, Goldberg AL. The origin of alanine produced in skeletal muscle. J Biol Chem 1978; 253: 3677–84.

413. Odessey R, Khairallah EA, Goldberg AL. Origin and possible significance of alanine production by skeletal muscle. J Biol Chem 1974; 249: 7623–9.

414. Chang TW, Goldberg AL. The metabolic fates of amino acids and the formations of glutamine in skeletal muscle. J Biol Chem 1978; 253: 3685–95.

415. Windmueller HG, Spaeth AE. Uptake and metabolism of plasma glutamine by the small intestine. J Biol Chem 1974; 249: 5070–9.

416. Shulman GI, Lacy WW, Liljenquist JE, Keller U, Williams PE, Cherrington AD. Effect of glucose, independent of changes in insulin and glucagon secretion, on alanine metabolism in the conscious dog. J Clin Invest 1980; 65: 496–505.

417. Aikawa T, Matsutaka H, Yamamoto H et al. Gluconeogenesis and amino acid metabolism. Interorgan relations and roles of glutamine and alanine in the amino acid metabolism of fasted rats. J Biochem 1973; 74: 1003–17.

418. Chiasson JL, Liljenquist JE, Sinclair-Smith BC, Lacy WW. Gluconeogenesis from alanine in normal postabsorptive man. Intrahepatic stimulatory effect of glucagon. Diabetes 1975; 24: 574–84.

419. Frame EG. The levels of individual free amino acids in the plasma of normal man at various intervals after a high-protein meal. J Clin Invest 1958; 37: 1710–23.

420. Consoli A, Nurjahn N, Capani F, Gerich J. Predominant role of gluconeogenesis in increased hepatic glucose production in NIDDM. Diabetes 1989; 38: 550–6.

421. Felig P, Wahren J, Hendler R. Influence of oral glucose ingestion on splanchnic glucose and gluconeogenic substrate metabolism. Diabetes 1975; 24: 468–75.

422. Chiasson JL, Atkinson RL, Cherrington AD et al. Effects of insulin at two dose levels on gluconeogenesis from alanine in fasting man. Metabolism 1980; 29: 810–18.

423. Carlsten A, Hallgren B, Jagenburg R et al. Amino acids and free fatty acids in plasma in diabetes. Acta Med Scand 1966; 179: 361–70.

424. Sherwin R, Rosenzweig J, Soman V, Hendler R, Felig P. Effect of insulin and diabetes on protein and branched chain amino acid utilization. Diabetes 1976; 25 (suppl 1): 332.

425. Chirgwin JM. Molecular biology for non-molecular biologists. Diabetes Care 1990; 13: 188–97.

28

The Assessment of Insulin Action *In Vivo*

M. Walker, G.R. Fulcher and K.G.M.M. Alberti

Human Diabetes and Metabolism Research Centre, University of Newcastle upon Tyne, UK

Diabetes mellitus encompasses several distinct clinical syndromes [1, 2]. Most patients have either insulin dependent diabetes mellitus (IDDM) or non-insulin dependent diabetes mellitus (NIDDM), in both of which conditions abnormalities of insulin secretion are found. In the former, insulin secretion is lacking and patients are prone to ketosis. In patients with NIDDM, insulin levels in absolute terms are often similar to, or greater than, the levels found in normal subjects [3, 4], suggesting that there is decreased responsiveness to insulin. More recently it has been recognized that insulin action is abnormal in both major forms of diabetes, and in patients with NIDDM it may be a fundamental metabolic abnormality. To document this, a quantitative relationship between plasma insulin levels and a measurable insulin-induced biological response must be established. The development of a sensitive radioimmunoassay for insulin [5, 6] and simple, accurate and reproducible tests of insulin action *in vivo* are the keys to this process. The pathophysiology of diminished insulin responsiveness is dealt with elsewhere in this book; this chapter focuses on the tests that have been used to quantitate insulin sensitivity. Almost without exception, these tests have assessed changes in blood glucose levels or changes in carbohydrate metabolism. This inherently provides a very narrow definition of insulin sensitivity.

Tests of insulin action can be broadly separated into those that measure insulin action indirectly, and those that provide direct measures. Indirect tests measure the action of endogenous insulin, usually in response to a glucose stimulus, whereas direct tests measure the metabolic responses to exogenous insulin (Table 1).

The development of these techniques has allowed insulin action to be quantitated *in vivo* and, as a result, changes in insulin action have been clearly documented in patients with diabetes. The advantages and disadvantages of the most commonly used methods are discussed below.

INDIRECT ASSESSMENT OF INSULIN SENSITIVITY

Basal (Fasting) Measurements of Plasma Glucose and Insulin Levels

Basal plasma glucose and insulin levels have been used to estimate insulin sensitivity. Two different approaches can be followed. First, the ratio of basal insulin to glucose concentrations has long been used but no attempts have been made to validate its use. Second, Turner and co-workers, in the late 1970s, constructed a mathematical model to predict the interaction of two potential determinants of glycaemia in diabetic patients, namely insulin deficiency and insulin resistance [7]. This was later termed the homeostatic model assessment (HOMA) [93], and has been reviewed recently [94]. This model was based upon the known characteristics of the B-cell response to glucose, together with the levels of basal plasma glucose and insulin concentrations. The two basic assumptions of the model were:

(1) The degree to which basal glucose concentration increased in response to insulin deficiency reflected the shape of the normal insulin secretory response to glucose.

International Textbook of Diabetes Mellitus, Second Edition. Edited by K.G.M.M. Alberti, P. Zimmet, R.A. DeFronzo, and H. Keen (Honorary)
© 1997 John Wiley & Sons Ltd

Table 1 Methods for studying human insulin sensitivity

Indirect	Direct
Measurement of circulating insulin and glucose:	Insulin tolerance test
	Euglycaemic hyperinsulinaemic clamp
	Insulin suppression test
Fasting values	
OGTT	
IVGTT	
Minimal model	
CIGMA	

(2)   Basal insulin levels were directly proportional to insulin resistance.

Plotting plasma insulin concentrations against plasma glucose levels predicted the proportion of insulin deficiency and insulin resistance present (Figure 1). This model has supported the view that insulin resistance is significant in NIDDM patients. It is not widely used, both because of the assumptions made, and also because it has not been possible to obtain independent validation of the accuracy of the values derived. There are, however, significant correlations with the euglycaemic clamp (see below), but such correlations are weak. This is not surprising in that basal insulin sensitivity is compared in the one case, with sensitivity at higher insulin levels in the other. The model is none the less important as one of the few attempts to assess insulin responsiveness in the basal state. We

have used the HOMA model in two population studies [8, 95], and found good correlations between HOMA measures of resistance and other metabolic variables, not found when insulin/glucose ratios or fasting insulin levels were used, thus suggesting some sort of validity.

One criticism has emerged and applies to all the methods dependent upon the measurement of endogenous insulin. It has been reported that conventionally measured immunoreactive insulin also measures the biologically less active proinsulin and proinsulin split products [9]. These make up approximately 10% of total insulin reactivity in normal individuals, but this may increase to 50% or more in NIDDM [9, 10]. Thus, apparently high insulin levels (which would be interpreted as showing insulin resistance) may be spurious. Studies must be repeated using more specific insulin assays. It is also worth adding that peripheral insulin levels are measured, whereas insulin is secreted into the portal vein with variable extraction by the liver. Hepatic insulin sensitivity is thus assessed indirectly, at best, by measuring peripheral venous insulin levels; C peptide-derived portal insulin levels should perhaps be calculated.

Postprandial Measurements of Plasma Glucose and Insulin Levels

Other attempts to measure insulin sensitivity have been made by taking simultaneous measurements of glucose

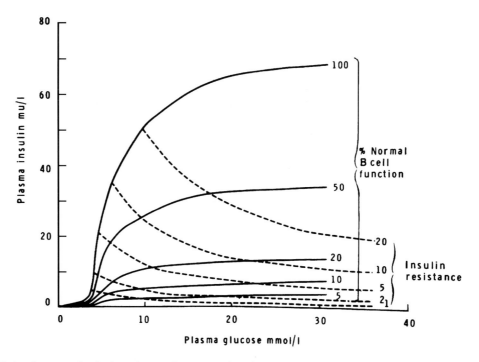

Figure 1   Relation between the fasting plasma glucose and insulin concentrations, appropriate for different degrees of insulin deficiency and insulin resistance. The continuous lines represent B-cell function with different degrees of B-cell deficit. From the graph it is theoretically possible to estimate directly the B-cell deficiency and insulin resistance from the basal plasma glucose and insulin concentrations of a patient. From reference 7, with permission

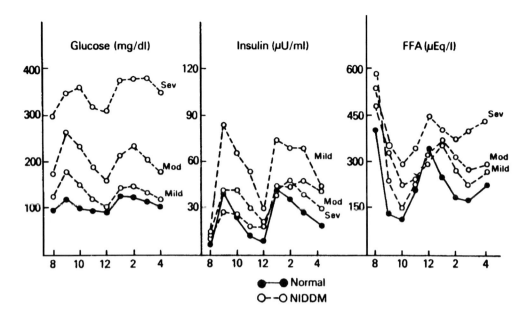

Figure 2 Mean fasting and postprandial plasma glucose, insulin and free fatty acid (FFA) concentrations in normal subjects (solid circles) and patients with NIDDM (open circles). The patients with NIDDM were divided into mild, moderate or severe, on the basis of fasting plasma glucose levels. From reference 4, with permission, © 1985 The Endocrine Society

and insulin across the day and comparing these estimations [4]. This approach has been used by Reaven and colleagues to clarify the metabolic characteristics of normal-weight and obese diabetic subjects [4, 11]. The clearest evidence of insulin resistance from these studies is found in patients with the lowest levels of plasma glucose (Figure 2). Thus, patients with 'mild' NIDDM (i.e. lesser degrees of hyperglycaemia) have postprandial plasma insulin levels that are higher than those of normal subjects throughout the day. This implies that insulin action is abnormal in these patients. The finding that plasma non-esterified fatty acids are also raised throughout the day, despite the absolute elevation in insulin levels, further supports this notion.

In general, static measures of glucose and insulin levels may be useful to establish metabolic patterns and relationships between variables, but provide only limited quantitative information concerning insulin action.

Oral Glucose Tolerance Test

One of the earliest tests of insulin action was the oral glucose tolerance test (OGTT) [6]. Although it was primarily used to measure and diagnose abnormalities of glucose tolerance [2], additional information can be obtained from the test if insulin levels are measured simultaneously with glucose levels at each time point. By comparing insulin responses at comparable levels of glycaemia, an indirect measure of insulin action is obtained. Thus, non-diabetic subjects of normal weight have widely variable insulin responses following a standard 75 g glucose load, despite very similar

glucose responses [12] (Figure 3). Assuming normal pancreatic secretory capacity, then insulin action must vary even in normal subjects; that is, the greater the insulin response to glucose, the more insulin-resistant the subject if glucose levels remain the same. Similarly, in obese non-diabetic subjects [13] and in patients with impaired glucose tolerance [14], cirrhosis [15] and uraemia [16], decreased insulin action has been documented, or at least inferred, by finding increased plasma insulin levels with simultaneous normal glucose tolerance curves.

Nevertheless, measuring insulin action in this way has major limitations. First, insulin resistance can be documented unequivocally only when insulin levels are elevated in the presence of normal or supranormal plasma glucose levels, i.e. when the pancreatic response to hyperglycaemia is preserved. Such is the case for each of the conditions listed above. By comparison, this is not usually seen in patients who are overtly diabetic [14]. As fasting plasma glucose levels rise toward diabetic levels, the mean plasma insulin response during an OGTT progressively falls, indicating the development of relative insulinopenia [17] (Figure 4). This is most pronounced in patients with higher levels of fasting plasma glucose (greater than 11.1 mmol/l, 200 mg/dl). In these subjects with more severe hyperglycaemia during an OGTT, plasma insulin responses are often less than normal in absolute terms [18]. These patients are unequivocally insulin deficient. Although these patients may also be insulin resistant, this cannot be stated on the basis of the OGTT data [14].

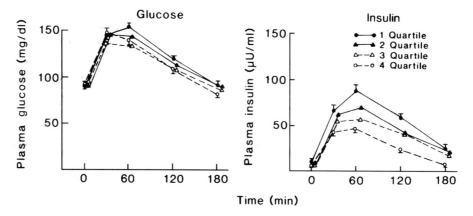

Figure 3 Plasma glucose (left) and insulin (right) responses to 75 g oral glucose challenge in normal subjects with differing sensitivity to insulin. From reference 12, with permission, © 1987 The Endocrine Society

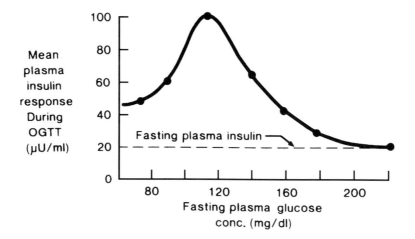

Figure 4 In normal-weight patients with impaired glucose tolerance and mild diabetes mellitus, plasma insulin responses to an oral glucose challenge progressively increase until fasting plasma glucose concentrations reach 120 mg/dl (6.7 mmol/1). Further increases in fasting glucose levels are associated with a progressive decline in insulin secretion. From reference 17, with permission

The usefulness of the OGTT as a measure of insulin action is limited. The test is poorly reproducible [19, 20] with a wide coefficient of variation (up to 40%) [21]. Variations in glucose absorption and gut hormone secretion are confounding variables [14]. Furthermore, during the OGTT, both plasma glucose and insulin levels are constantly changing due to a continuous feedback between the pancreatic B cells and plasma glucose levels. Nijpels and colleagues [96] compared various variables derived from the OGTT with insulin sensitivity measured with the hyperglycaemic clamp. Only the 2-hour post-glucose insulin level showed a significant correlation, and they concluded that data derived from the OGTT should be used with caution.

To determine the relative contributions of insulin resistance and decreased insulin secretion to OGTT glucose responses in diabetes, Bergman and co-workers used a computer model to account for five individual glucose tolerance patterns that had previously been reported in the literature [18, 22]. They concluded that subtle defects in insulin secretion and action could not be detected or differentiated reliably using the OGTT alone. Belfiore et al [97] have taken a different approach. They use an insulin infusion with computer control to maintain plasma glucose levels in the normal range after an oral glucose load. The insulin area is then used as a measure of insulin resistance. Interestingly, they have looked at suppression of circulating fatty acid (NEFA) levels as another measure of insulin sensitivity and showed clearer separation between groups with this. The method certainly distinguishes between groups in the expected manner, but it is complex and its relation to other tests of insulin sensitivity is uncertain, although the authors claim it is more 'physiological' than, for example, the clamp. Therefore, although the OGTT is still highly relevant to diabetic medicine, it has been replaced as a means of measuring insulin action.

Intravenous Glucose Tolerance Test

The intravenous glucose tolerance test (IVGTT) has advantages over the OGTT in that glucose absorption is not a significant variable, and gut factors are clearly no longer involved. Glucose disappearance is log-linear and can be expressed as percentage disappearance per minute (K_G). An index of whole body insulin sensitivity can be obtained by dividing the K_G by the increase in insulin area between 0 and 40 min as described by Galvin and colleagues [119]. This index correlates well with the glucose disposal rate (M) derived from the euglycaemic–hyperinsulinaemic clamp (see below) in subjects with varying degrees of glucose tolerance.

Bergman and his colleagues developed a model that derives a rather sophisticated measure of insulin sensitivity from a standard IVGTT with very frequent sampling (FSIGT) [22–25], eruditely discussed in Bergman and Ader [98]. Using 'physiologically' based models of glucose utilization and insulin kinetics, a computer-based measure of insulin sensitivity (S_I) and glucose effectiveness (S_G) (the ability of glucose to increase glucose uptake and suppress endogenous production) is obtained—the 'minimal model'. Problems arose in diabetic subjects because of poor insulin response to glucose, so that Bergman then introduced the 'modified minimal model' in which the glucose bolus was followed by tolbutamide 20 minutes later [26]. More recently, Alford and his colleagues further refined the model to measure insulin sensitivity in IDDM subjects by simultaneously infusing a constant background of insulin [27]. The key assumptions of the minimal models are:

(1) Glucose inhibits its own endogenous production and increases its utilization (by both insulin sensitive and insulin insensitive tissues) in proportion to its concentration in plasma (glucose effectiveness).
(2) Insulin acts with glucose to increase these effects.
(3) The effect of insulin on the promotion of glucose disappearance from plasma depends upon its concentration in a remote compartment now known to be interstitial fluid [28, 99].

These assumptions are represented by two equations that respectively describe the rate at which glucose is restored to basal after injection (equation 1) and the factors that determine the level of insulin in the interstitium (equation 2) (see references [24] and [28] for a full derivation of these equations).

$$dG/dt = -[S_G + X_{(t)}]G + C \qquad (1)$$

i.e. glucose restoration rate

$$= -(\text{glucose effectiveness} + \text{remote insulin effect})G + C$$

where dG/dt is the rate of restoration of plasma glucose to basal levels over time, S_G is the effectiveness of glucose to limit its own production and increase its own utilization, $X_{(t)}$ is the remote insulin level, G is glucose concentration, and C accounts for glucose production at basal levels.

In general, the restoration rate of glucose to basal levels depends on both the effect of glucose independent of an increase in insulin (S_G) and an effect of glucose that is enhanced by remote insulin ($X_{(t)}$). The factors influencing the level of insulin in the interstitium are described in equation 2:

$$dX_{(t)}/dt = k_a I_{(t)} - k_b X_{(t)} \qquad (2)$$

i.e. increase in remote insulin

$$= k_a(\text{plasma insulin}) - k_b(\text{remote insulin})$$

The level of insulin in the interstitium ($X_{(t)}$) is increased by plasma insulin ($I_{(t)}$, determined by k_a —the efficiency with which the remote compartment is filled), but decreased by a first-order process, proportional by k_b to interstitial insulin itself [$k_b X_{(t)}$].

The pattern of the FSIGT (modified) is shown in Figure 5 [29]. The time-course of plasma insulin and glucose concentrations in response to an intravenous injection of 0.3 g/kg of glucose (followed 20 minutes later by 100–300 mg tolbutamide) is analysed by computer. The prediction of the model is compared with the measured glucose levels and the values of the equation parameters are adjusted until the glucose pattern is fitted. Using these derived variables, S_G is calculated from equation 1, and insulin sensitivity (S_I), as the ratio of coefficients k_a and k_b [24]. In other words, the ratio $k_a/k_b = S_I$ defines the relationship between the rate of insulin leaving the plasma and entering the interstitial space, and the rate of insulin degradation. The efficiency of filling the interstitial compartment and the ability of insulin to remain there will determine, in part, the dynamic or steady-state ability of insulin to increase glucose disappearance. Usually 28 blood samples are taken over 180 minutes. A simplified version using only 12 samples has been developed for use in adults [100] and children [101]. This apparently works, but some accuracy is lost and the claim that this makes the test suitable for use in population studies [100] seems far-fetched. The day-to-day repeatability of S_I from the full test showed a coefficient of variation of 20%, compared with 27% for the 12-sample test [102]. It should be noted that this implies 95% confidence limits for a single test of 60–140%, a more than twofold range.

Insulin sensitivity so derived is strongly correlated with the insulin sensitivity index (S_{IP}) derived from the euglycaemic clamp [29] (see below), although we were not able to confirm this in the unmodified version

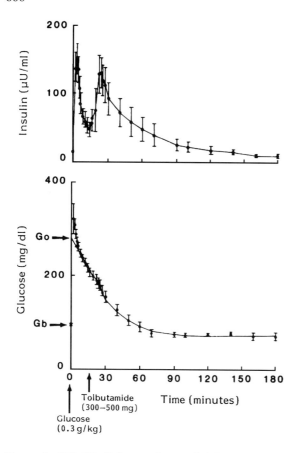

Figure 5 'Modified' frequently sampled intravenous glucose tolerance test. Glucose (0.3 g/kg) is injected over 1 min at time 0; tolbutamide is injected as a bolus 20 minutes later. G_b is the average basal (preinjection) glucose concentration; G_0 is the predicted value at time 0. From reference 29, by copyright permission of the American Society for Clinical Investigation

[103]. In practice, the estimate of insulin sensitivity derived from the FSIGT exceeds S_{IP} from the clamp by approximately 17%, and the reasons for this are currently being explored. One possible explanation is that whereas the euglycaemic clamp measures the effect of insulin on R_d (total glucose disappearance), the minimal model yields the total effect of insulin on glucose metabolism, including both glucose production (R_a) and utilization (R_d).

The minimal model approach, although clearly not the 'gold standard', has some particular advantages over the clamp techniques that warrant its further study as a method. It is independent of ambient glycaemia and insulin response, and (importantly) allows a simultaneous measurement of B-cell secretory function. Its accuracy and precision remain to be established, however, particularly in view of the heterogeneous material measured as 'insulin' (see above). It also fails to meet several of the criteria set by Groop et al [104] for an 'ideal' test of insulin sensitivity: (a) insulin levels must be high enough to stimulate glucose metabolism

and detect small differences; (b) it should be able to distinguish between hepatic and peripheral sensitivity; (c) measurements should be made under steady-state conditions; (d) model assumptions should be physiologically sound (thus glucose kinetics are clearly not monocompartmental); and (e) hyperglycaemia should be avoided as this will of itself have effects. No current tests meet all these criteria, the minimal model included.

Continuous Infusion of Glucose with Model Assessment (CIGMA)

In order to improve the precision of their HOMA method, the Oxford group introduced the CIGMA technique in 1985 [117]. This involves infusion of glucose at 5 mg/kg bodyweight per min for 1 hour. This is approximately 2.5 times basal hepatic glucose output. The mean of arterialized blood glucose after 50, 55 and 60 minutes is used as an estimate of insulin sensitivity. The level involves a compound of peripheral glucose uptake, the initial starting glucose and suppression of hepatic glucose output, all of which will be influenced by insulin secretion which is assessed from insulin and C-peptide levels. A model has been used to construct a chart from which a resistance index can be read, based on the final blood glucose and insulin concentrations.

The authors have reported good agreement between the CIGMA model and the euglycaemic and hyperglycaemic clamps [117]. Nijpels et al [96] obtained a reasonable correlation ($r = 0.66$; $p < 0.05$) with the M/I ratio from the clamp (see below), close to the value we found in our own comparisons (0.63) [103]. This was less good, however, than the correlations for the insulin tolerance test or insulin suppression test.

The advantage of the CIGMA test is that it is easy to do, and it assesses B-cell function as well as insulin sensitivity. It is certainly easier and cheaper than the minimal model. However, attained insulin levels are low (giving a low stimulus to peripheral glucose uptake), it does not achieve a real steady state, and it represents a pot-pourri of metabolic responses not allowing other aspects of metabolism or physiology to be investigated.

Glucagon Test

Recently Castillo et al [118] have published a modified glucagon test to assess insulin secretion and action simultaneously. In brief, 1 mg/m² glucagon was given as an i.v. bolus; 20 minutes later the Biostator (or artificial pancreas) was used to infuse insulin in a glucose dependent manner for a further 30 minutes. Insulin sensitivity was calculated as the rate of fall of blood glucose divided by the amount of insulin infused. The correlation with the euglycaemic clamp was good ($r = 0.82$) but in view of the much simpler other methods available, this new test is unlikely to gain widespread popularity.

DIRECT ASSESSMENT OF INSULIN SENSITIVITY

Insulin Tolerance Test

The response of plasma glucose to an intravenous bolus of insulin has long been used as a guide to human insulin sensitivity, and this forms the basis of the insulin tolerance test (ITT). Following an intravenous dose of insulin (0.1 U/kg), the exponential rate of decline in plasma glucose between 1 minute and 30 minutes can be measured (K_{ITT}) and is an estimate of tissue responsiveness to exogenous insulin. The test is attractive because it is simple to perform, but became unpopular both because of perceived problems that could confound the interpretation of the study, and potential morbidity. In particular, hypoglycaemia occurred, especially in insulin sensitive subjects. It was also considered that the counter-regulatory hormone secretion that occurs in response to hypoglycaemia would inhibit insulin action and thereby diminish glucose disposal; the slope of the glucose disappearance curve could be altered and insulin action underestimated. Furthermore, adverse cardiovascular responses to hypoglycaemia have been reported [30, 31] and care must be taken, particularly in patients with underlying coronary artery disease. Recent modifications have improved the safety profile of the ITT. First, the test can be terminated after 15 minutes, and the glucose fall between 3 and 15 minutes used to assess insulin sensitivity. Using this approach, insulin action has been measured in control subjects, diabetic patients and patients with impaired glucose tolerance [32]. We have compared the K_{ITT} values of normal and diabetic subjects with glucose disposal (M) values calculated from hyperinsulinaemic, euglycaemic clamps (see below). Overall, there was an excellent correlation between methods ($r = 0.81$; $p < 0.001$) [33]. These conclusions are similar to those reached by Bonora et al [34] and Grulet et al [105]. Similarly, good correlations have been found with the IVGTT [32]. Second, a smaller dose of insulin (0.05 U/kg) can be used, and this has allowed insulin action to be assessed in healthy pregnant women [106]. The ITT in this form also compares favourably with the hyperinsulinaemic–euglycaemic clamp [107]. Hirst et al [108] have shown a within-subject coefficient of variation of 13% (better than for the minimal model) and a between-subject value of 26%. These studies confirm the ITT to be an accurate and reliable method

for assessing insulin action, with particular suitability for testing large numbers of subjects. Currently, arterialized blood is recommended for sampling. We found poorer correlation of venous blood glucose with the 'clamp' [33], although Young et al [109] have found venous sampling to give reproducible results but did not validate their results against a reference method. Overall the ITT is nonetheless simple, and the major concern that counter-regulatory hormone secretion would occur to confound the results has not been confirmed [105]. It is, however, a non-steady state method and direct comparison of metabolic parameters with the other methods is difficult, although not impossible.

Glucose–Insulin Tolerance Test

Pioneering work on the role of insulin resistance in diabetes was carried out over 50 years ago by Himsworth and co-workers. They combined an intravenous bolus of insulin with an oral glucose load on separate occasions. On the first, 50 g of oral glucose was given and blood glucose measured at regular intervals for the following 60 minutes. On the second occasion, the same glucose load was given together with 5 U short-acting insulin intravenously. The test was based on the premise that in insulin sensitive subjects the exogenous insulin would attenuate the rise in plasma glucose levels following the oral load. By calculating the ratio of the areas under the two glucose tolerance curves, a quantitative measure of insulin action would be obtained. On the basis of this and other studies [35–38], patients with diabetes were classified as being either insulin sensitive (largely IDDM patients) or insulin insensitive (predominantly NIDDM patients). However, insulin action could not be quantified and, although of historical importance, the test is little used today.

Insulin Suppression Tests

The insulin suppression test (IST) was the first test to utilize *steady-state* plasma insulin levels to promote disposal of a glucose load. This test was developed by Reaven and co-workers in the early 1970s [39], and in its modern form it has become a widely used technique. In the original protocol exogenous glucose and insulin were infused together at a constant, predetermined rate (6 mg/kg per minute and 80 mU per minute, respectively), while endogenous insulin secretion was inhibited pharmacologically. To achieve this, adrenaline was infused at 6 µg per minute together with propranolol (0.08 mg/min) which stopped the occurrence of β-adrenergic side-effects [40]. Using this protocol, plasma insulin levels were raised to approximately 100 mU/1, significantly increasing insulin-stimulated glucose disposal. After a 90-minute equilibration period, plasma glucose levels reached steady state. For the purposes of calculation, the mean of plasma glucose levels measured between 90 minutes and 150 minutes (steady-state plasma glucose, SSPG) was used as a reflection of total-body insulin-stimulated glucose disposal [39–41]. The higher the SSPG concentration, the greater the degree of insulin resistance. Using this protocol, insulin resistance was documented and quantitated in patients with IGT [39] and NIDDM [18], and the values obtained have correlated well with the degree of glucose intolerance present. The risk of cardiac dysrhythmias with this method [42] led to the use of somatostatin (instead of adrenaline and propranolol) to inhibit endogenous insulin secretion. This was pioneered by Harano and colleagues [43], although concern remains about the potential effects of somatostatin on insulin sensitivity [22]. This does not appear to be a problem except in the basal state, although the clearly documented effects of somatostatin on hepatic blood flow (in animal models) raises other questions.

Subsequently, it has been shown that somatostatin can be omitted from this regimen and the assessment of insulin sensitivity is not affected. Thus, excellent correlations with the euglycaemic clamp technique (see below) have been obtained, using a fixed infusion rate of glucose and insulin alone [44], either at a single dose (50 mU/kg per hour of insulin plus 6 mg/kg per minute of glucose) or with stepwise increases [45], which allows dose–response curves to be constructed. We have confirmed the excellent correlation with the euglycaemic clamp in normal and diabetic subjects, with much better correlation than either the minimal model or CIGMA tests [103]. This modified Harano method is particularly simple, and the steady state glucose seems independent of starting plasma glucose levels. We have recently lengthened the test so that glucose levels are measured between 150 minutes and 180 minutes, which gives a better steady state.

The interpretation of SSPG values obtained using the IST has been analysed in some detail by Bergman and colleagues [22]. Although it is generally assumed that SSPG reflects sensitivity of the tissues to insulin, a number of important aspects of this measure must be remembered. First, insulin independent glucose clearance will have an important effect on final SSPG levels. Thus, under steady state conditions, the rate of glucose infusion must equal the sum of both insulin independent as well as insulin dependent glucose utilization. If the rate of insulin independent glucose disposal varies as plasma glucose and insulin levels vary, then SSPG as a measure of insulin-mediated glucose disposal will be

confounded. Similarly, it cannot be assumed that hepatic glucose output (HGO) is completely suppressed during the IST in all pathophysiological states; the SSPG will be increased by an amount proportional to the residual rate of HGO. The implication is that SSPG reflects both peripheral and hepatic insulin resistance, i.e. it is a measure of total insulin resistance *in vivo* as well as reflecting non-insulin-mediated glucose disposal [22]; this may not necessarily be a defect. Finally, when SSPG levels exceed the renal threshold, urinary glucose loss will influence final SSPG levels. Under these circumstances, urinary glucose levels should be measured and appropriate correction made. The somatostatin-free IST is easy to perform and indeed we have used it extensively in developing country settings. It fulfils three of the criteria of Groop et al [104], but the fact that plasma glucose may rise to quite high levels or drop into the hypoglycaemic range does cause concern when interpreting results from the very sensitive or the very resistant.

Glucose Clamp Techniques

The glucose clamp technique is the most widely used method of measuring insulin action *in vivo*, and was first introduced by DeFronzo et al in 1979 [46]. It resulted in an explosion of studies on insulin sensitivity. It is a method of quantifying the ability of either exogenous or endogenous insulin to stimulate glucose disposal under steady state conditions [40]. Patients can be studied in either euglycaemic or hyperglycaemic conditions. HGO can be measured simultaneously. Several detailed reviews are available [22, 110, 111, 112, 113].

Euglycaemic Clamp

In most cases the glucose clamp is performed under steady state euglycaemic, hyperinsulinaemic conditions. After basal blood sampling, insulin is administered intravenously, usually by an exponentially decreasing bolus [47] followed by a fixed-rate infusion (e.g. 50 mU/kg per hour) for the duration of the clamp (usually 2–3 hours). In conjunction with frequent sampling (every 5–10 minutes) and measurement of blood glucose levels, glucose is infused as a 20% (w/v) solution at a variable rate in order to maintain a predetermined blood glucose level (Figure 6) [46]. The amount of glucose that must be infused to maintain euglycaemic plasma glucose levels is a measure of the net effect of insulin to alter the production and peripheral disposal of glucose. It is assumed that endogenous insulin secretion is suppressed and that steady state levels of glucose and insulin are reached (although both

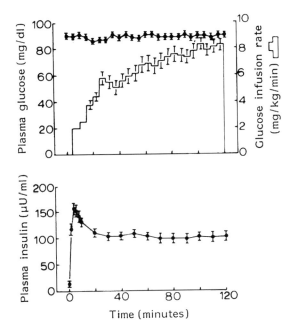

Figure 6 Time-course of plasma insulin, glucose and exogenous glucose infusion rate during the glucose clamp in humans. From reference 46, with permission

these points are debatable). When steady state conditions are reached, the rate of glucose infusion reflects the rate of insulin-stimulated glucose utilization, i.e. the rate of appearance of glucose (R_a) is equal to the total rate of disappearance of glucose from the plasma (R_d). The assumptions inherent in this generalization are, first, that urinary glucose loss is insignificant (and will continue to be, provided that the steady state glucose is less than the renal threshold, about 9 mmol/1, 162 mg/dl), and secondly that HGO is nil. Under some circumstances it can be reasonably assumed that HGO is completely suppressed (e.g. in normal subjects at high plasma insulin levels) [48]. When this assumption cannot be made, e.g. in most pathological states, then HGO must be measured using isotopically labelled glucose, and this value added to the rate at which glucose is being infused (G_{inf}), to obtain a true estimate of R_d. Similarly, if urinary glucose loss (U_{gl}) is significant, then this must be subtracted from R_d to estimate correctly the true rate of glucose utilization by tissues (M). Therefore, the equation for determining M from the clamp data becomes:

$$G_{inf} + HGO = M + U_{gl} \qquad (3)$$

$$M = G_{inf} + HGO - U_{gl} \qquad (4)$$

The interval during the clamp during which the G_{inf} is measured will vary depending upon the study design. Thus, in the original description, DeFronzo et al calculated the amount of glucose metabolized between 20 minutes and 2 hours of the study [46]. Quite clearly, steady state conditions did not apply over this period

and the value represented a mean estimate only. In general, most euglycaemic clamps are performed over at least 3 hours and calculations derived from measurements taken during the final 30 minutes. Although there is debate as to whether steady state conditions are ever achieved during a clamp, the coefficient of variation of plasma glucose and insulin values during this interval is low, and the values of M so derived are widely accepted.

The rates of glucose disposal calculated during a clamp can be compared directly, provided that the concentration of glucose perfusing muscle is the same in each case. This cannot be done with measurements based on venous samples. If patients with different levels of insulin sensitivity are clamped at similar venous glucose levels, then arterial concentrations will be higher in the more insulin-sensitive subjects. For these subjects, glucose disposal will be overestimated; this means that arterial blood sampling should be used. Because of the potential morbidity, particularly in subjects undergoing multiple studies, McGuire et al introduced the technique of arterialized venous blood sampling [49], and showed that glucose levels in arterialized venous blood were an accurate approximation of true arterial glucose. Wahab et al [114] have claimed that venous blood sampling for glucose measurement gives the same results as arterialized-venous blood sampling at both low and high insulin levels. Arteriovenous glucose differences were relatively small (maximum 0.4 mmol/l, 7.2 mg/dl) and confirmation of this interesting, practical suggestion is required.

There are a number of ways of controlling the glucose infusion rate during a clamp study. The simplest and probably most widely used method involves manual infusion control based empirically upon operator experience. The stability of blood glucose levels determined from the coefficient of variation of blood glucose levels during the steady state interval has been used to validate this approach. At the same time, it is recognized that this approach can be confounded by operator bias [50] and for this reason various 'objective' methods of determining glucose infusion rates have been devised. A mathematical algorithm proposed by DeFronzo [46] has been widely used but its usefulness has been questioned [50]. The Biostator can be used to adjust glucose infusion rates regularly, according to an algorithm using measurements obtained from continuously sampled venous blood [51]. An alternative approach uses an 'adaptive' computer program (PACBERG) that continually assesses the effect of insulin on glucose disappearance and, from this, calculates the glucose infusion rate [52]. Although it would seem logical for automatic clamp algorithms to be preferable to an empirical manual approach, there is no evidence to support this assumption and no single method currently enjoys universal acceptance.

Clamp-based Measures of Sensitivity

Metabolic clearance rate. The most widely used measure of insulin sensitivity is the rate of glucose disposal (M) at a fixed level of hyperinsulinaemia. Although there is little disagreement that this provides an excellent method of comparing insulin action between subjects with comparable basal glucose levels, difficulties arise when comparisons are made between subjects whose ambient blood glucose levels differ. The reason is that the rate of glucose uptake at any level of plasma insulin depends upon the levels of glucose in the blood [53–55]. That is, at higher levels of plasma glucose there will be a mass action effect which will act to increase glucose disposal. Under these circumstances two different approaches to allow a direct comparison between subjects have been suggested, although neither is entirely satisfactory. The first is to normalize blood glucose levels before the study, so that patients are compared at similar glucose levels. This is usually achieved either by an overnight insulin infusion or by allowing the glucose level to decline after the start of the insulin infusion before starting the glucose infusion. Both approaches have been criticized. Specifically, changes in insulin sensitivity can occur owing to either prolonged exposure to insulin or the counter-regulatory response to lowering blood glucose. A second approach is to relate the glucose disposal rate to the prevailing plasma glucose level (G) by calculating the metabolic clearance rate (MCR) for glucose (MCR $= M/G$). This ratio has been widely used as a measure of insulin sensitivity [22, 54, 56, 57]. It has been proposed that, whereas the glucose utilization rate increases with plasma glucose levels over a wide range of plasma glucose concentrations, MCR remains relatively constant [54, 56]. As such, MCR should theoretically provide a measure of insulin sensitivity independent of the level of glycaemia at which the subjects are being compared. This proposal has been challenged [23], as the ratio can be valid only if there is an identical proportional increase in both R_d and G as glucose levels rise. It has been pointed out, however, that this cannot be so [23, 55]; if non-insulin-mediated glucose uptake into the central nervous system is saturated at low levels of glycaemia, then identical proportional increases in glucose levels and total glucose disposal cannot occur. This means that if two individuals with identical insulin sensitivity are compared, the one clamped at higher glucose levels would have lower glucose clearance. In fact, a significant decline in MCR in patients clamped at hyperglycaemic plasma levels has been demonstrated

[58]. Thus, glucose clearance may be an inappropriate means for comparing insulin sensitivity in individuals with different levels of fasting glycaemia.

A further problem is that, for a fixed rate of insulin infusion, subjects will show quite wide variation in circulating insulin levels, due to differences in hepatic uptake, renal clearance and distribution volume. For peripheral glucose uptake it is the ambient insulin level which matters. Several workers have allowed for this by expressing sensitivity as M/I where I is the steady state insulin level [22, 115].

Insulin sensitivity index. The insulin sensitivity index (S_{IP}) was introduced by Bergman as a measure of insulin sensitivity independent of glycaemia. In essence, two isoglycaemic clamps are performed at different insulin infusion rates or, alternatively, a clamp is performed at two or more insulin levels. Insulin sensitivity is calculated as the difference between glucose clearance at the higher and lower glucose levels related to the increment in plasma insulin levels [59]. As the change in clearance is totally insulin mediated and therefore independent of the saturable non-insulin dependent component of glucose disposal (largely central nervous system uptake), it is directly proportional to the glucose concentration. Conversely, the slope of the relationship between clearance and insulin is theoretically independent of glycaemia.

$$S_{IP} = [(R_{d2}/G_2) - (R_{d1}/G_1)]/I_2 - I_1 \qquad (5)$$

where R_{d2} and R_{d1} are the glucose disposal rates in the two clamps, I_1 and I_2 are the measured steady state insulin values, and G_1 and G_2 are the two clamped glucose values.

Studies in normal individuals performed at euglycaemia and hyperglycaemia at both normal and elevated insulin levels have confirmed that the S_{IP} is independent of both insulin and glucose over a wide range [23]. Nonetheless there are problems even with this. If sequential clamps are done, there is likely to be a carry-over effect from one dose to the next [48,110], whilst doing them on separate days builds in a considerable variation.

Hyperglycaemic Clamp

The hyperglycaemic clamp technique was first developed to examine insulin secretion and to assess B-cell function. Glucose is elevated above basal levels either by an exponentially declining glucose infusion [22, 46] or by a bolus of intravenous glucose [60]. As a result, endogenous insulin secretion is stimulated. To maintain the elevated target level of glycaemia (usually approximately 7 mmol/l, 126 mg/dl, above baseline levels), glucose is infused at a variable rate for at least 120 minutes [46]. The amount of glucose infused approximates to the amount of glucose utilized while steady state plasma glucose concentrations are maintained.

There are several problems with the use of the hyperglycaemic clamp for measurement of insulin action *in vivo*. Endogenous insulin secretion can vary from subject to subject. Although this can be measured by calculating the area under the insulin response curve, and thus defects in insulin secretion can be quantitated and documented, the corollary is that patients are not necessarily studied under identical conditions. We have in fact found poor correlation between the *M* values using euglycaemic–hyperinsulinaemic and hyperglycaemic clamping [103]. In addition, we were unable to show a difference between NIDDM and normal subjects when this was clearly evident using the conventional euglycaemic clamp. Furthermore, insulin secretion can vary with time, making it difficult to achieve steady state insulin levels. For these reasons, somatostatin is usually administered to suppress endogenous insulin secretion, and insulin is infused to achieve the desired steady peripheral insulin levels. As previously discussed, however, somatostatin influences the release of other hormones and may exert an independent effect on insulin sensitivity which needs to be recognized when interpreting the data from such clamp studies. Hyperglycaemia *per se* is a powerful inhibitor of hepatic glucose production, and this effect is amplified in the presence of insulin [61]. Therefore, during a hyperglycaemic–hyperinsulinaemic clamp in a normal subject, hepatic glucose production will be completely suppressed, and the rate of glucose infusion will equal the rate of extrahepatic glucose uptake. Clearly, the rate of glucose disposal will need to be adjusted for urinary losses if the blood glucose concentration rises above the renal threshold.

It is important to recognize that the rates of both insulin-mediated and non-insulin-mediated glucose disposal increase during the hyperglycaemic clamp in the presence of insulin [62]. Therefore, it is necessary to repeat the hyperglycaemic clamp at the same plasma glucose concentration, but in the absence of insulin, in order to determine the rate of non-insulin-mediated glucose disposal alone. This value is then subtracted from the rate of total glucose disposal to give the true rate of insulin-mediated glucose uptake. With this technique, Baron and colleagues have demonstrated that the increase in non-insulin-mediated glucose disposal during hyperglycaemia is principally into skeletal muscle [62].

The hyperglycaemic clamp technique has been applied to other areas of glucose metabolism. It has been used to examine the separate effects of insulin and glycaemia on intracellular glucose metabolism [63–65]. From these studies it has been shown that glycaemia primarily stimulates non-oxidative glucose disposal, principally into glycogen storage.

Overall the euglycaemic–hyperinsulinaemic clamp remains the gold standard, although slightly tarnished. It fulfils most of the postulates of Groop et al [104], although many workers have underestimated how long it takes to reach steady state. Indeed it seems that there is a slight continued drift over many hours. There is also a tolerance on the method which allows different operators to infuse amounts of glucose differing by as much as 10–20% to achieve the same blood glucose level. It is also predominantly a test of peripheral (muscle) glucose uptake and tells you little about the basal state, other tissues, and aspects of metabolism other than glucose. Because the insulin infusion is systemic, it overestimates the contribution of peripheral tissues to glucose disappearance when compared with oral ingestion of glucose which stimulates portal insulin delivery [104]. Nonetheless it is robust, dose–response curves can be constructed, and it has greatly enhanced our knowledge of *in vivo* insulin action.

TISSUE INSULIN SENSITIVITY

The techniques that have been considered so far have examined whole-body insulin sensitivity, whereas information regarding the insulin sensitivity of specific tissues and metabolic processes is often desirable.

Hepatic Insulin Sensitivity

The glucose clamp technique measures the combined ability of insulin to promote peripheral glucose uptake, which is predominantly into skeletal muscle [66], and to suppress hepatic glucose output. As the portal vein cannot be cannulated in humans, there is no reliable or safe method of measuring hepatic glucose output directly [67]. Therefore, a technique has been developed which uses isotope-labelled glucose to measure hepatic glucose output indirectly. The rate of total glucose appearance (R_a) during a clamp is equal to the sum of the glucose infusion rate (G_{inf}) and the residual HGO:

$$R_a = \text{HGO} + G_{inf} \qquad (6)$$

Hence

$$\text{HGO} = R_a - G_{inf} \qquad (7)$$

The continuous infusion of isotope-labelled glucose allows R_a to be determined, and this is equal to the rate of total glucose disposal (R_d) when the plasma glucose concentration is constant. As a true steady state is never reached during clamps of the usual duration, Steele developed equations for calculating R_a and R_d for non-steady state conditions [68]. These equations are based on a model that assumes that the extracellular glucose occupies a single compartment of a constant volume, and that there is no metabolic discrimination between labelled and unlabelled glucose molecules. Both stable and radioisotope-labelled glucose preparations have been used. An important feature of the tracer is that the label must occupy a position in the glucose molecule so that it is irreversibly lost following the metabolism of glucose. If this is not the case, the labelled glucose moiety might be recycled at the liver and lead to an underestimation of R_a. The most commonly used tracers that satisfy the requirements of insignificant recycling are glucose labelled with tritium at the 3-carbon position [69], and glucose labelled with two deuterium atoms at the 6-carbon position [70].

The major problem with this method has been the frequent underestimation of R_a when used with the hyperinsulinaemic clamp, and this has given negative values for hepatic glucose output when the value for R_a has been substituted into equation 7. This is clearly nonsense, and there are several possible explanations that might account for this underestimation. First, a tritiated non-glucose contaminant has been identified in some preparations of tritiated glucose [71]. The accumulation of the contaminant during the clamp would contribute to the plasma radioactivity and result in the underestimation of the true R_a. Although this might contribute to the underestimation of R_a, another explanation is necessary, as not all preparations of tritiated glucose are contaminated [72] and the underestimation is still apparent when uncontaminated deuterium-labelled glucose is used [73]. An alternative explanation is that there is an 'isotope effect', and that the unlabelled glucose is preferentially metabolized leaving the labelled glucose to accumulate in the plasma. Such an effect has been described in work conducted in rats [74], although a significant isotope effect has not been identified in humans [72, 75]. The third (and most likely) explanation is that the one-compartment model originally proposed by Steele is inadequate for the conditions that prevail during a hyperinsulinaemic clamp, and it is probable that the distribution volume for glucose expands and the system becomes multicompartmental [76, 77]. The underestimation of R_a can be prevented by using a one-compartment model with a variable glucose pool size [77], although this requires data from two clamps instead of the usual one. Alternatively, a multicompartmental model can be used [78]; however, this is often imprecise because of the lack of the necessary physiological data required to define the parameters of the model [76]. A practical way to minimize the underestimation of R_a is to use a variable infusion of tracer to maintain basal plasma isotope concentrations during the clamp. This has been used

successfully with radio-isotope [75–77, 79] and stable-isotope [116] labelled glucose. The result of these considerations is that the suppressive action of insulin on HGO has probably been overestimated, under both normal and pathological conditions.

Extrahepatic Insulin Sensitivity

The insulin sensitivity of a specific tissue can also be assessed by measuring the rate of insulin-mediated glucose uptake across a tissue bed. Applying the Fick principle, the rate of glucose uptake is calculated from the product of the blood flow and the glucose arterio-venous concentration difference across the tissue bed. As glucose is not released by the peripheral tissues, the true rather than the net rate of glucose uptake is determined. However, the technique should be applied only when the blood flow and the arterio-venous concentration differences have reached steady state conditions [80], as failure to achieve this can lead to either under-estimation or overestimation of the true rate of glucose uptake.

The forearm method is probably the most widely used form of this technique, and was pioneered by Andres and colleagues [81]. The method is important as it allows the direct measurement of glucose uptake into skeletal muscle, which is the principal tissue for insulin-mediated glucose uptake [66] and is the major site of peripheral insulin insensitivity in NIDDM [82]. The most commonly used methods for measuring forearm blood flow are venous occlusion plethysmography [83] and the dye dilution technique [81]. The latter method requires arterial cannulation for the injection of a bolus of dye. Apart from the potential problems of arterial cannulation, errors in the measurement can arise if there is poor mixing of dye with arterial blood [81]; however, this method has the advantage of allowing direct measurement of the rate of blood flow through the muscle bed. This is not possible with venous occlusion plethysmography which measures total forearm blood flow, although the rate of muscle blood flow can be predicted using established equations [84]. However, this method is easy to perform and arterial cannulation can be avoided by measuring arterialized venous blood glucose concentrations, which are comparable to the true arterial values as previously discussed [49]. For deep venous blood sampling, a cannula is inserted retrogradely via the perforating vein at the antecubital fossa into a vein draining the forearm muscle bed [85]. The position of the cannula can be verified either by dye injection or by ensuring that the blood oxygen saturation is less than 55% [86, 87], and intermixing between the superficial and muscle venous systems can be minimized by arresting the hand circulation for 5 minutes before sampling from the deep venous cannula [87]. Other tissues are also amenable to investigation by this technique, and a method has recently been developed for examining substrate exchange across adipose tissue, which is another important site for the regulatory action of insulin [88].

Insulin Sensitivity: Wider Considerations

Several of the methods for assessing insulin sensitivity have been applied in conjunction with techniques that have been devised to examine specific metabolic pathways, so allowing the insulin sensitivity of these processes to be determined.

The most widely applied method has been the hyperinsulinaemic clamp, which has been used with stepwise incremental increases in the insulin infusion rate in order to provide dose–response characteristics for these pathways. The pathways of glucose oxidation, non-oxidative glucose disposal and glycogen synthesis have been examined in this way in normal human subjects [89, 90] and in patients with NIDDM [91, 92], and it has been established that all of these pathways are insensitive to the action of insulin in NIDDM.

This chapter has focused on the assessment of insulin sensitivity in the context of glucose metabolism. However, similar approaches have been used to examine the action of insulin on lipid and protein metabolism in man.

REFERENCES

1. National Diabetes Data Group. Classification and diagnosis of diabetes mellitus and other categories of glucose intolerance. Diabetes 1979; 28: 1039–57.
2. World Health Organization Expert Committee. Second report on diabetes mellitus. Technical Report Series 646. Geneva: WHO, 1980.
3. Golay A, Swislocki ALM, Chen Y-DI, Reaven GM. Relationships between plasma free-fatty acid concentration, endogenous glucose production, and fasting hyperglycaemia in normal and non-insulin-dependent individuals. Metabolism 1987; 36: 692–6.
4. Fraze E, Donner CC, Swislocki ALM, Chiou Y-AM, Chen Y-DI, Reaven GM. Ambient plasma free fatty acid concentrations in non-insulin dependent diabetes mellitus: evidence for insulin resistance. J Clin Endocrinol Metab 1985; 61: 807–11.
5. Yalow RS, Berson SA. Immunoassay of endogenous plasma insulin in man. J Clin Invest 1960; 39: 1157–75.
6. Yalow RS, Berson SA. Plasma insulin concentrations in nondiabetic and early diabetic subjects. Determinations by a new sensitive immunoassay technique. Diabetes 1960; 9: 254–60.
7. Turner RC, Holman RR, Matthews D, Hockaday TDR, Peto J. Insulin deficiency and insulin resistance interaction in diabetes: estimation of their relative contribution by feedback analysis from basal plasma insulin and glucose concentrations. Metabolism 1979; 28: 1086–96.
8. Dowse GK, Qin H, Collins VR et al. Determinants of estimated insulin resistance and B-cell function in Indian, Creole and Chinese Mauritians. Diabetes Res Clin Pract 1990; 10: 265–79.
9. Sobey WJ, Beer SF, Carrington CA et al. Sensitive and specific two-site immunoradiometric assays for human insulin, proinsulin, 65–66 split and 32–33 split proinsulins. Biochem J 1989; 260: 535–41.
10. Temple RC, Clark PMS, Nagi DK, Schneider AE, Yudkin JS, Hales CN. Radioimmunoassay may overestimate insulin in non-insulin-dependent diabetics. Clin Endocrinol 1990; 32: 689–93.
11. Golay A, Chen Y-DI, Reaven GM. Effect of differences in glucose tolerance on insulin's ability to regulate carbohydrate and free fatty acid metabolism in obese individuals. J Clin Endocrinol Metab 1986; 62: 1081–8.
12. Hollenbeck C, Reaven GM. Variations in insulin-stimulated glucose uptake in healthy individuals with normal glucose tolerance. J Clin Endocrinol Metab 1987; 64: 1169–73.
13. Karam JH, Grodsky GM, Forsham PH. Excessive insulin response to glucose in obese subjects as measured by immunochemical assay. J Am Diet Assoc 1963; 12: 197–204.
14. Reaven G, Miller R. Study of the relationship between glucose and insulin responses to an oral glucose load in man. Diabetes 1968; 17: 560–9.
15. Leatherdale BA, Chase RA, Rogers J, Alberti KGMM, Davies P, Record CO. Forearm glucose uptake in cirrhosis and its relationship to glucose tolerance. Clin Sci 1980; 59: 191–8.
16. Mondon CE, Dolkas CB, Reaven GM. The site of insulin resistance in acute uremia. Diabetes 1978; 27: 571–6.
17. DeFronzo RA. The triumvirate: B-cell, muscle, liver. A collusion responsible for NIDDM. Diabetes 1988; 37: 667–86.
18. Reaven GM, Bernstein R, Davis B, Olefsky JM. Nonketotic diabetes mellitus: insulin deficiency of insulin resistance. Am J Med 1976; 60: 80–8.
19. McDonald GW, Fisher GF, Burnham C. Reproducibility of the oral glucose tolerance test. Diabetes 1965; 14: 473–80.
20. Olefsky JM, Reaven GM. Insulin and glucose responses to identical oral glucose tolerance tests performed forty-eight hours apart. Diabetes 1974; 23: 449–53.
21. Home P. The OGTT: gold that does not shine. Diabet Med 1988; 5: 313–14.
22. Bergman RN, Finegood DT, Ader M. Assessment of insulin sensitivity *in vivo*. Endocr Rev 1985; 6: 45–86.
23. Bergman RN, Hope ID, Yang YJ et al. Assessment of insulin sensitivity *in vivo*: a critical review. Diabetes Metab Rev 1989; 5: 411–29.
24. Bergman RN, Ider YZ, Bowden CR, Cobelli C. Quantitative estimation of insulin sensitivity. Am J Physiol 1979; 236: E667–77.
25. Bergman RN, Phillips LS, Cobelli C. Physiologic evaluation of factors controlling glucose tolerance in man. Measurement of insulin sensitivity and beta-cell sensitivity from the response to intravenous glucose. J Clin Invest 1981; 68: 1456–67.
26. Beard JC, Bergman RN, Ward WK, Porte D. The insulin sensitivity index in nondiabetic man. Correlation between clamp-derived and IVGTT-derived values. Diabetes 1986; 35: 362–9.
27. Ward GM, Weber KM, Walters IM et al. A modified minimal model analysis of insulin sensitivity

and glucose-mediated disposal in insulin-dependent diabetes. Metabolism 1991; 40: 4-9.

28. Bergman RN. Lilly Lecture 1989. Toward physiological understanding of glucose tolerance. Minimal-model approach. Diabetes 1989; 38: 1512-27.

29. Bergman RN, Prager R, Volund A, Olefsky JM. Equivalence of the insulin sensitivity index in man derived by the minimal model method and the euglycaemic glucose clamp. J Clin Invest 1989; 79: 790-800.

30. Koh H, Nambu S, Tsushima M, Nishiohada Y, Murakami K, Ikada M. The effects of insulin on the cardiovascular system in patients with coronary heart disease. Arzneim Forsch 1984; 34: 185-90.

31. Shimada R, Nakashima T, Nunoi K, Kokno Y, Takeshita A, Omae T. Arrhythmia during insulin-induced hypoglycaemia in a diabetic patient. Arch Intern Med 1984; 144: 1068-9.

32. Alford FP, Martin FI, Pearson MJ. The significance and interpretation of mildly abnormal oral glucose tolerance. Diabetologia 1971; 7: 173-80.

33. Akinmokun A, Selby PL, Ramaiya K, Alberti KGMM. The short insulin tolerance test for determination of insulin sensitivity: a comparison with the euglycaemic clamp. Diabet Med 1992; 9: 432-7.

34. Bonora E, Moghetti P, Zancanaro C et al. Estimates of *in vivo* insulin action in man: comparison of insulin tolerance tests with euglycaemic and hyperglycaemic glucose clamp studies. J Clin Endocrinol Metab 1989; 68: 374-8.

35. Himsworth HP. Diabetes mellitus. Its differentiation into insulin-sensitive and insulin-insensitive types. Lancet 1936; i: 127-30.

36. Himsworth HP, Kerr RB. Insulin-sensitive and insulin-insensitive types of diabetes mellitus. Clin Sci 1939; 4: 119-52.

37. Himsworth HP. The syndrome of diabetes mellitus and its causes. Lancet 1949; ii: 465-72.

38. Himsworth HP, Kerr RB. Age and insulin sensitivity. Clin Sci 1939; 4: 153-7.

39. Shen SW, Reaven GM, Farquhar J. Comparison of impedence to insulin-mediated glucose uptake in normal subjects and in subjects with latent diabetes. J Clin Invest 1970; 49: 2151-60.

40. Reaven GM. Insulin resistance in noninsulin-dependent diabetes mellitus. Does it exist and can it be measured? Am J Med 1983; 3-17.

41. Ginsberg H, Olefsky JM, Reaven GM. Further evidence that insulin resistance exists in patients with chemical diabetes. Diabetes 1974; 23: 674-8.

42. Lampman RM, Santinga JT, Bassett DR, Savage PJ. Cardiac arrhythmias during epinephrine-propranolol infusions for measurement of *in vivo* insulin resistance. Diabetes 1981; 30: 618-20.

43. Harano Y, Ohgaku S, Hidaka H. Glucose, insulin and somatostatin infusion for the determination of insulin sensitivity. J Clin Endocrinol Metab 1977; 45: 1124-7.

44. Heine RJ, Home PD, Poncher M et al. A comparison of 3 methods for assessing insulin sensitivity in subjects with normal and abnormal glucose tolerance. Diabetes Res 1985; 2: 113-20.

45. Heine RJ, Bilo HJG, Van Der Meer J, Van Der Veen EA. Sequential infusions of glucose and insulin at prefixed rates: a simple method for assessing insulin sensitivity and insulin responsiveness. Diabetes Res 1986; 3: 453-61.

46. DeFronzo RA, Tobin JD, Andres R. Glucose clamp technique: a method for quantifying insulin secretion and resistance. Am J Physiol 1979; 237: E214-23.

47. Sherwin RS, Kramer KJ, Tobin JD et al. A model of the kinetics of insulin in man. J Clin Invest 1974; 53: 1481-92.

48. Rizza RA, Mandarino LJ, Gerich JE. Dose-response characteristics for effects of insulin on production and utilization of glucose in man. Am J Physiol 1981; 240: E630-69.

49. McGuire EAH, Helderman JH, Tobin JD, Andres R, Berman M. Effects of arterial versus venous sampling on analysis of glucose kinetics in man. J Appl Physiol 1976; 41: 565-73.

50. Greenfield MS, Doberne L, Kraemer F, Tobey T, Reaven G. Assessment of insulin resistance with the insulin suppression test and the euglycaemic clamp. Diabetes 1981; 30: 387-92.

51. Clemens AH, Hough DL, D'Orazio PA. Development of the Biostator glucose clamping algorithm. Clin Chem 1982; 28: 1899-904.

52. Pacini G, Bergman RN. PACBERG: an adaptive program for controlling the blood sugar. Comput Prog Biomed 1983; 16: 13-20.

53. Verdonk CA, Rizza RA, Gerich JE. Effects of plasma glucose concentration on glucose utilization and glucose clearance in normal man. Diabetes 1981; 30: 535-7.

54. Cherrington AD, Williams PE, Harris MS. Relationship between the plasma glucose level and glucose uptake in the conscious dog. Metabolism 1978; 27: 787-91.

55. Best JD, Taborsky GJ Jr, Halte JB, Porte D Jr. Glucose disposal is not proportional to plasma glucose level in man. Diabetes 1981; 30: 847-50.

56. Doberne L, Greenfield MS, Rosenthal M, Widstrom A, Reaven G. Effect of variations in basal plasma glucose concentrations on glucose utilization (M) and metabolic clearance rate (MCR) during insulin clamp studies in patients with noninsulin-dependent diabetes mellitus. Diabetes 1982; 31: 396-400.

57. Gottesman I, Mandarino L, Gerich J. Use of glucose uptake and glucose clearance for the evaluation of insulin action *in vivo*. Diabetes 1984; 33: 184-91.

58. DeFronzo RA, Ferrannini E. Influence of plasma glucose and insulin concentration on plasma glucose clearance in man. Diabetes 1982; 31: 683-8.

59. Ader M, Bergman RN. Insulin sensitivity in the intact organism. In Alberti KGMM, Home PD, Taylor R (eds) Baillière's clinical endocrinology and metabolism. Techniques for metabolic investigation in man. London: Baillière Tindall, 1987; 879-910.

60. Ferner RE, Ashworth L, Tronier B, Alberti KGMM. Effects of short-term hyperglycaemia on insulin secretion in normal humans. Am J Physiol 1986; 250: E655-61.

61. DeFronzo RA, Ferrannini E, Hendler R, Felig P, Wahren J. Regulation of splanchnic and peripheral glucose uptake by insulin and hyperglycaemia in man. Diabetes 1983; 32: 35-45.

62. Baron AD, Brechtel G, Wallace P, Edelman SV. Rates and tissue sites of non-insulin and insulin-mediated uptake in humans. Am J Physiol 1988; 255: E769-74.

63. Ferrannini E, Locatelli L, Jequier E, Felber JP. Differential effects of insulin and hyperglycaemia

on intracellular glucose disposition in humans. Metabolism 1989; 38: 459-65.

64. Thorburn AW, Gumbiner B, Brechtel G, Henry RR. Effect of hyperinsulinemia and hyperglycemia on intracellular glucose and fat metabolism in healthy subjects. Diabetes 1990; 39: 22-30.

65. Felley CP, Felley EM, van Melle GD, Frascarlo P, Jequier E, Felber JP. Impairment of glucose disposal by infusion of triglycerides in humans: role of glycemia. Am J Physiol 1989; 256: E747-52.

66. DeFronzo RA, Jacot E, Jequier E, Maeder E, Wahren J, Felber JP. The effect of insulin on the disposal of intravenous glucose. Results from indirect calorimetry and hepatic and femoral venous cannulation. Diabetes 1981; 30: 1000-1007.

67. DeFronzo RA. Use of the splanchnic hepatic balance technique in the study of glucose metabolism. In Alberti KGMM, Home PD, Taylor R (eds) Baillière's clinical endocrinology and metabolism. Techniques for metabolic investigation in man. London: Baillière Tindall, 1987; pp 837-62.

68. Steele R. Influences of glucose loading and injected insulin on hepatic glucose output. Ann NY Acad Sci 1959; 82: 420-30.

69. Altszuler N, Barkai A, Bjerknes C, Gottlieb B, Steele R. Glucose turnover values in the dog obtained with various species of labelled glucose. Am J Physiol 1975; 229: 1662-7.

70. Bier DM, Leake RD, Haymond MW et al. Measurement of 'true' glucose production rates in infancy and childhood with 6,6-dideutero-glucose. Diabetes 1977; 26: 1016-23.

71. Butler PC, Kryshak EJ, Schwenk WF, Haymond MW, Rizza RA. Hepatic and extrahepatic responses to insulin in NIDDM and nondiabetic humans. Diabetes 1990; 39: 217-25.

72. Yki-Jarvinen H, Consoli A, Nurjhan N, Young AA, Gerich JE. Mechanism for the underestimation of isotopically determined glucose disposal. Diabetes 1989; 38: 744-51.

73. Argoud GM, Schade DS, Eaton RP. Underestimation of hepatic glucose production by radioactive and stable tracers. Am J Physiol 1987; 252: E606-15.

74. Rose IA, Kellermeyer R, Stjernhold R, Wood HG. The distribution of C^{14} in glycogen from deuterated glycerol-C^{14} as a measure of the effectiveness of triosephosphate isomerase *in vivo*. J Biol Chem 1962; 237: 3325-31.

75. Molina JM, Baron AD, Edelman SV, Brechtel G, Wallace P, Olefsky JM. Use of a variable tracer infusion method to determine glucose turnover in humans. Am J Physiol 1990; 258: E16-23.

76. Levy JC, Brown G, Matthews DR, Turner RC. Hepatic glucose output in humans measured with labeled glucose to reduce negative errors. Am J Physiol 1989; 257: E531-40.

77. Finegood DT, Bergman RN, Vranic M. Modeling error and apparent isotope discrimination confound estimation of endogenous glucose production during euglycaemic clamps. Diabetes 1988; 37: 1025-34.

78. Ferrannini E, Smith JD, Cobelli C, Toffolo G, Pilo A, DeFronzo RA. Effect of insulin on the distribution and disposition of glucose in man. J Clin Invest 1985; 76: 357-64.

79. Finegood DT, Bergman RN, Vranic M. Estimation of endogenous glucose production during hyperinsulinemic euglycemic glucose clamps. Diabetes 1987; 36: 914-24.

80. Zierler KL. Theory of the use of arteriovenous concentration differences for measuring metabolism in steady and non-steady states. J Clin Invest 1961; 40: 2111-25.

81. Andres R, Cader G, Zierler KL. The quantitatively minor role of carbohydrate in oxidative metabolism by skeletal muscle in intact man in the basal state. J Clin Invest 1956; 35: 671-82.

82. DeFronzo RA, Gunnarsson R, Bjorkman O, Olsson M, Wahren J. Effects of insulin on peripheral and splanchnic glucose metabolism in non-insulin dependent (Type II) diabetes mellitus. J Clin Invest 1985; 76: 149-55.

83. Whitney RJ. The measurement of volume changes in human limbs. J Physiol 1953; 121: 1-27.

84. Cooper KE, Edholm OG, Mottram RF. The blood flow in skin and muscle of the human forearm. J Physiol 1955; 128: 258-67.

85. Mottram RF, Butterfield WJF. The human forearm as a preparation for metabolic investigations. Proc Roy Soc Med 1961; 54: 549-52.

86. Wahren J. Quantitative aspects of blood flow and oxygen uptake in the human forearm during rhythmic exercise. Acta Physiol Scand 1966; 67: 33-45.

87. Jackson RA, Hamling JB, Sim BM, Hawa MI, Blix PM, Nabarro JDN. Peripheral lactate and oxygen metabolism in man: the influence of oral glucose loading. Metabolism 1987; 36: 144-50.

88. Coppack SW, Fisher RM, Gibbons GF et al. Postprandial substrate deposition in human forearm and adipose tissue *in vivo*. Clin Sci 1990; 79: 339-48.

89. Thiebaud D, Jacot E, DeFronzo RA, Maeder E, Jequier E, Felber JP. The effect of graded doses of insulin on total glucose uptake, glucose oxidation and glucose storage in man. Diabetes 1982; 31: 957-63.

90. Yki-Jarvinen H, Mott D, Young AA, Stone K, Bogardus C. Regulation of glycogen synthase and phosphorylase activities by glucose and insulin in human skeletal muscle. J Clin Invest 1987; 80: 95-100.

91. Groop LC, Bonadonna C, DelPrato S et al. Glucose and free fatty acid metabolism in non-insulin dependent diabetes mellitus. J Clin Invest 1989; 84: 205-13.

92. Thorburn AW, Gumbiner B, Bulacan F, Brechtel G, Henry RR. Multiple defects in muscle glycogen synthase activity contribute to reduced glycogen synthesis in non-insulin dependent diabetes mellitus. J Clin Invest 1991; 87: 489-95.

93. Matthews DR, Hosker JP, Rudenski AS, Naylor BA, Treacher DF, Turner RC. Homeostasis model assessment: insulin resistance and beta-cell function from fasting plasma glucose and insulin concentrations in man. Diabetologia 1985; 28: 412-19.

94. Turner RC, Levy JC, Rudenski AS, Hammersley M, Page R. Measurement of insulin resistance and beta-cell function: the HOMA and CIGMA approach. In Belfiore F, Bergman RN, Molinatti GM (eds) Current topics in diabetes research, vol. 12. Basel: Karger, 1993; pp 66-75.

95. Winocour PH, Kaluvya S, Brown L et al. The association of different measures of insulinaemia with

vascular risk factors in normoglycaemic normotensive non-obese men and women. Q J Med 1991; 79: 539–60.

96. Nijpels G, Van Der Wal PS, Bouter LM, Heine RJ. Comparison of three methods for the quantification of β-cell function and insulin sensitivity. Diabetes Res Clin Pract 1994; 26: 189–95.

97. Belfiore F, Volpicelli G, Iannello S, Campione R. Computer-controlled OGTT. In Belfiore F, Bergman RN, Molinatti GM (eds) Current topics in diabetes research, vol. 12. Basel: Karger, 1993; pp 76–85.

98. Bergman RN, Ader M. Concepts emerging from the minimal model approach. In Belfiore F, Bergman RN, Molinatti GM (eds) Current topics in diabetes research, vol. 12. Basel: Karger, 1993; pp 39–65.

99. Ader M, Poulin RA, Yang YJ, Bergman RN. Dose-response relationship between lymph insulin and glucose uptake reveals enhanced insulin sensitivity of peripheral tissues. Diabetes 1992; 41: 241–53.

100. Steil GM, Volund A, Kahn SE, Bergman RN. Reduced sample numbers for calculation of insulin sensitivity and glucose effectiveness from the minimal model: suitability for use in population studies. Diabetes 1992; 42: 250–6.

101. Cutfield WS, Bergman RN, Menon RK, Sperling MA. The modified minimal model: application to measurement of insulin sensitivity in children. J Clin Endocrinol Metab 1990; 70: 1644–50.

102. Steil GM, Murray J, Bergman RN, Buchanan TA. Repeatability of insulin sensitivity and glucose effectiveness from the minimal model. Implications for study design. Diabetes 1994; 43: 1365–71.

103. Davis SN, Monti L, Piatti PM et al. Estimates of insulin action in normal, obese and NIDDM man: comparison of insulin and glucose infusion test, CIGMA, minimal model and glucose clamp techniques. Diabetes Res 1993; 23: 1–18.

104. Groop L, Widen E, Ferrannini E. Insulin resistance and insulin deficiency in the pathogenesis of type 2 (non-insulin dependent) diabetes mellitus: errors of metabolism or of methods. Diabetologia 1993; 36: 1326–31.

105. Grulet H, Durlach V, Hecart AC, Gross A, Leutenegger M. Study of the rate of early glucose disappearance following insulin injection: insulin sensitivity index. Diabetes Res Clin Pract 1993; 20: 201–7.

106. Dornhorst A, Edwards SGM, Nicholls JSD et al. A deficit in insulin release in women at risk of future non-insulin-dependent diabetes. Clin Sci 1991; 81: 195–9.

107. Gelding SV, Robinson S, Lowe S, Niththyananthan R, Johnston DG. Validation of low dose short insulin tolerance test for evaluation of insulin sensitivity. Clin Endocrinol 1994; 40: 611–15.

108. Hirst S, Phillips DIW, Vines SK, Clark PM, Hales CN. Reproducibility of the short insulin tolerance test. Diabet Med 1993; 10: 839–42.

109. Young RP, Critchley JAJH, Anderson PJ, Lau MSW, Lee KKC, Chan JCN. The short insulin tolerance test: feasibility study using venous sampling. Diabet Med 1996, 13: 429–33.

110. Waldhausl W. The glucose clamp technique. In Belfiore F, Bergman RN, Molinatti GM (eds) Current topics in diabetes research, vol. 12. Basel: Karger, 1993; pp 24–31.

111. Scheen AJ, Lefebvre PJ. Assessment of insulin resistance *in vivo*: application to the study of type 2 diabetes. Horm Res 1992; 38: 19–27.

112. Scheen AJ, Paquot N, Castillo MJ, Lefebvre PJ. How to measure insulin action *in vivo*. Diabetes Metab Rev 1994; 10: 151–88.

113. Beck-Nielsen H. Methodologies in characterization and classification of prediabetic states to non-insulin-dependent diabetes mellitus (NIDDM). In Mogensen CE, Standl E (eds) Research methodologies in human diabetes, vol. 5. Berlin: de Gruyter, 1994; 147–69.

114. Wahab PJ, Rijnsburger WE, Oolbekkink M, Heine RJ. Venous versus arterialised venous blood for assessment of blood glucose levels during glucose clamping: comparison in healthy men. Horm Metab Res 1992; 24: 576–9.

115. Ng LL. Application of modelling techniques to the assessment of insulin sensitivity in man. Diabet Med 1988; 5: 217–22.

116. Powrie JK, Smith GD, Hennessy TR et al. Incomplete suppression of hepatic glucose production in non-insulin dependent diabetes mellitus measured with [6.6-^{2}H$_2$] glucose enriched glucose infusion during hyperinsulinaemic euglycaemic clamps. Eur J Clin Invest 1992; 22: 244–53.

117. Hosker JP, Matthews DR, Rudenski AS et al. Continuous infusion of glucose with model assessment: measurement of insulin resistance and β-cell function in man. Diabetologia 1985; 28: 401–11.

118. Castillo MJ, Scheen AJ, Lefebvre PJ. Modified glucagon test allowing simultaneous estimation of insulin secretion and insulin sensitivity: application to obesity, insulin-dependent diabetes mellitus and non-insulin-dependent diabetes mellitus. J Clin Endocrinol Metab 1995; 80: 393–9.

119. Galvin P, Ward G, Walters J et al. A simple method for quantitation of insulin sensitivity and insulin release from an intravenous glucose tolerance test. Diabet Med 1992; 9: 921–8.

29

The Relationship between Obesity and Diabetes

Per Björntorp

Department of Heart and Lung Diseases, University of Göteborg, Sahlgren's Hospital, Göteborg, Sweden

INTRODUCTION

The close association between obesity and non-insulin dependent diabetes mellitus (NIDDM) is well known and long established. Clinicians also know that many obese subjects never develop NIDDM in spite of long-standing severe obesity, as if there were a protected subgroup who can resist the challenge of the diabetogenic trigger mechanism(s) of obesity. As a corollary, some subjects seem to be more prone to the precipitation of NIDDM than others. In general this has long been believed, and subgroups of obesity have been categorized according to various principles. Vague [1] was one of the early investigators who made such an attempt, which has proved to be valid when re-examined with more modern, precise techniques. Vague's subdivision takes into consideration the distribution of excess body fat, being either android (like that seen typically in men) or gynoid (like that seen typically in women). Subsequently, a more valid categorization of these distribution characteristics seems to be, respectively, abdominal (or, rather, visceral) and peripheral obesity.

It is now agreed that both genetic and environmental factors are important in the pathogenesis of NIDDM. There is much information to suggest that the genetic factor may comprise a tendency of the B cells to produce insufficient amounts of insulin. There also seems to be a consensus that an inadequate effect of insulin at the periphery—insulin resistance—is an important prerequisite for the precipitation of NIDDM.

This might be due to environmental factors, although genetic predisposition may have an important role.

It is well established that obesity is associated with increased insulin resistance. It therefore seems likely that the most important way in which obesity precipitates NIDDM is via an increase in insulin resistance. The following discussion is focused on this alternative in the light of recent observations on insulin resistance and its pathogenesis in subgroups of human obesity. This subgrouping has made it possible to see new explanations of insulin resistance in obesity, and therefore could be of considerable significance for the further understanding of the pathogenesis of NIDDM.

INSULIN SECRETION, METABOLISM AND EFFICACY IN OBESITY SUBGROUPS

Peripheral hyperinsulinemia during fasting and during oral or intravenous glucose challenge is clearly more pronounced in abdominal than in peripheral obesity [2–4]. The question arises whether this is a specific effect of the distribution of adipose tissue or if the increase of body fat mass plays an additional part. Statistical analyses suggest that the latter is indeed the case; in comparison with controls, subjects with peripheral obesity also develop slight hyperinsulinemia, which is proportional to the amount of total body fat [2, 4]. Obesity, defined as increased total mass of body fat, in addition to the distribution of this fat mass, is thus an important factor in hyperinsulinemia.

International Textbook of Diabetes Mellitus, Second Edition. Edited by K.G.M.M. Alberti, P. Zimmet, R.A. DeFronzo, and H. Keen (Honorary)
© 1997 John Wiley & Sons Ltd

The elevated insulin concentrations observed have all been measured in the peripheral circulation. These concentrations are the result of the secretion of insulin from the pancreatic B cells minus that taken up by the liver. Peripheral hyperinsulinemia might therefore be due to either increased insulin secretion or decreased hepatic uptake, or a combination of both these factors.

Studies by Peiris et al [3] have elucidated this important question. Utilizing C-peptide turnover as a measure of insulin secretion, it was shown that both factors have a role. Insulin secretion was found to be proportional to body mass index (BMI), whereas hepatic clearance of insulin was negatively correlated with the ratio of the waist circumference to the hip circumference (WHR). BMI is closely associated with total body fat mass, while WHR is a simple estimation of abdominally distributed fat mass.

The peripheral efficacy of insulin is usually estimated *in vivo* by the euglycemic glucose clamp. Such studies have shown that insulin resistance is clearly more pronounced in abdominal obesity than in peripheral obesity [2, 5]. It seems likely that there is also a moderate abnormality in peripheral obesity compared with controls. Thus it seems likely that insulin resistance is associated primarily with fat distribution, but also to a lesser degree with overall obesity. Thus examining insulin secretion and resistance according to abdominal and peripheral obesity suggests that distribution (abdominally localized adipose tissue) is associated with decreased hepatic clearance and more pronounced insulin resistance, while total obesity is more closely associated with increased insulin secretion and less with inefficient hepatic clearance and peripheral efficacy of insulin. Obviously, none of these are exclusive characteristics of either the distribution or the obesity factor. It is known that exposure of the insulin receptor to increased concentrations of insulin leads to less efficient insulin binding through downregulation [6]. Therefore, the increased insulin secretion found in obesity, irrespective of fat distribution, would presumably lead to a decreased hepatic clearance of insulin as well as defective peripheral insulin binding in comparison with normal subjects.

This new information may be useful from at least two aspects. First, in the search for pathogenetic mechanisms of NIDDM, future studies are probably more rewarding if focused on the most susceptible subgroup of obesity, i.e. subjects with abdominal obesity. Second, the thrust of further studies can now be directed towards defined abnormalities in insulin secretion, handling and efficacy in different types of obesity. Further studies on other characteristics of abdominal and peripheral obesity have already yielded information leading to new hypotheses for the pathogenesis of NIDDM, as reviewed in the following sections.

A major difficulty with the studies seeking the primary defect causing insulin resistance is that once hyperinsulinemia is established this will by itself cause a 'regulatory', secondary insulin resistance. Similarly, the decrease of hepatic insulin clearance may also be a secondary consequence of increased insulin secretion. In addition, with established peripheral insulin resistance, a compensatory increase of insulin secretion will follow. This means that the combination of increased insulin secretion, hyperinsulinemia, decreased hepatic insulin clearance and peripheral insulin resistance may have started at any of the above-mentioned points, perpetuating itself in a vicious circle. This in turn means that the cause of this chain of events, once established, cannot be determined. It is thus necessary to study the problem before this vicious circle is established.

INCREASED INSULIN SECRETION IN OBESITY

Increased peripheral insulin concentrations have long been observed in obesity [7]. More recent studies have also demonstrated increased peripheral C-peptide concentrations [8–10] and although not conclusive, due to possible differences in peripheral handling of C-peptide in obese and normal subjects, these studies again suggest increased insulin secretion. These observations have now been reinforced by measurements of C-peptide turnover. In addition, it has been shown that obesity as such is most strongly associated with this hypersecretion [3].

The mechanisms behind the increased insulin secretion remain elusive. Those suggested include central regulatory aberrations of appetite, primary increases in insulin secretion, primary peripheral insulin resistance, other endocrine aberrations, as well as intestinal hormones [7]. Recent developments make it more likely, however, that a major cause might be a central nervous system mechanism, causing an imbalance between the cholinergic and sympathetic nervous system, in turn caused by neuroendocrine mechanism(s) [11].

DECREASED HEPATIC CLEARANCE OF INSULIN IN ABDOMINAL OBESITY

Defective hepatic clearance may be an important factor in peripheral hyperinsulinemia of abdominal obesity [3]. The mechanism of regulation of insulin uptake by the liver is known to be dependent on the insulin concentration in the portal vein; thus, portal hyperinsulinemia decreases hepatic clearance of insulin [12].

In addition, free fatty acids (FFA) may play an important part in this process. In isolated hepatocytes

FFA cause a decrease of insulin binding, degradation and function. The inhibition of insulin binding is found with a number of physiologically occurring long-chain fatty acids, and at concentrations found in the portal vein [13]. This has also been found to occur in the rat liver perfused *in situ*, where an inhibition of insulin action is also found at physiological fatty acid concentrations, and is apparently specific for FFA because neither glucose nor lactate have such effects [14]. Furthermore, livers from rats rendered moderately obese by overfeeding show decreased insulin clearance, inversely proportional to the triglyceride content of the livers, which in turn is dependent on the portal concentrations of fatty acids [15]. When such rats are given Etomoxir, a compound inhibiting hepatic fatty acid oxidation, their hepatocytes bind insulin normally. Also, when fatty acid oxidation is prevented in hepatocytes *in vitro*, insulin binding is improved. The number of insulin receptors and their tyrosine kinase activity remain normal [16, 17]. Taken together, these studies suggest that insulin clearance by the liver is inhibited by the oxidation of fatty acids, either as FFA in the portal vein, or triglyceride fatty acids in the hepatocytes, while the number and function of the insulin receptors are unaffected. Fatty acid oxidation may cause an internalization of the insulin receptor, and in this way decrease insulin turnover at the level of the receptor [18].

No direct information is available on this mechanism in humans. Inhibition of hepatic insulin uptake by fatty acids is less pronounced in older than younger rats [14], which might be due to a higher triglyceride content in the liver of the former [15]. Whether the human liver is similar to that of older or younger rats has not been studied. It should be noted, however, that there is evidence for insulin resistance of hepatic glucose production in human obesity [19]. Furthermore, hepatic insulin extraction is markedly reduced in abdominal obesity [3]. This might at least partly be a consequence of elevated portal FFA or hepatic triglycerides, due to the effect described above.

These observations add a novel function of portal FFA in their influence on hepatic metabolism. It is of considerable interest that fatty acids have previously been shown to drive the synthesis of very low-density lipoproteins (VLDL), and of the apoprotein B100, the protein constituent of these lipoprotein particles. In addition, a series of previous studies have shown that fatty acid oxidation in the liver drives hepatic gluconeogenesis (reviewed in [20]).

The events here of particular interest in diabetes are the interactions between fatty acids and insulin uptake as well as gluconeogenesis. The net effect would be to increase concentrations of circulating glucose and

peripheral hyperinsulinemia, which might be considered as an early stage of diabetes when sufficiently pronounced. It might also be considered that portal fatty acids may in this way trigger the transition between the alimentary and postalimentary phase. After a meal insulin is needed for hepatic glycogen synthesis, and fatty acid mobilization is inhibited. In the postalimentary phase, or during fasting, fatty acid mobilization is pronounced, driving hepatic gluconeogenesis. Insulin is also removed from the site of gluconeogenesis by fatty acids.

Portal FFA are derived from the abdominal (visceral) fat depots. These depots have several specific characteristics which may be of importance in relation to their specific functions. First, the intrinsic metabolic activity of the adipocytes in these regions is greater than in other depots. Both lipid uptake [21] and mobilization occur at a higher rate in men and in abdominally obese men and women [22, 23]. The basis for this may well be a high density of glucocorticoid as well as androgen receptors [22, 24]. The effects of glucocorticoids in visceral adipose tissue mainly result in fat accumulation (cf. Cushing's disease) by expressing lipoprotein lipase activity [25, 26], while testosterone is mainly lipolytic through the expression of β-adrenergic receptors [27, 28]. Another important difference between subcutaneous and visceral adipocytes is the diminished antilipolytic effect of insulin in the latter [29], perhaps due to a lower density of insulin receptors [30].

In addition to these intrinsic characteristics of the adipocytes in these regions of adipose tissue, the surrounding conditions of these cells are well adapted to their high metabolic activity. Blood flow is higher than in other adipose tissue [31], which is of fundamental importance for both lipid uptake and mobilization. The rate of lipid uptake mediated via lipoprotein lipase is dependent on substrate availability, which in turn is dependent on the presentation of circulating triglyceride to the enzyme. This means that lipid uptake is not always dependent on the maximal activity of the enzyme, but rather on other conditions such as blood flow [32]. Furthermore, lipid mobilization is critically dependent on sufficient blood flow removing the hydrolysed fatty acids from the scene of lipolysis, which will otherwise be inhibited [33].

The lipolytic process is mainly regulated by catecholamines in human adipose tissue [34]. Recent studies have shown that visceral adipose tissue contains far more catecholamines and catecholaminergic nerves than other adipose tissues [35].

Thus, visceral fat is uniquely equipped in metabolic capacity, hormone receptor density, blood flow and innervation to form a metabolic center of adipose tissue. The high turnover of lipid in this store therefore most probably results in a high flow of FFA from the adipocytes into the portal vein. When visceral depots are enlarged this flow will be further augmented. This is of considerable potential importance in view of the effects of FFA on hepatic regulation of metabolism. With elevated flow of FFA in the portal vein, such as with enlarged visceral fat depots, these metabolic effects will be magnified and may reach harmful levels. It has indeed been shown that high portal FFA concentrations are able to produce hyperlipidemia and hyperglycemia [20].

There is an ongoing discussion about the relationship between hyperinsulinemia and hypertension, with evidence for a cause-and-effect relationship, i.e. hypertension follows from hyperinsulinemia [36, 37]. Exposure of the liver to elevated portal FFA concentrations may cause increased circulating concentrations of glucose, insulin, VLDL, LDL and apo-B100, as well as (in a second step) causing blood pressure elevation. The consequence would be the formation of a majority of well established risk factors, not only for NIDDM but also for cardiovascular disease. In this way one might actually see visceral adipose tissue as a generator for the established risk factors for both NIDDM and cardiovascular disease. This might explain the findings that expansion of visceral fat mass (increased WHR) is an independent risk factor for both NIDDM and cardiovascular disease. This hypothesis has been described in more detail elsewhere [20].

As mentioned above, it is not possible to determine the origin of insulin resistance once it is established, because of the fact that hyperinsulinemia causes a global insulin resistance via a vicious circle. It should be observed that a redistribution of fat from peripheral to central adipose tissue depots in the intra-abdominal regions may well be a primary event, followed by elevated portal FFA concentrations as a trigger for a subsequent peripheral hyperinsulinemia and insulin resistance. Therefore, factors regulating adipose tissue distribution to central depots become of considerable importance.

INSULIN RESISTANCE IN ABDOMINAL OBESITY

Increased insulin resistance occurs in abdominal obesity as measured by the 'clamp' [2, 5]. Such measurements examine the insulin sensitivity mainly of tissues other than liver, particularly muscle and adipose tissue. Adipose tissue has previously been thought to contribute only a small percentage of total glucose uptake. However, recent studies have shown that the uptake might well be of quantitative significance, particularly in obesity, if the large production of lactate in adipose tissue is taken into consideration [38]. However, in these studies there were no indications that glucose

uptake in adipose tissue varied with the distribution of adipose tissue. Therefore, peripheral insulin resistance in abdominal obesity seems most likely to be found in muscle tissue and/or the liver, judged from these studies.

The distribution of adipose tissue is of interest in NIDDM, where FFA concentrations in the circulation show reduced sensitivity to the inhibitory effects of insulin [39]. This might be interpreted as a diminished antilipolytic effect of insulin in adipose tissue in general, but an alternative possibility might be considered. Visceral accumulation of body fat is prevalent in NIDDM [40], and these depots are very sensitive to lipolytic stimuli, so they may contribute a significant fraction of the FFA in the systemic circulation. This fraction would be relatively 'insulin-resistant' because sensitivity to the antilipolytic effect of insulin is lower in visceral than other adipocytes [29]. The consequence would be an apparent insulin resistance of FFA release in NIDDM because of a higher contribution of FFA from visceral depots.

Insulin Resistance in the Liver

There is also considerable evidence that the liver is insulin-resistant in abdominal obesity. The inhibition of glucose production occurs at higher concentrations of insulin than normal [41]. This insulin resistance of the liver in abdominal obesity and perhaps in NIDDM may well be an effect of portal FFA [19, 41–43]. Again, this is of considerable importance as a primary defect, because it may be an early event caused by redistribution of adipose tissue lipid stores from the periphery to central visceral depots.

Insulin Resistance in Muscle

The inhibitory effects of FFA on glucose uptake in muscle are well known as the glucose–fatty acid cycle [44]. Increased concentrations [2] as well as fractional turnover rate [45] of systemic FFA have been observed in abdominal obesity. This may be followed by an increased resistance to the effects of insulin on muscle and could be one factor contributing to the insulin resistance in muscle observed with abdominal obesity.

There are, however, also other candidates for the production of this effect, notably steroid hormones (reviewed in the following section); the insight into this possibility has come from observations in muscle, the main site of insulin resistance in the periphery.

Interestingly, muscle of women with abdominal obesity is quite characteristic. First, the lean body mass of such women is elevated, probably because of an increase in total muscle mass [5]. Furthermore, the qualitative characteristics of their muscles seem to be specific. Such women have more fast twitch (white) fibers than women with peripheral obesity, more like muscle of obese men. Abdominally obese women thus have android features not only in their adipose tissue distribution, but also in the quantitative and qualitative characteristics of muscle.

It is of particular interest that muscles with white fibers seem to be less insulin-sensitive and bind less insulin than muscles with red fibers [46–48]. Muscle of abdominally obese women would thus be expected to be less insulin-sensitive, in agreement with the findings in glucose clamp measurements. These findings have been confirmed and found also in men [49].

Could a lower degree of physical conditioning be a common denominator for the relative shift between red and white muscle fibers, as well as for higher insulin levels, because insulin sensitivity increases in physically trained obese subjects [50]? The degree of physical conditioning was not lower in abdominally obese women than in peripherally obese women as measured by maximal oxygen uptake capacity. Furthermore, with physical training to the same degree of improvement in circulatory variables, insulin sensitivity increased more in abdominally obese women than in peripherally obese women [5]. These findings suggest that muscle factors other than degree of conditioning are the cause of the insulin resistance of women with abdominal obesity.

An explanation in terms of the muscles having a low number of insulin-sensitive, red fibers seems unlikely, because the contractile elements of muscle are unlikely to be associated with insulin regulation of glucose uptake. In addition, there are a number of unrelated conditions which are associated with, or followed by, changes in muscle fiber composition towards more white and less red fibers. These include physical inactivity [51], corticosteroid hormones [52, 53], and hyperandrogenicity in females [5], as well as hypogonadism in males [54]. All these conditions are characterized by insulin resistance and hyperinsulinemia. We therefore considered the possibility that hyperinsulinemia might be the primary factor, followed by muscle fiber changes, rather than the converse. Recent experiments suggest that this might indeed be correct. Rats were rendered chronically hyperinsulinemic while anti-insulin hormones were controlled. This was followed by a marked increase of white, at the expense of red, muscle fibers [55]. It seems possible that insulin is actually involved in the regulation of different muscle myosins, so that a change in muscle fiber composition towards more white fibers may be secondary to the prevalent hyperinsulinemia, rather than the reverse.

Another structural change of muscle is of interest in this connection. Several reports have shown strong direct statistical relationships between insulin sensitivity and capillary density in muscle [49, 56–58]; hormonal manipulations are followed by changes in capillary density in close association with insulin sensitivity [55, 59]. The low capillary density of muscle in insulin-resistant conditions is probably not a consequence of the hyperinsulinemia, because in the experiments with chronically hyperinsulinemic rats, capillary density actually increased, tightly associated with an increased insulin sensitivity [55]. It seems more likely that capillary density is involved in the regulation of insulin sensitivity.

The information supporting this possibility is as follows. Evidence for insulin binding to capillaries was found several years ago [60–62], and capillary endothelium binds insulin *in vitro* [63]. Insulin occupies a larger space in muscle than inulin, a molecule of similar diameter [64]. The insulin space was proportional to capillary density, suggesting insulin binding to capillaries. Recent studies have also demonstrated that the insulin effect on glucose transport in muscle is more closely associated with extravascular extracellular than intravascular insulin concentrations. Furthermore, extracellular concentrations rise more slowly than insulin concentrations in the circulation and never reach those found in the circulation [65]. Taken together this suggests that insulin is first taken up in an intermediary pool by binding to endothelial cells, and then released into the extracellular space of muscle tissue where it interacts with the insulin receptor.

This may provide an understanding of the close parallels between the capillary density and insulin sensitivity of muscle. The intermediary capillary pool of insulin may in fact regulate the availability of insulin for the insulin receptor on the muscle cells. The more capillary endothelium, the larger the intermediary pool of insulin. The regulation of capillary density and function may thus be important for muscle insulin sensitivity.

In view of the well-known capillary pathologies in different organs in diabetes, sometimes already visible at diagnosis of NIDDM, it is tempting to suggest that in the prediabetic state with insulin resistance there might already be functional changes in capillary endothelium or in the regulation of capillary density. In line with this possibility is the observation in NIDDM of an abnormal response of muscle capillaries to physical training [66], normally a potent stimulator of capillary growth [67].

Role of Steroid Hormones

The endocrine abnormalities associated with visceral obesity may well be involved in the creation of insulin resistance in this prediabetic condition. The aberrations seem to include a functional hypersensitivity of the hypothalamo–adrenal axis, probably resulting in bursts of hypercortisolemia, hyperandrogenicity in women, and relative hypogonadism in men. This will be discussed later in more detail.

The capacity of cortisol to induce insulin resistance is well known [68]. Androgens have been studied surprisingly little from this aspect and turn out to be of considerable interest. Recent studies have shown the pronounced effects of androgens in the regulation of peripheral insulin sensitivity, utilizing the glucose clamp technique in rats. Female rats were given testosterone to mimic the hyperandrogenic status of insulin-resistant women. This resulted in a marked insulin resistance, localized to muscle and found in both glucose transport and glycogen synthesis on the basis of glycogen synthase regulation, after only 48 hours of testosterone exposure [59, 69]. Other experiments (unpublished) indicate that the numbers and function of the insulin receptors, as well as the numbers of glucose transporter 4, seem unaltered. Capillary density is markedly diminished, and muscle fiber composition is changed towards more white and fewer red fibers [59]. As discussed above, the latter may well be secondary to the prevailing hyperinsulinemia.

The insulin resistance of the muscles in these rats is found only at submaximal insulin concentrations, and is overcome at maximal concentrations [59], suggesting that the lesion is localized at the level of the insulin receptor. Since the number and function of the insulin receptors appeared normal, it might be that the insulin receptor is not sufficiently stimulated, resulting in an abnormally weak signal to glucose transport and glycogen synthesis. This might be due to insufficient availability of insulin. If this is correct, then transcapillary transport might be the rate-limiting step for insulin action in this condition. This interpretation is supported by the parallel between insulin action and capillary density in muscle [59], and by the fact that the abnormalities are overcome by elevated insulin concentrations.

With this background information from females it is of obvious importance to examine the effects of testosterone on insulin effectiveness in male rats. Supraphysiological concentrations of testosterone seem to have the same effect as in female rats, creating insulin resistance at the level of the muscle. Interestingly, in male rats low testosterone levels induced by castration were followed by a similar picture, reversible by testosterone substitution to the levels of controls [70].

Female sex steroid hormones also regulate muscle insulin resistance. Oophorectomy was followed by decreased insulin sensitivity of muscle, fully restored by replacement therapy with 17-β-estradiol. Progesterone caused moderate insulin resistance. These effects seemed to be most marked on hexose transport as measured by 2-deoxyglucose uptake *in vivo*. In the liver glycogen synthesis was dependent on both estrogen and progesterone [71]. Estrogen replacement therapy has previously been described as improving insulin sensitivity in postmenopausal women [72]. At least part of the mechanism(s) responsible for this might thus be through effects on muscle and the liver.

Hypercortisolemia, like excess androgens in both sexes, is followed by insulin resistance. In all these conditions muscle fiber composition is changed towards more white and fewer red fibers, possibly secondary to hyperinsulinemia. Capillary density is diminished after exposure to excess steroid hormones [53, 59], suggesting that steroid hormones are of importance in the regulation of capillary density. Preliminary studies indicate that testosterone administration to female rats is followed by a severe inhibition of blood flow to muscles, in parallel with the low capillary density, measured with histochemical techniques, and also parallel with the insulin resistance of these muscles (unpublished).

Clearly, the status of steroid hormone secretion should be included in discussion of the pathogenesis of insulin resistant conditions in man. Table 1 summarizes factors considered to contribute to the hyperinsulinemia associated with obesity, particularly when this is localized to abdominal, visceral regions. Other unidentified factors may also be involved. The hyperinsulinemia resulting may well also amplify the perturbations at several sites.

Table 1 Contributing mechanisms resulting in peripheral hyperinsulinemia in obesity

Mechanism	Effector tissue	Hypothetical cause
Increased insulin secretion	Pancreas B cells	Imbalance in central autonomic nervous system
Decreased hepatic uptake	Liver	Androgens FFA
Decreased peripheral efficacy	Muscle Liver	Androgens Corticosteroids FFA

HORMONAL ABNORMALITIES IN ABDOMINAL OBESITY

Androgens

It is relevant, following the discussion above, to examine the secretion of steroid hormones in human obesity and the relationships to the aberrations found here, particularly as the steroid hormones exert marked effects on the regional distribution of adipose tissue.

Free testosterone has repeatedly been found to be elevated and sex hormone binding globulin concentration low in abdominal obesity [73]. Adrenal androgens such as androstenedione or dehydroepiandrosterone sulfate have been reported to have elevated or normal secretion or blood concentrations, while 17-β-estradiol and estrone were unchanged [73–75]. Progesterone production is probably diminished in abdominal obesity, because of the irregular ovulation seen in this condition [76].

Androgenicity seems to be the best documented of the steroid hormone aberrations in abdominal obesity in women. It is interesting to note the striking similarities between the syndrome of abdominal obesity in women and polycystic ovarian syndrome (PCOS). In comparison with normal women, in both these syndromes women have increased body fat mass, particularly in the abdominal region, while the characteristic increase of femoral fat-cell size and lipoprotein lipase activity seen in normal women is missing. Lean body mass is increased [77]. Free testosterone is elevated and sex hormone binding globulin low. Hirsutism and menstrual irregularities are frequently found, as well as hypertension and metabolic aberrations including hyperinsulinemia and NIDDM (for review, see [78]). The PCOS might therefore be considered as an interesting model for abdominal obesity in women. It should be mentioned that most of the abnormalities seen in the PCOS are found also in women with this syndrome without obesity, defined as enlargement of body fat mass [77]. In non-obese women [79] a high WHR is also associated with several of the metabolic aberrations. Such observations suggest that the obesity following abdominal distribution of body fat is not necessary for the development of the full-blown syndrome.

It has been suggested that hyperandrogenism follows hyperinsulinemia and insulin resistance, irrespective of the cause of the former, suggesting that insulin resistance and hyperinsulinemia are the primary factors [80]. In a few patients with varying backgrounds to their insulin resistance, catheterization of the adrenal and ovarian veins showed that the excess androgen production had an ovarian origin [80, 81].

The problem here is whether the hyperandrogenism is the primary factor causing insulin resistance, or *vice versa*. The first alternative seems to be strengthened by the effects of androgens on the insulin sensitivity of muscle tissue. Furthermore, administration of testosterone to trans-sexual women seems to be followed by insulin resistance (unpublished). In addition, treatment with estrogen and progesterone of a patient with PCOS caused remission of insulin resistance [82], and spironolactone, an androgen antagonist, lowers testosterone and insulin levels in women with PCOS [83]. On the other hand, inhibiting ovarian androgen secretion by other means in this syndrome was not effective [84].

The other possibility is that hyperinsulinemia and insulin resistance cause increased secretion of androgens. Although this cannot be reproduced experimentally with relatively short-term hyperinsulinemia [85], it might occur over a longer time. The main argument in favour of this hypothesis is the parallel between hyperinsulinemia and hyperandrogenism in a number of unrelated syndromes [80]. It is also known that insulin and insulin-like growth factors stimulate the production of several ovarian steroid hormones under tissue culture conditions, including progesterone [86], estrogen [87] and androstenedione [86]. The next question is how insulin stimulation would specifically cause hyperandrogenism. This might be due to inhibition of ovarian aromatase, transforming estrogen to androgens, a relative increase of the cell mass producing ovarian androgens, or a synergism between luteinizing hormone and insulin to produce excess androgens [88] (for detailed review see [89]). Recent data show that in normal women, selected at random, there is a correlation between insulin and free testosterone [90], suggesting perhaps that hyperinsulinemia may not be the primary factor, because these women were not hyperinsulinemic.

The importance of hyperandrogenicity for the development of NIDDM in women has recently been demonstrated in a prospective epidemiological study [91]. A low concentration of sex hormone binding globulin (SHBG) was found to be a strong independent risk factor for the development of NIDDM in women. The risk was concentrated below the lowest quintile of the distribution where a threshold value seemed to discriminate the women at risk. Below this quintile the risk seemed to increase exponentially up to at least tenfold in the lowest 5% of the distribution as compared with the rest of the population. Other studies in this population have shown that fasting plasma insulin and abdominal obesity are the two other strong independent risk factors for NIDDM [92, 93]. It seems reasonable to suggest that plasma insulin is an early sign of insulin resistance, and that factors associated with abdominal obesity might be responsible for the creation of insulin resistance. This might particularly be the case with low SHBG, probably a sign of relative hyperandrogenism, by analogy with the effects of testosterone on insulin resistance in female rats and trans-sexual women.

Recently we have also found that women with NIDDM are characterized by elevated testosterone values and low SHGB, in parallel with signs of insulin resistance [94]. When such women are given 17-β-estradiol to alleviate hyperandrogenicity, their diabetes seems to improve [95]. Taken together these studies suggest that hyperandrogenicity may be of hitherto underestimated importance for insulin resistance in women. Table 2 summarizes the findings in this area. It is tempting to suggest that hyperandrogenicity found in women in the non-selected population, as well as in women with visceral obesity or NIDDM, may actually cause muscle insulin resistance, particularly since muscle characteristics, when measured, seem to be identical to those seen after testosterone administration.

The situation in men is only partially congruent. It has been reported that the intake of excess androgens in male power-athletes is associated with pronounced insulin resistance [96]. In contrast, in middle-aged men selected from a health survey, insulin sensitivity was inversely correlated to the levels of free testosterone, suggesting that men with relative hypogonadism are also insulin-resistant. It should be noted that this was also associated with increased masses of visceral fat [97]. The finding of a statistical relationship between low testosterone values and insulin resistance in men has recently been confirmed [98, 99].

These observations indicate that relative hypogonadism in men is also followed by insulin resistance. These clinical observations of insulin resistance in men, following both supraphysiological and low testosterone concentrations, indicate that a 'window' of physiological testosterone concentrations is optimal for insulin sensitivity. This is in excellent agreement with the rat studies referred to above, showing that too high and too low testosterone levels in male rats are followed by insulin resistance [70].

We recently studied men with visceral obesity and the Metabolic Syndrome, and with relative hypogonadism, who were given supplementary testosterone up to normal juvenile concentrations. An improvement of their insulin resistance was an early consequence of treatment, and was rather pronounced. Furthermore, plasma lipids, blood pressure and visceral fat mass were also lowered, suggesting that the entire syndrome was improved by testosterone substitution [100, 101]. These findings further emphasize the significance of low testosterone values in men in relation to insulin resistance. Recent results suggest that men with clinically manifest NIDDM and insulin resistance also are relatively hypogonadal (unpublished observations), and substitution trials are taking place.

In summary, it seems that there are arguments for both the possibility that overproduction of androgens in women results in insulin resistance and hyperinsulinemia, and *vice versa*. Although it seems that the origin of the increased testosterone is the ovary in several related conditions, this has not been demonstrated in abdominal obesity. Furthermore, relative hypogonadism in men might be followed by insulin resistance. The experimental data referred to above clearly show that androgens are important regulators of peripheral insulin sensitivity. A primary change in androgen production may thus well result in the changes of insulin sensitivity seen with abdominal obesity in both men and women.

Corticosteroids

It is well known that cortisol has pronounced inhibitory effects on insulin sensitivity, resulting in hyperinsulinemia and NIDDM during exogenous or endogenous corticosteroid excess. There are several reports of an increased secretion of cortisol in obesity, but there are

Table 2 A summary of observations on the relationship between hyperandrogenicity and muscle characteristics in female rats and in women

	Hyperandrogenic status	Muscle characteristics				Risk for development of NIDDM
		Insulin resistance	Capillarization ↓	Glycogen synthase ↓	Glucose transport ↓	
Female rats	T administration	+ + +	+ + +	+ + +	+ +	?
Trans-sexual women	T administration	+ +	?	?	?	?
Women in population	SHBG ↓	+ +	?	?	?	+ +
Women with visceral obesity	SHBG ↓, T ↑	+ + +	+ +	+ +	?	+ + +
Women with NIDDM	SHBG ↓, T ↑	+ + +	+ +	+ + +	?	+ + +

T, testosterone; SHBG, sex hormone binding globulin; NIDDM, non-insulin dependent diabetes mellitus.

also several reports finding no abnormalities [102]. In some of the negative reports, increased production of cortisol was found which disappeared when corrected for the accompanying increase in creatinine excretion. This seems to be a questionable manoeuvre, however, since the effects of cortisol are mediated via the glucocorticoid receptor (GR) [103], and the ensuing results are those of the GR-cortisol complex interacting with the gene in question. It has been shown that these effects are quantitatively dependent on the traffic of cortisol over the available GRs; in other words, the more frequent the interactions between the GR-cortisol and the gene in question, the more pronounced will be the cortisol effects expected. Therefore, it seems to follow that with increased cortisol production, as reported in obesity, the impact of cortisol on the effector organs should be augmented. A correction of cortisol secretion by creatinine excretion seems to be irrelevant to this particular aspect of cortisol function.

A putative increase of cortisol secretion in obesity may well be different in abdominal and peripheral obesity, explaining the somewhat conflicting results when this question has been examined in mixed populations of obese humans. Only a few studies have so far addressed this question. Both Vague et al [74] and Krotkiewski et al [104] have in early studies reported increased production of corticosteroids and androgens in android obese women. We have studied this question further in several ways. First, urinary cortisol secretion shows a weak ($P < 0.05$) positive correlation with WHR in large populations. Secondly, plasma cortisol measured in the morning shows an inverse relationship with WHR, suggesting deranged diurnal secretion. This needs further studies for clarification. Furthermore, although the dexamethasone inhibition test did not show any abnormalities, it seems that ACTH stimulation of cortisol secretion shows an increased response with abdominal obesity. Furthermore, mental and physical stress-tests are followed by elevated cortisol secretion in abdominal obesity [105]. Thus a relative, perhaps functional, hypercortisolism may be a characteristic of abdominal obesity. Other observations, reviewed in a subsequent section, provide further circumstantial evidence that this might be the correct interpretation.

Growth Hormone

A recent study has suggested an additional endocrine abnormality, which is particularly pronounced in visceral obesity. Insulin-like growth factor I (IGF-I) is low in parallel with visceral fat mass in men [106]. IGF-I concentrations in the circulation are mainly dependent on growth hormone (GH) secretion [107] and, in harmony with low IGF-I concentrations, diurnal

GH secretion has recently been found to be severely diminished in abdominal obesity [108]. The previously known deficiency of GH secretion in obesity [109] thus seems to be particularly pronounced in visceral obesity.

GH is known to inhibit the effects of insulin in the periphery, and low GH secretion would consequently be expected to be followed by improved insulin sensitivity. However, in visceral obesity with low GH secretion, insulin resistance is clearly present. It may be that other factors, causing insulin resistance, prevail over the effects of diminished GH secretion. Another possibility seems to be that regulation of insulin sensitivity by GH is dependent on the secretion pattern rather than the total amount produced. These alternatives are currently being examined.

HORMONAL ABNORMALITIES AND ADIPOSE TISSUE DISTRIBUTION

Thus hormone abnormalities as well as abdominal fat mass may be of importance for the regulation of insulin homeostasis. The question is whether these two factors might be associated; could the endocrine aberrations explain the distribution of depot fat to central regions in abdominal obesity?

Cortisol hypersecretion is clearly followed by visceral obesity, as seen most dramatically in Cushing's syndrome. This is reversible after successful treatment (Sjöström, personal communication). The mechanisms for this phenomenon seem to be as follows. Cortisol stimulates the expression of lipoprotein lipase (LPL) activity in adipose tissue by interaction with a specific GR. The hormone–receptor complex then stimulates LPL-gene transcription. The enzyme protein is then also probably stabilized by cortisol. These effects are critically dependent on insulin, and dramatically inhibited by GH [25, 26, 53, 110, 111]. The combination of elevated cortisol secretion, hyperinsulinemia and low GH, as seen in visceral obesity, would thus result in markedly elevated activity of LPL, the enzyme which regulates triglyceride uptake in adipocytes.

These hormones, alone and in combination, also interfere markedly with the lipolytic cascade, regulating triglyceride mobilization. Cortisol alone seems to have inhibitory effects on lipolysis. However, in the presence of GH, cortisol clearly stimulates lipolysis. This process is markedly inhibited by insulin (M. Ottosson, unpublished). Taken together, increased cortisol secretion in the presence of hyperinsulinemia and diminished GH secretion, characteristics of visceral obesity, would be expected to result in a lipid mobilization machinery with low efficacy. In fact in Cushing's syndrome, the net effect of these hormonal abnormalities is elevated LPL activity and diminished lipolysis, which is found specifically in abdominal regions [53]. Why these hormonal effects on the balance of adipocyte lipid turnover should be most pronounced in visceral fat is not clear, but data suggest a particularly high density of the GR in this adipose tissue region [24], so cortisol effects would be expected to be most pronounced here. Other explanations are also possible, however.

Testosterone exerts several, pronounced effects on adipocyte metabolism, again in close concert with GH. LPL expression is inhibited by testosterone [112], more so in the presence of GH (unpublished observations). On the lipid mobilization side testosterone, exclusively in the presence of GH, stimulates the lipolytic cascade by increasing the number of β-adrenergic receptors as well as protein kinase A and/or the hormone-sensitive lipase [27, 28, 113, 114]. These are most likely again gene transcription effects via binding to a specific androgen receptor in adipose tissue. This receptor has the interesting characteristic of being upregulated in density by its ligand, testosterone [115].

These effects of testosterone-GH are amplified by the autoregulation by testosterone of the androgen receptor density. These are opposite effects to those of cortisol. GH inhibits the LPL expression by cortisol, and amplifies lipolysis in the presence of cortisol. In viscerally obese men with a tendency towards increased cortisol secretion and low testosterone and GH levels, LPL activity would therefore be expected to be high and lipolysis potential blunted. The balance between lipid uptake and mobilization is thus again shifted towards the former. Elevated insulin concentrations are also characteristic of abdominally obese men, tending to amplify effects of cortisol on LPL and inhibit lipolysis. The net effect of this multiple hormonal derangement is probably more pronounced in visceral than other adipose tissue regions, due to a higher density of androgen and glucocorticoid receptors in this tissue, although the evidence for this assumption is indirect [116].

The hyperandrogenicity in women with visceral obesity is more difficult to fit into this picture. Increased levels of testosterone in women would, by analogy with the situation in men, tend to mobilize visceral triglycerides. Testosterone effects in men might not, however, necessarily apply to women. Thus, testosterone administration to castrated female rats [117] is followed by different effects on lipolysis regulation than testosterone given to castrated male rats [118].

The effects of the female sex hormones are much less clear. Progesterone and estrogen seem to direct depot fat to the gluteal–femoral regions in women [119], but it is not clear how this is accomplished in the apparent absence of specific receptors for these hormones [120]. Furthermore, no direct effects of these hormones have been observed in human adipose tissue [121]. It seems clear that progesterone competes with

the GR at physiological concentrations [24, 122], so it may be that progesterone counteracts the effects of cortisol by this mechanism.

Table 3 provides a summary of the effects of cortisol, testosterone, insulin and GH on triglyceride balance at the adipocyte level. Viscerally obese men tend to secrete elevated concentrations of cortisol, are hyperinsulinemic and have low concentrations of testosterone and GH. It is clear from Table 3 that this combination of hormonal abnormalities would be expected to shift the balance towards accumulation of triglycerides. The effects of testosterone are amplified by the positive autoregulation of the androgen receptor. The detailed effects of these hormones in women and of female sex steroid hormones are not known. It is suggested that the more pronounced effects on visceral than other adipose tissues are due to a higher density of cortisol and androgen receptors in this tissue, but the evidence for this possibility cannot be considered conclusive. Other possible explanations include effects of circulatory and nervous factors, or simply the fact that visceral adipose tissue contains more adipocytes per unit mass, and is therefore more metabolically active [123, 124].

Table 3   A summary of effects of hormones on triglyceride balance in adipose tissue

	LPL	Lipolysis
Cortisol	0	−
Cortisol + insulin	+ + +	− − −
Cortisol+ GH	0	+ + +
Cortisol + insulin + GH	− − −	− − −
Testosterone	−	0
Testosterone + GH	− − −	+ + +
Testosterone + GH + insulin	?	− − −

LPL, lipoprotein lipase; GH, growth hormone.

ORIGIN OF THE ENDOCRINE ABNORMALITIES

The preceding sections have pointed out the possibility that the multiple endocrine abnormalities associated with visceral obesity may not only cause insulin resistance and its associated metabolic disturbances, but also direct depot fat to central, visceral adipose tissues. The metabolic abnormalities include those recently called syndrome X [125] or the Metabolic Syndrome. Visceral fat accumulation is thus an integral part of this syndrome. We have recently performed a quantitative analysis of the prevalence of abdominal obesity in the syndrome. Women selected at random were divided by quintiles of the WHR and BMI, and the percentage having one or more abnormalities characterizing the Metabolic Syndrome was calculated for each fifth of the distribution. The variables included elevations of insulin, blood pressure and plasma lipids, defined as being above 2 SD of the total cohort. One or more of these perturbations were found in about 90% of the women in the highest fifth of the distribution of WHR and BMI. The entire, full-blown syndrome, including all or most of the metabolic abnormalities, was not frequent, however, suggesting individual differences in its expression [126].

NIDDM is considered to be one of the consequences of the Metabolic Syndrome, triggered via insulin resistance. One may ask whether the endocrine abnormalities characterizing visceral obesity and the Metabolic Syndrome have been observed in patients with NIDDM. First, it should be noted that subjects with NIDDM often have visceral obesity [94, 127] and, in addition to insulin resistance, often also have other parts of the Metabolic Syndrome, including hypertension and hyperlipidemia. NIDDM and the Metabolic Syndrome are therefore largely overlapping conditions, separated mainly by the hyperglycemia of NIDDM.

Direct information on the presence in NIDDM of the endocrine perturbations of the Metabolic Syndrome is now partially available. The characteristic hyperandrogenicity of women with visceral obesity and the Metabolic Syndrome (see section above) has now also been found in women with NIDDM [94], as has relative hypogonadism in men with NIDDM [128]. The more subtle perturbations of the hypothalamo–adrenal axis have apparently not been rigorously studied in NIDDM, and might be difficult to trace in a condition with severely perturbed glucose homeostasis. It should be noticed, however, that trauma, disease and depression, conditions with elevated cortisol secretion, are followed by deterioration of glucose homeostasis, and occasionally by clinical onset of NIDDM [129]. In summary, the endocrine abnormalities of the Metabolic Syndrome seem to be important for the pathogenesis of the insulin resistance of that condition. When NIDDM is preceded by the Metabolic Syndrome, and there is considerable evidence that this is often the case, then the endocrine abnormalities are likely to be involved not only in the pathogenesis of the insulin resistance of the Metabolic Syndrome, but also in the precipitation of NIDDM via the impact of insulin resistance.

The evidence now available points to the possibility that the endocrine abnormalities of visceral obesity cause both cardinal symptoms of that condition, the insulin resistance and the accumulation of visceral fat. It therefore becomes of fundamental importance to try to understand why these endocrine perturbations occur.

The abnormalities include a sensitive hypothalamo–adrenal axis, inhibited sex steroid hormone secretion, and blunted GH secretion. In addition, there is evidence for abnormalities in the regulation of the autonomic nervous system [130]. Both the latter and the cortisol abnormalities can be amplified by mental stressors in the laboratory, and, probably, in every-day life [105], suggesting their central origin. There is evidence of gonadotropin abnormalities [94], and GH secretion is directly dependent on central regulatory mechanisms. Taken together, the multiplicity of the endocrine abnormalities, as well as the evidence of involvement of tropic hormones, strongly suggest that the endocrine aberrations have a central, neuroendocrine origin. The hyperandrogenicity of women cannot be directly included in this proposed view, however, mainly because of lack of information as to its origin.

Neuroendocrine abnormalities of this character are reminiscent of hypothalamic arousal described after certain types of stress [131, 132], as well as after tobacco smoking [133] and alcohol consumption [134]. Smoking and elevated consumption of alcohol have both been found to be associated with visceral accumulation of depot fat [79, 135].

The endocrine response to stress has been repeatedly studied in animal experiments [131, 132]. The outcome depends to a large extent on the ability of the individual to cope with the perceived stressful stimuli. The classical fight-or-flight reaction is characterized by activation of the sympathetic nervous system during a period of striving for control and, when control has been achieved, testosterone secretion becomes elevated. Under the pressure of a noncontrollable stress, however, a 'submissive', 'helplessness' reaction develops, whose endocrine counterparts are increased activity along the hypothalamo–adrenal axis, and depression of sex steroid hormone secretion. In addition, GH secretion becomes blunted, and hemodynamic responses abnormal. The similarity with the endocrine abnormalities of visceral obesity is striking, and is amplified by laboratory stress experiments [105, 130]. It may therefore be warranted to look for signs and symptoms of stressors of equivalent character to those causing submissive behaviour in animals in subjects with the syndrome in question. Evidence for such stressors has been obtained in standardized laboratory tests, although they are not as distinctly separable into defined categories as in the animal experiments [136]. A similarity of stress reactions among species may be expected, because the control mechanisms are localized in a common area of the brain, and are necessary for survival [137].

Although acute experiments in humans have shown essentially similar endocrine reactions to stress as in animal experiments [105, 130, 136], chronic, controlled induction of stress cannot be performed in humans for ethical reasons. There is a considerable literature on the reaction pattern of humans exposed to chronic stress due to psychosocial and socioeconomic conditions, or to life-events of a stressful nature [129], but detailed examinations of the metabolic consequences have seldom been performed.

A series of elegant studies has, however, recently been conducted in primates exposed to chronic, controlled stress of non-controllable, submissive type under strictly standardized conditions. The endocrine consequences were those already known from previous experiments, with enlarged adrenals and low sex hormone secretion. Additional studies revealed signs of insulin resistance, decreased glucose tolerance, and elevated blood pressure and plasma lipid concentrations. Furthermore, recent studies have shown an accumulation of visceral depot fat [138–141; also Shively, personal communication]. The disease consequences of this syndrome, induced by submissive stress during prolonged periods, have been found to be coronary arteriosclerosis, in addition to the development towards NIDDM suggested by the insulin resistance and decreased glucose tolerance. Similar observations, although less detailed, had previously been made by Mason [132]. The similarities with the Metabolic Syndrome, including visceral obesity and its endocrine associations are considerable. It does not seem unreasonable to suspect that a similar chain of events occurs in humans with similar endocrine, metabolic, body fat distribution and disease characteristics, particularly since the endocrine abnormalities can be amplified by acute stress tests.

The next question is which factors in the environment of subjects with visceral obesity and the Metabolic Syndrome might lead to a chronic stress reaction similar to that observed in the primate experiments. In population studies we found suggestive evidence for such connections in both men [135] and women [79], utilizing the WHR as indicator of the syndrome in question. Both men and women with elevated WHR were often on sick-leave and absent from work. They frequently used free health facilities such as X-ray and examinations at doctors' offices. The diseases included psychosomatic conditions such as peptic ulcer and gastrointestinal bleeding, but also infections and traumata. Men generally had a poor education, belonged to a low social class, and often had physical, relatively poorly paid work. In women psychological and psychiatric variables were also registered, and revealed frequent use of tranquilizers, anxiolytic and antidepressant drugs. Both men and women showed high scores in the question whether they 'felt to be stressed'. Both men and women were also frequently smokers, and consumed alcohol more frequently, often strong liquor in larger volumes than average.

In total these results seem to fit into a picture with subjects under psychosocial and socioeconomic pressures due to poor education and poorly paid work,

with the consequences of psychosomatic and psychiatric conditions, leading to frequent sick-leave and use of health facilities. It is of interest that subjects with elevated BMI, adjusted for the WHR factor, indicating generalized obesity, did not have these characteristics. In fact, such persons often had lower scores in several of the mentioned variables [79, 135].

From these observations we have suggested that subjects in the population with elevated WHR, signifying abdominal distribution of body fat stores, are subjected to a stressful environment with which they have deficient abilities to cope, leading to various psychological and somatic consequences [79, 135, 142, 143]. The endocrine perturbations of such a situation, reviewed above, were not measured in these individuals, but by analogy with other cross-sectional studies, it does not seem far-fetched to suggest that such abnormalities would have been found, had they been measured. Recent studies have confirmed these observations [144, 145].

GENERAL SUMMARY

The connection between obesity and NIDDM is clearly stronger in the subgroup of abdominal, visceral obesity. It seems probable that this is due to the more marked insulin resistance of this subgroup. Visceral obesity is also associated with the multiple metabolic derangements characterizing the Metabolic Syndrome. The insulin resistance is probably at least partly due to elevations of FFA concentrations in combination with a number of endocrine abnormalities. Evidence of insulin resistance is found both at the level of the liver and muscle. Recent and previous findings suggest the possibility that elevated FFA concentrations in the portal vein may generate several of the components of the Metabolic Syndrome. The endocrine abnormalities may well amplify insulin resistance in muscle, where decreased capillary density might be a central feature, leading to a diminished insulin signal to glucose transport and glycogen synthesis regulated by glycogen synthase. The endocrine abnormalities may also direct depot fat to centrally localized adipose tissues because of the high density of specific steroid hormone receptors in these tissues.

The multiple endocrine abnormalities are most likely of central origin, and may be the consequence of neuroendocrine disturbance(s) on the basis of a hypothalamic arousal syndrome. Indirect evidence suggests that this in turn may be caused by a combination of factors, where smoking, alcohol consumption and poor coping with stress are important ingredients. The endocrine aberrations are similar to those elicited by poor coping in a stressful environment. Such factors can be traced in the psychosocial and socioeconomic environment of

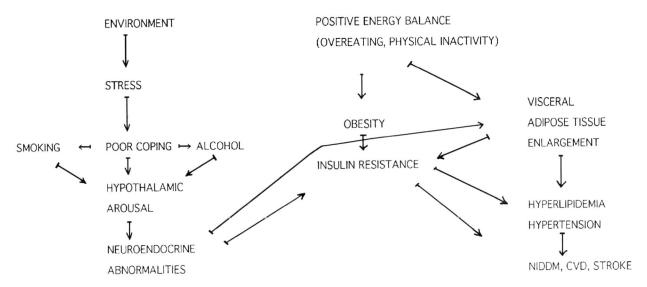

Figure 1 Proposed development of a 'Civilization Syndrome'. Primary factors are a positive energy balance leading to obesity, with excess depot fat directed to visceral adipose tissue by multiple endocrine abnormalities, due to neuroendocrine perturbations. These amplify insulin resistance, and are caused by a hypothalamic arousal syndrome. This in turn is based on environmental stress, leading to poor coping, smoking and alcohol consumption. Insulin resistance and visceral adipose tissue enlargement are followed by hyperlipidemia and hypertension, all established precursors to non-insulin dependent diabetes mellitus (NIDDM), cardiovascular disease (CVD) and stroke. Genetic susceptibility modifies the consequences at multiple, different levels

subjects with abdominally distributed adipose tissue in population studies.

This summary (Figure 1) is based on the results of cross-sectional and prospective epidemiological surveys, clinical case-control and intervention studies, as well as detailed cellular and molecular observations. Much more work is needed before this integrated hypothesis can be proven to be correct or will have to be refuted. An attractive feature of this approach to the pathogenesis of the Metabolic Syndrome seems to be that its putative pathogenetic factors embrace several unhealthy life-style components of urban, civilized society. These factors include overeating and physical inactivity (leading to obesity), stress, alcohol and smoking, presumably leading to insulin resistance (amplified by obesity), as well as visceral fat accumulation. This then might be considered as a 'Civilization Syndrome', as recently suggested [146]. The basic abnormalities may lead to different expressions of disease depending on genetic susceptibility. NIDDM, for example, might be particularly commonly expressed in individuals who are prone to develop insulin resistance and have insufficient capability for compensatory insulin secretion.

REFERENCES

1. Vague J. La differentiation sexuelle. Facteur determinant des formes de l'obesité. Presse Med 1947; 55: 339–41.
2. Kissebah AH, Evans DJ, Peiris A, Wilson CR. Endocrine characteristics of regional obesities: role of sex steroids. In Vague J et al (eds) Metabolic complications of human obesities. Amsterdam: Excerpta Medica, 1985: pp 115–30.
3. Peiris AN, Mueller RA, Struve MF, Smith GA, Kissebah AH. Relationships of androgenic activity to splanchnic insulin metabolism and peripheral glucose utilization in premenopausal women. J Clin Endocrinol Metab 1987; 64: 162–9.
4. Krotkiewski M, Björntorp P, Sjöström L, Smith U. Impact of obesity on metabolism in men and women. Importance of regional adipose tissue distribution. J Clin Invest 1983; 72: 1150–8.
5. Krotkiewski M, Björntorp P. Muscle tissue in obesity with different distribution of adipose tissue, effects of physical training. Int J Obesity 1986; 10: 331–41.
6. Olefsky JM. Decreased insulin binding to adipocytes and circulating monocytes from obese subjects. J Clin Invest 1976; 57: 1165–72.
7. Clark MG, Rattigan S, Clark DG. Obesity with insulin resistance: experimental insights. Lancet 1983; ii: 1236–40.
8. Bonora E, Zavaroni I, Coscelli C, Butturini U. Decreased hepatic insulin extraction in subjects with mild glucose intolerance. Metabolism 1983; 32: 438–44.
9. Faber OK, Christensen K, Kehlet H, Madsbad S, Binder C. Decreased insulin removal contributes to hyperinsulinemia in obesity. J Clin Endocrinol 1981; 53: 618–25.
10. Krotkiewski M, Lönnroth P, Mandroukas K et al. The effects of physical training on insulin secretion and effectiveness and on glucose metabolism in obesity and Type 2 (non-insulin dependent) diabetes mellitus. Diabetologia 1985; 28: 881–90.
11. Jeanrenaud B, Halimi S, van de Werve G. Neuroendocrine disorders seen as triggers of the triad obesity–insulin resistance–abnormal glucose tolerance. Diabetes Metab Rev 1985; 1: 261–91.

12. Karakash C, Assimacopoulos-Jeannet F, Jeanrenaud B. An anomaly of insulin removal in perfused livers of obese-hyperglycemic (Ob/ob) mice. J Clin Invest 1976; 57: 1117–23.

13. Svedberg J, Björntorp P, Smith U, Lönnroth P. Free-fatty acid inhibition of insulin binding, degradation, and action in isolated rat hepatocytes. Diabetes 1990; 39: 570–4.

14. Svedberg J, Strömblad G, Wirth A, Smith U, Björntorp P. Fatty acids in the portal vein regulate hepatic insulin clearance. J Clin Invest 1991; 88: 2054–8.

15. Strömblad G, Björntorp P. Reduced hepatic insulin clearance in rats with dietary-induced obesity. Metabolism 1986; 35: 323–7.

16. Svedberg J, Björntorp P, Lönnroth P, Smith U. Prevention of inhibitory effect of free fatty acids on insulin binding and action in isolated rat hepatocytes by etomoxir. Diabetes 1991; 40: 783–6.

17. Svedberg J, Björntorp P, Smith U, Lönnroth P. Effect of free fatty acids on insulin receptor binding and tyrosine kinase activity in hepatocytes isolated from lean and obese rats. Diabetes 1992; 41: 294–8.

18. Hennes MM, Shrago E, Kissebah AH. Receptor and postreceptor effects of free fatty acids (FFA) on hepatocyte insulin dynamics. Int J Obesity 1990; 14: 831–9.

19. Ferrannini E, Barrett EJ, Bevilaqua MP, DeFronzo RA. Effects of fatty acids on glucose production and utilization in man. J Clin Invest 1983; 72: 1737–44.

20. Björntorp P. 'Portal' adipose tissue as a generator of risk factors for cardiovascular disease and diabetes. Arteriosclerosis 1990; 10: 493–6.

21. Mårin P, Rebuffé-Scrive M, Björntorp P. Uptake of triglyceride fatty acids in adipose tissue *in vivo* in man. Eur J Clin Invest 1990; 20: 158–65.

22. Rebuffé-Scrive M, Andersson B, Olbe L, Björntorp P. Metabolism of adipose tissue in intra-abdominal depots in non-obese men and women. Metabolism 1989; 38: 453–8.

23. Rebuffé-Scrive M, Andersson B, Olbe L, Björntorp P, Metabolism of adipose tissue in intra-abdominal depots in severely obese men and women. Metabolism 1990; 139: 1021–5.

24. Rebuffé-Scrive, M, Lundholm K, Björntorp P. Glucocorticoid hormone binding to human adipose tissue. Eur J Clin Invest 1985; 15: 267–71.

25. Cigolini M, Smith U. Human adipose tissue in culture. VIII. Studies on the insulin-antagonistic effects of glucocorticoids. Metabolism 1979; 28: 502–10.

26. Ottosson M, Rebuffé-Scrive M, Björntorp P. Effects of glucocorticoids on human adipose tissue. Int J Obesity 1989; 13 (suppl. 1): 197.

27. Xu X, De Pergola G, Björntorp P. The effects of androgens on the regulation of lipolysis in adipose precursor cells. Endocrinology 1990; 126: 1229–34.

28. Xu X, De Pergola G, Björntorp P. Testosterone increases lipolysis and the number of β-adrenoceptors in male rat adipocytes. Endocrinology 1991; 128: 379–82.

29. Bolinder J, Engfeldt P, Östman J, Arner P. Site differences in insulin receptor binding and insulin action in subcutaneous fat of obese females. J Clin Endocr Metab 1983; 57: 455–60.

30. Bolinder J, Kager L, Östman J, Arner P. Differences at the receptor and postreceptor levels between human omental and subcutaneous adipose tissue in the action of insulin on lipolysis. Diabetes 1983; 32: 117–23.

31. West DB, Prinz WA, Greenwood MRC. Regional changes in adipose tissue, blood flow and metabolism in rats after a meal. Am J Physiol 1989; 257: R711–16.

32. Björntorp P. Adipose tissue distribution and function. Int J Obesity 1991; 15: 67–81.

33. Rosell R, Belfrage E. Blood circulation in adipose tissue. Physiol Rev 1979; 59: 1078–104.

34. Björntorp P, Östman J. Human adipose tissue. Dynamics and regulation. Adv Metab Dis 1971; 5: 277–327.

35. Rebuffé-Scrive M. Regional differences in visceral adipose tissue. Int J Obesity 1990; 14 (suppl. 2): 26.

36. Björntorp P. Hypertension in obesity. Acta Med Scand 1982; 211: 241–2.

37. Reaven GR, Hoffman BB. A role for insulin in the aetiology and course of hypertension? Lancet 1987; ii: 435–6.

38. Mårin P, Rebuffé-Scrive M, Smith U, Björntorp P. Glucose uptake in human adipose tissue. Metabolism 1987; 36: 1154–60.

39. Chen YD, Golay A, Swislocki ALM, Reaven GM. Resistance to insulin suppression of plasma free fatty acid concentrations and insulin stimulation of glucose uptake in non-insulin dependent diabetes mellitus. J Clin Endocr Metab 1987; 64: 17–21.

40. Shuman WP, Morris LN, Leonetti DL et al. Abnormal body fat distribution detected by computed tomography in diabetic men. Inv Radiol 1986; 21: 483–7.

41. Kissebah AH, Peiris AN. Biology of regional body fat distribution: relationship to non-insulin-dependent diabetes mellitus. Diabetes Metab Rev 1989; 5: 83–109.

42. Reaven G, Chang M, Ho H, Jeng CY, Hoffman BB. Lowering of plasma glucose in diabetic rats. Am J Physiol 1988; 254: E23–30.

43. Reaven G, Chang H, Hoffman BB. Additive hypoglycemic effects of drugs that modify free fatty acid metabolism by different mechanisms in rats with streptozocin-induced diabetes. Diabetes 1988; 37: 28–32.

44. Randle PJ, Garland PB, Hales CN, Newsholme EA. The glucose fatty acid cycle. Its role in insulin sensitivity and the metabolic disturbances of diabetes mellitus. Lancet 1963; i: 785–9.

45. Jensen MD, Haymond MW, Rizza RA, Cryer PE, Miles JM. Influence of body fat distribution on free fatty acid metabolism in obesity. J Clin Invest 1989; 83: 1168–73.

46. Bonen A, Tan MH, Watson-Wright WM. Insulin binding and glucose uptake in rodent skeletal muscle. Diabetes 1981; 30: 702–4.

47. James DE, Jenkins AB, Kraegen EW. Heterogeneity of insulin action in individual muscles *in vivo*: euglycemic clamp studies in rats. Am J Physiol 1985; 218: E567–74.

48. Richter EA, Garetto LP, Goodman MN, Ruderman NB. Enhanced muscle glucose metabolism after exercise: modulation by local factors. Am J Physiol 1984; 246: E476–82.

49. Lillioja S, Young AA, Culter CL et al. Skeletal muscle capillary density and fiber type are possible determinants of *in vivo* insulin resistance in man. J Clin Invest 1987; 80: 415–24.

50. Björntorp P, de Jounge K, Sjöström L, Sullivan L. The effect of physical training on insulin production in obesity. Metabolism 1970; 19: 631–8.

51. Saltin B, Henriksson J, Nygaard E, Andersen P. Fiber-types and metabolic potentials of skeletal muscle in sedentary man and endurance runners. Ann NY Acad Sci 1977; 30: 3-29.

52. Danneskiold-Samsøe B, Grimby G. The influence of prednisolone on the muscle morphology and muscle enzymes in patients with rheumatoid arthritis. Clin Sci 1986; 71: 693-701.

53. Rebuffé-Scrive M, Krotkiewski M, Elfversson J, Björntorp P. Muscle and adipose tissue morphology and metabolism in Cushing's syndrome. J Clin Endocrinol Metab 1988; 67: 1122-5.

54. Krotkiewski M, Kral JG, Karlsson J. Effects of castration and testosterone substitution on body composition and muscle metabolism in rats. Acta Physiol Scand 1980; 109: 233-7.

55. Holmäng A, Brzczinska Z, Björntorp P. Effects of hyperinsulinemia on muscle fiber composition and capillarization in rats. Diabetes 1993; 42: 1073-81.

56. Lithell H, Lindgärde F, Hellsing K, Lundqvist G, Nygaard E, Vessby B, Saltin B. Body weight, skeletal muscle morphology and enzyme activities in relation to fasting serum insulin concentration and glucose tolerance in 48-year-old men. Diabetes 1981; 30: 19-25.

57. Lindgärde F, Eriksson KF, Lithell H, Saltin B. Coupling between dietary changes, reduced body weight, muscle fiber size and improved glucose tolerance in middle-aged men with impaired glucose tolerance. Acta Med Scand 1982; 212: 99-106.

58. Krotkiewski M, Bylund-Fellenius A-C, Holm J, Björntorp P, Grimby G, Mandroukas K. Relationship between muscle morphology, and metabolism in obese women: the effects of long-term physical training. Eur J Clin Invest 1983; 13: 5-12.

59. Holmäng A, Svedberg J, Jennische E, Björntorp P. The effects of testosterone on muscle insulin sensitivity and morphology in female rats. Am J Physiol 1990; 259: E555-60.

60. Rasio EA, Mach E, Egdahl RM, Herrera MG. Passage of insulin across vascular membranes in the dog. Diabetes 1968; 17: 668-72.

61. Rasio EA. The displacement of insulin from blood capillaries. Diabetologia 1969; 5: 416-19.

62. Rasio EA. The capillary barrier to circulating insulin. Diabetes Care 1982; 5: 158-61.

63. King GL, Johnson SM. Receptor-mediated transport of insulin across endothelial cells. Science 1986; 227: 1583-6.

64. Holmäng A, Björntorp P, Rippe B. Tissue uptake of insulin and inulin in red and white skeletal muscle *in vivo*. Am J Physiol 1992; 263: H1170-76.

65. Yang YJ, Hope ID, Ader M, Bergman RN. Insulin transport across capillaries is rate-limiting for insulin action in dogs. J Clin Invest 1989; 84: 1620-28.

66. Allenberg K, Johansen K, Saltin B. Skeletal muscle adaptions to physical training in type 2 (non-insulin dependent) diabetes mellitus. Acta Med Scand 1988; 223: 365-73.

67. Andersen P, Henriksson J. Capillary supply of the quadriceps femoris muscle of man: adaptive response to exercise. J Physiol 1977; 270: 677-90.

68. Holmäng A, Björntorp P. The effects of cortisol on insulin sensitivity in muscle. Acta Physiol Scand 1992; 144: 425-31.

69. Holmäng A, Larsson BM, Brzezinska Z, Björntorp P. Effects of short-term testosterone exposure on insulin sensitivity of muscles in female rats. Am J Physiol 1992; 262: E851-5.

70. Holmäng A, Björntorp P. The effects of testosterone on insulin sensitivity in male rats. Acta Physiol Scand 1992; 146: 505-10.

71. Kumagai S, Holmäng A, Björntorp P. The effects of oestrogen and progesterone on insulin sensitivity in female rats. Acta Physiol Scand 1993 149: 91-7.

72. Kalkhoff R. Effects of oral contraceptive agents and sex steroids on carbohydrate metabolism. Am Rev Med 1972; 23: 429-38.

73. Evans PJ, Hoffman RG, Kalkhoff RK, Kissebah AH. Relationship of androgenic activity to body fat topography, fat cell morphology and metabolic aberrations in menopausal women. J Clin Endocrinol Metab 1983; 57: 304-10.

74. Vague J, Meignen JM, Negrin JF, Thomas M, Tramoni M, Jubelin J. La diabète de la femme androide. Trente-cinq ans après. Sem Hôp Paris 1985; 61: 1015-25.

75. Kurtz BR, Givens JR, Komindr et al. Maintenance of normal circulating levels of androstenedione and dehydroepiandrosterone in simple obesity despite increased metabolic clearance rates. Evidence for a servocontrol mechanism. J Clin Endocrinol Metab 1987; 64: 1261-7.

76. Hartz AJ, Rupley DC, Kalkhoff RD, Rimm AA. Relationship of obesity to diabetes: influence of obesity level and body fat distribution. Prev Med 1983; 12: 351-7.

77. Rebuffé-Scrive M, Cullberg G, Lundberg PA, Lindstedt G, Björntorp P. Anthropometric variables and metabolism in polycystic ovarian disease. Horm Metab Res 1989; 21: 391-7.

78. Yen SSC, Chaney C, Judd HL. Functional aberrations of the hypothalamic–pituitary system in polycystic ovary syndrome: a consideration of the pathogenesis. In James VHT, Serio M, Iusit G (eds) Endocrine function of the human ovary. New York: Academic Press, 1976: pp 373.

79. Lapidus L, Bengtsson C, Hällström T, Björntorp P. Obesity, adipose tissue distribution and health in women—results from a population study in Gothenburg, Sweden. Appetite 1989; 12: 25-35.

80. Taylor SJ, Dons RF, Hernandez E, Roth J, Gordon P. Insulin resistance associated with androgen excess in women with autoantibodies to the insulin receptor. Ann Intern Med 1982; 97: 851-61.

81. McNatty KP, Smith DM, Makris A et al. The intraovarian sites of androgen and estrogen formation of women with normal and hyperandrogenic ovaries as judged by *in vitro* experiments. J Clin Endocrinol Metab 1980; 50: 755-66.

82. Cole C, Kitabchi AE. Remission of insulin resistance with Orthonovum in a patient with polycystic ovarian disease and acanthosis nigricans. Clin Res 1978; 26: 412A (abstr).

83. Shoupe D, Lobo RA. The influence of androgens on insulin resistance. Fertil Steril 1984; 41: 385-92.

84. Geffner ME, Kaplan SA, Bersch N, Golde DW, Landaw EM, Chang RS. Persistence of insulin resistance in polycystic ovarian disease after inhibition of ovarian steroid secretion. Fertil Steril 1986; 45: 327-32.

85. Nester JE, Clove JN, Strauss JF, Blackard WG. The effects of hyperinsulinemia on serum testosterone, progesterone, dehydroepiandrosterone sulfate, and

cortisol levels in normal women and in women with hyperandrogenism, insulin resistance, and acanthosis nigricans. J Clin Endocrinol Metab 1987; 64: 180–92.

86. Barbieri RL, Makris A, Ryan KJ. Effects of insulin on steroid-genesis in cultured porcine ovarian theca. Fertil Steril 1983; 40: 237–49.

87. Davoren JB, Kasson BG, Li CH, Hsueh AJW. Specific insulin-like growth factor (IGF) I- and II-binding sites in rat granulosa cells: relation to IGF action. Endocrinology 1986; 119: 2155–67.

88. Erickson GF, Magoffin DA, Dyer CA, Hofeditz C. The ovarian androgen producing cells: a review of structure/function relationships. Endocr Rev 1985; 6: 371–402.

89. Poretsky L, Karlin MF. The gonadotropic function of insulin. Endocr Rev 1987; 8: 132–41.

90. Seidell J, Cigolini M, Ellsinger B-M et al. Androgenicity in relation to body fat distribution and metabolism in 38-year-old women—the European Fat Distribution Study. J Clin Epidemiol 1990; 42: 21–34.

91. Lindstedt G, Lundberg P-A, Lapidus L, Lundgren H, Bengtsson C, Björntorp P. Low sex-hormone binding globulin as independent risk factor for development of non-insulin dependent diabetes mellitus. 12-year follow-up of population study of women in Gothenburg, Sweden. Diabetes 1991; 40: 123–8.

92. Lundgren H, Bengtsson C, Blohmé G, Lapidus L. Adiposity and adipose tissue distribution in relation to incidence of diabetes in women: results from a prospective population study in Gothenburg, Sweden. Int J Obesity 1989; 13: 413–18.

93. Lundgren H, Bengtsson C, Blohmé G, Lapidus L, Waldenström J. Fasting serum insulin and early insulin response as risk determinants for developing diabetes. Results from a 12-year follow-up of women aged 50 in Gothenburg, Sweden. Diabet Med 1990; 7: 407–13.

94. Andersson B, Mårin P, Lissner L, Vermeulen A, Björntorp P. Testosterone concentrations in women and men with non-insulin dependent diabetes mellitus. Diabetes Care 1994; 17: 405–11.

95. Andersson B, Hahn L, Mattsson L-Å, Björntorp P. Female sex steroids and the metabolic syndrome. In Proceedings of the Novo Nordisk International Symposium, Copenhagen, Denmark. Novo Copenhagen: Wells Medical Ltd, 1993; pp 85–92.

96. Cohen JC, Hickman R. Insulin resistance and diminished glucose tolerance in power lifters ingesting anabolic steroids. J Clin Endocrinol Metab 1987; 64: 960–71.

97. Seidell JC, Björntorp P, Sjöström L, Kvist H, Sannerstedt R. Visceral fat accumulation in men is positively associated with insulin, glucose, and C-peptide levels but negatively with testosterone levels. Metabolism 1990; 39: 897–901.

98. Khaw KT, Chir MBB, Barrett-Connor E. Lower endogenous androgens predict central adiposity in men. Am J Epidem 1992; 2: 675–82.

99. Haffner SH, Waldez RA, Stern MP, Katz MS. Obesity, body fat distribution and sex hormones in men. Int J Obesity 1993; 17: 643–9.

100. Mårin P, Krotkiewski M, Björntorp P. Androgen treatment of middle-aged obese men: effects on metabolism, muscle, and adipose tissue. Eur J Med 1992; 1: 329–36.

101. Mårin P, Björntorp P. Androgen treatment of middle-aged obese men: effects on glucose tolerance, insulin

sensitivity, and fat distribution. Obesity Research 1993; 1: 245–51.

102. Jung R. Endocrinological aspects of obesity. Clin Endocrinol Metab 1984; 13: 597–612.

103. Baxter JD, Rousseau GG. Glucocorticoid hormone action. Monogr Endocrinol 1979; 12: 1–26.

104. Krotkiewski M, Butruk E, Zembrzuska Z. Les fonctions cortico-surrenales dans les divers types morphologiques d'obesité. Diabète 1966; 19: 229–33.

105. Mårin P, Darin N, Amemeiya T, Andersson B, Jern S, Björntorp P. Cortisol secretion in relation to body fat distribution in obese premenopausal women. Metabolism 1992; 41: 882–6.

106. Mårin P, Kvist H, Lindstedt G, Sjöström L, Björntorp P. Low concentrations of insulin-like growth factor I in abdominal obesity. Int J Obesity 1993; 17: 83–9.

107. Clemmons DA, Van Wyk JJ. Factors controlling blood concentrations of somatomedin C. J Clin Endocr Metab 1984; 13: 113–43.

108. Mårin P, Rosmond R, Bengtsson B-Å, Gustafsson C, Molin G, Björntorp P. Growth hormone secretion after testosterone administration to men with visceral obesity. Obesity Res 1994; 2: 263–70.

109. Rudingenau D, Kutner MH, Rogers CM, Lubin MF, Fleming GA, Brain RP. Impaired growth hormone secretion in the adult population: relation to age and adiposity. J Clin Invest 1981; 67: 1361–9.

110. Ottosson M, Vikman-Adolfsson K, Enerbäck S, Bengtsson-Olivecrona G, Björntorp P. The effects of cortisol on the regulation of lipoprotein lipase in human adipose tissue. J Clin Endocrinol Metab 1994; 79: 820–25.

111. Appel B, Fried SK. Effects of insulin and dexamethasone on lipoprotein lipase in human adipose tissue. Am J Physiol 1992; 262: E695–9.

112. Rebuffé-Scrive M, Mårin P, Björntorp P. Effect of testosterone on abdominal adipose tissue in men. Int J Obesity 1991; 15: 791–5.

113. Xu X, De Pergola G, Eriksson PS, Fu L, Carlsson B, Yang S, Edén S, Björntorp P. Post-receptor events involved in the up-regulation of β-adrenergic receptor mediated lipolysis by testosterone. Endocrinology 1993; 132: 1651–7.

114. Yang S, Xu X, Björntorp P, Edén S. Additive effects of growth hormone and testosterone on lipolysis in adipocytes of hypophysectomized rats. J Endocrinol 1995;147: 147–52.

115. De Pergola G, Xu X, Yang S, Giorgino R, Björntorp P. Up-regulation of androgen receptor binding in male rat fat pad adipose precursor cells exposed to testosterone: study in a whole cell assay system. J Ster Biochem Molec Biol 1991; 37: 553–8.

116. Björntorp P. Adipose tissue distribution and function. Int J Obesity 1991; 15 (suppl. 2): 67–81.

117. De Pergola G, Holmäng A, Svedberg J, Giorgino R, Björntorp P. Testosterone treatment of ovariectomized rats: effects on lipolysis regulation in adipocytes. Acta Endocrin (Copenh) 1990; 123: 61–6.

118. Xu X, De Pergola G, Björntorp P. Testosterone increases lipolysis and the number of β-adrenoceptors in male rat adipocytes. Endocrinology 1991; 128: 379–82.

119. Rebuffé-Scrive M, Björntorp P. Regional adipose tissue metabolism in man. In Vague J et al

(eds) Metabolic complications of human obesities. Amsterdam: Elsevier, 1985: pp 149–59.

120. Rebuffé-Scrive M, Brönnegård M, Nilsson A, Eldh J, Gustafsson J-Å, Björntorp P. Steroid hormone receptors in human adipose tissues. J Clin Endocrinol Metab 1990; 71: 1215–19.

121. Brönnegård M, Ottosson M, Böös J, Marcus C, Björntorp P. Lack of evidence for estrogen and progesterone receptors in human adipose tissue. J Steroid Biochem Mol Biol 1994; 51: 275–81.

122. Xu X, Hoebeke J, Björntorp P. Progestin binds to the glucocorticoid receptor and mediates antiglucocorticoid effect in rat adipose precursor cells. J Steroid Biochem 1990; 36: 465–70.

123. Salans LB, Cushman SW, Weismann RE. Studies on human adipose tissue. Adipose cell size and number in non-obese and obese patients. J Clin Invest 1973; 52: 929–41.

124. Li M, Yang S, Björntorp P. Metabolism of different adipose tissue *in vivo* in the rat. Obesity Research 1993; 1: 459–68.

125. Reaven GH. Role of insulin in human disease. Diabetes 1988; 37: 1595–1607.

126. Lapidus L, Björntorp P. The quantitative relationship between 'The Metabolic Syndrome' and abdominal obesity in women. Obesity Res 1994; 2: 372–7.

127. Bergström RW, Newell-Morris LL, Leonetti DL, Shuman WP, Wahl PW, Fujimoto WY. Association of elevated C-peptide level and increased intra-abdominal fat distribution with development of NIDDM in Japanese-American men. Diabetes 1990; 39: 104–11.

128. Barrett-Connor E, Khaw KT, Yen SSC. Endogenous sex hormone levels in older adult men with diabetes mellitus. Am J Epid 1990; 132: 895–901.

129. Wolf S. The role of the brain in bodily disease. In Weiner H, Hofer MA, Stunkard A (eds) Brain, behavior and bodily disease. New York: Raven Press, 1981: pp 1–9.

130. Jern S, Bergbrant A, Björntorp P, Hansson L. Relation of central hemodynamics to obesity and body fat distribution. Hypertension 1992; 19: 520–7.

131. Henry JP, Stephens PM. Stress, health, and the social environment. A sociobiological approach to medicine. New York: Springer, 1977.

132. Mason JW. Organization of the multiple endocrine responses to avoidance in the monkey. Psychosom Med 1967; 330: 774–90.

133. Gossain VV, Sherma NK, Srivastava L, Michelakis AM, Rovner DR. Hormonal effects of smoking. II: Effects on plasma, cortisol, growth hormone, and prolactin. Amer J Med Sci 1986; 291: 325–7.

134. Cicero TJ. Sex differences in the effects of alcohol and other psychoactive drugs on endocrine function. In Israel Y, Kalant O, Kalant H (eds) Research advances in alcohol and drug problems. New York: Plenum, 1980; pp 544–93.

135. Larsson B, Seidell J, Svärdsudd K, Welin L, Tibblin G, Björntorp P. Obesity, adipose tissue distribution and health in men. The study of men born in 1913. Appetite 1989; 13: 37–44.

136. Frankenhaeuser M. The sympathetic-adrenal and pituitary-adrenal response to challenge: Comparisons between the sexes. In Dombrowski TM, Schmidt TH, Blümchen G (eds) Biobehavioural bases of coronary heart disease, human psychophysiology. Biobehavioral Medicine Series, vol. 2. Basel: Karger, 1983: pp 91–105.

137. Folkow B. Stress, hypothalamic function and neuroendocrine consequences. In Björntorp P, Smith U, Lönnroth P (eds) Health implications of regional obesity. Acta Med Scand, Symposium Series no 4. Stockholm: Almqvist & Wiksell International, 1988; pp 61–9.

138. Kaplan JR, Adams MR, Clarkson TB, Koritnik DR. Psychosocial influences on female 'protection' among cynomolgus macaques. Atherosclerosis 1984; 53: 221–33.

139. Adams MR, Kaplan JR, Clarkson TB, Koritnik DR. Ovariectomy, social status and atherosclerosis in cynomolgus monkeys. Arteriosclerosis 1985; 5: 192–200.

140. Shively C, Clarkson TB, Miller CL, Weingard JW. Body fat as a risk factor for coronary artery atherosclerosis in female cynomolgus monkeys. Arteriosclerosis 1987; 7: 226–31.

141. Shively C, Clarkson TB. Regional adiposity, atherogenesis and atherosclerosis risk factors in a non-human primate model. In Björntorp P, Smith U, Lönnroth P (eds) Health implications of regional obesity. Acta Med Scand 1987; suppl. 723; 71–8.

142. Björntorp P. Possible mechanisms relating fat distribution and metabolism. In Bouchard C, Johnston F (eds) Fat distribution during growth and later health outcomes. New York: Alan R Liss, 1988; pp 175–91.

143. Björntorp P. The association between obesity, adipose tissue distribution and disease. Acta Med Scand 1987; suppl. 723: 121–34.

144. Leonetti DL, Bergström RW, Shuman WP, Wahl PW, Jenner DA, Harrison GA, Fujimoto WY. Urinary catecholamines, plasma insulin and environmental factors in relation to body fat distribution. Int J Obesity 1991; 15: 345–57.

145. Wing RR, Matthews KA, Kuller LH, Meilahn EN, Plantings P. Waist to hip ratio in middle-aged women. Association with behavioural and psychosocial factors and with changes in cardiovascular risk factors. Arterioscler Thromb 1991; 11: 1250–57.

146. Björntorp P. Visceral obesity: a 'Civilization Syndrome'. Obesity Res 1993; 1: 206–22.

30

Assays for Insulin and Precursors

P. M. S. Clark and C. N. Hales

Department of Clinical Biochemistry, University of Cambridge, UK

INTRODUCTION

Since the discovery of insulin in the 1920s much effort has been expended in developing assays for its measurement. Early assays, either chemical or bioassays, lacked sensitivity but were used to determine insulin concentrations in pharmaceutical preparations [1]. The introduction of radioimmunoassays (RIA) by Yalow and Berson in 1959 [2] paved the way for more specific, sensitive and faster assays for insulin in a variety of body fluids.

Assays for insulin and its precursors are now used for a variety of reasons. For diagnostic and forensic purposes these assays are used for the investigation of suspected insulinomas, neonatal hypoglycaemia and surreptitious administration of hypoglycaemic agents. More particularly it is hoped that the development of assays for insulin and its precursors will allow the further investigation of the pathogenetic mechanisms involved in non-insulin dependent diabetes (NIDDM, type 2 diabetes).

PROINSULIN(S) AND INSULIN

Insulin is synthesized from a precursor peptide, proinsulin [3] by a process of enzymatic cleavage (Figure 1). Cleavage at the AC junction (by endopeptidase II) yields 65–66 split proinsulin and cleavage at the BC junction (by endopeptidase I) yields 32–33 split proinsulin. Further processing by carboxypeptidase H results in a loss of a pair of basic amino acids to give the *des* forms of the partially processed proinsulins. C-peptide and insulin are produced when the enzymatic cleavage

is complete at both junctions. It is not yet clear which is the preferred processing pathway, but there is evidence for the control of the processing pathway through the effects of calcium and hydrogen ion concentration on the activity of the enzymes involved [4, 5].

In vertebrates there are minor differences in the primary structure of insulin, most variations occurring in positions 8, 9 and 10 of the loop bridged by the intra-chain disulphide bond of the A chain and in position 30 of the B chain. For C-peptide in mammals there is a high degree of interspecies variability. In particular, rats and mice are unusual in producing two different non-allelic proinsulins (I and II) which are processed to insulins I and II and C-peptide I and II. The difference in amino acid composition between the proinsulins, insulins and C-peptides are four, two and two respectively. These differences may be important in determining the specificity of assays for insulin which are based on monoclonal antibodies, as discussed later.

Thus it can be seen that there are marked similarities in structure between insulin and its precursors. This and the low concentrations of these peptides in the peripheral circulation pose the two main challenges in the design and development of assays.

CRITERIA FOR ASSESSING THE PERFORMANCE OF ASSAYS

There are a number of characteristics of an assay that can be measured and which will determine how well an assay performs. Generally these relate to the accuracy of the assay—how close the results are to the 'true'

International Textbook of Diabetes Mellitus, Second Edition. Edited by K.G.M.M. Alberti, P. Zimmet, R.A. DeFronzo, and H. Keen (Honorary)
© 1997 John Wiley & Sons Ltd

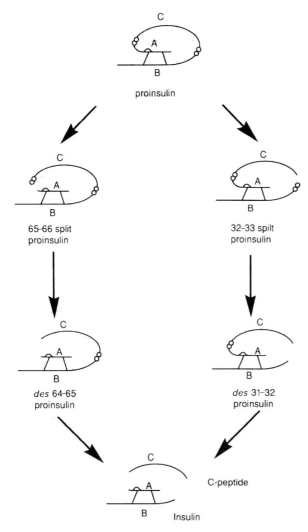

Figure 1   Processing of proinsulin to major intermediates and to insulin

Table 1   Validation of Immunoassays

Accuracy
  Linearity of response with analyte concentration
  Percentage recovery of added analyte
  Cross-reactivity of compounds with similar structure
  Comparison of sample results with those obtained by a
    reference or other method
  Internal and external quality control results

Precision
  Intra-assay imprecision
  Inter-assay imprecision
  Working range
  Sensitivity

Standards and reagents
  Source, method of preparation and stability

From reference 6, with permission.

result—and to the precision of the assay—how reproducible the results are. Some important characteristics are outlined in Table 1. Unfortunately these details are often not published or the data are presented in a nonstandard fashion. This may mean that published clinical studies are uninterpretable. It should also be noted that even seemingly minor changes in assay protocols, such as the use of half-volumes of sample and reagents, or changes in incubation times or labels, may influence the performance of the assays. For example, changes in incubation times/temperatures may affect the degree of cross-reactivity by affecting the relative amounts of primary and cross-reacting ligands that are antibody-bound at any given time [7].

BIOASSAYS

Proinsulin, intact and the split and *des* forms, are thought to have little biological activity and bioassays have only been used for the assay of insulin. A number of systems have been used, the commonest being the increase in the glycogen content of isolated rat diaphragm and glucose uptake by rat epididymal fat pad. Theoretically, bioassays will measure net insulin-like activity and may be affected by the insulin antagonists growth hormone and catecholamines. The assays are technically complex and laborious and their main use has been in the standardization of insulin preparations [8].

CHROMATOGRAPHIC ASSAYS

Chromatography as a general analytical technique has obvious applications in the analysis of insulin(s). Size exclusion, affinity and reversed-phase chromatography have been used and more recently these have been used as high performance liquid chromatography (HPLC). Where chromatography is used for the analysis of pharmaceutical preparations, sensitivity is not limiting and the methods are reported to be precise and accurate [9]. However, for the analysis of insulins and proinsulin(s) in biological fluids it is necessary to concentrate/purify the sample and then to use a non-specific immunoassay to detect the analyte in the separated fractions. Sample pretreatment that is frequently used is affinity chromatography followed by reversed phase HPLC [10, 11]. The technique is laborious, requires large sample volumes (for example up to 10 ml serum) and is time-consuming. Data on the recovery and precision of the complete analytical procedure is limited although recoveries of 99–105% have been reported for the chromatographic procedure [12]. Care must be taken in optimizing both the mobile and stationary phases for reversed-phase HPLC, as non-ideal behaviour of the C_{18} columns has been described [13].

Chromatographic techniques can be useful, particularly for the validation of immunoassays, for the analysis of plasma/serum samples from patients being investigated for the surreptitious injection of insulin where a number of animal insulins may be present (pork, beef, human) [14], and for the estimation of circulating insulin [15, 16].

IMMUNOASSAYS

Immunoassays are based on the reaction of analyte (antigen, Ag) with an immunoglobulin (for a review see [17]). Such immunoassays may be of two types. In the first, the antibody is used in limiting amounts so that the number of antigen binding sites on the antibody is less than the total number of antigen molecules (unlabelled antigen in sample or standard and reagent-labelled antigen). The amount of labelled antigen bound to antibody is measured and is inversely proportional to antigen concentration in the sample/standard. The label may be a radioisotope (radioimmunoassay, RIA) an enzyme (enzymeimmunoassay, EIA), a fluorescent compound (fluoroimmunoassay, FIA), and so on. Generally these assays have used polyclonal antisera and ^{125}I label. In contrast, in the second type of immunoassay (immunometric), the antigen reacts with an excess amount of antibody. The bound antigen–antibody complex is measured and the measured signal is proportional to the antigen concentration. There are a number of variations to this assay type. In particular the two-site assay [18], where two monoclonal antibodies form a 'sandwich' with the antigen in the middle, has advantages in terms of sensitivity and specificity.

Labels

The earlier immunoassays tended to use ^{125}I as the label, but more recently a host of non-isotopic labels have been employed, with the advantages of improved safety, longer shelf-life of reagents and in some cases improvements in sensitivity. More recently assays for insulin and proinsulin have been described using enzymes as labels: e.g. horseradish peroxidase [19], enzyme amplification [20, 21, 22] and time-resolved fluorescence [23]. It must be remembered, however, that the sensitivity of an assay will also be influenced by the affinity of the antibodies used and non-specific binding [25].

Antibodies

Radioimmunoassays for insulin and proinsulin have generally been based on polyclonal antisera and the problems of non-specificity, particularly the cross-reactivity of the 32–33, 65–66 split, and corresponding *des* proinsulins and intact proinsulin have increasingly been recognized [6]. The development of monoclonal antibody production [26, 27, 28] has meant that

more specific antibodies can be generated in larger quantities—a necessity for immunometric assays. In addition, the availability of biosynthetic proinsulin(s) has aided the production of monoclonal antibodies as well as the standardization of the assays.

The use of antibodies as analytical reagents can, however, under certain circumstances, introduce error. Some patients' samples contain antibodies that can bind non-specifically to the reagent antibodies or reagent antigen, causing falsely elevated or lowered results [29, 30]. The nature of the effect will depend on whether the assay is a competitive immunoassay or a reagent excess, immunometric assay. These so-called heterophilic antibodies may be polyspecific or anti-idiotypic antibodies and also autoantibodies such as the rheumatoid factor and antimitochondrial antibodies.

They may interfere by binding non-specifically to antigen, thus preventing specific binding, by cross-linking the solid phase and labelled antibodies in two-site immunometric assays, or by blocking the binding site of the antibody. A number of techniques has been used to minimize these effects, but the presence of these antibodies should be suspected if results appear to be inconsistent. It has been suggested that such antibodies might be found in as many as 15% of serum samples assayed [31].

Solid Phases

In both radioimmunoassays and immunometric assays there is a requirement to separate fractions of bound and 'free' label. A variety of means has been employed for this, from cellulose and magnetic particles to microtitre plates. The choice of solid phase will depend on the label used and available instrumentation.

IMMUNOASSAYS FOR INSULIN

As discussed previously, the first immunoassays for insulin were RIAs. With the discovery of proinsulin(s) and their production, it has become apparent that many RIAs show cross-reactivity in these assays. This is not surprising, as the polyclonal antisera used recognize many of the epitopes common to insulin, proinsulin and the partially processed proinsulins. Estimates of proinsulin cross-reactivity in insulin assays vary from 38% [32] to 100% [33]. Two-site immunometric assays have led to improvements in specificity [6, 19, 23, 24, 34, 35] and detection limits of less than 4 pmol/l have been described.

A number of broader issues should also be considered in relation to assay performance. Optimal sample collection conditions and type may vary between assays. Haemolysis should be avoided [36] as this results in the loss of insulin. An International Reference

Preparation of human insulin is available for the standardization of assays, although there is still wide variation in the performance of assays despite this. Whilst external quality assessment schemes are available, the materials used for quality assessment and control may not be suitable for all assays. Materials spiked with bovine or porcine insulin will not be of use for assessing the performance of assays for human insulin.

Diabetic patients treated with insulin, particularly non-human insulins, may develop antibodies to the insulin. The patients will thus have circulating 'free' and antibody-bound insulin. The degree to which different immunoassays will measure both forms may differ according to the relative affinity of the reagent antibody used. It is possible that immunometric assays may be less affected [35]. Methods involving polyethylene glycol precipitation or chromatographic separation have been developed to measure 'free' insulin in these cases [10]. Although the increasing use of human insulin in treatment should reduce this problem, it has been reported that such patients may also have circulating aggregates of insulin [15] and antibodies to these aggregates [16].

In normal, healthy individuals the plasma insulin concentration is influenced by the plasma glucose concentration and also by such factors as obesity, age and ethnic origin, in addition to the insulin assay used. Concentration ranges of 67–174 pmol/l (10–26 mU/l) have been reported, but with more specific assays with no significant cross-reactivity with proinsulin(s) a fasting plasma insulin concentration in a lean individual of less than 60 pmol/l (9 mU/l) is the rule.

IMMUNOASSAYS FOR PROINSULIN(S)

A number of radioimmunoassays for intact proinsulin have been described, with varying and often significant cross-reactivities with the split and *des* proinsulins [32, 35, 37–39]. More recently, using two-site assays, there have been improvements in specificity and sensitivity [34, 19–22].

Biosynthetic proinsulin is now available commercially for use as a standard or for immunization. However, there is no International Reference Preparation. Few laboratories perform this assay so that comparison of results has been limited and there is, as yet, no external quality assessment scheme, thus limiting the assessment of the accuracy of these assays.

The majority of assays for the split and *des* forms of proinsulin rely on chromatographic separation and concentration of precursors followed by immunoassay using a non-specific proinsulin assay as discussed earlier. One group [34] has described immunometric assays for the partially processed proinsulins. Though these assays cannot distinguish the *des* and split forms, it is thought that the main circulating form is the *des* and good agreement with a chromatographic method has been shown [40].

Elevations in circulating proinsulin (Table 2) and 32–33 split proinsulin have been identified in a number of clinical conditions. These changes may reflect the pathogenetic mechanisms of the diseases studied, but they may also have implications for the interpretation of diagnostic results. The measurement of insulin in these conditions needs caution as, for example, a specific insulin assay may not measure the excess proinsulin secreted by a proinsulinoma and only a 'normal' insulin concentration would be measured [49]. On the other hand, the use of a non-specific insulin assay may mask insulin deficiency in NIDDM [50].

In the latter study elevations of fasting proinsulin and of 32–33 split proinsulin (up to 54 pmol/l in obese NIDDM subjects) were found. For these reasons it is important to understand the assay characteristics used for any given study or investigation.

Table 2 Conditions associated with raised proinsulin

Condition	Proinsulin (pmol/l) Subjects	Controls	Definition of range	Cross-reactivity of 32–33 split proinsulins	Reference
Genetic hyperproinsulinaemia	173	–	One case	Chromatographic separation	[41]
First-degree relatives of IDDM	8(3.2–14)	1.7(1.7–4.0)	Median (25th–75th percentile)	80–100	[42]
Mothers of IDDM Impaired glucose tolerance (fasting)	4(2–68)	4(2–33)	Median (range)	60–100%	[43]
	4.5(1.0)	1.2(0.2)	Mean (SEM)	Non-detected	[44]
	3.2(0.9)	2.2(0.2)	Mean (SEM)	Non-detected	[45]
Polycystic ovary disease	3.0(1.5–7.0)	2.0(1.6–4.5)	Median (range)	Non-detected	[46]
Insulinoma	19–600	–	Range	3%	[47]
	43–780	–	Range	38%	[47]
	30–2300	–	Range	Not stated	[48]

CONCLUSIONS

Since the development of radioimmunoassay for insulin over 30 years ago, there have been significant improvements in the performance of the assays and in the understanding of the importance of proinsulin and its intermediates in assay design and in understanding disease processes.

However, as always, there is room for improvement. Increased sensitivity of all the assays would be useful in investigation of the control mechanisms involved in the suppression of insulin release, and improvements in the specificity of immunoassays for the partially processed proinsulins could increase our understanding of their role in the development of diabetes.

In terms of assay convenience it is interesting that 'dry chemistry' systems have been available for standard clinical chemistry tests for some years and more recently immunoassays have been adapted to this format [51]. Whether they will achieve the sensitivity required for insulin assays remains to be demonstrated.

It is a salutary lesson that the problems of assessing insulin release in the non-insulin dependent diabetic might have been anticipated from the early work of Yalow and Berson on a radioimmunoassay for plasma insulin reported in 1960 [52]. In this paper they state, 'However, the data at hand can only indicate that absolute insulin deficiency *per se* is not the cause of the hyperglycemia and suggest . . . (2) an abnormal insulin that acts poorly with respect to hormonal activity *in vivo* but reacts well immunologically *in vitro*'. Thus the presence of circulating proinsulins and the need for specific insulin assays has been recognized for some time.

REFERENCES

1. Stewart GA. Methods of insulin assay. Br Med Bull 1960; 16: 196–201.
2. Yalow RS, Berson SA. Assay of plasma insulin in human subjects by immunological methods. Nature 1959; 184: 1648–9.
3. Steiner DF, Oyer PE. The biosynthesis of insulin and a probable precursor of insulin by a human islet cell adenoma. Proc Natl Acad Sci USA 1967; 57: 473–80.
4. Davidson HW, Rhodes CJ, Hutton JC. Intraorganellar calcium and pH control proinsulin cleavage in the pancreatic β-cell via two distinct site-specific endopeptidases. Nature 1988; 333: 93–6.
5. Rhodes CJ, Lincoln B, Shoelson SE. Preferential cleavage of *des*-31,32-proinsulin over intact proinsulin by the insulin secretory granule type II endopeptidase. J Clin Invest 1985; 260: 535–41.
6. Temple R, Clark PMS, Hales CN. Measurement of insulin secretion in type 2 diabetes: problems and pitfalls. Diabet Med 1992; 9: 503–12.
7. Valdes R. Increasing the specificity of immunoassays. J Clin Immunoass 1992; 15: 87–96.
8. Bangham DR, Mussett MV. The Fourth International Standard for Insulin. Bull WHO/HIM Org 1959; 20: 1209–20.
9. Lookabaugh M, Biswas M, Krull IS. Quantitation of insulin injection by high-performance liquid chromatography and high performance capillary electrophoresis. J Chromatogr 1991; 549: 357–66.
10. Kuzuya H, Blix PM, Horwitz DL, Steiner DF, Rubenstein AH. Determination of free and total insulin and C-peptide in insulin-treated diabetes. Diabetes 1977; 26: 22–9.
11. Shoelson S, Haneda M, Blix P, Nanjo A, Sanke T, Inouye K, Steiner D, Rubenstein AH, Tager H. Three mutant insulins in man. Nature (Lond) 1983; 302: 540–3.
12. Linde S, Røder ME, Hartling SG, Binder C. Separation and quantitation of serum proinsulin and proinsulin intermediates in humans. J Chromatogr 1991; 548: 371–80.
13. Linde S, Welinder BS. Non-ideal behaviour of silica-based stationary phases in trifluoroacetic acid-acetonitrile-based reversed-phase high-performance liquid chromatographic separation of insulins and proinsulins. J Chromatogr 1991; 536: 43–55.
14. Given BD, Ostrega DM, Polonsky KS, Baldwin D, Kelley RI, Rubenstein AH. Hypoglycemia due to surreptitious injection of insulin. Identification of insulin species by high performance liquid chromatography. Diabetes Care 1991; 14: 544–7.
15. Robbins DC, Mead PM. Free covalent aggregates of therapeutic insulin in blood of insulin-dependent diabetics. Diabetes 1987; 36: 147–51.
16. Robbins DC, Cooper SM, Fineberg SE, Mead PM. Antibodies to covalent aggregates of insulin in blood of insulin-using diabetic patients. Diabetes 1987; 36: 838–41.
17. Clark PMS, Hales CN. Immunoassays. In Lachmann PJ, Peters K, Rosen FS, Walport MJ (eds) Clinical aspects of immunology. Boston: Blackwell Scientific Publications, 1993; pp 829–43.
18. Miles LEM, Hales CN. Labelled antibodies and immunological assay systems. Nature 1968; 219: 186–9.
19. Morris ER, Dinesen B, Burnett MA, Christopher P, Bassett PA, Manley SE. A new ELISA for specific insulin measurements in type 2 diabetic patients. Biochem Soc Trans 1992; 21: 25S.
20. Alpha B, Cox L, Crowther N, Clark PMS, Hales CN. Sensitive amplified immunoenzymometric assays (IEMA) for human insulin and intact proinsulin. Eur J Clin Chem Clin Biochem 1992; 30: 27–32.
21. Dahir FJ, Cook DB, Self CH. Amplified enzyme-linked immunoassay of human proinsulin in serum (diabetes limit 0–1 pmol/L). Clin Chem 1992; 38: 227–32.
22. Cook DB, Self CH. Determination of one thousandth of an attamole (1 Zeptomole) of alkaline phosphatase: application in an immunoassay of proinsulin. Clin Chem 1993; 39: 965–71.
23. Tolvonen E, Hemmilä I, Marnlemi J, Jorgensen PN, Zeuthen J, Lovgren T. Two-site time-resolved immunofluorometric assay of human insulin. Clin Chem 1986; 32: 637–40.
24. Storch MJ, Marbach P, Kerp L. A time resolved fluoroimmunoassay for human insulin based on two monoclonal antibodies. J Immunol Meth 1993; 157: 197–201.
25. Ekins R. Immunoassay design and optimisation. In Price CP, Newman DJ (eds) Principles and practice of immunoassay. London: Macmillan, 1991; pp 96–153.

26. Kohler G, Milstein C. Continuous cultures of fused cells secreting antibody of predefined specificity. Nature 1975; 256: 495–7.

27. Kohler G, Milstein C. Derivation of specific antibody-producing tissue culture and tumour lines by cell fusion. Eur J Immunol 1976; 6: 511–19.

28. Winter G, Milstein C. Man-made antibodies. Nature 1991; 349: 293–9.

29. Kohse KP, Wisser H. Antibodies as a source of analytical errors. J Clin Chem Clin Biochem 1990; 28: 881–92.

30. Levinson SS. The nature of heterophilic antibodies and their role in immunoassay interference. J Clin Immunoass 1992; 15: 108–115.

31. Boscato LM, Stuart MC. Incidence and specificity of interference in two-site immunoassays. Clin Chem 1986; 32: 1491–5.

32. Yoshioka N, Kuzuya T, Matsuda A, Taniguchi M, Iwamoto Y. Serum proinsulin levels at fasting and after oral glucose load in patients with type 2 (non-insulin dependent) diabetes mellitus. Diabetologia 1988; 31: 355–60.

33. Ward WK, Le Cava EC, Paquette TL, Beard JC, Wallum BJ, Porte D. Disproportionate elevations of immunoreactive proinsulin in type 2 (non-insulin dependent) diabetes mellitus and in experimental insulin resistance. Diabetologia 1987; 30: 698–702.

34. Sobey WJ, Beer SF, Carrington CA, Clark PMS, Frank BH, Gray IP, Luzio SD, Owens DR, Schneider AE, Siddle K, Temple RC, Hales CN. Sensitive and specific two-site immunoradiometric assays for human insulin, proinsulin, 65–66 split and 32–33 split proinsulins. Biochem J 1989; 260: 535–41.

35. Andersen L, Dinesen B, Jørgensen PN, Poulsen F, Røder ME. Enzyme immunoassay for intact human insulin in serum or plasma. Clin Chem 1992; 39: 578–82.

36. O'Rahilly S, Burnett MA, Smith RF, Darley JH, Turner RC. Haemolysis affects insulin, but not C-peptide immunoassay. Diabetologia 1987; 30: 394–6.

37. Deacon CF, Conlon JM. Measurement of circulating human proinsulin concentrations using a specific antiserum. Diabetes 1985; 34: 491–7.

38. Cohen RM, Given BD, Licinio-Paixao J, Provow SA, Rue PA, Frank BH et al. Proinsulin radioimmunoassay in the evaluation of insulinomas and familial hyperproinsulinaemia. Metabolism 1986; 35: 1137–46.

39. Hartling SG, Dinesen B, Kappelgård SM, Faber OK, Binder C. ELISA for human proinsulin. Clin Chim Acta 1986; 156: 289–98.

40. Ostrega D, Polonsky K, Nagi D, Yudkin J, Cox L, Clark PMS, Hales CN. Measurement of proinsulin and intermediates: validation of immunoassay methods by high performance liquid chromatography. Diabetes 1995; 44: 437–40.

41. Nakashima N, Sakamoto N, Umeda F, Hashimoto T, Hisatomi A, Umemura T, et al. Point mutation in a family with hyperproinsulinemia detected by single stranded conformational polymorphism. J Clin Endocrinol Metab 1993; 76: 633–6.

42. Spinas GA, Oberholzer M, Snorgaard O, Berger W, Hartling SG. Elevated proinsulin levels related to islet cell antibodies in first-degree relatives of IDDM patients. Diabetes Care 1992; 15; 632–7.

43. Lindren FA, Hartling SG, Persson BE, Røder ME, Snellman K, Binder C, Dahlquist G. Proinsulin levels in newborn siblings of type 1 (insulin-dependent) diabetic children and their mothers. Diabetologia 1993; 36: 560–3.

44. Krentz AJ, Clark PM, Cox L, Nattrass M. Hyperproinsulinaemia in impaired glucose tolerance. Clin Sci 1993; 85: 97–100.

45. Williams DRR, Byrne C, Clark PMS, Cox L, Day NE, Rayman G, Wong T, Hales CN. Raised proinsulin concentration as early indicator of B-cell dysfunction. Br Med J 1991; 303: 95–6.

46. Conway GS, Clark PMS, Wong D. Hyperinsulinaemia in the polycystic ovary syndrome confirmed with a specific immunoradiometric assay for insulin. Clin Endocrinol 1993; 38: 219–22.

47. Cohen RM, Given BD, Licinio-Paixao J, Provow SA, Rue PA, Frank BH, et al. Proinsulin radioimmunoassay in the evaluation of insulinomas and familial hyperproinsulinemia. Metabolism 1986; 35: 1137–46.

48. Hampton SM, Beyzavi K, Teale D, Marks V. A direct assay for proinsulin in plasma and its application in hypoglycaemia. Clin Endocrinol 1988; 29: 9–16.

49. Cohen RM, Camus F. Update on insulinomas or the case of the missing (pro)insulinoma. Diabetes Care 1988; 11: 506–8.

50. Temple RC, Carrington CA, Luzio SD, Owens DR, Schneider AE, Sobey WJ, Hales CN. Insulin deficiency in non-insulin dependent diabetes. Lancet 1989; 1: 293–5.

51. Morris DL, Ledden DJ, Boguslaski RC. Dry-phase technology for immunoassays. J Clin Lab Analysis 1987; 1: 243–9.

52. Yalow RS, Berson SA. Immunoassay of endogenous plasma insulin in man. J Clin Invest 1960; 39: 1157–75.

31

Pathogenesis of NIDDM

Ralph A. DeFronzo*, Riccardo C. Bonadonna† and Eleuterio Ferrannini††

*University of Texas Health Science Center, San Antonio, TX, USA; †University of Verona School of Medicine and Ospedale Civile Maggiore, Verona, Italy; and ††University of Pisa School of Medicine, Pisa, Italy

In the postabsorptive state the majority of total-body glucose disposal occurs in insulin independent tissues: brain (about 50%) and splanchnic organs (about 25%). The remaining 25% of glucose utilization occurs in insulin dependent tissues, primarily muscle [1–5]. Basal glucose uptake, which averages about 2 mg/kg/min, is precisely matched by the release of glucose from the liver [1–5] (Figure 1). Following glucose ingestion or infusion, this delicate balance between uptake and output is disrupted, and the maintenance of normal glucose homeostasis is dependent upon three processes that must occur simultaneously in a coordinated and tightly integrated fashion (Table 1). In response to the rise in plasma glucose concentration, insulin secretion by the pancreas is stimulated and the combination of hyperinsulinemia plus hyperglycemia must effectively promote glucose uptake by splanchnic (liver and gut) and peripheral (primarily muscle) tissues and suppress hepatic glucose production [1–9]. From this brief overview (see Chapter 24 for a more detailed discussion), it is obvious that defects at the level of the islet B cell, muscle and/or liver can lead to the development of glucose intolerance or overt diabetes mellitus. Although adipose and other tissues are responsive to insulin, from the quantitative standpoint they are responsible for the disposal of less than 5% of an ingested or infused glucose load [10–12]. Nonetheless, to the extent that adipocyte tissue is resistant to insulin [13], it will play a role, albeit small, in the defect in whole body glucose disposal. However, because of the important interaction between free fatty acid and glucose metabolism [14], insulin resistance in adipocytes with respect to free fatty acid metabolism [15, 16] can lead to the development of insulin resistance [1, 5, 17] and impaired insulin secretion [18, 19]. In this chapter the concept is developed that, in order to observe the full-blown syndrome of non-insulin dependent diabetes mellitus (NIDDM), two major defects—insulin resistance and impaired B-cell function—must be present simultaneously. In most populations with a high incidence of NIDDM, i.e. American Indians, Mexican-Americans, and Pacific islanders, the earliest discernible abnormality is an impairment in tissue (muscle and/or liver) sensitivity to insulin. When the islet B-cell no longer can maintain a sufficiently high rate of insulin secretion to offset the insulin resistance, fasting hyperglycemia and overt diabetes mellitus ensue. Such individuals typically are represented by the obese diabetic. In some type 2 diabetic patients the initial defect appears to start at the level of the B-cell and manifests itself as an impairment in insulin secretion, while insulin resistance develops concomitantly with, or subsequent to the disturbance in insulin secretion. If the defect in insulin secretion is sufficiently severe, overt diabetes can develop in the absence of insulin resistance. These individuals typically are lean and this type of diabetes has been described in a minority of Europid [20] and African-American [21, 22] individuals with NIDDM. However, even in the lean type 2 diabetic individual the majority of evidence indicates that insulin resistance, involving both muscle and liver, precedes the onset of, or occurs

International Textbook of Diabetes Mellitus, Second Edition. Edited by K.G.M.M. Alberti, P. Zimmet, R.A. DeFronzo, and H. Keen (Honorary)
© 1997 John Wiley & Sons Ltd

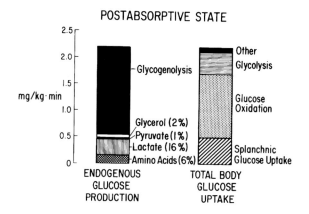

Figure 1 Schematic representation of glucose production and glucose utilization in the normal human in the postabsorptive state (drawn from data presented in references 2, 3, 4 and 365)

simultaneously with, the defect in insulin secretion. Since approximately 10% of 'NIDDM' subjects have slowly evolving IDDM [23], it is important to measure circulating islet cell and GAD antibodies to exclude type 1 diabetes mellitus masquerading as NIDDM. Maturity onset diabetes of the young (MODY) also has been cited as an example of pure insulin deficiency [24, 25] but recent evidence has demonstrated that defects in both hepatic glucose production and peripheral tissue sensitivity to insulin contribute to the impairment in glucose homeostasis [26]. It is important to emphasize that whichever defect (i.e. diminished insulin secretion or insulin resistance) initiates the development of NIDDM, it subsequently will lead to the emergence of the other abnormality. Again, it should be underscored that in the great majority of NIDDM individuals, defects in both insulin sensitivity and insulin secretion must be present simultaneously before significant glucose intolerance will ensue.

Table 1 Factors responsible for the maintenance of normal glucose tolerance in healthy subjects

1. Insulin secretion
2. Tissue glucose uptake
   (a) Peripheral (primarily muscle)
   (b) Splanchnic (liver plus gut)
3. Suppression of hepatic glucose production

From reference 1, with permission.

INSULIN SECRETION IN NIDDM

Overview

Considerable controversy continues to exist concerning B-cell function in NIDDM. However, in the great majority of type 2 diabetic subjects there has emerged a consistent pattern which reveals a complex interplay

between insulin secretion and both the magnitude of insulin resistance and severity of hyperglycemia. When normal weight type 2 diabetic subjects with mild fasting hyperglycemia (148 ± 8 mg/dl, 8.2 mmol/l) are given a standard (100 g) oral glucose tolerance test (OGTT), both the fasting and stimulated plasma insulin levels are higher in diabetic patients compared to age-matched and weight-matched control subjects (Figure 2). Evidence as simple and reproducible as this makes it obvious that the glucose intolerance in NIDDM subjects cannot result solely from an *absolute* deficiency of insulin. However, it is important to emphasize that the plasma insulin response, although increased in absolute terms, is not normal. It is well established that the B-cell response is, in large part, determined by the prevailing plasma glucose concentration [27, 28]. Thus, when the control subjects are restudied with the same OGTT but with a supplemental glucose infusion designed to mimic the plasma glucose profile observed in NIDDM individuals, it is obvious that the insulin response in the diabetic group is impaired (R.A. DeFronzo, unpublished results). Thus, when viewed in the context of the prevailing hyperglycemia, it is clear that in NIDDM there is a defect in the ability of the pancreas to secrete insulin. The defect in insulin secretion is readily evident if one calculates the early insulin response, i.e. increment in insulin divided by the increment in plasma glucose concentration at 30 min, as proposed by Hales [29].

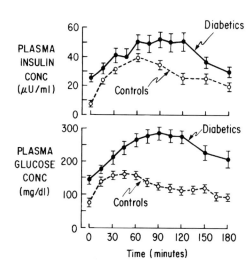

Figure 2 Plasma glucose (lower panel) and plasma insulin (upper panel) concentrations in control (open circles) and normal weight type 2 diabetic (solid circles) subjects during a 100 g oral glucose tolerance test (drawn from data presented in references 1, 4, 7, 30, 272, 340 and 341)

The English literature is replete with studies that have employed the OGTT and the intravenous glucose tolerance test (IVGTT) to examine insulin secretion in NIDDM patients. Table 2 summarizes the studies up to 1983 in which insulin secretion was examined in normal weight type 2 diabetic subjects with fasting hyperglycemia (see reference 30 for a complete listing of these 32 publications). Although many more studies examining insulin secretion in normal weight type 2 diabetic patients [29, 31–38] have appeared since this initial review, the basic findings have not been altered. Since obesity causes insulin resistance, which in turn elicits a compensatory increase in insulin secretion [1, 5, 39], we will focus on normal weight NIDDM patients in order to examine the impact of diabetes *per se* on insulin secretion. Several important points are obvious from the summary presented in Table 2.

Table 2 Summary of plasma insulin response during glucose tolerance tests in non-obese NIDDM subjects with fasting hyperglycemia, from publications up to 1983

	Fasting insulin	Plasma insulin response to glucose		
		Early*	Late	Total
Decreased	0	21	13	16
Normal	27	6	12	11
Increased	5	5	7	5

The 32 publications from which the above summary was prepared can be found in reference 30. *The early phase of insulin secretion refers to the 0–10 min period during the IVGTT and the 0–30 min period during the OGTT.

Fasting Insulin Concentration

In the postabsorptive state the plasma insulin concentration invariably has been found to be normal or increased (Table 2). Even in those studies where 'normal' fasting plasma insulin concentrations have been reported, the levels uniformly have been in the high normal range. This is not surprising, since diabetic subjects have fasting hyperglycemia which presents a persistent stimulus for insulin secretion throughout the day. When basal insulin secretion has been estimated in NIDDM patients using C peptide, it has been found to be increased [40, 41]. DeFronzo et al measured the fasting plasma insulin concentration and performed OGTTs in 77 normal weight NIDDM subjects [42]. As can be seen from Figure 3, the relationship between the fasting plasma glucose concentration and the fasting insulin level is complex, and resembles an inverted U or horseshoe. Because this curve closely resembles Starling's curve of the heart, DeFronzo has referred to it as Starling's curve of the pancreas [1, 5, 42]. As the fasting glucose level rises from 80 mg/dl to 140 mg/dl (4.4 to 7.8 mmol/l), there is a progressive rise in fasting plasma insulin concentration which peaks at a value which is 2–2.5 times greater than in normal weight, age-matched controls (Figure 3). This progressive rise in basal insulin secretion can be viewed

as an adaptive response by the pancreas to offset the progressive deterioration in glucose homeostasis. However, when the fasting glucose concentration exceeds 140 mg/dl, the B cell no longer can maintain its high rate of insulin secretion, and with increasing fasting hyperglycemia insulin secretion drops off precipitously. This decline in basal plasma insulin concentration has important pathophysiologic implications, because it is at this point that hepatic glucose production starts to increase and makes a major contribution to the elevated fasting glucose level [42]. It is noteworthy, however, that even in diabetic patients with fasting glucose levels in the range of 250–300 mg/dl (13.9–16.7 mmol/l) the basal plasma insulin concentration is similar to, or slightly greater than, that of the controls. The simultaneous presence of fasting hyperglycemia and elevated basal insulin levels indicates the presence of severe insulin resistance. As is discussed subsequently, both the liver [42, 43] and peripheral [1, 5] tissues share in this insulin resistance in the postabsorptive state.

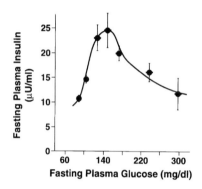

Figure 3 Relationship between the fasting plasma glucose concentration and the fasting plasma insulin concentration in normal weight controls, in individuals with impaired glucose tolerance, and in NIDDM subjects with varying degrees of fasting hyperglycemia. As the fasting plasma glucose concentration rises from baseline to 140 mg/dl, there is a progressive increase in the fasting insulin concentration. Thereafter, further rises in the fasting glucose level are associated with a progressive decline in fasting insulin concentration. In diabetic subjects with fasting glucose concentrations in excess of 200–220 mg/dl, the fasting insulin level declines to values observed in control subjects (from reference 42, with permission)

Glucose-stimulated Insulin Secretion

NIDDM with Hyperinsulinemia

From Table 2 it can be seen that in only half of the 32 reported series before 1983 (containing approximately 500 type 2 diabetic patients) was there a decrease in the absolute amount of insulin secreted in response to oral or intravenous glucose. In the other 16 series, the plasma insulin response to hyperglycemia was either normal (*n* = 11) or increased (*n* = 5). These observations are similar to those reported by DeFronzo [1, 5] (see Figure 2) and other investigators [29, 31, 32]. It should be emphasized, however, that the plasma insulin response, although normal or increased in absolute terms, is deficient when viewed relative to the level of hyperglycemia. Nonetheless, these results indicate that factors other than impaired insulin secretion must also contribute to the defect in glucose metabolism.

From the data summarized in Table 2 it is clear that the plasma insulin response to both oral and intravenous glucose is quite heterogeneous in NIDDM subjects. In part, this heterogeneity is explained by different etiologies of NIDDM, i.e. insulin resistance [1, 5] vs. impaired insulin secretion [20–22, 29, 31]. A large part of the variance, however, is explained by the complex relationship between the plasma insulin response to hyperglycemia and the severity of diabetes [1, 5, 44–54] (Figure 4). As was observed with the fasting insulin concentration (Figure 3), if the fasting plasma glucose concentration—an index of the severity of diabetes—is plotted against the mean plasma insulin response during a 100 g oral glucose load, the same inverted U-shaped curve is observed. The first point on the curve in Figure 4 represents a lean individual with perfectly normal glucose tolerance. This person, with a fasting glucose of 80 mg/dl (4.4 mmol/l), would be expected to have a mean plasma insulin concentration of approximately 50 μU/ml during the 2 hours following glucose ingestion. As this normal individual starts to become glucose-intolerant and the fasting plasma glucose concentration rises, albeit slightly, the B cell recognizes that the glucose homeostatic mechanism has become disrupted and it augments its insulin secretory capacity in an attempt to overcome the disturbance in glucose metabolism. Thus, an individual with a fasting plasma glucose of 120 mg/dl (6.7 mmol/l)—i.e. impaired glucose tolerance—will secrete approximately twice as much insulin as a normal person with a fasting glucose concentration of 80 mg/dl (Figure 4). As long as this high rate of insulin secretion can be maintained, glucose tolerance remains normal or only minimally impaired. However, when the fasting glucose level exceeds 120 mg/dl, the B cell can no longer maintain its accelerated rate of insulin secretion and further increases in plasma glucose are associated with a progressive decline in insulin secretion. Thus, a diabetic person with a fasting glucose of 150–160 mg/dl (8.3–8.9 mmol/l) secretes an amount of insulin that is quite similar to that in a normal, non-diabetic individual (Figure 4). However, a 'normal' insulin response in the presence of this degree of hyperglycemia is markedly abnormal. With further increments in the fasting glucose concentration above 150–160 mg/dl, the plasma insulin response, when viewed in absolute terms,

becomes insulinopenic. Finally, when the basal glucose level exceeds 200–220 mg/dl (11.1–12.2 mmol/l), the plasma insulin response to a glucose challenge is markedly blunted. Nevertheless, the postabsorptive rate of insulin secretion remains elevated and fasting hyperinsulinemia persists, even in diabetic patients with fasting plasma glucose concentrations as high as 250–300 mg/dl (13.9–16.7 mmol/l) [1, 5, 29, 31, 32, 40–42, 55] (Figure 4). Even in the face of severe fasting hyperglycemia, 24-hour insulin profiles in both lean and NIDDM subjects reveal normal integrated insulin and C-peptide values [56–58]. These normal values result from the combination of high fasting and decreased postprandial insulin and C-peptide secretory rates.

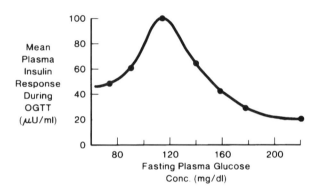

Figure 4 Starling's curve of the pancreas for insulin secretion. In normal weight patients with impaired glucose tolerance and mild diabetes mellitus, the plasma insulin response to ingested glucose (OGTT) increases progressively until the fasting glucose reaches 120 mg/dl. Thereafter, further increases in the fasting glucose concentration are associated with a progressive decline in insulin secretion (from reference 1, with permission)

The preceding synthesis is consistent with the natural history of the development of impaired glucose tolerance and type 2 diabetes mellitus in populations with a high incidence of NIDDM, i.e. American Indians, Mexican-Americans, and Pacific islanders [1, 48, 54, 59–68], and in the rhesus monkey [69, 70], an animal model that closely resembles type 2 diabetes mellitus in man. It should be pointed out that in all of these population studies, as well as in the rhesus monkey, NIDDM is closely associated with the presence of obesity. In these high-risk populations, as normal glucose-tolerant subjects progress to impaired glucose tolerance (IGT), there is a marked increase in both fasting and glucose-stimulated plasma insulin levels [1, 54, 59, 63] and a decrease in the body's sensitivity to insulin (Figure 5). It should be emphasized, however, that even though the plasma insulin response is increased 2–3-fold above that in normal glucose tolerant subjects, glucose intolerance would not develop

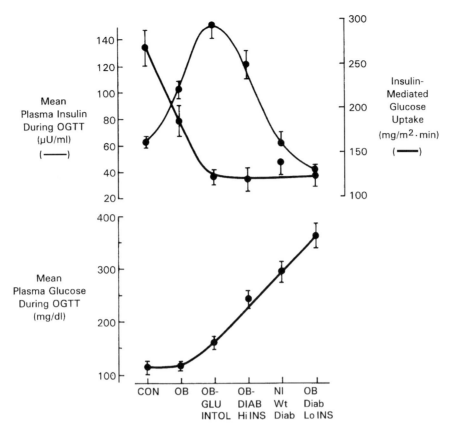

Figure 5 Summary of the plasma glucose (bottom panel) and plasma insulin (top panel, inverted U-shaped curve) responses during a 100 g OGTT, and tissue sensitivity to insulin (top panel) in control (CON), obese non-diabetic (OB), obese glucose intolerant (OB-GLU INTOL), obese hyperinsulinemic diabetic (OB-DIAB Hi INS), normal weight diabetic (NL Wt Diab) and obese hypoinsulinemic diabetic subjects (OB-DIAB Lo INS). See text for a detailed discussion (from reference 1, with permission)

if a concomitant defect in insulin secretion were not present. The defect in insulin secretion can be appreciated when B-cell function is viewed relative to the prevailing severity of insulin resistance. The progression from IGT to NIDDM with mild fasting hyperglycemia (120–140 mg/dl, 6.7–7.8 mmol/l) is heralded by an inability of the B-cell to maintain its previously high rate of insulin secretion in response to a glucose challenge [1, 54, 60, 62, 63] without any further deterioration in tissue sensitivity to insulin. It should be noted, however, that increased basal insulin secretion and fasting hyperinsulinemia are maintained until fasting plasma glucose levels exceed 140 mg/dl (Figure 3). A similar picture of insulin secretion is observed in the rhesus monkey [69, 70]. As monkeys age, they become obese and a high percentage develop typical NIDDM. Longitudinal, as well as cross-sectional, studies have documented that the earliest detectable abnormality that precedes the onset of diabetes mellitus is an increase in the fasting and glucose-stimulated plasma insulin concentration and a decrease in the body's sensitivity to insulin [69, 70]. With time, this high rate of insulin secretion cannot be maintained and the downward slope of Starling's curve commences (Figure 4). At this point

marked fasting hyperglycemia and glucose intolerance ensue. All of these studies [1, 54, 59, 62, 63, 65, 67] clearly demonstrate that hyperinsulinemia precedes the development of NIDDM. Consistent with this, a number of studies in high-risk ethnic groups [52, 54, 59, 68, 71–74] and in other populations [60, 75–78] have demonstrated that hyperinsulinemia predicts the development of IGT and NIDDM. However, these studies [1, 5, 62, 64] also demonstrate that overt NIDDM (fasting glucose >140 mg/dl) does not develop in the absence of a significant defect in B-cell function. The nature of this B-cell defect is considered in subsequent sections.

NIDDM with Hypoinsulinemia

Despite an impressive body of evidence that implicates the presence of hyperinsulinemia and insulin resistance as the antecedents of NIDDM, a number of studies have documented that absolute insulin deficiency with or without impaired tissue sensitivity to insulin can lead to the development of NIDDM. This is best exemplified by patients with maturity onset diabetes of the young (MODY), which represents a familial subtype of NIDDM, characterized by an early age of onset, autosomal dominant inheritance with high penetrance, mild-to-moderate fasting hyperglycemia, and impaired insulin secretion [26, 32].

The initial description of MODY was made by Fajans et al [79] in the RW family and the diabetes subsequently was shown by Bell et al [80] to be linked to a DNA polymorphism in the adenosine deaminase gene on chromosome 20 (MODY 1). The actual gene responsible for diabetes in this family has yet to be described. Subsequently, Froguel and colleagues [25, 26, 81, 82] demonstrated that MODY in French families is associated with mutations in the glucokinase gene on chromosome 7p (MODY 2). Since the original description by Froguel et al [25, 26, 81, 82], over 25 mutations in the glucokinase gene have been described but many of these are unlikely to cause a defect in insulin secretion. Most recently, a third type of MODY has been demonstrated and shown to be linked to a region of chromosome 12 [83–86]. MODY individuals are characterized by impaired insulin secretion in response to glucose and other stimuli [24–26, 31, 32, 87–89]. Although diminished insulin secretion clearly is the primary defect in MODY, a number of studies have demonstrated that peripheral tissue resistance to insulin [26, 90, 91] and disturbances in hepatic glucose metabolism [92, 93] also play a role in the development of impaired glucose homeostasis. Although glucokinase mutations leading to impaired insulin secretion are well established features of MODY 2, intensive investigations in typical older onset NIDDM individuals in a variety of ethnic populations have demonstrated that a mutation in the glucokinase gene can account for no more than 1% of the common form of type 2 diabetes [94–100] (see also Chapter 3).

It also has been suggested that insulin deficiency may represent the primary defect responsible for glucose intolerance in individuals who present with typical NIDDM and who do not have a glucokinase mutation. This view, which has been championed by Cerasi, Luft and colleagues, argues that a defect in early insulin secretion leads to an excessive rise in plasma glucose levels and that the resultant hyperglycemia is responsible for late hyperinsulinemia [34, 35, 38, 101]. Most recently, Hales et al [29, 33] have demonstrated that many lean Europid individuals with mild fasting hyperglycemia (<140 mg/dl, 7.8 mmol/l) are characterized by insulin deficiency at all time points during an OGTT. An impaired early insulin response also has been shown to be a characteristic finding in Japanese Americans who progress to NIDDM [102]. Unfortunately, all of these studies failed to provide information about insulin sensitivity. Arner et al [20] examined insulin secretion (IVGTT) and insulin sensitivity (euglycemic insulin clamp) in 28 untreated male NIDDM subjects. In the 16 who were obese, both impaired insulin secretion and diminished insulin action were present, whereas the 12 who were lean had normal insulin sensitivity with severely impaired insulin secretion. Similarly, Banerji and Lebovitz [21, 22] have demonstrated that up to 50% of black NIDDM individuals who reside in New York city are characterized by severely impaired insulin secretion and normal insulin sensitivity.

In summary, these results demonstrate that impaired insulin secretion—in the absence of insulin resistance—can lead to the development of full-blown NIDDM. However, several important questions remain to be answered. How frequently does a pure B-cell defect result in typical NIDDM? Why does insulin resistance not develop secondarily in these insulinopenic individuals, given that hyperglycemia (i.e. glucose toxicity) down-regulates the glucose transport system and causes other post-transport defects in insulin action.

First-phase Insulin Secretion

It is well established that in both humans [103] and animals [104], insulin is secreted in a biphasic pattern with an early burst of insulin release within the first 10 min, followed by a gradually increasing phase of insulin secretion which persists as long as the hyperglycemic stimulus is present (see also Chapter 15). Although this biphasic insulin response is not easily identifiable following oral glucose, it is readily demonstrable after intravenous glucose. It has been suggested that loss of the first phase of insulin secretion is the earliest detectable abnormality in patients who are destined to develop NIDDM [32, 35, 101, 105]. From the data in Table 2 it is obvious that the early phase of insulin secretion during the OGTT (0–30 min) and during the IVGTT (0–10 min) tends to be reduced in most NIDDM subjects with fasting plasma glucose levels above 110–120 mg/dl (6.1–6.7 mmol/l). During the OGTT the defect in early insulin secretion is most readily detected if one calculates incremental plasma insulin response at 30 min divided by the incremental plasma glucose response at 30 min ($\Delta I30/\Delta G30$). These results have been substantiated by more recent studies by Hales, Polonsky, Cerasi and others [29, 31–36, 38, 106].

The loss of the first phase of insulin secretion has important pathogenetic consequences, as this early burst of insulin release plays an important role in priming those insulin target tissues, especially the liver, that are responsible for the maintenance of normal glucose homeostasis [107–110]. However, a number of studies [59, 60] have shown that progression to IGT or NIDDM is associated with a reduction in insulin sensitivity and an increase in insulin secretion, including the first-phase response. Although the first-phase insulin secretory response is characteristically lost in NIDDM (Table 2), this defect does not occur until the fasting plasma glucose concentration rises to 115–120 mg/dl (6.4–6.7 mmol/l) [111]. Moreover, tight metabolic control partially restores the defect in first-phase insulin response [112–114], indicating that at least part of the defect is acquired, most likely secondary to glucotoxicity [115] or lipotoxicity [18, 19] (see subsequent discussion).

Pulsatile Insulin Secretion

Insulin is secreted in a pulsatile fashion in humans [31, 32, 36, 116–118] and animals [119, 120], and some evidence suggests that pulsatile insulin delivery is more biologically effective than continuous administration [121, 122]. Several recent studies have reported that loss of oscillatory insulin secretion is a characteristic feature of relatives of patients with NIDDM and in subjects with IGT [31, 32, 36, 123–125], and these investigators have suggested that abnormal oscillatory insulin secretion may be the earliest detectable lesion in the natural history of NIDDM.

In normal subjects insulin is secreted in pulses of rapid frequency that recur every 5–15 min. This pulsatility of insulin secretion is readily observed in the portal vein but is largely filtered out by hepatic extraction of insulin. It has been suggested that this portal pulsatility may play a role in the regulation of hepatic glucose production [122] but, because of their dampened effect in the periphery, these rapid insulin pulses are unlikely to have any influence on muscle insulin sensitivity. If healthy subjects are infused with glucose at a constant rate, regular oscillations in glucose and insulin secretion occur every 90–120 min. Oscillations occurring at this frequency are called ultradian oscillations. If the exogenous glucose infusion rate is either decreased or increased, the B cell responds by appropriately adjusting the periodicity of insulin secretion, a process termed 'entrainment'. In subjects with NIDDM or IGT, and in first-degree relatives of NIDDM individuals, the regular rapid oscillations are replaced by irregular cycles of shorter duration and the ultradian insulin oscillations became more irregular, are of diminished amplitude, and lose their phase relationship to the glucose oscillations [31, 32, 123–126]. In obese NIDDM subjects all of these defects in insulin pulsatility can be significantly improved by weight loss and the achievement of tight metabolic control, but they cannot be restored completely to normal [123]. In order to define at what stage in the natural history of NIDDM the oscillatory defects in insulin secretion became manifest, Polonsky has studied insulin resistant obese subjects with IGT and normal fasting glucose and glycohemoglobin concentrations [32]. These obese

subjects with IGT secreted less insulin in response to a stepped glucose infusion than did equally insulin resistant obese subjects with normal glucose tolerance (Figure 6) and they manifested a reduced ability to entrain the ultradian oscillations of insulin secretion. These results make several important points. First, with regard to the specific insulin secretory tests that were utilized, the defects in B-cell function were not present in obese subjects with normal glucose tolerance and became manifest only after the onset of IGT. This observation raises the issue as to whether the insulin oscillatory defects are primary, i.e. inherited, or acquired secondarily to poor metabolic control, i.e. glucotoxicity or lipotoxicity. Second, in absolute terms the amount of insulin secreted in the obese subjects with IGT is similar to that in controls (Figure 6). This indicates that in *absolute* terms, insulin secretion is not impaired in subjects with IGT. However, *relative* to the severity of insulin resistance and postprandial hyperglycemia—albeit mild—obese subjects with IGT do not secrete sufficient amounts of insulin. This finding is very similar to that described in ethnic populations that are characterized by a high incidence of NIDDM and obesity [1, 54, 59, 61, 62, 65, 67, 75]. Lastly, it remains to be defined whether similar defects in insulin secretory oscillations are present in lean type 2 patients, many of whom present with insulinopenia, and, if so, at what time in the natural history of NIDDM, i.e. IGT or pre-IGT, such abnormalities become manifest.

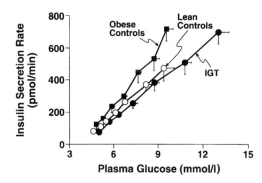

Figure 6 Relationship between average plasma glucose concentration and insulin secretion rate during graded intravenous glucose infusions ranging from 1 to 8 mg/kg/min (each infusion lasting for 40 min) in lean control subjects, in non-diabetic obese subjects, and in matched obese subjects with impaired glucose tolerance (IGT) (from reference 32, with permission)

Proinsulin

It has been suggested that NIDDM individuals may be more insulinopenic than previously appreciated because of the presence of high circulating levels of proinsulin and 32–33 split proinsulin, which are biologically much less active than insulin but cross-react substantially with insulin in the routine radioimmunoassay [29, 38] (see also Chapters 16 and 30). In normal subjects the amount of proinsulin secreted is small compared with insulin [29, 127, 128]. However, because its metabolic clearance rate is significantly less than that of insulin [129], it accounts for about 10% of the total amount of insulin that is measured in the basal and glucose-stimulated states [128]. Using a specific proinsulin assay [29, 38, 130–132], a number of laboratories have demonstrated that in NIDDM subjects with moderate to severe hyperglycemia, proinsulin makes up a significantly larger fraction of the immunoassayable insulin. This raises several important questions. When does the increase in proinsulin occur, and are subjects with IGT or NIDDM with mild fasting hyperglycemia characterized by 'true' insulin deficiency? Yoshioka et al [132] have measured both the insulin and proinsulin responses in normal healthy subjects, in subjects with IGT and in NIDDM patients with a wide range of fasting plasma glucose levels. Subjects with IGT and mild fasting hyperglycemia (<140 mg/dl, 7.8 mmol/l) demonstrated significant increases in both fasting and glucose-stimulated insulin and proinsulin levels. Although plasma proinsulin levels increased disproportionately to the plasma insulin concentration, resulting in an increase in the ratio of proinsulin to insulin, in absolute terms the amount of 'true' insulin secreted was nevertheless increased. Similar findings have been reported by Reaven, Polonsky and co-workers [133]. These observations indicate that during the earliest stages of development of NIDDM, the diabetic patients studied by Yoshioka et al [132] and Reaven et al [133] are characterized by hyperinsulinemia. Consistent with this, it should be noted that the diabetic patients reported by Temple et al [38] were severely hyperglycemic—fasting plasma glucose levels over 225 mg/dl (12.5 mmol/l)—and only the 30 min time point was analyzed. However, more recent studies by the same group have demonstrated a similarly increased ratio of proinsulin to insulin in mild diabetics with fasting plasma glucose concentrations less than 144 mg/dl (8.0 mmol/l) [29, 106]. It should be noted, however, that these subjects—in contrast to those reported by Yoshioka et al [132] and Reaven et al [133]—were very insulinopenic.

Recent investigations have demonstrated that human proinsulin processing is sequential and involves three enzymes: PC3 (type I) endopeptidase, PC2 (type II) endopeptidase, and carboxypeptidase H [29, 128]. PC3 and carboxypeptidase H convert proinsulin to des 31,32 proinsulin and subsequently to insulin plus C-peptide. Hyperglycemia is a potent stimulus for the synthesis of proinsulin and PC3, but not PC2 [29, 128, 134]. Short-term exposure (<2 h) to glucose stimulates the

biosynthesis of PC3 in concert with that of proinsulin at the translational level [134]. The synthesis of PC2 and carboxypeptidase H is not regulated by glucose. Nonetheless, proinsulin processing to insulin proceeds normally, indicating that sufficient amounts of PC2 and carboxypeptidase H normally are present within the B cell [29, 128]. During prolonged B-cell stimulation, as occurs in the presence of insulin resistance or chronic hyperglycemia, PC3 synthesis keeps pace with proinsulin biosynthesis but PC2 synthesis, which is not glucose-regulated, does not. This results in an increase in the ratio of des 31,32 proinsulin to insulin (as well as the ratio of proinsulin to insulin), as has been described in NIDDM [29]. Because most insulin radioimmunoassays cross-react with des 31,32 proinsulin and proinsulin, the concentration of true biologically active insulin may be overestimated. Highly specific and sensitive, two-site immunometric assays of insulin, proinsulin and proinsulin split products are now available. Using these specific two-site radiometric assays, the majority of NIDDM subjects with mild to moderate fasting hyperglycemia have been shown to have elevated plasma insulin concentrations in both the fasting and glucose-stimulated state [132, 133].

ETIOLOGY OF INSULIN DEFICIENCY IN NIDDM

Introduction

The progression from normal glucose tolerance to IGT to NIDDM with mild fasting hyperglycemia (<120–140 mg/dl) is characterized by hyperinsulinemia (Figures 3 and 4). However, once the basal glucose concentration exceeds 120 mg/dl (6.7 mmol/l) and 140 mg/dl (7.8 mmol/l), respectively, there is a progressive decline in fasting and glucose-stimulated plasma insulin levels. These observations suggest that the decline in B-cell function is acquired. This conclusion is supported by the recent studies of Polonsky, using more sophisticated techniques to evaluate insulin secretion [32] (Figure 6). In this section we will review the pathogenetic factors that have been implicated in the progressive impairment in insulin secretion.

B-cell Mass

The number of B cells is a critical determinant of the amount of insulin that is secreted by the pancreas. Most [135–140] but not all [141] studies have demonstrated a modest reduction (20–40%) in B-cell mass in patients with long-standing NIDDM. Morphologically, the islets of Langerhans appear normal and insulitis is not observed. At present the cause of decrease in B-cell mass remains undefined and cannot be explained simply by advancing age. Obesity, another insulin-resistant state, is characterized by a significant increase in B-cell mass [139]. Thus, the finding of even a modest reduction in B-cell mass in any insulin-resistant state is most impressive. Nonetheless, a greater than 80–90% decrease in B-cell mass is required before sufficient insulinopenia develops to cause overt diabetes mellitus [142]. Moreover, it is unknown whether, in the earliest stages of NIDDM, B-cell mass is diminished. It seems likely, therefore, that factors in addition to B-cell loss must be responsible for the impairment in insulin secretion.

Low Birthweight

Recent studies in a variety of populations have demonstrated an association between low birthweight and the development of IGT and NIDDM later in life [143–149]. In studies reported by Hales and colleagues [143, 144], men and women with IGT or newly diagnosed NIDDM had a mean birthweight that was 0.3 kg less than non-diabetic subjects, a higher placental-to-birthweight ratio, a smaller head circumference and a lower ponderal (weight/length) index. Developmental studies in animals and man have provided evidence that poor nutrition and impaired growth are associated with reduced insulin secretion and/or reduced B-cell mass [150]. Some studies have suggested that fetal malnutrition also may lead to the development of insulin resistance later in life [151]. One could postulate that an environmental influence, i.e. impaired fetal nutrition leading to an acquired defect in insulin secretion or reduced B-cell mass, when superimposed upon an inherited defect in insulin action, could result in NIDDM later in life. Thus, with the normal aging process, the onset of obesity or a worsening of the genetic component of the insulin resistance, the B cell would be called upon to augment its secretion of insulin to offset the defect in insulin action. If B-cell mass/function were reduced by an environmental insult during fetal life, the result would be the emergence of IGT or overt NIDDM. It should be noted, however, that although such a defect may place a limit on the maximum amount of insulin that is secreted, it would not explain the progressive decline in the absolute amount of insulin that is secreted as individuals progress from IGT to mild to moderately severe NIDDM (Figures 3 and 4).

Amylin, CGRP, Galanin, GLP-1

Amylin, or islet amyloid polypeptide (IAPP), is produced by the B cell, packaged with insulin in secretory granules, and co-secreted into the sinusoidal space [152–155] (see Chapter 19). This peptide has been shown to be the precursor for the amyloid deposits which frequently are observed in patients with NIDDM [154–158]. At very high doses amylin inhibits insulin secretion by the perfused rat pancreas *in vitro* [159], and pancreatic amylin deposits have been shown to precede the appearance of glucose intolerance in spontaneously diabetic monkeys [160]. In this latter model the severity of the diabetes is correlated closely with the amount of amylin which is deposited within the pancreas [160]. Elevated plasma amylin levels have been demonstrated in obese glucose-intolerant subjects [161], in glucose-intolerant first-degree relatives of NIDDM patients [162] and in animal models of diabetes [163]. Following its secretion, amylin accumulates extracellularly in close contact with the B cell and it has been suggested that these amylin deposits might cause B-cell dysfunction, and eventually death, by impairing the transport of nutrients from the plasma to the B cell or by interfering with the glucose-sensing and/or insulin-secreting apparatus of the B cell [154–160]. Although attractive, this theory has been seriously challenged by Bloom and co-workers [164, 165], who failed to find any inhibitory effect of amylin on insulin secretion when the peptide was infused in pharmacologic doses in rats, rabbits and humans. Using immunohistochemical and *in situ* hybridization techniques, islet amyloid polypeptide mRNA has been demonstrated by Westermark et al [166]. These authors reported varying degrees of islet amyloid polypeptide derived amyloid in pancreatic tissue from 6/7 NIDDM and 3/7 non-diabetic controls but there was considerable overlap between the two groups. Most recently, Hoppener et al [167] have generated transgenic mice with the gene encoding either human or rat islet amyloid polypeptide under control of an insulin promoter. Although pancreatic and plasma amyloid polypeptide levels were significantly elevated, hyperglycemia and hyperinsulinemia were not observed. In summary, at present the evidence that amylin is responsible for the defect in B-cell function in NIDDM in man is not very strong. Similarly, calcitonin gene-related peptide (CGRP), which shares a 46% homology with amylin, has been shown to have no effect on insulin secretion when infused intravenously in rats [168].

Glucagon-like peptide 1 (GLP-1) is synthesized and secreted by the small intestine in response to ingested nutrients [169, 170] and is a potent insulin secretagogue [171–173]. GLP-1 has a specific B-cell receptor that has been localized to chromosome 6 [174]. After binding of GLP-1 to the B-cell receptor, the adenylate cyclase system is stimulated, cyclic AMP levels rise, and cAMP-dependent protein kinase A augments glucose-induced insulin secretion by phosphorylation of key elements of the glucose signaling pathway, including the ATP-dependent K$^+$ channel, the voltage-dependent calcium channel and/or elements of the insulin secretory machinery. In NIDDM the gluco-incretin effect of GLP-1 is reduced [173, 175, 176], but GLP-1 levels are normal or increased [175], suggesting B-cell resistance to GLP-1. Pharmacologic doses of GLP-1, but not gastric inhibitory peptide (the other major intestinally secreted peptide that functions as an incretin and also works by activation of cAMP-dependent protein kinase A [173, 177]), can enhance the postprandial insulin secretory response and restore near-normal glycemia in NIDDM patients [178-181]. Conversely, elimination of the action of GLP-1 in baboons and rats has been shown to impair glucose tolerance and diminish insulin secretion, especially first phase insulin release [182-184]. In summary, GLP-1 is a novel incretin which deserves further investigation to define its role in the pathogenesis of decreased insulin secretion in NIDDM.

The newest hormone that has been implicated in the impairment of insulin secretion in NIDDM is galanin [185] (see also Chapter 18). This 29-amino acid peptide, which is released by pancreatic sympathetic nerve terminals in response to neural stimulation, has been shown to inhibit both basal and meal-stimulated insulin secretion in rodents and dogs [185]. However, infusion of porcine galanin into humans had no effect on glucose-stimulated insulin secretion [186]. Recently, human galanin has been synthesized and shown to have no effect on glucose-stimulated insulin secretion using the hyperglycemic clamp [187]. It seems unlikely, therefore, that galanin plays any role in impaired B-cell function in NIDDM.

Glucose Toxicity

The most likely explanation for the acquired defect in insulin secretion relates to the concept of 'glucose toxicity' [1, 115, 188, 189] discussed in Chapter 32. The consistent observation that tight metabolic control (however it is achieved—diet, insulin therapy, sulfonylureas) leads to an improvement in insulin secretion provides strong clinical support that hyperglycemia exerts a deleterious effect on the insulin secretion. In order to provide a more rigorous test of the 'glucose toxicity' hypothesis, it was necessary to lower the plasma glucose concentration without altering circulating substrate levels (other than glucose), and without administering any agent that has direct effect on cellular metabolism (which obviously excludes insulin). This goal was achieved by the chronic administration of phlorhizin, a potent inhibitor of renal tubular glucose transport [115], applied particularly to rats made diabetic by removal of 90% of the pancreas, as described in Chapter 32. On the basis of the *in vivo*

and *in vitro* studies reviewed in Chapter 32 it seems reasonable to postulate that chronic hyperglycemia is responsible, at least in part, for the inability of B cells to respond to an acute hyperglycemic challenge. Most recently, Robertson et al [210] have provided evidence that prolonged exposure of B cells to high glucose concentrations impairs insulin gene transcription, leading to decreased insulin synthesis and secretion, and they have suggested the term 'desensitization' to explain a temporary, readily induced, reversible state of impaired insulin secretion following chronic exposure to hyperglycemia, while reserving the term 'glucose toxicity' for an irreversible loss of B-cell secretory capacity [210]. Regardless of the terminology, the key concept is that chronic physiologic hyperglycemia, if not corrected, can cause the B-cell to progress from a state of temporary refractoriness to an irreversible loss of function. This has far-reaching implications. First, it means that hyperglycemia no longer simply can be viewed as a manifestation, i.e. a laboratory marker, of diabetes mellitus: rather, the hyperglycemia must be considered as a pathogenetic factor which impairs insulin secretion and, therefore, is responsible for the perpetuation of the diabetic state. Second, the concept of glucose toxicity has important therapeutic implications and may help to explain the uniform improvement in insulin secretion that has been observed after a number of diverse maneuvers, all of which have in common the ability to lower the plasma glucose concentration.

Lipotoxicity

Most recently, the concept of 'lipotoxicity' has been put forward to explain the progressive decline in B-cell function as individuals progress from IGT to overt NIDDM with fasting hyperglycemia [18, 19, 211]. Because many of the tenets of 'lipotoxicity' overlap with those of 'glucotoxicity', the term 'glucolipotoxicity' or 'lipoglucotoxicity'—depending upon one's perspective—may be more appropriate. To understand the potential far-reaching implications of the lipotoxicity concept, it is necessary to review the basic biochemical events involved in the process by which glucose stimulates insulin secretion (Figure 7) and to review how these intracellular steps interdigitate with the key processes involved in the regulation of lipid metabolism (Figure 8).

The biochemical and molecular events involved in glucose and lipid metabolism have been elegantly and exhaustively reviewed by Matschinsky [212], Unger [19], Prentki and Corkey [18] and Randle [14] and will be summarized briefly below. This review of B-cell function also will serve as a template upon which to explore potential candidate genes that might be

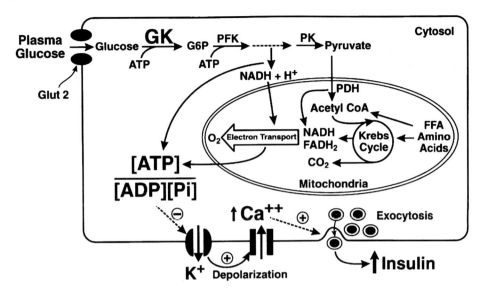

Figure 7 Key steps involved in glucose-stimulated insulin secretion by the pancreatic B cell. Glucokinase (GK) is the rate-limiting step for glucose metabolism by the islets. Generation of ATP from the electron transport chain closes an ATP-dependent potassium channel, which in turn opens a voltage-dependent calcium channel. The resultant increase in intracellular calcium leads to the stimulation of insulin secretion. See text for a more detailed discussion (adapted from reference 212, with permission)

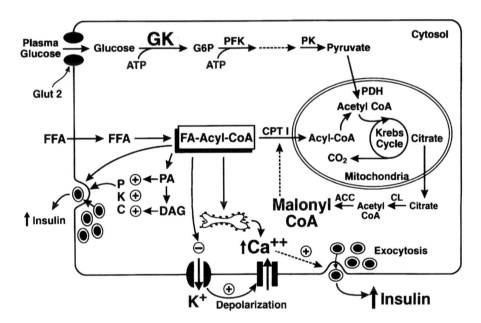

Figure 8 Relationship between lipid metabolism and insulin secretion. An increase in fatty acyl-CoA can augment insulin secretion by (a) increasing intracellular calcium which stimulates exocytosis of insulin containing granules; and/or (b) enhancing exocytosis directly or through protein kinase C (PKC). The latter mechanism involves generation of phosphatidic acid (PA) and diacylglycerol (DAG). It should be noted that malonyl-CoA generated from the metabolism of glucose is a potent inhibitor of carnitine palmitoyl transferase (CPT) I. Inhibition of CPT I increases fatty acyl-CoA, which contributes to the stimulation of insulin secretion. Thus, a mechanism exists via which increased lipid metabolism within the B cell potentiates glucose-stimulated insulin secretion (adapted from reference 212, with permission)

responsible for the genetic or inherited component of the B-cell defect in NIDDM.

Stimulation of insulin synthesis and secretion requires, not only the *entry* of glucose into the B cell, but its subsequent *metabolism*. Glucose enters the cell through the high capacity, low affinity Glut 2 transporter (Figure 7). The glucose transporter is highly efficient, responding rapidly to both increases and decreases in the plasma glucose concentration, and ensures almost instantaneous equilibration between the intracellular and extracellular glucose concentrations. Once glucose enters the cell, it is quickly phosphorylated to glucose-6-phosphate. Although the B cell contains hexokinase I, glucokinase is the major enzyme responsible for phosphorylating glucose and because of its unique characteristics, serves as the 'pacemaker' or 'glucose sensor' for insulin secretion [212, 213] (Figure 7). The K_m of glucokinase has been reported to range from 6 to 11 mmol/l, with a substrate concentration dependency that is sigmoidal with an inflection point of 2.5–4.0 mmol/l and a Hill number of 1.4–1.8. These characteristics ensure that glucose increments throughout the physiologic to pharmacologic range are rapidly sensed by the B cell with a prompt stimulation of insulin synthesis and secretion. Glucokinase is not subject to product inhibition and requires Mg^{++}-ATP, which normally is present within the B cell at near-saturation concentrations. Because the capacity of Glut 2 to transport glucose into the cell exceeds the capacity of glucokinase to phosphorylate it, glucokinase is the rate limiting step for insulin secretion and is believed to represent the glucose sensor [14, 212, 213].

The major intracellular fate of glucose-6-phosphate (G-6-P) within the B cell is glycolysis. Less than 10% of G-6-P enters the pentose phosphate shunt, the enzymatic machinery for glycogen synthesis is limited, and glucose-6-phosphatase is not present within the B cell [212–214]. The intermediates in the glycolytic pool from fructose-1,6-diphosphate to phosphoenol pyruvate are in equilibrium, such that pyruvate is formed at a rate that keeps pace with glucose phosphorylation [214]. Because lactate dehydrogenase activity is very low, lactate formation is negligible [215] (Figure 7). Hydrogen, which is generated in the cytosol, is nearly quantitatively channeled into the electron transport chain within the mitochondria via the α-glycero-phosphate and malate-aspartate shuttles [18, 212, 216]. Electron transport is tightly coupled to proton pumping across the mitochondrial membrane and the proton motive force thus generates the driving force for ATP synthesis [212, 217, 218] (Figure 7).

The pyruvate which is generated within the cytosol is transported into the mitochondria where it is converted to acetyl-CoA by the enzyme pyruvate dehydrogenase. Acetyl-CoA subsequently enters the Krebs (TCA) cycle, giving rise to NADH and reduced flavin adenine dinucleotide (FADH$_2$), which drives the electron transport chain [212, 219]. The metabolism of one glucose molecule generates 6–8 molecules of ATP and the ATP/ADP ratio increases [212]. There is evidence that both the increase in ATP and decline in ADP within the cytosol (resulting in an increase in the ATP/ADP ratio) lead to a closure of adenine nucleotide-sensitive potassium channels, which results in depolarization

of the plasma cell membrane (Figure 7) [18, 212, 220–224]. Only fuels that cause depolarization of the plasma cell membrane stimulate insulin secretion [18, 212, 224]. Depolarization of the cell membrane opens voltage-sensitive calcium channels, leading to a manifold increase in intracellular calcium concentration (Figure 7) [18, 212, 220, 225–227]. The rise in intracellular calcium is enhanced by the voltage-dependent release of calcium from intracellular stores [18, 212, 228].

A substantial body of evidence has accumulated to indicate that alterations in lipid metabolism play an important auxiliary role in glucose-induced insulin secretion (Figure 8) [18, 19, 211–213, 226]. Cytosolic long chain fatty acyl-CoA esters, which represent the activated energy-rich intracellular form of FFA and the substrate for FFA-metabolizing enzymes, appear to be the signal that triggers the secretion of insulin. Free fatty acids are transported into the B cell via the fatty acid binding protein 2 and within the cytosol are converted to their fatty acyl-CoA derivative. Under basal conditions, the fatty acyl-CoA molecule is transported into the mitochondria by carnitine palmitoyl transferase 1(CPT-1), where it enters the Krebs (TCA) cycle and undergoes β-oxidation. In the presence of an elevated glucose concentration this process is inhibited, the cytosolic concentration of long-chain fatty acyl-CoA rises, and this stimulates insulin secretion [18, 19, 211, 212, 226].

Malonyl-CoA, formed as the result of increased glucose metabolism, acts as the switch compound that facilitates the rise in cytosolic fatty acyl-CoA by inhibiting CPT-1. Increased intracellular glucose levels enhance substrate flux into the TCA cycle, leading to the accumulation of oxaloacetic acid which condenses with acetyl-CoA to form citrate. Citrate is then transported into the cytosol where it is converted to acetyl-CoA by citrate lysate. The acetyl-CoA subsequently is metabolized by acetyl-CoA carboxylase to malonyl-CoA, which inhibits CPT-1 and causes a rise in cytosolic long chain fatty acyl-CoA [18, 19, 211, 212, 226]. Long-chain fatty acyl-CoA esters and their products exert a wide range of effects on enzymes, ion channels, and genes [18, 19, 226] (Figure 8). Long-chain fatty acyl-CoA derivatives lead to the increased formation of phosphatidic acid and diacylglycerol, which can directly activate specific protein kinase C (PKC) isoforms, which are believed to participate in the exocytosis of insulin [18, 226, 229–232]. Long-chain fatty acyl-CoA also has been shown to directly enhance exocytosis [18] and to stimulate endoplasmic reticulum Ca^{++}-ATPase and increase intracellular calcium, thus augmenting insulin secretion [18, 226, 229–232]. Recent evidence indicates that long-chain fatty acyl-CoA esters stimulate closure of the

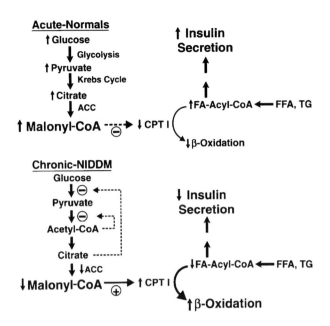

Figure 9 Potential mechanism for altered glucose sensing in NIDDM—'glucolipotoxicity'. In healthy normal subjects hyperglycemia augments glycolytic flux and malonyl-CoA accumulates. Malonyl-CoA inhibits carnitine palmitoyl transferase (CPT) I and fatty acyl-CoA accumulates, leading to a stimulation of insulin secretion. In subjects with NIDDM increased free fatty acid (FFA) oxidation by the B-cell and FFA-induced down-regulation of acetyl-CoA-carboxylase (ACC) lead to a decline in intracellular fatty acyl-CoA and·a reduction in insulin secretion. Increased FFA metabolism also inhibits glucose metabolism within the B-cell (Randle cycle). The decline in glycolytic flux has two consequences: (a) it further reduces malonyl-CoA, leading to an increase in CPT I activity and favoring FFA oxidation; and (b) it impairs ATP generation, leading to a reduction in insulin secretion (redrawn from reference 18, with permission)

K^+-ATPase channel [18]. All of these effects of long chain fatty acyl-CoA derivatives favor the stimulation of insulin secretion. From the above review, it is clear that both glucose (by stimulating glycolysis and the TCA cycle, leading to an increase in the ATP:ADP ratio) and FFA (by increasing fatty acyl-CoA esters) acutely augment insulin secretion. Indirectly, glucose contributes to the rise in intracellular fatty acyl-CoA by increasing malonyl-CoA. However, chronic exposure to FFA or glucose (by increasing long-chain fatty acyl-CoA) could lead to down-regulation or even an inhibition of insulin secretion via operation of the Randle cycle [14], in which increased β-oxidation increases acetyl-CoA, leading to an inhibition of pyruvate dehydrogenase and elevated citrate levels, which inhibit phosphofructokinase and subsequently glycolysis [14, 18, 226, 233, 234]. Thus, 'glucotoxicity' may be mediated via 'lipotoxicity'. Since impaired insulin secretion can persist for a considerable period after exposure of islets *in vitro* to glucose [211, 235] or to lipid [236–238], it is likely that alterations in intracellular lipid metabolism may alter the expression of genes encoding proteins that are involved in glucose-mediated insulin secretion. With regard to this, long-chain fatty acyl-CoA esters down-regulate acetyl-CoA carboxylase gene expression and up-regulate CPT-1 gene expression [14]. This would result in increased

transport of fatty acyl-CoA into the mitochondria for β-oxidation (leading to insulin resistance in muscle and stimulation of gluconeogenesis in liver) and to a decrease in cytosolic long-chain fatty acyl-CoA (leading to a decrease in insulin secretion) (Figure 9). It should be noted that chronic exposure of B cells to elevated FFA would be expected to reproduce the same scenario.

Mitochondrial Gene Mutation

As reviewed in the previous section, mitochondrial metabolism plays a crucial role in insulin secretion [14, 212] (Figure 7). Recently, a subtype of NIDDM has been described in which at least 10 distinct mitochondrial gene mutations have been shown to cause impaired insulin secretion due to a defect in mitochondrial energy metabolism [239–242]. Phenotypically, 50–70% of the affected individuals present with deafness and maternal transmission with or without other neurologic symptoms including encephalopathy, dementia and stroke-like episodes. Epilepsy, ragged red fiber muscle disease, lactic acidosis, hypothryoidism, and hypogonadism also are commonly observed.

Cells vary in their energy demands and possess hundreds to thousands of mitochondria, each containing 2–10 mitochondrial DNA molecules. The mitochondrial energy chain is encoded by both mitochondrial and nuclear genomes [239–242]. The mitochondrial DNA is a circular closed double-stranded DNA molecule that is maternally inherited [239–244] and encodes 13 of the proteins required for oxidative phosphorylation and 22 transfer RNAs and two ribosomal RNAs required for their translation. Mitochondrial DNA has a very high mutation rate, 10–20-fold higher than nuclear DNA [245]. This high mutation rate derives from the lack of protection from histones, absence of DNA repair mechanisms, and the production of highly energetic oxygen radicals from the electron transport chain. Despite its high mutation rate, mitochondrial DNA encodes highly conserved proteins and a change in phenotype becomes apparent only when the proportion of mutant DNA exceeds a threshold level which varies for each organ, depending upon its reliance on mitochondrial energy production which declines with age [246–248].

The mitochondrial tRNA$^{Leu(UUR)}$ gene has an especially high mutation rate and, of the 10 disease-related mutations that have been described, four have been associated with diabetes and various other symptoms [239–242, 249]. In 1992, two separate publications [250, 251] described an A/G exchange at np 3243 in the tRNA$^{Leu(UUR)}$ gene. These initial reports have been confirmed by a number of groups and recently summarized [241, 252, 253]. The tRNA$^{Leu(UUR)}$ mutation was found in approximately 1% of unselected diabetic patients, both type 1 and type 2. In diabetics with a positive family history, the incidence increases to about 10% [239, 241, 242, 252]. At least 10 distinct mitochondrial gene mutations have been described, each with varying phenotypic expressions [239–242, 246, 247, 252] depending upon the specific mutation, the organs involved, the energy requirements of the affected tissues, organ specific threshold, age of the involved family member, concomitant presence of nuclear gene abnormalities and other, as yet unidentified factors. Because of the frequent combination (~70%) of maternally inherited diabetes and deafness (MIDD), the mitochondrial mutation at np 3243 in the tRNA$^{Leu(UUR)}$ deserves recognition as a distinct entity [239–242, 246, 247, 252].

A mitochondrial mutation could present either as a defect in insulin secretion or as insulin resistance. Although extensive studies have yet to be carried out, individuals with the A/G point mutation at np 3243 in the tRNA$^{Leu(UUR)}$ gene appear to be characterized by a delayed and deficient plasma insulin response to a glucose challenge [253–256]. Insulin clamp studies have revealed either no impairment or a very mild impairment in insulin sensitivity [242, 257–259]. It seems likely, however, that in the future specific mitochondrial gene mutations will be described in which insulin resistance represents the major metabolic abnormality.

GENETIC BASIS OF DEFICIENT INSULIN SECRETION IN NIDDM

Considerable controversy has arisen about the primary genetic disturbance(s) responsible for impaired glucose homeostasis in patients with NIDDM [1, 5, 29, 31, 35, 60, 64–67, 78, 79, 260–263]. In the present section we will focus on studies performed in individuals with normal glucose tolerance who are genetically predisposed to develop NIDDM later in life in an attempt to define which defect, i.e. diminished insulin secretion or insulin resistance, occurs first in the natural history of NIDDM before the onset of abnormalities—hyperglycemia ('glucotoxicity') and hyperlipidemia ('lipotoxicity')—which are known to impair B-cell function. The following three groups will be examined: individuals with normal glucose tolerance who are followed prospectively and develop overt NIDDM; normal glucose-tolerant first-degree relatives of patients with NIDDM, including twins; and normal glucose-tolerant women with a history of gestational diabetes mellitus (GDM).

Prospective Studies

Fourteen studies have reported the incidence of NIDDM in individuals who were followed prospectively over a prolonged period of time (Table 3) [52, 54, 59, 65, 67, 102, 264–271]. They have provided evidence to support both impaired insulin secretion and insulin resistance as the primary factor responsible for the development of NIDDM, but criticisms can be raised about most of the studies: (a) only one of the studies quantified both insulin secretion and insulin sensitivity in the same individual; (b) the techniques used to measure insulin secretion and insulin sensitivity would be considered relatively primitive according to currently employed methods; (c) many subjects already had IGT at the time of entry into the study, and this recruitment bias would favor the selection of individuals with insulin secretion defects, since first-phase insulin response is lost when the fasting glucose concentration rises to 110–115 mg/dl [35, 101, 105]; (d) measurement of the 2 h plasma insulin response during an OGTT would tend to underestimate the importance of an insulin secretory defect since the 2 h value has been shown to be inversely related to the 30 min plasma insulin response [29]; (e) failure to control for body weight in individuals who progress to NIDDM vs. those who maintain normal glucose tolerance. Thus, the presence of obesity would tend to overemphasize the importance of insulin resistance [272, 273], whereas the inclusion predominantly of lean and older subjects would tend to favor the likelihood of finding a defect in insulin secretion [20, 35, 101, 105].

Table 3 Findings of the 14 studies which have examined insulin secretion and/or insulin sensitivity in normal glucose-tolerant subjects who were followed prospectively and developed NIDDM (see references 52, 54, 59, 65, 67, 68, 102, 264–271)

	Insulin secretion	Insulin resistance
Decreased	9	1
Normal	2	0
Increased	2	0
Not examined	1	13

In the one study which measured both insulin secretion (OGTT and IVGTT) and insulin sensitivity (insulin clamp) in the same group, insulin resistance was the major factor that predicted the later development of NIDDM in Pima Indians; the acute insulin response (whether viewed in absolute terms or as the incremental above baseline) had no predictive value for the development of NIDDM [67]. Likewise, the acute insulin response factored by the degree of insulin resistance (measured with the euglycemic insulin clamp) was not a predictor of NIDDM, and this index was virtually identical in subjects who progressed to NIDDM vs. those who did not. A slight decrease in the insulin response factored by percentage body fat (but not the severity of insulin resistance) was found in the progressors [67]. Since insulin resistance is a major determinant of insulin secretion [274, 275], the importance of this latter finding is of questionable physiological significance. Thus, in normal glucose tolerant Pima Indians who progress to NIDDM, pre-existing insulin resistance—not impaired insulin secretion—predicts the development of diabetes later in life.

The lack of any direct measurement of insulin resistance presents a major obstacle to the interpretation of the other 13 studies [52, 54, 59, 65, 68, 102, 264–271] summarized in Table 3. The pitfalls encountered in the interpretation of studies in which only insulin secretion is directly measured, is exemplified by the study of Haffner et al [65]. These investigators reported that 99 of 714 normal glucose tolerance Mexican-American subjects developed NIDDM after a mean follow-up period of 7 years. Insulin secretion was measured with the OGTT, while the fasting plasma insulin concentration was used as a surrogate measure of insulin resistance. From univariate and multivariate logistic regression analyses summarized in Table 4, the authors concluded that both impaired insulin secretion and insulin resistance contribute to the risk of development of NIDDM, with the greatest risk being present in individuals with both defects. On a relative scale, however, insulin resistance (inferred from the surrogate measure = fasting plasma insulin concentration) was 5–10-fold more predictive (depending upon

whether one uses univariate or multivariate analysis) than impaired early insulin secretion (absolute insulin concentration at 30 min, the incremental insulin concentration (ΔI) at 30 min, or the incremental insulin concentration factored by the incremental glucose concentration ($\Delta I/\Delta G$) at 30 min). Of these, $\Delta I30/\Delta G30$ had the greatest predictive value. Taken at face value, this conclusion is consistent with that of Lillioja et al [67] and indicates that insulin resistance is the major predictor of eventual progression to NIDDM. However, the fasting glucose concentration in the progressors described by Haffner et al [65] was significantly elevated and during multivariate analysis proved to be as great a predictor of progression to NIDDM as the fasting insulin concentration (Table 4). Since the plasma glucose concentration is the primary determinant of insulin secretion, it is obvious that one cannot use the fasting insulin concentration as a measure of insulin resistance to predict the progression of normal glucose tolerant subjects to NIDDM.

Table 4 Univariate logistic regression analysis (adjusted for age and sex) and multiple logistic regression analysis (adjusted for age, sex and body mass index) for conversion to NIDDM ($n = 99$) in 714 Mexican-Americans followed prospectively for 7 years.

Variable	Odds ratio Univariate	Multivariate
Insulin—fasting	5.43	2.57
Insulin—30 min	0.67	0.50
Δ Insulin—30 min	0.65	0.46
$\Delta I_{30}/\Delta G_{30}$	0.20	0.17
Glucose—fasting	2.43	2.57

All values presented in the table are statistically significant. It should be noted that the odds ratio for all parameters of insulin secretion, although statistically significant, is quite low. $\Delta I_{30}/\Delta G_{30}$ = increment in plasma insulin concentration at 30 min divided by the increment in plasma glucose concentration at 30 min (from reference 65, with permission)

Studies in First-degree Relatives

A number of investigators have examined insulin secretion and insulin sensitivity in first-degree relatives of NIDDM patients, with the assumption that observed disturbances are genetic in origin [23, 263, 276–280]. Although this assumption is likely to be true, at least in part, shared environmental factors amongst individuals growing up within the same family and in same societal structure (i.e. diet, physical activity, etc.) can exert significant influences on both insulin secretion and insulin sensitivity [261, 262]. In addition, most of these studies suffer from all of the criticisms described in the previous section, especially the failure to measure both insulin secretion and insulin resistance in the same individuals. Recently, Pimenta et al [260] have summarized the findings from 38 published studies which have examined insulin secretion and/or insulin sensitivity in first-degree relatives of NIDDM subjects. In addition to their own study [260], three other studies have been published subsequently [66, 281, 282], yielding a total of 42 studies (Table 5). About half of the studies report a defect in insulin secretion (20 of 42 publications) while two-thirds of the studies report the presence of insulin resistance (eight of 12 publications). It should be noted that in most of the studies demonstrating a decrease in insulin secretion, insulin resistance was not simultaneously measured, so it is not possible to define whether both defects were present in the first-degree relatives of NIDDM patients. Of note, seven studies report a significant *increase* in insulin secretion as the major abnormality.

Table 5 Findings of the 42 studies which have examined insulin secretion and/or insulin sensitivity in normal glucose-tolerant, first-degree relatives of NIDDM patients (summarized from the data in reference 260 plus references 66, 281 and 282)

	Insulin secretion ($n = 42$)	Insulin sensitivity ($n = 12$)
Reduced	19(20)*	8
Normal	16(17)	4
Increased	7	0

*Pimenta et al [262] reported normal insulin secretion with the OGTT but impaired insulin secretion with the hyperglycemic clamp

Several studies deserve special note. In the studies by Warram, Martin and colleagues [60, 78] 155 normal glucose tolerant offspring of 86 couples who both had NIDDM were compared with 186 control subjects without any family history of NIDDM. The minimal model technique (IVGTT) was used to evaluate insulin sensitivity and insulin secretion. Because the offspring of two diabetic parents are at very high risk to develop NIDDM later in life [60, 283–285], any observed abnormalities are very likely to represent genetic predispositions. In the 25-year follow-up, impaired insulin sensitivity, irrespective of changes in body weight, predicted which offspring developed NIDDM later in life (Figure 10); insulin secretion was increased and was appropriate for the degree of insulin resistance [78].

The study of Gulli et al [64] also is very informative. In this study 11 normal weight, normal glucose-tolerant offspring of two Mexican-American NIDDM parents (FPG = 5.0 ± 0.1 mmol/l, BMI = 25.3 ± 0.7 kg/m^2, IBW = $114 \pm 4\%$, age = 39 ± 3 years, fat free mass (FFM) = 45.4 ± 1.7 kg) and 10 age- and weight-matched control subjects were studied with highly sophisticated methods to evaluate insulin sensitivity (euglycemic insulin clamp with tritiated glucose), insulin secretion (+100 mg/dl hyperglycemic clamp) and lean body mass (tritiated water). Because of the high incidence of NIDDM in Mexican-American

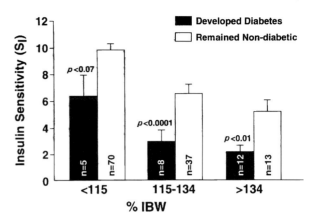

Figure 10 Long-term follow-up (25 years) of offspring who had two NIDDM parents. Decreased insulin sensitivity (minimal model technique) predicted which offspring developed NIDDM later in life and this was independent of body weight. IBW = ideal body weight (from reference 78, with permission)

families, it can be estimated that approximately 70% of the offspring will develop NIDDM later in life [64, 78, 283–285]. In the offspring the fasting plasma insulin concentration was significantly increased, and during the OGTT the absolute insulin/C-peptide responses, the incremental insulin/C-peptide responses, and the incremental insulin/C-peptide responses per incremental glucose response (at 30 min, at 120 min, and 0–120 min) were increased in the offspring (Figure 11). Similarly, the early (0–10 min), late (10–120 min), and total (0–120 min) plasma insulin/C-peptide responses during the hyperglycemic clamp were increased approximately twofold in the offspring. Because both the increment in glucose concentration above baseline (98 ± 2 vs. 97 ± 3 mg/dl) and absolute plasma glucose concentration (188 ± 2 vs. 185 ± 3 mg/dl) during the hyperglycemic clamp were virtually identical, it is obvious that this genetically predisposed group is characterized by fasting and glucose-stimulated hyperinsulinemia (Figure 12). During both the hyperglycemic and euglycemic insulin clamp studies, insulin-mediated glucose disposal was moderately to severely reduced (Figure 13). Thus, in Mexican-Americans, as well as in Pima Indians [54, 59, 67], insulin resistance (independent of obesity) and hyperinsulinemia are the characteristic features which precede the development of NIDDM later in life. It should be emphasized, however, that although these studies strongly argue against B-cell insufficiency, i.e. insulinopenia, as the initiating cause of glucose intolerance, they can not exclude more subtle defects in pulsatile insulin secretion [31, 32, 123].

Pimenta et al, in a largely Europid population, compared 50 individuals with and 50 individuals without a first-degree NIDDM relative [260]. All

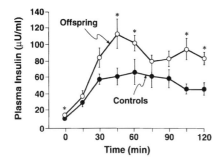

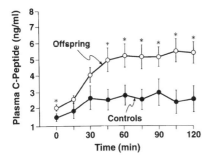

Figure 11 Plasma insulin (top) and plasma C-peptide (bottom) responses during an OGTT performed in normal glucose-tolerant offspring who had two Mexican-American parents with NIDDM, and in controls. $*p < 0.05$ (from reference 64, with permission)

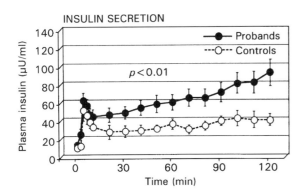

Figure 12 Plasma insulin response during a +100 mg/dl hyperglycemic clamp performed in control subjects (open circles) and in normal glucose-tolerant offspring who had two Mexican-American parents with NIDDM (solid circles) (drawn from data presented in reference 64)

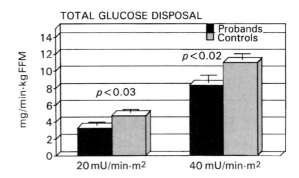

Figure 13 Whole-body insulin-mediated glucose disposal during a 20 mU/m² min (+40 μU/ml) and 40 mU/m² min (+80 μU/ml) euglycemic insulin clamp performed with indirect calorimetry in control subjects (shaded bars) and in normal glucose-tolerant offspring (probands) who had two diabetic parents (solid bars). FFM, fat-free mass (drawn from data presented in reference 64)

subjects had normal glucose tolerance and both groups were well matched for age, sex and degree of obesity. *Both groups also were matched for insulin sensitivity.* During the OGTT, insulin secretion (absolute, incremental, relative to glucose) was virtually identical in the first-degree relatives and controls. However, during the hyperglycemic clamp both the early and late phases of insulin secretion were significantly reduced in the relatives (although not necessarily in the same individuals), while insulin sensitivity (measured in all subjects by the hyperglycemic clamp and in about half

of the subjects with the euglycemic insulin clamp) was not significantly diminished in the group as a whole. The authors interpreted their results to indicate the primacy of impaired insulin secretion as the precursor of NIDDM. Unfortunately, there is a major flaw in the study design which clouds the interpretation of this paper [260]. Since the first-degree relatives and control subjects were matched *a priori* for insulin sensitivity, it would be impossible to discern whether a defect in insulin action also contributed to the predisposition to develop NIDDM later in life. Interestingly, in subjects from a Finnish European population who were studied with the insulin clamp, impaired insulin sensitivity with normal insulin secretion was observed in the first-degree relatives of NIDDM individuals [75].

Taken collectively, these studies indicate that insulin resistance is the earliest identifiable metabolic/endocrine abnormality in the first-degree relatives of NIDDM subjects in high risk populations, i.e. American Indians and Pima Indians, whereas both impaired insulin secretion and insulin resistance have been described in first-degree relatives of NIDDM patients of European ancestry.

Studies in Twins

Only five studies have examined identical twin pairs who are discordant for NIDDM [286–290]. Unfortunately, the total number of subjects combined was small ($n = 52$) and at least 18 of 52 twins had IGT. All five studies demonstrated a defect in insulin secretion, which is not surprising because of the large number of twins with IGT. In the only study that examined insulin sensitivity [286], an impairment in insulin action during the euglycemic insulin clamp was observed in the twins with normal glucose tolerance and IGT. Thus, these twin studies provide support for impairment of both insulin secretion and insulin action as early genetic lesions responsible for NIDDM, although the results are confounded to some extent by the presence of IGT.

Subjects with History of Gestational Diabetes Mellitus (GDM)

A number of studies have examined insulin secretion and insulin sensitivity in women with GDM after delivery and then followed them prospectively to define the incidence of NIDDM and the predisposing factors. These studies have been extensively reviewed by Pendergrass et al [291] and Buchanan and Catalano [292]. In an often quoted 15-year postpartum study, O'Sullivan [293] found that 26% of lean (1.1% per year) and 47% of obese (3.2% per year) women with GDM developed NIDDM, compared with only 5–10% of age-, weight- and ethnicity-matched women with normal glucose tolerance during pregnancy. In a recent study of 671 Latino women with a history of GDM and normal glucose tolerance documented 4–16 weeks postpartum Kjos et al [294] found a 47% cumulative incidence rate of NIDDM 5 years after delivery (or 9.4% per year). The postpartum OGTT provided the best discrimination between high-risk and low-risk individuals. Women who met the WHO criteria for IGT at early postpartum examination had an 84% risk of developing NIDDM at 5 years.

Women with a history of GDM, when studied postpartum at a time when glucose is normal, uniformly have been shown to be significantly more insulin resistant than women with normal glucose tolerance in prior pregnancies [292, 295–300]. Using the euglycemic clamp technique in conjunction with indirect calorimetry, Buchanan and Catalano and colleagues [292, 296] demonstrated the presence of insulin resistance in women with previous GDM when they were studied postpartum at a time when glucose tolerance was normal. The defect in insulin action was entirely accounted for by a decrease in non-oxidative glucose disposal, which primarily represents glycogen synthesis.

In the insulin-resistant women studied by Catalano et al [292, 296], insulin secretion was normal or increased. When compared with lean GDM patients, obese patients with previous GDM had an even greater insulin response during the OGTT. Other groups, however, have reported impaired insulin secretory responses in women with a history of GDM [297–303]. Several factors may explain these variable findings. Glucose tolerance was impaired in the majority of subjects studied by Efendic et al [300] and first-phase insulin secretion is known to be impaired in individuals with IGT [35]. In the studies by Ward and colleagues [297, 298], postpartum glucose tolerance was not evaluated, and it is likely that some of the women

had abnormal glucose tolerance. Moreover, since the patients of Efendic et al [300] and Ward and colleagues [297, 298] were studied many years after delivery, they may have been at a later stage in the natural history of NIDDM compared with those of Catalano et al [292, 296]. Ryan et al [299] also demonstrated impaired insulin secretion following delivery in normal glucose tolerant subjects with a history of GDM. The first-phase insulin secretory response was impaired primarily in lean subjects, while the obese subjects had equal or exaggerated first- and second-phase insulin responses relative to control subjects. Notably, the subjects with diminished insulin responses also had somewhat less severe insulin resistance compared with the groups with normal or augmented insulin responses. This suggests that there may be a subgroup of patients with prior GDM in whom impaired insulin secretion appears to play a more significant role in the development of diabetes. This variability in insulin secretory response, which ranges from subnormal to exaggerated in individuals with a prior history of GDM, underscores the dynamic interaction between insulin sensitivity and insulin secretion. Lastly, some women with GDM have been shown to have a glucokinase mutation [304].

In summary, insulin resistance appears to be the characteristic finding in normal glucose tolerant women with a history of GDM. It is only when the B cell can no longer compensate for the decrease in insulin sensitivity that overt diabetes ensues. Thus, both insulin resistance and impaired insulin secretion appear to be important precursors of eventual progression to overt NIDDM in women with GDM.

SUMMARY: INSULIN SECRETION

NIDDM involves defects in both insulin secretion and insulin action [1, 5]. In high risk ethnic populations, i.e. American Indians, Mexican-Americans and Pacific islanders, which have a high prevalence of diabetes, insulin secretion is enhanced and both fasting and glucose-stimulated plasma insulin levels are elevated during the earliest stages of the natural history of NIDDM, compared with age/weight-matched non-diabetic controls. Most of the available evidence suggests that in such populations insulin resistance is the primary genetic disturbance and that augmented B-cell function represents a compensatory adaptation to offset the defect in insulin action.

In contrast to the preceding scenario, there appears to be growing support for the primacy of insulin deficiency in the pathogenesis of NIDDM in certain subgroups. In a significant minority of reports, type 2 individuals with impaired insulin secretion and normal insulin sensitivity have been well described. These NIDDM patients generally are lean, older (>60 years of age at onset) and of European ancestry. In this group glucokinase and mitochondrial gene mutations are especially prevalent, but even when these are taken into account, the origin of the B-cell defect remains unexplained in the majority of these individuals. Although it has been estimated that as many as 10% of these diabetics may represent slowly evolving IDDM patients with positive GAD antibodies [23], there is mounting evidence for a primary non-immunologic B-cell defect in a significant number of lean, older NIDDM patients. Lastly, one cannot fail to be impressed by the large number of studies in which defects in both insulin secretion and insulin sensitivity have been reported simultaneously in the same genetically predisposed individual. This could imply a single underlying genetic abnormality in some key regulatory protein that is involved in both insulin action and insulin secretion. A more detailed schema about the pathogenesis of NIDDM, impaired insulin secretion and insulin sensitivity will be provided at the end of this chapter.

HYPERSECRETION OF INSULIN: A NEW HYPOTHESIS

The major focus of investigations about the etiology of NIDDM has been to define whether impaired insulin secretion or insulin resistance are the earliest precursors for the development of NIDDM later in life. However, one could suggest another equally plausible hypothesis: *hypersecretion of insulin is the primary defect in NIDDM and insulin resistance develops secondarily to the chronic hyperinsulinemia*. Within the normal population, DeFronzo et al [274, 305, 306] and Reaven et al [275, 307, 308] have shown that there is a fourfold range of insulin sensitivity. However, glucose tolerance remains perfectly normal because of the *dynamic interaction between insulin secretion and insulin sensitivity*. Thus, in normal glucose tolerance individuals the B-cell is able very precisely to perceive the degree of insulin resistance or insulin sensitivity and appropriately adjust its insulin secretory capacity to maintain normal glucose tolerance. This *dynamic interaction* is demonstrated graphically by the results of Diamond et al [274]. Thirty-two normally menstruating, normal glucose-tolerant women (age = 19–40 years; IBW <90–120%) received a euglycemic insulin clamp during the follicular phase of the menstrual cycle (documented by menstrual history and plasma progesterone levels <0.2 mg/dl) and they were stratified by quartiles based upon the rate of insulin-mediated glucose disposal during a 1 mU/kg/min euglycemic insulin clamp (Figure 14, upper panel). Insulin secretion was measured independently on a separate day with a +125 mg/dl hyperglycemic clamp (Figure 14, lower panel). Insulin secretion and insulin

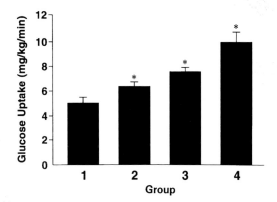

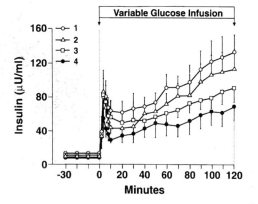

Figure 14 Upper panel, whole-body rate of glucose disposal during the euglycemic insulin clamp in 32 women divided into groups 1–4 by quartiles of insulin sensitivity (lowest in group 1). $^*p < 0.001$ for each group vs. the adjacent group. Lower panel, time course of plasma insulin response during the hyperglycemic clamp in the same 32 women. Insulin secretion rose progressively from the group with the highest to the group with the lowest insulin sensitivity ($p < 0.01$) (from reference 274, with permission)

resistance were strongly and positively correlated ($r = 0.79$, $p < 0.001$). Virtually identical results have been reported by Reaven et al [275, 307, 308].

Populations with a very high prevalence of NIDDM are characterized by hyperinsulinemia [44, 48, 51–54, 59, 62, 64–68], and it generally has been assumed that the hyperinsulinemia reflects a compensatory B-cell response to the underlying insulin resistance. However, in Pima Indians it is very obvious that the plasma insulin response to both oral and intravenous glucose administration is significantly greater than in Europids (Figure 15), even after matching for differences in plasma glucose levels, obesity, and insulin resistance (Figure 16) [309]. These results strongly suggest that *primary* (not compensatory) *hypersecretion* of insulin by the pancreatic B cells may represent the basic genetic defect responsible for NIDDM in this population. Consistent with this hypothesis, fasting and postprandial hyperinsulinemia have been shown to precede the development of insulin resistance in individuals

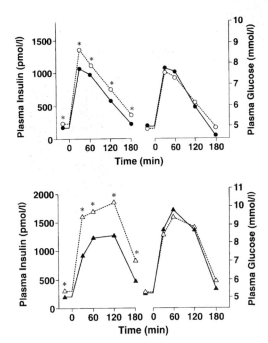

Figure 15 Upper panel, plasma insulin and glucose response in Europids (solid circles) and Pima Indians (open circles) with perfectly normal glucose tolerance. Lower panel, plasma insulin and glucose responses in Europids (solid triangles) and Pima Indians (open triangles) with impaired glucose tolerance. Pima Indians with normal and impaired glucose tolerance secrete significantly ($p < 0.05$) more insulin than Europids when matched for glucose tolerance (from reference 309, with permission)

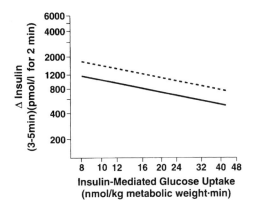

Figure 16 Incremental plasma insulin response during a 25 g IVGTT in 59 Europids (solid line) and 149 Pima Indians (dashed line) who also had a euglycemic insulin clamp to quantify whole-body insulin-mediated glucose uptake. The relationship between insulin secretion and insulin sensitivity was linear and parallel in Pima Indians and Europids. However, for any level of insulin sensitivity (resistance), Pima Indians secreted twice as much insulin as Europids ($p < 0.00001$) (from reference 309, with permission)

with juvenile onset obesity [310] and in a variety of animal models of obesity and diabetes, including VMH lesioned normal rats and the fa/fa rat (see review by

Jeanrenaud [311]). According to this hypothesis [311], alterations within the central nervous system (i.e. ventromedial hypothalamus, median eminence, and other as yet unidentified areas) increase the production of neuropeptide Y and/or other neuroregulatory peptides which are involved in food intake, thermogenesis, and regulation of sympathetic nervous system activity [312] and activate the vagus nerve, leading to an increase in insulin secretion [311, 312] (see also Chapter 18). It is noteworthy that in all human populations which are characterized by a very high incidence of diabetes and hyperinsulinemia, obesity is a common feature.

Recent studies in man by Del Prato et al [313] have conclusively demonstrated that chronic physiologic euglycemic hyperinsulinemia (insulin increment from 7 to 17 µU/ml) for as little as 3–5 days can induce severe insulin resistance in healthy young subjects with normal glucose tolerance and no family history of NIDDM (Figure 17). The hyperinsulinemia-induced insulin resistance was entirely explained by a defect in non-oxidative glucose disposal or glycogen synthesis in muscle (Figure 17). This pattern of insulin resistance closely resembles that observed in human NIDDM [1, 5]. Identical results have been reported by Jeanrenaud and colleagues in rats [314, 315].

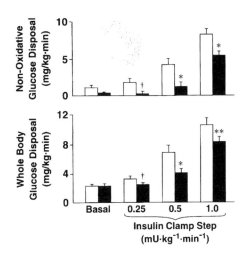

Figure 17 Lower panel, effect of chronic (72 h) sustained physiologic hyperinsulinemia (7–24 µU/ml) on whole-body insulin-mediated glucose disposal during the basal state and during a three-step euglycemic insulin clamp. *$p < 0.01$, **$p < 0.02$, †$p < 0.05$ for the insulin clamp performed after (solid bars) vs. before (open bars) the chronic insulin infusion. Upper panel, all of the impairment in insulin-mediated whole body glucose disposal was the result of a decrease in non-oxidative glucose disposal (glycogen synthesis). Whole-body insulin-mediated glucose oxidation (not shown) increased slightly following chronic insulin infusion (from reference 313, with permission)

The observation that sustained physiologic hyperinsulinemia of only 15–20 µU/ml can induce severe insulin resistance is a very provocative finding and provokes a novel hypothesis to explain the pathogenesis of NIDDM in certain high risk populations, i.e. American Indians, Mexican-Americans, and Pacific islanders, which are characterized by hyperinsulinemia, insulin resistance, obesity and a high prevalence of NIDDM. In this hypothesis primary hypersecretion of insulin represents the basic genetic disturbance, and the insulin resistance develops secondarily to downregulation of the insulin receptor signal transduction system, glucose transport, glucose phosphorylation, and/or glycogen synthase [311, 313]. At this juncture, the focus of this chapter will shift from the B cell to the insulin sensitive tissues, muscle and liver. However, it will return to the B cell to examine the dynamic interaction between insulin action and insulin secretion [1, 39, 42, 54, 59, 62–64, 67, 69, 70, 75, 274, 316, 317], as it is the disruption of this finely regulated balance that leads to the emergence of overt diabetes mellitus with fasting hyperglycemia.

INSULIN SENSITIVITY IN NIDDM

A number of longitudinal and cross-sectional studies conclusively have documented that hyperinsulinemia precedes the development of NIDDM in most ethnic populations with a high incidence of the disease [1, 5, 45–54, 59–75, 78, 261, 262, 268, 273, 309, 318, 319]. Moreover, recent studies employing the euglycemic insulin clamp and minimal model techniques have demonstrated that the progression from normal to impaired glucose tolerance is associated with the development of severe insulin resistance [1, 5, 54, 59, 60, 63, 64, 67, 75, 78, 309], whereas plasma insulin concentrations, both in the fasting state and in response to a glucose load (Figures 3 and 4), are markedly increased (see prior discussion about insulin secretion). These observations provide convincing evidence that insulin resistance, not impaired insulin secretion, initiates the process of NIDDM in these populations.

Over the years, there has accumulated an impressive body of evidence which demonstrates that insulin action is impaired in the great majority of individuals with type 2 diabetes. Himsworth and Kerr [320], using a combined oral glucose and intravenous insulin tolerance test, were the first to demonstrate that tissue sensitivity to insulin was diminished in diabetic patients. Subsequent investigators, using the insulin tolerance test, also documented a blunted decline in the plasma glucose concentration in NIDDM patients with fasting hyperglycemia [321–323].

Reaven and colleagues in 1970, using the quadruple (combined epinephrine, propranolol, insulin and glucose) infusion technique (also called the insulin suppression test), found that the ability of insulin to promote tissue glucose uptake in NIDDM was severely reduced [324–326], and the results of his work have been summarized more recently [327]. Subsequently, several groups [328, 329] substituted somatostatin for epinephrine and propranolol in the quadruple infusion cocktail to exclude any potential antagonistic effects of epinephrine on hepatic or peripheral tissues. Using this modification [328, 329], a major impairment in tissue sensitivity to insulin was observed in type 2 diabetic patients. A defect in insulin action in NIDDM also has been demonstrated with the forearm and leg catheterization technique [3–5, 330–332], as well as with radioisotope turnover studies [333, 334], the modified intravenous glucose tolerance test [335] and the minimal model technique [317, 336, 337] (see also Chapter 28).

DeFronzo and colleagues, using the more physiologic insulin clamp technique [103], have provided the most conclusive documentation of insulin resistance in NIDDM. In the largest published series involving *normal-weight* diabetic patients, DeFronzo and colleagues reported the results of euglycemic insulin clamp studies in over 50 lean NIDDM patients and in control subjects matched for age and weight [1, 4, 5, 30, 338–341]. Because obesity is an insulin-resistant state [39, 272, 273, 342, 343], it is important to exclude this metabolic disorder in order to define the true contribution of diabetes *per se* to the presence of insulin resistance. Most investigators have found that obese non-diabetic individuals are as insulin resistant as NIDDM subjects, and that the superimposition of obesity on diabetes causes only a modest (10–20%) worsening of the insulin resistance [1, 272, 343, 344]. However, even a modest deterioration in insulin action in an individual whose pancreatic B cells are operating at maximal capacity can lead to a major deterioration in glucose tolerance.

In the lean diabetics studied by DeFronzo and collaborators [1, 4, 5, 30, 272, 338–341] the fasting plasma glucose concentration (mean = 150 ± 8 mg/dl, 8.3 ± 0.4 mmol/l) was only mildly elevated. None of the diabetic patients was taking any medication and none had ever received insulin. Diabetic patients with more severe degrees of glucose intolerance were not included. Thus, the study population focused on the early stages of the evolution of NIDDM in normal weight subjects. Patients with more severe diabetes— fasting plasma glucose concentrations greater than 180–200 mg/dl (10.0–11.1 mmol/l) are known to be insulinopenic, and insulin deficiency is associated with the emergence of a number of intracellular defects in insulin action [345–348]. All diabetic and control subjects received a euglycemic insulin ($+100$ μU/ml) clamp study [103] in combination with tritiated glucose to quantitate rates of hepatic glucose production

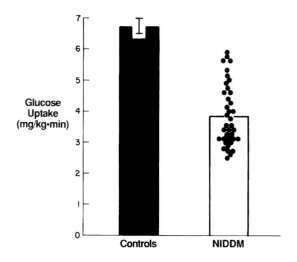

Figure 18 Insulin-mediated whole-body glucose uptake in 38 normal weight NIDDM patients (right panel) and in 33 control subjects matched for age and weight (left panel). Tissue sensitivity to insulin was reduced by approximately 40% in the NIDDM group; each individual diabetic subject is represented by a solid circle (drawn from data presented in references 1, 4, 30, 272, 340, 341 and 391)

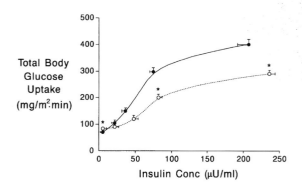

Figure 19 Dose-response curve relating the plasma insulin concentration to the rate of insulin-mediated whole-body glucose uptake in control (solid circles) and NIDDM (open circles) subjects. *$p < 0.01$ vs. controls (from reference 15, with permission)

[1, 4, 5, 30, 272, 338–341] (Figure 18). The mean rate of insulin mediated whole-body glucose disposal was reduced by 35–40% in NIDDM compared with control subjects. It is noteworthy that none of the diabetic patients fell within 2 standard deviations of the controls. Thus, not only is there a moderate to severe degree of insulin resistance in the NIDDM group, there is a complete separation between the diabetic and control subjects. Three additional points are worthy of comment: (a) in lean type 2 diabetic individuals with more severe fasting hyperglycemia (198 ± 10 mg/dl), the severity of insulin resistance is only slightly (10–20%) greater than in diabetic patients with mild fasting hyperglycemia [1, 272, 343, 344]; (b) the defect in insulin action is observed at all plasma

insulin concentrations, spanning the physiologic and pharmacologic range [15, 349, 350] (Figure 19); (c) in diabetic patients with overt fasting hyperglycemia, even maximally stimulating plasma insulin concentrations are not capable of eliciting a normal glucose metabolic response under euglycemic conditions [15, 349, 350]. With a few exceptions [20–22], the great majority of investigators have demonstrated that lean type 2 diabetics are resistant to the action of insulin [1, 4, 5, 66, 272, 316, 317, 327].

SITE OF INSULIN RESISTANCE IN NIDDM

The regulation of whole-body glucose homeostasis is primarily controlled by insulin and hyperglycemia (i.e. the mass action effect of glucose to promote its own uptake) and is dependent on three tightly coupled mechanisms (Table 1): (a) suppression of hepatic glucose production; (b) stimulation of glucose uptake by the splanchnic (hepatic plus gastrointestinal) tissues; and (c) stimulation of glucose uptake by peripheral tissues. Tissue glucose uptake, in turn, is dependent upon two major metabolic pathways: glucose oxidation and glucose storage or non-oxidative glucose disposal. Using nuclear magnetic resonance (NMR) spectroscopy [351], glucose storage has been shown to primarily reflect glycogen synthesis. In the subsequent discussion, the contribution of each of these processes to the insulin resistance in NIDDM is examined.

Hepatic Glucose Production

The use of tritiated glucose allows quantitation of the basal rate of HGP, as well as its suppression in response to hyperinsulinemia. DeFronzo and colleagues were amongst the first to demonstrate that in the basal, postabsorptive state the liver of healthy subjects produces glucose at the rate of approximately 1.8–2.0 mg/kg/min [1, 2, 4, 15, 30, 272, 338–341]. This glucose flux is critical to meet the obligatory needs of the brain and other neural tissues, which utilize glucose at a constant rate of about 1–1.2 mg/kg/min [3, 352]. It is important to note that brain glucose uptake accounts for approximately 50–60% of glucose disposal in the postabsorptive state; it is insulin independent and therefore occurs at the same rate during absorptive and postabsorptive periods, and is not altered in NIDDM [352]. Following the ingestion of a mixed meal or a glucose load, insulin is released into the portal vein and carried to the liver where it binds to specific receptors on the hepatocyte and suppresses hepatic glucose output. If the liver does not perceive this insulin signal and continues to produce glucose, there will be two inputs of glucose into the body, one from the liver and another from the gastrointestinal

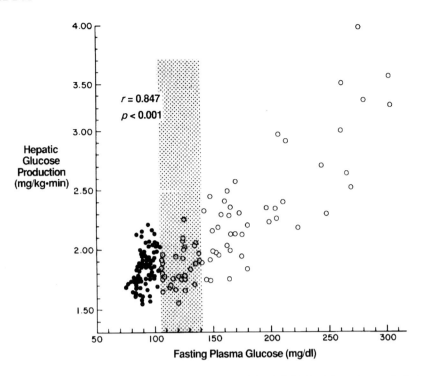

Figure 20 Summary of hepatic glucose production in 77 normal weight NIDDM subjects (open circles) with fasting plasma glucose concentrations ranging from 105 mg/dl to greater than 300 mg/dl; 72 controls matched for age and weight are shown by the solid circles. In the 33 diabetic subjects with fasting plasma glucose levels below 140 mg/dl (shaded area), the mean rate of HGP was identical to that of controls. In diabetic subjects with fasting plasma glucose concentrations >140 mg/dl, there was a progressive rise in hepatic glucose production that correlated closely ($r = 0.847$, $p < 0.001$) with the fasting plasma glucose concentration (from reference 1, with permission)

tract, and marked hyperglycemia will ensue. NIDDM subjects with moderate fasting hyperglycemia manifest a significant ($p < 0.001$) increase in basal HGP of about 0.5 mg/kg/min. Extrapolated over 24 h, the liver of a 70 kg diabetic individual with modest fasting hyperglycemia would be expected to add an additional 50 g of glucose to the systemic circulation. When all NIDDM subjects were considered, the increase in basal HGP was closely correlated ($r = 0.847$, $p < 0.001$) with the degree of fasting hyperglycemia [1, 2, 4, 5, 15, 30, 272, 338–341] (Figure 20). These findings indicate that in type 2 diabetic individuals with *overt fasting hyperglycemia* (>140 mg/dl, 7.8 mmol/l), an excessive rate of hepatic glucose output is a major factor responsible for the elevated fasting plasma glucose concentration. The close relationship between fasting plasma glucose concentration and HGP is consistent with results that have been published by a number of other investigators [44, 70, 197, 349–364].

It is noteworthy that, in the postabsorptive state, diabetic subjects manifest both elevated plasma insulin and glucose levels. In fact, the fasting plasma insulin concentration in the NIDDM subjects was more than twice that in controls (Figure 2). As hyperinsulinemia is a potent inhibitor of HGP [1, 2, 15, 349, 350, 365, 366], it is clear that significant *hepatic* resistance to the

action of insulin must be present in the postabsorptive state to explain the excessive output of glucose by the liver. Hyperglycemia *per se* also exerts a powerful suppressive action on HGP [365–368]. Therefore, there also may be 'glucose resistance' with respect to the inhibitory effect of hyperglycemia on hepatic glucose output. This latter possibility has received little attention in NIDDM.

All investigators consistently have found that basal HGP is elevated in NIDDM subjects with fasting glucose levels above 140 mg/dl, implying a significant degree of hepatic insulin resistance. However, apparently conflicting results have been reported concerning the response of the liver to an increment in plasma insulin concentration above baseline. In the diabetic subjects studied by DeFronzo et al [1, 2, 4, 15, 338–341], insulin infusion inhibited hepatic glucose production by over 90% and a similar degree of suppression was observed in controls. Others have reported that the ability of insulin to inhibit HGP is impaired in NIDDM [349, 350, 358, 369]. These apparently discrepant results are explained by more than one factor. First, the dose–response curve relating inhibition of HGP to the plasma insulin concentration is quite steep, with an ED_{50} of approximately 30–40 µU/ml [134] (Figure 21). Similar findings have been reported by Campbell et al [350]. Thus, the high plasma insulin concentrations (in excess of 100 μU/ml) employed by DeFronzo et al [1, 2, 4, 15, 338–346] approach the V_{max} for the suppressive effect of insulin on HGP, and a defect in insulin action might not be observed. Indeed, at lower plasma insulin concentrations an impaired suppression of HGP by insulin is readily demonstrable [15] (Figure 21). Second, the severity of the hepatic insulin resistance appears to be related to the severity of the diabetic state. In NIDDM individuals with mild fasting hyperglycemia, an increment in plasma insulin concentration of 100 μU/ml caused a complete suppression of HGP. However, in diabetic subjects with more severe fasting hyperglycemia, the ability of the same plasma insulin concentration to suppress HGP is impaired [15] (Figure 21). These results suggest that there is an acquired component of the hepatic insulin resistance and that this defect becomes progressively worse as the diabetic state decompensates over time.

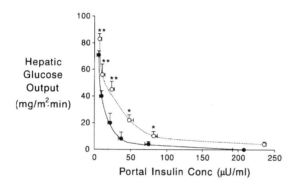

Figure 21 Dose–response curve relating the plasma insulin concentration to the suppression of hepatic glucose production in control (solid circles) and NIDDM (open circles) subjects with moderately severe fasting hyperglycemia. *p < 0.05, **p < 0.01 vs. controls (from reference 15, with permission)

The glucose released by the liver can be derived either from glycogenolysis or from gluconeogenesis [2, 367]. Studies by Waldhausl et al [370] have shown that uptake of gluconeogenic precursors, especially lactate, is increased in type 2 diabetic subjects. Consistent with this observation, Consoli and colleagues [371–373], using radiolabeled lactate, alanine and glycerol have shown that approximately 90% of the increase in HGP above baseline can be accounted for by accelerated gluconeogenesis (Figure 22). Moreover, the increase in gluconeogenesis was closely correlated with the elevated fasting plasma glucose concentration. Similar results have been reported by others [374–376] using radiolabeled lactate and glycerol. Most recently, Stumvoll et al [377] have shown that increased conversion of glutamine to glucose also contributes to the elevated rate of gluconeogenesis in NIDDM subjects. Using ^{13}C NMR, Magnusson et al

[378] have confirmed the important contribution of accelerated gluconeogenesis to the increase in HGP. The mechanisms responsible for the increase in hepatic gluconeogenesis have yet to be defined, but include hyperglucagonemia [379, 380], increased circulating levels of gluconeogenic precursors (lactate, alanine, glycerol) [371, 381], increased FFA oxidation [15–17, 272], enhanced sensitivity to glucagon, and/or decreased sensitivity to insulin [15, 349, 350, 369, 383].

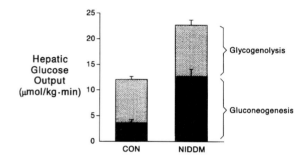

Figure 22 Contribution of gluconeogenesis and glycogenolysis in control (left panel) and NIDDM (right panel) subjects. All of the increase in total hepatic glucose production in NIDDM is accounted for by an excessive rate of gluconeogenesis (drawn from data presented in reference 371)

Less dramatic increases in gluconeogenesis have been reported by some investigators [359, 376]. Although the majority of evidence supports increased gluconeogenesis as the major cause of the increase in HGP in NIDDM subjects [371–373, 378], it is likely that accelerated glycogenolysis also contributes [359, 376]. In large part, the controversy concerning the precise contributions of increased gluconeogenesis vs. glycogenolysis to the enhanced rate of HGP in NIDDM relates to methodologic problems in quantitating the dilution of radiolabeled carbon in the TCA cycle [375]. Because of the inaccessibility of the liver in man, it has been difficult to assess the role of key enzymes involved in the regulation of gluconeogenesis (pyruvate carboxylase, phosphoenol pyruvate carboxykinase), glycogenolysis (glycogen phosphorylase) and net hepatic glucose output (glucokinase, glucose-6-phosphatase). With regard to this, it recently has been shown that transgenic mice overexpressing phosphoenol pyruvate carboxykinase develop a clinical phenotype that closely resembles NIDDM in man [384].

Splanchnic (Hepatic) Glucose Uptake

A second potential mechanism that could account for the impairment in insulin action during the insulin clamp is a decrease in glucose uptake by the liver. In humans it is difficult to catheterize the portal vein, and glucose disposal by the liver has not been examined directly. However, using the hepatic vein catheterization technique in combination with the euglycemic insulin clamp, DeFronzo et al [4] examined the contribution of the splanchnic (liver plus gastrointestinal) tissues to overall glucose homeostasis in 10 NIDDM subjects with mild to moderate fasting hyperglycemia. In the postabsorptive state there was a net release of glucose from the splanchnic area (i.e. negative balance) in both the control and NIDDM subjects (Figure 23), reflecting glucose production by the liver. In response to insulin there was a prompt suppression of splanchnic glucose output (reflecting the inhibition of hepatic glucose production) and by 20 min the net glucose balance across the splanchnic region was zero (i.e. there was no net uptake or release). After 2 h of sustained hyperinsulinemia, there was a small net uptake of glucose by the splanchnic area (i.e. positive balance), which averaged approximately 0.5 mg/kg/min. This uptake was virtually identical to the rate of splanchnic glucose uptake observed in the basal state, indicating that the splanchnic tissues, like the brain, are insensitive to insulin at least with respect to the stimulation of glucose uptake [2, 3, 365]. It is important to note that there was no difference between diabetic and control subjects in the amount of glucose that was taken up by the splanchnic tissues at any time during the insulin clamp study. Thus, a defect in splanchnic (hepatic) glucose uptake during intravenous glucose infusion could not be demonstrated in NIDDM.

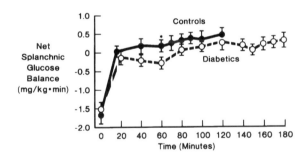

Figure 23 Time course of change in the net splanchnic glucose balance in NIDDM (open circles) and control (solid circles) subjects. The difference between diabetic and control subjects is small, statistically insignificant, and cannot account for the marked impairment in total-body glucose metabolism observed during the euglycemic insulin clamp study. Also note that the total amount of glucose disposed of by the splanchnic area represents less than 10% of the infused glucose load in both groups (from reference 4, with permission)

Figure 23 illustrates another important point: namely, that under conditions of *euglycemic hyperinsulinemia* very little of the infused glucose is taken up by the splanchnic (and, therefore, hepatic) tissues. During

the insulin clamp the rate of whole-body glucose uptake averaged 7 mg/kg/min and, of this, only 0.5 mg/kg/min or 7% was disposed of by the splanchnic region. As the difference in insulin mediated total-body glucose uptake between the NIDDM and control groups during the euglycemic clamp study was 2.5 mg/kg/min, from a purely quantitative standpoint it is clear that a defect in splanchnic (hepatic) glucose removal could never account for the magnitude of impairment in total body glucose uptake. However, following glucose ingestion, both the oral route of administration, as well as the resultant hyperglycemia conspire to enhance splanchnic (hepatic) glucose uptake [2, 365, 385], and under these conditions diminished hepatic glucose uptake may contribute to the impairment in glucose tolerance in NIDDM [2, 356, 386].

In summary, it can be concluded that in NIDDM individuals with modest fasting hyperglycemia (<160–180 mg/dl, 8.9–10.0 mmol/l), neither a defect in suppression of HGP nor a defect in hepatic glucose uptake can account for the major impairment (>40–50%) in tissue sensitivity to insulin which is observed during the euglycemic insulin clamp study. During insulin (+100 µU/ml) clamp studies performed at lower plasma insulin concentrations and in diabetics with more severe fasting hyperglycemia, impaired suppression of HGP will constitute a greater percentage of the observed total body insulin resistance.

Peripheral (Muscle) Glucose Uptake

During a euglycemic insulin clamp study, endogeneous insulin secretion is suppressed and the circulating plasma insulin concentration is virtually identical in diabetic and control subjects. Moreover, the suppression of HGP and splanchnic glucose uptake are similar in NIDDM subjects during the insulin clamp (see Figures 21 and 23). Therefore, by exclusion, peripheral tissues must be the primary site of insulin resistance. To address this question directly, the same 10 subjects who had the insulin clamp study performed in combination with hepatic venous catheterization, also had a catheter inserted into the femoral vein to quantify glucose exchange across the leg tissues [4] (Figure 24). In the basal state, leg glucose uptake was slightly but significantly ($p < 0.01$) increased in the diabetic group. A similar increase in basal glucose uptake by forearm muscle has been demonstrated in NIDDM subjects by other investigators [356, 387–389]. This increase in tissue glucose uptake is consistent with radioisotope turnover studies, which consistently have demonstrated a significant enhancement in the basal rate of tissue glucose disposal in NIDDM subjects [1, 2, 15, 30, 44, 197, 338–341, 353–364, 371, 387–389]. In the postabsorptive state this increase in tissue glucose uptake in NIDDM subjects is due to the mass action effect of hyperglycemia, which passively drives glucose into cells [2, 368, 390]. It must be emphasized, however, that the metabolic fate of the glucose which is taken up in increased amounts by peripheral tissues, primarily muscle, is not normal in type 2 diabetic patients. In the postabsorptive state, glucose oxidation is impaired in NIDDM subjects [273, 391] and there is no net flux of glucose into glycogen. Moreover, muscle glycogen synthase activity and glycogen synthesis have been shown to be impaired in NIDDM [392–394]. Therefore, a disproportionate amount of the excessive glucose which is taken up by the muscle in the postabsorptive state is converted to lactate [4, 395–397], which is subsequently released and can serve as a substrate to drive gluconeogenesis by the liver [370, 398]. A similar cycle also is likely to occur locally within the splanchnic region (i.e. gut glucose uptake and conversion to lactate, release of lactate into the portal vein, uptake of lactate by the liver, and conversion of lactate to glucose) [2], and this accelerated Cori cycle activity can be viewed as an important mechanism that provides substrate to sustain the accelerated rate of HGP in diabetic individuals with well-established fasting hyperglycemia.

glucose uptake was reduced by 50% in the NIDDM group. These results provide conclusive evidence that the primary site of insulin resistance during the euglycemic insulin clamp studies performed in NIDDM subjects resides in peripheral tissues. Using the forearm and leg catheterization techniques, a number of investigators [330, 332, 388, 399–405] also have demonstrated a decreased rate of insulin mediated glucose uptake by peripheral tissues. The use of PET scanning to quantitate leg glucose uptake in NIDDM subjects has provided additional support for the presence of severe muscle resistance to insulin [406]. In humans, adipocytes are quite inert and respond poorly to the stimulatory effect of insulin on glucose metabolism; less than 2–3% of an infused or ingested glucose load is taken up by adipose tissue [10–12, 407–410]. Thus, the leg and forearm tissue which is responsible for the majority (>95%) of glucose uptake is muscle. If it is assumed that all muscle tissue in the body has a response similar to that of leg muscle, it can be calculated that impaired muscle glucose uptake accounts for about 90% of the decrease in total body glucose disposal during the insulin clamp study in diabetic subjects [1, 4, 5].

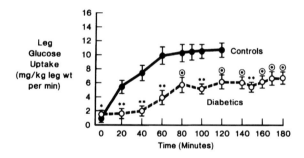

Figure 24 Time course of change in leg glucose uptake in NIDDM (open circles) and control (solid circles) subjects. In the postabsorptive state, glucose uptake in the diabetic group was significantly greater than that in controls. However, the ability of insulin (euglycemic insulin clamp) to stimulate leg glucose uptake was reduced by 50% in the diabetic subjects (from reference 4, with permission)

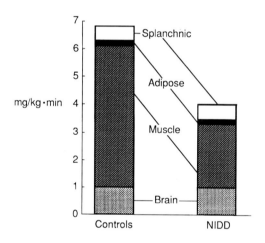

Figure 25 Summary of glucose metabolism during euglycemic insulin (+ 100 μU/ml) clamp studies performed in normal weight NIDDM and control subjects; see text for a more detailed discussion (from reference 1, with permission)

During the insulin clamp in control subjects, hyperinsulinemia elicited a prompt stimulation of leg glucose uptake, which reached a plateau value of approximately 10 mg/kg of leg weight per minute during the last hour of the study (Figure 24) [4]. By contrast, in NIDDM subjects the onset of insulin action was delayed for approximately 40 min and the ability of the hormone to stimulate leg glucose uptake was markedly blunted, even though the study was carried out for an additional 60 min in the NIDDM group in order to allow insulin to express its biologic effects more fully [4]. During the last hour of the insulin clamp study, the rate of

Insulin mediated whole-body glucose utilization during the euglycemic insulin clamp is summarized in Figure 25. The height of each bar represents the total amount of glucose taken up during the insulin clamp in control and NIDDM subjects. Net splanchnic glucose uptake quantitated by the hepatic venous catheterization technique is similar in both groups and averages 0.5 mg/kg/min. Adipose tissue glucose uptake, which was not directly measured, is assumed to represent 2–3% of total glucose disposal [10–12, 407–410]. Brain glucose uptake, estimated to be 1.0–1.2 mg/kg

Table 6 Balance sheet for the disposal of an oral glucose load in normal subjects

Glucose	Mean ± SEM (g)	Range (g)
A. Ingested	68 ± 3	55–93
B. Appearing in peripheral plasma (oral)	50 ± 4	32–56
C. Released by the liver	15 ± 2	5–20
D. Taken up by splanchnic tissues	19 ± 4	0.7–34
E. Taken up by peripheral tissues	48 ± 6	28–83
F. Remaining in the glucose space	2 ± 2	−2–+15
G. Unrecovered	18 ± 3	8–31
H. 'Saved' by the liver	18 ± 2	12–26
True net splanchnic balance (D − C)	4 ± 3	−17–+17
Splanchnic 'conversion' (D + H)	37 ± 4	20–62
Splanchnic overall contribution to glucose homeostasis (D + H − C)	22 ± 4	1–42

Summarized from reference 7

per minute in the postabsorptive state [352, 411, 412], is unaffected by hyperinsulinemia [352]. Muscle glucose uptake (extrapolated from leg catheterization data) in control subjects accounts for approximately 75% of the total glucose uptake. In NIDDM subjects, it is apparent that the largest part of the impairment in insulin-mediated glucose uptake can be accounted for by a defect in muscle glucose disposal. Even if adipose tissue of NIDDM subjects took up absolutely no glucose, it could, at best, explain only a small fraction of the defect in whole-body glucose metabolism.

GLUCOSE DISPOSAL DURING THE ORAL GLUCOSE TOLERANCE TEST

The OGTT has fallen into disfavor as a tool to examine the mechanisms responsible for impaired glucose metabolism in NIDDM subjects. The rate of glucose absorption varies considerably from one subject to another and cannot be quantified easily. Consequently, the rise in plasma glucose concentration differs markedly from one subject to another and is constantly changing. This presents an ever-fluctuating glycemic stimulus which, when combined with intrinsic differences in B-cell function from one individual to another, leads to large variations in the plasma insulin profile between subjects. Because the two primary variables of interest—plasma glucose and plasma insulin concentration—are changing simultaneously, it is difficult to draw any conclusions about insulin secretion or insulin sensitivity. Lastly, it is difficult to quantify changes in HGP following glucose ingestion, because the rate of entry of glucose into the systemic circulation is unknown.

Nevertheless, glucose ingestion represents the normal route by which glucose enters the body. Therefore it is important to examine whether the tissues and mechanisms responsible for diminished insulin mediated glucose disposal during the euglycemic insulin

clamp (see previous section) also contribute to impaired glucose tolerance following ingestion of an oral glucose load. To address this issue, Ferrannini, DeFronzo and colleagues administered an oral glucose load to healthy controls [6, 8, 386]. Studies were performed with hepatic vein catheterization to quantify the net splanchnic glucose balance, while the oral glucose load and endogenous glucose pool were labeled with 1-^{14}C-glucose and 3-^{3}H-glucose, respectively, to quantify total body glucose disposal (from tritiated glucose turnover) and endogenous hepatic glucose production (difference between the total rate of glucose appearance, as measured with tritiated glucose, and the rate of oral glucose appearance, as measured with 1-^{14}C-glucose). The balance sheet is shown in Table 6. During the 3.5 h following glucose ingestion, 28% was taken up by splanchnic tissues, 71% was disposed of by peripheral tissues (with the brain, an insulin-independent tissue, probably accounting for 22% of the total glucose load [352, 411, 412]), and basal HPG declined by 53%. Remarkably similar percentages have been reported for splanchnic glucose uptake (24–29%) and suppression of HGP (50–60%) in normal subjects by other investigators [7, 8, 356, 402, 413, 414]. Four studies [7, 413, 414, 416] have examined the contribution of skeletal muscle to the disposal of oral glucose and the results have varied from a low of 26% of the ingested glucose load [413] to a high of 56% [416], with a mean of 45%. These results emphasize several important differences between oral vs. i.v. glucose administration. Following glucose ingestion: (a) HGP is less completely suppressed: this may be related to activation of local sympathetic nerves which innervate the liver [417]; (b) peripheral tissue (primarily muscle) glucose uptake is quantitatively less important; (c) splanchnic glucose uptake is quantitatively much more significant.

Five studies have examined the disposal of an oral glucose load in type 2 diabetes [354, 356, 386,

Table 7 Summary of glucose metabolism following glucose ingestion in type 2 (non-insulin dependent) diabetic patients. The number of arrows indicates the magnitude of change

Author	Ref.	Test	Body weight	Insulin response*	Splanchnic glucose uptake	Suppression of HGP	Tissue R_d	Incremental tissue R_d	Glucose clearance	Forearm glucose uptake	Incremental forearm glucose uptake
Ferrannini	386	OGTT	Normal weight	sl↓	N	↓	↓↓	↓↓	↓↓	–	–
Firth	356	OGTT	Obese	↓	sl↓	↓↓	↑	↓↓	↓↓	N	sl↓
Mitrakou	402	OGTT	Obese	N, delayed	sl↓	↓↓	N	↓	↓↓	N	↓
Firth	354	MM	Obese	N	sl↓	↓↓	sl↑	↓↓	↓↓	N	↓
McMahon	418	MM	Obese	↓	↑↑	↓↓	↑	↓↓	↓↓	↑	↓

*In all studies the plasma insulin response was deficient when viewed relative to the plasma glucose concentration. OGTT, oral glucose tolerance test; MM, mixed meal; N, normal; sl, slight; HGP, hepatic glucose production; R_d, glucose disposal.

402, 418] and all have revealed very similar results (Table 7). As originally demonstrated by Ferrannini et al [386], the disturbance in glucose metabolism in type 2 diabetic patients is accounted for by two factors: (a) decreased tissue glucose uptake (44 vs. 60 over 3.5 h), (b) impaired suppression of HGP (17 vs. 10 g over 3.5 h). Splanchnic glucose uptake was similar in diabetic and control groups. Thus, inappropriate suppression of HGP (7 g over 3.5 h) accounts for approximately one-third of the defect in total body glucose homeostasis, while reduced peripheral (presumably muscle) glucose uptake (14 g over 3.5 h) accounts for the remaining two-thirds. Essentially identical results have been reported by others [356, 357, 402, 418]. It should be noted that the double tracer technique (^{14}C-glucose orally and 3-^{3}H-glucose intravenously) is associated with significant variability, since it involves the subtraction of two large numbers (rate of appearance (R_a) of 3-^{3}H-glucose minus R_a of ^{14}C-glucose). A similar conclusion can be drawn from the data of Chen et al [364], even though these investigators did not label the oral glucose load with 1-^{14}C-glucose to calculate the suppression of HGP. Therefore, small differences in suppression of HGP between laboratories are likely to have little physiologic meaning. The inherent variability of the double tracer method, variation in patients' characteristics and differences in insulin secretory response easily can explain the 10–20% differences in suppression of HGP reported by various investigators [354, 356, 386, 402, 418]. The important message is that everyone has found that suppression of HPG is impaired in type 2 diabetes and that this defect can account for about one-third to one-half of the disturbance in whole body glucose homeostasis. Splanchnic glucose uptake has been reported to be normal [386], slightly decreased [354, 356, 402] or increased [418], and does not appear to contribute significantly to the impairment in oral glucose tolerance.

Special comment is warranted concerning whole body tissue glucose disposal following glucose ingestion. In absolute terms most, but not all [386], studies

have shown it to be normal [402] or slightly increased [354, 356, 418] (Table 7). However, the efficiency of glucose disposal, i.e. the glucose clearance, is severely reduced. Most importantly, it is not the absolute glucose disposal rate, but rather the increment in glucose disposal above baseline which determines the rise in plasma glucose above the fasting value. In every published study [354, 356, 386, 402, 418] the incremental response in whole body glucose uptake was moderately to severely reduced in type 2 diabetes (Table 7). Similar results have been reported for forearm muscle glucose uptake [354, 356, 402, 418] (Table 7). Thus, all published results are very consistent and point out the important contribution of diminished muscle glucose disposal to impaired oral glucose tolerance in type 2 diabetes.

In summary, results of the OGTT indicate that both impaired suppression of hepatic glucose production and decreased tissue (muscle) glucose uptake contribute approximately equally to the glucose intolerance of type 2 diabetes. However, none of the currently available studies [354, 356, 386, 402, 418] allows one to define whether the defects in hepatic and peripheral (muscle) glucose metabolism are the result of insulin resistance, diminished insulin secretion, or an impairment in the mass action effect of glucose (i.e. glucose resistance) to promote its own uptake.

SUMMARY OF INSULIN RESISTANCE IN NIDDM

A large body of evidence firmly establishes insulin resistance as an important pathogenetic mechanism which contributes to the glucose intolerance of NIDDM. However, it must be kept clearly in mind that the tissues responsible for the insulin resistance in the postabsorptive state are very different from those responsible for the defect in insulin action in the insulin-stimulated state. In the *basal state* the liver represents the major site of insulin resistance and this is reflected by an *overproduction of glucose* despite the presence of fasting hyperinsulinemia and hyperglycemia. This accelerated rate of hepatic glucose output plays a critical role in maintaining fasting hyperglycemia in NIDDM individuals. Although tissue glucose uptake in the postabsorptive state is increased when viewed in absolute terms, the efficiency with which glucose is removed from the body, i.e. the glucose clearance, is diminished (see subsequent discussion). Following glucose infusion or ingestion, i.e. in the *insulin-stimulated state*, both decreased muscle glucose uptake and impaired suppression of HGP play major roles in the insulin resistance. From the quantitative standpoint the impairment in insulin-mediated glucose uptake by muscle and the defect in the suppression of HGP by insulin contribute approximately equally to the disturbance in whole-body glucose homeostasis in NIDDM following glucose ingestion. However, under *euglycemic* hyperinsulinemic conditions, HGP is largely suppressed and impaired muscle glucose uptake is primarily responsible for the insulin resistance.

FASTING HYPERGLYCEMIA IN NIDDM: ROLE OF PANCREAS, MUSCLE AND LIVER

All published studies, be they longitudinal or cross-sectional [1, 52, 54, 59, 60–72, 102, 309] in design, have demonstrated that an increase in basal plasma insulin concentration precedes the onset of fasting hyperglycemia in patients with impaired glucose tolerance and overt NIDDM. Such evidence provides overwhelming support for the theory that the primary disturbance responsible for the elevation in fasting glucose concentration must result from a decrease in tissue (i.e. liver or muscle) sensitivity to insulin. From the preceding sections it is clear that once overt fasting hyperglycemia (>140 mg/dl, 7.8 mmol/l) has developed, HGP is elevated and correlates well with the increase in basal glucose concentration [1, 2, 4, 5, 30, 44, 197, 273, 338–341, 350, 353–364]. However, by the time that the fasting glucose level has reached 140 mg/dl, the diabetic patient will have had the disease for a very long period, 5–10 years or more. Thus, these studies cannot answer the question as to whether, in the earliest stages of NIDDM, fasting hyperglycemia results from an excessive rate of HGP or from decreased tissue glucose uptake. To address this issue, DeFronzo and colleagues [42] quantified HGP and tissue glucose uptake (tritiated glucose turnover method) in the postabsorptive state in 77 normal weight ($110 \pm 2\%$ ideal body weight) NIDDM patients and 72 healthy subjects matched for age, sex and weight (Figure 20). All diabetic subjects had a diagnostic OGTT [420]. Thirty-three of the NIDDM subjects had

fasting plasma glucose levels below 140 mg/dl, which represents the level at which NIDDM is diagnosed according to the National Diabetes Data Group [420] and in NIDDM represents the top of Starling's curve of the pancreas, at which level the fasting plasma insulin concentration begins to decline (Figure 3). In these 33 NIDDM subjects (Figure 20), the mean rate of HGP (1.85 ± 0.03 mg/kg/min) is virtually identical to that of the control group (1.84 ± 0.02 mg/kg/min). However, this normal basal rate of HGP is maintained at the expense of a fasting insulin concentration that is twice as great in the diabetic patients as in the controls (20 ± 2 μU/ml vs. 11 ± 1 μU/ml, $p < 0.001$). A normal basal rate of hepatic glucose output in the presence of marked fasting hyperinsulinemia demonstrates that *hepatic resistance* to insulin already is well established early in the course of type 2 diabetes mellitus.

A number of other investigators have confirmed the close relationship between increased fasting plasma glucose concentrations and an elevated basal rate of HGP in NIDDM subjects (350, 351, 355–364, 415). Two groups have suggested that HGP may be increased in patients with IGT or mild type 2 diabetes (360, 415, 421). In the study of Gerich et al [421] the number of patients was small ($n = 10$), the patient population was obese, the fasting plasma insulin concentration was not provided, and OGTT results were not given. Most importantly, in six of ten individuals with fasting glucose levels between 6 and 7 mmol/l (108–126 mg/dl), HGP was within the normal range, and the mean HGP (11.7 ± 0.3 μmol/kg min) was not significantly elevated compared to 19 control subjects (11.2 ± 0.2 μmol/kg min) with fasting glucose between 5 and 6 mmol/l (90–108 mg/dl). Thus, the data of Gerich et al suggest that HGP is not significantly elevated in the early stages of type 2 diabetes. Fery has also suggested that HGP is increased in diabetic subjects with mild fasting hyperglycemia [360]. Again, NIDDM subjects with fasting glucose levels less than 140 mg/dl did not have an increased basal rate of HGP. One study [363] has suggested that the basal rate of HGP in NIDDM patients does not start to increase until the fasting plasma glucose concentration exceeds 180 mg/dl [363]. Although the authors of this paper studied 31 newly diagnosed NIDDM subjects, only five had a fasting glucose plasma concentration between 140 and 180 mg/dl. Of these five, three appeared to have an increased basal rate of HGP (see Figure 3 of reference 363). In diabetic people with a fasting glucose concentration less than 140 mg/dl, HGP was perfectly normal [363]. In summary, it appears that basal HGP remains within the normal range until the fasting glucose concentration exceeds ~140 mg/dl. At this level, the prevailing hyperglycemia and hyperinsulinemia are insufficient to restrain HGP, which then rises linearly with the increase in fasting plasma glucose concentration.

Chen, Reaven and colleagues [362, 364] have raised methodologic concerns about the measurement of HGP with tritiated glucose, citing insufficient time for tracer equilibration and an inappropriately low priming dose in diabetic subjects. It is, however, reasonably well established that the priming dose of radiolabeled glucose must be increased in proportion to the increase in fasting glucose concentration and that the tracer equilibration time must be prolonged from 2 to at least 3 h, as done in our own studies [42]. Chen, Reaven et al [362, 364] demonstrated that in NIDDM subjects with severe fasting hyperglycemia (274–329 mg/dl, 15.2–18.3 mmol/l), initiation of the fast at 1800 h and prolongation of the fast until 1300–1400 h (i.e. total period of fast = 20 h) resulted in basal rates of HGP that were similar to or only slightly increased compared to controls [362, 364]. There are a number of conceptual problems with these studies. Because of the long fast there is a progressive decline in HGP in the NIDDM group, whereas in the control group HGP will decrease minimally. This will serve to minimize the difference in HGP between the diabetic and control groups. In everyday life, people rarely fast for more than 10–12 h. Indeed, if one compares rates of HGP in diabetic and control subjects after 10–12 h in these studies, it can be seen that NIDDM individuals have an elevated rate of HGP which is nearly identical in magnitude to that reported by ourselves [42]. Also, by selecting NIDDM subjects with markedly elevated fasting glucose levels (274 mg/dl [362] and 329 mg/dl [364]), the investigators maximized the decline in fasting glucose concentration and HGP by prolonging the fast. When HGP in type 2 diabetic and control subjects is compared after 10–12 h of fasting, all investigators consistently have found a highly significant increase in HGP which correlates closely with the increase in fasting plasma glucose concentration [350, 351, 355, 359–364, 394, 421].

In the basal state the fasting plasma glucose concentration is constant and the rate of HGP equals the rate of tissue glucose uptake. It follows, therefore, that glucose disposal, when viewed in absolute terms, is increased. However, when viewed in the context of the elevated plasma glucose and insulin levels, it is clear that the efficiency of tissue glucose uptake must be reduced early in the course of NIDDM. This is best appreciated by plotting the metabolic clearance rate of glucose (i.e. total-body glucose uptake divided by fasting plasma glucose concentration) vs. the fasting plasma glucose concentration in diabetic individuals with mild fasting hyperglycemia (Figure 26). As the fasting plasma glucose concentration rises from 105 mg/dl to 140 mg/dl (5.8 to 7.8 mmol/l), the glucose clearance rate declines

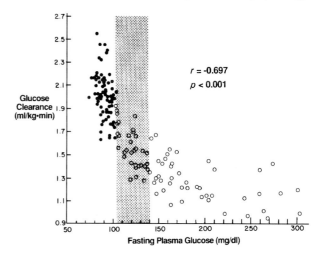

Figure 26 Summary of the metabolic clearance rate of glucose in 77 normal weight NIDDM subjects (open circles) with fasting plasma glucose concentrations ranging from 105 mg/dl to greater than 300 mg/dl; 72 controls matched for age and weight are shown by the closed circles. In the 33 diabetic subjects with fasting plasma glucose concentrations less than 140 mg/dl (shaded area), the glucose clearance rate fell precipitously and was inversely correlated ($r = -0.697$, $p < 0.001$) with the increase in plasma glucose concentration. At fasting plasma glucose levels above 140 mg/dl, the rate of decline in glucose clearance began to slow and reached a plateau at glucose levels above 180 mg/dl (from reference 1, with permission)

in a steeply progressive and linear ($r = 0.697$, $p < 0.001$) fashion, whereas HGP (shown in Figure 20) remains quite constant. Some investigators [423, 424], but not others [366, 425], have objected to the use of the glucose clearance to provide a quantitative measure of tissue glucose disposal. However, the controversy revolves around whether or not glucose uptake increases in direct proportion to the increase in plasma glucose concentration. Everyone would agree that some increase in the absolute rate of tissue glucose disposal should occur as the plasma glucose concentration increases [366, 423–425]. The failure to observe any increase in the basal rate of tissue glucose clearance whatsoever in the diabetic group, despite the presence of fasting hyperglycemia and fasting hyperinsulinemia, indicates that one of the earliest discernible abnormalities in NIDDM is a reduction in the efficiency with which tissues take up glucose. With progressing severity of diabetes, the contributions of excessive HGP and diminished tissue glucose clearance to fasting hyperglycemia reverse themselves. In NIDDM individuals with fasting plasma glucose levels above 140 mg/dl, the restraining effect of hyperinsulinemia on the liver is lost and HGP increases linearly ($r = 0.847$, $p < 0.001$) with the rise in fasting glucose concentration (Figure 20). In contrast, the decline in whole-body glucose clearance begins to level off at glucose values between 140 mg/dl and 180 mg/dl, and changes little at fasting glucose levels of 180–300 mg/dl (Figure 26). Stated otherwise, at glucose levels above 180 mg/dl (10.0 mmol/l), the whole-body glucose disposal rate rises in proportion to the increase in basal glucose concentration in such a manner that the glucose clearance remains constant, although reduced by about 40–50% compared with the postabsorptive state. This linear increase in glucose disposal at plasma glucose concentrations above 180 mg/dl can be viewed as a protective mechanism which prevents the further development of severe hyperglycemia and associated intracellular dehydration. It is noteworthy that the renal tubular threshold for maximum glucose reabsorption is approximately 180 mg/dl [426]. Thus, the development of glycosuria may, in large part, explain the parallel increases in plasma glucose concentration and whole-body glucose disposal rate when the plasma glucose concentration exceeds 180 mg/dl. The whole-body glucose clearance comprises two components—tissue glucose clearance and renal glucose clearance. If the constancy of whole-body glucose clearance at plasma glucose concentrations above 180 mg/dl is explained by glycosuria, then it follows that there must be a progressive decline in tissue glucose clearance, although the rate of decline at these higher plasma glucose levels would be less steep.

It is reasonable to ask why, in diabetic individuals with mild fasting hyperglycemia, the development of fasting hyperinsulinemia is sufficient to prevent overproduction of glucose by the liver but fails to maintain a normal basal rate of glucose clearance. This paradox is best understood by examining the dose–response relationship between the plasma insulin concentration vs. HGP and tissue glucose disposal [15, 39, 349, 350, 369]. When the plasma insulin concentration is increased from a basal level of 8 µU/ml to 15 µU/ml then to 27 µU/ml, by infusing insulin at rates of 0.1 µU/kg and 0.25 µU/kg per minute, respectively, in normal subjects, basal HGP is suppressed by 33% and 68%, respectively, whereas whole-body glucose uptake fails to increase above baseline (Figure 19). These results indicate that inhibition of HGP, in contrast to the stimulation of tissue glucose uptake, is exquisitely sensitive to small increments in the plasma insulin concentration. Thus, as the plasma glucose concentration increases, for whatever reason, insulin secretion is stimulated (Figure 3) and the resultant fasting hyperinsulinemia is sufficient to offset any hepatic insulin resistance and maintain a normal *absolute* rate of hepatic glucose output in the postabsorptive state. The situation regarding glucose utilization is quite different: because small increments in the plasma insulin concentration do not stimulate tissue glucose uptake [15, 427–429], the development of impaired tissue glucose

disposal in NIDDM subjects is not counteracted by the fasting hyperinsulinemia and the glucose clearance drops progressively (Figure 26).

The results summarized in Figures 20 and 26 clearly demonstrate that early in the course of NIDDM a decline in the basal rate of whole-body glucose clearance is present while the basal rate of HGP is normal despite fasting hyperinsulinemia [42]. These results are consistent with those of other investigators [360, 363, 364]. However, they do not establish which defect, i.e. hepatic insulin resistance or decreased efficiency of tissue glucose removal, developed first. *Three equally plausible sequences* can be envisioned. First, it is possible that both defects develop in parallel. As hyperglycemia ensues (owing both to excessive HGP and diminished tissue glucose uptake), basal insulin secretion is stimulated and the resultant hyperinsulinemia is sufficient to return HGP to basal levels. Because the small rise in plasma insulin concentration has no stimulatory effect on tissue glucose uptake, whole-body glucose clearance falls progressively. It could also be argued that the primary defect responsible for fasting hyperglycemia in NIDDM is a decreased efficiency of tissue glucose uptake, as reflected by a decrease in the glucose clearance. As the plasma glucose concentration rises and insulin secretion is enhanced, the resultant hyperinsulinemia has two opposing actions: (a) it induces a state of hepatic insulin resistance by down-regulating both receptor and postreceptor [313, 316, 430–434] events involved in insulin action; and (b) it has a direct suppressive effect on HGP. Because these two metabolic actions of insulin offset each other, the absolute basal rate of HGP remains unaltered. Lastly, it could be argued that the initial disturbance responsible for fasting hyperglycemia in NIDDM is the development of hepatic insulin resistance [43]. This leads to an imperceptible rise in plasma glucose concentration, which in turn stimulates insulin secretion and returns the elevated rate of HGP to basal levels. The persistent hyperinsulinemia causes a decline in the efficiency of tissue glucose removal by inducing both receptor and postreceptor defects [313, 316, 430–434]. Alternatively, hyperglycemia *per se* may be responsible for the development of impaired tissue glucose disposal by causing a down-regulation of the glucose transport system [115].

It is interesting to speculate about which factors might be responsible for the progressive rise in HGP at fasting plasma glucose concentrations above 140 mg/dl [1, 5, 42]. One obvious explanation is the progressive decline in basal plasma insulin levels that occur in NIDDM patients with fasting plasma glucose concentrations greater than 140 mg/dl. In this group, basal HGP and fasting insulin levels are inversely correlated, i.e., the decline in fasting plasma insulin concentration is closely related to the rise in HGP. A similar relationship between HGP and fasting insulin concentration has been reported by Fery [360]. Other factors that could account for the rise in HGP include a worsening of hepatic insulin resistance with progressive severity of diabetes or an accelerated rate of hepatic gluconeogenesis.

The defects in basal HGP and tissue glucose disposal are better appreciated by studying NIDDM subjects after an overnight infusion of insulin to normalize the basal rate of HGP [42]. In 19 normal weight NIDDM subjects a peripheral plasma insulin concentration of 24 μU/ml, a value more than double that in 72 age- and weight-matched controls, was required to reduce the basal rate of HGP to normal. In normal subjects a similar infusion of insulin has been shown to inhibit basal HGP by over 60% (see Figure 21). Despite similar rates of HGP in the NIDDM (1.77 mg/kg/min) and control (1.84 mg/kg/min) subjects, the fasting plasma glucose concentration remained elevated in the NIDDM group (105 ± 3 mg/dl vs. 92 ± 1 mg/dl, $p < 0.001$). This elevation in the basal plasma glucose concentration can only be explained by a decreased efficiency of glucose removal by all the tissues of the body, and this is reflected by a significant decrease in the rate of glucose clearance (1.71 ml/kg/min vs. 2.00 ml/kg/min, $p < 0.001$). Because HGP was reduced to normal, an elevated fasting plasma glucose concentration would not be anticipated if the metabolic machinery within the cells responsible for glucose uptake in the postabsorptive state was intact.

Further evidence to support the presence of a defect in tissue glucose uptake came from an extension of this study in which NIDDM individuals ($n = 11$) received an overnight infusion of insulin to normalize the fasting plasma glucose concentration [42]. Under conditions of normoglycemia, the rates of tissue glucose disposal can be directly compared in diabetic and control subjects without having to calculate the glucose clearance. At identical plasma glucose concentrations the rate of tissue glucose uptake was significantly reduced in the NIDDM subjects compared with control subjects (1.68 ml/kg/min vs. 1.84 ml/kg/min, $p < 0.01$), even though the plasma insulin concentration was more than doubled in the former group. These data conclusively demonstrate that, under comparable conditions of euglycemia, the tissues of NIDDM subjects are unable to metabolize glucose at rates comparable to those in control individuals. Virtually identical results and conclusions have been published by Chen et al [362, 364]. Using prolonged fasting, these investigators were able to reduce the elevated rate of HGP in NIDDM subjects to values observed in non-diabetic control subjects. Nonetheless, the fasting plasma glucose concentration

remained increased due to a decrease in whole body tissue glucose uptake.

At present the tissues responsible for the defect in glucose uptake in the postabsorptive state remain undefined. Leg glucose uptake was found by us to be significantly increased in NIDDM vs. control subjects (1.8 mg/kg/min vs. 1.1 mg/kg/min) in the postabsorptive state, but as the fasting plasma glucose concentration was proportionately increased (158 mg/dl vs. 99 mg/dl), the muscle glucose clearance was virtually identical in the two groups [4]. By contrast, Gerich et al [387] and Firth et al [356] have reported slightly decreased rates of glucose clearance by forearm muscle in the postabsorptive state. Using the hepatic vein catheter technique, at least part of the decline in whole-body glucose clearance has been shown to reside within the splanchnic tissues (liver plus gastrointestinal) [4]. However, from the quantitative standpoint it is clear that tissues in addition to those within the splanchnic region and muscle must contribute to the decline in whole-body glucose clearance.

As the brain and other neural tissues are responsible for 50–60% of total glucose disposal in the postabsorptive state, such tissues remain a likely source of the decrease in whole-body glucose clearance [387]. Consistent with this hypothesis, brain glucose uptake has been shown to be normal in NIDDM individuals despite the presence of fasting hyperglycemia [352]. It follows, therefore, that basal brain glucose clearance must be reduced in type 2 diabetic subjects. It is of note that chronic hyperglycemia has been shown to inhibit brain glucose transport [435, 436] through a mechanism that involves a down-regulation of the glucose transport system [437]; conversely, chronic hypoglycemia has been shown to enhance glucose transport by cerebral tissues [438]. From a purely teleologic standpoint, the ability of the plasma glucose concentration to directly regulate the glucose transport system in brain has important survival advantages. Thus, under conditions of hyperglycemia, excessive translocation of glucose and fluid into the brain is prevented and the development of cerebral edema is counteracted. Conversely, under conditions of chronic hypoglycemia the glucose transport system is up-regulated, thereby ensuring a continuous source of energy to the brain, which is dependent upon glucose for its metabolic needs.

In conclusion, the results summarized in this section indicate that in NIDDM subjects with mild fasting hyperglycemia (<140 mg/dl) the principal disturbance responsible for the elevated postabsorptive plasma glucose concentration is a defect in the efficiency of tissue glucose uptake (Figure 26). Hepatic glucose production, when viewed in *absolute* terms, is not increased because the increase in fasting plasma insulin concentration is sufficient to offset the hepatic insulin resistance. Nonetheless, a normal rate of HGP in the presence of fasting hyperinsulinemia establishes the presence of hepatic insulin resistance. By contrast, in NIDDM subjects with more severe fasting hyperglycemia (>140 mg/dl) an augmented rate of HGP is the major factor responsible for the progressive rise in fasting plasma glucose concentration (Figure 20). However, it is important to emphasize that in this latter diabetic group (FPG >140 mg/dl) tissue glucose uptake remains impaired and that this amplifies the deleterious impact of the elevated rate of HGP on the fasting glucose level.

DYNAMIC INTERACTION BETWEEN INSULIN SENSITIVITY AND INSULIN SECRETION IN NIDDM

In the preceding sections, evidence was presented to document that NIDDM subjects have readily demonstrable abnormalities in both tissue (muscle and liver) sensitivity to insulin and in pancreatic insulin secretion. In order to appreciate fully how these two metabolic disturbances conspire to produce the full-blown diabetic condition, it is necessary to understand the dynamic interaction between insulin action and insulin secretion. This requires quantitation of insulin action and insulin secretion in the same individual over a wide range of insulin sensitivity, and such studies have been reported by four groups of investigators [1, 54, 59, 62, 63, 67, 68, 272, 309, 316]. DeFronzo and colleagues [1] studied four groups of subjects. Group I comprised 47 obese subjects (age 33 years, 148% IBW), further subdivided into those with perfectly normal glucose tolerance (*n* = 24) and those with impaired glucose tolerance (*n* = 23) according to National Diabetes Data Group criteria [420]. Group II comprised 35 obese subjects (age 53 years, 147% IBW) with frank diabetes mellitus (fasting glucose >140 mg/dl), and was further subdivided into those with a hyperinsulinemic response and those with a hypoinsulinemic response during a 100 g OGTT. All the obese subjects were very similar in percentage IBW. Group III comprised 16 normal weight diabetic subjects (age 54 years, 109% IBW) and group IV consisted of 13 normal weight controls (age 53 years, 100% IBW), matched in age to the normal weight diabetic group. All subjects ingested 100 g glucose to provide a measure of glucose tolerance and insulin secretion. Whole-body insulin sensitivity was quantified with the euglycemic insulin (+100 μU/ml) clamp technique, which was performed with indirect calorimetry [439] to quantify rates of glucose oxidation and non-oxidative glucose disposal or glucose storage. This latter measure has been shown to primarily reflect glycogen synthesis [351, 392].

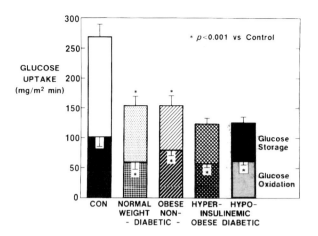

Figure 27 Insulin-mediated rates (+100 μU/ml euglycemic insulin clamp) of whole-body glucose uptake (total height of bar), glucose oxidation (lower portion of each bar), and non-oxidative glucose disposal (upper part of each bar) in control, normal weight diabetic, obese non-diabetic, and obese diabetic subjects. Obese diabetic patients were further subdivided into hyperinsulinemic and hypoinsulinemic groups, based upon their plasma insulin response during a 100 g OGTT. *p < 0.001 vs. controls (from reference 1, with permission)

In normal weight NIDDM subjects, insulin mediated whole-body glucose uptake was reduced by 40–50%, and this impairment in insulin action resulted from defects in both oxidative and non-oxidative glucose metabolism (Figures 5 and 27). It is noteworthy that the non-diabetic obese individuals were as insulin-resistant as the normal weight NIDDM subjects (Figures 5 and 27). Defects in both glucose oxidation and glucose storage contributed to the insulin resistance observed in the obese non-diabetic group (Figures 5 and 27). Thus, from the metabolic standpoint, obesity and NIDDM closely resemble each other. Similar results concerning whole-body insulin sensitivity in obese and NIDDM individuals have been reported by Reaven, Hollenbeck and colleagues [346, 440] and Bogardus, Lillioja and co-workers [44, 441, 442]. Despite nearly identical degrees of insulin resistance, normal weight diabetic subjects (Figures 5) manifested fasting hyperglycemia and marked glucose intolerance, whereas the obese non-diabetic individuals had normal or only minimally impaired oral glucose tolerance. This apparent paradox is explained by the plasma insulin response during the OGTT (Figure 28). Compared with controls, the obese non-diabetic group secreted more than twice as much insulin and this was sufficient to offset the insulin resistance. By contrast, in normal weight diabetics, the pancreas, when faced with the same challenge, was not able to augment its secretion of insulin sufficiently to compensate for the insulin resistance. This imbalance between insulin supply by the B cells and tissue insulin

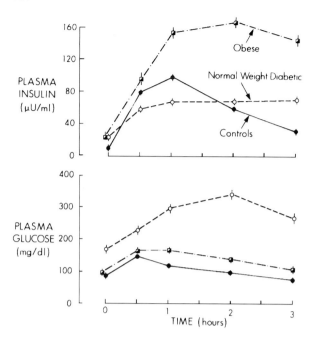

Figure 28 Plasma glucose and insulin concentrations during a 100 g OGTT in control (solid circles), normal weight diabetic (open circles), and obese non-diabetic (squares) subjects whose tissue sensitivity to insulin is shown in Figure 27 (drawn from data presented in references 1, 272, 341 and 391)

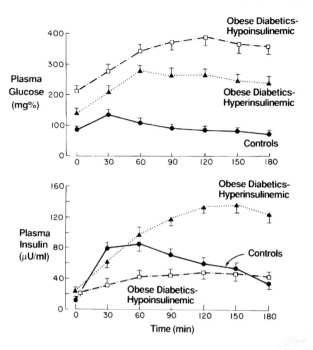

Figure 29 Plasma glucose and insulin concentrations in control (solid circles), obese hyperinsulinemic diabetic (solid triangles) and obese hypoinsulinemic diabetic (open squares) subjects whose tissue sensitivity to insulin is shown in Figure 27 (drawn from data presented in references 1, 272, 341 and 391)

requirements resulted in a frankly diabetic state, with fasting hyperglycemia and marked glucose intolerance.

When obesity and diabetes co-exist in the same individual, one might expect a precipitous decline in the rate of insulin-mediated glucose disposal. On the contrary, however, in obese diabetic subjects, whether hyperinsulinemic or hypoinsulinemic, the severity of insulin resistance was only slightly greater than that in either the normal weight diabetic or non-diabetic obese groups (Figures 5 and 27). Furthermore, the magnitude of the defects in glucose oxidation and non-oxidative glucose disposal were similar in all four obese and diabetic groups (Figures 5 and 27). Although hyperinsulinemic and hypoinsulinemic obese diabetic subjects were equally insulin-resistant, the severity of glucose intolerance was significantly worse in the hypoinsulinemic group and this was clearly related to the presence of insulin deficiency (Figure 29). Thus, the obese hyperinsulinemic diabetic group, which is able to sustain a high rate of insulin secretion, maintains a better degree of glucose tolerance than the obese insulinopenic diabetic group.

Figure 5 presents an integrated summary of the results which were discussed in the preceding paragraphs for the obese, diabetic and control groups. The mean plasma glucose concentration during the OGTT is displayed in the bottom panel, while the plasma insulin secretory response during the OGTT is shown in the top panel, along with the rate of insulin-mediated glucose

disposal (measured with the euglycemic insulin clamp technique). In obese non-diabetic subjects there is a dramatic decline in tissue sensitivity to insulin, but glucose tolerance remains perfectly normal because the B cells are able to appropriately augment their insulin secretory capacity to offset the defect in insulin action. As the obese individual becomes mildly glucose intolerant, there is a further reduction in insulin-mediated glucose disposal, which is primarily due to a decrease in glucose storage, i.e. glycogen synthesis. However, there is only a small additional impairment in glucose tolerance, because the B cell is able to augment further its secretion of insulin to counteract to a large extent the deterioration in insulin sensitivity. The progression of the obese, glucose intolerant person to overt diabetes mellitus is heralded by a decline in insulin secretion without any worsening of the insulin resistance. However, this modest decline in insulin secretion, in the presence of severe insulin resistance, is sufficient to cause marked glucose intolerance and frank diabetes mellitus (Figure 5). The obese diabetic person has tipped over the top of Starling's curve of the pancreas and is now on the descending portion (Figures 3 and 4). Even though the plasma insulin response is increased compared with that of controls, it is not elevated appropriately for the degree of insulin resistance. In the normal weight diabetic group, there was a greater decline in glucose tolerance; this was the result of a greater impairment in insulin secretion without any further deterioration in insulin sensitivity. Lastly, the obese diabetic group with a low insulin response manifested the greatest glucose intolerance; this was due entirely to the presence of marked insulin deficiency without any change in insulin sensitivity (Figures 5 and 27). The preceding sequence of events, leading from obesity with normal glucose tolerance to obesity with impaired glucose tolerance and then to obesity with diabetes, has been confirmed in a 6-year prospective study [63] involving the same subjects who previously participated in the cross-sectional study [1, 272, 341, 391].

The development of frank diabetes mellitus thus requires that a defect in insulin secretion be superimposed upon the presence of insulin resistance. This construct is consistent with the classic overfeeding studies of Sims and colleagues [443]. When healthy, lean subjects received an increased caloric intake and gained 20–30 lb (9–14 kg) over 3–5 months, moderate to severe insulin resistance in muscle tissue could be documented with the forearm perfusion technique. Nevertheless, glucose tolerance remained normal because the pancreas was able to augment its insulin secretory capacity to offset the impairment in insulin action.

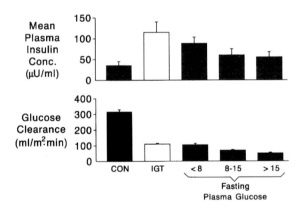

Figure 30 Insulin-mediated glucose clearance (measured with the insulin suppression test) and the plasma insulin response (measured with OGTT) in controls (CON), in subjects with impaired glucose tolerance (IGT) and in NIDDM individuals (shaded bars) with varying severity of glucose intolerance; see text for a more detailed discussion (drawn from data presented in reference 316)

The natural history of NIDDM described above is entirely consistent with results published by other investigators in both humans and monkeys [54, 59, 62–70, 309, 316]. Reaven et al [316] studied five groups of lean subjects with a wide range of glucose tolerance ranging from normal to severely impaired. The progression from normal to impaired glucose tolerance was marked by the development of severe insulin

resistance which was counterbalanced by a marked increase in insulin secretion (Figure 30). The development of NIDDM was associated with no (or only slight) deterioration in tissue sensitivity to insulin (Figure 30). Rather, there was a stepwise decline in insulin secretion, which paralleled the decrease in glucose tolerance (Figure 30). In a prospective study in Pima Indians [54, 59, 62, 316] a similar sequence of events has been documented.

It is important to recognize, however, that there are well described NIDDM populations in whom insulin sensitivity is normal at the onset of diabetes, whereas insulin secretion is severely impaired as discussed in the introduction [20–22].

CELLULAR MECHANISMS OF INSULIN RESISTANCE

In order for insulin to exert its biologic effects on glucose metabolism, it must first bind to specific receptors which are present on the cell surface of all insulin target tissues (see Chapter 21). The first step in insulin action involves activation of the insulin receptor tyrosine kinase, which is an integral part of the receptor itself. The second messengers subsequently generated initiate a series of events, involving a cascade of phosphorylation–dephosphorylation reactions that eventually result in the stimulation of intracellular glucose metabolism (see Chapters 21 and 22).

Insulin Receptor/Insulin Receptor Signal Transduction Defects in NIDDM

Insulin Receptor Number and Affinity

Both receptor and postreceptor defects have been shown to contribute to insulin resistance in NIDDM individuals. Some, but not all, studies have demonstrated that insulin binding to monocytes and adipocytes from NIDDM patients is modestly reduced, by approximately 20–30% [496–506]. The reduction in insulin binding is due to a decrease in the number of insulin receptors without change in insulin receptor affinity. In addition to the decreased number of cell surface receptors, a variety of defects in insulin receptor internalization and processing have been described [505, 507]. However, some caution should be employed in interpreting these studies. From the quantitative standpoint, the two major organs for insulin action *in vivo* are the liver and muscle, and few studies have examined insulin binding to these tissues in the human. With regard to this, insulin binding to solubilized receptors obtained from skeletal muscle biopsies and liver has been shown to be normal in obese and lean diabetic individuals when expressed per mg of protein

[500, 506, 508–513]. Several other lines of evidence indicate that decreased insulin binding cannot be the only factor responsible for the defect in insulin action in NIDDM. First, a decrease in insulin receptor number cannot be demonstrated in approximately one-third of all NIDDM subjects, especially those with high fasting plasma glucose levels [514–520]. Second, Lonnroth et al [521], Olefsky and Reaven [522] and others have been unable to find a correlation between insulin binding and the severity of insulin resistance in their NIDDM patients. Third, a number of groups [15, 349, 350, 369, 523], who have examined the dose–response relationship between insulin mediated glucose uptake and the plasma insulin concentration, have provided evidence to support the existence of a severe postreceptor (i.e. post-binding) defect in insulin action. In patients with impaired glucose tolerance and with very mild diabetes, the dose–response curve was shifted to the right, but very high plasma insulin concentrations elicited a normal glucose metabolic response. This is most consistent with a postreceptor (i.e. post-binding) defect in insulin action [524] which, indeed, has been documented in isolated adipocytes [369]. By contrast, in diabetic patients with moderate to severe fasting hyperglycemia, the dose–response curve was not only shifted to the right but also exhibited a decrease in maximally insulin-stimulated glucose disposal (Figure 19). These results also suggest a postreceptor (i.e. post-binding) defect in insulin action [524] and, consistent with this, no decrease in insulin binding could be demonstrated in diabetic patients with well-established fasting hyperglycemia [369].

Insulin Receptor Mutations

With the cloning of the human insulin receptor gene [463], a large number of point mutations have been identified [456, 463, 525]. Each is associated with a specific defect in insulin receptor function and several are characterized by impaired insulin receptor tyrosine kinase activity [456, 525] (see Chapter 21). Common to each of these insulin receptor gene defects is the presence of severe insulin resistance. Although overt NIDDM may occur, this is not a universal finding. Nonetheless, this raises the possibility that an abnormality in the insulin receptor gene may be responsible for typical NIDDM in humans. Although restriction fragment length polymorphisms in the insulin receptor gene have been reported in a small percentage of NIDDM subjects with insulin resistance [526–528], this has not been a reproducible finding [529–533]. Most recently, the insulin receptor gene has been directly sequenced in a large number of NIDDM patients from a wide diversity of ethnic populations using denaturing gradient gel electrophoresis or single

stranded conformational polymorphism analysis, and with very rare exceptions [534] mutations in the insulin receptor gene were not observed [535–537]. This excludes a structural gene abnormality in the insulin receptor as a cause of common type NIDDM.

Insulin Receptor Tyrosine Kinase Activity

Because of its central role in the insulin signal transduction cascade, a number of investigators have examined tyrosine kinase activity in a variety of cell types (skeletal muscle, adipocytes, hepatocytes and erythrocytes) from normal weight and obese diabetic subjects. Most [454, 500, 504, 506, 508, 513, 515, 516, 538–540, 542, 543], but not all [510, 544] investigators have found a significant reduction in tyrosine kinase activity which could not be explained by alterations in insulin receptor number or insulin receptor binding. The study of Freidenberg et al [540] is particularly informative because weight loss, which decreased the fasting glucose from 205 mg/dl to 118 mg/dl (11.4 to 6.6 mmol/l), led to a near-normalization of insulin receptor tyrosine kinase activity. These observations suggest that the defect in tyrosine kinase is acquired and results from some combination of hyperglycemia, defective intracellular glucose metabolism, hyperinsulinemia or insulin resistance—all of which improved following weight loss. Consistent with the observations of Freidenberg et al [540], a glucose-induced reduction in insulin receptor tyrosine kinase activity has been demonstrated in rat fibroblasts [545]. When insulin-stimulated tyrosine kinase activity was examined in normal glucose tolerant or impaired glucose tolerant individuals at high risk to develop NIDDM, a normal response was observed by Nyomba et al [539]. Again, this is consistent with the concept that the impairment in insulin receptor tyrosine kinase activity observed in overtly NIDDM patients is acquired secondarily to hyperglycemia or some other metabolic disturbance. Since the prediabetics studied by Nyomba et al [539] were both insulin resistant and hyperinsulinemic, these abnormalities are unlikely to explain the acquired defect in insulin receptor tyrosine kinase activity.

Because of tissue-specific alternative splicing of the mRNA of the proreceptor, the human insulin receptor exists as two isoforms, termed IR-A and IR-B [454, 465, 466, 548] (see Chapter 21). Several groups have provided evidence for an altered isoform pattern for both the protein and mRNA levels in NIDDM [454, 549, 550], but this has not been confirmed by other investigators [551, 552]. The significance, if any, of an altered isoform pattern in NIDDM remains to be defined.

Insulin Receptor Signal Transduction Defects

Because the key intracellular intermediates involved in insulin receptor signal transduction have only recently begun to be identified (see Chapter 21) and many important signaling molecules have yet to be defined, little information currently is available about these early steps of insulin action, either in healthy subjects or in individuals with NIDDM. Recently, two mutations of the gene for insulin receptor substrate 1 (IRS-1) were found with increased frequency in Danish subjects with NIDDM compared to controls, although each variant by itself was not significantly different from the frequency in the control group [553]. Similar mutations were not observed in Finnish diabetics, while in subjects from South India a slight, statistically insignificant increase in one of these two mutations was observed [554]. Although the current evidence is meager, it does not suggest that mutations in the IRS-1 gene are likely to explain the insulin resistance observed in NIDDM. No studies have yet examined the gene for PI 3-kinase which, together with IRS-1, forms a multicomponent signaling molecule that is essential for insulin's stimulatory action on glucose transport and glycogen synthesis.

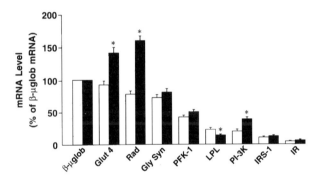

Figure 31 Muscle mRNA levels of target genes involved in glucose and lipid metabolism before and after a 3 h euglycemic insulin (2 mU/kg/min) clamp in healthy young subjects. Insulin increased the mRNA levels (expressed as a percentage of β-microglobulin mRNA) of Glut 4, Rad (Ras associated with diabetes), phosphatidylinositol (PI) 3-kinase, and lipoprotein lipase (LPL). Insulin had no effect on mRNA levels of phosphofructokinase (PFK)-1, insulin receptor substrate (IRS)-1, glycogen synthase (Gly Syn), and insulin receptor (IR) (from reference 555, by copyright permission of The American Society for Clinical Investigation)

One very recent study [555] has examined the effect of acute (3 h) pharmacologic hyperinsulinemia on muscle mRNA levels of six genes involved in insulin action including IRS-1, PI 3-kinase and Rad (Ras-associated with diabetes) in healthy non-diabetic subjects (Figure 31). Insulin caused a significant increase in the mRNA levels of PI 3-kinase and Rad, but had no effect on IRS-1 mRNA levels. There are, however, no

published studies in humans with NIDDM. Recently, we have shown that the ability of insulin to phosphorylate tyrosine residues on IRS-2 and to increase PI 3-kinase activity in muscle biopsy samples from Mexican-American NIDDM subjects is diminished (DeFronzo, Mandarino, Kahn; unpublished results). Using an anti-phosphotyrosine antibody, the amount of PI 3-kinase associated with IRS-1 was found to be reduced. Thus, these preliminary results suggest that major abnormalities in the insulin signal transduction pathway may be present in insulin resistant subjects with NIDDM. Similarly, in animal models of diabetes mellitus, an 80% decrease in IRS-1 phosphorylation and > 90% reduction in insulin-stimulated PI 3-kinase activity have been reported [556]. Rad, the protein identified by Reynet and Kahn using subtraction cloning [557], is overexpressed in the muscle of NIDDM patients, but the importance of this observation is not yet clear (see Chapter 21).

Glucose Transport

After the second messenger for insulin action has been generated, the glucose transport system is activated. As initially described by Cushman and Wardzala [458] and Kono et al [558], this effect of insulin is brought about by the translocation of a large intracellular pool of glucose transporters (associated with low-density microsomes) to the plasma membrane. It is now recognized that there are at least five different facilitative glucose transporters with distinctive tissue distributions [559–561] (Table 8). Glut 6 (renamed Glut 3P1) is a pseudogene which does not undergo translation into a functional protein because of the presence of multiple termination codons. Glut 4, the insulin-regulatable transporter, is found in the insulin-sensitive tissues (muscle and adipocytes), has a K_m of approximately 5 mmol/l (which is close to the plasma glucose concentration) [458–462, 559, 562], and is associated with hexokinase II [562, 563]. In adipocytes and muscle its concentration in the plasma membrane increases markedly after exposure to insulin and this increase is associated with a reciprocal decline in the intracellular Glut 4 pool. Glut 1 represents the predominant glucose transporter in the insulin independent tissues (brain and erythrocytes), but also is found in muscle and adipocytes. It is located primarily in the plasma membrane where its concentration changes little after the addition of insulin. It has a low K_m, approximately 1 mmol/l, and is well suited for its function which is to mediate basal glucose uptake. It is found in association with hexokinase I [563–565]. Glut 2 predominates in the liver and pancreatic B cells, where it is found in association with a specific hexokinase IV [563, 564, 566, 567]. In the B cell, hexokinase IV has

Table 8 Classification of glucose transport and hexokinase activity according to their tissue distribution and functional regulation

Organ	Glucose transporter	Hexokinase coupler	Classification
Brain	Glut 1	HK I	Glucose dependent
Erythrocyte	Glut 1	HK I	Glucose dependent
Adipocyte	Glut 4	HK II	Insulin dependent
Muscle	Glut 4	HK II	Insulin dependent
Liver	Glut 2	HK IV$_L$	Glucose sensor
B-cell	Glut 2	HK IV$_B$ (Glucokinase)	Glucose sensor
Gut	Glut 3—symporter	–	Sodium dependent
Kidney	Glut 3—symporter	–	Sodium dependent

been referred to as glucokinase [212, 213]. Glut 2 has a high K_m, approximately 15–20 mmol/l and, as a consequence, the glucose concentration in cells expressing this transporter rises in direct proportion to the increase in plasma glucose concentration. This characteristic allows these cells to respond as glucose sensors. Thus, the B cell senses the ambient glucose concentration and adjusts its output of insulin, whereas the liver reads the plasma glucose level and adjusts its output of glucose. However, because glucose transport exceeds glucose phosphorylation, glucokinase is believed to be the glucose sensor for insulin secretion [212, 213]. In summary, each tissue has a specific glucose transporter and associated hexokinase which allows it uniquely to carry out its specialized function to maintain whole-body glucose economy.

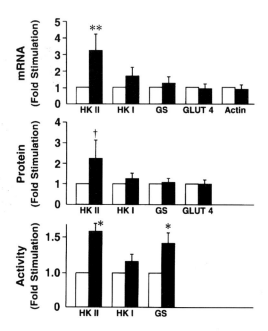

Figure 32 Effect of euglycemic hyperinsulinemia (63 μU/ml) for 4 h on hexokinase (HK), glycogen synthase (GS), and Glut 4 mRNA levels (upper panel) and protein content (middle panel), and on activity of HK and GS (lower panel) in healthy young subjects. $**\,p < 0.05$, $*\,p < 0.01$, $\dagger\,p = 0.10$. (from reference 585, with permission)

A number of investigators have examined glucose transport activity in NIDDM and have found it to be uniformly decreased in both adipocytes [515, 516, 523, 562, 568–571] and muscle [562, 572–577]. Using cytochalasin B binding, Garvey et al [570] were amongst the first to demonstrate that adipocytes from NIDDM subjects demonstrated a marked depletion of intracellular glucose transporters and a diminished ability of insulin to elicit a normal translocation response. Moreover, the 'intrinsic activity' of the transporters after their insertion into the plasma cell membrane was impaired [570]. It was therefore assumed that a decrease in the expression of the Glut 4 transporter was responsible for the insulin resistance of NIDDM. This was consistent with observations in alloxan diabetic rats [562, 578, 579]. In this *insulinopenic* model, a pretranslational defect in the Glut 4 transporter was demonstrated in adipocytes, as manifested by a severe reduction in Glut 4 mRNA and a generalized decrease in Glut 4 protein in all subcellular fractions. Similar decreases in Glut mRNA and protein were observed in muscle [578]. However, a number of groups [580–585] subsequently demonstrated that muscle tissue obtained from lean and obese NIDDM subjects contained normal or increased basal levels of Glut 4 mRNA and normal levels of Glut 4 protein. Moreover, in muscle acute (2–4 h) physiologic hyperinsulinemia does not increase the number of Glut 4 transporters in either healthy subjects (Figure 32) or NIDDM subjects [579–585], and in one study a decrease in Glut 4 protein was observed [586]. In response to insulin several studies have demonstrated an increase in muscle Glut 4 mRNA levels in control subjects [555, 582, 587]. In the only published study that simultaneously measured muscle Glut 4 mRNA and protein levels in response to insulin, the increment in mRNA levels was significantly decreased in NIDDM patients and first-degree relatives of NIDDM patients compared to controls; Glut 4 protein failed to increase in either control or diabetic groups [582], suggesting insulin resistance at the level of gene transcription. However, the physiologic significance (with regard to impaired insulin-mediated glucose disposal) of the blunted increase in muscle Glut 4 mRNA levels in NIDDM subjects is unclear since both basal and insulin-stimulated Glut 4 protein levels were normal.

Because muscle insulin resistance is the hallmark feature of NIDDM and since glucose transport is the first committed step for intracellular glucose metabolism, investigators have screened large populations of NIDDM patients for mutations in the Glut 4 gene [588, 589]. In one study a single point mutation was found in 1 of 60 NIDDM subjects [588] and the same mutation was found in 3 of 190 NIDDM subjects in another study [589]. The functional significance of this mutation is uncertain at present, but it is clear that the vast majority of cases of NIDDM cannot be explained by alterations in the Glut 4 gene.

The results summarized above indicate that the genetic material encoding the major insulin-responsive glucose transporter, as well as the transcription and translation of the Glut 4 gene, are not impaired in NIDDM. However, they do not exclude a defect in the intrinsic activity of the glucose transporter (see subsequent discussion).

In contrast to the normal levels of Glut 4 protein and mRNA in muscle of NIDDM patients, every study that has examined adipose tissue has reported reduced basal and insulin-stimulated Glut 4 mRNA levels, decreased Glut 4 transporter number in all subcellular fractions, diminished Glut 4 translocation, and impaired intrinsic activity of Glut 4 [562, 569, 570, 584, 590, 591]. These observations demonstrate that: (a) Glut 4 expression in man is subject to tissue-specific regulation, and (b) regulation of Glut 4 expression exhibits marked species variation (i.e. normal muscle Glut 4 protein/mRNA levels in human NIDDM vs. decreased muscle Glut 4 protein/mRNA levels in animal models of diabetes). In man the marked difference between adipocyte and muscle Glut 4 transporter levels in the basal and insulin-stimulated states and the observation that muscle Glut 4 protein levels in normal subjects either do not change [579, 585] or decrease slightly [586] in response to acute insulin infusion emphasizes the need to measure glucose transport *in vivo in muscle*, the primary tissue responsible for glucose disposal [1, 3, 4, 5].

Using a novel triple tracer technique which employs the simultaneous injection of ^{12}C-mannitol, ^{14}C-3-*O*-methylglucose, and 3-^{3}H-glucose into the brachial artery, Bonadonna, Cobelli, DeFronzo and colleagues [592, 593] have defined the *in vivo* dose–response curve for the action of insulin on glucose transport in human skeletal muscle of healthy subjects [594] and demonstrated that the ability of insulin to stimulate inward glucose transport was severely impaired in NIDDM subjects who were studied under euglycemic

conditions. Basal glucose transport was similar in control and diabetic subjects [595, 596] (Figure 33). The defect in glucose transport could be overcome by studying the diabetic subjects at their normal level of fasting hyperglycemia (Figure 33). Since the number of Glut 4 transporters in the muscle of diabetic subjects is normal [579–585], yet muscle glucose transport is severely impaired [595, 596], either glucose transporter translocation [597, 598] and/or the intrinsic activity of the glucose transporter [599, 600] must be impaired. Unfortunately, quantitative techniques to examine these two important processes in man are lacking. However, one recent study [598] using a qualitative method has provided evidence which indicates that the stimulation of glucose transporter translocation by insulin is impaired in NIDDM subjects. No published studies have examined the effect of insulin on the intrinsic activity of the Glut 4 transporter in human muscle.

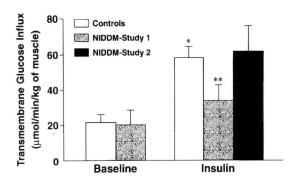

Figure 33 Rates of transmembrane glucose influx into forearm muscle at baseline and during the insulin clamp (~65 μU/ml). Study 1 was performed in the NIDDM patients at euglycemia (~5.0 mmol/l) as in the controls, whereas study 2 was performed at hyperglycemia (~13 mmol/l). $^*p < 0.01$ insulin clamp vs. baseline in controls, $^{**}p < 0.05$ NIDDM vs. controls (from reference 596, with permission)

Recently, Carey et al [577] have provided some insight into the biochemical basis of the defect in glucose transport in muscle of NIDDM subjects. A number of intracellular proteins are phosphorylated on tyrosine and on serine/threonine residues (see Chapter 21). To examine whether decreased phosphorylation of signaling peptides by a defective insulin receptor tyrosine kinase was responsible for the impairment in glucose transport, these investigators [577] employed inhibitors of serine/threonine phosphatase and inhibitors of tyrosine phosphatase. Both classes of inhibitors improved 2-deoxyglucose transport in insulin resistant muscle of NIDDM subjects but did not return it to normal. These observations suggest that defects in the insulin receptor-stimulated phosphorylation–dephosphorylation cascade are responsible, in part, for the impairment in glucose transport.

Glucose Phosphorylation

Glucose phosphorylation and glucose transport are tightly coupled phenomena. Isoenzymes of hexokinase (HKI–HKIV) catalyze the first committed intracellular step of glucose metabolism, the conversion of glucose to glucose-6-phosphate [563–567, 585, 601, 602] (Table 8). Hexokinase I, II and III are single-chain peptides which have a number of properties in common, including a molecular weight of approximately 100 kDa, a very high affinity for glucose, and product inhibition by glucose-6-phosphate (G-6-P). Hexokinase IV, also called glucokinase, has a molecular weight of about 50 kDa, a lower affinity for glucose, and is not inhibited by G-6-P. Glucokinase (HK-IVB) is believed to be the glucose sensor in the B cell (see prior discussion), while HK-IVL plays an important role in the regulation of hepatic glucose metabolism. By comparing the rat glucokinase [603] and human hexokinase II genes, Granner and colleagues [601] have provided evidence that HKI-II arose from a duplication and tandem ligation of a glucokinase-like precursor. HKII is predominantly expressed in insulin sensitive tissues, including skeletal and cardiac muscle and adipocytes [562, 563, 585, 604–606]. In both rat [601, 606] and human [555, 585] skeletal muscle, HKII transcription is regulated by insulin. In response to physiologic euglycemic hyperinsulinemia, HKII cytosolic activity and total HKII protein content and mRNA levels increased by 59%, 47% and 180%, respectively; insulin had no effect on mitochondrial HKII activity. Hexokinase I (HKI) is also present in human skeletal muscle, but insulin had no effect on HKI activity, protein content, or mRNA levels [585].

Over the years there has been considerable debate about the rate-limiting step for glucose utilization in muscle. Because of the inability to detect significant amounts of free glucose in muscle, it has been assumed that glucose transport (Glut 4)—not HKII—is rate-limiting for insulin action. However, as pointed out by Saccomani et al [593], the measurement of intracellular free glucose concentration with the muscle biopsy technique is based upon a number of assumptions that are not correct. Using the triple tracer technique, it has been shown that the intracellular muscle glucose concentration (in the space which is available to glucose) in the basal state in healthy subjects is about 1 mmol/l and decreases to approximately 0.5 mmol/l in response to insulin [593]. In lean NIDDM subjects a very different picture is observed [596]. In response to euglycemic hyperinsulinemia, inward glucose transport in muscle is markedly impaired (Figure 33). However, the rate of intracellular glucose phosphorylation is impaired to an even greater extent (Figure 34) and as a result the intracellular free glucose concentration

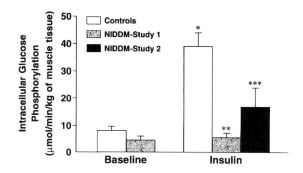

Figure 34 Rates of intracellular glucose phosphorylation in forearm muscle at baseline and during the insulin clamp ($\sim$65 μU/ml) study. Study 1 was performed in NIDDM patients at euglycemia ($\sim$5 mmol/l) as in controls, whereas study 2 was performed at hyperglycemia ($\sim$13 mmol/l). $^*p < 0.05$ insulin clamp vs. baseline in controls, $^{**}p < 0.01$ NIDDM vs. controls during insulin clamp, $^{***}p < 0.05$ NIDDM vs. controls during insulin clamp (from reference 596, with permission)

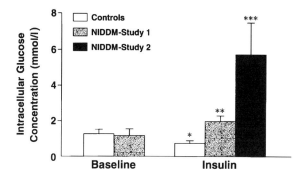

Figure 35 Glucose concentration in the available intracellular glucose space in forearm muscle at baseline and during the insulin clamp ($\sim$65 μU/ml) study. Study 1 was performed in NIDDM patients at euglycemia ($\sim$5 mmol/l) as in controls, whereas study 2 was performed at hyperglycemia ($\sim$13 mmol/l). $^*p < 0.05$ insulin clamp vs. baseline in controls, $^{**}p < 0.01$ NIDDM vs. controls during insulin clamp, $^{***}p < 0.05$ study 2 vs. study 1 in NIDDM patients (from reference 596, with permission)

rises (Figure 35). By performing the insulin clamp at the diabetic subjects' normal level of fasting hyperglycemia, one can elicit a normal rate of whole body glucose disposal and a normal rate of glucose influx into muscle (Figure 33). However, the rate of intracellular glucose phosphorylation increases only modestly and remains markedly less than in controls (Figure 34). This results in a dramatic rise in the free glucose concentration within the intracellular space that is accessible to glucose (Figure 35). These observations indicate that, while both glucose transport and glucose phosphorylation are severely resistant to the action of insulin in NIDDM individuals, impaired glucose phosphorylation (HKII) is the rate limiting step for insulin action in such individuals. These findings are entirely consistent with ^{31}P-NMR studies by Rothman et al [607], who demonstrated that during hyperinsulinemia muscle G-6-P concentrations were reduced in NIDDM versus control subjects. This observation is consistent with an early defect in insulin action, although it cannot distinguish between a defect in glucose phosphorylation vs. glucose transport. Using the triple tracer technique, Pendergrass et al [608] have shown that a similar pattern of impaired muscle glucose phosphorylation and transport is present in the normal glucose tolerant offspring of two diabetic parents. Rothman et al [609] also have shown decreased muscle G-6-P concentrations during hyperinsulinemia in the normal glucose tolerant offspring of two diabetic parents. These observations indicate that the defects in glucose phosphorylation/transport are established early in the natural history of NIDDM and cannot be explained solely by 'glucose toxicity' [115]. It is noteworthy that under certain metabolic and hormonal conditions glucose phosphorylation has been shown to be rate-limiting for insulin action [605, 610].

Because of the severe defect in muscle glucose phosphorylation demonstrated in NIDDM subjects with the triple tracer technique [596], Pendergrass et al examined the effect of euglycemic hyperinsulinemia on HKII activity, gene transcription and translation in lean NIDDM individuals [611]. Compared to controls, HKII activity and mRNA levels were reduced by 30% and 50%, respectively (Figure 36). A similar impairment in muscle HKII activity and mRNA levels in NIDDM subjects has been reported by Vestergaard et al [612]. Decreased insulin-stimulated muscle HKII activity also has been reported in subjects with impaired glucose tolerance [613].

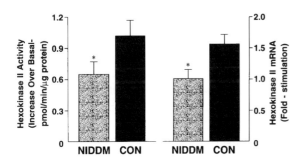

Figure 36 Increase in muscle hexokinase (HK) II activity and mRNA level and protein after a 4 h euglycemic insulin clamp performed in control and NIDDM subjects. *$p < 0.01$ vs. controls (drawn from data presented in reference 611)

The human HKII gene has been localized to chromosome 2p13 [614] and its complete structure has been characterized [602]. Because of its central role in insulin-mediated muscle glucose metabolism and impaired activity in NIDDM subjects, several groups have looked for associations between HKII polymorphisms and NIDDM [615] and for point mutations in the HKII gene in individuals with NIDDM [613, 616–619]. Although a number of nucleotide substitutions have been found, none were located close to the glucose- and ATP-binding sites and none were associated with insulin resistance. Thus, an abnormality in the HKII gene is unlikely to explain the inherited insulin resistance in common variety NIDDM. No linkage between HKII and MODY has been described [84].

Glycogen Synthesis

The two major intracellular pathways of glucose disposal are oxidation and glycogen formation (Figure 27). In the low range of physiologic hyperinsulinemia, these pathways are of equal quantitative importance. With increasing plasma insulin concentrations, glycogen synthesis becomes predominant [429]. Using indirect calorimetry [439], total-body glucose oxidation can be measured directly [1, 2, 272, 341, 343, 391, 429]. If the rate of glucose oxidation is subtracted from the rate of whole-body insulin mediated glucose disposal (which is determined from the insulin clamp), the difference represents glucose storage or non-oxidative glucose disposal. The latter primarily reflects glycogen synthesis [3, 272, 351, 392, 394, 621–623], since glucose conversion to lipid accounts for less than 5–10% of total glucose disposal [10–12, 407–410] and little of the glucose taken up by muscle is released as lactate [3, 395, 396, 624]. As can be seen in Figure 27, a major defect in glucose storage is a characteristic finding in all insulin resistant states, including obesity, diabetes and the combination of obesity plus diabetes. Consistent with this, Lillioja et al [442] have shown that impaired glucose storage represents the major determinant of insulin resistance *in vivo* in obese subjects with normal or only slightly impaired glucose tolerance. These findings are consistent with those of Golay et al [272]. In a group of 173 obese individuals, encompassing a wide spectrum of glucose tolerance, these investigators [272] found that the development of obesity with normal or impaired glucose tolerance was characterized by the emergence of a severe defect in glucose storage under euglycemic hyperinsulinemic conditions. However, the defect could be overcome by hyperglycemia (i.e. in an OGTT). The further progression of obesity with IGT to overt diabetes mellitus was associated with the inability of hyperglycemia to compensate for the defect in insulin-mediated glucose storage during an OGTT. These results demonstrate that the impaired ability of insulin to promote glucose storage (glycogen synthesis) represents a characteristic and early defect in the development of insulin resistance in both obesity and type 2 diabetes mellitus. The emergence of overt diabetes mellitus with fasting hyperglycemia is associated with a major reduction in insulin mediated glucose storage or non-oxidative glucose disposal [15, 272, 343]. A number of studies have confirmed that a defect in non-oxidative glucose disposal or glycogen synthesis is a characteristic feature of NIDDM in all ethnic races [625–633]. Impaired non-oxidative glucose disposal also has been demonstrated in the normal glucose tolerant offspring of two diabetic parents [64, 609], in the first-degree relatives of NIDDM individuals [75, 626, 634] and in the normoglycemic individual whose monozygotic twin has NIDDM [286].

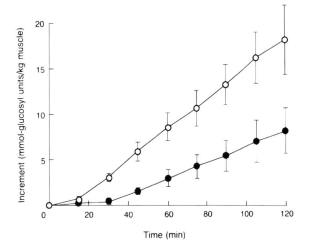

Figure 37 Effect of combined hyperinsulinemia (100 μU/ml) and hyperglycemia (200 mg/dl) on muscle glycogen synthesis in control (open circles) and NIDDM (solid circles) subjects. The ability of insulin to stimulate glycogen formation was delayed and markedly decreased in diabetic patients. The time course and magnitude of decrease in leg muscle glycogen formation closely parallel that of total leg glucose uptake (see Figure 24) (from reference 351, with permission)

Shulman et al [351], using NMR imaging spectroscopy to quantify glycogen synthesis directly in the gastrocnemius muscle of the leg, demonstrated decreased incorporation of [^{1}H, ^{13}C]-glucose into muscle glycogen of NIDDM subjects under steady-state conditions of hyperglycemia and hyperinsulinemia (Figure 37). In all subjects, the rate of non-oxidative glucose disposal (glucose storage) correlated closely with the rate of glycogen synthesis, as determined by NMR ($r = 0.89$, $p < 0.001$). These results indicate that the measurement of non-oxidative glucose disposal using indirect calorimetry closely reflects muscle glycogen synthesis. In the NIDDM subjects, however, there was a marked lag in the onset of insulin-stimulated glycogen synthesis (Figure 37) that was

similar to the delay observed in glucose uptake in the leg (see Figure 24). The rate of glycogen synthesis in NIDDM subjects was decreased by approximately 50%, paralleling the decrease in total glucose uptake in the leg (see Figure 24), and accounted for essentially all of the defect in whole body glucose disposal since glucose oxidation was normal under the experimental conditions of combined hyperglycemia and hyperinsulinemia.

The results summarized above provide convincing evidence that impaired glycogen synthesis represents a major defect in normal, glucose tolerant obese subjects, in individuals with IGT and in patients with overt diabetes mellitus. Moreover, the studies of Gulli et al [64] and others [75, 278, 392, 394, 442, 609, 626, 634] suggest that the earliest detectable metabolic defect responsible for the insulin resistance in normal glucose tolerant individuals who are destined to develop NIDDM is an impairment in glycogen synthesis.

Glycogen synthase (GS) is the key insulin-regulated enzyme which controls the rate of muscle glycogen formation [480, 481, 585, 623, 635]. Insulin enhances GS activity by stimulating a cascade of phosphorylation–dephosphorylation reactions which ultimately lead to the activation of protein phosphatase type 1 (PP1, also called glycogen synthase phosphatase) [480, 481]. The regulatory subunit of PP1 has two serine phosphorylation sites, called site 1 and site 2, and phosphorylation of site 1 of PP1 (which activates PP1 and hence stimulates GS) is catalyzed by an insulin-stimulated protein kinase 1 (ISPK-1) [636–638]. Considerable attention has been focused on the three enzymes, GS, PP1 and ISPK-1 in the pathogenesis of the insulin resistance in individuals with NIDDM.

Under basal conditions the total GS activity in NIDDM subjects is reduced and the ability of insulin to activate GS is severely impaired [625, 631, 632, 639–651]. The reduction in GS activity correlates closely with the defect in insulin-stimulated non-oxidative glucose disposal [5, 44, 351, 394, 585, 625, 628, 631, 646, 651], which primarily reflects glycogen formation [351]. A similar defect in the ability of insulin to activate GS has been demonstrated in the normal glucose-tolerant relatives of NIDDM individuals [75, 286, 626, 634]. Additional evidence in support of a defect in insulin-mediated activation of GS comes from the study of cultured myocytes and fibroblasts from NIDDM subjects [652–654]. Following multiple culture passages, basal, as well as insulin-stimulated GS activity, is severely reduced. Studies in insulin resistant non-diabetic as well as diabetic Pima Indians have demonstrated that the ability of insulin to activate muscle PP1 is severely impaired.

Several studies [555, 585, 611, 625, 628] have examined the effect of insulin on GS gene transcription and translation. In normal subjects acute physiologic hyperinsulinemia increases muscle GS mRNA [555, 585, 625] without any change in GS protein content [585, 625]. The disparity between the mRNA and protein expression suggests either that the period of hyperinsulinemia was not sufficient to detect an increase in translational activity or that there were different turnover rates for GS mRNA and protein. In NIDDM subjects the ability of insulin to increase muscle GS mRNA levels was severely impaired [611, 625, 628]; insulin had no effect on GS protein content [611, 628], although the basal level was decreased in one study [628] and normal in another [611].

Because impaired muscle glycogen synthesis and GS activity are characteristic features of NIDDM and have been demonstrated early in the natural history of diabetes at a time when glucose tolerance is normal, the GS gene [655] has been the subject of intensive investigation (see Chapter 3), but this has proved unable to explain the defect in insulin-stimulated glycogen synthase. It is possible that another gene close to the GS gene may be involved in the development of NIDDM. Most recently, the genes encoding the catalytic subunits of PP1 [665, 666] and ISPK-1 [667] have been examined in insulin-resistant Pima Indians and Danes with NIDDM. Several silent nucleotide substitutions were found in the PP1 and ISPK-1 genes in the Danish population; the mRNA levels of both genes in skeletal muscle were normal [665, 666]. No structural gene abnormalities in the catalytic subunit of PP1 were detected in Pima Indians [667]. Thus, neither abnormalities in the PP1 and ISPK-1 genes nor in their translation can explain the impaired enzymatic activities of GS and PP1 that have been observed *in vivo*. Similarly, there is no evidence that an alteration in glycogen phosphorylase plays any role in the abnormality in glycogen formation in NIDDM [626].

Glycolysis/Glucose Oxidation

The other major pathway of insulin-mediated glucose disposal, namely glycolysis/glucose oxidation, also has been shown to be impaired in many individuals with NIDDM (5, 395, 396). However, some investigators have demonstrated a normal rate of glucose oxidation in NIDDM subjects [628]. Glucose oxidation accounts for approximately 90% of total glycolytic flux, while anaerobic glycolysis accounts for the other 10% [5, 395, 396]. Two enzymes, phosphofructokinase (PFK) and pyruvate dehydrogenase (PDH), play central roles in the regulation of glycolysis and glucose oxidation, respectively. Although one study has suggested that the activity of PFK is modestly reduced in muscle biopsies from NIDDM subjects [668], most evidence indicates that it is normal [628, 653]. Insulin has no effect on muscle PFK activity, mRNA levels, or protein content in either non-diabetic or diabetic individuals [628]. PDH is a key insulin-regulated enzyme whose activity in muscle is acutely stimulated by a physiologic increment in the plasma insulin concentration [639]. Two previous studies have examined PDH activity in type 2 diabetic patients. In one study the ability of insulin to activate muscle PDH was not impaired [641]. In the other study the ability of insulin to stimulate this enzyme complex in adipocytes was found to be impaired [642]. However, it should be remembered that muscle, not fat, tissue is the major site of glucose disposal and represents the tissue that is primarily responsible for the defect in insulin action in insulin-resistant states [1, 5]. Moreover, both obesity and moderate to severe diabetes mellitus are associated with accelerated FFA turnover and oxidation [15, 272] which, according to the Randle cycle [14, 669, 670], would be expected to inhibit PDH and consequently glucose oxidation (see subsequent discussion). Thus, any observed defect in glucose oxidation or PDH activity could be acquired secondarily to increased FFA oxidation and feedback inhibition of PDH by elevated intracellular levels of acetyl-CoA and reduced availability of NAD. Consistent with this observation, the rate of basal and insulin-stimulated glucose oxidation has been shown to be normal in the normal glucose-tolerant offspring of two diabetic parents [64] and in the first-degree relatives of type 2 diabetic subjects [75, 626], while it may be decreased in overtly diabetic subjects [5, 395, 396]. Additional studies examining PDH activity in muscle tissue from lean diabetics with mild fasting hyperglycemia are needed before the role of this enzyme in the development of insulin resistance in NIDDM can be established or excluded.

In summary, it appears that postbinding defects in insulin action primarily are responsible for the insulin resistance in NIDDM. Diminished insulin binding, when present, occurs primarily in individuals with IGT or very mild diabetes, and results secondarily from down-regulation of the insulin receptor by chronic, sustained hyperinsulinemia. Moreover, even in such circumstances the decrease in insulin receptor number is small and cannot explain the marked degree of insulin resistance. In type 2 diabetic patients with fasting glucose levels in excess of 140 mg/dl (7.8 mmol/l), postbinding defects primarily account for the insulin resistance. A number of postbinding defects have been documented, including diminished insulin receptor tyrosine kinase activity, abnormalities in the insulin receptor signal transduction system, decreased glucose transport, reduced glucose phosphorylation, and impaired GS activity. The glycolytic/glucose oxidative pathway appears to be largely intact and, when defects are observed, they appear to be acquired secondarily to enhanced FFA/lipid oxidation. From the quantitative standpoint, impaired glycogen synthesis represents the major pathway responsible for the insulin resistance in NIDDM, and family studies suggest that a defect in the glycogen synthetic pathway represents the earliest detectable abnormality in NIDDM. However, at present it cannot be determined whether the primary defect is caused by the production of some gene product that directly alters the activity of GS or by an abnormality in some insulin-regulated step (i.e. signal transduction, glucose transport, glucose phosphorylation) proximal to GS.

OTHER MECHANISMS OF INSULIN RESISTANCE

In addition to the cellular mechanisms of insulin resistance described above, a number of other potentially interesting hypotheses have been proposed to explain the defect in insulin action in NIDDM.

Lipid Oxidation and Insulin Resistance in NIDDM

More than three decades ago, Randle et al [14, 669, 670] proposed that increased FFA oxidation restrains glucose oxidation in muscle by altering the redox potential of the cell and by inhibiting several key enzymatic steps within the glycolytic cascade (Figure 38). The excessive FFA oxidation leads to the intracellular accumulation of acetyl-CoA, which is a powerful inhibitor of PDH [669–672], and increases the NADH/NAD ratio, resulting in a slowing of the TCA cycle and accumulation of citrate. Citrate is a potent inhibitor of PFK [14, 669, 670, 673] and inhibition of this enzyme leads to product inhibition of the early steps involved in glucose metabolism. G-6-P eventually builds up and inhibits HK, causing a decrease in glucose transport into the cell. The sequence of events described above impairs both glucose oxidation (direct inhibition of PDH and TCA cycle) and glycogen formation (secondary to decreased glucose transport). Increased FFA oxidation also has been shown directly to inhibit GS activity in liver [674] and muscle [675–677] by causing a dissociation of its subunits [674]. Thus, an elevated rate of FFA oxidation can reproduce all of the major intracellular abnormalities (decreased glucose transport and phosphorylation, decreased glycogen synthesis, decreased glucose oxidation) that have been described in NIDDM. Recently, Roden et al [675] have challenged the biochemical basis of the Randle cycle. Using the euglycemic clamp in combination with indirect calorimetry and $^{13}C/^{31}P$

NMR spectroscopy, they demonstrated that FFA infusion in normal subjects inhibited both glycogen synthesis and glucose oxidation. However, muscle G-6-P concentrations (measured by ^{31}P NMR spectroscopy) declined, and the decrease preceded the FFA-mediated inhibition of glycogen synthesis. This led the investigators [675] to postulate that the primary effect of elevation in plasma FFA concentration is to inhibit glucose transport and/or phosphorylation which, in combination with the decrease in G-6-P (an allosteric activator of GS), leads to a reduction in glycogen synthesis. Regardless of the mechanism, much evidence demonstrates that elevated plasma FFA/FFA oxidation impairs insulin-mediated glucose disposal *in vivo*.

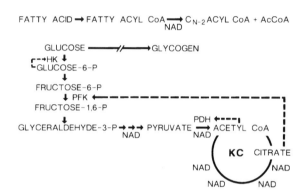

Figure 38 Randle cycle. Enhanced free fatty acid oxidation depletes NAD stores, leading to an inhibition of the Krebs (TCA) cycle (KC) and resultant increase in intracellular citrate and acetyl-CoA concentrations. Accumulation of acetyl-CoA and citrate leads to the inhibition of pyruvate dehydrogenase (PDH) and phosphofructokinase (PFK), respectively. Build-up of glucose-6-phosphate (glucose-6-P) inhibits hexokinase, leading to an inhibition of glucose transport into the cell. The decrease in glucose transport, in combination with an inhibitory effect of fatty acetyl-CoA on glycogen synthase, results in diminished glycogen formation. Dashed and interrupted lines represent sites of inhibition of glucose metabolism. See text for a more detailed description

Experimental validation of the Randle cycle has been provided in healthy humans [14, 17, 272, 675–683]. Physiologic elevation of the plasma FFA concentration stimulates FFA oxidation, which in turn inhibits both glucose oxidation and non-oxidative glucose disposal (glycogen synthesis). In normal subjects physiologic hyperinsulinemia (+100 µU/ml euglycemic insulin clamp) caused a 50–60% decline in plasma FFA concentration and a parallel decline in lipid oxidation. When Intralipid was infused during the insulin clamp to maintain or increase the plasma FFA concentration, the insulin-mediated stimulation of both glucose oxidation and glucose storage was significantly reduced (Figure 39).

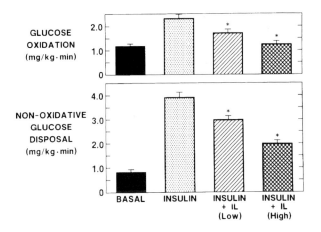

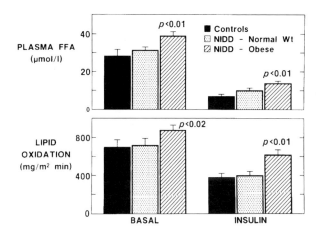

Figure 39 Inhibitory effect of Intralipid infusion and enhanced lipid oxidation on insulin-mediated rates of glucose oxidation and non-oxidative glucose disposal (glycogen synthesis). A +100 μU/ml euglycemic insulin clamp was performed with and without Intralipid (IL) infusion. Intralipid was infused at two rates in order to maintain (low IL infusion) or increase (high IL infusion) the basal plasma FFA concentration (drawn from data presented in reference 678)

Figure 40 Plasma free fatty acid (FFA) concentration and total-body lipid oxidation in the basal and insulin-stimulated (+100 μU/ml euglycemic insulin clamp) states in control (solid bars), normal weight NIDDM (stippled bars) and obese NIDDM (cross-hatched bars) subjects. Elevated basal plasma FFA concentration and lipid oxidation, as well as impaired suppression of plasma FFA and lipid oxidation by insulin, were observed only in obese NIDDM subjects (drawn from data presented in references 272, 341 and 391)

Felber and co-workers [684–687] were amongst the first to demonstrate that basal plasma FFA levels and lipid oxidation are elevated in human obesity and diabetes and fail to suppress normally following glucose ingestion. The results of insulin clamp studies [1, 15, 272, 343, 391] performed in obese non-diabetic, obese diabetic, and lean diabetic subjects are in agreement with those of Felber et al [684–687]. In obese non-diabetic, obese glucose intolerant, and obese diabetic individuals, the fasting plasma FFA concentration and basal rate of lipid oxidation are elevated compared with controls and fail to suppress normally during the euglycemic insulin clamp (Figure 40). Lipid and glucose oxidation were strongly and inversely correlated during both the basal state and the insulin clamp ($r = -0.80$, $p < 0.001$). An inverse relationship between lipid oxidation and glucose storage during the insulin clamp ($r = -0.35$, $p < 0.05$) also was observed, although the correlation was much weaker than that between lipid and glucose oxidation. Increased postabsorptive plasma FFA concentrations and lipid oxidation, as well as impaired suppression of FFA/lipid oxidation in response to insulin, have been reported by others in obese non-diabetic and obese diabetic individuals [44, 688–690]. Recently, Reaven has emphasized that adipose tissue is severely resistant to the effects of insulin on lipid metabolism and that the impairment in lipolysis results in elevated plasma FFA concentrations which are closely linked to glucose intolerance and insulin resistance in obese and diabetic individuals [16]. Phillips et al [691] have shown that elevated intramuscular triglyceride concentrations are closely correlated with impaired insulin action in

non-diabetic subjects. This observation is consistent with those of Bonadonna et al [692, 693], who demonstrated that only half of total body lipid oxidation can be accounted for by circulating plasma FFA. Since muscle triglyceride content is markedly increased in NIDDM subjects [668], a local intramuscular Randle cycle also may contribute to the defect in insulin-mediated glucose disposal. When viewed collectively, these results indicate that elevated rates of lipid oxidation contribute to the defects in glucose oxidation and glucose storage in insulin resistant *obese* diabetic individuals. By contrast, in *normal weight* NIDDM subjects with mild fasting hyperglycemia, basal rates of lipid oxidation have been reported to be normal and to suppress normally in response to insulin [272, 341, 694] (Figure 40). Thus, increased Randle cycle activity is less likely to explain the insulin resistance in *normal weight* diabetic patients. In such individuals a normal fat mass and the presence of basal and meal-stimulated hyperinsulinemia appear to be sufficient to prevent any increase in lipid oxidation. However, as insulinopenia develops, the restraining effect of insulin on lipolysis is lost, plasma FFA levels rise, and even normal weight NIDDM subjects eventually manifest an increase in lipid oxidation [15, 683, 695]. Interestingly, an elevated rate of basal lipid oxidation has been described in lean, normal glucose-tolerant, insulin-resistant offspring of two Mexican-American diabetic parents [64]. Such individuals are at extremely high risk to develop NIDDM later in life. Thus, in certain high risk populations it is possible that an elevated rate of lipid oxidation might contribute to the insulin resistance.

An elevated rate of FFA oxidation also augments hepatic glucose production. Studies *in vitro* have demonstrated that FFA stimulate gluconeogenesis [696, 697]. Furthermore, FFA infusion in normal humans, under conditions that simulate the diabetic state [679], and in obese insulin-resistant subjects [698], enhances HGP, probably secondarily to stimulation of gluconeogenesis. In NIDDM subjects the basal plasma FFA level and basal rate of lipid oxidation are increased, and both are strongly correlated with the increase in fasting plasma glucose concentration and the increased basal rate of HGP [15, 16, 44, 272, 343, 695, 699]. The following sequence can be offered to explain the relationship between plasma FFA concentration, lipid oxidation and HGP in obesity and NIDDM: (a) increased plasma FFA concentration, by mass action, enhances cellular FFA uptake; this, in turn, leads to an increase in lipid oxidation and the accumulation of acetyl-CoA, which stimulates pyruvate carboxylase, the rate-limiting enzyme for gluconeogenesis [700]; (b) the augmented rate of lipid oxidation provides a continued source of energy (ATP) and reduced nucleotides to drive gluconeogenesis; (c) the hepatic uptake of circulating gluconeogenic precursors is elevated in obesity [701] and NIDDM [370]; (d) NIDDM subjects have increased plasma glucagon levels [702–705], and hepatic sensitivity to the stimulatory effect of glucagon on glucose production may be increased [383]; (e) lastly, the inhibitory influence of insulin on gluconeogenesis is much more resistant than its restraining action on glycogenolysis [367]. Consistent with this thesis, Puhakainen and Yki-Jarvinen [706] have shown that a reduction in plasma FFA concentration with acipimox in NIDDM subjects caused a decline in basal hepatic gluconeogenesis. However, there was a reciprocal rise in glycogenolysis, such that total HPG did not change. Saloranta et al [707] have shown that a reduction in plasma FFA levels with acipimox improves the insulin-mediated suppression of HGP.

In summary, an increase in body fat mass in obese individuals, both diabetic and non-diabetic, is associated with an accelerated rate of lipolysis and an increase in the plasma FFA concentration. By mass action effect, the elevated plasma FFA level enhances its cellular uptake and stimulates lipid oxidation. In muscle the accelerated rate of fat oxidation impairs insulin-mediated glucose disposal by inhibiting both glucose oxidation and glycogen synthesis, while at the level of the liver it stimulates gluconeogenesis and increases hepatic glucose output. Operation of the Randle cycle within the B cell also may contribute to impaired insulin secretion [18]. However, despite an impressive amount of evidence implicating altered FFA/lipid metabolism in the pathogenesis of the insulin

resistance in NIDDM, normalization of the plasma FFA levels by lipid-lowering medications has not consistently led to an improvement in glycemic control and insulin resistance [707, 708]. Therefore, the precise clinical importance of the Randle cycle in the development of NIDDM remains to be defined.

Several recent provocative studies [709, 710] have demonstrated that insulin sensitivity is closely related to the fatty acid composition of serum lipids and skeletal muscle phospholipids. In particular, an increase in palmitic acid has been shown to predict the presence of insulin resistance in non-diabetic subjects, while similar changes in the fatty acid composition of serum cholesterol esters predict the development of NIDDM in Swedish men [711].

Skeletal Muscle Capillary Density, Fiber Type and Endothelial Transport

Recent studies have suggested that skeletal muscle capillary density and fiber type also may be a determinant of insulin sensitivity (712) and contribute to the insulin resistance in type 2 diabetic individuals [713] (see also Chapter 29). In Europids and Pima Indians with a wide range of insulin sensitivity, insulin-mediated glucose disposal correlated closely with capillary density, and the authors suggested that the diffusion distance from capillary to muscle cells, or some associated biochemical change related to the diffusion distance, contributed to the insulin resistance [713]. A positive correlation between the severity of insulin resistance (insulin clamp technique) and the decrease in the number of type 1, oxidative slow-twitch fibers also was reported [713]. Type 1 fibers are very sensitive to insulin, and appear to be genetically determined and relatively fixed in number [713]. Conversely, insulin-mediated glucose uptake was inversely related to the number of type 2b, fast-twitch glycolytic fibers which are insulin-resistant. These findings suggest an anatomic/histologic basis for the insulin resistance in NIDDM. However, these findings could not be reproduced by Garvey et al [584], who found no differences in muscle fiber composition between lean control subjects, obese subjects with normal glucose tolerance, subjects with IGT, and lean and obese NIDDM individuals.

The diffusion of insulin across the vascular endothelium also has been suggested to be a potential rate-limiting step for insulin action [317]. King and Johnson have shown that transport of insulin across the capillary endothelial cell *in vitro* is receptor-mediated and rapid [714]. Bergman and colleagues demonstrated a positive correlation in dogs between the insulin concentration in thoracic duct lymph and glucose utilization during the insulin clamp [715]. On the basis of this observation they suggested that transcapillary insulin transport is responsible for the normal delay in the onset of insulin action in healthy subjects and may contribute to the excessive delay observed in NIDDM subjects [715, 716]. Unfortunately, the great majority of thoracic duct lymph is derived from the splanchnic area and this is confirmed by the authors' findings of higher glucose concentrations (the liver produces glucose) and much lower insulin concentrations (the liver extracts insulin) in thoracic duct lymph compared with plasma [715]. This observation raises questions about the physiologic significance of the positive correlation between thoracic duct lymph insulin levels and whole-body (which primarily reflects muscle) insulin-mediated glucose disposal. More recently, the same investigators have measured the insulin concentration in hind limb lymph of the dog and observed a strong correlation between the time course of increase in hind limb insulin and whole body glucose disposal [717]. Further support for the hypothesis that trans-endothelial passage of insulin into the interstitial space plays an important role in regulating glucose metabolism has been provided by Miles et al [718]. These investigators demonstrated that the time course of action of insulin to stimulate whole body glucose uptake and to enhance muscle insulin receptor tyrosine kinase activity were similar to the time course of build-up of insulin concentration in thoracic duct lymph. However, this study also suffers from the measurement of thoracic duct, not muscle, insulin concentrations. In addition, a major criticism of all of these papers [715–718] is that lymph insulin concentrations may not reflect those in interstitial fluid.

Jansson et al [719] have tried to examine the importance of an endothelial barrier to insulin action by measuring simultaneously the interstitial and plasma insulin concentrations. At both physiologic and pharmacologic plasma insulin concentrations, the interstitial insulin levels were ~50% lower than those in plasma. On the basis of this observation, the authors suggested the presence of an endothelial barrier to the passage of insulin and to the ability of insulin to stimulate glucose disposal. This conclusion is, however, difficult to accept, since at steady-state pharmacologic insulin concentrations an endothelial barrier to insulin diffusion cannot explain the lower interstitial insulin concentrations. It seems more likely that increased clearance of insulin from the interstitial compartment explains the lower insulin concentration. Most recently, Prakash et al [720] also have measured simultaneously plasma and interstitial insulin concentrations during a euglycemic insulin clamp performed in lean and obese subjects. They found that steady-state insulin concentrations were achieved in plasma and in thigh and abdominal interstitial fluid within 10 minutes after the start of insulin infusion and within 10 minutes after discontinuation of the insulin infusion. This argues against a major barrier to the diffusion of insulin into the interstitial fluid. Moreover, in obese subjects plasma and interstitial insulin concentrations were virtually identical in both abdominal and thigh lymph, whereas in lean subjects the interstitial insulin concentration was only 10–15% lower than in plasma. These findings are strikingly different from those reported by Jansson et al [719]. Since the time course of insulin concentration in interstitial and plasma compartments was similar in lean and obese subjects, it is difficult to explain the insulin resistance in the latter group by a difference in trans-capillary insulin transport. No other group has measured the interstitial insulin concentration and related it to insulin action. However, Castillo et al [721] have shown that in both lean and obese subjects lymph insulin concentrations in the lower limb are ~30–40% lower than in arterial plasma, rise much more slowly than arterial insulin concentrations, and are closely correlated with glucose uptake. Of particular note, obese subjects had much higher lymph and arterial insulin concentrations but much lower rates of glucose uptake than controls. Thus, even if insulin diffusion into the interstitial fluid compartment is rate-limiting for insulin action, a defect in cellular glucose metabolism must be responsible for the insulin resistance in obese individuals.

In summary, the available evidence—although still scant in amount—suggests that there may be a trans-capillary barrier for insulin diffusion, but that a cellular defect rather than a diffusion defect is responsible for the insulin resistance in commonly encountered metabolic disorders such as obesity and diabetes. The capillary endothelium as a barrier to insulin action is an interesting concept which is deserving of further investigation to clarify its role in the insulin resistance of NIDDM.

Blood Flow

The effect of insulin on blood flow to peripheral tissues, i.e. muscle, and the role of alterations in insulin-mediated blood flow in the well documented insulin resistance observed in NIDDM and obesity, has become a topic of much controversy. Baron has championed the concept that physiologic levels of hyperinsulinemia increase muscle blood flow in a dose-dependent fashion in lean normal subjects [722–742] and that approximately 50% of the impairment in insulin-mediated whole body and leg glucose uptake (both of which primarily reflect glucose disposal in muscle under conditions of euglycemic hyperinsulinemia) in NIDDM [726] and normal glucose-tolerant obese subjects [727, 728] is related to a defect in

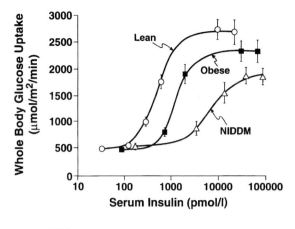

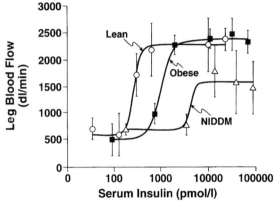

Figure 41 Dose–response curves relating whole-body glucose uptake (upper panel) and leg blood flow (lower panel) to the serum insulin concentration during euglycemic insulin clamp studies performed in lean control subjects, normal glucose-tolerant obese subjects, and subjects with non-insulin dependent diabetes mellitus (NIDDM). To convert insulin concentrations from pmol/l to μU/ml divide by 7.175 (from reference 722, with permission)

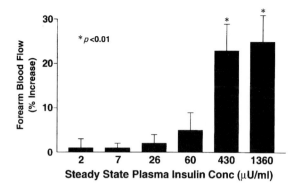

Figure 42 Dose–response curve relating forearm blood flow and plasma insulin concentration during euglycemic insulin clamps performed for 130 min in healthy control subjects. The rise in forearm blood flow was significant only at the two highest (pharmacologic) plasma insulin concentrations. The data are expressed as the mean of the increase above baseline for each individual subject (drawn from data presented in references 592–596)

insulin's vasodilatory action (Figure 41). A number of other studies have provided support for the concept that insulin causes vasodilation and augments muscle blood flow in normal subjects [729–733]. However, for every study that has demonstrated that insulin augments blood flow to peripheral tissues *in vivo*, there are at least as many—if not more—studies which have failed to demonstrate any stimulatory effect of insulin on blood flow to a variety of tissues, including leg and forearm muscle, splanchnic tissues, and kidney [3, 4, 350, 365, 400, 404, 416, 428, 443, 592–596, 611, 624, 631, 641, 694, 734–738]. The reasons for these discrepant findings are not clear. However, as reviewed by Yki-Jarvinen and colleagues [739], a number of factors may be involved. The level of hyperinsulinemia and duration of insulin infusion are most important. When insulin is infused to achieve pharmacologic levels of hyperinsulinemia (>100 μU/ml) a modest dose–response rise in forearm blood flow can uniformly be demonstrated [594] (Figure 42). Within

the physiologic range of hyperinsulinemia, prolonging the insulin infusion for more than 2 hours leads to a time-related increase in leg blood flow (reviewed in references 739 and 740). Since in the studies of Baron and colleagues [722] the blood flow measurements are made after 2–3 hours of hyperinsulinemia, one can question the physiologic significance of their findings. Another problem with the blood flow measurements during insulin infusion is the great individual variability which can range from −12% to +60% [740]. The reasons underlying this large between-individual variation are not known but clearly make it difficult to interpret experimentally induced changes in muscle blood. The discrepant findings concerning the effect of insulin on muscle blood flow cannot be explained by the methods employed to measure blood flow, i.e. dye dilution, plethysmography, thermodilution, PET scanning [1, 3, 4, 611, 739, 740], but may be related to differences in experimental design and patient characteristics.

Recently, Yki-Jarvinen et al [739] have provided data which strongly argue against a role for increased blood flow in the regulation of muscle glucose uptake. These investigators infused bradykinin, an endothelium (nitric oxide) dependent vasodilator, locally into the femoral artery of normal subjects under basal and under euglycemic hyperinsulinemic conditions. Despite a ~60% increase in leg blood flow, leg muscle glucose uptake did not increase because of a proportional and opposite decline in arterio-venous glucose concentration difference. Similar results have been reported by Natali et al [741] who used adenosine to increase forearm blood flow by 100%, yet observed no rise in forearm glucose uptake. These results indicate that blood flow *per se* is not an important regulator of tissue glucose disposal.

In studies demonstrating an insulin-induced increase in blood flow, this has been shown to be endothelium (i.e. nitric oxide) dependent. Thus, N-monomethyl-L-arginine, a specific inhibitor of the synthesis of endothelium-derived nitric oxide, has been shown to block completely the insulin-induced rise in forearm blood flow [723, 724, 742]. In one study, L-NMMA caused a 20% decrease in basal forearm blood flow [723], while in another study L-NMMA had no effect on basal forearm blood flow [742]. Thus, it is unclear what component, if any, of resting muscle blood flow is endothelium-dependent. Even more conflicting are the results obtained concerning the effect of L-NMMA on muscle glucose uptake [723, 724, 742]. Sherrer et al [742] have shown that L-NMMA infusion into the brachial artery completely blocked vasodilation and the increase in forearm blood flow during a euglycemic insulin clamp. Even though insulin-induced vasodilation was totally inhibited, insulin-stimulated forearm glucose uptake was unaffected. Thus, this study [742] demonstrates that the effect of insulin on muscle blood flow and glucose uptake are completely dissociable and argues against any role of increased blood flow in insulin's stimulatory effect on muscle glucose uptake. In marked contrast to these results, Baron and colleagues [723, 724] have shown that the inhibition of insulin-stimulated leg blood flow by L-NMMA significantly reduces leg glucose uptake. However, the inhibitory effect of L-NMMA on glucose uptake was much more apparent at pharmacologic than at physiologic plasma insulin concentrations [724].

In the studies by Baron and colleagues [726–728] NIDDM subjects were more resistant than non-diabetic obese individuals and this was largely accounted for by a greater impairment of insulin-stimulated blood flow. Intensive insulin treatment and improved glycemic control partially reversed the defects in insulin-stimulated blood flow and whole body insulin-mediated glucose disposal [726]. In contrast to the results of Baron and co-workers, Neahring et al [743] failed to find any impairment in insulin-stimulated blood flow in non-diabetic obese subjects.

In summary, there is evidence to suggest a potential role for impaired insulin-stimulated muscle blood flow in the insulin resistance observed in NIDDM, but these results must be viewed with some degree of caution for a number of reasons: (a) many investigators have failed to demonstrate any increase in muscle, splanchnic, or renal blood flow in response to physiologic hyperinsulinemia [3, 4, 350, 365, 400, 404, 416, 428, 443, 592-596, 611, 624, 631, 641, 684, 734-738]; (b) inhibition of insulin-stimulated blood flow has been shown to have no effect on muscle glucose uptake by some investigators [742]; (c) the use of vasodilators to augment muscle blood flow is not associated with an increase in muscle glucose uptake either under basal or insulin-stimulated conditions [739, 741]; (d) many investigators have documented a number of primary cellular defects (i.e. insulin receptor tyrosine kinase, insulin receptor signal transduction, glucose transport, glucose phosphorylation, glycogen synthase) which can account for the majority, if not all, of the insulin resistance *in vivo* in NIDDM patients. Moreover, these basic cellular defects in insulin-mediated muscle and adipose tissue metabolism persist *in vitro*, making it difficult to envision how a reduction in insulin-stimulated blood flow can contribute to the insulin resistance in NIDDM patients.

One last issue needs to be addressed when interpreting the effect of any vasoactive molecule on muscle blood flow and glucose uptake. In such circumstances one would expect that the increase in muscle blood flow would be offset precisely by a decrease in the arteriovenous glucose concentration difference and that glucose uptake would remain unchanged. This is exactly what has been demonstrated in man by Nuutila et al [739]. On the other hand, if the increase in blood flow resulted in the opening of previously closed vascular beds and the recruitment of new muscle fibers, muscle glucose uptake would increase, even though the plasma insulin concentration remained unchanged. This important distinction has yet to be addressed by any published articles. Clearly, much more scientific investigation will be needed to resolve the current controversy concerning the role of insulin-induced changes in blood flow on the regulation of glucose utilization in healthy and NIDDM subjects.

Amylin and Calcitonin Gene-related Peptide

Although amylin (IAPP) was initially thought to be responsible for the defect in insulin secretion in NIDDM (see earlier discussion), more recently it has been suggested to be responsible for the impairment in insulin sensitivity. Studies both *in vivo* and *in vitro* have demonstrated that amylin causes insulin resistance by interfering with glycogen synthesis [745–748]. A similar defect in insulin action has been reported with CGRP [746, 748]. Unfortunately, all of these infusion studies [191, 745–750] have employed pharmacologic levels of amylin and CGRP, and recent investigations have failed to demonstrate any difference in either basal or meal-stimulated plasma amylin concentrations between type 2 diabetic and control subjects [192]. Since amylin is not known to be concentrated in muscle, its role in the insulin resistance of NIDDM seems remote [162, 193]. Moreover, a recent study using the insulin clamp failed to demonstrate any effect of amylin on insulin sensitivity despite a 100-fold increase in the plasma amylin concentration

[194]. By contrast, local concentrations of CGRP in skeletal muscle may be considerably higher than the simultaneous plasma concentration, because it is secreted by sensory afferent nerve fibers [195], which are abundant in skeletal muscle [196]. This raises the possibility that part of the insulin resistance in NIDDM may be neurogenic in origin and related to an excessive secretion of CGRP. Surprisingly little work has appeared on the role, if any, of CGRP in the insulin resistance of NIDDM since the last edition of this textbook.

Tumor Necrosis Factor-alpha (TNF-α)

TNF-α, previously called cachexin, was initially isolated and identified as the active factor which induced tissue necrosis in animals infected with bacteria [198, 199]. Circulating TNF-α subsequently was shown to be elevated in a variety of catabolic states, including cancer and infection, which were associated with severe wasting, i.e. the 'cachexia' syndrome. It is now recognized that TNF-α is a cytokine which has many diverse functions, including modulation of the immune system, apoptosis, tumor cell lysis and others. Most recently, TNF-α has been shown to have profound effects on whole body lipid metabolism and on the regulation of glucose metabolism.

Studies in animal models of NIDDM and obesity have suggested that TNF-α plays a role in the development of insulin resistance in these two metabolic disorders [198–203]. TNF-α inhibits insulin-stimulated glucose uptake in adipose and muscle tissue [202, 203]. Although it originally was thought that TNF-α induced insulin resistance by down-regulating Glut 4 mRNA and protein levels in fat cells and myocytes [200, 204, 205], more recent information indicates that TNF-α works more proximally by inhibiting the phosphorylation of insulin receptor tyrosine kinase and IRS-1 [198, 201, 202, 206], as well as other intracellular proteins that have been implicated in insulin action. A similar inhibition of tyrosine kinase in liver also has been demonstrated [207].

In non-diabetic, insulin-resistant obese human subjects mRNA levels of TNF-α in adipose tissue have been shown to be increased 2.5-fold [202] and similar observations have been made in muscle from NIDDM individuals [208]. In obesity, circulating TNF-α concentrations have been shown to be very low [202, 209], while one study demonstrated increased TNF-α production in NIDDM subjects [382]. Of great interest, Garvey et al have shown a very strong correlation between the amount of TNF-α mRNA in muscle and the rate of insulin-mediated whole body glucose disposal in NIDDM subjects [208]. Unfortunately, plasma TNF-α levels were not measured in this study. At present, there is no evidence that TNF-α produced within cells has an effect on cellular function. Most authorities believe that the action of the cytokine is mediated via specific TNF-α receptors on the cell surface [208, 209].

In a rodent model of obesity, Hotamisligil et al [200–202] showed that treatment with an antibody against TNF-α improved the insulin resistance and lowered plasma glucose and FFA levels. In an attempt to define the role of TNF-α in the insulin resistance observed in obese NIDDM humans, Ofei et al [209] utilized a recombinant-engineered human TNF-α neutralizing antibody. Six weeks after treatment with the antibody, which was shown to reduce the circulating TNF-α concentration to unmeasurable levels, no effect on insulin sensitivity or glucose homeostasis was observed. However, a definite conclusion about the role, if any, of TNF-α in the insulin resistance of NIDDM must await the development of a specific inhibitor of TNF-α biosynthesis.

In summary, although there is good evidence to implicate TNF-α in the development of insulin resistance in certain rodent models of obesity and NIDDM, and the findings of Garvey and co-workers [208] in human diabetes are provocative, the presently available data in man are too meager to allow any definite conclusion about the pathogenetic role of TNF-α in the insulin resistance of obesity and NIDDM.

Hyperglycemia and Glucose Toxicity

A number of studies, employing both *in vivo* and *in vitro* techniques, have demonstrated that chronic physiologic hyperglycemia can lead to the development of insulin resistance, which results from down-regulation of the glucose transport system as well as from post glucose transport steps. This is discussed in detail in Chapter 32.

GENETIC DEFECTS IN NIDDM

An overwhelming amount of evidence has been provided to support a genetic basis for NIDDM, although the number of genes involved and the mode of inheritance remains unclear [23, 279, 280, 444–450] (see Chapter 3). The simplest and most straightforward approach to identifying genes that are associated with NIDDM is to examine loci which encode proteins that are known to play an important role in glucose homeostasis (i.e. the candidate gene approach).

At present over 250 candidate genes have been examined for linkage or association to NIDDM. Although individual investigators have claimed linkage or association to specific candidate genes, none of these linkages/associations have been shown to be significant within a given ethnic group or different across ethnic backgrounds [32, 239, 278–280, 419, 444, 445, 451–453, 455, 457, 464, 467–474].

Because the candidate gene approach has proven unsuccessful to date, a number of investigators have undertaken genome-wide searches to identify potential susceptibility loci for NIDDM in man. Such studies are possible because of the identification of satellite markers spaced at 1–5 cM intervals throughout the human genome [280, 445–447, 475, 476]. Using this approach, evidence for linkage to markers on chromosome 2 (in Mexican-Americans) [452], on chromosomes 6 and 11 (in Mexican-Americans) [477], on chromosomes 1, 4, and 7 (in Pima Indians) [473, 478, 479, 482, 483], on chromosome 7 in Europids [484] and on chromosome 12 (in Finns) [485] has been reported. Although these results are very exciting, it is obvious that different investigators have found linkage to different chromosomal regions, even within the same ethnic population [452, 477]. It also is somewhat surprising that different chromosomal regions have been linked to NIDDM in Pima Indians [473, 478, 479, 482, 483] and Mexican-Americans [452, 477], two populations which are believed to have been derived from a common ancestry. Even after such linkage studies have been confirmed, the task of identifying the specific gene(s) in a given chromosomal region that is responsible for NIDDM remains daunting. Recent advances in positional cloning [486, 487] offer promise for the eventual identification of the gene(s) responsible for human NIDDM.

ACQUIRED DETERMINANTS OF INSULIN RESISTANCE

Within the normal population, there is a 4–5-fold variation in insulin sensitivity [274, 307–309, 327]. However, normal glucose tolerance is maintained because the pancreas is able to increase its secretion of insulin to precisely compensate for the defect in insulin action [274, 307–309, 327] (Figure 14). It is now clear that both acquired and genetic factors contribute to the development of insulin resistance. In this section we will review the contribution of acquired factors that can cause or are associated with insulin resistance. These acquired factors, which lead to the development of insulin resistance in the normal population, also contribute to the insulin resistance in NIDDM subjects, and make it difficult to differentiate between what is inherited and what is acquired in patients with NIDDM.

Age [308, 309, 488] and *obesity* [1, 39, 63, 190, 197, 272, 273, 343, 344, 391, 441, 443] are major factors which contribute to the development of insulin resistance. Yki-Jarvinen has estimated that 35% of the variability in insulin action in the normal population can be explained by these two factors alone [261]. A number of investigators have shown that with advancing age there is a progressive decline in insulin sensitivity, although in absolute terms, this aging effect is modest [308, 309, 488]. In contrast, obesity has been shown to exert a major negative effect on insulin sensitivity [1, 39, 63, 190, 197, 272, 273, 343, 344, 391, 441, 443]. Both the total amount of fat in the body, as well as its distribution [22, 489–492], have a negative impact on insulin sensitivity. Intra-abdominal fat accumulation, manifested by an increased waist to hip ratio (i.e. male type obesity), has an especially deleterious effect on insulin sensitivity. By contrast, accumulation of fat in the buttock region (i.e. female type obesity) has a relatively minor effect on insulin sensitivity. The deleterious effect of intra-abdominal fat tissue has been related to the high lipolytic rate of this adipose tissue depot [489, 492, 493]; this results in elevated portal and peripheral FFA levels, leading to hepatic and muscle resistance, respectively. The mechanisms via which increased plasma FFA concentrations and elevated rates of lipid oxidation contribute to the development of insulin resistance were discussed in an earlier section. It is of interest that, when insulin-mediated whole-body glucose metabolism (expressed as mg/kg of body weight/min) is compared in normal weight men and women who are equally physically fit, no significant difference between genders is noted [494, 495]. However, the failure to observe any gender-related difference in insulin sensitivity results from two opposing effects in women: decreased muscle mass (which is associated with a decreased rate of whole body glucose uptake) and a smaller intra-abdominal fat mass (which increases whole body glucose disposal) [261].

Decreased *physical activity* is another acquired factor that has been shown to be associated with insulin resistance [264, 541, 546]. Conversely, physical training has been shown to improve insulin action [541, 547, 620, 656]. Not surprisingly, a close correlation between the maximum aerobic power (VO_{2max}) and whole body insulin-mediated glucose disposal has been demonstrated in both non-diabetic and diabetic subjects [261, 276, 541, 656]. With regard to this, it is noteworthy that NIDDM subjects uniformly have been demonstrated to have a lower VO_{2max} than non-diabetic subjects of similar age and body weight [261, 541, 656], and part of the insulin resistance in NIDDM individuals is the result of decreased physical training.

Recently, smoking has been shown to be associated with the development of insulin resistance and this can be reversed by cessation of smoking [657, 658]. The mechanisms responsible for the deleterious effect of smoking on insulin sensitivity have yet to be defined. Alterations in sympathetic nervous system activity have been suggested as the cause of the insulin resistance, but one also could argue that decreased physical activity due to the adverse effects of smoking on the cardiovascular and pulmonary systems is responsible for the impairment in insulin sensitivity.

Most recently, non-diabetic subjects with essential hypertension have been shown to be resistant to insulin [327, 488, 659] and some investigators have suggested that the combination of hypertension plus microalbuminuria explains the majority of the insulin resistance in NIDDM [660]. This latter suggestion seems untenable since most NIDDM subjects are neither hypertensive nor have microalbuminuria, yet they are resistant to insulin. Although hypertension *per se* is not an acquired disease, the insulin resistance in hypertensive individuals could be acquired secondarily to alterations in the cardiovascular system, muscle blood flow, or muscle fiber type. With regard to this, two recent studies have demonstrated that when patients with essential hypertension and a decrease in VO_{2max} are matched with non-hypertensive control subjects who have a similarly low VO_{2max}, no or very little difference in insulin sensitivity between the two groups could be demonstrated [661, 662]. This suggests that it is the decrease in VO_{2max} and not the hypertension *per se* that is responsible for the insulin resistance.

Thus, when evaluating the etiology of insulin resistance in NIDDM subjects, it is essential to consider both acquired and genetic factors. It also should be remembered that some of the 'acquired' factors considered above also may have an inherited or genetic component, i.e. obesity, decreased VO_{2max}, and essential hypertension. Moreover, the development of NIDDM can lead to acquired defects in thermogenesis [663, 664, 744], which in turn can contribute to the development of obesity. One could argue that the reduced VO_{2max} found in NIDDM subjects results secondarily to the diabetic state or some associated condition, i.e. impaired cardiovascular function or insulin resistance. Thus, in any given NIDDM patient the component of insulin resistance that is acquired vs. that which is genetic is difficult to ascertain.

PATHOGENESIS OF NIDDM: SUMMARY AND SYNTHESIS

The maintenance of normal glucose homeostasis is dependent upon a finely balanced dynamic interaction between tissue (muscle and liver) sensitivity to insulin and insulin secretion. Even in the presence of severe insulin resistance, a perfectly normal B cell is capable of secreting sufficient amounts of insulin to offset the defect in insulin action. Thus, *the evolution of NIDDM requires the presence of defects in both insulin secretion and in insulin action* and both of these defects can have a genetic as well as an acquired component. When NIDDM patients initially present to the physician, they will have had their diabetes for many

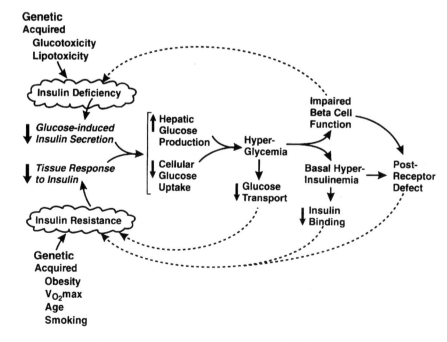

Figure 43 Pathogenetic sequence of events leading to the development of insulin resistance in NIDDM. Note that whether the primary defect initiating the glucose intolerance resides in the B-cell or in peripheral tissues, development of insulin resistance eventually will ensue or become aggravated, respectively. By the time that overt fasting hyperglycemia (>140 mg/dl) develops, both impaired insulin secretion and severe insulin resistance are present. Broken arrows represent positive feedback loops, which result in self-perpetuation of primary defects (adapted from reference 1, with permission)

years, and defects in both insulin action and insulin secretion will be well established [1, 5]. At this stage it is not possible to define which defect came first in the natural history of the disease. Nevertheless, it is now clear that, in any given diabetic patient, whatever defect (i.e. insulin resistance or impaired insulin secretion) initiates the disturbance in glucose metabolism, it eventually will be followed by the emergence of its counterpart. Figure 43 represents an attempt to integrate the principal pathogenetic factors responsible for the development of NIDDM as we currently understand them. It should be noted that the sequence of events outlined in Figure 43, like the development of NIDDM, is still in a state of dynamic evolution that is meant to be altered as new data become available. However, this hypothesis has as its foundation a large body of existing experimental evidence. Much knowledge has been gained in the short period since this topic was last reviewed [1, 5], and the explosion in molecular biology has added tremendously to this knowledge. The following discussion emphasizes two points: (a) individuals who are destined to develop NIDDM inherit a gene (or set of genes) that confers insulin resistance; and (b) the full-blown diabetic syndrome with overt fasting hyperglycemia develops only in those subjects in whom a concomitant insulin secretory defect, be it acquired (as through glucolipotoxicity) or inherited, also is present.

Primary Defect in Insulin Sensitivity

Insulin resistance is a nearly universal finding in patients with established NIDDM. In normal weight and obese individuals with impaired glucose tolerance, in NIDDM subjects with mild fasting hyperglycemia (110–140 mg/dl, 6.1–7.8 mmol/l) both the basal and glucose-stimulated plasma insulin levels are increased. Although the first-phase insulin response may be decreased in some of these subjects, the total insulin response is increased. In each of these groups, tissue sensitivity to insulin, measured with the insulin clamp technique, has been shown to be diminished. Prospective studies have conclusively demonstrated that hyperinsulinemia and insulin resistance precede the development of IGT, and that IGT represents the forerunner of NIDDM [1, 52, 54, 59, 60, 62, 63, 66–70, 72, 73, 78, 309, 316]. This scenario has been well documented in Pima Indians, Mexican-Americans and Pacific islanders. It is noteworthy that all of these populations are characterized by obesity and a younger onset of diabetes. Such results provide conclusive evidence that insulin resistance is the inherited defect that initiates the diabetic condition in the majority of type 2 diabetic patients. Recent studies in normal glucose-tolerant first-degree relatives of diabetic individuals,

and in the offspring of two diabetic parents, indicate that the inherited defect in insulin action most likely results from an abnormality in the glycogen synthetic pathway in muscle [64, 75, 77, 626]. Hepatic glucose production (HGP) is also resistant to the suppressive action of fasting hyperinsulinemia in these groups. Because of the compensatory increase in insulin secretion, initially the insulin resistance by itself is not sufficient to impair glucose uptake by muscle or to cause an increase in HGP. As the insulin resistance progresses and muscle glucose uptake becomes further impaired, the postprandial rise in plasma glucose concentration becomes excessive but the increase in basal hyperinsulinemia is sufficient to maintain the fasting plasma glucose concentration and HGP within the normal range. Nonetheless, there is an excessive postprandial rise in plasma glucose concentration and a longer time is required to restore normoglycemia after each meal. Eventually the insulin resistance becomes so severe that the compensatory hyperinsulinemia is no longer sufficient to maintain the fasting glucose concentration at the basal level. The development of hyperglycemia further stimulates B-cell secretion of insulin, and the resultant hyperinsulinemia causes a down-regulation both of insulin receptor number and the intracellular events involved in insulin action, thus exacerbating the insulin resistance. Initially, the hyperglycemia-induced increase in insulin secretion serves a compensatory function to maintain near-normal glucose tolerance. In some individuals the persistent stimulus to the B cell to over-secrete insulin leads to a progressive loss of B-cell function (see Figures 3 and 4). In this regard, recent studies have indicated that chronic hyperglycemia (glucose toxicity) or disturbances in lipid metabolism (lipotoxicity) may be responsible for the defect in insulin secretion. It is likely that those individuals in whom 'glucolipotoxicity' leads to a progressive impairment in insulin secretion have an underlying genetic defect in B-cell function that is unmasked by the persistent hyperglycemia and/or derangement in lipid metabolism. The resultant insulinopenia leads to the emergence of, or exacerbation of, postreceptor defects in insulin action. Many of the intracellular events involved in glucose metabolism are dependent upon the surge of insulin that occurs 3–4 times per day in response to nutrient ingestion. When the insulin response becomes deficient, the activity of the glucose transport system becomes severely impaired, and a number of key intracellular enzymatic steps involved in glucose metabolism become depressed. Additionally, when severe insulinopenia ensues, plasma FFA levels rise and fatty acid oxidation increases, further contributing to the defects in intracellular glucose disposal. In addition there is compelling evidence that hyperglycemia *per se* can down-regulate the glucose transport system, as well as a number of other intracellular events involved in insulin action (glucose toxicity) and a similar argument can be made concerning the intracellular derangement in lipid metabolism (Randle cycle). This pathogenetic sequence can explain all of the clinical and laboratory features observed in NIDDM patients. Insofar as the cellular defect is generalized, both hepatic and peripheral tissues (and possibly the B cells themselves) would manifest the insulin resistance, and the numerous metabolic alterations characteristic of the diabetic state could be related to one and the same primary defect.

At present the basic defect responsible for the insulin resistance remains unknown. Although diabetologists traditionally have tended to focus their attention on intracellular defects involving glucose metabolism—i.e. insulin receptor signal transduction, glucose transport, glucose phosphorylation, glycogen synthase—a number of other explanations are equally plausible (Figure 44). Thus, abnormalities in intracellular lipid metabolism, enhanced sympathetic nervous system activity, alterations in muscle blood flow or fiber type, disturbances in ion pump activity, etc., all could represent the primary or inherited (genetic) defect in NIDDM. The B cell would respond to the insulin resistance regardless of its etiology by augmenting its secretion of insulin. The resultant hyperinsulinemia, in turn, would serve as a self-amplifying factor to further worsen the insulin resistance. Eventually, B-cell exhaustion would ensue, reproducing the sequence of events outlined in Figure 43.

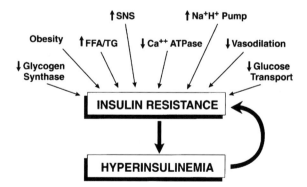

Figure 44 Schematic representation of potential defects that can lead to the development of insulin resistance in NIDDM. Regardless of the etiology of the insulin resistance, the B cell will enhance its secretion of insulin to offset the defect in insulin action. The resultant compensatory hyperinsulinemia will down-regulate a variety of intracellular events involved in insulin action and thus serve as a self-perpetuating cause of the insulin resistance. FFA, free fatty acids; SNS, sympathetic nervous system activity; TG, triglycerides

Primary Defect in Insulin Secretion

Most evidence indicates that hyperinsulinemia precedes the development of IGT and NIDDM [1, 52, 54, 59, 60, 62, 63, 66–70, 72, 73, 78, 309, 316]. Moreover, in populations that are genetically predisposed to develop NIDDM, hyperinsulinemia is a common finding. Such observations strongly argue against insulinopenia as the initiating cause of NIDDM in the majority of individuals. However, there clearly are some diabetic subjects in whom the first and/or second phases of insulin secretion are impaired. In such individuals the defect in insulin secretion will result in an excessive, prolonged rise in plasma glucose concentration. The postprandial hyperglycemia will present a persistent stimulus to the B-cell and the total amount of insulin secreted in response to the meal may actually be increased early in the development of diabetes. Initially, this postprandial hyperinsulinemia may even be sufficient to return the fasting plasma glucose concentration to normal. As the diabetes becomes more severe (as a consequence of the progressive nature of the B-cell defect), the plasma insulin response (although still increased in absolute terms) will become insufficient to return the plasma glucose concentration to its basal level and fasting hyperglycemia will ensue. Fasting hyperglycemia will present a persistent stimulus to the pancreas to over-secrete insulin throughout the day and fasting hyperinsulinemia will result. The elevated fasting insulin concentration will lead to a decrease in the number of insulin receptors on insulin target tissues and a down-regulation of the intracellular events involved in insulin action. This pathogenetic sequence of events could explain all of the laboratory features in the patient with impaired glucose tolerance (i.e. fasting euglycemia, an impaired but not overtly diabetic glucose tolerance test, fasting hyperinsulinemia, an increased insulin response to glucose) and in the patient with early diabetes mellitus (mild fasting hyperglycemia, a diabetic glucose tolerance test, fasting hyperinsulinemia, normal or increased plasma insulin response to glucose). In such an individual the basal rate of HGP would remain within the normal range because of the restraining effects of fasting hyperglycemia and fasting hyperinsulinemia on glucose release by the liver, whereas the efficiency of tissue glucose uptake would be markedly reduced.

As the plasma insulin response becomes progressively more impaired, as a result of the genetic B-cell defect, 'pancreatic exhaustion', or 'glucose toxicity', both the early and late phases of insulin secretion will become absolutely deficient. However, the basal plasma insulin level will remain elevated because of the persistent stimulus presented to the B cell by the fasting hyperglycemia. With the onset of insulinopenia, be it relative or absolute, marked fasting hyperglycemia will ensue because of excessive glucose production by the liver and a further reduction in tissue glucose clearance. Another important pathogenetic disturbance that emerges with the development of insulinopenia is a postreceptor defect in insulin action. The eventual clinical picture would be that of a typical NIDDM patient.

In summary, the sequence of events, starting with a defect in insulin secretion and leading to the emergence of insulin resistance, appears to be quite plausible on the basis of the information currently available. What remains to be determined is how commonly a primary B-cell defect and resultant insulinopenia initiates the sequence of events leading to the development of NIDDM in humans.

Combined Defects in Insulin Sensitivity and Insulin Secretion

Lastly, it is possible the defects in insulin action (involving both muscle and liver) and insulin secretion result from the same, as of yet unidentified genetic abnormality, and that insulin resistance and impaired B-cell function evolve in parallel.

REFERENCES

1. DeFronzo RA. Lilly Lecture. The triumvirate: beta cell, muscle, liver. A collusion responsible for NIDDM. Diabetes 1988; 37: 667–87.
2. DeFronzo RA, Ferrannini E. Regulation of hepatic glucose metabolism in humans. Diabetes Metab Rev 1987; 3: 415–59.
3. DeFronzo RA, Jacot E, Jequier E, Maeder E, Wahren J, Felber JP. The effect of insulin on the disposal of intravenous glucose: results from indirect calorimetry. Diabetes 1981; 30: 1000–1007.
4. DeFronzo RA, Gunnarsson R, Bjorkman O, Olsson M, Wahren J. Effects of insulin on peripheral and splanchnic glucose metabolism in non-insulin dependent diabetes mellitus. J Clin Invest 1985; 76: 149–55.
5. DeFronzo RA. Pathogenesis of type 2 (non-insulin dependent) diabetes mellitus: a balanced overview. Diabetologia 1992; 35: 389–97.
6. Mari A, Wahren J, DeFronzo RA, Ferrannini E. Glucose absorption and production following oral glucose: comparison of compartmental and arteriovenous-difference methods. Metabolism 1994; 43: 1419–25.
7. Katz LD, Glickman MG, Rapoport S, Ferrannini E, DeFronzo RA. Splanchnic and peripheral diposal of oral glucose in man. Diabetes 1983; 32: 675–9.
8. Ferrannini E, Bjorkman O, Reichard GA Jr et al. The disposal of an oral glucose load in healthy subjects. Diabetes 1985; 34: 580–8.
9. Taylor R, Magnusson I, Rothman DL et al. Direct assessment of liver glycogen storage by ^{13}C nuclear magnetic resonance spectroscopy and regulation of glucose homeostasis after a mixed meal in normal subjects. J Clin Invest 1996; 97: 126–32.
10. Bjorntorp P, Sjostrom L. Carbohydrate storage in man: speculations and some quantitative considerations. Metabolism 1978; 27(suppl. 2): 1853–65.
11. Bjorntorp P, Berchtold P, Holm J. The glucose uptake of human adipose tissue in obesity. Eur J Clin Invest 1971; 1: 480–5.
12. Jansson P-A, Larsson A, Smith U, Lonroth P. Lactate release from the subcutaneous tissue in lean and obese men. J Clin Invest 1994; 93: 240–6.
13. Kalant N, Leibovici D, Fukushima J, Kuyumjian J, Ozaki S. Insulin responsiveness of superficial forearm tissues in type 2 (non-insulin dependent) diabetes. Diabetologia 1982; 22: 239–44.
14. Randle PJ. Glucokinase and candidate genes for type 2 (non-insulin-dependent) diabetes mellitus. Diabetologia 1993; 36: 269–75.
15. Groop LC, Bonadonna RC, Del Prato S et al. Glucose and free fatty acid metabolism in non-insulin dependent diabetes mellitus. Evidence for multiple sites of insulin resistance. J Clin Invest 1989; 84: 205–15.
16. Reaven GM. The fourth Musketeer—from Alexandre Dumas to Claude Bernard. Diabetologia 1995; 38: 3–13.
17. Foley JE. Rationale and application of fatty acid oxidation inhibitors in treatment of diabetes mellitus. Diabetes Care 1992; 15: 773–84.
18. Prentki M, Corkey BE. Are the beta cell signaling molecules malonyl-CoA and cytosolic long-chain acyl-CoA implicated in multiple tissue defects of obesity and NIDDM? Diabetes 1996; 45: 273–83.
19. Unger RH. Lipotoxicity in the pathogenesis of obesity-dependent NIDDM. Genetic and clinical implications. Diabetes 1995; 44: 863–70.
20. Arner P, Pollare T, Lithell H. Different aetiologies of Type 2 (non-insulin-dependent) diabetes mellitus in obese and non-obese subjects. Diabetologia 1991; 34: 483–7.
21. Banerji MA, Lebovitz HE. Insulin action in black Americans with NIDDM. Diabetes Care 1992; 15: 1295–302.
22. Banerji MA, Chaiken RL, Gordon D, Kral JG, Lebovitz HE. Does intra-abdominal adipose tissue in black men determine whether NIDDM is insulin-resistant or insulin-sensitive? Diabetes 1995; 44: 141–6.
23. Zimmet PZ. The pathogenesis and prevention of diabetes in adults. Diabetes Care 1995; 18: 1050–64.
24. Byrne MM, Sturis J, Fajans SS et al. Altered insulin secretory responses to glucose in subjects with a mutation in the MODY1 gene on chromosome 20. Diabetes 1995; 44: 699–704.
25. Sturis J, Kurland IJ, Byrne MM et al. Compensation in pancreatic β-cell function in subjects with glucokinase mutations. Diabetes 1994; 43: 718–23.
26. Clement K, Pueyo ME, Vaxillaire M et al. Assessment of insulin sensitivity in glucokinase-deficient subjects. Diabetologia 1996; 39: 82–90.
27. Halter JB, Graf RJ, Porte D. Potentiation of insulin secretory responses by plasma glucose levels in man: evidence that hyperglycemia in diabetes compensates for impaired glucose potentiation. J Clin Endocrinol Metab 1979; 48: 946–54.
28. Ward WK, Bolgiano DC, McKnight B, Halter J, Porte D. Diminished beta cell secretory capacity in patients with non-insulin-dependent diabetes mellitus. J Clin Invest 1984; 74: 1318–28.
29. Hales CN. The pathogenesis of NIDDM. Diabetologia 1994; 37(suppl. 2): S162–8.

30. DeFronzo RA, Ferrannini E, Koivisto V. New concepts in the pathogenesis and treatment of non-insulin-dependent diabetes mellitus. Am J Med 1983; 74 (IA): 52–81.

31. Polonsky KS, Sturis J, Bell GI. Non-insulin-dependent diabetes mellitus—a genetically programmed failure of the beta cell to compensate for insulin resistance. New Engl J Med 1996; 334: 777–83.

32. Polonsky KS. Lilly Lecture 1994. The beta cell in diabetes: from molecular genetics to clinical research. Diabetes 1995; 44: 705–17.

33. Davies MJ, Metcalfe J, Gray IP, Day JL, Hales CN. Insulin deficiency rather than hyperinsulinaemia in newly diagnosed type 2 diabetes mellitus. Diabet Med 1993; 10: 305–12.

34. Nesher R, Della Casa L, Litvin Y et al. Insulin deficiency and insulin resistance in type 2 (non-insulin-dependent) diabetes: quantitative contributions of pancreatic and peripheral responses to glucose homeostasis. Eur J Clin Invest 1987; 17: 266–74.

35. Cerasi E. Insulin deficiency and insulin resistance in the pathogenesis of NIDDM: is a divorce possible? Diabetologia 1995; 38: 992–7.

36. O'Rahilly SP, Turner RC, Matthews DR. Impaired pulsatile secretion of insulin in relatives of patients with non-insulin-dependent diabetes. New Engl J Med 1988; 318: 1225–30.

37. O'Rahilly SP, Nugent Z, Rudenski AS et al. B-cell dysfunction, rather than insulin insensitivity, is the primary defect in familial type 2 diabetes. Lancet 1986; 2: 360–64.

38. Temple RC, Carrington Ca, Luzio SD et al. Insulin deficiency in non-insulin-dependent diabetes. Lancet 1989; 1: 293–5.

39. Bonadonna RC, Groop L, Kraemer N, Ferrannini E, Del Prato S, DeFronzo RA. Obesity and insulin resistance in man. A dose response study. Metabolism 1990; 39: 452–9.

40. Faber OK, Damsgaard EM. Insulin secretion in type II diabetes. Acta Endocrinol 1984; 262(suppl.): 47–50.

41. Faber OK, Hagen C, Binder C et al. Kinetics of human connecting peptide in normal and diabetic subjects. J Clin Invest 1978; 62: 197–203.

42. DeFronzo RA, Ferrannini E, Simonson DC. Fasting hyperglycemia in non-insulin-dependent diabetes mellitus: contributions of excessive hepatic glucose production and impaired tissue glucose uptake. Metabolism 1989; 38: 387–95.

43. Matsuda M, DeFronzo RA. Isolation of hepatic and peripheral insulin sensitivity: application to the investigation of inherited or acquired defects in NIDDM. Diabetes 1996; 45(suppl. 1): 17A.

44. Bogardus C, Lillioja S, Howard BV, Reaven G, Mott D. Relationships between insulin secretion, insulin action, and fasting plasma glucose concentration in non-diabetic and non-insulin-dependent subjects. J Clin Invest 1984; 74: 1238–46.

45. Reaven GM, Miller R. Study of the relationship between glucose and insulin responses to an oral glucose load in man. Diabetes 1968; 17: 560–69.

46. Welborn TA, Stenhouse NS, Johnson CJ. Factors determining serum insulin response in a population sample. Diabetologia 1969; 5: 263–6.

47. Savage PJ, Dippe SE, Bennett PH et al. Hyperinsulinemia and hypoinsulinemia. Diabetes 1975; 24: 362–8.

48. Zimmet P, Whitehouse S, Alford F, Chisholm D. The relationship of insulin response to a glucose stimulus over a wide range of glucose tolerance. Diabetologia 1978; 15: 23–7.

49. Reaven GM, Miller RG. An attempt to define the nature of chemical diabetes using a multidimensional analysis. Diabetologia 1979; 16: 17–24.

50. Martin FIR, Wyatt GB, Griew AR, Hauranelia M, Higginbotham LI. Diabetes mellitus in urban and rural communities in Papua New Guinea: studies of prevalence and plasma insulin. Diabetologia 1980; 18: 369–74.

51. Zimmet P, Whitehouse S. Biomodality of fasting and two-hour glucose tolerance distributions in a Micronesian population. Diabetes 1978; 27: 793–800.

52. Sicree RA, Zimmet P, King HO, Coventry JO. Plasma insulin response among Nauruans. Prediction of deterioration in glucose tolerance over 6 years. Diabetes 1987; 36: 179–86.

53. Zimmet P, Whitehouse S, Kiss J. Ethnic variability in the plasma insulin response to oral glucose in Polynesian and Micronesian subjects. Diabetes 1979; 28: 624–8.

54. Saad MF, Knowler WC, Pettitt DJ, Nelson RG, Mott DM, Bennett PH. Sequential changes in serum insulin concentration during development of non-insulin-dependent diabetes. Lancet 1989; i: 1356–9.

55. Kingston ME, Skoog WC. Maintenance of basal insulin secretion in severe non-insulin dependent diabetes. Diabetes Care 1986; 9: 232–5.

56. Reaven GM, Hollenbeck C, Jeng C-Y, Wu MS, Chen Y-DI. Measurement of plasma glucose, free fatty acid, lactate, and insulin for 24 hours in patients with NIDDM. Diabetes 1988; 37: 1020–24.

57. Garvey WT, Olefsky JM, Rubenstein AH, Kolterman OG. Day-long integrated serum insulin and C-peptide profiles in patients with NIDDM: correlation with urinary C-peptide excretion. Diabetes 1988; 37: 590–96.

58. Liu G, Coulston A, Chen Y-DI, Reaven GM. Does day-long absolute hypoinsulinemia characterize the patient with non-insulin-dependent diabetes mellitus? Metabolism 1983; 32: 754–6.

59. Lillioja S, Mott DM, Howard BV et al. Impaired glucose tolerance as a disorder of insulin action. Longitudinal and cross-sectional studies in Pima Indians. New Engl J Med 1988; 318: 1217–25.

60. Warram JH, Martin BC, Krolewski AS, Soeldner JS, Kahn CR. Slow glucose removal rate and hyperinsulinemia precede the development of type II diabetes in the offspring of diabetic parents. Ann Intern Med 1990; 113: 909–15.

61. Yudkin JS, Alberti KGMM, McLarty DG, Swai ABM. Impaired glucose tolerance—is it a risk factor for diabetes or a diagnostic ragbag? Br Med J 1990; 301: 397–401.

62. Saad MF, Knowler WC, Pettitt DJ, Nelson RG, Mott DM, Bennett PH. The natural history of impaired glucose tolerance in the Pima Indians. New Engl J Med 1988; 319: 1500–505.

63. Jallut D, Golay A, Munger R et al. Impaired glucose tolerance and diabetes in obesity: a 6 year follow-up study of glucose metabolism. Metabolism 1990; 39: 1068–75.

64. Gulli G, Ferrannini E, Stern M, Haffner S, DeFronzo RA. The metabolic profile of NIDDM is

fully established in glucose-tolerant offspring of two Mexican-American NIDDM parents. Diabetes 1992; 41: 1575–86.

65. Haffner SM, Miettinen H, Gaskill SP, Stern MP. Decreased insulin secretion and increased insulin resistance are independently related to the 7-year risk of NIDDM in Mexican-Americans. Diabetes 1995; 44: 1386–91.

66. Haffner SM, Miettinen H, Stern MP. Insulin secretion and resistance in non-diabetic Mexican-Americans and non-hispanic whites with a parental history of diabetes. J Clin Endocrinol Metab 1996; 81: 1846–51.

67. Lillioja S, Mott DM, Spraul M et al. Insulin resistance and insulin secretory dysfunction as precursors of non-insulin-dependent diabetes mellitus. New Engl J Med 1993; 329: 1988–92.

68. Dowse GK, Zimmet PZ, Collins VR. Insulin levels and the natural history of glucose intolerance in Nauruans. Diabetes 1996; 45: 1367–72.

69. Hansen BC, Bodkin NH. Heterogeneity of insulin responses: phases leading to type 2 (non-insulin-dependent) diabetes mellitus in the rhesus monkey. Diabetologia 1986; 29: 713–19.

70. Bodkin NL, Metzger BL, Hansen BC. Hepatic glucose production and insulin sensitivity preceding diabetes in monkeys. Am J Physiol 1989; 256: E676–81.

71. Haffner SM, Stern MP, Hazuda HP, Pugh JA, Patterson JK. Hyperinsulinemia in a population at high risk for non-insulin-dependent diabetes mellitus. New Engl J Med 1986; 315: 220–24.

72. Haffner SM, Stern MP, Mitchell BD, Hazula HP, Patterson JK. Incidence of type II diabetes in Mexican-Americans predicted by fasting insulin and glucose levels, obesity, and body-fat distribution. Diabetes 1990; 39: 283–8.

73. Haffner SM, Stern MP, Hazuda HP, Mitchell BD, Patterson JK. Increased insulin concentrations in non-diabetic offspring of diabetic parents. New Engl J Med 1988; 319: 1297–301.

74. Balkau B, King H, Zimmet P, Raper LR. Factors associated with the development of diabetes in the Micronesian population of Nauru. Am J Epidemiol 1985; 122: 594–605.

75. Eriksson J, Franssila-Kallunki A, Ekstrand A et al. Early metabolic defects in persons at increased risk for non-insulin-dependent diabetes mellitus. New Engl J Med 1989; 321: 337–43.

76. Efendic S, Luft R, Wajngot A. Aspects of the pathogenesis of type 2 diabetes. Endocr Rev 1984; 5: 395–419.

77. Ho LT, Chang ZY, Wang JT et al. Insulin insensitivity in offspring of parents with type 2 diabetes mellitus. Diabet Med 1990; 7: 31–4.

78. Martin BC, Warram JH, Krolewski AS, Bergman RN, Soeldner JS, Kahn RC. Role of glucose and insulin resistance in development of type 2 diabetes mellitus: results of a 25-year follow-up study. Lancet 1992; 340: 925–9.

79. Fajans SS. Maturity-onset diabetes of the young (MODY). Diabetes Metab Rev 1989; 5: 579–606.

80. Bell GI, Zian K, Newman M et al. Gene for non-insulin-dependent diabetes mellitus (maturity-onset diabetes of the young subtype) is linked to DNA polymorphism on human chromosome 20q. Proc Natl Acad Sci USA 1991; 88: 1484–8.

81. Froguel Ph, Vaxillaire M, Sun F et al. Close linkage of glucokinase locus on chromosome 7p to early-onset non-insulin-dependent diabetes mellitus. Nature 1992; 356: 162–4.

82. Froguel Ph, Zouali H, Vionnet N et al. Familial hyperglycaemia due to mutations in glucokinase: definition of a subtype of diabetes mellitus. New Engl J Med 1993; 328: 697–702.

83. Menzel S, Yamagata K, Trabb JB et al. Localization of MODY3 to a 5-cM region of human chromosome 12. Diabetes 1995; 44: 1408–13.

84. Vaxillaire M, Vionnet N, Vigouroux C et al. Search for a third susceptibility gene for maturity-onset diabetes of the young: studies with eleven candidate genes. Diabetes 1994; 43: 389–95.

85. Lesage S, Hani E, Phippi, A et al. Linkage analyses of the MODY3 locus on chromosome 12q with late-onset NIDDM. Diabetes 1995; 44: 1243–7.

86. Zhang Y, Warren-Perry M, Saker PJ et al. Candidate gene studies in pedigrees with maturity-onset diabetes of the young not linked with glucokinase. Diabetologia 1995; 38: 1055–66.

87. Herman WH, Fajans SS, Ortiz FJ et al. Abnormal insulin secretion, not insulin resistance, is the genetic or primary defect of MODY in the RW pedigree. Diabetes 1994; 43: 40–46.

88. Hager J, Blanché H, Sun F et al. Six mutations in the glucokinase gene identified in MODY by using a non-radioactive sensitive screening technique. Diabetes 1994; 43: 730–3.

89. Wajngot A, Alvarsson M, Glaser A, Efendic S, Luthman H, Grill V. Glucose potentiation of arginine-induced insulin secretion is impaired in subjects with a glucokinase Glu256Lys mutation. Diabetes 1994; 43: 1402–6.

90. Beck-Nielsen H, Nielsen OH, Pedersen O, Bak J, Faber O, Schmitz O. Insulin action and insulin secretion in identical twins with MODY: evidence for defects in both insulin action and insulin secretion. Diabetes 1988; 37: 730–35.

91. Mohan V, Sharp PS, Aber VR, Mather HM, Kohner EM. Insulin resistance in maturity-onset diabetes of the young. Diabète Métab 1988; 13: 193–7.

92. Velho G, Petersen K, Perseghin G et al. Impaired hepatic glycogen synthesis in glucokinase-deficient (MODY-2) subjects. J Clin Invest 1996; 98: 1755–61.

93. Clement K, Pueyo ME, Vaxillaire M et al. Assessment of insulin sensitivity in glucokinase-deficient subjects. Diabetologia 1996; 39: 82–90.

94. Kazuhiro E, Sakura H, Shimokawa K et al. Sequence variations of the glucokinase gene in Japanese subjects with NIDDM. Diabetes 1994; 43: 730–33.

95. Zouali H, Vaxillaire M, Lesage S et al. Linkage analysis and molecular scanning of glucokinase gene in NIDDM families. Diabetes 1993; 42: 1238–45.

96. Elbein SC, Hoffman M, Chiu K, Tanizawa Y, Permutt MA. Linkage analysis of the glucokinase locus in familial type 2 (non-insulin-dependent) diabetic pedigrees. Diabetologia 1993; 36: 141–5.

97. Tanizawa Y, Chiu KC, Province MA et al. Two microsatellite repeat polymorphisms flanking opposite ends of the human glucokinase gene: use in haplotype analysis of Welsh Caucasians with type 2 (non-insulin-dependent) diabetes mellitus. Diabetologia 1993; 36: 409–13.

98. Shimada E, Makino H, Hashimoto N et al. Type 2 (non-insulin-dependent) diabetes mellitus associated

with a mutation of the glucokinase gene in a Japanese family. Diabetologia 1993; 36: 433–7.

99. Elbein SC, Hoffman M, Qin H, Chiu K, Tanizawa Y, Permutt MA. Molecular screening of the glucokinase gene in familial type 2 (non-insulin-dependent) diabetes mellitus. Diabetologia 1994; 37: 182–7.

100. Chiu KC, Tanizawa Y, Permutt MA. Glucokinase gene variants in the common form of NIDDM. Diabetes 1993; 42: 579–82.

101. Efendic S, Grill V, Luft R, Wajngot A. Low insulin response: a marker of pre-diabetes. Adv Exp Med Biol 1988; 246: 167–74.

102. Chen K-W, Boyko EJ, Bergstrom RW et al. Earlier appearance of impaired insulin secretion than of visceral adiposity in the pathogenesis of NIDDM. 5-year follow-up of initially non-diabetic Japanese-American men. Diabetes Care 1995; 18: 747–53.

103. DeFronzo RA, Tobin JD, Andres R. Glucose clamp technique: a method for quantifying insulin secretion and resistance. Am J Physiol 1979; 6: E214–23.

104. Curry DL, Bennett LL, Grodsky GM. Dynamics of insulin secretion by the perfused rat pancreas. Endocrinology 1968; 83: 572–84.

105. Cerasi E, Luft R, Efendic S, Decreased sensitivity of the pancreatic beta cells to glucose in pre-diabetic and diabetic subjects. Diabetes 1972; 21: 224–34.

106. Temple R, Clark PMS, Hales CN. Measurement of insulin secretion in type 2 diabetes: problems and pitfalls. Diabet Med 1992; 9: 503–12.

107. Calles-Escandon J, Robbins DC. Loss of early phase of insulin release in humans impairs glucose tolerance and blunts thermic effect of glucose. Diabetes 1987; 36: 1167–72.

108. Bruce DG, Chisholm DJ, Storlien LH, Kraegen EW. Physiological importance of deficiency in early prandial insulin secretion in non-insulin dependent diabetes. Diabetes 1988; 37: 736–44.

109. Steiner KE, Bowles CR, Mouton SM, Williams PE, Cherrington AD. The relative importance of first and second phase insulin secretion in countering the action of glucagon on glucose turnover in the conscious dog. Diabetes 1982; 31: 964–72.

110. Luzi L. Effect of the loss of first phase insulin secretion on glucose production and disposal in man. Am J Physiol 1989; 257: E241–6.

111. Brunzell JD, Robertson RP, Lerner RL et al. Relationships between fasting plasma glucose levels and insulin secretion during intravenous glucose tolerance tests. J Clin Endocrinol 1976; 46: 222–9.

112. Vague P, Moulin J-P. The defective glucose sensitivity of the B cell in insulin dependent diabetes. Improvement after twenty hours of normoglycaemia. Metabolism 1982; 31: 139–42.

113. Savage PJ, Bennion LJ, Flock EV. Diet-induced improvement of abnormalities in insulin and glucagon secretion and in insulin receptor binding in diabetes mellitus. J Clin Endocrinol Metab 1979; 48: 999–1007.

114. Kosaka K, Kuzuya T, Akanuma Y, Hagura R. Increase in insulin response after treatment of overt maturity onset diabetes mellitus is independent of the mode of treatment. Diabetologia 1980; 18: 23–8.

115. Rossetti L, Giaccari A, DeFronzo RA. Glucose toxicity. Diabetes Care 1990; 13: 610–30.

116. Lang DA, Matthews DR, Peto J, Turner RC. Cyclic oscillations of basal plasma glucose and insulin concentrations in human beings. New Engl J Med 1979; 301: 1023–7.

117. Simon C, Follenius M, Brandenberger G. Postprandial oscillations of plasma glucose, insulin, and C-peptide in man. Diabetologia 1987; 30: 769–73.

118. Polonsky KS, Given BD, Van Cauter E. Twenty-four-hour profiles and pulsatile patterns of insulin secretion in normal and obese subjects. J Clin Invest 1988; 81: 442–8.

119. Goodner CJ, Walike BC, Koerker DJ et al. Insulin, glucagon, and glucose exhibit synchronous, sustained oscillations in fasting monkeys. Science 1977; 195: 177–9.

120. Chou HF, Ipp E. Pulsatile insulin secretion in isolated rat islets. Diabetes 1990; 39: 112–17.

121. Paolisso G, Sgambato S, Passariello N, Sheen A, D'Onofrio F, Lefebvre PJ. Greater efficacy of pulsatile insulin in type I diabetes critically depends on plasma glucose levels. Diabetes 1987; 36: 566–70.

122. Sturis J, Scheen AJ, Leproult R, Polonsky KS, Van Cauter E. 24-hour glucose profiles during continuous or oscillatory insulin infusion: demonstration of the functional significance of ultradian insulin oscillations. J Clin Invest 1995; 95: 1464–71.

123. Gumbiner B, Van Cauter E, Beltz WF et al. Abnormalities of insulin pulsatility and glucose oscillations during meals in obese non-insulin-dependent diabetic patients: effects of weight reduction. J Clin Endocrinol Metab 1996; 81: 2061–8.

124. O'Meara NM, Sturis J, Van Cauter E, Polonsky KS. Lack of control by glucose of ultradian insulin secretory oscillations in impaired glucose tolerance and in non-insulin-dependent diabetes mellitus. J Clin Invest 1993; 92: 262–71.

125. Polonsky KS, Given BD, Hirsch LJ, Tillil H, Shapiro ET. Abnormal patterns of insulin secretion in non-insulin dependent diabetes mellitus. New Engl J Med 1988; 318: 1231–9.

126. O'Rahilly S, Turner RC, Matthews DR. Impaired pulsatile secretion of insulin in relatives of patients with non-insulin-dependent diabetes. New Engl J Med 1988; 318: 1225–30.

127. Horowitz DL, Starr JI, Mako ME, Blackard WG, Rubenstein AH. Pro-insulin, insulin, and C-peptide concentrations in human portal and peripheral blood. J Clin Invest 1975; 55: 1278–83.

128. Rhodes CJ, Alarcon C. What beta cell defect could lead to hyperproinsulinemia in NIDDM? Diabetes 1994; 43: 511–17.

129. Glauber HS, Revers RR, Henry R et al. *In vivo* glucose deactivation of pro-insulin action on glucose disposal and hepatic glucose production in normal man. Diabetes 1986; 35: 311–17.

130. Ward WK, LaCava EC, Paquette TL, Beard JC, Wallum BJ, Porte D. Disproportionate elevation of immunoreactive pro-insulin in type 2 (non-insulin-dependent) diabetes mellitus and in experimental insulin resistance. Diabetologia 1987; 30: 698–702.

131. Deacon CF, Schleser-Mohr S, Ballmann M, Willms B, Conlon JM, Creutzfeldt W. Preferential release of pro-insulin relative to insulin in non-insulin-dependent diabetes mellitus. Acta Endocrinol 1988; 119: 549–54.

132. Yoshioka N, Kuzuya T, Matsuda A, Taniguchi M, Iwamoto Y. Serum proinsulin levels at fasting and after oral glucose load in patients with type 2 (non-insulin-dependent) diabetes mellitus. Diabetologia 1988; 31: 355–60.

133. Reaven GM, Chen YD, Hollenbeck CB, Sheu WH, Ostrega D, Polonsky KS. Plasma insulin, C-peptide and proinsulin concentrations in obese and non-obese individuals with varying degrees of glucose tolerance. J Clin Endocrinol Metab 1993; 76: 44–8.

134. Alarcon C, Lincoln B, Rhodes CJ. The biosynthesis of the subtilisin-related proprotein convertase PC3, but not that of the PC2 convertase, is regulated by glucose in parallel to proinsulin biosynthesis in rat pancreatic islets. J Biol Chem 1993; 268: 4276–80.

135. Westermark P, Wilander E. The influence of amyloid deposits on the islet volume in maturity onset diabetes mellitus. Diabetologia 1978; 15: 417–21.

136. Gepts W, Lecompte PM. The pancreatic islets in diabetes. Am J Med 1981; 70: 105–14.

137. Maclean N, Ogilvie RF. Quantitative estimation of the pancreatic islet tissue in diabetic subjects. Diabetes 1955; 4: 367–76.

138. Saito K, Yaginuma N, Takahashi T. Differential volumetry of alpha, beta, and delta cells in the pancreatic islets of diabetic and non-diabetic subjects. Tohoku J Exp Med 1979; 129: 273–83.

139. Kloppel G, Lohr M, Habich K, Oberholzer M, Heitz PU. Islet pathology and the pathogenesis of type I and type 2 diabetes mellitus revisited. Surv Synth Path Res 1985; 4: 110–25.

140. Clark A, Wells CA, Buley ID et al. Islet amyloid, increased alpha-cells, reduced beta-cells and exocrine fibrosis: quantitative changes in the pancreas in type 2 diabetes. Diabetes Res 1988; 9: 151–9.

141. Stefan Y, Orci L, Malaisse-Lagae F, Perrelet A, Patel Y, Unger R. Quantitation of endocrine cell content in the pancreas of non-diabetic and diabetic humans. Diabetes 1982; 31: 694–700.

142. Eisenbarth GS, Connelly J, Soeldner JS. The 'natural' history of type I diabetes. Diabetes Metab Rev 1987; 3: 873–91.

143. Hales CN, Barker DJP, Clark PM et al. Fetal and infant growth and impaired glucose tolerance at age 64 years. Br Med J 1991; 303: 1019–22.

144. Phipps K, Barker DJP, Hales CN, Fall CH, Osmond C, Clark PM. Fetal growth and impaired glucose tolerance in men and women. Diabetologia 1993; 36: 225–8.

145. Barker DJ, Hales CN, Fall CH, Osmond C, Phipps K, Clark PM. Type 2 (non-insulin-dependent) diabetes mellitus, hypertension and hyperlipidaemia (syndrome X): relation to reduced fetal growth. Diabetologia 1993; 36: 62–7.

146. Athens M, Valdez R, Stern M. Effect of birthweight on future development of 'syndrome X' in adult life. Diabetes 1993; 42(suppl. 1): 61A.

147. McCance DR, Pettitt DJ, Hanson RL, Jacobson LT, Knowler WC, Bennett PH. Birth weight and non-insulin dependent diabetes: thrifty genotype, thrifty phenotype, or surviving small baby genotype? Br Med J 1994; 308: 942–5.

148. Purdy LP, Metzger BE. Influences of the intrauterine metabolic environment on adult disease: what may we infer from size at birth? Diabetologia 1996; 39: 1126–30.

149. Eriksson UJ. Lifelong consequences of metabolic adaptations *in utero*? Diabetologia 1996; 39: 1123–5.

150. Hales CN, Barker DJP. Type 2 (non-insulin-dependent) diabetes mellitus: the thrifty phenotype hypothesis. Diabetologia 1993; 35: 595–601.

151. Phillips DIW. Insulin resistance as a programmed response to fetal undernutrition. Diabetologia 1996; 39: 1119–22.

152. Lukinius A, Willander E, Westermark GT, Engstrom U, Westermark P. Co-localization of islet amyloid polypeptide and insulin in the beta cell secretory granules of the human pancreatic islets. Diabetologia 1989; 32: 240–44.

153. Ogawa A, Harris V, McCorkle SK, Unger RH, Luskey KL. Amylin secretion from the rat pancreas and its selective loss after streptozotocin treatment. J Clin Invest 1990; 85: 973–6.

154. Johnson KH, O'Brien TD, Betysholtz C, Westermark P. Islet amyloid, islet-amyloid polypeptide, and diabetes mellitus. New Engl J Med 1989; 321: 513–18.

155. Clark A. Islet amyloid and type 2 diabetes. Diabet Med 1989; 6: 561–7.

156. Nishi M, Sanke T, Nagamatsu S, Bell GI, Steiner DF. Islet amyloid polypeptide. A new beta cell secretory product related to islet amyloid deposits. J Biol Chem 1990; 265: 4173–6.

157. Westermark P, Wernstedt C, Wilander E, Hayden DW, O'Brien TD, Johnson KH. Amyloid fibrils in human insulinoma and islets of Langerhans of the diabetic cat are derived from a neuropeptide-like protein also present in normal islet cells. Proc Natl Acad Sci USA 1987; 84: 3881–5.

158. Cooper GJS, Willis AC, Clark A, Turner RC, Sim RB, Reid KBM. Purification and characterization of a peptide from amyloid-rich pancreases of type 2 diabetic patients. Proc Natl Acad Sci USA 1987; 84: 8628–32.

159. Ohsawa H, Kanatsuka A, Yamaguchi T, Makino H, Yoshida S. Islet amyloid polypeptide inhibits glucose-stimulated insulin secretion from isolated rat pancreatic islets. Biochem Biophys Res Comm 1989; 160: 961–7.

160. Howard CF. Longitudinal studies on the development of diabetes in individual *Macaca nigra*. Diabetologia 1986; 29: 301–6.

161. Hartter E, Svoboda T, Ludvik B et al. Basal and stimulated plasma levels of pancreatic amylin indicate its co-secretion with insulin in humans. Diabetologia 1991; 34: 52–4.

162. Eriksson J, Nakazato M, Miyazato M, Shiomi K, Matsukura S, Groop L. Islet amyloid polypeptide: plasma-concentrations in individuals at increased risk of developing type 2 (non-insulin-dependent) diabetes mellitus. Diabetologia 1992; 35: 292–3.

163. Bretherton-Watt D, Ghatei MA, Bloom SR et al. Altered islet amyloid polypeptide (amylin) gene expression in rat models of diabetes. Diabetologia 1989; 32: 881–3.

164. Ghatei MA, Datta HK, Zaidi M, et al. Amylin and amylin-amide lack an acute effect on blood glucose and insulin. J Endocrinol 1990; 124: R9–11.

165. Bretherton-Watt D, Gilbey SG, Ghatei MA, Beacham J, Bloom SR. Failure to establish islet amyloid polypeptide (amylin) as a circulating beta cell inhibiting hormone in man. Diabetologia 1990; 33: 115–17.

166. Westermark GT, Christmanson L, Terenghi G et al. Islet amyloid polypeptide: demonstration of mRNA in human pancreatic islets by *in situ* hybridization in islets with and without amyloid deposits. Diabetologia 1993; 36: 323–8.

167. Hoppener JWM, Verbeek JS, de Koning EJP et al. Chronic overproduction of islet amyloid polypeptide-amylin in transgenic mice: lysosomal localization of human islet amyloid polypeptide and lack of marked hyperglycaemia or hyperinsulinaemia. Diabetologia 1993; 36: 1258–65.

168. Yamaguchi A, Chiba T, Morishita T et al. Calcitonin gene-related peptide and induction of hyperglycemia in conscious rats *in vivo*. Diabetes 1990; 39: 168–74.

169. Drucker D. Glucagon and the glucagon-like peptides. Pancreas 1990; 5: 484–8.

170. Goke R, Fehmann H-C, Goke B. Glucagon-like peptide-1 (7-36) amide is a new incretin/enterogastrone candidate. Eur J Clin Invest 1991; 21: 135–44.

171. Mojsov S, Weir GC, Habener JF. Insulinotropin: glucagon-like peptide 1 (7-37) co-encoded in the glucagon gene is a potent stimulator of insulin release in the perfused rat pancreas. J Clin Invest 1987; 79: 616–19.

172. Kreymann B, Ghatei MA, Williams G, Bloom SR. Glucagon-like peptide-1 7-36: a physiological incretin in man. Lancet 1987; 2: 1300–303.

173. Thorens B, Waeber G. Glucagon-like peptide-1 and the control of insulin secretion in the normal state and in NIDDM. Diabetes 1993; 42: 1219–25.

174. Stoffel M, Espinosa R III, Le Beau MM, Bell GI. Human glucagon-like peptide-1 receptor gene. Localization to chromosome band 6p21 by fluorescence *in situ* hybridization and linkage of a highly polymorphic simple tandem repeat DNA polymorphism to other markers on chromosome 6. Diabetes 1993; 42: 1215–18.

175. Nauck M, Stockmann F, Ebert R, Creutzfeld W. Reduced incretin effect in type II (non-insulin-dependent) diabetes. Diabetologia 1986; 29: 46–52.

176. Suzuki S, Kawai K, Ohashi S, Mukai H, Murayama Y, Yamashita K. Reduced insulinotropic effects of glucagon-like peptide I(7-36)-amide and gastric inhibitory polypeptide in isolated perfused diabetic rat pancreas. Diabetes 1990; 39: 1320–25.

177. Ebert R, Creutzfeld W. Gastrointestinal peptides and insulin secretion. Diabetes Metab Rev 1987; 3: 1–6.

178. Nanauck MA, Kleine N, Orskov C, Holst JJ, Willms B, Creutzfeldt W. Normalization of fasting hyperglycaemia by exogenous glucagon-like peptide 1 (7-36 amide) in type 2 (non-insulin-dependent) diabetic patients. Diabetologia 1993; 36: 741–4.

179. Nathan DM, Schreiber E, Fogel H, Mojsov S, Habener JF. Insulinotropic action of glucagon-like peptide 1(7-37) in diabetic and nondiabetic subjects. Diabetes Care 1992; 15: 270–76.

180. Gutniak M, Orskov C, Holst JJ, Ahren B, Efendic S. Antidiabetogenic effect of glucagon-like peptide I(7-36)amide in normal subjects and patients with diabetes mellitus. New Engl J Med 1992; 326: 1316–22.

181. Nauck MA, Heimesaat MM, Orskov C, Holst JJ, Ebert R, Creutzfeld W. Preserved incretin activity of glucagon-like peptide I(7-36)amide but not of synthetic human gastric inhibitory polypeptide in patients with type II diabetes mellitus. J Clin Invest 1993; 91: 301–7.

182. D'Alessio DA, Vogel R, Prigeon R et al. Elimination of the action of glucagon-like peptide 1 causes an impairment of glucose tolerance after nutrient ingestion by healthy baboons. J Clin Invest 1996; 97: 133–8.

183. Wang Z, Wang RM, Owji AA, Smith DM, Ghatei MA, Bloom SR. Glucagon-like peptide 1 is a physiologic incretin in rat. J Clin Invest 1995; 95: 417–21.

184. Kolligs F, Fehmann H-C, Goke R, Goke B. Reduction of the incretin effects in rats by the glucagon-like peptide 1 receptor antagonist exendin (9-39) amide. Diabetes 1995; 44: 16–19.

185. Dunning BE, Taborsky GJ. Galanin-sympathetic neurotransmitter in endocrine pancreas. Diabetes 1988; 37: 1157–62.

186. Gilbey SG, Stephenson J, O'Halloran DJ, Burrin JM, Bloom SR. High-dose porcine galanin infusion and effect on intravenous glucose tolerance in humans. Diabetes 1989; 38: 1114–16.

187. Holst JJ, Bersani M, Hvidberg A et al. On the effects of human galanin in man. Diabetologia 1993; 36: 653–7.

188. Unger RH, Grund S. Hyperglycaemia as an inducer as well as a consequence of impaired islet cell function and insulin resistance: implications for the management of diabetes. Diabetologia 1985; 28: 119–21.

189. Leahy JL. Natural history of beta cell dysfunction in non-insulin-dependent diabetes mellitus. Diabetes Care 1990; 13: 992–1010.

190. McCance DR, Pettitt DJ, Hanson RL, Jacobsson LTH Bennett PH, Knowler WC. Glucose, insulin concentrations and obesity in childhood and adolescence as predictors of NIDDM. Diabetologia 1994; 37:617–23.

191. Frontoni S, Choi SB, Banduch D, Rossetti L. *In vivo* insulin resistance induced by amylin primarily through inhibition of insulin-stimulated glycogen synthesis in skeletal muscle. Diabetes 1991; 40: 568–73.

192. Butler PC, Chou J, Carter WB et al. Effects of meal ingestion on plasma amylin concentration in NIDDM and non-diabetic humans. Diabetes 1990; 39: 752–5.

193. Westermark P, Johnson KH, O'Brien TD, Betsoltz C. Islet amyloid polypeptide—a novel controversy in diabetes research. Diabetologia 1992; 35: 297–303.

194. Wilding JPH, Khandan-Nia N, Bennet WM et al. Lack of acute effect of amylin (islet associated polypeptide) on insulin sensitivity during hyperinsulinaemic euglycaemic clamp in humans. Diabetologia 1994; 37: 166–9.

195. Mitchell JH, Schmidt RF. Cardiovascular reflex control by afferent fibers from skeletal muscle receptors. In Shepherd JT, Abboud FM (eds) Handbook of physiology: the cardiovascular system, peripheral and organ blood flow, sect. 2, vol. 3. Bethesda, MD: Am Physiol Soc, 1983; pp 623–58.

196. Xiao-Ying H. Tachykinins and calcitonin gene-related peptide in relation to peripheral functions of capsaicin-sensitive sensory neurons. Acta Physiol Scand 1986; suppl. 551: 1–45.

197. Henry RR, Wallace P, Olefsky JM. Effects of weight loss on mechanisms of hyperglycemia in obese non-insulin dependent diabetes mellitus. Diabetes 1986; 35: 990–98.

198. Hotamisligil GS, Spiegelman BM. Tumor necrosis factor alpha: a key component of the obesity–diabetes link. Diabetes 1994; 43: 1271–8.

199. Spiegelman BM, Hotamisligil GS. Through thick and thin: wasting, obesity, and TNF-α. Cell 1993; 73: 625–7.

200. Hotamisligil GS, Shargill NS, Spiegelman BM. Adipose expression of tumor necrosis factor-alpha: direct

role in obesity-linked insulin resistance. Science 1993; 259: 87–91.

201. Hotamisligil GS, Murray DL, Choy LN, Spiegelman BM. TNF-α inhibits signaling from insulin receptor. Proc Natl Acad Sci USA 1994; 91: 4854–8.

202. Hotamisligil GS, Budavari A, Murray DL, Spiegelman BM. Reduced tyrosine kinase activity of the insulin receptor in obesity-diabetes: central role of tumor necrosis factor-α. J Clin Invest 1995; 95: 2409–15.

203. Lang CH, Dobrescu C, Bagby GJ. Tumor necrosis factor impairs insulin action on peripheral glucose disposal and hepatic glucose output. Endocrinology 1992; 130: 43–52.

204. Stephens JM, Pekala PH. Transcriptional repression of the GLUT4 and C/EBP genes in 3T3-L1 adipocytes by tumor necrosis factor-alpha. J Biol Chem 1991; 266: 21839–45.

205. Feinstein R, Kanety H, Papa MZ, Lunenfeld B, Karasik A. Tumor necrosis factor-α suppresses insulin-induced tyrosine phosphorylation of insulin receptor and its substrates. J Biol Chem 1993; 268: 26055–8.

206. Kroder G, Bossenmaier B, Kellerer M, et al. Tumor necrosis factor-a and hyperglycemia-induced insulin resistance. Evidence for different mechanisms and different effects on insulin signaling. J Clin Invest 1996; 97: 1471–7.

207. Cornelius P, Lee MD, Marlowe M, Pekala PH. Monokine regulation of glucose transporter mRNA in L6 myotubes. Biochem Biophys Res Commun 1989; 165: 429–36.

208. Saghizadeh M, Ong JM, Garvey WT, Henry RR, Kern PA. The expression of TNF-alpha by human muscle. Relationship to insulin resistance. J Clin Invest 1996; 97: 1111–16.

209. Ofei F, Hurel S, Newkirk J, Sopwith M, Taylor R. Effects of an engineered human anti-TNF-α antibody (CDP571) on insulin sensitivity and glycemic control in patients with NIDDM. Diabetes 1996; 45: 881–5.

210. Robertson RP, Olson IK, Zhang H-J. Differentiating glucose toxicity from glucose desensitization: a new message from the insulin gene. Diabetes 1994; 43: 1085–9.

211. Chen S, Ogawa A, Ohneda M, Unger RH, Foster DW, McGarry JD. More direct evidence for a malonyl-CoA-carnitine palmitoyltransferase I interaction as a key event in pancreatic beta cell signaling. Diabetes 1994; 43: 878–83.

212. Matchinsky FM. Banting Lecture 1995. A lesson in metabolic regulation inspired by the glucokinase glucose sensor paradigm. Diabetes 1996; 45: 223–41.

213. Matschinsky FM, Liang Y, Kesavan P et al. Glucokinase as pancreatic beta cell glucose sensor and diabetes gene. J Clin Invest 1993; 92: 2092–8.

214. Perales MA, Sener A, Malaisse WJ. Hexose metabolism in pancreatic islets: the glucose-6-phosphatase riddle. Mol Cell Biochem 1991; 101: 67–71.

215. Sekine N, Circulli V, Regazzi R et al. Low lactate dehydrogenase and high mitochondrial glycerol phosphate dehydrogenase in pancreatic beta cells. J Biol Chem 1994; 269: 4895–902.

216. MacDonald MJ. Elusive proximal signals of beta cells for insulin secretion. Diabetes 1990; 39: 1461–6.

217. Dukes ID, McIntyre MS, Mertz RJ et al. Dependence of NADH produced during glycolysis for beta cell glucose signaling. J Biol Chem 1994; 269: 10979–82.

218. McCormack JG, Denton RM. Mammalian mitochondrial metabolism and its regulation in mitochondria. In Darley-Usmar V, Schapira AHV (eds) DNA, proteins and disease. Chapel Hill, NC: Portland, 1994; pp 81–112.

219. Lehninger AL, Nelson DL, Cox MM. Oxidative phosphorylation and photo phosphorylation. In Principles of Biochemistry, New York: Worth, 1993; pp 542–97.

220. Ashcroft FM, Ashcroft SJH. Mechanisms of insulin secretion. In Ashcroft FM, Ashcroft SJH (eds) Insulin. Oxford, Oxford University Press, 1992; pp 97–150.

221. Gilon P, Henquin JC. Influence of membrane potential changes on cytoplasmic Ca^{++} concentration in an electrically excitable cell, the insulin secreting pancreatic beta cell. J Biol Chem 1992; 267: 20713–720.

222. Hopkins WF, Fatherazi J, Peter-Reisch B, Corkey BE, Cook DL. Two sites for adenine-nucleotide regulation of ATP-sensitive potassium channels in mouse pancreatic beta cells and HIT cells. J Membr Biol 1992; 129: 287–95.

223. Ghosh A, Ronner P, Cheong E, Khaid P, Matschinsky FM. The role of ATP and free ADP in metabolic coupling during fuel-stimulated insulin release from islet beta-cells in the isolated perfused rat pancreas. J Biol Chem 1991; 266: 22887–92.

224. Hedeskov CJ. Mechanism of glucose-induced insulin secretion. Physiol Rev 1980; 60: 442–509.

225. Wollheim CB, Sharp GWG. Regulation of insulin release by calcium. Physiol Rev 1981; 61: 914–73.

226. Newgard CB, McGarry JD. Metabolic coupling factors in pancreatic beta cell signal transduction. Ann Rev Biochem 1995; 64: 689–719.

227. Corkey BE, Deeney JT, Glennon MC, Matschinsky FM, Prentki M. Regulation of steady-state free Ca^{++} levels by the ATP/ADP ratio and orthophosphate in permeabilized RINm5F insulinoma cells. J Biol Chem 1988; 263: 4247–53.

228. Cook DL, Satin LS, Hopkins WF. Pancreatic beta cells are bursting, but how? Trends Neurosci 1991; 14: 411–14.

229. Dunlop ME, Larkins RG. Pancreatic islets synthesize phospholipids *de novo* from glucose via acyl-dihydroxyacetone phosphate. Biochem Biophys Res Commun 1985; 132: 467–73.

230. Nishizuka Y. Intracellular signaling by hydrolysis of phospholipids and activation of protein kinase C. Science 1992; 258: 607–14.

231. Deeney JT, Tornheim K, Korschak HM, Prentki M, Corkey BE. Acyl-CoA esters modulate intracellular Ca^{++} handling by permeabilized clonal pancreatic beta cells. J Biol Chem 1992; 267: 19840–845.

232. Corkey BE, Deeney JT. Acyl-CoA regulation of metabolism and signal transduction. Prog Clin Biol Res 1990; 321: 217–32.

233. Zhou YP, Grill VE. Long-term exposure of rat pancreatic islets to fatty acids inhibits glucose-induced insulin secretion and biosynthesis through a glucose fatty acid cycle. J Clin Invest 1994; 93: 870–76.

234. Yaney GC, Schultz V, Cunningham BA, Dunaway GA, Corkey BE, Tornheim K. Phosphofructokinase isozymes in pancreatic islets and clonal beta cells (INS-1). Diabetes 1995; 44: 1285–9.

235. Sweet IR, Matschinsky FM. Mathematical model of beta-cell glucose metabolism and insulin release.

I. Glucokinase as glucosensor hypothesis. Am J Physiology 1995; 268: E775-8.

236. Sako Y, Grill VE. A 48-hour lipid infusion in the rat time-dependently inhibits glucose-induced insulin secretion and B cell oxidation through a process likely coupled to fatty acid oxidation. Endocrinology 1990; 127: 1580-89.

237. Capito K, Hansen SE, Hedeskov CJ, Islin H, Thams P. Fat-induced changes in mouse pancreatic islet insulin secretion, insulin biosynthesis and glucose metabolism. Acta Diabetol 1992; 28: 193-8.

238. Zhou Y-P, Ling Z-C, Grill VE. Inhibitory effects of fatty acids on glucose-regulated beta cell function: association with increased islet triglyceride stores and altered effect of fatty acid oxidation on glucose metabolism. Metabolism 1996; 45: 981-6.

239. Gerbitz K-D, Gempel K, Brdiczka D. Mitochondria and diabetes. Genetic, biochemical, and clinical implications of the cellular energy circuit. Diabetes 1996; 45: 113-26.

240. Maassen JA, Kadowaki T. Maternally inherited diabetes and deafness: a new diabetes subtype. Diabetologia 1996; 39: 375-82.

241. Gerbitz K-D, van den Ouweland JMW, Maassen JA, Jaksch M. Mitochondrial diabetes mellitus: a review. Biochem Biophys Acta 1995; 1271: 253-60.

242. van den Ouweland JMW. A new subtype of non-insulin-dependent diabetes mellitus is associated with a mitochondrial gene mutation. Doctoral thesis, University of Leiden, The Netherlands, 1994, pp 1-127.

243. Andersen S, Bankier AT, Barrell BGH et al. Sequence and organisation of the human mitochondrial genome. Nature 1981; 290: 457-65.

244. Attardi G, Schatz G. Biogenesis of mitochondria. Ann Rev Cell Biol 1988; 4: 289-333.

245. Richter C, Park JW, Ames BN. Normal oxidative damage to mitochondrial and nuclear DNA is extensive. Proc Natl Acad Sci USA 1988; 85: 6465-7.

246. Wallace DC. Diseases of the mitochondrial DNA. Ann Rev Biochem 1992; 61: 1175-212.

247. Wallace DC. Mitochondrial DNA sequence variation in human evolution and disease. Proc Natl Acad Sci USA 1994; 91: 8739-46.

248. Trounce I, Byre E, Marzuki S. Decline in skeletal muscle mitochondrial respiratory chain function: possible factor in ageing. Lancet 1989; I: 637-9.

249. Moraes CT, Ciacci F, Bonilla E et al. Two novel pathogenic mitochondrial DNA mutations affecting organelle number and protein synthesis: is the transfer RNALeu(UUR) gene an etiologic hot spot? J Clin Invest 1993; 92: 2909-15.

250. van den Ouweland JMW, Lemkes HHPJ, Ruitenbeek W et al. Mutation in mitochondrial tRNALeu (UUR) gene in a large pedigree with maternally transmitted type II diabetes mellitus and deafness. Nature Genet 1992; 1: 368-71.

251. Reardon W, Ross RJM, Sweeney MG et al. Diabetes mellitus associated with a pathogenic point mutation in mitochondrial DNA. Lancet 1992; 340: 1376-9.

252. van den Ouweland JMW, Lemkes HHPJ, Gerbitz KD, Maassen JA. Maternally inherited diabetes and deafness (MIDD): a distinct subtype of diabetes associating with a mitochondrial tRNALeu gene point mutation. Muscle Nerve 1995; (suppl. 3): S124-30.

253. Gerbitz K-D, Paprotta A, Jaksch M, Zierz S, Drechsel J. Diabetes is one of the heterogeneous phenotypic features of a mitochondrial DNA point mutation within the tRNA$^{Leu(UUR)}$ gene. FEBS Lett 1993; 321: 194-6.

254. Katagiri H, Asano T, Ishihara H et al. Mitochondrial diabetes mellitus: prevalence and clinical characterization of diabetes due to mitochondrial tRNALeu (UUR) gene mutation in Japanese patients. Diabetologia 1994; 37: 504-10.

255. Okay Y, Katagiri H, Tshihara H, Asan T, Kikuchi M, Kobayashi T. Mitochondrial diabetes mellitus glucose-induced signaling defects and beta-cell loss. Muscle Nerve 1995; (suppl. 3): S131-6.

256. Suzuki S, Hinokio Y, Hirai S et al. Pancreatic beta-cell secretory defect associated with mitochondrial point mutation of the tRNALeu gene: a study in seven families with mitochondrial encephalomyopathy, lactic acidosis and stroke-like episodes (MELAS). Diabetologia 1994; 37: 818-25.

257. Vionnet N, Passa P, Froguel P. Prevalence of mitochondrial gene mutations in families with diabetes mellitus. Lancet 1993; 342: 1429-30.

258. Kadowaki T, Kadowaki H, Mori Y et al. A subtype of diabetes associated with a mutation of the mitochondrial DNA. New Engl J Med 1994; 330: 962-8.

259. Tanabe Y, Miyamoto S, Kinoshita Y et al. Diabetes in Kearns-Sayre syndrome. Eur Neurol 1988; 28: 34-8.

260. Pimenta W, Korytkowski M, Mitrakou A et al. Pancreatic beta-cell dysfunction as the primary genetic lesion in NIDDM. Evidence from studies in normal glucose-tolerant individuals with a first-degree NIDDM relative. JAMA 1995; 273: 1855-61.

261. Yki-Jarvinen H. Role of insulin resistance in the pathogenesis of NIDDM. Diabetologia 1995; 38: 1378-88.

262. Groop LC, Widen E, Ferrannini E. Insulin resistance and insulin deficiency in the pathogenesis of type 2 (non-insulin-dependent) diabetes mellitus: errors of metabolism or of methods. Diabetologia 1993; 36: 1326-31.

263. Kahn CR. Insulin action, diabetogenes, and the cause of type II diabetes. Diabetes 1994; 43: 1066-84.

264. Eriksson K-F, Lindgarde F. Poor physical fitness, and impaired early insulin response but late hyperinsulinaemia, as predictors of NIDDM in middle-aged Swedish men. Diabetologia 1996; 39: 573-9.

265. Danowski T, Lambardo Y, Mendelsohn L, Corredor D, Morgan C, Sabeh G. Insulin patterns prior to and after onset of diabetes. Metabolism 1969; 18: 731-40.

266. Charles MA, Fontbonne A, Thibult N, Warnet J-M, Rosselin GE, Eschwege E. Risk factors for NIDDM in white population. Paris Prospective Study. Diabetes 1991; 40: 769-99.

267. Savage P, Bennett P, Gorden P, Miller M. Insulin responses to oral carbohydrate in true prediabetic and controls. Lancet 1975; 1: 300-302.

268. Strauss W, Hales C. Plasma insulin in minor abnormalities of glucose tolerance: a 5-year follow-up. Diabetologia 1974; 10: 237-43.

269. Cerasi E, Luft R. Follow-up of non-diabetic subjects with normal and decreased insulin response to glucose infusion—first report. Horm Metab Res 1974; 6: 113-20.

270. Lundgren H, Bengtsson C, Blohme G, Lapidus L, Waldenstrom J. Fasting serum insulin concentration and early insulin response as risk determinants for developing diabetes. Diabet Med 1990; 7: 407–13.

271. Skarfors E, Selinus K, Lithell H. Risk factors for developing non-insulin dependent diabetes: a 10-year follow-up of men in Uppsala. Br Med J 1991; 303: 755–60.

272. Golay A, Felber JP, Jequier E, DeFronzo RA, Ferrannini E. Metabolic basis of obesity and non-insulin-dependent diabetes mellitus. Diabetes Metab Rev 1988; 4: 727–47.

273. Lillioja S, Bogardus C. Obesity and insulin resistance: lessons learned from the Pima Indians. Diabetes Metab Rev 1988; 4: 515–40.

274. Diamond MP, Thornton K, Connolly-Diamond M, Sherwin RS, DeFronzo RA. Reciprocal variations in insulin-stimulated glucose uptake and pancreatic insulin secretion in women with normal glucose tolerance. J Soc Gynecol Invest 1995; 2: 708–15.

275. Reaven GM, Brand RJ, Chen Y-DI, Mathur AK, Goldfine I. Insulin resistance and insulin secretion are determinants of oral glucose tolerance in normal individuals. Diabetes 1993; 42: 1324–32.

276. Lillioja S, Mott DM, Zawadzki JK et al. *In vivo* insulin action is a familial characteristic in non-diabetic Pima Indians. Diabetes 1987; 36: 1329–35.

277. Schumacher MC, Hasstedt SJ, Hunt SC, Williams RR, Elbein SC. Major gene effect for insulin levels in familial NIDDM pedigrees. Diabetes 1992; 41: 416–23.

278. Mitchell BD, Kammerer CM, Hixson JE et al. Evidence for a major gene affecting post-challenge insulin levels in Mexican-Americans. Diabetes 1995; 44: 284–9.

279. Elbein SC, Hoffman MD, Bragg KL, Mayorga RA. The genetics of NIDDM. An update. Diabetes Care 1994; 17: 1523–33.

280. Ghosh S, Schork NJ. Perspectives in diabetes. Genetic analysis of NIDDM. The study of quantitative traits. Diabetes 1996; 45: 1–14.

281. Gelding S, Nithyananthan R, Chan S et al. Insulin sensitivity in non-diabetic relatives of patients with non-insulin-dependent diabetes from two ethnic groups. Clin Endocrinol 1994; 40: 55–62.

282. Birkeland K, Torjesen P, Eriksson J, Valler S, Groop L. Hyperproinsulinemia of type 2 diabetes is not present before the development of hyperglycemia. Diabetes Care 1994; 17: 1307–10.

283. Kobberling J. Tillil H. Empirical risk figures for first-degree relatives of non-insulin-dependent diabetics. In Kobberling J, Tattersall R (eds) The genetics of diabetes mellitus. London: Academic Press, 1982; pp 201–10.

284. Viswanathan M, Mohan V, Snehalatha C, Ramachandran A. High prevalence of type 2 (non-insulin-dependent) diabetes among the offspring of conjugal type 2 diabetic parents in India. Diabetologia 1985; 28: 907–10.

285. Knowler WC, Pettitt DJ, Saad MF, Bennett PH. Diabetes mellitus in the Pima Indians: incidence, risk factors and pathogenesis. Diabetes Metab Rev 1990; 6: 1–27.

286. Vaag A, Henriksen JE, Madsbad S, Holm N, Beck-Nielsen H. Insulin secretion, insulin action, and hepatic glucose production in identical twins discordant for non-insulin-dependent diabetes mellitus. J Clin Invest 1995; 95: 690–98.

287. Gottlieb MS, Soeldner JS, Kyner JL, Gleason RE. Oral glucose-stimulated insulin release in non-diabetic twin siblings of diabetic twins. Diabetes 1974; 23: 684–92.

288. Barnett AH, Spilipoulos AJ, Pyke DA, Stubbs WA, Burrin J, Alberti KGMM. Metabolic studies in unaffected co-twins of non-insulin-dependent diabetics. Br Med J 1981; 282: 1656–8.

289. Pyke DA, Taylor KW. Glucose tolerance and serum insulin in unaffected identical twins of diabetics. Br Med J 1967; 4: 21–2.

290. Cerasi E, Luft R. Insulin response to glucose infusion in diabetic and non-diabetic monozygotic twin pairs. Genetic control of insulin response? Acta Endocrinol 1967; 55: 330–45.

291. Pendergrass M, Fazioni E, DeFronzo RA. Non-insulin dependent diabetes mellitus and gestational diabetes mellitus: same disease, another name? Diabetes Rev 1995; 3: 566–83.

292. Buchanan TA, Catalano PM. The pathogenesis of GDM: implications for diabetes after pregnancy. Diabetes Rev 1995; 3: 584–601.

293. O'Sullivan JB. Diabetes mellitus after GDM. Diabetes 1991; 40(suppl. 2): 131–5.

294. Kjos SL, Peters RK, Xiang A, Henry QA, Montoro M, Buchanan TA. Predicting future diabetes in Latino women with gestational diabetes, utility of early postpartum glucose tolerance testing. Diabetes 1995; 44: 586–91.

295. Catalano PM, Tyzbir ED, Wolfe RR et al. Carbohydrate metabolism during pregnancy in control subjects and women with gestational diabetes. Am J Physiol 1993; 264: E60–67.

296. Catalano PM, Bernstein IM, Wolfe RR, Srikanta S, Tyzbir E, Sims EAH. Subclinical abnormalities of glucose metabolism in subjects with previous gestational diabetes. Am J Obstet Gynecol 1986; 155: 1255–62.

297. Ward WK, Johnston CLW, Beard JC, Benedetti TJ, Halter JB, Porte D Jr. Insulin resistance and impaired insulin secretion in subjects with histories of gestational diabetes mellitus. Diabetes 1985; 34: 861–9.

298. Ward WK, Johnston CL, Beard JC, Benedetti TJ, Porte D Jr. Abnormalities of islet beta cell function, insulin action, and fat distribution in women with histories of gestational diabetes: relationship to obesity. J Clin Endocrinol Metab 1985; 61: 1039–45.

299. Ryan EA, Imes S, Liu D et al. Defects in insulin secretion and action in women with a history of gestational diabetes. Diabetes 1995; 44: 506–12.

300. Efendic S, Hanson U, Persson B, Wajngot A, Luft R. Glucose tolerance, insulin release, and insulin sensitivity in normal-weight women with previous gestational diabetes mellitus. Diabetes 1987; 36: 413–19.

301. Dornhorst A, Edwards SGM, Nichols JSD et al. A defect in insulin release in women at risk of future non-insulin-dependent diabetes mellitus. Clin Sci 1991; 81: 195–9.

302. Damm P, Kuhl C, Hornnes P, Molsted-Pedersen L. A longitudinal study of plasma insulin and glucagon in women with previous gestational diabetes. Diabetes Care 1995; 18: 654–65.

303. Swinn RA, Wareham NJ, Gregory R et al. Excessive secretion of insulin precursors characterizes and predicts gestational diabetes. Diabetes 1995; 44: 911–15.

304. Stoffel M, Bell KL, Blackburn CL et al. Identification of glucokinase mutations in subjects with gestational diabetes mellitus. Diabetes 1993; 42: 937–40.

305. DeFronzo RA. Glucose intolerance and aging. Evidence for tissue insensitivity to insulin. Diabetes 1979; 28: 1095–1109.

306. DeFronzo RA. Glucose intolerance and aging. Diabetes Care 1981; 4: 483–501.

307. Reaven GM, Olefsky JM. Relationship between heterogeneity of insulin responses and insulin resistance in normal subjects and patients with chemical diabetes. Diabetologia 1977; 13: 201–6.

308. Hollenbeck CB, Reaven GM. Variations in insulin-stimulated glucose uptake in healthy individuals with normal glucose tolerance. J Clin Endocrinol Metab 1987; 64: 1169–73.

309. Lillioja S, Nyomba BL, Saad MF et al. Exaggerated early insulin release and insulin resistance in a diabetes-prone population: a metabolic comparison of Pima Indians and Caucasians. J Clin Endocrinol Metab 1991; 73: 866–76.

310. Le Stunff C, Bougneres P. Early changes in postprandial insulin secretion, not in insulin sensitivity, characterize juvenile obesity. Diabetes 1994; 43: 696–702.

311. Jeanrenaud B. Central nervous system and peripheral abnormalities: clues to the understanding of obesity and NIDDM. Diabetologia 1994; 37(suppl. 2): S169–78.

312. Williams G, McKibbin PE, McCarthy HD. Hypothalamic regulatory peptides and the regulation of food intake and energy balance: signals or noise? Proc Nutr Soc 1991; 50: 527–44.

313. Del Prato S, Leonetti E, Simonson DC, Sheehan P, Matsuda M, DeFronzo RA. Effect of sustained physiologic hyperinsulinaemia and hyperglycaemia on insulin secretion and insulin sensitivity in man. Diabetologia 1994; 37: 1025–35.

314. Cusin I, Terrettaz J, Rohner-Jeanrenaud F, Jeanrenaud B. Metabolic consequences of hyperinsulinaemia imposed on normal rats on glucose handling by white adipose tissue, muscles and liver. Biochem J 1990; 267: 99–103.

315. Cusin I, Terrettaz J, Rohner-Jeanrenaud F, Zarjevski N, Asimacopoulos-Jeannet F, Jeanrenaud B. Hyperinsulinemia increases the amount of GLUT4 mRNA in white adipose tissue and decreases that of muscles: a clue for increased fat depot and insulin resistance. Endocrinology 1990; 127: 3246–8.

316. Reaven GM, Hollenbeck CB, Chen Y-DI. Relationship between glucose tolerance, insulin secretion, and insulin action in non-obese individuals with varying degrees of glucose tolerance. Diabetologia 1989; 32: 52–5.

317. Bergman RN. Lilly Lecture. Toward physiological understanding of glucose tolerance—minimal-model approach. Diabetes 1989; 38: 1512–26.

318. Hara H, Egusa G, Yamakido M, Kawate R. The high prevalence of diabetes mellitus and hyperinsulinemia among the Japanese-Americans living in Hawaii and Los Angeles. Diabetes Res Clin Pract 1994; (suppl.): S37–42.

319. Berrish TS, Hetherington CS, Alberti KGMM, Walker M. Peripheral and hepatic insulin sensitivity in subjects with impaired glucose tolerance. Diabetologia 1995; 38: 699–704.

320. Himsworth HP, Kerr RB. Insulin-sensitive and insulin-insensitive types of diabetes mellitus. Clin Sci 1939; 4: 120–52.

321. Alford FP, Martin FI, Pearson MF. The significance of interpretation of mildly abnormal oral glucose tolerance. Diabetologia 1971; 7: 173–80.

322. Beck-Nielsen H, Pedersen O, Sorensen NS. Effects of dietary changes on cellular insulin binding and *in vivo* insulin sensitivity. Metabolism 1980; 29: 482–7.

323. Bonora E, Moghetti P, Zancanaro C et al. Estimates of *in vivo* insulin action in man: comparison of insulin tolerance tests with euglycemic and hyperglycemic glucose clamp studies. J Clin Endocrinol Metab 1989; 68: 374–8.

324. Shen SW, Reaven GM, Farquhar JW. Comparison of impedance to insulin-mediated glucose uptake in normal subjects and in subjects with latent diabetes. J Clin Invest 1970; 49: 2151–60.

325. Ginsberg H, Kimmerling G, Olefsky JM, Reaven GM. Demonstration of insulin resistance in untreated adult-onset diabetic subjects with fasting hyperglycemia. J Clin Invest 1975; 55: 454–61.

326. Kimmerling G, Javorski C, Olefsky JM, Reaven GM. Locating the site(s) of insulin resistance in patients with non-ketotic diabetes mellitus. Diabetes 1976; 25: 673–8.

327. Reaven GM. Banting Lecture. Role of insulin resistance in human disease. Diabetes 1988; 37: 1595–607.

328. Harano Y, Ongaku S, Hidaka H et al. Glucose, insulin, and somatostatin infusion for the determination of insulin sensitivity. J Clin Endocrinol Metab 1977; 45: 1124–7.

329. Ratzman KP, Besch W, Witt S, Schulz B. Evaluation of insulin resistance during inhibition of endogenous insulin and glucagon secretion by somatostatin in non-obese subjects with impaired glucose tolerance. Diabetologia 1981; 21: 192–7.

330. Butterfield WJH, Whichelow MJ. Peripheral glucose metabolism in control subjects and diabetic patients during glucose, glucose-insulin, and insulin sensitivity tests. Diabetologia 1965; 1: 43–53.

331. Zierler KL, Rabinowitz D. Roles of insulin and growth hormone, based on studies of forearm metabolism in man. Medicine 1963; 42: 385–402.

332. Beck-Nielsen H, Hother-Nielsen O, Vaag A, Alford F. Pathogenesis of type 2 diabetes mellitus (NIDDM): the role of skeletal muscle glucose uptake and hepatic glucose production in the development of hyperglycaemia. A critical comment. Diabetologia 1994; 37: 217–221.

333. Bowen HF, Moorhouse JA. Glucose turnover and disposal in maturity-onset diabetes. J Clin Invest 1973; 52: 3033–45.

334. Katz H, Homan M, Jensen M, Caumo A, Cobelli C, Rizza R. Assessment of insulin action in NIDDM in the presence of dynamic changes in insulin and glucose concentration. Diabetes 1994; 43: 289–96.

335. Wangot A, Roovete A, Vranic M, Luft R, Efendic S. Insulin resistance and decreased insulin response to glucose in lean type II diabetes. Proc Natl Acad Sci USA 1982; 79: 4432–7.

336. Welch S, Gebhart SSP, Bergman RN, Phillips LS. Minimal models analysis of intravenous glucose tolerance test-derived insulin sensitivity in diabetic subjects. J Clin Endocrinol Metab 1990; 71: 1508–18.

337. Coates PA, Ollerton RL, Luzio SD, Ismail IS, Owens DR. Reduced sampling protocols in estimation of insulin sensitivity and glucose effectiveness using the minimal model in NIDDM. Diabetes 1993; 42: 1635–41.

338. DeFronzo RA, Deibert D, Hendler R, Felig P. Insulin sensitivity and insulin binding to monocytes in maturity-onset diabetes. J Clin Invest 1982; 63: 939–46.

339. DeFronzo RA, Simonson D, Ferrannini E. Hepatic and peripheral insulin resistance: a common feature in non-insulin-dependent and insulin-dependent diabetes. Diabetologia 1982; 23: 313–19.

340. Simonson DC, Ferrannini E, Bevilacqua S et al. Mechanism of improvement in glucose metabolism following chronic glyburide therapy. Diabetes 1984; 33: 838–45.

341. Golay A, DeFronzo RA, Ferrannini E et al. Oxidative and non-oxidative glucose metabolism in non-obese type 2 (non-insulin dependent) diabetic patients. Diabetologia 1988; 31: 585–91.

342. DeFronzo RA, Sherwin RS, Hendler R, Felig P. Insulin binding to monocytes and insulin action in human obesity, starvation, and refeeding. J Clin Invest 1978; 62: 204–13.

343. Felber JP, Golay A, Jequier E et al. The metabolic consequences of long-term human obesity. Int J Obesity 1988; 12: 377–89.

344. Hollenbeck CB, Chen Y-DI, Reaven GM. A comparison of the relative effects of obesity and non-insulin dependent diabetes mellitus on *in vivo* insulin-stimulated glucose utilization. Diabetes 1984; 33: 622–4.

345. Karnieli E, Armoni M, Cohen P, Kanter Y, Rafaeloff R. Reversal of insulin resistance in diabetic rat adipocytes by insulin therapy. Diabetes 1987; 36: 925–31.

346. Dall'Aglio E, Chang H, Hollenbeck CB, Mondon CE, Sims C, Reaven GM. *In vivo* and *in vitro* resistance to maximal insulin-stimulated glucose disposal in insulin deficiency. Am J Physiol 1985; 249: E312–16.

347. Mäkimattila S, Virkamäki A, Malmström R, Utriainen T, Yki-Järvinen H. Insulin resistance in type I diabetes mellitus: a major role for reduced glucose extraction. J Clin Endocrinol Metab 1996; 81: 707–12.

348. Vuorinen-Markkola H, Koivisto VA, Yki-Järvinen H. Mechanisms of hyperglycemia-induced insulin resistance in whole body and skeletal muscle of type 1 diabetic patients. Diabetes 1992; 41: 571–80.

349. Firth R, Bell P, Rizza R. Insulin action in non-insulin-dependent diabetes mellitus: the relationship between hepatic and extrahepatic insulin resistance and obesity. Metabolism 1987; 36: 1091–5.

350. Campbell PJ, Mandarino LJ, Gerich JE. Quantification of the relative impairment in actions of insulin on hepatic glucose production and peripheral glucose uptake in non-insulin dependent diabetes mellitus. Metabolism 1988; 37: 15–21.

351. Shulman GI, Rothman DL, Jue T, Stein P, DeFronzo RA, Shulman RG. Quantitation of muscle glycogen synthesis in normal subjects and subjects with non-insulin-dependent diabetes by ^{13}C nuclear magnetic resonance spectroscopy. New Engl J Med 1990; 322: 223–8.

352. Grill V. A comparison of brain glucose metabolism in diabetes as measured by positron emission tomography or by arteriovenous techniques. Ann Med 1990; 22: 171–5.

353. Kurtz F. Mechanism of metformin action in non-insulin-dependent diabetes mellitus. Diabetes 1987; 36: 632–40.

354. Firth RG, Bell PM, Rizza RA. Effects of tolazamide and exogenous insulin on insulin action in patients with non-insulin-dependent diabetes mellitus. New Engl J Med 1986; 314: 1280–86.

355. Best JD, Judzewitsch RG, Pfeiffer MA, Beard JC, Halter JB, Porte D. The effect of chronic sulfonylurea therapy on hepatic glucose production in non-insulin-dependent diabetes mellitus. Diabetes 1982; 31: 333–8.

356. Firth RG, Bell PM, Marsh HM, Hansen I, Rizza RA. Postprandial hyperglycemia in patients with non-insulin-dependent diabetes mellitus. J Clin Invest 1986; 77: 1525–32.

357. Jackson RA, Hawa MI, Jaspan JB et al. Mechanisms of metformin action in non-insulin dependent diabetes mellitus. Diabetes 1987; 36: 632–40.

358. Garvey WT, Olefsky JM, Griffin J, Hamman RF, Kolterman OG. The effect of insulin treatment on insulin action in type II diabetes mellitus. Diabetes 1985; 34: 222–34.

359. Tayek JA, Katz J. Glucose production, recycling, and gluconeogenesis in normals and diabetics: a mass isotopomer [U-^{13}C] glucose study. Am J Physiol 1996; 270: E709–17.

360. Fery F. Role of hepatic glucose production and glucose uptake in the pathogenesis of fasting hyperglycemia in type 2 diabetes: normalization of glucose kinetics by short-term fasting. J Clin Endocrinol Metab 1994; 78: 536–42.

361. Clore JN, Blackard WG. Suppression of gluconeogenesis after a 3-day fast does not deplete liver glycogen in patients with NIDDM. Diabetes 1994; 43: 256–62.

362. Chen Y-DI, Swislocki ALM, Jeng C-Y, Juang J-H, Reaven GM. Effect of time on measurement of hepatic glucose production. J Clin Endocrinol Metab 1988; 67: 1084–8.

363. Jeng C-Y, Sheu WH-H, Fuh MM-T, Chen Y-DI, Reaven GM. Relationship between hepatic glucose production and fasting plasma glucose concentration in patients with NIDDM. Diabetes 1994; 43: 1440–44.

364. Chen Y-DI, Jeng C-Y, Hollenbeck CB, Wu M-S, Reaven GM. Relationship between plasma glucose and insulin concentration, glucose production, and glucose disposal in normal subjects and patients with non-insulin-dependent diabetes. J Clin Invest 1988; 82: 21–5.

365. DeFronzo RA, Ferrannini E, Hendler R, Felig P, Wahren J. Regulation of splanchnic and peripheral glucose uptake by insulin and hyperglycemia. Diabetes 1983; 32: 35–45.

366. DeFronzo RA, Ferrannini E. Influence of plasma glucose and insulin concentration on plasma glucose clearance in man. Diabetes 1982; 31: 683–8.

367. Cherrington AD, Stevenson RW, Steiner KE et al. Insulin, glucagon, and glucose as regulators of hepatic glucose uptake and production *in vivo*. Diabetes Metab Rev 1987; 3: 307–32.

368. Bergman RN, Bucolo RJ. Interaction of insulin and glucose in the control of hepatic glucose balance. Am J Physiol 1974; 227: 1314–22.

369. Kolterman OG, Gray RS, Griffin J et al. Receptor and postreceptor defects contribute to the insulin resistance in non-insulin-dependent diabetes mellitus. J Clin Invest 1981; 68: 957–69.

370. Waldhausl W, Bratusch-Marrain P, Gasic S, Korn A, Nowotny P. Insulin production rate, hepatic insulin retention, and splanchnic carbohydrate metabolism after oral glucose ingestion in hyperinsulinemic type II (non-insulin dependent) diabetes mellitus. Diabetologia 1982; 23: 6–15.

371. Consoli A, Nurjahn N, Capani F, Gerich J. Predominant role of gluconeogenesis in increased hepatic glucose production in NIDDM. Diabetes 1989; 38: 550–56.

372. Nurjhan N, Consoli A, Gerich J. Increased lipolysis and its consequences on gluconeogenesis in non-insulin-dependent diabetes mellitus. J Clin Invest 1992; 89: 169–75.

373. Consoli A, Nurjhan N, Reilly J, Bier D, Gerich J. Mechanism of increased gluconeogenesis in non-insulin dependent diabetes mellitus: role of alterations in systemic, hepatic and muscle lactate and alanine metabolism. J Clin Invest 1990; 86: 2038–45.

374. Puhakainen I, Koivisto V, Yki-Jarvinen H. Lipolysis and gluconeogenesis from glycerol are increased in patients with non-insulin-dependent diabetes mellitus. J Clin Endocrinol Metab 1992; 75: 789–94.

375. Landau BR. Estimating gluconeogenic rates in NIDDM. Adv Exp Med Biol 1993; 334: 209–20.

376. Cusi K, Consoli A, DeFronzo RA. Metabolic effects of metformin on glucose and lactate metabolism in NIDDM. J Clin Endocrinol Metab (in press).

377. Stumvoll M, Perriello G, Nurjhan N, Bucci A, Welle S, Jansson P-A et al. Glutamine and alanine metabolism in NIDDM. Diabetes 1996; 45: 863–8.

378. Magnusson I, Rothman D, Katz L, Shulman R, Shulman G. Increased rate of gluconeogenesis in type II diabetes: a ^{13}C nuclear magnetic resonance study. J Clin Invest 1992; 90: 1323–7.

379. Unger RH, Aguilar-Parada E, Mueller WA, Eisentraut AM. Studies of pancreatic alpha-cell function in normal and diabetic subjects. J Clin Invest 1970; 49: 837–45.

380. Baron AD, Schaeffer L, Shragg P, Kolterman OG. Role of hyperglucagonemia in maintenance of increased rates of hepatic glucose output in type II diabetics. Diabetes 1987; 36: 274–83.

381. Felig P, Wahren J, Hendler R. Influence of maturity-onset diabetes on splanchnic balance after oral glucose ingestion. Diabetes 1978; 27: 121–6.

382. Ohno Y, Aoki N, Nishimura A. *In vitro* production of interleukin-1, interleukin-6, and tumor necrosis factor-α in insulin-dependent diabetes mellitus. J Clin Endocrinol Metab 1993; 77: 1072–7.

383. Matsuda M, Consoli A, Bressler P, DeFronzo RA, Del Prato S. Sustained response of hepatic glucose production (HGP) to glucagon in type 2 diabetic subjects. Diabetologia 1992; 35 (suppl. 1): A37.

384. Valera A, Pujol A, Pelegrin M, Bosch F. Transgenic mice overexpressing phosphoenolpyruvate carboxykinase develop non-insulin-dependent diabetes mellitus. Proc Natl Acad Sci USA 1994; 91: 9151–4.

385. Adkins BA, Myers SR, Hendrik GK, Stevenson RW, Williams PE, Cherrington AD. Importance of the route of glucose delivery to hepatic glucose balance in the conscious dog. J Clin Invest 1987; 79: 557–65.

386. Ferrannini E, Simonson DC, Katz LD et al. The disposal of an oral glucose load in patients with non-insulin dependent diabetes. Metabolism 1988; 37: 79–85.

387. Gerich JE, Mitrakou A, Kelley D et al. Contribution of impaired muscle glucose clearance to reduced postabsorptive systemic glucose clearance in NIDDM. Diabetes 1990; 39: 211–16.

388. Revers R, Fink R, Griffin J, Olefsky J, Kolterman O. Influence of hyperglycemia in insulin's *in vivo* effects in type II diabetes. J Clin Invest 1984; 73: 664–72.

389. Capaldo B, Santoro D, Riccardi G, Perrotti N, Sacca L. Direct evidence for a stimulatory effect of hyperglycemia *per se* on peripheral glucose disposal in type II diabetes. J Clin Invest 1986; 77: 1285–90.

390. Best JD, Kahn SE, Ader M, Watanabe RM, Ni T-C, Bergman RN. Role of glucose effectiveness in the determination of glucose tolerance. Diabetes Care 1996; 19: 1018–30.

391. Felber JP, Ferrannini E, Golay A et al. Role of lipid oxidation in the pathogenesis of the insulin resistance of obesity and type II diabetes. Diabetes 1987; 36: 1341–50.

392. Young A, Bogardus C, Wolfe-Lopez D, Mott D. Muscle glycogen synthesis and disposition of infused glucose in humans with reduced rates of insulin-mediated carbohydrate storage. Diabetes 1988; 37: 303–7.

393. Kida Y, Esposito-DelPuente A, Bogardus C, Mott D. Insulin resistance is associated with reduced fasting and insulin-stimulated glycogen synthase phosphatase activity in human skeletal muscle. J Clin Invest 1990; 85: 476–81.

394. Bogardus C, Lillioja A, Stone K, Mott D. Correlation of muscle glycogen synthase activity and *in vivo* insulin action in man. J Clin Invest 1984; 73: 1185–90.

395. Avogaro A, Toffolo G, Miola M et al. Intracellular lactate- and pyruvate-interconversion rates are increased in muscle tissue of non-insulin-dependent diabetic individuals. J Clin Invest 1996; 98: 108–15.

396. Del Prato S, Bonadonna RC, Bonora E et al. Characterization of cellular defects of insulin action in type 2 (non-insulin-dependent) diabetes mellitus. J Clin Invest 1993; 91: 484–94.

397. Zawadzki JK, Wolfe RR, Mott DM, Lillioja S, Howard B, Bogardus C. Increased rate of Cori cycle in obese subjects with NIDDM and effect of weight reduction. Diabetes 1988; 37: 154–9.

398. Davis MA, Williams PE, Cherrington AD. The effect of glucagon on lactate metabolism in conscious dog. Am J Physiol 1985; 248: E463–70.

399. Kalant N, Leibovici D, Fukushima J, Ozaki S. Insulin responsiveness of superficial forearm tissues in type II (non-insulin-dependent) diabetes. Diabetologia 1982; 22: 239–44.

400. Campbell P, Mandarino L, Gerich J. Quantification of the relative impairment in actions of insulin on hepatic glucose production and peripheral glucose intake in non-insulin-dependent diabetes mellitus. Metabolism 1988; 37: 15–22.

401. Jackson RA, Perry G, Rogers J, Advoni U, Pilkington TRE. Relationship between the basal glucose concentration, glucose tolerance, and forearm glucose

uptake in maturity onset diabetes. Diabetes 1973; 22: 751–61.

402. Mitrakou A, Kelley D, Veneman T et al. Contribution of abnormal muscle and liver glucose metabolism to postprandial hyperglycemia in NIDDM. Diabetes 1990; 39: 1381–90.

403. Butterfield WJH, Whichelow MJ. Peripheral glucose metabolism in control subjects and diabetic patients during glucose, glucose-insulin and insulin sensitivity tests. Diabetologia 1965; 1: 43–53.

404. Zierler KL, Rabinowitz D. Roles of insulin and growth hormone, based on studies of forearm metabolism in man. Medicine 1963; 42: 385–402.

405. Capaldo B, Napoli R, Dimarino L, Picardi A, Riccardi G, Sacca L. Quantitation of forearm glucose and free fatty acid (FFA) disposal in normal subjects and type 2 diabetic patients: evidence against an essential role for FFA in the pathogenesis of insulin resistance. J Clin Endocrinol Metab 1988; 67: 893–8.

406. Utriainen T, Nuutila P, Takala T et al. Direct quantitation of regional muscle glucose uptake and blood flow using ^{18}FDG and $H_2^{15}O$ in NIDDM (abstr). Diabetologia 1996; 39(suppl. 1): A45.

407. Frayn KN, Coppack SW, Humphreys SM, Whyte PL. Metabolic characteristics of human adipose tissue *in vivo*. Clin Sci 1989; 76: 509–16.

408. Jansson P-A, Smith U, Lonnroth P. Evidence for lactate production by human adipose tissue *in vivo*. Diabetologia 1990; 33: 253–6.

409. Coppack SW, Fisher RM, Gibbons GF et al. Postprandial substrate deposition in human forearm and adipose tissue *in vivo*. Clin Sci 1990; 79: 339–48.

410. Marin P, Rebuffe-Scrive M, Smith U, Bjorntorp P. Glucose uptake in human adipose tissue. Metab Clin Exp 1987; 36: 1154–60.

411. Reinmuth OM, Schienberg P, Bourne B. Total cerebral blood flow and metabolism. Arch Neurol 1965; 12: 49–66.

412. Huang SC, Phelps ME, Hoffman EJ, Sideris K, Selin CJ, Kuhl DE. Non-invasive determination of local cerebral metabolic rate of glucose in man. Am J Physiol 1980; 238: E69–82.

413. Kelley D, Mitrakou A, Marsh H et al. Skeletal muscle glycolysis, oxidation, and storage of an oral glucose load. J Clin Invest 1988; 81: 1563–71.

414. Jackson RA, Roshania RD, Hawa MI, Sim BM, DiSilvio L. Impact of glucose ingestion on hepatic and peripheral glucose metabolism in man: an analysis based on simultaneous use of the forearm and double isotope techniques. J Clin Endocrinol Metab 1986; 63: 541–9.

415. Mitrakou A, Kelley D, Mokan M et al. Role of reduced suppression of glucose production and diminished early insulin release in impaired glucose tolerance. New Engl J Med 1992; 326: 22–9.

416. Jackson RA, Perry G, Rogers J, Advoni U, Pilkington TRE. Relationship between the basal glucose concentration, glucose tolerance, and forearm glucose uptake in maturity onset diabetes. Diabetes 1973; 22: 751–61.

417. Shimazu T. Neuronal regulation of hepatic glucose metabolism in mammals. Diabetes Metab Rev 1987; 3: 185–206.

418. McMahon V, Marsh HM, Rizza RA. Effects of basal insulin supplementation on disposition of mixed meal in obese patients with NIDDM. Diabetes 1989; 38: 291–303.

419. Jansen RC, Bogardus C, Takeda J, Knowler WC, Thompson CB. Linkage analysis of acute insulin secretion with GLUT2 and glucokinase in Pima Indians and the identification of a missense mutation in GLUT2. Diabetes 1994; 43: 558–63.

420. National Diabetes Data Group. Classification and diagnosis of diabetes mellitus and other categories of glucose intolerance. Diabetes 1979; 28: 1039–57.

421. Gerich JE. Is muscle the major site of insulin resistance in type 2 (non-insulin-dependent) diabetes mellitus? Diabetologia 1991; 34: 607–10.

422. Ferrannini E, Del Prato S, DeFronzo RA. Glucose kinetics: tracer methods. In Larner J, Pohl S (eds) Methods in diabetes research, vol. II. New York: John Wiley, 1985; pp 62–84.

423. Gottesman I, Mandarino L, Gerich J. Use of glucose uptake and glucose clearance for the evaluation of insulin action *in vivo*. Diabetes 1984; 33: 184–91.

424. Best J, Taborsky G, Halter J, Porte D. Glucose disposal is not proportional to plasma glucose level in man. Diabetes 1981; 30: 847–50.

425. Doberne L, Greenfield MS, Rosenthal M, Didstrom A, Reaven G. Effects of variation in basal plasma glucose concentration on glucose utilization and metabolic clearance rate during insulin clamp studies in patients with non-insulin-dependent diabetes mellitus. Diabetes 1982; 31: 396–400.

426. DeFronzo RA, Their SO. Inherited disorders of renal tubular function. In Brenner BM, Rector FC (eds) The kidney. Philadelphia: WB Saunders, 1986; pp 1297–340.

427. Zierler KL, Rabinowitz D. Effect of very small concentrations of insulin on forearm metabolism. Persistence of its action on potassium and free fatty acids without its side effect on glucose. J Clin Invest 1964; 43: 950–62.

428. Andres R, Baltzan MA, Cader G, Zierler KL. Effect of insulin on carbohydrate metabolism and on potassium in the forearm of man. J Clin Invest 1962; 41: 108–14.

429. Thiebaud D, Jacot E, DeFronzo RA, Maeder E, Jequier E, Felber JP. The effect of graded doses of insulin on total glucose uptake, glucose oxidation, and glucose storage in man. Diabetes 1982; 31: 957–63.

430. Marshall S, Olefsky J. Effect of insulin incubation on insulin binding, glucose transport, and insulin degradation by isolated adipocytes. Evidence of hormone-induced desensitization at the receptor and post-receptor level. J Clin Invest 1980; 66: 763–72.

431. Amatruda JM, Newmeyer HW, Chang CL. Insulin-induced alterations in insulin binding and insulin action in primary cultures of rat hepatocytes. Diabetes 1982; 31: 145–8.

432. Mandarino L, Baker B, Rizza R, Genest J, Gerich JE. Infusion of insulin impairs human adipocyte glucose metabolism *in vitro* without decreasing adipocyte insulin receptor binding. Diabetologia 1984; 27: 358–63.

433. Rizza RA, Mandarino LA, Genest J, Baker BA, Gerich JE. Production of insulin resistance by hyperinsulinemia in man. Diabetologia 1985; 28: 70–75.

434. Marangou AG, Weber KM, Boston RC et al. Metabolic consequences of prolonged hyperinsulinemia in humans. Evidence for induction of insulin insensitivity. Diabetes 1986; 35: 1383–9.

435. Gjedde A, Crone C. Blood–brain glucose transfer: repression in chronic hyperglycemia. Science 1981; 214: 456–7.

436. McCall AL, Millington WR, Wurtman RJ. Metabolic fuel and amino acid transport into the brain in experimental diabetes mellitus. Proc Natl Acad Sci USA 1982; 79: 5406–10.

437. Matthaei S, Horuk R, Olefsky JM. Blood–brain glucose transfer in diabetes mellitus. Diabetes 1986; 35: 1181–4.

438. McCall AL, Fixman LB, Fleming N, Tornheim K, Chick W, Ruderman NB. Chronic hypoglycemia increases brain glucose transport. Am J Physiol 1986; 251: E442–7.

439. Simonson DC, DeFronzo RA. Measurement of substrate oxidation and energy expenditure in man by indirect calorimetry: practical and theoretical consideration. Am J Physiol 1990; 258: E399–412.

440. Reaven GM, Chen Y-DI, Donner CC, Fraze E, Hollenbeck CB. How insulin resistant are patients with non-insulin-dependent diabetes mellitus? J Clin Endocrinol Metab 1985; 61: 32–6.

441. Bogardus C, Lillioja S, Mott D, Reaven GR, Kashiwagi A, Foley J. Relationship between obesity and maximal insulin-stimulated glucose uptake *in vivo* and *in vitro* in Pima Indians. J Clin Invest 1984; 73: 800–805.

442. Lillioja A, Mott DM, Zawadzki JK, Young AA, Abbott WG, Bogardus C. Glucose storage is a major determinant of *in vivo* 'insulin resistance' in subjects with normal glucose tolerance. J Clin Endocrinol Metab 1986; 62: 922–7.

443. Sims EAH, Danford E, Horton ES, Bray GA, Glennon JA, Salans LB. Endocrine and metabolic effects of experimental obesity in man. Rec Prog Horm Res 1973; 29: 457–96.

444. Hamman RF. Genetic and environmental determinants of non-insulin-dependent diabetes mellitus (NIDDM). Diabetes Metab Rev 1992; 8: 287–338.

445. Aitman TJ, Todd JA. Molecular genetics of diabetes mellitus. Baillière's Clin Endocrinol Metab 1995; 9: 631–56.

446. Turner RC, Hattersley AT, Shaw JTE, Levy JC. Type II diabetes: clinical aspects of molecular biological studies. Diabetes 1995; 44: 1–10.

447. McCarthy MI, Froguel P, Hitman GA. The genetics of non-insulin-dependent diabetes mellitus: tools and aims. Diabetologia 1994; 37: 959–68.

448. Cook JTE, Shields DC, Page RCL et al. Segregation analysis of NIDDM in Caucasian families. Diabetologia 1994; 37: 1231–40.

449. Granner DK, O'Brien RM. Molecular physiology and genetics of NIDDM. Diabetes Care 1992; 15: 369–95.

450. Cook JTE, Hattersley AT, Levy JC et al. Distribution of type II diabetes in nuclear families. Diabetes 1993; 42: 106–12.

451. Froguel P, Velho G, Passa P, Cohen D. Genetic determinants of type 2 diabetes mellitus: lessons learned from family studies. Diabète Métab 1993; 19: 1–10.

452. Hanis CL, Boerwinkle E, Chakroborty R et al. A genome-wide search for human non-insulin-dependent (type 2) diabetes genes reveals a major susceptibility locus on chromosome 2. Nature Genetics 1996; 13: 161–6.

453. Elbein SC, Chiu KC, Hoffman MD, Mayorga RA, Bragg KL, Leppert MF. Linkage analysis of 19 candidate regions for insulin resistance in familial NIDDM. Diabetes 1995; 44: 1259–65.

454. Haring HU, Mehnert H. Pathogenesis of type 2 (non-insulin-dependent) diabetes mellitus: candidates for a signal transmitter defect causing insulin resistance of the skeletal muscle. Diabetologia 1993; 36: 176–82.

455. Elbein SC, Bragg KL, Hoffman MD, Mayorga RA, Leppert MF. Linkage studies of NIDDM with 23 chromosome 11 markers in a sample of whites of northern European descent. Diabetes 1996; 45: 370–75.

456. Taylor SI, Kadowaki T, Kadowaki H, Accili D, Cama A, McKeon C. Mutations in insulin receptor gene in insulin-resistant patients. Diabetes Care 1990; 13: 257–75.

457. Tsaur M-L, Menzel S, Lai F-P et al. Isolation of a cDNA clone encoding a K_{ATP} channel-like protein expressed in insulin-secreting cells, localization of the human gene to chromosome band 21q22.1, and linkage studies with NIDDM. Diabetes 1995; 44: 592–6.

458. Cushman SW, Wardzala LJ. Potential mechanism of insulin action on glucose transport in the isolated rat adipose cell. Apparent translocation of intracellular transport systems to the plasma membrane. J Biol Chem 1980; 255: 4758–62.

459. Klip A, Paquet MR. Glucose transport and glucose transporters in muscle and their metabolic regulation. Diabetes Care 1990; 13: 228–40.

460. Kasanicki MA, Pilch PF. Regulation of glucose transporter function. Diabetes Care 1990; 13: 219–25.

461. Thorens B, Charron MJ, Lodish HF. Molecular physiology of glucose transporters. Diabetes Care 1990; 13: 209–16.

462. Kahn BB, Flier JS. Regulation of glucose transporter gene expression *in vitro* and *in vivo*. Diabetes Care 1990; 13: 548–60.

463. Seino S, Seino M, Bell GI. Human insulin-receptor gene. Diabetes 1990; 39: 129–33.

464. Zhang Y, Warren-Perry M, Sakura H et al. No evidence for mutations in a putative beta cell ATP-sensitive K^+ channel subunit in MODY, NIDDM, or GDM. Diabetes 1995; 44: 597–600.

465. Seino S, Bell GI. Alternative splicing of human insulin receptor messenger RNA. Biochem Biophys Res Commun 1989; 159: 312–16.

466. McClain DA. Insulin action in cells expressing truncated or kinase-defective insulin receptors: dissection of multiple hormone signaling pathways. Diabetes Care 1990; 13: 302–14.

467. Tanizawa Y, Riggs AC, Chiu KC et al. Variability of the pancreatic islet beta cell/liver (GLUT2) glucose transporter gene in NIDDM patients. Diabetologia 1994; 37: 420–27.

468. Orho M, Carlsson M, Kanninen T, Groop LC. Polymorphism at the rad gene is not associated with NIDDM in Finns. Diabetes 1996; 45: 429–33.

469. Stirling B, Cox NJ, Bell GI, Hanis CL, Spielman RS, Concannon P. Linkage studies in NIDDM with markers near the sulphonylurea receptor gene. Diabetologia 1995; 38: 1479–81.

470. Stirling B, Cox NJ, Bell GI, Hanis CL, Spielman RS, Concannon P. Identification of microsatellite markers near the human ob gene and linkage studies in NIDDM-affected sib pairs. Diabetes 1995; 44: 999–1001.

471. Gambino V, Menzel S, Trabb JB et al. An approach for identifying simple sequence repeat DNA polymorphisms near cloned cDNAs and genes. Linkage studies of the islet amyloid polypeptide/amylin and liver glycogen synthase genes and NIDDM. Diabetes 1996; 45: 291-4.

472. Ferrer J, Wasson J, Salkoff L, Permutt MA. Cloning of human pancreatic islet large conductance Ca^{++} activated K^+ channel (hSlo) cDNAs: evidence for high levels of expression in pancreatic islets and identification of a flanking genetic marker. Diabetologia 1996; 39: 891-8.

473. Prochazka M, Lillioja S, Tait JF et al. Linkage of chromosomal markers on 4q with a putative gene determining maximal insulin action in Pima Indians. Diabetes 1993; 42: 514-19.

474. Humphreys P, McCarthy M, Tuomilehto J et al. Chromosome 4q locus associated with insulin resistance in Pima Indians. Diabetes 1994; 43: 800-814.

475. Hanis CL. Genetics of non-insulin-dependent diabetes mellitus among Mexican-Americans: approaches and perspectives. In: Berg K, Boulyjekov V, Christen Y (eds) Genetic approaches to noncommunicable diseases. Berlin: Springer-Verlag, 1996; pp 65-77.

476. Lander E, Kruglyak L. Genetic dissection of complex traits: guidelines for interpreting and reporting linkage results. Nature Genet 1995; 11: 241-7.

477. Stern MP, Duggirala R, Mitchell BD et al. Evidence for linkage of regions on chromosomes 6 and 11 to plasma glucose concentrations in Mexican-Americans. Genome Res 1996; 724-34.

478. Thompson DB, Janssen RC, Ossowski VM, Prochazka M, Knowler WC, Bogardus C. Evidence for linkage between a region on chromosome 1p and the acute insulin response in Pima Indians. Diabetes 1995; 44: 478-81.

479. Baier LJ, Sacchettini JC, Knowler WC et al. An amino acid substitution in the human intestinal fatty acid binding protein is associated with increased fatty acid binding, increased fat oxidation, and insulin resistance. J Clin Invest 1995; 95: 1281-7.

480. Dent P, Lavoinne A, Nakielny S, Caudwell FB, Watt P, Cohen P. The molecular mechanisms by which insulin stimulates glycogen synthesis in mammalian skeletal muscle. Nature 1990; 348: 302-7.

481. Cohen P. The structure and regulation of protein phosphatases. Ann Rev Biochem 1989; 58: 453-508.

482. Baier L. The Pima Diabetes Genes Group. Suggestive linkage of genetic markers on chromosome 4q.12 to NIDDM and insulin action in Pima Indians: new evidence to extend associations reported in other populations (abstr). Diabetes 1996; 45(suppl. 2): 30A.

483. Tsui LC, Donis-Keller H, Grzeschik K-H. Report of the second international workshop on human chromosome 7 mapping. Cytogenet Cell Genet 1995; 71: 2-31.

484. Elbein SC, Hoffman M, Mayorga R, Wegner K, Miles C, Leppert M. Evidence for an NIDDM susceptibility locus in Caucasians at a reported Pima Indian diabetes locus (abstr). Diabetes 1996; 45(suppl. 2): 231A.

485. Mahtani MM, Widen E, Lehto M et al. Mapping of a gene for type 2 diabetes associated with an insulin secretion defect by a genome scan in Finnish families. Nature Genet 1996; 13: 90-94.

486. Collins FS. Positional cloning: let's not call it reverse anymore. Nature Genet 1992; 1: 3-6.

487. Collins FS. Positional cloning moves from perditional to traditional. Nature Genet 1995; 9: 347-50.

488. DeFronzo RA, Ferrannini E. Insulin resistance: a multifaceted syndrome responsible for NIDDM, obesity, hypertension, dyslipidemia, and ASCVD. Diabetes Care Rev 1991; 14: 173-94.

489. Peiris AN, Struve MF, Mueller RA, Lee MB, Kissebah AH. Glucose metabolism in obesity: influence of body fat distribution. J Clin Endocrinol Metab 1988; 67: 760-67.

490. Bjorntorp P. Abdominal obesity and the development of non-insulin-dependent diabetes mellitus. Diabetes Metab Rev 1988; 4: 615-22.

491. Bonora E, Del Prato S, Bonadonna RC et al. Total body fat content and fat topography are associated differently with *in vivo* glucose metabolism in non-obese and obese non-diabetic women. Diabetes 1992; 41: 1151-9.

492. Kissebah AH. Central obesity: measurement and metabolic effects. Diabetes Rev.

493. Lonnqvist F, Thorne A, Nilsell K, Hoffstedt J, Arner P. A pathogenetic role of visceral beta-adrenoreceptors in obesity. J Clin Invest 1995; 95: 1109-16.

494. Yki-Jarvinen H. Sex and insulin sensitivity. Metabolism 1984; 30: 1011-15.

495. Nuutila P, Knuuti MJ, Maki M et al. Gender and insulin sensitivity in the heart and in skeletal muscles. Studies using positron emission tomography. Diabetes 1995; 44: 31-6.

496. Olefsky JM. Insulin resistance and insulin action. An *in vitro* and *in vivo* perspective. Diabetes 1981; 30: 148-62.

497. Rizza RA, Mandarino LJ, Gerich JE. Mechanism and significance of insulin resistance in non-insulin-dependent diabetes mellitus. Diabetes 1981; 30: 990-95.

498. DePirro R, Fusco A, Lauro R, Testa I, Ferreti F, DeMartinis C. Erythrocyte insulin receptors in non-insulin-dependent diabetes mellitus. Diabetes 1980; 29: 96-9.

499. Pederson O. Studies of insulin receptor binding and insulin action in humans. Danish Med Bull 1984; 31: 1-32.

500. Caro JF, Ittoop O, Pories WJ et al. Studies on the mechanism of insulin resistance in the liver from humans with non-insulin-dependent diabetes. Insulin action and binding in isolated hepatocytes, insulin receptor structure, and kinase activity. J Clin Invest 1986; 78: 249-58.

501. Comi RJ, Grunberger G, Gorden P. Relationship of insulin binding and insulin-stimulated tyrosine kinase activity is altered in type II diabetes. J Clin Invest 1987; 79: 453-62.

502. Freidenberg GR, Henry RR, Klein HH, Reichart DR, Olefsky JM. Decreased kinase activity of insulin receptors from adipocytes of non-insulin-dependent diabetic studies. J Clin Invest 1987; 79: 240-50.

503. Takayama S, Kahn CR, Kubo K, Foley JE. Alterations in insulin receptor autophosphorylation in insulin resistance: correlation with altered sensitivity to glucose transport and antilipolysis to insulin. J Clin Endocrinol Metab 1988; 66: 922-9.

504. Thies RS, Molina JM, Ciaraldi TP, Freidenberg GR, Olefsky JM. Insulin-receptor autophosphorylation and

endogenous substrate phosphorylation in human adipocytes from control, obese and NIDDM subjects. Diabetes 1990; 39: 250-58.

505. Trichitta V, Brunetti A, Chiavetta A, Benzi L, Papa V, Vigneri R. Defects in insulin-receptor internalization and processing in monocytes of obese subjects and obese NIDDM patients. Diabetes 1989; 38: 1579-84.

506. Caro JF, Sinha MK, Raju SM et al. Insulin receptor kinase in human skeletal muscle from obese subjects with and without non-insulin dependent diabetes. J Clin Invest 1987; 79: 1330-37.

507. Molina JM, Ciaraldi TP, Brady D, Olefsky JM. Decreased activation rate of insulin-mediated glucose transport in adipocytes from obese and NIDDM subjects. Diabetes 1989; 38: 991-5.

508. Arner P, Pollare T, Lithell H, Livingston JN. Defective insulin receptor tyrosine kinase in human skeletal muscle in obesity and type II (non-insulin-dependent) diabetes mellitus. Diabetologia 1987; 30: 437-40.

509. Dohm GL. Insulin receptor kinase in human skeletal muscle from obese subjects with and without non-insulin-dependent diabetes. J Clin Invest 1987; 79: 1330-37.

510. Klein HH, Vestergaard H, Kotzke G, Pedersen O. Elevation of serum insulin concentration during euglycemic hyperinsulinemic clamp studies leads to similar activation of insulin receptor kinase in skeletal muscle of subjects with and without NIDDM. Diabetes 1995; 344: 1310-17.

511. Grasso G, Frittitta L, Anello M, Russo P, Sesti G, Trischitta V. Insulin receptor tyrosine-kinase activity is altered in both muscle and adipose tissue from non-obese normoglycaemic insulin-resistant subjects. Diabetologia 1995; 38: 55-61.

512. Haring HU, Obermaier B, Ermel B et al. Insulin receptor kinase defects as a possible cause of cellular insulin resistance. Diabète Métab 1987; 13: 284-93.

513. Obermaier-Kusser B, White MF, Pongratz DE et al. A defective intramolecular autoactivation cascade may cause the reduced kinase activity of the skeletal muscle insulin receptor from patients with non-insulin-dependent diabetes mellitus. J Biol Chem 1989; 264: 9497-503.

514. Arner P, Einarsson K, Ewerth S, Livingston J. Studies on the human liver insulin receptor in non-insulin-dependent diabetes mellitus. J Clin Invest 1986; 77: 1716-18.

515. Kashiwagi A, Verso MA, Andrews J, Vasquez B, Reaven G, Foley JE. In vitro insulin resistance of human adipocytes isolated from subjects with non-insulin-dependent diabetes mellitus. J Clin Invest 1983; 72: 1246-54.

516. Bolinder J, Ostman J, Arner P. Postreceptor defects causing insulin resistance in normo-insulinemic non-insulin-dependent diabetes mellitus. Diabetes 1982; 31: 911-16.

517. Hidaka H, Nagulesparan M, Klimes I et al. Improvement of insulin secretion but not insulin resistance after short-term control of plasma glucose in obese type II diabetes mellitus. J Clin Endocrinol Metab 1982; 54: 217-22.

518. Nankervis A, Proietto J, Aitken P, Harwood M, Alford F. Differential effects of insulin therapy on hepatic and peripheral insulin sensitivity in type II (non-insulin-dependent) diabetes. Diabetologia 1982; 23: 320-25.

519. Okamoto M, Kuzuya H, Seino Y, Ikeda M, Imura H. Insulin binding to erythrocytes in diabetic patients. Endocrinol J 1981; 28: 169-73.

520. Seltzer H. Are insulin receptors clinically significant? J Lab Clin Med 1982; 100: 821-51.

521. Lonnroth P, Digirolamo M, Krotkiewski M, Smith U. Insulin binding and responsiveness in fat cells from patients with reduced glucose tolerance and type II diabetes. Diabetes 1983; 32: 748-54.

522. Olefsky JM, Reaven GM. Insulin binding in diabetes. Relationships with plasma insulin levels and insulin sensitivity. Diabetes 1977; 26: 680-88.

523. Mandarino LJ, Campbell PJ, Gottesman IS, Gerich JE. Abnormal coupling of insulin receptor binding in non-insulin-dependent diabetes. Am J Physiol 1984; 247: E688-92.

524. Kahn CR. Role of insulin receptors in insulin resistant state. Metabolism 1980; 29: 455-66.

525. Kadowaki T, Kadowaki H, Rechler MM et al. Five mutant alleles of the insulin receptor gene in patients with genetic forms of insulin resistance. J Clin Invest 1990; 86: 254-62.

526. McClain DA, Henry RR, Ullrich A, Olefsky JM. Restriction-fragment-length polymorphism in insulin-receptor gene and insulin resistance in NIDDM. Diabetes 1988; 37: 1071-5.

527. Raboudi SH, Mitchell BD, Stern MP et al. Type II diabetes mellitus and polymorphisms of insulin-receptor gene in Mexican-Americans. Diabetes 1989; 38: 975-9.

528. Xiang KS, Cox NJ, Sanz N, Huang P, Karan JH, Bell GI. Insulin receptor and apolipoprotein genes contribute to development of NIDDM in Chinese-Americans. Diabetes 1989; 38: 17-23.

529. Elbein SC, Borecki I, Corsetti L et al. Linkage analysis of the human insulin receptor gene and maturity onset diabetes of the young. Diabetologia 1987; 30: 641-7.

530. O'Rahilly S, Trembath RC, Patel P, Galton DJ, Turner RC, Wainscoat JS. Linkage analysis of the human insulin receptor gene in type II (non-insulin-dependent) diabetic families and a family with maturity onset diabetes of the young. Diabetologia 1988; 31: 797-7.

531. Elbein SC, Ward WK, Beard JC, Permutt MA. Familial NIDDM: molecular-genetic analysis and assessment of insulin action and pancreatic beta-cell function. Diabetes 1988; 37: 337-82.

532. Cox NJ, Epstein PA, Spielman RS. Linkage studies on NIDDM and the insulin and insulin receptor genes. Diabetes 1989; 38: 653-8.

533. Li SR, Oelbaum RS, Stocks J, Galton DJ. DNA polymorphisms of the insulin-receptor gene in Japanese subjects with non-insulin-dependent diabetes mellitus. Hum Hered 1988; 38: 273-6.

534. Moller DE, Yakota A, Flier JS. Normal insulin receptor cDNA sequence in Pima Indians with non-insulin-dependent diabetes mellitus. Diabetes 1989; 38: 1496-500.

535. O'Rahilly S, Choi WH, Patel P, Turner RC, Flier JS, Moller DE. Detection of mutations in insulin-receptor gene in NIDDM patients by analysis of single-stranded conformation polymorphisms. Diabetes 1991; 40: 777-82.

536. Kusari J, Verma US, Buse JB, Henry RR, Olefsky JM. Analysis of the gene sequences of the insulin

receptor and the insulin-sensitive glucose transporter (GLUT4) in patients with common-type non-insulin-dependent diabetes mellitus. J Clin Invest 1991; 88: 1323-30.

537. Cocozza S, Procellini A, Riccardi G, et al. NIDDM associated with mutation in tyrosine kinase domain of insulin receptor gene. Diabetes 1992; 41: 521-6.

538. Brillon DJ, Freidenberg GR, Henry RR, Olefsky JM. Mechanism of defective insulin-receptor kinase activity in NIDDM. Evidence for two receptor populations. Diabetes 1989; 38: 397-403.

539. Nyomba BL, Ossowski VM, Bogardus C, Mott DM. Insulin-sensitive tyrosine kinase: relationship with *in vivo* insulin action in humans. Am J Physiol 1990; 258: E964-/4.

540. Freidenberg GR, Reichart D, Olefsky JM, Henry RR. Reversibility of defective adipocyte insulin receptor kinase activity in non-insulin dependent diabetes mellitus. Effect of weight loss. J Clin Invest 1988; 82: 1398-406.

541. Koivisto VA, DeFronzo RA. Physical training and insulin sensitivity. Diabetes Metab Rev 1986; 1: 445-81.

542. Maegwa H, Shigeta Y, Egawa K, Kobayshai M. Impaired autophosphorylation of insulin receptors from abdominal skeletal muscles in non-obese subjects with NIDDM. Diabetes 1993; 40: 815-19.

543. Nolan JJ, Freidenberg G, Henry R, Reichart D, Olefsky JM. Role of human skeletal muscle insulin receptor kinase in the *in vivo* insulin resistance of non-insulin-dependent diabetes and obesity. J Clin Endocrinol Metab 1994; 78: 471-7.

544. Bak JF, Moller N, Schmitz O, Saaek A, Pedersen O. *In vivo* insulin action and muscle glycogen synthase activity in type 2 (non-insulin dependent) diabetes mellitus: effects of diet treatment. Diabetologia 1992; 35: 777-94.

545. Kellerer M, Kroder G, Tippmer S et al. Troglitazone prevents glucose-induced insulin resistance of insulin receptor in rat-1 fibroblasts. Diabetes 1994; 43: 447-53.

546. Rosenthal M, Haskell WL, Solomon R, Widstrom A, Reaven GM. Demonstration of a relationship between physical training and insulin-stimulated glucose utilization in normal humans. Diabetes 1983; 32: 408-11.

547. Eriksson K-F, Lindgarde F. Prevention of type 2 (non-insulin-dependent) diabetes mellitus by diet and physical exercise. The 6-year Malmo feasibility study. Diabetologia 1991; 34: 891-8.

548. Moller DE, Yakota A, Caro JF, Flier JS. Tissue-specific expression of two alternatively spliced insulin receptor mRNAs in man. Mol Endocrinol 1989; 3: 1263-9.

549. Mosthaf L, Vogt B, Haring HU, Ullrich A. Altered expression of insulin receptor types A and B in the skeletal muscle of non-insulin-dependent diabetes mellitus patients. Proc Natl Acad Sci USA 1991; 88: 4728-30.

550. Sesti G, Marini MA, Tullio AN et al. Altered expression of the two naturally occurring human insulin receptor variants in isolated adipocytes of non-insulin-dependent diabetes mellitus patients. Biochem Biophys Res Commun 1991; 181: 1419-24.

551. Benecke H, Flier JS, Moller DE. Alternatively spliced variants of the insulin receptor protein. Expression in normal and diabetic human tissues. J Clin Invest 1992; 89: 2066-70.

552. Hansen T, Bjoerbaek C, Vestergaard H, Bak JF, Pedersen O. Expression of insulin receptor spliced variants and their functional correlates in muscle from patients with non-insulin dependent diabetes mellitus. J Clin Endocrinol Metab 1993; 77: 1500-505.

553. Almind K, Bjorbaek C, Vestergaard H, Hansen T, Echwald S, Pederson O. Amino acid polymorphisms of insulin receptor substrate-1 in non-insulin dependent diabetes mellitus. Lancet 1993; 342: 828-32.

554. Hitman GA, Hawrami K, McCarthy MI et al. Insulin receptor substrate-1 gene mutations in NIDDM; implications for the study of polygenic disease. Diabetologia 1995; 38: 481-6.

555. Laville M, Auboeuf D, Khalfallah Y, Vega N, Riou JP, Vidal H. Acute regulation by insulin of phosphatidylinositol-3-kinase, Rad, Glut 4, and lipoprotein lipase mRNA levels in human muscle. J Clin Invest 1996; 98: 43-9.

556. Folli F, Saad JA, Backer JM, Kahn CR. Regulation of phosphatidylinositol 3-kinase activity in liver and muscle of animal models of insulin-resistant and insulin-deficient diabetes mellitus. J Clin Invest 1993; 92: 1787-94.

557. Reynet C, Kahn CR. Rad: a member of the *ras* family overexpressed in muscle of type II diabetic humans. Science 1993; 262: 1441-4.

558. Kono T, Robinson FW, Blevins TL, Ezaki O. Evidence that translocation of the glucose transport activity is the major mechanism of insulin action on glucose transport fat cells. J Biol Chem 1982; 257: 10942-7.

559. Bell GI, Kayano T, Buse JB et al. Molecular biology of mammalian glucose transporters. Diabetes Care 1990; 13: 198-200.

560. Mueckler MM, Caruso C, Baldwin SA et al. Sequence and structure of a human glucose transporter. Science 1985; 229: 941-5.

561. Birnbaum MJ, Haspel HC, Rosen OM. Cloning and characterization of cDNA encoding the rat brain glucose transporter protein. Proc Natl Acad Sci USA 1986; 83: 5784-8.

562. Kahn BB. Facilitative glucose transporters: regulatory mechanisms and dysregulation in diabetes. J Clin Invest 1992; 89: 1367-74.

563. Colowick SP. The hexokinases. In Boyer PD (ed.) The enzymes, vol. 9. New York: Academic Press, 1973; pp 1-48.

564. Nishi S, Susumu S, Bell GI. Human hexokinase: sequences of amino-and carboxyl-terminal halves are homologous. Biochem Biophys Res Commun 1988; 157: 937-43.

565. Schwab DA, Wilson JE. Complete amino acid sequence of rat brain hexokinase, deduced from the cloned cDNA, and proposed structure of a mammalian hexokinase. Proc Natl Acad Sci USA 1989; 86: 2563-7.

566. Magnuson MA, Andreone IL, Printz RL, Koch S, Granner DK. The glucokinase gene: structure and regulation by insulin. Proc Natl Acad Sci USA 1989; 86: 4838-42.

567. Magnuson MA, Shelton KD. An alternate promoter in the glucokinase gene is active in the pancreatic beta cell. J Biol Chem 1989; 264: 15936-42.

568. Ciaraldi TP, Kolterman OG, Scarlett JA, Kao M, Olefsky JM. Role of the glucose transport system

in the postreceptor defect of non-insulin-dependent diabetes mellitus. Diabetes 1982; 31: 1016–22.

569. Foley JE, Kashawagi A, Verso MA, Reaven G, Andrews J. Improvement in *in vitro* action after one month of insulin therapy in obese non-insulin-dependent diabetes. J Clin Invest 1983; 72: 1901–9.

570. Garvey WT, Huecksteadt TP, Mattaei S, Olefsky JM. Role of glucose transporters in the cellular insulin resistance of type II non-insulin dependent diabetes mellitus. J Clin Invest 1988; 81: 1528–36.

571. Scarlett JA, Kolterman OG, Ciaraldi TP, Kao M, Olefsky JM. Insulin treatment reverses the postreceptor defect in adipocyte 3-*O*-methylglucose transport in type II diabetes mellitus. J Clin Endocrinol Metab 1983; 56: 1195–201.

572. Dohm GL, Tapscott EB, Pories WJ et al. An *in vitro* human muscle preparation suitable for metabolic studies: decreased insulin stimulation of glucose transport in muscle from morbidly obese and diabetic subjects. J Clin Invest 1988; 82: 486–94.

573. Andreasson K, Galuska D, Thorne T, Sonnenfeld T, Wallberg-Henriksson H. Decreased insulin-stimulated 3-*O*-methylglucose transport in *in vitro* incubated muscle strips from type II diabetic subjects. Acta Physiol Scand 1991; 142: 255–60.

574. Zierath JR, Galuska D, Nolte LA, Thorne A, Kristensen JS, Wallberg-Henriksson H. Effects of glycaemia on glucose transport in isolated skeletal muscle from patients with NIDDM: *in vitro* reversal of muscular insulin resistance. Diabetologia 1994; 37: 270–77.

575. Henry RR, Abrams L, Nikoulina S, Ciaraldi TP. Insulin action and glucose metabolism in non-diabetic control and NIDDM subjects. Diabetes 1995; 44: 936–46.

576. Ciaraldi TP, Abrams L, Nikoulina S, Mudaliar S, Henry RR. Glucose transport in cultured human skeletal muscle cells. J Clin Invest 1995; 96: 2820–27.

577. Carey JO, Azevedo JL Jr, Morris PG, Pories WJ, Dohn GL. Okadaic acid, vanadate and phenylarsine oxide stimulate 2-deoxyglucose transport in insulin-resistant human skeletal muscle. Diabetes 1995; 44: 682–8.

578. Kahn BB, Shulman GI, DeFronzo RA, Cushman SW, Rossetti L. Normalization of blood glucose in diabetic rats with phlorizin treatment reverses insulin-resistant glucose transport in adipose cells without restoring glucose transporter gene expression. J Clin Invest 1991; 87: 561–70.

579. Handberg A, Vaag A, Damsbo P, Beck-Nielsen H, Vinten J. Expression of insulin regulatable glucose transporters in skeletal muscle from type 2 (non-insulin-dependent) diabetic patients. Diabetologia 1990; 33: 625–7.

580. Pedersen O, Bak J, Andersen P, Lund S, Moller DE, Flier JS, Kahn BB. Evidence against altered expression of GLUT1 or GLUT4 in skeletal muscle of patients with obesity or NIDDM. Diabetes 1990; 39: 865–70.

581. Eriksson J, Koranyi L, Bourey R et al. Insulin resistance in type 2 (non-insulin-dependent) diabetic patients and their relatives is not associated with a defect in the expression of the insulin-responsive glucose transporter (GLUT-4) gene in human skeletal muscle. Diabetologia 1992; 35: 143–7.

582. Schalin-Jantti C, Yki-Jarvinen H, Koranyi L et al. Effect of insulin on GLUT-4 mRNA and protein

concentrations in skeletal muscle of patients with NIDDM and their first-degree relatives. Diabetologia 1994; 37: 401–7.

583. Lund S, Vestergaard H, Andersen PH, Schmitz O, Gotzsche LBH, Pedersen O. Glut-4 content in plasma membrane of muscle from patients with non-insulin-dependent diabetes mellitus. Am J Physiol 1993; 265: E889–97.

584. Garvey WT, Maianu L, Hancock JA, Golichowski AM, Baron A. Gene expression of Glut4 in skeletal muscle from insulin-resistant patients with obesity, IGT, GDM, and NIDDM. Diabetes 1992; 41: 465–75.

585. Mandarino LJ, Printz RL, Cusi KA et al. Regulation of hexokinase II and glycogen synthase mRNA, protein, and activity in human muscle. Am J Physiol 1995; 269: E701–8.

586. Andersen P, Lund S, Vestergaard H, Junker S, Kahn B, Pedersen O. Expression of the major insulin regulatable glucose transporter (GLUT4) in skeletal muscle of non-insulin-dependent diabetic patients and healthy subjects before and after insulin infusion. J Clin Endocrinol Metab 1993; 77: 27–32.

587. Yki-Jarvinen H, Vuorinen-Markkola H, Koranyi L et al. Defect in insulin action on expression of the muscle/adipose tissue glucose transporter gene in skeletal muscle of type 1 diabetic patients. J Clin Endocrinol Metab 1992; 75: 795–9.

588. Kusari J, Verma US, Buse JB, Henry RR, Olefsky JM. Analysis of the gene sequences of the insulin receptor and the insulin-sensitive glucose transporter (GLUT 4) in patients with common-type non-insulin-dependent diabetes mellitus. J Clin Invest 1991; 88: 1323–30.

589. Choi WH, O'Rahilly S, Rees A, Morgan R, Flier JS, Moller DE. Molecular scanning of the insulin-responsive glucose transporter (GLUT 4) gene in patients with non-insulin dependent diabetes mellitus. Diabetes 1991; 40: 1712–18.

590. Sinha M, Raineri-Maldonado C, Buchanan C et al. Adipose tissue glucose transporters in NIDDM: decreased levels of muscle/fat isoform. Diabetes 1991; 40: 474–7.

591. Garvey W, Maianu L, Huecksteadt T, Molina J, Ciaraldi T. Pretranslational suppression of a glucose transporter protein causes cellular insulin resistance in non-insulin-dependent diabetes mellitus and obesity. J Clin Invest 1991; 87: 1072–81.

592. Cobelli C, Saccomani MP, Ferrannini E, DeFronzo RA, Gelfand R, Bonadonna R. A compartmental model to quantitate *in vivo* glucose transport in the human forearm. Am J Physiol 1989; 257: E943–58.

593. Saccomani MP, Bonadonna RC, Bier DM, DeFronzo RA, Cobelli C. A model to measure insulin effects on glucose transport and phosphorylation in muscle: a three-tracer study. Am J Physiol 1996; 270 (Endocrinol Metab 33): E170–85.

594. Bonadonna RC, Saccomani MP, Seely L et al. Glucose transport in human skeletal muscle. The *in vivo* response to insulin. Diabetes 1993; 42: 191–8.

595. Bonadonna RC, Del Prato S, Saccomani MP et al. Transmembrane glucose transport in skeletal muscle of patients with non-insulin-dependent diabetes. J Clin Invest 1993; 92: 486–94.

596. Bonadonna RC, Del Prato S, Bonora E et al. Roles of glucose transport and glucose phosphorylation in

muscle insulin resistance of NIDDM. Diabetes 1996; 45: 915–25.

597. Guma A, Zierath JR, Wallberg-Henriksson H, Klip A. Insulin induces translocation of GLUT-4 glucose transporters in human skeletal muscle. Am J Physiol 1995; 268: E613–22.

598. Kelley DE, Mintun MA, Watkins SC, Simoneau J-A, Jadali F, Fredrickson A. The effect of non-insulin-dependent diabetes mellitus and obesity on glucose transport and phosphorylation in skeletal muscle. J Clin Invest 1996; 97: 2705–13.

599. Goodyear LJ, Hirshman MF, Napoli R et al. Glucose ingestion causes GLUT4 translocation in human skeletal muscle. Diabetes 1996; 45: 1051–6.

600. Napoli R, Hirshman MF, Horton FS. Mechanisms of increased skeletal muscle glucose transport activity after an oral glucose load in rats. Diabetes 1995; 44: 1362–8.

601. Printz RL, Koch S, Potter LR et al. Hexokinase II mRNA and gene structure, regulation by insulin, and evolution. J Biol Chem 1993; 268: 5209–19.

602. Printz RL, Ardehali H, Koch S, Granner DK. Human hexokinase II mRNA and gene structure. Diabetes 1995; 44: 290–94.

603. Magnuson MA, Andreone TL, Printz RL, Koch S, Granner DK. Rat glucokinase gene: structure and regulation by insulin. Proc Natl Acad Sci USA 1989; 86: 4838–42.

604. Katzen HM. The multiple forms of mammalian hexokinase and their significance to the action of insulin. Adv Enzyme Regul 1967; 5: 335–56.

605. Manchester J, Kong X, Nerbonne J, Lowry OH, Lawrence JC Jr. Glucose transport and phosphorylation in single cardiac myocytes: rate-limiting steps in glucose metabolism. Am J Physiol 1994; 266: E326–33.

606. Postic CA, Leturque A, Rencurel F et al. The effect of hyperinsulinemia and hyperglycemia on GLUT4 and hexokinase II mRNA and protein in rat skeletal muscle and adipose tissue. Diabetes 1993; 42: 922–9.

607. Rothman DL, Shulman RG, Shulman GI. ^{31}P nuclear magnetic resonance measurements of muscle glucose-6-phosphate. Evidence for reduced insulin-dependent muscle glucose transport or phosphorylation activity in non-insulin-dependent diabetes mellitus. J Clin Invest 1992; 89: 1069–75.

608. Pendergrass M, Fazioni E, Saccomani MP et al. *In vivo* glucose transport and phosphorylation in skeletal muscle is impaired in insulin resistant, normal glucose-tolerant offspring of two NIDDM parents. Diabetes 1995; 44(suppl. 1): 197A.

609. Rothman DL, Magnusson I, Cline G et al. Decreased muscle glucose transport/phosphorylation is an early defect in the pathogenesis of non-insulin-dependent diabetes mellitus. Proc Natl Acad Sci USA 1995; 92: 983–7.

610. Kubo K, Foley JE. Rate-limiting steps for insulin-mediated glucose uptake into perfused rat hindlimb. Am J Physiol 1986; 250: E100–102.

611. Pendergrass M, Koval J, Collins D et al. Insulin-induced hexokinase II (HKII) expression is reduced in obesity and NIDDM. Diabetes 1996; 45(suppl. 2): 19A.

612. Vestergaard H, Bjorbaek C, Hansen T, Larsen FS, Granner DK, Pedersen O. Impaired activity and gene

expression of hexokinase II in muscle from non-insulin-dependent diabetes mellitus patients. J Clin Invest 1995; 96: 2639–45.

613. Lehto M, Huang X, Davis EM et al. Human hexokinase II gene: exon–intron organization, mutation screening in NIDDM, and its relationship to muscle hexokinase activity. Diabetologia 1995; 38: 1466–74.

614. Lehto M, Xiang K, Stoffel M et al. Human hexokinase II: localization of the polymorphic gene to chromosome 2. Diabetologia 1993; 36: 1299–1302.

615. Laakso M, Malkki M, Kekalainen P, Kuusito J, Deeb SS. Polymorphisms of the human hexokinase II gene: lack of association with NIDDM and insulin resistance. Diabetologia 1995; 38: 617–22.

616. Taylor RW, Printz RL, Armstrong M et al. Variant sequences of the hexokinase II gene in familial NIDDM. Diabetologia 1996; 39: 322–8.

617. Laakso M, Malkki M, Deeb SS. Amino acid substitutions in hexokinase II among patients with NIDDM. Diabetes 1995; 44: 330–34.

618. Echwald SM, Bjorbaek C, Hansen T et al. Identification of four amino acid substitutions in hexokinase II and studies of relationships to NIDDM, glucose effectiveness, and insulin sensitivity. Diabetes 1995; 44: 347–53.

619. Vidal-Puig A, Printz RL, Stratton IM, Granner DK, Moller DE. Analysis of the hexokinase II gene in subjects with insulin resistance and NIDDM and detection of a Gln142 His substitution. Diabetes 1995; 44: 340–46.

620. Helmrich SP, Ragland DR, Leting RW, Patfenbarger RS. Physical activity and reduced occurrence of non-insulin-dependent diabetes mellitus. New Engl J Med 1991; 325: 147–52.

621. Bogardus C. Skeletal muscle and insulin action *in vitro* in man. Upjohn, Kalamazoo, MI: Current Concept Series, 1987; pp 1–28.

622. Nilsson LH, Hultman E. Liver glycogen in man—the effect of total starvation and the effects of a carbohydrate-poor diet followed by carbohydrate refeeding. Scand J Lab Invest 1973; 32: 325–30.

623. Nilsson LH, Hultman E. Liver and muscle glycogen in man after glucose and fructose ingestion. Scand J Lab Invest 1974; 33: 5–10.

624. Natali A, Buzzigoli G, Taddei S et al. Effects of insulin on hemodynamics and metabolism in human forearm. Diabetes 1990; 39: 490–98.

625. Vestergaard H, Lund S, Bjorbaek C, Pedersen O. Unchanged gene expression of glycogen synthase in muscle from patients with NIDDM following sulfonylurea-induced improvement of glycaemic control. Diabetologia 1995; 38: 1230–38.

626. Schalin-Jantti C, Harkonen M, Groop LC. Impaired activation of glycogen synthase in people at increased risk for developing NIDDM. Diabetes 1992; 41: 598–604.

627. Boden G, Ray TK, Smith RH, Owen OE. Carbohydrate oxidation and storage in obese non-insulin-dependent diabetic patients: effects of improving glycemic control. Diabetes 1983; 32: 982–7.

628. Vestergaard H, Lund S, Larsen FS, Bjerrum OJ, Pedersen O. Glycogen synthase and phosphofructokinase protein and mRNA levels in skeletal muscle from insulin-resistant patients with non-insulin-dependent diabetes mellitus. J Clin Invest 1993; 91: 2342–50.

629. Mandarino LJ, Consoli A, Kelley DE, Reilly JP, Nurjhan N. Fasting hyperglycemia normalizes oxidative

and non-oxidative pathways of insulin-stimulated glucose metabolism in non-insulin-dependent diabetes mellitus. J Clin Endocrinol Metab 1990; 71: 1544–51.

630. Vaag A, Damsbo P, Hother-Nielsen O, Beck-Nielsen H. Hyperglycemia compensates for the defect in insulin-mediated glucose metabolism and in the activation of glycogen synthase in the skeletal muscle of patients with type 2 (non-insulin-dependent) diabetes mellitus. Diabetologia 1992; 35: 80–88.

631. Kelley DE, Mandarino LJ. Hyperglycemia normalizes insulin-stimulated skeletal muscle glucose oxidation and storage in non-insulin-dependent diabetes mellitus. J Clin Invest 1990; 86: 1999–2007.

632. Damsbo P, Vaag A, Hother-Nielsen O, Beck-Nielsen H. Reduced glycogen synthase activity in skeletal muscle from obese patients with and without type 2 (non-insulin-dependent) diabetes mellitus. Diabetologia 1991; 34: 239–45.

633. Nyomba BL, Freymond D, Raz I, Stone K, Mott DM, Bogardus C. Skeletal muscle glycogen synthase activity in subjects with non-insulin-dependent diabetes mellitus after glyburide therapy. Metabolism 1990; 39: 1204–10.

634. Vaag A, Henriksen JE, Beck-Nielsen H. Decreased insulin activation of glycogen synthase in skeletal muscles in young non-obese Caucasian first-degree relatives of patients with non-insulin-dependent diabetes mellitus. J Clin Invest 1992; 89: 782–8.

635. Yki-Jarvinen H, Mott D, Young AA, Stone K, Bogardus C. Regulation of glycogen synthase and phosphorylase activity by glucose and insulin in human skeletal muscle. J Clin Invest 1987; 80: 95–100.

636. Stralfors P, Hiraga A, Cohen P. The protein phosphatases involved in cellular regulation: purification and characterization of the glycogen-bound form of protein phosphatase-1 from rabbit skeletal muscle. Eur J Biochem 1985; 149: 295–303.

637. Hubbard MJ, Cohen P. Regulation of protein phosphatase-1G from rabbit skeletal muscle. Eur J Biochem 1989; 186: 711–16.

638. Sutherland C, Campbell DG, Cohen P. Identification of insulin-stimulated protein kinase-1 as the rabbit equivalent of rsk-mo-2. Eur J Biochem 1993; 212: 581–8.

639. Mandarino LJ, Wright KS, Verity LS et al. Effects of insulin infusion on human skeletal muscle pyruvate dehydrogenase, phosphofructokinase, and glycogen synthase. Evidence for their role in oxidative glucose metabolism. J Clin Invest 1987; 80: 655–63.

640. Thorburn AW, Gumbiner B, Bulacan F, Wallace P, Henry RR. Intracellular glucose oxidation and glycogen synthase activity are reduced in non-insulin-dependent (type II) diabetes independent of impaired glucose uptake. J Clin Invest 1990; 85: 522–9.

641. Mandarino LJ, Consoli A, Jain A, Kelley DE. Interaction of carbohydrate and fat fuels in human skeletal muscle: impact of obesity and NIDDM. Am J Physiol 1996; 270: E463–70.

642. Mandarino LJ, Madar Z, Kolterman OG, Bell JM, Olefsky JM. Adipocyte glycogen synthase and pyruvate dehydrogenase in obese and type II diabetic patients. Am J Physiol 1986; 251: E489–96.

643. Wright KS, Beck-Nielsen H, Kolterman OG, Mandarino LJ. Decreased activation of skeletal muscle glycogen synthase by mixed-meal ingestion in NIDDM. Diabetes 1988; 37: 436–40.

644. Thorburn AW, Gumbiner B, Bulacan R, Brechtel G, Henry RR. Multiple defects in muscle glycogen synthase activity contribute to reduced glycogen synthesis in non-insulin dependent diabetes mellitus. J Clin Invest 1991; 87: 489–95.

645. Johnson AB, Argyraki M, Thow JC, Broughton D, Jones IR, Taylor R. Effects of intensive dietary treatment on insulin-stimulated skeletal muscle glycogen synthase activation and insulin secretion in newly presenting type 2 diabetic patients. Diabet Med 1990; 7: 420–28.

646. Beck-Nielsen H, Vaag A, Damsbo P et al. Insulin resistance in skeletal muscle in patients with NIDDM. Diabetes Care 1992; 15: 418–29.

647. Vestergaard H, Bjorbaek C, Andersen PH, Bak JF, Pedersen O. Impaired expression of glycogen synthase mRNA in skeletal muscle of NIDDM patients. Diabetes 1991; 40: 1740–45.

648. Johnson AB, Argyraki M, Thow JC et al. Impaired activation of skeletal muscle glycogen synthase in non-insulin-dependent diabetes mellitus is unrelated to degree of obesity. Metabolism 1991; 40: 252–60.

649. Johnson AB, Argyraki M, Thow JC et al. The effect of sulphonylurea therapy on skeletal muscle glycogen synthase activity and insulin secretion in newly presenting type 2 (non-insulin-dependent) diabetic patients. Diabet Med 1990; 8: 243–53.

650. Bak JF, Moller N, Schmitz O, Saaek A, Pedersen O. *In vivo* insulin action and muscle glycogen synthase activity in type 2 (non-insulin-dependent) diabetes mellitus: effects of diet treatment. Diabetologia 1992; 35: 777–84.

651. Freymond C, Bogardus C, Okubo M, Stone K, Mott D. Impaired insulin-stimulated muscle glycogen synthase activation *in vivo* in man is related to low fasting glycogen synthase phosphatase activity. J Clin Invest 1988; 82: 1503–9.

652. Henry RR, Ciaraldi TP, Mudaliar S, Abrams L, Nikoulina SE. Acquired defects of glycogen synthase activity in cultured human skeletal muscle cells. Influence of high glucose and insulin levels. Diabetes 1996; 45: 400–407.

653. Wells AM, Sutcliffe IC, Johnson AB, Taylor R. Abnormal activation of glycogen synthesis in fibroblasts from NIDDM subjects. Evidence for an abnormality specific to glucose metabolism. Diabetes 1993; 42: 583–9.

654. Henry RR, Ciaraldi TP, Abrams-Carter L, Mudaliar S, Park KS, Nikoulina SE. Glycogen synthase activity is reduced in cultured skeletal muscle cells of non-insulin-dependent diabetes mellitus subjects. J Clin Invest 1996; 98: 1231–6.

655. Browner MF, Nakano K, Bang AG, Fleffenzk RJ. Human muscle glycogen synthase with DNA sequence: a negatively charged protein with asymmetric charge distribution. Proc Natl Acad Sci USA 1989; 86: 1443–7.

656. Schneider Sh, Morgado A. Effects of fitness and physical training on carbohydrate metabolism and associated cardiovascular risk factors in patients with diabetes. Diabetes Rev 1995; 3: 379–403.

657. Faccini FS, Hollenbeck CB, Jeppesen J, Chen YD, Reaven GM. Insulin resistance and cigarette smoking. Lancet 1992; 339: 1128–30.

658. Attorall S, Fowelin J, Lager I, Smith U. Smoking induces insulin resistance—a potential link with the

insulin resistance syndrome. J Int Med 1993; 233: 327–33.

659. Ferrannini E, Buzzigoli G, Bonadonna R et al. Insulin resistance in essential hypertension. New Engl J Med 1987; 317: 350–57.

660. Groop L, Ekstrand A, Forslbom C et al. Insulin resistance, hypertension, and microalbuminuria in patients with type 2 (non-insulin-dependent) diabetes mellitus. Diabetologia 1993; 36: 642–7.

661. Nuutila P, Maki M, Laine H et al. Insulin action on heart and skeletal muscle glucose uptake in essential hypertension. J Clin Invest 1995; 96: 1003–9.

662. Dengel DR, Pratley RE, Hagberg JM, Goldberg AP. Impaired insulin sensitivity and maximal responsiveness in older hypertensive men. Hypertension 1994; 23: 320–24.

663. Fontvieille AM, Lillioja S, Ferraro RT, Schulz LO, Rising R, Ravussin E. Twenty-four-hour energy expenditure in Pima Indians with type 2 (non-insulin-dependent) diabetes mellitus. Diabetologia 1992; 35: 753–9.

664. Golay A, Schutz Y, Felber JP, DeFronzo RA, Jequier E. Lack of thermogenic response to glucose/insulin infusion in obese diabetic subjects. Int J Obesity 1986; 10: 107–16.

665. Bjorbaek C, Fik TA, Echward SM et al. Cloning of human insulin-stimulated protein kinase (ISPK-1) gene and analysis of coding regions and mRNA levels of the ISPK-1 and the protein phosphatase-1 genes in muscle from NIDDM patients. Diabetes 1995; 44: 90–97.

666. Chen YH, Hansen L, Chen MX et al. Sequence of the human glycogen-associated regulatory subunit of type 1 protein phosphatase and analysis of its coding region and mRNA level in muscle from patients with NIDDM. Diabetes 1994; 43: 1234–41.

667. Procharzka M, Michizuki H, Baier LJ, Cohen PTW, Bogardus C. Molecular and linkage analysis of type-1 protein phosphatase catalytic beta-subunit gene: lack of evidence for its major role in insulin resistance in Pima Indians. Diabetologia 1995; 38: 461–6.

668. Falholt K, Jensen I, Lindkaer Jensen S et al. Carbohydrate and lipid metabolism of skeletal muscle in type 2 diabetic patients. Diabet Med 1988; 5: 27–31.

669. Randle PJ, Garland PB, Hales CN, Newsholme EA. The glucose fatty acid cycle. Its role in insulin sensitivity and the metabolic disturbances of diabetes mellitus. Lancet 1963; 1: 785–9.

670. Randle PJ, Newsholme EA, Garland PB. Regulation of glucose uptake by muscle. Effects of fatty acids, ketone bodies and pyruvate, and of alloxan-diabetes and starvation on the uptake and metabolic fate of glucose in rat heart and diaphragm muscles. Biochem J 1964; 93: 652–65.

671. Taylor SI, Mukherjee C, Jungas RL. Regulation of pyruvate dehydrogenase in isolated rat liver mitochondria. J Biol Chem 1975; 250: 2028–35.

672. Taylor SI, Mukherjee C, Jungas RL. Studies on the mechanism of activation of adipose tissue pyruvate dehydrogenase by insulin. J Biol Chem 1973; 248: 73–81.

673. Jeanrenaud B, Halimi S, van de Werve G. Neuroendocrine disorders seen as triggers of the triad: obesity–insulin resistance–abnormal glucose tolerance. Diabetes Metab Rev 1985; 1: 261–92.

674. Wititsuwannakul D, Kim K. Mechanism of palmityl coenzyme A inhibition of liver glycogen synthase. J Biol Chem 1977; 252: 7812–17.

675. Roden M, Price TB, Perseghin G et al. Mechanism of free fatty acid-induced insulin resistance in humans. J Clin Invest 1996; 97: 2859–65.

676. Ebeling P, Koivisto VA. Non-esterified fatty acids regulate lipid and glucose oxidation and glycogen synthesis in healthy man. Diabetologia 1994; 37: 202–9.

677. Kelley DE, Mokan M, Simoneau JA, Mandarino LJ. Interaction between glucose and free fatty acid metabolism in human skeletal muscle. J Clin Invest 1993; 92: 91–8.

678. Thiebaud D, DeFronzo RA, Jacot E et al. Effect of long-chain triglyceride infusion on glucose metabolism in man. Metabolism 1982; 31: 1128–36.

679. Ferrannini E, Barrett EJ, Bevilacqua S, DeFronzo RA. Effect of fatty acids on glucose production and utilization in man. J Clin Invest 1983; 72: 1737–47.

680. Felber JP, Vannotti A. Effect of fat infusion on glucose tolerance and insulin plasma levels. Med Exp 1964; 10: 153–6.

681. Rousselle J, Buckert A, Pahud P, Jequier E, Felber JP. Relationship between glucose oxidation and glucose tolerance in man. Metabolism 1982; 31: 866–70.

682. Vouillamoz D, Temler E, Jequier E, Felber JP. Importance of substrate competition in the mechanism of insulin resistance in man. Metabolism 1987; 36: 715–20.

683. Piatti PM, Monti LD, Davis SN et al. Effects of an acute decrease in non-esterified fatty acid levels on muscle glucose utilization and forearm indirect calorimetry in lean NIDDM patients. Diabetologia 1996; 39: 103–12.

684. Meyer HU, Curchod B, Maeder E, Pahud P, Jequier E, Felber JP. Modifications of glucose storage and oxidation in non-obese diabetics, measured by continuous indirect calorimetry. Diabetes 1980; 29: 752–6.

685. Golay A, Felber JP, Meyer HU, Curchod B, Maeder E, Jequier E. Study on lipid metabolism in obesity diabetes. Metabolism 1984; 33: 111–16.

686. Felber JP, Meyer HU, Curchod B et al. Glucose storage and oxidation in different degrees of human obesity measured by continuous indirect calorimetry. Diabetologia 1981; 20: 39–44.

687. Felber JP, Magnenat G, Casthelaz M et al. Carbohydrate and lipid oxidation in normal and diabetic subjects. Diabetes 1977; 26: 693–9.

688. Taskinen MR, Bogardus C, Kennedy A, Howard BV. Multiple disturbances of free fatty acid metabolism in non-insulin dependent diabetes. J Clin Invest 1985; 76: 637–44.

689. Lillioja S, Bogardus C, Mott DM et al. Relationship between insulin mediated glucose disposal and lipid metabolism in man. J Clin Invest 1985; 75: 1106–15.

690. Chen Y-DI, Golay A, Swislocki ALM, Reaven GM. Resistance to insulin suppression of plasma free fatty acid concentrations and insulin stimulation of glucose uptake in non-insulin dependent diabetes mellitus. J Clin Endocrinol Metab 1987; 64: 7–21.

691. Phillips DIW, Caddy S, Illic V et al. Intramuscular triglyceride and muscle insulin sensitivity: evidence for a relationship in non-diabetic subjects. Metabolism 1996; 45: 947–50.

692. Bonadonna RC, Zych K, Boni C, Ferrannini E, De-Fronzo RA. Time dependence of the interaction between lipid and glucose metabolism in humans. Am J Physiol 1989; 20: E49–56.

693. Bonadonna RC, Groop LC, Zych K, Shank M, De-Fronzo RA. Dose dependent effect of insulin on plasma free fatty acid turnover and oxidation in humans. Am J Physiol 1990; 22: 736–50.

694. Capaldo B, Napoli R, DiMarino L, Picardi A, Riccardi G, Sacca L. Quantitation of forearm glucose and free fatty acid (NEFA) disposal in normal subjects and type II diabetic patients. Evidence against an essential role for NEFA in the pathogenesis of insulin resistance. J Clin Endocrinol Metab 1988; 67: 893–8.

695. Groop L, Saloranta C, Shank M, Bonadonna RC, Ferrannini E, DeFronzo RA. The role of free fatty acid metabolism in the pathogenesis of insulin resistance in obesity and non-insulin dependent diabetes mellitus. J Clin Endocrinol Metab 1991; 72: 96–107.

696. Ruderman NB, Toeus CJ, Shafir E. Role of free fatty acids in glucose homeostasis. Arch Intern Med 1969; 123: 299–313.

697. Blumenthal SA. Stimulation of gluconeogenesis by palmitic acid in rat hepatocytes: evidence that this effect can be dissociated from provision of reducing equivalents. Metabolism 1983; 32: 971–5.

698. Bevilacqua S, Bonadonna R, Buzzigoli G et al. Acute elevation of free fatty acid levels leads to hepatic insulin resistance in obese subjects. Metabolism 1987; 36: 502–6.

699. Golay A, Swislocki ALM, Chen Y-DI, Reaven GM. Relationships between plasma free fatty acid concentration, endogenous glucose production, and fasting hyperglycemia in normal and non-insulin-dependent diabetic individuals. Metabolism 1987; 36: 692–6.

700. Williamson JR, Kreisberg RA, Felts PW. Mechanism for the stimulation of gluconeogenesis by fatty acids in perfused rat liver. Proc Natl Acad Sci USA 1966; 56: 247–54.

701. Felig P, Wahren J, Hendler R. Splanchnic glucose and amino acid metabolism in obesity. J Clin Invest 1974; 53: 582–90.

702. Baron AD, Schaeffer L, Shragg P, Kolterman OG. Role of hyperglucagonemia in maintenance of increased rates of hepatic glucose output in type II diabetics. Diabetes 1987; 36: 274–83.

703. Reaven GM, Chen Y-DI, Golay A, Swislocki AL, Jaspan JB. Documentation of hyperglucagonemia throughout the day in non-obese and obese patients with non-insulin dependent diabetes mellitus. J Clin Endocrinol Metab 1987; 64: 106–10.

704. Unger RH, Aguilar-Parada E, Mueller WA, Eisentrant AM. Studies of pancreatic alpha cell function in normal and diabetic subjects. J Clin Invest 1970; 49: 837–9.

705. Boden JG, Soriano M, Hoeldtke RD, Owen GE. Counter-regulatory hormone release and glucose recovery after hypoglycemia in non-insulin dependent diabetic patients. Diabetes 1983; 32: 1055–9.

706. Puhakainen I, Yki-Jarvinen H. Inhibition of lipolysis decreases lipid oxidation and gluconeogenesis from lactate but not fasting hyperglycemia or total hepatic glucose production in NIDDM. Diabetes 1993; 42: 1694–9.

707. Saloranta C, Franssila-Kallunki A, Ekstrand A, Taskinen M-R, Groop LC. Modulation of hepatic glucose production by non-esterified fatty acids in type 2 (non-insulin-dependent) diabetes mellitus. Diabetologia 1991; 34: 409–15.

708. Jeng C-H, Sheu WH-H, Fug MM-T, Shieh S-M, Chen Y-DI, Reaven GM. Gemfibrozil treatment of endogenous hypertriglyceridemia: effect on insulin-mediated glucose disposal and plasma insulin concentrations. J Clin Endocrinol Metab 1996; 81: 2550–58.

709. Bjorkman M, Storlien LH, Pan DA, Jenkins AB, Chisholm DJ, Campbell LB. The relationship between insulin sensitivity and the fatty acid composition of skeletal-muscle phospholipids. N Engl J Med 1993; 328: 238–44.

710. Vessby B, Tengblad S, Lithell H. Insulin sensitivity is related to the fatty acid composition of serum lipids and skeletal muscle phospholipids in 70-year-old men. Diabetologia 1994; 37: 1044–50.

711. Vessby B, Aro A, Skarfors E, Berglund L, Salminen I, Lithell H. The risk to develop NIDDM is related to the fatty acid composition of the serum cholesterol esters. Diabetes 1994; 43: 1353–7.

712. Krotkiewski M, Seidell JC, Bjorntorp P. Glucose tolerance and hyperinsulinemia in obese women: role of adipose tissue distribution, muscle fiber characteristics and androgens. J Intern Med 1990; 228: 385–92.

713. Lillioja S, Young AA, Culter CL et al. Skeletal muscle capillary density and fiber type are possible determinants of *in vivo* insulin resistance in man. J Clin Invest 1987; 80: 415–24.

714. King GL, Johnson SM. Receptor-mediated transport of insulin across endothelial cells. Science 1985; 227: 1583–6.

715. Yeon JY, Hope ID, Ader M, Bergman RN. Insulin transport across capillaries is rate limiting for insulin action in dogs. J Clin Invest 1989; 84: 1620–28.

716. Ader M, Poulin RA, Yang YJ, Bergman RN. Dose-response relationship between lymph insulin and glucose uptake reveals enhanced insulin sensitivity of peripheral tissues. Diabetes 1992; 41: 241–53.

717. Poulin RA, Steil GM, Moore DM, Ader M, Bergman RN. Dynamics of glucose production and uptake are more closely related to insulin in hindlimb lymph than in thoracic duct lymph. Diabetes 1994; 43: 180–90.

718. Miles PDG, Levisetti M, Reichart D, Khoursheed M, Moossa AR, Olefsky JM. Kinetics of insulin action *in vivo*. Identification of rate-limiting steps. Diabetes 1995; 44: 947–53.

719. Jansson PE, Fowelin JP, Henning F, Von Schenck P, Smith UP, Lonnroth PN. Measurement by microdialysis of the insulin concentration in subcutaneous interstitial fluid. Diabetes 1993; 42: 1469–73.

720. Prakash S, Mokshagundam L, Peiris AN, Stagner JI, Gingerich RL, Samols E. Interstitial insulin during euglycemic–hyperinsulinemic clamp in obese and lean individuals. Metabolism 1996; 45: 951–6.

721. Castillo C, Bogardus C, Bergman R, Thuillez P, Lillioja S. Interstitial insulin concentrations determine glucose uptake rates but not insulin resistance in lean and obese men. J Clin Invest 1994; 93: 10–16.

722. Baron AD. Hemodynamic actions of insulin. Am J Physiol 1994; 267: E187–202.

723. Steinberg HO, Brechtel G, Johnson A, Fineberg N, Baron AD. Insulin-mediated skeletal muscle vasodilation is nitric oxide dependent. A novel action of insulin

to increase nitric oxide release. J Clin Invest 1994; 94: 1172-9.

724. Baron AD, Steinberg HO, Chaker H, Leaming R, Johnson A, Brechtel G. Insulin-mediated skeletal muscle vasodilation contributes to both insulin sensitivity and responsiveness in lean humans. J Clin Invest 1995; 96: 786-92.

725. Baron AD, Brechtel G. Insulin differentially regulates systemic and skeletal muscle vascular resistance. Am J Physiol 1993; 265: E61-7.

726. Baron AD, Laakso M, Brechtel G, Edelman SV. Reduced capacity and affinity of skeletal muscle for insulin-mediated glucose uptake in non-insulin-dependent diabetic subjects. Effects of insulin therapy. J Clin Invest 1991; 87: 1186-94.

727. Laakso M, Edelman SV, Brechtel G, Baron AD. Decreased effect of insulin to stimulate skeletal muscle blood flow in obese man. A novel mechanism for insulin resistance. J Clin Invest 1990; 85: 1844-52.

728. Steinberg HO, Chaker H, Leaming R, Johnson A, Brechtel A, Baron AD. Obesity/insulin resistance is associated with endothelial dysfunction. Implications for the syndrome of insulin resistance. J Clin Invest 1996; 97: 2601-10.

729. Anderson EA, Hoffman RP, Balon TW, Sinkey CA, Mark AL. Hyperinsulinemia produces both sympathetic neural activation and vasodilation in normal humans. J Clin Invest 1991; 87: 2246-52.

730. Creager MA, Liang C-S, Coffman JD. Beta adrenergic-mediated vasodilator response to insulin in the human forearm. J Pharmacol Ther 1985; 235: 709-14.

731. Jamerson KA, Julius S, Gudbrandsson T, Andersson O, Brant DO. Reflex sympathetic activation induces acute insulin resistance in the human forearm. Hypertension 1993; 21: 618-23.

732. Neahring JM, Stepniakowski K, Green AS, Egan BM. Insulin does not reduce forearm alpha-vasoreactivity in obese hypertensive or lean normotensive men. Hypertension 1993; 22: 584-90.

733. Vollenweider P, Tappy L, Randin O et al. Differential effects of hyperinsulinemia and carbohydrate metabolism on sympathetic nerve activity and muscle blood flow in humans. J Clin Invest 1993; 92: 147-54.

734. Buchanan TA, Thawani H, Kades W et al. Angiotensin II increases glucose utilization during acute hyperinsulinemia via a hemodynamic mechanism. J Clin Invest 1993; 92: 720-26.

735. Capaldo B, Napoli R, DiBonito RP, Albano G, Sacca L. Glucose and gluconeogenic substrate exchange by the forearm skeletal muscle in hyperglycemia and insulin treated type II diabetic patients. J Clin Endocrinol Metab 1990; 71: 1220-23.

736. Kelley DE, Reilly JP, Veneman T, Mandarino LJ. Effects of insulin on skeletal muscle glucose storage, oxidation and glycolysis. Am J Physiol 1990; 258: E923-9.

737. Yki-Jarvinen H, Young AA, Lamkin C, Foley JE. Kinetics of glucose disposal in whole body and across the forearm in man. J Clin Invest 1987; 79: 1713-19.

738. DeFronzo RA, Cooke CR, Andres R, Faloona GR, Davis PJ. The effect of insulin on renal handling of sodium, potassium, calcium and phosphate in man. J Clin Invest 1975; 55: 845-55.

739. Nuutila P, Raitakari M, Laine H et al. Role of blood flow in regulating insulin-stimulated glucose uptake in humans. J Clin Invest 1996; 97: 1741-7.

740. Utriainen T, Malmstrom R, Makimattila S, Yki-Jarvinen H. Methodological aspects, dose-response characteristics and causes of interindividual variation in insulin stimulation of limb blood flow in normal subjects. Diabetologia 1995; 38: 555-64.

741. Natali A, Bonadonna R, Santoro D et al. Insulin resistance and vasodilation in essential hypertension. Studies with adenosine. J Clin Invest 1994; 94: 1570-76.

742. Scherrerr U, Randin D, Vollenweider P, Vollenweider L, Nicod P. Nitric oxide release accounts for insulin's vascular effects in humans. J Clin Invest 1994; 94: 2511-15.

743. Neahring JM, Stepniakowski K, Greene AS, Egan BM. Insulin does not reduce forearm alpha-vasoreactivity in obese hypertensive or lean normotensive men. Hypertension 1993; 22: 584-90.

744. Ravussin E. Energy expenditure and obesity. Diabetes Rev 1996 (in press).

745. Cooper GJS, Leighton B, Dimitriadis GD et al. Amylin found in amyloid deposits in human type II diabetes mellitus may be a hormone that regulates glycogen metabolism in skeletal muscle. Proc Natl Acad Sci USA 1988; 85: 7763-6.

746. Cooper GJS, Leighton B. Pancreatic amylin and calcitonin gene-related peptide cause resistance to insulin in skeletal muscle *in vitro*. Nature 1988; 335: 632-5.

747. Sowa R, Sanke T, Hirayama J et al. Islet amyloid polypeptide amide causes peripheral insulin resistance *in vivo* in dogs. Diabetologia 1990; 33: 118-20.

748. Molina JM, Cooper GJS, Leighton B, Olefsky JM. Induction of insulin resistance *in vivo* by amylin and calcitonin gene-related peptide. Diabetes 1990; 39: 260-64.

749. Koopmans SJ, van Mansfeld ADM, Jansz HS et al. Amylin-induced *in vivo* insulin resistance in conscious rats: the liver is more sensitive to amylin than peripheral tissues. Diabetologia 1991; 34: 218-24.

750. Zierath JR, Galuska D, Engstrom A et al. Human islet amyloid polypeptide at pharmacological levels inhibits insulin and phorbol ester-stimulated glucose transport in *in vitro* incubated human muscle strips. Diabetologia 1992; 35: 26-31.

32

Glucose Toxicity

Donald C. Simonson*, Luciano Rossetti**, Andrea Giaccari† and Ralph A. DeFronzo†

**Joslin Diabetes Center, Harvard Medical School, Boston, MA,* ***Albert Einstein College of Medicine, Bronx, New York, and* †*University of Texas Health Science Center and Audie L. Murphy Veterans Administration Hospital, San Antonio, TX, USA*

The hallmark of diabetes mellitus is the presence of hyperglycemia. In addition to the two common naturally occurring forms of the disease—type 1 (insulin dependent, IDDM) and type 2 (non-insulin dependent, NIDDM) diabetes—a variety of other disorders may lead to an elevation of the plasma glucose level and result in a similar clinical syndrome. Thus, if the pancreas is surgically removed or destroyed by inflammation, tumor infiltration or toxins, most of the signs, symptoms and complications of diabetes will ultimately develop. Since the principal abnormality common to all of these clinical syndromes is hyperglycemia, it has been suggested (and widely accepted) that the exposure to high levels of glucose is responsible for these sequelae. During the past decade, the term 'glucose toxicity' has been used to describe this pathophysiologic sequence of events [1, 2]. In the most general terms, glucose toxicity can be defined as the acute and chronic adverse effects of hyperglycemia on cellular structure and function.

The spectrum of glucose toxicity is quite broad. Indeed, there is now considerable evidence that hyperglycemia plays an important role in the pathogenesis of all the major complications of diabetes, including nephropathy, retinopathy, neuropathy and macrovascular disease. In addition to these microvascular and macrovascular complications, hyperglycemia is also closely linked with other physiologic, biochemical and anatomic complications, including basement membrane thickening, protein glycosylation, impaired cellular immunity and abnormalities in cell growth and differentiation (Table 1). For a more complete discussion of these areas, the reader is referred to other chapters of this text that are devoted to these topics.

Table 1 Pathogenetic consequences of hyperglycemia

Microvascular complications
  Nephropathy
  Retinopathy
  Neuropathy
Macrovascular disease
  Coronary
  Cerebral
  Peripheral
Basement membrane thickening
Protein glycosylation
Impaired cellular immunity
Disordered cell growth and differentiation
Abnormal carbohydrate metabolism ('glucose toxicity')
  Impaired insulin secretion
  Impaired insulin sensitivity

In this chapter, we will focus specifically on the effects of hyperglycemia on insulin secretion and insulin action. Evidence will be presented to support the hypothesis that hyperglycemia sustains and exacerbates the insulin secretory defects observed in type 2 diabetes, and contributes to insulin resistance in both type 2 and type 1 diabetes. When viewed in these terms, hyperglycemia not only represents

International Textbook of Diabetes Mellitus, Second Edition. Edited by K.G.M.M. Alberti, P. Zimmet, R.A. DeFronzo, and H. Keen (Honorary)
© 1997 John Wiley & Sons Ltd

a manifestation of diabetes mellitus, but is a self-perpetuating factor that is responsible for sustaining the diabetic state. The role of intensive glycemic control—including diet, exercise, oral hypoglycemic medications and insulin—in reversing the toxic effects of glucose will also be discussed.

INSULIN SECRETION

Physiology of Insulin Secretion

Glucose has long been recognized as the major physiologic stimulus of insulin secretion in humans [3]. In addition to directly stimulating insulin release from the pancreas, glucose also modulates the B-cell response to non-glucose secretagogues, regulates proinsulin synthesis and processing, and influences B-cell growth [4–8]. Primary defects in insulin secretion, whether partial or complete, are clearly capable of producing the clinical syndrome of diabetes mellitus. However, it is now apparent that hyperglycemia *per se* plays an important role in exacerbating and sustaining these defects, thus leading to a vicious cycle of further hyperglycemia and more profound deficiencies in insulin secretion.

Leahy, Bonner-Weir and Weir were among the first to systematically examine the deleterious effects of chronic hyperglycemia on islet cell function [8–11]. They initially used the neonatal streptozotocin rat model to produce an animal with glucose intolerance analogous to human type 2 diabetes. In this model, after a brief initial period of hyperglycemia due to pancreatic B-cell destruction, there is partial regeneration of B-cell mass accompanied by a return of the plasma glucose concentration towards normal at 7–10 days of life. By 6 weeks of age, however, these animals develop persistent fasting and postprandial hyperglycemia with a marked impairment in glucose-stimulated insulin secretion. Of particular importance, the reduction in insulin secretory capacity is substantially greater than that which could be attributed solely to the reduction in B-cell mass. Thus, these data suggested that chronic hyperglycemia *per se* may induce a functional defect in insulin release.

Although this model provided good circumstantial evidence for an acquired defect in glucose-induced insulin secretion, concern was raised as to whether the abnormal function in the remaining B cells may be due to a potential toxic effect from exposure to streptozotocin, rather than simply exposure to hyperglycemia. To circumvent this problem, the partial pancreatectomy model was developed and has become widely adopted by other researchers in this field [8,

12–14]. With this technique, 80–90% of the pancreas is surgically removed, leading to mild elevations in the fasting glucose with more severe postprandial hyperglycemia—a state resembling mild to moderate type 2 diabetes in humans. An important advantage of this approach is that insulin secretion in the pancreatic remnant (expressed per residual B-cell mass) should be normal unless an acquired defect has occurred in response to the presence of chronic hyperglycemia. Although substantial regeneration of B cells in the pancreatic remnant can be observed within 4–5 weeks, the animals continue to exhibit fasting and postprandial hyperglycemia. Importantly, defects in both the first and second phases of glucose-induced insulin secretion again exceeded those which would be expected based on the volume and cellular composition of the remaining islets (Figure 1), again suggesting that a toxic effect of glucose was present [13].

More recently, an alternative approach using the chronic glucose infusion technique has confirmed the results of these earlier studies [15–18]. When healthy rats were infused with a 50% dextrose solution for 48 h to produce severe hyperglycemia (>350 mg/dl, 19.4 mmol/l), insulin secretion in response to glucose was severely impaired. This defect was less pronounced in rats with more moderate hyperglycemia ($\approx$ 180 mg/dl, 10.0 mmol/l). It is noteworthy that rats maintained at a mildly hyperglycemic level (150–160 mg/dl, 8.3–8.9 mmol/l) actually exhibited a significant potentiation of insulin secretion in response to glucose [15]. These data suggest that there may be a threshold of glycemia above which the inhibitory effects of glucose on insulin secretion become evident. In support of this observation, 2 days of glucose infusion designed to raise circulating glucose levels to 6.0 mmol/l (108 mg/dl) in normal humans produced significant potentiation, not impairment, of glucose-stimulated insulin secretion [19].

Although mild transient hyperglycemia may acutely enhance insulin secretion, it is possible that a similar mild hyperglycemic stimulus might have the opposite effect when present chronically. To address this question, rats were subjected to a 60% pancreatectomy and fed tap-water or 10% sucrose in addition to their normal rat chow [16]. Plasma glucose levels in the partially pancreatectomized rats consuming tap-water were similar to controls; in contrast, in partially pancreatectomized sucrose-fed rats the mean non-fasting plasma glucose concentration was slightly, but significantly, elevated (by 15 mg/dl, 0.8 mmol/l) compared to partially pancreatectomized animals drinking tap-water. Importantly, in the tap-water group, insulin secretion per residual B-cell mass was comparable to that in sham-operated controls. By contrast, in the partially pancreatectomized rats with mild hyperglycemia,

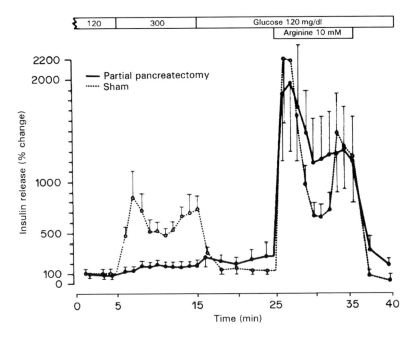

Figure 1 Insulin secretory response to glucose and arginine in the perfused pancreatic remnant of 90% pancreatectomized diabetic rats (solid line) and controls (dotted line). Studies were performed 8–11 weeks after pancreatectomy or sham operation (from reference 13, with permission)

insulin secretion by the perfused remnant was reduced by 75% (Figure 2). These results provide support for the concept that a chronic mild elevation in the mean plasma glucose concentration, in the presence of a reduced B-cell mass, can lead to a significant impairment in insulin secretion by the remaining pancreatic tissue.

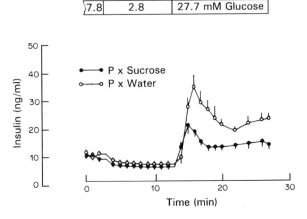

Figure 2 Effect of an acute reduction and then an increase in perfusate glucose concentration on insulin secretion in partially pancreatectomized rats maintained on tap-water (open circles) or tap-water supplemented with sucrose (closed circles) to chronically elevate the plasma glucose concentration (from reference 14, with permission)

Similar findings have been reported by Imamura et al [20]. They surgically reduced the pancreatic

mass by 50–84% in dogs and studied them for up to 250 days. No evidence of diabetes mellitus was observed. However, a similar reduction in pancreatic mass combined with sustained hyperglycemia (induced by glucose infusion) led to severe diabetes within 2 weeks. There was no evidence of improvement in the diabetic state during the 6–10-week period of observation after discontinuation of the glucose infusion. During this period, the ability of an acute hyperglycemic challenge to stimulate insulin secretion was markedly impaired, indicating that the initial insult to the B-cell may persist unless glucose is actively lowered by some non-pharmacologic or pharmacologic intervention.

An alternative approach to unraveling the mechanism of B-cell dysfunction during hyperglycemia is to examine changes in the insulin secretory response to an acute reduction in the ambient glucose level. Leahy et al [21] were among the first to demonstrate that exogenous insulin administration did not appropriately inhibit endogenous insulin release in the neonatal streptozotocin rat. In an analogous study, fasting in normal rats led to a reduced insulin response to glucose, whereas fasting in 90% pancreatectomized diabetic rats enhanced the B-cell response to glucose and increased B-cell insulin content [22]. Dimitriadis et al [23] have also reported that exposure of islets to hyperglycemia affects both B- and A-cell responses to a subsequent reduction in the plasma glucose concentration. These findings are consistent with the hypothesis that the B-cell is 'overworked' in diabetes and, thus, can regain some function after a period of rest.

Non-glucose Secretagogues

In addition to the abnormalities in glucose-stimulated insulin secretion, chronic hyperglycemia also leads to profound alterations in the B-cell response to non-glucose secretagogues [9, 15, 24, 25]. There are several natural dietary amino acids (e.g. leucine or arginine) as well as synthetic compounds (e.g. isoproterenol, sulfonylureas, or 3-isobutyl-1-methylxanthine (IBMX)) which are potent stimulators of insulin secretion. In healthy animals and humans these substances provoke an acute insulin response at normal glucose levels, and their potency is significantly enhanced by hyperglycemia. In the presence of diabetes, however, at least two important functional derangements are observed: (a) there may be an exaggerated response to the non-glucose secretagogue under ambient glycemic conditions; and (b) the potentiating effect of hyperglycemia is reduced. Thus, although these substances clearly maintain their capability of eliciting an insulin secretory response in the diabetic state, the ability of glucose to modulate this response is impaired. The importance of the role of amino acids and other dietary constituents in regulating insulin secretion is also underscored by the fact that more than half of the 24-hour insulin secretion in healthy individuals occurs in the postprandial period, whereas in the patient with type 2 diabetes, most insulin is secreted basally [26, 27]. Thus, loss of glucose potentiation has important clinical implications in the maintenance of diurnal glucose homeostasis in type 2 diabetes.

This phenomenon was nicely demonstrated in a series of studies using both the partially pancreatectomized and neonatal streptozotocin rat models to produce a state of mild fasting hyperglycemia [9, 11, 13, 14, 25]. When the pancreatic remnant was perfused *in vitro,* the insulin response to hyperglycemia was markedly impaired, while the secretory response to arginine, IBMX and isoproterenol was either normal or enhanced (Figure 1). Similar findings were observed after a chronic (72 h) glucose infusion in normal rats [15–17]. During the initial 48 h of glucose infusion the mean plasma glucose concentration was quite high (200–300 mg/dl, 11.1–16.7 mmol/l), but returned toward baseline levels during the 48–72 h period. When the pancreases from these rats were removed after 72 h and perfused *in vitro,* the insulin response to glucose was significantly impaired, whereas arginine-induced insulin secretion remained intact.

The studies of Giroix et al [24], Kergoat et al [28], and Grill et al [29] are in agreement with those of Leahy, Weir and colleagues regarding the effects of hyperglycemia on the insulin response to non-glucose secretagogues. Using the same neonatal streptozotocin diabetic rat model, these investigators also observed a markedly impaired insulin response to glucose in the perfused pancreas preparation, whereas the insulin response to a variety of non-glucose stimuli (including acetylcholine, isoproterenol, tolbutamide, α-ketoisocaproic acid, leucine, arginine and IBMX) was either normal or potentiated. Importantly, prior treatment of the diabetic rats with insulin to normalize the plasma glucose concentration [28] or lowering of the perfusate glucose concentration *in vitro* [29] improved both the deficient plasma insulin response to glucose and the exaggerated plasma insulin response to the non-glucose stimuli. Similarly, in perfused pancreases of the SHR/N-cp obese diabetic rat [30], insulin secretion is markedly impaired and the defect can be restored to normal by antecedent perfusion with a normal glucose concentration. In analogous models, when fetal mouse islets are incubated in a high glucose medium before transplantation [31], or when islets from normal rats are grafted under the kidney capsule of alloxan diabetic rats [32], the subsequent insulin secretory response of the previously normal islets is severely impaired. Insulin treatment partially normalized the deficient insulin response in the transplanted islets [32], again demonstrating that improvement in the metabolic milieu of the B-cell can partially correct these acquired defects.

More recently, the temporal sequence for development of these alterations in insulin secretion has been elucidated. Using the 90% pancreatectomy model, Leahy et al [33] measured insulin secretion to glucose and glucose + arginine at weekly intervals. Of interest, the B cells initially exhibited increased sensitivity to glucose (i.e. a shift of the ED_{50} to a lower glucose level) before eventually displaying the impaired responsiveness and altered potentiation to arginine [33, 34]. This is consistent with the hypothesis that the islets in the remnant were operating at nearly 100% of their individual capacity vs. the usual 10% of capacity when the full complement of B cells were present. These observations, plus similar findings from other investigators [35–39], provide a mechanism to explain how minimal hyperglycemia can produce exhaustion of B cells and altered potentiation when B-cell mass is reduced.

Finally, one must consider the importance of these observations to the natural history of insulin secretion in NIDDM in humans. Since no thorough prospective studies of the pathophysiology of insulin secretion in spontaneous human diabetes have been performed, and since it is obviously unethical to induce the disease in humans, our inferences must be drawn from cross-sectional or observational studies. Despite this weakness in methodology, several marked similarities between the experimentally induced disease in animals and the spontaneous disease in man are apparent [8,

40]. First, a severe defect in the first phase of glucose-induced insulin secretion is apparent in humans with very mild NIDDM (i.e. fasting plasma glucose of only 100–114 mg/dl, 5.6–6.3 mmol/l) or in first-degree relatives of patients with NIDDM [41–43]. Second, the ability of hyperglycemia to potentiate the stimulatory effects of arginine or isoproterenol on insulin secretion in early NIDDM or in family members of NIDDM patients is defective [44–47]. Finally, autopsy studies indicate that pancreatic insulin content in NIDDM patients is not reduced to a sufficient degree to explain the defect in insulin secretion unless some other factor, e.g. hyperglycemia, is causing a functional impairment of insulin release [48, 49]. Thus, to the extent that our experimental models reflect human pathophysiology, we may conclude that hyperglycemia is the cause, as well as the result, of defective insulin secretion [50].

Reversibility by Correction of Hyperglycemia

As the regulation of insulin secretion and its alteration in diabetes have become better defined, it is important to examine whether these defects are reversible. Although disturbances in insulin secretion and insulin action are both clearly present once NIDDM is established [9, 10, 51–61], it is still not clear which defect is the primary initiating event. In fact, it is becoming more evident that NIDDM is quite heterogeneous, with defects in insulin secretion, insulin action, and hepatic glucose production all potentially contributing to different degrees in different patients. Nevertheless, current thinking suggests that regardless of which defect arises first, the resulting hyperglycemia will play a central role in initiating and sustaining all of the defects [50, 60–62]. Evidence in support of this hypothesis derives from the observation that strict metabolic control—whether it be achieved by diet (weight loss), sulfonylureas, biguanides or insulin therapy—leads to improvements in both insulin secretion and insulin sensitivity [63–91]. This initially may appear somewhat paradoxical since weight loss and biguanides have no known direct effect on B-cell function, sulfonylureas enhance insulin secretion, and insulin administration suppresses endogenous insulin release. However, all of these therapies lower the plasma glucose concentration. Thus, it appears that an underlying mechanism common to each of these treatment modalities—i.e., reversal of hyperglycemia—is responsible for the improvements in endogenous insulin release (also see subsequent discussion of therapy of NIDDM).

Although insulin secretion can be improved by these diverse therapeutic modalities, complete restoration of B-cell function is rarely achieved. In particular, the impairment in the first phase of insulin secretion typically remains severely deficient. There are several potential explanations for this inability to completely reverse these defects. First, our therapeutic interventions are rarely capable of completely normalizing the plasma glucose concentration. The chronic exposure to residual mild hyperglycemia may be sufficient to perpetuate the impairment in insulin secretion. Second, it is possible that after diabetes has been present for many years, permanent structural or functional defects occur in the B cell such that restoration of normal insulin secretion is not possible. Finally, it is conceivable that the loss of insulin secretion (particularly the first phase) is a primary pathogenetic mechanism in the etiology of NIDDM and thus cannot be reversed by correction of hyperglycemia. This is supported by the observation that defects in islet cell function can be demonstrated in relatives of patients with NIDDM, suggesting the existence of an underlying genetic defect [47].

In contrast to the failure to restore insulin secretion in diabetic humans, animal studies indicate that nearly complete reversal may be achieved. After 48 h of high-dose glucose infusion, the acquired defects in insulin secretion are completely reversed within 72 h of discontinuing the infusion [15] or within 6 h of insulin administration [92]. It is of interest that the first phase of insulin secretion can be restored in less than 1 h, suggesting that protein synthesis is probably not required, as it would be for the recovery of second phase secretion [29, 93]. However, the period of hyperglycemia in all of these models is quite brief and the results may not be applicable to diabetes in humans.

Some of the most compelling evidence for improvement in insulin secretion by correction of hyperglycemia is the work of Rossetti et al [94]. They established an animal model of diabetes in which the plasma glucose concentration could be normalized by administering a drug, phlorhizin, that (a) does not alter other circulating substrate levels, (b) does not directly stimulate tissue glucose uptake, or (c) does not stimulate insulin secretion. Phlorhizin is a potent inhibitor of renal tubular glucose transport, and blocks proximal tubular glucose reabsorption when the plasma glucose concentration is increased above the basal level. The persistent glycosuria leads to a normalization of the plasma glucose level without causing hypoglycemia or altering plasma insulin, amino acid, free fatty acid, or other substrate/hormone concentrations [94–96]. At the doses employed in these studies, phlorhizin has no effect on gut or muscle glucose transport.

To examine the effects of phlorhizin treatment on insulin secretion, three groups of rats were studied [94]. Group I underwent a sham pancreatectomy. Group II received a partial (90%) pancreatectomy as described above [13] to produce a state of mild fasting hyperglycemia and severe glucose intolerance. Finally,

Group III was partially pancreatectomized and then received a continuous infusion of phlorhizin via an implantable pump. After 6 weeks, the rats were challenged with a meal tolerance test. As can be seen in Figure 3, phlorhizin treatment resulted in normalization of the glucose profile during the meal tolerance test.

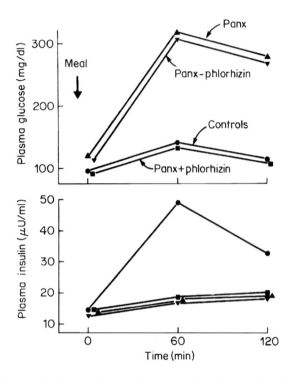

Figure 3 Plasma glucose (upper panel) and plasma insulin (lower panel) responses during a meal tolerance test performed in four groups of awake, unstressed, chronically catheterized rats: sham-operated controls (circles), 90% pancreatectomized (Panx) diabetic rats (triangles), pancreatectomized rats treated with phlorhizin (squares), pancreatectomized rats treated with phlorhizin in which the phlorhizin was stopped for 2 weeks (inverted triangles) (drawn from data presented in reference 94)

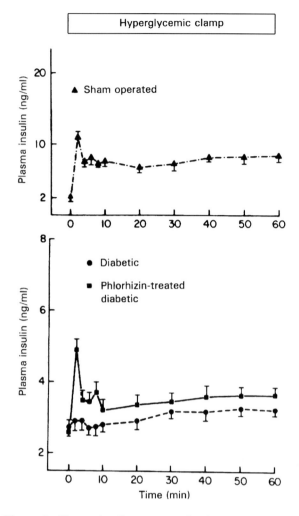

Figure 4 Plasma insulin responses in sham-operated controls (triangles, upper panel) and in 90% pancreatectomized diabetic rats with (squares) or without (circles) phlorhizin treatment (lower panel) (drawn from data presented in reference 94)

To further examine the effect of the improved glycemic milieu on glucose-induced insulin secretion, rats also received a hyperglycemic clamp in which the plasma glucose concentration was acutely raised and maintained at 100 mg/dl (5.6 mmol/l) above the baseline level for 60 minutes, and the plasma insulin concentration was measured at frequent intervals thereafter (Figure 4) [94]. In control rats the typical biphasic insulin secretory response was observed, with an early burst of insulin release within the first 10 minutes followed by a progressive increase in insulin release over the subsequent 50 minutes. In the partially pancreatectomized rats the first phase of insulin secretion was totally absent and the second phase was markedly impaired. When the chronic hyperglycemia was corrected by phlorhizin treatment of the partially

pancreatectomized animals, both the first and second phases of insulin secretion were significantly enhanced.

Since 90% of the pancreas was removed in groups II and III, it is not surprising that the absolute plasma insulin response did not return to normal. To account for differences in pancreatic mass between control and pancreatectomized rats, the plasma insulin response was normalized per gram of residual pancreatic tissue (Figure 5). When viewed in these terms, it can be seen that improved glycemic control after phlorhizin administration completely restored both first and second phase insulin responses to normal. Similar results are obtained if the plasma insulin response is expressed per unit of pancreatic insulin content [94].

These results clearly indicate that the impaired B-cell response in partially pancreatectomized animals is functional and cannot be attributed to B-cell death. If the latter were true, one would not expect to observe a

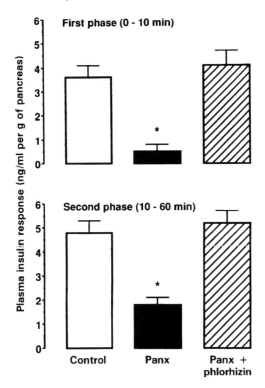

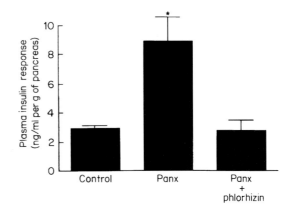

Figure 5 Mean early (0–10 min; top panel) and late (10–60 min; bottom panel) plasma insulin responses expressed per gram of pancreatic tissue during a +100 mg/dl hyperglycemic clamp study performed in sham-operated controls (open bars), 90% pancreatectomized diabetic rats (Panx) (solid bars), and pancreatectomized rats treated with phlorhizin (cross-hatched bars) (drawn from data presented in reference 94)

Figure 6 Mean plasma insulin response to a prime-continuous arginine infusion (plasma arginine concentration – 2.3 mmol/l) in sham-operated controls (left bar), 90% pancreatectomized diabetic rats (Panx) (middle bar), and pancreatectomized rats treated with phlorhizin (right bar) (drawn from data presented in reference 94)

recovery of B-cell function during improved glycemic control. To further determine whether B-cell function was fully normalized, the effect of arginine infusion on insulin secretion was also examined. As can be seen in Figure 6, the plasma insulin response to arginine was increased threefold in diabetic rats, and this potentiated insulin response was restored to normal following correction of the hyperglycemia with phlorhizin [94].

At least two recent studies have examined the effects of high glucose exposure in cultured human islets [97, 98]. When cadaveric islets were incubated in 11 mmol/l or 28 mmol/l glucose media, insulin content and glucose-stimulated insulin release were significantly less than when islets were cultured in 5.6 mmol/l glucose. The high glucose exposure also reduced rates of glucose oxidation, proinsulin synthesis, and total protein synthesis, but did not alter islet DNA content or induce morphologic change [97].

In summary, the results described above and depicted in Figures 1–6 establish the following principles: (a) chronic hyperglycemia *in vivo* in the setting of a reduced B-cell mass markedly impairs the ability of the remaining pancreatic tissue to respond to an acute glucose stimulus; (b) the refractoriness of the response to glucose involves both the first and second phases of insulin secretion; (c) chronic hyperglycemia induces a state of B-cell 'potentiation' to non-glucose secretagogues such as arginine; and (d) all of the preceding alterations in insulin secretion can be reversed by correction of the hyperglycemia.

Effects of Hyperglycemia on Cellular Mechanisms of Insulin Secretion

The cellular mechanism(s) via which sustained hyperglycemia alters the B-cell response to glucose are not yet fully defined. It was initially proposed that chronic hyperglycemia may cause a generalized down-regulation of glucose transport and metabolism in all cells of the body [60, 61]. This could account for such diverse observations as insulin resistance in peripheral and hepatic tissues, impaired insulin secretion in response to glucose but normal or enhanced responses to non-glucose stimuli, and the development of symptoms of neuroglycopenia at 'normal' plasma glucose levels in poorly controlled diabetic individuals. Although this is an attractive unifying hypothesis that may also explain the defect in insulin action (discussed below), recent studies suggest that many other mechanisms may also contribute.

Colella et al [99] compared glucose utilization in islets isolated from the neonatal streptozotocin diabetic rat and from control rats who received a 48 h glucose infusion. In both models, glucose-stimulated insulin secretion *in vivo* was significantly reduced. However, when islets were cultured *in vitro* at both low (0.5 mmol/l) and high (10 mmol/l) glucose concentrations, glucose metabolism (measured by ^3H_2O

release from [5-³H]-glucose) was either normal (in the streptozotocin diabetic model) or increased (in the 48 h glucose-infused model) (Figure 7). These results suggest that glucose transport into the B cell and its metabolism to triose compounds is normal and cannot account for the impaired insulin response in these two models.

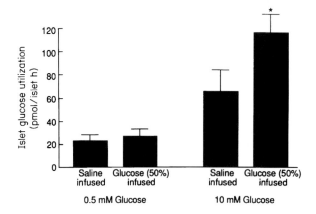

Figure 7 Glucose utilization rates at low (0.5 mmol/l: left bars) and high (10 mmol/l: right bars) medium glucose concentration from pancreatic islets isolated from control rats exposed to 72 hours of hyperglycemia *in vivo* (created by a continuous infusion of 50% glucose). *p < 0.01 vs. saline (drawn from data presented in reference 99)

Hoenig et al [100], Grodsky and colleagues [101–104], and others [105] have employed a perifusion system to study the mechanism(s) by which continuous glucose infusion impairs insulin secretion in freshly isolated islets. During the initial 4 h of continuous glucose (11 mmol/l) infusion, there was a progressive rise in insulin secretion (Figure 8); thereafter, insulin secretion gradually decreased, reaching a nadir between 16 and 20 h. Importantly, a similar 'desensitization' was observed with non-glucose metabolites, including α-ketoisocaproate and arginine, as well as synthetic insulin secretagogues including sulfonylureas, phorbol esters, and IBMX (Figure 8) [103]. It appears unlikely that the cyclic AMP system is involved in this desensitization, since neither IBMX nor forskolin (cyclic AMP generators) influenced the desensitization process [100, 103, 104] and islet ATP levels remained unchanged [99]. Furthermore, the desensitization was not related to changes in cellular NAD content and could not be prevented by the addition of amino acids, phosphate, arachidonic acid or myoinositol [100].

It seems unlikely that the acute desensitization effect of glucose occurs at an early step of insulin biosynthesis [105]. Glucose is known to increase insulin mRNA levels by enhancing transcription and/or mRNA stability [101]. However, subsequent studies have shown that

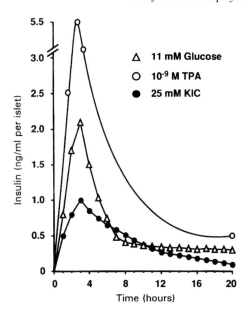

Figure 8 Desensitization of islets from non-diabetic rats after 20 hours of continuous perfusion *in vitro* with 11 mmol/l glucose (triangles), 25 mmol/l keto-isocaproic acid (KIC, solid circles), or 10⁻⁹ mol/l tetradecanoyl phorbol acetate (TPA, open circles) (adapted from data presented in reference 103)

islets cultured with glucose (11 mmol/l) for 24 hours contain insulin mRNA levels similar to those in acutely stimulated islets [101–103]. The acute desensitization of insulin secretion in cultured islets occurs in the absence of any change or with a slight decrease in proinsulin synthesis coupled with an increased conversion of proinsulin to insulin [102, 106, 107]. Moreover, Orland et al [106] also demonstrated a marked increase in proinsulin mRNA in islets from 90% pancreatectomized rats and a loss of the normal close relationship between insulin synthetic rate and insulin secretion [108]. In contrast, Robertson et al [109] have reported that serial passage of HIT-T15 cells in a high glucose medium (11.1 mmol/l) leads to a marked reduction in insulin responsivity, insulin content and insulin mRNA. A follow-up study from the same group [110] suggested that part of this effect may be mediated by the ability of glucose to alter a regulatory protein that consequently decreases insulin gene transcription [110]. These results indicate that glucose metabolism by the B-cell and the subsequent stimulation of insulin synthesis is not down-regulated during acute exposure to a hyperglycemic stimulus, even though insulin secretion is drastically reduced. However, the results do suggest that the mechanism(s) which couple glucose metabolism in the islet to the insulin secretory process are altered during more chronic exposure to hyperglycemia, and some of these effects may be mediated at the transcriptional level.

The dose–response curve for B-cell function is steepest at the high physiologic range of plasma glucose levels (10–12 mmol/l), whereas the normal fasting glucose is at the very low end of the curve (5–6 mmol/l). Because of the sigmoid shape of the dose–response curve, the B-cell has a 10-fold or greater capacity to augment insulin secretion in response to glucose. Perhaps most significant, however, is the observation that the ED_{50} of the B-cell dose–response curve corresponds to the ED_{50} of glucokinase. This has led to the hypothesis that B-cell glucokinase is at least one key regulator of insulin secretion, and abnormalities in its regulation can explain the alterations in insulin secretion observed in diabetes [111, 112]. However, since glucokinase level and activity is increased in individual islets from hyperglycemic models, the precise role of glucokinase remains unclear [113–115].

Recently, it has been proposed that in addition to the lower ED_{50} for glucokinase in diabetes, a corresponding increase in the K_m of hexokinase (the other major enzyme responsible for glucose phosphorylation in the islet) may also contribute to the dysregulation of insulin secretion in diabetes [113–115]. According to this hypothesis, hexokinase—which normally has a K_m of approximately 1 mmol/l and therefore contributes little to the regulation of islet glucose metabolism—would now be able to modulate the effect of glucose on insulin secretion. This hypothesis would also help explain why fasting enhances insulin secretion in diabetic animals while it inhibits insulin secretion in normal animals. Fasting reduces glucokinase activity in both normal and diabetic models, thereby reducing the ability of the islet to respond to an acute glucose challenge, whereas hexokinase activity is not affected [115–117]. However, since hexokinase activity is increased in the diabetic islets, they appear to paradoxically increase their insulin secretory ability compared to normal islets.

Recently, considerable attention also has focused on the role of the islet glucose transporter (Glut 2) as a potential site of the defective regulation of glucose-stimulated insulin secretion in diabetes. Several investigators have reported that exposure of rodent islets to hyperglycemia results in decreased levels of Glut 2 protein and mRNA [118–121], although another study in cultured HIT-T15 cells showed no reduction in Glut 2 after incubation in 11.1 mmol/l glucose [109]. In some studies, milder hyperglycemia has been shown to increase the activity of B-cell Glut 2 [122, 123]. However, since the reduction in Glut 2 (if it indeed occurs) is, at most, rather modest, and since glucose transport capacity normally exceeds B-cell glucose metabolism by as much as 50-fold [124], it is not readily apparent how the change in Glut 2 could produce a meaningful effect on insulin secretion. Moreover, at least one recent study suggests that human B cells may contain much less Glut 2 than rodent islets [125].

A number of studies also have provided evidence for a primary role of phosphoinositol metabolism and activation of protein kinase C in the final secretory processes that regulate insulin release [126, 127]. According to this schema (Figure 9), glucose, after interacting with a specific site on the surface of the B cell, activates phospholipase C. This enzyme catalyzes the hydrolysis of membrane phosphoinositides, producing

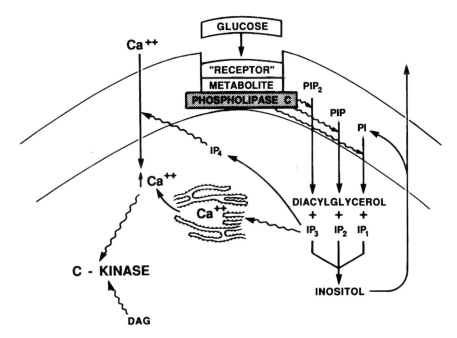

Figure 9 Representation of the role of phosphoinositide metabolism in glucose-stimulated insulin secretion. DAG, diacylglycerol; IP, inositol phosphate (adapted from references 126 and 127)

diacylglycerol and inositol phosphate. The latter, in turn, increases intracellular calcium and activates protein kinase C, both of which have been implicated in the insulin secretory process. Zawalich et al [128] have provided evidence that the inability of islets to maintain a sustained insulin response following chronic exposure *in vivo* to hyperglycemia results from impaired membrane phosphoinositide hydrolysis, with a resultant decrease in islet cell diacylglycerol and inositol phosphate concentrations. In support of this hypothesis, the defect in insulin secretion can be offset by inhibiting diacylglycerol kinase [129]. Further investigation is needed to explore these interesting findings.

Other alternative hypotheses also have been proposed for the desensitization of B cells during chronic glucose exposure. Bedoya and Jeanrenaud [130] reported that B-cell tolerance to chronic hyperglycemia may be mediated by adaptation of the metabolically regulated potassium channel in the cell membrane. This idea is further supported by observations that diazoxide, which normally inhibits insulin secretion by hyperpolarizing potassium channels, prevents glucose-induced B-cell desensitization [131] and depletion of B-cell insulin stores [34, 132]. Other investigators have proposed that defects in glucose oxidation [105] or transfer of reducing equivalents into the mitochondria of the B-cell [133] may contribute to the desensitization process. Finally, Robertson [62] has suggested three additional mechanisms which might account for the B-cell desensitization: increased α-adrenergic tone, augmented endogenous opioid action, and excessive islet prostaglandin E_2 (PGE$_2$) synthesis. The first two of these possibilities seem less likely, since the downregulation of insulin secretion can be shown in isolated perfused islets [100–104]. Since glucose stimulates PGE$_2$ synthesis in B cells, and since PGE$_2$ can inhibit insulin secretion [134, 135], excess local prostaglandin production remains a possible mediator of the desensitization phenomenon.

Chronic hyperglycemia also alters the ratio of proinsulin to insulin in the circulation [136–139]. It is of note that the hyperproinsulinemia is not present before the development of hyperglycemia (e.g. it is not observed in non-diabetic obese insulin-resistant patients), and it is reversible with control of the glucose level [140, 141]. It remains unclear why the increased proinsulin:insulin ratio occurs. Some studies have demonstrated a decrease in proinsulin synthesis and mRNA in neonatal streptozotocin diabetic rats, suggesting that an additional defect in the processing of proinsulin to insulin must also be present [142, 143]. However, others have reported that proinsulin synthesis and mRNA are increased while intra-islet levels of insulin are decreased in the partially pancreatectomized

diabetic rat model [144, 145]. This would be more consistent with a high demand for proinsulin production and premature insulin release from the islet to meet an increased demand—i.e. the overworked B cell. Subsequent studies will be needed to distinguish between these alternative hypotheses.

Finally, it should be mentioned that the nomenclature for describing the various changes in the B-cell during chronic exposure to hyperglycemia is still evolving. Specifically, Robertson et al [146] have proposed that a distinction be made between 'glucose toxicity' and 'glucose desensitization' (Figure 10). They have suggested that the former term be reserved for the irreversible alterations in B-cell function (e.g. insulin gene transcription and translation), whereas 'glucose desensitization' would be used to describe the inducible and reversible changes in insulin storage, exocytosis and the metabolic pathways of glucose metabolism that control them. As our knowledge of this field expands, it is quite likely that further differentiation of these processes will be appreciated [147].

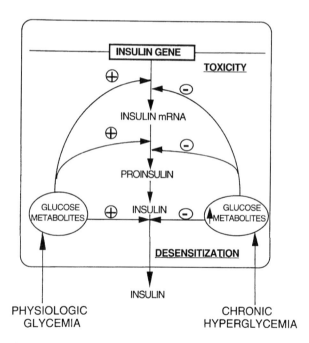

Figure 10 Differentiation of glucose toxicity from glucose desensitization (reproduced from reference 146, with permission)

GLUCOSE METABOLISM

Insulin Action and Glucose Uptake in Diabetes

It is now well established that patients with diabetes are resistant to the action of insulin [61]. By this we mean that the ability of insulin to elicit its normal physiologic responses (e.g. stimulation of glucose transport, glucose oxidation, glycogen synthesis, lipogenesis, etc.) is defective in patients with diabetes mellitus. This fact was first noted by Himsworth and Kerr [148] in the early 1940s using the combined intravenous insulin tolerance test and oral glucose tolerance test. Over the subsequent decades, this observation has been confirmed by a variety of more sophisticated means, including the forearm perfusion technique [149, 150], the insulin suppression test [151], the insulin clamp technique [152, 153] and the minimal model technique [154] (see Chapter 28). It is now known that this insulin resistance is characterized by (a) an over-production of glucose by the liver in the basal state, despite the presence of normal or elevated fasting plasma insulin and glucose levels, both of which should suppress hepatic glucose production, and (b) a substantial defect in glucose uptake by muscle and other insulin-sensitive tissues in the postprandial or insulin-stimulated state [61, 153, 155].

It is important to note that insulin resistance is observed in both type 2 and type 1 diabetes mellitus as well as secondary forms of the disease [52, 53, 56, 60, 61, 153, 156]. In type 2 diabetic patients, the defect in insulin action is thought to be inherited [157–159], while in type 1 and secondary diabetes it is acquired [156, 160, 161]. It has been suggested that hyperglycemia may be responsible, in part, for exacerbating the defect in insulin-mediated glucose disposal in all forms of the disease [50, 61]. In diabetic animals it has been clearly demonstrated that an initial defect in insulin secretion produced by pancreatectomy, B-cell toxins or spontaneous immune destruction of B cells can lead to the development of insulin resistance [55, 57, 94, 95, 162, 163]. For example, when dogs are made diabetic with streptozotocin, moderate to severe fasting hyperglycemia ensues and insulin-mediated glucose uptake (measured by the insulin clamp technique) becomes markedly impaired (Figure 11) [162]. However, it is not clear whether insulin deficiency or some other metabolic derangement that occurs as a result of the insulinopenia is responsible for the defect in insulin action.

Despite the well recognized presence of insulin resistance, only recently has it been appreciated that the

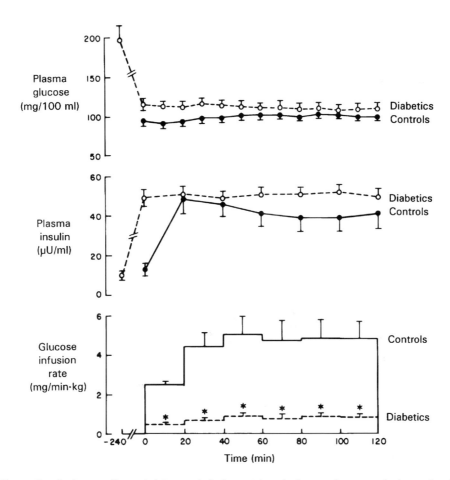

Figure 11 Insulin-mediated glucose disposal (glucose infusion rate) and plasma glucose and plasma insulin concentrations in control (solid line) and streptozotocin-induced diabetic (dashed lines) dogs. $^*p < 0.001$ vs. control (reproduced from reference 162, with permission)

ability of glucose *per se* to promote its own uptake into cells is also impaired in the patient with diabetes [164]. Under normal physiologic circumstances, glucose uptake across the cell membrane occurs by a facilitated transport mechanism [166, 167]. The movement of glucose into the cell occurs via a specific family of proteins in the cell membrane known as glucose transporters. The seven currently known glucose transporters (Glut 1–Glut 7) are present in different amounts in different tissues, and vary in their ability to respond to insulin. Under the influence of insulin, the number of insulin-sensitive glucose transporters (Glut 4) in the cell membrane increases as additional transporters are recruited from the interior of the cell [167]. However, even in the presence of low levels of insulin, some glucose is still able to enter the cell due to a mass action effect, because the concentration of glucose outside the cell exceeds its concentration on the inside. In fact, it has been proposed by some investigators that the hyperglycemia of diabetes is a compensatory mechanism to ensure that adequate amounts of glucose are able to enter the cell [168–170].

Studies in humans have examined the ability of glucose to stimulate its own uptake. We investigated this question in patients with type 1 and type 2 diabetes as well as in healthy control subjects [164]. All subjects had their basal insulin level maintained at 10–15 μU/ml by an infusion of somatostatin in combination with basal replacement doses of insulin and glucagon. The plasma glucose concentration was then sequentially increased by 50, 100 and 200 mg/dl (2.8, 5.6 and 11.1 mmol/l) above the fasting level using the hyperglycemic clamp technique. In response to this hyperglycemic stimulus in the presence of basal levels of

insulin, normal subjects displayed a characteristic dose-related increase in total body glucose disposal. In contrast, the ability of glucose to enhance its own uptake was significantly impaired in both IDDM and NIDDM patients. Thus, one might say that diabetes is characterized by 'glucose resistance' as well as insulin resistance.

Yki-Jarvinen et al [171] also examined this question in well-controlled IDDM patients who were receiving chronic subcutaneous insulin infusion therapy. Subjects participated in two euglycemic insulin clamp procedures on successive days. During the initial study the plasma glucose concentration was maintained at the basal level (approximately 100 mg/dl, 5.6 mmol/l) for the 24 h before the insulin clamp, whereas prior to the second study the plasma glucose concentration was elevated to approximately 280 mg/dl (15.6 mmol/l) for 24 h. As can be seen in Figure 12, 24 h of hyperglycemia was sufficient to induce a 20% decline in the rate of insulin-mediated glucose disposal. Using a more physiologic increment in plasma glucose concentration (20–40 mg/dl, 1.1–2.2 mmol/l) for 3 days, we have demonstrated a similar impairment in insulin action in healthy young subjects (Figure 13) [172]. It is of interest that the development of insulin resistance was associated with a defect in non-oxidative glucose disposal, suggesting that both glucose transport and post-glucose transport abnormalities contribute to the defect in insulin action, and could not be explained by changes in other substrates or counter-regulatory hormones.

Data obtained from animal studies also support this concept. Rats who are chronically maintained in a hyperglycemic state exhibit a significant reduction in glucose transport activity [173, 174], whereas animals who are rendered chronically hypoglycemic display

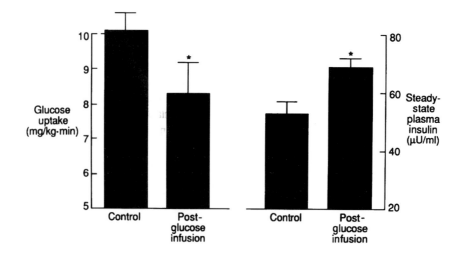

Figure 12 Effect of short-term (24-hour) hyperglycemia on whole body insulin-mediated glucose disposal (left bars) in well-controlled insulin-dependent diabetic subjects. Steady-state plasma insulin levels during the insulin clamp studies performed after the 24-hour period of hyperglycemia are shown in the two right-hand bars. * $p < 0.01$ vs. control (drawn from data presented in reference 171)

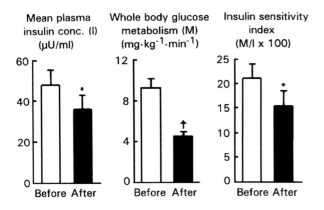

Figure 13 Plasma insulin (I) response, whole body glucose metabolism (M), and insulin sensitivity index (M/I ratio × 100) during hyperglycemic clamp studies carried out before (open bars) and after (solid bars) 96-hour constant glucose infusion. $*p < 0.05$, $†p < 0.001$ (reproduced from reference 172, with permission)

enhanced glucose uptake [175]. Thus, the regulation of glucose transport by glucose itself is analogous in some ways to the manner in which many hormones regulate their receptors—high levels of the hormone lead to down-regulation of activity, while low levels produce an up-regulation of activity.

Not all tissues in the body exhibit glucose resistance when diabetes is present. For example, in normal humans high levels of circulating glucose are capable of directly inhibiting hepatic glucose release [176, 177]. This autoregulatory response appears to be preserved in both IDDM and NIDDM patients. If the plasma glucose concentration is increased by 50, 100 or 200 mg/dl, while pancreatic insulin secretion is inhibited with somatostatin, hepatic glucose production is inhibited to a similar degree in diabetic and healthy subjects [164].

The clinical implications of these observations have become increasingly important in recent years. For example, the beneficial effect of diverse therapeutic regimens (e.g. diet, sulfonylureas, biguanides or insulin) on glucose metabolism may, in part, be related to improvements in 'glucose resistance' as well as insulin resistance. Furthermore, since glucose appears to be capable of regulating its own transport into cells, this opens new avenues of research for pharmacologic means of improving glycemic control. Finally, alterations in glucose transport activity may help to explain the frequent clinical observation that diabetic patients in poor control appear to have symptoms of hypoglycemia at relatively 'normal' glucose levels (80–100 mg/dl, 4.4–5.6 mmol/l) while patients in very good glycemic control may not have any symptoms in the presence of frank biochemical hypoglycemia (40–50 mg/dl, 2.2–2.8 mmol/l) [178–183]. If glucose transport is inhibited by high ambient levels of glucose

and enhanced by low levels of circulating glucose, then the intracellular concentration of glucose may actually be lower in the former case than in the latter. Further study using non-invasive imaging techniques (e.g. positron emission tomography (PET) scanning) [184] to examine brain glucose metabolism under differing glycemic conditions should provide important insights in this area.

Reversibility by Correction of Hyperglycemia

Although the studies cited above suggest that hyperglycemia *per se* is capable of regulating glucose transport, it must be remembered that in most cases the improvement in glycemic control was simultaneously accompanied by administration of exogenous insulin or a drug that enhances insulin secretion or insulin sensitivity. Thus, it is conceivable that insulin, not glucose, was primarily responsible for amelioration of the defects in insulin secretion or insulin action.

Rossetti et al [95] were among the first to provide experimental proof in a diabetic animal model of NIDDM that hyperglycemia *per se* plays a central role in the development of insulin resistance following insulin deficiency. They studied four groups of chronically catheterized, awake, unstressed rats: Group 1, sham-operated controls; Group 2, 90% surgically pancreatectomized rats; Group 3, 90% pancreatectomized rats treated with phlorhizin (an inhibitor of renal tubular glucose transport) to normalize the plasma glucose level; Group 4, diabetic rats treated with phlorhizin for 6 weeks and subsequently restudied 2 weeks after discontinuation of the phlorhizin. Groups 1–3 were studied 6 weeks after pancreatectomy or sham pancreatectomy. The pancreatectomized rats all had mild fasting hyperglycemia and an abnormal meal tolerance test compared with the control rats. Insulin secretion during the mixed meal was markedly impaired in the diabetic group. Phlorhizin treatment normalized the fasting plasma glucose concentration and the post-meal glucose profile without altering plasma insulin or other hormone/substrate levels. When the phlorhizin was discontinued, glucose intolerance returned and the plasma insulin response remained markedly impaired.

If hyperglycemia *per se* were an important regulator of insulin action *in vivo*, the diabetic animals should be insulin resistant and phlorhizin would be expected to improve the defect in insulin-mediated glucose disposal even though total insulin secretion remained markedly deficient. To examine this question, rats were studied using the euglycemic insulin clamp technique. Not only was insulin sensitivity improved in phlorhizin-treated diabetic rats, it was completely returned to normal (Figure 14). As further proof of the deleterious effect of hyperglycemia on insulin sensitivity, discontinuation of phlorhizin therapy was associated with a return of the insulin resistance. Since phlorhizin did not enhance insulin sensitivity in sham-operated rats, the improvement in insulin action in diabetic rats cannot be attributed to a non-specific effect of phlorhizin [95]. Similar data have been reported by Blondel et al [185].

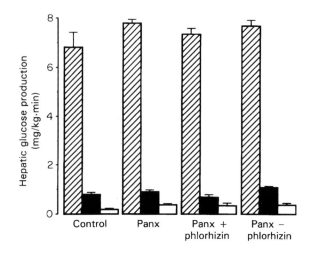

Figure 15 Hepatic glucose production during the basal state (hatched bars) and during +80 μU/ml (solid bars) and +160 μU/ml (open bars) euglycemic insulin clamp studies performed in four groups of rats: sham-operated controls, 90%-pancreatectomized diabetic rats (Panx), and partially pancreatectomized rats treated with phlorhizin for 6 weeks (Panx + phlorhizin) and again after discontinuation of phlorhizin for 2 weeks (Panx − phlorhizin) (adapted from data presented in reference 95)

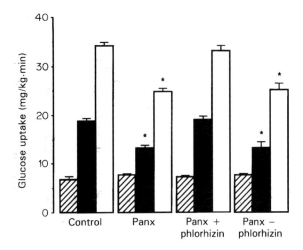

Figure 14 Whole-body insulin-mediated glucose uptake during the basal state (hatched bars) and during +80 μU/ml (solid bars) and +160 μU/ml (open bars) euglycemic insulin clamp studies performed in four groups of awake, unstressed, chronically catheterized rats: sham-operated controls, 90%-pancreatectomized diabetic rats (Panx), and partially pancreatectomized diabetic rats treated with phlorhizin for 6 weeks (Panx + phlorhizin) and again after discontinuation of the phlorhizin for 2 weeks (Panx − phlorhizin) (adapted from data presented in reference 95)

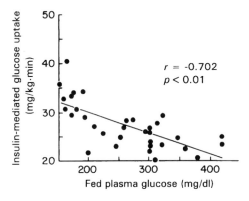

Figure 16 Relationship between the fed (meal tolerance test) plasma glucose concentration and the rate of whole-body insulin-mediated glucose uptake during +160 μU/ml euglycemic insulin clamp studies performed in control, partially pancreatectomized diabetic rats, and partially pancreatectomized rats treated with phlorhizin (reproduced from reference 95, with permission)

Under euglycemic hyperinsulinemic conditions, the majority (>80–90%) of an infused glucose load is disposed of by peripheral tissues, primarily muscle, in both normal individuals and patients with type 2 diabetes [61, 155, 177, 186]. Therefore, these results in partially pancreatectomized diabetic rats suggest that muscle is the major site responsible for the development of insulin resistance following exposure to chronic hyperglycemia. Consistent with this, basal hepatic glucose production (measured with [3-^{3}H]-glucose), as well as its suppression during the insulin clamp, was not significantly different in diabetic vs. control animals, and was not altered by phlorhizin treatment (Figure 15). These data also demonstrate a close inverse relationship between the defect in total body (primarily muscle) glucose uptake and the plasma glucose level during the meal tolerance test (Figure 16),

indicating a link between the severity of the hyperglycemia and the severity of the insulin resistance in muscle.

Cellular Mechanisms

Many studies have suggested that a defect in the glucose transport system plays an important role in the insulin resistance of NIDDM [187, 188]. In most insulin-sensitive tissues, glucose transport is the rate-limiting step in glucose metabolism [169, 189,

190]. In order to define the mechanism(s) responsible for the insulin resistance observed following chronic hyperglycemia in partially pancreatectomized diabetic rats, Kahn et al [191] measured 3-*O*-methylglucose transport in isolated adipose cells 6 weeks after pancreatectomy. This metabolite of glucose is transported into cells, but is not phosphorylated and does not undergo further metabolism. The results indicated that insulin-stimulated glucose transport is impaired in diabetic rats and that the defect in glucose transport is restored to normal with phlorhizin treatment. Moreover, the improvement in glucose transport activity was closely correlated with the improvement in *in vivo* insulin sensitivity.

These observations in the phlorhizin treated diabetic rats are in agreement with a large number of *in vitro* and *in vivo* studies. Incubation of muscle cells and adipocytes with a high glucose concentration (10–20 mmol/l) leads to a progressive decline in glucose transport activity, loss of cytochalasin B binding activity in both plasma and low-density microsomal membrane fractions, and the development of insulin resistance. Conversely, glucose starvation leads to an up-regulation of the glucose transport system in cultured muscle cells, adipocytes and fibroblasts [192–213]. Sasson and Cerasi [192] reported that when rat soleus muscle or rat skeletal myocytes were incubated for 24 h in a high glucose concentration, a progressive decline in insulin-mediated glucose transport was evident. This effect of hyperglycemia was both dose- and time-dependent, and was fully reversible. Because the development of insulin resistance involves a decrease in both the number and activity of glucose transport units, one might expect that the ability of glucose to enhance its own uptake, i.e. the mass action effect of hyperglycemia, also would be impaired. This possibility was explored by incubating myocytes with different glucose concentrations and then examining the effect of hyperglycemia (in the absence of insulin) to stimulate its own uptake [192]. As can be seen in Figure 17, incubation of myocytes in hyperglycemic conditions impaired the ability of both physiologic and pharmacologic levels of glucose to enhance its own uptake. Of note, several studies have confirmed that insulin enhances the ability of hyperglycemia to down-regulate its own transport [196, 214, 215].

Chronic hyperglycemia also has been shown to inhibit glucose transport in insulin-independent tissues, such as brain [173, 216], through mechanism(s) that involve a down-regulation of the glucose transport system [217, 218] or post-transcriptional inhibition of glucose transporter mRNA translation [219]. Conversely, chronic hypoglycemia has the opposite effect on brain glucose transport [175]. However, it should be noted that many of the cell lines studied to date have had

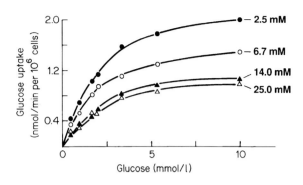

Figure 17 Dose–response relationships between glucose concentration in the medium and glucose uptake by myocytes cultured at different glucose concentrations (reproduced from reference 192, with permission)

a preponderance of Glut 1 (which is not regulated by insulin) vs. Glut 4, the insulin-sensitive glucose transporter [2, 205, 220, 221]. Thus, one needs to be cautious in applying the findings from these cell culture studies to human physiology.

Although correction of hyperglycemia with phlorhizin is capable of normalizing meal tolerance, total body insulin-mediated glucose disposal, and glucose adipocyte transport activity in diabetic animals, one cannot conclude that all of the intracellular pathways of glucose metabolism are necessarily intact. To examine this question Rossetti et al [96] contrasted the effects of vanadate (an insulinomimetic agent) and phlorhizin on whole body and muscle glucose metabolism in 90% pancreatectomized rats (Figure 18). As previously described, diabetic rats manifested a 30% reduction in whole body sensitivity to insulin, and this was corrected by phlorhizin treatment. A similar improvement in insulin action was observed with vanadate; however, vanadate, unlike phlorhizin, also corrected the defect in muscle glycogen synthesis. Consistent with this observation, the V_{max} of muscle glycogen synthase was reduced in diabetic rats and returned to normal with vanadate, but not with phlorhizin [96]. These results indicate that correction of hyperglycemia in diabetic rats normalizes the defect in glucose transport but does not necessarily improve the intracellular abnormality in glycogen synthesis. Thus, the 'glucose toxicity' effect in muscle appears to be directed specifically against the glucose transport system.

There is also an important temporal component to regulation of the glucose transport system. For example, in L6 myocytes, glucose deprivation leads to up-regulation of glucose transport with a $t_{1/2}$ of 15 min, and a maximal effect at 2 h, suggesting that increased protein synthesis is probably not the major mechanism involved [209]. Conversely, down-regulation of glucose transport is initially apparent within 30 min and becomes maximal at 4 h [205]. The effect of glucose

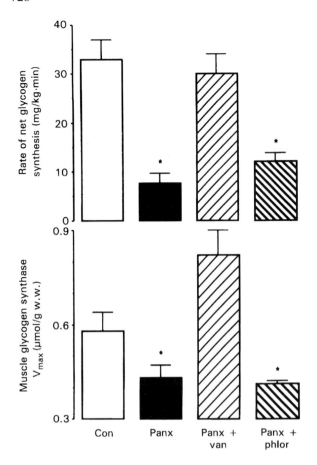

Figure 18 Muscle glycogen synthesis rate (upper panel) and the V_{max} for glycogen synthase (lower panel) in control (Con, open bars) and 90% pancreatectomized rats before (Panx) and after treatment with vanadate (Panx + van) or phlorhizin (Panx + phlor). $*p < 0.01$ vs. controls (redrawn from reference 96, with permission)

on its own transport system is mediated through the distribution of transporters between the plasma membrane and intracellular vesicles as well as changes in the intrinsic rate at which the transporter carries glucose across the cell membrane. The regulation of glucose transport by the ambient glucose concentration also occurs at the transcriptional level. Glucose deprivation for more than 6 h in either L6 myocytes [209, 210] or 3T3 L1 adipocytes [212] increases Glut 1 mRNA, although it has been proposed that this up-regulation represents a more generalized 'survival' response by the cell to a stressful environment [222].

In contrast to cultured cell lines where Glut 1 is often the predominant glucose transporter, Glut 4 is quantitatively the most important in most mammalian models *in vivo*. In rat adipose tissue [191, 223–226] and muscle [226, 227], hyperglycemia decreased Glut 4 mRNA, although Glut 4 protein has been reported either to decrease [225, 226] or remain unchanged [228]. The inhibitory effect on glucose transport can be reversed by prior insulin therapy to normalize glucose [223, 225, 226], but not by phlorhizin [191]. Thus, the particular response may depend on the diabetic model employed, the tissue being studied, and whether insulin is used in the therapeutic regimen. The regulation of Glut 4 in human physiologic and pathophysiologic states has recently begun to be addressed. Glut 4 mRNA in the basal state has been reported as normal in IDDM [229] and either normal or increased in NIDDM [230, 231]. However, the role of hyperglycemia and hyperinsulinemia in regulating Glut 4 in normal and diabetic states remains to be fully elucidated.

The metabolic pathways regulating the changes in glucose transport have been the subject of intense recent investigation. It is known that down-regulation of the transport system cannot be induced by L-glucose (which is not transported) [194, 206], 3-O-methylglucose (which is transported but not phosphorylated) [214, 232], or fructose (which enters glycolysis at the fructose-6-phosphate level) [194, 195, 206, 214, 232]. However, it has been shown that certain amino acids, particularly glutamine, appear to be essential for down-regulation of the transport system to occur [214]. Based on this initial observation, Marshall and Traxinger [214, 232, 233] proposed that a quantitatively minor pathway of glucose metabolism involving the conversion of fructose-6-phosphate and glutamine to glucosamine-6-phosphate via the enzyme glutamine:fructose-6-phosphate amidotransferase (GFAT) might be a critical regulatory step in this process.

To explore this hypothesis, they demonstrated that blocking GFAT activity with azaserine could prevent the down-regulation of glucose transport by hyperglycemia, and that down-regulation was restored when D-glucosamine was added in the presence of azaserine [233]. When RNA synthesis was inhibited, the activity of GFAT was blocked and desensitization was, again, impaired, suggesting that there is some control at the transcriptional level [234]. Importantly, more recent studies have shown that incubation of islet cells or fibroblasts with glucosamine, or infusion of glucosamine *in vivo* in rats, can induce defects in insulin secretion and insulin action (Figure 19) [232–241]. Thus, glucosamine is a possible candidate for the molecular basis of glucose toxicity, but more studies are clearly needed in this area.

Among the many other potential mechanisms that have been proposed, perhaps one of the more attractive hypotheses involves the regulation of glucose transport by glycosylation of the transporter protein. One study has shown that glucose transport activity is decreased when the transporter is glycated [242], although another study in humans showed that poor glycemic control is associated with an increase in

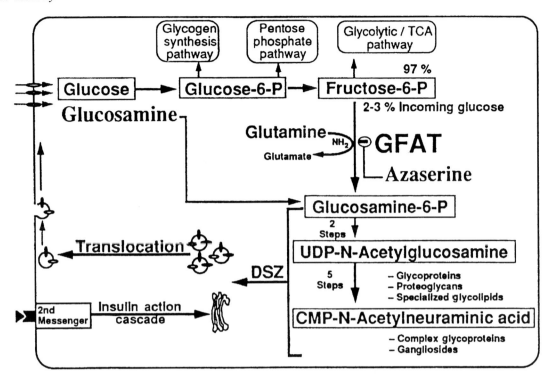

Figure 19 Metabolic pathway mediating desensitization of the insulin-responsive glucose transport system (reproduced from reference 235, with permission)

the density of transporters on circulating erythrocytes [243]. Additional studies should help resolve this issue.

Clinical Implications

If the concept of glucose toxicity is correct and if hyperglycemia contributes to the insulin resistance observed in human diabetes mellitus, one would expect that normalization of the plasma glucose profile, regardless of the therapeutic modalities involved, should lead to an improvement in insulin sensitivity. Using the insulin clamp technique a number of investigators have examined the effect of diet (weight loss) [69, 244–246], sulfonylureas [70–73, 247, 248], biguanides [87–91], and insulin therapy [73, 77, 81–83, 244, 249, 250] on insulin action in IDDM and NIDDM individuals. The results of these studies provide a number of interesting insights.

First, all therapeutic interventions are effective in reducing the fasting and/or postprandial plasma glucose concentration and improving glucose tolerance. However, in most of these studies the improvement in insulin sensitivity is small compared to the nearly complete normalization of insulin-mediated glucose disposal following restoration of normoglycemia with phlorhizin in experimental diabetes in the rat.

Second, strict glycemic control with insulin in IDDM patients [84, 85, 251–255] uniformly improves insulin sensitivity, whereas a similar degree of

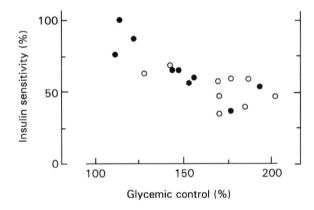

Figure 20 Relationship between insulin sensitivity and glycemic control in studies performed in patients with IDDM (filled circles) and NIDDM (open circles). Insulin sensitivity is expressed as a percentage of that measured in non-diabetic subjects. Glycemic control is expressed as a percentage of the non-diabetic glycated hemoglobin where 100% is the upper limit of the mean normal range (reproduced from reference 2, with permission)

glycemic control has less of an effect on insulin action in NIDDM subjects [2, 73, 77, 81–83, 244, 249, 250] (Figure 20). In NIDDM subjects insulin sensitivity is reduced on average by approximately 40% compared to controls. Improved glycemic control with insulin causes a quantitatively small, albeit frequently statistically significant, rise in tissue sensitivity to insulin. The lack of more dramatic improvement is to be contrasted with a more consistent enhancement of insulin action observed in IDDM individuals (Figure 20). Thus, the failure to observe a significant amelioration of the insulin resistance in NIDDM cannot be attributed to insulin therapy itself [256, 257].

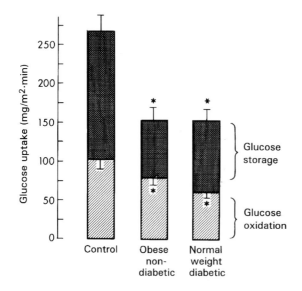

Figure 21 Whole-body insulin-mediated glucose uptake in control (left), normal-weight diabetic (right), and obese non-diabetic subjects (middle) during a +100 µU/ml euglycemic insulin clamp. Rates of glucose oxidation (hatched portion) and glucose storage (glycogen formation; shaded portion) are also shown. *$p < 0.01$ vs. controls (reproduced from reference 60, with permission)

One might initially interpret these results in NIDDM as evidence against the glucose toxicity hypothesis. However, it should be remembered that a primary abnormality that is inherited in NIDDM is insulin resistance, and that the defect in insulin action becomes maximally manifest early in the natural history of NIDDM [61, 258–261]. Thus, even when another state of severe insulin resistance such as obesity is superimposed upon NIDDM, the insulin resistance is only slightly greater than with diabetes alone or obesity alone [56, 60, 61] (Figure 21). By analogy, if one were to superimpose insulin resistance from 'glucose toxicity' upon the insulin resistance that is inherited in NIDDM, one would not expect much of an additional deterioration in insulin action. Thus, normalization of the plasma glucose concentration and removal of glucose toxicity would not be expected to produce a major improvement in insulin sensitivity in these patients, since a substantial component of the insulin resistance is inherited. Conversely, in IDDM in humans and in experimental animal models of diabetes—where the insulin resistance is acquired, not inherited—glycemic control, however achieved, would

be expected to lead to an improvement in insulin-mediated glucose disposal.

Lastly, it should be noted that the effect of strict glycemic control with insulin in NIDDM subjects consistently enhanced insulin secretion [77, 78, 81, 83, 86, 244, 262, 263]. In one study in which the plasma insulin response failed to increase significantly, the fasting glucose concentration remained above 140 mg/dl (7.8 mmol/l) [244].

THERAPEUTIC APPROACH TO GLUCOSE TOXICITY

Based upon the preceding discussion, it is of interest to examine what features the standard therapies of NIDDM (weight loss, exercise, sulfonylureas, biguanides or insulin) have in common (Figure 22).

Sulfonylurea therapy exerts its beneficial effects on glucose tolerance primarily by augmentation of insulin secretion. To a lesser degree, enhanced peripheral, primarily muscle, glucose uptake and suppression of the elevated rate of hepatic glucose production may also contribute to the ability of sulfonylureas to lower glucose levels. The increase in portal vein insulin concentration during sulfonylurea therapy directly suppresses hepatic glucose production (HGP), and the increase in circulating insulin level enhances muscle glucose uptake. It is the former effect, however, that is primarily responsible for the decline in fasting glucose concentration and overall improvement in glucose tolerance [61, 264]. As HGP declines and the fasting glucose level falls, 'glucose toxicity' is lessened; the removal of the inhibitory effect of hyperglycemia ultimately is responsible for long-term beneficial action of the sulfonylureas on insulin secretion and tissue sensitivity to insulin.

Weight reduction also has a major effect to decrease HGP [67–69, 265] (Figure 22). In NIDDM increased HGP is primarily due to excessive gluconeogenesis [266–268]. Nonetheless, a significant portion of HGP still derives from glycogenolysis [268]. With caloric deprivation and the attendant weight loss, liver glycogen stores are depleted and total HGP declines. This leads to a reduction in the fasting glucose concentration and the deleterious effects of hyperglycemia are removed. As glucose toxicity is ameliorated, insulin secretion and insulin sensitivity improve, and overall glucose tolerance is enhanced.

Exercise, in contrast to sulfonylureas and weight loss, usually does not have a major effect on the fasting plasma glucose concentration or on overall glucose tolerance [269–273]. The most notable effect of chronic exercise is to enhance peripheral, primarily muscle, tissue glucose uptake [269]. However, it has little effect on basal HGP. Consequently, the fasting

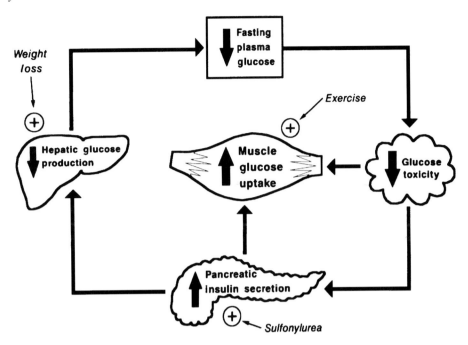

Figure 22 Mechanism of improved glucose tolerance after sulfonylureas, weight loss and exercise. Sulfonylureas, by enhancing insulin secretion into the portal circulation, suppress hepatic glucose output and thus lower the fasting plasma glucose concentration. Weight loss, by depleting liver glycogen stores, also leads to a decrease in hepatic glucose output and a fall in the fasting plasma glucose concentration. The resultant decline in fasting glucose, by removing the deleterious effects of hyperglycemia (glucose toxicity) on B-cell and muscle cell function, leads to improvements in insulin secretion and insulin sensitivity, respectively. Exercise acts primarily on muscle to augment insulin sensitivity. However, this has little effect on the fasting glucose concentration, which is largely determined by the rate of hepatic glucose production. Because neither the fasting plasma glucose nor the mean plasma glucose concentration throughout the day is significantly decreased, glucose toxicity is not ameliorated, insulin secretion does not increase, and major improvements in glucose tolerance usually are not observed (reproduced from reference 1, with permission)

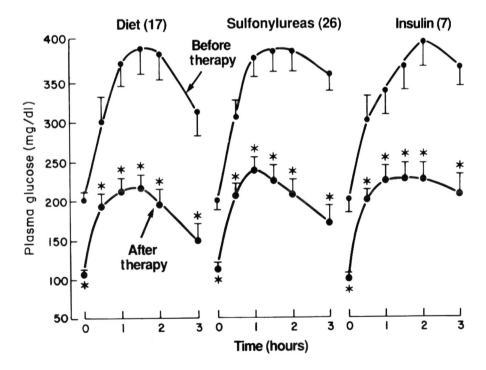

Figure 23 Effect of treatment with diet (weight loss), sulfonylureas and insulin on the plasma glucose concentration during an oral glucose tolerance test in non-insulin-dependent diabetic subjects. $^*p < 0.01$ vs. before therapy. Numbers in parentheses indicate number of subjects (reproduced from reference 86, with permission)

plasma glucose concentration, which is primarily determined by the rate of basal HGP, declines minimally or not at all. Not surprisingly, insulin secretion fails to increase (due to the improved insulin sensitivity) and a major improvement in glucose tolerance usually is not observed. It should be emphasized, however, that the improved peripheral tissue sensitivity to insulin has a number of other beneficial effects which improve the atherogenic profile.

From the above discussion it is clear that the various therapeutic interventions work by different mechanisms of action, but all are accompanied by improved insulin secretion (Figures 23 and 24). Although these observations do not constitute proof of the glucose toxicity hypothesis, they are certainly consistent with the concept that any treatment which lowers the fasting glucose concentration (which is the primary determinant of the mean glucose concentration throughout the day) will lead to an improvement in B-cell function. Moreover, suppression of the augmented rate of glucose output by the liver is critical if one wishes to achieve normoglycemia.

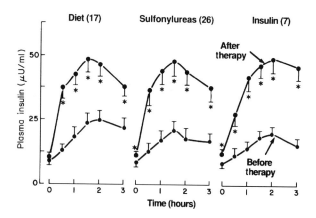

Figure 24 Effect of glycemic control with diet (weight loss), sulfonylureas and insulin on the plasma insulin response during an oral glucose tolerance test in non-insulin-dependent diabetic subjects. *$p < 0.01$ vs. before therapy. Numbers in parentheses indicate number of subjects (reproduced from reference 86, with permission)

The results of intensified insulin therapy in NIDDM are also consistent with the sequence of events outlined above. Although insulin augments glucose uptake by peripheral tissues, its main action in achieving normoglycemia is a suppression of hepatic glucose output [61, 268]. That correction of the hyperglycemia is associated with a significant improvement in insulin secretion is consistent with amelioration of the deleterious effects of glucose on B-cell function (Figures 23 and 24). Since insulin resistance is, in large part, genetically determined in NIDDM [61, 258–261], and since hyperinsulinemia *per se* can induce insulin resistance, it is

not surprising that intensified insulin therapy fails to achieve a substantial improvement in tissue sensitivity to insulin in individuals with NIDDM.

PATHOGENESIS OF NIDDM: ROLE OF GLUCOSE TOXICITY

In view of the evidence presented in this chapter, it is reasonable to ask what factor(s) is (are) responsible for the development of NIDDM with overt fasting hyperglycemia and severe glucose intolerance. To the extent that hyperglycemia contributes to a deterioration of insulin action, it will lead to a worsening of glucose tolerance. However, since the genetic component of the insulin resistance is established early in the course of NIDDM, the superimposition of glucose toxicity is unlikely to cause a further substantial decline in tissue sensitivity to insulin. Once the insulin resistance becomes fully established, however, the maintenance of normal glucose tolerance becomes critically dependent upon the ability of the B cells to augment insulin secretion in an attempt to offset the peripheral defect in insulin action. As long as the pancreas can maintain a high rate of insulin secretion, glucose tolerance will remain normal or only slightly impaired. Thus, in individuals with impaired glucose tolerance and in diabetic patients with mild fasting hyperglycemia (110–140 mg/dl, 6.1–7.8 mmol/l), the plasma insulin response to glucose is uniformly increased [61, 258–262, 265, 274–287].

The available data in man indicate that islet mass is reduced by no more than 30–40% in NIDDM [48, 49]. A decrease of this degree cannot account for the marked insulinopenia observed in many type 2 diabetic patients, especially those with fasting glucose levels above 200 mg/dl (11.1 mmol/l) [61]. In general, a greater than 80–90% reduction in B-cell mass is required before sufficient insulinopenia develops to result in overt diabetes mellitus [288]. It seems likely, therefore, that factors in addition to the loss of B cells must be responsible for the impairment in insulin secretion. On the basis of animal studies and the large number of *in vitro* studies reviewed above, it seems reasonable to postulate that chronic hyperglycemia is responsible, at least in part, for the inability of the B cells to respond to an acute glycemic challenge.

The relationship between insulin secretion and insulin sensitivity is depicted in Figure 25 for the obese diabetic patient [60]. As a lean individual gains weight, glucose tolerance initially remains normal because the obesity-related increase in insulin resistance [60, 61, 289] is counterbalanced by an increase in insulin secretion. Progression to impaired glucose tolerance is accompanied by a worsening of the insulin resistance, but because of further augmentation in both fasting and

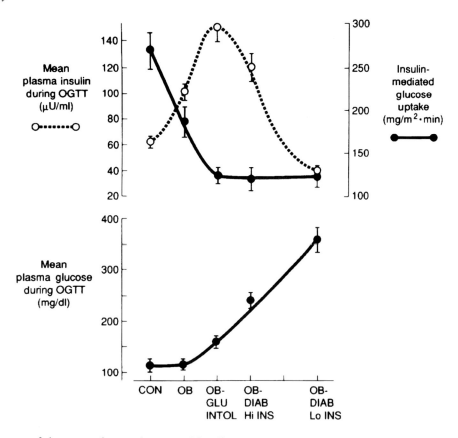

Figure 25 Summary of the mean plasma glucose and insulin responses during a 100 g oral glucose tolerance test (OGTT) and tissue sensitivity to insulin (top) in control (CON), obese non-diabetic (OB), obese glucose-intolerant (OB-GLU INTOL), obese hyperinsulinemic diabetic (OB-DIAB Hi INS), and obese hypoinsulinemic diabetic (OB DIAB Lo INS) subjects. Note the inverted U-shaped curve for insulin secretion (adapted from reference 60, with permission)

glucose-stimulated insulin secretion, only a minimal impairment in glucose tolerance ensues (Figure 25). It is at this point, i.e. impaired glucose tolerance, that the individual is most dependent upon sustaining this high rate of insulin secretion to maintain nearly normal carbohydrate tolerance. Even the slightest decline in insulin secretion at a time when the insulin resistance is maximally established will result in marked deterioration of glucose tolerance. Although the plasma insulin response remains significantly increased compared to the normal weight control group, it is no longer appropriately elevated for the degree of insulin resistance. The series of events depicted schematically in Figure 25 has been documented by both cross-sectional and prospective studies in Europids, in Pima Indians and in the Rhesus monkey [60, 61, 285, 287, 290–292]. It is important to emphasize that no study has documented a decrease in total insulin secretion prior to the development of NIDDM.

One key question, however, remains unanswered: what factor(s) is (are) responsible for the inability of the pancreas to maintain its augmented rate of insulin secretion indefinitely in response to insulin resistance?

In the past this has been referred to by the term 'B-cell exhaustion'. Evidence presented earlier in this chapter suggests that at least one factor (and by no means the only factor) responsible for 'B-cell exhaustion' is 'glucose toxicity'. Inherent to this hypothesis is the concept that, in addition to the defect in insulin resistance, type 2 diabetic patients also have inherited a second abnormality that limits the pancreas's ability to maintain a high rate of insulin secretion for a prolonged period of time when faced with hyperglycemia. This could result from a genetically determined decrease in the number of islets within the pancreas, from an inherent biochemical defect in the insulin biosynthetic/secretory apparatus, or other factors. In the absence of any superimposed metabolic stress (e.g. the development of insulin resistance from obesity, a high fat diet, or other factors) such a B-cell defect would be clinically quiescent. However, once hyperglycemia, albeit minimal, becomes established, it inhibits the B cell's ability to respond to subsequent hyperglycemia which, in a predisposed individual, may lead to B-cell exhaustion. Such a sequence of events would explain why normalization of the plasma glucose concentration via a variety of diverse therapeutic modalities uniformly leads to an improvement in insulin secretion and glucose tolerance that often persists for some time after the therapy has been discontinued (Figure 24).

CLINICAL IMPLICATIONS AND SUMMARY

The observation that sustained, physiologic elevation in the plasma glucose concentration leads to an impairment in insulin secretion has several implications for understanding the pathogenesis of type 2 diabetes.

First, it means that hyperglycemia can no longer be viewed merely as a manifestation, i.e. a laboratory marker, of diabetes mellitus. Rather, hyperglycemia must be considered as a pathogenetic factor which impairs insulin secretion and insulin action and, therefore, is responsible for the perpetuation of the diabetic state. Thus, hyperglycemia, in addition to being implicated in the microvascular, macrovascular and other complications of diabetes, must also be considered as an important factor that leads to metabolic decompensation.

Second, the glucose toxicity hypothesis has important therapeutic implications and may help to explain the uniform improvement in insulin secretion that has been observed after a number of diverse maneuvers, all of which have in common the ability to lower the plasma glucose concentration. Thus, acute and chronic caloric restriction, intensified insulin therapy, sulfonylureas and biguanides all result in a significant lowering of the plasma glucose concentration and a concomitant improvement in the insulin secretory profile, which may be sustained even after the therapy is discontinued. The results of Kosaka et al [86] are particularly relevant to this argument. In that study, weight loss (which has no known direct effect on insulin secretion), exogenous insulin (which inhibits insulin secretion), and sulfonylureas (which augment insulin secretion) all improved B-cell function (Figure 24). The one feature common to all three therapeutic interventions is a reduction in the plasma glucose concentration (Figure 23), suggesting that normalization of the plasma glucose and removal of glucose toxicity is responsible for the improvement in insulin secretion.

A third consequence of the glucose toxicity hypothesis relates to the pathophysiology of secondary failure to pharmacologic therapy. Approximately 10–20% of diabetic patients who are started on sulfonylureas fail to respond and are considered to be primary treatment failures [293–295]. In the remaining patients, the failure rate is about 5–10% per year. These secondary failures often are attributed to weight gain, although this observation has been poorly documented. B-cell desensitization *in vitro* has been shown to occur in response to a wide variety of insulin secretagogues,

including sulfonylureas [103]. For example, Karam et al [296] have demonstrated a selective unresponsiveness of the pancreatic B cells to acute sulfonylurea stimulation in NIDDM during chronic sulfonylurea therapy (Figure 26). These results suggest that many cases of secondary failure may be due to a desensitization of the B-cell to the stimulatory effect of the sulfonylurea. Further, they raise the interesting possibility that chronic exposure of the B cell to any given secretagogue will lead to down-regulation of the insulin secretory response only to that specific stimulus. As a result, one might suggest that such desensitization will occur only in individuals with a reduced B-cell mass or a pre-existing defect in B-cell function. If this hypothesis is correct, it logically follows that aggressive treatment of decompensated patients with an intensified insulin regimen or severe caloric restriction, by acutely lowering and maintaining a reduced plasma glucose concentration, will remove the toxic effect of hyperglycemia and, after a period of tight glycemic control, allow the successful reinstitution of sulfonylurea therapy.

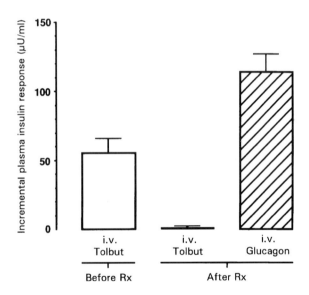

Figure 26   Peak incremental insulin response to acute intravenous (i.v.) tolbutamide (Tolbut; 1 g) in seven NIDDM subjects before and after 4–6 weeks of tolazamide treatment (Rx). The incremental insulin response to acute intravenous glucagon (1 mg) after tolazamide treatment (4–6 weeks) is shown in the same seven NIDDM subjects (drawn from the data presented in reference 296, with permission)

A fourth consequence of the glucose toxicity hypothesis centers on the cause of the 'honeymoon period' in patients with newly diagnosed type 1 diabetes. It is well known that after newly diagnosed IDDM patients are started on insulin treatment, a decrease in insulin requirement often is observed, and some patients may be taken off insulin entirely [297]. A likely explanation

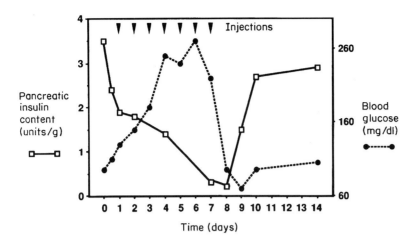

Figure 27 Effect of anterior pituitary extract and insulin therapy on the pancreatic insulin content (squares) and blood glucose level (circles) in partially pancreatectomized dogs. Arrows indicate insulin injections (reproduced from reference 165, with permission)

for this common phenomenon is the reversal of glucose toxicity that occurs with normalization of the blood glucose concentration. It is known that at the time of initial presentation, most patients with IDDM have significant residual B-cell mass [288]. However, current thinking suggests that there is an additional functional impairment resulting from the chronic hyperglycemia that is superimposed on the reduced B-cell mass. This can be improved by aggressive insulin therapy. As evidence for this hypothesis, IDDM children who were in remission and who displayed only mild glucose intolerance had first-phase insulin responses to intravenous glucose that were totally absent, whereas significant insulin responses to intravenous arginine, tolbutamide and glucagon persisted [298]. These results are consistent with the animal models, in which mild glucose intolerance has been shown to impair the B cell's response to glucose but not to non-glucose stimuli.

Lastly, we should note that the concept of glucose toxicity is not new, but was initially suggested by results of Haist, Campbell and Best [165] in 1940. These authors concluded that 'although many years may be required to complete the obvious extension of the present experiments, sufficient information is now available to show that the production of diabetes in partially pancreatectomized animals (dogs) by administration of pituitary diabetogenic substances may be prevented by dietary means or by the administration of large doses of insulin'. In their classic study they noted that partially pancreatectomized dogs did not develop diabetes unless there was a progressive loss of insulin secretory capacity by the remnant pancreas (Figure 27). Further, they noted that daily insulin injections, which created near-normal glycemia, maintained insulin stores within the remaining pancreatic tissue

and prevented the development of permanent diabetes. Perhaps the most compelling part of their conclusion was that 'many years may be required to complete the obvious extension of the present experiments'. Although it has taken almost half a century, it appears that the concept of glucose toxicity has finally become established and its molecular mechanisms are beginning to be defined.

In summary, a large amount of data from animal and human models of diabetes has been generated in support of the glucose toxicity hypothesis. Chronic hyperglycemia is capable of altering the B cell's insulin secretory response as well as tissue glucose uptake. These results are consistent with a number of *in vivo* observations, which demonstrate that correction of the hyperglycemia in diabetes, regardless of the therapeutic intervention, leads to an improvement in insulin secretion and glucose uptake which may be sustained even after the initial therapy has been removed. In this pathogenetic sequence, hyperglycemia must be considered not only as a manifestation of NIDDM, but also as its cause. On the basis of these observations, the arguments for tight metabolic control in all patients with diabetes are even more compelling.

REFERENCES

1. Rossetti L, Giaccari A, DeFronzo RA. Glucose toxicity. Diabetes Care 1990; 13: 610–30.
2. Yki-Jarvinen H. Glucose toxicity. Endocrine Rev 1992; 13: 415–31.
3. Grodsky GM, Batts AA, Bennett LL, Vicella C, McWilliams NB, Smith DF. Effects of carbohydrates on secretion of insulin from isolated rat pancreas. Am J Physiol 1963; 205: 638–44.
4. Levin SR, Grodsky GM, Hagura R, Smith DF, Forsham PH. Relationships between arginine and glucose

in the induction of insulin secretion from the isolated perfused rat pancreas. Endocrinology 1972; 90: 624–31.

5. Pagliara A, Stillings S, Hover B, Martin D, Matschinsky F. Glucose modulation of amino acid-induced glucagon and insulin release in the isolated perfused rat pancreas. J Clin Invest 1974; 54: 819–32.

6. Gerich J, Charles M, Grodsky G. Characterization of the effects of arginine and glucose on glucagon and insulin release from the perfused rat pancreas. J Clin Invest 1974; 54: 833–42.

7. Porte D. Beta-cells in type II diabetes mellitus. Diabetes 1991; 40: 166–80.

8. Leahy JL, Bonner-Weir S, Weir GC. Beta-cell dysfunction induced by chronic hyperglycemia: current ideas on the mechanism of the impaired glucose-induced insulin secretion. Diabetes Care 1992; 15: 442–55.

9. Weir GC, Clore ET, Zmachinski CJ, Bonner-Weir S. Islet secretion in a new experimental model for non-insulin-dependent diabetes. Diabetes 1981; 30: 590–95.

10. Bonner-Weir S, Trent DF, Honey RN, Weir GC. Responses of neonatal rat islets to streptozotocin: limited B-cell regeneration and hyperglycemia. Diabetes 1981; 30: 64–9.

11. Leahy JL, Bonner-Weir S, Weir GC. Abnormal insulin secretion in a streptozocin model of diabetes. Diabetes 1985; 34: 660–66.

12. Martin JM, Lacy PE. The prediabetic period in partially pancreatectomized rats. Diabetes 1963; 12: 238–42.

13. Bonner-Weir S, Trent DF, Weir GC. Partial pancreatectomy in the rat and subsequent defect in glucose-induced insulin release. J Clin Invest 1983; 71: 1544–53.

14. Leahy JL, Bonner-Weir S, Weir GC. Minimal chronic hyperglycemia is a critical determinant of impaired insulin secretion after an incomplete pancreatectomy. J Clin Invest 1988; 81: 1407–14.

15. Leahy JL, Cooper HE, Deal DA, Weir GC. Chronic hyperglycemia is associated with impaired glucose influence on insulin secretion: a study in normal rats using chronic *in vivo* glucose infusions. J Clin Invest 1986; 77: 908–15.

16. Leahy JL, Cooper HE, Weir GC. Impaired insulin secretion associated with near normoglycemia. Diabetes 1987; 36: 459–64.

17. Leahy JL, Weir GC. Evolution of abnormal insulin secretory responses during 48-h *in vivo* hyperglycemia. Diabetes 1988; 37: 217–22.

18. Leahy JL. Natural history of beta-cell dysfunction in NIDDM. Diabetes Care 1990; 13: 992–1010.

19. Flax H, Matthews DR, Levy JC, Coppack SW, Turner RC. No glucotoxity after 53 hours of 6.0 mmol/l hyperglycaemia in normal man. Diabetologia 1991; 34: 570–75.

20. Imamura T, Koffler M, Helderman JH et al. Severe diabetes induced in subtotally depancreatized dogs by sustained hyperglycemia. Diabetes 1988; 37: 600–609.

21. Leahy JL, Weir GC. Unresponsiveness to glucose in a streptozotocin model of diabetes: inappropriate insulin and glucagon responses to a reduction of glucose concentration. Diabetes 1985; 34: 653–9.

22. Hosokawa YA, Hosokawa H, Chen C, Leahy JL. Mechanism of impaired glucose-potentiated insulin

23. Dimitriadis G, Cryer P, Gerich J. Prolonged hyperglycaemia during infusion of glucose and somatostatin impairs pancreatic A- and B-cell responses to decrements in plasma glucose in normal man: evidence for induction of altered sensitivity to glucose. Diabetologia 1985; 28: 63–9.

24. Giroix MH, Portha B, Kergoat M, Bailbe D, Picon L. Glucose insensitivity and amino acid hypersensitivity of insulin release in rats with non-insulin-dependent diabetes: a study with the perfused pancreas. Diabetes 1983; 32: 445–51.

25. Leahy JL, Bonner-Weir S, Weir GC. Abnormal glucose regulation of insulin secretion in models of reduced B-cell mass. Diabetes 1984; 33: 667–73.

26. Reaven GM, Chen YDI, Hollenbeck CB, Sheu WHH, Ostrega D, Polonsky KS. Plasma insulin, c-peptide, and proinsulin concentrations in obese and non-obese individuals with varying degrees of glucose tolerance. J Clin Endocrinol Metab 1993; 76: 44–8.

27. Polonsky KS, Gumbiner B, Ostrega D, Griver K, Tager H, Henry RR. Alterations in immunoreactive proinsulin and insulin clearance induced by weight loss in NIDDM. Diabetes 1994; 43: 871–7.

28. Kergoat M, Bailbe D, Portha B. Insulin treatment improves glucose-induced insulin release in rats with NIDDM induced by streptozocin. Diabetes 1977; 36: 971–7.

29. Grill V, Westberg M, Ostenson CG. Beta-cell insensitivity in a rat model of non-insulin-dependent diabetes. J Clin Invest 1987; 80: 664–9.

30. Voyles NNR, Powel AM, Timmers KI et al. Reversible impairment of glucose-induced insulin secretion in SHR/N-cp rats. Diabetes 1988; 37: 398–404.

31. Collier SA, Mandel TE, Carter WM. Detrimental effect of high medium glucose concentration on subsequent endocrine function of transplanted organ-cultured foetal mouse pancreas. Aust J Exp Biol Med Sci 1982; 60: 437–45.

32. Korsgren O, Jansson L, Anderson A. Effects of hyperglycemia on function of isolated mouse pancreatic islets transplanted under kidney capsule. Diabetes 1989; 38: 510–15.

33. Leahy JL, Bumbalo LM, Chen C. Beta-cell hypersensitivity for glucose precedes loss of glucose-induced insulin secretion in 90% pancreatectomized rats. Diabetologia 1993; 36: 1238–44.

34. Leahy JL, Bumbalo LM, Chen C. Diazoxide causes recovery of β-cell glucose responsiveness in 90% pancreatectomized diabetic rats. Diabetes 1994; 43: 173–9.

35. Marynissen G, Leclercq-Meyer V, Sever A, Malaisse WJ. Perturbation of pancreatic islet function in glucose-infused rats. Metabolism 1990; 39: 87–95.

36. Thibault C, Guettel C, Lowry MC et al. *In vivo* and *in vitro* increased pancreatic beta-cell sensitivity to glucose in normal rats submitted to a 48-h hyperglycemic period. Diabetologia 1993; 36: 589–95.

37. Chen N-G, Tassava TM, Romsos DR. Threshold for glucose-stimulated insulin secretion in pancreatic islets of genetically obese (ob/ob) mice is abnormally low. J Nutr 1993; 123: 1567–74.

38. Jia X, Elliot R, Kwok YN, Pederson RA, McIntosh CHS. Altered glucose dependence of glucagon-like

peptide I(7-36)-induced insulin secretion from the Zucker (fa/fa) rat pancreas. Diabetes 1995; 44: 495–500.

39. Teruya M, Takei S, Forrest LE, Grunewald A, Chan EK, Charles MA. Pancreatic islet function in non-diabetic and diabetic BB rats. Diabetes 1993; 42: 1310–17.

40. Ostenson CG, Khan A, Efendic S. Impaired glucose-induced insulin secretion: studies in animal models with spontaneous NIDDM. Adv Exp Med Biol 1993; 334: 1–11.

41. Brunzell JD, Robertson RP, Lerner RL et al. Relationships between fasting plasma glucose levels and insulin secretion during intravenous glucose tolerance tests. J Clin Endocrinol Metab 1976; 42: 222–9.

42. Saad MF, Knowler WC, Pettit DJ, Nelson RG, Charles MA, Bennett PH. A two-step model for the development of non-insulin-dependent diabetes. Am J Med 1991; 90: 229–35.

43. Beck-Nielsen H, Groop LC. Metabolic and genetic characterization of prediabetic state. Sequence of events leading to non-insulin-dependent diabetes mellitus. J Clin Invest 1994; 94: 1714–21.

44. Palmer JP, Benson JW, Walter RM, Ensinck JW. Arginine-stimulated acute phase of insulin and glucagon secretion in diabetic subjects. J Clin Invest 1976; 58: 565–70.

45. Halter JB, Graf RJ, Porte D. Potentiation of insulin secretory responses by plasma glucose levels in man: evidence that hyperglycemia in diabetes compensates for impaired glucose potentiation. J Clin Endocrinol Metab 1979; 48: 946–54.

46. Ward WK, Bolgiano DC, McKnight B, Halter JB, Porte D. Diminished B-cell secretory capacity in patients with non-insulin dependent diabetes mellitus. J Clin Invest 1984; 74: 1318–28.

47. Johnston C, Raghu P, McCulloch DK et al. β-cell function and insulin sensitivity in non-diabetic HLA-identical siblings of insulin-dependent diabetes. Diabetes 1987; 36: 829–37.

48. Westermark P, Wilander E. The influence of amyloid deposits on the islet volume in maturity-onset diabetes mellitus. Diabetologia 1978; 15: 417–21.

49. Gepts W, Lecompte PM. The pancreatic islets in diabetes. Am J Med 1981; 70: 105–14.

50. Unger RH, Grundy S. Hyperglycemia as an inducer as well as a consequence of impaired islet cell function and insulin resistance: implications for the management of diabetes. Diabetologia 1985; 28: 119–21.

51. Cerasi E, Luft R, Efendic S. Decreased sensitivity of the pancreatic beta cells to glucose in prediabetic and diabetic subjects. Diabetes 1972; 21: 224–34.

52. Kolterman OG, Gray RS, Griffin J, Olefsky JM. Receptor and postreceptor defects contribute to insulin resistance in non-insulin dependent diabetes mellitus. J Clin Invest 1981; 68: 957–69.

53. DeFronzo RA, Hendler R, Simonson DC. Insulin resistance is a prominent feature of insulin dependent diabetes. Diabetes 1982; 31: 795–801.

54. DeFronzo RA, Ferrannini E, Koivisto V. New concepts in the pathogenesis of non-insulin-dependent diabetes mellitus. Am J Med 1983; 74: 52–81.

55. Levy J, Gavin JR, Fausto A, Gingerich RL, Avioli L. Impaired insulin action in rats with non-insulin dependent diabetes. Diabetes 1984; 33: 901–8.

56. Hollenbeck CB, Chen Y-DI, Reaven GM. A comparison of the relative effects of obesity and non-insulin-dependent diabetes mellitus on in vivo insulin-stimulated glucose utilization. Diabetes 1984; 33: 622–6.

57. Dall'Aglio E, Chang H, Hollenbeck CB, Mondon CE, Sims C, Reaven GM. *In vivo* and *in vitro* resistance to maximal insulin stimulated glucose disposal in insulin deficiency. Am J Physiol 1985; 249: E312–16.

58. Weir GC, Leahy JL, Bonner-Weir S. Experimental reduction of beta-cell mass. Implications for the pathogenesis of diabetes. Diabetes Metab Rev 1986; 2: 125–61.

59. Ward WK, Beard JC, Porte D. Clinical aspects of islet beta-cell function in non-insulin dependent diabetes mellitus. Diabetes Metab Rev 1986; 2: 297–313.

60. DeFronzo RA. The triumvirate: beta cell, muscle, liver. A collusion responsible for NIDDM. Diabetes 1990; 37: 667–87.

61. DeFronzo RA, Bonadonna RC, Ferrannini E. Pathogenesis of NIDDM. A balanced overview. Diabetes Care 1992; 15: 318–68.

62. Robertson RP. Type II diabetes, glucose 'non-sense', and islet cell desensitization. Diabetes 1989; 38: 1501–5.

63. Savage PJ, Bennion LJ, Flock EV et al. Diet-induced improvement of abnormalities in insulin and glucagon secretion and in insulin receptor binding in diabetes mellitus. J Clin Endocrinol Metab 1979; 48: 999–1007.

64. Stanik S, Marcus R. Insulin secretion improves following dietary control of plasma glucose in severely hyperglycemic obese patients. Metabolism 1980; 29: 346–50.

65. Beck-Nielsen H, Pedersen O, Sorensen NS. Effects of dietary changes on cellular insulin binding and in vivo insulin sensitivity. Metabolism 1980; 29: 482–7.

66. Nagulesparan N, Savage PJ, Bennion LJ, Unger RH, Bennett PH. Diminished effect of caloric restriction on control of hyperglycemia with increasing duration of type II diabetes mellitus. J Clin Endocrinol Metab 1981; 53: 560–68.

67. Henry RR, Scheaffer L, Olefsky JM. Glycemic effects of intensive caloric restriction and isocaloric refeeding in non-insulin-dependent diabetes mellitus. J Clin Endocrinol Metab 1985; 61: 917–25.

68. Henry RR, Wiest-Kent TA, Scheaffer L, Kolterman OG, Olefsky JM. Metabolic consequences of very-low-calorie diet therapy in obese non-insulin-dependent diabetic and non-diabetic subjects. Diabetes 1986; 35: 155–164.

69. Henry RR, Wallace P, Olefsky JM. Effects of weight loss on mechanisms of hyperglycemia in obese non-insulin dependent diabetes mellitus. Diabetes 1986; 35: 990–98.

70. Simonson DC, Ferrannini E, Bevilacqua S et al. Mechanism of improvement in glucose metabolism after chronic glyburide therapy. Diabetes 1984; 33: 838–45.

71. Mandarino LJ, Gerich JE. Prolonged sulfonylurea administration decreases insulin resistance and increases insulin secretion in non-insulin-dependent diabetes mellitus: evidence for improved insulin action at a postreceptor site in hepatic as well as extrahepatic tissues. Diabetes Care 1984; 7 (suppl. 1): 89–99.

72. Kolterman OG, Gray RS, Shapiro G, Scarlett JA, Griffin J, Olefsky JM. The acute and chronic effects

of sulfonylurea therapy in type II diabetes. Diabetes 1984; 33: 346–54.

73. Firth RG, Bell PM, Rizza RA. Effects of tolazamide and exogenous insulin on insulin action in patients with non-insulin-dependent diabetes mellitus. New Engl J Med 1986; 314: 1280–6.

74. Turner RC, McCarthy ST, Holman RR, Harris E. Beta-cell function improved by supplementing basal insulin secretion in mild diabetes. Br Med J 1976; 1: 1252–4.

75. Vague P, Moulin JP. The defective glucose-sensitivity of the β-cell in non-insulin dependent diabetes: improvement after twenty hours of normoglycemia. Metabolism 1982; 31: 139–42.

76. Nankervis A, Proietto J, Aitken P, Harewood M, Alford F. Differential effects of insulin therapy on hepatic and peripheral insulin sensitivity in type 2 (non-insulin-dependent) diabetes. Diabetologia 1982; 23: 320–5.

77. Hidaka H, Nagulesparan M, Klimes I et al. Improvement of insulin secretion but not insulin resistance after short-term control of plasma glucose in obese type II diabetics. J Clin Endocrinol Metab 1982; 54: 217–22.

78. Scarlett JA, Garvey RS, Griffin J, Olefsky JM, Kolterman OG. Insulin treatment reverses the insulin resistance of type II diabetes mellitus. Diabetes Care 1982; 5: 353–63.

79. Scarlett JA, Kolterman OG, Ciaraldi TP, Kao M, Olefsky JM. Insulin treatment reverses the postreceptor defect in adipocyte 3-O-methylglucose transport in type II diabetes mellitus. J Clin Endocrinol Metab 1983; 56: 1195–201.

80. Foley J, Kashiwagi A, Verso MA, Reaven G, Andrews J. Improvement in *in vitro* insulin action after one month of insulin therapy in obese non-insulin-dependent diabetics. J Clin Invest 1983; 72: 1901–9.

81. Andrews WJ, Vasquez B, Nagulesparan M et al. Insulin therapy in obese, non-insulin-dependent diabetes induces improvements in insulin action and secretion that are maintained for two weeks after insulin withdrawal. Diabetes 1984; 33: 634–42.

82. Garvey WT, Olefsky JM, Griffin J, Hamman RF, Kolterman OG. The effect of insulin treatment on insulin secretion and action in type II diabetes mellitus. Diabetes 1985; 34: 222–34.

83. Gormley MJ, Hadden DR, Woods R, Sheridan B, Andrews WJ. One month's insulin treatment of type II diabetes: the early and medium-term effects following insulin withdrawal. Metabolism 1986; 35: 1029–36.

84. Beck-Nielsen H, Richelsen B, Hasling C, Nielsen OH, Heding L, Sorensen NS. Improved *in vivo* insulin effect during continuous subcutaneous insulin infusion in patients with IDDM. Diabetes 1984; 33: 832–7.

85. Simonson DC, Tamborlane WV, Sherwin RS, DeFronzo RA. Improved insulin sensitivity in patients with type I diabetes mellitus after CSII. Diabetes 1985; 34 (suppl. 3): 80–6.

86. Kosaka K, Kuzuya T, Akanuma Y, Hagura R. Increase in insulin response after treatment of overt maturity-onset diabetes is independent of the mode of treatment. Diabetologia 1980; 18: 23–8.

87. Jackson RA, Hawa MI, Jaspan JB et al. Mechanism of metformin action in non-insulin-dependent diabetes. Diabetes 1987; 36: 632–40.

88. DeFronzo RA, Barzilai N, Simonson DC. Mechanism of metformin action in obese and lean non-insulin-dependent diabetic subjects. J Clin Endocrinol Metab 1991; 73: 1294–1301.

89. Johnson AB, Webster JM, Sum CF et al. The impact of metformin therapy on hepatic glucose production and skeletal muscle glycogen synthase activity in overweight type II diabetic patients. Metabolism 1993; 42: 1217–22.

90. Perriello G, Misericordia P, Volpi E et al. Acute antihyperglycemic mechanisms of metformin in NIDDM. Evidence for suppression of lipid oxidation and hepatic glucose production. Diabetes 1994; 43: 920–8.

91. Stumvoll M, Nurjhan N, Perriello G, Dailey G, Gerich JE. Metabolic effects of metformin in non-insulin-dependent diabetes mellitus. New Engl J Med 1995; 333: 550–4.

92. Leahy JL, Weir GC. B-cell dysfunction in hyperglycemic rat models. Recovery of glucose-induced insulin secretion with lowering of the ambient glucose level. Diabetologia 1991; 34: 640–7.

93. Chen C, Thorens B, Bonner-Weir S, Weir GC, Leahy JL. Recovery of glucose-induced insulin secretion in a rat model of NIDDM is not accompanied by return of the B-cell GLUT2 glucose transporter. Diabetes 1992; 41: 1320–7.

94. Rossetti L, Shulman GI, Zawalich W, DeFronzo RA. Effect of chronic hyperglycemia on *in vivo* insulin secretion in partially pancreatectomized rats. J Clin Invest 1987; 80: 1037–44.

95. Rossetti L, Smith D, Shulman GI, Papachristou D, DeFronzo RA. Correction of hyperglycemia with phlorizin normalizes tissue sensitivity to insulin in diabetic rats. J Clin Invest 1987; 79: 1510–15.

96. Rossetti L, Laughlin MR. Correction of chronic hyperglycemia with vanadate but not with phlorizin, normalizes *in vivo* glycogen repletion and *in vitro* glycogen synthase activity in diabetic skeletal muscle. J Clin Invest 1989; 84: 892–9.

97. Eizirik DL, Korbutt GS, Hellerstrom C. Prolonged exposure of human pancreatic islets to high glucose concentrations *in vitro* impairs the β-cell function. J Clin Invest 1992; 90: 1263–8.

98. Davalli AM, Ricordi C, Socci C et al. Abnormal sensitivity to glucose of human islets cultured in a high glucose medium: partial reversibility after an additional culture in a normal glucose medium. J Clin Endocrinol Metab 1991; 72: 202–8.

99. Colella RM, May JM, Bonner-Weir S, Leahy JL, Weir GC. Glucose utilization in islets of hyperglycemic rat models with impaired glucose-induced insulin secretion. Metabolism 1987; 36: 335–7.

100. Hoenig M, MacGregor LC, Matschinsky FM. *In vitro* exhaustion of pancreatic beta cells. Am J Physiol 1986; 250: E502–11.

101. Bolaffi JL, Heldt A, Lewis LD, Grodsky GM. The third phase of *in vitro* insulin secretion—evidence for glucose insensitivity. Diabetes 1986; 35: 370–3.

102. Nagamatsu S, Bolaffi JL, Grodsky GM. Direct effects of glucose on proinsulin synthesis and processing during desensitization. Endocrinology 1987; 120: 1225–31.

103. Bolaffi JL, Bruno L, Heldt A, Grodsky GM. Characteristics of desensitization of insulin secretion in fully *in vitro* systems. Endocrinology 1988; 122: 1801–9.

104. Grodsky GM. Perspectives in diabetes—a new phase of insulin secretion. How will it contribute to our understanding of beta cell function? Diabetes 1989; 38: 673–8.

105. Bedoya FJ, Jeanrenaud B. Evolution of insulin secretory response to glucose by perifused islets from lean (FA/FA) rats chronically infused with glucose. Diabetes 1991; 40: 7–14.

106. Orland MJ, Chyn R, Permutt MA. Modulation of proinsulin messenger RNA after partial pancreatectomy in rats. J Clin Invest 1984; 75: 2047–55.

107. Portha B. Decreased glucose-induced insulin release and biosynthesis by islets of rats with non-insulin-dependent diabetes: effect of tissue culture. Endocrinol 1985; 117: 1735–41.

108. Orland MJ, Permutt MA. Comparative modulations of insulin secretion, pancreatic insulin content, and proinsulin mRNA in rats: effects of 50% pancreatectomy and dexamethasone administration. Diabetes 1991; 40; 181–9.

109. Robertson RP, Zhang HJ, Pyzdrowski KL, Walseth TF. Preservation of insulin mRNA levels and insulin secretion in HIT cells by avoidance of chronic exposure to high glucose concentrations. J Clin Invest 1992; 90: 320–5.

110. Olson LK, Redmon JB, Towle HC, Robertson RP. Chronic exposure of HIT cells to high glucose concentrations paradoxically decreases insulin gene transcription and alters binding of insulin gene regulatory protein. J Clin Invest 1993; 92: 514–19.

111. Meglasson MD, Matschinsky FM. Pancreatic islet glucose metabolism and regulation of insulin secretion. Diabetes Metab Rev 1986; 2: 163–214.

112. Matschinsky FM. Glucokinase as glucose sensor and metabolic generator in pancreatic β-cells and hepatocytes. Diabetes 1990; 39: 647–52.

113. Chen C, Bumbalo LM, Leahy JL. Increased catalytic activity of glucokinase in isolated islets from hyperinsulinemic rats. Diabetes 1994; 43: 684–9.

114. Liang Y, Bonner-Weir S, Wu YJ et al. *In situ* glucose uptake and glucokinase activity of pancreatic islets in diabetic and obese rodents. J Clin Invest 1994; 93: 2473–81.

115. Hosokawa H, Hosokawa YA, Leahy JL. Upregulated hexokinase activity in isolated islets from diabetic 90% pancreatectomy rats. Diabetes 1995; 44: 1328–33.

116. Malaisse WJ, Sener A, Levy J. The stimulus-secretion coupling of glucose-induced insulin release. Fasting-induced adaptation of key glycolytic enzymes in isolated islets. J Biol Chem 1976; 251: 1731–7.

117. Burch PT, Trus MD, Berner DK, Leontire A, Zawalich KC, Matschinsky FM. Adaptation of glycolytic enzymes: glucose use and insulin release in rat pancreatic islets during fasting and refeeding. Diabetes 1981; 30: 923–8.

118. Johnson JH, Ogawa A, Chen L et al. Underexpression of B-cell high K_m glucose transporters in non-insulin-dependent diabetes. Science 1990; 250: 546–9.

119. Milburn JL, Ohneda M, Johnson JH, Unger RH. Beta-cell GLUT-2 loss and non-insulin-dependent diabetes mellitus: current status of the hypothesis. Diabetes Metab Rev 1993; 9: 231–6.

120. Orci L, Unger RH, Ravazzola M et al. Reduced β-cell glucose transporter in new onset diabetic BB rats. J Clin Invest 1990; 86: 1615–22.

121. Thorens B, Weir GC, Leahy JL, Lodish HF, Bonner-Weir S. Reduced expression of the liver/beta-cell glucose transporter isoform in glucose-insensitive pancreatic beta cells of diabetic rats. Proc Natl Acad Sci USA 1990; 87: 6492–6.

122. Chen L, Alam T, Johnson JH, Hughes S, Newgard CB, Unger RH. Regulation of β-cell glucose transporter gene expression. Proc Natl Acad Sci USA 1990; 87: 4088–92.

123. Yasuda K, Yamada Y, Inagaki N et al. Expression of GLUT1 and GLUT2 glucose transporter isoforms in rat islets of Langerhans and their regulation by glucose. Diabetes 1992; 41: 76–81.

124. Tal M, Liang Y, Najafi H, Lodish HF, Matschinsky FM. Expression and function of GLUT-1 and GLUT-2 glucose transporter isoforms in cells of cultured rat pancreatic islets. J Biol Chem 1992; 267: 17241–7.

125. De Vos A, Heimberg H, Quartier E et al. Human and rat beta cells differ in glucose transporter but not in glucokinase gene expression. J Clin Invest 1995; 96: 2489–95.

126. Zawalich WS. Modulation of insulin secretion from beta cells by phosphoinositide-derived second-messenger molecules. Diabetes 1988; 37: 137–41.

127. Rasmussen H, Zawalich KC, Ganesan S, Calle R, Zawalich WS. Physiology and pathophysiology of insulin secretion. Diabetes Care 1990; 13: 655–66.

128. Zawalich WS, Zawalich KC, Shulman GI, Rossetti L. Chronic *in vivo* hyperglycemia impairs phosphoinositide hydrolysis and insulin release in isolated perfused rat islets. Endocrinology 1990; 126: 253–60.

129. Bishop WR, Ganong BR, Bell RM. Attenuation of sn-1,2-diacylglycerol second messengers by diacylglycerol kinase. J Biol Chem 1986; 261: 6993–7000.

130. Bedoya FJ, Jeanrenaud B. Insulin secretory response to secretagogues by perifused islets from chronically glucose-infused rats. Diabetes 1991; 40: 15–19.

131. Sako Y, Grill VE. Coupling of beta-cell desensitization by hyperglycemia to excessive stimulation and circulating insulin in glucose-infused rats. Diabetes 1990; 39: 1580–3.

132. Sako Y, Grill VE. Diazoxide infusion at excess but not at basal hyperglycemia enhances β-cell sensitivity to glucose *in vitro* in neonatally streptozotocin-diabetic rats. Metabolism 1992; 41: 738–43.

133. Giroix MH, Rasschaert J, Bailbe D et al. Impairment of glycerol phosphate shuttle in islets from rats with diabetes induced by neonatal streptozocin. Diabetes 1991; 40: 227–32.

134. Robertson RP. Arachidonic acid metabolite regulation of insulin secretion. Diabetes Metab Rev 1986; 2: 261–96.

135. Robertson RP. Eicosanoids as pluripotential modulators of pancreatic islet function. Diabetes 1988; 37: 367–70.

136. Ward WK, La Cava EC, Paquette TL, Beard JC, Wallum BJ, Porte D. Disproportionate elevation of immunoreactive proinsulin in type II (non-insulin-dependent) diabetes mellitus and in experimental insulin resistance. Diabetologia 1987; 30: 698–702.

137. Yoshioka N, Kuzuya T, Matsuda A, Taniguchi M, Iwamoto Y. Serum proinsulin levels at fasting and after oral glucose load in patients with type II (non-insulin-dependent) diabetes mellitus. Diabetologia 1988; 31: 355–60.

138. Saad MF, Kahn SE, Nelson RG et al. Disproportionately elevated proinsulin in Pima Indians with non-insulin-dependent diabetes mellitus. J Clin Endocrinol Metab 1990; 70: 1247–53.

139. Rhodes CJ, Alarcon C. What beta-cell defect could lead to hyperproinsulinemia in NIDDM? Some clues from recent advances made in understanding the proinsulin-processing mechanism. Diabetes 1994; 43: 511–17.

140. Yoshioka N, Kuzuya T, Matsuda A, Iwamoto Y. Effects of dietary treatment on serum insulin and proinsulin response in newly diagnosed NIDDM. Diabetes 1989; 38: 262–6.

141. Birkeland KI, Torjesen PA, Eriksson J, Vaaler S, Groop L. Hyperproinsulinemia of type II diabetes is not present before the development of hyperglycemia. Diabetes Care 1994; 17: 1307–10.

142. Permutt MA, Kakita K, Malinas P. An *in vivo* analysis of pancreatic protein and insulin biosynthesis in a rat model for non-insulin-dependent diabetes. J Clin Invest 1984; 73: 1344–50.

143. Giddings SJ, Orland MJ, Weir GC, Bonner-Weir S, Permutt MA. Impaired insulin biosynthetic capacity in a rat model for non-insulin-dependent diabetes. Studies with dexamethasone. Diabetes 1985; 34: 235–40.

144. Sako Y, Eizirik D, Grill V. Impact of uncoupling glucose stimulus from secretion on β-cell release and biosynthesis. Am J Physiol 1992; 262: E150–54.

145. Leahy JL. Increased proinsulin/insulin ratio in pancreas extracts of hyperglycemic rats. Diabetes 1993; 42: 22–7.

146. Robertson RP, Olson LK, Zhang HJ. Differentiating glucose toxicity from desensitization: a new message from the insulin gene. Diabetes 1994; 43: 1085–9.

147. Timmers KI, Powell AM, Voyles NR et al. Multiple alterations in insulin responses to glucose in islets from 48-h glucose-infused non-diabetic rats. Diabetes 1990; 39: 1436–44.

148. Himsworth HP, Kerr RB. Insulin-sensitive and insulin-insensitive types of diabetes mellitus. Clin Sci 1942; 4: 120–52.

149. Zierler KL, Rabinowitz D. Roles of insulin and growth hormone based on studies of forearm metabolism in man. Medicine 1963; 42: 385–402.

150. Jackson RA, Perry G, Rogers J, Advani U, Pilkington TR. Relationship between the basal glucose concentration, glucose tolerance and forearm glucose uptake in maturity-onset diabetes. Diabetes 1973; 22: 751–61.

151. Ginsberg H, Kimmerling G, Olefsky JM, Reaven GM. Demonstration of insulin resistance in untreated adult-onset diabetic subjects with fasting hyperglycemia. J Clin Invest 1975; 55: 454–61.

152. DeFronzo RA, Tobin JD, Andres R. Glucose clamp technique: a method for quantifying insulin secretion and resistance. Am J Physiol 1979; 237: E214–23.

153. DeFronzo RA, Simonson D, Ferrannini E. Hepatic and peripheral insulin resistance: a common feature in non-insulin dependent and insulin dependent diabetes. Diabetologia 1982; 23: 313–19.

154. Bergman RS. Toward physiological understanding of glucose tolerance: minimal model approach. Diabetes 1989; 38: 1512–27.

155. DeFronzo RA, Gunnarsson R, Bjorkman O, Olsson M, Wahren J. Effects of insulin on peripheral and splanchnic glucose metabolism in non-insulin-dependent (type II) diabetes mellitus. J Clin Invest 1985; 76: 149–55.

156. Yki-Jarvinen H, Koivisto VA. Natural course of insulin resistance in type I diabetes. New Engl J Med 1986; 315: 224–30.

157. Kobberling J, Tillil H. Empirical risk figures for first-degree relatives of non-insulin-dependent diabetics. In Kobberling J, Tattersall R (eds) The genetics of diabetes mellitus. London: Academic Press, 1982; pp 201–10.

158. Newman B, Selby JV, King MC, Slemenda C, Fabisitz R, Friedman GDL. Concordance for type 2 (non-insulin-dependent) diabetes mellitus in male twins. Diabetologia 1987; 30: 763–8.

159. Barnett AH, Eff C, Leslie RD, Pyke DA. Diabetes in identical twins: a study of 200 pairs. Diabetologia 1981; 20: 87–93.

160. Yki-Jarvinen H, Taskinen MR, Kiviluoto T et al. Site of insulin resistance in type 1 diabetes: insulin-mediated glucose disposal *in vivo* in relation to insulin binding and action in adipocytes *in vitro*. J Clin Endocrinol Metab 1984; 59: 1183–92.

161. Vuorinen-Markkola H, Koivisto VA, Yki-Jarvinen H. Mechanisms of hyperglycemia-induced insulin resistance in whole body and skeletal muscle of type 1 diabetic patients. Diabetes 1992; 41: 571–80.

162. Bevilacqua S, Barrett EJ, Smith D et al. Hepatic and peripheral insulin resistance following streptozotocin-induced insulin deficiency in the dog. Metabolism 1985; 34: 817–25.

163. Reaven GM, Sageman WS, Swenson RS. Development of insulin resistance in normal dogs following alloxan-induced insulin deficiency. Diabetologia 1977; 13: 459–62.

164. DeFronzo RA, Simonson DC, DelPrato S. Glucose resistance in diabetes: evidence for impaired insulin-independent glucose uptake. Diabetes 1985; 34 (suppl. 1): 87A.

165. Haist RE, Campbell J, Best CH. The prevention of diabetes. New Engl J Med 1940; 223: 607–15.

166. Baldwin S, Leinhard G. Glucose transport across plasma membranes: facilitated diffusion system. Trends Biochem Sci 1981; 6: 208–11.

167. Garvey WT, Maianu L, Hancock JA, Golichowski AM, Baron A. Gene expression of GLUT4 in skeletal muscle from insulin-resistant patients with obesity, IGT, GDM, and NIDDM. Diabetes 1992; 41: 465–75.

168. Cherrington AD, Williams P, Harris M. Relationship between the plasma glucose level and glucose uptake in the conscious dog. Metabolism 1978; 27: 787–91.

169. Yki-Jarvinen H, Sahlin K, Ren JM, Koivisto VA. Localization of rate-limiting defect for glucose disposal in skeletal muscle of insulin-resistant type I diabetic patients. Diabetes 1990; 39: 157–67.

170. Henry RR, Gumbiner B, Flynn T, Thorburn AW. Metabolic effects of hyperglycemia and hyperinsulinemia on fate of intracellular glucose in NIDDM. Diabetes 1990; 39: 149–56.

171. Yki-Jarvinen H, Helve E, Koivisto VA. Hyperglycemia decreases glucose uptake in type I diabetes. Diabetes 1987; 36: 892–6.

172. DelPrato S, Leonetti F, Simonson DC, Sheehan P, Matsuda M, DeFronzo RA. Effect of sustained physiologic hyperinsulinemia and hyperglycemia on

insulin secretion and insulin sensitivity in man. Diabetologia 1994; 37: 1025–35.

173. Gjedde A, Crone C. Blood–brain glucose transfer: repression in chronic hyperglycemia. Science 1981; 214: 456–7.

174. McCall AL, Gould JB, Ruderman NB. Diabetes-induced alterations of glucose metabolism in rat cerebral microvessels. Am J Physiol 1984; 247: E462–7.

175. McCall AL, Fixman LB, Fleming N, Tornheim K, Chick W, Ruderman NB. Chronic hypoglycemia increases brain glucose transport. Am J Physiol 1986; 251: E442–7.

176. Sacca L, Hendler R, Sherwin RS. Hyperglycemia inhibits glucose production in man independent of changes in glucoregulatory hormones. J Clin Endocrinol Metab 1978; 47: 1160–7.

177. DeFronzo RA, Ferrannini E, Hendler R, Felig P, Wahren J. Regulation of splanchnic and peripheral glucose uptake by insulin and hyperglycemia in man. Diabetes 1983; 32: 35–45.

178. Simonson DC, Tamborlane WV, DeFronzo RA, Sherwin RS. Intensive insulin therapy reduces counter-regulatory hormone responses to hypoglycemia in patients with type I diabetes. Ann Intern Med 1985; 103: 184–90.

179. Amiel SA, Tamborlane WV, Simonson DC, Sherwin RS. Defective glucose counterregulation after strict glycemic control of insulin-dependent diabetes mellitus. New Engl J Med 1987; 316: 1376–83.

180. Widom B, Simonson DC. Glycemic control and neuropsychologic function during hypoglycemia in patients with insulin-dependent diabetes mellitus. Ann Intern Med 1990; 112: 904–12.

181. Kinsley BT, Widom B, Simonson DC. Differential regulation of counter-regulatory hormone secretion and symptoms during hypoglycemia in IDDM. Effect of glycemic control. Diabetes Care 1995; 18: 17–26.

182. Weinger K, Jacobson AM, Draelos MT, Finkelstein DM, Simonson DC. Blood glucose estimation and symptoms during hyperglycemia and hypoglycemia in patients with insulin-dependent diabetes mellitus. Am J Med 1995; 98: 22–31.

183. Boyle PJ, Kempers SF, O'Connor AM, Nagy RJ. Brain glucose uptake and unawareness of hypoglycemia in patients with insulin-dependent diabetes mellitus. New Engl J Med 1995; 333: 1726–31.

184. Gutniak M, Blomqvist G, Widen L, Stone-Elander S, Hamberger B, Grill V. D-[U-^{11}C]glucose uptake and metabolism in the brain of insulin-dependent diabetic subjects. Am J Physiol 1990; 258: E805–12.

185. Blondel O, Bailbe D, Portha B. Insulin resistance in rats with non-insulin-dependent diabetes induced by neonatal (5 days) streptozotocin: evidence for reversal following phlorizin treatment. Metabolism 1990; 39: 787–93.

186. DeFronzo RA, Jacot E, Jequier E, Maeder E, Wahren J, Felber JP. The effect of insulin on the disposal of intravenous glucose: results from indirect calorimetry and hepatic and femoral venous catheterization. Diabetes 1981; 30: 1000–1007.

187. Garvey WT, Huecksteadt TP, Matthaei S, Olefsky JM. Role of glucose transporters in the cellular insulin resistance of type II non-insulin-dependent diabetes mellitus. J Clin Invest 1988; 81: 1528–36.

188. Garvey WT, Kolterman OG. Correlation of *in vivo* and *in vitro* actions of insulin in obesity and non-insulin dependent diabetes mellitus: role of the glucose transport system. Diabet Metab Rev 1988; 4: 543–69.

189. Katz A, Nyomba BL, Bogardus C. No accumulation of glucose in skeletal muscle during euglycemic hyperinsulinemia. Am J Physiol 1988; 255: E942–5.

190. Klip A, Marette A. Acute and chronic signals controlling glucose transport in skeletal muscle. J Cell Biochem 1992; 48: 51–60.

191. Kahn BB, Shulman GI, DeFronzo RA, Cushman SW, Rossetti L. Normalization of blood glucose in diabetic rats with phlorizin treatment reverses insulin resistant glucose transport in adipose cells without restoring glucose transporter gene expression. J Clin Invest 1990; 87: 561–70.

192. Sasson S, Cerasi E. Substrate regulation of the glucose transport system in rat skeletal muscle. J Biol Chem 1986; 261: 16827–33.

193. Sasson S, Edelson D, Cerasi E. *In vitro* autoregulation of glucose utilization in rat soleus muscle. Diabetes 1987; 36: 1041–6.

194. Garvey WT, Olefsky JM, Matthaei S, Marshall S. Glucose and insulin co-regulate the glucose transport system in primary cultured adipocytes. J Biol Chem 1987; 262: 189–97.

195. Van Putten JPM, Krans HMJ. Glucose as a regulator of insulin-sensitive hexose uptake in 3T3 adipocytes. J Biol Chem 1985; 260: 7996–8001.

196. Marshall S. Kinetics of insulin action on protein synthesis in isolated adipocytes. J Biol Chem 1989; 264: 2029–36.

197. Traxinger RR, Marshall S. Recovery of maximal insulin responsiveness and insulin sensitivity after induction of insulin resistance in primary cultured adipocytes. J Biol Chem 1989; 264: 8156–63.

198. Richter EA, Hansen BF, Hansen SA. Glucose-induced insulin resistance of skeletal muscle glucose transport and uptake. Biochem J 1988; 252: 733–7.

199. Whitesell RR, Regen DM, Pelletier D, Abumrad NA. Evidence that downregulation of hexose transport limits intracellular glucose in 3T3-L1 fibroblasts. Diabetes 1990; 39: 1228–34.

200. Kletzien RF, Perdue JF. Induction of sugar transport in chick embryo fibroblasts by hexose starvation: evidence for transcriptional regulation of transport. J Biol Chem 1985; 250: 593–600.

201. Ullrey D, Gammon BMT, Kalckar HM. Uptake patterns and transport enhancements in cultures of hamster cells deprived of carbohydrates. Arch Biochem Biophys 1975; 167: 410–16.

202. Ullrey DB, Kalckar HM. The nature of regulation of hexose transport in cultured mammalian fibroblasts: aerobic 'repressive' control by D-glucosamine. Arch Biochem Biophys 1981; 209: 168–74.

203. Haspel C, Wilk EW, Birnbaum MJ, Cushman SW, Rosen OM. Glucose deprivation and hexose transporter polypeptides of murine fibroblasts. J Biol Chem 1986; 261: 6778–89.

204. Lemmon SK, Sens DA, Buse MG. Insulin stimulation of glucose transport and metabolism in a human Wilms' tumor-derived myoblast-like cell line: modulation of hormone effects by glucose deprivation. J Cell Physiol 1985; 125: 456–64.

205. Klip A, Paquet MR. Glucose transport and glucose transporters in muscle and their metabolic regulation. Diabetes Care 1990; 13: 228–43.

206. Germinario RI, Roekman H, Oliveira M, Manuel S, Taylor M. Regulation of sugar transport in cultured diploid human skin fibroblasts. J Cell Physiol 1982; 112: 367–72.

207. Yamada K, Tillotson LG, Isselbacher KJ. Regulation of hexose carriers in chicken embryo fibroblasts. Effect of glucose starvation and role of protein synthesis. J Biol Chem 1983; 258: 9786–92.

208. Tillotson LG, Yamada K, Isselbacher KJ. Regulation of hexose transporters of chicken embryo fibroblasts during glucose starvation. Fed Proc 1984; 43: 2262–4.

209. Walker PS, Ramlal R, Donovan JA et al. Insulin and glucose-dependent regulation of the glucose transport system in the rat L6 skeletal muscle cell line. J Biol Chem 1989; 264: 6587–95.

210. Walker PS, Ramlal R, Sarabia V et al. Glucose transport activity in L6 muscle cells is regulated by the coordinate control of subcellular glucose transporter distribution, biosynthesis, and mRNA transcription. J Biol Chem 1990; 265: 1516–23.

211. Wertheimer E, Sasson S, Cerasi E. Regulation of hexose transport in myocytes by glucose: possible sites of interaction. J Cell Physiol 1990; 143: 330–6.

212. Tordjman KM, Leingang KA, Mueckler M. Differential regulation of the HepG2 and adipocyte/muscle glucose transporters in 3T3L1 adipocytes. Effect of chronic glucose deprivation. Biochem J 1990; 271: 201–7.

213. Sarabia V, Ramlal T, Klip A. Glucose uptake in human and animal muscle cells in culture. Biochem Cell Biol 1990; 68: 536–42.

214. Traxinger RR, Marshall S. Role of amino acids in modulating glucose-induced desensitization of the glucose transport system. J Biol Chem 1989; 264: 20910–16.

215. Traxinger RR, Marshall S. Glucose regulation of insulin receptor affinity in primary cultured adipocytes. J Biol Chem 1990; 265: 18879–83.

216. McCall AL, Millington WR, Wurtman RJ. Metabolic fuel and amino acid transport into the brain in experimental diabetes mellitus. Proc Natl Acad Sci USA 1982; 79: 5406–10.

217. Matthaei S, Horuk R, Olefsky JM. Blood–brain glucose transfer in diabetes mellitus. Diabetes 1986; 35: 1181–4.

218. Pelligrino DA, Lipa MD, Albrecht RF. Regional blood–brain glucose transfer and glucose utilization in chronically hyperglycemic, diabetic rats following acute glycemic normalization. J Cereb Blood Flow Metab 1990; 10: 774–80.

219. Pardridge WM, Triguero D, Farrell CR. Downregulation of blood–brain barrier glucose transporter in experimental diabetes. Diabetes 1990; 39: 1040–4.

220. Kern M, Wells JA, Stephens JM et al. Insulin responsiveness in skeletal muscle is determined by glucose transporter (GLUT4) protein level. Biochem J 1990; 270: 397–400.

221. Koranyi L, Bourey RE, Vuorinen-Markkola H et al. Level of skeletal muscle glucose transporter protein correlates with insulin-stimulated whole body glucose disposal in man. Diabetologia 1991; 34: 763–5.

222. Wertheimer E, Sasson S, Cerasi E, Ben-Neruah Y. The ubiquitous glucose transporter GLUT1 belongs to the glucose-regulated protein family of stress-inducible proteins. Proc Natl Acad Sci USA 1991; 88: 2525–9.

223. Kahn BB, Charron MI, Lodish HF, Cushman SW, Flier JS. Differential regulation of two glucose transporters in adipose cells from diabetic and insulin-treated diabetic rats. J Clin Invest 1989; 84: 404–11.

224. Berger J, Biswas C, Vicario PP, Strout HV, Saperstein R, Pilch PF. Decreased expression of the insulin-responsive glucose transporter in diabetes and fasting. Nature 1989; 340: 70–72.

225. Sivitz WI, DeSautel SL, Kayano T, Bell GI, Pessin JAE. Regulation of glucose transporter messenger RNA in insulin-deficient states. Nature 1989; 340: 72–4.

226. Garvey WT, Huecksteadt TP, Birnbaum MI. Pretranslational suppression of an insulin-responsive glucose transporter in rats with diabetes mellitus. Science 245: 60–3.

227. Bourey RE, Koranyi L, James DE, Mueckler M, Permutt MA. Effects of altered glucose homeostasis on glucose transporter expression in skeletal muscle of the rat. J Clin Invest 1990; 86: 542–7.

228. Kahn BB, Rossetti L, Lodish HF, Charron MJ. Decreased *in vivo* glucose uptake but normal expression of GLUT1 and GLUT4 in skeletal muscle of diabetic rats. J Clin Invest 1991; 87: 2197–206.

229. Yki-Jarvinen H, Vuorinen-Markkola H, Koranyi L et al. Defect in insulin action on expression of the muscle/adipose tissue glucose transporter gene in skeletal muscle of type 1 diabetic patients. J Clin Endocrinol Metab 1992; 75: 795–9.

230. Pedersen O, Bak JF, Andersen PH et al. Evidence against altered expression of GLUT1 or GLUT4 in skeletal muscle of patients with obesity or NIDDM. Diabetes 1990; 39: 865–70.

231. Eriksson J, Koranyi L, Bourey R et al. Insulin resistance in type 2 (non-insulin-dependent) diabetic patients and their relatives is not associated with a defect in the expression of the insulin-responsive glucose transporter (GLUT4) gene in human skeletal muscle. Diabetologia 1992; 35: 143–7.

232. Traxinger RR, Marshall S. Coordinated regulation of glutamine:fructose-6-phosphate amidotransferase activity by insulin, glucose, and glutamine. Role of hexosamine biosynthesis in enzyme regulation. J Biol Chem 1991; 266: 10148–54.

233. Marshall S, Bacote V, Traxinger RR. Discovery of a metabolic pathway mediating glucose-induced desensitization of the glucose transport system. Role of hexosamine biosynthesis in the induction of insulin resistance. J Biol Chem 1991; 266: 4706–12.

234. Marshall S, Bacote V, Traxinger RR. Complete inhibition of glucose-induced desensitization of the glucose transport system by inhibitors of mRNA synthesis. Evidence for rapid turnover of glutamine:fructose-6-phosphate amidotransferase. J Biol Chem 1991; 266: 10155–61.

235. Marshall S, Garvey WT, Traxinger RR. New insights into the metabolic regulation of insulin action and insulin resistance: role of glucose and amino acids. FASEB J 1991; 5: 3031–6.

236. Traxinger RR, Marshall S. Insulin regulation of pyruvate kinase activity in isolated adipocytes. Crucial role of glucose and the hexosamine biosynthesis pathway in the expression of insulin action. J Biol Chem 1992; 267: 9718–23.

237. Zawalich WS, Zawalich KC. Glucosamine-induced desensitization of beta-cell responses: possible

involvement of impaired information flow in the phosphoinositide cycle. Endocrinology 1992; 130: 3135–42.

238. Robinson KA, Sens DA, Buse MG. Pre-exposure to glucosamine induces insulin resistance of glucose transport and glycogen synthesis in isolated rat skeletal muscles. Study of mechanisms in muscle and rat-1 fibroblasts overexpressing the human insulin receptor. Diabetes 1993; 42: 1333–46.

239. Crook ED, Daniels MC, Smith TM, McClain DA. Regulation of insulin-stimulated glycogen synthase activity by overexpression of glutamine : fructose-6-phosphate amidotransferase in rat-1 fibroblasts. Diabetes 1993; 42: 1289–96.

240. Giaccari A, Morviducci L, Zorretta D et al. *In vivo* effects of glucosamine on insulin secretion and insulin sensitivity in the rat: possible relevance to the maladaptive responses to chronic hyperglycemia. Diabetologia 1995; 38: 518–24.

241. Crook ED, Zhou J, Daniels M, Neigih JL, McClain DA. Regulation of glycogen synthase by glucose, glucosamine, and glutamine : fructose-6-phosphate amidotransferase. Diabetes 1995; 44: 314–20.

242. Bilan PJ, Klip A. Glycation of the human erythrocyte glucose transporter *in vitro* and its functional consequences. Biochem J 1990; 268: 661–7.

243. Harik SI, Behmand RA, Arafah BM. Chronic hyperglycemia increases the density of glucose transporters in human erythrocyte membranes. J Clin Endocrinol Metab 1991; 72: 814–18.

244. Laakso M, Uusitupa M, Takala J, Majander H, Reijonen T, Penttila I. Effects of hypocaloric diet and insulin therapy on metabolic control and mechanisms of hyperglycemia in obese non-insulin-dependent diabetic subjects. Metabolism 1988; 37: 1092–1100.

245. Zawadski JK, Bogardus C, Foley JE. Insulin action in obese non-insulin-dependent diabetics and in their isolated adipocytes before and after weight loss. Diabetes 1987; 36: 227–36.

246. Walshe K, Andrews WJ, Sheridan B, Woods R, Hadden DR. Three months energy restricted diet does not induce peripheral insulin resistance in new diagnosed non-insulin dependent diabetics. Horm Metab Res 1987; 19: 197–200.

247. Ma A, Kamp M, Bird D, Howlett V, Cameron DP. The effects of long-term gliclazide administration on insulin secretion and insulin sensitivity. Aust NZ J Med 1989; 19: 44–9.

248. Groop L, Schalin C, Franssila-Kallunki A, Widen E, Ekstrand A, Eriksson J. Characteristics of non-insulin-dependent diabetic patients with secondary failure to oral antidiabetic therapy. Am J Med 1989; 87: 183–90.

249. Castillo M, Scheen AJ, Paolisso G, Lefebvre PJ. The addition of glipizide to insulin therapy in type II diabetic patients with secondary failure to sulfonylureas is useful only in the presence of a significant residual insulin secretion. Acta Endocrinol 1987; 116: 364–72.

250. Yki-Jarvinen H, Nikkila E, Eero H, Taskinen MR. Clinical benefits and mechanisms of a sustained response to intermittent insulin therapy in type 2 diabetic patients with secondary drug failure. Am J Med 1988; 84: 185–92.

251. Yki-Jarvinen H, Koivisto VA. Continuous subcutaneous insulin infusion therapy decreases insulin resistance in type I diabetes. J Clin Endocrinol Metab 1984; 58: 659–66.

252. Yki-Jarvinen H, Koivisto VA. Insulin sensitivity in newly diagnosed type I diabetics after ketoacidosis and after three months of insulin therapy. J Clin Endocrinol Metab 1984; 59: 371–8.

253. Lager I, Lonnroth P, Von Schenck H, Smith U. Reversal of insulin resistance in type I diabetes after treatment with continuous subcutaneous insulin infusion. Br Med J 1983; 287: 1001–4.

254. Kruszynska YT, Petranyi G, Home PD, Taylor R, Alberti KGMM. Muscle enzyme activity and insulin sensitivity in type I (insulin-dependent) diabetes mellitus. Diabetologia 1986; 29: 699–705.

255. Gray RS, Cowan P, Duncan LJP, Clarke BF. Reversal of insulin resistance in type I diabetes following initiation of insulin treatment. Diabet Med 1986; 3: 18–23.

256. Garvey WT, Olefsky JM, Marshall S. Insulin receptor down-regulation is linked to an insulin-induced postreceptor defect in the glucose transport system in rat adipocytes. J Clin Invest 1985; 76: 22–30.

257. Rizza RA, Mandarino LJ, Genest J, Baker BA, Gerich JE. Production of insulin resistance by hyperinsulinemia in man. Diabetologia 1985; 28: 70–5.

258. Lillioja S, Mott DM, Zawadski JK et al. *In vivo* insulin action is a familial characteristic in non-diabetic Pima Indians. Diabetes 1987; 36: 1329–35.

259. Lillioja S, Bogardus C. Obesity and insulin resistance: lessons learned from the Pima Indians. Diabetes Metab Rev 1988; 4: 515–40.

260. Eriksson J, Franssila-Kallunki A, Edstrand A et al. Early metabolic defects in persons at increased risk of non-insulin-dependent diabetes mellitus. New Engl J Med 1989; 321: 337–43.

261. Gulli G, Haffner S, Ferrannini E, DeFronzo RA. What is inherited in NIDDM? Diabetes 1990; 39 (suppl. 1): 116A.

262. Samanta A, Burden AC, Jones GR, Clarkson L. The effect of short-term intensive insulin therapy in non-insulin-dependent diabetics who had failed on sulphonylurea therapy. Diabetes Res 1986; 3: 269–71.

263. Hollenbeck CB, Reaven GM. Treatment of patients with non-insulin-dependent diabetes mellitus: diabetic control and insulin secretion and action after different treatment modalities. Diabet Med 1987; 4: 311–16.

264. DeFronzo RA, Ferrannini E, Simonson DC. Fasting hyperglycemia in non-insulin dependent diabetes mellitus: contributions of excessive hepatic glucose production and impaired tissue glucose uptake. Metabolism 1989; 38: 387–95.

265. Golay A, Felber JP, Jequier E, DeFronzo RA, Ferrannini E. Metabolic basis of obesity and non-insulin dependent diabetes mellitus. Diabetes Metab Rev 1988; 4: 727–47.

266. Consoli A, Kennedy F, Miles J, Gerich J. Determination of Krebs cycle metabolic carbon exchange *in vivo* and its use to estimate the individual contributions of gluconeogenesis and glycogenolysis to overall glucose output in man. J Clin Invest 1987; 80: 1303–10.

267. Waldhausl W, Bratusch-Marrain P, Gasic S, Korn A, Nowatony P. Insulin production rate, hepatic insulin retention, and splanchnic carbohydrate metabolism after oral glucose ingestion in hyperinsulinemic

type 2 (non-insulin dependent) diabetes mellitus. Diabetologia 1982; 23: 6–15.

268. DeFronzo RA, Ferrannini E. Regulation of hepatic glucose metabolism in humans. Diabetes Metab Rev 1987; 3: 415–59.

269. Koivisto V, DeFronzo RA. Physical training and insulin sensitivity. Diabetes Metab Rev 1986; 1: 445–81.

270. Koivisto V, DeFronzo RA. Exercise in the treatment of type II diabetes. Acta Endocrinol 1984; (suppl. 262): 107–11.

271. Schneider SH, Vitug A, Ruderman N. Atherosclerosis and physical activity. Diabetes Metab Rev 1986; 1: 513–53.

272. Wallberg-Henriksson H, Gunnarson R, Henriksson J et al. Increased peripheral insulin sensitivity and muscle mitochondrial enzymes but unchanged blood glucose control in type I diabetes after physical training. Diabetes 1982; 31: 1044–50.

273. Bogardus C, Ravussin E, Robbins DC, Wolfe RR, Horton ES, Sims EAH. Effects of physical training and diet therapy on carbohydrate metabolism in patients with glucose intolerance and non-insulin dependent diabetes mellitus. Diabetes 1984; 33: 311–18.

274. Lillioja S, Mott DM, Howard BV et al. Impaired glucose tolerance as a disorder of insulin action —longitudinal and cross-sectional studies in Pima Indians. New Engl J Med 1988; 318: 1217–25.

275. Reaven GM, Hollenbeck CB, Chen Y-DI. Relationship between glucose tolerance, insulin secretion, and insulin action in non-obese individuals with varying degrees of glucose tolerance. Diabetologia 1989; 32: 52–5.

276. Zimmet P, Whitehouse S, Kiss J. Ethnic variability in the plasma insulin response to oral glucose in Polynesian and Micronesian subjects. Diabetes 1979; 28: 624–8.

277. Sicree RA, Zimmet PZ, King HOM, Coventry JO. Plasma insulin response among Nauruans: prediction of deterioration in glucose tolerance over 6 yr. Diabetes 1987; 36: 179–86.

278. Zimmet P, Whitehouse S. Bimodality of fasting and two-hour glucose tolerance distributions in a Micronesian population. Diabetes 1978; 27: 793–800.

279. Martin FIR, Wyatt GB, Griew AR, Haurahelia M, Higginbothan L. Diabetes mellitus in urban and rural communities in Papua New Guinea: studies of prevalence and plasma insulin. Diabetologia 1980; 18: 369–74.

280. Reaven GM, Miller RG. An attempt to define the nature of chemical diabetes using a multidimensional analysis. Diabetologia 1979; 16: 17–24.

281. Zimmet P, Whitehouse S, Alford F, Chisholm D. The relationship of insulin response to a glucose stimulus over a wide range of glucose tolerance. Diabetologia 1978; 15: 23–7.

282. Savage PJ, Dippe SE, Bennet PH et al. Hyperinsulinemia and hypoinsulinemia: insulin responses to oral carbohydrate over a wide spectrum of glucose tolerance. Diabetes 1975; 24: 362–8.

283. Welborn TA, Stenhouse NS, Johnson CJ. Factors determining serum insulin response in a population sample. Diabetologia 1969; 5: 263–6.

284. Reaven G, Miller R. Study of the relationship between glucose and insulin responses to an oral glucose load in man. Diabetes 1968; 17: 560–69.

285. Bogardus C, Lillioja S, Howard BV, Reaven G, Mott D. Relationships between insulin secretion, insulin action and fasting plasma glucose concentration in non-diabetic and non-insulin dependent diabetic subjects. J Clin Invest 1984; 74: 1238–46.

286. Haffner SM, Stern MP, Hazuda HP, Mitchell BD, Patterson JK. Increased insulin concentrations in non-diabetic offspring of diabetic parents. New Engl J Med 1988; 319: 1297–1301.

287. Saad MF, Knowler C, Pettit J, Nelson G, Mott M, Bennett PH. Sequential changes in serum insulin concentration during development of non-insulin-dependent diabetes. Lancet 1989; 1: 1356–9.

288. Eisenbarth GS, Connelly J, Soeldner JS. The 'natural' history of type I diabetes. Diabetes Metab Rev 1987; 3: 873–91.

289. Sims EAH, Danforth E, Horton ES, Bray GA, Glennon JA, Salans LB. Endocrine and metabolic effects of experimental obesity in man. Recent Prog Horm Res 1973; 29: 457–96.

290. Felber JP, Jallut D, Golay A, Munger R, Francarolo P, Jequier E. Obesity to diabetes. A longitudinal study of glucose metabolism in man. Diabetes 1989; 38 (suppl. 1): 221A.

291. Hansen BC, Bodkin NL. Heterogeneity of insulin responses: phases leading to type 2 (non-insulin-dependent) diabetes mellitus in the rhesus monkey. Diabetologia 1986; 29: 713–19.

292. Bodkin NL, Metzger BL, Hansen BC. Hepatic glucose production and insulin sensitivity preceding diabetes in monkeys. Am J Physiol 1989; 256: E676–81.

293. Marble A. Incidence and causes of secondary failure in treatment with tolbutamide: experience with 2500 patients treated up to 5 years. JAMA 1962; 181: 1–4.

294. Haupt E, Laube F, Loy H, Schoffing K. Secondary failures in modern therapy of diabetes mellitus with blood glucose lowering sulfonamides. Med Klin 1977; 72: 1529–36.

295. Groop L, Schalin C, Franssila-Kalolunki A, Widen E, Ekstrand A, Eriksson J. Characteristics of non-insulin dependent diabetic patients with secondary failure to oral antidiabetic therapy. Am J Med 1989; 87: 183–90.

296. Karam JH, Sanz N, Salamon E, Nolte MS. Selective unresponsiveness of pancreatic beta cells to acute sulfonylurea stimulation during sulfonylurea therapy in NIDDM. Diabetes 1986; 35: 1314–20.

297. Madsbad S. Prevalence of residual B-cell function and its metabolic consequences in type 1 (insulin-dependent) diabetes. Diabetologia 1983; 24: 141–7.

298. Ganda OP, Srikanta S, Brink SJ et al. Differential sensitivity to beta cell secretagogues in 'early' type I diabetes mellitus. Diabetes 1984; 33: 516–21.

33

Glycation of Macromolecules

Michael Brownlee

Albert Einstein College of Medicine, New York, USA

The primary causal factor responsible for the development of most diabetic complications is prolonged exposure to hyperglycemia [1–4, 90] (Figure 1). The pathologic and clinical consequences of tissue exposure to hyperglycemia reflect both acute, insulin-reversible abnormalities and chronic, irreversible abnormalities [2, 5]. Among the reversible abnormalities are increased polyol pathway and protein kinase C activity in target tissue cells, elevated hydrostatic pressure in the microcirculation, and greater formation of early glycosylation products on matrix, cellular and plasma proteins [5–10]. These insulin-reversible abnormalities are associated with the intermittent increases in vascular permeability and protein leakage that characterize early diabetes, as well as with early increases in extracellular matrix production [2, 11, 12]. Chronic, irreversible abnormalities unaffected by normalization of blood glucose levels primarily involve long-lived molecules such as extracellular matrix components and chromosomal DNA. Relevant examples *in vitro* of hyperglycemia-induced irreversible abnormalities include disordered three-dimensional structure of both basement membrane and collagen [13, 14], impaired matrix-binding of heparan sulfate proteoglycan [15, 16], and increased rates of genetic mutation [17, 18].

The work reviewed in this chapter suggests that hyperglycemia-accelerated formation of non-enzymatic advanced glycosylation end-products (AGE) on tissue macromolecules is the common underlying biochemical basis for deposition of extravasated plasma proteins, expansion of extracellular matrix and abnormal growth of cells. Together, the cumulative effect of these shared pathologic processes is progressive narrowing of diabetic vascular lumina, with inadequate perfusion of critical segments of target organs.

CHEMICAL PROPERTIES OF ADVANCED GLYCOSYLATION PRODUCTS

Advanced products of non-enzymatic glycosylation play a critical part in the evolution of diabetic complications because of their characteristic chemical properties. As discussed below, these slowly formed glucose-derived compounds are chemically irreversible, and thus accumulate continuously with time. The degree of this accumulation in patients' dermal collagen has been shown to correlate with the severity of diabetic retinopathy [19]. These products participate in the critical process of glucose-derived crosslink formation [20–22], and by so doing alter the structure and function of the vascular wall. In addition, these products are recognized by specific cell surface receptors, an event that stimulates local cytokine growth factor production. Finally, formation of these products on DNA may result in altered structure and function of genetic elements.

The formation of advanced glycosylation products begins with the formation of the more familiar early glycosylation products (Figure 2), when glucose attaches to amino groups to form unstable Schiff base adducts. Levels of the labile Schiff base increase rapidly, and equilibrium is reached after several hours [23]. Ambient glucose concentration over that brief period determines the steady state level of Schiff base adducts.

International Textbook of Diabetes Mellitus, Second Edition. Edited by K.G.M.M. Alberti, P. Zimmet, R.A. DeFronzo, and H. Keen (Honorary)
© 1997 John Wiley & Sons Ltd

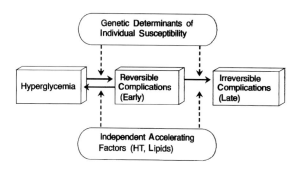

Figure 1 Schematic representation of the relationship between hyperglycemia and secondary risk factors in the evolution of reversible and irreversible diabetic complications. HT, hypertension

Once formed, Schiff base adducts of glucose and protein amino groups undergo a slow chemical rearrangement over a period of weeks to form a more stable (but still chemically reversible) sugar–protein adduct, the Amadori product [24, 25].

Equilibrium of Amadori glycosylation products is reached over a period of approximately 28 days. Thus, even on very long-lived proteins, the total amount of Amadori product is only proportional to the integrated glucose concentration of the preceding 4 weeks. After the relatively brief period of time necessary to attain equilibrium, measured levels of Amadori products reach a constant steady state value which does not increase as a function of time beyond that point.

As these early glycosylation products increase when blood glucose is high, return towards normal when blood glucose levels are optimized, and do not continue to accumulate on stable tissue molecules over years of chronic diabetes, it is not surprising that their randomly measured concentration does not correlate with either the presence or severity of diabetic retinopathy

[26]. However, intermittent increases in Schiff base and Amadori product concentration can rapidly alter the function of some modified molecules, and thereby can contribute to some of the acute, reversible abnormalities induced by hyperglycemia.

Advanced glycosylation products form on molecules having low physiologic turnover rates, such as matrix protein components and DNA in terminally differentiated cells. Here, Amadori products slowly undergo an extensive series of dehydrations, oxidations, and rearrangements to form complex AGEs from reactive dicarbonyl sugars such as 3-deoxyglucosone and methylglyoxal [22]. These are frequently pigmented or fluorescent, and—most importantly for diabetic complications—they participate in glucose-derived crosslink formation [20, 21]. In contrast to the Amadori product, which is in equilibrium with glucose, AGEs are irreversibly attached to proteins. Consequently, the level of AGEs in diabetic tissue does not return to normal when hyperglycemia is corrected, but instead these products continue to accumulate over the lifetime of the vessel wall [27].

Specific chemical characterization of AGE proteins has been difficult, as Amadori products can theoretically undergo a large number of potential rearrangements, and many AGEs may be unstable to hydrolysis. Studies with antibodies to AGEs suggest that immunologically similar structures form from the incubation of different sugars with different proteins [28–31]. Alternatively, compounds such as 3-deoxyglucosone can be reduced to more inactive metabolites such as 3-deoxyfructose by the activity of specific reductase enzymes. The nature and efficiency of such enzymes could be an important determinant of the amount of AGEs that form at a given level of hyperglycemia. The kinetics of AGE formation with respect to glucose

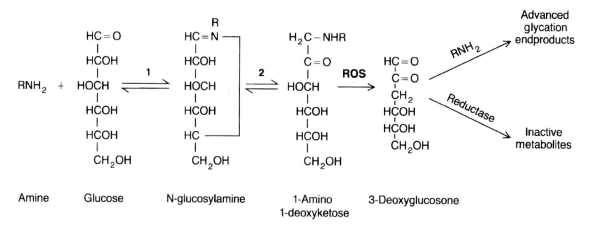

Figure 2 Formation of advanced glycation endproducts (AGEs) from glucose. Reversible early products give rise to irreversible advanced products through generation of highly reactive carbonyl compounds such as 3-deoxyglucosone. AGE formation *in vivo* may be retarded by the action of reductase enzymes. ROS, reactive oxygen species (Modified from reference 110, with permission of American Diabetes Association.)

concentration have not been rigorously characterized, but preliminary experiments suggest that AGE formation over time is exponential. Since the rate of AGE formation appears to be nearly second order with respect to the ambient glucose concentration (i.e. it is proportional to [glucose concentration]^2), even modest elevations of blood glucose could result in significant AGE accumulation.

Non-enzymatic glycosylation products are also formed by biologically relevant non-glucose reducing sugars, including most of the glycolytic intermediates that are elevated in diabetic target tissues [36]. As nearly all of these sugars are much more reactive than glucose, they may be responsible for significant modification of long-lived intracellular components.

AGE-INDUCED ALTERATIONS IN VESSEL WALL PROTEIN COMPONENTS

Accumulation of Extravasated Plasma Proteins

Both large and small blood vessels of diabetics characteristically show early and continuous accumulation of a variety of plasma proteins. In the arterial subintima, extracellular accumulation of extravasated low-density lipoprotein (LDL) makes up the bulk of such material, whereas in arterial media PAS-positive plasma glyco-protein deposits are most prominent [37]. In atherosclerotic plaques, this accumulated lipoprotein can only be released from lesions by treatment with proteolytic enzymes, suggesting that it is chemically attached to vessel wall matrix components [38].

Hyperglycemia could enhance such extracellular immobilization of lipoproteins by accelerating the formation of AGE crosslinks. This would promote excessive plaque formation at any given level of plasma LDL by preventing diffusion out of the intima, permitting oxidative modification of lipids by endothelial cells.

In vitro, human LDL covalently binds to collagen having preformed AGE [39]. AGE-formation on both lipid and apolipoprotein components of LDL may further accelerate this process [32].

In the diabetic microcirculation, deposition of PAS-positive material occurs in retinal, glomerular and endoneurial arterioles with basement membrane accumulation of plasma proteins such as IgG, albumin and IgM [40–43]. These proteins remain tightly bound to matrix components during disruptive isolation procedures, and cannot be extracted with either high salt buffers or thiocyanate treatment [43]. Similarly, the experimental addition of serum albumin or IgG to non-enzymatically glycosylated collagen or basement membrane washed free of glucose results in covalent binding of both these proteins to matrix [44, 45].

Once normally short-lived plasma proteins such as LDL and IgG become covalently attached to vascular matrix through reaction with AGE, new AGEs form on these incorporated proteins, which can then serve as attachment sites for additional molecules of extravasated plasma protein.

In the walls of both large and small blood vessels, continued accumulation of deposited plasma proteins by AGE crosslinking would contribute directly to progressive luminal narrowing over time [46].

Accumulation of Modified Matrix Proteins

Vascular wall accumulation of plasma protein deposits through crosslinking by glycosylation products on matrix is only one element in the progressive luminal narrowing that occurs in all diabetic vessels. In addition, AGEs on matrix proteins contribute to the formation of thickened vascular walls by crosslinking adjacent matrix components.

Collagen was the first matrix protein used to demonstrate unequivocally that glucose-derived AGEs form covalent, heat-stable intermolecular bonds [47, 48]. The collagen samples were analyzed after being digested by cyanogen bromide. SDS gels showed that the amount of crosslinked collagen peptides formed increased as a function of both time and glucose concentration [47]. Crosslinks derived from AGEs were found throughout the collagen molecule, in marked contrast to normal crosslinks generated by the enzyme lysyl oxidase, which occur only on two peptides at the N-terminal and C-terminal ends of the molecule [49]. The degree of AGE-derived crosslink formation was unchanged after selective enzymatic removal of lysyl oxidase-generated crosslinks [47, 50]. Similar changes were found *in vivo* where aortic collagen from diabetic rats was three times more crosslinked than aortic collagen from non-diabetic animals [47].

Matrix components crosslinked by glucose accumulate in diabetic vessel walls because they are less susceptible to normal enzymatic degradation. *In vitro*, non-enzymatically glycosylated glomerular basement membrane is considerably more resistant to digestion by pepsin, papain, trypsin and endogenous glomerular proteases than is normal basement membrane [51, 52]. Similarly, non-enzymatically glycosylated diabetic collagen shows significantly reduced susceptibility to digestion by pepsin and collagenase [53]. *In vivo*, reduced physiologic degradation of diabetic capillary basement membrane and arterial matrix molecules due to excessive non-enzymatic glycosylation would contribute to thickening of these structures over time.

Functional Abnormalities of Modified Matrix Proteins

In addition to reducing the susceptibility of matrix proteins to removal by enzymes, crosslinking by AGE induces abnormalities in critical matrix protein functions such as basement membrane self-assembly and binding of growth-modulating heparan sulfate proteoglycans (HSPGs). These changes may contribute to distorted three-dimensional matrix structure with increased effective intermolecular pore size, cellular hypertrophy and hyperplasia.

Normal development and maintenance of basement membrane structure involve a geometrically ordered self-assembly process involving site-specific end-to-end and lateral interactions of type IV collagen, laminin, HSPG and entactin. With AGE formation, however, an impairment of the associative properties of basement membrane components occurs which reduces the ability of these molecules to interact with each other to form an ordered polymeric complex. Following AGE formation, distinctive changes in basement membrane molecular morphology have been observed by rotary shadowing electron microscopy, including increased crosslinking of type IV collagen and impaired site-specific end-to-end and lateral interactions, which as stated above are essential for normal basement membrane self-assembly. Similarly, X-ray diffraction studies of AGE crosslinked type I collagen have demonstrated that AGE formation causes an increase in intermolecular spacing [13–16, 54]. Such changes in AGE collagens would lead to permanent increases in the size selectivity of matrix pores in diabetic vessels.

The anionic proteoglycan components of vascular matrix, particularly heparan sulfate, may have a particularly critical role in the pathogenesis of diabetic vascular disease because these molecules are a major component of the charge-selective matrix filtration barrier. In addition, they appear to downmodulate the proliferative activity of adherent cells [55], either through direct transmembrane inhibition of cellular activation via specific glycosaminoglycan (GAG) receptors, or indirectly via sequestration of growth factors such as fibroblast growth factor (bFGF). In diabetes of long duration, basement membrane content of anionic proteoglycan is markedly decreased in several tissues including the renal glomerulus [56–58], and there is evidence suggesting that loss of this inhibitory matrix signal results in a compensatory increase in basement membrane production [59].

Accumulation of AGE on collagen and basement membrane contributes to this permanent loss of proteoglycan by reducing the ability of these long-lived matrix proteins to bind heparin [16, 60–62]. A similar reduction in heparin binding has been reported

with AGE-modified laminin [15]. These glycosylation-induced matrix defects would both increase leakage of plasma proteins and stimulate matrix overproduction.

Recent studies have defined a lysine-containing amino acid sequence within the A chain of the laminin molecule that promotes neurite outgrowth [33]. Modification of this sequence by AGE formation inhibits neurite outgrowth by 55–65%. Similarly, modification of the cell-binding domains of type IV collagen causes decreased endothelial cell adhesion [34, 35].

AGE-induced conformational changes in matrix components are also likely to cause further abnormalities in diabetic blood vessels by altering matrix interactions with platelets and vascular wall cells. These abnormalities, mediated by specific transmembrane signalling receptors called integrins [63], may result in microthrombus formation, hyper-responsiveness to growth factors, enhanced secretion of vasoconstrictor molecules and abnormalities in cell adhesion [92, 93].

AGE formation on intact matrix also affects biologic functions important to normal vascular tissue integrity. The endothelium-derived relaxing factor and antiproliferative factor nitric oxide is quenched by AGEs in a dose-dependent fashion. In diabetic animals, defects in the vasodilatory response to nitric oxide correlate with the level of accumulated AGEs and are prevented by inhibition of AGE formation. In cell culture, AGEs block the cytostatic effect of nitric oxide on aortic smooth muscle cells and mesangial cells. In large arteries from diabetic rats, AGEs decrease elasticity even after abolition of vascular tone, and increase fluid filtration across the carotid artery significantly [69–71].

AGE-INDUCED ALTERATIONS IN VESSEL WALL CELLULAR COMPONENTS

Stimulation of Growth-promoting Cytokine Production

Expansion of diabetic vascular matrix is due in part to the decreased degradation of AGE crosslinked plasma and matrix proteins discussed previously, and in part to a significant increase in the synthesis of matrix components themselves [8, 11]. The most likely chronic stimulus for these processes is increased local production of such growth-promoting factors as insulin-like growth factor I (IGF-I) [64, 65], tumour necrosis factor (TNF), interleukin-1 (IL-1) and platelet-derived growth factor (PDGF) [66].

Both murine and human monocyte-macrophages have been shown to have a previously undescribed high-affinity receptor for AGE proteins [67], which also exists on endothelial cells [68]. There are 1.5×10^5 macrophage receptors for AGE-modified proteins per cell, with a binding affinity of 1.75×10^7 M^{-1}. This receptor has a unique biological significance, as it is the first receptor to recognize a ligand known to form extensively *in vivo*. A 60 kDa and a 90 kDa AGE-binding protein have been isolated from rat liver [72]. Both proteins are present on monocyte/macrophages, and antiserum to either protein blocks AGE binding to macrophages. AGE receptors have been identified on glomerular mesangial cells using antisera against these two proteins, and interaction with AGE proteins increases PDGF-mediated mesangial cell production of type IV collagen, laminin, and HSPG [73, 74].

When AGE protein binds to its macrophage receptor, it induces production of IL-1 and IGF-I in addition to TNFα. The concentrations of these induced cytokines have been shown to be sufficient to stimulate proliferation of glomerular mesangial cells and arterial smooth muscle cells, and to increase glomerular synthesis of type IV collagen [66, 75] (Figure 3).

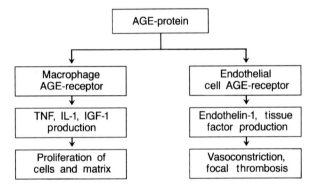

Figure 3 Schematic representation of the mechanisms by which AGE-protein binding to specific receptors on macrophages and endothelial cells may cause pathologic changes in diabetic vessels. (From reference 110, with permission)

Endothelial cells also express AGE-specific receptors. Ligand binding to this receptor on macrovascular endothelial cells induces two additive procoagulatory changes in the endothelial surface [76]. One such change is a fast reduction in thrombomodulin activity, which prevents activation of the protein C pathway. The other procoagulatory change is a rise in tissue factor activity, which activates coagulation factors IX and X through factor VIIa binding. In addition to these changes, AGE-protein binding to the endothelial cell AGE-receptor also causes increased production of the vasoconstrictor peptide endothelin-1 [77]. The overall consequences of these AGE-induced changes in endothelial function are focal thrombosis and marked vasoconstriction (Figure 3).

Two endothelial cell AGE-binding proteins have recently been isolated and characterized [78–80], a 35 kDa and a 46 kDa protein, which were purified to

homogeneity. The N-terminal sequence of the 35 kDa protein was identical to lactoferrin. The 46 kDa protein, for which a full-length 1.5 kb cDNA was cloned, was novel. It proved to be an integral membrane protein and a member of the superfamily of immunoglobulin-related proteins, with 3 disulfide-bonded immunoglobulin homology units.

The binding of AGEs can be blocked by antibodies to either protein. Immunoelectronmicroscopy suggests that the two proteins are closely associated on the cell surface, whilst *in vitro* the two purified proteins bind together with high affinity ($k_d = 100$ pmol/l). Cross-linking studies with endothelial cells show formation of a new higher molecular weight band that reacts with antibodies to both proteins. In human monocytes there are two AGE-binding proteins that are related to the endothelial cell receptor [81]. Antibodies to either protein block AGE-induced chemotaxis. Figure 4 shows a model of AGE binding to a receptor composed of the integral membrane protein and its non-covalently associated 'lactoferrin-like polypeptide'.

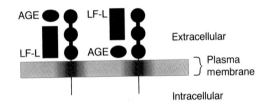

Figure 4 Model of AGE binding to a receptor composed of an integral membrane protein and its non-covalently associated 'lactoferrin-like polypeptide' (LF-L) (see text for details). (From reference 111, with permission of American Diabetes Association)

The generation of oxygen free radicals appears to mediate signal transduction by the AGE receptor: thus AGE binding to endothelial cells results in oxidant stress that is blocked by antibodies to either of the AGE-receptor components [82]. Receptor-mediated oxidant stress is also blocked by antibodies to AGEs themselves.

The transcription factor NF-kappaB, a pleiotropic regulator of many 'response-to-injury' genes, is activated by infusion of AGE-albumin. In endothelial cells, these genes include several induced by AGEs, including tissue factor and endothelin-1. Such activation can be inhibited by pretreatment of animals with antibodies to the AGE-receptor. These results suggest that interaction of AGEs with their cellular receptor leads to oxidant stress which causes potentially damaging changes in gene expression [66, 67, 72–82].

Modification of DNA Function

Although the primary amino groups of nucleotides are chemically less reactive nucleophiles than the ε-amino groups of lysine, studies with nucleic acids *in vitro* have demonstrated that reducing sugars found intracellularly can react with amino groups on DNA nucleotides in a manner analogous to the non-enzymatic glycosylation of amino groups on proteins [83]. The spectral and fluorescent properties of these AGEs on DNA are similar to those of AGEs on proteins. AGEs also form readily on all classes of histones, suggesting that hyperglycemia may result in crosslinking of DNA with nucleoproteins as well [84].

Formation of AGEs on DNA is associated with mutations and altered gene expression in prokaryotic cells and may cause deleterious DNA transpositions in mammalian cells [91]. Non-enzymatic glycosylation of double-stranded DNA in a prokaryotic system causes mutations that are associated with both insertions and deletions of the DNA [17, 18]. After non-enzymatic glycosylation accomplished either *in vitro* or *in vivo* (using *E. coli* mutants that accumulate glucose 6-phosphate), tetracycline resistance genes in the plasmid pBR322 and the β-galactosidase gene in the plasmid pAM006 no longer function in their *E. coli* host. The glycosylation-induced mutations in the tetracycline resistance gene of pBR322 appear to arise during attempted enzymatic repair of DNA segments that have been modified by AGE, as glycosylated pBR322 DNA functions normally in mutant bacteria lacking the repair enzyme uvrABC excision nuclease. The rate of mutations in pAM006 was shown to be proportional to the degree to which glucose 6-phosphate was elevated. This is consistent with the observation that the hyperglycemia-induced tissue damage of diabetes occurs primarily in insulin-independent cells, where the intracellular concentration of glucose and (even more reactive) glycolytic intermediates is proportional to the level of hyperglycemia [36].

Non-enzymatic glycosylation of DNA also appears to cause decreased gene expression by direct inhibition of template function [83]. Accumulation of advanced glycosylation products on single-stranded f1 bacteriophage DNA reduces its ability to transfect *E. coli* at a rate proportional to both incubation time and sugar concentration. When lysine is present in the incubation mixture, the rate of glucose-induced reduction in DNA function is accelerated nearly twentyfold, after a lag period of several days. This observation suggests that an amino acid glycosylation adduct can form first, which is then highly reactive toward DNA. Direct evidence for the formation of reactive glucose 6-phosphate/lysine intermediates capable of covalently binding protein to DNA has recently been obtained, and it is likely that similar AGE–protein intermediates react with DNA *in vivo* [85].

Hyperglycemia also affects DNA from eukaryotic cells [86, 87]. When human endothelial cells are cultured in 30 mmol/l glucose, there is an increase in single-strand breaks and an increase in DNA repair synthesis. Increased single-strand breaks in DNA also occur in lymphocytes from chronically hyperglycemic diabetic patients. Advanced glycosylation end-products have not yet been quantitated in these human DNA preparations, however. Accumulation of AGE on nucleic acids of diabetic vascular wall cells may eventually interfere with normal physiology. Clinically, the early loss of pericytes from diabetic retinal capillaries may be one irreversible consequence of AGE-induced nucleic acid alterations, and the expression of transforming genes by human coronary artery plaque cells may be another [88].

Modification of Intracellular Proteins

AGEs also form on intracellular proteins *in vivo*. In erythrocytes, AGE-hemoglobin accounts for 0.42% of circulating hemoglobin in normal subjects and 0.75% in diabetics [94]. More striking is the observation that in endothelial cells cultured in high glucose-containing media for only 1 week, intracellular AGE content increases 13.8-fold. The major AGE-modified protein is basic fibroblast growth factor (bFGF). Anti-bFGF antibody completely neutralizes cytosolic mitogenic activity at both 5 mmol/l and 30 mmol/l glucose, demonstrating that all mitogenic activity is due to bFGF. At 30 mmol/l glucose, mitogenic activity of endothelial cell cytosol is reduced 70%. Quantitation by ELISA showed that 30 mmol/l glucose did not decrease the level of bFGF protein, suggesting that the marked decrease in bFGF mitogenic activity resulted from post-translational modification of bFGF by AGEs. Cytosolic AGE-bFGF was increased 6.1-fold [98]. These data are consistent with the hypothesis that AGE modification of intracellular proteins can alter vascular cell function.

PHARMACOLOGICAL MODULATION OF ADVANCED GLYCOSYLATION REACTIONS

As the chemical determinants and the biological consequences of AGE formation appear to explain many of the features of diabetic complications, pharmacologic agents were sought that could inhibit this process by selectively blocking reactive carbonyls on early glycosylation products and on their derivatives 3-deoxyglucosone and glycoaldehyde. The essentially non-toxic nucleophilic hydrazine compound aminoguanidine HCl (LD$_{50}$ 1800 mg/kg in rodents) was selected as the prototype inhibitor. Importantly, this compound does not interfere with the formation of normal, enzymatically derived collagen crosslinks, as determined both indirectly [47] and by direct quantitation of lysyl oxidase-dependent crosslink products (M. Yamin et al, unpublished data).

The mechanism by which aminoguanidine prevents AGE formation does not involve adduct formation with Amadori products on proteins. Rather, aminoguanidine reacts mainly with non-protein-bound derivatives of early glycation products such as 3-deoxyglucosone [99]. Thus, potentially antigenic aminoguanidine adducts do not appear to form on proteins. More detailed mechanistic studies [100] using NMR, mass spectroscopy and X-ray diffraction have shown that aminoguanidine reacts with the AGE-precursor 3-deoxyglucosone to form 3-amino-5- and 3-amino-6-substituted triazines. These triazines are produced as a result of initial hydrazone formation at either C-1 or C-2 (Figure 5).

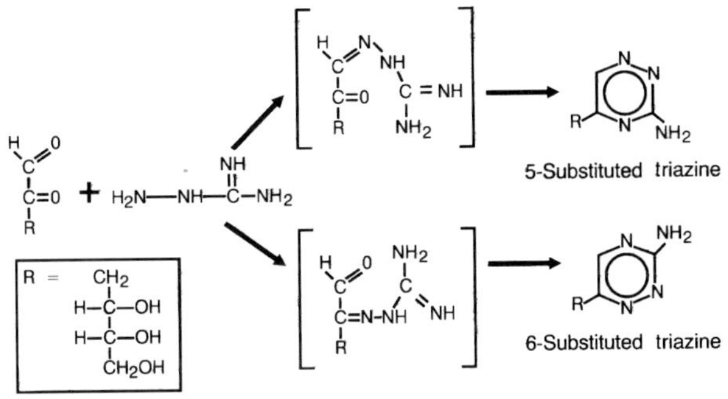

Figure 5 Aminoguanidine prevents AGE formation by reacting with 3-deoxyglucosone to form substituted triazines. (From reference 100, with permission of Macel Dekker Inc)

In vitro, aminoguanidine effectively inhibits the formation of AGE, and inhibits AGE crosslinking of soluble proteins to matrix. In addition, this compound inhibits AGE crosslinking of collagen, and prevents crosslink-induced defects both of heparin binding to collagen/fibronectin and of HSPG binding to basement membrane ([47, 61, 89] and M. Brownlee et al, unpublished data).

In vivo, in animal models of diabetes, the effect of aminoguanidine on early vascular lesions has been examined in retina, renal glomerulus, nerve and artery. In the retina, aminoguanidine treatment prevents increases in vascular permeability [95], AGE formation, and the subsequent intercapillary deposition of extravasated proteins in long-term diabetic rats. In addition, there is a significant reduction of the diabetes-induced PAS-positive deposits at branching sites of precapillary arterioles in aminoguanidine-treated animals. Overall, these findings suggest that AGE accumulation precedes the occurrence of vascular damage and capillary occlusion [96, 97]. In keeping with this conclusion, pathologic development of retinal microaneurysms and an 18-fold increase in acellular capillaries are dramatically reduced by aminoguanidine in long-term diabetic rats, and the endothelial : pericyte cell ratio which is increased in untreated diabetic animals remains nearly normal [96]. Aminoguanidine treatment also inhibits the development of accelerated diabetic retinopathy in the spontaneous hypertensive rat model, suggesting that hypertension-induced deposition of AGEs in the retinal vasculature plays an important role in the acceleration of diabetic retinopathy by hypertension [101, 102].

In animal models of diabetic kidney disease, similar results have been obtained [103–105]. Diabetes increases AGEs in the renal glomerulus, and aminoguanidine treatment prevents this diabetes-induced increase. Untreated diabetic animals develop the characteristic structural feature of human diabetic nephropathy, increased fractional mesangial volume. When diabetic animals are treated with aminoguanidine, this increase in fractional mesangial volume is completely prevented. Untreated diabetic animals also developed albuminuria that averaged 30 mg/24 hours by 32 weeks. This was more than a ten-fold increase above control levels. In aminoguanidine-treated diabetic rats, the level of albumin excretion was reduced nearly 90%. In hypertensive diabetic rats, aminoguanidine treatment also prevented albuminuria without affecting blood pressure.

Aminoguanidine treatment also improves abnormalities of diabetic peripheral nerve in animal models. After eight weeks of diabetes, both motor nerve and sensory nerve conduction velocity are decreased. These decreases are prevented by aminoguanidine treatment [106]. After 24 weeks of diabetes, nerve action-potential amplitude was decreased by 37%, and peripheral nerve blood flow by 57%. Aminoguanidine treatment normalized both [107].

Inhibition of AGE formation by aminoguanidine treatment also ameliorates the effects of diabetes on large arteries. In animal models, aminoguanidine treatment increased elasticity as measured by static compliance, aortic input impedance, and left ventricular power output. Abnormal increases in fluid filtration across the carotid wall were also significantly reduced [71].

In vivo, inhibition of AGE formation appears to be the predominant mechanism by which diabetic pathology is prevented by aminoguanidine treatment, but an additional *in vivo* inhibitory effect on the inducible form of nitric oxide synthase has been hypothesized [108]. An effect of aminoguanidine on this enzyme is unlikely to play a role in the prevention of diabetic pathology, however, since an aminoguanidine derivative with no *in vitro* effect on nitric oxide synthase activity (morpholino–ethyl–aminoguanidine) inhibits both AGE formation and the development of diabetic pathology [109].

From the biochemical, cell and animal studies described in this chapter, it is known that AGEs accumulate as a function of the level of chronic hyperglycemia and that this AGE accumulation causes dysfunctional changes in extracellular matrix, abnormal receptor-mediated production of cytokines, and altered function of intracellular proteins. Most importantly, it has been established that pharmacologic inhibition of AGEs prevents diabetic complications in animal models. What is not known is whether AGE inhibition will prevent diabetic complications in humans. To answer this question, a multi-centered, randomized, double-blind study is currently in progress examining the effects of aminoguanidine on various endpoints in different stages of diabetic nephropathy. There are two major components to the study.

One component is an Overt Diabetic Nephropathy protocol, in which adult insulin-dependent patients will be randomized to either placebo or one of two different aminoguanidine dosage treatment groups. Entry criteria include diabetes onset prior to age 25, proteinuria >500 mg/day, and creatinine clearances between 40 and 90 ml/min. Decline in GFR and changes in urinary protein excretion will be sequentially evaluated. The other component is an End Stage Renal Disease protocol, in which diabetic patients with end-stage renal failure who have been on chronic hemodialysis less than three months will be randomized to either placebo or one of two aminoguanidine dosage treatment groups. The primary endpoints in this portion of the study are cardiovascular morbidity and mortality. Additional clinical studies focused on non-renal endpoints will follow in the near future. The results of these definitive clinical trials will define the place of AGE inhibitors in the prevention and treatment of diabetic complications.

Acknowledgments

This chapter is dedicated to my mentor, friend, and collaborator Dr Anthony Cerami. His guidance, enthusiasm, and scientific interactions have made working together in this area both intellectually stimulating and great fun.

REFERENCES

1. Nathan D. Relationship between metabolic control and long-term complications of diabetes. In Kahn CR, Weir G (eds) Joslin's diabetes. Philadelphia: Lea & Febiger, 1994.
2. Brownlee M, Cerami A. The biochemistry of the complications of diabetes mellitus. Ann Rev Biochem 1981; 50: 385–432.
3. The Diabetes Control and Complications Trial Research Group. The effect of intensive treatment of diabetes on the development and progression of long-term complications in insulin-dependent diabetes mellitus. New Engl J Med 1993; 329: 977–86.
4. Kuusisto J, Mykkänen, L, Pyörälä K, Laakso M. NIDDM and its metabolic control predict coronary heart disease in elderly subjects. Diabetes 1994; 43: 960–7.
5. Ruderman NB, Williamson JR, Brownlee M. Glucose and diabetic vascular disease. FASEB J 1992; 6: 2905–14.
6. Greene DA, Lattimer SA, Sima AAF. Sorbitol, phosphoinositides, and sodium-potassium-ATPase in the pathogenesis of diabetic complications. New Engl J Med 1987; 316: 599–606.
7. Winegrad AI. Does a common mechanism induce the diverse complications of diabetes? Diabetes 1987; 36: 396–406.
8. Lee TS, Saltsman KA, Ohashi H, King GL. Activation of protein kinase C by elevation of glucose concentration: proposal for a mechanism in the development of diabetic vascular complications. Proc Natl Acad Sci USA 1989; 86(13): 5141–5.
9. Brownlee M, Vlassara H, Cerami A. Non-enzymatic glycosylation and the pathogenesis of diabetic complications. Ann Intern Med 1989; 101: 527–37.
10. Witztum JL, Mahoney EM, Branks MJ et al. Nonenzymatic glucosylation of low-density lipoprotein alters its biologic activity. Diabetes 1982; 3: 283–91.
11. Brownlee M, Spiro RG. Glomerular basement membrane metabolism in the diabetic rat. *In vivo* studies. Diabetes 1979; 28: 121–5.
12. Brownlee M, Cahill GF Jr. Diabetic control and vascular complications. Atheroscler Rev 1979; 4: 29–70.
13. Tsilibary EC, Charonis AS, Reger LA, Wohlhueter RM, Furcht LT. The effect of non-enzymatic glucosylation on the binding of the main non-collagenous NCl domain to type IV collagen. J Biol Chem 1988; 263: 4302–8.
14. Tanaka S, Avigad G, Brodsky B, Eikenberry EF. Glycation induces expansion of the molecular packing of collagen. J Mol Biol 1988; 203: 495–505.
15. Tarsio JF, Reger LA, Furcht LT. Molecular mechanisms in basement membrane complications of diabetes: alterations in heparin, laminin, and type IV collagen association. Diabetes 1988; 37: 532–40.
16. Tarsio JF, Reger LA, Furcht LT. Decreased interaction of fibronectin, type IV collagen, and heparin, due to nonenzymatic glycosylation. Implications for diabetes mellitus. Biochemistry 1987; 26: 1014–20.
17. Bucala R, Model P, Russel M, Cerami A. Modification of DNA by glucose-6-phosphate induces DNA rearrangements in an *E. coli* plasmid. Proc Natl Acad Sci USA 1985; 82: 8439–42.
18. Lee AT, Cerami A. Elevated glucose 6-phosphate levels are associated with plasmid mutations *in vivo*. Proc Natl Acad Sci USA 1987; 84: 8311–14.
19. Monnier VM, Vishwanath V, Frank KE et al. Relation between complications of type I diabetes mellitus and collagen-linked fluorescence. New Engl J Med 1986; 314: 403–8.
20. Reynolds TM. Chemistry of non-enzymatic browning I. Adv Food Res 1963; 12: 1–52.
21. Reynolds TM. Chemistry of non-enzymatic browning II. Adv Food Res 1965; 14: 167–283.
22. Monnier VM, Cerami A. Non-enzymatic glycosylation and browning of proteins *in vivo*. In Waller GR,

Feather MS (eds) The Maillard reaction in foods and nutrition. Symposium Series no. 215. Washington: American Chemical Society, 1983: pp 431-9.

23. Baynes JW, Thorpe SR, Murtiashaw MH. Non-enzymatic glucosylation of lysine residues in albumin. In Wold F, Moldave K (eds) Methods in enzymology: post-translational modifications, Vol. 106. New York: Academic Press, 1984: pp 88-98.

24. Higgins PJ, Bunn HF. Kinetic analysis of the non-enzymatic glucosylation of hemoglobin. J Biol Chem 1981; 256: 5204-8.

25. Mortensen HB. Christophersen C. Glucosylation of human haemoglobin A in red blood cells studied *in vitro*. Kinetics of the formation and dissociation of haemoglobin A_{1c}. Clin Chim Acta 1983; 134: 317-26.

26. Vishwanath V, Frank KE, Elmets CA et al. Glycation of skin collagen in type 1 diabetes mellitus: correlation with long-term complications. Diabetes 1986; 35: 916-21.

27. Monnier VM, Kohn RR, Cerami A. Accelerated age-related browning of human collagen in diabetes mellitus. Proc Natl Acad Sci USA 1984; 81: 583-7.

28. Araki N, Ueno N, Chakrabarti B, Morino Y, Horiuchi S. Immunochemical evidence for the presence of advanced glycation end products in human lens protein and its positive correlation with aging. J Biol Chem 1992; 267: 10211-14.

29. Dyer DG, Blackledge JA, Thorpe SR, Baynes JW. Formation of pentosidine during non-enzymatic browning of proteins by glucose: identification of glucose and other carbohydrates as possible precursors of pentosidine *in vivo*. J Biol Chem 1991; 266: 11654-60.

30. Horiuchi S, Araki N, Morino Y. Immunochemical approach to characterize advanced glycation end products of the Maillard reaction: evidence for the presence of a common structure. J Biol Chem 1991; 266: 7329-32.

31. Makita Z, Vlassara H, Cerami A, Bucala R. Immunochemical detection of advanced glycosylation end products *in vivo*. J Biol Chem 1992; 267: 5133-8.

32. Bucala R, Makita L, Koschinsky T, Cerami A, Vlassara H. Lipid advanced glycosylation: pathway for lipid oxidation *in vivo*. Proc Natl Acad Sci 1993; 90: 6434-8.

33. Tashiro K, Sephel GC, Weeks B, Sasaki M, Martin GR, Kleinman HK, Yamada Y. A synthetic peptide containing the IKVAV sequence from the A chain of laminin mediates cell attachment, migration, and neurite outgrowth. J Biol Chem 1990; 264: 16174-82.

34. Federoff HJ, Lawrence D, Brownlee M. Non-enzymatic glycosylation of laminin and the laminin peptide CIKVAVS inhibits neurite outgrowth. Diabetes 1993; 42: 509-13.

35. Haitoglou CS, Tsilibary EC, Brownlee M, Charonis AS. Altered cellular interactions between endothelial cells and non-enzymatically glucosylated laminin/type IV collagen. J Biol Chem 1992; 267: 12404-7.

36. Stevens VD, Vlassara H, Abati A, Cerami A. Nonenzymatic glycosylation of hemoglobin. J Biol Chem 1977; 252: 2998-3004.

37. Dybdahl H, Ledet TS. Diabetic macroangiopathy: quantitative histopathological studies of the extramural coronary arteries from Type 2 diabetic patients. Diabetologia 1987; 30: 882-6.

38. Smith EB, Massie IB, Alexander KM. The release of an immobilized lipoprotein fraction from atherosclerotic lesions by incubation with plasmin. Atherosclerosis 1986; 25: 71-84.

39. Brownlee M, Vlassara H, Cerami A. Non-enzymatic glycosylation products on collagen covalently trap low-density lipoprotein. Diabetes 1985; 34: 938-41.

40. Graham AR, Johnson PC. Direct immunofluorescence findings in peripheral nerve from patients with diabetic neuropathy. Ann Neurol 1985; 17: 450-4.

41. Miller K, Michael AF. Immunopathology of renal extracellular membranes in diabetes: specificity of tubular basement-membrane immunoflorescence. Diabetes 1976; 25: 701-8.

42. Cohn RA, Mauer SM, Barbosa J, Michael AF. Immunofluorescence studies of skeletal muscle extracellular membranes in diabetes mellitus. Lab Invest 1978; 39: 13-16.

43. Michael AF, Brown DM. Increased concentration of albumin in kidney basement membranes in diabetes mellitus. Diabetes 1981; 30: 843-6.

44. Brownlee M, Pongor S, Cerami A. Covalent attachment of soluble proteins by non-enzymatically glycosylated collagen: role in the *in situ* formation of immune complexes. J Exp Med 1983; 158: 1739-44.

45. Sensi M, Tanzi P, Bruno MR et al. Human glomerular basement membrane: altered binding characteristics following *in vitro* non-enzymatic glycosylation. Ann NY Acad Sci 1986; 488: 549-52.

46. Parving HH. Microvascular permeability to plasma proteins in hypertension and diabetes mellitus in man—on the pathogenesis of hypertensive and diabetic microangiopathy. Dan Med Bull 1975; 22: 217-33.

47. Brownlee M, Vlassara H, Kooney T, Ulrich P, Cerami A. Aminoguanidine prevents diabetes-induced arterial wall protein cross-linking. Science 1986; 232: 1629-32.

48. Kent MJC, Light ND, Bailey AJ. Evidence for glucose-mediated covalent cross-linking of collagen after glycosylation in vitro. Biochem J 1985; 225: 745-52.

49. Miller EJ, Gay S. Collagen: an overview. In Cummingham LW, Frederiksen DW (eds) Methods in enzymology, 82A. New York: Academic Press, 1982: pp 3-32.

50. Miller EJ, Rhodes RK. Preparation and characterization of the different types of collagen. In Cummingham LW, Frederiksen DW (eds) Methods in enzymology, 82A. New York: Academic Press, 1982; pp 33-52.

51. Lubec G, Pollak A. Reduced susceptibility of nonenzymatically glucosylated glomerular basement membrane to proteases: is thickening diabetic glomerular basement due to reduced proteolytic degradation? Renal Physiol 1980; 3: 4-8.

52. Knecht R, Leber R, Hasslacher C. Degradation of glomerular basement membrane in diabetes. Susceptibility of diabetic and nondiabetic basement membrane to proteolytic degradation of isolated glomeruli. Res Exp Med 1987; 187: 323-8.

53. Schnider SL, Kohn RR. Effects of age and diabetes mellitus on the solubility and non-enzymatic glucosylation of human skin collagen. J Clin Invest 1982; 67: 1630-5.

54. Yurchenco PD, Tsilibary EC, Charonis AS, Furthmayr H. Models of the self assembly of basement membrane. J Histochem Cytochem 1986; 34: 93–102.

55. Klahr S, Schreiner G, Ichikawa I. The progression of renal disease. New Engl J Med 1988; 318: 1657–66.

56. Klein DJ, Brown DM, Oegema TR. Glomerular proteoglycans: partial structural characterization and metabolism of de novo synthesized heparan-^{35}SO$_4$ proteoglycan in streptozotocin-induced diabetic rats. Diabetes 1986; 35: 1130–42.

57. Saraswathi S, Vasan NS. Alterations in the rat renal glycosaminoglycans in streptozotocin-induced diabetes. Biochim Biophys Acta 1983; 755: 237–43.

58. Shimomura H, Spiro RG. Studies on macromolecular components of human glomerular basement membrane and alterations in diabetes: decreased levels of heparan sulfate proteoglycan and laminin. Diabetes 1987; 36: 374–81.

59. Rohrbach DH, Hassel JR, Kleinman HK, Martin GR. Alterations in basement membrane (heparan sulfate) proteoglycan in diabetic mice. Diabetes 1982; 31: 185–8.

60. Tarsio JF, Wigness B, Rhode TD, Rupp WM, Buchwal H, Furcht LT. Non-enzymatic glycation of fibronectin and alterations in the molecular association of cell matrix and basement membrane components in diabetes mellitus. Diabetes 1985; 34: 477–84.

61. Brownlee M, Vlassara H, Cerami A. Aminoguanidine prevents hyperglycemia-induced defect in binding of heparin by matrix molecules. Diabetes 1987; 36: 85A.

62. Klein DJ, Brown DM, Oegema TR. Glomerular proteoglycans in diabetes: partial structural characterization and metabolism of de novo synthesized heparan-^{35}SO$_4$ and dermatan-^{35}SO$_4$ proteoglycans in streptozotocin-induced diabetic rats. Diabetes 1986; 35: 1130–42.

63. Ruoslahti E, Pierschbacher MD. New perspectives in cell adhesion: RGD and integrins. Science 1987; 238: 491–7.

64. King GL, Goodman AD, Buzney S, Moses A, Kahn CR. Receptors and growth-promoting effects of insulin and insulin-like growth factors on cells from bovine retinal capillaries and aorta. J Clin Invest 1985; 75: 1028–36.

65. Grant M, Russell B, Fitzgerald C, Merimee TJ. Insulin-like growth factors in vitreous studies in control and diabetic subjects with neovascularization. Diabetes 1986; 35: 416–20.

66. Vlassara H, Brownlee M, Monogue K et al. Cachectin / TNF and IL-1 induced by glucose-modified proteins: role in normal tissue remodeling. Science 1988; 240: 1546–8.

67. Vlassara H, Brownlee M, Cerami A. High-affinity receptor-mediated uptake and degradation of glucose-modified proteins: a potential mechanism for the removal of senescent macromolecules. Proc Natl Acad Sci USA 1985; 82: 5588–92.

68. Esposito C, Gerlach H, Brett J, Stern D, Vlassara H. Endothelial receptor mediated binding of glucose modified albumin is associated with increased monolayer permeability and modulation of cell surface coagulant properties. J Exp Med 1989; 170: 1387–1407.

69. Bucala R, Tracey KJ, Cerami A. Advanced glycosylation products quench nitric oxide and mediate defective endothelium-dependent vasodilation in experimental diabetes. J Clin Invest 1991; 87: 432–8.

70. Hogan M, Cerami A, Bucala R. Advanced glycosylation end products block the antiproliferative effect of nitric oxide. J Clin Invest 1992; 90: 1110–15.

71. Huijberts MSP, Wolffenbuttel BRH, Struijker Boudier HAJ, Crijns FRL, Neiuwenhiujzen Kruseman AC, Poitevin P, Levy BI. Aminoguanidine treatment increases elasticity and decreases fluid filtration of large arteries from diabetic rats. J Clin Invest 1993; 92: 1407–11.

72. Yang Z, Makita Z, Horii Y, Brunelle S, Cerami A, Sehajpal P, Suthanthiran M, Vlassara H. Two novel rat liver membrane proteins that bind advanced glycosylation endproducts: relationship to macrophage receptor for glucose-modified proteins. J Exp Med 1991; 174: 515–24.

73. Skolnik EY, Yang Z, Makita Z, Radoff S, Kirstein M, Vlassara H. Human and rat mesangial cell receptors for glucose-modified proteins: potential role in kidney tissue remodelling and diabetic nephropathy. J Exp Med 1991; 174: 931–9.

74. Doi T, Vlassara H, Kirstein M, Yamada Y, Striker GE, Striker LJ. Receptor-specific increase in extracellular matrix productions in mouse mesangial cells by advanced glycosylation end-products is mediated via platelet-derived growth factor. Proc Natl Acad Sci USA 1992; 89: 2873–7.

75. Kirstein M, Aston C, Hintz R, Vlassara H. Receptor-specific induction of insulin-like growth factor I in human monocytes by advanced glycosylation end product-modified proteins. J Clin Invest 1992; 90: 439–46.

76. Esposito C, Gerlach H, Brett J, Stern D, Vlassara H. Endothelial receptor-mediated binding of glucose-modified albumin is associated with increased monolayer permeability and modulation of cell surface coagulant properties. J Exp Med 1992; 170: 1387–407.

77. Nawroth PP, Stern D, Bierhaus A, Lu J, Lin R, Ziegler R. Diabetes Stoffwechsel 1992; 1 (suppl. 1): 153.

78. Schmidt AM, Vianna M, Gerlach M, Brett J, Ryan J, Kao J et al. Isolation and characterization of two binding proteins for advanced glycosylation end products from bovine lung which are present on the endothelial cell surface. J Biol Chem 1992; 267: 14987–97.

79. Neeper M, Schmidt AM, Brett J, Du Yan S, Wang F, Yu-Ching EP et al. Cloning and expression of RAGE: a cell surface receptor for advanced glycosylation end-products of proteins. J Biol Chem 1992; 267: 14998–15004.

80. Schmidt AM, Mora R, Cao K, Yan SD, Brett J, Ramakrishnan R et al. The endothelial cell binding site for advanced glycation endproducts consists of A complex: an integral membrane protein and a lactoferrin-like polypeptide. J Biol Chem 1994; 269: 9882–8.

81. Schmidt AM, Yan SD, Brett J, Mora R, Nowygrod R, Stern D. Regulation of human mononuclear phagocyte migration by cell suface-binding proteins for advanced glycation end-products. J Clin Invest 1993; 91(5): 2155–68.

82. Yan SD, Schmidt AM, Anderson GM, Zhang J, Brett J, Zou YS et al. Enhanced cellular oxidant stress

by the interaction of advanced glycation end products with their receptors/binding proteins. J Biol Chem 1994; 269: 9889–97.

83. Bucala R, Model P, Cerami A. Modification of DNA by reducing sugars: a possible mechanism for nucleic acid aging and age-related dysfunction in gene expression. Proc Natl Acad Sci USA 1984; 81: 105–9.

84. De Bellis D, Horowitz MI. *In vitro* studies of histone glycation. Biochim Biophys Acta 1987; 926: 365–8.

85. Lee AT, Cerami A. The formation of reactive intermediate(s) of glucose 6-phosphate and lysine capable of rapidly reacting with DNA. Mutat Res 1987; 179: 151–8.

86. Lorenzi M, Montisano DF, Toledo S, Barrieux A. High glucose and DNA damage in endothelial cells. J Clin Invest 1986; 77: 322–5.

87. Lorenzi M, Montisano DF, Toledo S, Wong HCH. Increased single strand breaks in DNA of lymphocytes from diabetic subjects. J Clin Invest 1987; 79: 653–6.

88. Penn A, Garte SJ, Warren L, Nesta D, Mindich B. Transforming gene in human atherosclerotic plaque DNA. Proc Natl Acad Sci USA 1986; 83: 7951.

89. Brownlee M, Vlassara H, Kooney A, Cerami A. Inhibition of glucose-derived protein crosslinking and prevention of early diabetic changes in glomerular basement membrane by aminoguanidine. Diabetes 1986; 35 (suppl. 1): 42A.

90. Brownlee M, Sherwood LM (eds) Diabetes Mellitus and its Complications: Pathogenesis and Treatment. Philadelphia: Hanley & Belfus, 1990: 1–300.

91. Bucala R, Lee AT, Rourke L, Cerami A. Transposition of an Alu-containing element induced by DNA-advanced glycosylation endproducts. Proc Natl Acad Sci USA 1993; 90: 2666–70.

92. Tsilibary EC, Charonis AS. The effect of non-enzymatic glucosylation on cell and heparin-binding microdomains from type IV collagen and laminin. Diabetes 1990; 39 (suppl. 1): 194A (abstr).

93. Crowley S, Brownlee M, Edelstein D, Satriano J, Mori T, Singhal P, Schlondorff D. Effects of non-enzymatic glucosylation of mesangial matrix on proliferation of mesangial cells. Diabetes 1991; 40: 540–7.

94. Makita Z, Vlassara H, Rayfield E, Cartwright K, Friedman E, Rodby R et al. Hemoglobin-AGE: a circulating marker of advanced glycosylation. Science 1992; 258: 651–3.

95. Tilton RG, Chang K, Ostrow E, Allison W, Williamson JR. Invest Ophthal 1990; 31: 3 (abstr).

96. Hammes HP, Martin, S, Federlin K, Geisen K, Brownlee M. Aminoguanidine treatment inhibits the development of experimental diabetic retinopathy. Diabetes 1990; 39 (suppl. 1): 62A (abstr).

97. Hammes HP, Federlin K, Brownlee M. Aminoguanidine treatment inhibits advanced glycosylation product accumulation in diabetic retinal vessels. International Diabetes Federation Congress 1991; (abstr).

98. Giardino I, Edelstein D, Brownlee M. Non-enzymatic glycosylation *in vitro* and in bovine endothelial cells alters basic fibroblast growth factor activity: a model for intracellular glycosylation in diabetes. J Clin Invest 1994; 94: 110–117.

99. Edelstein D, Brownlee M. Mechanistic studies of advanced glycosylation end-product inhibition by aminoguanidine. Diabetes 1992; 41: 26–9.

100. Hirsch J, Baines CL, Feather MS. X-ray structures of a 3-amino-5- and a 3-amino-6-substituted triazine, produced as a result of a reaction of 3-deoxy-D-erythro-hexos-2-ulose (3-deoxyglucosone) with aminoguanidine. J Carbohyd Chem 1992; 11: 891–901.

101. Hammes H-P, Martin S, Federlin K, Geisen K, Brownlee M. Aminoguanidine treatment inhibits the development of experimental diabetic retinopathy. Proc Natl Acad Sci USA 1991; 88: 11555–8.

102. Hammes H-P, Brownlee M, Edelstein D, Saleck M, Martin S, Federlin K. Aminoguanidine inhibits the development of accelerated diabetic retinopathy in the spontaneous hypertensive rat. Diabetologia 1994; 37: 32–5.

103. Soules-Liparota T, Cooper M, Papazoglou D, Clarke B, Jerums G. Retardation by aminoguanidine of development of albuminuria, mesangial expansion, and tissue fluorescence in streptozocin-induced diabetic rat. Diabetes 1991; 40: 1328–35.

104. Edelstein D, Brownlee M. Aminoguanidine ameliorates albuminuria in diabetic hypertensive rats. Diabetologia 1992; 35: 96–7.

105. Ellis EN, Good BH. Prevention of glomerular basement membrane thickening by aminoguanidine in experimental diabetes mellitus. Metabolism 1991; 40: 1016–19.

106. Cameron NE, Cotter MA, Dines K, Love A. Effects of aminoguanidine on peripheral nerve function and polyol pathway metabolites in streptozotocin-diabetic rats. Diabetologia 1992; 35: 946–50.

107. Kihara M, Schmelzer JD, Poduslo JF, Curran GL, Nickander KK, Low PA. Aminoguanidine effects on nerve blood flow, vascular permeability, electrophysiology and oxygen free radicals. Proc Natl Acad Sci USA 1991; 88: 6107–11.

108. Corbett JA, Tilton RG, Chang K, Hasan KS, Ido Y, Wang JL et al. Aminoguanidine, a novel inhibitor of nitric oxide formation, prevents diabetic vascular dysfunction. Diabetes 1992; 41: 552–6.

109. Mallon VM, Ulrich PC, Boyd TA, Miyauchi Y, Takasu T, Yamin M. N[2-(4 Morpholino) ethyl]N' aminoguanidine (MEAG) inhibits AGE formation *in vitro* and diabetic changes in STZ diabetic rats without inhibiting diamine oxidase (DAO) in nitric oxide sythetase (NOS). Diabetes 1993; 42 (suppl. 1): 106A.

110. Brownlee M. Glycation products and the pathogenesis of diabetic complications. Diabetes Care 1992; 15: 1835–43.

111. Brownlee M. Glycation and diabetic complications. Diabetes 1994; 43: 836–41.

Management of Diabetes

34a

Dietary Management of Diabetes Mellitus in Europe and North America

J.I. Mann and N.J. Lewis-Barned

Departments of Human Nutrition and Medicine, University of Otago, and Diabetes Service, Dunedin Hospital, Dunedin, New Zealand

INTRODUCTION

Dietary modification is the mainstay of treatment for non-insulin dependent diabetes (NIDDM). A large proportion of patients with NIDDM who comply with dietary advice will show improvement in the major metabolic abnormalities associated with this condition to an extent that will obviate the need for oral agents and insulin. For those who cannot be managed without drug therapy, attention to dietary advice may modify blood lipids in a way which would be expected to reduce lipoprotein-mediated risk of coronary heart disease (CHD) and further improve glycaemic control. In insulin dependent diabetes (IDDM) the role of diet is twofold: firstly, to help minimize the short-term fluctuations in blood glucose (especially to reduce any tendency towards hypoglycaemia); secondly, to reduce risk of long-term complications by helping to achieve optimal glycaemic control and satisfactory levels of blood lipids. Dietary advice for those with NIDDM and IDDM is similar and the major principles resemble those for entire populations at high risk of CHD. There is therefore no need for diabetic patients to be given meals which differ from those eaten by the rest of the family. Dietary recommendations for people with diabetes have been made in many countries. It is reassuring that those of the Diabetes and Nutrition Study Group of the European Association for the Study of Diabetes, representing the majority of European countries [1], and the American Diabetes Association [2] are remarkably consistent. Readers are particularly advised to refer to the supporting paper associated with the American recommendations [3]. Table 1 summarizes the basic principles of diabetic dietary recommendations.

TOTAL ENERGY INTAKE

The majority of people with NIDDM are overweight. Successful weight reduction, at least in part as a consequence of reduced insulin resistance, will result in lowering of blood glucose, and a reduction in triglyceride and triglyceride-rich very low density lipoprotein (VLDL). The reduction in triglyceride and VLDL is particularly important since levels are elevated in NIDDM and obesity, and in NIDDM raised levels of triglycerides in VLDL may be more important risk indicators of CHD than in non-diabetics (Table 2). Weight reduction will also help to reduce blood pressure levels which are often elevated in NIDDM. Even modest weight reduction is associated with a reduction in insulin resistance, a reduction in hepatic glucose production, and perhaps an improvement in islet B-cell function [4]. It is generally accepted that total energy should be reduced so that body mass index (BMI) moves towards the desirable range (20–25 kg/m^2). However, despite advice and support

International Textbook of Diabetes Mellitus, Second Edition. Edited by K.G.M.M. Alberti, P. Zimmet, R.A. DeFronzo, and H. Keen (Honorary)
© 1997 John Wiley & Sons Ltd

Table 1 Nutritional recommendations for individuals with diabetes mellitus, 1994

Energy
   Achieve or maintain ideal body weight (BMI < 25)
Carbohydrate
   Approx. 50% total energy, more if high in soluble fibre
Fibre
   Increase soluble fibre, e.g. dried beans, lentils, peas,
   oats, barley. Also increase wholegrain cereals, green
   leafy and root vegetables
Glycaemic index
   May identify useful foods
Alcohol
   Reduce in general, avoid in hypertriglyceridaemia,
   overweight and hypertension
Fat
   Total: usually 30% total energy*
   Saturated ≤ 10% total energy
   Polyunsaturated ≤ 10% total energy
   Mono-unsaturated ≤ 10% total energy*
Protein
   Reduce towards requirement, maximum 20% total
   energy
Sucrose
   < 30 g/day as table sugar
Sodium
   < 6 g/day in general
   < 3 g/day with hypertension

*Total fat may be increased beyond 30% in those who choose to have a higher
intake of mono-unsaturated fatty acids of *cis* configuration.

Table 2 Lipid and lipoprotein-mediated risk of coronary heart disease in those with and without diabetes

	Non-diabetics	IDDM	NIDDM
Total cholesterol	+ + +	+ + +	+
LDL-cholesterol	+ + +	+ + +	+
Triglyceride	+	+	+ + +
VLDL	+	+	+ + +
HDL-cholesterol (low levels)	+ +	+	+ + +
Remnant particles	+ +	?	+ +

+ + + = Appreciable risk.
+ + = Moderate risk.
+ = Some risk.

many people with NIDDM are unable to achieve this target. It is important therefore to set realistic goals for weight reduction and to provide intermediate as well as long-term targets. Despite the strong evidence that central distribution of obesity is particularly associated with an increased risk of diabetes and the range of metabolic derangements associated with the condition [5], there is insufficient evidence to suggest that advice regarding energy intake should be influenced by distribution of body fat. There is now considerable evidence to support the suggestion that a diet low in fat and relatively high in fibre-rich carbohydrate is more appropriate for achieving and maintaining weight reduction than other dietary prescriptions [6, 7, 8].

Very low calorie diets (VLCDs) have been the subject of considerable controversy, which has centred around concerns about reductions in resting metabolic rate and in lean body mass. They can be used either as total diet replacement for short periods (not usually more than 4 weeks) or as meal replacement incorporated into more conventional weight reduction regimens. There is no doubt that when used as total diet replacement they result in striking improvements in the metabolic profile for NIDDM patients [9–11]. These changes are attributed to improved insulin sensitivity [12]. The long-term benefits of these diets have been less certain, however, although in some studies a high proportion of individuals show benefit after up to 18 months [13–15], especially when combined with behaviour modification approaches. One study has suggested that the metabolic benefits of VLCD used for induction of weight loss are greater at 1 year than for a conventional weight reduction regimen, despite similar amounts of weight lost, and this requires further investigation. While some authorities believe that this approach has a place for some patients [16], such diets are not generally recommended. When they are used by people with diabetes, it should always be under close medical supervision and with long-term dietary support.

It is widely accepted that a sustained weight loss of 1–2 kg/month (which can usually be achieved by a reduction of about 500 kcal below that required for weight maintenance) is the preferred means of weight loss. Regular physical activity enhances weight loss and is particularly important in weight maintenance when targets have been achieved. In addition exercise increases insulin action, the glucose transporter Glut4 in muscle, and HDL (especially HDL_2), whereas triglycerides, LDL-cholesterol and blood pressure are reduced [17, 18]. Further evidence for the benefit of exercise comes from a recent study demonstrating appreciable reduction in mortality in physically active compared with sedentary people with diabetes [19].

The most appropriate approach to achieving weight reduction depends upon the requirements of individual patients. For some it may be sufficient to advise the restriction of energy-dense foods and provide advice with regard to appropriate food types, as well as to provide some general guidance concerning increased physical activity. For those unable to lose weight, a more prescriptive approach based on calorie-counting as well as an exercise prescription may be helpful, especially when this approach is used in conjunction with behavioural modification techniques.

For those with NIDDM who are not overweight, and for the majority of those with IDDM, self-selected energy intakes are appropriate. It is important to ensure that energy intake is sufficient to achieve growth and development in childhood and adolescence. The prescription of insulin in excess of requirements may lead to weight gain. Overweight patients with IDDM can often appreciably improve glycaemic control and at the same time reduce insulin requirements if they are able to lose weight.

QUANTITY AND NATURE OF DIETARY FAT

In most Western countries fat provides 36–40% total energy and saturated fatty acids 13–18%. The modification of quantity and nature can favourably influence several important lipoprotein-mediated predictors of CHD (Table 2). The recommendation that saturated fatty acids (SAFA) and *trans* isomers of unsaturated fatty acids be restricted is almost universal [1–3] and has a several-fold justification. Fat is the most energy-rich of all nutrients and reduction helps to reduce total energy intake which is important for many people with NIDDM and some with IDDM. Much epidemiological evidence suggests that people with diabetes (as is the case with non-diabetics) in populations consuming a low saturated fat diet have reduced incidence and mortality from CHD, compared with those living in countries with a high intake of saturated fat. Reduced saturated fat intake is associated with reduced levels of LDL-cholesterol. These attributes may not be associated with all saturated fatty acids. Thus, in non-diabetics, stearic and lauric acids do not have as striking an effect on LDL as do myristic and palmitic acids [20]. However, because these fatty acids coexist in foods and it is difficult to disentangle separate effects, for the purpose of recommendations they are generally considered as a group. Recent evidence suggests that the *trans* isomers of unsaturated fatty acids, which are produced in a range of manufacturing processes, have a similar adverse effect to that of saturated fatty acids on LDL [21, 22]. In addition, they result in lowering of HDL [22] and an increase of lipoprotein (a) (Lp(a)), which may further contribute to the lipoprotein-mediated risk of CHD [23, 24, 25]. It is for all these reasons that restriction of saturated and *trans* unsaturated fatty acids to 10% or less of total energy has been advised. For those with elevated levels of LDL-cholesterol a lower level of intake (i.e. 8% or less of total energy) may be advised.

n-6 Polyunsaturated fatty acids (chiefly linoleic acid) may help to reduce LDL-cholesterol, but in large quantities (i.e. more than 10% of total energy) can reduce HDL [26]. n-3 Polyunsaturated fatty acids (eicosapentaenoic and docosahexaenoic acids), chiefly derived from oily fish, can help to reduce triglycerides and VLDL as well as reduce the risk of thrombosis as a result of reduced platelet aggregation [27–29]. However, these fatty acids have a variable effect on LDL [30, 31] and the most appropriate ratio of n-3 to n-6 unsaturated fatty acids has yet to be established. Total intake of polyunsaturated fatty acids is very low in most European countries and some increase may be appropriate, though total intake should not exceed 8% total energy. Fish oil supplements are not advised, though increased intake of fish will facilitate the reduction of saturated fat as well as increase intake of naturally occurring n-3 fatty acids, especially if oily fish is eaten regularly.

Mono-unsaturated fatty acids with a *cis* configuration (principally oleic acid from olive oil and the rapeseed oil derivative, canola) on the other hand appear not only to facilitate the reduction of saturated fatty acids, but also help to decrease LDL-cholesterol, increase HDL-cholesterol and may also have antioxidant properties which reduce oxidizability of LDL. Compared with high carbohydrate–low soluble fibre diets, high mono-unsaturated fat diets are associated with improved peripheral insulin sensitivity and improved glycaemic control [32–34]. A fairly wide range of intakes is considered acceptable.

Substantial reduction of saturated fat will almost invariably be associated with a reduction of dietary cholesterol to 300 mg or less per day. There is no good evidence to suggest that a further reduction of dietary cholesterol confers additional benefit when intake of saturated fat is already low.

CARBOHYDRATE, FIBRE AND GLYCAEMIC INDEX

Carbohydrate and Fibre

Traditionally in many affluent societies, low carbohydrate diets (i.e. carbohydrate providing 40% or less total energy) were recommended for people with diabetes. It is now widely accepted that this was unnecessary and undesirable, especially when associated with a high intake of saturated fatty acids [35]. European and North American recommendations suggest that the amount of carbohydrate could be liberalized so that about half of total daily energy is derived from carbohydrate and that an appropriate intake of dietary fibre might be around 20 g/1000 kcal or, on average, about 40 g per day. It is acceptable for the amount of carbohydrates to be even higher than this provided that the foods providing the carbohydrates are also rich in soluble fibre. Much research and a little dissension lie behind this recommendation.

High carbohydrate diets are certainly not new to diabetes. They have been recommended intermittently for at least 2000 years. However, recent interest stems from the work of Anderson who, in uncontrolled studies in the mid-1970s, showed that patients with NIDDM, but treated with insulin, who were given a diet high in carbohydrate and fibre required less insulin [36] (Figure 1). At about the same time Jenkins and colleagues showed that the addition of guar, a viscous fibre, to a test meal reduced postprandial glucose and insulin responses [37] (Figure 2). In order to appreciate some of the subsequent, apparently conflicting, research findings, it is necessary to appreciate

the complexity of the components of dietary fibre. For convenience, dietary fibre may be divided into two broad classes: soluble fibre, which includes gums, gels, mucilages and pectic substances, and insoluble fibre including lignin, cellulose and some of the hemicelluloses. Soluble fibre is broken down in the large bowel by fermentation to produce gas and short-chain fatty acids, and this type of fibre influences carbohydrate and lipid metabolism. Insoluble fibre increases faecal bulk and has little metabolic effect. Two principal approaches have been used to study the effects of increasing carbohydrate and fibre in diabetes: in some studies purified forms of soluble fibre are given as a supplement; in others, foods high in dietary fibre have been increased.

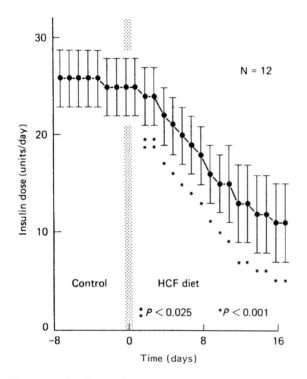

Figure 1 Insulin requirements of NIDDM patients before and after the introduction of a high-carbohydrate, high-fibre (HCF) diet

Purified Forms of Soluble Fibre

Reports from Jenkins' group that the regular addition of guar, pectin and other soluble fibres may improve glycaemic control and in addition lower cholesterol levels have now been confirmed [38]. At first it was thought that the main effect of these fibres was to reduce postprandial glycaemia by slowing absorption. However, a Finnish study has suggested that much of the apparent improvement in postprandial levels is explained by the fall in basal (fasting) glucose levels [39]. Failure of some researchers to confirm the beneficial effect of these substances has been a result of failure to appreciate that all fibres are not equally effective (those with the highest viscosity appear to be most potent in altering blood glucose and lipid profiles), that the fibres need to be incorporated into foods and that the beneficial effect is only apparent when the substances are taken as part of a high-carbohydrate diet (carbohydrate providing at least 50% total energy). These issues have been reviewed in detail by Vinik and Jenkins [40]. Equally important is the fact that until recently many of the commercially available preparations of soluble fibre have been unpalatable and were undoubtedly associated with poor compliance. Different preparations appear to have different potencies and a dose–response effect may operate. The effect of different preparations on glucose and cholesterol is shown in Figure 3. Relatively acceptable preparations are now available and these may have a role in NIDDM patients who have not responded adequately to dietary modification alone, as well as in those with NIDDM or IDDM already on tablets or insulin whose glycaemic control remains unsatisfactory [41]. This form of therapy should be regarded as pharmacological rather than dietary, and although it seems very unlikely that significant side-effects will occur when used in the recommended doses, longer-term studies, continued for years

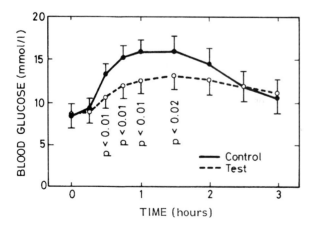

Figure 2 Mean blood glucose levels (mmol/l) of eight non-insulin-requiring diabetic patients after taking control and fibre-enriched test meals (from reference 37, with permission)

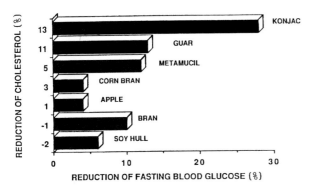

Figure 3 Effect of different types of fibre on cholesterol and glucose levels

rather than months, are desirable in order to establish safety as well as long-term benefits.

Dietary Fibres Fed as Part of a Mixed Diet

Studies to establish conclusively the benefit of increasing fibre in ordinary foods are even more difficult to carry out than studies of fibre supplementation. Carefully controlled studies have shown that increasing carbohydrate to the recommended level by increasing the intake of foods high in soluble fibre (e.g. legumes, lentils, some fruits, oats and barley) can produce an appreciable improvement in glycaemic control and a reduction in low-density lipoprotein (LDL)-cholesterol without an increase in triglycerides or a reduction in the ratio of high-density lipoprotein (HDL) to LDL. Table 3 shows the results of one study in which relatively poorly controlled patients with NIDDM on maximum doses of oral therapy were randomized to receive either reinforced advice concerning their low-carbohydrate diets or advice to change to a high-carbohydrate/high-fibre diet. After 6 weeks a metabolic profile was carried out and the diets were reversed for a further 6 weeks before a final metabolic profile. The

reinforced low-carbohydrate diet produced little benefit, whereas an appreciable improvement was observed on the experimental diet [42]. Some other foods such as pasta, although not necessarily containing as much dietary fibre, may be associated with a similar beneficial effect [43]. Many of the experimental studies have also included substantial quantities of root and green leafy vegetables as well as grain cereals, and these foods may have conferred some additional benefit.

There is no doubt that increasing carbohydrate *per se* without a parallel increase in dietary fibre gives no overall benefit and is associated with several potential disadvantages, despite a slight fall in fasting and overnight glucose levels on such dietary regimens. Glucose levels throughout the day are the same as, or higher than, on a low-carbohydrate diet, HDL-cholesterol levels fall and there may be an increase in triglyceride levels. There is thus no merit in increasing carbohydrate without fibre [43, 44].

Two potential problems remain with regard to extrapolating the findings of the various high-fibre experiments into clinical practice. First, the majority of the studies have used extremely large quantities of dietary fibre which are most unlikely to be acceptable in clinical practice. One study showing a most impressive effect of a diet high in soluble fibre involved participants taking up to 90 g/day [45]! However, other studies appear to show benefits with amounts ranging from 35 to 50 g/day. Vegetarians usually have an intake of around 40 g/day and studies in Oxford suggest that well-instructed and reasonably well-motivated people with diabetes attending outpatient clinics can achieve an intake in this range [46]. Second, it has been correctly argued that, as with the pharmacological preparations of guar and other soluble fibres, the experimental studies of high-fibre foods have been carried out over periods of months rather than years. One of the few relatively long-term studies to be carried out, which claims to show no benefit of a

Table 3 Indices of diabetes control in NIDDM patients unsatisfactorily controlled on maximum doses of oral hypoglycaemic agents (from reference 42, with permission)

	After 6 weeks on a reinforced low-carbohydrate diet	After 6 weeks on a high-carbohydrate/high-fibre diet
HbA$_1$ (%)	** 10.3 ± 2.2	** 8.5 ± 1.9
Fasting glucose (mmol/l)	** 8.4 ± 2.8	** 6.8 ± 2.8
Average preprandial blood glucose (mmol/l)	*** 9.5 ± 2.9	*** 7.5 ± 3.1
Average 2-hour postprandial blood glucose (mmol/l)	11.4 ± 3.5	* 10.8 ± 2.8
Mean 24-hour blood glucose (mmol/l)	** 10.8 ± 1.3	*** 9.3 ± 1.7

* $P < 0.5$.
** $P < 0.01$.
***$P < 0.001$.

high-fibre diet in terms of glycaemic control, had various flaws in experimental design: in particular there was remarkably little difference in achieved intake of dietary fibre between experimental and control groups [47]. Appropriate long-term studies would clearly be of considerable benefit, but there is widespread acceptance that the present experimental data supported by epidemiological evidence are sufficient to justify the recommendations to increase fibre to around 20 g per 1000 kcal, to encourage the use of fibre-rich foods mentioned above and to justify the suggestion that carbohydrates provide around 50% total energy. Such advice is regarded as being appropriate for those with NIDDM and IDDM, though the importance of not increasing fibre-depleted starchy foods, especially in the presence of hypertriglyceridaemia or unsatisfactory glycaemic control, must be emphasized.

Concerns have been expressed regarding the vitamin and mineral status of people who take large quantities of fibre-rich food. There is certainly no evidence that diets such as those recommended cause significant malabsorption of macronutrients or micronutrients. Such diets are not different from those traditionally eaten by some populations; however, it may be prudent to ensure adequate intakes of both macronutrients and micronutrients in the elderly as well as in growing children who are taking large quantities of fibre-rich foods.

Simple Sugars

Simple sugars naturally present in milk and fruits have not usually been restricted provided they are included in the energy allowance, but sucrose has traditionally been restricted. A number of studies have now shown that at least under certain circumstances, monosaccharides and disaccharides do not result in deterioration of glycaemic control or elevated lipid levels. The results of one study in which 45 g of sucrose replaced an isocaloric amount of carbohydrate (mostly bread and potato) are shown in Table 4 [48]. As a result of this and other similar studies the recommendations do not preclude the use of limited quantities (up to 30 g/day) of sucrose as a sweetener, provided that the energy content is taken into account and it does not replace foods high in fibre.

Fructose is another naturally occurring sweetener, sweeter than sucrose, which has been widely used for people with diabetes in the past. However, fructose may increase fasting triglyceride and VLDL, and can cause gastrointestinal disturbances when taken in large amounts, and concerns have also been expressed regarding protein fructosylation. Thus, while there is no concern about fructose which occurs naturally (e.g. in fruits) there is at present no strong case to suggest

Table 4 Indices of glycaemic control from diurnal profiles for IDDM patients. Similar results were observed in NIDDM patients

	Plasma glucose (mmol/l)	
	Control diet	Sucrose diet
Fasting	10.5 ± 1.8	10.3 ± 1.5
Preprandial mean	10.5 ± 1.3	10.0 ± 1.3
Incremental postprandial mean	3.3 ± 0.7	3.7 ± 0.8
Mean daily	11.4 ± 1.0	11.4 ± 1.2
HbA_1 (%)	9.9 ± 0.3	10.3 ± 0.6

that fructose has advantages over sucrose as a nutritive sweetener for people with diabetes [49–52]. The same is probably also true of other nutritive sweeteners, including sugar alcohols such as sorbitol and xylitol, which have been recommended because they have lower glycaemic responses than sucrose and a slightly lower energy value.

Glycaemic Index

One approach to looking at physiological responses to different types of ingested carbohydrate has been the use of the glycaemic index (GI). Classifying foods according to their GI has been suggested as an appropriate means of identifying the optimal carbohydrate-containing foods [53]. The GI has been defined as the ratio of the incremental blood glucose area after food to the corresponding area after a glucose load or portion of white bread containing an equal quantity of carbohydrate. It is usually expressed as a percentage. The suggestion is that foods with a low GI may be the most appropriate carbohydrate-containing foods for people with diabetes; regular use of such foods has also been shown to improve glycaemic control over a period of several weeks.

The main objections to the GI approach were identified in a National Institutes of Health Consensus Conference on diet and exercise, and include the large individual variation in responses, lack of agreement among centres, lack of difference between mixed meals including foods of different GI, and lack of studies showing long-term benefits of low-GI foods [54]. To these might be added the fact that different researchers have used different mathematical approaches in the calculation of GI. These criticisms have been addressed in detail in three reviews [53, 55, 56]. Whilst these criticisms are acknowledged, it does appear that many of the foods with low GIs (e.g. legumes, pasta, grains such as oats and barley, cracked wheat) when incorporated into diets are associated with reduction in LDL-cholesterol and improved glycemic control. Provided that it is conceded that acceptability of food should not be determined solely on the basis of having a low GI (e.g. many high-fat foods, undesirable for other reasons, have a low GI) it seems reasonable to use GI as a means of ranking starchy foods. The GI of a range of foods is shown in Table 5. Longer-term studies in which a range of low-GI foods are recommended to patients are presently being undertaken. Studies of GI need to be carried out in different countries in order to investigate local foods, because processing as well as composition of foods, which can profoundly influence GI, differs from country to country.

Table 5 Mean glycaemic index (GI) of a range of foods studied by various investigators and adjusted so that GI of white bread = 100 (from reference 53, with permission)

Food	Mean GI
Breads	
Rye	
Crispbread	95
Wholemeal	89
Pumpernickel (wholegrain)	68
Wheat	
White	100
Wholemeal	100 ± 2
Pasta	
Macaroni	64
Spaghetti	38–61
Cereal grains	
Barley	31
Buckwheat	74
Bulgar	65
Millet	103
Breakfast cereals	
All Bran	74 ± 1
Cornflakes	115 ± 4
Porridge oats	87 ± 6
Weetabix	109
Root vegetables	
Potatoes	
Mashed	100
Boiled (new)	80 ± 7
Sweet	70
Yam	74
Legumes	
Canned baked beans	60
Butter beans	46
Chick peas	49
Green peas	65
Haricot beans	57 ± 10
Kidney beans	45 ± 11
Red lentils	37 ± 6
Soya beans (dried)	20
Fruit	
Apple	53
Banana	84 ± 7
Orange	
Whole	59 ± 8
Juice	67
Dairy products	
Skimmed milk	46
Whole milk	49
Yoghurt	52

DIETARY PROTEIN

The WHO recommends 0.6 g/kg/day of protein as a safe intake, although it is clear that measured intakes are frequently greater than this in diabetes. The low-carbohydrate diabetic dietary prescription of the past was associated with relatively high intakes of protein (as much as 20% or more of total energy). There is now a reasonable body of evidence to suggest that reducing protein intake to the levels recommended by the WHO can reduce albuminuria and improve renal haemodynamics in IDDM patients with incipient and established nephropathy [57–62]. Such diets do not necessarily worsen blood glucose control [63], and protein undernutrition appears only to occur during the first three months [64]. In patients with advanced nephropathy the benefits of even very-low-protein diets are more limited [65]. While there is limited evidence concerning the extent to which partial or total substitution of animal protein by vegetable protein may reduce proteinuria [66], vegetable proteins are generally less bioavailable, and more vegetarian-type diets may allow liberalization of overall protein intake in those with early nephropathy. Overall, while there is no confirmation of early suggestions that a high-protein diet contributes to the pathogenesis of early diabetic nephropathy, there is certainly no need for a high-protein diet among people with diabetes in general.

DISTRIBUTION OF ENERGY FROM MACRONUTRIENTS

The major dietary restriction is that of saturated and *trans*-unsaturated fatty acids to no more than 10% total energy or 8% if LDL-cholesterol is raised. If energy restriction is not required (i.e. if BMI is in the satisfactory range) the lost energy may be replaced by either an increase in *cis*-mono-unsaturated fatty acids from vegetable sources (e.g. olive oil, canola) or carbohydrates rich in soluble fibre; both these nutrients have a wide acceptable range of intakes (*cis*-mono-unsaturated fatty acid 10–20% total energy, total carbohydrates 50–60% total energy). This involves a restriction of fatty meat and meat products as well as high-fat dairy products, confectionery and high-fat manufactured foods, which are replaced by mono-unsaturated vegetable oils and spreads and fibre-rich carbohydrate derived from a range of lightly processed cereals, pulses, vegetables and fruits. Such substitution will ensure that sucrose remains well below the maximum recommended intake (10% of total energy), and the overall distribution of macronutrients is no different from that widely advised for the population as a whole in countries with high CHD risk. For those who are overweight it is appropriate to recommend only partial replacement of energy lost by reduced intake of saturated and *trans*-unsaturated fatty acids.

MICRONUTRIENTS: VITAMINS AND MINERALS

A whole range of micronutrients have at one time or another been the focus of attention in diabetes. In particular chromium, zinc and magnesium have received special attention. However, apart from the possibility of chromium deficiency leading to glucose intolerance in association with inappropriate parenteral nutrition prescriptions, the occasional need for magnesium replacement in patients with persistently poor diabetes control (associated with osmotic diuresis) or those on diuretic therapy, and the possibility that zinc supplementation may occasionally aid the healing of venous leg ulcers, there is little evidence that those with diabetes have different requirements for vitamins and minerals than those who do not have diabetes [67]. Nonetheless, because of the increased frequency of hypertension and the increased cardiovascular risk in diabetes, advice concerning some micronutrients is especially relevant. As in the general population, people with diabetes should be advised to restrict sodium intake to under 6 g/day. Those with even modestly raised blood pressure should be encouraged to aim for an intake of 3 g/day or less [68]. Increased potassium intake and sometimes supplementation is particularly important when those with diabetes are treated with thiazide and loop-acting diuretics, whereas hyperkalaemia requiring dietary restriction may occur in those taking potassium-sparing diuretics, ACE inhibitors or in patients with renal failure.

There is powerful epidemiological evidence that a range of antioxidant nutrients (e.g. tocopherols, carotenoids, vitamin C, flavenoids) protect against CHD and certain cancers in non-diabetic people. There is a disturbed equilibrium between pro- and anti-oxidants in diabetes and there is no doubt that increased oxidative stress can adversely influence cardiovascular risk (e.g. increased oxidation of low-density lipoproteins). In the past many people with diabetes may have had a low intake of dietary anti-oxidants as a result of restriction of fruit and some vegetables. Although no intervention studies have been carried out in people with diabetes, the circumstantial evidence is sufficiently strong to recommend an increase in foods rich in anti-oxidant nutrients (a wide range of vegetables and fruits). Pharmacological doses of some of these nutrients have been shown to influence risk indicators in diabetes, but the evidence is insufficient to routinely recommend supplements at present [69–71].

ALCOHOL

The same caution regarding alcohol intake which applies to the general population applies to those with diabetes. Alcohol consumption should be eliminated as far as possible in those with hypertriglyceridaemia, those who are overweight and those with hypertension. When alcohol is taken by those on insulin or tablets, it should be taken with meals because of its potentially profound hypoglycaemic effect, which can be prolonged or delayed. There is evidence, principally in people who do not have diabetes, that a modest intake of alcohol, in particular wine, may reduce cardiovascular risk because of a beneficial effect on HDL-cholesterol, reduced coagulability, and reduced lipid oxidation. For those who choose to drink alcohol and do not have the complications listed above, a quantity equivalent to two glasses of wine/day is acceptable [72, 73].

SWEETENERS

A range of non-nutritive sweeteners (including saccharin, aspartame, cyclamate, acesulphame K) are available and may be useful in drinks and for cooking. Aspartame may be considered in this category, although it is a dipeptide, because it is so intensely sweet that only minute quantities are required. These sweeteners provide a useful means of reducing energy intake.

Several nutritive sweeteners (notably fructose and sorbitol) have been recommended for use by people with diabetes when required in baking as an alternative to sucrose. They are also used extensively in so-called 'diabetic foods'. They generally have the same energy content as sucrose and may be associated with untoward effects (e.g. in large quantities fructose may cause hypertriglyceridaemia and diarrhoea). However, while they have no proven advantage over sucrose, moderate intakes (up to a maximum of 50 g/day) do not appear to have adverse gastrointestinal or metabolic effects.

'Diabetic foods' are not an essential part of the diabetic diet. Some may be convenient, but they are usually expensive and often relatively high in energy. Low-calorie and sugar-free drinks usually contain no nutritive sweeteners and are useful for many people with diabetes.

IMPLEMENTATION OF DIET THERAPY

The diabetic dietary prescription often involves a major change in lifestyle, and physicians are rarely competent

Table 6 Guidelines for optimal food choices

Eat regularly (foods high in soluble fibre and especially beneficial are marked*)	Eat in moderate amounts		Avoid (foods in this column are high in saturated fat and/or sugar)
	More often	Occasionally	
Pulses			
*Beans, e.g. baked, red kidney, haricot, black-eyed, soya *Lentils *Chick-peas		Nuts—peanuts	
Fruit and vegetables			
*Fruit (with skin where possible) Peas, sweetcorn, potatoes (with skin) Fresh or frozen vegetables of all kinds, e.g. carrots, cauliflower, cabbage, spinach, frozen beans, parsnips, etc. All salad vegetables, e.g. tomato, cucumber, radish, celery, etc.	Fruit canned in water or in fruit juice	Dried fruit Nuts, e.g. walnuts, Brazil nuts, almonds Fruit juice Chips or roast vegetables cooked in polyunsaturated fats	Canned sweetened fruit Crystallized fruit Crisps, chips or vegetables cooked in dripping or lard
Cereals			
Wholemeal bread and rolls Wholemeal biscuits, e.g. crispbread Wholegrain cereals, e.g. Allbran, Weetabix, unsweetened muesli Brown rice Wholemeal pasta Wholemeal flour *Oats, e.g. porridge, oatcakes, oatmeal		White bread White flour Unsweetened breakfast cereals e.g. Special K, rice bubbles, cornflakes, Krispies Pudding cereals, e.g. sago, custard powder	Sugar-coated breakfast cereals, e.g. Sugar Puffs, Frosties, Coco Pops Croissants, brioches
Meat and fish			
	Lean meat Poultry White fish Tinned fish Shellfish		Meat fat Poultry fat Duck, goose Fried fish Fish and meat paté Luncheon meat Corned beef Fatty bacon
Dairy foods			
Low-fat Quark Skimmed milk Cottage cheese Curd cheese Low-fat/low-sugar yoghurt	Medium fat cheeses, e.g. mozzarella, Gouda, Edam, Brie Egg whites	Cheddar and blue cheeses Whole milk Plain ice cream Whole eggs or egg yolk	Cream, cream cheese, condensed milk, full-fat sweetened yoghurt

continued overleaf

Table 6   (*continued*)

Eat regularly (foods high in soluble fibre and especially beneficial are marked*)	Eat in moderate amounts		Avoid (foods in this column are high in saturated fat and/or sugar)
	More often	Occasionally	
Fats and oils			
	cis mono-unsaturated or polyunsaturated oils or margarine	Butter	Lard, suet, dripping Oils: coconut palm oil, hydrogenated fats and oils
Made-up dishes			
Vegetable or clear soups		Pastry made with polyunsaturated margarine Plain biscuits	Pork pie, sausage-rolls, pastry
			Sweet pastries Desserts Cream soups and sauces
Drinks, etc.			
Tea or coffee Tomato juice, sugar-free drinks, e.g. soda water, sugar-free squashes Sugar-free sweeteners Herbs and spices		Spirits, beer, dry wine and sherry Champagne French dressing made with olive or polyunsaturated oils	Irish coffee, drinking chocolate, malted milk Sweet wine, liqueurs, sweet sherry Sweetened fruit drink, sweetened fizzy drinks
Sweets and preserves			
Marmite, Vegemite		Jam, marmalade	Sugar, glucose, honey, syrup, treacle Boiled sweets Lemon curd, mincemeat Chocolates, fudge, butterscotch

Table prepared by Alex Chisholm, Registered Dietitian, Otago University.

to be the sole providers of appropriate advice. The help of an experienced dietitian is important in order to give the individual help required by the great majority of patients. Where a dietitian is not available, a trained nurse specialist can provide valuable assistance. The diet must be tailored to suit individual and family food, culture, and economic and cooking conditions. The techniques of implementation differ from country to country. For example, in the UK patients with NIDDM are usually provided with dietary principles, and guidelines as to how they might be implemented. Sometimes precise energy intakes are advised, but frequently even this is achieved by the provision of lists including foods to be eaten regularly, to be taken in moderation and to be avoided. Such lists also facilitate recommendations concerning the relative proportions of macronutrients, and an example is shown in Table 6. Carbohydrate exchanges are used only for patients on insulin. Those on oral therapy are simply advised to have regular meals. In other countries a more prescriptive approach is used. Precise energy intakes are prescribed and carbohydrate exchange lists are

used for those on insulin as well as some NIDDM patients on sulphonylureas. There are unfortunately few comparative studies of different techniques of implementing dietary advice.

Whereas advice for older people may concentrate on energy balance and restriction of rapidly absorbed carbohydrate, younger people are encouraged to pay attention to all aspects of the recommendations. Exchange systems are still widely recommended for insulin-requiring patients who need to ensure consistency and regularity of carbohydrate intake to balance injected insulin and exercise. Exchange lists are at present being developed which encourage patients to select the most beneficial carbohydrate-containing foods.

New techniques of food preparation often need to be learned. The provision of recipes and cookery demonstrations are helpful aids to compliance and it is very helpful if other family members can be persuaded to eat the same meals. With appropriate and enthusiastic instruction, many diabetic patients can be persuaded to make the changes which are often more effective than oral hypoglycaemic therapy in improving

Table 7 A sample eating plan for a patient requiring 2200 kcal/day. Carbohydrate provides 58%, protein 16% and fat 26% of total energy

Breakfast	
Porridge	200 g
Milk	200 ml
Sugar	10 g
Toast	80 g
Margarine	10 g
Mid-morning	
Bran muffin	×1
Margarine	5 g
Mid-day	
Home-made vegetable soup	250 ml
Barley	50 g
Bread roll	90 g
Margarine	10 g
Jam	10 g
Macaroni cheese	100 g
Lettuce	20 g
Orange	100 g
Mid-afternoon	
Fruit bread	60 g
Evening	
Beef stew	100 g
Haricot beans	50 g
Potatoes	140 g
Peas	75 g
Carrots	100 g
Apple charlotte	1 serving
Milk	400 ml
Before bed	
Banana	100 g
Bread	50 g
Margarine	5 g
Energy	2200 kcal
Carbohydrate	58% of total energy
Protein	16%
Fat	26%
Saturated fat 7%, Polyunsaturated fat 8%, Mono-unsaturated fat 11%	
Fibre	20 g per 1000 kcal
Sugar and jam	20 g total

Sample diet prepared by Alex Chisholm, Registered Dietitian, Otago University.

glycaemic control and blood lipids. A daily meal plan complying with current dietary recommendations is shown in Table 7.

REFERENCES

1. Diabetes and Nutrition Study Group of the European Association for the Study of Diabetes. Nutritional recommendations for individuals with diabetes mellitus. Diabet Nutr Metab 1995; 8: 1–4.
2. American Diabetes Association. Nutrition recommendations and principles for people with diabetes mellitus. Diabetes Care 1994; 17: 519–22.
3. Franz MJ, Horton ES Sr, Bantle JP, Beebe CA, Brunzell JD, Coulston AM et al. Nutrition principles for the management of diabetes and related complications. Diabetes Care 1994; 17: 490–518.
4. Goldstein DJ. Beneficial health effects of modest weight loss. Int. J Obesity 1992; 16: 397–415.
5. Yudkin JS. How can we best prolong life? The benefits of coronary risk factor reduction in non-diabetic and diabetic subjects. Br Med J 1993; 306: 1313–18.
6. Prewitt TE, Schmeisser D, Bowen PE, Aye P, Dolecek TA, Langenberg, P et al. Changes in body weight, body composition, and energy intake in women fed high- and low-fat diets. Am J Clin Nutr 1991; 54: 304–10.
7. Miller WC, Linderman AK, Wallace J, Niederpruem M. Diet composition, energy intake, and exercise in relation to body fat in men and women. Am J Clin Nutr 1990; 52: 426–30.
8. Dreon DM, Frey-Hewitt B, Ellsworth N, Williams PT, Terry RB, Wood PD. Dietary fat : carbohydrate ratio and obesity in middle-aged men. Am J Clin Nutr 1988; 47: 995–1000.
9. Henry RR, Wallace P, Olefsky JM. Effects of weight loss on mechanisms of hyperglycaemia in obese non-insulin dependent diabetes mellitus. Diabetes 1986; 35: 990.
10. Henry RR, Schaeffer L, Olefsky JM. Glycaemic effects of intensive calorie restriction and iso-caloric refeeding in non-insulin dependent diabetes mellitus. J Clin Invest 1985; 61: 917.
11. Henry RR, Wiest-Kent TA, Schaeffer L et al. Metabolic consequences of very-low-calorie diet therapy in obese non-insulin dependent diabetic and non-diabetic subjects. Diabetes 1986; 35: 155.
12. Olefsky J, Reaven GM, Farquhar JW. Effects of weight reduction on obesity: studies of lipid and carbohydrate metabolism in normal and hyperlipidaemic subjects. J Clin Invest 1974; 53: 64.
13. Kern PA, Trozzolino L, Wolfe G, Purdy L. Combined use of behaviour modification and very-low-calorie diet in weight loss and weight maintenance. Am J Med Sci 1994; 307: 325–8.
14. Anderson JW, Hamilton CC, Brinkman-Kaplan V. Benefits and risks of an intensive very-low-calorie diet program for severe obesity. Am J Gastroenterol 1992; 87: 6–15.
15. Wing RR, Marcus MD, Blair EH, Burton LR. Psychological responses of obese type 2 diabetic subjects to very-low-calorie diet. Diabetes Care 1991; 14: 596–9.
16. Henry RR, Gumbiner B. Benefits and limitations of very-low-calorie diet therapy in obese NIDDM. Diabetes Care 1991; 14: 802–23.
17. Hughes VA, Fiatarone MA, Fielding RA, Kahn BB et al. Exercise increases muscle Glut-levels and insulin action in subjects with impaired glucose tolerance. Am J Physiol 1993; 264: E855–62.
18. Barnard RJ, Ugianskis EJ, Martin DA, Inkeles SB. Role of diet and exercise in the management of hyperinsulinemia and associated atherosclerotic risk factors. Am J Cardiol 1992; 69: 440–44.
19. Moy CS, Songer TJ, LaPorte RE et al. Insulin dependent diabetes mellitus, physical activity and death. Am J Epid 1993; 137: 74–81.
20. Zock PL, de Vries HM, Katan MB. Impact of myristic acid versus palmitic acid on serum lipid and lipoprotein levels in healthy women and men. Arterioscler Thromb 1994; 14: 567–75.

21. Mensink RP, Katan MB. Effect of dietary *trans* fatty acids on high-density lipoprotein cholesterol levels in healthy subjects. New Engl J Med 1990; 323: 439–45.

22. Zock PL, Katan MB. Hydrogenation alternatives: effects of *trans* fatty acids and stearic acid versus linoleic acid on serum lipids and lipoprotein in humans. J Lipid Res 1992; 33: 399–410.

23. Mensink RP, Zock PL, Katan MB, Hornstra G. Effect of dietary *cis* and *trans* fatty acids on serum lipoprotein(a) levels in humans. J Lipid Res 1992; 33: 1493–1501.

24. Nestel P, Noakes M, Belling B, McArthur R, Clifton P, Janus E, Abbey M. Plasma lipoprotein lipid and Lp(a) changes with substitution of elaidic acid for oleic acid in the diet. J Lipid Res 1992; 33: 1029–36.

25. Willett WC, Stampfer MJ, Manson JE, Colditz GA et al. Intake of *trans* fatty acids and risk of coronary heart disease among women. Lancet 1993; 341: 581–5.

26. Foley M, Ball M, Chisholm A, Duncan A, Spears G, Mann J. Should mono- or polyunsaturated fats replace saturated fat in the diet? European J Clin Nutr 1992; 46: 429–36.

27. Rillaerts EG, Engelmann GJ, van Camp KM, De Leeuw I. Effect of omega-3 fatty acids in diet of type 1 diabetic subjects on lipid values and haemorrheological parameters. Diabetes 1989; 38: 1412–16.

28. Popp-Snijders C, Schouten JA, Heine RJ, van der Meer J, van der Veen EA. Dietary supplementation of omega-3 polyunsaturated fatty acids improves insulin sensitivity in non-insulin dependent diabetes. Diabetes Res 1987; 4: 141–7.

29. Jones DB, Haitas B, Bown EG, Carter RD, Barker K, Jelfs R, Turner RC, Mann JI, Prescott RJ. Platelet aggregation in non-insulin dependent diabetes in association with platelet fatty acids. Diabetic Medicine 1986; 3: 52–5.

30. Mori, TA, Vandongen R, Masarei JR, Stanton KG, Dunbar D. Dietary fish oil increases serum lipids in insulin-dependent diabetes compared with healthy controls. Metabolism 1989; 38: 404–9.

31. Schetchman G, Kaul S, Kissebah AH. Effect of fish oil concentrate on lipoprotein composition in NIDDM. Diabetes 1988; 37: 1567–73.

32. Garg A, Bonanome A, Grundy SM, Zhang Z-J, Unger RH. Comparison of a high-carbohydrate diet with a high-monounsaturated-fat diet in patients with non-insulin dependent diabetes mellitus. New Engl J Med 1988; 391: 829–34.

33. Garg A, Reaven GM, Bantle JP, Griver K. Multi centre diet study group. Long-term effects of high carbohydrate versus high MUFA diets in NIDDM. Diabetes 1992; 41 (suppl. 1): 72A.

34. Parillo M, Rivellese AA, Ciardullo AV, Capaldo B, Giacco A, Genovese S, Riccardi G. A high-monoun-saturated-fat/low-carbohydrate diet improves peripheral insulin sensitivity in non-insulin dependent diabetic patients. Metabolism 1992; 41: 1373–8.

35. Mann JI. Diet and diabetes. Diabetologia 1980; 18: 89–95.

36. Kiehm TG, Anderson JW, Ward K. Beneficial effects of a high carbohydrate, high fibre diet on hyperglycaemic men. Am J Clin Nutr 1976; 29: 895–9.

37. Jenkins DJA, Wolever TMS, Haworth R, Leeds AR, Hockaday TDR. Guar gum in diabetes. Lancet 1976; 2: 1086–7.

38. Jenkins DJA, Leeds AR, Gassull MA, Cochet B, Alberti KGMM. Decrease in postprandial insulin and glucose concentrations for guar and pectin. Ann Intern Med 1977; 86: 20–23.

39. Aro A, Uusitupa M, Voutilainen E et al. Improved diabetic control and hypocholesterolaemic effect induced by long-term supplementation with guar in type 2 diabetics. Diabetologia 1981; 21: 29.

40. Vinik AI, Jenkins DJA. Dietary fibre in the management of diabetes. Diabetes Care 1988; 11: 160–73.

41. Peterson DB, Mann JI. Guar: pharmacological fibre or food fibre? Diabet Med 1985; 2: 345–7.

42. Lousley, SE, Jones DB, Slaughter P, Carter RD, Jelfs R, Mann JI. High carbohydrate/high fibre diets in poorly controlled diabetes. Diabet Med 1984; 1: 21–5.

43. Riccardi G, Rivellese A, Pacioni D, Genovese D, Mastranzo P, Mancini M. Separate influence of dietary carbohydrate and fibre on the metabolic control in diabetes. Diabetologia 1984; 26: 116–21.

44. Simpson HCR, Carter RD, Lousley S, Mann JI. Digestible carbohydrate—an independent effect on diabetic control in type 2 (non-insulin dependent) diabetic patients? Diabetologia 1982; 23: 235–9.

45. Simpson HCR, Simpson RW, Lousley S, Carter RD, Geekie M, Hockaday TD, Mann JI. A high carbohydrate leguminous fibre diet improves all aspects of diabetic control. Lancet 1981; 1: 1–5.

46. Geekie MA, Porteous J, Hockaday TDR, Mann JI. Acceptability of high-fibre diets in diabetic patients. Diabet Med 1986; 3: 52–5.

47. McCulloch DK, Mitchell RD, Ambler J, Tattersall RB. A prospective comparison of 'conventional' and high carbohydrate/high fibre/low fat diets in adults with established type 1 (insulin-dependent) diabetes. Diabetologia 1985; 28: 208.

48. Peterson DB, Lambert J, Gerring S et al. Sucrose in the diabetic diet—just another carbohydrate? Diabet Med 1986; 2: 345.

49. Anderson JW, Story LJ, Zettwoch NC, Gustafson NJ, Jefferson BS. Metabolic effects of fructose supplementation in diabetic individuals. Diabetes Care 1989; 12: 337–44.

50. Crapo PA, Kolterman OG, Henry RR. Metabolic consequence of two-week fructose feeding in diabetic subjects. Diabetes Care 1986; 9: 111–19.

51. Born P, Eimiller A, Paul F. High rate of gastrointestinal side effects in fructose-consuming patients. Diabetes Care 1987; 10: 376–7.

52. Dills WL. Protein fructosylation: fructose and the Maillard reaction. Am J Clin Nutr 1993; 58 (suppl.): 779S–87S.

53. Jenkins DJA, Wolever TMS, Jenkins AL. Starchy foods and glycemic index. Diabetes Care 1988; 11: 149–59.

54. Kolata G. Diabetics should lose weight, avoid fad diets. Science 1987; 235; 163–4.

55. Thorburn AW, Brand JC, Truswell AS. The glycaemic index of foods. Med J Austr 1986; 144: 580–82.

56. Gannon MC, Nuttall FQ. Factors affecting interpretation of postprandial glucose and insulin areas. Diabetes Care 1987; 10: 754–63.

57. Dullaart RP, Beusekamp BJ, Meijer S, van-Doormaal JJ, Sluiter WJ. Long-term effects of protein-restricted diet on albuminuria and renal function in IDDM patients without clinical nephropathy and hypertension. Diabetes Care 1993; 16: 483–92.

58. Jones SL, Kontessis P, Wiseman M, Dodds R, Bognetti E, Pinto J, Viberti G. Protein intake and blood

glucose as modulators of GFR in hyperfiltering diabetic patients. Kidney Int 1992; 41: 1620–8.

59. Keller K, Whittaker E, Sullivan L, Raskin P, Jacobson HR. Effect of restricting dietary protein on the progression of renal failure in patients with insulin-dependent diabetes mellitus. New Engl J Med 1991; 324: 78–84.

60. Evanoff G, Thompson C, Brown J, Weinman E. Prolonged dietary protein restriction in diabetic nephropathy. Arch Intern Med 1989; 149: 1129–33.

61. Walker JD, Bending JJ, Dodds RA, Mattock MB, Murrells TJ, Keen H, Viberti GC. Restriction of dietary protein and progression of renal failure in diabetic nephropathy. Lancet 1989; 2(8677): 1411–15.

62. Ciavarella A, Di Mizio G, Stefoni S et al. Reduced albuminuria after dietary protein restriction in insulin dependent diabetic patients with clinical nephropathy. Diabetes Care 1987; 10: 407.

63. Pomerleau J, Verdy M, Garrel DR, Nadeau MH. Effect of protein intake on glycaemic control and renal function in type 2 (non-insulin dependent) diabetes mellitus. Diabetologia 1993; 36: 829–34.

64. Brodsky IG, Robbins DC, Hiser E, Fuller SP, Fillyaw M, Devlin JT. Effects of low-protein diets on protein metabolism in insulin-dependent diabetes mellitus patients with early nephropathy. J Clin Endocrinol Metab 1992; 75: 351–7.

65. Klahr S, Levey AS, Beck GJ, Caggiula AW, Hunsicker L, Kusek JW, Striker G. The effects of dietary protein restriction and blood-pressure control on the progression of chronic renal disease. Modification of Diet in Renal Disease Study Group. New Engl J Med 1994; 330: 877–84.

66. Jibani MM, Bloodworth LL, Foden E, Griffiths KD, Galpin OP. Predominantly vegetarian diet in patients with incipient and early clinical diabetic nephropathy: effects on albumin excretion rate and nutritional status. Diabet Med 1991; 8: 949–53.

67. Walter RM, Uriu-Hare JY, Lewis Olin K, Oster MH, Anawalt BD, Critchfield JW, Keen CL. Copper, zinc, manganese, and magnesium status and complications of diabetes mellitus. Diabetes Care 1991; 14: 1050–56.

68. American Diabetes Association. Treatment of hypertension in diabetes: consensus statement. Diabetes Care 1993; 16: 1394–1401.

69. Rimm EB, Stampfer MJ, Ascherio A, Giovannucci E. Colditz GA, Willett WC. Vitamin E consumption and risk of coronary heart disease in men. New Engl J Med 1993; 328: 1450–6.

70. Paolisso G, D'Amore A, Galzerano D, Balbi V et al. Daily vitamin E supplements improve metabolic control but not insulin secretion in elderly type 2 diabetic patients. Diabetes Care 1993; 16: 1433–7.

71. Ceriello A, Guigliano D, Quatraro A, Donzella C, Dipalo G, Lefebvre PJ. Vitamin E reduction of protein glycosylation in diabetes. Diabetes Care 1991; 14: 68–72.

72. Christiansen C, Thomsen C, Rasmussen O, Balle M, Hauerslev C, Hansen C, Hermansen K. Wine for type 2 diabetic patients? Diabet Med 1993; 10: 958–61.

73. Koivisto VA, Tulokas S, Toivonen M, Haapa E, Pelkonen R. Alcohol with a meal has no adverse effects on post-prandial glucose homeostasis in diabetic patients. Diabetes Care 1993; 16: 1612–14.

34b

Dietary Management of Diabetes Mellitus in India and South East Asia

A. Ramachandran and M. Viswanathan

Diabetes Research Centre, Madras, India

DIETARY THERAPY IN DIABETES MELLITUS—A HISTORICAL BACKGROUND

Attempts to alleviate diabetes mellitus by diet were first made by the Egyptians as early as 3500 BC. In India, about 2500 years ago, Susruta and Charaka had recognized the importance of dietary regulation in the treatment of diabetes and many of the principles suggested by these eminent physicians hold good even today. They adopted measures to correct obesity in subjects with diabetes, advised feeding of lean diabetic individuals and prohibited the use of sugar, jaggery (unrefined cane sugar), wines, ghee (clarified butter), butter and meat [1].

In the eighteenth century, John Rollo [2] observed that glycosuria could be decreased by moderation in the quantity of food taken by diabetic individuals and by restriction of the diet to animal foods. In the twentieth century, prior to the discovery of insulin, the treatment of diabetes mellitus included intermittent fasting, undernutrition and carbohydrate restriction. With the advent of insulin and the oral hypoglycaemic drugs, there was a tendency to prescribe liberal diets. Nevertheless, several long-term studies have unequivocally proved the prime importance of a calorie-restricted well-balanced diet in the treatment of diabetes.

Dietary Pattern in India and South East Asia

For the acceptance of a diet and adherence to it by a diabetic individual, it is necessary that the diet advised closely resembles that to which he and his family are accustomed. A high degree of patient acceptability ensures long-term compliance and thus, better metabolic control. This helps in achieving the main objective of successful dietary therapy in diabetes. Fortunately, the food consumption patterns seen in India and other countries of South East Asia do not present any major obstacles to acceptance of the diet prescribed for a diabetic subject.

Data available from the National Nutritional Monitoring Bureau (NNMB) show that in recent years in India there has been a moderate increase in the average energy consumption from 2000 kcal to 2400 kcal/person/day, which has been attributed mainly to an increased intake of rice and vegetables with no appreciable change in the intake of sugar and fats (oils) [3]. There is a fairly consistent and comparable pattern of consumption of food which is mainly cereal-based, with rice and wheat being consumed as the staple items of food in the southern and northern states of India, respectively.

Determination of the proximate principles in the food indicates that 70–75% of the total energy intake is being derived from complex carbohydrates, 12% from proteins and 14% from fats. The common Indian diet is made up of whole-grain cereals, pulses (legumes), leafy vegetables, fruits, milk and milk products. The majority of the population in India are vegetarians, and even in so-called non-vegetarians the actual intake of meat, eggs and poultry is restricted to once or twice a week. Vegetable oils are the main source of fat. The

International Textbook of Diabetes Mellitus, Second Edition. Edited by K.G.M.M. Alberti, P. Zimmet, R.A. DeFronzo, and H. Keen (Honorary)
© 1997 John Wiley & Sons Ltd

Table 1 Proximate principles in the common pulses and legumes used in the Indian diet*

Foodstuff	Protein (N × 6.25) (g)	Fat (g)	Minerals (g)	Fibre (g)	Carbohydrates (g)	Energy (kcal)
Bengal gram, dhal	30.8	5.6	2.2	1.2	59.8	372
Black gram, dhal	24.0	1.4	3.2	0.9	59.6	347
Green gram, dhal	24.5	1.2	3.5	0.8	59.9	348
Lentil	25.1	0.7	2.1	0.7	59.0	343
Moth beans	23.6	1.1	3.5	4.5	56.5	330
Peas, green	7.2	0.1	0.8	4.0	15.9	93
Rajmah	22.9	1.3	3.2	(4.8)	60.6	346
Red gram, dhal	22.3	1.7	3.5	1.5	57.6	335
Soyabean	43.2	19.5	4.6	3.7	20.9	432

*All values are per 100 g of edible portion.

traditional diet of the majority of the population in India and South East Asia is rich in whole-grain cereals and complex carbohydrates, low in animal proteins and saturated fats, and rich in unsaturated fats from vegetable oils. The overall energy content is fairly restricted, with a high intake of fibre-rich food and a low intake of free sugar.

DIET IN THE MANAGEMENT OF DIABETES MELLITUS

The importance of the diet in the management of diabetes has been recognized for centuries. Diet is the main pillar in the treatment and control of diabetes, but successful dietary therapy depends as much on the patient as on the physician. Although dietary goals are often dismissed as impossible to achieve, intensive education and motivation of the diabetic patient has convinced us that dietary therapy can be successful. Furthermore, the traditional diets consumed in India offer specific advantages in the dietary management of diabetes.

The Evolution of the High-carbohydrate High-fibre Diet

In the late 1950s, the diet advised for diabetic patients was based on the Western diet pattern, in which a marked reduction in carbohydrate content and a high fat intake were advised. This restricted carbohydrate diet provided only about 33% of the calories from carbohydrate. Such a diet was not suitable for the Indian diabetic patient, as the diet of an average Indian has very high carbohydrate content. For better and sustained dietary compliance, the Indian diabetic patient had to be given enough carbohydrate in his diet. The only advice given at that time was to avoid free sugar completely and reduce the total intake of calories in the diet. As early as 1958, Viswanathan and his co-workers evolved the 'High Carbohydrate Diet', which provided

about 60% of the calories in the form of complex carbohydrates [4]. Contrary to existing beliefs, the diet did not worsen carbohydrate tolerance, neither was the control of diabetes difficult. Indeed, the dose of drugs required to control diabetes was very small [5]. The diet was further modified around 1968 by increasing the protein content to 20% and reducing the fat content to 13% [6]. As the traditional Indian diet is vegetarian, the protein content of the diabetic diet was increased by increasing the content of pulses and legumes. Table 1 shows the proximate principles in some of the commonly used pulses and legumes, the most popular of which are bengal gram, green gram and black gram. This change further increased the fibre content of the diet. Analysis showed that the diet provided 52 g of fibre, which is almost double that in the standard American Diabetes Association diet. Hence the diet is now called 'The high-carbohydrate high-fibre (HCHF) diet' (Table 2).

Table 2 Composition of the high-carbohydrate high-fibre (HCHF) diet of the Diabetes Research Centre, Madras, for a patient requiring 1800 kcal/day

	Weight (g)	Energy (kcal)
Carbohydrate	301	1204(67%)
Protein	86	344(19%)
Fat	28	252(14%)

*From reference 6, with permission.

Our observations on a large number of patients in the Diabetes Research Centre, Madras, seen during the last three decades show that the diet is acceptable to the patients, which ensures long-term compliance [7, 8]. There is rapid and sustained control of hyperglycaemia [5] with lowering of plasma cholesterol and triglyceride levels [9]. It does not reduce the level of HDL-cholesterol, the protective factor for cardiovascular complications [10], and it improves peripheral sensitivity to insulin [11].

Principles of the HCHF Diet

The total calories advised will vary with each patient. The calories are restricted much more in the obese patient who is required to reduce his body weight. Carbohydrates are mainly derived from cereals like rice and wheat. Refined sugars are totally prohibited. Proteins prescribed are mainly vegetable proteins derived from pulses (legumes) like bengal gram, green gram and black gram, and fresh vegetables. The proteins of cereals and pulses have mutual supplementary effects, a deficiency of any particular amino acid in the one being made good by an excess in the other if both are consumed at the same time. The fat content of the diet is restricted to the oil used in cooking. By prescribing vegetables containing 3–4% carbohydrate, like greens, cucumber, drumstick, bitter gourd, banana flower, banana stem, cabbage, cauliflower and ash pumpkin, the bulk of the meal is increased and the patient's hunger satisfied without appreciably increasing the total calories.

Therapeutic Benefits of Dietary Fibre in the Indian Diet

Dietary fibre comprises those components of plant cells, which are present as part of the diet yet are resistant to digestive secretions of the gastrointestinal tract. It is not a single entity but includes a wide range of complex polysaccharides, consisting of a mixture of cellulose, lignin, hemicellulose, plant gums, pectins and mucin. A number of studies [12, 13] have established that intake of a high-fibre diet has definite therapeutic benefits for diabetic patients. A high-fibre diet can help the diabetic patient in reducing postprandial hyperglycaemia [14] and insulin secretion [15], and in decreasing the raised plasma lipids (triglycerides and cholesterol, particularly LDL-cholesterol), and also helps in the reduction of body weight. Although it is not entirely clear how all these effects are produced, possible mechanisms that have been suggested include (a) delayed gastric emptying time [16], (b) increased intestinal transit time, and (c) alterations in the rate and site of nutrient absorption in the gut, possibly as a result of a release of gut hormones [17].

The fact that a HCHF diet is the ideal diet for diabetic patients has gained acceptance all over the world. This is further substantiated by the recommendations made by the WHO study group in 1985 [18]. During the 1980s many Western diabetologists were recommending that high-carbohydrate diets for their patients be supplemented with artificial fibres in the form of bran, guar gum and pectins. In India, since natural foods are rich in soluble fibre, addition of artificial fibre is rarely indicated or necessary. While artificial fibres are good for research purposes, the addition of fibre-containing natural foods to the diet in communities in the developing world is preferable for achieving better metabolic control and is also cost-effective.

Dietary Protein

Dietary protein should contribute about 15% of total energy intake and is mainly derived from vegetable sources. A high-protein diet may accelerate the progression of diabetic nephropathy. Currently, a protein intake of 0.6–0.8 g/kg body weight/day is recommended for the diabetic patient [19].

Dietary Fat

Sustained hyperglycaemia and hyperlipidaemia have been implicated as factors in the aetiology of the long-term micro- and macrovascular complications of diabetes. Presence of diabetes in the absence of other risk factors has been linked to a two- to threefold increase in cardiovascular disease risk, and diabetic patients often have hypercholesterolaemia and hypertriglyceridaemia [19]. The control of plasma lipids and lipoprotein profile is a prime objective when considering the dietary management of diabetes.

It is recommended that about 15% of the total calories allowed should be derived from fats. About one-third of the total fat content of the diet can be in the form of saturated fats and the rest is to be contributed by polyunsaturated (e.g. vegetable and fish oils) and mono-unsaturated fats (e.g. olive oil). This has been found to improve the lipaemic profile, reducing atherogenic LDL-cholesterol levels and increasing the cardioprotective HDL-cholesterol levels [19].

Several reports have indicated antiatherogenic benefits of omega-3-fatty acids in normal and hyperlipidaemic individuals [20]. Increased intake of this type of fatty acid, which is widely present in some of the common food items of Indians (fish oil, wheat-germ oil, green leafy vegetables, common beans, etc.) is believed to exert a protective effect against cardiovascular diseases in diabetic individuals [21]. However, the clinical utility of omega-3-fatty acids has been questioned in relation to glucose metabolism following the demonstration of possible pro-atherogenic effects [19]. A number of reports have found that fish oil supplementation may impair overall glycaemic control in NIDDM subjects and thus negate the beneficial effects on plasma triglycerides and VLDL-cholesterol.

Meal Planning

Daily energy requirements are calculated taking into consideration the following points: (a) type of diabetes; (b) ideal body weight to be achieved and maintained;

(c) special requirements such as optimal growth and development in children; and (d) pregnancy and lactation in women. The distribution of energy intake between carbohydrates, protein and fats must closely match the distribution of these proximate principles in the traditional diet. The food exchange system practised in Western societies helps to keep the diet varied to prevent monotony, while maintaining the daily pattern of food intake. However, exchanges based on whole meals are preferable to those concentrating on the carbohydrate content of different foods. The glycaemic index may be useful as it takes into account factors which reduce absorption rate, such as the nature of the starch, fibre and antinutrients (e.g. phytate, lectins, tannins and saponins). At present, it may prove a useful addition to dietary management in identifying how particular foods might be used in the diabetic diet. A low glycaemic index staple food forming the basic and major component of each meal may offer advantages. Thus, an approximately equivalent amount of cereal, bread or rice may be suggested as a basis for a meal-planning approach to diabetic diets, together with appropriate guidelines about cooking and the use of fresh vegetables.

NUTRITIONAL COUNSELLING AND PATIENT EDUCATION FOR DIETARY COMPLIANCE

Nutritional Counselling

Effective nutritional counselling must take into consideration the social, cultural and religious aspects of food consumption. It is widely believed in the Orient that certain food items have to be restricted or totally avoided in diseased states. Therefore most patients do expect physicians to advise them regarding the food items that are to be restricted or prohibited. Physicians rarely have enough time to be the sole providers of appropriate and balanced advice on nutrition because of their heavy clinical workload. Hence experienced dietitians are essential to provide individual guidance. Training programmes and learning experiences for the health care providers constitute an essential strategy for diabetes care. Health care providers must render appropriate nutritional counselling so as to enable the diabetic patients to follow religious practices without unduly disturbing their metabolic control. Frequent intervals of follow-up, individualization of diet prescription, and family involvement are some of the factors which contribute to the success of diet therapy.

Patient Education

Patient education regarding the dietary management of diabetes mellitus in developing countries poses a variety of difficulties. The two major handicaps that one faces in patient education are (a) the existence of a multilingual society, and (b) the large number of adults with low standards of literacy [22]. Printed pamphlets and materials are of only limited use. Teaching sessions that include the use of food models that exhibit the model diet plan for an entire day, simple pictorial charts and other audio-visual aids, and demonstration of household measures for food exchanges do help in motivating the patient to achieve a high level of dietary compliance [23, 24]. Wherever possible the spouse and other family members must also take part in the education programmes. Experience at the Diabetes Research Centre, Madras has convinced us of the usefulness of this approach in Indian diabetic subjects.

CONCLUDING REMARKS

The objectives and goals of diet therapy in diabetes mellitus are: (a) to achieve and maintain normal blood glucose levels, lipid profile and ideal body weight; (b) to maintain optimal nutrition; and (c) to relieve obvious symptoms and minimize chronic degenerative vascular complications. Nutritional requirements and dietary recommendations to diabetic patients are not different from those of the general population, although the emphasis and practical approaches may be different. In our experience, as the diet in India and South East Asia is essentially cereal-based and rich in fibre, the prescription of a high-carbohydrate high-fibre diet presents few practical difficulties and dietary compliance is easily achieved. However, constant motivation through nutrition counselling and education imparted in an appropriate way goes a long way in achieving these goals.

Acknowledgements

The authors wish to thank profusely Dr L. Susheela for her assistance in the preparation of the manuscript.

REFERENCES

1. Frank LL. Diabetes mellitus in the texts of old Hindu medicine (Charaka, Susruta, Vagbhata). Am J Gastroenterol 1957; 27: 76.
2. Joslin EP. Development of the present treatment of diabetes. J Am Diet Assoc 1949; 25: 213.
3. ICMR. National Institute of Nutrition, Hyderabad—Annual Report 1985–86, pp 105–35.
4. Viswanathan M. High carbohydrate diet in diabetes. J Diab Assoc India 1968; 8: 353–60.
5. Viswanathan M, Snehalatha C, Ramachandran A, Mohan V. Rapid control of diabetes with high carbohydrate diet and combination of glibenclamide and phenformin. J Diab Assoc India 1978; 18: 119–23.

6. Viswanathan M, Ramachandran A, Mohan V, Snehalatha C. High-carbohydrate, high-fibre diet in diabetes. J Diab Assoc India 1981; 21 (suppl. 1): 90–96.

7. Viswanathan M, Mohan V, Ramachandran A, Snehalatha C, Anderson JW. Long-term experience with high carbohydrate high fibre diets in Indian diabetic patients. Diabetologia Croat 1984; 13: 163–74.

8. Viswanathan M, Snehalatha C, Ramachandran A, Mohan V. High-carbohydrate diet in diabetes: long-term experience. Proceedings of the International Diabetes Federation Congress, Vienna. Amsterdam: Excerpta Medica, 1979; p 84.

9. Viswanathan M, Snehalatha C, Ramachandran A, Mohan V, Shobana R. Effect of a calorie-restricted, high-carbohydrate, high-protein, low-fat diet on serum lipids: a follow-up study. J Assoc Phys India 1978; 26: 163–8.

10. Susheela L, Shyamsundar R, Ramachandran A, Mohan V, Viswanathan M. Favourable alterations in serum total/HDL and LDL/HDL cholesterol ratios after glucoregulation in newly diagnosed NIDDM. Diabetologia Croat 1983; 12: 17–33.

11. Viswanathan M, Snehalatha C, Ramachandran A, Mohan V. Effect of high-carbohydrate, high-fibre diet on immunoreactive insulin level in diabetes. J Diab Assoc India 1983: 23: 45–8.

12. Crapo PA, Reaven G, Olefsky J. Postprandial plasma glucose and insulin responses to different complex carbohydrates. Diabetes 1977: 26: 1178–83.

13. Crapo PA, Kolterman OG, Waldeck N, Reaven GM, Olefsky JM. Postprandial hormonal responses to different types of complex carbohydrate in individuals with impaired glucose tolerance. Am J Clin Nutr 1980; 33: 1723–8.

14. Vinik AI, Jenkins DJA. Dietary fiber in management of diabetes. Diabetes Care 1988; 11: 160–72.

15. Viswanathan M, Ramachandran A, Mohan V, Snehalatha C. Effect of ingestion of natural food fibre on glucose tolerance and plasma immunoreactive insulin response. Biomedicine 1980; 1: 43–6.

16. Holt S, Heading RC, Carter DC, Prescott LF, Tothill P. Effect of gel fibre on gastric emptying and absorption of glucose and paracetamol. Lancet 1979; i: 636–9.

17. Morgan LM, Goulder TJ, Tsiolakis D, Marks V, Alberti KGMM. The effect of unabsorbable carbohydrate on gut hormones: modification of postprandial GIP secretion by guar. Diabetologia 1979; 17: 85–9.

18. WHO Study Group. Diabetes Mellitus. Technical Report Series 727. Geneva: WHO, 1985: p 77.

19. Boctor DL, Jenkins DJA. Trends in dietary management of diabetes mellitus: an update. In Alberti KGMM, Krall LP (eds) The diabetes annual vol 6. Amsterdam; Elsevier Science, 1991: pp 105–36.

20. Stacpoole PW, Alig J, Ammon L, Crockett SE. Dose-response effects of dietary marine oil on carbohydrate and lipid metabolism in normal subjects and patients with hypertriglyceridaemia. Metabolism 1989; 38: 946–56.

21. Raheja BS. Indian diet—diabetes and its complications. IDF Bull 1988; 33: 14–7.

22. Shobana R, Indira P, Ramachandran A, Mohan V, Viswanathan M. Effectiveness of patient education in a multilingual, multiliterate population. J Med Assoc Thai 1987; 70 (suppl. 2): 219–22.

23. Bajaj JS. Dietary therapy: principles and practice. In Diabetes health care: trainers' manual for allied health professionals. Srinagar: Vishwanath Press, 1982: pp 34–7.

24. Shobana R, Premila L, Shyamala P, Mohan V, Ramachandran A, Viswanathan M. Assessment of background knowledge of diabetes mellitus in diabetic patients. J Diab Assoc India 1989; 29: 70–3.

34c

Dietary Management of Diabetes Mellitus in Japan

Shigeaki Baba

International Institute for Diabetes Education and Study, Kobe, Hyogo, Japan

When considering dietary therapy for Japanese diabetic patients, the remarkable social and environmental changes since World War II (1945) need to be understood. In particular, there have been marked changes in various demographic factors, including aging of the population, urbanization, changes in meal content and popular foods, a decrease in daily exercise, and an increase in stress. Similarly, major changes have occurred in concepts of dietary therapy for diabetes, together with the development of new pharmaceutical products, such as alpha-glucosidase inhibitors, and advances in diagnostic and investigative techniques.

In the present review, the recent changes in the Japanese diet will be summarized first and then dietary therapy for diabetic patients will be discussed with references to the guidelines of the Japanese Diabetes Society. It is of interest that the incidence of cardiovascular disease is lower in Japan than in the Western world, and this is generally thought to be at least partially attributable to the Japanese diet [1].

CHANGES IN THE JAPANESE DIET

Table 1 shows the changes in the Japanese per capita daily intake of various nutrients in the period between 1975 and 1990, based on data published by the Japanese Ministry of Health and Welfare [2]. Cereals accounted for 66.3% of the overall energy intake in 1960, decreasing gradually to 47.9% in 1988 and to 45.5% in 1990. On the other hand, the intake of animal products including fats and oils has increased considerably and now makes up a much higher percentage of the total energy intake.

Among the various nutrients, the biggest increase has been in the total intake of fats in the postwar period since 1945. Recent data show a daily per capita fat intake of 55–58 g. Vegetable fats derived from cereals and beans accounted for 42.2% of fat intake in 1955. However, this percentage had decreased to 18.1% by 1990, while fats derived from oils and animal products increased from 52.4% to 56.9%. As shown in Figure 1, the ratio of animal fats (excluding those derived from fish) to fish and vegetable fats was 0.62 in 1990 compared with 0.16 in 1955. Nonetheless this is still significantly lower than in Westernized countries. In addition, the sugar intake has been decreasing gradually, while the intake of alcohol has tended to increase recently.

These changes suggest that the traditional Japanese-style diet has been gradually changing to a Western-style diet together with various social changes.

With respect to calcium intake, the consumption of cows' milk and dairy products has increased markedly, but the total calcium intake, 550–580 mg/day, remains only 80% of the recommended level. Cows' milk, dairy products and sugar are mainly used for Western-style dishes, while the Japanese diet usually includes no milk or dairy products but typically uses soy sauce, miso (fermented soybean paste), and soup stock made from seaweed and dried small fishes. The lack of calcium in the Japanese diet may be explained by these features. In

International Textbook of Diabetes Mellitus, Second Edition. Edited by K.G.M.M. Alberti, P. Zimmet, R.A. DeFronzo, and H. Keen (Honorary)
© 1997 John Wiley & Sons Ltd

Table 1 Changes in the Japanese per capita daily intake of various nutrients between 1975 and 1990

		1975	1980	1985	1987	1989	1990
Energy	kcal	2226	2119	2088	2053	2061	2026
Protein	g	81.0	78.7	79.0	78.5	80.2	78.7
Animal protein	g	38.9	39.2	40.1	40.1	42.4	41.4
Fat	g	55.2	55.6	56.9	56.6	58.9	56.9
Animal fat	g	26.2	26.9	27.6	27.6	28.3	27.5
Carbohydrate	g	335	309	298	291	290	287
Calcium	mg	552	539	553	551	540	531
Iron	mg	10.8	10.4	10.7	10.5	11.4	11.1
Salt (Na × 2.54/1000)	g	13.5	12.9	12.1	11.7	12.2	12.5
Vitamin A	IU	1889	1986	2188	2119	2687	2567
Vitamin B1	mg	1.39	1.37	1.34	1.34	1.26	1.23
Vitamin B2	mg	1.23	1.21	1.25	1.25	1.36	1.33
Vitamin C	mg	138	123	128	122	123	120

From reference 2, with permission.

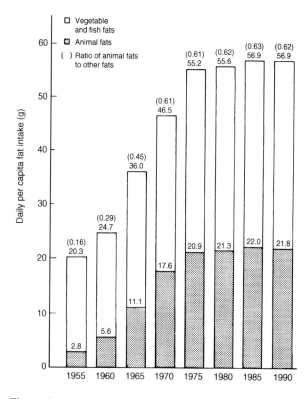

Figure 1 Changes in animal and vegetable fat content of the Japanese diet [1955–1990]. Animal fats exclude those derived from fish. Other fats includes vegetable and fish fats. Height of bars indicates total fat content. From reference 2

addition, salt intake by the Japanese is higher than the average world level, with a mean daily intake of 12.5 g.

CHANGE OF DISEASE PATTERNS AND DIET IN JAPAN

Stroke and related conditions were the leading cause of death before 1980, while cancer-related mortality became the leading cause after this time [3]. Heart disease-related mortality has increased with the aging of society, while stroke-related mortality is tending

to decline. Factors involved in these mortality trends include not only an increase in the elderly population but also a rise in serum cholesterol and triglyceride levels, an increase in obesity or overweight, a decrease in exercise, and an increase in social stresses among younger Japanese.

The number of diabetic patients continues to increase in Japan. The incidence of hepatitis, liver cirrhosis and liver cancer related to HBV or HCV (hepatitis B and C virus) infection has also increased [3], and since the increase in these diseases in unique to this country, they are sometimes called the 'national diseases'.

In 1993, the Science and Technology Agency of Japan extensively amended its List of Food Ingredients because the nutrients and vitamins contained in agricultural products and other natural foods have decreased [4]. Also, since the consumption of imported foods and synthetic foods has increased and new additives such as preservatives are being used, there have been many changes in the ingredients of various foods. In addition, the contents of cholesterol, dietary fiber, minerals and vitamins have been newly specified for a total of 1621 foods that are commonly eaten by the Japanese. Although the Japanese diet has changed remarkably, as mentioned above, it is still closer to the recommended healthy diet than is a Western-style diet.

JAPANESE DIETARY CULTURE

What is the essence of Japanese dietary culture? Food, clothing and shelter are the basic necessities of life, but these necessities have developed cultural associations which improve the quality of life. The concept of creation of a better quality of life should also be the basis for preparing a therapeutic diet.

Japanese-style cuisine is said to have developed by the late Edo era, about 200 years ago. Japanese-style cuisine originally developed as court cooking and used to be eaten according to a strict etiquette. However, cookery books were published in the eighteenth century after printing became available, as a result of which the court-style diet became popular among the general population and is similar to that eaten now. Current cooking methods have become established through increasing sophistication with respect to taste, flavor, color, size, shape and texture, so that the effects on several senses are taken into consideration in the present dietary style. It can also be said that the Japanese diet is intended to harmonize natural resources and human skills in order to increase the joy of eating.

In the Japanese diet, food is cooked not only for taste but also as an expression of nature. The cooked food is then placed in a bowl, dish or plate which matches it in size, color and nature. Numerous dishes are arranged together at mealtimes, and the harmony of the arranged dishes is also appreciated.

These features of the dietary culture should be taken into consideration when dietary therapy is designed for diabetic patients.

GUIDANCE FOR A DIABETIC DIET

The Japan Diabetes Society and the Japanese Society of Nutrition recommend that a diabetic diet should not be specially regulated but should be an ordinary healthy diet, and they have proposed the following requirements for a healthy diet:

(1) A variety of foods which are well balanced nutritionally should be eaten, and at least 30 kinds of food should comprise one day's meals.

(2) Three meals should be eaten daily at regular times, and the calorie intake should be equally divided between them.

(3) The intake of animal fat should be decreased and that of vegetable fat should be increased. Fish and fish products should be eaten rather than meat. Less than 30% of the total dietary energy should come from saturated fats, with the balance provided by mono- and polyunsaturated fatty acids.

(4) Green and yellow vegetables should be eaten and dietary fiber should be increased.

(5) The intake of carbohydrates should be mainly as unrefined carbohydrates (polysaccharide, starch and dietary fiber, etc.) rather than as refined sugars, and should provide 55–65% of total energy.

(6) Protein should not exceed requirements, and should provide no more than 15% of total energy.

(7) A target weight should be set (e.g. the weight of a patient during their 20s) and patients should try to avoid obesity. For patients who have been slim since a young age, it is not necessary to try to gain weight.

(8) It is recommended that patients take alcohol only with meals, and excessive alcohol intake is to be avoided.

(9) Salt intake should be limited to less than 10 g/day.

(10) In order to increase the daily calcium intake, it is recommended that patients eat more small fish, cabbage, milk and other calcium-rich foods. Pregnant women are in particular need of more calcium and the elderly should take more iron-rich foods.

In addition to these basic requirements for a healthy diet, specific instructions should be provided separately for patients with insulin dependent diabetes mellitus (IDDM) and non-insulin dependent diabetes mellitus (NIDDM). Thus, if an IDDM patient is receiving insulin on a daily basis, instructions should be given to prevent hypoglycemia.

IDDM patients should be advised to take a snack before retiring to bed so as to prevent nocturnal hypoglycemia. When these patients feel very hungry, they can eat a low-calorie snack such as konnyaku (made from the dietary fiber, glucomannan, of the konnyaku plant), tofu, seaweed, vegetables or crackers. Since dietary therapy should not be a cause of stress for the diabetic patient, it is necessary for psychological support to be given by the patient's family members and by society as a whole.

PATIENT EDUCATION AND UTILIZATION OF THE FOOD EXCHANGE LISTS

Patient education is very important in the treatment of diabetes. The specific points regarding diabetic education are as follows:

(1) It should be performed periodically.

(2) Patients should record their health status in a diabetes diary with a set format, and IDDM patients should be instructed to record the blood glucose levels that they measure.

(3) Healthy diet, exercise and rest (i.e. physical, mental and social relaxation) are the major principles of diabetic therapy, but excessive exercise should be avoided. The managing physicians should provide the necessary instructions to prevent the development or progression of complications.

(4) To facilitate dietary therapy, the Japanese Food Exchange Lists should be utilized to allow more enjoyable dishes to be prepared. Adequate nutritional education should also be provided.

The following tests should be performed: body weight, blood pressure, microalbuminuria, HbA$_{1c}$, blood lipid levels and ECG. The blood glucose level and HbA$_{1c}$ are to be recorded by the patients themselves and the data are to be checked by the doctor at the outpatient department.

DIETARY THERAPY UTILIZING THE JAPANESE FOOD EXCHANGE LISTS

Clinical practice in Japan requires unique recommendations, so the Japan Diabetes Society (JDS) compiled the 5th Edition of the Food Exchange Lists in 1993 [5]. The six lists divide foods according to nutritional content (Table 2). For example, the intake of 1600 kcal is met by choosing food scores from the lists that supply 80 kcal each. Additional scores can be added to meet the individual patient's energy needs. The physician specifies how much of the daily diet should be drawn from each list. The index diet draws 11 scores from list 1, 1 from list 2, 4 from list 3, 1.4 from list 4, 1 from list 5, 1 from list 6 and 0.6 from seasonings, for a total of 20 scores and 1600 kcal (Table 3). These 20 scores will provide 76 g of protein, 254 g of carbohydrate and about 33 g of fat, 2700 IU of vitamin A, 182 mg of vitamin C, 206 mg of cholesterol, 9 g of saturated fat, 11 g of polyunsaturated fat and 23 g of dietary fiber, in 32 kinds of food. Dietary fiber content is calculated from the list of foods rich in dietary fiber, shown in Table 4.

The JDS lists are presented in simple language. They provide guideline weights for each food score as well as photographs of each food for easy comprehension. The lists have been designed for ease and flexibility, and have so far produced good compliance.

The general therapeutic goal for all diabetic patients in Japan includes: (a) the obvious goal of a nutritionally adequate diet; (b) an attempt at normalizing the

Table 2 Food exchange lists for diabetic treatment

Category of food	List of foods	Average amount of nutrition contained per basic score (80 kcal)		
		Protein (g)	Fats (g)	Carbohydrates (g)
I. Foods that primarily supply carbohydrates	1. Grain, potatoes, beans (excluding soybeans and their products)	2	–	18
	2. Fruits	–	–	20
II. Foods that primarily supply protein	3. Fish and seafood; meat, poultry and whalemeat and their products; eggs, cheese and soybeans and their products	9	5	–
	4. Milk and dairy products (excluding cheese)	4	5	6
III. Foods that primarily supply fats	5. Oils, fats and fatty foods	–	9	–
IV. Foods that primarily supply vitamins and minerals	6. Vegetables (excluding those with high sugar content), seaweeds, mushrooms and konnyaku (a gelatinous food made from the tuber of the konnyaku plant)	5	1	13

From reference 5, with permission.

Table 3 An example showing the distribution of 20 scores in a daily food intake of 1600 kcal

	List of foods						
	1	2	3	4	5	6	
Food component	Grain Potatoes Beans, etc.	Fruits	Fish Meat Eggs	Milk	Oil Fats	Vegetables Seaweeds Konnyaku	Seasoning
Daily scores	11	1	4	1.4	1	1	0.6
Distribution of scores							
Breakfast	3		1			0.3	
Lunch	4		1		1	0.3	0.6
Dinner	4		2			0.4	
A between-meal snack		1		1.4			

Table 4 Foods rich in dietary fiber

List of foods	1 Score of 80 kcal (g)	Dietary fiber/ 80 kcal (g)
Grain, potatoes & beans (excluding soybeans and their products)		
Green peas	90	6.8
Pumpkin (Japanese)	220	5.1
Kidney beans (dried)	25	4.3
Red beans 'Azuki' (dried)	25	4.5
Peas (dried)	25	4.4
Pumpkin	110	3.1
Broad beans	70	3.1
Corn (raw)	80	2.7
Chestnuts	50	2.5
Taros	130	2.5
Fruits		
Kiwifruit	150	4.4
Navel orange	200	3.4
Strawberries	250	3.3
Loquat (Japanese medlar)	200	3.2
Hassaku orange	200	3.0
Peach	200	2.4
Persimmon	150	2.4
Plum (Japanese)	150	2.4
Pineapple	150	2.3
Summer orange	200	2.0
Apple 'Kougyoku'	150	2.0
Soybeans and their products		
'Okara' (bean curd refuse)	100	9.8
Green soybeans (raw)	60	6.1
Fermented soybeans	40	2.7
Soybean flour	20	3.4
Soybeans (dried)	20	3.4
Foods that primarily supply carbohydrates		
Brown rice	25	0.9
White rice	55	0.2
Rice with germ	55	0.3
White bread	30	0.7
Japanese noodle (dried)	20	0.5
Japanese vermicelli (dried)	20	0.5
Macaroni, spaghetti (dried)	20	0.5
Buckwheat noodles (raw)	30	0.8
Chinese noodles (raw)	30	0.6
Barley	25	2.0
French bread	30	0.9
Oatmeal (dried)	25	1.7
Cornflakes	20	0.5
White flour	20	0.5

From reference 4, with permission.

metabolic abnormalities as far as possible, to prevent or delay the complications associated with diabetes; (c) pleasing the patient and making the diet possible to live with, i.e. enhancing quality of life and culture.

With the aim of keeping the diet nutritionally adequate, the physician tailors the prescription to the individual's medication schedule, ideal weight, energy needs and diabetic condition. Advice to the patient generally includes the following: eat all the food in your daily plan; be sure not to exceed your daily plan; check your measurements often; have meals at regular hours (this is especially important for diabetic patients on insulin treatment); avoid hypoglycemic episodes and be aware of hypoglycemic symptoms; ask your doctor what to do if you are very active on special occasions (sports, marathon running, etc.); ask your doctor what to do if traveling and changing time zones is going to confuse your routine.

The popular Japanese diet [6] is, in many respects, a 'thinking diet'. Our recommendations as clinicians must reflect this situation. The JDS lists provide a clinical tool to achieve this. Regular and well-balanced meals, rest, exercise and education continue to be the goals for keeping our diabetic patients healthy.

REFERENCES

1. Matsuzaki T. Epidemiological trends and statistical data of atherosclerosis in Japan. Nihonrinsho 1988; 46: 508–14 (in Japanese).

2. Ministry of Health and Welfare, Japan. Changes in the Japanese per capita daily intake of various nutrients. Present National Nutritional Condition. Tokyo: Daiichi-Shuppan, 1992; p 29 (in Japanese).

3. Ministry of Health and Welfare, Japan. Annual Report on Health and Welfare 1991–1992. Kosei-Hakusho, 1992 (in Japanese).

4. The Science and Technology Agency, Japan. The list of food ingredients, 1993 (in Japanese).

5. Japan Diabetes Society. Food exchange lists for diabetic treatment, 5th edn. Tokyo: Bunkodo, 1993 (in Japanese).

6. Konishi K. Japanese cooking for health and fitness. Tokyo: Gakken, 1983.

34d

Dietary Management of Diabetes Mellitus in Africa

Jean-Claude Mbanya and Sarah T. Gwangwa'a*

*Department of Internal Medicine, University of Yaounde I, and *Centre for Nutrition, Ministry of Scientific and Technical Research, Yaounde, Cameroon*

Most countries in Africa are undergoing a demographic transition, and African urban societies are increasingly coming within the sphere of influence of Western market economies. The style of life of city dwellers tends to be material-behavioural, with the adoption of cosmopolitan behaviour (travel, mass media exposure) and the consumption of material (radios, televisions, etc.) and food culture. This has led to an increase in the consumption of fat, sugar and salt. Rural African societies, however, have seen an increase in nutritional deficiencies, which appear to be related to drought, poverty, war and socioeconomic deprivation rather than to culture or religion. In these rural areas, the focus has been on maintaining food availability rather than equitable distribution.

These lifestyle changes have evolved against a background of increasing prevalence of diabetes mellitus and diabetic complications in Africa [1, 2]. Certainly, there is a demand for more nutrition education to a more cosmopolitan diabetic population by a limited number of poorly equipped staff who need to formulate new approaches more relevant to the needs of their patients.

CHARACTERISTICS OF THE AFRICAN DIET

The dietary patterns found in Africa differ from country to country and from region to region, with large differences in agricultural practices in the north, south, east and west. The very rapid increase in the population of Africa has led to inadequate production of local cereals and plant products like sorghum, millet, maize, yam and plantain, whereas cassava production has become more and more important. This phenomenon has led to many countries having low daily per caput dietary energy supplies (Table 1) [3].

In Africa, adults are usually short with a low body weight [3]. Although the population of Africa is physically more active, particularly in rural areas, its men and women usually have a lower energy requirement than North Americans simply because their body weight is lower [4]. Average daily energy intake is shown in Table 1.

The main parts of the traditional African meals are staples consisting of cereals (rice, cornmeal or flour, sorghum and millet), roots and tubers (yams, plantains, potatoes and cassava), which accompany meat, fish or vegetable dishes. A variety of vegetables, pulses, beans, groundnuts, herbs and spices are used frequently as 'onepot' meals, for example soup or rice dishes containing meat, pulses and vegetables.

Protein requirements are generally met in Africans since most of their diets are based predominantly on cereals and pulses, which provide on the average 10–15% of the total daily energy. The rest of the dietary energy intake is derived from carbohydrates and fats. In practice, the diets are low in fat and high in

International Textbook of Diabetes Mellitus, Second Edition. Edited by K.G.M.M. Alberti, P. Zimmet, R.A. DeFronzo, and H. Keen (Honorary)
© 1997 John Wiley & Sons Ltd

Table 1 Daily per caput dietary energy supplies for some African countries

<2000 kcal	2001–2300 kcal	>2300 kcal
Burkina Faso	Cameroon	Algeria
Ghana	Ethiopia	Angola
Mali	Kenya	Cote d'Ivoire
Mozambique	Malawi	Madagascar
Uganda	Zaire	Morocco
	Zambia	Nigeria
	Zimbabwe	Senegal
		Tanzania
		Tunisia
		South Africa
		Sudan

Adapted from reference 3, by kind permission of the authors, with slight modifications.

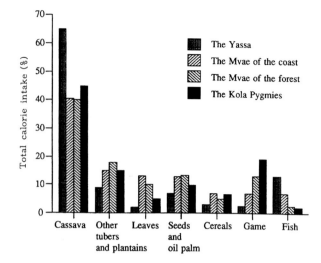

Figure 1 Percentage of total calorie intake provided by various food classes in four populations of Southern Cameroon (adapted from reference 7, by kind permission of UNESCO)

bulky foods, and concern exists that the total volume of food may restrict energy intake in special groups [5]. In general, pulses, nuts and seeds contribute about 5.6% of the daily energy intake while cereals, potatoes, roots, tubers, fish and meat provide the rest (Table 2 and Figure 1). Thus, the diet in Africa in general is characterized by frequent consumption of vegetables, fruits, cereals, tubers and legumes [6, 7].

Nevertheless, rapid increase in the urban population of Africa has led to a difference in food patterns between the urban and rural dwellers. The

Table 2 Nutrient composition of African staples per 100 g of edible portion

Foods		Energy (kcal)	Carbohydrate (g)	Protein (g)	Fat (g)	Fiber (g)
(a)	Starchy roots and tubers					
	Plantain	112	29.7	0.9	0.2	0.4
	Banana	110	28.7	1.4	0.2	0.5
	Yam	108	25.1	2.0	0.1	0.5
	Cassava	136	32.8	1.0	0.3	1.0
	Cocoyam	145	33.6	2.3	0.4	1.8
	Sweet Potato	112	25.6	1.0	0.3	0.8
	Potato	82	18.7	1.2	0.1	0.4
	Taro (*Colocosia esculenta*)	94	21.0	2.2	0.1	0.8
(b)	Cereals					
	Millet	335	70.2	11.4	5.0	1.5
	Sorghum	364	72.7	10.0	2.7	2.2
	Maize	349	71.7	9.1	9.2	2.3
	Rice	366	80.4	6.4	0.8	0.3
	Wheat	360	74.5	11.3	1.5	0.3
(c)	Protein foods					
	Insects fresh	356	4.2	20.4	28.0	2.7
	dried	656	3.5	35.7	54.3	–
	Fish fresh	103	–	18.8	2.5	–
	dried	269	–	47.3	7.4	–
	Game fresh	147	–	16.8	8.3	–
	dried	447	–	66.3	18.2	–
(d)	Legumes and seeds					
	Groundnuts	548	21.6	23.4	45.3	2.1
	Beans	366	62.7	20.3	1.2	4.8
	Cassava leaves	91	18.0	7.0	1.0	4.0
	Cocoyam leaves	34	5.3	2.5	1.0	2.1
(e)	Fats and oils					
	Palm oil	875	0.3	–	98.9	0.1
	Cotton oil	884	–	–	99.9	–
	Groundnut oil	884	–	–	99.9	–

(Adapted from reference 6, by kind permission of Institut de Recherches Médicales et d'Etudes des Plantes Médicinales; Ministry of Scientific Research, Yaounde, Cameroon.)

Table 3 Daily per caput energy supplies for major nutrients in various areas in Kenya

Nutrient	Vihiga Area (kcal)	(%)	Kilifi Area (kcal)	(%)	Coast Area (kcal)	(%)
Carbohydrate	1832	73	2116	80	1926	64
Fat	411	15	247	10	763	18
Protein	288	12	276	10	656	18
Total	2492	100	2637	100	3601	100

Adapted from reference 8, by kind permission of the authors, with slight modification.

Table 4 Percentage of energy obtained from different food components and salt and fibre intakes of different human groups in Africa

Food component	Hunter-gatherers	Peasant farmers	Modern affluent African societies
Fat (%)	15–20	10–15	>40
Sugar (%)	0	5	20
Starch (%)	50–70	60–75	25–30
Protein (%)	15–20	10–15	12
Salt (g/day)	1	5–15	10
Fibre (g/day)	40	60–120	20

Modified from reference 3, by kind permission of the authors.

rural population has maintained the traditional diet, while as urban societies grow and generate money, they perceive the diet, similar to that of other affluent communities, as a symbol of their newly acquired status. They move towards high-fat, energy-rich, high-salt and processed sugar-based items. Soft drinks, alcohol and 'fast' foods are popular, taking the place of traditional home-based diets.

Clearly, there are striking differences in the dietary patterns of different groups of Africans, even within one country [3, 8]. As you move from the coastal affluent communities to the distant rural communities in Kenya (Table 3), the consumption of complex carbohydrates and fibers increases while that of fat, protein and simple sugars decreases [8]. There are clear differences in food consumption between hunter-gatherers of the desert or rain forest, peasant farmers of the forest or savannah regions, and modern affluent societies in Africa as a whole (Table 4). However, except among modern affluent community dwellers, food composition falls within that recommended by the World Health Organization (WHO) [3].

Food choice in Africa is determined not only by tradition, knowledge and experience but also by social and economic factors, including family size, availability and seasonal variations. There are many different religious denominations in Africa and, within each, a wide range of beliefs concerning diets.

Seasonal variation of food supply has been observed in several regions of Africa, although with apparently less drastic consequences in some areas [7]. Although some staples, especially cassava, are available throughout the year, plant products such as groundnuts, seeds and, to a lesser extent, palm nuts are subject to seasonal

cycles [7]. As a result, there are variations of different degrees throughout the year in meeting calorie requirements among several ethnic groups of Africa [9].

To a large extent, food intake is dependent on social organization at meal times. There are many ways of organizing meals in Africa. Often, in several ethnic groups of Africa, adult men eat separately, with the food shared in an informal way or according to seniority. Women, together with their small children, constitute another food consumption group. Children, before they reach puberty, receive their personal helping of staple but sometimes they all share one portion of relish. Adolescents of both sexes often use independent dishes. In other areas of Africa, meals are taken with the whole family group. However, in the affluent societies of Africa, the organization of meals is similar to that of Western society.

Meal patterns are usually related to occupation. In practice there are two to three meals per day for office employees and businessmen of the urban communities, who may also have snacks in between meals. The majority of the population, however, have one bulky meal a day which is usually supplemented with fruits, tubers and roots as 'snacks'. Also, in most areas, some form of alcohol is easily available during and outside mealtimes.

DIETARY MANAGEMENT OF AFRICAN DIABETIC PATIENTS

The dietary management of diabetes mellitus in Africa must be seen against the background of the diet of the local population, which has been discussed in the previous section. Obviously, it is important,

Table 5 Daily per caput energy supplies for major nutrients in the general and diabetic populations of Kilifi District, Kenya

Nutrients	General population (kcal)	(%)	Diabetic population (kcal)	(%)
Carbohydrates	2115	80	2436	69
Fat	248	10	531	15
Protein	274	10	576	16
Total	2637	100	3543	100

Adapted from reference 8, by kind permission of the authors.

more so in the African context, to take into account food perceptions, prohibitions and prescriptions, and economic factors, while adjusting dietary advice in particular to suit each individual.

DIET OF AFRICAN DIABETIC PATIENTS

In most places in Africa, diabetic diets are based on the old approach of a restrictive special diet which inevitably stigmatizes the diabetic patient and isolates him from the rest of the population. This includes strict instruction regarding totally forbidden foods, including common staples such as cassava, yams, maize and alcoholic drinks. Whereas carbohydrates are restricted from the diets, milk and eggs are encouraged in large amounts. Unfortunately, this prescribed diet is expensive and deviates from the traditional diet of the general population [8]. There is a decrease in the intake of carbohydrate staples in favour of fat and protein, with a resultant increase in dietary energy intake in these patients (Table 5).

The traditional African diet, for the most part, is similar to the dietary recommendations of the British Diabetic Association [10] and the American Diabetes Association [11] for people with diabetes, and the WHO healthy nutrition recommendations for the general population [12]. Thus, with slight modification of the traditional African diets, it is relatively easy to draw up dietary guidelines in this region. Moreover, the difficulty involved in making permanent changes to entrenched eating habits may be avoided, especially in patients living in rural areas. There is an ever-growing recognition in Africa of the need for dietary education of diabetic patients by all members of diabetes health care teams.

DIETARY EDUCATION

The aim of diabetic dietary education is to help the person with diabetes to achieve and maintain good glucose control and lipid profiles [13, 14, 15]. Patients receive inadequate dietetic treatment in most African countries because very few health institutions have dietitians. Therefore physicians, nurses or medical assistants

advise patients about diet, and they may merely advise the avoidance of sugar and the limitation of starch intake. However, in some centres, specialized dietary education is available.

Dietary Assessment

During the initial dietary assessment, the various circumstances affecting food choices made by the patient and family should be detailed. In Africa, these include life-style and work routine, availability of foodstuffs, seasonal variations, educational status and the economic, cultural and religious factors influencing the choice of food. On the basis of this information, the eating plan, which should be as close as possible to that of the household, should be discussed with the diabetic patient and the family member who does the food shopping and cooking. This eating plan should be both desirable and acceptable, hence attainable. The level of change, and appropriate realistic short- and long-term targets for body weight should be agreed with the patient.

Dietary Advice

In most African countries, calorie counts for portions of traditional foods are not available. Furthermore, very few homes have kitchen scales. It is necessary for the educator to have food models of various sizes of the local staple diets which should be shown to the patients during dietary counselling.

Nutritional goals for insulin dependent diabetes mellitus (IDDM), non-insulin dependent diabetes mellitus (NIDDM), and malnutrition-related diabetes mellitus are the same. However, emphasis should be laid on the pursuit of weight loss in overweight and weight gain in underweight diabetic patients through appropriate dietary prescription. The major topics for dietary education in African diabetic patients are listed in Table 6. Some of these topics, especially regarding refined carbohydrates, fat and protein, have been discussed in Chapter 34a of this book, and these recommendations are not different in African diabetic patients. Also, the African diet, which is mainly high in starch and dietary fibre and low in fat and sugar, indeed approaches the

Table 6 Major topics for dietary education in African diabetic patients

1. Avoid major sources of refined carbohydrates
2. Distribution of starch-containing foods throughout the day
3. Avoid major sources of fat
4. How to select meals and snacks from a food exchange list
5. Exercise, illness and diets
6. Eating out and alcohol
7. Special situations; feasts, fasting, etc.
8. Hypoglycemia

ideal diabetic diet [16, 17]. The recommendations of expert groups in Europe [10] and the USA [11] on the low-fat, high-carbohydrate diet are impressive and are applicable to all populations whatever their usual dietary habits.

Distribution of Starch-containing Foods Throughout the Day

Carbohydrate intake should be distributed throughout the day even in patients who are used to eating one staple dish a day, and it should not vary widely from day to day. Carbohydrate intake should be in the form of snacks of boiled or roast cassava, maize or plantain outside the main staple dish. Whole fruits should be eaten in moderation and are ideal as snack substitutes. Artificial sweeteners like saccharin or aspartame, if available, can be used as sugar substitutes in tea and coffee.

Exercise, Illness and Diet

Regular exercise helps to maintain muscle mass and promotes the preferential loss of adipose tissue [18] and is particularly advantageous in NIDDM since it improves insulin sensitivity and glucose disposal [19]. Patients should be reminded to eat a starch snack of fruit, roast or boiled cassava, maize or plantain after strenuous exercise or physical activity, including farm work, in order to replenish glycogen stores and avoid late hypoglycemia. During illness, extra food intake of tea or coffee with sugar, or of foods and drinks containing sugar, is recommended.

Eating Out and Alcohol

Local beer brewed from corn or millet is drunk in varying quantity in most places in Africa [20, 21]. Alcohol, unless medically or religiously contra-indicated, may be consumed in moderation along with food or shortly before it, provided it is part of the total energy intake. When alcoholic drinks are consumed the usual dietary carbohydrate should always be eaten in addition, because alcohol-induced hypoglycemia may occur. The same precautions regarding the use of alcohol that apply to the general population apply to people with diabetes.

Special Situations

Eating patterns change during religious fasting, so a redistribution of the daily carbohydrate and energy intake within the allowed meals is necessary. During Ramadan, insulin-treated patients should take the usual morning insulin dose at sunset before their meal and the evening dose at dawn with a lighter meal.

The general principles of healthy diet described above are appropriate for pregnant and lactating mothers with diabetes. In young IDDM patients, diets should be adapted to accommodate the special needs of growth and development. For some IDDM patients, food may be required every 2–3 hours through the day and sometimes more than one snack may be helpful if the interval is long. Also, drug and insulin dosages should be tailored to the meals, and not the reverse.

PROBLEMS TO BE OVERCOME IN DIETARY MANAGEMENT OF DIABETES IN AFRICA

Dietitians play an important role in the diabetes health care delivery team. Unfortunately, they are in chronic short supply in most African countries [22]. There is, therefore, a need for local training of dietitians and where this is not possible, therapeutic dietetics should be a strong component in the curriculum of nursing and medical schools.

Food exchange charts, food models and portion sizes of common local staples adapted to kitchen and home measures, for example the use of kitchen spoons or cups, are urgently needed. These nutrition education materials are more useful than diet sheets in a region where most of the diabetic patients are illiterate.

The overall diabetes prevalence in most African communities is low but that of impaired glucose tolerance is high [2] and will rise even further because of the demographic transition taking place in Africa. Community-based programmes must be developed in each country to change the 'affluent' dietary pattern and sedentary lifestyle that tends to accompany socioeconomic development.

Because of the diversity and complexity of diets in Africa, there is no prescribed diet for the management of diabetes in the region. Nevertheless, whatever the individual patient's dietary targets, successful implementation depends on the acceptability of the prescribed diet and on continuous counselling. The traditional high-carbohydrate African diets, based on readily available local foods, are more acceptable and compatible with the African diabetic patients' eating habits, cultures and tradition.

REFERENCES

1. Yajnik CS. Diabetes in tropical developing countries. In Alberti KGMM, Krall LP (eds) Diabetes annual 5. Amsterdam: Elsevier, 1990: pp 72–87.

2. King H, Rewers M. Global estimates for prevalence of diabetes mellitus and impaired glucose tolerance in adults. Diabetes Care 1993; 16: 157–77.

3. WHO. Diet, nutrition, and the prevention of chronic diseases. Report of a WHO study group. WHO Technical Report Series 797. Geneva: WHO, 1990.

4. James WPT, Schoefield EC. Human energy requirements: a manual for planners and nutritionists. Oxford: Oxford Medical Publications, 1990.

5. FAO. Dietary fats and oils in human nutrition. Report of an expert consultation. FAO Food and Nutrition Series 20. Geneva: FAO, 1980.

6. Ngo Som J, Abondo A. Les resources alimentaires du Cameroun: repartition ecologique, classification et valeur nutritive. Cahiers de l'IMPM 7. Yaounde: 1989.

7. Koppert G, Hladik CM. Measuring food consumption. In Hladik CM, Bahuchet S, de Garine I (eds) Food and nutrition in the African rainforest. Paris: UNESCO/MAB 1990; pp 59–61.

8. Kishida KRD, Kinyari TN, Mngola EN. A dietary survey of diabetic patients before diagnosis compared with non-diabetic controls in various General Hospitals in Kenya 1991–92. In Abstracts of the 3rd PanAfrican Diabetes Study Group Congress. Tunis: PADSG, 1993; p 93.

9. FAO/WHO. Energy and protein requirements. Report of a joint FAO/WHO/UNU expert consultation. WHO Technical Report Series 724. Geneva: WHO, 1986.

10. Nutrition Subcommittee, British Diabetic Association. Dietary recommendations for people with diabetes: an update for the 1990s. Diabet Med 1992; 9: 189–202.

11. Committee on Food and Nutrition of the American Diabetes Association. Nutritional recommendations and principles for individuals with diabetes mellitus. Diabetes Care 1992; 15(suppl. 2): 21–8.

12. WHO Regional Office for Europe. Healthy nutrition: preventing nutrition-related diseases in Europe. WHO European Series 24. Copenhagen: WHO Publications for Europe, 1988.

13. D'Antonio JA, Ellis D, Doft BH, Becker DJ, Drash AL, Kuller LH et al. Diabetes complications and glycemic control. The Pittsburgh prospective insulin dependent diabetes cohort study status report after 5 years of IDDM. Diabetes Care 1989; 12: 694–700.

14. Feinstein AR. How good is the statistical evidence against oral hypoglycemia agents? Adv Intern Med 1979; 24: 71–95.

15. Seviour PW, Teal TK, Richmond W, Elkeles RS. Serum lipids, lipoproteins and macrovascular disease in non-insulin dependent diabetics; a possible new approach to prevention. Diabet Med 1988; 5: 166–71.

16. Simpson HCR, Simpson RW, Lousley S, Carter RD, Geekie M, Hockaday TDR et al. A high carbohydrate leguminous fibre diet improves all aspects of diabetic control. Lancet 1981; 1: 1–5.

17. Riccardi G, Rivellese A, Pacioni D, Genovese S, Mastranzo P, Mancini M. Separate influence of dietary carbohydrate and fibre on the metabolic control in diabetes. Diabetologia 1984; 26: 116–21.

18. Stern JS, Titchenal CA, Johnson PR. Obesity: does exercise make a difference? In Berry EM, Blondheim SH, Eliahou HE, Shafrir E (eds) Recent advances in obesity research, V. London: J Libbey 1987; 352–64.

19. Delvin JT, Horton ES. Glucose metabolism and thermogenesis in lean, obese, and non-insulin dependent diabetic men following exercise. In Berry EM, Blondheim SH, Eliahou HE, Shafrir E (eds) Recent advances in obesity research, V. London: J Libbey 1987; 365–72.

20. Desta B. A survey of the alcohol content of traditional beverages. Ethiop Med J 1977; 15: 2.

21. Raikes A. Women's health in East Africa. Soc Sci Med 1989; 28: 457–9.

22. Netherlands International Nutrition Institute. International Course in Food Science and Nutrition. Institutional feeding in the region Eastern, Central and Southern Africa. Workshop Report 3. Wageningen: NINI, 1985.

34e

Dietary Management of Diabetes Mellitus in China

Pan Xiao-Ren

China-Japan Friendship Hospital, Beijing, P R China

The prevalence of diabetes and the rate of macrovascular complications in China are lower than in Western countries [1-4]. A major reason is that the life-style of Chinese people is different from that of Western people. The Chinese have lower caloric intake, relatively high complex carbohydrate, high fibre, and low fat in the diet compared with most Western societies (Table 1) [5], and take more exercise. Overweight and obesity are not as common in the Chinese as among Western people. The prevalence of diabetes among Chinese with a Western life-style is also higher, as seen in Singapore, Taiwan and Mauritius [2]. Chinese people in rural areas have relatively higher complex carbohydrate and lower fat in the diet and do more physical work than those in urban areas, and the prevalence of diabetes is lower in rural than in urban areas [1]. In 1994, we conducted a survey in 19 provinces of a population of 250 000 aged 25 years and over. The prevalence of diabetes and IGT was 2.8% and 2.7%, respectively, which was 2.7 to 3 times higher than that found ten years earlier. A logistic model with stepwise analysis showed that age, obesity, higher income, less physical exercise, hypertension, and family history of diabetes were independent risk factors for diabetes (unpublished data). Thus, in the context of socioeconomic development, it is very important for the prevention and treatment of diabetes that Chinese people keep to their traditional lifestyle.

COMMON TYPES OF FOOD FOR THE CHINESE DIABETIC PERSON

According to Chinese life-style and clinical practice, the dietary management of diabetes is as follows: total calories of about 25-30 kcal/kg body weight for adults with normal weight (BMI 22.5-23.5 kg/m^2) and mild physical activity (Table 2). Carbohydrate, protein and fat provide about 55-65%, 10-15% and 25-30% of total energy, respectively. This dietary composition is similar to that recommended by the American, Canadian and British diabetes associations.

People with overweight or obesity should take fewer calories (about 20-25 kcal/kg body weight/day). For normal growth and development of children, younger people and people with heavier physical work, more energy is needed (>30 kcal/kg body weight/day). Energy intake should also be based on the previous diet and life-style of an individual patient, taking into account other factors such as gender, occupation and the presence of hypertension, dyslipidaemia or medical conditions such as diabetic nephropathy.

Carbohydrate

Cereals in the form of rice or wheat are the staple foods for Chinese people. Patients are advised to take semi-polished cereals and some foods containing more fibre with a lower glycaemic index (such as oat flakes,

International Textbook of Diabetes Mellitus, Second Edition. Edited by K.G.M.M. Alberti, P. Zimmet, R.A. DeFronzo, and H. Keen (Honorary)
© 1997 John Wiley & Sons Ltd

Table 1   Comparison of diet in developed countries, developing countries and China

	Total calories (kcal)	Protein (g)	Protein (%)	Fat (g)	Fat (%)
Developed countries (1979–1981)	3385	98.9	11.7	120.4	31.9
Developing countries (1979–1981)	2350	57.5	9.8	40.6	15.5
China (1982)					
Urban areas	2446	66.7	10.9	68.2	25.0
Rural areas	2615	68.8	10.5	41.3	14.3
DaQing (1986)	2459	71.3	11.6	69.4	25.4

%, Percentage of total calories. (From reference 5, with permission.)

Table 2   Dietary reference values for adults of normal weight and mild physical activity

Height (cm)	Energy (kcal)	Cereals (mg)	Vegetable (mg)	Meat (mg)	Milk (ml)	Vegetable oil (9-mg spoonfuls)
155	1500	200–225	500	150	250	14
160	1650	225–250	500	175	250	14
165	1800	250–275	500	175	250	18
170	1950	275–325	500	200	250	22
180	2250	325–375	500	225	250	22
185	2400	375–400	500	250	250	27

A food exchange list, including these five groups of foods (40 g bean = 250 ml milk) is used to help patients to eat a wide variety of foods of their choice.

cornmeal, buckwheat meal, soybean meal) [6]. Simple sugar should not exceed 25 g/day (fruit mainly contains simple sugar).

Protein

Protein intake is 1.0–1.2 g/kg body weight/day. Protein for the majority of Chinese people is mainly of vegetable origin (cereals and soybean). Based on the dietary recommendations (Table 2), most diabetic patients are advised to take more animal protein (lean meat, especially chicken, and fish). Patients with lower income are advised to take more soybean and its products. High protein may, however, accelerate the progression of diabetic nephropathy [7]. Patients with nephropathy should therefore take less protein (0.8 g/kg body weight/day) containing relatively more animal protein (more essential amino acids). Diabetic people with malnutrition, pregnant diabetic women, and diabetic children or adolescents need more protein (about 1.5 g/kg body weight/day).

Fat and Cholesterol

About 70% of the fat content in the diet is derived from the vegetable oil used in cooking. Patients are advised to take lean meat and not more than one egg yolk per day. The daily cholesterol intake should be controlled to less than 300 mg. Usually the ratio of polyunsaturated to saturated fatty acids in Chinese food

is 1.5–2.0 [6]. The ratio should not be less than 1.0 for diabetic patients.

Vegetables

Diabetic patients are encouraged to take more non-starchy vegetables, which contain only 3–4% carbohydrate and satisfy hunger. Large amounts of vegetables are also helpful in increasing the fibre content of the diet. It is not difficult for Chinese diabetic subjects to take more vegetables since this is the cultural norm. Diabetic patients usually do not like to add artificial or purified fibre to their diet.

Salt, Alcohol and Sweeteners

Daily salt intake should be less than 6 g for diabetic patients, and less than 3 g for those with hypertension. In China it is recommended that alcohol intake should be less than 3 units/week. One unit is equivalent to 285 ml beer, or 115 ml wine, or 25 ml spirits. Xylitol has been used as a sweetener, but intake should be not more than 20–30 g/day. Smoking should be actively discouraged.

NON-INSULIN DEPENDENT DIABETES

Of Chinese patients with newly diagnosed NIDDM, 54% are overweight or obese (BMI > 25 kg/m^2) [8], which suggests a considerable contribution from insulin resistance. Diet should be the first consideration in treating NIDDM. The aim of dietary treatment for obese NIDDM is gradually to reduce the excessive weight (by 1–2 kg/month) by reducing energy intake (by about 300–400 kcal/day) and increasing exercise, which will decrease glycaemia and blood pressure, improve dyslipidaemia and reduce the incidence of diabetes in subjects with IGT (unpublished data). Most NIDDM patients should reduce carbohydrate intake, and some of them should reduce fat and protein intake, but the team should emphasize that it is not correct to take a low-carbohydrate, high-protein and high-fat diet. Patients with non-obese NIDDM (some of whom may actually have IDDM) need a normal energy intake to maintain ideal body weight, as well as normal physical activity. Non-obese NIDDM patients should not reduce necessary energy intake in order to avoid insulin injections.

INSULIN-DEPENDENT DIABETES

Most children and adolescents with IDDM are non-obese. The formula used to calculate calorie intake for patients under 18 years old is: $90 - (3 \times age)$ kcal/kg body weight/day in order to achieve normal growth and development. It is very important to adjust diet, physical activity and insulin treatment together. In order to flatten the plasma glucose profile, dietary carbohydrate should be divided into six portions: breakfast (1/10), mid-morning snack (1/10), lunch (3/10), mid-afternoon snack (1/10), supper (3/10) and bed-time snack (1/10). Breakfast should be taken 45–90 minutes after giving the morning dose of insulin, which is injected at 0600–0630 h in order to control morning hyperglycaemia. The time of taking meals and the quantity of food ingested at each meal should be kept constant, but flexibility is also important, such as increasing the amount of food taken before or during exercise in order to avoid hypoglycaemia.

REFERENCES

1. Cooperative Diabetic Research Group in China. Report on the screening for diabetes in Chinese population of 300 000. Chinese Med J 1981; 20: 678–83 (in Chinese).
2. King H, Rewers M. Global estimates for prevalence of diabetes mellitus and impaired glucose tolerance in adults. Diabetes Care 1993; 16: 157–77.
3. Pan XR, Hu YH, Li GW, Liu PA, Bennett PH, Howard BV. Impaired glucose tolerance and its relationship to ECG-indicated coronary heart disease and risk factors among Chinese: Da Qing IGT and Diabetes Study. Diabetes Care 1993; 16: 150–6.
4. Chi ZS. Study on the cardiovascular complications of diabetes mellitus in Beijing and Tianjing. In Mimura G et al (eds) Diabetes mellitus in East Asia. Amsterdam: Excerpta Medica, 1988: pp 23–8.
5. Institute of Health, China National Center for Preventive Medicine. National Nutrition Survey, 1982.
6. Du S, Sun Q et al. Postprandial plasma glucose and insulin response to different kinds of foods. Physiol Sci Basic Clin 1986; 6: 462–70.
7. Ciavarella A, Di Mizio G, Stefoni S, Borgnino LC, Vannini P. Reduced albuminuria after dietary protein restriction in insulin-dependent diabetic patients with clinical nephropathy. Diabetes Care 1987; 10: 407–13.
8. Hu YH, Pan XR, Liu PA, Li GW, Bennett PH, Howard BV. Coronary heart disease and diabetic retinopathy in newly diagnosed diabetes in Da Qing, China: the Da Qing IGT and Diabetes Study. Acta Diabetol 1991; 28: 169–73.

34f

Dietary Management of Diabetes Mellitus in the Middle East

Morsi Arab

University of Alexandria, Egypt

HISTORICAL

The history of medicine, like the history of many other aspects of civilization, started in the Middle East. Knowledge about diabetes, and even attempts to treat it by diet, were no exception [1]. As many as 3500 years ago the Ancient Egyptians gave a description of diabetes, though not complete, in the Ebers Papyrus (1550 BC). 'Where the body shrinks... with no apparent disease of the body... it is decay inside...'. They treated that disease with 'ground dragon's blood from Elephantine, flexseed, colocynth, boiled with honey...'. [2]. Later Arab physicians, who knew about diabetes from Greco-Roman medicine, gave a comprehensive description of the disease and its complications, and treated it empirically with medicines and diet. Among the remedies they described were acacia (gum arabic), dry rose, balaustrus and seeds of psyllium (which contain 10% mucilage, xylose, arabinose, galactose, galacturonic acid, oil, protein and salts). They also recommended eating beans, fruits and 'cold pulps which do not cause diuresis' [3]. Thus, we may trace the empirical use of fibre (both soluble and insoluble forms) in the diabetic diet back to those times.

PATTERNS OF FOOD CONSUMPTION IN THE MIDDLE EAST

Total Caloric Intake

Total energy intake has prime importance in the dietary management of diabetes, especially NIDDM, which is commonly associated with obesity. In this case, reduction of body weight by restriction of total caloric intake will improve metabolic control, even with only modest weight loss. In addition, weight reduction may be accompanied by several other beneficial effects, such as lowering of raised blood pressure, correcting in part dyslipidaemia and improving cardiac performance [4].

Total energy intake is closely related to the pattern of food consumption. Although food consumption in the Middle East area has common features, individual countries may differ according to both the specific stage of their economic development and cultural factors [5].

In most of the Middle Eastern countries, the total caloric intake is at acceptable levels from the nutritional view point, approaching 3000 kcal/day. In North African countries it may be about 12% less [5]. A steady change has been observed in the Middle East during recent years, with an increase in the average total consumption per capita from 2650 to 3100 kcal between the 1970s and the 1990s. This has been more prominent in certain countries, e.g. Saudi Arabia, Tunisia and Algeria. Increasing prevalence of overweight was a natural consequence of this, especially when combined with the lower physical activity resulting from changes in lifestyle during these years [6].

Sources of Energy: Ratio of Carbohydrate to Fat

Carbohydrate and fat are the main sources of food energy. Carbohydrate constitutes the cheaper source, while fat and protein are costly. So, in this part of the world, with predominantly low incomes, cost becomes of prime importance. Fortunately, recent trends in the management of diabetes encourage more liberal consumption of carbohydrate than was considered before [7]. Therefore, the recommendation that about 65% of non-protein energy should be provided from carbohydrate and 35% at most from fat, fits with the available dietary composition of developing countries. In countries of the Middle East there are still, however, some regional differences. In North Africa, carbohydrate provides 72% of food energy, while in the Mediterranean islands it provides only 52%, which is nearer to the general Westernized model [5]. Fat provides about 37% of food energy in the more economically developed areas, but only 19% in the lower income countries of the East Mediterranean and African coasts.

The Complex Carbohydrate to Sugar Ratio, Glycaemic Index and Fibre Content

It is now established that more complex carbohydrates, i.e. polysaccharides, should form the main bulk of the total carbohydrate intake, with some degree of limitation (but not complete restriction) of simple sugars. This will ensure a better glycaemic response and will have other beneficial effects on different aspects of both carbohydrate and lipid metabolism in diabetic people. The total content of fibre, both soluble and insoluble forms, has also been recognized as an important factor in lowering the glycaemic index of the diet. Fibre, particularly the soluble form, may have some beneficial effects on hyperinsulinaemia, insulin resistance and the serum lipid profile [7].

The Middle Eastern diet pattern, especially with more consumption of traditional foods, more than adequately matches current trends to encourage the intake of more fibre in the diabetic diet. This is because of its higher content of vegetables and fruits and because of the habit of consumption of bread which commonly contains a reasonable amount of bran. However, it is unfortunate that rapid changes in lifestyle in certain Middle Eastern countries include an increasing consumption of white bread with less fibre. This trend should be discouraged.

At present, the general consensus on sugar consumption is towards an allowance within a limit of at most 10% of the total caloric intake for diabetic subjects. In most Middle Eastern countries the estimated average consumption of sugar by the general population is around this level. Only in the Mediterranean islands, with their Westernized lifestyle, and in the countries with rapidly developing economies, are higher levels of sugar consumption observed [5].

Specific Types of Fat in the Middle Eastern Diet

In the Middle East, where on average incomes are low, consumption of animal fat, and hence saturated fats, is on the low side compared to the Western world. However, again the rapidly changing lifestyle in certain high-income Middle Eastern countries is associated with an increasing tendency to consume more animal fat. This almost certainly contributes to the increasing occurrence of macrovascular disease. Certain countries in the Middle East consume more mono-unsaturated fatty acids from olive oil, which is abundant locally and constitutes a common item of traditional food. This is an advantage, since the addition of a mono-unsaturated fat supplement has been recommended as a way of improving the lipid metabolic profile, particularly in people with diabetes. Several studies indicate that it is effective in lowering serum LDL without decreasing HDL levels [8].

Alternative sources of dietary fat in the Middle Eastern diet also come from other vegetable oils which provide polyunsaturated fatty acids. Among the locally produced and much consumed oils are cotton seed oil, less commonly corn oil, while sunflower and soya bean oils, which are imported, are consumed in smaller amounts.

Fish oil, with its high content of omega-3 fatty acids, has been recommended in diabetes because of its effect in ameliorating the risk factors for atherosclerosis and lowering the incidence of coronary heart disease mortality [9]. Fish consumption is not at a high level in most Middle Eastern countries in spite of wide availability, and this is even the case in the Mediterranean islands. However, it may be noted that in certain coastal cities, like Alexandria, Damietta, Rashid and Port Said in the north of the Egyptian Nile Delta, more fish is eaten as a common food tradition.

Proteins

In the more industrialized countries protein may provide up to 25% of the caloric energy of the diet, and most of this protein is of animal origin (average intake 98 g/day, of which 57 g is animal protein). This is in contrast to developing countries, with an average intake of 53 g/day of which 10 g is animal protein [5]. In the Middle East less animal protein is consumed in several countries, but this is compensated for by consumption of more plant protein. Thus, in most of the Middle East, total protein intake is quite satisfactory from the nutritional point of view. Special consideration should be made whenever more protein is required, e.g. for growth, pregnancy, and wound healing. On the other hand, protein restriction may be required in impending or established nephropathy [7].

Traditional Foods and Dietary Habits

Certain areas of the Middle East have characteristic traditional meals, and the consumption of these in abundance may influence the balance of the diabetic diet. Thus the rice and meat meal is traditional in most of the Arab Gulf countries. Egyptians consume a lot of beans and bread which provide an adequate source of total protein. The fish and rice meal is traditional in the Mediterranean coastal cities in the north of Egypt. Dates, with their high content of carbohydrate, are particularly consumed in excess, but this is tradition which is hard to restrict, especially among Bedouin tribes of the rural areas. Honey, although not much consumed, requires special consideration because of the widespread belief in its nutritional value and its remedial effects. It has a high content of fructose. Therefore, its consumption as food or as a sweetener, should be carefully guided to avoid the side-effects of excessive intake on glycaemic control and on the gastrointestinal tract. Pork, ham and and other pig meat products are traditionally absent from the Moslem diet because they are prohibited by religion. Vegetarianism is quite uncommon in the Middle East. Coffee and tea drinking are very common. Their intake throughout the day is a frequent social habit. Heavily sugared tea may also be taken by the poorer classes as replacement for dessert or fruits at the end of their meals.

There have been a number of recent studies to determine the glycaemic indices of various traditional foods [10]. Also, several studies investigated the possible hypoglycaemic value of particular foods and beverages, but there were no outstanding or unexpected findings [11].

Food exchange lists evaluating local foods, including the traditional items, are available. However, in practice few diabetes care centres use them effectively and few individuals are acquainted with their proper utilization.

Dietary Education

As in most of the developing countries, diabetes education is inadequate, not only because of lack of facilities but also because of lack of educators. This is particularly observed in the field of dietary guidance. Few countries in the Middle East have facilities to provide this education through professional dietitians. Even when such facilities are available, there is maldistribution, with great deficiencies particularly in the rural communities.

Misconceptions among the population may have adverse effects on dietary management in diabetes, and have to be specially considered. Examples are the misconception that sugar intake may induce diabetes,

or that diabetic subjects should be totally prevented from consuming sugar. More seriously, the belief in the remedial effects of certain foods or beverages to control or cure diabetes may lead to a serious neglect of treatment by insulin or oral agents when required.

Alcohol

Because alcohol is prohibited in the Moslem religion, it does not usually constitute a common diet problem. However, if alcohol is taken, its caloric content should be considered. It should be eliminated from diets of hypertensive hypertriglyceridaemic obese diabetic patients and in chronic hepatic diseases which are quite common in the Middle East.

Sweeteners

Both nutritive and non-nutritive sweeteners are available in the Middle East. Natural fructose is most commonly consumed, either in special commercial preparations or as honey, which contains mainly fructose. Saccharin is the most commonly used artificial sweetener. Aspartame, which is more expensive, is less commonly used. In general, the use of artificial sweeteners is not as widespread as in Western countries, by either diabetic or non-diabetic people. Thus, they are not to be expected to be routinely present on the tables of restaurants and cafeterias as is commonly the habit in Western communities.

Diabetic Foods

Diabetic foods are also available in the Middle East, but mainly in the larger cities. They are not common constituents of the diet of poorer people because they are usually expensive and because of lack of information. However, it must be noted that their use is not an essential element in the dietary management of diabetes. This is particularly true with the current trend for liberal allowance of total carbohydrate and a reasonable allowance of natural sucrose when this is evenly distributed and mixed with meals. This may be a relief from the economic burden of diet planning in the great majority of the diabetic population.

SPECIFIC CONSIDERATIONS IN DIETARY MANAGEMENT

Insulin Dependent Diabetes

As in other regions, insulin administration should be coordinated with the distribution of meals, and hypoglycaemia should be prevented and special extra caloric allowances made for growth and physical activity of children. Prevalent habits in the Middle East do not encourage the frequent recommendation of multi-dose insulin injections, while insulin pumps are only very rarely used. Self-monitoring of blood glucose is also not a common practice. All these factors make it imperative for the practising physician to depend more on his judgement for careful distribution of the caloric intake, with periodic revision to ensure adequate glycaemic control, free from episodes of hypoglycaemia.

Obese NIDDM

Those patients who require body weight reduction present a real problem for the practice of diabetes care in the Middle East. Again, this is due to prevailing habits, together with inadequate diabetes education. Seldom does an overweight, mildly diabetic patient who simply requires dietary restriction alone to reduce weight in order to achieve glycaemic control, comply with this regimen. Patients, and very frequently also physicians, start oral agents or insulin prematurely, which may lead to further gain of body weight and more difficulty in achieving metabolic control.

Weight Reduction Planning by Diet and Exercise

The practice of weight reduction by moderate caloric restriction (e.g. 1200–1500 kcal/day) is commonly tried. On the other hand, a more stringent dietary restriction (400–600 kcal/day) is not common practice as it is risky and requires in-hospital management or very careful out-patient monitoring, and furthermore, it is not socially welcomed.

Supplementing dietary restriction with exercise, to ensure more lasting effects, is widely recommended and should be encouraged. Success depends on careful consideration of individual differences in age, physical capacity and educational background.

The combination of dietary planning with the recent trends to involve behavioural modification can produce more lasting effects than diet education alone [12]. This may improve compliance with long-term regimens.

Strategies for behavioural modification involve eating habits, food purchase, self-monitoring of food consumption and weight changes, family involvement, etc. In all such strategies, success depends on careful consideration of the socio-economic background (e.g. individual resources), the prevalent ethnic and cultural factors (e.g. traditional foods), and social customs (e.g. eating on special social occasions). In a region such as the Middle East, which is very rich in customs and traditions, a diabetes care physician will be faced with a continuous but very interesting challenge.

REFERENCES

1. Mashaly ME, Arab MM, Rifaie M. History of diabetes mellitus. MS thesis in medicine. University of Alexandria, 1984.
2. Kamal H. Dictionary of pharaonic medicine. Cairo: The National Publication House, 1967; p 134.
3. Ali Ibn El Hussein Ibn Sina. Al Quanoon Fi Al Tibb, Vol. 3. Cairo: Government Press, 1877; pp 320, 526–8 (in Arabic).
4. Vinik A, Wing RR. Nutritional management of the person with diabetes. In Rifkin H, Porte D (eds) Diabetes mellitus, 4th edn. New York, Amsterdam, London: Elsevier 1990; pp 464–96.
5. PC Globe. 4.0, Computer Programme. Tempe, AZ, USA: PC Globe Inc, 1990.
6. United Nations ACC/SCN. Second report on the World Nutrition Situation 1992. Regional Trends in nutrition, vol. 1. pp 17–28.
7. American Diabetes Association. Clinical Practice Recommendations 1992–1993. Diabetes Care 1993; 16 (suppl. 2): 22–9.
8. Grundy S. In Simopoulos AP, Kifer RR, Martin RE (eds) Health effects of polyunsaturated fatty acids in seafood. Orlando, FL: Academic Press, 1986; pp 14–17.
9. Axelrod L. Omega-3 fatty acids in diabetes mellitus: a gift from the sea? Diabetes 1989; 38: 539–43.
10. Khater R, Elsawy A, Sheta M et al. Glycaemic index of some Egyptian foods. J Egyp Soc End Met Diabet 1987; 19: 87–90.
11. Rassad M, Arab MM. Effect of common Egyptian beverages on glucose tolerance. MS thesis in medicine. University of Alexandria, 1989.
12. Hynes RB. In Hynes RB, Taylor DN, Sackett DL (eds) Compliance in health care. Baltimore: Johns Hopkins University Press, 1979.

35

Exercise

Friedrich W. Kemmer, Uwe Gudat and Michael Berger

Department of Metabolic Diseases and Nutrition, Heinrich-Heine-University Düsseldorf, Germany

During the last two decades the popularity of active participation in various kinds of physical exercise and training has grown rapidly for several reasons. On the one hand, a large part of the population considers exercise to be an integral part of recreational and social activities, while on the other many people of all ages want to take advantage of the possible somatic and psychological benefits of physical activity. From a medical point of view such activities are most welcome, as there is no doubt about the importance of exercise in promoting physical and mental health and, perhaps, even in preventing and helping to cure disease [1]. In the case of diabetes the ability of exercise either to improve or to impair the metabolic situation has been recognized long before our century, thus triggering contradictory recommendations concerning the benefit of exercise in the treatment of this particular disease. It was after the discovery of insulin, in particular, that exercise was strongly recommended as a cornerstone in the treatment of diabetes [2, 3]. For almost half a century this dogmatic opinion appeared to be irrefutable. However, during the last two decades our knowledge of the physiology and pathophysiology of exercise and training [4–7], the different types of diabetes and the problems encountered by patients when trying to follow the recommendation of their physicians to exercise for therapeutic purposes, has increased tremendously. As a consequence we have had to revise the opinion that physical activity can be used as a special form of treatment for diabetic patients [6, 8–10]. The story has not yet come to an end but at present the following picture can be drawn. First, it must be realized that the particular effects of physical exertion differ fundamentally between type 1 and type 2 diabetes. Second, it has emerged that defined physical activity prescribed as a means of improving metabolic control in type 1 diabetic patients should nowadays be regarded as obsolete. Third, the overall results from a large number of elaborate investigations are rather disappointing as far as the beneficial effects of physical activity on improvement of glucose tolerance in non-insulin treated type 2 diabetic patients are concerned. Fourth, physical activity may have a role in the prevention of type 2 diabetes in high risk individuals, albeit prospective intervention studies are yet to be performed.

These insights should not lead to the conclusion that type 1 and many type 2 diabetic patients should be advised not to exercise, but rather that although exercise is no cure-all, it does have specific indications. Indeed, diabetic patients should be encouraged to exercise for the same reasons as the non-diabetic population. However, on the basis of our current concepts of the physiologic and pathophysiologic mechanisms involved in the regulation of fuel homeostasis during exercise, and the knowledge of numerous complications associated with exercise such as hypoglycemia and coronary events, modern diabetes treatment should be aimed at teaching diabetic patients how to reduce or prevent such exercise-associated complications. As many of the physiologic and pathophysiologic mechanisms operative during exercise in diabetes have been reviewed in detail previously [4–7, 11, 12], we concentrate here on updating the theoretical concepts and review the practical aspects of exercise in the management of diabetes.

International Textbook of Diabetes Mellitus, Second Edition. Edited by K.G.M.M. Alberti, P. Zimmet, R.A. DeFronzo, and H. Keen (Honorary)
© 1997 John Wiley & Sons Ltd

FUEL SUPPLY AND REGULATION OF FUEL FLUXES IN NORMAL HUMANS

Fuel Sources

The successful performance of exercise requires a drastic increase of energy and oxygen supply to the working muscle while, at the same time, energy and oxygen supply to the brain and other vital organs must be maintained. The increase in oxygen supply is mainly provided by increased respiration and cardiovascular output, while the adjustment of fuel supply is a more complex procedure. The major energy-yielding substrates for the resting and working muscle are glucose and free fatty acids (FFA). To a lesser extent, amino acids and ketone bodies may be used as fuel, particularly when the availability of other substrates is limited. Glucose and FFA are derived from the circulation, and from depots in the muscle itself and in liver and adipose tissue.

The relative contribution of the different substrates to the energy needs of the muscle depends on the state of nutrition and training as well as the duration and intensity of exercise. Whereas in the postabsorptive state the resting muscle mainly burns FFA stemming from adipose tissue [13], the muscle shifts from using primarily FFA to using a blend of FFA, extramuscular glucose and glycogen during the transition from rest to moderate-intensity exercise. During the initial exercise period, glucose is mainly derived from glycogen stores in the working muscle. As exercise continues, the contributions of circulating glucose and particularly of FFA become of increasing importance because glycogen depots in the working muscles are gradually depleted. Initially, circulating glucose is supplied by enhanced hepatic glucose output which slowly shifts from hepatic glycogenolysis to gluconeogenesis. Substrates for increased gluconeogenesis are derived from increased breakdown of glycogen in non-exercising muscle to lactate, which is then increasingly taken up by the liver [14], and from other 3-carbon molecules which are channelled into gluconeogenesis by intrahepatic mechanisms. However, during prolonged exercise, hepatic glucose production fails to keep pace with the increased peripheral glucose uptake [14], and declining blood glucose levels ensue. Consequently, it has been suggested that the availability of circulating glucose could be a limiting factor for endurance exercise. Interestingly, it could be demonstrated in normal humans [15] that maintenance of euglycemia by ample supply of oral glucose could not delay exhaustion, indicating that hypoglycemia is not the only limiting factor for performance of endurance exercise.

Regulation of Fuel Fluxes

Regulation of fuel fluxes during exercise is mainly achieved by the combined action of insulin, glucagon, catecholamines, cortisol and other hormones [6, 16–20]. In general, endogenous insulin secretion is suppressed during exercise while circulating levels of glucagon, catecholamines and cortisol rise [5, 9] depending on the workload employed, the duration of physical activity and the state of training. In addition to these hormones, other factors such as shifts in blood flow [18], subtle changes in glycemia [21, 22] or other metabolic factors [23, 24], as well as muscle contractions *per se* [25], appear to play a part in controlling fuel supply to the working muscle.

Control of Glucose Uptake

Chaveau and Kaufmann [26] revealed more than a century ago that skeletal muscle is able to increase glucose uptake from the circulation while contracting. Nevertheless, the precise mechanism by which this takes place is still not completely understood. Although several potential amplifiers of glucose uptake have been proposed [4], only muscle contraction and insulin appear to be the most relevant stimuli for enhanced glucose uptake during exercise. From earlier experiments in animals *in vitro* [27] and *in vivo* [28] it was concluded that the presence of minute amounts of insulin is essential for the stimulation of peripheral glucose uptake during exercise. However, recent studies *in vitro* in isolated rat muscles and isolated perfused rat hindquarters have demonstrated that muscle contraction *per se* may stimulate glucose uptake even without presence of insulin [29–32]. Depending on the type of muscle, the stimulatory effects of muscle contraction can even exceed maximal effects of insulin [33, 34]. However, results obtained *in vitro* cannot automatically be extrapolated to the situation *in vivo* in which factors such as catecholamine action antagonizing glucose uptake occur. Observations in completely insulin-deprived [35, 36] or severely underinsulinized depancreatized dogs [28], in which exercise induced only small increments of whole-body metabolic clearance of glucose, are in support of the 'permissive role' of insulin.

Although the studies *in vitro* document that exercise and maximal insulin stimulus have additive effects on glucose transport, it appears that, *in vivo*, exercise may act synergistically with insulin. Thus, it could be shown that a bout of exercise superimposed on a hyperinsulinemic euglycemic clamp increased leg glucose uptake to a greater extent than the sum of these two stimuli independently [18]. Nevertheless, circulating levels of insulin usually are low during exercise and it has been suggested that factors such as augmented muscle blood flow [18] and enlarged muscular capillary area [37] increased neuromotor tone [38]. Metabolic factors such as oxygen availability [24, 39] and changes in insulin affinity to its receptor could be involved in increasing the efficacy of insulin during exercise.

As far as changes in insulin binding are concerned, it was first suggested from studies with human erythrocytes and monocytes that insulin affinity to its receptor was enhanced during exercise [40, 41]. While more recent experiments in humans showed a bidirectional alteration of insulin binding to monocytes depending on the work intensity [42], affinity of insulin to its muscle receptor did not increase with acute exercise in humans [43]. Furthermore, studies in animals have been inconclusive, showing no change [42, 44] or an increase [45] in insulin binding. Hence, it seems unlikely that insulin action during exercise is influenced by alterations in the binding of insulin to its skeletal muscle receptor.

Glucose uptake by muscle is controlled not only by insulin but also by catecholamines. Epinephrine inhibits insulin-mediated glucose uptake in skeletal muscle, as shown in experiments in animals [46–48] and humans [49, 50]. This inhibitory effect of epinephrine appears to be mediated through an inhibition of glucose phosphorylation [46]. During exercise, epinephrine stimulates glycogenolysis from exercising [51] and resting muscles [14, 52, 53] through a β-receptor mechanism. The enhanced glycogenolysis leads to the accumulation of glucose 6-phosphate, which inhibits hexokinase and hence glucose phosphorylation. The importance of catecholamines in controlling this mechanism is supported by the observation that β-blockade lowers the intramuscular concentration of the glycolytic intermediate glucose 6-phosphate. This mechanism to limit glucose uptake may become of importance during prolonged exercise, to prevent a premature collapse of glucose supply.

After cessation of exercise, glucose uptake remains increased as glycogen stores are depleted and glucose fluxes are directed toward rapid replenishment of glycogen stores [54–57]. Mechanisms involved in the increased uptake of glucose during the postexercise period have predominantly been investigated in rats and only to a minor extent in humans. First, experiments in fed rats suggested that such increased glucose uptake and glycogen synthesis after exercise may be due to increased insulin sensitivity [58]. Almost at the same time, Ivy and Holloszy [59] reported that glucose uptake by perfused rat muscle from starved and markedly glycogen-depleted animals increased in the absence of insulin. It could then be demonstrated that glycogen repletion after voluntary exercise occurs in

two phases [60]: in phase I, in which muscular glycogen is still depleted, glucose utilization and glycogen synthesis are enhanced both in the presence and absence of insulin, while in phase II, when glycogen levels have been restored, only the increase in insulin sensitivity persists. Increased binding of insulin to its muscle receptor could be excluded as a reason for the enhanced insulin sensitivity after exercise [61]. Further, it was suggested that glycogen depletion solely acts as an initiator of enhanced muscle glucose uptake after exercise [61], but that persistent glycogen depletion is not able to maintain increased glucose transport into the muscle in the absence of insulin [34]. Finally, it appears that increased insulin-mediated glucose utilization and glycogen synthesis in muscle after exercise are modulated by local contraction-induced factors, as glucose is predominantly utilized by muscle that had been active [62]. As no doubts exist that insulin sensitivity is enhanced during the post-exercise period in humans [63, 64] the same mechanisms may be found in man. This hypothesis finds support from the most recent observation that enhanced insulin-stimulated glucose utilization after a single prolonged bout of exercise is limited to the previously active muscle [156].

Control of Fuel Supply

The increasing amounts of FFA oxidized by the muscle during endurance exercise originate from lipolysis which is regulated by the combined action of insulin and catecholamines. Both the exercise-induced fall of serum insulin and the increase in circulating catecholamines stimulate the release of FFA from muscle and adipose tissue. The stimulatory effect of catecholamines is mediated through a β-adrenergic mechanism, as α-blockade enhances and β-blockade attenuates the lipolytic response to exercise [49] and the β-blocking effects predominate during combined α- and β-blockade [16, 49]. As suggested recently, this mechanism may be due to postreceptor adrenergic events [65]. In any case, the increase of FFA concentration in blood is associated with a proportional uptake of FFA by the working muscle because this process is not insulin dependent [66] and thus provides the necessary fuel to spare glucose and prevent premature exhaustion during long-term physical activity.

As mentioned above, the increase in catecholamines stimulates glycogenolysis during exercise [51]. Studies *in vitro* suggest that, in addition to epinephrine, contractions *per se* can stimulate muscle glycogenolysis even in the absence of catecholamines [67]. Thus, it is possible that catecholamines and muscle contractions exert a dual control over muscle glycogenolysis, at least at the onset of exercise, to cover the drastically increased fuel demands of the working muscle during the initial period of physical activity. However, recent experiments also document the importance of epinephrine in mobilizing glycogen from inactive muscles during prolonged exercise [14, 52, 53], which can then serve as fuel for the working muscle via gluconeogenesis in the liver.

Without timely and adequate glucose replacement from the liver or intestinal absorption, the glucose circulating in blood would be rapidly consumed and exercise would come to a halt because of failure of glucose-dependent vital organs such as the brain. In the fed state, glucose from exogenous sources is oxidized almost completely during exercise, provided that sufficient insulin is available [68]. Even after exercise, orally administered glucose is preferentially used to replete muscle glycogen stores [55, 69]. Thus, glucose stemming from intestinal absorption contributes to the maintenance of glucose homeostasis during exercise, if available.

In the postabsorptive state, normoglycemia is maintained by precise coordination of hepatic glucose production and peripheral glucose utilization during and after exercise in the normal human. The appropriate increase of hepatic glucose production during exercise is regulated by the interplay of insulin, glucagon, catecholamines and, to a lesser extent, cortisol and growth hormone [6, 9]. With the onset of exercise, insulin secretion decreases almost instantaneously [70–72], leading to portal and peripheral hypoinsulinemia and, consequently, relative hyperglucagonemia. In principle, this change in the ratio of glucagon to insulin appears to be one major determinant of increased hepatic glucose production during exercise. It could then be demonstrated in experiments in animals [17, 19, 73, 74] and humans [16, 20, 75] that not only the reduction of portal insulin levels but also the presence of glucagon was essential to facilitate increased hepatic glucose output. When glucagon secretion was suppressed below basal by somatostatin in dogs, this was associated with attenuated hepatic glucose production during exercise [19]. In human studies, endogenous insulin and glucagon release were prevented with somatostatin and the pancreatic hormones were replaced via a peripheral vein so that the normal arterial levels of these hormones and euglycemia were maintained [16]. Under these conditions hepatic glucose production responded normally to exercise. As the physiological portoperipheral insulin gradient is lost with infusion of insulin and glucagon, the liver may still be hypoinsulinemic, facilitating the increase in hepatic glucose output. To overcome this problem, increased rates of insulin were infused to create portal euinsulinemia (albeit peripheral hyperinsulinemia) and euglycemia was maintained with glucose infusion. When exercise was performed

under these conditions, hepatic glucose production was attenuated [20, 75].

Although these experiments support the importance of the physiological changes in pancreatic hormones for normal glucose kinetics during exercise, it seems likely that the increase in hepatic glucose production with the onset of exercise is dependent not only on a change in the glucagon:insulin ratio but also on the activation of the sympathetic nervous system [19]. In fact, recent studies in normal and bilaterally adrenalectomized humans demonstrated that epinephrine is an unimportant determinant of glucose production during exercise [76]. On the other hand, sympathetic neural norepinephrine appears to be the operative catecholamine in stimulating glucose output during exercise in humans and thus it could provide the signal for the instantaneous increase of hepatic glucose production at the onset of exercise [76].

Whereas during the initial phase of exercise the presence of basal glucagon levels appears to be an important factor for an adequate increase of hepatic glucose production, increased levels of glucagon together with cortisol, growth hormone and catecholamines are apparently necessary to maintain increased hepatic glucose output during prolonged exercise [5]. The importance of increased glucagon levels could be shown in depancreatized dogs in which intraportally infused insulin preventing the fall of intraportal insulin levels during exercise was associated with a blunted increase in glucagon secretion [77]. The failure of insulin to

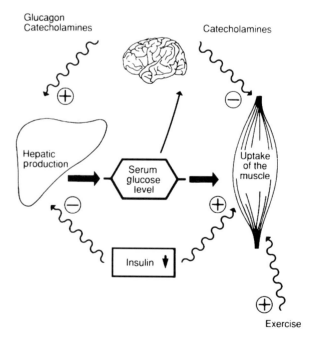

Figure 1 Schema of glucose homeostasis during exercise under physiological conditions. Straight arrows indicate fuel fluxes; wavy arrows indicate stimulatory and inhibitory effects

fall and glucagon to rise led to an 80% reduction in glucose output from the liver. When normal exercising glucagon levels were restored in the presence of unchanged portal insulin, hepatic glucose production was 50% of the normal response, whereas the gluconeogenic conversion rate was normalized [78]. These findings suggest further that the fall in insulin and the rise in glucagon together mainly control liver glycogenolysis, while the rise in glucagon is critical for the increase in gluconeogenesis during endurance exercise.

Thus, under physiologic conditions, the interactions of insulin, glucagon and catecholamines and other hormones coordinate and maintain the fuel supply to the working muscle and the brain while glucose homeostasis is preserved (Figure 1).

EXERCISE IN INSULIN-TREATED DIABETICS

Pathophysiology of Fuel Fluxes

Type 1 diabetes represents a conceptually simple disorder characterized by the cessation of endogenous insulin secretion. This insulin deficit is replaced by subcutaneous administration of exogenous insulin using various types of modern intensified insulin therapy. Nevertheless, even recent advances in insulin substitution cannot fully restore physiological changes in portal and peripheral insulin levels as seen in normal humans. Consequently, various states of insulin deficiency or excess in peripheral or portal blood may occur. Considering the complexity of fuel fluxes and the central role of insulin in its regulation, it is not surprising that in type 1 diabetes the basic mechanism of glucoregulation during exercise is upset. On the basis of the prevailing insulin levels, two classic phenomena associated with physical activity, i.e. deterioration and improvement of metabolic control, can be observed [79].

During insulin-deficient states, severe ketoacidosis and/or hyperglycemia is likely to occur. Tracer studies in depancreatized dogs [28] and type 1 diabetic patients [80] indicated that insulin deficiency facilitates an enhanced liver glucose output during exercise although it does not permit an adequate uptake of glucose into the working muscle. As a consequence, progressive hyperglycemia ensued (Figure 2). Although insulin deficiency appears to have the central role in deterioration of blood glucose levels during exercise in diabetic patients, this process may be aggravated by excessive increments in glucagon [79, 81, 82], catecholamines [83, 84], growth hormone [84, 85] and cortisol [79]. For instance, it could be shown in totally insulin-deprived dogs that β-blockade markedly reduced increments in glucose production

during exercise [35]. In addition, insulin deficiency and elevated levels of counter-regulatory hormones will further enhance FFA and ketone body levels with exercise [82].

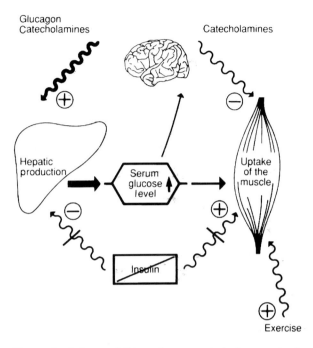

Figure 2 Schema of glucose homeostasis during exercise in presence of insulin lack. Straight arrows indicate fuel fluxes, wavy arrows indicate stimulatory and inhibitory effects

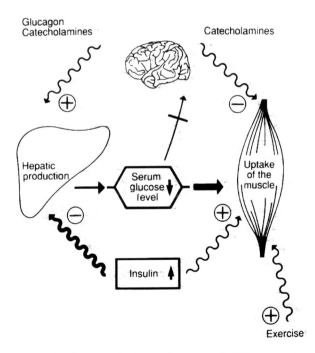

Figure 3 Schema of glucose homeostasis during exercise in presence of hyperinsulinemia. Straight arrows indicate fuel fluxes; wavy arrows indicate stimulatory and inhibitory effects

The currently available strategies of insulin substitution are associated with peripheral hyperinsulinemia [86, 87] which may be aggravated by accelerated absorption of insulin when injected into a moving part of the body [88, 89]. When exercise is performed under these conditions the excess insulin will prevent an adequate rise in hepatic glucose production but promote an enhanced peripheral glucose utilization which may even be aggravated by increased insulin sensitivity during exercise [80, 90]. As a consequence, a fall in glycemia and possibly hypoglycemia will develop (Figure 3).

Clinical Implications of Impaired Glucoregulation in Exercising Diabetic Patients

The ability of exercise to decrease circulating blood glucose levels in insulin-treated diabetic patients was observed shortly after insulin had been introduced in the therapy of diabetes mellitus [91]. This observation gave rise to the earlier recommendation [2, 3] to use physical activity in addition to insulin and diet in the treatment of diabetes mellitus, because it was thought that exercise could play the part of a third important element in normalizing glycemia and maintaining good metabolic control. However, during the last decade it was realized that physical activity prescribed as a means to improve glycemic control in type 1 diabetic patients should be regarded as obsolete, for the following reasons:

(1) Relatively precise concepts on the complexity of fuel fluxes and its regulation during physical activity in normal and diabetic individuals have been developed, and leave no doubt that the use of physical exercise as a therapeutic tool meets almost unsurmountable problems in clinical practice.

(2) Numerous studies have shown that exercise programs are not helpful when used to improve metabolic control on a long-term basis [92–95].

(3) Glycemic control may very well be optimized and near-normoglycemia be maintained by intensified treatment and teaching programs *per se* [96–98].

The principal problem with the use of exercise to improve metabolic control is that the net effect of exercise on blood glucose is unpredictable in type 1 diabetic patients because of the many variables influencing glucose supply and utilization: these include the state of nutrition and of metabolic control, before and at the onset of exercise; the time of day that exercise is begun; the duration and intensity of exercise; the state of physical training of the patient; and the type, dose and site of insulin injection. Thus, in clinical practice the patient who wants to take advantage of exercise to improve metabolic control on a long-term basis would be faced with the problem of coordinating meals, insulin injections and exercise. If, for instance, this patient were to exercise to attenuate the postprandial rise in glycemia, he or she would have to exercise regularly for a defined period of time and at a defined workload. The majority of diabetic patients would consider this procedure as a further and unnecessary burden, as their daily schedule is already largely determined by insulin injections and meal-times. As no evidence for a beneficial role in treatment of type 1 diabetes on a long-term basis could be provided [92–95], only a few type 1 diabetic patients may decide to adhere to an exercise program for the sake of improving metabolic control alone.

Very much like the non-diabetic population, an ever-growing proportion of type 1 diabetic patients intend to take up or to intensify their leisure-time physical activity for a number of motivations which mainly are not health-related. This means that, like anybody else, diabetic patients exercise mainly at weekends, in the evening and during holidays. Under these conditions, physical activity is largely spontaneous, and time, duration and intensity of exercise are variable; hence the metabolic effects of exercise are difficult to predict. Although such factors are of no importance for the non-diabetic population, diabetic patients may abstain from participating in physical activity for fear of experiencing acute complications, such as hypoglycemia. As participation in exercise and games has become an important facet of the social structure of our societies, it is the obligation of all diabetologists to enable type 1 diabetic patients to perform physical activity with a minimal risk of acute complications. Any effective prevention of much-feared exercise-associated complications in insulin-treated diabetic patients may best be achieved in the context of an intensive diabetes treatment and teaching program. The efficacy and long-term safety of such programs, aiming at far-reaching independence of the patient from physicians and clinics, has been documented even for unselected patients [98].

First of all, before taking on regular physical activities or increasing habitual physical activity, type 1 diabetic patients need to be examined carefully for the presence of retinal and neurological complications. Exercise-induced increases of blood pressure may cause acute complications in certain stages of pre-proliferative or proliferative retinopathy. Thus, hypertension must be treated adequately and laser treatment may be needed before participation in physical exercise can be recommended. Patients with autonomic neuropathy may be at risk of disturbed cardiovascular function during or after exercise. Loss of sensory function due to peripheral polyneuropathy may create a serious risk of foot injury.

Type 1 diabetic patients who wish to participate in exercise must also be cognizant of measures to prevent further increase of hyperglycemia or severe ketoacidosis. Blood glucose levels of about 300 mg/dl (16.7 mmol/l) associated with significant acetonuria indicate insulin deficiency. If exercise is performed under such conditions, metabolic control is likely to deteriorate further [79]; therefore, patients who detect these indices of insulin deficiency should be warned against exercise. Instead, it is important that they inject adequate amounts of insulin to restore good metabolic control before starting to exercise again. At this point it must be mentioned that further deterioration of metabolic control may also occur during the initial period after a short bout of maximal exercise as seen in normal subjects [99] and diabetic patients on continuous subcutaneous insulin infusion (CSII) [100]. Depending on the pre-exercise blood glucose levels, the rise in glycemia may be considerable, possibly requiring an adaptation of the insulin dose after short bouts of exhaustive exercise.

Hypoglycemia, the most feared and more frequent complication of physical activity in diabetes, is mainly caused by hyperinsulinemia and the loss of physiological adaptation of insulin needs to exercise. As exercise may accelerate the absorption of regular insulin injected in the thigh immediately before the onset of exercise, it was felt at one time that injection of insulin into a non-moving part of the body might prevent or at least reduce the risk of exercise-induced hypoglycemia [88]. Shortly after this idea was put forward, however, it was demonstrated that this measure could not effectively prevent hypoglycemia during exercise [101, 102]. From a physiological point of view it would be logical to mimic the situation that obtains in normal subjects, by reducing the insulin dose before exercise. However, this approach is of value only when the time, duration and intensity of exercise can be defined. In cases when insulin already has been injected, or when duration and intensity of exercise are unforeseeable, the only measure to prevent hypoglycemia is to supplement hepatic glucose production by increasing carbohydrate ingestion before, during and after the physical activity.

This principal recommendation to prevent exercise-induced hypoglycemia meets with a number of difficulties when it comes to the determination of the insulin dose reduction or the additional amount of carbohydrate to be consumed. The adjustments in insulin dose and carbohydrate supplements undoubtedly depend on the duration and intensity of the workload and the level of glycemia before exercise, as well as the time of day that exercise is begun. Thus, only general recommendations can be given which can serve as a starting point from which patients must find the optimal measure for their individual situation.

If a patient plans to exercise for a longer period of time, e.g. cross-country skiing, marathon running, hiking or bicycling, the insulin dose should be reduced if possible. If such exercise is performed in the morning after the usual breakfast and normoglycemia is found before exercise, a reduction of more than 50% of the morning insulin dose may be necessary to prevent hypoglycemia [103, 104]. At blood glucose levels above 200 mg/dl (11.1 mmol/l) a lesser reduction in the insulin dose was sufficient to prevent hypoglycemia. Similar results were found in patients participating in a ski race over a distance of 75 km [105]. In diabetic patients participating in a marathon run [106], insulin was withheld altogether for 16–26 hours prior to the race; nevertheless, the patients were not deprived of insulin, as shown by circulating free insulin levels and normal plasma free fatty acids and blood ketone bodies. Only when blood glucose levels were near 300 mg/dl (16.7 mmol/l) initially did all patients complete the race without complications, achieving normoglycemia during the final third of the race. As shown in the skiers, this type of endurance exercise increased insulin sensitivity after the race. This effect should be taken into consideration when endurance exercise has been performed, and reduced insulin doses may be necessary even on the day after such physical activity.

The time of day at which exercise is performed, and the prevailing insulin levels, may be of importance for consideration of the appropriate measure to prevent hypoglycemia during exercise. In a recent study it was suggested that the risk of exercise-induced hypoglycemia was lowest when exercise was performed in the morning before breakfast and insulin injection, when low insulin levels prevailed [157]. However, when taking this approach, hypoglycemia may be prevented at the cost of inducing hyperglycemia. In particular, physical activity performed in the evening or afternoon carries the risk of nocturnal hypoglycemia [107, 108]. As enhancement of insulin sensitivity extends beyond the exercise period [63, 64] and muscle continues to take up substantial amounts of glucose from the circulation to replenish glycogen stores, an adequate supply to the circulation must be guaranteed. At night the liver is the main source of glucose and hyperinsulinemia would block this source. Therefore, even after physical exercise in the evening, the insulin dose must be reduced substantially and additional amounts of carbohydrates must be taken [107]. Although all these studies are far from providing precise guidelines for the reduction of insulin in association with exercise, they indicate clearly that a dose reduction of only 1–4 U of insulin would be useless to prevent exercise-induced hypoglycemia under those circumstances.

When exercise is spontaneous, only ingestion of extra carbohydrates can prevent hypoglycemia. No doubt exists about the efficacy of this measure, because glucose stemming from exogenous sources is oxidized almost completely by the working muscle if sufficient amounts of insulin are available. The additional carbohydrates should be ingested in small amounts to avoid exercising on a full stomach. Additional carbohydrates may also be sufficient to maintain an adequate supply of glucose to the working muscle before and/or after relatively short and mild physical exercise. However, in association with short periods of exhaustive exercise, additional carbohydrates may be disadvantageous as under such conditions glycemia may increase, as observed in diabetic patients treated with CSII [100]. Similar increments in glycemia were seen in cross-country skiers during the initial phase of the race [105].

Continuous subcutaneous insulin infusion (CSII) is now an established form of insulin therapy and many patients use it as their preferred form of treatment. In principle, patients using CSII therapy should also follow guidelines such as reduction of the insulin bolus in anticipation of postprandial exercise [104] and adaptation of the insulin infusion rate [158]. As demonstrated recently, patients on CSII treatment planning to perform long-term physical activity could best prevent acute exercise-induced hypoglycemia by reducing the pre-meal insulin bolus by 50% and stopping the basal insulin infusion rate while exercising [159]. In order to reduce the risk of late-onset hypoglycemia, reduction of the basal insulin infusion rate by 25% for several hours after the exercise period appeared to be the appropriate measure [159].

These general guidelines can only serve as a starting point for individual patients to discover their personal reaction to the physical exercise of their choice under varying conditions. Thus, diabetic patients who want to exercise must be offered an intensive and comprehensive teaching program for self-management of their metabolic control [109]. As the personal experience of the patient grows and success in preventing hypoglycemia and other exercise-related complications increases, exercise can be performed safely and with optimal physical performance. The success of diabetic athletes and the activities of the International Diabetic Athletes Association have impressively documented that this is undoubtedly possible.

EXERCISE IN TYPE 2 DIABETES

Type 2 (non-insulin dependent) diabetes mellitus represents a complex syndrome of hyperglycemia, insulin resistance [110] and often a variety of interrelated cardiovascular risk factors [111] such as hypertension and hyperlipoproteinemia. In addition, patients with type 2 diabetes are usually obese and characterized by reduced physical activity. Furthermore, for most of the 3–4% of our population currently known as type 2 diabetics, this disorder develops after the age of 60 years, and very often as just one aspect of a multifaceted geriatric morbidity. As a consequence, for the majority of these patients, macrovascular disease and its complications rather than diabetic microvascular disease are the major determinant of their longevity. Only in those patients who manifest type 2 diabetes at a younger age must the prevention of microangiopathy by strict normalization of glycemia be regarded as a primary therapeutic goal. In parallel to the obvious heterogeneity of type 2 diabetes and the individual therapeutic goals for these patients, there is a diversity of treatment strategies such as a low-energy diet, oral antidiabetic drugs and/or insulin. Despite all of these aspects of heterogeneity of this disease, insulin resistance associated with a relative deficiency of insulin secretory capacity is thought to be the basic defect for all stages and subgroups of type 2 diabetes mellitus [110, 112]. Therefore, any treatment of this metabolic syndrome should aim at increasing insulin sensitivity. From a pathophysiologic point of view, such a therapeutic approach would be fundamental, as opposed to any treatment involving β-cytotropic drugs. Therefore, together with weight reduction, physical exercise training must *a priori* be regarded as a rational approach to the treatment of type 2 diabetes mellitus.

As certain metabolic derangements precede the manifestation of overt type 2 diabetes, the metabolic benefits of regular physical activity theoretically represent a preventive strategy against progressive glucose intolerance.

Effects of Acute Exercise

Despite the high prevalence of type 2 diabetes, only a few studies have examined the effects of exercise on glucoregulatory hormones and glucose kinetics in this population. It is now a decade since a group of obese type 2 diabetic patients treated with diet or diet plus sulfonylurea was investigated while exercising for 45 min on a cycle ergometer [113]. The patients had postabsorptive hyperglycemia (about 200 mg/dl, 11.1 mmol/l) and normal basal insulin levels. Exercise did not suppress circulating insulin levels and glycemia fell by approximately 50 mg/dl (2.8 mmol/l) during the exercise period. In type 2 diabetic patients with moderate fasting hyperglycemia (140 mg/dl, 7.8 mmol/l) and hyperinsulinemia, prolonged exercise reduced glycemia by 40 mg/dl (2.2 mmol/l) and decreased the elevated insulin levels to a certain extent [114].

It could be shown that the drop in glycemia was caused by an attenuated rise in hepatic glucose production while glucose utilization increased normally. At least two factors, i.e. unaltered insulin levels and

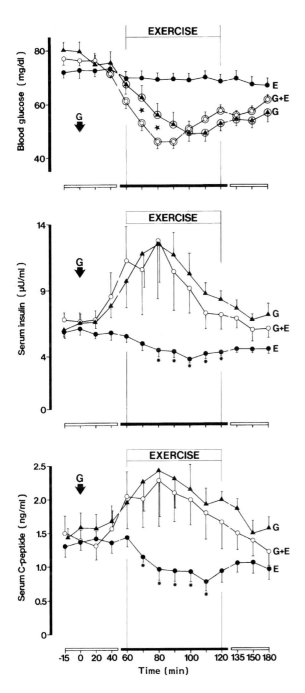

Figure 4 Mean blood glucose, plasma insulin, and C-peptide concentrations in 9 healthy men after oral administration of 1.75 mg glyburide (glibenclamide) with (G + E) and without (G) performance of exercise and during performance of exercise alone (E). ° significant differences vs. 0 min ($P < 0.01$); *, significant differences vs. 60 min, $P < 0.01$; ⋆, significant differences between G and G + E, $P < 0.01$ (from reference 114, with permission)

hyperglycemia, are likely to have contributed to the reduced response in hepatic glucose production. The failure of exercise to suppress insulin secretion, as in normal subjects, may be a consequence of the prevailing hyperglycemia or a defective control of insulin secretion in type 2 diabetic patients. In addition to the defective control of insulin secretion in type 2 diabetes mellitus, persisting hyperinsulinemia during exercise could be the consequence of sulfonylurea treatment. As was shown recently in normal humans [115], 1 hour of moderate-intensity exercise was not able to blunt glyburide-stimulated insulin secretion and thus enhanced the hypoglycemic action of this sulfonylurea (Figure 4). The same mechanism is likely to be operative in sulfonylurea-treated patients with type 2 diabetes mellitus. Thus, complications such as exercise-induced hypoglycemia must be taken into account in diabetic patients treated with oral sulfonylureas. These studies suggest that physiological alterations of hormones and glucoregulation in response to exercise are abnormal in type 2 diabetic patients with hyperglycemia, hyperinsulinemia and sulfonylurea treatment. On the other hand, no evidence has been provided as yet that any difference exists in hormonal and metabolic responses to physical exercise between healthy subjects and type 2 diabetic patients who are treated with diet alone and are metabolically well controlled.

Effects of Training on Insulin Sensitivity and Glucose Tolerance

As insulin resistance is the primary defect in type 2 diabetic patients, the main interest has been directed towards effects of acute and chronic exercise on insulin sensitivity and metabolic control (for a more detailed review of the effects of physical training on cardiovascular risk factors, see reference 116). The evidence in support of beneficial effects of physical training on glucose tolerance and insulin sensitivity has been largely derived from experiments in non-diabetic animals and humans. In normal rats, mild physical exercise of approximately 2 weeks improved intravenous glucose tolerance [117] (Figure 5). This improvement in glucose tolerance was associated with a marked reduction of basal and glucose-stimulated insulin levels, indicating an increased sensitivity to insulin. Similarly, studies in obese non-diabetic subjects [118] as well as in trained athletes [119–121] have clearly demonstrated an association between physical training and increased insulin sensitivity. In addition, it was shown that insulin resistance in obese subjects with normal glucose tolerance could be reversed by a moderate-intensity physical conditioning program [122].

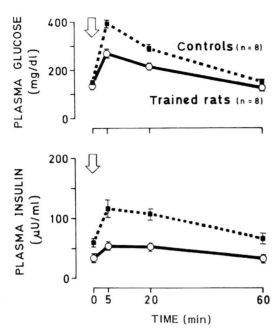

Figure 5 Effect of swim training for 2 weeks on intravenous glucose tolerance test in normally fed rats. The arrow indicates the time of glucose injection. Plasma glucose and insulin levels are significantly different between trained animals (O——O) and the controls (■- - -■) at all time points (from reference 117, with permission)

Considering the fundamental role of skeletal muscle during exercise and the fact that it represents the bulk of insulin-sensitive tissue, it is likely that muscle is the major site of the increased insulin sensitivity that occurs with training. Earlier experiments *in vitro* revealed that the insulin-stimulated glucose uptake of skeletal muscle was enhanced in trained rats [117, 123] while hepatic glucose uptake of such animals was reduced as compared with sedentary controls [123]. More recently, it could be shown in isolated muscles [124, 125] that the increase in insulin action on glucose uptake of the muscle is mainly due to increased glucose oxidation. In several experiments the glucose metabolism of adipose tissue has also been shown to be sensitized to insulin after training [124, 126, 127], which is consistent with the finding that trained rats have a greater number of glucose transporters in fat cell membranes [128]. These results suggest that, at least in animals, skeletal muscle is the major site of increased insulin sensitivity after training, with adipose tissue contributing to a lesser extent to the increased whole-body insulin sensitivity associated with physical training [124].

In humans, the sensitivity of different tissues to physiological insulin levels has been assessed in trained long-distance runners [121] using a euglycemic clamp with insulin infusions maintaining circulating insulin at levels of 10 μU/ml and 50 μU/ml. At either insulin

concentration, trained subjects had markedly increased insulin-stimulated glucose uptake while their hepatic glucose production was much lower than in controls. Thus, both an increased peripheral and hepatic sensitivity to insulin may be present in trained subjects. In addition, it has been shown that a close relationship exists between the level of physical training and insulin-stimulated glucose utilization [129]. These effects of training are probably specific for aerobic exercise, as strength training is associated with increased muscle mass. Thus, in heavy athletes, the decreased response of insulin to a glucose challenge [120], the net increase in insulin-stimulated glucose disposal [130] and the improved glucose tolerance [131] are probably due to this enlarged muscle mass rather than an increase in insulin sensitivity *per se*.

The increase in insulin action in skeletal muscle during physical training could be mediated by several factors. Thus it may in part be due to an increase of insulin binding to its skeletal muscle receptor [132, 133]. On the other hand, an increase in the number of insulin receptors may occur as well, as demonstrated in rats after a 4-week training program [133]. Furthermore, activities of cytoplasmic and mitochondrial enzymes such as muscle citrate synthase and succinate dehydrogenase increase in parallel to insulin sensitivity in diabetic rats [134] and insulin dependent diabetes mellitus patients during training [98]. In addition, increased muscle capillary density, which is associated with physical training in normal subjects [37] but not in diabetic patients [135, 136], has been considered to be operative in enhancing insulin sensitivity by augmenting the exposure of muscle to insulin and glucose. More recently, it has been shown that the expression of insulin-regulatable glucose transporters (IRGT) can be increased in skeletal muscle of rats by exercise training [160]. Thus, exercise may enhance insulin sensitivity, at least in part, through increased production of glucose transporters.

Much of the enhanced insulin sensitivity associated with physical training is lost if physical activity is discontinued for several days, as shown in trained athletes [137, 138]. However, insulin sensitivity can be largely restored by a single intensive bout of exercise to the supranormal, trained level [138]. In untrained, insulin-resistant, obese non-diabetic subjects, an acute bout of high-intensity cycle exercise was associated with significant increases in submaximal and maximal rates of insulin-mediated glucose utilization 12–16 hours after exercise [139]. This increase was accounted for totally by increased rates of non-oxidative glucose disposal, possibly reflecting increased glucose storage as glycogen during the postexercise period. The same mechanism appears to be operative in non-insulin dependent diabetic patients [140].

Training in Treatment of Type 2 Diabetic Patients

Until recently, only a few studies in diabetic animals and humans suggested that physical training might be used successfully for the treatment of type 2 diabetes mellitus. In fact, only one prospective study in obese Zucker rats, which have a syndrome that is similar to type 2 diabetes mellitus [141, 142], has documented that physical training initiated at an early age can in part prevent the development of insulin resistance, glucose intolerance (Figure 6), hyperlipidemia and obesity [143]. On the other hand, epidemiological studies are suggestive of a possible role of physical inactivity in increasing the incidence of type 2 diabetes mellitus [144, 145, 161]. Beyond this theoretical anticipation of the beneficial effects of physical training programs on glucose tolerance, no unequivocal evidence for the effectiveness of such a therapeutic approach, based upon prospective controlled trials, has been provided so far. In contrast, a multitude of investigations have been carried out in glucose-intolerant and/or type 2 diabetic patients, with the aim of demonstrating an improvement in glucose tolerance or glycemic control,

along with improvements of body mass index and lipidemia by regular physical exercise.

Clinical studies in middle-aged men with impaired glucose tolerance [146] and type 2 diabetes mellitus [147] have demonstrated a slight improvement in glucose tolerance after a 6-month training program. In another small group of type 2 diabetic patients [148], participation in a training program resulted only in a transient improvement of intravenous glucose tolerance but not of oral glucose tolerance. In several more recent studies in non-insulin dependent diabetic patients [149–152], such training programs were associated with a decrease in fasting blood glucose levels and an improvement of hemoglobin A_{1c}. At present, HbA_{1c} is considered to represent the most reliable index of the current state of metabolic control in diabetic patients. Therefore the decline in HbA_{1c} provides some evidence that physical training might be used successfully to improve overall metabolic control in type 2 diabetic patients. More detailed investigations in some of these studies support the view that the improved metabolic control is related to increased insulin sensitivity of skeletal muscle. Using the euglycemic insulin

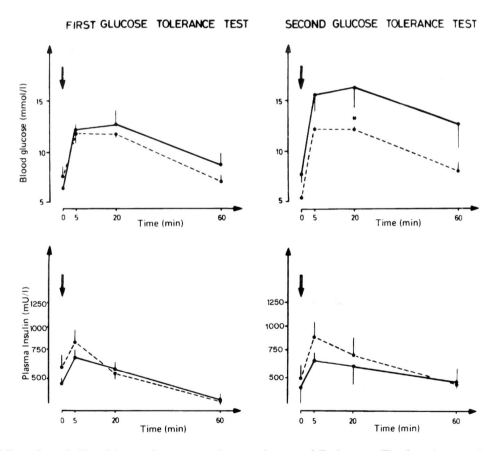

Figure 6 Effect of treadmill training on intravenous glucose tolerance of Zucker rats. The first glucose tolerance test was performed in 7-week-old animals: ●————● 6 control rats; ●- - - -● 5 training rats. The second glucose tolerance test was performed following a 9-week training or control period; * indicates significant difference between training and control group ($P < 0.05$) (from reference 143, with permission)

clamp technique, Reitman et al [150] and Bogardus et al [152] have shown that, following a physical training program, peripheral glucose uptake is increased. Furthermore, it could be demonstrated that these increased amounts of glucose taken up by peripheral tissues were channelled into storage, presumably as glycogen, rather than oxidation. Thus, while these and other studies [153] are suggestive of a beneficial effect of a training program on overall metabolic control and insulin sensitivity, they fail to provide evidence for the anticipated beneficial effect on glucose tolerance. Even when a small group of selected type 2 diabetic men participated in regular physical exercise over a period of 2 years, no improvement of glucose tolerance could be achieved [154]. Moreover, as in trained non-diabetic patients, the enhanced insulin sensitivity associated with physical training is lost in diabetic patients if they stop exercising on a regular basis.

The critical evaluation of these overall rather disappointing results from a large number of most elaborate investigations, at a recent National Institutes of Health Consensus Conference [155], gave rise to some sceptical conclusions as to the general beneficial effects of physical training programs as part of the treatment of type 2 diabetes mellitus. In addition, the study by Skarfors et al [154], investigating effects of regular physical exercise in type 2 diabetic patients over a period of 2 years, has cast doubts on the feasibility and efficacy of such training programs. Thus, from this study a number of problems emerged which had been encountered to a certain extent in previous investigations. These include difficulties in separating dietary from exercise effects, heterogeneity of the initial hormonal–metabolic status of the patients, the appearance or aggravation of coronary heart disease, the deterioration of diabetes and (last but not least) the apparent lack of motivation of patients to participate in physical training over a period lasting more than 3–6 months.

Against the therapeutic benefits of physical training yet to be proven in type 2 diabetics, one has to balance possible risks associated with training programs in elderly populations with major cardiovascular risks and very often manifest atherosclerosis and coronary heart disease. As with comparable groups, type 2 diabetic patients need to be screened specifically for cardiovascular risks and diseases before participation in any such training program. In addition, these training programs should be designed and carried out under professional and medical supervision, taking into account that the majority of these elderly type 2 diabetic patients have not been physically active for quite some time and are thus particularly vulnerable to all kinds of injuries. Finally, patients treated with insulin and/or oral sulfonylureas are prone to develop exercise-induced hypoglycemia [115]. Thus, such patients must be advised to adapt their insulin dose and/or to reduce the dose of the sulfonylurea before exercise.

It appears that only in a few selected subgroups of type 2 diabetic patients, i.e. the relatively healthy, hyperinsulinemic patients below the age of 60 years, can clear-cut positive effects of physical activity upon glucose tolerance be anticipated. Nevertheless, even before recommendation of physical training programs for treatment of this minority of type 2 diabetic patients can be made, considerably more research is needed.

Physical Activity and Prevention of Type 2 Diabetes

Epidemiological studies in Pacific populations—when based on the presumption that the major difference between rural and urban populations is their degree of everyday physical activity—suggest that exercise confers a protective influence toward the manifestation of type 2 diabetes [144, 145]. Similar evidence has recently been presented from a Pima Indian population. Self-reported life-time physical activity correlated inversely with manifestation of diabetes [162].

Helmrich et al (161) used questionnaires to examine patterns of physical activity in relation to the subsequent development of type 2 diabetes in 5990 male alumni of the University of Pennsylvania. Type 2 diabetes developed in a total of 202 men during 98 524 man years of follow-up from 1962 to 1976. The protective influence of physical activity was highest in persons at greatest risk of type 2 diabetes, defined as those with a high body mass index, a history of hypertension or a parental history of diabetes. In addition to weight gain since college graduation, these items were predictive of type 2 diabetes.

Manson et al [163] correlated self-reported participation in vigorous physical exercise in a prospective cohort of 87 253 nurses (US Nurses Health Study), aged 34–59 years and free of cardiovascular disease and cancer in 1980, with manifestation of type 2 diabetes. During 8 years of follow-up, 1303 cases of type 2 diabetes occurred. Women who had engaged in vigorous exercise at least once a week had an age adjusted relative risk (RR) of type 2 diabetes equal to 0.67 ($P < 0.0001$) compared to women who did not exercise at least once weekly. After adjustment for body mass index, the reduction in risk was attenuated but remained statistically significant ($RR = 0.84$; $P < 0.005$). Among women who exercised at least once weekly, there was no clear-cut dose–response gradient according to the frequency of exercise. Multivariate adjustments for age, body mass index, family history of diabetes and other variables did not alter the reduced risk associated with regular exercise.

In a further report, Manson et al [164] presented data from the physicians' health study. Originally designed to assess the cardioprotective benefit of aspirin or β-carotene, 21 271 male physicians were asked, among other things: 'How often do you exercise vigorously enough to work up a sweat?' The answers were correlated with the incidence of type 2 diabetes during the five-year follow-up period, which summed up to 105 141 person-years. Overall, 285 cases of type 2 diabetes were reported. Physicians who worked up a sweat at least once a week showed a relative risk of manifesting type 2 diabetes of 0.64 (confidence interval 0.51–0.82) with respect to those exercising less. Although the raw data suggested a dose–response relationship, when corrected for age and body mass index this effect was no longer statistically significant.

In summary, we have circumstantial evidence (descriptive associations in defined ethnic groups such as Pima Indians or Nauru islanders, cohort studies in nurses, physicians or alumni) that physical activity of even a low intensity and/or frequency may reduce the incidence of NIDDM in those at greatest risk, especially individuals with a positive family history, high body mass index or a history of hypertension. However, in the absence of a proper intervention study this evidence must be considered preliminary. On a practical note it seems prudent, if physical activity interventions are to be used, that they should be targeted at high-risk individuals. In contrast, in the moderately active individual of normal weight additional activity probably does not make diabetes more unlikely.

REFERENCES

1. Smith T. Exercise: cult or cure-all? Br Med J 1983; 286: 1637–9.
2. Joslin EP. The treatment of diabetes mellitus. In Joslin EP, Root HF, White P, Marble A (eds) Treatment of diabetes mellitus, 10th edn. Philadelphia: Lea & Febiger 1959: pp 243–300.
3. Katsch G. Arbeitstherapie der Zuckerkranken. Erg Physikal Diät Ther 1939; 1: 1–36.
4. Vranic M, Berger M. Exercise and diabetes mellitus. Diabetes 1979; 28: 147–67.
5. Kemmer FW, Vranic M. The role of glucagon and its relationship to other glucoregulatory hormones in exercise. In Orci L, Unger RH (eds) Glucagon. Contemporary endocrinology series. New York: Elsevier/North Holland, 1981: pp 297–331.
6. Kemmer FW, Berger M. Exercise and diabetes mellitus: physical activity as a part of daily life and its role in the treatment of diabetic patients. Int J Sports Med 1983; 4: 77–88.
7. Richter EA, Ruderman NB, Schneider SH. Diabetes and exercise. Am J Med 1981; 70: 201–9.
8. Kemmer FW, Berger M. Exercise in therapy and the life of diabetic patients. Clin Sci 1984; 67: 279–83.
9. Kemmer FW, Berger M. Therapy and better quality of life: the dichotomous role of exercise in diabetes mellitus. Diabetes Metab Rev 1986; 2: 53–68.
10. Berger M, Kemmer FW. Discussion: exercise, fitness, and diabetes. In Bouchard C, Shepard RJ, Stepehens Th. Sutton JR, McPherson BD (eds) Exercise, fitness, and health: a consensus of current knowledge. Champaign, IL: Human Kinetics Books, 1990: pp 491–5.
11. Galbo H. Endocrinology and metabolism in exercise. Int J Sports Med 1981; 2: 203–11.
12. Wasserman DH, Vranic M. Exercise and diabetes. In Alberti KGMM, Krall LP (eds) Diabetes annual 3. Amsterdam: Elsevier, 1987: pp 527–59.
13. Ahlborg G, Felig P, Hagenfeldt L, Hendler R, Wahren J. Substrate turnover during prolonged exercise. J Clin Invest 1974; 53: 1080–90.
14. Ahlborg G, Felig P. Lactate and glucose exchange across the forearm, legs and splanchnic bed during and after prolonged exercise. J Clin Invest 1982; 69: 45–54.
15. Felig P, Cherif A, Minagawa A, Wahren J. Hypoglycemia during prolonged exercise in normal man. New Engl J Med 1982; 306: 895–900.
16. Hoelzer D, Dalsky G, Clutter W et al. Glucoregulation during exercise: hypoglycemia is prevented by redundant glucoregulatory systems during exercise: sympathochromaffin activation, and changes in hormone secretion. J Clin Invest 1986; 77: 212–21.
17. Issekutz B, Vranic M. Significance of glucagon in the control of glucose production during exercise. Am J Physiol 1980; 238: E13–20.
18. DeFronzo RA, Ferrannini E, Sato Y et al. Synergistic interaction between exercise and insulin on peripheral glucose uptake. J Clin Invest 1981; 68: 1468–74.
19. Wasserman DH, Lickley HLA, Vranic M. Interactions between glucagon and other counter-regulatory hormones during normoglycemic and hypoglycemic exercise. J Clin Invest 1984; 74: 1404–13.
20. Wolfe RR, Nadel ER, Shal JHF et al. Role of changes in insulin and glucagon in glucose homeostasis in exercise. J Clin Invest 1986; 77: 900–7.
21. Jenkins AB, Furler SM, Chisholm DJ et al. Regulation of hepatic glucose output during exercise by circulating glucose and insulin in humans. Am J Physiol 1986; 250: R411–17.
22. Jenkins AB, Chisholm DJ, James DE et al. Exercise induced hepatic glucose output is precisely sensitive to the rate of systemic glucose supply. Metabolism 1985; 34: 431–6.
23. Katz A, Brobert S, Sahlin K et al. Leg glucose uptake during maximal dynamic exercise in humans. Am J Physiol 1986; 251: E65–70.
24. Cooper DM, Wasserman DH, Vranic M et al. Glucose turnover in response to exercise during high- and low-F_IO_2 breathing in humans. Am J Physiol 1986; 14: E209–14.
25. Wallberg-Henriksson H. Glucose transport into skeletal muscle. Influence of contractile activity, insulin, catecholamines and diabetes mellitus. Acta Physiol Scand 1987; (suppl. 564): 1–80.
26. Chaveau MA, Kaufmann M. Experiences pour la determination du coefficient de l'activité nutritive et respiratorie des muscles en repos et en travail. Compt Rend Ac Sci 1887; 104: 1126–32.
27. Berger M, Hagg SA, Ruderman NB. Glucose metabolism in perfused skeletal muscle. Interaction of insulin and exercise on glucose uptake. Biochem J 1975; 146: 231–8.

28. Vranic M, Kawamori S, Pek S, Kovacevic N, Wrenshall GA. The essentiality of insulin and the role of glucagon in regulating glucose utilization and production during strenuous exercise in dogs. J Clin Invest 1976; 57: 245-55.

29. Wallberg-Henriksson H, Holloszy JO. Contractile activity increases glucose uptake by muscle in severely diabetic rats. J Appl Physiol 1984; 57: 1045-9.

30. Wallberg-Henriksson H, Holloszy JO. Activation of glucose transport in diabetic muscle: responses to contraction and insulin. Am J Physiol 1985; 249: C233-7.

31. Nesher R, Karl IE, Kipnis KM. Dissociation of the effect(s) of insulin and contraction on glucose transport in rat epitrochlearis muscle. Am J Physiol 1985; 249: C226-32.

32. Richter EA, Ploug T, Galbo H. Increased muscle glucose uptake after exercise. No need for insulin during exercise. Diabetes 1985; 34: 1041-8.

33. James DE, Kraegen EW, Chisholm DJ. Muscle glucose metabolism in exercising rats: comparison with insulin stimulation. Am J Physiol 1985; 248: E575-80.

34. Ploug T, Galbo H, Vinten J et al. Kinetics of glucose transport in rat muscle: effects of insulin and contractions. Am J Physiol 1987; 253: E12-20.

35. Bjorkman O, Miles P, Wasserman DH et al. Muscle glucose uptake during exercise in total insulin deficiency: effect of beta adrenergic blockade. J Clin Invest 1988; 81: 759-67.

36. Vranic M, Wrenshall GA. Exercise, insulin and glucose turnover in dogs. Endocrinology 1969; 85: 165-71.

37. Lilloja S, Young AA, Cutler CL et al. Skeletal muscle capillary density and fiber type are possible determinants of *in vivo* insulin resistance in man. J Clin Invest 1987; 80: 415-24.

38. James DE, Burleigh KM, Storlien LH, Bennett SP, Kraegen EW. Heterogeneity of insulin action in muscle: influence of blood flow. Am J Physiol 1986; 251: E422-30.

39. Wasserman DH, Lickley HLA, Vranic M. Effect of hematocrit reduction on hormonal and metabolic responses to exercise. J Appl Physiol 1985; 58: 1257-62.

40. Koivisto AA, Soman VR, Conrad P, Hendler R, Nadel E, Felig P. Insulin binding to monocytes in trained athletes: changes in the resting state and after exercise. J Clin Invest 1979; 64: 1011-15.

41. Pedersen O, Beck-Nielsen H, Heding L. Increased insulin receptors after exercise in patients with insulin dependent diabetes mellitus. New Engl J Med 1980; 302: 886-9.

42. Michel G, Vocke T, Fiehn W et al. Bi-directional alteration of insulin receptor affinity by different forms of physical exercise. Am J Physiol 1984; 246: E153-9.

43. Bonen A, Tan MH, Clune P et al. Effects of exercise on insulin binding to human muscle. Am J Physiol 1985; 248: E403-8.

44. Zorzano A, Balon TW, Garetto LP et al. Muscle alpha aminoisobutyric acid transport after exercise: enhanced stimulation by insulin. Am J Physiol 1985; 248: E546-52.

45. Webster B, Vigna SR, Panquette T. Acute exercise, epinephrine, and diabetes enhance insulin binding to skeletal muscle. Am J Physiol 1986; 250: E186-97.

46. Chiasson JL, Shikama H, Chu DTW et al. Inhibitory effect of epinephrine on insulin-stimulated glucose uptake by rat skeletal muscle. J Clin Invest 1981; 68: 706-13.

47. Kemmer FW, Lickley HLA, Gray DE, Perez G, Vranic M. State of metabolic control determines role of epinephrine-glucagon interaction in glucoregulation in diabetes. Am J Physiol 1982; 242: E428-36.

48. Wasserman DH, Lickley HLA, Vranic M. Role of beta-adrenergic mechanisms during exercise in poorly-controlled insulin deficient diabetes. J Appl Physiol 1985; 59: 1282-9.

49. Simonson DC, Koivisto V, Sherwin RS et al. Adrenergic blockade alters glucose kinetics during exercise in insulin-dependent diabetics. J Clin Invest 1984; 73: 1648-58.

50. Rizza R, Haymond M, Cryer P, Gerich J. Differential effects of epinephrine on glucose production and disposal in man. Am J Physiol 1979; 237: E356-62.

51. Jansson E, Hjemdahl P, Kaijser L. Epinephrine induced changes in muscle carbohydrate metabolism during exercise in male subjects. J Appl Physiol 1986; 60: 1466-70.

52. McDermott JC, Elder GC, Bonen A. Adrenal hormones enhance glycogenolysis in non-exercising muscle during exercise. J Appl Physiol 1987; 63: 1275-82.

53. Ahlborg G. Mechanism for glycogenolysis in non-exercising human muscle during and after exercise. Am J Physiol 1985; 248: E540-5.

54. Conlee RK, Hickson RC, Winder WW, Hagberg JM, Holloszy JO. Regulation of glycogen resynthesis in muscle of rats following exercise. Am J Physiol 1978; 235: R145-50.

55. Maehlum S, Felig P, Wahren J. Splanchnic glucose and muscle glycogen metabolism after glucose feeding during post-exercise recovery. Am J Physiol 1978; 235: E255-60.

56. Maehlum S, Hermansen L. Muscle glycogen concentrations during recovery after prolonged severe exercise in fasting subjects. Scand J Clin Lab Invest 1978; 38: 557-60.

57. Maehlum S, Horstmark AT, Hermansen L. Synthesis of muscle glycogen during recovery after prolonged severe exercise in diabetic and non-diabetic subjects. Scand J Clin Lab Invest 1977; 37: 309-16.

58. Richter EA, Garetto LP, Goodman MN, Ruderman NB. Muscle glucose metabolism following exercise in the rat. Increased sensitivity to insulin. J Clin Invest 1982; 69: 785-93.

59. Ivy JL, Holloszy JO. Persistent increase in glucose uptake by rat skeletal muscle following exercise. Am J Physiol 1981; 241: C200-3.

60. Garetto LP, Richter EA, Goodman MN et al. Enhanced muscle glucose metabolism after exercise in the rat: the two phases. Am J Physiol 1984; 246: E471-5.

61. Zorzano A, Balon TW, Goodman MN et al. Glycogen depletion and increased insulin sensitivity and responsiveness in muscle after exercise. Am J Physiol 1986; 251: E664-9.

62. Richter EA, Garetto LP, Goodman MN, Ruderman NB. Enhanced muscle glucose metabolism after exercise: modulation by local factors. Am J Physiol 1984; 246: E476-82.

63. Bogardus C, Thuillez P, Ravussin E et al. Effect of muscle glycogen depletion on *in vivo* insulin action in man. J Clin Invest 1983; 72: 1605-10.

64. Ivy JL, Frishberg BA, Farrell SW et al. Effects of elevated and exercise-reduced muscle glycogen levels on insulin sensitivity. J Appl Physiol 1985; 59: 154–9.

65. Wahrenberg H, Engfeldt P, Bolinder J et al. Acute adaptation in adrenergic control of lipolysis during physical exercise in humans. Am J Physiol 1987; 253: E383–90.

66. Hagenfeld L. Metabolism of free fatty acids and ketone bodies during exercise in normal and diabetic man. Diabetes 1979; 28 (suppl 1): 66–70.

67. Richter EA, Ruderman NB, Gavras H et al. Muscle glycogenolysis during exercise: dual control by epinephrine and contractions. Am J Physiol 1982; 242: E25–32.

68. Krzentkowski G, Pirnay F, Pallikarakis N, Luyckx AS, Lacroix M, Mosora F, Lefebvre PJ. Glucose utilization during exercise in normal and diabetic subjects: the role of insulin. Diabetes 1981; 30: 983–9.

69. Costill DL, Sherman WM, Fink WJ, Maresh C, Witten M, Miller JM. The role of dietary carbohydrates in muscle glycogen resynthesis after strenuous running. Am J Clin Nutr 1981; 34: 1831–6.

70. Hermansen L, Pruett EDR, Cosnes JB, Giere FA. Blood glucose and plasma insulin in response to maximal exercise and glucose infusion. J Appl Physiol 1970; 29: 13–16.

71. Kemmer FW, Berchtold P, Berger M, Starke A, Cüppers HJ, Gries FA, Zimmermann H. Exercise induced fall of blood glucose in insulin treated diabetics unrelated to alteration of insulin mobilization. Diabetes 1979; 28: 1131–7.

72. Wahren J, Felig P, Ahlborg G, Jorfeldt L. Glucose metabolism during leg exercise in man. J Clin Invest 1971; 50: 2715–25.

73. Richter EA, Galbo H, Holst JJ et al. Significance of glucagon for insulin secretion and hepatic glycogenolysis during exercise in rats. Horm Metab Res 1981; 13: 323–6.

74. Wasserman DH, Lickley HLA, Vranic M. Important role of glucagon during exercise and diabetes. J Appl Physiol 1985; 59: 1272–81.

75. Shilo S, Sotsky M, Shamoon. Effect of plasma insulin on glucose kinetics in exercising non-diabetic and type I diabetic man. Diabetes 1987; 36 (suppl 1): 16A.

76. Hoelzer DR, Dalsky GP, Schwartz NS et al. Epinephrine is not critical to prevention of hypoglycemia during exercise in humans. Am J Physiol 1986; 251: E104–10.

77. Wasserman DH, Goldstein R, Donahue P et al. Importance of the exercise-induced fall in insulin to the regulation of hepatic carbohydrate metabolism. Diabetes 1987; 36 (suppl 1): 39A.

78. Wasserman DH, Lacy DB, Goldstein R et al. Role of the exercise-induced fall in insulin independent of the effects of glucagon. Med Sci Sports Exer 1988; 20: 84.

79. Berger M, Berchtold P, Cüppers HJ et al. Metabolic and hormonal effects of muscular exercise in juvenile type diabetics. Diabetologia 1977; 13: 355–65.

80. Zinman B, Murray FT, Vranic M, Albisser AM, Leibel BS, McClean PA, Marliss EB. Glucoregulation during moderate exercise in insulin treated diabetics. J Clin Endocrinol Metab 1977; 45: 641–52.

81. Wahren J, Hagenfeldt L, Felig P. Splanchnic and leg exchange of glucose, amino acids, and free fatty acids during exercise in diabetes mellitus. J Clin Invest 1975; 55: 1303–14.

82. Wahren J, Sato Y, Ostman J et al. Turnover and splanchnic metabolism of free fatty acids and ketones in insulin-dependent diabetics during exercise. J Clin Invest 1984; 73: 1367–76.

83. Christensen NJ. Abnormally high plasma catecholamines at rest and during exercise in ketonic juvenile diabetics. Scand J Clin Lab Invest 1970; 26: 343–4.

84. Tamborlane WV, Sherwin RS, Koivisto V et al. Normalization of the growth hormone and catecholamine response to exercise in juvenile-onset diabetic subjects treated with a portable insulin infusion pump. Diabetes 1979; 28: 785–8.

85. Hansen AP. Abnormal serum growth hormone response to exercise in juvenile diabetics. J Clin Invest 1970; 49: 1467–78.

86. Kemmer FW, Bisping R, Steingrüber HJ, Baar H, Hardtmann F, Schlaghecke R, Berger M. Psychological stress and metabolic control in patients with type-I diabetes mellitus. New Engl J Med 1986; 314: 1078–84.

87. Berger M, Cüppers HJ, Hegner H, Jörgens V, Berchtold P. Absorption kinetics and biological effects of subcutaneously injected insulin preparations. Diabetes Care 1982; 5: 77–91.

88. Koivisto V, Felig P. Effects of leg exercise on insulin absorption in diabetic patients. New Engl J Med 1978; 298: 77–83.

89. Berger M, Halban PA, Assal JP, Offord RE, Vranic M, Renold AE. Pharmacokinetics of subcutaneously injected tritiated insulin: effects of exercise. Diabetes 1979; 28 (suppl 1): 53–7.

90. Kawamori R, Vranic M. Mechanisms of exercise induced hypoglycemia in depancreatized dogs maintained on long acting insulin. J Clin Invest 1977; 59: 331–7.

91. Lawrence RD. The effect of exercise on insulin action in diabetes. Br Med J 1926; 1: 648–52.

92. Landt KW, Campaigne BN, James FW, Sperling MA. Effects of exercise training on insulin sensitivity in adolescents with Type I diabetes. Diabetes Care 1985; 8: 461–5.

93. Wallberg-Henriksson H, Gunnarson R, Henriksson J, DeFronzo RA, Felig P, Östman J, Wahren J. Increased peripheral insulin sensitivity and muscle mitochondrial enzymes but unchanged blood glucose control in Type I diabetics after physical training. Diabetes 1982; 31: 1044–50.

94. Yki-Järvinen H, DeFronzo RA, Koivisto VA. Normalization of insulin sensitivity in Type I diabetic subjects by physical training during insulin pump therapy. Diabetes Care 1984; 7: 520–7.

95. Zinman B, Zuniga-Guajardo S, Kelly D. Comparison of the acute and long-term effects of exercise on glucose control in type I diabetes. Diabetes Care 1984; 7: 515–19.

96. Assal JP, Mülhauser I, Pernet A, Gfeller R, Jörgens V, Berger M. Patient education as the basis for diabetes care in clinical practices and research. Diabetologia 1985; 28: 602–13.

97. Jörgens V, Grüsser M, Bott U, Mühlhauser I, Berger M. Effective and safe translation of intensified insulin therapy to general internal medicine departments. Diabetologia 1993; 36: 99–105.

98. Mühlhauser I, Bruckner I, Berger M et al. Evaluation of an intensified insulin treatment and teaching program as routine management of Type I (insulin dependent) diabetes. The Bucharest–Düsseldorf Study. Diabetologia 1987; 30: 681–91.

99. Hermansen L, Pruett EDR, Osnes JB, Giere FA. Blood glucose and plasma insulin in response to maximal exercise and glucose infusion. J Appl Physiol 1970; 29: 13–16.

100. Mitchell TH, Gebrehiwot A, Schiffrin A, Leiter LA, Marliss EB. Hyperglycemia after intense exercise in IDDM subjects during continuous subcutaneous insulin infusion. Diabetes Care 1988; 11: 311–17.

101. Kemmer FW, Berchtold P, Berger M, Starke A, Cüppers HJ, Gries FA, Zimmermann H. Exercise induced fall of blood glucose in insulin treated diabetics unrelated to alteration of insulin mobilization. Diabetes 1979; 28: 1131–7.

102. Süsstrunk H, Morell B, Ziegler WH, Froesch ER. Insulin absorption from the abdomen and the thigh in healthy subjects during rest and exercise: blood glucose, plasma insulin, growth hormone, adrenaline and noradrenaline levels. Diabetologia 1982; 22: 171–4.

103. Kemmer FW, Sonnenberg GE, Cüppers HJ, Berger M. Prevention of exercise induced hypoglycaemia in diabetes. In Serrano-Rios M, Lefèbvre PJ (eds) Diabetes 1985. Amsterdam: Elsevier, 1986: pp 963–7.

104. Shiffrin A, Parikh S. Accommodating planned exercise in type I diabetic patients on intensive treatment. Diabetes Care 1985; 8: 337–42.

105. Sane T, Helve E, Pelkonen R, Koivisto VA. The adjustment of diet insulin dose during long-term endurance exercise in Type 1 (insulin-dependent) diabetic men. Diabetologia 1988; 31: 35–40.

106. Meinders AE, Willekens FLA, Heere LP. Metabolic and hormonal changes in IDDM during long-distance run. Diabetes Care 1988; 11: 1–7.

107. Campaigne BN, Wallberg-Henriksson H, Gunnarsson R. Glucose and insulin response in relation to insulin dose and caloric intake 12 h after acute physical exercise in men with IDDM. Diabetes Care 1987; 10: 716–21.

108. MacDonald MJ. Postexercise late-onset hypoglycemia in insulin-dependent diabetic patients. Diabetes Care 1987; 10: 584–8.

109. Berger M. Adjustment of insulin therapy. In Ruderman NB, Devlin JT (eds) The health professional's guide to diabetes and exercise. Alexandria, VA, USA: American Diabetes Association, 1995: pp 115–23.

110. Reaven GM. Insulin-independent diabetes mellitus: metabolic characteristics. Metabolism 1980; 29: 445–54.

111. Panzram G. Mortality and survival in Type 2 (non-insulin-dependent) diabetes mellitus. Diabetologia 1987; 30: 123–32.

112. Weir GC. Non insulin dependent diabetes mellitus: interplay between B-cell inadequacy and insulin resistance. Am J Med 1982; 73: 461–4.

113. Minuk HL, Hanna AK, Marliss EB, Vranic M, Zinman B. Metabolic response to moderate exercise in obese man during prolonged fasting. Am J Physiol 1980; 238: E322–9.

114. Kemmer FW, Tacken M, Berger M. On the mechanism of exercise induced hypoglycemia during sulfonylurea treatment. Diabetes 1987; 36: 1178–87.

115. Koivisto V, DeFronzo RA. Exercise in the treatment of Type II diabetes. Acta Endocrinol 1984; 107 (suppl. 1): 107–11.

116. Schneider SH, Vitug A, Ruderman NB. Atherosclerosis and physical activity. Diabetes Metab Rev 1986; 1: 514–53.

117. Berger M, Kemmer FW, Becker K, Herberg L, Schwenen M, Gjinovci A, Berchtold P. Effect of physical training on glucose tolerance and on glucose metabolism of skeletal muscle in anaesthetized normal rats. Diabetologia 1979; 16: 179–84.

118. Björntorp P, De Jounge K. Sjöström L, Sullivan L. The effect of physical training on insulin production in obesity. Metabolism 1970; 19: 631–7.

119. Lohmann D, Leibold F, Heilmann W. Senger H, Pohl A. Diminished insulin response in highly trained athletes. Metabolism 1978; 27: 521–42.

120. Cüppers HJ, Erdmann D, Schubert H, Berchtold P, Berger M. Glucose tolerance, serum insulin and serum lipids in athletes. In Berger M, Christacopoulos P, Wahren J (eds) Diabetes and exercise. Bern: Huber, 1982: pp 155–65.

121. Rodnick KJ, Haskell WL, Swislocki ALM et al. Improved insulin action in muscle, liver, and adipose tissue in physically trained human subjects. Am J Physiol 1987; 253: E489–95.

122. DeFronzo RA, Sherwin RS, Kraemer N. Effect of physical training on insulin action in obesity. Diabetes 1987; 36: 1379–85.

123. Mondon CE, Dolkas B, Reaven GM. Site of enhanced insulin sensitivity in exercise-trained rats at rest. Am J Physiol 1980; 239: E169–77.

124. James DE, Kraegen EW, Chisholm DJ. Effects of exercise training on in vivo insulin action in individual tissues of the rat. J Clin Invest 1985; 76: 657–66.

125. Davis TA, Klahr S, Tegtmeyer ED et al. Glucose metabolism in epitrochlearis muscle of acutely exercised and trained rats. Am J Physiol 1986; 250: E137–43.

126. Craig BW, Garthwaite SM, Holloszy JO. Adipocyte insulin resistance: effects of aging, obesity, exercise, and food restriction. J Appl Physiol 1987; 62: 95–100.

127. Wardzala LJ, Horton ES, Crettaz M et al. Physical training of lean and genetically obese Zucker rats: effect on fat cell metabolism. Am J Physiol 1982; 243: E418–26.

128. Vinten J, Norgaard Petersen L, Sonne B et al. Effect of physical training on glucose transporters in fat cell fractions. Biochim Biophys Acta 1985; 841: 223–7.

129. Rosenthal M, Haskall WL, Solomon R, Widstrum A, Reaven G. Demonstration of a relationship between level of physical training and insulin-stimulated glucose utilization in normal humans. Diabetes 1983; 32: 408–11.

130. Yki-Järvinen H, Koivisto V. Effects of body composition on insulin sensitivity. Diabetes 1983; 32: 965–9.

131. Miller WJ, Sherman WM, Ivy JL. Effect of strength training on glucose tolerance and post-glucose insulin response. Med Sci Sports Exer 1984; 16: 539–43.

132. Bonen A, Clune PA, Tan MH. Chronic exercise increases insulin binding in muscles but not liver. Am J Physiol 1987; 251: E196–203.

133. Dohm GI, Sinha MK, Caro JF. Insulin receptor binding and protein kinase activity in muscles of trained rats. Am J Physiol 1987; 252: E170–5.

134. Noble EG, Ianuzzo CD. Influence of training on skeletal muscle enzymatic adaptions in normal and diabetic rats. Am J Physiol 1985; 249: E360–5.

135. Wallberg-Henriksson H, Gunnarsson R, Henriksson J et al. Influence of physical training on formation of muscle capillaries in type I diabetes. Diabetes 1984; 33: 851–7.

136. Lithell H, Krotkiewski M, Kiens B et al. Non-response of muscle capillary density and lipoprotein-lipase activity to regular training in diabetic patients. Diabetes Res 1985; 2: 17–22.

137. Burstein R, Polychronakos C, Toews CJ, MacDougall JD, Guyda HJ, Posner BI. Acute reversal of the enhanced insulin action in trained athletes: association with insulin receptor changes. Diabetes 1985; 34: 756–60.

138. Heath GW, Gavin JR, Hinderliter JM, Hagberg JM, Bloomfield SA, Holloszy JO. Effects of exercise and lack of exercise on glucose tolerance and insulin sensitivity. J Appl Physiol 1983; 55: 512–17.

139. Devlin JT, Horton ES. Effects of prior high-intensity exercise on glucose metabolism in normal and insulin-resistant men. Diabetes 1985; 34: 973–9.

140. Devlin JT, Hirshman M, Horton ES et al. Enhanced peripheral and splanchnic insulin sensitivity in NIDDM men after single bout of exercise. Diabetes 1987; 36: 434–9.

141. Crettaz M, Prentki M, Zaninetti D, Jeanrenaud B. Insulin resistance in soleus muscle from obese Zucker rats. Biochem J 1980; 186: 525–34.

142. Kemmer FW, Berger M, Herberg L, Gries FA, Wirdeier A, Becker K. Glucose metabolism in perfused skeletal muscle: demonstration of insulin resistance in the obese Zucker rat. Biochem J 1979; 178: 733–41.

143. Becker-Zimmermann K, Berger M, Berchtold P, Gries FA, Herberg L, Schwenen M. Treadmill training improves intravenous glucose tolerance and insulin sensitivity in fatty Zucker rats. Diabetologia 1982; 22: 468–74.

144. King H, Zimmet P, Raper LR, Balkau B. Risk factors for diabetes in three Pacific populations. Am J Epidemiol 1984; 119: 396–409.

145. Zimmet P, Faaiuso S, Ainuu J, Whitehouse S, Milne B, DeBoer W. The prevalence of diabetes in the rural and urban Polynesian population of Western Samoa. Diabetes 1981; 30: 45–51.

146. Saltin B, Lindgarde F, Housten M, Horlin R, Nygaard E, Gad P. Physical training and glucose tolerance in middle-aged men with chemical diabetes. Diabetes 1979; 28 (suppl 1): 30–2.

147. Saltin B, Lindgarde F, Lithell H, Erisson KF, Gad P. Metabolic effects of longterm physical training in maturity onset diabetes. In Waldhäusl WK (ed.) Diabetes. Amsterdam: Excerpta Medica, 1980: p 345.

148. Ruderman NB, Ganda OP, Johansen K. The effects of physical training on glucose tolerance and plasma lipids in maturity onset diabetes. Diabetes 1979; 28 (suppl 1): 89–92.

149. Schneider SH, Amorosa LF, Khachadurian AK, Ruderman NB. Studies on the mechanism of improved glucose control during regular exercise in type-2 (non-insulin-dependent) diabetes. Diabetologia 1984; 26: 355–60.

150. Reitman JS, Vasquez B, Klimes I, Nagulesparan M. Improvement of glucose homeostasis after exercise training in non-insulin-dependent diabetes. Diabetes Care 1984; 7: 434–41.

151. Trovati M, Darta O, Cavalot F et al. Influence of physical training on blood glucose control, glucose tolerance, insulin secretion, and insulin action in non-insulin-dependent diabetic patients. Diabetes Care 1984; 7: 416–20.

152. Bogardus C, Ravussin E, Robbins DC, Wolfe RR, Horton ED, Sims EAH. Effects of physical training and diet therapy on carbohydrate metabolism in patients with glucose intolerance and non-insulin-dependent diabetes mellitus. Diabetes 1984; 33: 311–18.

153. Krotkiewski M, Lönnroth P, Mandroukas K et al. The effects of physical training on insulin secretion and effectiveness and on glucose metabolism in obesity and Type 2 (non-insulin dependent) diabetes. Diabetes 1985; 28: 881–90.

154. Skarfors ET, Wegener TA, Lithell H, Selinus I. Physical training as treatment for Type 2 (non-insulin-dependent) diabetes in elderly men. A feasibility study over 2 years. Diabetologia 1987; 30: 930–3.

155. National Institutes of Health. Consensus development conference on diet and exercise in non-insulin-dependent diabetes mellitus. Diabetes Care 1987; 10: 639–44.

156. Annuzzi G, Riccardi G, Capaldo B, Kaijser L. Increased insulin stimulated glucose uptake by exercised human muscle one day after prolonged physical exercise. Eur J Clin Invest 1991; 21: 6–12.

157. Ruegemer J, Squires RW, Marsh HM, Haymond MW, Cryer PE, Rizza RA, Miles JM. Differences between prebreakfast and late afternoon glycemic response to exercise in IDDM patients. Diabetes Care 1990; 13: 104–10.

158. Poussier P, Zinman B, Marliss EB, Albisser M, Perlman K, Caron D. Open-loop intravenous insulin waveforms for postprandial exercise in type I diabetes. Diabetes Care 1983; 6: 129–34.

159. Sonnenberg GE, Kemmer FW, Berger M. Exercise in type 1 (insulin dependent) diabetic patients treated with continuous subcutaneous insulin infusion: prevention of exercise induced hypoglycemia. Diabetologia 1990; 33: 696–703.

160. Wake SA, Sowden JA, Storlien LH, James DE, Clark PW, Shine J, Chisholm DJ, Kraegen EW. Effects of exercise training and dietary manipulation on insulin-regulatable glucose-transporter mRNA in rat muscle. Diabetes 1991; 40: 275–9.

161. Helmrich SP, Ragland DR, Leung RW, Paffenbarger RS. Physical activity and reduced occurrence of non-insulin dependent diabetes mellitus. New Engl J Med 1991; 325: 147–52.

162. Kriska AM, LaPorte RE, Pettit DJ, Charles MA, Nelson RG, Kuller LH et al. The association of physical activity with obesity, fat distribution and glucose intolerance in Pima Indians. Diabetologia 1993; 36: 863–9.

163. Manson JE, Rimm EB, Stampfer MJ, Colditz GA, Willett WC, Krolewski AS, et al. Physical activity and incidence of non-insulin dependent diabetes mellitus in women. Lancet 1991; 338: 774–8.

164. Manson JE, Nathan DM, Krolewski AS, Stampfer MJ, Colditz GA, Willett WC, Hennekens CH. A prospective study of exercise and incidence of diabetes among US male physicians. JAMA 1992; 268: 63–7.

36

Sulfonylureas: Basic Aspects and Clinical Uses

H.E. Lebovitz* and A. Melander †

*Department of Medicine, State University of New York, Brooklyn, NY, USA, and †The NEPI Foundation, Medical Research Centre, University Hospital, Malmö, Sweden

After 45 years of clinical use, and despite having been the subject of thousands of investigative studies, the role of sulfonylureas in the management of non-insulin dependent diabetes mellitus (NIDDM) remains enigmatic. Some clinicians are convinced that sulfonylureas are drugs of convenience and would not be needed if patients were compliant with non-pharmacologic therapy. Others are certain that these drugs help to ameliorate basic defects of NIDDM and that most patients can benefit from their judicious use. The NIDDM Policy Group of the European Association for the Study of Diabetes (EASD) has recognized 'that (except in emergency cases) if diet and exercise treatment fails, sulfonylureas are generally the first choice for additional treatment'. The number of diabetic patients taking oral sulfonylureas is increasing: the percentage of diabetic patients taking sulfonylureas in the USA has increased from 29.5% in 1982 to 35.7% in 1986 [1].

Several questions about sulfonylureas remain to be answered. Why do some NIDDM patients fail to respond to sulfonylureas initially, whereas others respond remarkably well? Why do some patients who respond well to sulfonylurea therapy later lose their responsiveness? What are the relative contributions of pancreatic vs. extrapancreatic actions of sulfonylureas in the treatment of NIDDM? What is the role of the B-cell plasma membrane sulfonylurea binding site in the physiological regulation of insulin secretion and the pharmacological actions of sulfonylureas? What

are the mechanisms responsible for the extrapancreatic effects of sulfonylureas? Can intervention in prediabetic states with sulfonylureas prevent the development of NIDDM and its complications? Do combinations of sulfonylureas with other antidiabetic agents have a role in current therapy?

This review examines the contemporary knowledge of these issues as well as current views on the relative merits and disadvantages of the various sulfonylureas and their clinical use.

PHARMACOLOGY AND CLINICAL PHARMACOLOGY

Chemistry and Structure of Sulfonylureas

All sulfonylureas are sulfonamide derivatives (Figure 1). It seems likely that the sulfonylurea moiety is responsible for the distribution of these drugs to the B cell, if not for their binding to the B-cell surface and for their insulin releasing activity (see below). Certain non-sulfonylurea analogs of glibenclamide and gliquidone mimic the effects *in vitro* and *in vivo* of their parent compounds on pancreatic B-cell function and insulin release, indicating that the sulfonylurea moiety may not be the only one capable of activating the 'sulfonylurea receptor' [2, 3].

The 'first-generation' sulfonylureas, such as tolbutamide and chlorpropamide, have a phenyl ring with simple substituent groups at one end and an aliphatic

International Textbook of Diabetes Mellitus, Second Edition. Edited by K.G.M.M. Alberti, P. Zimmet, R.A. DeFronzo, and H. Keen (Honorary)

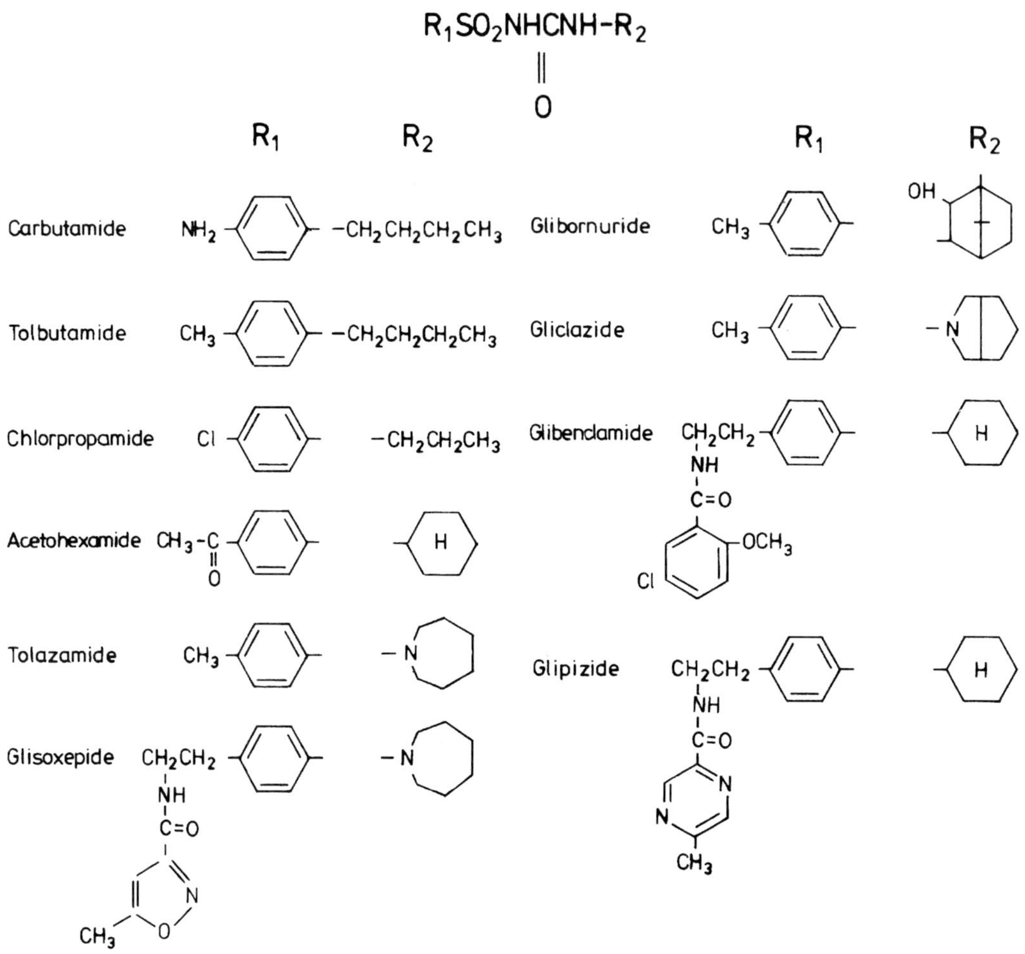

$$R_1SO_2NHCNH\text{-}R_2$$
$$\|$$
$$O$$

Figure 1   Chemical structures of sulfonylureas (from reference 59, with permission)

side-chain at the other end of the molecule (Figure 1). In 'second-generation' sulfonylureas, such as gliben-clamide (glyburide in the USA) and glipizide, the aliphatic side-chain has been replaced by a cyclo-hexyl group, and the substituent group at the other end is a more complex structure than in the 'first-generation' agents (Figure 1). These substitutions have markedly increased the molecular affinity to bind-ing sites on the B cells, and this probably explains the higher intrinsic activity and higher potency of these 'second-generation' sulfonylureas (see below). Detailed descriptions and comparisons of the differ-ent sulfonylureas are given later in the chapter. A new sulfonylurea, glimepiride, has recently been marketed. Its structure is shown in Figure 5 of Chapter 38.

Mechanisms of Action

The main effect of sulfonylureas is to reduce fasting and non-fasting blood glucose levels. This follows from their effects on insulin secretion, insulin action and, possibly, on systemic availability of insulin.

Pancreatic Effects of Sulfonylureas

Acute effects on insulin secretion   Insulin secretion is stimulated by sulfonylureas, and a functional pancreas is necessary to exert this action [4]. Sulfonylurea administration is without effect on blood glucose in pancreatectomized [5] or alloxan-diabetic [6] animals, or in patients with well-established insulin dependent diabetes mellitus (IDDM) [7] or pancreatic diabetes [8]. Acute intravenous or oral administration of sulfonylurea leads to a rapid rise in portal and then peripheral plasma insulin levels and C-peptide levels in normal or NIDDM humans or animals [9]. Direct stimulation of insulin release by sulfonylureas has been demonstrated *in vitro* utilizing perfused pancreas preparations, isolated islets and B-cell cultures [10, 11]. Sulfonylurea stimulation of insulin secretion from normal B cells is usually weaker than nutrient stimulation, but the reverse is frequently true with diabetic B cells.

Although it has been known for over 30 years that sulfonylureas acutely release insulin from the B cell, it is only recently that the mechanism of this effect has become more clearly defined. The current hypothesis (Figure 2) is that sulfonylureas cause the closure of specific potassium ion channels located in the B-cell plasma membrane. Inhibition of potassium efflux from the B cell depolarizes the plasma membrane, and this leads to gating of voltage-dependent plasma membrane calcium ion channels resulting in facilitated influx of calcium ions into the B cell. The increase in cytosolic calcium ion concentration activates a cytoskeletal system which is responsible for the translocation of secretory granules to the cell surface and extrusion of insulin via exocytosis [11–14].

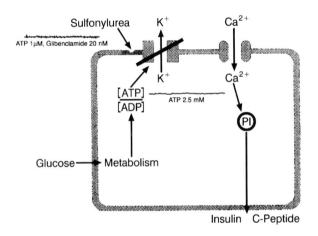

Figure 2 Scheme of a stimulated B cell. Sulfonylureas stimulate by binding to plasma membrane receptors that are coupled to ATP-dependent K$^+$ channels. This inhibits efflux of K$^+$, causing depolarization of the plasma membrane. As a consequence, voltage-dependent Ca^{2+} channels open, causing influx of Ca^{2+} into the cytosol, which stimulates extrusion of both mature and immature insulin granules. ATP-dependent K$^+$ channels can also be inhibited by intracellular metabolic events that increase the ATP:ADP ratio. Typical recorded transmembrane voltage patterns from patch clamps from Schmid-Antomarchi et al [22] are illustrated. PI, proinsulin (from reference 14, with permission)

A number of observations suggest that the initial event in this process is binding of the sulfonylurea molecule to a specific site on the B-cell plasma membrane. Early studies of the distribution of tolbutamide *in vivo* concluded that this drug was restricted to the extracellular compartment, with the possible exception of the liver [15]. The uptake of [^{35}S]tolbutamide into microdissected pancreatic islets was found to be

identical to that of markers known to equilibrate with the extracellular space [16]. When perfused through isolated rat pancreas, dextran-linked tolbutamide was shown to be as effective as tolbutamide in stimulating first-phase insulin release [17].

Recently, several groups of investigators have demonstrated that radiolabelled sulfonylureas such as [^{3}H]glipizide or [^{3}H]glibenclamide bind to purified plasma membranes from either rat insulinoma or transformed hamster tumor B cells with characteristics that are compatible with specific receptor binding [13, 14]. Displacement by sulfonylureas occurs in proportion to their activity (Figure 3). Table 1 lists the characteristics reported by different investigators for the presumed sulfonylurea B-cell binding site. Although many data support the concept of a sulfonylurea receptor, these findings need to be interpreted with some caution for the following reasons: (a) in contrast to other sulfonylureas, glibenclamide enters B cells, and approximately 75% binds to B-cell granules [18, 19]; (b) sulfonylureas bind to artificial multilamellar liposomes with criteria that are somewhat characteristic of membrane receptors [20]; (c) several synthetic sulfonylurea analogs dissociate binding and insulin secretory activity [21]. Those who believe in a specific B-cell plasma membrane sulfonylurea receptor indicate that it is clearly linked, but not identical, to an ATP-sensitive K$^+$ channel which closes when the sulfonylurea molecule binds to its receptor [12, 13].

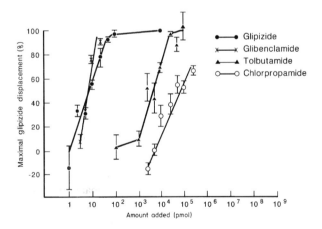

Figure 3 Displacement of [^{3}H]glipizide from purified plasma membranes from RINm5F-generated insulinomas by glipizide (●), glyburide (×), tolbutamide (▲) and chlorpropamide (○). Data are mean ± SE of 3 determinations (from reference 14, with permission)

ATP-sensitive K$^+$ channels have been identified in the plasma membrane of B cells [12]. The channel density ranges from 1.5 to 8 per mm^2. The resting

Table 1 Studies demonstrating sulfonylurea plasma membrane binding sites

Ligand	Binding site	K_d (nmol/l)	R_o (pmol/mg)
[³H]Glipizide	Rat insulinoma purified plasma membranes	7.0	0.93
[³H]Glibenclamide	RINm5F cell microsomes	0.3	0.15
[³H]Glibenclamide	HIT cell membrane pellet	0.76	1.09
[³H]Glibenclamide	Rat insulinoma crude membranes	0.01–0.05 0.24–0.32	0.29–0.52 0.75–1.29
[³H]Gliquidone	Rat brain crude membrane preparation	0.9	
[³H]Glipizide	Rat cerebral cortex membranes	1.5	0.11
[³H]Glibenclamide	Rat cerebral cortex membranes	0.041–0.1 0.05–0.4	0.013–0.024 0.030–0.034

R_o, number of binding sites

B-cell K^+ permeability is primarily determined by the ATP-dependent K^+ channel, and this is closed by increased ATP concentrations at the intracellular surface or by sulfonylureas at the extracellular surface [11–13]. Using patch-clamp techniques, an order of glibenclamide > glipizide > tolbutamide has been established as to the inhibition of the ATP-dependent K^+ current in insulin secreting cells [22].

Evidence for the subsequent ionic events postulated in sulfonylurea-mediated insulin release has been obtained with various islet cell or tumor B-cell preparations *in vitro*. Sulfonylureas inhibit the $^{86}Rb^+$ efflux (used as a tracer for K^+ movement) from islets incubated at basal glucose concentrations [11, 23]. The stimulatory effect of sulfonylureas on insulin secretion is abolished in Ca^{2+}-deprived media [11, 24], and blockage of Ca^{2+} entry by agents such as verapamil causes a dose-dependent inhibition of sulfonylurea-mediated insulin secretion [24]. Additional experimental observations utilizing radiolabelled Ca^{2+} indicate that entry into the cell is required for the insulinotrophic action of insulin-releasing sulfonylureas [24]. Some data suggest that this Ca^{2+} entry is in part mediated through Ca^{2+} channels. Sulfonylureas cause a twofold to threefold increase in cytosolic Ca^{2+} in B cells as determined by quin-2 fluorescence [11, 24]. The rise in cytosolic Ca^{2+} activates the microtubular-microfilamentous system in B cells through one or more of several proposed mechanisms involving protein kinase phosphorylation [11].

The proposed model raises several questions. How does sulfonylurea stimulation of insulin secretion differ from that evoked by nutrient stimulation? Can the model explain all the observed phenomena? If a specific sulfonylurea receptor exists, what is its natural ligand? How is it regulated? Does the receptor or its natural ligand have a role in the pathogenesis of NIDDM?

D-Glucose is thought to stimulate insulin secretion by increasing ATP and/or modifying other factors that close the ATP-sensitive K^+ channel from the cytoplasmic surface of the membrane [11, 12]. Sulfonylureas differ from D-glucose in that they do not increase intracellular ATP or increase the efflux of radioactive phosphate from prelabelled islets [11]. Similarly, they do not stimulate proinsulin biosynthesis, neither do they inhibit [2-³H]-adenosine efflux from prelabelled islets [11]. Sulfonylureas only stimulate first-phase insulin secretion [11, 23]. Thus there are many differences between sulfonylurea-mediated and nutrient-mediated insulin secretion.

It has been pointed out that the proposed mechanism of action does not explain all observations. In contrast to glucose, sulfonylureas decrease K^+ inflow into islet cells, increase their Na^+ content and lower their intracellular pH [11]. It has also been questioned how the postulated hypothesis could account for sulfonylurea-mediated insulin release at glucose concentrations at or below 8.3 mmol/l (150 mg/dl), as the majority of ATP-responsive channels are apparently closed already at this glucose level [11]. Obviously, much is still to be learned about sulfonylurea-mediated insulin secretion.

Chronic effects on insulin secretion Assessments of the chronic effects of sulfonylureas on insulin secretion in patients with NIDDM have been complex and confusing. Factors that appear to influence insulin secretion during chronic sulfonylurea therapy are: (a) the intrinsic effect of sulfonylureas on B-cell insulin secretion; (b) the level of glycemia attained during the stimulus for secretion; (c) the degree of fasting hyperglycemia which itself may cause inhibition of insulin secretion, and (d) tachyphylaxis to sulfonylureas during chronic continuous therapy.

Many studies in NIDDM patients indicate that chronic sulfonylurea treatment increases the ability of the B cell to respond to a fixed stimulus. Porte and colleagues have defined the insulin secretory responses of non-glucose stimuli at different ambient glycemic levels in normal subjects and in patients with NIDDM [25]. Normal individuals have an increase in insulin secretion stimulated by intravenous arginine or isoproterenol during an acute intravenous tolbutamide infusion provided that the plasma glucose level is clamped, but not if it is allowed to fall [25]. It was also shown that 4 of 9 NIDDM patients treated with chlorpropamide for 12 to 16 weeks had an increase in non-glucose-mediated insulin secretion when their pretreatment glycemic values were restored [26]. The same phenomenon may explain why NIDDM patients on chronic sulfonylurea therapy will show a rise in nutrient-mediated insulin responses immediately following discontinuation of sulfonylurea therapy [27]. A chronic effect of sulfonylurea therapy to increase the insulin secretory capacity of laboratory animal pancreas to stimuli has not been observed; rather, nutrient-stimulated insulin secretion is decreased.

Studies in NIDDM patients with normal or mildly elevated fasting plasma glucose concentrations show that the degree of the nutrient-evoked rise in plasma glucose is a major determinant of insulin secretion [28]: thus, a lesser rise such as occurs during chronic sulfonylurea therapy will result in less secretion.

The level of fasting hyperglycemia is as important as the nutrient-evoked rise in plasma glucose in determining insulin secretion. In this case, however, the higher the fasting plasma glucose value the lower the nutrient-mediated insulin secretion. A reduction in fasting hyperglycemia by any form of therapy (diet, drugs or insulin) results in increased glucose-mediated insulin secretion [29]. Extensive experimental and clinical data support the concept that chronic hyperglycemia itself inhibits glucose-mediated insulin secretion [30]. Apparently, reduction of fasting and postprandial hyperglycemia in NIDDM patients by any modality can either increase or decrease glucose-mediated insulin secretion.

The question of sulfonylurea tachyphylaxis has been raised by Karam et al [31], who studied the acute insulin secretory response to intravenous tolbutamide or glucagon in 10 NIDDM patients both before and during tolazamide therapy. They found that chronic tolazamide therapy abolished the insulin secretory response to tolbutamide but not to glucagon, and they also showed that the acute response to tolbutamide reappeared after cessation of tolazamide therapy. They concluded that chronic continuous sulfonylurea therapy may blunt the acute insulin secretory response to sulfonylurea. If the concept of the sulfonylurea receptor is valid, this phenomenon could be explained by downregulation of this receptor. Support for this assumption can be obtained from two studies described below under 'Kinetic–Dynamic Relations' showing that increases of dosage and sulfonylurea steady state

concentrations over a certain level impaired rather than improved glucose and insulin responses.

This complexity explains why so much controversy exists as to whether the primary action of chronic sulfonylurea therapy is increased insulin secretion.

Effects on the secretion of insulin precursors There is increasing evidence that small amounts of insulin precursors, particularly intact proinsulin and 32/33 split proinsulin, are released along with insulin, and that the proportions of these precursors are increased in NIDDM subjects [32]. In addition, the levels of 32/33 split proinsulin correlate more closely with cardiovascular risk factors in NIDDM than do those of insulin itself. If the increased levels of 32/33 split proinsulin were to be causally related to the cardiovascular complications in NIDDM, and if sulfonylurea treatment further enhanced the levels of 32/33 split proinsulin, sulfonylurea treatment could be detrimental. However, a recent study indicates that such treatment does not increase the concentrations of 32/33 split proinsulin in NIDDM subjects, although insulin and proinsulin levels are enhanced [32].

Effects on proinsulin biosynthesis A major difference between sulfonylurea-stimulated insulin secretion and nutrient-stimulated insulin secretion is that sulfonylureas cause only first-phase insulin release (preformed insulin) whereas nutrients stimulate both first-phase and second-phase insulin release. Second-phase insulin release consists largely of newly synthesized insulin. The explanation for the failure of sulfonylureas to stimulate second-phase insulin release might be found in studies utilizing models *in vivo* and *in vitro* of animal perfused pancreas, isolated islets or islet cell cultures which have shown that sulfonylureas inhibit the biosynthesis of proinsulin [33–34].

Effects on glucagon and somatostatin secretion Although animal studies show some effects of sulfonylureas on glucagon secretion, neither acute nor chronic sulfonylurea therapy consistently alters glucagon secretion in normal individuals or in patients with NIDDM [35]. Sulfonylureas stimulate pancreatic D-cell somatostatin release [35], but it is not clear whether this plays any part in their antidiabetic actions.

Extrapancreatic Effects of Sulfonylureas

Sulfonylurea drugs have been investigated extensively for extrapancreatic actions. Most studies demonstrating such actions have utilized organ perfusion, cell culture or subcellular preparations from laboratory animals. Some have shown extrapancreatic effects with concentrations of sulfonylureas far in excess of ordinarily attainable therapeutic plasma levels. Studies *in vivo* have frequently failed to validate that the action

Table 2 Extrapancreatic actions of sulfonylurea drugs

Probably related to antidiabetic action
1. Potentiation of insulin stimulation of carbohydrate transport in skeletal muscle and adipose tissue
2. Potentiation of insulin-mediated translocation of glucose transport molecules
3. Potentiation of insulin-mediated activation of hepatic glycogen synthase and glycogen synthesis
4. Potentiation of insulin-mediated hepatic lipogenesis

Possibly related to antidiabetic action
1. Direct effects on the liver
    a. Increase in fructose 2,6-biphosphate
    b. Increase in glycolysis
    c. Decrease in gluconeogenesis
    d. Decrease in long-chain fatty acid oxidation
2. Direct effects on skeletal muscle
    a. Increase in amino acid transport
    b. Increase in fructose 2,6-biphosphate
3. Inhibition of insulinase

Unlikely to be related to antidiabetic action
1. Direct effects on adipose tissue
    a. Increase in glycogen synthase
    b. Activation of adenosine $3',5'$-monophosphate diesterase and inhibition of lipolysis
2. Direct effects on myocardial tissue
    a. Increase in contractility, oxygen consumption, glycogenolysis and decrease in sarcolemmal Ca^{2+}-ATPase
    b. Increase in glucose transport, glycolysis, phosphofructokinase activity and pyruvate oxidation
3. Increase in synthesis and secretion of plasminogen activator from endothelial cells

From reference 35, with permission.

is a primary one rather than a consequence of better glycemic regulation due to increased insulin secretion.

Table 2 summarizes some extrapancreatic effects. As sulfonylureas lower blood glucose only in the presence of a functioning pancreas, it is difficult to attribute a meaningful antidiabetic action to an extrapancreatic effect that occurs in the absence of insulin [36]. Thus, a primary action in increasing fructose 2,6-bisphosphate in the liver with subsequent stimulation of glycolysis and inhibition of gluconeogenesis, although of interest, is unlikely to explain the antidiabetic action [37]. A similar analysis can be made for primary actions on muscle or adipose tissue [37].

Effects on insulin action The main extrapancreatic action of sulfonylureas that is likely to have a meaningful antidiabetic effect is involved in the potentiation of insulin action. Such an action was described in 1955 and has been controversial ever since. The clearest demonstrations of sulfonylurea potentiation of insulin action have been in animal models. Experiments on mouse diaphragm and on organ culture with rat adipose tissue have demonstrated that ordinary doses or concentrations of sulfonylureas will potentiate insulin-mediated 2-deoxy-D-glucose uptake after a latent period of about 12 hours [38]. One study has suggested that this is attributable to sulfonylurea potentiation of insulin-mediated translocation of the glucose transporter from intracellular storage sites to the plasma membrane [39]. This needs to be confirmed and extended, as the genes for the insulin-sensitive and

insulin-insensitive glucose transport molecules now have been cloned.

Putnam et al [40] utilized the euglycemic insulin clamp at physiological insulin levels in normal dogs and showed that 2 weeks' treatment with glipizide caused a twofold increase in insulin-mediated glucose disposal. The chronic treatment caused no significant alterations in plasma glucose or insulin.

Studies in patients with NIDDM that have attempted to demonstrate whether sulfonylureas potentiate insulin-mediated glucose disposal have reported diverse results. Some show that sulfonylurea treatment increased insulin-mediated glucose disposal, but only in patients who have increased insulin secretion [41, 42]; the improved glucose disposal is attributed to higher plasma insulin levels. In a study on insulin-treated NIDDM-subjects who had little or no remaining endogenous insulin, sulfonylurea failed to evoke any glucose reduction [43]. Other studies also show that sulfonylurea treatment increases insulin-mediated glucose disposal, but the improvement is attributed to the effect of better glycemic regulation. Finally, there are studies in which sulfonylurea treatment improves glycemic control, increases insulin-mediated glucose disposal and yet does not correlate with improved insulin secretion, suggesting that true sulfonylurea-induced potentiation of insulin action does occur in some patients with NIDDM [44–46].

Apart from muscle and adipose tissue, the liver may be a site of sulfonylurea potentiation of insulin action. Sulfonylureas have been reported to potentiate insulin-mediated glycogen and lipid synthesis. These effects have been well described in hepatic cell cultures [37]. Clinical studies suggest that the reduction in fasting hyperglycemia during sulfonylurea treatment can be attributed in large part to potentiation of insulin action on glycogen synthesis and gluconeogenesis [47]. Detailed discussions of the relative roles of pancreatic versus extrapancreatic mechanisms in the antidiabetic action of sulfonylureas are available in several recent reviews [37, 48, 49].

The mechanisms of the various extrapancreatic actions of sulfonylureas have not been defined. Specific plasma membrane sulfonylurea binding sites have not been found on liver or muscle cells, but have been discovered in crude membranes isolated from cerebral cortex [14]; the significance of the latter is unknown. There is no evidence to suggest that ionic fluxes have any role in mediating the extrapancreatic effects. The insulin-potentiating action of sulfonylureas has a latent period of several hours, and this effect is blocked by cycloheximide, indicating that new protein synthesis may be necessary for the effect to occur [50].

The effect of sulfonylureas in potentiating insulin action on muscle, adipose tissue and liver has raised the issue of whether these effects are mediated by a direct action in increasing insulin binding by the insulin receptor (either an increase in receptor number or in affinity) or through postreceptor mechanisms. Studies *in vivo* in which insulin binding is assessed are invalid to answer this question because changes in plasma insulin levels will influence the number of insulin receptors, and measurements of insulin binding to circulating monocytes or adipose tissues may not reflect what is occurring at liver and muscle cells. Assessment of insulin binding to fibroblasts in culture has little physiologic meaning. Several studies *in vitro* indicate that the effect occurs at a postreceptor site [35].

Effect on systemic availability of insulin One of the earliest extrapancreatic actions of sulfonylureas to be described was inhibition of insulinase, particularly in the liver [51]. Later studies disputed these data, and the idea was abandoned. However, several recent studies suggest that at least glipizide [52–55] and glibenclamide [56] may increase the systemic availability of insulin through reduction of the hepatic extraction of insulin secreted from the pancreas. It is not known whether the effect is a primary one, e.g. inhibition of hepatic insulinase [51] or displacement of insulin from hepatic binding sites, or is secondary to the increased rate of insulin secretion subsequent to sulfonylurea stimulation of the B cells [55]. If the increased systemic availability were attributable to displacement of

insulin from hepatic insulin receptors, it is also possible that such displacement might reduce the effect of insulin exerted on the liver and hence would lead to an increased hepatic output of glucose, provided that the displacement was extensive enough. Such a phenomenon would help to explain why high doses of sulfonylurea may impair instead of improve blood glucose control [57, 58].

Effects on blood lipids Sulfonylurea treatment has been reported to have beneficial, neutral or adverse effects on blood lipids [59]. It seems unlikely, therefore, that sulfonylureas have direct effects on very low-density lipid triglycerides, low-density lipid cholesterol or high-density lipid cholesterol.

Effect on fibrinolysis A recent study on bovine aortic endothelial cells indicated that certain sulfonylureas may enhance fibrinolysis and that the fibrinolytic mechanism is associated with sulfonylurea-enhanced production of plasminogen activator [60].

Differences in extrapancreatic effects Some extrapancreatic effects of sulfonylureas are related to parts of the molecule other than the sulfonylurea core and are therefore unrelated to the antidiabetic action. These extrapancreatic effects may confer unique advantages or disadvantages to a particular sulfonylurea. Chlorpropamide facilitates both the release and the tubular action of vasopressin, causing water retention and hyponatremia in certain patients [61]. Sulfonylureas increase the synthesis and secretion of plasminogen activator from bovine aortic endothelial cells, but the potency is unrelated to the blood glucose lowering activity [60]. The spectrum of action of glibenclamide on the myocardium differs from that of tolbutamide [37]. The clinical potential of many of these differences has yet to be explored.

Clinical Effects

Sulfonylureas decrease fasting and postprandial hyperglycemia in patients with NIDDM. These effects result from reduction of the elevated fasting hepatic glucose production and an increased peripheral glucose disposal through enhanced insulin secretion and possibly some potentiation of insulin action [28, 44, 62–64]. The early clinical studies that documented the beneficial effects of sulfonylurea drugs in NIDDM patients were, for the most part, poorly designed and inadequately implemented. Frequently, they did not have a proper dietary run-in period. The large trials were rarely double blind and placebo controlled. Only the more recent short-term clinical pharmacologic studies utilizing small numbers of patients have been adequately controlled. Table 3 lists the results reported from several large open-labelled studies which examined the

Table 3 Effect of sulfonylurea treatment on glycemic control in NIDDM patients

Sulfonylurea (ref. no.)	No. of patients	Duration of treatment (years)	Glycemic control*		
			Excellent	Good	Unsatisfactory
Tolbutamide [65]	1812	1–5	43	23	34
Chlorpropamide [66]	339	1–6	30	28	42
Glibenclamide [67]	3440	0.6**	37	32	31
Glipizide [68]	1015	0.6**	25	34	41

*Criteria for glycemic control are as follows:

Blood glucose levels	Excellent	Good
Fasting mmol/l (mg/dl)	≤5.6 (100)	≤ 7.2 (130)
1 h postprandial mmol/l (mg/dl)	≤8.3 (150)	≤10.0 (180)
2 h postprandial mmol/l (mg/dl)	≤7.2 (130)	≤ 8.3 (150)

** Average duration of treatment.

effects of different sulfonylureas on glycemic control in NIDDM patients [65–68]. The criteria for glycemic control in these older studies varied a little, but generally 'excellent control' signified that 70% of blood glucose measurements showed fasting, 1-hour and 2-hour postprandial levels that did not exceed 5.6, 8.3 and 7.2 mmol/l (100, 150 and 130 mg/dl), respectively. In 'good control', 70% of blood glucose measurements showed fasting, 1-hour and 2-hour postprandial levels not exceeding 7.2, 10.0 and 8.3 mmol/l (130, 180 and 150 mg/dl), respectively. 'Unsatisfactory control' meant values exceeding those for good control. The effects of the various sulfonylureas on glycemic control in these studies do not differ to any relevant extent, and they suggest that approximately 60–65% of NIDDM patients might be expected to achieve excellent or good glycemic control on sulfonylurea therapy.

An initially successful therapeutic response to sulfonylurea treatment is often followed by secondary failure. The data on the frequency with which secondary failure occurs are limited, as few long-term data on sulfonylurea treatment have been reported [69]. Approximately 20% of patients treated with tolbutamide for 1–5 years develop secondary failure (4% in the first year and about 9% per year in years 2 to 5) [63]. Of patients taking the drug for 6–9 years, 26% develop secondary failure [70]. The secondary failure rates for chlorpropamide and other sulfonylureas are probably similar to that for tolbutamide [66, 69].

Sulfonylurea treatment has been shown to cause a near-euglycemic remission which persists for at least several months and possibly years after the drugs have been discontinued. This was well documented by Singer and Hurwitz in 1967 [71] following tolbutamide (31% of patients) or chlorpropamide treatment (17% of patients), and later confirmed by Lev-Ran [72]. It is likely that the remission is related to excellent glycemic regulation rather than to a specific effect of sulfonylurea treatment, but this concept needs more verification.

Patients who are most likely to show an excellent or good glycemic response to sulfonylurea therapy are those who have relatively recently diagnosed NIDDM, have mild to moderate fasting hyperglycemia (fasting plasma glucose levels below 12.5 mmol/l) on dietary management, have a good B-cell reserve as reflected by high C-peptide levels, have a normal weight or are moderately obese, and have either never been treated with insulin or are taking less than 30 U of insulin daily.

One large, randomized, double-blind, placebo-controlled study of tolbutamide treatment for 8 years was the University Group Diabetes Program (UGDP) [73]. A total of 823 patients were randomly assigned initially to one of four treatments: placebo, tolbutamide 1.5 g per day, a fixed dose of insulin, or a variable insulin dose adjusted to achieve normal blood glucose levels. This controversial study indicated that the fixed dose of tolbutamide decreased fasting blood glucose levels by 20% in the first year of treatment. Over the ensuing 4 years the fasting blood glucose values increased, and by 5 years they were the same as before treatment and no different from those of the placebo-treated group. The significance of these data is obscured by the lack of intention to treat to a specific glycemic end-point.

A large, prospective, randomized study comparing diet, sulfonylurea, insulin or biguanide therapy in the treatment of newly diagnosed NIDDM patients has been in progress in the UK since the early 1980s. Several thousand patients have entered the study. Its goal is to compare the effects of different treatments on metabolic regulation and the development of chronic complications. With the exception of those patients who are primary failures, sulfonylurea treatment has been found to control glycemia and to reduce hemoglobin A_{1c} in a manner comparable to that of insulin treatment for the first years of treatment [74, 75]. This study should provide more definitive data on the long-term effectiveness of sulfonylurea therapy.

Similarities and Differences Between Sulfonylureas

It is generally assumed that all sulfonylureas have the same mechanism of action, and this may relate to (receptor) binding on the B-cell surface (see above). However, as all sulfonylureas have not been tested or compared in similar pharmacodynamic systems *in vitro* and *in vivo*, it cannot be excluded that there may be qualitative pharmacodynamic differences between them. One such difference might reside in the ability of sulfonylureas to penetrate the B cell; in contrast to most other sulfonylureas, glibenclamide may accumulate within the B cells [18]. On the other hand, as both glibenclamide and other sulfonylureas seem to release insulin by an interaction with the surface of the B cell, the relevance of the B-cell penetrating ability of glibenclamide remains uncertain.

All sulfonylureas are weak acids. Some of them are highly lipophilic, e.g. glibenclamide and glipizide, whereas chlorpropamide is rather hydrophilic. Most sulfonylureas seem to be extensively absorbed, some of them completely. However, the rates of absorption differ between agents, formulations and individuals, and this may be clinically important (see below). All have a small distribution volume, signifying that most of the drug is contained within blood plasma; they are extensively bound to plasma albumin, the most lipophilic ones to the greatest extent [59]. All sulfonylureas are metabolized, the more lipophilic ones virtually completely, whereas the more hydrophilic chlorpropamide is partially excreted unchanged through the kidneys [59, 76]. All sulfonylureas have a low clearance [59, 76]. Some, but not all, sulfonylureas have active metabolites that may depend upon renal function for their elimination. There is no evidence of any relevant first-pass metabolism of any sulfonylurea [59, 76]. A detailed description of the pharmacokinetics of the different sulfonylureas is given later in the chapter.

Potency and Intrinsic Molecular Activity

Although the sulfonylureas may have identical or similar pharmacodynamics, they have different potencies and intrinsic activities, related to the variations in chemical structure (see Figure 1). These structural variations are associated with variations in sulfonylurea binding to the B cell, and, as these binding differences vary with differences in the effective plasma concentrations, it is likely that variations in intrinsic activity are consequent on variations in the affinity of different sulfonylureas to binding sites in the B cell [14, 21]. The highest affinity to B-cell binding sites has been observed for glibenclamide and glipizide [14], and these two sulfonylureas also have the highest activity in terms of their minimum effective plasma concentrations, which are 50–100 nmol/l [59]. At the other end of the binding spectrum are tolbutamide and chlorpropamide, which have a B-cell affinity and intrinsic activity that are only about 1/1000 of that of glibenclamide and glipizide, as expressed by their minimum effective plasma concentrations, which are 50–100 μmol/l [59]. Acetohexamide and tolazamide seem to be active in the latter range [59, 76], whereas glibornuride, gliclazide and gliquidone seem to have an intermediate activity [59, 76]. The new sulfonylurea, glimepiride, is comparable to glibenclamide and glipizide in these respects.

As the common daily dose of chlorpropamide is 250–500 mg, whereas that of tolbutamide is 1500–3000 mg, it may be said that chlorpropamide is more potent than tolbutamide. However, the reason why a lower daily dose of chlorpropamide can be used is that the elimination of this compound is very slow, allowing a high degree of accumulation of the drug. Indeed, at a similar degree of glucose control, the plasma levels of chlorpropamide are higher than those of tolbutamide, suggesting that the intrinsic activity of the chlorpropamide molecule is, in fact, lower than that of tolbutamide [77].

The issue of potency and activity may be mainly academic, as no appropriately controlled study has shown that any sulfonylurea, in appropriate dosage, is clinically more effective than any other. However, the differences in potency and intrinsic activity may be relevant from the safety aspect, including the issues of hypoglycemia and interactions (see later).

Rate of Onset and Duration of Action

The structural variations between the different sulfonylureas are associated with differences in pharmacokinetics, i.e. in the rate and extent of absorption, distribution, biotransformation and excretion. These differences, in turn, lead to variations in the rate of onset and in the duration of action of the sulfonylureas, and these variations may be clinically more relevant than the differences in potency and intrinsic activity (pharmacodynamics).

Rate and timing of onset of sulfonylurea action The rate of onset is relevant as it relates to the capacity to improve the acute insulin release in response to meals, which is impaired in patients with NIDDM as well as in subjects with impaired glucose tolerance (IGT) [59, 78–81]. Indeed, a recent study, employing a highly selective insulin assay, indicates that a delayed and reduced insulin response to glucose challenge is a dominant feature in both NIDDM and IGT [81]. Accordingly, a rapid onset of sulfonylurea action may be important. The most rapidly acting sulfonylurea currently available is glipizide [59], and it has been shown that glipizide is able to increase the rate of insulin release in response to meals, both acutely and chronically [59, 82, 83]. Moreover, glipizide may rapidly enhance the systemic availability of insulin by reducing its first-pass hepatic clearance [52-55]. The importance of the rate of absorption and onset of action is also apparent from the fact that the efficacy of glipizide is directly dependent upon its absorption rate: the time to reach the threshold concentration of this drug correlates with the time to reach the nadir of blood glucose concentration [84].

Chlorpropamide is the most slowly absorbed sulfonylurea [59]. Glibenclamide is slower in onset than glipizide, partly because it is more slowly and incompletely absorbed, at least from the non-micronized formulation that is the only one available in North and South America, Asia, Australia and in the tropical areas [59, 85]. In Germany, Scandinavia and the UK this formulation has been replaced by a micronized one from which glibenclamide is more rapidly and more completely absorbed [85]. However, glibenclamide is slower in onset than glipizide even when infused at an equal rate and to a similar plasma level [86].

For several sulfonylureas, e.g. glibenclamide [76, 87], gliclazide [76, 88] and glipizide [76, 89], it has been shown that certain individuals are 'slow absorbers', leading to extensive delays in their uptake of these drugs. This may be clinically important, but the long-term relevance has not been elucidated.

Another potentially important finding is the recent observation that hyperglycemia may affect sulfonylurea absorption [90]; indeed, this might help to explain some primary and secondary failures in NIDDM patients who have pronounced hyperglycemia.

From the above it follows that the timing of sulfonylurea dosing relative to the time of meal intake would be important. It may, in fact, be more relevant than the dose size: 2.5 mg glibenclamide half an hour before breakfast was found to be more effective than 7.5 mg taken with breakfast [91]. Glipizide [92] and tolbutamide [93] are also more effective when given half an hour before, rather than with, a meal. These findings emphasize the relevance of developing optimum biopharmaceutic formulations of at least some of the sulfonylureas [85]. For a slow, long-acting agent such as chlorpropamide, which accumulates extensively, the timing of the dose would seem to be irrelevant.

Duration of sulfonylurea action The duration of action is important as it may relate to the probability of certain adverse effects, such as long-lasting hypoglycemia [59, 76, 94, 95], and also relates to the issue of discontinuous sulfonylurea exposure. As sulfonylureas may act via B-cell receptors, it is possible that continuous exposure may desensitize the B cells (see below).

The short-acting sulfonylureas include glipizide, which has the shortest half-life (1-5 hours) and no active metabolites; other sulfonylureas with short half-lives are glibornuride (5-12 hours), gliclazide (6-15 hours), tolazamide (4-7 hours) and tolbutamide (6-12 hours), and these also have metabolites with little or no activity [59, 76].

Chlorpropamide has the longest elimination half-life (24-48 hours, or longer in subjects with renal impairment) of all sulfonylureas currently in use, and is very long acting [59, 76]. This is a probable explanation of the fact that chlorpropamide is one of the sulfonylureas most likely to provoke long-lasting (and hence dangerous) hypoglycemic reactions [59, 76, 96]. Gliquidone has the next-longest elimination half-life (24 hours) reported, but little is known of its clinical duration of action and the risk of long-lasting hypoglycemia, mainly because the use of this sulfonylurea has so far been very limited.

While previous studies have reported a short elimination half-life of glibenclamide (2-10 hours), a recent study, employing a more sensitive HPLC method, showed that the elimination half-life is rather long, 15-20 hours [97]. This is also in agreement with the impression that this drug seems to have a rather long duration of action and may have been implicated in more cases of long-lasting hypoglycemic reactions than other sulfonylureas [59, 76, 94, 95]. This is not only because glibenclamide is the most widely used sulfonylurea in many countries; the number of long-lasting cases is higher, even after correction for number of patients on the drug and the number of doses prescribed [94, 95, 98]. A possibility not yet examined is that glibenclamide is slowly distributed; another possibility is accumulation of polar, active metabolites [99]; a recent study shows that both metabolites of glibenclamide are active in man [100]. Yet another possibility relates to the observation that glibenclamide, in contrast to other sulfonylureas, may accumulate within B cells [18].

Kinetic–Dynamic Relations

The kinetic–dynamic relations of sulfonylureas are complex. Firstly, as glucose is the major stimulator of insulin secretion, differences in dietary regimens, amount of food and time of food intake hinder the establishment of a relation between the plasma level of the sulfonylurea in question and the reductions of blood glucose and HbA_{1c}. Secondly, differences in the severity of diabetes will further confound this relation; indeed, as most doctors assume that progressive dose increase will bring about a progressive reduction of blood glucose levels, the most severely hyperglycemic patients will be given the highest doses, with the result that high sulfonylurea levels will be associated with high glucose levels. In this context, it is of particular interest that pronounced hyperglycemia may delay the absorption of sulfonylurea [90]. Thirdly, as blood glucose reduction by any therapeutic means will gradually improve B-cell function and insulin action [83, 101], there may not exist any stable relation between the plasma drug level and its effect. Fourthly, a sulfonylurea with a long elimination half-life, such as chlorpropamide, will show little fluctuation in the diurnal concentration profile of the drug, whereas a sulfonylurea with a short half-life, e.g. glipizide, will not only show large fluctuations in its plasma concentration but the level may fall to zero before the next dose [54, 59, 89]. Finally, there is evidence to suggest that chronic, continuous sulfonylurea exposure over a certain level may lead to desensitization of the insulin-releasing effect [31], and there is also evidence that very high drug levels may impair instead of improve glucose control [57, 58]. What is needed in order to establish a relationship between possible dose, plasma drug level and effect is long-term, strictly dietary regulated, placebo-controlled studies at several dose levels of the various sulfonylureas given to NIDDM patients with a uniform degree of metabolic disturbance and of sulfonylurea sensitivity. Such studies are exceedingly difficult to perform. The same applies to appropriate comparisons between different sulfonylureas.

Characteristics and Comparisons of Different Sulfonylureas

In this section relevant pharmacokinetic and pharmacodynamic data are given for different sulfonylureas, and mention is also made of comparative studies.

Tolbutamide Having been available since 1955, tolbutamide is still in use in many countries, given in various formulations from different manufacturers. There are differences in absorption rate between formulations [76, 102] and this may be important, as more rapid absorption may signify a higher efficacy in reducing postprandial hyperglycemia (see above). Tolbutamide is more rapidly absorbed than chlorpropamide [59], but less rapidly than glipizide. Many, but not all, tolbutamide formulations have a high degree of absorption, but there are no appropriate estimates of the absolute bioavailability of this drug.

Concomitant food intake may not delay the absorption of tolbutamide, but its efficacy may be improved if the drug is given half an hour before meals rather than with meals [93].

The volume of distribution of tolbutamide is small, like that of all other sulfonylureas. It is highly bound to plasma albumin, but the extent of protein binding

decreases with age, roughly in parallel with decreasing plasma albumin levels [76]. Tolbutamide is completely metabolized, mainly to hydroxytolbutamide and subsequently to carboxytolbutamide, both of which have little or no activity. Metabolism occurs by oxidation, and it has been suggested that the first oxidative step to hydroxytolbutamide is genetically polymorphic with a trimodal distribution [103]. Phenylbutazone [76] and cimetidine [76] may inhibit the metabolism of tolbutamide.

Little, if any, tolbutamide is excreted unchanged. The metabolites are excreted by the kidney [76].

The usual dosage of tolbutamide is 0.5–1.0 g three times daily. It has not been ascertained whether or not its efficacy may be maintained on a once-daily basis.

Chlorpropamide Chlorpropamide has been available almost as long as tolbutamide, and it has been extensively used all over the world. Chlorpropamide is more slowly absorbed than tolbutamide and has the longest elimination half-life of all sulfonylureas. This leads to pronounced accumulation with very small fluctuations over the day within the individual [77]. Therefore, the elimination rate is the major determinant of its effect, whereas variations in its rate of absorption are unimportant. Hence the timing of the daily dose is irrelevant, and it is also irrelevant whether chlorpropamide is ingested before or with breakfast. There are no data on the absolute bioavailability of chlorpropamide. Like that of all other sulfonylureas, the volume of distribution is small, but its binding to plasma albumin is less pronounced.

In contrast to widespread belief, chlorpropamide undergoes extensive, albeit slow, metabolic transformation. This occurs by oxidation to 2-hydroxychlorpropamide, 3-hydroxychlorpropamide and p-chlorobenzene sulfonylurea [76]. It is not clear whether the hydroxylated metabolites are active; however, they are more rapidly eliminated than the parent drug, at least in subjects with normal renal function, and would hence add little to the overall activity except perhaps in patients with renal insufficiency.

A significant portion of chlorpropamide is excreted unchanged by the kidneys [76]; this proportion can be increased by alkalinization and reduced by acidification of the urine [59, 76, 104]. The elimination half-life of chlorpropamide is long but variable (24–48 hours), partly because of variations in the excretion rate of the unchanged compound, partly because of variations in the metabolic turnover rate. This also helps to explain why there is a very large interindividual variation in the steady state plasma concentrations of chlorpropamide during treatment [77].

The usual dosage of chlorpropamide is 250–500 mg once daily.

Given intravenously, tolbutamide and chlorpropamide have shown similar acute blood glucose reductions. As they differ in both rates of absorption and rates of elimination it is difficult to make appropriate comparisons during long-term treatment. This is also evident from the previously mentioned fact that, although a larger tolbutamide dose is needed to maintain the same degree of blood glucose control, the steady state levels of chlorpropamide become higher than those of tolbutamide because of more extensive accumulation [77].

Chlorpropamide is more commonly associated with long-lasting hypoglycemic events than are most other sulfonylureas, possibly with the exception of glibenclamide (see below); this is probably related to the slow elimination and pronounced accumulation of the drug. On the other hand, chlorpropamide is the only sulfonylurea with elimination that can be enhanced by forced diuresis and urine alkalinization [59, 76, 104]. The pronounced accumulation may also help to explain why chlorpropamide, more often than other sulfonylureas, is involved in events of ethanol-provoked facial flushing (see below).

Comparisons between chlorpropamide and glibenclamide have given a variety of results, depending upon the design of the studies: in some of these, chlorpropamide has tended to promote lower fasting blood glucose levels but higher non-fasting ones; other studies have failed to show any difference [76].

Acetohexamide The absorption of acetohexamide appears to be almost complete, but its absolute bioavailability is not known [76].

There are no reports on its volume of distribution or its degree of protein binding, but it may be assumed that the distribution volume is small and the extent of protein binding great, like those of all other sulfonylureas.

Acetohexamide undergoes metabolic reduction to hydroxyhexamide; this is an active metabolite responsible for a significant part of the clinical effect. Other metabolites are inactive, and part of acetohexamide is eliminated unchanged through the kidneys.

Acetohexamide has a very limited use nowadays. The recommended dosage is 125–750 mg twice daily.

Tolazamide Tolazamide is absorbed relatively slowly, and its absorption rate is formulation sensitive [76]. It is not known whether its effect is improved if the drug is taken before rather than with meals. There are no reported estimates of its absolute bioavailability, nor of its volume of distribution or degree of protein binding. However, the latter are probably similar to those of other sulfonylureas.

Tolazamide is almost completely metabolized, mainly by oxidative hydroxylation. The hydroxylated

metabolite is active, but it is uncertain to what extent the metabolite adds to the clinical effect [76]. One may assume that it would accumulate in patients with renal impairment, as most of the tolazamide metabolites are eliminated by renal excretion. Little if any tolazamide is excreted unchanged. Its elimination rate is relatively high, with a half-life of about 4–7 hours.

The common dose range is 250–500 mg once or twice daily.

A comparison between tolazamide and tolbutamide showed no difference in the effect on fasting blood glucose levels [76].

Glibenclamide The most extensively used sulfonylurea in many parts of the world is glibenclamide (called glyburide in the USA). It was the first 'second-generation' sulfonylurea to be introduced in clinical practice, and it is one of the most potent.

The absorption of glibenclamide is rather slow and incomplete from the non-micronized formulation used on the American continents and in Asia and Australia, whereas the rate and degree of absorption are higher from the micronized formulation available in Germany, the UK and Scandinavia [85]. Both non-micronized and micronized generic formulations have appeared, but it is not clear whether they are fully equivalent to the original products. Although concomitant food intake does not seem to delay the absorption of glibenclamide, its efficacy may be increased if given before meals, at least in the short term. Indeed, as previously mentioned, 2.5 mg given half an hour before breakfast was more effective than 7.5 mg given together with breakfast [91]. The rate of absorption varies extensively between individuals [87], and this may be important at least during short-term conditions.

Like other sulfonylureas, glibenclamide has a small volume of distribution, and it is very extensively bound to albumin.

Glibenclamide is completely metabolized, mainly by oxidation to two hydroxylated metabolites, both of which have blood glucose-reducing activity [100].

About half of a given dose of glibenclamide is eliminated by renal excretion of metabolites, and a significant portion is excreted through the bile. Although renal insufficiency should not alter the elimination rate of this very lipophilic and completely metabolized drug, it may nevertheless increase the risk of hypoglycemia [76, 99]. This may be because renal insufficiency is associated with reduced drug binding to albumin; in addition, renal impairment may lead to accumulation of polar, active metabolites [99, 100]. Surprisingly, severe renal impairment in one subject has been associated with delayed elimination of glibenclamide itself [76].

Both clinical experience and various studies support the view that glibenclamide should be classified as a long-acting sulfonylurea. Indeed, glibenclamide has been associated with long-lasting (and hence dangerous) hypoglycemic reactions more often than other sulfonylureas except, perhaps, chlorpropamide [59, 76, 92, 95, 98]. There may be various reasons for this, including the now recognized fact that glibenclamide's elimination half-life is longer than previously assumed [97] and that both its main metabolites are active in man [100] (see also above).

The usual daily dose of glibenclamide is 1.75–14 mg (micronized) or 2.5–20 mg (non-micronized), given in a single morning dose or split in a morning and an evening dose.

Studies comparing glibenclamide and chlorpropamide have been commented upon above. Glibenclamide and glipizide have also been compared, but the comparisons suffer from various problems. Some studies have used only one fixed-dose level; some have involved patients whose clinical responses have been minute and hence were unsuitable for study; some have been too short to allow for the progressive improvement of blood glucose levels that follows the improved B-cell function and insulin action secondary to the reduction of hyperglycemia. It appears quite certain, however, that glipizide releases insulin more rapidly than glibenclamide [54, 86, 105], and that glibenclamide suppresses hepatic glucose output more than does glipizide [86].

In a placebo-controlled study wherein glibenclamide and glipizide were given in a crossover fashion for 6 months, and in which most patients were continuously exposed to either drug, there was no difference in the final mean daily dose, nor in final mean blood glucose or hemoglobin A_{1c} levels. Moreover, although fasting blood glucose values tended to be lower in patients on glibenclamide and postprandial blood glucose values lower in those on glipizide, neither difference was significant [54].

In one short-term study with fixed doses (10 mg of each drug), fasting blood glucose values were lower after glibenclamide [105], whereas in another short-term study postprandial glucose was more reduced by glipizide [106]. Together with the findings in the long-term study [54], and in view of the different rates of onset and different durations of action of the two compounds, it is possible that glibenclamide is slightly more able to reduce fasting blood glucose levels and glipizide slightly more able to reduce non-fasting blood glucose levels. This would also be in accord with the findings that glibenclamide suppresses hepatic glucose output more than glipizide does [86], and that glipizide is more able to enhance acute insulin release than is glibenclamide [86]. However, this would be clinically relevant only when the dosage is such that it generates discontinuous exposure to the sulfonylurea (see below).

Differences between glibenclamide and glipizide with regard to the risk of causing long-lasting hypoglycemia are discussed at the end of the chapter.

Gliclazide Gliclazide is a rapid-acting and short-acting sulfonylurea that is widely used in some countries, among them France and the UK. It is rapidly absorbed, but its absolute bioavailability is not known. Absorption is slower in the elderly [107]. Like other sulfonylureas, gliclazide is extensively bound in plasma and has a small volume of distribution [76, 88]. It is not known whether intake before meals makes gliclazide more effective than does intake together with meals.

Gliclazide is almost completely metabolized, and the metabolites seem to be inactive [76].

Most gliclazide is eliminated by excretion of the inactive metabolites through the kidneys, but a small fraction is eliminated by the bile [76]. The elimination half-life is short but variable, between 6 hours and 15 hours. Although this might not be expected for a completely metabolized drug, the elimination half-life might be increased in subjects with renal insufficiency [76].

It has been argued that gliclazide offers an advantage over other sulfonylureas in being able to reduce platelet aggregation [108]. However, it is most likely that all sulfonylureas are able to improve platelet aggregation as an indirect effect of improved blood glucose control [59]. There are no comparative studies showing that gliclazide is superior to other sulfonylureas in reducing platelet aggregation. In terms of blood glucose control, gliclazide seems to be as effective as other sulfonylureas [76].

The usual daily dose is 40–320 mg, given in a single morning dose or morning and evening.

Glipizide Glipizide is widely used in the USA and in several European countries. It is the most rapidly acting sulfonylurea available, and is also one of the most short-acting [59, 76]. Its potency and intrinsic activity are in the same range as those of glibenclamide.

The absorption and bioavailability of glipizide are fast and complete [59, 89]. It is more rapidly absorbed when taken before breakfast than when ingested together with breakfast, and intake before breakfast is also associated with a more appropriate timing of insulin release relative to the meal, and with an enhanced efficacy of the drug [92]. Its absorption rate correlates with its efficacy [82, 84], and pronounced hyperglycemia may reduce the absorption rate [90].

Glipizide has been shown to improve the acute insulin release in response to a meal [82], and this capacity may be maintained during long-term therapy, at least when the exposure is discontinuous [83]. This is interesting in view of the possibility that chronic, continuous sulfonylurea exposure may desensitize the B cell to sulfonylurea stimulation [31, 59].

The volume of distribution of glipizide is small, like that of other sulfonylureas, and the binding to albumin is very extensive [76].

Glipizide is completely metabolized, mainly by oxidative hydroxylation [76]. The metabolites appear to be inactive [76].

Glipizide is rapidly eliminated with a half-life of 1–5 hours. The half-life does not seem to increase with age [109]. Renal insufficiency does not seem to alter the elimination rate of glipizide. These facts may explain why glipizide seems to carry a lower risk of long-lasting hypoglycemia than do glibenclamide and chlorpropamide (see end of chapter).

Although glipizide is rapidly eliminated, a morning dose of 7.5 mg or more maintains effective plasma concentrations for more than 12 hours [59, 95, 110]. This may help to explain why glipizide, despite its short half-life, can be equally effective when given once daily or three times daily [110]. Based upon available documentation, dosage should be in the range of 2.5–10 mg daily, either as a single morning dose half an hour before breakfast or divided in a morning and an evening dose. In the USA the official maximum dose is 40 mg, but there is very limited support for increased efficacy with daily doses over 10–15 mg. Instead, dose increase from 15 mg to 25 mg per day has been found to impair rather than improve glucose control [57], and a placebo-controlled study using 3-month periods of glipizide at 10, 20 and 40 mg daily showed impaired glucose and insulin responses above 10 mg daily [58]. On the other hand, ethnic differences may exist in the disposition and effect of sulfonylureas, and hence in appropriate dosage (see below).

Comparisons between glipizide and glibenclamide have been commented upon above.

Gliquidone   The absorption of gliquidone seems to be rapid but formulation-dependent [76]. Data on its absolute bioavailability have not been found. It is not known whether the efficacy of gliquidone is improved by intake before meals.

Gliquidone is extensively bound in plasma. Its volume of distribution is not known but is presumably small.

The drug is almost completely metabolized by oxidation to demethylated and hydroxylated products. One of the latter is active, but reaches only low plasma concentrations [76].

Gliquidone has a terminal elimination half-life of about 24 hours; nevertheless, it is recommended that the daily dose (which may range from 15 mg to 180 mg) should be divided, being given two or even three times daily [76].

There are no controlled comparative studies showing any therapeutic advantage of gliquidone over more commonly used sulfonylureas such as tolbutamide, chlorpropamide, glibenclamide, gliclazide or glipizide.

Glibornuride   Glibornuride is rapidly absorbed, but there are no data on its absolute bioavailability. It is not known whether the efficacy of glibornuride is improved by intake before meals.

Like that of other sulfonylureas, its volume of distribution is small, and the drug is extensively bound in plasma.

Glibornuride is metabolized by oxidative processes to metabolites that seem to be inactive.

Its elimination is rapid, with an elimination half-life of 5–12 hours [76].

The recommended dose is 12.5–25 mg, and it may be given once or twice daily.

Glisoxepide   Glisoxepide is a high-potency sulfonylurea that is not well characterized from the pharmacokinetic point of view and is not much used.

Glimepiride   Glimepiride has recently been marketed. It is similar to glibenclamide and glipizide in potency and intrinsic activity, and is rapid-acting. It may be more selective for B-cell binding than other sulfonylureas, but it remains unclear whether this confers any clinical benefit.

Selection of Sulfonylureas for Therapeutic Use

As emphasized earlier, there is little or no evidence that one sulfonylurea is therapeutically more effective than another, at least not when used to promote continuous sulfonylurea exposure, and when dosage is adjusted on the basis of the individual control of blood glucose. A well-nourished, middle-aged individual with NIDDM (but otherwise healthy) can be treated effectively with any one of the available sulfonylureas. A rapid-acting sulfonylurea may improve acute insulin release and promote better control of postprandial blood glucose, whereas a long-acting sulfonylurea may give better control of overnight glycemia. A short-acting agent may allow a better chance of maintaining the insulinotrophic effect through discontinuous exposure, and carries a lower risk of provoking long-lasting hypoglycemia. High-potency sulfonylureas may reduce the risk of drug–drug interactions compared with low-potency agents, because many fewer molecules are needed to achieve blood glucose control (see later). An old NIDDM patient, particularly if poorly nourished and having other chronic ailments, is at considerable risk of developing long-lasting, severe hypoglycemia and should be treated (if at all) with a sulfonylurea with short action and inactive metabolites.

NIDDM patients with impaired renal function should be treated with a short-acting sulfonylurea, the elimination of which is entirely dependent upon hepatic metabolic degradation to inactive metabolites. The use of chlorpropamide might be discouraged because of its very long duration of action, high incidence of alcohol-induced flushing, considerable water retention with subsequent hyponatremia, dependence upon renal function for elimination, and high prevalence for long-lasting hypoglycemic reactions (see later).

WHEN AND HOW TO USE SULFONYLUREAS

Indications

The primary indication for sulfonylurea therapy is NIDDM in which optimum blood glucose control has not been achieved by dietary regulation and exercise [111, 112]. Presumed advantages of oral sulfonylurea therapy are delivery of insulin through the physiologic route (portal vein), less hyperinsulinemia than that occurring from insulin treatment, and possible extrapancreatic actions. In rare instances, sulfonylurea therapy may be indicated because of insulin allergy or hypersensitivity, or severe insulin resistance [113].

Early Intervention

The chronic hyperglycemia of NIDDM evolves slowly, and subjective symptoms of the disease usually occur only after several years. However, at least some complications may occur in the early phase of NIDDM, and the risk of cardiovascular complications is increased even in the pre-NIDDM phase of IGT [114–118]. Retinopathy may be present in 20% of NIDDM patients at the time of diagnosis [119]. Accordingly, there is reason to assume that therapeutic intervention should be introduced in the early stages of NIDDM. Indeed, there is reason to argue that efforts should be made to find NIDDM subjects before they experience symptoms that spontaneously bring them to medical care [83]. Detection programs can be made very simple: a random blood sample of non-fasting glucose may suffice for NIDDM screening [83, 120].

A most important reason for early detection and intervention is the increasingly recognized fact that chronic hyperglycemia is a self-perpetuating condition: it not only results from, but may also exacerbate, impaired insulin secretion and impaired insulin action [30]; in other words, chronic hyperglycemia generates a vicious circle. Conversely, reduction of chronic hyperglycemia has been shown to improve both insulin secretion and insulin action [28, 29, 37, 101]. Hence, it seems logical that therapeutic intervention should start

as soon as persistent hyperglycemia has been recorded, and, with due reservations for individual needs, euglycemia should be the principal goal of therapy (see below).

Therapeutic intervention should always start with dietary regulation, and the importance of persistence in dietary regulation should be emphasized at regular intervals (see Chapter 34a). The same applies for regular exercise (see Chapter 35). If euglycemia is not achieved after 2–3 months of dietary regulation and increased regular exercise, addition of a sulfonylurea is usually indicated. However, sulfonylureas must not be used instead of dietary regulation but always as a supplement; otherwise, secondary sulfonylurea failure is likely to ensue, and even primary sulfonylurea failure may occur [59, 83] (see below).

Critics of the sulfonylureas often argue that sulfonylurea treatment could be counterproductive because it may lead to weight increase, chronic hyperinsulinemia and more severe insulin resistance, and it has also been claimed that long-term sulfonylurea treatment might cause B-cell exhaustion. However, there is little scientific support for these views. On the contrary, early sulfonylurea introduction may be able to reverse the vicious circle of hyperglycemia and thereby improve insulin secretion and insulin action. There is even evidence to suggest that sulfonylurea treatment in combination with dietary restriction might delay the development of IGT to manifest NIDDM and reduce the increased risk of cardiovascular morbidity and mortality [121]. As for B-cell exhaustion by sulfonylurea treatment, there is no support for this in the literature; instead, the blood glucose reduction subsequent to sulfonylurea treatment improves B-cell function [28, 29, 101]. Finally, even though chronic hyperinsulinemia might occur during treatment with long-acting sulfonylureas, treatment with a rapid-acting and short-acting sulfonylurea in combination with hypocaloric dietary regulation can attain and maintain near-normal blood glucose levels for years without provoking chronic hypersecretion of insulin or chronic hyperinsulinemia [83]. The concept of discontinuous sulfonylurea exposure is of particular interest in this context (see below).

Discontinuous Exposure

As sulfonylureas may release insulin by activation of a receptor-mediated mechanism in the B cell [11–14], it is possible that chronic, continuous exposure to sulfonylurea at or over a certain level may desensitize the B cell by down-regulation of the putative receptors. This hypothesis may draw support from a recent study showing that the insulin-releasing effect of a single dose of sulfonylurea (tolbutamide) vanished during chronic treatment with another sulfonylurea (tolazamide). In addition, the acute insulinotrophic effect of tolbutamide reappeared after cessation of the chronic tolazamide treatment [31]. Further support for this idea may be found in the fact that high concentrations of sulfonylureas inhibit proinsulin biosynthesis *in vitro* [32, 33] and attenuate insulin secretion *in vitro* [122]. Furthermore, dosage increase of glipizide from 15 mg daily to 25 mg daily has been associated with impaired instead of improved blood glucose control in NIDDM subjects [57]. In addition, treatment with glipizide at 10, 20 and 40 mg daily for 3-month periods was accompanied by reduced instead of increased insulin and glucose responses at the 20 and 40 mg dose levels [58]. Conversely, acute insulin release could be maintained in NIDDM patients during low-dose, once-daily glipizide treatment [83]. The validity of this concept remains to be proved. Numerous studies *in vitro* suggest that desensitization may occur with many different insulin secretagogues and that desensitization may also result from the insulin secreted in response to the secretagogues [122, 123]. The significance of desensitization therefore needs to be clarified, but it may add to the arguments for low-dose sulfonylurea therapy (see below).

Therapeutic Goals in Practice

The management of patients with NIDDM should have three major goals: to alleviate symptoms, to improve the sense of well-being, and to prevent the development of chronic complications.

The alleviation of symptoms such as polyuria, polydipsia, polyphagia, weight loss and recurrent infections can usually be achieved by reducing the fasting plasma glucose level to, or below, 10 mmol/l (180 mg/dl). The sense of well-being of NIDDM patients is usually maximal at a fasting plasma glucose value of 7.5–8.0 mmol/l (135–145 mg/dl). The prevention of chronic complications, however, requires achievement of near-euglycemia (fasting plasma glucose values below 7 mmol/l (125 mg/dl); hemoglobin A_{lc} at upper limit of normal), maintenance of normal blood pressure and normal serum lipid levels [111, 112].

The goal for the management of the individual NIDDM patient must be individually defined. The prevention of chronic complications can only occur in an individual who will live long enough potentially to develop the complications and does not already have severe complications. Thus, in new-onset, elderly NIDDM patients, or in those with a complicating life-threatening illness, control aimed at preventing chronic complications is unjustified. In contrast, a newly diagnosed 40-year-old NIDDM patient with no other complications is an ideal candidate for intensive metabolic

regulation. The therapeutic treatment program is developed for NIDDM patients after the goals of treatment have been defined.

Dose and Dosage of Sulfonylureas

Dose Size and Dose Change

Regardless of the compound chosen, sulfonylurea therapy should always be started with the lowest effective dose. Moreover, as the blood glucose reduction evoked by this initial low dose may secondarily improve B-cell function and insulin action, the dosage should be only slowly increased. It is often recommended that dose increase be carried out after 1–2 weeks, but it is quite possible that monthly or even longer intervals are preferable. As a matter of fact, there are very few clinical dose–response studies that show any therapeutic improvement by dose increases within the dose intervals officially recommended for the various sulfonylureas. In addition, little is known about the different dosage needs between different ethnic groups and between lean, overweight and grossly obese patients. As an illustration of the problem, one of the authors has the experience that very high doses of, for example, glipizide (up to 40 mg) may be needed in certain black or Hispanic patients, whereas the other author has the experience that doses beyond 10–15 mg of glipizide add little benefit in Scandinavian patients; higher doses may actually impair blood glucose control [57, 58]. More studies are needed to define the appropriate dose range for sulfonylureas in different ethnic groups.

Dosage Intervals

It is well known that patient adherence to chronic pharmacotherapy improves if the medication is given only once or (at most) twice daily. Owing to its very long half-life, chlorpropamide can be given once daily without loss of efficacy. In fact, the half-life is long enough to suggest that the dosage interval should be longer than 24 hours.

Glibenclamide can also be given once or twice daily, owing to its rather long duration of action, even though this has not seemed to correspond to its elimination half-life (see above). Gliclazide may also be given once or twice daily. Although glipizide is short-acting, it is so potent that a single dose of 5 mg maintains effective concentrations for 8–10 hours, and a single dose of 7.5–15 mg maintains effective concentrations for 16 hours or more [89, 110]. Once-daily glipizide at this dose level has also been shown to be as effective as dosage three times daily [110]. No such comparisons are known to exist for tolbutamide, but by inference from pharmacokinetic data this agent also might be given once or twice daily.

If after-breakfast or after-lunch hypoglycemic reactions occur during once-daily dosage of sulfonylureas, the daily dose should be split in two, the latter dose being given before dinner. A dose before lunch does not add effectiveness for any sulfonylurea.

SULFONYLUREA FAILURES

The concept of sulfonylurea failure arose from initial clinical observations which indicated that about 10–20% of patients initially treated with sulfonylureas failed to show a significant decrease in hyperglycemia (primary failure) and an additional 20–30% lost their initial satisfactory decrease in hyperglycemia after 6 months or more of treatment (secondary failure) [65–70].

The cause of primary failure, although not extensively studied, would seem most probably attributable to a marked deficiency in insulin secretory capacity. These individuals generally have fasting plasma glucose values in excess of 15 mmol/l (270 mg/dl), and some may prove to be slowly evolving IDDM patients [124].

Secondary failure has been attributed to a variety of causes. Groop et al have divided the causes of secondary failure in NIDDM into patient-related factors (failure to follow a reasonable dietary program, poor knowledge about diabetes, lack of exercise, stress and intercurrent illnesses), disease-related factors (increasing insulin deficiency or increasing insulin resistance) and therapy-related factors (inadequate drug dosage, desensitization to chronic sulfonylurea exposure, impaired absorption of sulfonylurea due to hyperglycemia, concomitant therapy with diabetogenic drugs) [125, 126].

The practical questions raised by sulfonylurea failure are:

(1)   How do we define failure in the 1990s?
(2)   Can we predict sulfonylurea failures?
(3)   Can we reverse or prevent secondary failures?

The definition of primary or secondary sulfonylurea failure has never been standardized. Previously it was arbitrarily defined by the level of glycemic control achieved. A positive response to therapy was considered to be the attainment of 'excellent' or 'good' control. When that level of control could no longer be maintained, the patient was defined as a sulfonylurea failure. In the 1990s, when the goal of treatment of NIDDM is to minimize chronic complications (which means achieving near-euglycemia), the concept of sulfonylurea failure needs to be revised; a patient who fails to achieve any significant degree of glycemic control

should be defined as a sulfonylurea failure; a patient who achieves near-euglycemia on diet and sulfonylureas should be defined as a sulfonylurea success; if diet and sulfonylureas achieve only partial restoration of glycemia to normal, this might be called 'sulfonylurea inadequacy' [127]. The cause of such 'sulfonylurea inadequacy' should be evaluated, and appropriate measures added to achieve the appropriate glycemic goals defined for the specific individual. These might involve additional dietary management, treatment of an intercurrent illness, reduction of diabetogenic drugs, temporary treatment with insulin, or combination therapy with insulin or biguanides.

SULFONYLUREAS OR BIGUANIDES?

In many, but not all, countries, biguanides are available as alternative antihyperglycemic oral agents. In several of these countries metformin is the only biguanide available. The doctor hence has the option of using either a sulfonylurea or metformin as the first choice. Many studies have compared the therapeutic efficacy of sulfonylurea with that of metformin (see Chapter 37). However, many of these studies suffer from various flaws. In general, blood glucose control has been equal following the two treatments.

The advantages of sulfonylureas are that the mechanisms of action are better known, that sulfonylurea-induced enhancement of insulin release corrects one of the primary disturbances in NIDDM in a physiologic manner, and that lactic acidosis is avoided. The advantages with metformin are that obese patients tend to lose weight during metformin treatment, that this drug seems to have beneficial effects on plasma lipids, and that hypoglycemia can be avoided. As sulfonylureas and metformin have different mechanisms of action, they may be therapeutically combined on a rational basis.

SULFONYLUREA AND BIGUANIDE IN COMBINATION

Several studies suggest that the combination of a sulfonylurea and a biguanide can be very effective, and recent findings from a placebo-controlled randomized study gives further support to this view. While sulfonylurea (glibenclamide) and biguanide (metformin) were equally effective in reducing glucose levels, primary or secondary combination of the two drugs promoted better control than single-drug treatment [128]. Mean fasting blood glucose levels following treatment with high-dose combination were reduced from 13.3 to 7.8 mmol/l (240 to 140 mg/dl) [128], and there was little or no weight increase and little or no accentuation of hyperinsulinemia [128]. The study also suggested that body weight is not a predictor of therapeutic outcome or an indicator of which drug to select [129]; however, low initial blood glucose and high initial C-peptide levels predicted successful treatment [129].

SULFONYLUREAS OR INSULIN?

It is a common view that insulin therapy is able to achieve euglycemia in most, if not all, patients with NIDDM. If this is correct, one may question the rationale in using xenobiotic antihyperglycemic drugs such as sulfonylureas or metformin. On the other hand, insulin therapy by subcutaneous injections in the arm or the leg administers insulin in a unphysiological manner: whereas the endogenous insulin levels following a meal normally are very much higher in the portal than in the systemic circulation, the situation is reversed following subcutaneous, systemic administration of exogenous insulin. Furthermore, it is well established that many NIDDM patients require large doses of insulin and a daily multiple injection program if they are to achieve a satisfactory control of blood glucose by exogenous insulin [35]. Insulin therapy is frequently associated with increased body weight and an increased requirement of insulin. This may be due to decreased glucosuria or to an increased appetite (perhaps secondary to frequent episodes of hypoglycemia). Irrespective of the mechanism involved, insulin therapy must be accompanied by considerable dietary energy restriction if it is to be successful. Moreover, all patients with NIDDM who are treated with insulin have chronic systemic hyperinsulinemia. This should be borne in mind because hyperinsulinemia may be an independent risk factor for the development of atherosclerotic disease [118].

Sulfonylureas, on the other hand, enhance insulin secretion and improve insulin action in muscle tissue, adipose tissue and the liver. If used appropriately, sulfonylureas may attain and maintain euglycemia without causing hyperinsulinemia [59].

Clinical studies indicate that, in NIDDM patients who respond to sulfonylureas, sulfonylurea therapy and insulin therapy are essentially equal in controlling blood glucose levels. Thus, unless a true sulfonylurea failure has developed, there is no apparent disadvantage in using a sulfonylurea, and sulfonylurea therapy may in fact be advantageous from both a practical and a physiological point of view.

SULFONYLUREA AND INSULIN IN COMBINATION

Sulfonylurea–insulin therapy has been studied extensively [130, 131]. Simultaneous treatment with both agents can significantly improve glycemia in about 20–30% of mildly to moderately obese NIDDM patients who have adequate endogenous insulin secretory reserves and are in poor glycemic control (fasting plasma glucose values above 11 mmol/l) despite twice-daily insulin administration of more than 70 U/day and a history of inadequate glycemic control on diet and sulfonylurea. Most patients on combination sulfonylurea–insulin therapy will require 20–50% less insulin for the same level of glycemic control as when given insulin alone.

A sulfonylurea–insulin combination that appears to be more effective in improving glycemic control in NIDDM patients is the administration of NPH or Lente insulin at 10 p.m. to achieve normal fasting plasma glucose levels, and sulfonylurea therapy during the day to improve postprandial glycemia. This sequential therapy has been evaluated extensively in the last few years [132–134]. It results in decreases of glycosylated hemoglobin between 1.0 and 2.0% and fasting plasma glucose of 2 to 3 mmol/l (35–50 mg/dl) [132–134]. Bedtime insulin–sulfonylurea combinations are superior to daytime insulin–sulfonylurea combinations [132]. In short-term studies (3 months), bedtime insulin–sulfonylurea combination is as effective as multiple injections of insulin in controlling glycemia and does so with less hyperinsulinemia and less weight gain [132, 133]. Sequential insulin sulfonylurea therapy has been effective in controlled studies for more than one year [134]. One report claims that initial hypertriglyceridemia predicts a poor long-term outcome.

SULFONYLUREA AND ALPHA-GLUCOSIDASE IN COMBINATION

Combination sulfonylurea–α-glucosidase inhibitor therapy improves glycemic control in sulfonylurea-treated patients by a mean decrement of plasma glucose levels of about 1.5–2.0 mmol/l (27–36 mg/dl) and a mean decrease of hemoglobin A_{lc} of about 1% [135]. The major effect of adding the α-glucosidase inhibitor is to decrease further the postprandial plasma glucose rise.

The advantage of combining sulfonylurea therapy with other antidiabetic agents results from the differing mechanisms of antidiabetic action of these agents.

ADVERSE EFFECTS OF SULFONYLUREAS

The overall frequency of adverse effects is low, in the range of 2–5%, and most adverse effects are mild and reversible upon withdrawal. However, sulfonylureas are able to cause serious and even fatal complications, usually through provoking hypoglycemia.

Hypoglycemia

Whereas slight and short-lasting episodes of hypoglycemia may seem natural and negligible when using blood glucose-lowering drugs, sulfonylureas may sometimes cause very serious, long-lasting hypoglycemic reactions. There is also reason to suspect that long-lasting hypoglycemia in the elderly may be misdiagnosed as a cerebrovascular insult, and the number of sulfonylurea-induced hypoglycemic reactions is certainly under-reported. The prevalence of sulfonylurea-associated hypoglycemia requiring hospital treatment has been reported as 0.38 per 1000 treatment years in Switzerland [95], 0.19 per 1000 treatment years in Sweden [94] and 4.2 per 1000 treatment years in the Swedish island of Gotland where the use of sulfonylurea is particularly common [98]. The Swiss survey reported a fatality rate of 4.3% among the hospital-admitted patients [95]. In a US survey, 10% of hypoglycemic patients referred to hospital died, and 3% had permanent neurologic damage [136].

Long-lasting, and hence serious, hypoglycemia occurs more often with long-acting sulfonylureas, such as glibenclamide and chlorpropamide, than with short-acting ones, such as glipizide and tolbutamide [95, 98, 137]. The numbers of serious cases in the Swiss review were 0.38, 0.34, 0.15 and 0.07 per 1000 treatment years for glibenclamide, chlorpropamide, glipizide and tolbutamide, respectively [95]. Figures from Sweden for the period 1975–85 show that the number of long-lasting hypoglycemic cases per million defined daily doses were 0.195 for glibenclamide and 0.184 for chlorpropamide, but only 0.004 for glipizide and 0.072 for tolbutamide [98].

A predisposing factor is age: most serious cases in Sweden were patients over 75 years old, 21% of whom were over 85 years old [94]. Other predisposing factors are reduced food intake, intercurrent illness, renal disease, hepatic disease and cardiovascular disease [94, 95]. There is no apparent dose relation: severe and fatal hypoglycemia may occur with low doses of the offending sulfonylurea. Drug interactions frequently may be involved, often involving aspirin, salicylate or alcohol (see below).

The occurrence of severe sulfonylurea-induced hypoglycemia is minimized by avoiding sulfonylureas, particularly long-acting ones, in patients with predisposing conditions or who are taking potentially interacting drugs. When such cases do occur, the patients should be hospitalized. A bolus of 50% glucose should be given intravenously and should be followed by continuous infusion of 10% or 20% glucose. Blood glucose levels should be monitored for at least 3 days and maintained at 6–8 mmol/l (110–145 mg/dl). If intravenous glucose treatment is insufficient, hydrocortisone and/or glucagon administration may be useful.

A somatostatin analog (octreotide) has been shown to reverse sulfonylurea-induced hyperinsulinemia and hypoglycemia and might be useful in intractable cases [138].

Interactions

Several drugs interfere with the efficacy of sulfonylureas, by influencing their pharmacokinetics or pharmacodynamics, or both. As the majority of NIDDM patients are elderly subjects or are in late middle age, they are liable to be exposed to other medication in addition to sulfonylurea. Thus, the risk of interactions is considerable. Two of the most important interactions may occur with alcohol and with aspirin, both of which may provoke, prolong and/or deepen a hypoglycemic reaction [59, 76, 84, 94]. Plausible and/or documented interactions are listed in Table 4. It should be noted that the degree and extent of a certain interaction may vary between the different sulfonylureas.

Toxicity

Hypoglycemic reactions have been commented upon above. Most other adverse effects are said to appear within the first 2 months of treatment, and they include the following.

Blood Agranulocytosis, thrombocytopenia, bone marrow aplasia, red cell aplasia, hemolytic anemia.

Skin Rashes, pruritus, erythema nodosum, erythema multiforme, Stevens–Johnson syndrome, exfoliative dermatitis, purpura, photosensitivity.

Gastrointestinal tract Nausea, vomiting, heartburn.

Liver Abnormal function tests, jaundice, cholestasis, granulomatous hepatitis.

Lung Possible diffuse pulmonary reaction.

Thyroid Weak antithyroid activity.

Kidney Antidiuresis, water retention (chlorpropamide).

Vasomotor Alcohol flush, tachycardia, headache (mainly chlorpropamide).

Cardiovascular Vasculitis.
The most frequently debated adverse sulfonylurea reaction is that of an alleged mortality increase in subjects treated with tolbutamide (the UGDP study) [139]. It seems likely that this was based on a spuriously low mortality rate in the placebo group [140]. Currently, most authorities maintain that the risk of increased cardiovascular mortality is unfounded.

Table 4 Mechanisms of drug interactions with sulfonylureas

---

*Agents that augment sulfonylurea action and may cause
profound hypoglycemia*:

A. Displacers of sulfonylureas from albumin-binding sites
   1. Aspirin and salicylic acid
   2. Other non-steroidal anti-inflammatory drugs
   3. Sulfonamides
   4. Trimethoprim
   5. Fibrates
B. Competitive inhibitors of sulfonylurea metabolism
   1. Alcohol
   2. H_2-blockers
   3. Sulfonamides
   4. Anticoagulants
   5. Pyrazolone derivatives (phenylbutazone,
      oxiphenbutazone, sulfinpyrazone)
   6. Monoamine oxidase (MAO) inhibitors
C. Inhibitors of urinary excretion of sulfonylurea and
   active metabolites
   1. Probenecid
   2. Aspirin and salicylic acid
   3. Other non-steroidal anti-inflammatory drugs
   4. Allopurinol
   5. Sulfonamides
D. Augmentors of the effect of sulfonylurea
   1. Alcohol
   2. Aspirin and salicylic acid
   3. Guanethidine and betanidine
   4. Monoamine oxidase (MAO) inhibitors
E. Antagonists of endogenous hyperglycemic hormones
   1. Beta blockers
   2. Sympatholytic drugs

*Agents that attenuate sulfonylurea action and may
counteract the antihyperglycemic effect*:

A. Enzyme inducers that increase sulfonylurea elimination
   1. Alcohol (chronic, moderate use)
   2. Barbiturates (chronic, moderate use)
   3. Rifampicin
B. Agents that antagonize sulfonylurea action
   1. Beta blockers
C. Inhibitors of insulin secretion or insulin action
   1. Thiazides and loop diuretics
   2. Diazoxide
   3. Beta blockers
   4. Phenytoin
   5. Corticosteroids
   6. Estrogens
   7. Indomethacin
   8. Isoniazid
   9. Nicotinic acid
D. Mechanism obscure
   1. Phenothiazines
   2. Acetazolamide

CONTRAINDICATIONS

The following patients should not be treated with
sulfonylureas:

(1) patients with IDDM or 'pancreatic' diabetes;

(2) pregnant women;

(3) patients with severe infections, stress or trauma;

(4) patients with a history of severe adverse reactions
to sulfonylureas;

(5) patients particularly prone to develop hypoglycemia, e.g. with liver or kidney disease.

CONCLUSION

Sulfonylureas have a definite and important role in the
management of NIDDM. They are able to counteract
several metabolic disturbances of this disease and may
help to reduce the risk of certain complications, provided that they are introduced early in the course of
NIDDM. However, they must not be introduced until
intense and persistent treatment with dietary regulation and regular exercise has proved to be insufficient,
and they should never be used instead of such treatment. When used appropriately, sulfonylureas are safe,
particularly the short-acting ones.

REFERENCES

1. Kennedy DL, Piper JM, Baum C. Trends in the use
   of oral hypoglycemic agents. Diabetes Care 1988; 11:
   558–62.
2. Ribes G, Trimble ER, Blayac JP, Wollheim CB,
   Puech R, Loubatières-Mariani MM. Effect of a new
   hypoglycaemic agent (HB 699) on the *in vivo*
   secretion of pancreatic hormones in the dog.
   Diabetologia 1981; 20: 501–5.
3. Garrino M-G, Meissner H-P, Henquin J-C. The non-
   sulphonylurea moiety of gliquidone mimics the effects
   of the parent molecule on pancreatic B-cells. Eur J
   Pharmacol 1986; 124: 309–16.
4. Levine R. Sulfonylureas: Background development of
   the field. Diabetes Care 1984; 7 (suppl. 1): 3–7.
5. Loubatières A. Analyse du mécanisme de l'action
   hypoglycémiante du *p*-aminobenzène-sulfamidothio-
   diazol. Compt Rend Soc Biol 1944; 138: 766–7.
6. Mirsky IA, Perisutti G, Jinks R. Ineffectiveness of
   sulfonylureas in alloxan diabetic rats. Proc Soc Exp
   Biol Med 1956; 91: 475–7.
7. Parker ML, Pildes RS, Chao K, Cornblath M, Kipnis DM. Juvenile diabetes mellitus. A deficiency in
   insulin. Diabetes 1968; 17: 27–32.
8. Joffe BI, Jackson WPU, Bank S, Vinik AI. Effect of
   oral hypoglycemic agents on glucose tolerance in
   pancreatic diabetes. Gut 1972; 13: 285–7.
9. Yalow RS, Black H, Villazon M, Berson SA. Comparison of plasma insulin levels following administration of tolbutamide and glucose. Diabetes 1960; 9:
   356–62.
10. Hellman B, Täljedal I-B. Effects of sulphonylurea
    derivatives on pancreatic beta cells. In Dorzbach E
    (ed.) Insulin, pt 2. Berlin: Springer, 1975: pp 175–94.
11. Malaisse WJ, Lebrun P. Mechanisms of sulfonylurea-
    induced insulin release. Diabetes Care 1990; 13
    (suppl. 3): 9–17.
12. Cook DL, Satin LS, Ashford MLJ, Hales CN. ATP-
    sensitive K^+ channels in pancreatic B-cells. Spare
    channel hypothesis. Diabetes 1988; 37: 495–8.

13. Boyd AE III. Sulfonylurea receptors, ion channels, and fruit flies. Diabetes 1988; 37: 847–50.

14. Siconolfi-Baez L, Banerji MA, Lebovitz HE. Characterization and significance of sulfonylurea receptors. Diabetes Care 1990; 13 (suppl. 3): 2–8.

15. Wick AN, Britton B, Gabowski R. The action of a sulfonylurea hypoglycemic agent (Orinase) in extrahepatic tissues. Metabolism 1956; 5: 739–43.

16. Hellman B, Sehlin J, Täljedal I-B. The pancreatic B cell recognition of insulin secretagogues. II Sites of action of tolbutamide. Biochem Biophys Res Comm 1971; 45: 1384–8.

17. Bowen V, Lazarus NR. Insulin release from the perfused rat pancreas. Biochem J 1974; 142: 385–9.

18. Hellman B, Sehlin J, Täljedal I-B. Glibenclamide is exceptional among hypoglycaemic sulphonylureas in accumulating progressively in B-cell rich pancreatic islets. Acta Endocrinol 1984; 385–90.

19. Carpentier J-L, Sawano F, Ravazzola M, Malaisse WJ. Internalization of [³H]glibenclamide in pancreatic islet cells. Diabetologia 1986; 29: 259–61.

20. Deleers M, Malaisse WJ. Binding of hypoglycaemic sulphonylureas to an artificial phospholipid bilayer. Diabetologia 1984; 26: 55–9.

21. Geisen K, Hitzel V, Okomonpoloulos R, Punter J, Weyer R, Summ H-D. Inhibition of ³H-glibenclamide binding to sulfonylurea receptors by oral antidiabetics. Arzneim Forsch 1985; 35: 707–12.

22. Schmid-Antomarchi H, De Weille J, Fosset M, Lazdunski M. The receptor for antidiabetic sulphonylureas controls the activity of the ATP-modulated K⁺ channel in insulin secreting cells. J Biol Chem 1987; 262: 15840–4.

23. Gylfe E, Hellman B, Sehlin J, Täljedal I-B. Interaction of sulphonylurea with the pancreatic B-cell. Experientia 1984; 40: 1126–34.

24. Boyd AE III, Hill RS, Oberwetter JM, Berg M. Calcium dependency and free calcium concentrations during insulin secretion in a hamster beta cell line. J Clin Invest 1986; 77: 774–81.

25. Pfeifer MA, Halter JB, Graf R, Porte D Jr. Potentiation of insulin secretion to non-glucose stimuli in normal man by tolbutamide. Diabetes 1980; 29: 335–40.

26. Judzewitsch RG, Pfeifer MA, Best JD, Beard JC, Halter JB, Porte D Jr. Chronic chlorpropamide therapy of non-insulin-dependent diabetes augments basal and stimulated insulin secretion by increasing islet sensitivity to glucose. J Clin Endocrinol Metab 1982; 55: 321–7.

27. Sumi S, Ichihara K, Nonaka K, Tauri S. Effect of the discontinuation of long-term sulfonylurea treatment on blood glucose and insulin secretion in non-insulin-dependent diabetes mellitus. Endocrinol Jpn 1982; 29: 41–7.

28. DeFronzo RA. The triumvirate: B-cell, muscle, liver. A collusion responsible for NIDDM. Diabetes 1988; 37: 667–87.

29. Kosaka K, Kuzuya T, Akanuma Y, Hagura R. Increase in insulin response after treatment of overt maturity onset diabetes mellitus is independent of the mode of treatment. Diabetologia 1980; 18: 23–8.

30. Unger RH, Grundy S. Hyperglycaemia as an inducer as well as a consequence of impaired islet cell function and insulin resistance: implication for the management of diabetes. Diabetologia 1985; 28: 119–21.

31. Karam JH, Sanz N, Salamon E, Nolte MS. Selective unresponsiveness of pancreatic B-cells to acute sulfonylurea stimulation during sulfonylurea therapy in NIDDM. Diabetes 1986; 35: 1314–20.

32. Davies MJ, Metcalf J, Day JL, Greenfell A, Hales CN, Gray IP. Effect of sulphonylurea therapy on plasma insulin, intact and 32/33 split proinsulin in subjects with type 2 diabetes mellitus. Diabet Med 1994; 11: 293–8.

33. Levy J, Malaisse WJ. The stimulus–secretion coupling of glucose-induced insulin release. XVII. Effects of sulfonylureas and diazoxide on insular biosynthetic activity. Biochem Pharmacol 1975; 24: 235–9.

34. Duckworth WC, Solomon SS, Kitabchi AE. Effect of chronic sulfonylurea therapy on plasma insulin and proinsulin levels. J Clin Endocrinol Metab 1972; 35: 585–91.

35. Lebovitz HE. Oral hypoglycemic agents. In Rifkin H, Porte D Jr (eds) Diabetes mellitus: theory and practice, 4th edn. New York: Excerpta Medica, 1990: pp 554–75.

36. Lebovitz HE, Feinglos MN. Sulfonylurea drugs: mechanism of antidiabetic action and therapeutic usefulness. Diabetes Care 1978; 1: 189–97.

37. Lebovitz HE. Oral hypoglycemic agents. In Alberti KGMM, Krall LP (eds) Diabetes annual 3. Amsterdam: Elsevier, 1987: pp 72–93.

38. Lebovitz HE. Cellular loci of sulfonylurea actions. Diabetes Care 1984; 7 (suppl. 1): 67–71.

39. Jacobs DB, Hayes GR, Lockwood DH. *In vitro* effects of sulfonylurea on glucose transport and translocation of glucose transporters in adipocytes from streptozotocin-induced diabetic rats. Diabetes 1989; 38: 205–10.

40. Putnam WS, Andersen DK, Jones RS, Lebovitz HE. Selective potentiation of insulin-mediated glucose disposal in normal dogs by the sulfonylurea, glipizide. J Clin Invest 1981; 67: 1016–23.

41. Firth RG, Bell PM, Rizza RA. Effects of tolazamide and exogenous insulin on insulin action in patients with non-insulin-dependent diabetes mellitus. New Engl J Med 1986; 314: 1280–6.

42. Simonson DC, Delprato S, Castellino P, Groop L, DeFronzo RA. Effect of glyburide on glycemic control, insulin requirement, and glucose metabolism in insulin-treated diabetic patients. Diabetes 1987; 36: 136–46.

43. Sartor G, Ursing D, Nilsson-Ehle P, Wåhlin-Boll E, Melander A. Lack of primary effect of sulphonylurea (glipizide) on plasma lipoproteins and insulin action in former type 2 diabetics with attenuated insulin secretion. Eur J Clin Pharmacol 1987; 33: 279–82.

44. Lebovitz HL, Feinglos MN, Bucholtz HK, Lebovitz FL. Potentiation of insulin action: a probable mechanism for the antidiabetic action of sulfonylurea drugs. J Clin Endocrinol Metab 1977; 45: 601–4.

45. Kolterman OG, Gray RS, Shapiro G, Scarlett JA, Griffin J, Olefsky JM. The acute and chronic effects of sulfonylurea therapy in type II diabetic subjects. Diabetes 1984; 33: 346–54.

46. Ward G, Harrison LC, Proietto J, Aitken P, Nankervis A. Gliclazide therapy is associated with potentiation of postbinding insulin action in obese, non-insulin-dependent diabetic subjects. Diabetes 1985; 34: 241–5.

47. Faber OK, Beck-Nielsen H, Binder C et al. Acute actions of sulfonylurea drugs during long-term

treatment of NIDDM. Diabetes Care 1990; 13 (suppl. 3): 26–31.

48. Lebovitz HE. Oral hypoglycemic sulfonylureas: pancreatic vs extrapancreatic actions. In Shigeta Y, Lebovitz HE, Gerich JE, Malaisse WJ (eds) Best approach to ideal therapy of diabetes mellitus. Amsterdam: Excerpta Medica, 1987: pp 21–6.

49. Beck-Nielsen H, Hother-Hielsen O, Pedersen O. Mechanism of action of sulphonylureas with special reference to the extrapancreatic effect: an overview. Diabet Med 1988; 5: 613–20.

50. Wang PH, Beguinot F, Smith RJ. Augmentation of the effects of insulin and insulin-like growth factors I and II on glucose uptake in cultured rat skeletal muscle cells by sulfonylureas. Diabetologia 1987; 30: 797–803.

51. Mirsky IA, Perisutti G, Diengatt D. The inhibition of insulinase by hypoglycemic sulfonamides. Metabolism 1956; 5: 138–43.

52. Almér L-O, Johansson E, Melander A, Wåhlin-Boll E. Influence of sulphonylureas on the secretion, disposal and effect of insulin. Eur J Clin Pharmacol 1982; 22: 27–32.

53. Scheen AJ, Lefebvre PJ, Luyckx AS. Glipizide increases plasma insulin but not C-peptide level after a standardized breakfast in type 2 diabetic patients. Eur J Clin Pharmacol 1984; 26: 471–4.

54. Groop L, Groop P-H, Stenman S, Saloranta C, Tötterman K-J, Fyhrquist F, Melander A. Comparison of pharmacokinetics, metabolic effects and mechanisms of action of glyburide and glipizide during long-term treatment. Diabetes Care 1987; 10: 671–8.

55. Groop L, Groop P-H, Stenman S, Saloranta C, Tötterman K-J, Fyhrquist F, Melander, A. Do sulfonylureas influence hepatic insulin clearance? Diabetes Care 1988; 11: 689–90.

56. Beck-Nielsen H, Hother Nielsen O, Andersen PH, Pedersen O, Schmitz O. *In vivo* action of glibenclamide. Diabetologia 1986; 29: 515A (abstr 26).

57. Wåhlin-Boll E, Sartor G, Melander A, Schersten B. Impaired effect of sulphonylurea following increased dosage. Eur J Clin Pharmacol 1982; 22: 21–5.

58. Stenman S, Melander A, Groop P-H, Groop L. What is the benefit of increasing the sulphonylurea dose? Ann Int Med 1993; 118: 169–72.

59. Melander A, Bitzén P-O, Faber O, Groop L. Sulphonylurea antidiabetic drugs: an update of their clinical pharmacology and rational therapeutic use. Drugs 1989; 37: 58–72.

60. Kuo BS, Korner G, Bjornsson TD. Effects of sulfonylureas on the synthesis and secretion of plasminogen activator from bovine aortic endothelial cells. J Clin Invest 1988; 81: 730–7.

61. Moses AM, Numann P, Miller M. Mechanism of chlorpropamide-induced antidiuretics in man. Evidence for release of ADH and enhancement of peripheral action. Metabolism 1973; 22: 59–66.

62. Greenfield MS, Doberne L, Rosenthal M, Schulz B, Widström A, Reaven GM. Effect of sulfonylurea treatment on *in vivo* insulin secretion and action in patients with non-insulin-dependent diabetes mellitus. Diabetes 1982; 31: 307–12.

63. Best JD, Judzewitsch RG, Pfeifer MA, Beard JC, Halter JB, Porte D Jr. The effect of chronic sulfonylurea therapy on hepatic glucose production in non-insulin-dependent diabetes mellitus. Diabetes 1982; 31: 333–8.

64. Lebovitz HE, Feinglos MN. Mechanism of action of the second generation sulfonylurea glipizide. Am J Med 1983; 75 (suppl. 5B): 46–54.

65. Camerini-Davalos R, Lozano-Castaneda O, Marble A. Five years experience with tolbutamide. Diabetes 1962; 11 (suppl.): 74–80.

66. Cervantes-Amezeua A, Naldjian S, Camerini-Davalos R, Marble A. Long-term use of chlorpropamide in diabetes. JAMA 1965; 193: 759–62.

67. Muller R, Bauer G, Schroder R, Saito S. Summary report of clinical investigation of the oral antidiabetic drug HB 419 (glibenclamide). Horm Metab Res 1969; 1 (suppl.): 88–92.

68. Emanueli A, Molari E, Colombo A, Pirola L, Caputo G. Glipizide, a new sulfonylurea in the treatment of diabetes mellitus. Arzneim Forsch (Drug Res) 1972; 22: 1881–5.

69. Rizza RA. Is secondary failure inevitable? In Cameron D, Colagiuri S, Heding L, Kuhl C, Ma A, Mortimer R (eds) Non-insulin-dependent diabetes mellitus. Hong Kong: Excerpta Medica, 1989: pp 57–61.

70. Balodimos MC, Camerini-Davalos R, Marble A. Nine years experience with tolbutamide in the treatment of diabetes. Metabolism 1966; 11: 957–70.

71. Singer DL, Hurwitz D. Long-term experience with sulfonylureas and placebo. New Engl J Med 1967; 277: 450–6.

72. Lev-Ran A. Trial of placebo in long-term chlorpropamide-treated diabetics. Diabetologia 1974; 10: 197–200.

73. University Group Diabetes Program. Effects of hypoglycemic agents on vascular complication in patients with adult-onset diabetes. III Clinical implications of UGDP results. JAMA 1971; 218: 1400–10.

74. UK Prospective Study of Therapies of Maturity-onset Diabetes. I. Effect of diet, sulphonylurea, insulin or biguanide therapy on fasting plasma glucose and body weight over one year. Diabetologia 1983; 24: 404–11.

75. UK Prospective Diabetes Study. II. Reduction in HbA$_{1c}$ with basal insulin supplement, sulfonylurea or biguanide therapy in maturity-onset diabetes. Diabetes 1985; 34: 793–8.

76. Ferner RE, Chaplin S. The relationship between the pharmacokinetics and pharmacodynamic effects of oral hypoglycaemic drugs. Clin Pharmacokin 1987; 12: 379–401.

77. Melander A, Sartor G, Wåhlin E, Schersten B, Bitzén P-O. Serum tolbutamide and chlorpropamide concentrations in patients with diabetes mellitus. Br Med J 1978; 1: 142–4.

78. Cerasi E, Efendic S, Luft R. Dose response relation between insulin and blood glucose levels during oral glucose loads in prediabetic and diabetic subjects. Lancet 1973; i: 794–7.

79. Luft R, Wajngot A, Efendic S. On the pathogenesis of maturity-onset diabetes. Diabetes Care 1981; 4: 58–63.

80. DeFronzo RA, Ferrannini E, Koivisto V. New concepts in the pathogenesis and treatment of noninsulin-dependent diabetes mellitus. Am J Med 1983; 74 (suppl. 1A): 52–81.

81. Temple RC, Carrington CA, Luzio SD, Owens DR, Schneider AE, Sobey WJ, Hales CN. Insulin deficiency in non-insulin-dependent diabetes. Lancet 1989; i: 293–5.

82. Bitzén P-O, Melander A, Scherstén B, Wåhlin-Boll E. The influence of glipizide on early insulin release and glucose disposal before and after diet regulation in diabetic patients with different degrees of hyperglycaemia. Eur J Clin Pharmacol 1988; 35: 31–7.

83. Bitzén P-O. On the early detection and treatment of non-insulin-dependent diabetes mellitus in primary health care. PhD Thesis 1988. University of Lund, Sweden.

84. Hartling SG, Faber OK, Wegmann M-L, Wåhlin-Boll E, Melander A. Interaction of ethanol and glipizide in humans. Diabetes Care 1987; 10: 683–6.

85. Arnqvist HJ, Karlberg BE, Melander A. Pharmacokinetics and effects of glibenclamide in two formulations, HB419 and HB420, in type 2 diabetics. Ann Clin Res 1983; 15 (suppl. 37): 21–5.

86. Groop L, Luzi L, Melander A, Groop P-H, Ratheiser K, Simonson DC, DeFronzo RA. Different effects of glyburide and glipizide on insulin secretion and hepatic glucose production in normal and NIDDM subjects. Diabetes 1987; 36: 1320–8.

87. Ikegawi H, Shima K, Tanaka A, Tahara Y, Hirota M, Kumahara Y. Interindividual variation in the absorption of glibenclamide in man. Acta Endocrinol 1986; 111: 528–32.

88. Campbell DB, Adriaenssens P, Hopkins YW, Gordon B, Williams JRB. Pharmacokinetics and metabolism of gliclazide: a review. In Keen H et al (eds) Gliclazide and the treatment of diabetes. International Congress and Symposium Series 20. London: Academic Press, 1980: pp 71–82.

89. Wåhlin-Boll E, Almér L-O, Melander A. Bioavailability, pharmacokinetics and effects of glipizide in type 2 diabetics. Clin Pharmacokin 1982; 7: 363–72.

90. Eriksson J, Franssila-Kalluni A, Ekstrand A, Saloranta C, Widén E, Schalin C, Groop L. Early metabolic defects in persons at increased risk for non-insulin-dependent diabetes mellitus. New Engl J Med 1989; 321: 337–43.

91. Sartor G, Lundquist I, Melander A, Scherstén B, Wåhlin-Boll E. Improved effect of glibenclamide on administration before breakfast. Eur J Clin Pharmacol 1982; 21: 403–8.

92. Wåhlin-Boll E, Melander A, Sartor G, Scherstén B. Influence of food intake on the absorption and effect of glipizide in diabetics and in healthy subjects. Eur J Clin Pharmacol 1980; 18: 279–83.

93. Silins RA, Butcher MA, Marlin GE. Improved effect of tolbutamide when given before food in patients on long-term therapy (letter). Br J Clin Pharmacol 1984; 18: 647–8.

94. Asplund K, Wiholm B-E, Lithner F. Glibenclamide-associated hypoglycaemia. A report on 57 cases. Diabetologia 1983; 24: 412–17.

95. Berger W, Cardiff F, Pasquel M, Rump A. Die relative Häufigkeit der schweren Sulfonylharnstoff-Hypoglykämie in den letzten 25 Jahren in der Schweiz. Schweiz Med Wschr 1986; 116: 145–51.

96. Seltzer HS. Severe drug-induced hypoglycemia. A review. Comp Ther 1979; 5: 21–9.

97. Jönsson A, Rydberg T, Ekberg G, Hallengren B, Melander A. Slow elimination of glyburide in NIDDM subjects. Diabetes Care 1994; 17: 142–5.

98. Statistics from the Department of Drugs, Swedish Board of Health and Welfare, Uppsala, Sweden.

99. Behrle M. Untersuchung zur Pharmakokinetik von Glibenclamid bei nierengesunden und niereninsuffizienten Diabetikern. Thesis 1980, Ruprecht-Karl-Universität, Heidelberg, Germany.

100. Rydberg T, Jönsson A, Røder M, Melander A. Hypoglycemic activity of glyburide (glibenclamide) metabolites in man. Diabetes Care 1994; 17: 1026–30.

101. Ferner R, Rawlins MD, Alberti KGMM. Impaired B-cell responses improve when fasting blood glucose concentration is reduced in non-insulin-dependent diabetes. Quart J Med 1988; 66: 137–46.

102. Olson SC, Ayres JW, Antal EJ, Albert KS. Effect of food and tablet age on relative bioavailability and pharmacodynamics of two tolbutamide products. J Pharmaceut Sci 1985; 74: 735–9.

103. Scott J, Poffenbarger PL. Pharmacodynamics of tolbutamide metabolism in humans. Diabetes 1979; 28: 41–51.

104. Neuvonen PJ, Kärkkäinen S. Effects of charcoal, sodium bicarbonate and ammonium chloride on chlorpropamide kinetics. Clin Pharmacol Ther 1983; 33: 386–93.

105. Groop L, Wåhlin-Boll E, Groop P-H, Tötterman K-J, Melander A, Tolppanen E-M, Fyhrqvist F. Pharmacokinetics and metabolic effects of glibenclamide and glipizide in Type 2 diabetics. Eur J Clin Pharmacol 1985; 28: 697–704.

106. Taylor R, Isles TE, MacLaren S, Stevenson IH, Newton RW. Comparison of metabolic profiles in non-obese non-insulin-dependent diabetics receiving glipizide and glibenclamide. Diabetologia Croatica 1983; 12: 279–92.

107. Forette B, Rolland A, Hopkins Y, Gordon B, Campbell B. Gliclazide kinetics in the elderly. In Alberti KGMM, Ogada T, Aluoch JA, Mngola EN (eds) 11th Congress of the International Diabetes Federation. Amsterdam: Excerpta Medica, 1982: p 9.

108. Holmes B, Heel RC, Brogden RN, Speight TM, Avery GS. Gliclazide. A preliminary review of its pharmacodynamic properties and therapeutic efficacy in diabetes mellitus. Drugs 1984; 27: 301–27.

109. Kradjian W, Kobayashi KA, Bauer LA, Horn JR, Opheim K, Wood F Jr. Glipizide pharmacokinetics: effects of age, diabetes and multiple dosing (in press).

110. Wåhlin-Boll E, Groop L, Karhumaa S, Groop P-H, Tötterman K-J, Melander A. Therapeutic equivalence of once- and thrice-daily glipizide. Eur J Clin Pharmacol 1986; 31: 95–9.

111. Alberti KGMM, Gries FA. Management of non-insulin-dependent diabetes mellitus in Europe: a consensus view. Diabet Med 1988; 5: 275–81.

112. Lebovitz HE (ed) Physician's guide to non-insulin dependent (type II) diabetes: diagnosis and treatment, 2nd edn. Washington, DC: American Diabetes Association, 1988; pp 37–46.

113. Rendell M, Slevin D, Meltz G, Simpson J, Barquet A. A case of maturity-onset diabetes mellitus resistant to insulin but responsive to tolbutamide. Arch Int Med 1979; 90: 195–7.

114. Persson G. Cardiovascular complications in diabetics and subjects with reduced glucose tolerance. Acta Med Scand 1977; suppl. 605.

115. Donahue RP, Abbott RD, Reed DM, Katsuhiko Y. Postchallenge glucose concentration and coronary heart disease in men of Japanese ancestry. Honolulu Heart Program. Diabetes 1987; 36: 689–92.

116. Fuller JH, Shipley MJ, Rose G, Jarrett RJ, Keen H. Coronary-heart-disease risk and impaired glucose tolerance. Lancet 1980; i: 1373–6.

117. Jarrett RJ, McCartney P, Keen H. The Bedford Survey. Ten year mortality rates in newly diagnosed diabetics, borderline diabetics and normoglycaemic controls and risk indices for coronary heart disease in borderline diabetics. Diabetologia 1982; 22: 79–84.

118. Eschwège E, Richard JL, Thibault N et al. Coronary heart disease mortality in relation with diabetes, blood glucose and plasma insulin levels. The Paris prospective study, ten years later. Horm Metab Res 1985; 15 (suppl.): 41–6.

119. Owens DR, Dolben J, Vora JP et al. Retinopathy and nephropathy in relation to metabolic status in newly diagnosed NIDDM. In Cameron D, Colagiuri S, Heding L, Kuhl C, Ma A, Mortimer R (eds) Non-insulin-dependent diabetes mellitus. Hong Kong: Excerpta Medica, 1989; pp 11–19.

120. Bitzén P-O, Schersten B. Assessment of laboratory methods for detection of unsuspected diabetes in primary health care. Scand J Primary Health Care 1986; 4: 85–95.

121. Sartor G, Schersten B, Carlström S, Melander A, Nordén Å, Persson G. Ten-year follow-up of subjects with impaired glucose tolerance. Prevention of diabetes by tolbutamide and diet regulation. Diabetes 1980; 29: 41.

122. Bailey TS, Lebovitz HE. Continuous sulfonylurea exposure desensitizes beta cell insulin secretion at a distal site. Diabetes 1990; 39 (suppl. 1): 137A (abstr 548).

123. Grodsky GM. A new phase of insulin secretion. How will it contribute to our understanding of B-cell function? Diabetes 1989; 38: 673–8.

124. Groop LC, Bottazzo GF, Doniach D. Islet cell antibodies identify latent type I diabetes in patients aged 35–75 years at diagnosis. Diabetes 1986; 35: 237–41.

125. Groop LC, Eriksson J, Schalin C, Ahola A. Does secondary oral failure represent slowly evolving type I diabetes? In Cameron D, Colagiuri S, Heding L, Kuhl C, Ma A, Mortimer R (eds) Non-insulin dependent diabetes mellitus. Hong Kong: Excerpta Medica, 1989: pp 48–51.

126. Groop LC, Pelkonen R, Koskimies S, Bottazzo GF, Doniach D. Secondary failure to treatment with oral antidiabetic agents in non-insulin-dependent diabetes. Diabetes Care 1986; 9: 129–33.

127. Turner RC, Holman RR, Matthews DR. Sulfonylurea failure and inadequacy. In Cameron D, Colagiuri S,

Heding L, Kuhl C, Ma A, Mortimer R (eds) Non-insulin dependent diabetes mellitus. Hong Kong: Excerpta Medica, 1989: pp 52–6.

128. Hermann LS, Schersten B, Bitzén P-O, Kjellström T, Lindgärde F, Melander A. Therapeutic comparison of metformin and sulfonylurea, alone and in various combinations: a double-blind controlled study. Diabetes Care 1994; 17: 1100–1109.

129. Hermann LS, Schersten B, Melander A. Antihyperglycaemic efficacy, response prediction and dose-response relations of treatment with metformin and sulphonylurea, alone and in primary combination. Diabet Med 1994; 11: 953–60.

130. Lebovitz HE, Pasmantier RM. Combination insulin-sulfonylurea therapy. Diabetes Care 1990; 13: 667–75.

131. Groop LC, Groop P-H, Stenman S. Combined insulin-sulfonylurea therapy in treatment of NIDDM. Diabetes Care 1990; 13 (suppl. 3): 47–52.

132. Yki-Järvinen H, Kauppila M, Kusansuu E et al. Comparisons of insulin regimens in patients with non-insulin-dependent diabetes mellitus. New Engl J Med 1992; 327: 1426–33.

133. Pugh JA, Wagner ML, Sawyer J, Ramirez G, Tuley M, Friedberg SJ. Is combination sulfonylurea and insulin therapy useful in NIDDM patients? A meta-analysis. Diabetes Care 1992; 15: 953–8.

134. Sane T, Helve E, Yki-Järvinen H, Taskinen MR. One year response to evening insulin therapy in non-insulin dependent diabetes. J Int Med 1992; 231: 253–60.

135. Reaven GM, Lardinois CB, Greenfield MS, Schwartz HC, Vreman HJ. Effect of acarbose on carbohydrate and lipid metabolism in NIDDM patients poorly controlled by sulfonylureas. Diabetes Care 1990; 13 (suppl. 3): 32–6.

136. Seltzer HS. Drug-induced hypoglycemia: a review based on 473 cases. Diabetes 1972; 21: 955–66.

137. Seltzer HS. Drug-induced hypoglycemia. Endocrinol Metab Clin North Am 1989; 18: 163–83.

138. Boyle PJ, Justice K, Krentz AJ, Nagy RJ, Schade DS. Octreotide reverses hyperinsulinemia and prevents hypoglycemia induced by sulfonylurea overdoses. J Clin Endocrinol Metab 1993; 76: 752–6.

139. University Group Diabetes Program. A study of the effects of hypoglycemic agents on vascular complications in patients with adult-onset diabetes. Diabetes 1970; 19 (suppl. 2).

140. Williamson JR, Kilo C. Effect of tolbutamide (TOLB) treatment on cardiovascular (CV) mortality in the University Group Diabetes Program (UGDP). Abstracts of 10th Congress of the International Diabetes Federation no. 663F. Amsterdam: Excerpta Medica; 1979; p 255. International Congress Series 481.

37

Biguanides: Basic Aspects and Clinical Uses

Leif Sparre Hermann and Arne Melander

Swedish Network for Pharmacoepidemiology, Malmö, Sweden

The biguanide drugs phenformin, buformin and metformin were introduced in the late 1950s [1]. However, the history of these guanidine derivatives can be traced back to medieval times, when extracts of goat's rue were used in the treatment of diabetes. The preparation *Galega officinalis* contains isoamylene guanidine. In the 1920s diguanidines (Synthalin A) were used as antihyperglycaemic agents, but were soon withdrawn because of hepatotoxic effects. During the 1960s and 1970s phenformin was studied intensively, especially in the USA, while fewer experimental studies were carried out with buformin (in Germany) and metformin (in France). The mode of action of biguanides was shown to be multifactorial, and for a long time it remained essentially unknown.

The relation to lactate metabolism was acknowledged early, and lactic acidosis became associated with biguanides, especially phenformin [2]. Later this drug and buformin were withdrawn in most countries. Metformin was kept on the market, because few cases of lactic acidosis were associated with this biguanide. Nevertheless, the use of metformin became infrequent, as the differences between phenformin and metformin were not recognized.

During the 1980s and recently there has been a renewed interest in metformin, as it was increasingly realized that this biguanide offers several therapeutic advantages. Its specific documentation was reviewed [3] and the mode of action re-evaluated [4]. Since the survey in the first edition of this book (1992), updated reviews on the pharmacology and therapeutic action in NIDDM have been published [5, 113, 114, 151, 162]. The safety of metformin has also been reconsidered and assessed in relation to sulphonylureas [6]. The mortality risks of metformin-associated lactic acidosis and glibenclamide-associated hypoglycaemia seem to be comparable [7, 8]. Metformin is included in the large United Kingdom Prospective Diabetes Study (UKPDS) [9, 163] concerning long-term benefits, and new studies have been performed for registration of the drug in the USA [164]. There is an increasing interest in the effect of metformin on insulin resistance, hyperinsulinaemia and other components of the metabolic syndrome or 'syndrome X' [6, 151, 165]. Metformin is included as the sole biguanide recommended for treatment of non-insulin dependent diabetes mellitus (NIDDM) in the proposal issued by the European NIDDM Policy Group. There is current interest in combination therapy and a recent study has documented a high therapeutic efficacy of combined treatment with metformin and sulphonylurea [114, 115].

This chapter is mainly restricted to metformin, and is particularly concerned with recent literature. References to earlier studies are given in previous reviews of biguanides [1, 113, 151] and metformin [3, 4, 5, 10, 114]. When appropriate, reference is also made to other biguanides. The review deals mainly with studies in humans, but some new animal experiments have been quoted for clarification of the mechanism of action.

International Textbook of Diabetes Mellitus, Second Edition. Edited by K.G.M.M. Alberti, P. Zimmet, R.A. DeFronzo, and H. Keen (Honorary)
© 1997 John Wiley & Sons Ltd

CHEMISTRY

Biguanides are derived from guanidine. The chemical structure is shown in Figure 1. Metformin (*N*-1, 1-dimethylbiguanide) is bisubstituted, and the side-chain is short. Phenformin (β-phenethylbiguanide) and buformin (*n*-butylbiguanide) are monosubstituted compounds and have longer side-chains. This difference leads to important pharmacokinetic and clinical differences (see below).

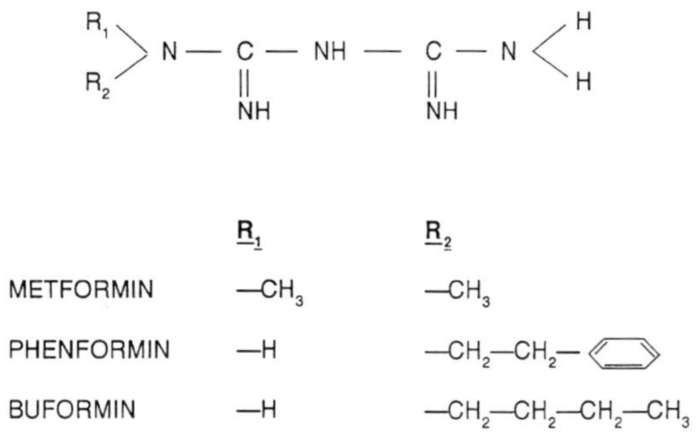

	$\underline{R_1}$	$\underline{R_2}$
METFORMIN	—CH_3	—CH_3
PHENFORMIN	—H	—CH_2—CH_2— (phenyl)
BUFORMIN	—H	—CH_2—CH_2—CH_2—CH_3

Figure 1 Chemical structure of biguanides. Because of the guanidine structure, common to all biguanides, these compounds are strong bases and exist as positively charged protonated forms under physiological conditions. The side chain (R), which differs for the various biguanides, determines the degree of lipophilia and membrane binding

Two properties of biguanides are probably important for their metabolic effects: the non-polar hydrocarbon side-chain (R in Figure 1) and the strong basic character of the polar guanidine moiety. The side-chain determines the degree of lipophilia of the molecule and allows the drug to bind to hydrophobic structures, especially phospholipids of biological and artificial membranes [1]. The affinity to membranes is directly correlated to the partition coefficient between organic solvent and water. Phenformin is more lipophilic than metformin and has a higher affinity for mitochondrial membranes. Biguanides are strong bases ($pK_a = 11.5$ for metformin at pH 8) and exist as positively charged protonated forms under physiological conditions. This hydrophilic part of the molecule accounts for the changes in surface potential [1].

PHARMACODYNAMICS

Mode of Action

The precise mechanism of action of biguanides is unknown. A multifactorial action has been proposed [1, 3–5] and the drugs labelled "pleiotropic", but the contribution of various suggested mechanisms in the overall effect remains unsettled. The mode of action has been investigated in a large number of clinical and metabolic studies [1, 5, 10, 113, 114, 151, 165, 166].

The cellular mechanism of action of metformin has been reviewed [5, 11, 166], suggesting that a major effect of the drug is on glucose utilization.

Biguanides lower blood glucose in diabetic patients and often reduce body weight and elevated blood lipids, but so far the long-term efficacy is unknown. With the final results from the UKPDS this problem should be clarified. Some long-term results have already been published [163].

Various processes in glucose, lactate and lipid metabolism have been investigated by quantifying substrates and hormones under different experimental conditions. Animal experiments have often yielded conflicting results, and human pharmacological studies have been difficult to perform and interpret. A common error has been to use results from studies with one biguanide to make conclusions about others [12]. Another mistake has been to draw conclusions regarding therapeutic effects from animal studies using supraphysiological biguanide doses and concentrations.

Human studies have shown that, in contrast to sulphonylureas, biguanides reduce elevated blood glucose concentrations and improve glucose tolerance in NIDDM patients without any increase in insulin secretion. The latter is probably the reason why biguanides do not cause hypoglycaemia. Accordingly, these drugs should be considered as antihyperglycaemic rather than hypoglycaemic agents [4, 5]. In further contrast to the sulphonylureas there is no blood glucose lowering effect in non-diabetic subjects, i.e. the efficiency of biguanides in reducing blood glucose levels is specific for the hyperglycaemic state. In non-diabetic subjects, biguanides initiate counter-regulatory mechanisms [5, 10, 13, 114], whereby the blood glucose level is unaffected.

Recent studies with metformin as presented in the following sections and reviewed separately [165] show that metformin can ameliorate insulin resistance in NIDDM. Although the binding of insulin to its receptors may be increased, the main effect appears to be directed at postreceptor sites. The major consequences of the enhanced insulin action are increased insulin-mediated peripheral glucose uptake and metabolism, and potentiation of insulin-mediated suppression of hepatic gluconeogenesis. Whereas the peripheral effect appears to be most important for the chronic therapeutic effect [5, 11, 14], there is evidence that the hepatic action accounts for the acute antihyperglycaemic mechanism of metformin in NIDDM [152]. Biguanides may also influence glucose metabolism independently of insulin [5, 11, 15, 114, 165, 166], and it is possible that insulin resistance can be reduced secondarily subsequent to the blood glucose reduction from such direct effects, whether in the periphery or in the liver. The influence of metformin on intestinal glucose absorption seems less important in humans [5, 11, 12,

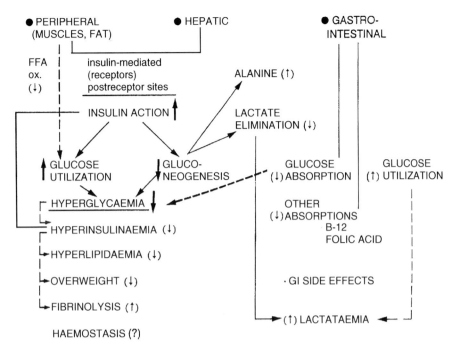

Figure 2 Metabolic and clinical effects of metformin. Binding to phospholipid membranes and changes in surface potential elicit a multifactorial metabolic response. The main clinical consequence in patients with NIDDM is a reduction of elevated blood glucose concentrations (antihyperglycaemic effect). This is caused predominantly by amelioration of insulin resistance, especially through increased muscular glucose utilization, but to a certain extent also through a hepatic effect resulting in inhibition of hypergluconeogenesis. The insulin-mediated effects are exerted on postreceptor sites, and to some extent even on insulin receptors. Glucose utilization can also be affected independently of insulin, e.g. via decreased FFA oxidation. As a consequence of the decreased gluconeogenesis, concentrations of gluconeogenic precursors (e.g. alanine and lactate) may be slightly elevated. Increase of blood lactate concentration is derived from the decreased lactate elimination and also from increased intestinal glucose utilization. A decreased or delayed intestinal glucose absorption may contribute to the reduction of blood glucose concentration, but seems to be of minor importance in the overall effect. Other gastrointestinal effects account for various unwanted effects, e.g. on vitamin B_{12} and folic acid absorption and on secretion and motility (causing gastrointestinal side-effects). The improved insulin action with decreased glycaemia and without stimulation of insulin secretion favours a reduction of hyperinsulinaemia; this may lead to decreased lipid levels, weight stabilization and increased fibrinolysis. A direct effect on VLDL synthesis has also been suggested as an explanation for the reduction of hyperlipidaemia (especially hypertriglyceridaemia). Effects on haemostasis (platelet aggregation) have been proposed

14, 16]. However, stimulation of intestinal glucose utilization by metformin has been proposed as a source of lactate formation [5, 113]. Increased gluconeogenesis from lactate represents a counter-regulatory mechanism against hypoglycaemia in diabetics [113, 114].

Biguanides can exert a variety of metabolic effects via alteration of biological membrane functions [1]. Phospholipids are considered to be the primary binding sites for the non-polar hydrocarbon side-chain at the membrane/solution interface. The accumulation of positive charges evokes a change in the electrostatic surface potential, and various metabolic responses subsequently can be elicited. This unifying concept may explain the diversity of biguanide effects, but it does not allow prediction of the overall response of the integrated organism. Membrane binding must be regarded as the primary or fundamental (and unspecific) action at the molecular level, but the link between alterations in membrane properties and changes in glucose metabolism remains to be established [5].

Biguanide metabolites show no membrane binding and have no antihyperglycaemic effect. The effects of metformin at the clinical and metabolic level are discussed in the following sections and are summarized in Figure 2.

Glucose Levels

Normal blood glucose concentrations remain unaffected by metformin [3, 12]. This has been demonstrated following an intravenous bolus dose [17]; no significant changes in fasting blood glucose, C-peptide, insulin, glucagon or growth hormone were noticed up to 30 minutes after injection. Neither are there any acute metabolic effects of metformin after intravenous infusion in diabetic subjects [116]. Chronic therapy with metformin reduces elevated fasting blood glucose concentrations in NIDDM patients, sometimes to normal values, but never to hypoglycaemic levels [3, 10, 14, 16–26]. Concurrently, intravenous glucose tolerance is improved [12, 25, 26]. Metformin also improves oral glucose tolerance in diabetics [3, 16, 18, 22, 23, 26, 115]. Three months of metformin treatment [26] improved both oral and intravenous glucose tolerance in NIDDM subjects, while having no effect in an obese non-diabetic control group. Metformin also improves daytime plasma glucose levels [10, 14, 21].

Insulin Levels

Several early studies on plasma insulin concentrations after glucose stimulation have shown that metformin can reduce hyperinsulinaemia both in obese non-diabetics [3, 10, 26] and diabetics [26], but this has not been confirmed in a study of borderline diabetic males [27] and in some other studies in diabetics [16, 18, 22, 23]. In studies where only the fasting plasma insulin concentration was measured, unchanged [24, 28, 29] or reduced [20, 30–32] levels after metformin treatment were found. Both fasting and postprandial insulin and C-peptide levels were unchanged by metformin in a further study [14]. Compared with gliclazide [33, 117] and other sulphonylureas [10], metformin treatment has been associated with lower insulin levels. Fasting insulin was unchanged both by metformin and tolbutamide in another comparative study [34]. Meal-stimulated insulin and C-peptide increased after 6 months of glibenclamide treatment but were unchanged after metformin in a recent double-blind, comparative study [115]. Metformin lowered daytime plasma insulin in NIDDM patients in some new studies, both as monotherapy [21, 118, 119] and in combination with sulphonylurea [120, 153]. Concomitantly, glucose and free fatty acid levels decreased. Thus, metformin never increases insulin levels, but on the contrary may reduce hyperinsulinaemia (see Tables 1 and 2).

Insulin Secretion

It is well established that biguanides do not stimulate insulin secretion [1, 3, 12]. Basal and stimulated C-peptide levels are unchanged [14, 16, 18, 28, 115, 121–124, 152], and intravenous metformin does not affect the levels of C-peptide, insulin or other hormones [17, 116]. The glucagon-induced rise in insulin and C-peptide was reduced by metformin in diabetic patients [35]. The glucagon-provoked hyperglycaemia was not significantly lowered, but fasting blood glucose was reduced, while the C-peptide/insulin ratio was unchanged. These effects were considered to be a consequence of improved glucose utilization. Other data [36] indicate that B-cell function in NIDDM improves secondarily when fasting blood glucose is reduced, whether by metformin or other measures. Both B-cell function and insulin action were improved by

metformin in a recent placebo-controlled study [125]. The metabolic clearance rate of glucose correlated with the change in fasting plasma glucose.

Insulin Action and Peripheral Glucose Utilization

While insulin secretion can be secondarily improved [36, 125], the main effect of metformin is exerted on insulin action as described in the section 'Mode of action'. Insulin requirements in IDDM are reduced when metformin is added [37, 38], and the same has been found in a study where obese diabetics were treated with insulin infusion [39] and in a controlled study in NIDDM patients [144]. Three days' treatment with phenformin, buformin or metformin increased insulin sensitivity (K_{IRR}) in those NIDDM patients who were classified as biguanide responders on the basis of their long-term blood glucose response to biguanide therapy [40].

Studies on insulin receptor binding and on insulin-stimulated metabolic processes using human cell systems are summarized in Table 1. The table also includes some animal experiments. The first study which was performed on erythrocytes from non-diabetic subjects [28], showed that metformin could increase the low affinity, high capacity receptors. This could be interpreted as unmasking of receptors already present [12] rather than synthesis *de novo*. These results have been confirmed on cultured cells [29], and in further studies with erythrocytes [22, 24] and monocytes [23, 29]. The effects depended upon the metabolic status of the subject [23, 24, 29]. No effect of metformin was seen on circulating cells in some other studies [18–20]. Studies on adipocytes have generally failed to confirm an increased receptor binding of insulin by metformin [41–43]. However, metformin increased adipocyte receptor binding, when insulin receptors were down-regulated [44]. Metformin is able to increase insulin receptor binding in mouse hepatocytes, depending on the metabolic state of the animal [45]. Increased binding to mouse soleus muscle has also been demonstrated [46], but in a study *in vivo* [47] there was no effect of metformin on insulin binding in muscle tissue from diabetic rats, whereas a slight effect was seen with liver receptors.

Only few studies have evaluated insulin receptors and insulin-mediated metabolic pathways simultaneously. In adipocytes from non-diabetic humans, metformin *in vitro* stimulated glucose conversion to both triglycerides and CO_2 without an effect on receptors [43], whereas no such metabolic effects were found in another study [41] using adipocytes both from non-diabetics (*in vitro*) and obese diabetics (*in vivo*). In rat adipocytes, metformin increased hexose transport

Table 1 Pharmacodynamic studies with metformin on insulin receptor binding and insulin-stimulated metabolic processes in human cell systems and some animal experiments. *In vitro* studies (above broken line) were performed by incubation and *in vivo* studies (below broken line) after treatment. Design and treatment time is given and number of patients/subjects (*n*) and type (e.g. normal, diabetic, etc.). Some clinical effects are included from *in vivo* studies (glycaemia, insulin levels etc). The studies are listed in chronological order. Abbreviations: d, days; w, weeks; mo, months; eryt., erythrocytes; mono., monocytes; hepat., hepatocytes; adip., adipocytes; cult., cultured; N, normal; O, obese; D, diabetic; ODM, NIDDM-obese; IDM, IDDM; DM, NIDDM; DB, double-blind; XO, crossover; rand., randomized; PLAC, placebo; FBG, fasting blood glucose; FPG, fasting plasma glucose; ppBG, postprandial glucose; INS, insulin; CP, C-peptide; TG, triglycerides; CH, total cholesterol; BW, body weight; LACT, lactate; rec., insulin receptors

Authors, year [ref. no.]	Methods *in vitro* / *in vivo*	*n* type	Results rec.	Results other	
Holle et al, 1981 [28]	eryt.	6 N	↑		
	open 2d	4 N	↑	FBG, INS, CP	0
Lord et al, 1983 [22]	eryt. open 4 w	8 ODM	↑	FBG, ppBG, HbA₁ BW, INS	↓ 0
Prager & Schernthaner, 1983 [18]	mono. DBXO PLAC 2/2 w	10 DM	0	FBG gluc. tolerance BW, INS, CP	↓ ↑ 0
Lord et al, 1983 [45]	hepat.	mice N mice D (ob/STZ)	↑ ↑/0	hypoglyc. response to ins.	0/↑
Vigneri et al, 1984 [29]*	cult. cells mono. open 4 d	human 6 N 8 O 6 DM	↑ 0 ↑ ↑↑		
Cigolini et al, 1984 [43]	adip.	16 N	0	FBG ↓ INS, LACT 0 gluc. oxidation lipogenesis antilipolysis	↑ ↑ 0
Cigolini et al, 1986 [44]	adip.	20 N	↑	(in downreg. cells)	
Rizkalla et al, 1986 [24]	eryt. DBXO PLAC rand. 2/2 w	5 N 5 O 6 ODM 5 IDM	↑ ↑ ↑↑ 0	FBG ↓ INS 0	
Prager et al, 1986 [19]	mono. open 4 w clamp	12 DM	0	gluc. utilization FPG, HbA₁c BW	↑ ↓ 0
Fantus & Brosseau, 1986 [23]	adip. mono. open 1 w	rats N 18 DM	↑ (↑)	gluc. oxidation gluc. tolerance FPG ↓ INS 0	↑ ↑
Jacobs et al, 1986 [42]	adip.	rats N	0	rec. tyrosine kinase hexose transport	0 ↑

continued overleaf

Table 1 (*continued*)

Authors, year [ref. no.]	Methods *in vitro* — — — — — — *in vivo*	*n* type	Results rec.	Results other	
Bailey & Puah, 1986 [46]	— — — — — — soleus muscle	diab. mice	(↑)	gluc. uptake and oxid. glycogen synthesis hexokinase activity lactate formation	↑ ↑ ↑ 0
Nosadini et al, 1987 [20]	eryt. mono. open 4 w clamp	7 DM 5 O (contr.)	0	gluc. disposal hep. gluc. output FPG, fast. INS BW	↑ (↓) ↓ 0
Pedersen et al, 1989 [41]	adip. — — — — — — adip. DBXO PLAC 4/4 w clamp	4 N — — — — — — 10 ODM	0 — — — 0	gluc. transp. and metabol. - - - - - - - - - - - - - - - - - - periph. gluc. uptake hep. gluc. output FPG, PG day profile lactate INS, CP	0 - - - ↑ 0 ↓ (↑) 0
Wu et al, 1990 [21]	— — — — — — mono. open 3 mo clamp	12 DM	(↑)	internalization glucose uptake hep. gluc. prod. FPG, PG day profile INS, TG, CH, FFA LDL 0 HDL ↑ VLDL ↓	0 0 0 ↓ ↓
Rossetti et al, 1990 [47]	hepat. muscle — — — — — — 6 w clamp	rats — — — — — — rats (diab.) (norm.)	(↑) 0 — — —	rec. tyrosine kinase - - - - - - - - - - - - - - - - - - gluc. disposal glycogen synthesis hep. gluc. prod. insulin secretion	↑ - - - ↑ ↑ 0 0

*Also published elsewhere: R. Vigneri et al, J Clin Endocrinol Metab 1982; 54: 95–100; V. Pezzino et al, Diabetologia 1982; 23: 131–5; V. Trischitta et al, J Clin Endocrinol Metab 1983; 57: 713–18.

but did not affect insulin binding or insulin receptor tyrosine kinase [42]. In mouse soleus muscle, glucose uptake and oxidation, glycogen formation and hexokinase activity were increased after metformin treatment [46]. The increased receptor binding was considered doubtful for the various metabolic effects demonstrated. In contrast to the observation in adipocytes from normal rats [42], muscle insulin receptor tyrosine kinase activity increased (to supranormal levels) after 6 weeks of metformin treatment of diabetic rats [47]. This was correlated with an increase in glucose disposal and muscle glycogen synthesis. Although one of these studies [41] did not demonstrate any effect of the drug on insulin-stimulated metabolic processes in adipocytes, other results of the study [14] showed a peripheral effect pointing at skeletal muscle as the prime target for the antihyperglycaemic action of metformin. The other four studies [42, 43, 46, 47] all indicate an effect of metformin on postreceptor sites, as

suggested by others [18–20]. This might be the basis for the improved insulin action, whereas insulin receptor binding might be affected secondarily [23, 29].

In accordance with an effect of metformin on postreceptor sites, studies with the euglycaemic–hyperinsulinaemic clamp technique have confirmed that metformin increases insulin-stimulated peripheral glucose disposal [165] in both NIDDM [14, 19, 20, 48, 119–121, 124, 154, 155] and IDDM subjects [38], and in diabetic rats [47]. Glucose utilization was improved by 20–30% at submaximal and maximal insulin concentrations and was correlated with improved metabolic control [19]. This shows that metformin is able to reduce insulin resistance in NIDDM. This has also been shown by clamp technique in non-diabetic subjects [70, 123, 126]. The improved insulin action was correlated to weight loss in one of these studies [123] and to reduced fasting insulin concentration in another investigation [70]. In a further study in diabetic patients

[119] only the obese group showed improved glucose utilization by euglycaemic clamp. In a clamp study of the acute effect of metformin [152] glucose uptake did not increase, but glucose oxidation increased slightly as mentioned below. The clamp studies mentioned above indicate an effect on insulin-stimulated glucose disposal, but this could not be confirmed in two other clamp studies [21, 118], where glycaemia improved after 3 months of metformin treatment in the absence of any change in insulin action. This suggests a non-insulin mediated mechanism of the drug. A direct effect of biguanides on glucose utilization has been demonstrated *in vitro* [15], and an insulin independent effect of metformin on glucose transporters has been proposed, based on experiments with human muscle cells in culture [11, 156]. Another possibility of affecting glucose utilization independently of insulin is through an influence on free fatty acids (FFA).

Inhibition of FFA oxidation has been suggested as an explanation for biguanide actions [10] (see also the section on lipid metabolism, below). Such an effect is in accordance with the findings of reduced plasma FFA levels in the above studies [21, 118] and in other recent investigations [152–154]. An accentuated FFA suppression during insulin clamp was found in patients treated with a combination of glibenclamide and metformin [48]. In this study, basal lipid oxidation was reduced and insulin-stimulated glucose disposal increased (by 32%), mainly as enhanced non-oxidative glucose metabolism. Insulin and C-peptide levels remained unaffected. Evidence that biguanides act on non-oxidative pathways of glucose metabolism also comes from animal studies showing increased glycogen synthesis [11, 46, 47]. The action of the drug on non-oxidative glucose metabolism has been confirmed in NIDDM patients [124] and their relatives [126]. Increased glucose oxidation after metformin has been found in animal studies [23, 46], human adipose tissue [43] and in non-diabetic, obese women [70]. This clinical finding was not confirmed in another study in diabetics [124]. A study of the acute effect of orally administered metformin in NIDDM [152] showed enhanced glucose oxidation, but no effect on the non-oxidative pathway.

It appears that the action of metformin and other biguanides cannot be regarded merely as a consequence of an effect on glucose uptake [11]. The effect on glucose utilization varies in different tissues depending on several factors, e.g. the propensities for aerobic and anaerobic glucose metabolism, insulin dependency and intracellular drug concentrations [49]. Species differences and pathophysiological changes are also important. The action must be viewed as multifactorial [1, 3–5] (see also the three sections following). In any case, an effect on muscular glucose uptake

and metabolism [14, 46, 47] seems more important than a similar effect in adipose tissue [41, 43], and is in accordance with earlier theories [1, 3, 10, 13] and new evidence [11]. Metformin has been shown to increase glucose uptake *in vitro* in human skeletal muscle [50], but only when glucose metabolism was inhibited and insulin was available. An effect on insulin-resistant human skeletal muscle *in vitro* has been demonstrated by using muscle strip preparations and relatively high (0.1 mmol/l) metformin concentrations in the incubation medium [127]. This finding was not confirmed at therapeutic (0.01 mmol/l) metformin concentrations [128]. The results of these two studies, investigating insulin-stimulated 3-0-methylglucose transport, suggested an effect of the drug due either to accumulation in the extracellular space of muscle tissue, or an effect distal to the glucose transport step. An effect on glycogen synthesis has been suggested from experiments with erythrocytes from NIDDM patients [129], but muscle glycogen synthase was unchanged in another study [124]. An effect of metformin has been demonstrated on glucose transporters [11, 130, 131] and on glucose transporter gene expression [132].

Hepatic Glucose Production

In clamp studies including measurement of hepatic glucose production (HGP) conflicting results have been obtained after chronic metformin treatment. Suppression of HGP was seen in some studies [20, 119, 120, 124], but not in others [14, 21, 48, 118, 121, 126]. In two studies [119, 124] the reduction of HGP was correlated to the decrease in fasting glucose concentration. One study [122] showed a fall in HGP only at high initial fasting plasma glucose, and no effect on glucose utilization. On the other hand, an increased hepatic insulin sensitivity with reduced basal hepatic glucose output was found in a placebo-controlled study on 10 non-obese NIDDM patients after treatment with metformin (added to glibenclamide) for several months [16]. However, the overall suppression of hepatic glucose output after glucose loading was similar with metformin and placebo. Forearm glucose uptake was reduced in the basal state and was unaffected after glucose loading. Peripheral insulin sensitivity and disappearance of radiolabelled glucose was also unaffected, as was the B-cell response to glucose. This study implicates the liver as the primary site of metformin action in the basal state, but does not preclude a peripheral action of the drug. Whereas interpretation of these results could be difficult, a hepatic effect of metformin is supported by animal experiments. A primary hepatic antihyperglycaemic action of the drug has been proposed again recently [152, 167]. Acute oral administration of metformin suppressed HGP compared to placebo [152]. The influence of long-term unspecific effects of removal of glucotoxicity was eliminated in this study, which also showed a suppression of FFA levels and lipid oxidation correlating with the effect on HGP.

Suppression of hepatic glucose output can be caused by inhibition of gluconeogenesis. Metformin and other biguanides inhibit this process in animals [1, 3–5, 12, 13] and in humans when this process is accelerated [10]. Studies on 12-hour plasma concentrations of gluconeogenic precursors (lactate, pyruvate, alanine) in NIDDM [51, 52] have shown slight elevations during exposure to phenformin and metformin as compared with glibenclamide. This indicates inhibition of gluconeogenesis, but that has not been confirmed in another study [53]. A further study of metformin-treated diabetics showed higher levels of alanine than in a diet-treated group, and elevations of both alanine and other gluconeogenic amino acids when compared with non-diabetic controls [54]. Alanine increased slightly after metformin in the acute study described above [152]. One theory is that metformin acts synergistically with physiological concentrations of insulin to suppress hepatic gluconeogenesis [4, 5, 113]. However, in an investigation of diabetic rats using the clamp technique, no effect of metformin on hepatic glucose production and its suppression by insulin could be demonstrated [47]. In a recent chronic study [167] metformin decreased gluconeogenesis from lactate by 37% in obese NIDDM patients without affecting systemic glucose clearance. Metformin may also influence the effect of glucagon, and a yet unpublished study has indicated inhibition of glycogenolysis following 3 months of treatment (R DeFronzo, personal communication). It should be noted that the liver is not necessary for the antihyperglycaemic effect of biguanides [12].

Lactate Metabolism

The relationship between biguanides and lactate metabolism is the basis of a potential adverse effect [13]. Comparative studies show higher lactate levels after phenformin than after metformin [3, 10, 51, 55, 133]. Commonly, blood lactate concentrations are within the normal range during metformin therapy [3, 53, 119, 124]. In a crossover study on 6 NIDDM patients [51], phenformin was followed by metformin and then by glibenclamide in 1-month periods. Fasting blood lactate and pyruvate did not differ, but the mean 12-hour concentrations were slightly elevated by both biguanides. However, the value during metformin therapy (1.2 mmol/l) was still within the normal range. Similarly, lactate and pyruvate levels were slightly raised during combined metformin–sulphonylurea

therapy compared with sulphonylurea alone [52]. In a group of unselected NIDDM patients, fasting blood lactate concentrations were slightly higher when biguanides were added to sulphonylurea [56], but again the median value for metformin (1.4 mmol/l) was within the normal range. The mean daytime plasma lactate concentration increased slightly after 4 weeks of metformin treatment in a placebo-controlled study [14], but fasting lactate was unchanged. Lactate levels were higher during therapy with metformin than with gliclazide in a crossover study [33], whereas no differences were found between metformin and tolbutamide in another study [34]. In a comparative study with glibenclamide [114, 115] there was a slight increase in meal-stimulated lactate after metformin, but there was no difference between the two drugs and there were no changes in fasting lactate concentrations. Lactate increased after metformin at the high-dose insulin step during the clamp in the acute study [152], whereas plasma pyruvate was unchanged.

In various tolerance tests with induced hyperlactataemia, minor changes in lactate levels after metformin have often been recorded [3, 10]. Such studies have been performed during muscular exercise or loading with glucose, fructose, lactate, pyruvate, ethanol or glucocorticoids [3, 10, 13, 55]. Biguanides, especially phenformin, may decrease the elimination of lactate accumulated under such experimental conditions. Metformin can enhance the rise in lactate levels after glucose ingestion and increase peripheral lactate uptake [16]. This indicates an increased splanchnic lactate output, probably from increased splanchnic glucose uptake and subsequent metabolism to lactate and glycogen. This might reflect a partial normalization of impaired hepatic glucose utilization in NIDDM [16]. An increased glucose utilization in the digestive tract after metformin treatment has been demonstrated in obese rats [57], and it has been suggested that increased lactate production by the jejunum makes an important contribution to postprandial hyperlactataemia during metformin treatment [5, 49, 113].

Studies on lactate turnover and glucose–lactate interconversion by isotope technique have shown that phenformin increases these processes in non-diabetics [13], i.e. it accelerates recycling in the Cori cycle. An increased recycling (enhanced glucose utilization and production) was also demonstrated after metformin in the above study [57]. Diabetic subjects are probably more or less unable to effect this counter-regulation, and thus gluconeogenesis from lactate can be reduced as confirmed recently [167]. In this study metformin increased lactate oxidation (by 25%), while plasma lactate concentration and turnover and muscle lactate release remained unchanged.

Lipid Metabolism

It is often noticed that patients lose weight and that elevated serum lipid concentrations are reduced during biguanide therapy [1, 3, 58]. Moreover, extensive animal experiments indicate an antiatherogenic effect of metformin [1, 3, 12, 58]. Studies in patients with type IV hyperlipoproteinaemia demonstrate a considerable decrease in triglyceride levels after metformin therapy [3, 26, 58, 59]. The reduction in cholesterol is more modest; this indicates a preferential decrease in very low-density lipoprotein (VLDL) levels [59]. About two-thirds of the subjects with type IV and type IIB hyperlipoproteinaemia showed a triglyceride decrease of more than 30% and could be characterized as 'responders' [58]. The effect was independent of any antihyperglycaemic effect [58], in accordance with other findings [3, 26]. A direct effect on VLDL metabolism has been proposed [58], and the hypotriglyceridaemic effect of metformin has been associated with a decrease in plasma VLDL concentrations [21, 60, 118, 120, 153] and compositional changes in lipoprotein particles [134].

The triglyceride-lowering effect of metformin was confirmed in obese, non-diabetic females in a short-term study [32], where the effect was related to reduced insulin levels. In NIDDM patients the effect has been demonstrated repeatedly [21, 26, 60–63, 118, 125, 153–155]. In one of these studies [60] the effect was observed only in a subgroup with serum cholesterol concentrations above 6.5 mmol/l (250 mg/dl) and in another study [62] only in the more obese patients. In a 12-month prospective study [61] the patients were newly detected diabetics treated primarily with diet alone, followed by glibenclamide or metformin if necessary. Metformin had a more favourable effect on serum triglycerides than had glibenclamide, and decreased triglycerides more in males than in females. Apolipoprotein B was reduced by metformin in males. Total cholesterol also decreased in males, whereas high-density lipoprotein (HDL) cholesterol was unaffected. Finally, metformin increased apolipoprotein A1 in females.

In a double-blind crossover study on male patients with peripheral vascular disease and varying degrees of glucose intolerance and hyperlipoproteinaemia, metformin increased apolipoprotein A1 and caused a highly significant increase of HDL-cholesterol [58]. In a crossover study [62] neither metformin nor glibenclamide affected HDL-cholesterol and its subfractions, but total cholesterol and LDL-cholesterol were significantly reduced by metformin. The reduction of LDL-cholesterol has been confirmed in recent investigations [115, 119, 125, 135] and seems to be maintained with long-term therapy [64]. LDL-cholesterol was unaffected by metformin in some other studies [21,

111, 118, 120] where HDL-cholesterol was increased. Total cholesterol has been unchanged [32, 53, 60, 111, 115, 155] or reduced [21, 26, 61–63, 118, 125, 135] Metformin and gliclazide reduced triglycerides and cholesterol equally in a randomized study [65], whereas neither metformin nor tolbutamide affected these lipids in another comparative study [34]. There were no intra- or inter-group differences in triglycerides and total cholesterol in another comparative study of metformin and gliclazide [117]. Unchanged triglycerides has also been reported by others [53, 111, 117] and both triglycerides and cholesterol remained constant after a combination of metformin and sulphonylureas [48, 66]. In another study on oral combination therapy [120], metformin + glipizide improved triglycerides, cholesterol and several lipoprotein fractions. This was confirmed in a further study from the same group [153], where the effect of metformin on postprandial lipidaemia was highlighted. By measuring retinyl ester concentrations it was found that the levels of triglyceride-rich lipoproteins of intestinal origin were lowered when metformin was added to sulphonylurea-treated NIDDM patients with less than optimal glycaemic control. The findings in comparative clinical studies are summarized in Table 2.

The mechanism by which metformin influences lipid metabolism is not clear. Aortic lesions induced by cholesterol-rich diet in rabbits are reduced independently of the cholesterol lowering effect [3, 12]. In this model the aortic uptake of VLDL was reduced and the turnover of VLDL accelerated [58]. A direct effect on lipid biosynthesis in the liver and intestine has also been postulated [12] and hepatic steatosis may be prevented [12]. Lipoproteins of lower atherogenicity may be formed by an effect on VLDL metabolism. The effect of metformin on lipid metabolism and lipoproteins varies under different circumstances, but is a potential clinical advantage and needs to be elucidated further.

There are only few studies on the effect of biguanides on lipolysis. The concentrations of free fatty acids (FFA) and glycerol have been determined in plasma during metformin treatment, but the results have been inconclusive [3, 10, 16, 30, 31, 51–53]. In an early study with infusion of [^{14}C]palmitate in NIDDM patients [30, 31], metformin reduced the concentration, turnover and oxidation of FFA, and this was correlated to an increased glucose disappearance rate and a reduction of basal insulin levels. The inhibitory effect on FFA oxidation has been confirmed in a recent study [154] and has been regarded as a central effect in biguanide action [10, 152] because of the interrelations between FFA and glucose metabolism. A proposed antilipolytic action of metformin [3] could be secondary to an effect on FFA oxidation [10] but has

Table 2 Clinical efficacy studies with metformin. The table contains three classical studies from Edinburgh [87] and other studies using comparative agents. The table is not a complete list of all controlled clinical studies with metformin. Studies with placebo are not included. Some are referred to in Table 1 [18, 24, 41] and others only in the reference list [16, 27, 32, 90, 125, 140, 144]. Number and type of patients are given, as well as design and treatment time and group (comparative drug). The results are expressed in terms of changes in glycaemia, body weight, insulin levels, lipids, etc. Blood glucose concentrations are given as mean values (mmol/l). Early clinical trials are cited in a previous review article [3] and studies with biguanides in combination with sulphonylureas have been reviewed separately [89, 114]. The studies are listed in chronological order. Ref. 87 is based on the following original references: Clarke BF, Duncan LJP, Lancet 1965; i: 1248–51; Clarke BF et al. In Butterfield WJH & Westering W (eds) Tolbutamide—after ten years. New York: Excerpta Medica, 1967; Clarke BF, Duncan LJP, Lancet 1968, i: 123–6; Clarke BF, Campbell, IW, Br Med J 1977: 2: 1576–8. Abbreviations: MET, metformin; CHLO, chlorpropamide; GLIB, glibenclamide; GLIC, gliclazide; SU, sulphonylurea; INS, insulin; mo, months; yr, year(s); incl., included; compl., completed; fail., failure; XO, crossover; par., parallel groups; DB, double-blind; rand., randomized; BG, blood glucose concentration (mmol/l); FBG, fasting blood glucose; FPG, fasting plasma glucose; ppBG, postprandial blood glucose; BW, body weight; BMI, body mass index; INS, plasma insulin level; LACT, lactate; TG, triglycerides; CH, total cholesterol; VLDL, LDL, HDL, lipoproteins; apo-A1, apo-B, apolipoproteins; succ., success rate; sec. fail., secondary failure rate

Authors, year [ref. no.]	Patients incl./compl. (type)	Design, treatment time	Group (comparative drug)	Results: Glycaemia, body weight, lipids, other
Clarke et al, 1965/67 [87]	200/184 (non-ob., SU-fail.)	open, 3 yr	MET + CHLO	age (yr): 20–39, 40–59, 60–74; succ. %: 11.5, 47.3, 64.6; BW (kg): +1.4, +0.6, +0.3; sec. fail %: 42.3, 42.2, 24.5
Clarke & Duncan, 1968 [87]	139/124 (obese); 77 (obese)	open, par. 1 yr; open, XO 1/1 yr	MET; CHLO	ppBG ($n = 77$): 16.6 → 9.3, 16.7 → 9.5; succ. %: 94, 80.7; BW (kg): −1.2, +5.3; sec. fail %: 3, 14
Clarke & Campbell, 1977 [87]	216/189 (non-ob.); 58 (non-ob.)	open, par. 1 yr; open, XO 1/1 yr	MET; CHLO	ppBG ($n = 58$): 17.6 → 8.9, 17.4 → 8.5; succ. %: 82.7, 82.4; BW (kg): −1.5, +4.6; sec. fail %: 5.1, 7.7
Taylor et al, 1982 [61]	131/115 (newly diagn.)	open par. 1 yr	MET (obese); GLIB (non-ob.)	sex/n: M 10, F 13, M 24, F 7; FBG: 11.1 → 6.8, 12.5 → 6.3, 12.2 → 6.7, 13.4 → 6.4; BW: →, →, →, →; TG: →, →, 0, 0; CH: →, →, 0, 0; HDL: 0, 0, 0, 0; Apo-B: 0, →, 0, →; Apo-A1: 0, ←, 0, ←
UKPDS 1985 [9]	195 (newly diagn.)	open par. rand. 1 yr	MET (obese); DIET; SU; INS	n: 16, 57, 72, 50; FPG: 8.6 → 7.2**, 8.6 → 9.3ns, 8.3 → 6.7***, 8.6 → 6.8***; HbA$_{1c}$ (%): 8.8 → 8.0*, 8.8 → 9.1ns, 9.1 → 7.8***, 9.1 → 8.1***; Results after 9 years (1996) in ref. [163]
Rains et al, 1982 [62]	35/34 (new + diet treat.)	open XO rand. 3/3 mo	MET; GLIB	HbA$_1$: −1.53%, −2.05%; FBG: −3 mmol/l, −3 mmol/l (from Figure 1 in ref. [62]); BW: 0, ←; TG: 0, 0; CH: →, →; HDL: 0, 0; LDL: →, 0; HDL$_{2/3}$: 0, 0

Study	Patients	Design	Drugs	BG day profile / HbA1	FBG	BW	TG	INS	CH / HDL / LDL etc.	LACT / other
McAlpine et al, 1988 [33]	27/21 (on MET mean 3 yr, obese)	open, XO 3/3 mo (MET → GLIC)	MET / GLIC	M = G	FBG (↓) / ↓	↓ / ↑		INS G > M		LACT M > G
Collier et al, 1989 [65]	24 (newly diagn., non-ob.)	open par. rand. 6 mo	MET / GLIC	HbA₁ −4.7% / −4.7%	FPG 11.8 → 7.5 / 12.2 → 6.4	BMI 0 / ↑	TG ↓ / ↓	CH ↓ / ↓		Platelet var. towards norm. (no diff.)
Wilson et al, 1989 [66]	15/12 (non-ob, on max SU)	open XO rand. 2/2 mo	MET / GUAR	BG day profile ↓ / 0	FBG 12.9 → 11.6 / 12.9 → 13.7	BW 0 / 0	TG 0 / 0	CH 0 / 0 — HDL 0 / 0	LDL 0 / 0 — HbA₁ 0 / 0	
Lalor et al, 1990 [60]	26/19 (obese)	DBXO rand. 3/3 mo	MET / GUAR	VLDL ↓ / 0	FBG 11.4 → 8.6 / 11.4 → 9.5	BW 0 / 0	TG ↓ / 0	CH ↓ / 0 — LDL ↓ / 0	Apo-B 0 / 0 — HDL 0 / 0	
patients with CH > 6.5 mmol/l										
Josephkutty & Potter, 1988 [34]	21/20 (elderly, 65–95 yr)	DBXO rand. 3/3 mo	MET / TOLB	HbA₁ +0.6 % ns / −0.1%	FPG 8.0 → 9.1 ns / 8.3 → 8.3	BW −2.0 kg / +1.6 kg		LACT 1.33 → 1.77 ns / 1.49 → 1.46		TG, CH, INS no diff.
Hermann et al, 1991 [111]	25/22	open, XO rand. 6/6 mo	MET / GLIB	HbA₁ M = G	FBG M = G	BW M vs. G −2.6 kg		HDL M vs. G +0.14 mmol/l		TG, CH, LDL no diff.
Noury & Nandeuil 1991 [117]	60/57	open, par. rand. 3 mo	MET / GLIC	HbA₁ 9.8 → 8.5 / 9.7 → 9.0	FBG 9.7 → 8.3 / 9.8 → 8.1	BW ↓ / 0	TG 0 / 0	INS ↓ / (↑)	CH 0 / 0 — HDL ↓ / (↑)	
Chan et al, 1993 [135]	12	XO rand. 1/1 mo	MET / GLIB	HbA₁c M = G	FPG M = G	BMI ↓ / 0	TG 0 / 0	CH ↓ / 0 — LDL (↓) / 0	HDL 0 / 0	
Hermann et al, 1994 [112, 115]	45/33	DB, par. rand. 6 mo	MET / GLIB	HbA₁c 6.9 → 5.8 / 6.7 → 5.3	FBG 9.3 → 6.9 / 8.6 → 6.6	BW 0 / ↑	LDL ↓ / 0	INS 0 / 0	TG, CH, HDL, LACT, Apo-Al, Apo-B no diff.	

Not included in the table: Long-term results from UKPDS [163], US pivotal studies [164] and comparative studies with acarbose (e.g. Chiasson J L et al., Ann Intern Med 1994; 121: 928–35) and other new antidiabetic agents.

not been confirmed in studies on human adipocytes [41, 43]. Plasma glycerol concentration was unaffected by metformin in the recent acute study [152]. Results of studies on ketone bodies are also inconclusive [30, 31, 51–53, 152]. Recently, a possible effect of metformin on FFA has received increased attention after the demonstration of reduced daytime plasma FFA levels after 3 months of metformin treatment as monotherapy [21, 118], and in combination with sulphonylurea [120, 153]. These findings were accompanied by changes in insulin (see section on insulin levels) and lipids (see above). A somewhat similar finding was observed after combined oral treatment [48] with an influence of the drugs on FFA and lipid oxidation (see section on insulin action and peripheral glucose utilization).

Haemorheology, Haemostasis, and Blood Pressure

Disturbances in blood flow properties and haemostatic functions are often but not always corrected when metabolic control is improved in diabetics. Early studies on fibrinolysis showed inconsistent effects of metformin [3], but an increased fibrinolytic activity has been demonstrated in a randomized, double-blind, placebo-controlled study on 18 obese, non-diabetic females compared with age-matched, non-obese controls [32]. Metformin significantly decreased plasminogen activator inhibition (PAI-1) and increased euglobulin fibrinolytic activity. This was correlated with decreased plasma levels of insulin and triglycerides. Reduced PAI-1 after metformin treatment has also been demonstrated in patients with NIDDM in a recent double-blind, placebo-controlled study [125]. In non-diabetic, hypertensive men fibrinolytic activity (t-PA antigen) was increased by metformin compared to placebo and metoprolol [137, 157]. Low plasma fibrinogen concentrations have been found in biguanide-treated patients compared with other treatment groups [67]. No correlation has been observed between fibrinogen and blood glucose. Fibrinogen was not affected by metformin and gliclazide in a randomized study [65] or by metformin in the above study [125]. Several platelet variables returned towards normal when glycaemic control was improved with metformin and gliclazide [65]. Otherwise, the effect of metformin on platelet aggregation has been only sporadically investigated; an antiplatelet action has been proposed [68] but has not been proved [125].

Improvements in certain cardiovascular parameters have been noticed during long-term therapy [3], and in a controlled study metformin increased arterial blood flow in male patients with peripheral arterial disease [58]. Metformin may also improve red cell flow [136].

The clinical relevance of these potentially beneficial effects remains to be clarified. Blood pressure and heart rate were not affected by metformin in a study on diabetics [53], but systolic and diastolic blood pressure decreased in a pilot study on insulin-resistant non-diabetic, non-obese hypertensive men [69]. However, this finding could not be reproduced in a controlled study by the same authors [137]. The subjects in this study were not insulin-resistant, and glucose disposal was unchanged after metformin. On the other hand, blood pressure did decrease after metformin in an uncontrolled study in diabetic patients [63] and in a recent randomized, placebo-controlled, crossover study in non-diabetic, hypertensive, obese women [70]. This latter study also showed an improvement of the insulin resistance in these patients and improvements in lipids. After 3 months of metformin treatment there was a decrease in fasting insulin, fibrinogen, plasma norepinephrine and even in left ventricular mass. In the above study [137] in non-obese hypertensive men, catecholamines and other hormones were unchanged after metformin [157]. Metformin reduced insulin resistance, hyperandrogenaemia and systolic blood pressure in a recent uncontrolled study in patients with polycystic ovary syndrome [158]. Diastolic blood pressure was decreased by metformin in a comparative study with glibenclamide [135], showing a difference between the drugs in systemic vascular resistance, which was increased slightly by glibenclamide but was unchanged after metformin. The impression from these studies is that metformin may have a blood pressure lowering effect in patients with insulin resistance, whether diabetic or not. On the other hand, phenformin therapy was associated with an increase in blood pressure and heart rate in the University Group Diabetes Program (UGDP) study [13]. Metformin may have a positive effect in controlling microalbuminuria [70, 71, 125].

Gastrointestinal Function

Inhibition of intestinal glucose absorption by biguanides has been demonstrated in animals [3, 12, 72], but in humans only by phenformin [1, 13, 72]. Inhibition of glucose absorption by metformin has been observed in non-diabetic human subjects after a single dose [73]. The clinical relevance of this study is doubtful, and the findings have not been confirmed. In a study with radiolabelled glucose [16] the systemic appearance of ingested glucose was unaffected by metformin in diabetics, indicating no effect of the drug on glucose absorption. Whereas increased intestinal glucose utilization in response to metformin has been proposed as a source of lactate formation [16, 57, 113], an intestinal effect seems insignificant for the antihyperglycaemic action of metformin in NIDDM patients.

Biguanides inhibit absorption of various actively transported substances, such as hexoses, amino acids, calcium and bile acids [72]. This effect has been attributed to an interaction with transport systems in the intestinal brush border [72]. Enzyme activities in intestinal epithelium might be affected [3, 72]. Intestinal effects of biguanides might also affect the levels of cholesterol and apoproteins.

The effect of metformin on vitamin B_{12} absorption has been demonstrated using conventional Schilling tests, but was not confirmed by a whole-body technique [3]. Vitamin B_{12} malabsorption was found in 30% of diabetic patients during long-term metformin treatment [74]. Although it was reversible in this study, it may be persistent [75]. Megaloblastic anaemia due to malabsorption associated with long-term metformin treatment has been reported [76]; B_{12} treatment was successful in this and a similar Danish case. The mechanism of biguanide-induced B_{12} malabsorption remains uncertain, but it may be attributed to direct intestinal effects or bacterial overgrowth with binding of the intrinsic factor–B_{12} complex [72, 75]. Results of studies with metformin and D-xylose absorption are inconsistent [25, 74]. Serum folic acid concentration might also be affected by metformin [3].

Biguanides can inhibit gastric emptying and delay small intestine motility in animals [72]. Metformin reduced gastric emptying in patients with partial gastrectomy [3, 72], but not in normal individuals [3, 72, 77]. Metformin has been found to relieve the dumping syndrome and symptoms of reactive hypoglycaemia [3, 72]. Gastric acid secretion and gastrointestinal hormone levels have been measured after metformin treatment for 2 weeks in healthy non-diabetic subjects [78]. Maximal and peak acid output were increased. Vasoactive intestinal peptide (VIP) and glucagon-like immunoreactivity were also increased, whereas insulin, gastric inhibitory polypeptide (GIP) and secretin levels were unchanged. The main conclusion from this study is that metformin can act as a weak histamine (H_2) agonist. However, this could not be confirmed in another study [75]. In a further study [77] metformin did not modify salivary and gastric secretions but induced a duodenogastric reflux in healthy volunteers. Effects on gastric secretion and motility might explain the gastrointestinal side-effects, including anorexia.

PHARMACOKINETICS

Differences in the chemical structure of biguanides lead to important differences in their pharmacokinetic properties. For example, the monosubstituted and more long-chained, lipophilic phenformin is metabolized by aromatic hydroxylation in the liver and can accumulate in subjects with a low hydroxylation capacity (see section on lactic acidosis). The bisubstituted and more short-chained, hydrophilic metformin escapes metabolism almost entirely, and is eliminated by renal excretion; hence, it accumulates only in subjects with renal impairment.

Biguanides can be determined in biological fluids by various methods. Early assays were based on colorimetry and had a low specificity and sensitivity. Modern techniques include liquid chromatography [54, 79, 80], gas–liquid chromatography [81–83] and mass fragmentography [84]. Liquid scintillation counting has been used for the analysis of ^{14}C-labelled metformin [85]. Radioimmunoassay has been used to measure phenformin and its metabolite.

Absorption

Metformin is incompletely absorbed [77, 81, 82], the faecal recovery being about 20–30% of an oral dose [77, 82]. The absorption is slower than the elimination [83, 85], and the elimination half-life reported after oral administration is more likely to reflect (slow) absorption than true elimination [81, 85]. Peak plasma concentrations of about 2 µg/ml are reached after 2 hours [81, 82, 85] or later [83]. The absorption is completed within 6 hours [82] and is presumably confined to the upper part of the intestine [82]. However, the results of another investigation [77] suggest that the whole intestine is necessary for sufficient absorption of the drug. Metformin is poorly absorbed from the stomach [77]. The absorption seems to be reduced in patients with renal failure [82]. Guar gum decreases the absorption of metformin in healthy subjects [86]. Food may slightly decrease the extent and slow the rate of absorption [168].

The oral bioavailability of usual doses is 50–60% [77, 82–85]. Higher doses are proportionally less available [82, 83]. This has tentatively been explained by an active, saturable absorption process [83]. The difference between absorbed and available drug might reflect minor presystemic clearance [82] or binding to the intestinal wall [84]. The slow and incomplete absorption in combination with a rapid elimination makes the rationale for sustained-release preparations less obvious. The bioavailability is also impaired with such formulations [81, 83], and they have not been shown to have fewer side-effects.

Distribution

The distribution of metformin is rapid [82], but a slow transfer to a deep compartment seems to occur [83].

The mean apparent volume of distribution ranges from 63 to 276 litres [82–85]. Metformin accumulates in the alimentary tract (especially in tissues of the small intestine), salivary glands and kidneys [1, 5] and is also present in the liver [16]. There is no binding to plasma proteins [82, 84, 85], but a slowly increasing binding to blood cells [82]. The concentration in saliva is lower than that in plasma.

Elimination

The mean plasma elimination half-life of metformin ranges from 1.5 hours to 4.5 hours [1, 81–85] and is shorter after intravenous than after oral administration [82, 85]. It is prolonged in patients with renal impairment and is correlated with creatinine clearance [84]. Urinary excretion data have disclosed a quantitatively minor terminal elimination phase with a longer mean half-life, ranging from 8.9 hours to 19 hours [81–83, 85]. This suggests a small deep compartment with a slow elimination which might contribute to prolonged action of metformin under certain circumstances.

Metformin is rapidly eliminated by renal excretion [81–85]. Although it was completely excreted unchanged in one study [85], only 80% of an intravenous dose was recovered as unchanged drug in the urine in two other studies [82, 84]. Mean values for renal clearance were 544 ml/min [82], 335 ml/min [84] and 454 ml/min [85], and for total clearance were 706 ml/min [82], 441 ml/min [84] and 459 ml/min [85]. This indicates active tubular secretion of metformin. Renal clearance of metformin is correlated with creatinine clearance [82, 84], but total clearance is a more appropriate (inverse) predictor of accumulation [82]. After intravenous administration, most of the drug is excreted within 8 hours [82]. After oral administration of 0.5 g metformin, 50% was recovered in urine and 27% in faeces [82]. No metformin seems to be exhaled by the lungs [85]. There are no data on breast milk levels of metformin in humans.

Metabolism

Metformin is excreted unmetabolized in laboratory animals [1]. This was also stated to be the case for humans, based on early studies [3] and a study with radiolabelled metformin [85]. However, the data from another study [84] showed incomplete recovery of metformin in the urine after intravenous administration, in accordance with a further study [82] in which 20% of the dose was not accounted for. Some metabolic transformation of metformin may therefore occur in humans, but neither conjugates nor other metabolites have been identified [82]. In contrast, phenformin is metabolized by all species including humans, in whom the

only metabolite is the inactive 4'-hydroxy-phenformin [1]. Hydroxylation follows the pattern of debrisoquine, which implies genetic polymorphism with a risk of impaired hydroxylative capacity in some individuals and accumulation of phenformin.

Dose–Response Relationship

Once absorbed, metformin displays log-linear pharmacokinetics [82], and a correlation between dose and plasma concentration in the therapeutic range has been demonstrated [83, 84, 138]. Absorption is dose-dependent [82, 83]. In a study in NIDDM patients on long-term therapy, metformin levels were inversely correlated with serum triglycerides and directly with HDL (and HDL_2) cholesterol, but not with fasting plasma glucose concentration, metformin dose and other parameters [79, 80]. No correlation was found between plasma amino acids and metformin dose or plasma concentration in another study from the same group [54]. A recent study by these authors [138] showed higher diurnal plasma metformin concentrations and lower diurnal glucose concentrations at high dose (1.7 g daily) compared with low dose (1.0 g daily). Mean blood lactate (but not alanine, glycerol and β-hydroxybutyrate) correlated with plasma metformin concentration. A dose–effect relationship has also been observed in three other studies [121, 139, 169]. In the study from our group [139] a dose–effect relationship over the whole dose range of metformin was observed, whereas maximum effect of glibenclamide was reached at low dose levels. Therapeutic levels may be 1–2 µg/ml (approximately 10 µmol/l) or even lower [79, 80], but level monitoring has little clinical value, except when lactic acidosis is suspected or present (below).

THERAPEUTIC USE

Results from Clinical Trials

The antihyperglycaemic effect of biguanides has been documented in a great number of therapeutic trials. Most of the early studies [3] were uncontrolled, and many are inadequate by modern standards. Patient selection has been questionable and confounding factors may have affected the results. Usually, metabolic control (i.e. blood and urine glucose) has been compared only before and after treatment, and few studies have used randomization, blinding and comparison with other therapies. However, many uncontrolled studies have given detailed descriptions of a large number of patients. During the last decade several new studies have been performed, using a more controlled design and including other measures of outcome than blood glucose (see Table 2).

The effect of metformin has been investigated both as monotherapy and in combination with sulphonylurea (mainly chlorpropamide or glibenclamide) or insulin [3–6, 113, 114]. The studies include both newly diagnosed and previously treated diabetics, almost exclusively NIDDM. Treatment periods have ranged from a few months to several years. On average, metformin has exerted an appropriate antihyperglycaemic effect in about 80% of the patients, the fasting blood glucose reduction being 1.4–3.9 mmol/l (25–70 mg/dl) in placebo-controlled studies [16, 18, 24, 41, 60, 115, 124, 125, 140]. Discontinuation of biguanide treatment leads to deterioration of metabolic control [10, 112, 115]. The effect of metformin on glycaemic control in NIDDM has appeared equivalent to that of sulphonylureas [3, 114], as demonstrated specifically with tolbutamide [3, 34, 36], chlorpropamide [87, 88], glibenclamide [61, 62, 111, 112, 115, 135] and gliclazide [33, 65, 117], and as confirmed in a recent meta-analysis [170]. Metformin has a better effect on glycaemic control than guar [60, 66]. Metformin has also been compared with glipizide [71], showing a better effect on glycaemia and weight [161]. Three major studies in Edinburgh have been reviewed [6, 87]. Data from these and some new studies are summarized in Table 2.

The long-term effects of metformin are currently being investigated in the UKPDS [9, 141]. Results after 1 year of treatment showed that 16 patients randomized to metformin had lower values of fasting blood glucose concentration and glycated haemoglobin than those treated with diet alone, but slightly higher values than patients treated with sulphonylurea [9]. Long-term results from this study are now available, showing that metformin is as effective as insulin and sulphonylureas at 3, 6 and 9 years [163].

The effect of biguanides and sulphonylureas as combination therapy in NIDDM has been reviewed recently [89, 114] and has been the subject of a recent double-blind, placebo-controlled 6-months study [115, 139]. In an open long-term study of metformin plus chlorpropamide in 200 non-obese sulphonylurea failures [87], 184 patients completed 3 years of treatment with a success rate of 50% (depending on age). In a randomized, double-blind, placebo-controlled crossover trial in 17 NIDDM patients inadequately controlled by diet and glibenclamide, addition of a low dose of metformin improved metabolic control considerably [90] without causing side-effects. In another study on newly diagnosed obese NIDDM patients [91], improved diurnal profiles of blood glucose were seen when metformin or phenformin was added to glibenclamide. A more favourable circadian variation of glucose, insulin and FFA has also been demonstrated after long-term metformin treatment compared with sulphonylurea [3]. In a randomized, double-blind study, long-term metformin treatment was compared with placebo, glibenclamide and the combination of metformin and glibenclamide in male patients with borderline impairment of glucose tolerance [27]. Metformin promoted weight loss but had no significant effect on fasting blood glucose and oral glucose tolerance, or on plasma insulin. In a randomized crossover study [92], glycaemic control was only slightly improved when metformin was added to sulphonylureas in patients with hyperglycaemia on maximal dose of these drugs. Insulin was more effective, but caused hypoglycaemia in some cases. A simple insulin regimen is not always efficacious in such patients [142]. Combined treatment with metformin plus glibenclamide was as effective as insulin in reducing glycaemia in another study [48], and more effective in reducing postprandial glycaemia [143]. Combined with glipizide, metformin improved glycaemia, lipids and FFA [120]. A recent controlled, double-blind study [115, 139] showed a high antihyperglycaemic efficacy of primary (n = 65) and early secondary add-on (n = 26) combination therapy with metformin + glibenclamide. Near-normal glycaemia was obtained in a majority of the patients, even in advanced NIDDM, and there was no increase in weight and insulin levels after 6 months of maintenance treatment with individually target-titrated doses.

In contrast to sulphonylureas, weight reduction following metformin has often been noticed [3, 10, 27, 33, 34, 61, 87, 88, 111, 117, 135, 161] but weight loss is not consistent [3, 9, 60, 62, 65, 66, 70, 112, 115, 137, 154]. Metformin is weight-stabilizing rather than weight-reducing [6]. During combined metformin and sulphonylurea treatment, body weight appears to be unchanged in NIDDM patients [48, 90, 92, 115, 120, 142, 143, 153, 155]. Lean body mass may decrease slightly [48], but the clinical significance of this finding, which is unconfirmed [167], remains uncertain. From animal experiments [47], a thermogenic effect of metformin cannot be excluded. Weight loss during metformin may also be related to reduction of hyperinsulinaemia, and seems to be more frequent in diabetics than in non-diabetics with obesity [3]. There is no difference between sulphonylureas and metformin regarding effects on energy expenditure [93], which, however, decreased after combined oral treatment in the above study [48]. Total energy expenditure was unaffected by metformin in the acute study mentioned previously [152] and in a recent 4-month study [167]. There are few published data on the effect of the drug on fat distribution, showing either unchanged [69, 125, 137] or decreased [158] waist–hip ratio.

Indications and Treatment Schedules

Buformin is no longer used in clinical practice except in a few countries. Phenformin is still used in several countries [114, 133]. The main indications for metformin are NIDDM uncontrolled by diet alone and sulphonylurea failure. The drug has also been used as adjuvant therapy in combination with insulin in IDDM patients, whose insulin requirements can then be reduced [37, 38]. However, this mode of use cannot be recommended generally because of the potential risk of lactic acidosis superimposed on the risk of ketosis. The use of metformin combined with insulin in NIDDM is a therapy of current interest. In a recent randomized, double-blind, placebo-controlled trial [144] this combination was shown to improve glycaemic control and cardiovascular risk factor profile after 6 months. The insulin dose was reduced and body weight remained stable; blood pressure decreased.

The mode of use of metformin in NIDDM is still a matter of debate. Treatment schedules are based on clinical experience and opinions rather than on controlled clinical trials. Adequate diet regulation should always be tried for 2–3 months before drug therapy is instituted. However, some patients are unable to improve metabolic control and require oral agents at an earlier time. There is no universal agreement on 'first-line' drugs, although sulphonylureas are usually preferred. As metformin may reduce hyperinsulinaemia and promote weight reduction or stabilize body weight, it would be more appropriate as first-line therapy in obese NIDDM patients [3, 6]. Many patients can be well controlled with metformin alone, and sulphonylurea can be added if metabolic control deteriorates [89]. Metformin is also effective in non-obese NIDDM patients. The degree of obesity does not predict the antihyperglycaemic response [62, 115, 139, 152]. The combination of metformin and sulphonylurea as primary drug treatment seems to be very effective [115, 139].

According to the European NIDDM Policy Group, the main indication for metformin is 'NIDDM associated with obesity and/or hyperlipidaemia'. An age limit of 65 years is also recommended, but the biological rather than the numerical age should guide therapy decisions. In this respect renal function seems more important than age when deciding to initiate treatment in elderly patients [145]. The potential use of metformin in IGT and other insulin-resistant conditions in non-diabetic subjects has been discussed recently [151].

Contraindications and Precautions

The contraindications generally agreed upon are shown in Table 3. These contraindications are justified by the

Table 3 Contraindications for metformin

Ketosis-prone diabetes
Pregnancy
Acute complications (severe infections, major operations and trauma)
Diabetes with significant late complications (nephropathy, retinopathy)
Before intravenous urography or aortography
Impaired renal function
Liver damage
Alcoholism
Severe cardiovascular or respiratory disease
Deficiencies of vitamin B_{12}, folic acid and iron
Bad general condition (e.g. malnutrition, dehydration)
Old age

risk of lactic acidosis in these conditions. Impaired renal function is of particular importance [84]. Serum creatinine concentrations should be normal when starting treatment and should be monitored regularly. Creatinine clearance may be estimated from nomograms [94]. Liver function should also be monitored during therapy, and serum vitamin B_{12} concentrations should be measured annually during long-term treatment. Metformin does not increase blood pressure [53, 63, 69, 70, 125, 135, 137, 144], and uncomplicated hypertension is not a contraindication [69]. Caution is recommended in cardiac disease.

Drug Interactions

An increased elimination of phenprocoumon (Marcoumar) has been reported during metformin treatment [95]. The basis of this interaction is uncertain, but it seems to be related to increased liver blood flow [95]. An interaction with cimetidine has been reported [96]: cimetidine increased the availability of metformin and reduced its renal clearance over 24 hours by 27%, and the peak concentration was also increased. The lactate–pyruvate ratio increased when both drugs were given. The results indicated a competitive inhibition of renal tubular secretion. The dose of metformin should be reduced if cimetidine is coprescribed. The mechanism is probably via the organic cation system. An interaction between metformin and guar gum at the level of absorption has been described [86] (see section on absorption).

Alcohol Interaction

Alcohol potentiates the blood glucose-lowering and hyperlactataemic effect of biguanides [10], and hence alcohol should be avoided during treatment.

Pregnancy

Metformin is contraindicated in pregnancy; insulin should be given. However, metformin has been used in pregnant NIDDM patients during the second and third trimester without any particular problems [97, 98]. There is no suspicion of teratogenic effect of metformin from retrospective studies [3]. Metformin does not pass through the placental barrier in mice, and no serious malformations are observed in rats following high doses. Metformin is not recommended during breast feeding.

Dosage

Treatment with metformin is usually initiated with a low dose in order to avoid gastrointestinal side-effects (0.5–1.0 g daily). If necessary, the dose is increased gradually. There is a dose–effect increase up to 3 g/day [139, 168]. When added to sulphonylurea therapy, a small dose is often sufficient.

The daily dose needed to obtain satisfactory metabolic control varies, depending mainly on the degree of metabolic disturbance. No further effect can be expected on blood glucose by doses above 3 g daily. However, higher doses have been used for blood lipid reduction in non-diabetics [58].

The optimal number of daily doses has not been assessed specifically, but there seems to be little or no difference in metabolic control between a single and divided dose schedule [3]. Metformin is usually given in two or three daily doses with meals in order to avoid gastrointestinal side-effects. Sufficient blood glucose control may not be apparent until after 1–2 weeks, but is sometimes evident already on the first day of treatment [4, 5]. When good control has been established over a longer period, the dose may be gradually reduced. This is especially important to attempt in elderly patients.

ADVERSE REACTIONS

Symptomatic Side-effects

Gastrointestinal side-effects of metformin have been reported to occur in 5–20% of all cases [1, 3, 6, 87]. In general, the symptoms are transient, and do not necessitate discontinuation of therapy [3, 87]. Clinical experience shows that side-effects can be avoided or minimized by gradual dose increase. However, a dose relationship for side-effects was not confirmed in a recent study [139]. The most frequently reported symptoms are metallic taste, anorexia, nausea, vomiting, abdominal distension or pain, and diarrhoea. The prevalence of diarrhoea was 20% in patients treated with metformin, compared with 6% in other treatment groups in a study on 285 randomly selected diabetics [99]. There was no difference between monotherapy and combination with sulphonylurea, and diarrhoea did

not appear to be dose-related in this study. It is often acute and disturbing and incontinence may occur, but it always disappears after cessation of therapy. The frequency was 8% in a non-diabetic control group. In the experience of others [6], a 20% frequency of diarrhoea might be an overestimate of the problem. Gastrointestinal side-effects may be related to changes in gastrointestinal motility and/or the proposed H_2-agonist capacity of metformin (see section on gastrointestinal function).

Very rarely, metformin has given rise to cutaneous hypersensitivity [3, 100]. A single case of vasculitis and pneumonitis [6] and three cases of hyponatraemia have been described. It seems that hypoglycaemia does not occur when metformin is given alone [3–6] (see also section on mode of action), but it has been described in a few cases in the UKPDS [163] and in a recent double-blind study [115], probably provoked by rapid glucose reduction.

Malabsorption of Vitamin B_{12}

Malabsorption of vitamin B_{12} may occur during long-term metformin treatment (see section on gastrointestinal function).

Lactic Acidosis

The association of biguanides with lactic acidosis is well established. The first cases were published in 1959 (phenformin), 1970 (buformin) and 1972 (metformin). A review of 330 cases [2] showed that the great majority of cases are associated with phenformin. It has been observed that lactic acidosis disappeared when treatment was changed from phenformin to metformin [3]. Phenformin-induced cases still occur [159] as this drug is available in some countries [114] and can be present in others through non-conventional channels and immigrants [159].

Metformin provokes lactic acidosis very rarely [2, 3, 6–8, 101]. Twenty-five cases have been reviewed earlier [3]. A 1972–82 review [7] revealed 42 cases with 43% mortality. A later review [101] describes 55 well-documented cases during 1972–84, with a mortality of 53%. A few cases have been associated with accidental or voluntary overdose [3, 7, 101], whereas conditions contraindicating the drug have been present in almost all other cases [3, 6–8, 101]. Impaired renal function is the precipitating factor encountered most frequently in metformin-associated lactic acidosis (MALA).

At present, a total of 120 cases of MALA have been reported in published papers. A recent review [171] presents details of 110 cases. The cases reviewed earlier [3, 7] are included in a French review of 55 cases

[101], except for six Swedish cases [7, 8]. A prospective study reports 20 French cases [102], and six further French cases (1 + 5) have been published separately [103, 146]. The literature contains three papers from the UK [104, 105, 147] comprising five cases (1 + 3 + 1), the most recent one from 1993 [147]. A Danish survey [106] reports five cases, but two of these have been published previously [3, 101]. A recent Swedish review [107] describes 18 cases reported during the period 1977–1991. This survey includes the seven cases reviewed earlier [7, 8], one of these being published separately [94] and also included in the French review [101]. The recent British case [147] was a patient on regular peritoneal dialysis, and a similar case has also been reported from Taiwan [148]. A patient with end-stage renal failure developed MALA in the USA [149]. The above publications [101–107, 146–149] describe a total of 111 cases of MALA. As two French cases seem to be identical in two publications [101, 102], and one other French case also appears to have been reported twice [101, 146], and double reporting is evident for two Danish cases [101,106] and one Swedish case [101, 107], six cases should be deducted from the 111 reported in the literature. A recent fatal case [172] was attributed to reinstatement of metformin too early after a major operation. A further 14 cases are described in a very recent publication from France [160] (see below), giving a total of 120 cases of MALA. There are additional cases not published in the literature, but reported to regulatory authorities. Three-quarters of the known cases have occurred in France, where metformin has a relatively high share of the market for oral antidiabetic agents.

The true frequency of MALA is not known. In the UK, metformin use has been 500 000 patient-years in 1970–85, with only 3 episodes of MALA recorded [104]; one of these cases was due to deliberate overdose. In Canada, clinical experience in 1972–83, including intensified monitoring since 1978, covered about 56 000 patient-years without a single documented MALA case [108]. In Sweden, 0.13 case per million defined daily doses was found during 1975–77 for metformin and 1.76 for phenformin [100]. On the basis of these Swedish data, together with Swiss [109] and French [101, 102] data, the incidence would be approximately 1:25 000 patient-years. The frequency in Sweden during the period 1987–1991 was 0.24 cases per 10 000 patient-years [107], which corresponds to a figure of approximately 1:40 000 patient-years. It was stated that this incidence is rather low and probably decreasing. An official figure for the frequency of MALA accepted by the Food and Drug Administration is 0.03/1000 patient-years (i.e. 1:33 000 patient-years).

Not all cases of MALA are, in fact, caused or precipitated by metformin. In a prospective study [102], plasma metformin concentrations were determined in 20 metformin-treated diabetics admitted to an intensive care unit with hyperlactataemia (arterial blood lactate values over 5 mmol/l) and a serious acute condition (coma, shock, respiratory distress, anuria). Two groups could be distinguished, one with high metformin levels (7 patients) and another with therapeutic or near-zero levels (13 patients). Both groups were given the same treatment and compared with a control group. In the first group the hyperlactataemia was ascribed to toxic accumulation of metformin secondary to a treatment error (i.e. failure to observe a contraindication, or overdosage) or to an intercurrent pathological factor affecting the renal elimination of metformin. Acute renal failure was predominant in this group and the prognosis was good (6 recovered from the hyperlactataemia). In the second group the hyperlactataemia was ascribed to 'anoxaemic aggressions in susceptible patients', i.e. not related to accumulation of metformin but to the occurrence during treatment of one or more aetiological factors for lactic acidosis, independent of metformin. Acute renal failure was common but inconstant in this group, and the prognosis was bad (only 3 recovered). In a recent study [160] 14 diabetic patients with MALA and acute renal failure were analysed. Ten had metformin accumulation as judged from drug concentrations in plasma, but hypoxia rather than metformin accumulation (and the degree of renal failure) determined the prognosis. In agreement with the above prospective study [102], the early mortality was highest in the subgroup without accumulation of the drug.

When lactic acidosis occurs in metformin-treated patients, early determination of the metformin concentration in plasma appears to be the best criterion for assessing the responsibility of the drug for this condition [94, 101, 102, 105]. The concentration of metformin in erythrocytes seems to be a good indicator of drug accumulation and a guide for repeat of haemodialysis [103]. It is more persistent than the plasma concentration, and blood levels can remain abnormally high at the end of dialysis [146].

Lactic acidosis is a very serious condition with a high mortality. The cases associated with biguanides have a better prognosis than others; for MALA, mortality is about 50%. The comparative mortality risks for MALA and glibenclamide-induced hypoglycaemia have been calculated from Swedish data [7, 8]: they were found to be almost identical (0.0240 versus 0.0332 per 1000 patient-years). Similar comparative data (metformin 0.024 versus sulphonylurea 0.020) are available from Switzerland [110].

The pathogenesis of MALA is usually complex, with several contributing factors. Diabetes itself predisposes to hyperlactataemia [149]. Lactate accumulation is due to increased production (hypoxia) and/or decreased elimination. A major precipitating factor (in 80–90% of the cases) is impaired renal function [3, 7, 8, 94, 101, 102, 107, 109, 146–149], either as a primary acute renal failure or a decompensation of chronic failure. Renal impairment may also be a consequence of lactic acidosis. Hepatic dysfunction is another important factor [101]. Other factors are alcohol, cardiac decompensation and serious infections. Pancreatitis was present in 2 Danish cases [3, 106], and splanchnic hypoxia is a conceivable pathogenetic factor in these cases. Old age can be regarded as a predisposing factor because glomerular filtration decreases with age. MALA has been reported even in the absence of pre-existing risk factors [105]. In the MALA cases the mean age has been 65 years (range 35–84 years) with an equal sex distribution.

In a recent retrospective survey of emergency admissions in Mexico [150] the odds ratio of lactic acidosis during a severe associated disease in a NIDDM patient treated with phenformin, sulphonylurea or insulin was the same. No metformin cases were found in this study, which also confirmed the significance of associated conditions. There are no data comparing the age-specific mortality rate from lactic acidosis with that occurring in the diabetic population not receiving biguanides.

It is evident that MALA might be prevented by proper prescribing of the drug and patient education (see above). Careful observation should be kept for early symptoms with sudden onset or aggravation (nausea, vomiting, diarrhoea, lower abdominal and muscular pain). Thus, the symptoms mimic some side-effects of the drug. Acidosis with hyperventilation, drowsiness and coma can develop within a few hours. The diagnosis should be confirmed by lactate determination. Calculation of the anion gap might also be useful [2, 13, 94, 102].

The treatment is complicated and often unsuccessful. The aim is to counter shock, hypoxia and acidosis, and to eliminate accumulated lactate and drug. The use of moderate alkalinization is advocated [102]. Glucose and insulin may increase lactate elimination, but the treatment is questionable [101, 102, 106]. Experience with dichloroacetate is limited [146, 149]. Extracorporeal dialysis provides both symptomatic and aetiological treatment by eliminating lactate and metformin, particularly as renal failure is often present. Haemodialysis is the most efficient method and may be repeated. Dialysis has been used in about two-thirds of the reported cases [101–103, 146].

CONCLUSION

Today, metformin is the only biguanide recommended for the treatment of NIDDM. The drug has a favourable pharmacokinetic profile and exerts an antihyperglycaemic effect without causing hypoglycaemia. Hyperinsulinaemia may be reduced. The mode of action involves amelioration of insulin resistance by improved insulin action through a multifactorial mechanism probably mediated via membrane-binding properties. An insulin-independent effect on glucose utilization has also been suggested, and insulin action may be improved indirectly by the blood glucose reduction from such an effect. Lipid metabolism is influenced in a favourable way, and metformin is particularly justified in NIDDM patients with obesity or hyperlipidaemia. Combination therapy with sulphonylurea may be highly effective. Lactate metabolism may be affected, rarely leading to lactic acidosis and then only in special circumstances; this complication can be prevented by proper use of the drug. Gastrointestinal side-effects are fairly common, and vitamin B_{12} malabsorption may occur during long-term treatment.

REFERENCES

1. Schäfer G. Biguanides: A review of history, pharmacodynamics and therapy. Diabète Métab 1983; 9: 148–63.
2. Luft D, Schmulling RM, Eggstein M. Lactic acidosis in biguanide-treated diabetics. A review of 330 cases. Diabetologia 1978; 14: 75–87.
3. Hermann LS. Metformin: a review of its pharmacological properties and therapeutic use. Diabète Métab 1979; 5: 233–45.
4. Bailey CJ. Metformin revisited; its actions and indications for use. Diabet Med 1988; 5: 315–20.
5. Bailey CJ. Metformin—an update. Gen Pharmacol 1993; 24: 1299–1309.
6. Campbell IW. Sulphonylureas and metformin: efficacy and inadequacy. In Bailey CJ, Flatt PR (eds) New antidiabetic drugs. London: Smith-Gordon, 1990: pp 33–51.
7. Campbell IW. Metformin and the sulphonylureas: the comparative risk. Horm Metab Res 1985; (suppl) 15: 105–11.
8. Campbell IW. Metformin and glibenclamide: comparative risks. Br Med J 1984; 289: 289.
9. UK Prospective Diabetes Study. II. Reduction in HbA_{1c} with basal insulin supplement, sulfonylurea, or biguanide therapy in maturity-onset diabetes. Diabetes 1985; 34: 793–8.
10. Hermann LS. Metabolic effects of metformin in relation to clinical effects and side-effects. In van der Kuy A, Hulst SGT (eds) Biguanide therapy today. Royal Society of Medicine International Congress and Symposium Series 48. London: Academic Press, 1981: pp 17–48.
11. Klip A, Leiter LA. Cellular mechanism of action of metformin. Diabetes Care 1990; 13: 696–704.
12. Sterne J, Junien JL. Metformin: pharmacological mechanisms of the antidiabetic and antilipidic effect and clinical consequences. In van der Kuy A, Hulst SGT (eds) Biguanide therapy today. Royal Society of Medicine International Congress and Symposium Series 48. London: Academic Press, 1981: pp 3–13.

13. Hermann LS. Biguanides and lactate metabolism; a review. Dan Med Bull 1973; 20: 65–79.

14. Hother-Nielsen O, Schmitz O, Andersen PH, Beck-Nielsen H, Pedersen O. Metformin improves peripheral but not hepatic insulin action in obese patients with type II diabetes. Acta Endocrinol 1989; 120: 257–65.

15. Purrello F, Gullo D, Brunetti A, Buscema M, Italia S, Goldfine ID, Vigneri R. Direct effects of biguanides on glucose utilization *in vitro*. Metabolism 1987; 36: 774–6.

16. Jackson RA, Hawa MI, Jaspan JW, Sima BM, Disilvio L, Featherbe D, Kurtz AB. Mechanism of metformin action in non-insulin-dependent diabetes. Diabetes 1987; 36: 632–40.

17. Bonora E, Cigolini M, Bosello O et al. Lack of effect of intravenous metformin on plasma concentrations of glucose, insulin, C-peptide, glucagon and growth hormone in non-diabetic subjects. Curr Med Res Opinion 1984; 9: 47–51.

18. Prager R, Schernthaner G. Insulin receptor binding to monocytes, insulin secretion, and glucose tolerance following metformin treatment. Diabetes 1983; 32: 1083–6.

19. Prager R, Schernthaner G, Graf H. Effect of metformin on peripheral insulin sensitivity in non insulin dependent diabetes mellitus. Diabète Métab 1986; 12: 346–50.

20. Nosadini R, Avogaro A, Trevisan R et al. Effect of metformin on insulin-stimulated glucose turnover and insulin binding to receptors in type II diabetes. Diabetes Care 1987; 10: 62–7.

21. Wu M-S, Johnston P, Sheu WH-H et al. Effect of metformin on carbohydrate and lipoprotein metabolism in NIDDM patients. Diabetes Care 1990; 13: 1–8.

22. Lord JM, White SI, Bailey CJ, Atkind TW, Fletcher RF, Taylor KG. Effect of metformin on insulin receptor binding and glycaemic control in type II diabetes. Br Med J 1983; 286: 830–1.

23. Fantus IG, Brosseau R. Mechanism of action of metformin: insulin receptor and postreceptor effects *in vitro* and *in vivo*. J Clin Endocrinol Metab 1986; 63: 898–905.

24. Rizkalla SW, Elgrably F, Tchobroutsky G, Slama G. Effects of metformin treatment on erythrocyte insulin binding in normal weight subjects, in obese non diabetic subjects, in type 1 and type 2 diabetic patients. Diabète Métab 1986; 12: 219–24.

25. Frayn KN, Adnitt PI, Turner P. The hypoglycaemic action of metformin. Postgrad Med J 1971; 47: 777–80.

26. Caporicci D, Mori A, Pepi R, Lapi E. Effetti della dimetilbiguanide (metformina) sulla clearance periferica dell'insulina e sulla biosintesi lipidica in pazienti obesi dislipidemici con e senza malatta diabetica. Clin Terapeut 1979; 88: 371–86.

27. Papoz L, Job D, Eschwège E et al. Effect of oral hypoglycaemic drugs on glucose tolerance and insulin secretion in borderline diabetic patients. Diabetologia 1978; 15: 373–80.

28. Holle A, Mangels W, Dreyer M, Kühnau J, Rüdiger W. Biguanide treatment increases the number of insulin-receptor sites on human erythrocytes. New Engl J Med 1981; 305: 563–6.

29. Vigneri R, Gullo D, Pezzino V. Metformin and insulin receptors. Diabetes Care 1984; 7 (suppl. 1): 113–17.

30. Schönborn J, Heim K, Rabast U, Kasper H. Oxidation rate of plasma free fatty acids in maturity-onset diabetics. Effect of metformin. Diabetologia 1975; 11: 375.

31. Heim K. Die Wirkung des Biguanides Metformin auf den Stoffwechsel der freien Plasmafettsäuren beim Altersdiabetiker (inaugural dissertation), University of Würzburg. Würzburg: Schmitt & Meyer, 1979: pp 1–56.

32. Vague PH, Juhan-Vague I, Alessi MC, Badier C, Valadier J. Metformin decreases the high plasminogen activator inhibition capacity, plasma insulin and triglyceride levels in non-diabetic obese subjects. Thromb Haemost 1987; 57: 326–8.

33. McAlpine LG, McAlpine CH, Waclawski ER, Storer AM, Kay JW, Frier BM. A comparison of treatment with metformin and gliclazide in patients with non-insulin-dependent diabetes. Eur J Clin Pharmacol 1988; 34: 129–32.

34. Josephkutty S, Potter JM. Comparison of tolbutamide and metformin in elderly diabetic patients. Diabet Med 1990; 7: 510–14.

35. Ferlito S, Del Campo F, Di Vincenzo S, Damante G, Coco R, Branca S, Fichera C. Effect of metformin on blood glucose, insulin and C-peptide responses to glucagon in non-insulin dependent diabetics. Il Farmaco 1983; 38: 248–54.

36. Ferner RE, Rawlins MD, Alberti KGMM. Impaired B-cell responses improve when fasting blood glucose concentration is reduced in non-insulin-dependent diabetes. Quart J Med 1988; 66: 137–46.

37. Pagano G, Tagliaferro V, Carta Q et al. Metformin reduces insulin requirement in type I (insulin-dependent) diabetes. Diabetologia 1983; 24: 351–4.

38. Gin H, Messerschmitt C, Brottier E, Aubertin J. Metformin improved insulin resistance in type I, insulin-dependent diabetic patients. Metabolism 1985; 34: 923–5.

39. Leblanc H, Marre M, Billault B, Passa PH. Intérêt de l'association infusion sous-cutanée d'insuline et metformine chez 10 diabétiques insulino-nécessitants obèses. Diabète Métab 1987; 13: 613–17.

40. von Lisch H-J, Sailer S, Braunsteiner H. Die Wirkung von Biguaniden auf die Insulinempfindlichkeit von Altersdiabetikern. Wiener Klin Wschr 1980; 92: 266–9.

41. Pedersen O, Hother Nielsen O, Bak J, Richelsen B, Beck-Nielsen H, Schwartz Sørensen N. The effects of metformin on adipocyte insulin action and metabolic control in obese subjects with type 2 diabetes. Diabet Med 1989; 6: 249–56.

42. Jacobs DB, Hayes GR, Truglia JA, Lockwood DH. Effects of metformin on insulin receptor tyrosine kinase activity in rat adipocytes. Diabetologia 1986; 29: 798–801.

43. Cigolini M, Bosello O, Zancanaro C, Orlandi PG, Fezzi O, Smith U. Influence of metformin on metabolic effect of insulin in human adipose tissue *in vitro*. Diabète Métab 1984; 19: 311–15.

44. Cigolini M, Zancanaro C, Benati D, Cavallo E, Bosello O, Smith U. Metformin enhances insulin binding to 'in vitro' down-regulated human fat cells. Diabète Métab 1987; 13: 20–2.

45. Lord JM, Atkins TW, Bailey CJ. Effect of metformin on hepatocyte insulin receptor binding in normal, streptozotocin diabetic and genetically obese diabetic (ob/ob) mice. Diabetologia 1983; 25: 108-13.

46. Bailey CJ, Puah JA. Effect of metformin on glucose metabolism in mouse soleus muscle. Diabète Métab 1986; 12: 212-18.

47. Rossetti L, DeFronzo RA, Gherzi R et al. Effect of metformin treatment on insulin action in diabetic rats: *in vivo* and *in vitro* correlations. Metabolism 1990; 39: 425-35.

48. Groop L, Widén E, Franssila-Kallunki A, Ekstrand A, Saloranta C, Schalin C, Eriksson J. Different effects of insulin and oral antidiabetic agents on glucose and energy metabolism in type 2 (non-insulin-dependent) diabetes mellitus. Diabetologia 1989; 32: 599-605.

49. Wilcock C, Bailey CJ. Sites of metformin-stimulated glucose metabolism. Biochem Pharmacol 1990; 39: 1831-4.

50. Frayn KN, Adnitt PI, Turner P. The use of human skeletal muscle *in vitro* for biochemical and pharmacological studies of glucose uptake. Clin Sci 1973; 44: 55-62.

51. Nattrass M, Todd PG, Hinks L, Lloyd B, Alberti KGMM. Comparative effects of phenformin, metformin and glibenclamide on metabolic rhythms in maturity-onset diabetics. Diabetologia 1977; 13: 145-52.

52. Nattrass M, Hinks L, Smythe P, Todd PG, Alberti KGMM. Metabolic effects of combined sulphonylurea and metformin therapy in maturity-onset diabetics. Horm Metab Res 1979; 11: 332-7.

53. Campbell IW, Duncan C, Patton NW, Broadhead T, Tucker GT, Woods HF. The effect of metformin on glycaemic control, intermediary metabolism and blood pressure in non-insulin dependent diabetes mellitus. Diabet Med 1987; 4: 337-41.

54. Marchetti P, Masiello P, Benzi L et al. Effects of metformin therapy on plasma amino acid pattern in patients with maturity-onset diabetes. Drugs Exper Clin Res 1989; 15: 565-70.

55. Björntorp P, Carlström S, Fagerberg SE, Hermann LS, Holm AGL, Scherstén B, Östman J. Influence of phenformin and metformin on exercise induced lactataemia in patients with diabetes mellitus. Diabetologia 1978; 15: 95-8.

56. Bruneder H, Klein HJ. Blutlaktat und Biguanidtherapie. Vergleich zwischen Phenformin, Metformin und Buformin bei 408 Altersdiabetikern. Acta Med Aust 1978; 5: 88-90.

57. Pénicaud L, Hitier Y, Ferré P, Girard J. Hypoglycaemic effect of metformin in genetically obese (fa/fa) rats results from an increased utilization of blood glucose by intestine. Biochem J 1989; 262: 881-5.

58. Sirtori CR, Lovati MR, Franceschini G. Management of lipid disorders and prevention of atherosclerosis with metformin. In Krans HMJ (ed.) Diabetes and metformin. A research and clinical update. RSM International Congress and Symposium Series, 79. London: Royal Society of Medicine, 1985: pp 33-44.

59. Gustafson A, Björntorp P, Fahlén M. Metformin administration in hyperlipidaemic states. Acta Med Scand 1971; 190: 491-4.

60. Lalor BC, Bhatnagar D, Winocour PH, Ishola M, Arrol S, Brading M, Durrington PN. Placebo-controlled trial of the effects of guar gum and metformin on fasting blood glucose and serum lipids in obese, type 2 diabetic patients. Diabet Med 1990; 7: 242-5.

61. Taylor KG, John WG, Matthews KA, Wright AD. A prospective study of the effect of 12 months treatment on serum lipids and apolipoproteins A-I and B in type 2 (non-insulin dependent) diabetes. Diabetologia 1982; 23: 507-10.

62. Rains SGH, Wilson GA, Richmond W, Elkeles RS. The effect of glibenclamide and metformin on serum lipoproteins in type 2 diabetes. Diabet Med 1988; 5: 653-8.

63. Haupt E, Knick B, Koschinsky T, Liebermeister H, Schneider J, Hirche H. Oral antidiabetic combination therapy with sulphonylureas and metformin. Results of a three-month general practice study. Medizin Welt 1989; 40: 118-23.

64. Rains SGH, Wilson GA, Richmond W, Elkeles RS. The reduction of low density lipoprotein cholesterol by metformin is maintained with long-term therapy. J Roy Soc Med 1989; 82: 93-4.

65. Collier A, Watson HHK, Patrick AW, Ludlam CA, Clarke BF. Effect of glycaemic control, metformin and gliclazide on platelet density and aggregability in recently diagnosed type 2 (non-insulin-dependent) diabetic patients. Diabète Métab 1989; 15: 420-5.

66. Wilson JA, Scott MM, Gray RS. A comparison of metformin versus guar in combination with sulphonylureas in the treatment of non-insulin dependent diabetes. Horm Metab Res 1989; 21: 317-19.

67. De Silva SR, Shawe JEH, Patel H, Cudworth AG. Plasma fibrinogen in diabetes mellitus. Diabète Métab 1979; 5: 201-6.

68. Gin H, Freyburger C, Boisseau M, Aubertin J. Study of the effect of metformin on platelet aggregation in insulin-dependent diabetics. Diabetes Res Clin Pract 1989; 6: 61-7.

69. Landin K, Tengborn L, Smith U. Treating insulin resistance in hypertension with metformin reduces both blood pressure and metabolic risk factors. J Internal Med 1991; 229: 181-7.

70. Giugliano D, DeRosa N, DiMario G et al. Metformin improves glucose, lipid metabolism, and reduces blood pressure in hypertensive, obese women. Diabetes Care 1993; 16: 1387-90.

71. Campbell IW, Menzies DG, McBain AM, Brown IRF. Effects of metformin on blood pressure and microalbuminuria in diabetes mellitus. Diabète Métab 1988; 14: 613-17.

72. Caspary WF. Biguanides and intestinal absorptive function. Acta Hep Gastr 1977; 24: 473-80.

73. Berger W, Künzli H. Effect of dimethylbiguanide on insulin, glucose and lactic acid contents observed in portal vein blood and peripheral venous blood in the course of intraduodenal glucose tolerance tests. Diabetologia 1970; 6: 37.

74. Tomkin GH, Hadden DR, Weaver JA, Montgomery DAD. Vitamin B_{12} status of patients on long-term metformin therapy. Br Med J 1971; 2: 685-7.

75. Adams JF, Clark JS, Ireland JT, Kesson CM, Watson WS. Malabsorption of vitamin B_{12} and intrinsic factor secretion during biguanide therapy. Diabetologia 1983; 24: 16-18.

76. Callaghan TS, Hadden DR, Tomkin GH. Megaloblastic anaemia due to vitamin B_{12} malabsorption associated with long-term metformin treatment. Br Med J 1980; 280: 1214-15.

77. Vidon N, Chaussade S, Noel M, Franchisseur C, Huchet B, Bernier JJ. Metformin in the digestive tract. Diabetes Res Clin Pract 1988; 4: 223–9.
78. Molloy AM, Ardill J, Tomkin GH. The effect of metformin treatment on gastric acid secretion and gastrointestinal hormone levels in normal subjects. Diabetologia 1980; 19: 93–6.
79. Marchetti P, Benzi L, Cecchetti P et al. Plasma biguanide levels are correlated with metabolic effects in diabetic patients. Clin Pharmacol Ther 1987; 41: 450–4.
80. Marchetti P, Benzi L, Cerri M et al. Effect of plasma metformin concentrations on serum lipid levels in type II diabetic patients. Acta Diabet Lat 1988; 25: 55–62.
81. Pentikäinen PJ. Bioavailability of metformin. Comparison of solution, rapidly dissolving tablet, and three sustained release products. Int J Clin Pharm Ther Toxicol 1986; 24: 213–20.
82. Tucker GT, Casey C, Phillips PJ, Connor H, Ward JD, Woods HF. Metformin kinetics in healthy subjects and in patients with diabetes mellitus. Br J Clin Pharmacol 1981; 12: 235–46.
83. Noel M. Kinetic study of normal and sustained release dosage forms of metformin in normal subjects. Res Clin Forums 1979; 1: 35–44.
84. Sirtori CR, Franceschini G, Gallikienle M, Cighetti G, Galli G, Bondioli A, Conti F. Disposition of metformin (N,N-dimethylbiguanide) in man. Clin Pharmacol Ther 1978; 24: 683–93.
85. Pentikäinen PJ, Neuvonen PJ, Penttilä A. Pharmacokinetics of metformin after intravenous and oral administration to man. Eur J Clin Pharmacol 1979; 16: 195–202.
86. Gin H, Orgerie MB, Aubertin J. The influence of guar gum on absorption of metformin from the gut in healthy volunteers. Horm Metab Res 1989; 21: 81–3.
87. Clarke BF, Duncan LJP. Biguanide treatment in the management of insulin independent (maturity-onset) diabetes: clinical experience with metformin. Res Clin Forums 1979; 1: 53–63.
88. Wales JK. Treatment of the obese diabetic patient. In Björntorp P, Cairella M, Ikiward AN (eds) Recent advances in obesity research. Proceedings of the 3rd International Congress on Obesity, 1980: pp 184–9.
89. Hermann LS. Biguanides and sulfonylureas as combination therapy in NIDDM. Diabetes Care 1990; 13 (suppl. 3): 37–41.
90. Higginbotham L, Martin FIR. Double-blind trial of metformin in the therapy of non-ketotic diabetics. Med J Aust 1979; 2: 154–6.
91. Capretti L, Bonora E, Coscelli C, Butturini U. Combined sulfonylurea–biguanide therapy for non-insulin dependent diabetics. Metabolic effects of glibenclamide and metformin or phenformin in newly diagnosed obese patients. Curr Med Res Opinion 1982; 7: 677–83.
92. Holman RR, Steemson J, Turner RC. Sulphonylurea failure in type 2 diabetes: treatment with a basal insulin supplement. Diabet Med 1987; 4: 457–62.
93. Leslie P, Jung RT, Isles TE, Baty J. Energy expenditure in non-insulin dependent diabetic subjects on metformin or sulphonylurea therapy. Clin Sci 1986; 73: 41–5.
94. Hermann LS, Magnusson S, Möller B, Casey C, Tucker GT, Woods HF. Lactic acidosis during metformin treatment in an elderly diabetic patient with impaired renal function. Acta Med Scand 1981; 209: 519–20.
95. Ohnhaus EE, Berger W, Duckert F, Oesch F. The influence of dimethylbiguanide on phenprocoumon elimination and its mode of action. Klin Wochenschr 1983; 61: 851–8.
96. Somogyi A, Stockley C, Keal J, Rolan P, Bochner F. Reduction of metformin renal tubular secretion by cimetidine in man. Br J Clin Pharmacol 1987; 23: 545–51.
97. Coetzee EJ, Jackson WPU. Metformin in the management of pregnant insulin-independent diabetics. Diabetologia 1979; 16: 241–5.
98. Coetzee EJ, Jackson WPU. The management of non-insulin dependent diabetes during pregnancy. Diabetes Res Clin Pract 1986; 1: 281–7.
99. Dandona P, Fonseca V, Mier A, Beckett AG. Diarrhoea and metformin in a diabetic clinic. Diabetes Care 1983; 6: 472–4.
100. Bergman U, Boman G, Wiholm B-E. Epidemiology of adverse drug reactions to phenformin and metformin. Br Med J 1978; 2: 464–6.
101. Perrot D, Claris O, Guillaume C, Bouffard Y, Laisne H. Metformine et acidose lactique. Revue de la littérature. Réanim Soins Int Méd Urgence 1986; 2: 85–91.
102. Lambert H, Isnard F, Delorme N, Claude D, Bollaert PE, Straczek J, Larcan A. Approche physiopathologique des hyperlactatémies pathologiques chez le diabetique. Intéret de la metforminémie. Ann Fr Anesth Réanim 1987; 6: 88–94.
103. Lacroix C, Hermelin A, Gerson M, Nouveau J, Guiberteau R. Acidose lactique imputable à la metformine: Intéret des taux intraérythrocytaires. Press Méd 1988; 17: 1158.
104. Hutchison SMW, Catterall JR. Metformin and lactic acidosis—a reminder. Br J Clin Pract 1987; 41: 673–4.
105. Tymms DJ, Leatherdale BA. Lactic acidosis due to metformin therapy in a low risk patient. Postgrad Med J 1988; 64: 230–1.
106. Lebech M, Olesen LL. Metforminassocieret laktatacidose. Ugeskr Laeger 1990; 152: 2511–12.
107. Wiholm B-E, Myrhed M. Metformin-associated lactic acidosis in Sweden 1977–1991. Eur J Clin Pharmacol 1993; 44: 589–91.
108. Lucis OJ. The status of metformin in Canada. Can Med Assoc J 1983; 128: 24–6.
109. Berger W. Incidence of severe side-effects during therapy with sulfonylureas and biguanides. Horm Metab Res 1985; (suppl) 15: 111–15.
110. Berger W. Present status of biguanides. Pharmakritik 1979; 1: 9–12.
111. Hermann LS, Karlsson J-E, Sjöstrand Å. Prospective comparative study in NIDDM patients of metformin and glibenclamide with special reference to lipid profiles. Eur J Clin Pharmacol 1991; 41: 263–5.
112. Hermann LS, Bitzén P-O, Kjellström T, Lindgarde F, Scherstén B. Comparative efficacy of metformin and glibenclamide in patients with non-insulin-dependent diabetes mellitus. Diabète Métab 1991; 17: 201–8.
113. Bailey CJ. Biguanides and NIDDM. Diabetes Care 1992; 15: 755–72.
114. Hermann LS. Metformin as monotherapy and combined with glibenclamide in patients with non-insulin dependent diabetes mellitus (thesis). Lund: Studentlitteratur, 1994; pp 38–62.

115. Hermann LS, Scherstén B, Bitzén P-O, Kjellström T, Lindgärde F, Melander A. Therapeutic comparison of metformin and sulphonylurea, alone and in various combinations: a double-blind controlled study. Diabetes Care 1994; 17: 1100-9.

116. Sum C-F, Webster JM, Johnson AB, Catalano C, Cooper BG, Taylor R. The effect of intravenous metformin on glucose metabolism during hyperglycaemia in type 2 diabetes. Diabet Med 1992; 9: 61-5.

117. Noury J, Nandeuil A. Comparative three-month study of the efficacies of metformin and gliclazide in the treatment of NIDD. Diabète Métab 1991; 17: 209-12.

118. Hollenbeck CB, Johnston P, Varasteh BB, Ida Chen Y-D, Reaven GM. Effects of metformin on glucose, insulin and lipid metabolism in patients with mild hypertriglyceridaemia and non-insulin dependent diabetes by glucose tolerance test criteria. Diabète Métab 1991; 17: 483-9.

119. DeFronzo RA, Barzilai N, Simonson DC. Mechanism of metformin action in obese and lean noninsulin-dependent diabetic subjects. J Clin Endocrinol Metab 1991; 73: 1294-1301.

120. Reaven GM, Johnston P, Hollenbeck CB, Skowronski R, Zhang J-C, Goldfine ID, Ida Chen Y-D. Combined metformin-sulfonylurea treatment of patients with non-insulin dependent diabetes in fair to poor glycemic control. J Clin Endocrinol Metab 1992; 74: 1020-26.

121. McIntyre HD, Paterson CA, Ma A, Ravenscroft PJ, Bird DM, Cameron DP. Metformin increases insulin sensitivity and basal glucose clearance in type 2 (non-insulin dependent) diabetes mellitus. Aust NZ J Med 1991; 21: 714-19.

122. Boyd K, Rogers C, Boreham C, Andrews WJ, Hadden DR. Insulin, glibenclamide or metformin treatment for non-insulin dependent diabetes: heterogenous responses of standard measures of insulin action and insulin secretion before and after differing hypoglycaemic therapy. Diabet Res 1992; 19: 69-76.

123. Fendri S, Debussche X, Puy H, Vincent O, Marcelli JM, Dubreuil A, Lalau JD. Metformin effects on peripheral sensitivity to insulin in non-diabetic obese subjects. Diabète Métab 1993; 19: 245-9.

124. Johnson AB, Webster JM, Sum C-F, Heseltine L, Argyraki M, Cooper BG, Taylor R. The impact of metformin therapy on hepatic glucose production and skeletal muscle glycogen synthase activity in overweight type II diabetic patients. Metabolism 1993; 42: 1217-22.

125. Nagi DK, Yudkin JS. Effects of metformin on insulin resistance, risk factors for cardiovascular disease, and plasminogen activator inhibitor in NIDDM subjects. A study of two ethnic groups. Diabetes Care 1993; 16: 621-9.

126. Widén EIM, Eriksson JG, Groop LC. Metformin normalizes non-oxidative glucose metabolism in insulin-resistant normoglycaemic first-degree relatives of patients with NIDDM. Diabetes 1992; 41: 354-8.

127. Galuska D, Zierath J, Thörne A, Sonnenfeld T, Wallberg-Henriksson H. Metformin increases insulin-stimulated glucose transport in insulin-resistant human skeletal muscle. Diabète Métab 1991; 17: 159-63.

128. Galuska D, Nolte LA, Zierath JR, Wallenberg-Henriksson H. Effect of metformin on insulin-stimulated glucose transport in isolated skeletal muscle obtained from patients with NIDDM. Diabetologia 1994; 37: 826-32.

129. Yoa RG, Rapin JR, Wiernsperger NF, Martinand A, Belleville I. Demonstration of defective glucose uptake and storage in erythrocytes from non-insulin dependent diabetic patients and effects of metformin. Clin Exp Pharmacol Physiol 1993; 20: 563-7.

130. Hundal HS, Ramlal T, Reyes R, Leiter LA. Cellular mechanism of metformin action involves glucose transporter translocation from an intracellular pool to the plasma membrane in L6 muscle cells. Endocrinology 1992; 131: 1165-73.

131. Matthaei S, Reibold JP, Hamann A, Benecke H, Häring HU, Greten H, Klein HH. *In vivo* metformin treatment ameliorates insulin resistance: evidence for potentiation of insulin-induced translocation and increased functional activity of glucose transporters in obese (fa/fa) Zucker rat adipocytes. Endocrinology 1993; 133: 304-11.

132. Hamann A, Benecke H, Greten H, Matthaei S. Metformin increases glucose transporter protein and gene expression in human fibroblasts. Biochem Biophys Res Com 1993; 196: 382-7.

133. Cavallo-Perin P, Aluffi E, Estivi P, Bruno A, Carta Q, Pagano G, Lenti G. The hyperlactatemic effect of biguanides: a comparison between phenformin and metformin during a 6-month treatment. Eur Rev Med Pharmacol Sci 1989; 11: 45-9.

134. Schneider J. Effects of metformin on dyslipoproteinemia in non-insulin dependent diabetes mellitus. Diabète Métab 1991; 17: 185-90.

135. Chan JCN, Tomlinson B, Critchley JAJH, Cockram CS, Walden RJ. Metabolic and hemodynamic effects of metformin and glibenclamide in normotensive NIDDM patients. Diabetes Care 1993; 16: 1035-8.

136. Barnes AJ, Willars EJ, Clark PA, Hunt WB, Rampling M. Effects of metformin on haemorrheological indices in diabetes. Diabète Métab 1988; 14: 608-9.

137. Landin K, Tengborn L, Smith U. Metformin and metoprolol CR treatment in non-obese men. J Int Med 1994; 235: 335-41.

138. Marchetti P, Gregorio F, Benzi L, Giannarelli R, Cecchetti P, Villani G, Di Cianni G, Di Carlo A, Brunetti P, Navalesi R. Diurnal pattern of plasma metformin concentrations and its relation to metabolic effects in type 2 (non-insulin-dependent) diabetic patients. Diabète Métab 1990; 16: 473-8.

139. Hermann LS, Scherstén B, Melander A. Antihyperglycaemic efficacy, response prediction and dose-response relations of treatment with metformin and sulphonylurea, alone and in primary combination. Diabet Med 1994; 11: 953-60.

140. Dornan TL, Heller SR, Peck GM, Tattersall RB. Double-blind evaluation of efficacy and tolerability of metformin in NIDDM. Diabetes Care 1991; 14: 342-4.

141. UK Prospective Diabetes Study Group. UK Prospective Diabetes Study (UKPDS) VIII. Study design, progress and performance. Diabetologia 1991; 34: 877-90.

142. Peacock I, Tattersall RB. The difficult choice of treatment for poorly controlled maturity onset diabetes: tablets or insulin? Br Med J 1984; 288: 1956-9.

143. Trischitta V, Italia S, Mazzarino S, Buscema M, Rabuazzo AM, Sangiorgio L, Squatritio S, Vigneri R. Comparison of combined therapies in treatment of

secondary failure to glyburide. Diabetes Care 1992; 15: 539–42.

144. Giugliano D, Quatraro A, Consoli G, Minei A, Ceriello A, De Rosa N, D'Onofrio F. Metformin for obese, insulin-treated diabetic patients: improvement in glycaemic control and reduction of metabolic risk factors. Eur J Clin Pharmacol 1993; 44: 107–12.

145. Chalmers J, McBain AM, Brown IRF, Campbell IW. Metformin: is its use contraindicated in the elderly? Pract Diabetes 1992; 9: 51–3.

146. Lalau JD, Westeel PF, Debussche X, Dkissi H, Tolani M, Coevoet B, Temperville B, Fournier A, Quichaud J. Bicarbonate haemodialysis: an adequate treatment for lactic acidosis in diabetics treated by metformin. Intens Care Med 1987; 13: 383–7.

147. Khan IH, Catto GRD, MacLeod AM. Severe lactic acidosis in patient receiving continuous ambulatory peritoneal dialysis. Br Med J 1993; 307: 1056–7.

148. Lim P-S, Huang C-C, Wei JS. Metformin-induced lactic acidosis: report of a case. J Formosan Med Assoc 1992; 91: 374–6.

149. Gan SC, Barr J, Arieff AI, Pearl RG. Biguanide-associated lactic acidosis. Case report and review of the literature. Arch Intern Med 1992; 152: 2333–6.

150. Aguilar C, Reza A, Garcia JE, Rull JA. Biguanide-related lactic acidosis: incidence and risk factors. Arch Med Res 1992; 23: 19–24.

151. Widén E, Groop L. Biguanides: metabolic effects and potential use in the treatment of the insulin resistance syndrome. In Marshall SM, Home PD (eds) The diabetes annual 8. Amsterdam: Elsevier, 1994; pp 227–41.

152. Perriello G, Misericordia P, Volpi E et al. Acute antihyperglycemic mechanisms of metformin in NIDDM. Evidence for suppression of lipid oxidation and hepatic glucose production. Diabetes 1994; 43: 920–28.

153. Jeppesen J, Zhou M-Y, Ida Chen Y-D, Reaven GM. Effect of metformin on postprandial lipemia in patients with fairly to poorly controlled NIDDM. Diabetes Care 1994; 17: 1093–9.

154. Riccio A, Del Prato S, Vigili de Kreutzenberg S, Tiengo A. Glucose and lipid metabolism in non-insulin dependent diabetes. Effect of metformin. Diabète Métab 1991; 17: 180–84.

155. Marena S, Tagliaferro V, Montegrosso G et al. Metabolic effects of metformin addition to chronic glibenclamide treatment in type 2 diabetes. Diabète Métab 1994; 20: 15–19.

156. Sarabia V, Lam L, Burdett E, Leiter LA, Klip A. Glucose transport in human skeletal muscle cells in culture. Stimulation by insulin and metformin. J Clin Invest 1992; 90: 1386–95.

157. Landin K, Tengborn L, Smith U. Effects of metformin and metoprolol CR on hormones and fibrinolytic variables during a hyperinsulinemic, euglycemic clamp in man. Thromb Haemost 1994; 71: 783–7.

158. Velazquez EM, Mendoza S, Hamer T, Sosa F, Glueck CJ. Metformin therapy in polycystic ovary syndrome reduces hyperinsulinemia, insulin resistance, hyperandrogenemia, and systolic blood pressure, while facilitating normal menses and pregnancy. Metabolism 1994; 43: 647–54.

159. McGuinness ME, Talbert RL. Phenformin-induced lactic acidosis: a forgotten adverse drug reaction. Ann Pharmacother 1993; 27: 1183–6.

160. Lalau JD, Lacroix C, Compagnon P et al. Role of metformin accumulation in metformin-associated lactic acidosis. Diabetes Care 1995; 18: 779–84.

161. Campbell IW, Menzies DG, Chalmers J, McBain AM, Brown IRF. One year comparative trial of metformin and glipizide in type 2 diabetes mellitus. Diabète Métab 1994; 21: 394–400.

162. Dunn CJ, Peters DH. Metformin. A review of its pharmacological properties and therapeutic use in non-insulin-dependent diabetes mellitus. Drugs 1995; 49: 721–49.

163. Turner R, Cull C, Holman R. United Kingdom Prospective Diabetes Study 17: A 9-year update of a randomized, controlled trial on the effect of improved metabolic control on complications in non-insulin-dependent diabetes mellitus. Ann Intern Med 1996; 124: 136–45.

164. DeFronzo RA, Goodman AM, the Multicenter Metformin Study Group. Efficacy of metformin in patients with non-insulin-dependent diabetes mellitus. N Engl J Med 1995; 333: 541–9.

165. Hermann LS. Clinical pharmacology of biguanides. In: Kuhlmann J, Puls W (eds) Oral antidiabetics. Handbook of experimental pharmacology. Berlin, Springer-Verlag, 1996; pp 373–407.

166. Wiernsperger N. Preclinical pharmacology of biguanides. In: Kuhlmann J, Puls W (eds) Oral antidiabetics. Handbook of experimental pharmacology. Berlin, Springer-Verlag, 1996; pp 305–58.

167. Stumvoll M, Nurjhan N, Perriello G, Dailey G, Gerich JE. Metabolic effects of metformin in non-insulin-dependent diabetes mellitus. N Engl J Med 1995; 333: 550–4.

168. Brookes LG, Sambol NC, Lin ET, Gee W, Benet LZ. Effect of dosage form, dose and food on the pharmacokinetics of metformin. Pharm Res Oct 8, 1991, Suppl: 320.

169. Grant PJ. The effects of high- and medium-dose metformin therapy on cardiovascular risk factors in patients with type II diabetes. Diabetes Care 1996; 19: 64–6.

170. Campbell IW, Howlett HCS. Worldwide experience of metformin as an effective glucose-lowering agent: A meta-analysis. Diab Metab Rev 1995; 11: S57–S62.

171. Sirtori CR, Pasik C. Re-evaluation of a biguanide, metformin: Mechanism of action and tolerability. Pharmacol Res 1994; 30: 187–228.

172. Gowardman JR, Havill J. Fatal metformin induced lactic acidosis: case report. N Z Med J 1995; 108: 230–1.

38

New Drugs for the Treatment of Diabetes Mellitus

Clifford J. Bailey

Department of Pharmaceutical and Biological Sciences, Aston University, Birmingham, UK

New agents being considered or recently introduced for the treatment of hyperglycaemia are reviewed in this chapter. Control of blood glucose is a key objective in the management of IDDM and NIDDM [1, 2], and compelling evidence now testifies that better control helps to defer the onset and reduce the severity of microvascular complications [3, 4]. However, limitations in the use of existing drugs make it difficult to achieve near-normal blood glucose control. Moreover, existing drugs fail to reinstate entirely normal glucose homeostasis [5, 6].

Hyperglycaemia is typically a sign of impaired cellular glucose utilization *and* excessive glucose production, consequent to defects in the secretion and actions of insulin. Thus, the basis for relieving the hyperglycaemia should address the underlying defects of glucose metabolism. Any new drug should ideally offer some advantage over existing therapies, not only in efficacy, tolerability and safety, but in mode of action and effects on accompanying disorders (e.g. dyslipidaemia) that might benefit a particular subpopulation of patients. A distinction exists between antihyperglycaemic and hypoglycaemic drugs—only the latter carrying the risk of clinical hypoglycaemia [7, 8]. Hence it is prudent that hypoglycaemic drugs should not compromise the mechanisms for counter-regulation.

Preclinical studies provide valuable guidance in the selection of compounds for clinical evaluation, and in determining their mode of action [9]. However, glucose-lowering activity in animal models does not predict efficacy in clinical diabetes, and animal studies may not reveal safety issues implicit in very long-term clinical treatment. Many compounds possess blood glucose-lowering properties, as described elsewhere [7–13], but only those presently attractive to pharmaceutical development are discussed herein. It is impossible to include all potential drugs, and inevitably this 'snap-shot' of the field will soon be superseded. For convenience the various agents have been grouped according to their main site of action or cellular target, as summarized in Table 1, although it

Table 1 Sites of action of blood glucose-lowering agents

Intestine
    Inhibitors of carbohydrate digestion
    Inhibitors of glucose absorption
Insulin supply
    Insulin analogues with 'selected' pharmacokinetics
    Insulin delivery routes and gene therapy
    Insulin secretagogues
Insulin action
    Insulin mimetics
    Insulin potentiators
Hepatic glucose output and peripheral glucose utilization
    Inhibitors of counter-regulatory hormones
    Antilipolytic agents
    Inhibitors of long-chain fatty acid oxidation
    Inhibitors of gluconeogenic enzymes
    Inhibitors of VLDL synthesis
    Stimulants of glucose metabolism
    Stimulants of glycogenesis
    Inhibitors of glycogenolysis

International Textbook of Diabetes Mellitus, Second Edition. Edited by K.G.M.M. Alberti, P. Zimmet, R.A. DeFronzo, and H. Keen (Honorary)
© 1997 John Wiley & Sons Ltd

will be appreciated that some agents exert effects on several different targets.

INHIBITORS OF CARBOHYDRATE DIGESTION AND ABSORPTION

Treatments which slow the rate of glucose absorption from the intestinal tract can delay and reduce post-prandial excursions of hyperglycaemia. This has been achieved by reducing the rate of carbohydrate diges-tion, altering the rate of gastrointestinal transit, and physically trapping nutrients within the lumen so as to restrict access to the intestinal epithelium.

Alpha-glucosidase Inhibitors

The term alpha-glucosidase inhibitor has been applied to inhibitors of alpha-amylase (which digests starch) and of brush-border oligosaccharidases and disaccharidases (e.g. maltase, glucoamylase and sucrase) which cleave off glucose. Agents directed primarily against alpha-amylase have been difficult to

adapt to the digestive process [14]. Alpha-amylase is delivered in both saliva and pancreatic juice, and acts rapidly, often completing starch hydrolysis with salivary amylase alone. Brush-border alpha-glucosidases have proved to be a more amenable target. However, the use of inhibitors against these enzymes still requires careful titration of dosage in relation to the quality and quantity of the diet. The inhibitory activity should be sufficient to extend the course of digestion along the intestinal tract, but not to prevent the completion of digestion and absorption before passage into the large bowel. Sugars entering the large bowel can be osmotically active and fermented by the local flora, causing diarrhoea and flatulence.

Acarbose (BAY g5421) is a pseudotetrasaccha-ride produced by Actinomycetes (Figure 1). It com-petitively inhibits mainly brush-border glucoamylase, sucrase and maltase, with a slight inhibition of alpha-amylase. Acarbose delays and reduces postprandial hyperglycaemia after a carbohydrate meal (14–16). It has been used effectively in NIDDM as a monotherapy and in combination with sulphonylureas. Acarbose

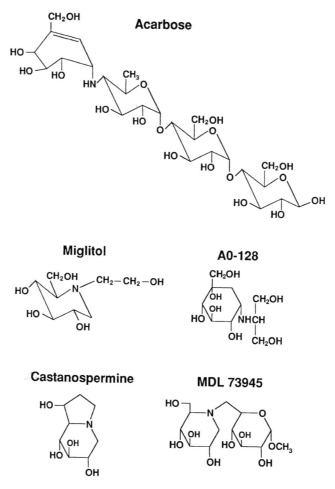

Figure 1 Molecular structures of alpha-glucosidase inhibitors: acarbose, miglitol, A0-128 (voglibose), castanospermine and MDL 73945

has also been used in combination with insulin in IDDM. Treatment with acarbose can reduce the insulin response in NIDDM and reduce the dosage of insulin required in IDDM [17, 18]. In some patients the anti-hyperglycaemic effect has been protracted, resulting in a lower basal glycaemia the following morning. However, reductions in glycated haemoglobin have been variable and usually modest. The effectiveness of acarbose is enhanced by good dietary compliance and by consumption of the drug together with each meal. However, the therapeutic index is relatively narrow and evidence of malabsorption is not uncommon. Acarbose therapy is often accompanied by a reduction in VLDL-triglyceride concentrations, but the mechanism is uncertain.

More than 75% of an oral dose of acarbose is broken down by amylases in the small intestine and by bacteria in the large bowel. Some metabolites and a little acarbose itself are absorbed and rapidly excreted in the urine. Acarbose is now available in the USA and many European countries.

Several derivatives of desoxynojirimycin are competitive inhibitors of alpha-glucosidases with similar activity to acarbose. Amongst these miglitol (BAY m1099) (Figure 1) has attracted interest because it is short-acting and appears to reduce the occurrence of malabsorption [14, 19–21]. Miglitol is almost completely absorbed by the intestine and rapidly eliminated unchanged in the urine. It may also exert a blood glucose-lowering effect that is independent of its alpha-glucosidase inhibition [22].

Derivatives of valiolamine inhibit alpha-glucosidase activity [23], and one member of this series with potent anti-sucrase activity, A0-128 (voglibose), has shown encouraging results in preclinical studies [24]. A long-acting inhibitor of sucrase with an inhibitory effect on most alpha-glucosidases is the alkaloid castanospermine [25], also renowned for its inhibitory effect on the growth of the human immunodeficiency virus (HIV). Another long-acting inhibitor of brush-border alpha-glucosidase activity is MDL 73945, which has shown a marked reduction in the glycaemic response to sucrose during preclinical tests [26].

Plant Fibre Supplements

Non-digestible plant fibres, mainly non-starch polysaccharides and lignin, present a diffusional barrier by entrapping carbohydrates within their matrix. This reduces the rate of carbohydrate digestion by luminal amylases and impedes the interaction of carbohydrates with brush-border enzymes. By restricting diffusional movement adjacent to the intestinal epithelium, fibrous materials also slow the rate of glucose absorption [27, 28].

Bulky viscous soluble fibres such as guar (Figure 2) prolong gastric emptying and extend intestinal transit time, whereas insoluble fibres such as wheat bran can reduce transit times, depending on fibre coarseness. Both types of fibre reduce postprandial glycaemia in diabetic patients. They can also reduce the insulin response in NIDDM and the insulin requirement in IDDM. Taken as a dietary supplement, soluble fibre appears to produce a greater antihyperglycaemic effect than insoluble fibre, provided that the supplements are thoroughly mixed with the food. Soluble fibre also reduces circulating LDL-cholesterol concentrations, and there are reports of a decrease in VLDL-triglyceride during long-term use [27, 28].

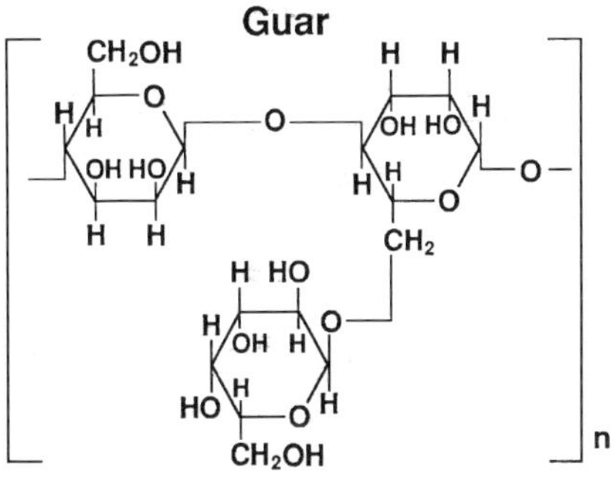

Figure 2 Molecular structure of guar gum, a soluble galactomannan polysaccharide fibre derived from the cluster bean *Cyamopsis tetragonolobus*

Various fibre supplements are available, of which guar has been studied most extensively. Soluble fibre supplements should be taken with ample water and preferably mixed with or consumed at the same time as a meal. Unpalatability, abdominal distension and flatulence are drawbacks, and there have been isolated accounts of intestinal obstruction. The possibility that some types of fibre might interfere with the absorption of other medicines or micronutrients should be borne in mind.

Plants rich in fibre are widely used as traditional treatments for diabetes [29]. Interestingly, some of their polysaccharide fibre components have been reported to lower blood glucose concentrations after intraperitoneal administration to animals, raising the possibility of activity that is independent of an intestinal fibre effect [30]. This effect has been substantiated with a synthetic branching glucopyranan polysaccharide which shows hypoglycaemic activity after intraperitoneal administration [31].

NEW APPROACHES TO INSULIN THERAPY

Other chapters review recent developments with insulin analogues (Chapter 40), oral and nasal insulin preparations (Chapter 41), islet transplants (Chapter 45) and the possibility of an implantable bioartificial pancreas (Chapter 43).

Gene Therapy

Somatic cell gene therapy offers a further means of insulin replacement therapy without daily intervention by the patient. In principle, a chosen type of somatic cell (not an islet B cell) could be taken from a diabetic donor, genetically engineered to produce insulin and returned to the donor (Figure 3). This might be accomplished by introducing and activating new copies of the genes encoding preproinsulin plus the enzymes required for processing to insulin. Additional genes encoding regulatory elements might also confer glucose sensitivity [42]. Implants of insulin-secreting pituitary cells and proinsulin-secreting fibroblasts have been shown to influence glycaemic control in diabetic animals [43, 44], and glucose sensitivity in the millimolar range has been conferred on pituitary cells by 'engineering' them to express Glut-2 [45].

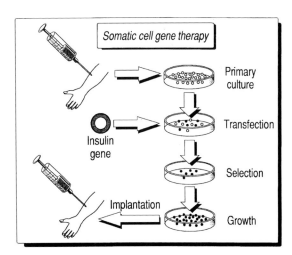

Figure 3 Schematic representation of *ex-vivo* somatic cell gene therapy applied to the delivery of insulin

By selecting a readily accessible and robust cell type such as a fibroblast, somatic cell gene therapy offers the potential advantage of requiring minimum surgical intervention. Also it does not require immunosuppression, since the patient's own cells would be implanted. The performance of the 'engineered' cells can be assessed *in vitro* before implantation, and extra cells can be cryopreserved for future use. Cells for implantation could be encapsulated to guard against uncontrolled growth and to facilitate retrieval at a later time [42].

INSULIN SECRETAGOGUES

Abnormalities of insulin secretion occur early in the pathogenesis of IDDM and NIDDM, but the therapeutic use of insulin secretagogues is confined to NIDDM patients, since these patients (by definition) retain a working B cell population. A notable feature of NIDDM is that the acute insulin response to glucose is impaired, and the later phase of glucose-induced insulin secretion becomes impaired as the diabetic condition worsens. However, the insulin responses to arginine, glucagon, sulphonylureas, gastrointestinal hormones and beta-adrenoreceptor agonists are well preserved, at least until hyperglycaemia becomes severe [46] (see Chapter 31).

The pathway of glucose-induced insulin secretion within the islet B cell (see Chapter 15) is illustrated in Figure 4. Glut-2 transfers glucose into the cell in direct proportion to the extracellular glucose concentration. Glucose phosphorylation by glucokinase is the rate-limiting step for commitment of glucose into glycolysis, resulting mainly in increased aerobic glucose metabolism and ATP production. An increase in the ATP:ADP ratio closes ATP-sensitive potassium efflux channels, thereby decreasing potassium efflux and facilitating membrane depolarization. Membrane depolarization activates voltage-dependent calcium influx channels and the consequent rise in cytosolic calcium activates calcium-dependent regulatory proteins. Calcium itself, and intracellular messengers activated by the calcium-dependent regulatory proteins activate the contractile proteins responsible for movement of beta-granules to the membrane for exocytosis of insulin.

Targeting Insulin Secretagogues

Figure 4 identifies the many different locations at which potential pharmaceutical insulin secretagogues could be targeted. These can induce insulin secretion, potentiate nutrient-induced insulin secretion or antagonize inhibitors of insulin secretion [47]. The selection of targets remains an open question, since the primary defects within islets B cells of human NIDDM patients have not been clarified. Abnormalities of the ATP-sensitive potassium channels and more distal events have been observed: a defect of glucose sensing is known to occur in a proportion of patients with maturity onset diabetes of the young (MODY) due to a glucokinase gene defect: and defects of islet glucose metabolism have been identified in some animal models of NIDDM [48].

Irrespective of the targets chosen, it would be advantageous for insulin secretagogue therapy to restore B-cell responsiveness to glucose while preserving the regulatory effects of other nutrients, ions, hormones and neurotransmitters. It is also necessary to ensure

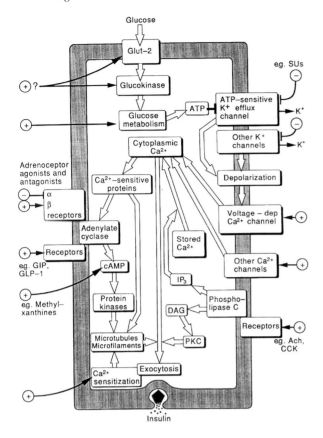

Figure 4 The pathway of glucose-induced insulin secretion by an islet B cell, showing sites at which insulin secretagogues can be targeted. Glut-2 = glucose transporter isoform 2; ATP = adenosine triphosphate; IP_3 = inositol-1,4,5-trisphosphate; DAG = diacylglycerol; PKC = protein kinase C; cAMP = cyclic $3',5'$-adenosine phosphate; SUs = sulphonylureas; Ach = acetylcholine; CCK = cholecystokinin; GIP = gastric inhibitory polypeptide; GLP-1 = glucagon-like peptide-1. Sites at which insulin-secretagogues can be targeted are shown with either ⊕ (stimulatory action) or ⊖ (inhibitory action)

adequate insulin biosynthesis, which is strongly influenced by glucose uptake and metabolism in the B cell [49]. It has recently been noted that glyceraldehyde phosphate and succinate esters are potent stimulants of B cell tricarboxylic acid (TCA) cycle activity, insulin secretion and insulin biosynthesis, whereas other glycolytic intermediates and esters of other TCA cycle intermediates are ineffective [50, 51]. This may be relevant to the targeting of new insulin secretagogue drugs.

ATP-sensitive Potassium Channel Inhibitors

Sulphonylureas such as tolbutamide and glibenclamide close ATP-sensitive potassium channels, causing membrane depolarization leading to insulin release, especially the acute phase [52]. They require the presence of sufficient glucose to support the metabolic needs of

the B cells, but they do not actually restore responsiveness to glucose *per se*. Additions to the existing range of sulphonylureas, such as glimepiride (amaryl), show the same actions as related compounds [53].

Benzoic acid derivatives such as HB699 (meglitinide), which is the non-sulphonylurea portion of glibenclamide (Figure 5), also interact with ATP-sensitive potassium channels to stimulate insulin release. Particularly potent derivatives are receiving scrutiny as prodrugs, including repaglinide (AGEE623ZW) and KAD-1229 [47, 154]. Several other agents which stimulate insulin secretion by

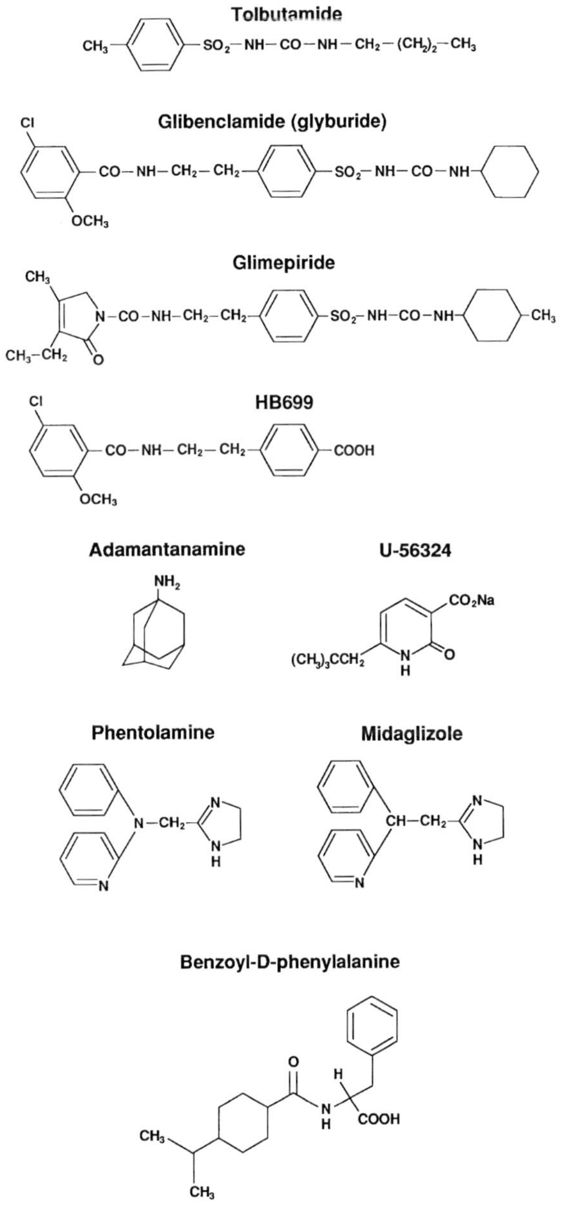

Figure 5 Molecular structures of insulin secretagogues: tolbutamide, glibenclamide, glimepiride (amaryl), HB699 (meglitinide), adamantanamine, U-56324, phentolamine, midaglizole, benzoyl-D-phenylalanine (A-4166)

closure of potassium channels have attracted pharmaceutical interest. These include adamantanamine, U-56324 (nicotinic acid derivative) [54], the amino acid derivative benzoyl-DL-phenylalanine (A-4166) [59], quinine derivatives, sparteine, and disopyramide [47].

Calcium, Cyclic AMP and Adrenoreceptor Manipulators

Agonists of L-type voltage-dependent calcium channels on islet B cells will stimulate insulin secretion, as will agents which mobilize intracellular stores of calcium, but compounds that act on the B cells with high specificity have not been forthcoming. Other nonspecific stimulants which await a tailored analogue include inhibitors of cyclic AMP phosphodiesterases (e.g. methylxanthines) and inhibitors of prostaglandin synthesis (e.g. salicylates).

Receptors coupled to adenylate cyclase have been identified as potentially selective sites for stimulating cyclic AMP, which in turn will potentiate insulin release induced by other agents. Analogues of 'incretins' (insulinotropic gut hormones released during feeding), principally glucagon-like-peptide 1 (7–36) amide and gastric inhibitory polypeptide (GIP), have been contemplated in this respect [55]. Beta-adrenoreceptor agonists, which stimulate insulin release, are probably not specific to the B cell (see Beta$_3$-adrenoreceptor Agonists, below). It has been mooted that selective antagonism of alpha-adrenoreceptors might lift the tonic suppression of insulin secretion normally mediated via these receptors, but achieving selectivity will be difficult. Moreover, several alpha-adrenoreceptor antagonists examined, notably the imidazole derivatives (phentolamine, idazoxan, efaroxan and midaglizole), also appear to bind at other sites on the B cell membrane, and probably stimulate insulin release by closing ATP-sensitive potassium channels [47, 56, 57].

Other Insulin Secretagogues

A number of insulin secretagogues have been considered in a pharmaceutical context, but their mechanism of action has not been clarified, for example the isoxazoyl indole SaRI 59-801 [58].

Several insulin secretagogues previously considered as potential drugs have not proceeded in development. These include the oxazolidinediones and oxazoleacetic acid derivative AD-4610, which showed insufficient activity in man; the benzylalcohol TA-078, which produced cardiovascular side-effects; and the guanidine derivatives linogliride and pirogliride,

which showed CNS and hepatic side effects, respectively [47, 60].

INSULIN MIMETICS

An orally active substitute for insulin has long been sought. Some traditional treatments have claimed to achieve this, but none has stood the test of thorough scrutiny [29]. Many substances can act independently of insulin to lower blood glucose levels and mimic some effects of insulin on cellular metabolism. Thus vitamin K$_5$, certain polyamines such as spermine (Figure 6), and deoxyfrenolicin increase glucose metabolism, but mainly by the pentose phosphate pathway [61]. Oxidants such as diamide, peroxides and phenazine methosulphate increase glucose oxidation, but they do not lend themselves to pharmaceutical development.

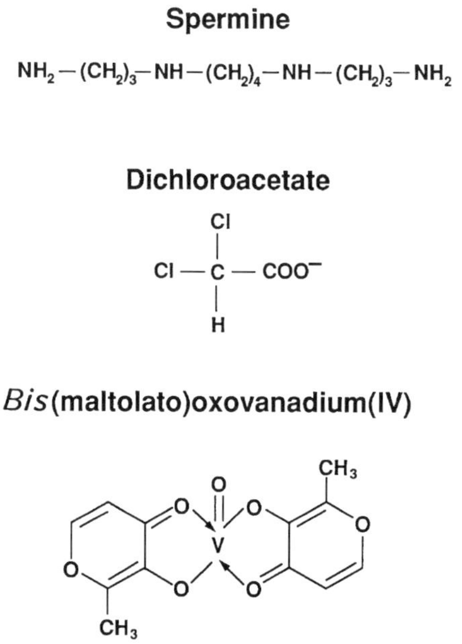

Figure 6 Molecular structures of insulin mimetic agents: spermine, dichloroacetate, a vanadium complex (*bis*-maltolato-oxovanadium IV) (from reference 67, with permission)

Dichloroacetate (Figure 6) and its esters stimulate pyruvate dehydrogenase activity, causing increased glucose oxidation [62]. Hepatic gluconeogenesis is suppressed in part by interrupting the supply of substrate (e.g. lactate), and also because dichloroacetate is metabolized to glyoxylate and then oxalate, which inhibits pyruvate carboxylase. Animal studies have indicated that chronic use of dichloroacetate adversely affects nerve function and lens structure, possibly as a consequence of the oxalate formation.

Vanadium Compounds

The trace element vanadium, and various vanadyl and vanadate salts exert insulin-like effects on glucose metabolism [63, 64]. These agents lower blood glucose levels to near-normal in both obese-hyperinsulinaemic and non-obese-hypoinsulinaemic animal models of diabetes [65, 66]. They act independently of insulin to stimulate glucose uptake, oxidation and glycogenesis in skeletal muscle, and increase glucose uptake, oxidation and lipogenesis in adipocytes. This may result in part from increased phosphorylation of insulin receptors, associated with inhibition of phosphotyrosine phosphatases and stimulation of tyrosine kinases. Effects distal to the insulin receptor have also been reported, and some vanadium compounds (e.g. pervanadates) appear to exert effects that are additive to insulin. Vanadium compounds additionally act as appetite suppressants: they decrease the rate of intestinal glucose absorption and may weakly facilitate insulin release by increasing phosphoinositide turnover and intracellular calcium mobilization in islet B cells.

Vanadium compounds are poorly absorbed from the alimentary tract, and there is only a narrow therapeutic index before toxic effects ensue. Thus more potent, less toxic and more readily absorbed vanadium-containing compounds are under investigation (Figure 6) [64, 67].

Other Trace Elements

Other trace metals have been ascribed some insulin-like properties, and have been considered as potential therapeutic interventions where trace element deficiencies exist. Lowered intracellular concentrations of chromium, magnesium and zinc have been noted in some diabetic patients, but dietary supplementation with these elements has not consistently improved glycaemic control [68–70].

In hypoinsulinaemic diabetic animals, magnesium and zinc have shown a more convincing antihyperglycaemic effect, and insulin-like effects on glucose metabolism have been noted with these elements in muscle and fat *in vitro* [71, 72]. Chromium (the so-called glucose tolerance factor) appears to be required for full expression of insulin-stimulated glucose uptake [73]. Magnesium is required for insulin receptor tyrosine kinase activity, while zinc can stimulate glucose uptake independently of insulin receptor binding or receptor tyrosine kinase activity [72, 74, 75].

Lithium salts stimulate glycogenesis *in vitro* and improve glucose homeostasis in hypoinsulinaemic diabetic animals [76]. However, improved glucose homeostasis has not been confirmed in human NIDDM, possibly because lithium salts also suppress insulin secretion. There have been reports that salts of manganese and selenium can exert insulin-like effects *in vivo* and *in vitro* [77, 78].

POTENTIATORS OF INSULIN ACTION

Insulin resistance is a feature of both IDDM and NIDDM, but is of particular pathogenetic importance in the latter [79, 80]. Cellular lesions in the pathways of insulin action appear to vary with the severity of the diabetes. Differences have also been observed between different tissues, possibly reflecting aetiologically and pathogenetically different subpopulations amongst NIDDM patients. Defects of insulin receptor binding occur in NIDDM, and there is often evidence of impaired receptor phosphorylation and tyrosine kinase activity [81–83]. However, these defects may not be rate-limiting for biological actions of insulin, indicating that critical defects are located at more distal steps in the pathways of insulin action [84]. Although insulin-mediated glucose transport into peripheral tissues is impaired, the production of glucose transporters is not consistently deficient, at least not in muscle. This leaves open the possibility that rate-limiting defects can also occur in the mobility and intrinsic activity of glucose transporters [84–87].

Many potential target sites are already apparent for agents designed to improve insulin action (Figure 7), but the identity of the most purposeful targets must wait until the crucial defects in the insulin signalling pathways become resolved [88]. Among presently used orally active treatments for NIDDM, metformin has an important effect to enhance insulin action, and the chronic efficacy of sulphonylureas involves the potentiation of insulin action through effects at unspecified sites within the postreceptor signalling pathways [89].

Thiazolidinediones

Starting with ciglitazone in the early 1980s, many and varied derivatives of the thiazolidinedione family (Figure 8) have been considered for the treatment of insulin resistance [90–93]. The effects of pioglitazone and CS-045 (troglitazone) have been reported in detail, and appear to offer representative information for this family [94–97]. Thiazolidinediones exert an antihyperglycaemic effect in animal models of NIDDM. They act without increasing insulin release, and typically lower plasma insulin concentrations in conditions of hyperinsulinaemia. They also afford protection against the progressive loss of B cell function and islet degeneration in advanced NIDDM in animals. The presence of insulin is required for the antihyperglycaemic effect, and there is little activity in

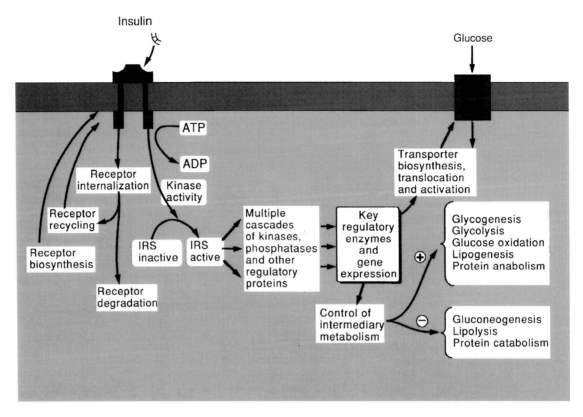

Figure 7 Pathways of insulin action showing sites at which potentiating agents could be targeted. IRS = insulin receptor substrate; positive (⊕) or negative (⊖) influence

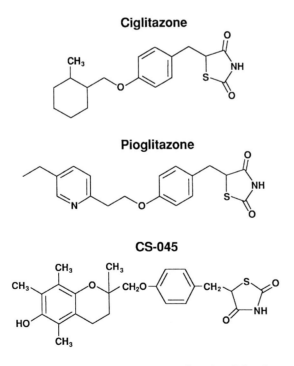

Figure 8 Molecular structures of thiazolidinediones: ciglitazone, pioglitazone, CS-045

conditions of severely insulinopenic diabetes. Thiazolidinediones improve insulin action through an effect distal to insulin receptor binding, possibly by enhancing insulin receptor tyrosine kinase activity and promoting insulin-sensitive transcription events. Preclinical studies have shown that thiazolidinediones increase insulin-stimulated glucose disposal, associated with an increase of insulin-stimulated glucose uptake and metabolism by muscle and fat. Hepatic glucose production is also suppressed, with restored sensitivity to insulin's inhibitory effect on the production of phosphoenolpyruvate carboxykinase. There is a reduction in plasma triglycerides attributed to increased clearance of lipids from the circulation, and an antihypertensive effect has been noted.

As more analogues of the thiazolidinedione family are being synthesized and screened, preliminary clinical trials with CS-045 (troglitazone) are yielding encouraging results in NIDDM patients [98, 99]. However, it must be borne in mind that the development of ciglitazone was discontinued due to limited efficacy in man, and the perfluoro anilides, which are hypoglycaemic analogues of ciglitazone, incur hepatomegaly [100]. Preliminary evidence of anaemia and cardiac hypertrophy has been noted with the thiazolidinedione TA-174 during studies in dogs, and the long-term safety of other thiazolidinediones is receiving careful scrutiny.

Human Growth Hormone Fragments

Human growth hormone (hGH) exerts both insulin-like and insulin-antagonistic effects, the latter usually predominating in the long term [101]. Insulin-like activity is conferred by a hexapeptide sequence near the amino terminal (hGH 8-13; Arg, Leu, Phe, Asp, Asn, Ala) [102]. A slightly extended fragment with greater stability (hGH 6-13) has confirmed that the insulin-like activity is mainly due to the potentiation of insulin action [103]. The fragment increased insulin-mediated glucose uptake, oxidation and glycogenesis in muscle and fat, but was not effective in the absence of insulin. Although insulin receptor binding was increased, the predominant site of action appeared to be distal to the insulin receptor. The ability of hGH 6-13 to improve glucose tolerance may include a component of activity that is independent of insulin, and there may also be modest assistance from increased glucose-induced insulin release, associated with increased islet oxidation of glucose [103]. Analogues with the minimum structure required to retain an insulin-like effect are now being considered [104].

INHIBITORS OF COUNTER-REGULATORY HORMONES

Key hormones that bring about a rise in blood glucose concentrations are glucagon, adrenaline, growth hormone and glucocorticoids [105]. Inappropriately raised concentrations of these hormones can occur in diabetic states [106-108], and the use of specific inhibitors against glucagon and growth hormone has been considered as an approach to improve glycaemic control. However, moderation is essential to preserve an adequate counter-regulatory response to hypoglycaemia [105].

A sulphonamido-benzamide (M & B 39890A) that inhibits glucagon secretion has been shown to exert a hypoglycaemic effect in diabetic animals [109, 110]. Some glucagon analogues have also been shown to exert an antihyperglycaemic effect in animal studies. These peptides compete with native glucagon for receptor binding sites but fail to elicit at least some of the biological effects [111-114]. This raises the possibility that the amino acids primarily responsible for receptor binding are different from those which actually stimulate receptor signalling, offering an interesting mechanism to block glucagon action. However, longer-acting analogues are required to pursue the therapeutic application of this approach.

Somatostatin Analogues

Somatostatin reduces intestinal motility, delays nutrient absorption, and inhibits the secretion of growth hormone and glucagon. Exploitation of these effects in the treatment of diabetic hyperglycaemia is restricted by the short half-life of the molecule; hence longer-acting analogues have been sought [108, 115, 116]. Since somatostatin inhibits insulin secretion, a selective analogue would be advantageous, but this does not present a problem with IDDM patients. The main analogue to receive detailed clinical evaluation, octreotide (Sandostatin, SMS 201-995) (Figure 9), rapidly suppresses growth hormone and glucagon secretion. In IDDM patients there is often a decrease in postprandial glycaemia when the analogue is injected subcutaneously before the meal, and the daily insulin requirement can be reduced by up to 30% [115-117]. Currently available analogues also improve basal metabolic control for up to 6 hours, and reduce ketonaemia [118].

Somatostatin

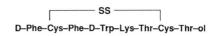

Ala–Gly–Cys–Lys–Asn–Phe–Phe–Trp–Lys–Thr–Phe–Thr–Ser–Cys

Octreotide

D–Phe–Cys–Phe–D–Trp–Lys–Thr–Cys–Thr–ol

Figure 9 Amino acid sequences of somatostatin-14 and the somatostatin analogue octreotide (Sandostatin, SMS 201-995)

It has been suggested that growth hormone-stimulated insulin-like growth factor I production may aggravate proliferative microvascular disease of the diabetic retina. Preliminary evidence has indicated some arrest of proliferative retinopathy during treatment with somatostatin analogues [108]. Reductions of renal hyperfiltration in diabetic patients have also been reported, with a delay in the progression of advanced diabetic nephropathy [108, 119].

MANIPULATORS OF LIPID METABOLISM

Dyslipidaemia occurs commonly in both IDDM and NIDDM, typically including raised plasma concentrations of VLDL-triglycerides and free fatty acids (FFA) (see Chapter 39). Drugs designed primarily to lower blood lipids, and other agents which act via their effects on lipid metabolism, have been considered as potential blood glucose-lowering entities. The rationale for this resides with the glucose–fatty acid (Randle) cycle, which dictates that the rate of glucose metabolism is inversely linked with the rate of fatty acid metabolism [120]. The increased rates of fatty acid oxidation and re-esterification in diabetic states throw the cycle out of balance and contribute to impaired glucose utilization and increased gluconeogenesis [121, 122].

Increased fatty acid oxidation raises the mitochondrial concentration of acetyl CoA, which suppresses the activity of pyruvate dehydrogenase. Fatty acid oxidation also creates a more reduced NADH:NAD ratio and increases citrate production. NADH further suppresses pyruvate dehydrogenase, and citrate inhibits phosphofructokinase. The net result in muscle is a decrease in glucose oxidation, reduced glycolysis and a decrease in glucose uptake. Raised acetyl-CoA stimulates pyruvate carboxylase, and in the liver these combined factors favour gluconeogenesis (Figure 10). Thus, interventions which limit the availability of fatty acids or inhibit

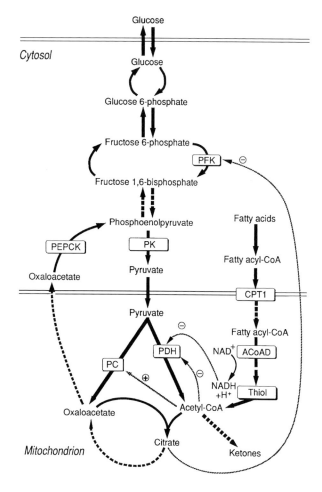

Figure 10 Pathway of long-chain fatty acid oxidation, and its implications for glycolysis, glucose oxidation and gluconeogenesis. ACoAD = acyl-CoA dehydrogenase; Thiol = thiolase; CPT1 = carnitine palmitoyl transferase 1; PDH = pyruvate dehydrogenase; PC = pyruvate carboxylase; PK = pyruvate kinase; PFK = phosphofructokinase; PEPCK = phosphoenolpyruvate carboxykinase; NAD = nicotinamide adenine dinucleotide; NADH = reduced NAD; → single step pathway; - - - → multiple step pathway; ·····→ positive (⊕) or negative (⊖) influence

their oxidation offer a means of increasing glucose utilization and inhibiting gluconeogenesis [123].

Antilipolytic Agents

Nicotinic acid acutely inhibits lipolysis by adipose tissue and lowers plasma FFA [124]. In diabetic states this is accompanied by increased glucose disposal, reduced hepatic glucose output and a lowering of plasma glucose [80]. These actions are short-lived and there is usually a rebound increase in plasma FFA within 3 h, which tends to aggravate the long-term control of hyperglycaemia [123].

The nicotinic acid analogue acipimox (Figure 11) is more potent, longer acting and better tolerated [124, 125]. It exerts a more protracted acute effect on glucose homeostasis, but a significant long-term improvement of glucose homeostasis in NIDDM patients has not been consistently observed [123]. Acipimox may directly enhance glucose utilization independently of its effect on plasma FFA and lipid oxidation [126].

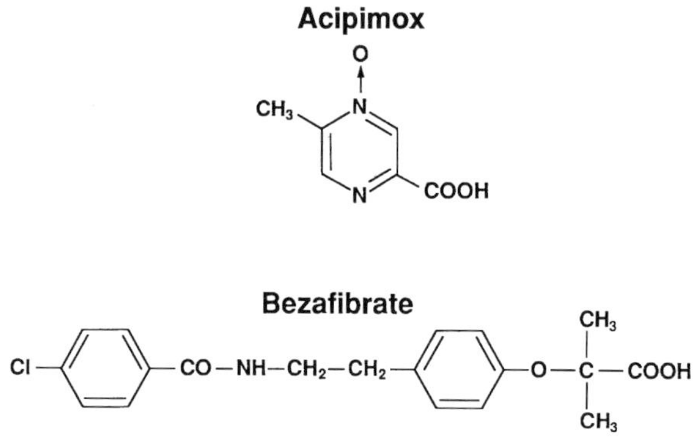

Figure 11 Molecular structures of antilipolytic agents: acipimox, bezafibrate

Lipid-lowering fibric acid derivatives such as clofibrate, and more recently bezafibrate and gemfibrozil, reduce plasma FFA and have been found to improve glucose tolerance in some studies [123, 127, 128].

Adenosine reduces lipolysis in adipocytes partly by inhibiting cAMP formation and possibly also by improving insulin sensitivity. The adenosine agonist phenylisopropyladenosine (PIA) reduced plasma FFA in mildly STZ-diabetic rats, associated with an increase in glucose disposal [80].

Inhibitors of Fatty Acid Oxidation

While agents which lower plasma FFA show a modicum of glucose-lowering activity, agents which directly inhibit the oxidation of long-chain fatty acids appear to be more powerful, and these have received considerable attention. Their major impact on glycaemic control is by suppressing hepatic gluconeogenesis, and they also increase peripheral glucose utilization due to the reduced formation of acetyl-CoA and NADH. A further important effect of reduced fatty acid oxidation is a decrease in ketogenesis. Most inhibitors of long-chain fatty acid oxidation act by inhibiting the enzyme carnitine palmitoyltransferase 1 (CPT1), which is rate-limiting for the transfer of long-chain fatty acyl-CoA into the mitochondria [129, 130]. Other inhibitors of long-chain fatty acid oxidation have been targeted against enzymes which regulate the intramitochondrial beta-oxidation pathway of acyl-CoA, such as acyl-CoA dehydrogenase and thiolase [130].

Aryl-substituted 2-oxirane carboxylic acids such as clomoxir (POCA) and etomoxir (Figure 12) are converted intracellularly to CoA esters which act as irreversible inhibitors of CPT1 [130]. Etomoxir is the more active compound and its hypoglycaemic activity has been demonstrated in preclinical and clinical trials. It is more effective when fatty acid oxidation is raised, notably during fasting and in diabetic states. The hypoglycaemic activity is due to a stronger antigluconeogenic effect than increased peripheral glucose utilization, and occurs without raising insulin [130–132]. Etomoxir is also effective at decreasing ketogenesis, and during chronic (but not acute) treatment there is a decrease in plasma triglycerides.

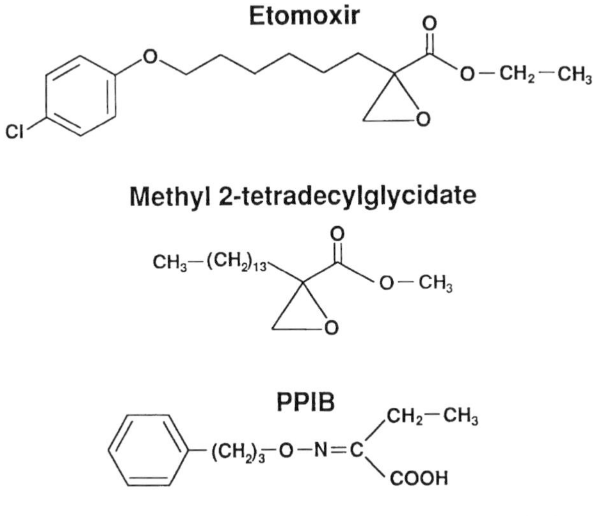

Figure 12 Molecular structures of inhibitors of fatty acid oxidation: etomoxir, methyl 2-tetradecylglycidate (MeTDGA), 2-(3-phenylpropoxyimino)-butyric acid (PPIB)

Closely related to the oxirane carboxylic acids are the alkylglycidates, of which methyl 2-tetradecylglycidate (methyl palmoxirate; MeTDGA) has been studied extensively [133–136]. The intracellularly formed CoA ester irreversibly inhibits CPT1 and produces a

hypoglycaemic effect, due mainly to reduced hepatic glucose production. MeTDGA is potent in conditions of severe hyperglycaemia and insulinopenia, and is especially effective as an antiketogenic agent. It can reduce insulin requirements in IDDM, but it also causes rapid depletion of hepatic glycogen reserves, which enhances vulnerability to precipitous hypoglycaemia. Whether MeTDGA has a role as an adjunct to insulin for the control of ketonaemia remains to be established pending more detailed toxicological considerations.

Hydrazonopropionic acid derivatives are competitive inhibitors of CPT1, lowering blood glucose concentrations by a combination of reduced hepatic gluconeogenesis, increased peripheral glucose utilization and suppression of intestinal glucose absorption [137–139]. There is also a reduction of ketogenesis. In general these compounds do not cause such a strong blockade of long-chain fatty acid oxidation as irreversible CPT1 inhibitors, which may reduce the risk of side effects. Particular interest has been shown in the clinical evaluation of a related compound, 2-(3-phenylpropoxyimino)-butyric acid (PPIB), which offers the advantage of greater stability [139].

ANTI-OBESITY AGENTS

Various compounds designed primarily as anti-obesity agents have proven themselves to have useful blood glucose-lowering and lipid-lowering effects. Treatment with the appetite suppressant fenfluramine was found to improve glycaemic control without stimulating insulin release in obese and non-obese NIDDM patients who were not severely hyperglycaemic. This effect was at least partly independent of any effect on food intake and body weight control [140]. A related compound, benfluorex (Figure 13), which is establishing itself as an antihypertriglyceridaemic agent, also enhances glucose utilization and improves glycaemic control in non-severe NIDDM, often accompanied by a reduction in hyperinsulinaemia [140].

Long-chain dicarboxylic acids such as Medica 16 are lipid-lowering compounds which inhibit hepatic VLDL synthesis and promote adipose tissue lipolysis [141]. They also improve glucose tolerance, apparently by relieving insulin resistance, and are being considered as a potential treatment against the multiple-pathology syndrome of obesity, diabetes, dyslipidaemia and hypertension.

The aetiocholanolones, which are metabolites of dehydroepiandrosterone (DHEA), decrease adiposity in obese-diabetic animals [142]. This often occurs without a change in food consumption, indicating a decrease in metabolic efficiency which has been attributed to increased substrate cycling in the liver [143]. Aetiocholanolones also reduce or prevent hyperglycaemia

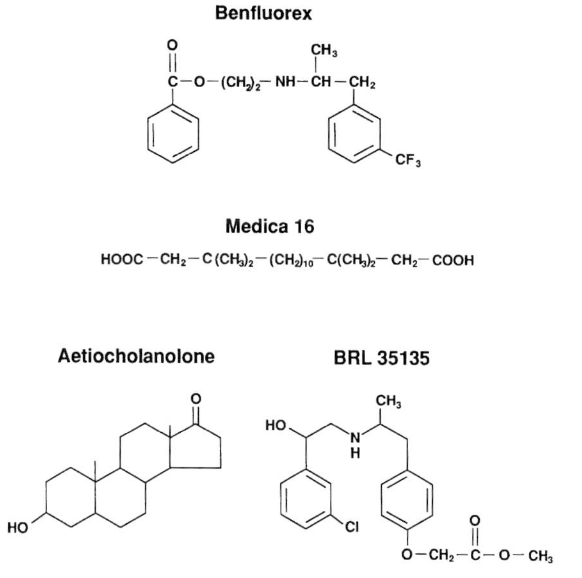

Benfluorex

Medica 16

$HOOC - CH_2 - C(CH_3)_2 - (CH_2)_{10} - C(CH_3)_2 - CH_2 - COOH$

Aetiocholanolone   **BRL 35135**

Figure 13 Molecular structures of anti-obesity agents: benfluorex, medica 16, aetiocholanolone, BRL 35135

in these animals, while lowering plasma insulin concentrations [144]. Improved insulin action, increased hepatic glucose oxidation and a reduction in gluconeogenesis have been considered as possible explanations for the lowering of blood glucose.

Beta₃-adrenoreceptor Agonists

Selective agonists of the beta₃-adrenoreceptors (e.g. BRL 35235 and its metabolite BRL 37344) increase energy expenditure by stimulating thermogenesis in brown adipose tissue. They also increase lipolysis in white adipose tissue and reduce the white adipose tissue mass during chronic treatment in obese animals [145, 146]. Although a single dose of BRL 35135 provokes insulin secretion in obese-diabetic animals, it has no effect or impairs glucose tolerance, possibly due to increased hepatic glucose output. However, chronic treatment improves glucose tolerance at doses which do not affect food intake, body weight or body composition, due mainly to increased insulin-mediated glucose disposal [145, 146]. Preliminary evidence during subchronic trials with NIDDM patients substantiates animal data, although a weak interaction with other beta-adrenoreceptors may cause transient cardiac effects and muscle tremor. Other selective beta₃-adrenoreceptor agonists are planned to enter clinical trial, namely an ethanolamine derivative (ZD 2079) and a benzodioxole dicarboxylate (CL 316,243) [147].

OTHER AGENTS

Many new compounds offer properties that may deserve consideration as potential antidiabetic drugs,

but their evaluation is preliminary as yet. Some of these compounds are considered below to illustrate the diversity of chemical types and biological actions.

Phenacyl imidazolium compounds (e.g. LY177507) show an antihyperglycaemic effect in obese-diabetic animals with increased hepatic glycogenesis due to activation of glycogen synthase and inactivation of glycogen phosphorylase [148, 149]. Glucose analogues are being designed as inhibitors of glycogen phosphorylase [150], and an inhibitor of glucose-6-phosphatase is being sought in the traditionally used antidiabetic plant *Coccinia indica* [151]. Variously modified biguanides are under investigation to increase glucose utilization and reduce hepatic gluconeogenesis [152], and certain carboximidamides, which are related to the guanidine insulin-secretagogue linogliride, have recently been shown to offer potential for development as hypoglycaemic agents [153]. Thiopyranopyrimidine derivatives have been identified with extra-pancreatic (e.g. MTP-3631) and also insulin-releasing (MTP-1307) activity [32, 33], while an antioxidant derivative of probucol (MDL 29311) shows both lipid-lowering and glucose-lowering activity in streptozotocin-diabetic rodents [34]. A non-androgenic analogue of dehydroepiandrosterone has been found to improve glucose homeostasis in obese-diabetic mice [35], and new inhibitors of fatty acid oxidation are being evaluated, such as the dioxolane compound SDZ 51641 [36]. A beta-adrenoreceptor agonist (Ro 16-8714) has been shown to decrease hepatic glucose production and increase glucose oxidation in some types of muscle [37], and interest continues in the possibility of increasing insulin release by antagonizing B cell alpha-adrenoreceptors [38].

Amylin Agonists and Antagonists

Islet amyloid polypeptide (IAPP or amylin) (see also Chapter 19) has been implicated in the pathogenesis of NIDDM [39, 40]. The peptide is produced by islet B cells and co-secreted with insulin. Fibrils produced by self-aggregation of IAPP occur intracellularly and accumulate extracellularly in the islets of ageing NIDDM patients. IAPP is believed to act as an autocrine and paracrine inhibitor of glucose-induced insulin secretion. Recently an IAPP antagonist (IAPP 8-37) has been reported to improve insulin secretion by rat islets [41], but its effect on fibril accumulation is difficult to test, since rodent IAPP has a slightly different structure and does not self-aggregate. The use of transgenic mice with the human IAPP gene may help to address this problem. Very high concentrations of IAPP impair insulin action but this does not appear to be relevant to the usual circulating concentrations of IAPP. Agents are contemplated that could prevent the synthesis of IAPP, possibly at the level of transcription. Interestingly, low dosages of the human IAPP analogue AC137 (pramlintide) improved glycaemic control when administered in combination with insulin to IDDM and NIDDM patients.

CONCLUSIONS

The scientific literature and patent files contain numerous accounts of blood glucose-lowering agents. Many are described as potential new drugs, but they have not proceeded into pharmaceutical development for reasons that are never disclosed. Others are known to be excluded by limitations of efficacy in man, or by toxicological, pharmacokinetic or formulation problems. Some continue in development pending attempts to improve potency, enhance specificity or eliminate untoward side effects. Which new entities will eventually find a place in the future routine management of diabetes is impossible to predict. There are many different potential target sites, but given the heterogeneity and multiple pathologies of diabetic syndromes, there is ample scope for therapeutic attack on several 'fronts'. As the basis for effective relief of hyperglycaemia, ideal treatments will contribute to the restoration of a normal physiological process of glucose homeostasis.

REFERENCES

1. Cahill GF, Etzwiler DD, Freinkel N. 'Control' and diabetes. New Engl J Med 1976; 294: 1004-5.
2. Alberti KGMM, Gries FA, Jervell J, Krans HMJ. A desktop guide for the management of non-insulin-dependent diabetes mellitus (NIDDM): an update. Diabetic Med 1994; 11: 899-909.
3. Singh BM, Nattrass M. Diabetes mellitus and the control of hyperglycaemia. In Bailey CJ, Flatt PR (eds) New antidiabetic drugs. London: Smith-Gordon, 1990; pp 1-18.
4. The Diabetes Control and Complications Trial Research Group. The effect of intensive treatment of diabetes on the development and progression of long-term complications in insulin dependent diabetes mellitus. New Engl J Med 1993; 329: 977-86.
5. Zinman B. The physiologic replacement of insulin. An elusive goal. New Engl J Med 1989; 321: 363-70.
6. Bilous RW, Alberti KGMM. Insulin treatment: efficacy and inadequacy. In Bailey CJ, Flatt PR (eds) New antidiabetic drugs. London: Smith-Gordon, 1990; pp 19-32.
7. Bailey CJ, Flatt PR, Marks V. Drugs inducing hypoglycemia. Pharmac Ther 1989; 42: 361-84.
8. Bailey CJ. Hypoglycaemic, antihyperglycaemic and antidiabetic drugs. Diabet Med 1992; 9: 482-3.
9. Bailey CJ, Flatt PR. Models for testing new hypoglycemic drugs. In Bailey CJ, Flatt PR (eds) New antidiabetic drugs. London: Smith-Gordon, 1990; pp 65-82.
10. Steiner KE, Lien EL. Hypoglycemic agents which do not release insulin. Prog Med Chem 1987; 24: 209-48.
11. Srivastava KV, Pandeya SN. Recent trends in hypoglycemic research. J Sci Indust Res 1988; 47: 706-21.
12. Atta-ur-Rahman, Zaman K. Medicinal plants with hypoglycemic activity. J Ethnopharmacol 1989; 26: 1-55.
13. Bressler R, Johnson DG. New pharmacological approaches to therapy of NIDDM. Diabetes Care 1992; 15: 792-805.
14. Taylor RH. Alpha-glucosidase inhibitors. In Bailey CJ, Flatt PR (eds) New antidiabetic drugs. London: Smith-Gordon, 1990; pp 119-32.
15. Jenkins DJA, Taylor RH, Goff DV, Fielden H, Misiewicz JJ, Sarson DL et al. Scope and specificity of acarbose in slowing carbohydrate absorption in man. Diabetes 1981; 30: 951-4.
16. Clissold SP, Edwards C. Acarbose, a preliminary review of its pharmacodynamic and pharmacokinetic properties, and therapeutic potential. Drugs 1988; 35: 214-43.
17. Dimitriadis GD, Tessari P, Go VLW, Gerich JE. α-Glucosidase inhibition improves postprandial hyperglycaemia and decreases insulin requirements in insulin dependent diabetes mellitus. Metabolism 1985; 34: 261-5.
18. Hotta N, Kakuta H, Sano T, Matsumae H, Yamada H. Long-term effect of acarbose on glycaemic control in non-insulin dependent diabetes mellitus: a placebo-controlled double-blind study. Diabet Med 1993; 10: 134-8.
19. Taylor RH, Barker HM, Bowey EA, Canfield JE. Regulation of the absorption of dietary carbohydrate in man by two new glucosidase inhibitors. Gut 1986; 27: 1471-8.
20. Holt PR, Thea D, Yang MY, Kotler DP. Intestinal and metabolic responses to an alpha-glucosidase inhibitor in normal volunteers. Metabolism 1988; 37: 1163-70.
21. Kingma PJ, Menheere PP, Sels JP, Kruseman AC. Alpha-glucosidase inhibition by miglitol in NIDDM patients. Diabetes Care 1992; 15: 478-83.
22. Joubert PH, Foukaridis GN, Bopape ML. Miglitol may have a blood glucose lowering effect unrelated to inhibition of alpha glucosidase. Eur J Clin Pharmacol 1987; 31: 723-4.
23. Horii S, Fukase H, Matsuo T, Kameda Y, Asano N, Matsui K. Synthesis and α-D-glucosidase inhibitory activity of N-substituted valiolamine derivatives as potential oral antidiabetic agents. J Med Chem 1986; 29: 1038-46.
24. Odaka H, Shino A, Ikeda H, Matsuo T. Antiobesity and antidiabetic actions of a new potent disaccharide inhibitor in genetically obese-diabetic mice KKA(y). J Nutr Sci Vitaminol 1992; 38: 27-37.
25. Rhinehart BL, Robinson KM, Payne AJ, Wheatley ME, Fisher JL, Liu PS, Cheng W. Castanospermine blocks the hyperglycaemic response to carbohydrates in vivo: a result of intestinal disaccharidase inhibition. Life Sci 1987; 41: 2325-31.
26. Robinson KM, Begovic ME, Rhinehart BL, Heineke EW, Ducep JB, Kastner PR et al. New potent α-glucohydrolase inhibitor MDL 73945 with long duration of action in rats. Diabetes 1991; 40: 825-30.
27. Vinik AI, Jenkins DJA. Dietary fiber in management of diabetes. Diabetes Care 1988; 11: 160-73.
28. Nuttall FQ. Dietary fiber in the management of diabetes. Diabetes 1993; 42: 503-8.

29. Bailey CJ, Day C. Traditional plant medicines as treatments for diabetes. Diabetes Care 1989; 12: 553–64.

30. Day C. Hypoglycaemic compounds from plants. In Bailey CJ, Flatt PR (eds) New antidiabetic drugs. London: Smith-Gordon, 1990; pp 267–78.

31. Hakanka K, Song SC, Maruyama A, Kobayashi A, Kuzuhara H, Akaike T. A new synthetic hypoglycemic polysaccharide. Biochem Biophys Res Commun 1992; 188: 16–19.

32. Kunoh Y, Ogawa H, Nagasaka M, Asai H, Iguchi A, Niki A, Sakamoto N. Pharmacological studies on the hypoglycemic effect of 7,8-dihydro-2-(4-methylpiperazinyl)-4-(1(1-pyrrolidinyl)-6H-thiopyrano ⟨3,2−D⟩ pyrimidine dimaleate (MTP-1307), a novel hypoglycaemic agent. Arch Int Pharmacodyn 1989; 298: 276–87.

33. Ogawa H, Kunoh Y, Sugiura T, Nagasaka M. Hypoglycaemic activities of MTP-3631, a novel thiopyranopyrimidine derivative. Life Sci 1992; 50: 375–81.

34. Johnson MB, Heineke EW, Rhinehart BL, Sheetz MJ, Barnhart RL, Robinson KM. MDL 29311. Antioxidant with marked lipid- and glucose-lowering activity in diabetic rats and mice. Diabetes 1993; 42: 1179–86.

35. Pashko L, Schwartz AG. Antihyperglycemic effect of dehydroepiandrosterone analogue 16α-fluoro-5-androsten-17-one in diabetic mice. Diabetes 1993; 42: 1105–8.

36. Young DA, Ho RS, Bell PA Cohen DK, McIntosh R, Nadelson J, Foley JE. Inhibition of hepatic glucose production by SDZ 51641. Diabetes 1990; 39: 1408–13.

37. Ferre P, Penicaud L, Hitier Y, Meier M, Girard J. Hypoglycemic effects of a beta-agonist, RO 16-8714, in streptozotocin diabetic rats: decreased hepatic glucose production and increased glucose utilization in oxidative muscles. Metabolism 1992; 41: 180–3.

38. Ortiz-Alonso FJ, Herman WH, Gertz BJ, Williams VC, Smith MJ, Halter JB. Effect of an oral α-adrenergic blocker (MK-912) on pancreatic islet function in non-insulin dependent diabetes mellitus. Metabolism 1991; 40: 1160–7.

39. Steiner DF, Ohagi S, Nagamatsu, Bell GI, Nishi M. Is islet amyloid a significant factor in pathogenesis or pathophysiology of diabetes? Diabetes 1991; 40: 305–9.

40. Westermark P, Johnson KH, O'Brien TD, Betsholtz C. Islet amyloid polypeptide: a novel controversy in diabetes research. Diabetologia 1991; 35: 297–303.

41. Wang ZL, Bennet WM, Ghatei MA, Byfield PGH, Smith DM, Bloom SR. Influence of islet amyloid polypeptide and the 8–37 fragment of islet amyloid polypeptide on insulin release from perifused rat islets. Diabetes 1993; 42: 300–35.

42. Bailey CJ, Docherty K. Exploring the feasibility of insulin gene therapy. In Flatt PR, Lenzen S (eds) Frontiers of insulin secretion and pancreatic B cell research. London: Smith-Gordon, 1994; pp 613–20.

43. Selden RF, Skoskiewicz MJ, Russell PS, Goodman HM. Regulation of insulin gene expression. Implications for gene therapy. New Engl J Med 1987; 317: 1067–76.

44. Stewart C, Taylor NA, Docherty K, Bailey CJ. Insulin delivery by somatic cell gene therapy. J Mol Endocrinol 1993; 11: 335–41.

45. Hughes SD, Johnson JH, Quaade C, Newgard CB. Engineering of glucose-stimulated insulin secretion and biosynthesis in non-islet cells. Proc Natl Acad Sci USA 1992; 89: 688–92.

46. Flatt PR, Bailey CJ, Berggren PO, Herberg L, Swanson-Flatt SK. Defective insulin secretion in diabetes and insulinoma. In Flatt PR (ed.) Nutrient regulation of insulin secretion. London: Portland Press, 1992; pp 341–86.

47. Henquin JC. Established, unsuspected and novel pharmacological insulin secretagogues. In Bailey CJ, Flatt PR (eds) New antidiabetic drugs. London: Smith-Gordon, 1990; pp 93–106.

48. Bailey CJ, Flatt PR. Islet defects and insulin resistance in models of obese non-insulin dependent diabetes. Diabet Metab Rev 1993; 9 (suppl. 1): 43S–50S.

49. Docherty K, Clark AR. Nutrient regulation of insulin gene expression. FASEB J 1994; 8: 20–7.

50. MacDonald MJ, Fahien LA. Glyceraldehyde phosphate and methyl esters of succinic acid. Two new potential insulin secretagogues. Diabetes 1988; 37: 997–9.

51. Malaisse WJ, Sener A. Metabolic effects and fate of succinate esters in pancreatic islets. Am J Physiol 1993; 264: E434–40.

52. Panten U, Burgfeld J, Goerke F, Rennicke M, Schwanstecher M, Wallasch A et al. Control of insulin secretion by sulfonylureas, meglitinide, and diazoxide in relation to their binding to the sulfonylurea receptor in pancreatic islets. Biochem Pharmacol 1989; 38: 1217–25.

53. Geisen K. Special pharmacology of the new sufonylurea glimepiride. Arzneimittelforschung 1988; 38: 1120–30.

54. Hopkins WF, Fatherazi S, Cook DL. The oral hypoglycaemic agent, U56324, inhibits the activity of ATP-sensitive potassium channels in cell-free membrane patches from cultured mouse pancreatic B-cells. FEBS Lett 1990; 277: 101–4.

55. Thorens B, Waeber G. Glucagon-like peptide-1 and the control of insulin secretion in the normal state and in NIDDM. Diabetes 1993: 42: 1219–25.

56. Chan SLF, Morgan NG. Stimulation of insulin secretion by efaroxan may involve interaction with potassium channels. Eur J Pharmacol 1990; 176: 87–101.

57. Ohneda K, Ohneda A, Koizumi F. Mechanism of insulin secretion by midaglizole. Diabet Res Clin Pract 1993; 19: 127–32.

58. Hanson RL, Isaacson CM. Stimulation of insulin secretion from isolated rat islets by SaRI 59-801. Relation to cAMP concentration and Ca^{2+} uptake. Diabetes 1985; 34: 691–5.

59. Shinkai H, Sato Y. Hypoglycaemic action of phenylalanine derivatives. In Bailey CJ, Flatt PR (eds) New antidiabetic drugs. London: Smith-Gordon, 1990; pp 249–54.

60. Tuman RW, Tutwiler GF, Bowden CR. Linogliride: a guanidine insulin secretagogue. In Bailey CJ, Flatt PR (eds) New antidiabetic drugs. London: Smith-Gordon, 1990; pp 163–9.

61. Czech MP, Lawrence JC, Lynn WS. Hexose transport in isolated brown fat cells. A model system for investigating insulin action on membrane transport. J Biol Chem 1974; 249: 5421–7.

62. Stacpoole PW, Greene YJ. Dichloroacetate. Diabetes Care 1992; 15: 785–91.
63. Shechter Y. Insulin-mimetic effect of vanadate: possible implications for future treatment of diabetes. Diabetes 1990; 39: 1–5.
64. Posner BI, Shaver A, Fantus IG. Insulin mimetic agents: vanadium and peroxovanadium compounds. In Bailey CJ, Flatt PR (eds) New antidiabetic drugs. London: Smith-Gordon, 1990; pp 107–18.
65. Meyerovitch J, Farfel Z, Sack J, Shechter Y. Oral administration of vanadate normalises blood glucose levels in streptozotocin-treated rats. J Biol Chem 1987; 262: 6658–62.
66. Brichard SM, Bailey CJ, Henquin JC. Marked improvement of glucose homeostasis in diabetic ob/ob mice given oral vanadate. Diabetes 1990; 39: 1326–32.
67. McNeill JH, Yuen VG, Hoveyda HR, Orvig C. *Bis*-(maltolato)oxovanadium(IV) is a potential insulin mimic. J Med Chem 1992; 35: 1489–91.
68. Mertz W. Chromium and its relation to carbohydrate metabolism. Med Clin N Amer 1976; 60: 739–44.
69. Kinlaw WB, Levine AS, Morley JE. Abnormal zinc metabolism in type II diabetes mellitus. Am J Med 1983; 75: 273–7.
70. Paolisso G, Sgambato S, Giugliano D, Torella R, Varricchio M, Scheen AJ et al. Impaired insulin-induced erythrocyte magnesium accumulation is correlated to impaired insulin-mediated glucose disposal in type 2 (non-insulin-dependent) diabetic patients. Diabetologia 1988; 31: 910–15.
71. Rossetti L, Giaccari A, Klein-Robbenhaar E, Vogel LR. Insulinomimetic properties of trace elements and characterization of their *in vivo* mode of action. Diabetes 1990; 39: 1243–50.
72. Shisheva A, Gefel D, Shechter Y, Insulin-like effect of zinc ion *in vitro* and *in vivo*. Diabetes 1992; 41: 982–8.
73. Offenbacher EG, Pi-Sunyer X. Beneficial effect of chromium-rich yeast on glucose tolerance and blood lipids in elderly subjects. Diabetes 1980; 29: 919–25.
74. Sacks DB, McDonald JM. Insulin-stimulated phosphorylation of calmodulin by rat liver insulin receptor preparations. J Biol Chem 1988; 263: 2377–83.
75. Ezaki O. IIb group metal ions (Zn^{2+}, Cd^{2+}, Hg^{2+}) stimulate glucose transport activity by post-insulin receptor kinase mechanism in rat adipocytes. J Biol Chem 1989; 264: 1618–22.
76. Rossetti L. Normalization of insulin sensitivity with lithium in diabetic rats. Diabetes 1992; 38: 648–52.
77. Rubenstein AH, Levin NW, Elliott GA. Manganese-induced hypoglycaemia. Lancet 1962; ii: 1348–51.
78. McNeill JH, Delgatty HLM, Battell ML. Insulin-like effects of sodium selenate in streptozotocin-induced diabetic rats. Diabetes 1991; 40: 1675–8.
79. DeFronzo RA. The triumvirate: B cell, muscle, liver. A collusion responsible for NIDDM. Diabetes 1988; 37: 667–87.
80. Reaven GM. Role of insulin resistance in human disease. Diabetes 1988; 37: 1595–1607.
81. Arner P, Pollare T, Lithell H, Livingston JN. Defective insulin receptor tyrosine kinase in human skeletal muscle in obesity and type 2 (non-insulin dependent) diabetes mellitus. Diabetologia 1987; 30: 437–40.
82. Caro JF, Sinha MK, Raju SM, Ittoop O, Pories WJ, Flickinger EG et al. Insulin receptor kinase in human skeletal muscle from obese subjects with and without non-insulin dependent diabetes. J Clin Invest 1987; 79: 1330–7.
83. Haring HU. The insulin receptor: signalling mechanism and contribution to the pathogenesis of insulin resistance. Diabetologia 1991; 34: 848–61.
84. Haring HU, Mehnert H. Pathogenesis of type 2 (non-insulin dependent) diabetes mellitus: candidates for a signal transmitter defect causing insulin resistance of the skeletal muscle. Diabetologia 1993; 36: 176–82.
85. Pedersen O, Bak JF, Andersen PH, Lund S, Moller DE, Flier JS, Khan BB. Evidence against altered expression of GLUT1 or GLUT4 in skeletal muscle of patients with obesity of NIDDM. Diabetes 1990; 39: 865–70.
86. Sinha MK, Raineri-Maldonado C, Buchanan C, Pories WJ, Carter-Su C, Pilch PF, Caro JF. Adipose tissue glucose transporters in NIDDM. Decreased levels of muscle/fat isoform. Diabetes 1991; 40: 472–7.
87. Pessin JE, Bell GI. Mammalian facilitative glucose transporter family: structure and molecular regulation. Ann Rev Physiol 1992; 54: 911–30.
88. Myers MG, White MF. The new elements of insulin signaling. Insulin receptor substrate-1 and proteins with SH2 domains. Diabetes 1993; 42: 643–50.
89. Bailey CJ. Hypoglycaemic and anti-hyperglycaemic drugs for the control of diabetes. Proc Nutr Soc 1991; 50: 619–30.
90. Colca JR, Morton DR. Antihyperglycaemic thiazolidinediones: ciglitazone and its analogues. In Bailey CJ, Flatt PR (eds) New antidiabetic drugs. London: Smith-Gordon, 1990; pp 255–61.
91. Stevenson, RW, Hutson NJ, Krupp MN, Volkmann RA, Holland GF, Eggler JF et al. Actions of novel antidiabetic agent englitazone in hyperglycemic hyperinsulinemic ob/ob mice. Diabetes 1990; 39: 1218–27.
92. Hofmann CA, Colca JR. New oral thiazolidinedione antidiabetic agents act as insulin sensitizers. Diabetes Care 1992; 15: 1075–8.
93. Sohda T, Mizuno K, Momose Y, Ikeda H, Fujita T, Meguro K. Studies on antidiabetic agents. 11. Novel thiazolidinedione derivatives as potent hypoglycemic and hypolipidemic agents. J Med Chem 1992; 35: 2617–26.
94. Hofmann C, Lorenz K, Colca JR. Glucose transport deficiency in diabetic animals is corrected by treatment with the oral antihyperglycemic agent pioglitazone. Endocrinology 1991; 129: 1915–25.
95. Hofmann CA, Edwards CW, Hillman RM, Colca JR. Treatment of insulin-resistant mice with the oral antidiabetic agent pioglitazone: evaluation of liver GLUT2 and phosphoenolpyruvate carboxykinase expression. Endocrinology 1992; 130: 735–40.
96. Fujiwara T, Wade M, Fukuda K, Fukami M, Yoshioka S, Yoshioka T, Horikoshi H. Characterization of CS-0 45, a new oral antidiabetic agent. II. Effects on glycaemic control and pancreatic islet structure at a late stage of the diabetic syndrome in C57BL/KsJ-db/db mice. Metabolism 1991; 40: 1213–18.
97. Yoshioka S, Nishino H, Shiraki T, Ikeda K, Koike H, Okuno A et al. Antihypertensive effects of CS-045 treatment in obese Zucker rats. Metabolism 1993; 42: 75–80.
98. Iwamoto Y, Kuzuya T, Matsuda A, Awata T, Kumakura S, Inooka G, Shiraishi I. Effect of new oral

antidiabetic agent CS-045 on glucose tolerance and insulin secretion in patients with NIDDM. Diabetes Care 1991; 14: 1083–6.

99. Suter SL, Nolan JJ, Wallace P, Gumbiner B, Olefsky JM. Metabolic effects of new oral hypoglycemic agent CS-045 in NIDDM subjects. Diabetes Care 1992; 15: 193–203.

100. Steiner KE, McCaleb ML, Kees KL. Perfluoro anilides: new tools for the study of insulin resistant states. In Bailey CJ, Flatt PR (eds) New antidiabetic drugs. London: Smith-Gordon, 1990; pp 237–44.

101. Wallis M. Mechanism of action of growth hormone. In Cooke BA, King RJB, van der Molen HV (eds) Hormones and their actions, part II. Oxford: Elsevier, 1988: pp 265–94.

102. Ng FM, Bornstein J, Pullin CO, Bromley JO, Macaulay L. The minimal amino acid sequence of the insulin potentiating fragments of human growth hormone—its mechanism of action. Diabetes 1980; 29: 782–7.

103. Ng FM. Human growth hormone fragments. In Bailey CJ, Flatt PR (eds) New antidiabetic drugs. London: Smith-Gordon, 1990; pp 197–206.

104. Ede NJ, Lim N, Rae ID, Ng FM, Hearn MTW. Synthesis and evaluation of constrained peptide analogs related to the N-terminal region of human growth hormone. Peptide Res 1991; 4: 171–6.

105. Cryer PE, Gerich JE. Glucose counterregulation, hypoglycemia, and intestine insulin therapy in diabetes mellitus. New Engl J Med 1985; 313: 232–41.

106. Christensen NJ. Plasma norepinephrine and epinephrine in untreated diabetes during fasting and after insulin administration. Diabetes 1974; 23: 1–8.

107. Unger R, Orci L. Glucagon and the A-cells. Physiology and pathophysiology. New Engl J Med 1981; 304: 1518–24, 1575–80.

108. Harris AG, Gutniak M, Efendic S. Somatostatin analogue therapy of diabetes mellitus. In Bailey CJ, Flatt PR (eds) New antidiabetic drugs. London: Smith-Gordon, 1990; pp 279–88.

109. Tadayyon M, Green I, Cook D, Pratt J. Effect of hypoglycaemic agent M & B 39890A on glucagon secretion in isolated rat islets of Langerhans. Diabetologia 1987; 30: 41–3.

110. Yen TT, Schmiegel KK, Gold G, Williams GD, Dininger NB, Broderick CL, Gill AM. Compound M&B 39890A [N-(3-imidazol-1-ylpropyl)-2-(3-trifluoromethylbenzensulphonamido)-benzamide hydrochloride], a glucagon and insulin secretion inhibitor, improves insulin sensitivity in viable yellow obese mice. Arch Int Pharmacodyn 1991; 310: 162–74.

111. Johnson DG, Goebel CU, Hruby VJ, Bregman MD, Trivedi D. Hyperglycemia of diabetic rats decreased by a glucagon receptor antagonist. Science 1982; 215: 115–16.

112. Corversa S, Huerta-Bahena J, Pelton JT, Hruby VJ, Trivedi D, Garcia-Sainz JA. Metabolic effects and cyclic AMP levels produced by glucagon (1-N^X-trinitrophenylhistidine, 12-homo-arginine)-glucagon and forskolin in isolated rat hepatocytes. Biochim Biophys Acta 1984; 804: 434–41.

113. Unson CG, Gurzenda EM, Iwasa K, Merrifield RB. Glucagon antagonists: contribution to binding and activity of the amino-terminal sequence 1–5, position 12, and the putative α-helical segment 19–27. J Biol Chem 1989; 264: 789–94.

114. Unson CG, MacDonald D, Ray K, Durrah TL, Merrifield RB. Position 9 replacement analogs of glucagon uncouple biological activity and receptor binding. J Biol Chem 1991; 266: 2763–6.

115. Davies RR, Turner SJ, Alberti KGMM, Johnston DG. Somatostatin analogues in diabetes mellitus. Diabet Med 1989; 6: 103–11.

116. Williams G, Bloom SR. Regulatory peptides, the hypothalamus and diabetes. Diabet Med 1989; 6: 472–85.

117. Grossman LD, Shumak SL, George SR. The effects of SMS 201-995 (Sandostatin) on metabolic profiles in insulin-dependent diabetes mellitus. J Clin Endocrinol Metab 1989; 68: 63–7.

118. Scheen AJ, Gillet J, Rosenthaler J. Sandostatin, a new analogue of somatostatin reduces the metabolic changes induced by the nocturnal interruption of continuous subcutaneous insulin infusion in type 1 (insulin-dependent) diabetic patients. Diabetologia 1989; 32: 801–9.

119. Pederson MM, Christensen SE, Christensen JS. Acute effects of a somatostatin analogue on kidney function in type 1 diabetic patients. Diabète Métab 1990; 7: 304–9.

120. Randle PJ, Garland PB, Hales CN, Newsholme EA. The glucose–fatty acid cycle. Its role in insulin sensitivity and the metabolic disturbances of diabetes mellitus. Lancet 1963; i: 785–9.

121. Felber J-P, Ferrannini E, Golay A, Meyer HU, Theibaud D, Curchod B et al. Role of lipid oxidation in pathogenesis of insulin resistance of obesity and type II diabetes. Diabetes 1987; 36: 1341–50.

122. Groop LC, Bonadonna RC, Del Prato S, Ratheiser K, Zyck K, Ferrannini E, DeFronzo RA. Glucose and fatty acid metabolism in non-insulin dependent diabetes mellitus. Evidence for multiple sites of insulin resistance. J Clin Invest 1989; 84: 205–13.

123. Fulcher GR, Alberti KGMM. Hypoglycaemic action of antilipolytic agents. In Bailey CJ, Flatt PR (eds) New antidiabetic drugs. London: Smith-Gordon, 1990; pp 143–55.

124. Fuccella LM, Goldaniga G, Louislo P, Maggi E, Musatti L, Mandelli V, Sirtori CR. Inhibition of lipolysis by nicotinic acid and by acipimox. Clin Pharmacol Ther 1980; 28: 790–5.

125. O'Connor P, Feely J, Shepherd J. Lipid lowering drugs. Br Med J 1990; 300: 667–72.

126. Fulcher GR, Walker M, Farrer M, Johnson AS, Alberti KGMM. Acipimox increases glucose disposal in normal man independent of changes in plasma non-esterified fatty acid concentration and whole body lipid oxidation. Metabolism 1993; 42: 308–14.

127. Jones IR, Swai A, Taylor R, Miller M, Laker MF, Alberti KGMM. Lowering of plasma glucose concentrations with bezafibrate in patients with moderately controlled NIDDM. Diabetes Care 1990; 13: 855–63.

128. Winocour PH, Durrington PN, Bhatnagar D, Ishola M, Arrol S, Lalor BC, Anderson DC. Double-blind placebo-controlled study of the effects of bezafibrate on blood lipids, lipoproteins, and fibrinogen in hyperlipidaemic type 1 diabetes mellitus. Diabetic Med 1990; 7: 736–43.

129. McGarry JW, Foster DW. Regulation of hepatic fatty acid oxidation and ketone body production. Ann Rev Biochem 1980; 49: 395–420.

130. Wolf HPO. Aryl-substituted 2-oxirane carboxylic acids: a new group of antidiabetic drugs. In Bailey CJ,

Flatt PR (eds) New antidiabetic drugs. London: Smith-Gordon, 1990; pp 217–29.

131. Kruszynska YT, Sherratt HSA. Glucose kinetics during acute and chronic treatment of rats with 2-[6-(4-chlorophenoxy)hexyl]oxirane-2-carboxylate, etomoxir. Biochem Pharmacol 1987; 36: 3917–21.

132. Ratheiser K, Schneeweiss B, Waldhausl W, Fasching P, Korn A, Nowotny P et al. Inhibition by etomoxir of carnitine palmitoyltransferase I reduces hepatic glucose production and plasma lipids in non-insulin dependent diabetes mellitus. Metabolism 1991; 40: 1185–90.

133. Lee SM, Bahl JJ, Bressler R. Prevention of the metabolic effects of 2-tetradecylglycidate by octanoic acid in the genetically diabetic mouse (db/db). Biochem Med 1985; 33: 104–9.

134. Ho W, Tutwiler GF, Cottrell SC, Morgans DJ, Tarhan D, Mohbacher RJ. Alkylglycidic acids: potential new hypoglycemic agents. J Med Chem 1986; 29: 2184–90.

135. Tuman RW, Tutwiler GF, Joseph JM, Wallace NH. Hypoglycaemic and hypoketonaemic effects of single and repeated oral doses of methyl palmoxirate (methyl 2-tetradecylglycidate) in streptozotocin/alloxan-induced diabetic dog. Br J Pharmacol 1988; 94: 130–6.

136. Bailey CJ, Flatt PR. Alkylglycidates. In Bailey CJ, Flatt PR (eds) New antidiabetic drugs. London: Smith-Gordon, 1990; pp 231–6.

137. Beneking M, Oellerich M, Haeckel R, Binder L. Inhibition of mitochondrial carnitine acylcarnitine translocase-mediated uptake of carnitine by 2-(3-methyl-cinnamyl-hydrazono)-propionate. J Clin Chem Clin Biochem 1987; 25: 467–71.

138. Binder L, Oellerich M, Haeckel R, Beneking M. Effects of 2-(3-methyl-cinnamyl-hydrazono)-propionate on fatty acid and glucose oxidation in the isolated rat hemidiaphragm using ^{14}C-labelled substrates. J Clin Chem Clin Biochem 1988; 26: 815–19.

139. Haeckel R, Oellerich M, Binder L. Hydrazonopropionic acid derivatives. In Bailey CJ, Flatt PR (eds) New antidiabetic drugs. London: Smith-Gordon, 1990; pp 207–16.

140. Arnaud O, Nathan C. Antiobesity and lipid-lowering agents with antidiabetic activity. In Bailey CJ, Flatt PR (eds) New antidiabetic drugs. London: Smith-Gordon, 1990; pp 133–42.

141. Bar-Tana J, Ben-Shoshan S, Blum J, Migron Y, Hertz R, Pill J et al. Synthesis, hypolipidemic and antidiabetogenic activities of B,B′-tetra-substituted, long-chain dioic acids. J Med Chem 1989; 32: 2072–84.

142. Coleman DL. Antiobesity effects of etiocholanolones in diabetes (db), viable yellow (A^{vy}) and normal mice. Endocrinology 1985; 117: 2279–83.

143. McIntosh MK, Berdanier CD. Antiobesity effects of dehydroepiandrosterone are mediated by futile substrate cycling in hepatocytes of BHE/cdb rats. J Nutr 1991; 121: 2037–43.

144. Coleman DL. Hypoglycaemic action of the aetiocholanolones in mice. In Bailey CJ, Flatt PR (eds) New antidiabetic drugs. London: Smith-Gordon, 1990; pp 191–6.

145. Smith SA, Sennitt MV, Cawthorne MA. BRL 35135: an orally active antihyperglycaemic agent with weight-reducing effects. In Bailey CJ, Flatt PR (eds) New antidiabetic drugs. London: Smith-Gordon, 1990; pp 177–89.

146. Cawthorne MA, Sennit MV, Arch JRS, Smith SA. BRL 3515, a potent and selective atypical B-adrenoceptor agonist. Am J Clin Nutr 1992; 55: 252S–257S.

147. Bloom JD, Dutia MD, Johnson BD, Wissner A, Burns MG, Largis EE et al. Disodium (R,R)-5-[2-[[2-(3-chlorophenyl)-2-hydroxyethyl]amino]propyl]-1,3-benzodioxole-2,2-dicarboxylate (CL 316,243). A potent β-adrenergic agonist virtually specific for β_3 receptors. A promising antidiabetic and antiobesity agent. J Med Chem 1992; 35: 3081–4.

148. Harris R, Yamanouchi K, Roach P, Yen T, Dominianni S, Stephens T. Stabilization of glycogen stores and stimulation of glycogen synthesis in hepatocytes by phenacyl imidazolium compounds. J Biol Chem 1989; 264: 14674–80.

149. Guo ZK, Wals PA, Katz J. Stimulation of glycogen synthesis by proglycosyn (LY 177507) by isolated hepatocytes of normal and streptozotocin diabetic rats. J Biol Chem 1991; 266: 22323–7.

150. Martin JL, Veluraja K, Ross K, Johnson LN, Fleet GW, Ramsden NG et al. Glucose analogue inhibitors of glucogen phosphorylase: the design of potential drugs for diabetes. Biochemistry 1991; 30: 10101–6.

151. Hossain MZ, Shibib BA, Rahman R. Hypoglycemic effects of *Coccinia indica*: inhibition of key gluconeogenic enzyme, glucose-6-phosphatase. Indian J Exp Biol 1992; 30: 418–20.

152. Reitz AB, Tuman RW. Carbohydrate biguanides as potential antidiabetic drugs. In Bailey CJ, Flatt PR (eds) New antidiabetic drugs. London: Smith-Gordon, 1990; pp 171–6.

153. Breslin HJ, Kukla MJ, Tuman RW, Rebarchak MC, Bowden CR. A novel series of N-(1-aminoalkylidene) carboximidamides as potential hypoglycaemic agents. J Med Chem 1993; 36: 1597–1603.

154. Malaisse WJ. Stimulation of insulin release by non-sulfonylurea hypoglycemic agents: the meglitinide family. Horm Metab Res 1995; 27: 263–6.

39

Hypolipidemic Agents: Their Role in Diabetes Mellitus

M.-R. Taskinen* and P.J. Nestel†

University of Helsinki, Finland, and †Flinders University, Adelaide, Australia

Epidemiological and clinical studies have repeatedly demonstrated that diabetic individuals have a 2–4 times higher risk of developing atherosclerotic cardiovascular disease than non-diabetic individuals [1, 2]. The development of atherosclerosis is accelerated, and the condition is more severe and affects both sexes with equal severity in diabetes [1, 3]. The increased risk is particularly striking in women. Common coronary heart disease (CHD) risk factors (hypertension, smoking and dyslipidemias) are operative in diabetes but cannot fully explain the excess risk of CHD [1]. In the Multiple Risk Factor Intervention Trial (MRFIT) the risk of cardiovascular disease (CVD) death was significantly higher at every level of the three major risk factors (serum cholesterol, systolic blood pressure, cigarette smoking) in diabetic than in non-diabetic men [2]. Interestingly, CVD mortality rose much more steeply with higher serum cholesterol in diabetic than non-diabetic men. Thus the absolute risk of CVD death became greater with increasing cholesterol. Although baseline lipoprotein abnormalities predicted CVD mortality in NIDDM patients over 10 years of follow-up, the most powerful predictor of CVD mortality was blood glucose [4]. Diabetes is thus a powerful independent risk factor for CVD mortality. Recent studies have conclusively demonstrated that lowering of serum cholesterol is associated with reduction in CHD risk in the general population [5–7, 8]. The most convincing evidence has emerged from secondary prevention trials which have conclusively shown the benefits of cholesterol lowering [8]. Therefore the treatment of

diabetic patients with high CHD risk should not be neglected; the management of dyslipidemias should be mandatory and even more aggressive in diabetic than in non-diabetic populations.

LIPOPROTEIN PHENOTYPES

Diabetes mellitus is the great imitator and almost all commonly occurring lipoprotein phenotypes have been observed in diabetes. The possibility of diabetes must therefore always be entertained in the differential diagnosis of hyperlipidemia. A further important consideration is the coexistence of two metabolic disorders, diabetes mellitus and hyperlipidemia. The genes that determine both are commonly distributed in many populations. Failure of reasonable diabetic treatment to control hyperlipidemia is not infrequently due to the independent presence of both disorders. This leads to the generalization that diabetic hyperlipidemia should be approached initially as a problem of diabetic control, and that specific lipid-lowering therapy should be considered as part of the evaluation of persisting hyperlipidemia.

Quantitative Changes of Lipoprotein Abnormalities

Diabetes mellitus can result in a profound disturbance of overall lipoprotein metabolism [9, 10, 11]. Characteristic changes of serum lipids and lipoproteins in

International Textbook of Diabetes Mellitus, Second Edition. Edited by K.G.M.M. Alberti, P. Zimmet, R.A. DeFronzo, and H. Keen (Honorary)

Table 1 Serum lipoproteins and apoproteins in treated diabetic patients

	IDDM		NIDDM	
	Good control	Poor control	Good control	Poor control
Chylomicrons	Absent	Minor increase	Absent or minor increase	Increased
VLDL	Normal or minor decrease	Increased	Slightly increased	Increased
IDL	Normal	Increased	Slightly increased	Increased
LDL	Normal or minor decrease	Normal or increased	Normal	Increased
HDL	Normal or increased	Minor decrease	Minor decrease	Reduced
Apoprotein-B	Reduced	Increased	Normal	Increased
Apoprotein-A1	Normal or increased	Reduced	Minor decrease	Reduced
Apoprotein-A2	Normal	Normal or minor decrease	Normal or minor decrease	Reduced
Lp(a)	Normal	Normal or increased	Normal	Normal

Note: at least 25% of all diabetics show some abnormality; frequently several lipoproteins are present in abnormal concentration, giving rise to a variety of phenotypes (e.g. high VLDL + high LDL; high VLDL + low HDL).

both types of diabetes are depicted in Table 1. The lipid abnormalities are most frequent in poorly controlled NIDDM patients who have an atherogenic lipid profile with an increase of both very low-density (VLDL) and low-density lipoproteins (LDL) and low levels of high-density lipoproteins (HDL). In contrast, IDDM patients with good metabolic control exhibit a near-normal lipoprotein profile. Many IDDM patients with intensive insulin treatment and tight control actually have subnormal concentrations of VLDL and LDL. Interestingly, data from the DCCT study indicated that elevations of total and LDL-cholesterol and lower HDL-cholesterol are common in young female IDDM patients [12].

Comprehensive reviews have recently highlighted lipoprotein lipid values in diabetes [13, 14]. The variability stems not only from the degree of severity of the diabetic condition and the adequacy of treatment, but also from the type of diabetes, the nature of therapy and the coexistence of other factors that influence lipid metabolism, such as glycemic control, nephropathy and obesity. The route of insulin delivery in IDDM patients is physiologically important and influences lipoprotein values [15, 16, 17]. Additional interactions may also be important. For instance, the failure of sulfonylurea to raise the HDL concentration in NIDDM [18], in contrast to the beneficial consequence of insulin in IDDM [19], may be attributable as much to the differing metabolic states of the two forms of diabetes as to the treatments.

The degree of derangement is roughly proportional to the severity of other metabolic distortions in both IDDM and NIDDM. Nevertheless, some aspects of lipoprotein regulation are more variable than others, leading to the development of characteristic lipoprotein phenotypes which parallel the progressive deterioration in the diabetic state. Thus, plasma triglyceride levels rise quite early and correlate with indices of diabetic disturbance, such as glycated Hb in both types of diabetes [12, 20, 21, 22]. The hypertriglyceridemia

is initially confined mainly to VLDL, reflecting overproduction of hepatic triglyceride [9, 10, 11]. In more severe NIDDM, clearance of triglyceride also deteriorates [9, 10, 11], leading to the retention of chylomicron remnants [23]. Interestingly a heterozygote state of lipoprotein lipase (LPL) deficiency has been associated with diabetic lipemia in two recent reports [24, 25]. A clearance defect of triglyceride-rich particles is also present in untreated insulin-deficient or ketoacidotic IDDM patients [10]. Overall improvement of glycemic control, regardless of the method of treatment, is associated with beneficial changes of both VLDL and LDL in both types of diabetes.

Winocour et al [26] reported that in adults with IDDM, hypertriglyceridemia occurred in 31% and hypercholesterolemia in 27% of cases. Compared with IDDM patients, hypertriglyceridemia is more common in NIDDM patients, varying between 20% and 60% in different studies. In the San Antonio Heart Study, 23% of diabetic patients had hypertriglyceridemia or low HDL independently of racial background [27]. Salomaa et al [28] have reported the prevalence of hypertriglyceridemia in a Finnish population to be 47.6% in NIDDM men and 21.9% in IGT men, compared to 15.4% in men with normal OGTT results. Overall the elevation of serum triglycerides is only moderate, the values being 1.5–3 times higher than in sex-, age- and BMI-matched non-diabetic subjects. The plasma total and LDL concentrations are generally normal in 'mild' NIDDM and in well controlled NIDDM and IDDM, but rise if glycemic control deteriorates [9, 10, 12, 14]. Overall the prevalence of hypercholesterolemia is lower in IDDM patients than in non-diabetic subjects if glycemic control is tight [14]. By contrast, data from the Second National Health and Nutrition Examination Survey (NHANES II) in the USA indicate that high or borderline-high total and LDL-cholesterol levels are found in 70% and 67% of adults with diagnosed diabetes, and the majority have clinical coronary heart disease (CHD) or two or more risk factors for CHD [29].

Circulating HDL levels also become disturbed, in particular if diabetic control is poor. However, in most studies no correlation exists between measures of glycemic control and plasma HDL concentration in IDDM [9, 12, 14, 18, 20]. In NIDDM the most common finding is that of reduced HDL concentration, reflecting the hypertriglyceridemic state [9,13, 14, 18]. HDL apo-A1 levels also tend to be reduced in NIDDM, but not as much as HDL-cholesterol. In contrast to NIDDM, HDL levels are normal in IDDM patients with good to moderate glycemic control [14], and may even be raised with optimal insulin treatment [19, 30]. In IDDM changes of HDL generally relate to the HDL_2 subfraction [9, 10, 18, 31]. In line with this we have recently reported that the concentration of HDL particles containing only apoprotein A1 (Lp A1) is elevated in IDDM patients [31].

Because high Lp(a) has been identified as an independent risk factor for CHD [32, 33] much interest has recently been focused on Lp(a) in diabetes. The available information has recently been highlighted by Haffner [34]. Substantial evidence indicates that in IDDM patients without microalbuminuria, nephropathy or macroangiopathy, the concentration of Lp(a) is comparable to that in the non-diabetic population [34, 35, 36, 37, 38], although elevation of Lp(a) has been found in some studies [39, 40, 41]. The data on whether glycemic control influences plasma Lp(a) levels are inconsistent [34]. Evidence from several studies has confirmed the observation by Jenkins et al [42] that in IDDM patients with microalbuminuria and macroalbuminuria, plasma Lp(a) levels are increased [34, 38, 43, 44]. So far the data are insufficient to determine whether or not high Lp(a) levels are a CHD risk factor in IDDM patients [34]. Preliminary data suggested that Lp(a) may be increased in NIDDM patients, but more recent data from studies including altogether more than 600 patients indicate that Lp(a) levels in NIDDM patients are similar to those as in non-diabetic populations [34]. Substantial evidence indicates that improvement of glycemic control has no effect on Lp(a) levels in NIDDM patients [34]. Current evidence also suggests that Lp(a) may not be a risk factor for CHD in diabetes, but more work is required before firm conclusions can be drawn [45, 46].

Dyslipidemia is a core component of the Metabolic Syndrome [47, 48]. The characteristic features are moderate hypertriglyceridemia, lowering of HDL-cholesterol and preponderance of small dense LDL [49]. The association between the combination of high triglycerides with low HDL and insulin resistance has been demonstrated in several studies. Emerging evidence indicates that insulin resistance precedes the development of dyslipidemia [50]. Importantly, individuals at high risk of developing NIDDM (such as normoglycemic relatives of NIDDM patients) have higher triglycerides and lower HDL-cholesterol than individuals without a family history of NIDDM [51, 52]. Similarly, family members of primary hypertriglyceridemic patients are at increased risk of NIDDM [53]. Altogether, the data indicate that dyslipidemia is an early marker of the insulin resistance syndrome.

Qualitative Abnormalities of Lipoproteins

All major lipoproteins (VLDL, IDL and LDL) demonstrate structural heterogeneity and comprise different subclasses. In diabetes multiple abnormalities of both surface and core lipid composition exist in VLDL, LDL and HDL particles and these changes are also reflected in their subclass distribution [14]. Although the concentrations of lipoproteins in IDDM patients with fair to good glycemic control are closely similar to those in the respective non-diabetic populations, VLDL subclasses show a shift toward VLDL particles of smaller size which are triglyceride-poor but cholesteryl-ester rich [54]. Small dense VLDL is considered to be atherogenic [55]. In IDDM patients with poor glycemic control, all three VLDL subclasses (VLDL1 Sf > 100, VLDL2 Sf 60–100 and VLDL3 Sf 20–60) are increased and contain a relative excess of non-apo-B apolipoproteins (apo-Cs and apo-E)[56]. These compositional changes are corrected but not fully restored by intensive insulin regimens [56, 57]. IDDM patients with good glycemic control have large buoyant LDL, but it should be recognized that the size of LDL is closely related to serum triglyceride levels [58]. In line with this, IDDM patients with poor glycemic control or with albuminuria tend to have a preponderance of small dense LDL [56, 58].

In addition to quantitative changes of lipoproteins, NIDDM patients display multiple compositional changes of all major lipoproteins [14]. Recently, James and Pometta reported that all VLDL subclasses are elevated and enriched in free and esterified cholesterol [59]. Triglycerides also accumulate in other lipoproteins, LDL and HDL, reflecting the transfer of these lipids from the primary triglyceride-rich lipoproteins. In line with this, LDL subfractions revealed an aberrant profile with elevation of the small dense LDL subclass (LDL3 fraction) [59]. Emerging evidence indicates that NIDDM subjects do indeed have a high prevalence of small dense LDL and this represents phenotype pattern B, which is highly atherogenic [60, 61, 62, 63]. The clustering of hypertriglyceridemia, low HDL-cholesterol and small dense LDL has been termed the atherogenic lipid profile [64]. However, the size of LDL particles is closely related to the ambient concentration of

VLDL-triglycerides in NIDDM patients, as in non-diabetic populations [62, 63]. Again the compositional alterations of lipoproteins are improved but not fully corrected with improvement of glycemic control, although the concentrations of lipoproteins are normalized [59, 65]. Importantly, these compositional abnormalities cannot be detected by measuring the concentrations of serum cholesterol, triglycerides and HDL-cholesterol. Consequently, the question has been raised whether the threshold values for initiating treatment should be lower in diabetic than in non-diabetic populations.

RATIONALE FOR LIPID-LOWERING AGENTS IN DIABETES MELLITUS

Recent consensus statements for the diagnosis and management of dyslipidemias in diabetes not only focus on the treatment of LDL-cholesterol levels as the primary aim but also acknowledge the combination of high triglycerides with low HDL-cholesterol as a CHD risk factor in diabetes and an indication for treatment with or without elevation of LDL-cholesterol in patients with established CHD [66, 67, 68, 69]. Recent data from the Prospective Cardiovascular Munster (PROCAM) study and from subgroup analysis of the Helsinki Heart Study have shown that hypertriglyceridemia is a powerful CHD risk factor in individuals with high ratios of total cholesterol to HDL-cholesterol and LDL-cholesterol to HDL-cholesterol [70, 71, 72]. Importantly, treatment with gemfibrozil in the subgroup with LDL-cholesterol : HDL-cholesterol ratio above 5.0 was associated with a 70% of lowering of the CHD risk [71]. Recently, Criqui et al [73] reported that plasma triglyceride level was associated with CHD mortality in a cohort with low levels of both HDL- and LDL-cholesterol. Of note is the observation that the association was dependent on plasma glucose level. The recognition of the fact that even moderate hypertriglyceridemia is associated with metabolic abnormalities of other lipoproteins (Table 2), which can be atherogenic, further emphasizes the significance of dyslipidemia as a CHD risk factor in both diabetes and the insulin resistance syndrome.

Table 2 Metabolic associations of hypertriglyceridemia

- Excessive postprandial lipemia
- Lowering of HDL and compositional changes of HDL
- Preponderance of small dense LDL
- Enhancement of thrombogenesis

At the moment we have no prospective intervention studies in diabetic patients; the strategy for treatment of lipid disorders in diabetes is therefore based on data from non-diabetic populations. However, there are no studies to suggest that diabetic populations would not benefit from adequate treatment of lipid disorders. Data from a subgroup analysis of diabetic patients included in the Helsinki Heart Study suggest that gemfibrozil reduced the elevated CHD risk similarly in diabetic patients and the non-diabetic population [74]. However, the evidence is not conclusive because of the small number of diabetic subjects included in the cohort. It is rational to assume that adequate control of serum lipids is warranted even more in diabetic patients than in the non-diabetic population. This is particularly true for patients with NIDDM, who often have manifest CHD at the time of diagnosis and also show the clustering of multiple risk factors associated with the insulin resistance syndrome. Studies are urgently needed to determine the benefits of both lowering triglycerides and raising HDL-cholesterol, and of aggressive lowering of LDL-cholesterol in diabetic populations. The Diabetes Atherosclerosis Intervention Study (DAIS) is a current international multicenter angiographic study addressing this question in 300 NIDDM patients, but the answer will not be available for 4–5 years [75]. Extensive studies are also required to determine the benefits of multiple risk factor intervention and changes of life style in diabetic populations.

MANAGEMENT OF HYPERLIPIDEMIAS IN DIABETES

Guidelines for Treatment of Dyslipidemias

Table 3 defines the guidelines for the management of dyslipidemias in diabetes. The guidelines identify diabetic patients with established CHD as the primary target group for intervention and recognize both the combination of hypertriglyceridemia with low HDL-cholesterol as well as elevation of LDL-cholesterol as targets for therapy. A second feature is that all diabetic patients (men and women) with LDL-cholesterol above 4.1 mmol/l (160 mg/dl) are considered to be at high risk and consequently treatment is recommended. Whether the therapeutic goal for optimal LDL values should be even lower (< 3.4 mmol/l or 130 mg/dl) in diabetic than in non-diabetic individuals is unresolved [76]. The rationale for this proposal is based on the fact that lipoproteins in diabetes show specific features (compositional changes, enhanced modification and oxidation) which may render particles, of LDL in particular, atherogenic even when the concentration is within the normal range [76, 77]. The deleterious joint effect of hypertriglyceridemia and low HDL-cholesterol is recognized in diabetic patients without existing CHD, and the level of triglycerides at which it

Table 3 Guidelines for intervention in NIDDM

NIDDM patient with clinical CHD
  • Triglycerides > 1.7 mmol/l (150 mg/dl)
    and
    HDL-cholesterol < 1.1 mmol/l (40 mg/dl)
NIDDM patient with clinical CHD
  • LDL-cholesterol > 3.5 mmol/l (135 mg/dl)
    or
  • Cholesterol/HDL-cholesterol > 5.0
NIDDM patient without evidence of CHD
  • LDL-cholesterol > 4.1 mmol/l (160 mg/dl)
  • Triglycerides > 2.8 mmol/l (250 mg/dl)
    and
    HDL-cholesterol < 1.1 mmol/l (40 mg/dl)

is recommended that treatment be considered is lower than in the non-diabetic population (Table 3) [66, 68].

If diabetic control is good and the patient has abnormal lipid values, the required actions are the same as for a non-diabetic patient at high risk (Table 4). If serum lipid levels do not respond to a lipid-lowering diet the institution of drug therapy is recommended. The choice of drug should be determined by the characteristics of the lipoprotein abnormality and its pathophysiology (Table 5). The therapy should be individualized and it should not evoke any serious side-effects or impair diabetic control.

Table 4 Management of dyslipidemias in diabetes

Poor glycemic control
  Optimize glucose control
  Make dietary adjustments
  Encourage weight reduction
  Check other CHD risk factors

Good glycemic control
  Check other CHD risk factors
  Optimize body weight
  Start lipid-lowering diet

Re-assess plasma lipids after 3 months

The combination of abnormal lipid values with poor glycemic control is probably the most common problem, particularly in NIDDM patients. First-line measures in the management of dyslipidemias in these patients include optimization of diabetic control and encouragement of dietary therapy, where caloric restriction to attain desirable weight and daily modest exercise are cornerstones for success (Table 4). The response of serum lipids to improvement of glycemic control should be followed over 3–6 months to ensure benefits.

Optimization of Diabetic Treatment

IDDM

It is well established that in chronically insulin-treated diabetic patients the lipoprotein profile is influenced by the degree of glycemic control and by the mode of insulin administration [10, 12, 19, 30, 78]. If glycemic control is adequate, the lipoprotein pattern is generally normal and not atherogenic (Table 1). Recent data from the DCCT indicated that lipid and lipoprotein levels in healthy IDDM patients were closely similar to those in the non-diabetic population [12]. Moderate deterioration in glycemic control is associated only with an increase of serum triglycerides, whereas there is no significant change in either LDL or HDL concentration [79]. Poor glycemic control with severe insulin deficiency and diabetic ketoacidosis is frequently associated with marked hypertriglyceridemia and lipemia due to reduced LPL activity, as well as with an elevation of LDL and a reduction in HDL. Optimization of insulin therapy rapidly restores LPL activity and normalizes VLDL metabolism but the response of HDL occurs more slowly. Ostlund et al [78] estimated that

Table 5 Drug treatment of dyslipidemias in NIDDM

• HDL-cholesterol < 0.9 mmol/l (35 mg/dl) and triglycerides > 2.8 mmol/l (250 mg/dl) (> 1.7 mmol/l, 150 mg/dl if CHD)	Fibrates Acipimox (?)
• LDL-cholesterol > 3.5–5.5 mmol/l (135–215 mg/dl) and triglycerides > 2.8 mmol/l (250 mg/dl) (> 1.7 mmol/l, 150 mg/dl if CHD)	Fibrates HMG-CoA reductase inhibitors
• LDL-cholesterol 3.5–4.5 mmol/l (135–175 mg/dl)	HMG-CoA reductase inhibitors Guar gum, acarbose, metformin
• LDL-cholesterol > 4.5 mmol/l (175 mg/dl)	HMG-CoA reductase inhibitors Resins

overall concentration of cholesterol fell by 0.1 mmol/l (2.2%) and plasma triglyceride level by 0.08 mmol/l (8%) for each percentage-point fall of glycohemoglobin in a US IDDM population. Intensive insulin therapy by continuous subcutaneous insulin infusion (CSII) or with multiple injections significantly lowers VLDL-triglyceride by reducing VLDL-triglyceride production [19, 30]. Notably, even subnormal VLDL levels can be achieved by rigorous insulin therapy [10, 30]. Improvement of glycemic control by intensive insulin therapy is commonly associated with a decrease in LDL-cholesterol and a rise in HDL-cholesterol levels, particularly in patients who initially had poor glycemic control [10, 30]. Long duration of intensive insulin therapy is accompanied by a rise in HDL (HDL$_2$) cholesterol, even in patients who initially have fair glycemic control and serum lipid and lipoprotein values within the normal range [30]. Thus the lipoprotein pattern in IDDM patients with strict glycemic control is actually anti-atherogenic because VLDL and LDL levels are subnormal and HDL levels are often increased. Furthermore, Rosenstock et al [30] showed that, if near-normoglycemia can be maintained, the favorable lipid changes persist over 3 years of follow-up.

NIDDM

An abnormal lipoprotein pattern occurs more frequently in NIDDM than in IDDM. The mean plasma triglyceride concentration is generally higher in NIDDM than in non-diabetic subjects of similar age and sex [9, 10, 14]. Lipoprotein abnormalities are frequent both in patients with newly diagnosed diabetes and in patients with previously known disease. In general there is no association between the type of therapy (diet, oral agents, conventional insulin therapy) and prevalence of dyslipidemia [80]. Since, in the majority of patients with NIDDM, glycemic control is not optimal, the first step to correcting lipid abnormalities is to intensify antidiabetic treatment. As a rule, any remedy that improves glycemic control is associated with a fall in serum triglycerides and often a slight rise in HDL [81, 82, 83, 84, 85, 86]. Nevertheless, the HDL concentration tends to remain subnormal [82, 86]. An important question is, how often does glycemic control strategy improve diabetic dyslipidemia in clinical practice? Recent data from Stern et al [87] suggest that glycemic control achieved in general practice by diabetic patients does not suffice to control dyslipidemia satisfactorily. Since in many cases neither euglycemia nor correction of lipid profile is achievable with appropriate conventional therapy, additional therapeutic approaches are needed. We and others have demonstrated that rigorous insulin therapy has multiple beneficial effects on lipoprotein metabolism in NIDDM if good glycemic

control is achieved [82, 85]. The concentrations of serum total and VLDL-triglyceride, total and LDL-cholesterol and apo-B fell during insulin therapy over 1 month (Figure 1). We also observed a significant rise of apo-A1 associated with a rise in HDL$_2$ but a fall in HDL$_3$, so that the total HDL-cholesterol concentration remained unchanged. Consequently, short-term intensified insulin therapy may in some NIDDM patients correct both insulin resistance and lipid abnormalities. Different insulin regimens show no differences in the lowering of VLDL-triglycerides if glycemic control is improved to same extent [85, 86].

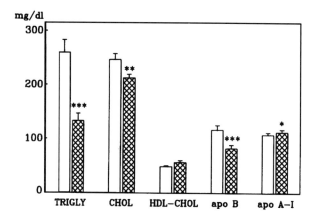

Figure 1 Effect of insulin therapy over 1 month on serum lipids and apoproteins in patients with NIDDM ($n = 18$) who were poorly controlled with oral agents. Open bars, before insulin; crosshatched bars, after insulin

Treatment of Hypercholesterolemia

As the primary objective in treating diabetic hyperlipidemia is to achieve full control of glucose and insulin metabolism, consideration of hypercholesterolemia is usually secondary. It becomes relevant when (a) optimal diabetic control cannot be achieved, or (b) hypercholesterolemia persists despite excellent diabetic control, indicating a primary form of the disorder. Both circumstances are common and pose very real difficulties. A recent survey in the USA revealed that high or borderline-high total cholesterol is present in 70% of adults with diabetes [29].

With suboptimal control of diabetes the hypercholesterolemia usually reflects excess VLDL as well as LDL. The abnormalities at this stage usually result from failure to catabolize VLDL remnants and LDL. Insulin resistance is the presumed reason for the failure of lipoprotein removal. By now, appropriate dietary management is assumed to have been fully implemented and weight reduction instituted if necessary.

Conventional cholesterol-lowering drugs can be considered on the grounds that upregulation of LDL receptors would accelerate clearance of particles containing apo-B and apo-E, provided that other impediments, such as glycosylation and abnormal conformation, are not the prime cause. VLDL remnants and intermediate-density lipoproteins (IDL), as well as LDL, can be cleared by LDL receptors.

Neither nicotinic acid nor the bile acid-sequestering drugs are totally appropriate. Nicotinic acid can adversely affect the diabetic state [88] and is contraindicated. The resins stimulate VLDL production [89], which is undesirable in a metabolic state characterized by VLDL accumulation. The use of resins is therefore limited to the less common circumstance of independent primary hypercholesterolemia coexisting with fully controlled diabetes. The only caution in its use then concerns the timing of the taking of the resin in relation to any hypoglycemic drug.

The inhibitors of hydroxymethyl glutaryl CoA reductase (HMG CoA reductase)—the 'statins'—offer attractive possibilities. Treatment results in substantial reduction of LDL levels but the VLDL concentration is also lowered, presumably through increased clearance of VLDL remnants or IDL [90]. Increased receptor-mediated clearance of LDL has been demonstrated (Table 6) [91, 92]. An additional effect, reduction of LDL production, has also been reported [91] and probably reflects increased uptake of IDL, the precursor of LDL. The inhibition of cholesterol synthesis in the liver, which is responsible for the heightened receptor activity, appears to have a profound effect on the metabolism of apo-B-containing particles [93]. Recently Gaw et al [94] demonstrated that simvastatin markedly increased the catabolism of apo-B-containing particles in the VLDL–IDL–LDL cascade by direct removal of particles, by promoting the activity of apo-B/E receptors. However, increased catabolism of apo-B-containing particles cannot fully explain the marked reduction of LDL pool size in moderately hypercholesterolemic subjects. Thus HMG CoA reductase inhibitors seem to have multiple actions at different steps in the VLDL–IDL–LDL cascade [93, 94].

So far relatively few data are available on the treatment of diabetic patients with HMG CoA reductase inhibitors. Extensive drug trials have not revealed adverse effects on glucose or insulin metabolism in non-diabetic populations [95]. Garg and Grundy [96] have reported beneficial cholesterol-lowering in NIDDM patients treated with lovastatin. In line with this, simvastatin and pravastatin have been demonstrated to be effective in diabetic subjects and to have no adverse effects on glycemic control [97, 98, 99]. T. Kazumi et al (personal communication) have recently reported that pravastatin (10 mg/day) reduced LDL cholesterol by 29% in non-diabetic hypercholesterolemic subjects (n = 137) and by 25% in hypercholesterolemic NIDDM patients (n = 51). HMG CoA reductase inhibitors also lower triglycerides and raise HDL-cholesterol in a dose-dependent manner. Since statins have marked therapeutic efficacy, a low incidence of adverse effects, and are easy to administer, HMG CoA reductase inhibitors are a drug of choice for reducing LDL-cholesterol in diabetic subjects (Table 5).

Probucol is another LDL-lowering drug (Table 6). However, it has the disadvantage that it also lowers the concentration of HDL due to inhibition of HDL apo-A synthesis [100]. The recent discovery that probucol prevents the peroxidation of LDL lipids [101] suggests that it may confer antiatherogenic properties. If this is confirmed in clinical trials, probucol may deserve consideration in the treatment of diabetic hypercholesterolemia.

Treatment of Hypertriglyceridemia

Although evidence directly linking increased triglyceride levels with high CHD risk is inconclusive, data from epidemiological studies indicate that the association between triglycerides and CHD is stronger in diabetic than in non-diabetic populations [102, 103, 104]. Recently Laakso et al [105] reported that high VLDL-triglycerides and VLDL-cholesterol as well as low HDL-cholesterol at the baseline were powerful risk

Table 6 Modes of action of recommended lipid-lowering drugs

Fibrates	↑ VLDL clearance; ↓ VLDL synthesis ↓ LDL synthesis ↑ HDL apoprotein-A synthesis
Cholestyramine and colestipol	↑ Bile acid excretion ↑ LDL receptor-mediated clearance
HMG CoA reductase inhibitors	↓ Cholesterol synthesis ↑ LDL receptor-mediated clearance ↓ LDL production
Probucol	↑ ? LDL clearance ↓ HDL apoprotein-A synthesis ↓ Production of oxidized LDL (which bypass LDL regulation and are atherogenic)

indicators for CHD events in NIDDM patients over 7 years of follow-up. The recognition that hypertriglyceridemia is commonly associated with metabolic consequences (Table 2), has reinforced the argument that it is important to treat hypertriglyceridemia. Consequently, both low HDL and high triglycerides are considered to warrant therapeutic intervention in NIDDM patients [66, 67, 68, 69]. Non-pharmacological measures are recommended as the primary therapeutic approach in patients without known CHD or concomitant elevation of LDL-cholesterol. A clear indication for drug therapy is severe hypertriglyceridemia (plasma triglycerides in excess of 1000 mg/dl or 11.3 mmol/l) [66, 68] because this is commonly associated with clinical symptoms or danger of pancreatitis.

Recent consensus statements have recognized the combination of high triglycerides with low HDL as warranting intervention in NIDDM patients with established CHD, even in the absence of elevated LDL-cholesterol (Table 3) [66, 68]. However, the decision when to start drug therapy is still arbitrary because there are no clinical drug trials on the efficacy of lowering triglycerides and raising HDL-cholesterol in either diabetic or non-diabetic populations selected on the basis of high triglycerides and low HDL-cholesterol (Table 5). Optimal treatment for hypertriglyceridemia should not only lower serum triglyceride levels but also have beneficial effects on the metabolic consequences of hypertriglyceridemia listed in Table 2. Thus it should:

(1) Lower postprandial lipemia;
(2) Normalize LDL subclass distribution;
(3) Raise HDL-cholesterol;
(4) Correct the adverse effects of hypertriglyceridemia on thrombogenic factors.

To achieve these aims the major action of the drug should be on VLDL metabolism [106]. Lowering of VLDL-triglycerides and apo-B can be established by drugs that reduce VLDL production and/or improve its clearance. Nicotinic acid is theoretically an ideal drug because it acts beneficially on both processes [107] and is effective in lowering both VLDL- and LDL-cholesterol and raising HDL. Unfortunately, nicotinic acid therapy seems to have adverse effects on glucose metabolism, and in NIDDM patients has been found to worsen glycemic control, raise uric acid levels and impair insulin sensitivity [76]. Consequently, nicotinic acid is not recommended for treatment of hypertriglyceridemia in NIDDM patients or in subjects with the metabolic syndrome. However, nicotinic acid can be used in IDDM patients and in NIDDM patients treated with insulin.

Acipimox is a new derivative of nicotinic acid with a longer duration of action. Available data indicate that acipimox has no adverse effect on glycemic control in NIDDM patients, at least in short-term studies [108, 109, 110, 111, 112, 113]. Results from a recent multicenter study of 82 NIDDM patients indicated that on average acipimox lowered triglycerides by 28% and cholesterol by 14% over three months of therapy [112]. The data indicate that acipimox may be less effective than nicotinic acid but it provides an alternative treatment for dyslipidemia in diabetic patients.

At the moment fibric acid derivatives are the drugs of choice for treatment of hypertriglyceridemia in diabetes (Table 5). As the newer agents (gemfibrozil, bezafibrate, fenofibrate and ciprofibrate) are more effective, we recommend the use of these fibric acid derivatives instead of clofibrate. Currently the most widely used fibrates are gemfibrozil, bezafibrate and fenofibrate. Fibric acid derivatives reduce serum total and VLDL-triglyceride by 40–60% on average [114, 115, 116]. All agents have been shown to increase HDL-cholesterol by 8–20%. Although data from clinical trials in diabetic patients are still limited, the available evidence indicates that fibrates are as effective and safe in diabetic as in non-diabetic populations [74, 117, 118, 119]. In a recent multicenter study including 442 NIDDM patients randomized to receive either gemfibrozil or placebo in double-blind fashion for 20 weeks, triglycerides fell by 26.4% and HDL-cholesterol rose by 12.2% in the gemfibrozil group [119]. Interestingly, there is emerging evidence that fibric acid derivatives may also reverse the adverse metabolic effects of hypertriglyceridemia (Table 7). We have shown that gemfibrozil markedly lowers postprandial lipemia in NIDDM patients [120]. Furthermore, we and others have reported that fibrates can normalize LDL subclass distribution with an increase in LDL size and a shift towards more buoyant and less dense LDL particles [121, 122, 123]. Taken together, fibrates seem to reverse the atherogenic lipid profile in NIDDM patients. Whether the observed alterations are beneficial with respect to CHD risk remains to be established in prospective studies. Subgroup analysis by Koskinen et al [74] of diabetic subjects included in the Helsinki Heart Study found that gemfibrozil treatment reduced CHD events, although the difference was not significant because of the small number of diabetic subjects and events. The effect on LDL concentration is variable in hypertriglyceridemia,

Table 7   Effects of treatment with fibrates on lipoproteins

- Lowers VLDL-triglycerides
- Lowers postprandial lipemia
- Increases the size of LDL particles
- Increases HDL concentration

and seems to be dependent on triglyceride and LDL-cholesterol levels [124]. Fibrates seem to lower LDL-cholesterol only in subjects with low baseline serum triglycerides, but to increase the initially low LDL-cholesterol values in severe hypertriglyceridemia [124, 125, 126]. Since NIDDM subjects commonly have only moderate hypertriglyceridemia the response of LDL-cholesterol concentration to fibrate treatments has been non-significant [127].

The precise mechanisms of action behind the lipid-lowering effects of fibric acid derivatives are not fully understood and seem to be multifactorial (Table 6). The primary action of fibric acid derivatives is stimulation of lipoprotein lipase activity and consequently increased catabolism of triglyceride-rich particles [126, 128, 129]. In line with this, data from kinetic studies have shown that both gemfibrozil and bezafibrate increase the fractional removal rate of VLDL [130, 131]. In addition, different fibrates seem to have a variable action on VLDL production. Gemfibrozil has been shown to decrease the production of VLDL-triglyceride and VLDL apo-B. This effect of gemfibrozil has been attributed to the suppression of free fatty acid release from adipose tissue and consequently reduced free fatty acid flux to the liver [131]. Recently we evaluated the possibility that gemfibrozil may be antilipolytic, but were unable to observe any changes in free fatty acid transport rate or metabolism during gemfibrozil treatment as compared to placebo [127].

The action of fibrates on LDL metabolism is complex, and depends on the initial plasma triglyceride level. The compounds seem to shift the metabolic routing of apo-B-containing particles [131, 132]. In hypertriglyceridemia fibrates reduce the initially high fractional clearance rate (FCR) of LDL by suppressing the removal of LDL via the receptor-independent pathway [132]. By contrast, in hypercholesterolemia patients the initially low FCR of LDL is increased due to activation of the receptor-mediated pathway. These paradoxical responses are explained by putative effects of fibrates on the size of VLDL particles released from the liver and consequently on changes in LDL subclasses and their ligand characteristics [132].

The HDL-cholesterol-raising action of fibric acid analogues has been attributed to the induction of lipoprotein lipase by these agents [126, 128]. However, gemfibrozil increases mainly preferable HDL_3 cholesterol, apo-A2 and LpA1:A2 particles [133]. The data suggest that gemfibrozil may have multiple sites of action on HDL metabolism [133]. Accordingly gemfibrozil has been demonstrated to increase apo-A1 synthesis [134]. The fact that gemfibrozil has been documented to reduce the incidence of CHD, particularly in patients with LDL-cholesterol:HDL-cholesterol ratio above 5.0

and triglycerides above 2.3 mmol/l (which is a common combination in NIDDM patients), makes fibrates the drugs of first choice for treating hypertriglyceridemia. Substantial evidence indicates that fibrates are well tolerated and do not adversely affect glucose metabolism [127, 135, 136].

Other Pharmacological Agents

Metformin was introduced as an antihyperglycemic agent long ago, but recently its therapeutic profile has been extended. Metformin has been shown to ameliorate insulin resistance and also to have beneficial effects on the metabolic alterations clustered with insulin resistance [137, 138, 139]. There is substantial evidence that metformin lowers total and LDL-cholesterol whereas alterations of serum triglycerides are less consistent [139, 140, 141, 142]. Interestingly, some studies indicate that metformin may also lower blood pressure [138, 139, 143]. These beneficial effects on CHD risk factors are welcome as adjuncts to its antihyperglycemic effect in the treatment of NIDDM patients.

Alpha-glucosidase inhibitors have recently been introduced into diabetic therapy because of their effects on glucose absorption from the gut. Concomitantly, beneficial effects on triglyceride metabolism and hypertriglyceridemia have been reported. Nestel et al [144] have shown by measuring triglyceride kinetics that the production of triglyceride can be significantly reduced with acarbose. Triglyceride clearance was not affected. This effect has been shown to result in a lowering of VLDL-triglyceride in hypertriglyceridemic patients in some but not all clinical trials [145, 146]. The effect on LDL-cholesterol is very much less. Further trials are justified.

Dosages and Possible Side Effects of Recommended Hypolipidemic Drugs

Table 8 outlines the daily dosages for the recommended drugs and possible side effects. Several drugs are administered twice daily (colestipol, cholestyramine, probucol, gemfibrozil). Bezafibrate (200 mg) and fenofibrate (100 mg) are generally given three times a day. Etofibrate can be given in a single dose in the evening. Recently long-acting preparations of bezafibrate, gemfibrozil and fenofibrate have become available and these are administered in a single dose.

All the recommended drugs are generally well tolerated and compliance in clinical studies with fibric acid derivatives has been good [115, 116, 147]. Although side effects of resins are not very serious, they can be irritating enough to decrease compliance. Long-term safety of HMG CoA reductase inhibitors remains to be confirmed, but so far clinical trials with different compounds have not revealed any serious side effects

Table 8 Recommended daily doses of hypolipidemic drugs and possible side effects

	Recommended doses	Possible side effects
HMG CoA reductase inhibitors		Sporadic rises of transaminases, muscle pains and cramps, rare cases of myopathy
Lovastatin	20-80 mg/day	
Simvastatin	10-40 mg/day	
Pravastatin	20-40 mg/day	
Resins		Gastrointestinal symptoms, interference with the absorption of anionic drugs
Colestipol	15-30 g/day	
Cholestyramine	12-24 g/day	
Probucol	1.0 g/day	Gastrointestinal symptoms (diarrhea)
Fibric acid derivatives		Gastrointestinal symptoms, sporadic transient increases in transaminases, rare cases of myopathy with an increase in creatine kinase
Gemfibrozil	1200 mg/day	
Bezafibrate	600 mg/day	
Fenofibrate	300 mg/day	
Etofibrate	500 mg/day	
Ciprofibrate	100 mg/day	

[148, 149, 150]. The currently registered drugs have been associated with occasional increases in abnormal liver function tests and rare increases in creatine kinase levels, possibly related to skeletal muscle damage. Elevations of liver enzymes above values greater than 3 times the upper limit of normal have been reported, with a prevalence of 0.4-0.9% [148, 149]. Development of muscle pains and cramps may occur, although a true myopathy is uncommon [148]. These side effects appear to reflect high circulating levels of these drugs, apparently brought about through combined treatment with several drugs including cyclosporin, gemfibrozil and nicotinic acid. Consequently, the combination therapy of statins with nicotinic acid or fibrates is not recommended. If combination therapy is requested in severe cases with familial combined hyperlipidemia (FCH) and mixed hyperlipidemia, monitoring should be frequent and take place in a special lipid clinic.

Bile acid sequestrants cause upper and lower gastrointestinal symptoms (constipation, bloating, gastrointestinal irritation) which are dose-dependent. If the therapy is begun at a low dose and increased gradually to the full dose, side effects are fewer and compliance will improve. However, it is not unusual for patients to interrupt medication because of intolerable side effects.

All fibric acid derivatives may cause upper gastrointestinal complaints (dyspepsia and gastric pain, nausea and, less frequently, vomiting and diarrhea), but compliance is better than in the case of resins. However, some patients (5-10%) may stop the medication because they cannot tolerate the side effects. It is important to note that fibric acid derivatives (fenofibrate, gemfibrozil) may influence the composition of bile and therefore predispose to gallstone formation [151], although to a lesser extent than clofibrate. Consequently, long-term studies are needed to evaluate the risk of gallstone formation in relation to these hypolipidemic drugs.

REFERENCES

1. Pyörälä K, Laakso M, Uusitupa K. Diabetes and atherosclerosis: an epidemiologic view. Diabetes Metab Rev 1987; 3: 463-524.
2. Stamler J, Vaccaro O, Neaton JD, Wentworth D. Diabetes, other risk factors, and 12-year cardiovascular mortality for men screened in the multiple risk factor intervention trial. Diabetes Care 1993; 16: 434-44.
3. Bierman EL. Atherogenesis in diabetes. Arterioscler Thromb 1992; 12: 647-56.
4. Uusitupa MIJ, Niskanen LK, Siitonen O, Voutilainen E, Pyörälä K. Ten-year cardiovascular mortality in relation to risk factors and abnormalities in lipoprotein composition in type 2 (non-insulin-dependent) diabetic and non-diabetic subjects. Diabetologia 1993; 36: 1175-84.
5. Lipid Research Clinics Program. The Lipid Research Clinics coronary primary prevention trial results. II. The relationship of reduction in incidence of coronary heart disease to cholesterol lowering. JAMA 1984; 251: 365-74.
6. Canner PL, Berge KG, Wenger NK, Stamler J, Friedman L, Prineas RJ et al. Fifteen-year mortality in coronary drug project patients: long-term benefit with niacin. J Am Coll Cardiol 1986; 8: 1245-55.
7. Frick MH, Elo O, Haapa K, Heinonen OP, Heinsalmi P, Helo P et al. Helsinki Heart Study: primary-prevention trial with gemfibrozil in middle-aged men with dyslipidemia. Safety of treatment, changes in risk factors, and incidence of coronary heart disease. New Engl J Med 1987; 317: 1237-45.
8. Rossouw JE. The effects of lowering serum cholesterol on coronary heart disease risk. Med Clin North Am 1994; 78: 181-95.
9. Howard BV. Lipoprotein metabolism in diabetes mellitus. J Lipid Res 1987; 28: 613-28.
10. Taskinen M-R. Hyperlipidemia in diabetes. Baillière's Clin Endocrin Metab 1990; 4: 743-75.
11. Ginsberg HN. Lipoprotein physiology in non-diabetic and diabetic states. Diabetes Care 1991; 14: 839-55.
12. The DCCT Research Group. Lipid and lipoprotein levels in patients with IDDM: diabetes control and complications trial experience. Diabetes Care 1992; 15: 886-94.

13. Stern MP, Haffner SM. Dyslipidemia in type II diabetes: implications for therapeutic intervention. Diabetes Care 1991; 14: 1144–59.

14. Taskinen M-R. Quantitative and qualitative lipoprotein abnormalities in diabetes mellitus. Diabetes 1992; 41 (suppl 2): 12–17.

15. Selam J-L, Kashyap M, Alberti KGMM, Lozano J, Hanna M, Turner D et al. Comparison of intraperitoneal and subcutaneous insulin administration on lipids, apolipoproteins, fuel metabolites, and hormones in type 1 diabetes mellitus. Metabolism 1989; 38: 908–12.

16. Ruotolo G, Micossi P, Galimberti G, Librenti MC, Petrella G, Marcovina S et al. Effects of intraperitoneal versus subcutaneous insulin administration on lipoprotein metabolism in type 1 diabetes. Metabolism 1990; 39: 598–604.

17. Ruotolo G, Parlavecchia M, Taskinen M-R, Galimberti G, Zoppo A, Le N-A et al. Normalization of lipoprotein composition by intraperitoneal insulin in IDDM. Diabetes Care 1994; 17: 6–12.

18. Chen Y-DI, Jeng C-Y, Reaven GM. HDL metabolism in diabetes. Diabetes Metab Rev 1987; 3: 653–68.

19. Helve E. High density lipoprotein subfractions during continuous insulin infusion therapy. Atherosclerosis 1987; 64: 173–80.

20. Lopes-Virella M, Wohltmann HJ, Loadholt C, Buse MG. Plasma lipids and lipoproteins in young insulin-dependent diabetic patients: relationship with control. Diabetologia 1981; 21: 216–23.

21. Schernthaner G, Kostner GM, Dieplinger H, Prager R, Muhlhauser I. Apo-lipoproteins (A1, A2, B), Lp(a) lipoprotein and lecithin:cholesterol acyltransferase activity in diabetes mellitus. Atherosclerosis 1983; 49: 277–93.

22. Pfeifer MA, Brunzell JD, Best JD, Judzewitsch RG, Halter JB, Porte D Jr. The response of plasma triglyceride, cholesterol, and lipoprotein lipase to treatment in non-insulin-dependent diabetic subjects without familial hypertriglyceridemia. Diabetes 1983; 32: 525–31.

23. Bagdade JD, Porte D, Bierman EL. Diabetic lipemia. A form of acquired fat-induced lipemia. New Engl J Med 1967; 276: 427–33.

24. Wilson DE, Hata A, Kwong LK, Lingam A, Shuhua J, Ridinger DN et al. Mutations in exon 3 of the lipoprotein lipase gene segregating in a family with hypertriglyceridemia, pancreatitis, and non-insulin dependent diabetes. J Clin Invest 1993; 92: 203–11.

25. Tenkanen H, Taskinen M-R, Antikainen M, Ulmanen I, Kontula K, Ehnholm C. A novel amino acid substitution (His183→Gln) in exon 5 of the lipoprotein lipase gene results in loss of catalytic activity: phenotypic expression of the mutant gene in a heterozygous state. J Lipid Res 1994; 35: 220–8.

26. Winocour PH, Durrington PN, Ishola M, Hillier VF, Anderson DC. The prevalence of hyperlipidaemia and related clinical features in insulin-dependent diabetes mellitus. Q J Med 1989; 70: 265–76.

27. Stern MP, Patterson JK, Haffner SM, Hazuda HP, Mitchell BD. Lack of awareness and treatment of hyperlipidemia in type II diabetes in a community survey. JAMA 1989; 262: 360–4.

28. Salomaa VV, Tuomilehto J, Jauhiainen M, Korhonen HJ, Stengård J, Uusitupa M et al. Hypertriglyceridemia in different degrees of glucose intolerance in a Finnish population-based study. Diabetes Care 1992; 15: 657–65.

29. Harris MI. Hypercholesterolemia in diabetes and glucose intolerance in the US population. Diabetes Care 1991; 14: 366–74.

30. Rosenstock J, Strowig S, Cercone S, Raskin P. Reduction in cardiovascular risk factors with intensive diabetes treatment in insulin-dependent diabetes mellitus. Diabetes Care 1987; 10: 729–34.

31. Kahri J, Groop P-H, Viberti GC, Elliott T, Taskinen M-R. Regulation of apolipoprotein A1 containing lipoproteins in insulin dependent diabetes mellitus. Diabetes 1993; 42: 1281–8.

32. Loscalzo J. Lipoprotein(a): a unique risk factor for atherothrombotic disease. Arteriosclerosis 1990; 10: 672–9.

33. Scanu AM, Lawn RM, Berg K. Lipoprotein(a) and atherosclerosis. Ann Intern Med 1991; 115: 209–18.

34. Haffner SM. Lipoprotein(a) and diabetes. Diabetes Care 1993; 16: 835–40.

35. Gall MA, Rossing P, Hommel E, Voldsgaard AI, Anderson P, Nielsen FS et al. Apolipoprotein(a) in insulin-dependent diabetic patients with and without nephropathy. Scand J Clin Lab Invest 1992; 52: 513–22.

36. Klausen IC, Berg Schmidt E, Lervang HH, Gerdes LU, Ditzel J, Faergeman O. Normal lipoprotein(a) concentrations and apolipoprotein(a) isoforms in patients with insulin-dependent diabetes mellitus. Eur J Clin Invest 1992; 22: 538–41.

37. Austin A, Warty V, Janosky J, Arslanian S. The relationship of physical fitness to lipid and lipoprotein(a) levels in adolescents with IDDM. Diabetes Care 1993; 16: 421–5.

38. Groop P-H, Viberti GC, Elliott T, Friedman R, Mackie A, Ehnholm C et al. Lipoprotein(a) in type 1 diabetic patients with renal disease. Diabetic Med 1994; 11: 961–7.

39. Guillauseau PJ, Peynet J, Chanson P, Legrand A, Altman JJ, Poupon J et al. Lipoprotein(a) in diabetic patients with and without chronic renal failure. Diabetes Care 1992; 15: 976–9.

40. Nagashima K, Yutani S, Miyake H, Onigata K, Yagi H, Kuroume T. Lipoprotein(a) levels in Japanese children with IDDM. Diabetes Care 1993; 16: 846.

41. Couper JJ, Bates DJ, Cocciolone R, Magarey AM, Boulton TJC, Penfold JL et al. Association of lipoprotein(a) with puberty in insulin dependent diabetes. Diabetes Care 1993; 16: 869–73.

42. Jenkins AJ, Steele JS, Janus ED, Best JD. Increased plasma apolipoprotein(a) levels in IDDM patients with microalbuminuria. Diabetes 1991; 40: 787–90.

43. Kapelrud H, Bansgted HJ, Dahl Jorgensen K, Berg K, Hansen KF. Serum Lp(a) lipoprotein concentrations in insulin-dependent diabetic patients with microalbuminuria. Br Med J 1991; 303: 675–8.

44. Winocour PH, Bhatnagar D, Ishola M, Arrol S, Durrington PH. Lipoprotein(a) and macrovascular disease in type 1 (insulin-dependent) diabetes. Diabet Med 1991; 8: 922–7.

45. Haffner SM, Klein BEK, Moss SE, Klein R. Lack of association between Lp(a) concentrations and coronary heart disease mortality in diabetes: the Wisconsin Epidemiologic Survey of Diabetic Retinopathy. Metabolism 1992; 41: 194–7.

46. Niskanen L, Mykkänen L, Karonen SL, Uusitupa M. Apoprotein(a) levels in relation to coronary heart

disease and risk factors in type II (non-insulin-dependent) diabetes. Cardiovasc Risk Factors 1993; 13: 205-10.

47. Reaven GM. Role of insulin resistance in human disease. Diabetes 1988; 37: 1595-607.

48. Frayn KN. Insulin resistance and lipid metabolism. Curr Opin Lipidol 1993; 4: 197-204.

49. Taskinen M-R. Strategies for the diagnosis of metabolic syndrome. Curr Opin Lipidol 1993; 4: 434-43.

50. Haffner SM, Valdez RA, Hazuda HP, Mitchell BD, Morales PA, Stern MP. Prospective analysis of the insulin-resistance syndrome (syndrome X). Diabetes 1992; 41: 715-22.

51. Schumacher MC, Maxwell TM, Wu LL, Hunt SC, Williams RR, Elbein SC. Dyslipidemias among normoglycemic members of familial NIDDM pedigrees. Diabetes Care 1992; 15: 1285-9.

52. Eriksson J, Taskinen M-R, Nissén M, Forsén B, Ehrnström B-O, Snickars B et al. The Botnia Study: factors associated with insulin resistance in first-degree relatives of type 2 diabetic patients. Diabetes 1992; 41 (suppl 1): 4A(13).

53. Sane T, Taskinen M-R. Does familial hypertriglyceridemia predispose to NIDDM? Diabetes Care 1993; 16: 1494-501.

54. Patti L, Romano G, DiMarino L, Annuzzi G, Mancini M, Riccardi G et al. Abnormal distribution of VLDL subfractions in type 1 (insulin-dependent) diabetic patients: could plasma lipase activities play a role? Diabetologia 1993; 36: 155-60.

55. Klein RL, Lyons TJ, Lopes-Virella MF. Interaction of very low-density lipoprotein isolated from type 1 (insulin-dependent) diabetic subjects with human monocyte-derived macrophages. Metabolism 1989; 38: 1108-14.

56. James R, Pometta D. Differences in lipoprotein subfraction composition and distribution between type 1 diabetic men and control subjects. Diabetes 1990; 39: 1158-64.

57. Rivellese A, Riccardi G, Romano G, Giacco R, Patti L, Marotta G et al. Presence of very low density lipoprotein compositional abnormalities in type 1 (insulin-dependent) diabetic patients: effects of blood glucose optimisation. Diabetologia 1988; 31: 884-8.

58. Lahdenperä S, Groop P-H, Tilly-Kiesi M, Kuusi T, Elliott TG, Viberti GC et al. LDL subclasses in IDDM patients; relation to diabetic nephropathy. Diabetologia 1994; 37: 681-8.

59. James RW, Pometta D. The distribution profiles of very low density and low density lipoproteins in poorly-controlled male, type 2 (non-insulin-dependent) diabetic patients. Diabetologia 1991; 34: 246-52.

60. Feingold KR, Grunfeld C, Pang M, Doerrler W, Krauss RM. LDL subclass phenotypes and triglyceride metabolism in non-insulin-dependent diabetes. Arterioscler Thromb 1992; 12: 1496-1502.

61. Selby JV, Austin MA, Newman B, Zhang D, Quesenberry CP, Mayer EJ et al. LDL subclass phenotypes and the insulin resistance syndrome in women. Circulation 1993; 88: 381-7.

62. Stewart MW, Laker MF, Dyer RG, Mitcheson GJ, Winocour PH, Alberti KGMM. Lipoprotein compositional abnormalities and insulin resistance in type II

diabetic patients with mild hyperlipidemia. Arterioscler Thromb 1993; 13: 1046-52.

63. Lahdenperä S, Sane T, Vuorinen-Markkola H, Knudsen P, Taskinen M-R. LDL particle size in moderately hypertriglyceridemic subjects: relation to insulin resistance and diabetes. Atheroscler 1995; 113: 227-36.

64. Austin MA, King M-C, Vranizan KM, Krauss RM. Atherogenic lipoprotein phenotype: a proposed genetic marker for coronary heart disease risk. Circulation 1990; 82: 495-506.

65. Bagdade JD, Buchanan WE, Kuusi T, Taskinen M-R. Persistent abnormalities in lipoprotein composition in non-insulin-dependent diabetes after intensive insulin therapy. Arteriosclerosis 1990; 10: 232-9.

66. Garber AJ, Vinik AI, Crespin SR. Detection and management of lipid disorders in diabetic patients. Diabetes Care 1992; 15: 1068-74.

67. Dunn FL. Managements of hyperlipidemia in diabetes mellitus. Endocrin Metab Clin North Am 1992; 21: 395-414.

68. American Diabetes Association. Detection and management of lipid disorders in diabetes. Diabetes Care 1993; 16: 828-34.

69. Brown WV. Lipoprotein disorders in diabetes mellitus. Med Clin North Am 1994; 78: 143-62.

70. Assmann G, Schulte H. Relation of high-density lipoprotein cholesterol and triglycerides to incidence of atherosclerotic coronary artery disease (the PROCAM experience). Am J Cardiol 1992; 70: 733-7.

71. Manninen V, Tenkanen L, Koskinen P, Huttunen JK, Mänttäri M, Heinonen OP et al. Joint effects of serum triglyceride and LDL-cholesterol and HDL-cholesterol concentrations on coronary heart disease risk in the Helsinki Heart Study. Circulation 1992; 85: 37-45.

72. Assmann G, Schulte H, von Eckardstein A. Hypertriglyceridemia/low high-density lipoprotein cholesterol syndrome. Nutr Metab Cardiovasc Dis 1993; 3: 1-4.

73. Criqui MH, Heiss G, Cohn R, Cowan LD, Suchindran CM, Bangdiwala S et al. Plasma triglyceride level and mortality from coronary heart disease. New Engl J Med 1993; 328: 1220-5.

74. Koskinen P, Mänttäri M, Manninen V, Huttunen JK, Heinonen OP, Frick MH. Coronary heart disease incidence in NIDDM patients in the Helsinki Heart Study. Diabetes Care 1992; 15: 820-5.

75. Steiner G. Lipoproteins and NIDDM. 62nd EAS Congress, Jerusalem, Israel, September 5-9, 1993. Abstracts, p 2.

76. Garg A, Grundy SM. Management of dyslipidemia in NIDDM. Diabetes Care 1990; 13: 153-69.

77. Taskinen M-R. Why and how to treat hyperlipidemia in diabetic patients. Nutr Metab Cardiovasc Dis 1991; 1: 201-6.

78. Ostlund RE, Semenkovich CF, Scechtman KB. Quantitative relationship between plasma lipids and glycohemoglobin in type I patients. Diabetes Care 1989; 12: 332-6.

79. Taskinen M-R, Kuusi T, Nikkilä EA. Regulation of HDL and its subfractions in chronically insulin treated patients with type 1 diabetes. In Crepaldi A, Tiengo A, Baggio G (eds) Diabetes, obesity and hyperlipidemias. Amsterdam: Elsevier Science Publishers, 1985; pp 251-9.

80. Laakso M, Voutilainen E, Sarlund H, Aro A, Pyörälä K, Penttilä I. Serum lipids and lipoproteins in middle-aged non-insulin-dependent diabetics. Atherosclerosis 1985; 56: 271–81.

81. Taskinen M-R, Beltz WF, Fields RM, Schonfeld G, Grundy SM, Howard BV. Effects of NIDDM on very-low-density lipoprotein triglyceride and apolipoprotein B metabolism. Diabetes 1986; 35: 1268–77.

82. Taskinen M-R, Kuusi T, Helve E, Nikkilä EA, Yki-Järvinen H. Insulin therapy induces antiatherogenic changes of serum lipoproteins in non-insulin-dependent diabetes. Arteriosclerosis 1988; 8: 168–77.

83. Uusitupa MIJ, Laakso M, Sarlund H, Majander H, Takala J, Penttilä I. Effects of a very-low-calorie diet on metabolic control and cardiovascular risk factors in the treatment of obese non insulin-dependent diabetics. Am J Clin Nutr 1990; 51: 768–73.

84. Taskinen M-R, Packard CJ, Shepherd J. Effect of insulin therapy on metabolic fate of apolipoprotein B-containing lipoproteins in NIDDM. Diabetes 1990; 39: 1017–27.

85. Lindström T, Arnqvist HJ, Olsson AG. Effect of different insulin regimens on plasma lipoprotein and apolipoprotein concentrations in patients with non-insulin-dependent diabetes mellitus. Atherosclerosis 1990; 81: 137–44.

86. Yki-Järvinen H, Kauppila M, Kujansuu E, Lahti J, Marjanen T, Niskanen L et al. Comparison of insulin regimens in patients with non-insulin-dependent diabetes mellitus. New Engl J Med 1992; 327: 1426–33.

87. Stern MP, Mitchell BD, Haffner SM, Hazuda HP. Does glycemic control of type II diabetes suffice to control diabetic dyslipidemia? Diabetes Care 1992; 15: 638–44.

88. Garg A, Grundy SM. Nicotinic acid as therapy for dyslipidemia in non-insulin-dependent diabetes mellitus. JAMA 1990; 264: 723–6.

89. Clifton-Bligh P, Miller NE, Nester PJ. Changes in plasma lipoprotein lipids in hypercholesterolemic patients treated with the bile acid-sequestering resin, colestipol. Clin Sci Mol Med 1974; 47: 547–57.

90. Simons LA, Nestel PJ, Calvert GD, Jennings GL. Effects of MK-733 on plasma lipid and lipoprotein levels in subjects with hypercholesterolemia. Med J Austr 1987; 147: 65–8.

91. Grundy SM, Vega GL. Influence of mevinolin on metabolism of low density lipoproteins in primary moderate hypercholesterolemia. J Lipid Res 1985; 26: 1464–75.

92. Reihnér E, Rudling M, Ståhlberg D, Berglund L, Ewerth S, Björkhem I et al. Influence of pravastatin, a specific inhibitor of HMG-CoA reductase, on hepatic metabolism of cholesterol. New Engl J Med 1990; 323: 224–8.

93. Arad Y, Ramakrishnan R, Ginsberg HN. Lovastatin therapy reduces low density lipoprotein apo-B levels in subjects with combined hyperlipidemia by reducing the production of apo-B-containing lipoproteins: implications for the pathophysiology of apo-B production. J Lipid Res 1990; 31: 567–82.

94. Gaw A, Packard CJ, Murray EF, Lindsay GM, Griffin BA, Caslake MJ et al. Effects of simvastatin on apo-B metabolism and LDL subfraction distribution. Arterioscler Thromb 1993; 13: 170–89.

95. The Lovastatin Study Group II. Therapeutic response to lovastatin (Mevinolin) in non-familial hypercholesterolemia. JAMA 1986; 256: 2829–34.

96. Garg A, Grundy SM. Lovastatin for lowering cholesterol levels in non-insulin-dependent diabetes mellitus. New Engl J Med 1988; 318: 81–6.

97. Yoshino G, Kazumi T, Iwai M, Matsushita M, Matsuba K, Uenoyama R et al. Long-term treatment of hypercholesterolemic non-insulin-dependent diabetic (NIDDM) patients with pravastatin (CS-514). Atherosclerosis 1989; 75: 67–72.

98. Kjær K, Hangaard J, Petersen NE, Hagen C. Effect of simvastatin in patients with type I (insulin-dependent) diabetes mellitus and hypercholesterolemia. Acta Endocrinol 1992; 126: 229–32.

99. Cassader M, Ruiu G, Gambino R, Alemanno N, Veglia F, Pagano G. Hypercholesterolemia in non-insulin-dependent diabetes mellitus: different effect of simvastatin on VLDL and LDL cholesterol levels. Atherosclerosis 1993; 99: 47–53.

100. Nestel PJ, Billington T. Effects of probucol on low density lipoprotein removal and high density lipoprotein synthesis. Atherosclerosis 1981; 38: 203–9.

101. Parthasarathy S, Young SG, Witztum JL, Pittman RC, Steinberg D. Probucol inhibits oxidative modification of low density lipoprotein. J Clin Invest 1986; 77: 641–4.

102. Fontbonne A, Eschwége E, Cambien F, Richard J-L, Ducimetière P, Thibult N et al. Hypertriglyceridaemia as a risk factor of coronary heart disease mortality in subjects with impaired glucose tolerance or diabetes. Diabetologia 1989; 32: 300–4.

103. Austin MA. Plasma triglyceride and coronary heart disease. Arterioscler Thromb 1991; 11: 2–14.

104. Castelli WP. Epidemiology of triglycerides: a view from Framingham. Am J Cardiol 1992; 70: 3H–9H.

105. Laakso M, Lehto S, Penttilä I, Pyörälä K. Lipids and lipoproteins predicting coronary heart disease mortality and morbidity in patients with non-insulin-dependent diabetes. Circulation 1993; 88(part 1): 1421–30.

106. Grundy SM, Vega GL. Two different views of the relationship of hypertriglyceridaemia to coronary heart disease. Arch Intern Med 1992; 152: 28–34.

107. Fattore PC, Sirtori CR. Nicotinic acid derivatives. Curr Opin Lipidol 1991; 2: 43–7.

108. Walldius G. Probucol and nicotinic acid: old drugs, new findings and new derivatives. Curr Opin Lipidol 1992; 3: 34–9.

109. Tornvall P, Walldius G. A comparison between nicotinic acid and acipimox in hypertriglyceridaemia—effects on serum lipids, lipoproteins, glucose tolerance and tolerability. J Intern Med 1991; 230: 415–21.

110. Fulcher GR, Catalano C, Walker M, Farrer M, Thow J, Whately-Smith CR et al. A double blind study of the effect of acipimox on serum lipids, blood glucose control and insulin action in non-obese patients with type 2 diabetes mellitus. Diabet Med 1992; 9: 901–14.

111. Dean JD, McCarthy S, Betteridge DJ, Whately-Smith C, Powell J, Owens DR. The effect of acipimox in patients with type 2 diabetes and persistent hyperlipidaemia. Diabetic Med 1992; 9: 611–15.

112. Koev D, Zlateva S, Susic M, Babic D, Profozic V, Skrabalo Z et al. Improvement of lipoprotein lipid

composition in type II diabetic patients with concomitant hyperlipoproteinemia by acipimox treatment. Diabetes Care 1993; 16: 1285–90.

113. Saloranta C, Groop L, Ekstrand A, Franssila-Kallunki A, Eriksson J, Taskinen M-R. Different acute and chronic effects of acipimox treatment on glucose and lipid metabolism in patients with type 2 diabetes. Diabet Med 1993; 10: 950–7.

114. Brown WV, Dujovne CA, Farquhar JW et al. Effects of fenofibrate on plasma lipids. Double-blind, multicenter study in patients with type IIA or IIB hyperlipidemia. Arteriosclerosis 1986; 6: 670–8.

115. Manninen V, Elo O, Frick MH, Haapa K, Heinonen OP, Heinsalmi P et al. Lipid alterations and decline in the incidence of coronary heart disease in the Helsinki Heart Study. JAMA 1988; 260: 641–51.

116. Jones PH. A clinical overview of dyslipidemias: treatment strategies. Am J Med 1992; 93: 187–98.

117. Jones IR, Swai A, Taylor R, Miller M, Laker MF, Alberti KGMM. Lowering of plasma glucose concentrations with bezafibrate in patients with moderately controlled NIDDM. Diabetes Care 1990; 13: 855–63.

118. Winocour PH, Durrington PN, Bhatnagar D, Ishola M, Arrol S, Lalor BC et al. Double-blind placebo-controlled study of the effects of bezafibrate on blood lipids, lipoproteins, and fibrinogen in hyperlipidaemic type 1 diabetes mellitus. Diabet Med 1990; 7: 736–43.

119. Vinik AI, Colwell JA. Effects of gemfibrozil on triglyceride levels in patients with NIDDM. Diabetes Care 1993; 16: 37–44.

120. Syvänne M, Vuorinen-Markkola H, Hilden H, Taskinen M-R. Gemfibrozil reduces postprandial lipemia in non-insulin-dependent diabetes. Arterioscler Thromb 1993; 13: 286–95.

121. Tsai MY, Yuan J, Hunninghake DB. Effect of gemfibrozil on composition of lipoproteins and distribution of LDL subspecies. Atherosclerosis 1992; 95: 35–42.

122. Lahdenperä S, Tilly-Kiesi M, Vuorinen-Markkola H, Kuusi T, Taskinen M-R. Effects of gemfibrozil on low-density lipoprotein particle size, density distribution, and composition in patients with type II diabetes. Diabetes Care 1993; 16: 584–92.

123. Bruckert E, Dejager S, Chapman MJ. Ciprofibrate therapy normalises the atherogenic low-density lipoprotein subspecies profile in combined hyperlipidemia. Atherosclerosis 1993; 100: 91–102.

124. Mänttäri M, Koskinen P, Manninen V, Huttunen JK, Frick MH, Nikkilä EA. Effect of gemfibrozil on the concentration and composition of serum lipoproteins. Atherosclerosis 1990; 81: 11–17.

125. Shepherd J, Caslake MJ, Lorimer AR, Vallance BD, Packard JC. Fenofibrate reduces low density lipoprotein catabolism in hypertriglyceridemic subjects. Arteriosclerosis 1985; 5: 162–8.

126. Gaw A, Shepherd J. Fibric acid derivatives. Curr Opin Lipidol 1991; 2: 39–42.

127. Vuorinen-Markkola H, Yki-Järvinen H, Taskinen M-R. Lowering of triglycerides by gemfibrozil affects neither the glucoregulatory nor antilipolytic effect of insulin in type 2 (non-insulin-dependent) diabetic patients. Diabetologia 1993; 36: 161–9.

128. Vessby B, Lithell H. Interruption of long-term lipid-lowering treatment with bezafibrate in hypertriglyceridaemic patients. Atherosclerosis 1990; 82: 137–43.

129. Grundy SM, Vega GL. Fibric acids: effects on lipids and lipoprotein metabolism. Am J Med 1987; 83 (suppl 5B): 9–20.

130. Kesäniemi A, Grundy SM. Influence of gemfibrozil and clofibrate on metabolism of cholesterol and plasma triglycerides in man. JAMA 1984; 251: 2241–6.

131. Shepherd J, Packard CJ. An overview of the effects of *P*-chlorophenoxy-isobutyric acid derivatives on lipoprotein metabolism. In Fears R, Prous JR (eds) Pharmacological control of hyperlipidemia. Barcelona: Science Publishers, SA, 1986; pp 135–44.

132. Caslake MJ, Packard CJ, Gaw A, Murray E, Griffin BA, Vallance BD et al. Fenofibrate and LDL metabolic heterogeneity in hypercholesterolemia. Arterioscler Thromb 1993; 13: 702–11.

133. Kahri J, Vuorinen-Markkola H, Tilly-Kiesi M, Lahdenperä S, Taskinen M-R. Effect of gemfibrozil on high density lipoprotein subspecies in non-insulin-dependent diabetes mellitus. Atherosclerosis 1993; 102: 79–89.

134. Saku K, Gartside PS, Hynd BA, Kashyap ML. Mechanism of action of gemfibrozil on lipoprotein metabolism. J Clin Invest 1985; 75: 1702–12.

135. Karhapää P, Uusitupa M, Voutilainen E et al. Effects of bezafibrate on insulin sensitivity and glucose tolerance in subjects with combined hyperlipidemia. Clin Pharmacol Ther 1992; 52: 620–26.

136. Sane T, Knudsen P, Vuorinen-Markkola H, Yki-Järvinen H, Taskinen M-R. Lowering of triglycerides by gemfibrozil affects neither the glucoregulatory nor antilipolytic effect of insulin in non-diabetic subjects with hypertriglyceridemia. Metabolism 1995; 220–228.

137. Wu M-S, Johnston P, Sheu WH-H, Hollenbeck CB, Jeng CY, Goldfine ID et al. Effect of metformin on carbohydrate and lipoprotein metabolism in NIDDM patients. Diabetes Care 1990; 13: 1–8.

138. Giugliano D, De Rosa N, Di Maro G, Marfella R, Acampora R, Buoninconti R et al. Metformin improves glucose, lipid metabolism, and reduces blood pressure in hypertensive, obese women. Diabetes Care 1993; 16: 1387–90.

139. Nagi DK, Yudkin JS. Effects of metformin on insulin resistance, risk factors for cardiovascular disease, and plasminogen activator inhibitor in NIDDM subjects. Diabetes Care 1993; 16: 621–9.

140. Pentikäinen PJ, Voutilainen E, Aro A, Uusitupa M, Penttilä I, Vapaatalo H. Cholesterol lowering effect of metformin in combined hyperlipidemia: placebo-controlled double-blind trial. Ann Med 1990; 22: 307–12.

141. Schneider J, Erren T, Zöfel P, Kaffarnik H. Metformin-induced changes in serum lipids, lipoproteins, and apoproteins in non-insulin-dependent diabetes mellitus. Atherosclerosis 1990; 82: 97–103.

142. Hermann LS, Karlsson J-E, Sjöstrand Å. Prospective comparative study in NIDDM patients of metformin and glibenclamide with special reference to lipid profiles. Eur J Clin Pharmacol 1991; 41: 263–5.

143. Landin K, Tengborn L, Smith U. Treating insulin resistance in hypertension with metformin reduces both blood pressure and metabolic risk factors. J Intern Med 1991; 229: 181–7.

144. Nestel PJ, Bazelmans J, Reardon MF, Boston RC. Lower triglyceride production during carbohydrate-rich diets through acarbose. A glucoside hydrolase inhibitor. Diabète Métab 1985; 11: 316–17.

145. Hillebrand I, Philipp E, Katsimantis D et al. Acarbose (BAY g 5421), a possible treatment for patients with type IV hyperlipoproteinemia. In Fidge NH, Nestel PJ (eds) Atherosclerosis VII. Amsterdam: Excerpta Medica, 1986.

146. Jenney A, Proietto J, O'Dea K, Nankervis A, Trajanedes K, D'Embden H. Low-dose acarbose improves glycemic control in NIDDM patients without changes in insulin sensitivity. Diabetes Care 1993; 16: 499–502.

147. Brown WV, Dujovne CA, Farquhar JW et al. Effects of fenofibrate on plasma lipids. Double-blind, multicenter study in patients with type IIA or IIB hyperlipidemia. Arteriosclerosis 1986; 6: 670–8.

148. Boccuzzi SJ, Bocanegra TM, Walker JF, Shapiro DR, Keegan ME. Long-term safety and efficacy profile of simvastatin. Am J Cardiol 1991; 68: 1127–31.

149. Shear CL, Franklin FA, Stinnett S, Hurley DP, Bradford RH, Chremos AN et al. Expanded clinical evaluation of lovastatin (EXCEL) study results. Circulation 1992; 85: 1293–1303.

150. Bradford RH, Downtown M, Chremos AN, Langendorfer A, Stinnett S, Nash DT et al. Efficacy and tolerability of lovastatin in 3390 women with moderate hypercholesterolemia. Ann Intern Med 1993; 118: 850–5.

151. Einarsson K, Angelin B. Hyperlipoproteinemia, hypolipidemic treatment, and gallstone disease. Atheroscler Rev 1986; 15: 67–97.

40

Insulin Therapy

P.D. Home

Newcastle Diabetes Services and Department of Medicine, University of Newcastle upon Tyne, UK

The introduction of insulin therapy remains the single most important milestone in the history of diabetes. Indeed, over the seven decades since subcutaneous insulin injections were first given, no other therapeutic or ancillary development has displaced insulin therapy as the most important treatment for diabetes. This status, increasingly extraordinary in the history of therapeutics, does not reflect a lack of commercial and research interest in the hormone, which has often been at the forefront of the application of new biochemical techniques to medicine. Furthermore, the insulin market, never insignificant in the industrialized nations, has continued to expand both with the increasing use of injection therapy in the type 2 (non-insulin dependent) diabetic patient, and with increasing recognition of insulin-requiring diabetes in less-developed areas of the world. Unless other therapeutic advances diminish the need for insulin injection therapy, it can be expected that insulin will be used by up to 30 million people world wide.

The lack of progress in developing alternatives to insulin therapy is in large part a testimonial to its chemical and metabolic complexity as a large peptide hormone. This has prevented, until recently, modification to improve its properties when delivered subcutaneously, and has posed apparently insurmountable difficulties in obtaining a preparation with sufficient efficiency when given by a non-parenteral route. Furthermore, the kinetics of the physiological insulin secretion/receptor system are very fast, allowing rapid fine-tuning to changing metabolic requirements, but thus posing major limitations on the development of any kind of new drug designed to replace the insulin molecule. Nevertheless, it is perhaps surprising that the twentieth-century pot-pourri of drug design has not delivered any agent that convincingly stimulates the insulin receptor.

The peptide nature of the insulin molecule, and its instability, were in part responsible for the difficulty in isolating the hormone from animal pancreas, despite many attempts between 1905 and 1920. It may have been the case that Zuelzer's preparation was simply severely hypoglycaemic (it was abandoned as 'toxic') [1], that Scott's superiors were wrong in dismissing his approach and progress in preparing alcoholic pancreatic extracts [2], and that Paulesco might have obtained therapeutically useful preparations with time. Nevertheless, as Banting's failing surgical practice gave him time to muse on the role of the pancreas, MacLeod's earlier contributions to the understanding of pancreatic function and carbohydrate metabolism allowed him to consider supporting and funding that scientific novice in what must have seemed an unlikely project. The involvement of Best in the project, and perhaps more importantly Collip, only serve to emphasize the role of fate and chance in one of the most significant medical advances of all time [2].

The complex nature and the instability of the insulin molecule have another grave therapeutic consequence. Pancreatic insulin is relatively expensive to produce, necessitating bulk storage and transport of deep-frozen animal pancreases, complex and large-scale extraction procedures, and then repeated purification procedures even for less pure preparations. High states of purification require technology that multiplies the cost to a level comparable with production by fermentation

International Textbook of Diabetes Mellitus, Second Edition. Edited by K.G.M.M. Alberti, P. Zimmet, R.A. DeFronzo, and H. Keen (Honorary)
© 1997 John Wiley & Sons Ltd

using genetically engineered organisms. As a consequence, therapy with insulin is expensive, outweighing all other aspects together of the costs of the day-to-day management of someone with insulin-requiring diabetes. Indeed, insulin injection therapy for an individual costs more than the average income of many citizens of our planet, posing major long-term problems in making the advances of 1920–21 available to all those who need them in 1995–2000.

CHEMISTRY AND MANUFACTURE OF INSULIN

Insulin Chemistry: Consequences for Pharmacokinetics

The insulin molecule was confirmed to be a polypeptide for the first time in 1928, but its amino acid sequence defied analysis until 1952 [3], partly because of the problems of analysing a dipeptide linked by disulphide bridges. Sanger's sequence has stood the test of time, although it was eventually recognized that the explanation for the dipeptide structure was the removal of a connecting sequence (hence 'C peptide') from the precursor molecule, proinsulin [4]. Details of the pancreatic synthesis of insulin, precursors to proinsulin, and proinsulin derivatives, are discussed in Chapter 14.

Sanger's *tour de force* sadly contributed very little to our understanding of the chemical properties of the insulin molecule, for the complexities of its three-dimensional structure could not be derived from knowledge of the sequence and properties of its constituent 51 amino acids. Even though the work of Hodgkin and her collaborators was already in hand at the time of Sanger's success, it was to be another 17 years before the folding of the peptide chains and position of the amino acid side-arms were fully determined (Figure 1) [5]. Even with this knowledge, which explained the solubility of the molecule in aqueous and alcoholic media, and defined the residues concerned with dimerization and hexamerization, our understanding of the active (receptor binding) site has remained incomplete.

The chemistry of insulin has a number of consequences for its therapeutic use:

(1) As a protein it is digested in the gut and is hence totally inactive by mouth.

(2) With a molecular weight of 5802, insulin is too large to cross any mucosal epithelium reliably, unless the integrity of that epithelium is disrupted.

(3) Its size means that, even in the monomeric form, diffusion in tissues is slow, and absorption through the endothelium of blood vessels delayed.

(4) At higher concentrations, including those found in tissue depots after injection, insulin forms dimers and hexamers, slowing diffusion further.

(5) In even higher concentrations, as found in pharmaceutical preparations, the molecule is present almost entirely as hexamers, which break down to dimers only after injection as they slowly diffuse out into the subcutaneous tissue.

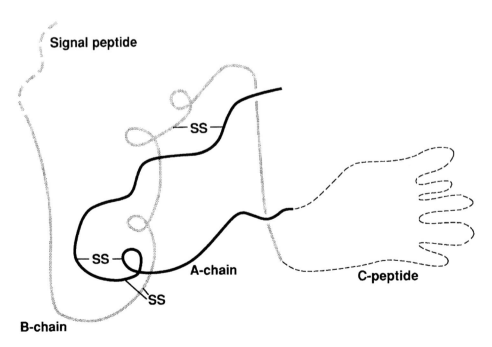

Figure 1   Diagram of the preproinsulin molecule to show the origin of the relationship between the A and B chains of insulin after removal of the signal and connecting peptides (C peptide)

Purification from Animal Pancreas

The insulin molecule bears many ionizable groups on its surface, but with a net charge tending to zero at pH 5.5 in water it is most soluble below pH 4.0 and above pH 7.0. This solubility is enhanced by divalent cations, in particular Zn^{2+}. At high pH, however, the molecule tends to degrade, because of instability of the cystine residues. It may be precipitated from solution by adjusting the pH to around its isoelectric point, and in quite low concentrations can also be precipitated by high concentrations of NaCl. Additionally, the relatively high content of hydrophobic amino acids renders the protein unusually soluble in alcohol–water mixtures.

These properties form the basis of the techniques developed from the pioneering efforts of Banting, Best and Collip for the commercial production of insulin [6]. Animal pancreas containing around 0.2 g/kg of insulin is deep-frozen until required. After homogenization it is extracted into acid ethanol/water, thus immediately separating it from most cellular proteins, including degrading enzymes. Neutralization and evaporation of the alcohol then removes further impurities, including fatty materials, by precipitation. The insulin itself is then precipitated from the extract with NaCl, the precipitate achieving a purity of some 20%. Further purification can be achieved by redissolving in acid and further judicious salting-out, before repeated recrystallization through precipitation at its isoelectric point. With careful choice of precipitation conditions, purity can be raised to around 90% insulin, the principal contaminants being proinsulin, proinsulin derivatives, insulin derivatives and other pancreatic peptides. In therapeutic use such a preparation has surprisingly little antigenicity of any clinical significance in the majority of patients.

Nevertheless, such preparations can hardly be described as pure, and some patients will develop significant levels of circulating insulin antibodies and immune complications (e.g. injection site lipoatrophy) when using such conventionally purified insulins. Methods based on gel filtration (separation by molecular size) and ion-exchange chromatography (separation by charge) were therefore developed, potentially reducing contaminants to less than 1 part in 10^6 [7]. Such methods remained the basis of highly purified insulin preparations until the advent of bioengineering.

Direct Synthesis of Insulin

Although direct synthesis of polypeptide chains became possible in the 1950s, the problems of achieving appropriate chemical combination of the A and B chains delayed total chemical synthesis of the molecule from its constituent amino acids until 1966 [8]. Even then the preparation was probably only around 70% pure, and yields of the order of 1–2% were obtained. Indeed, human insulin was first synthesized by building up the A and B chains around an already formed A20-B19 disulphide bridge, and enough of such a preparation was made to permit limited clinical studies in humans [9].

Experience with such methods also allowed the development of enzymatic techniques for the conversion of porcine insulin to human sequence insulin. This is possible because the amino acid sequence of these molecules differs by only a single residue (B30) at the end of the B chain.

The tedious synthesis and low yields have condemned such procedures to history, although the experience gained in combining A and B chains later proved useful in the early years of insulin production from bacteria. This became possible after the pioneering work of Ullrich et al in isolating rat insulin mRNA, synthesizing DNA using this template, and engineering the appropriate sequence into a bacterial plasmid [10]. Gilbert and colleagues were later able to control expression of such an engineered insulin gene [11], although the genes eventually used commercially were synthesized in the laboratory on the basis of the known amino acid sequence of human insulin. Early commercial methods used separate synthesis of A and B chains in *Escherichia coli*, with subsequent combination of the chains by chemical means. Later methods have employed synthesis of the human proinsulin molecule in yeast, and enzymatic cleavage of the C peptide as occurs in the islet B cell, but some chemical processing is still required to remove sequences necessary for the secretion of the end product.

Most insulin consumed around the world is now manufactured by such methods. There is no evidence that the introduction of the new technology has given rise to any problems in clinical practice. Genetic engineering has, however, allowed the synthesis of insulin derivatives with entirely novel amino acid sequences, and hence new chemical properties (see below).

IMMUNOGENICITY OF INJECTED INSULIN

Introduction and History

To a major extent the history of insulin therapy until the early 1980s is of continuing research into, and development of, ever purer insulin preparations. Although it might be considered that this interest ceased with the production of human sequence insulin, which is only clinically insignificantly antigenic, prospects for the introduction of entirely new insulin-like peptides may mean that the importance of minor degrees of immunogenicity again receive attention.

It seems likely that a large part of the toxicity of the early pancreatic extracts tested by Paulesco and others may have been due to immune reactions to their very high content of contaminants. The earliest extract used in the famous study on Leonard Thompson in Toronto was given only once, the 'thick brown muck' causing a sterile abscess at the injection site. Early commercial preparations caused a high incidence of reactions at injection sites in particular. Nevertheless, the key advance which allowed translation of the Toronto method to commercial production was the discovery of precipitation of insulin from aqueous solution at pH 5.5 by Walden in Indianapolis in late 1922 [2]. It was this recrystallization process, used repeatedly, that allowed the production of insulin preparations with no significant antigenicity in the majority of patients.

The first formal study of the relationship between the purity and antigenicity of insulin preparations is usually credited to Jorpes [12], who showed that the number of recrystallizations was inversely related to immunogenicity. Circulating insulin antibodies were subsequently demonstrated by Berson et al [13], while the advent of disc electrophoresis allowed Mirsky and Kawamura [14] to demonstrate that contemporary preparations of commercial insulin contained many components. It was with gel filtration, however, that Steiner and colleagues [15] were able to separate these components by molecular size, and quickly demonstrate the predominance of proinsulin, proinsulin derivatives and the covalent insulin dimer. Further refinement of electrophoresis led to the identification of monodesamido insulin as the first insulin-like impurity, but it is only with the advent of high-performance liquid chromatography (HPLC) that even some of the purest preparations currently available have been shown to contain small amounts of a range of insulin derivatives [16].

The presence of small amounts of other islet hormones, particularly glucagon and pancreatic polypeptide, and to a lesser extent somatostatin and vasoactive intestinal peptide, in conventionally purified insulin preparations of pancreatic origin has never been shown to be of any clinical significance.

That human insulin preparations could be immunogenic was demonstrated with insulin prepared in small amounts from human pancreas and used (therapeutically) in psychiatric patients. Such preparations would, however, contain other pancreatic contaminants and, in particular, human proinsulin derivatives, which might be expected to induce antibodies cross-reacting with insulin itself. It is, however, now clear that even highly purified human insulin prepared by semisynthesis from porcine insulin, or by recombinant DNA technology, is to some extent antigenic when injected subcutaneously, as demonstrated by detectable levels of insulin antibodies in 40–50% of patients despite the insensitive nature of the antibody assay. Indeed, studies suggest that whereas there are major differences in antigenicity between conventionally purified and highly purified insulin preparations, the differences between highly purified insulins of different species (especially porcine and human) are small and clinically insignificant [17].

Why should 'human' insulin be antigenic in human beings? Insulin is not entirely stable in solution, and it appears that a range of derivatives may form during the manufacturing and purification processes whatever methodology is followed. Futhermore, insulin is generally injected into subcutaneous tissue, often in forms designed to reside there for considerable periods of time, and it may be that insulin itself or its derivatives can undergo further degradation in the injection depot into forms that may be recognized by the body as foreign proteins. However, there is no evidence that systemic reactions occur as a result of this residual antigenicity, or that local reactions as a result interfere significantly with insulin absorption or contribute to local tissue damage.

Circulating Insulin Antibodies

With the advent of highly purified and human insulin preparations, it is no longer the case that all insulin-treated patients have detectable circulating insulin antibodies, as previously established by Berson and Yalow in the 1950s [13]. However, considerable non-specific binding is a problem in insulin antibody assays, making them insensitive to low antibody levels. This is not of any clinical consequence, except in so far as insulin antibodies interfere with assay of insulin in plasma. Even in patients in whom antibody-bound insulin in plasma is in similar concentration to unbound ('free') insulin, insulin antibody may not be detectable by current methods, and insulin antibody assays cannot therefore be used to select patients for assay of insulin levels by direct methods. Such low levels of antibodies are not otherwise of clinical significance (see below).

Significant circulating insulin antibody levels may, however, be found in patients on highly purified insulin preparations if they have previously been treated with conventionally purified animal insulins. Nevertheless, the majority of such patients will have shown a rapid decline in insulin antibodies to clinically insignificant but measurable levels at the time that their insulin preparations were changed [17]. Management of such change is now rarely needed in industrialized nations, and detailed guidelines are given elsewhere [18, 19]. Where insulin dosage is less than 1.0 U/kg per day, the patient has access to self-monitoring of blood glucose, and injection site lipoatrophy is not present, no prospective dose reduction is advised on changing to a highly purified preparation from recrystallized insulin. However, there may still be a significant fall in insulin antibody titres over the following months, and a gradual reduction in insulin dose will then be necessary, in line with monitoring results. Where there is evidence of high levels of serum insulin antibodies, then there is a risk of differential binding between beef and porcine/human insulin, so that a prospective dose reduction of up to 25% of the previous dose should be advised. However, in many patients this will prove to be unnecessary, and again the real need for less insulin will only be felt more gradually over the ensuing weeks and months.

About 40% of patients started on the newer insulin preparations will develop detectable plasma insulin antibodies by 6 months, with a small decline thereafter [20]. Factors that tend to enhance the antigenicity of insulin include the presence of other disease (e.g. foot ulceration) and intermittent therapy. In countries where highly purified preparations are in short supply, these patients, and pregnant women, should be given priority.

Insulin autoantibodies may also be detected in people in the prodrome of type 1 diabetes (Chapter 5). There are rare reports of non-diabetic people suffering hypoglycaemia as a result of extremely high plasma insulin antibody concentrations, and this may be a problem in the neonatal offspring of such women [21]. In many of these cases the presence of antibodies to bovine insulin and C peptide suggests the problem to be iatrogenic misuse of insulin.

Circulating insulin antibody is mostly present as IgG. Some patients also have detectable levels of anti-insulin IgE, and this is thought to be of significance in those with systemic immune reactions [22]. Insulin antibody levels can be measured by gel diffusion methods, immunochemical methods and enzyme-linked immunosorbent assays (ELISA). These methods correlate well in expert hands, but attention must be paid to problems of non-specific interference, especially with ELISA methods [23].

Clinical Significance of the Immunogenicity of Injected Insulin

Insulin Resistance

Immunological insulin resistance with a dose requirement greater than 1.4 U/kg body weight was already rare before the introduction of the highly purified insulin preparations in the mid-1970s [24]. Indeed, probably few patients using conventional preparations had any detectable increase in insulin dose as a result of circulating antibodies. Other causes of high dose requirement are now much more common (see below), and immunological resistance is easily excluded by laboratory assay of insulin antibodies.

Prolonged Insulin Action

Moderate insulin antibody levels, above those now commonly found in patients, do probably prolong the effect of a subcutaneous injection of insulin. The mechanism was probably that of delayed absorption, as the circulating antibody pool was rarely large enough to sequester (and subsequently to release) significant amounts of insulin. Placental passage of insulin antibodies may, however, be an additional factor contributing to the risk of hypoglycaemia in the hyperinsulinaemic neonate [25].

Injection Site Lipoatrophy

There is no evidence that the antigenicity of insulin contributes to injection site lipohypertrophy, which is thought to reflect the growth factor and anabolic properties of insulin. Lipoatrophy, however, correlates with high circulating insulin antibody levels, and immune complexes containing insulin can be demonstrated at the site of such skin problems [26]. Injection well away from the affected area, and dispersion of injection sites should be recommended. Lipoatrophy is very rarely seen in patients treated only with highly purified or human insulin, and appears then not to have an immune pathogenesis.

Injection Site Reactions

Problems of redness, soreness or swelling at insulin injection sites should initially suggest the use of inappropriate solutions to clean the skin, or an inappropriate (too superficial) injection technique. Immunological problems are rare, and skin testing kits are available from the manufacturers to test specifically for reactions to insulin itself or the other contents of the insulin vial. If the insulin itself is not at fault, it may then be possible to choose an insulin preparation that does not contain the incriminated vehicle or substance (see below). If the insulin does appear to be the cause, a change to a human insulin preparation is recommended, and injection technique should be reviewed to ensure placement of the depot deep in the subcutaneous tissue.

Systemic Insulin Allergy

Systemic reactions to injected insulin are now rare, and very rare without exposure to conventionally purified animal insulin under provocative conditions (see above). Such reactions are associated with raised plasma IgE levels, and unlike anti-insulin IgG this often shows differential binding between human and animal insulin [22]. Some insulin manufacturers will measure anti-insulin IgE on request. A change to human insulin is therefore indicated. Schedules for desensitization have been published [24] (see also Chapter 44).

Other Aspects

There is no solid evidence that the presence of circulating insulin antibodies is associated with better blood glucose control, development of diabetic complications, inhibition of endogenous insulin secretion or preservation of residual islet B-cell function [19].

PHARMACEUTICAL PREPARATIONS OF INSULIN

Short-acting Insulin; Unmodified Insulin

The earliest pharmaceutical preparations of insulin from early 1923, after Walden's discovery of the process of recrystallization (see above), were of insulin dissolved in acid solution. In 1926 Abel discovered that it was possible to prepare insulin crystals in the presence of zinc ions, and from that time the acid solution of insulin was termed 'crystalline insulin', 'soluble insulin' or 'regular insulin'. None of these terms was ever strictly accurate or helpful, and they are even less true now that manufacturers bypass the preparation of insulin crystals in any form. The term 'unmodified insulin' is currently creeping into the literature, and has the added benefit of distinguishing native insulin from both complexed forms and the newer insulin analogues (see below). On clinical grounds it is misleading

to term the unmodified formulations 'rapid-acting insulin'.

Acid solutions are mildly irritant, and cannot be mixed with neutral suspension insulin preparations in the syringe. Furthermore, insulin degrades more quickly in acid than in neutral solutions [27], and is hence rather more antigenic. There is, however, no evidence for differences in pharmacokinetics.

Neutral preparations (Table 1) made from acid-dissolved crystalline insulin will have a significant salt content, and sodium chloride is often added to these solutions so that they are isotonic with tissue fluids. More recently, however, glycerol has become the principal agent for adjusting osmolality. Some manufacturers have buffered neutral insulin solutions with acetate or phosphate; the latter is of practical significance in that it is inappropriate to mix such insulin with the insulin–zinc suspensions (see below). More recent formulations tend not to contain buffers.

Preparations containing up to 4 g/l Zn^{2+} will retain insulin in solution up to around 20 g/l (500 U/ml) [27]. This is the highest concentration of unmodified insulin generally available from manufacturers, although, in the absence of zinc, concentrations some ten times higher may be attained.

As aqueous isotonic solutions containing significant amounts of protein, insulin solutions in multiple-use vials would be ideal culture media in the absence of preservatives. By tradition, the preservatives used have been methyl 4-hydroxybenzoate, phenol or *m*-cresol. Studies have suggested that the last two are more effective, and phenol has become the standard for newer insulin preparations. These additives give insulin formulations their familiar odour, do not appear

Table 1 The characteristics of commercially available insulin preparations world wide

Insulin type	Synonyms	Retardant	Preservative	Buffers/salts	Species available	Timing of effect (hours)		
						Onset	Peak	Duration
Unmodified	Soluble Regular Short-acting	None	Methyl-*p*-benzoate *m*-Cresol Phenol	NaCl Glycerol Na(H)PO$_4$ Na acetate	Human Porcine Bovine	0.25–1	1.5–4	5–9
NPH	Isophane	Protamine	*m*-Cresol/ phenol	Glycerol Na(H)PO$_4$	Human Porcine Bovine	0.5–2	3–6	8–14
Lente	Insulin–zinc suspension (mixed)	Zinc	Methyl-*p*-benzoate	Na acetate NaCl	Human Porcine Bovine	1–2 1–2 1.5–3	3–8 3–8 5–10	7–14 7–16 10–24
Ultralente	Insulin–zinc suspension (crystalline)	Zinc	Methyl-*p*-benzoate	Na acetate NaCl	Human Bovine	2–3 3–4	4–8 6–12	8–14 12–28

to affect insulin absorption, and may improve the solubility of insulin in neutral solution.

Extended-acting Insulin Preparations Not in General Use

Earliest attempts to extend the duration of effect of subcutaneously injected unmodified insulin involved the addition of additives to the insulin solution. Examples tried without useful clinical effect included gum arabic, oils, tannin, cholesterol, lecithin and even (for pharmacological effect on local vasculature) adrenaline and vasopressin [28]. Attempts to reduce the solubility of insulin at neutral pH in tissue fluids involved the addition of basic organic compounds to the acid insulin solution, and it was this approach that set the use of protamine on the road to clinical dominance (see below). Globin, histones and surfen (1,3-bis(4-amino-2-methyl-6-quinolyl) urea) were further examples; the latter is still available in some countries. However, surfen appears to be more antigenic than protamine, and a significant cause of immunogenicity of insulin preparations.

A second approach involved the derivatization of insulin with phenylisocyanate (iso-insulin), probably resulting in the formation of non-covalent dimers, which cause a substantial change in solubility of the preparation. More recently, genetic engineering has been used to alter solubility (see below).

Isophane (NPH) and Protamine–Zinc Insulin

Protamine is a very basic protein found in large quantities in fish sperm nuclei, where it has a role in stabilizing DNA. Its basic properties stem from a high content of arginine residues, also resulting in a smooth sheet-like structure which is essentially non-immunogenic. Hagedorn and colleagues [29] used protamine to precipitate insulin at neutral pH, but the preparation was not stable, and was supplied as two vials which the patient mixed and then used for a few days. Scott and Fisher [30] noted that excess protamine and small quantities of zinc (2 μg/U) would stabilize the neutral insulin protaminate, the amorphous precipitate of which then evolves slowly into a crystalline form.

This protamine–zinc insulin has a very long absorption profile from subcutaneous tissue, perhaps because the zinc inhibits the tissue proteinases which digest the protamine. It is difficult to manufacture consistently, despite recent attempts to produce more useful versions of the complex, and now is little used. Antigenicity of the preparation was high, at least in its conventionally purified form, with a high prevalence of injection site lipoatrophy. Absorption tended to be very erratic, consistent with the very long duration of absorption.

Neutral protamine Hagedorn (NPH) insulin (Table 1) was developed as a stable insulin protaminate [31]. At neutral pH, in the obligatory presence of *m*-cresol and low concentrations of Zn^{2+} (two atoms per hexamer), insulin and protamine solutions are mixed in stoichiometric proportions (hence 'isophane'). The amorphous precipitate evolves with time to form tetragonal crystals. The purity and source of the protamine used, and details of the manufacturing process, significantly affect the final form of the crystals and hence insulin absorption, so that preparations from different manufacturers are not necessarily pharmacologically identical.

Insulin–Zinc Suspensions

Zinc concentrations above 0.5 μg/l significantly reduce the solubility of insulin, particularly at neutral pH [32]. If acetate rather than phosphate or citrate buffer is used (to avoid precipitation of zinc), stable precipitates of insulin can then be formed.

Ultralente insulin is prepared by first crystallizing insulin at pH 5.5 in its rhombohedral form with four Zn^{2+} per hexamer, and then adjusting to pH 7.4 in the presence of excess zinc. In the process the hexamer structure changes to the two Zn^{2+} form, but binds further zinc on its surface. Careful attention to crystal seeding and size is needed to obtain consistent preparations. Ultralente insulin is slowly absorbed from subcutaneous tissue, but the rate of absorption is highly dependent on the species of insulin used (Table 1).

If, however, the insulin solution is adjusted to pH 7.4 in the presence of excess zinc without previous crystallization, an amorphous precipitate is formed, and will resist crystallization for many years. This form is known as semilente insulin. Lente insulin is a 30:70 mixture of semilente and ultralente insulin preparations.

Phenol and its derivatives destroy the stability of these insulin crystals. Methyl 4-hydroxybenzoate is therefore used as preservative, but the excess zinc is also highly bacteriostatic.

Novel Insulin Derivatives

A number of attempts have been made in recent decades to design newer insulin derivatives to replace the extended-acting preparations in general use. Most of these have been founded on the old principles of zinc and protamine (or other binding proteins or substances), and while some have found their way into patient trials, their success has been so limited that not even preliminary reports have appeared in the literature.

In the last 5–10 years attention turned to the use of insulin analogues modified to reduce solubility in the subcutaneous tissue and thus delay absorption. This approach has seen limited success to date and is discussed below.

Very recently, novel insulin derivatives have been produced (and at the time of writing tested in pigs) by acylation of the amino group of the B29 lysine residue [122, 123]. Unlike acylation of the available amino groups at the N-terminal ends of the peptide chains [124], acylation at this site does not interfere with either potency or hexamerization (useful for stability) to any significant extent. The idea behind acylation is that the aliphatic chain will bind to albumin, and that absorption from the subcutaneous site will then be delayed by this attachment to the much larger albumin molecule.

Studies of different chain lengths have suggested that a 10-carbon chain provided the best compromise between albumin binding and receptor affinity [122]. Subcutaneous absorption time in pigs correlated with albumin binding, and is usefully longer than for NPH insulin. Intravenous clearance is also delayed.

This approach needs further testing in non-diabetic and diabetic man. While the very large number of binding sites of human albumin suggests that competition will not give problems (with drugs or non-esterified fatty acids for example) [125], there are also questions to be answered in people with high vessel wall permeability to albumin (microalbuminuria), and concerning pharmacokinetics and growth factor activity.

Premixed Formulations of Insulin

When unmodified (soluble, regular) insulin is mixed with an extended-acting preparation there is always some interaction between the free (dissolved) insulin and the complexing agent (zinc or protamine) (see below). Where manufacturers mix unmodified and isophane (NPH) insulin preparations, often in a 30:70 ratio, over one-half of the free insulin is not recoverable in the supernatant [33]. However, it is generally accepted that the complex formed between the added insulin and the crystals is a loose one (provided that there is no excess of protamine), and that after dilution in tissue fluid after injection this insulin is, for the most part, immediately available for absorption.

Such an approach is not possible with the insulin–zinc suspensions, owing to the relatively high free zinc concentrations in solution. An aproach to this problem (Rapitard, Novo), using the differential solubility of porcine (as unmodified) and bovine (as ultralente) insulins at particular conditions of zinc concentration and pH, did not gain a significant share of the market.

INSULIN ANALOGUES

The techniques of genetic engineering (see above) allow substitution or addition of any of the amino acid residues of insulin at will, simply by changing the nucleic acid sequence of the insulin gene. This contrasts with the difficulties inherent in chemical manipulations of the insulin molecule. The properties of the insulin molecule are diverse (including receptor binding, growth factor activity, covalent polymerization and antigenicity), and it is possible to produce derivatives of human insulin in which any of the characteristics are altered. Not surprisingly, it is difficult to change a single property only.

Two approaches have been followed in attempting to produce insulins with a shorter or longer duration of absorption compared to human insulin or current extended-acting insulin preparations respectively. For faster-absorbed insulin the thrust has been to produce insulin analogues which less readily associate into dimers and hexamers at the concentrations found in the subcutaneous depot [34, 35]. As the endothelial pore size is close to that of the insulin monomer, dimers and hexamers are absorbed very much more slowly than the monomer, and thus effectively are not available for absorption as such. Furthermore the very equilibrium between monomer↔dimer↔hexamer will be subject to conditions in the subcutaneous tissue, and might therefore be a source of variable absorption rates of the monomer.

For novel extended-acting preparations, which represent the greater clinical need, the approach has been to reduce solubility by introducing or adding hydrophobic amino acids to the insulin molecule [126, 127]. The general approach has been to produce a molecule whose pK was so shifted that it was soluble at pH 3.0–4.0 in buffer, but precipitated in the tissues at pH 7.2–7.4 after injection [126, 127].

Short-acting Analogues

Many of the sites involved in dimerization and hexamerization of insulin are on the B chain, particularly its terminal eight amino acids, although other residues on the A chain are also involved [35]. Indeed, it has been known for some time that removal of the last five amino acids of the B chain stops association while retaining potency, but the resulting despentapeptide insulin has poor chemical stability. Methods of interfering with association include substituting amino acids with negatively-charged aspartate or glutamate (positive charge would increase pK and therefore lead to precipitation near physiological pH), increasing solubility through substituting hydrophilic glutamate into hydrophobic interfaces, physical (steric) obstruction using an amino acid with a larger side chain, and removal of the histidines necessary for Zn^{2+} binding [35].

A very large number of insulin analogues have now been manufactured, but consideration has to be given to matters of potency (to some degree), antigenicity, and stability, in selecting those for studies in humans. In practice, *in vitro* potency is maintained with many such substitutions, and as insulin clearance is via its receptor, potency in laboratory assays within a range of 20–500% leads to *in vivo* potency indistinguishable from native insulin [128]. Stability is more of a problem, as fibril formation occurs through polymerization of the monomer, and is therefore a much greater problem with some of the analogues. Furthermore, the chemical reactivity of insulin is reduced in its associated states. Accordingly, these matters have dictated choice of insulin analogues for clinical development, favouring those which tend to dimerize and even hexamerize at the high concentrations and more acid pH of the insulin vial.

Immunogenicity of insulin analogues might be thought to be a potential problem. In practice minor substitutions which leave the overall structure of the molecule intact (necessary for receptor interaction and thus potency) cause little or no insulin antibody production in animal models or in humans compared to human insulin [129, 130].

An initial assumption was that, as minor derivatives of insulin, any such analogues would have little or no toxicity, but in the event toxicity has proved to be a major problem. An early candidate insulin analogue, B_{10}-Asp, entered trials in patients before being found to promote the formation of mammary tumours when administered at high concentrations to susceptible strains of rats [131]. This effect did not seem to be due to statistical chance, and subsequent investigation has demonstrated the mitogenicity of this analogue in *in vitro* assays. The effect seems to be related in some way to failure to dissociate from the insulin receptor, and to high tyrosine kinase stimulatory activity, and has led to new insights into insulin receptor function.

At present two candidate analogues are under investigation for clinical efficacy in people with diabetes. Lispro is a B_{28}-lysine, B_{29}-proline substituted analogue with reduced association properties, which can nevertheless be crystallized at high concentrations [132]. The unnamed 'X14' analogue is also B_{28} substituted, but with aspartate.

Long-acting Analogues

The principle employed in the development of long-acting analogues has been to reduce solubility at the pH of subcutaneous tissue fluid. Examples are the substitution of hydrophobic amino acids within the insulin

monomer [126], or the addition of arginine residues to the end of the B chain [127], this echoing one of the intermediates found in the conversion of proinsulin to insulin. The first approach, producing an insulin soluble in the insulin vial at pH 3.0, but precipitating in the tissues, has since been abandoned as a candidate for commercial development due to poor efficacy in patients [133], probably due to poor bioavailability after precipitation. The latter insulin analogue (B_{31}-B_{32}-diarginine) initially had poor chemical stability, but this has been enhanced by A_{21} glycine substitution, and the resulting analogue is undergoing clinical investigation at the time of writing [134].

STORAGE AND STANDARDIZATION OF INSULIN

Storage and Stability

A variety of reactions occur in insulin solutions and crystals with time, predominantly deamidation and polymerization (non-covalent). These changes will produce a gradual loss of potency, but this loss is highly temperature dependent. Thus, at 4°C a loss of potency of 2% will take decades for both complexed and dissolved insulin, whereas at 25°C such a loss will take about 6 months [27]. At higher temperatures (40°C) a 2% loss occurs in about 1 week, and a 5% loss in a month. This assumes that the insulin is kept in the dark. Sunlight increases the degradation rate many hundreds of times.

Freezing will damage the crystal structure of the complexed preparations, and must be avoided. Dissolved insulin will precipitate on freezing, and will slowly go back into solution after thawing.

Standardization of Insulin Preparations

Standardization of insulin was necessary from the beginnings of insulin manufacture to ensure consistency from batch to batch, and a rabbit hypoglycaemia test was used by Eli Lilly for this purpose from 1922. A mouse convulsion assay was employed as an alternative in Europe, and is perhaps to be preferred as being less time-dependent. Both these bioassays have wide confidence limits unless enormous numbers of animals are used, and nitrogen content eventually became the internal standard used by most manufacturers.

In the first international standard 1 U of insulin (mixed species) was defined as 0.125 mg, but this can only have been 28% pure. Later standards reached 24 U/mg, but improvements in purification techniques tracked against bioassays by nitrogen estimation suggest that salt-free human insulin is 28.9–29.0 U/mg [36]. More recently, HPLC techniques have superseded nitrogen estimation for quality control of potency of commercial insulin preparations [27], but it must be recognized that the range of potency accepted for different batches of insulin is around ±5%. In the first international standard for human insulin [37] there are 26.0 U/mg, but after allowing for the salt water content this suggests that there are 28.7 U/mg protein, or 6.00 nmol/U [38].

ABSORPTION OF INJECTED INSULIN

Subcutaneous injection was a common route of drug delivery at the time that insulin therapy was introduced, the few effective therapies then available often being toxic or ineffective by mouth. Although the nature of insulin was unknown at the time, preparations were soon shown not to be active by mouth, a property understood when insulin was shown to be a peptide. Very early attempts [39] were made to deliver insulin by application to various mucosal surfaces, but it is now clear that peptides with molecular weights above 1000 Da are not significantly absorbed, even across simple columnar epithelia [40]. Attention in the last decade has focused on the use of adjuvants to enhance absorption across mucosae, and on transperitoneal and intravenous insulin delivery. These are described in Chapter 41.

In contrast to insulin, most drugs now given by depot injection are given intramuscularly. Muscle gives more reliable absorption, and through its bulk allows more consistent placement of injection depots. The retention of subcutaneous tissue as a site for insulin injection largely reflects the needs of patients to self-inject, although recent research has suggested that with current insulin preparations there may be other advantages of the subcutaneous over the intramuscular route in day-to-day treatment (see below). However, in situations where the subcutaneous circulation may be compromised (ketoacidosis, circulatory collapse), intramuscular injection of insulin is to be preferred.

The primary aim of insulin injection therapy, at least in patients with type 1 diabetes, must be to replace as closely as possible the plasma insulin concentration profile that would have been provided by the islet B cell (see below). Apart from the problems of subcutaneous insulin pharmacokinetics (discussed below), a number of factors militate against this:

(1) Secretion of insulin is controlled on a minute-to-minute basis by complex interrelated mechanisms (Chapter 15), whereas injection must be of a depot given before requirements are known. This is a major therapeutic problem.

(2) Absorption of insulin is into the peripheral circulation, not the portal vein. Together with the high hepatic clearance rate of insulin, this results in a much lower portal to peripheral insulin concentration ratio than is found physiologically. The clinical significance of this remains obscure.

(3) Physiological insulin secretion appears to be pulsatile, with secretion periods of around 4 minutes in every 12 minutes [41]. The physiological importance of this remains to be established, but is probably of little importance compared with pulsatile delivery of other hormones.

The Absorption Process

Unmodified Insulin

At the insulin concentration in a standard vial (10^{-4} mol/l), unmodified insulin will be almost entirely in the hexameric state, with a molecular weight of around 35 000, and a molecular diffusion radius of 2.3 nm [42]. After injection, some dilution will occur, dependent on dispersion of the depot, and thus in different parts of the depot monomeric, dimeric and hexameric insulin molecules will be found in varying ratios. This ratio would also be expected to change with time, owing to further dispersion of the depot, and eventually as the depot approaches exhaustion. The molecular radius of monomeric insulin is around 1.2 nm. This is significantly different from the hexameric form, as the principal influence on absorption for molecules of this size will be the capillary pore radius, allowing virtually free diffusion below 1.0 nm but forming a nearly complete barrier at only 4.0 nm. As the capillary pore is the critical barrier, its numbers are also important, and hence the number of capillaries through which blood is flowing. The actual blood flow *per se* in those open capillaries will not be of importance; nor, under normal conditions, is lymph flow or lymphatic absorption of any significance [43]. It can be seen from the above that a number of variables will affect subcutaneous insulin absorption:

(1) Dispersion of the injected volume will increase dilution by tissue fluid, and hence increase the proportion of smaller molecular weight species, and also will increase the capillary area available for absorption.

(2) Diffusion should be relatively constant within tissue fluid, but may be affected by the ratio of cells to intercellular space in the subcutaneous tissue. Diffusion will be important immediately after injection in allowing the insulin to reach the capillary pores.

(3) Actual capillary density should be important, and may be expected to be reduced with obesity, for example.

(4) The proportion of capillaries open or closed will significantly affect the number of capillary pores available for absorption.

(5) Injected volume (and therefore concentration in the vial) would be expected to affect dispersion.

(6) The rate of removal (by diffusion and absorption) of zinc will affect the polymeric state of the insulin.

After absorption of insulin into the circulation, the kinetics of insulin clearance are very rapid compared with its absorption [44]. Although this high metabolic clearance rate is important in determining the concentrations of insulin reached at any one time, the shape of the absorption profile from an injection depot will be largely determined by the absorption rate rather than the clearance rate after the first half-hour.

The first phase of absorption after injection of unmodified insulin is, however, the lag period, representing the time for the first molecules to diffuse to the capillary pores for absorption. This phase lasts for approximately 10 minutes. If this was consistent throughout the depot plasma concentrations would then rise to a peak over the next 20–30 minutes (corresponding to five times the plasma half-life, as occurs with a square wave intravenous insulin infusion). In practice the peak is delayed to 45–180 minutes, reflecting the variable length of the diffusion path to the endothelial cells (Figure 2). Once past peak concentrations, the absorption rate and therefore the plasma concentration will fall exponentially with a half-time $(0.693/k)$ of 60–120 minutes as the depot is progressively exhausted. This exponential fall will, however, be interrupted by any change in available capillary surface area for absorption. The half-time of steady state absorption should not be confused with the $T_{1/2}$ beloved of those measuring disappearance times of radioactive insulin from subcutaneous depots: this latter is the time to half the original activity, and is hence affected by the lag time and tissue diffusion times as well as the steady state absorption rate.

The physiological effects of insulin will not, however, parallel the plasma concentration profile. Thus, even after a bolus intravenous injection of insulin, peak depression of blood glucose levels occurs at 30–40 minutes, after insulin concentrations have returned to near normal. This is generally conceptualized as insulin acting at a site remote from the plasma compartment [45]. Furthermore, the dose–response relationship for insulin is logarithmic for concentrations of physiological importance, and is left-shifted for tissues sensitive to insulin (adipocytes, liver) relative to skeletal muscle.

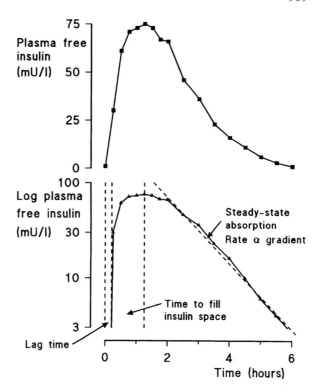

Figure 2 The incremental plasma insulin profile after injection of unmodified insulin plotted on a linear scale (top), with a logarithmic scale below to aid interpretation of the absorption process. Note the brief lag phase of around 10 minutes before any insulin appears in the plasma. This is followed by a period of rapid absorption during which a high proportion of the insulin entering the plasma goes to fill the insulin space to a high concentration. Peak levels are, however, delayed beyond what would be expected by this mechanism alone (5 plasma half-times), presumably while the insulin depot further diffuses within the subcutaneous tissue. From peak levels, relatively steady state absorption is encountered, and plasma concentrations then fall exponentially (straight line on the log scale) with a half-time of clearance of the depot of 60–120 minutes

Short-acting Insulin Analogues

Insulin analogues engineered to prevent formation of covalent hexamers and/or dimers will be subject to the same influences of dispersion as native human insulin, and will diffuse only a little faster (in terms of clinical significance) within the tissue. The absence of the hexamer will have marked effects on diffusion rate into the capillary, however, so that the steady state absorption rate will be around twice that of insulin. The plasma concentration profile will be further altered by the different metabolic clearance rate (some higher, some lower) of these analogues [35]. However, this is of little physiological significance as it is changes in removal of insulin through its receptor that determine the clearance rate, and thus, for example, decreased clearance results in higher concentrations being needed to have the same physiological effect.

Complexed Insulin Preparations

For complexed insulin preparations—isophane (NPH), insulin–zinc suspensions—a further factor in the absorption process will be dissolution of the complex to provide 'free' insulin, which will then be absorbed in the same way, and subject to the same influences, as unmodified insulin. Understanding of dissolution of the complexes is, however, poor, and the process is unlikely to be simple. Zinc–insulin complexes can be assumed to dissolve at the surface of the crystals [43], but the insulin and zinc concentrations at the surface will be high, and it is therefore likely that association states similar to semilente insulin (see above) as well as insulin hexamers will form. It is highly likely that these processes will be affected by changes in local conditions, such as tissue pH. The high free zinc concentrations of insulin–zinc suspensions will also form loose complexes with any unmodified insulin mixed with them at the time of injection, a problem that will assume clinical significance if there is delay between mixing and injection, and if high ratios of complexed to unmodified insulin are used with lower-strength insulin formulations (e.g. 40 U/ml) [46].

Isophane (NPH) insulin crystals have been assumed to dissociate largely through the action of local tissue proteases [47], but here also simple physical dissolution plays a part. As diffusion away from the crystals will be slow, there is again the likelihood of local interactions between the protamine and insulin, and all these processes will be affected by tissue state. Recent studies have shown that dissolution of isophane (NPH) complexes is indeed accelerated by some of the influences (temperature, exercise) that affect absorption of unmodified insulin [48]. The interaction between an isophane insulin preparation and added unmodified insulin is not thought to be clinically significant.

Although it will be clear from the above that the absorption of all insulin preparations is likely to be erratic (Figure 3), this is a particular problem for the extended-acting preparations. Indeed, the clinical impression is that unpredictable absorption increases in proportion to duration of effect, with the long-acting preparations (bovine ultralente, protamine–zinc insulin) most marked in this respect. With these preparations, and in some patients using intermediate-acting insulin preparations, insulin dose is also higher, suggesting that bioavailability is significantly reduced, in contrast to unmodified insulin where bioavailability is 90–100%. Although insulin-degrading proteases can be found in subcutaneous tissue it is not clear whether these mainly intracellular enzymes are responsible for the decreased bioavailability of long-resident insulin, or whether other scavenging mechanisms are at work.

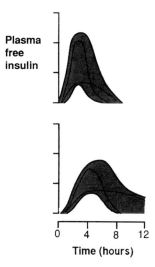

Figure 3 Diagrammatic plasma free insulin levels in diabetic patients after injection of unmodified (top) or intermediate-acting insulin subcutaneously. The grey areas represent the 95% confidence limits of insulin concentration, which can be seen to vary very widely. The light lines within the grey areas represent hypothetical absorption curves in the same individual on different days

Factors Affecting Insulin Absorption

Physiological Factors and Exercise

It is evident from the description of the absorption process above that the major variable is the capillary surface area available to the injection depot. In the subcutaneous plexus many capillaries will be closed at any one time, but this can change greatly if body temperature rises, local skin temperature is increased by external influences (e.g. local warming) [49], or through effects of vasodilating drugs (e.g. ethanol). Marked effects on absorption of unmodified insulin have been demonstrated, particularly with hot baths [50], and lesser effects can be demonstrated for complexed insulin preparations with local warming [48]. Opposite effects are to be expected with local or systemic cooling, vasoconstrictors (including smoking), dehydration or circulatory collapse. Hypoglycaemia will thus affect insulin absorption in normal subjects, although the effects are less easily demonstrable in diabetic patients. This may reflect the loss of autoregulatory control of skin blood flow in diabetes, perhaps as a result of the earliest processes of microangiopathy. However, the influence of basement membrane thickening and subcutaneous microvascular disease on insulin absorption remains obscure.

Massage has also been shown to increase absorption of unmodified insulin [51], presumably through dispersion of the depot, but is not used therapeutically on a wide scale. Massage may be relevant during exercise, when it is possible that the injection site could be effectively 'massaged' from beneath. This may partly explain the lesser changes in insulin absorption that occur with leg exercise if insulin is given into the anterior abdominal wall rather than the subcutaneous tissues of the thigh. Exercise, however, will have other effects on subcutaneous physiology, principally through increases in blood flow as body temperature rises. In the non-diabetic subject, insulin concentrations fall during exercise, mainly through the direct inhibition of insulin secretion by adrenaline, so the insulin-treated diabetic patient is doubly disadvantaged by plasma insulin concentrations tending to rise.

Structural Factors and Lipohypertrophy

Discussion of the structural factors affecting insulin absorption is relevant only when insulin is being given consistently into the subcutaneous tissue, and not into the dermis or underlying muscle (see below). Different regions used for insulin injection differ in their subcutaneous capillary density, which is highest for anterior abdominal wall and lowest for the thigh, with the upper arm intermediate between these [52]. More rapid absorption of insulin from the abdominal wall implies a faster rise to peak concentrations, and a faster fall towards baseline, both desirable features for short-acting insulins. Extended-acting insulin preparations are also absorbed more quickly from the same site, however, a feature less desirable in the majority of patients when trying to obtain reasonable overnight blood glucose control.

Less well studied is the effect of obesity on insulin absorption, but subcutaneous blood flow does decrease with the thickness of adipose tissue [53], and delayed insulin absorption has been described in subjects with increased adiposity. The effects are presumably due to decreased capillary density with displacement by adipocytes. Whether the advantage to insulin absorption rate of the anterior abdominal wall is lost in those patients with central obesity is not known.

A common form of local obesity at injection sites is lipohypertrophy, nearly always occurring as a result of recurrent injection into a closely circumscribed area. The form of lipohypertrophy varies from large bulges mainly composed of fat, to barely evident thickening. In the latter case ultrasonography reveals not just increased adipose tissue but also disorganization and scarring of the subcutis, presumably as the result of recurrent injection trauma. Such damage can be detected over quite large areas of a well-used injection site. Studies of insulin pharmacokinetics in these areas demonstrate both decreased and more erratic absorption [54].

Insulin Antibodies

Circulating insulin antibodies are now of little clinical significance in many patients (see above), but several authors have suggested that these could affect insulin absorption at higher levels by acting as a buffer or store of circulating insulin. There is, however, little evidence that the stock of circulating and exchangeable insulin was great enough for this, except in a very small minority of patients; it certainly could not explain insulin resistance. There is, however, some evidence that higher circulating insulin antibody titres cause a delayed rise in insulin concentrations [55], as some of the absorbed insulin is taken up by insulin antibodies (Figure 4).

Intramuscular Injections

In the 1980s it was generally advised that insulin injections should be given to the full depth of a 12.5-mm needle, to ensure consistent placement below the dermis. Towards the end of the decade it was pointed

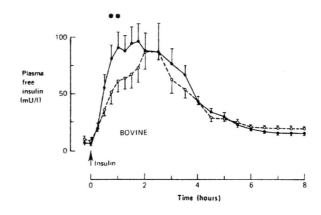

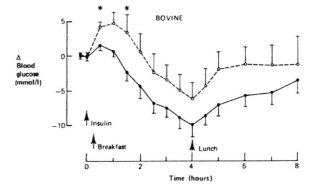

Figure 4 Experimental demonstration of the effect of high circulating insulin antibody levels (open circles) compared with more usual titres (solid circles) on the absorption of bovine unmodified insulin. The delayed rise in plasma insulin concentrations is likely to be due to the increase in the apparent insulin space resulting from circulating antibodies taking up insulin (from reference 55, with permission)

out that this would very often imply intramuscular injection, particularly in men injecting over the thigh [56]. Furthermore, many of the so-called subcutaneous absorption studies performed in the 1980s did utilize that injection technique, and were often performed in young men. Re-examination of the comparative effects of intramuscular and true subcutaneous (ultrasonographically guided) injection has confirmed that absorption from an intramuscular depot is faster for both short-acting and extended-acting insulin preparations [57]. This may be desirable for short-acting preparations, but the intramuscular depot is markedly affected by exercise, as may be expected. Furthermore, it is clearly undesirable to shorten the duration of effect of the intermediate-acting preparations, particularly for overnight use.

Examination of patient injection technique will reveal that, despite careful instruction, the majority of injections are not in practice given through the fascia over the muscle, which is well endowed with pain receptors.

INSULIN INJECTION REGIMENS

Design of insulin injection regimens depends both on a knowledge of an individual patient's requirements, in terms of eating and activities in particular, and on a knowledge of insulin pharmacokinetics. Furthermore, the pharmacokinetics of injected insulin vary markedly between patients, as does sensitivity to insulin. Because of these three variables (life-style, pharmacokinetics, sensitivity) it is impossible to specify regimens for

individual patients *a priori*. However, with the aid of reliable self-monitoring of blood glucose (Chapter 51), and a knowledge of these factors, it should be possible to optimize individual insulin dosage with time. Even within the individual these three factors do not remain constant, with changes in short-term and long-term life-style, and pharmacokinetics and sensitivity changing with puberty, pregnancy, obesity, illness and renal function. As a result, the optimization of insulin regimens is a continuing process.

In the overwhelming majority of patients, very good control of blood glucose levels (average within normal range) can be accomplished with insulin injection therapy only if multiple injections (more than four daily) are given, each dose is adjusted for current blood glucose level, and meals and snacks are taken at specified intervals [58]. Unfortunately, for many patients the quality of life lost by such a regimen far outweighs the average quality of life lost through the late complications of less well-controlled diabetes. Tolerance of strict insulin regimens, tolerance of symptomatic hypoglycaemia, and ease of blood glucose control all vary considerably between patients, so that the final level of control achieved will always be a matter for sympathetic discussion between patient and care advisers.

Physiological Plasma Insulin Profiles

Under the standardized conditions of fixed mealtimes, physiological insulin delivery results in the peripheral venous concentration profile given in Figure 5 [59]. Plasma C-peptide concentrations are also

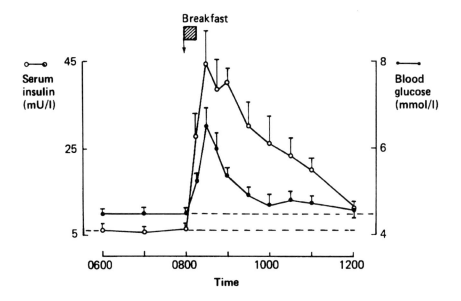

Figure 5   The blood glucose (solid circles) and serum insulin (open circles) profiles (±SE) of healthy normal subjects given a standard breakfast. Note the rapid rise in serum insulin concentrations to a peak about 30–45 minutes after the meal, and that this constrains the rise in mean blood glucose concentrations to around 2.0 mmol/l (36 mg/dl); peak postprandial 6.5 ± 0.5 (±SE) mmol/l. Insulin concentrations also fall rapidly after the early peak

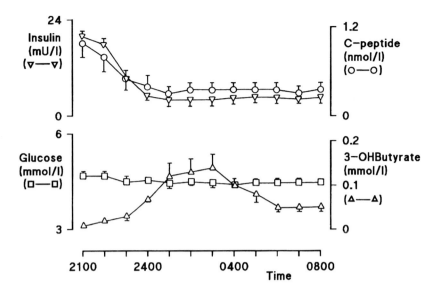

Figure 6 Overnight serum insulin and C-peptide levels (upper panel), and resulting blood glucose and ketone body levels (lower panel) in healthy normal subjects. Note the lack of change in insulin levels overnight, the C-peptide levels confirming this to be due to unchanging insulin secretion and clearance. Blood glucose levels are also constant right through to breakfast, but ketone body levels show a characteristic peak in the early hours (after reference 60, with permission)

given (Figure 6), because these more closely reflect insulin secretion rate as C peptide is not cleared by the liver. The profiles of plasma glucose and blood 3-hydroxybutyrate (ketone body) concentrations (Figures 5 and 6) emphasize that:

(1) Physiologically, blood glucose concentrations change very little at meal-times, peak concentrations in individuals rarely exceeding 7.0 mmol/l (125 mg/dl).

(2) Blood glucose concentrations overnight are very stable, with no tendency to a nadir in the middle of the night or rise towards morning being found in any individual.

(3) Although ketone body concentrations rise in the middle of the night, they fall towards dawn, remaining below 0.40 mmol/l.

The plasma insulin and C-peptide profiles show that this is achieved by:

(1) A rapid rise in insulin secretion at meal-times, sufficient to raise the concentration in the insulin space to a peak by 30–40 minutes after beginning the meal, despite continuing clearance.

(2) A rapid fall in insulin secretion even while absorption of food from the gut is still continuing, so that concentrations are only 30% of peak by 2 hours, and completely returned to baseline by 4 hours.

(3) Absolutely stable insulin delivery and clearance overnight.

Although, logically, the aim of insulin therapy should be to return insulin delivery profiles to those found in non-diabetic people, the constraints of variation in eating habits and activity must be borne in mind. Furthermore, it is possible that imperfect control of blood glucose levels in itself may result in a different pattern of insulin requirement. Thus, it has been suggested that if relative hypoinsulinaemia pertains overnight, then the effects of the burst of growth hormone secretion in the early phase of sleep may be to require increased insulin delivery towards the end of the night [61, 62]. Peripheral versus portal insulin delivery might also be of significance in terms of basal versus prandial insulin requirement, but as yet any possible effect is ill-defined.

Choice of Insulin Preparation

Short-acting Preparations

Species differences between natural insulins when injected subcutaneously are small, but probably significant between bovine and human insulin [63], in favour of a more rapid, and therefore more desirable, steady state absorption of the latter. Although there is also evidence for more rapid absorption of human than porcine unmodified insulin [64] and, indeed, there is a small difference in association state at depot concentrations between the two species [35], this is unlikely to be detectable in clinical practice.

Description of duration of action of any insulin preparation is not simple, as it depends on what other insulin injection depots are contributing to insulin delivery at the time. It should be remembered, when interpreting absorption curves, that infusion studies show that peripheral plasma free insulin concentrations of around 10–15 mU/l are needed simply to control basal (fasting) blood glucose concentrations. If, for example, basal blood glucose levels are normalized by insulin infusion or an extended-acting preparation, then an injection of short-acting human or porcine insulin will contribute extra insulin from 10 minutes after injection, peaking at 1.5–3 hours, remaining at 50% of peak levels until 2.5–5 hours, and returning to near-zero delivery (less than 10% of peak) at 5–9 hours (see Figure 2).

If, however, an injection of short-acting insulin takes over regulation of blood glucose levels from already deficient insulin delivery, for example at the end of the night, then at the same dose it would be 45–90 minutes before insulin delivery is sufficient even to control basal glucose concentrations, and insulin delivery will again be unable to suppress hepatic glucose production after 3.5–7 hours.

Duration of action also depends on the dose delivered. Thus, if twice the normal dose is given in an attempt to control high pre-breakfast blood glucose levels, then the duration of effect is extended by a further absorption half-time, 60–120 minutes. The major clinical consequences of this are:

(1) The maximum effects of an injection of short-acting insulin occur after absorption of a normal meal has been completed, if the injection is given at the start of the meal.

(2) If another meal and injection is taken within 4–6 hours, this second insulin dose will have to be very significantly reduced to allow for continuing insulin action from the first injection. This will be particularly true for a lunch-time injection following a large pre-breakfast injection.

(3) In many patients a preprandial dose of short-acting insulin will adequately control basal blood glucose levels for up to 8 hours after the last injection.

(4) Basal insulin supply can be provided by multiple preprandial injections of short-acting insulin during the day.

(5) When combined with an extended-acting preparation, an evening injection of short-acting insulin will contribute very significantly to depression of blood glucose levels in the first few hours of the night.

Insulin Analogues

Observations from both normal subjects and people with diabetes have confirmed that, under the conditions of a clinical study, short-acting insulin analogues are absorbed faster than native insulin, with a half-time of steady state absorption that is probably about 50% of that of insulin [135, 136]. Accordingly, when given with a meal in equimolar dosage, blood glucose profiles under these conditions are clearly improved, in that overall blood glucose concentrations are lower [137].

By contrast, clinical trials have been disappointing, and give little support for the use of these new insulins instead of human insulin. The situation has been further confused by attempts to perform studies under conditions that were not comparable (and hence not double-blind) [138, 139], on the incorrect assumption that human insulin is normally given by patients 30 minutes before meals, while the absorption profile of short-acting analogues suggests they should be given immediately before meals. Furthermore these studies have been embarked upon before experience has been gained in appropriate use of analogues, so that their possible advantages could not be exploited.

Accordingly overall blood glucose control was not found to be improved in a 2-month cross-over study, any gain in morning blood glucose control being lost through greater hyperglycaemia during the night [140]. In a series of studies in insulin-treated type 1 and type 2 diabetes, lispro insulin when combined with conventional NPH insulin failed to improve blood glucose control, while hypoglycaemia rates were improved in only some studies, and then only marginally [138, 139].

As a result, at the time of writing there is only preliminary support for assertions that short-acting analogues improve blood glucose control in clinical practice [142], or give an advantage in allowing more convenient timing of insulin injections. It may be, however, that patients suffering hypoglycaemia in the late morning would benefit from their use before breakfast, and similarly that patients suffering early night nocturnal hypoglycaemia while using large pre-dinner unmodified insulin doses might suffer fewer problems. One might also expect that patients with a large gap between lunch and dinner would suffer deterioration of metabolic control on insulin analogues in the hours before dinner.

At present there is no useful experience with the longer-acting insulin analogues, or newer insulin derivatives.

Extended-acting Insulin Preparations

The manufacture, chemical nature and absorption processes of extended-acting insulin preparations are described above.

True long-acting insulin preparations (bovine ultralente, protamine–zinc insulin) have found little clinical application outside the hands of a few enthusiasts [65].

Theoretically a long-acting preparation would be the ideal means of providing basal insulin supply, but, in practice, erratic absorption [43, 66] and poor bioavailability [67] result in unsatisfactory control in patients with type 1 diabetes and hence absolute insulin deficiency. Additional problems with these preparations include poor miscibility of protamine–zinc insulin with unmodified insulin due to its high zinc content, and the difficulty of initiating and altering insulin dosage when true duration of action is over 24 hours.

Bovine lente insulin is still available commercially, but is little used. As lente insulin preparations are 70% identical to ultralente, their properties will be not dissimilar. Porcine ultralente insulin is not commercially available. Human ultralente should be regarded as an intermediate-acting insulin, as should other human species crystalline insulin–zinc suspensions. This reflects evidence that human ultralente, like all other extended-acting insulin preparations, cannot achieve satisfactory overnight blood glucose control, and that its absorption rate after injection is about twice that of bovine ultralente [66]. Direct pharmacokinetic studies of human ultralente after injection into normal subjects are difficult to interpret, with peak concentrations at the highest dose barely adequate for basal blood glucose control, and the contribution of endogenous insulin secretion remaining a significant part of measured insulin concentrations [68]. Clinical studies have demonstrated that fasting blood glucose concentrations can be maintained below a mean of 7.0 mmol/l (125 mg/dl) in a population of C peptide-deficient patients, but only at the expense of an unacceptable rate of night-time hypoglycaemia [69].

Human and porcine lente insulin preparations are similar, although distinguishable in large numbers of patients [17]. Accumulated evidence suggests that human lente insulin preparations are absorbed significantly more slowly than human isophane (NPH) preparations [68], but in large, formal clinical trials they give similar overnight and daytime blood glucose control (Figure 7) [70]. Peak insulin concentrations are reached 3–6 hours after injection of human lente preparations, but fairly large doses (more than 20 U) are needed to give insulin concentrations high enough to control hepatic glucose output, and even with a half-time of absorption of 6–12 hours [68] levels quickly fall below those needed to maintain normal basal blood glucose levels.

Both lente and ultralente insulin preparations need to have high supernatant zinc concentrations (50 mg/l) to maintain integrity of the zinc–insulin complexes. When mixed with unmodified insulin, this will precipitate in a loose complex not dissimilar to semilente insulin. The effects are clearly demonstrable in formal studies with 40 U/ml insulin, and will be most significant

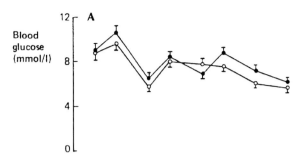

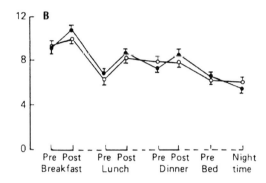

Figure 7 Blood glucose profiles in the last month (upper panel) and last 3 months (lower panel) of a cross-over study of twice-daily injection regimens in which the intermediate-acting insulin used was human NPH (open circles) or human lente (solid circles). No evidence was found of differing duration of action overnight, or of blunting of the action of the unmodified insulin after breakfast and dinner (from reference 70, with permission)

where the ratio of complexed to unmodified insulin is high [46]. Although demonstrable in pharmacokinetic studies [71], this appears not to be a significant clinical problem with 100 U/ml insulin when the mixture is immediately injected, post-injection blood glucose concentrations being similar to those of unmodified/isophane (NPH) mixtures [70].

Human and porcine isophane (NPH) insulin preparations are indistinguishable in formal absorption studies [72], although clinical studies showed large differences in effectiveness overnight in favour of porcine NPH [73]. This may reflect differences between preparations from different manufacturers. Absorption of isophane (NPH) insulin preparations appears to begin quite quickly after injection, with peak concentrations being reached at 2–4 hours, and with an absorption half-time of around 6 hours thereafter. The absorption of isophane insulin is known to be very erratic [74], but its very similar clinical efficacy to lente preparations [70], despite more rapid absorption, suggests a smaller problem than with the insulin–zinc suspensions.

In summary, there is little to choose at present between human or porcine ultralente, lente or isophane (NPH) insulin preparations for the provision of basal insulin supply. It is possible that some patients may benefit from the use of one or another, but guidelines to identify such individuals are not available, and in clinical practice changes between them are disappointing. On *a priori* grounds it would seem logical to use ultralente rather than lente when a bedtime injection is used to achieve overnight blood glucose control. Isophane (NPH) insulin may, however, be a better choice, particularly before breakfast when combined with a small dose of short-acting insulin in patients on twice-daily insulin injection regimens.

Semilente insulin preparations have no obvious role in clinical practice.

Design of Insulin Regimens

Once-daily Regimens

It is obvious from the complex form of the physiological plasma insulin profile (see above, and Figure 8) that, in the completely insulin-deficient patient, it is impossible to provide satisfactory insulin delivery from one injection a day. Satisfactory control (glycated haemoglobin below mean+4SD of normal) on such a regimen is uncommon, and will suggest periods of unrecognized hypoglycaemia. Even the provision of basal insulin supply alone is not possible with human or porcine intermediate-acting preparations given once daily, while the problems of erratic absorption and poor bioavailability severely restrict the usefulness of the long-acting bovine insulin preparations (see above).

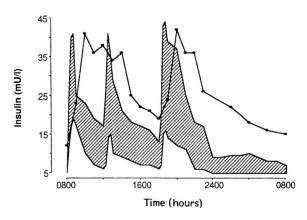

Figure 8 Twenty-four-hour plasma free insulin profiles of normal subjects (mean ± SE, hatched area), and of type 1 diabetic patients (solid circles) on a twice-daily insulin regimen using unmodified and NPH insulin. Note the abnormally high insulin levels, particularly in the late morning and around midnight, with the consequent problem of a high risk of hypoglycaemia. Although insulin levels may still appear high at the end of the night, the combination of peripheral insulin delivery and insulin insensitivity results in under-insulinization of the liver, with increased hepatic glucose output and hence hyperglycaemia

Once-daily injection regimens are therefore not recommended even for patients with significant endogenous insulin secretion, for example after partial pancreatectomy, or in the 'honeymoon' phase of type 1 diabetes.

A better case has been made for use of an evening injection of intermediate-acting insulin in the type 2 diabetic patient with moderate, but significant, hyperglycaemia (fasting plasma glucose concentration greater than 6.0 mmol/l, 110 mg/dl) [75]. This depends on control of overnight blood glucose levels by effective suppression of hepatic glucose output to provide an optimum starting concentration before breakfast, and improved islet B-cell function to cope with meals during the day, aided at first by whatever continuing insulin absorption may still be occurring. This regimen is not suitable in less well-controlled type 2 diabetes, when supplementary insulin is needed throughout the day, but has been advocated by some authors in combination with short-acting sulphonylureas (tolbutamide, glipizide) taken preprandially. It is not generally recommended [76].

Twice-daily Regimens

Twice-daily insulin injection regimens are attractive in that they can provide some semblance of appropriate insulin supply throughout the day for a minimum number of injections. Evidence from carefully conducted studies suggests that, under typical conditions of patient self-management, overall blood glucose concentrations are as good on twice-daily injection regimens as on multiple-injection regimens or subcutaneous pump therapy [77].

At its simplest, some patients with considerable endogenous insulin secretion who remain insulin sensitive (after partial pancreatectomy or with other early pancreatic damage, in the honeymoon phase of type 1 diabetes, or the thin, elderly type 2 diabetic patient) can often be managed successfully (glycated haemoglobin levels within target range without troublesome hypoglycaemia) on two injections a day of intermediate-acting insulin. Although there are differences in pharmacokinetics between isophane (NPH) and lente insulin preparations (see above), there is no evidence to favour one over the other for this purpose. A combination of glycated haemoglobin estimation and self-monitoring of blood glucose will determine when unmodified (soluble, regular) insulin should be added to the regimen.

If a twice-daily injection regimen is to be used in patients with more complete insulin deficiency, the less well-controlled insulin-insensitive type 2 diabetic patient, or in pregnancy, then a combination of unmodified and intermediate-acting insulin is essential.

Although this provides more complete insulin replacement, the resulting profile is still highly unphysiological (Figure 8), and it can be predicted that there will be problems of hypoglycaemia towards the end of the morning and in the early part of the night, and hyperglycaemia towards the end of the night and hence over breakfast (Figure 7). Clinical experience would suggest that, in the easily controlled patient, insulin doses tend to distribute 30:70 between unmodified and intermediate-acting insulin, and 50:50 between morning and evening. However, blood glucose control problems when using these regimens often result in deviations from this dose distribution, with nocturnal hypoglycaemia or fasting hyperglycaemia resulting in changes in the evening intermediate-acting insulin dose, and poor control around breakfast time resulting in a higher morning unmodified insulin dose. The carbohydrate distribution of the meals will also influence the appropriateness of this regimen, which in many patients will give acceptable control only with a large and early lunch.

Detailed clinical studies have shown no advantage between lente and isophane (NPH) insulin preparations when used in this type of regimen [70]. Indeed, human ultralente probably would give equivalent control as an alternative [69].

Where fasting hyperglycaemia and nocturnal hypoglycaemia are troublesome, and perhaps the basis of poor control for the rest of the day, then moving the second intermediate-acting insulin dose from the main evening meal to bedtime can improve pre-breakfast blood glucose levels by around 2.0 mmol/l (36 mg/dl) [78]. No prospective change in insulin dose is required. This manoeuvre may give improved pre-breakfast blood glucose levels in most patients using human/porcine insulin.

A special form of twice-daily injection therapy that can be useful in patients with intermediate degrees of insulin deficiency, or who need less tight control, is the use of premixed unmodified and isophane (NPH) insulin. Often, these mixtures are used in elderly type 2 diabetic patients with the 30:70 mix, although other ratios are available, from 50:50 to 10:90 unmodified to isophane insulin. More recently, these preparations have become available in pen-injectors, which can be advantageous in patients with difficulties in manipulating syringes, or with poor eyesight, and which are convenient to use.

Basal/Bolus Injection Regimens

The concept of providing separately preprandial insulin delivery and basal insulin requirement is attractive, although unfortunately to a large degree flawed by the absence of a true basal insulin preparation and the slow and prolonged absorption of so-called short-acting insulin (see above). As a result, under equivalent conditions of care, basal/bolus insulin regimens give no better blood glucose control than twice-daily injection regimens in the ordinary population of type 1 diabetic patients [79]. Nevertheless, it is much easier to understand and vary insulin dosage when meal-time injections are given separately, and this can be done without adverse effects on blood glucose control. The advent of the pen-injector [80, 81] has meant that pre-lunch injections are no longer a major inconvenience to patients, and as a result many patients have found their quality of life to be improved [82].

Basal insulin supply in the normal human represents about 50% of daily insulin secretion. On pharmacokinetic grounds (see above), human ultralente insulin given at bedtime is often chosen for basal insulin supply overnight. Nevertheless, the use of isophane (NPH) or even lente insulin at this time has its advocates, and the alternative of human ultralente before the evening meal has not been formally tested. None of these alternatives will produce satisfactory blood glucose control before breakfast in the overwhelming majority of patients, and as a result a relatively large dose of unmodified insulin from the pen-injector may be required at this time. As this dose will still be being absorbed at lunchtime, this second dose will need to be reduced (Figure 9). Typical insulin dose distributions therefore work out as 50% basal, with 20%, 10% and 20% before the three main meals. As with all insulin regimens, individual habits and metabolism will require tailoring of these averages.

Little formal guidance is available on adjustment of preprandial insulin dosage when meal food intake is varied. In general, however, as any dose is 50% basal supply, adjustment should be in proportion to the 50% of the normal dose used to control prandial carbohydrate disposal. At lunchtime, allowance should be made for the continuing absorption from the pre-breakfast insulin dose, as discussed above.

The putative role of insulin analogues in multiple injection regimens is discussed above.

Insulin Regimens in Special Groups of Patients

The elderly The elderly are discussed above under twice-daily injection regimens. Their needs vary according to the balance of insulin sensitivity and insulin deficiency, which can often be loosely assessed by body habitus. Goals of therapy may also be different where life expectancy is short, or where the patient's social functioning adds to the risks of hypoglycaemia.

In renal failure Patients in renal failure often require considerable reductions in insulin dose, for

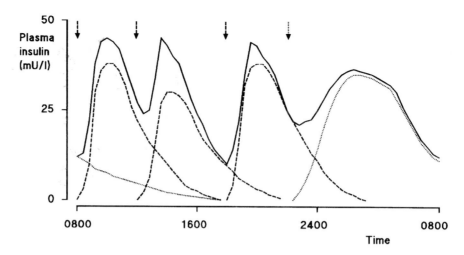

Figure 9 Composition of a multiple injection regimen, with unmodified insulin (broken line) before meals and intermediate-acting insulin (dotted line) before bed. Note the contribution of the bedtime insulin to the post-breakfast insulin peak (solid line), and that a smaller lunchtime insulin dose is needed because of continuing absorption from the breakfast dose

reasons which remain obscure. However, twice-daily or basal/bolus injection therapy should be continued.

Recurrent hypoglycaemia The management of hypoglycaemia in insulin-treated patients is discussed in Chapter 60. There is little evidence that any one insulin regimen benefits patients with recurrent hypoglycaemic problems, provided that insulin dose distribution has been properly optimized. The need for unusually high doses of intermediate-acting insulin can, however, suggest poor bioavailability and erratic absorption, indicating a move to a regimen based more on unmodified insulin. Empirically, it can be worth changing types of intermediate-acting insulin in patients with recurrent nocturnal hypoglycaemia, but the results are often disappointing. Moving the time of the evening intermediate-acting insulin injection to bedtime is often more helpful, allowing a reduction in dose without deterioration in fasting blood glucose control (see above).

Children Children should broadly be managed with the same insulin regimens as adults, although in the youngest children the shorter day limits the use of some multiple regimens. Some of the problems of insulin pharmacokinetics may be worse in children, in whom absorption of intermediate-acting preparations may be faster than in adults [83]. Basal/bolus regimens are usually well tolerated, but may give problems if the midday injection has to be self-administered at school. In some young patients pen-injector use has been associated with increased food abuse and hence poorer control and weight gain [84]. Semilente-based insulin regimens have been used in children, but have little to recommend them.

Pancreatic diabetes Patients with partial pancreatic deficiency can often be very well controlled on a twice-daily intermediate-acting insulin regimen. Patients with more complete insulin deficiency lack glucagon secretion in addition, and will require small doses of a twice-daily or basal/bolus regimen. If alcohol abuse is a continuing problem, then good blood glucose control will be almost impossible to obtain.

Steroid and endocrine diabetes These patients have massive insulin insensitivity but often considerable endogenous insulin secretion. Considerable doses of insulin may be required, but cessation of steroid therapy will often allow the patient to come off insulin again. A useful regimen in these patients uses twice-daily injections of the insulin premixes.

Obese type 2 diabetic patients As with patients on steroids, the middle-aged, obese type 2 diabetic patient will be secreting very large amounts of insulin (often more than 200 U per day) already. Large doses of exogenous insulin are usually needed to make any impression on blood glucose control in these people, who will also have a severe defect in insulin action. As insulin therapy is often started late in these patients, the reduction in urinary glucose loss with insulin therapy can result in significant weight gain. Interprandial snacks may be unnecessary in many of these insulin-insensitive patients with less than ideal control, and may also contribute to weight gain.

Pregnancy and prepregnancy Women already treated with insulin can often (but not always) manage some improvement in blood glucose control before conception on their usual twice-daily or basal/bolus regimen. During pregnancy, insulin dosage will increase, with the balance of insulin dose changing to greater daytime requirement compared with the basal requirement [85]. Patients with type 2 diabetes who become pregnant will need changing to the regimens used for type 1 diabetic women. If diabetes is diagnosed in pregnancy, insulin therapy may often not be required, but if it is, then a formal twice-daily injection regimen is indicated in the majority, or a basal/bolus regimen for the younger, thinner women likely to be in the prodrome of type 1 diabetes (see Chapter 57).

Patients with hepatic cirrhosis These patients are often severely insulin insensitive during the day, but have difficulty in maintaining glucose concentrations overnight, because of impaired gluconeogenesis. Insulin is therefore required for disposal of ingested carbohydrate, but little or none is needed overnight. In these circumstances a preprandial injection regimen from a pen-injector can be helpful.

Adjustment of Insulin Dosage

The literature on adjustment of insulin dosage is almost entirely opinion and prejudice. This section inevitably falls into the same trap, but tries to combine clinical observation with knowledge of insulin pharmacokinetics, as described above. The most common error, beloved of the pharmaceutical companies and followed by too many authors, is to assume that each insulin preparation works in a defined time period without overlap [86], and that extended-acting preparations provide some sort of constant basal insulin supply.

Some principles which should be applied to each dose adjustment are as follows:

(1) Reliable self-monitoring of blood glucose is necessary for dose adjustment. A discrepancy between this and glycated haemoglobin estimations needs investigation before dosage changes can be reliably made.

(2) Blood glucose levels measured on different days, even at any one time, have a coefficient of variation of 30–50% in the average patient. A considerable number of glucose measurements may therefore be needed to initiate dose changes, to judge the effect of dose changes, or simply to judge the safety of dose changes.

(3) Any individual's life-style varies from day to day. The impact of this on blood glucose records must be understood in making dose adjustments, and perhaps in tailoring dose adjustments to different types of activity and eating patterns.

(4) Erratic blood glucose levels and poor control overall may be due to overinsulinization. If this is suspected, then reduction of insulin dose is a necessary prerequisite to optimization of insulin dose distribution.

(5) A common form of overinsulinization occurs through gross maldistribution of insulin dosage when compared with the average distributions described above. This is most often seen when evening insulin doses are continually decreased because of night-time hypoglycaemia, or when fasting hyperglycaemia is treated by increasing the pre-breakfast insulin dose. In these circumstances, reduction in the higher doses is often needed before rebalancing the regimen.

(6) Control is often difficult to optimize in one time period of the day if it has been poor at the end of the previous period. Thus, in dealing with an inappropriate regimen, initial efforts will be directed into control of pre-breakfast blood glucose levels, then to the morning, and so to the rest of the day.

(7) Insulin absorption profiles overlap enormously. This needs particular consideration in the period after lunch. Perhaps the most common error, however, is to fail to recognize that if the morning intermediate-acting insulin dose is double the evening dose, then it may be contributing more to night-time hypoglycaemia than the later dose. Similarly, a large unmodified insulin dose in the evening will contribute significantly to hypoglycaemia in the early part of the night.

(8) As insulin absorption is erratic, small changes in dosage are likely to have undetectable effects. Changes should be 15–25% of any one preparation, and 10–20% of the total dose given at any one time.

(9) All insulin dose changes should be regarded as a trial, and the lessons from each change used in optimizing further changes.

(10) Blood glucose control can never be perfect, given currently available insulin preparations. Changes in insulin dose should be to meet a particular target, but if this is unattainable, stabilization on the best dose distribution does not benefit from continuing adjustment of doses.

(11) Insulin doses may be adjusted by informed patients in the light of anticipated changes in meal intake and activity, or on the basis of blood glucose tests, to optimize control.

(12) Adjustment of food intake may be more appropriate than adjustment of insulin dosage, if the new food energy distribution suits the patient.

Special Aspects of Insulin Therapy

Dietary Management

The balance of dietary constituents should not be different with insulin therapy, whatever the type of diabetes, from that in any other patient with the condition. However, insulin therapy imposes four limitations on the ideal pattern of food intake:

(1) The unphysiological insulin profiles, particularly in the late postprandial periods (see Figures 2 and 8), result in rapidly falling blood glucose concentrations and hence the need for interprandial snacks. If weight gain is to be avoided, then the energy content of these must be subtracted from main meals.

(2) Where insulin doses are given some hours before the meal that they are intended to cover, or where insulin doses cover more than one meal, it can be difficult to vary the dose to suit desired changes in energy intake. Basal/bolus regimens are an advantage in these circumstances.

(3) Hypoglycaemia, if allowed to become inappropriately frequent, or if very frightening for the patient, can result in considerable extra carbohydrate intake and thus weight gain.

(4) Unless insulin doses are reduced prospectively before exercise, hypoglycaemia can occur in the well-controlled patient, due to continued suppression of hepatic glucose production. Considerable extra carbohydrate may therefore be needed before marked exertion, the amount to be learnt by self-monitoring of blood glucose.

Insulin Injection Technique

Because of the risk of intramuscular insulin injection, with undesirable effects on insulin absorption (see above), it is now recommended that injections should be given into a lifted skin flap, with the syringe angled to ensure deep subcutaneous injection. This is not necessary in the obese patient, in whom injection to the full depth of the needle is preferable. Swabbing the skin with alcohol is not recommended, as injection site infections are rare, probably due to the bactericidal contents of the insulin vial (see above). Insulin injection technique should be reviewed yearly.

In view of the pharmacokinetics of insulin preparations (see above), unmodified insulin is best injected in the abdominal wall, where it is absorbed most quickly [141]. By contrast, extended-acting preparations will be best given into the subcutaneous tissue of the thigh, to reduce peak concentrations at night

and prolong their action as far as possible into the later hours of the night [97]. In both cases it is important to emphasize the need to rotate injection sites widely within one region, particularly as use of one single site leads not only to scarring but also to reinforcement of its use through relative anaesthesia. It is probably unrealistic to expect most people with diabetes to be able to give injections more than 5 minutes before meals, particularly as without routine self-monitoring there will be a risk of inducing hypoglycaemia on occasion.

Psychological Aspects of Insulin Therapy

The psychological impact of self-injection on patients is difficult to distinguish from the psychosocial effects of 'loss of healthy self', fear of hypoglycaemia, restrictions on dietary freedom and changed family priorities. True phobia severe enough to interfere with self-injection is not uncommon, but is generally manifest as poor control through the resulting poor technique rather than absolute refusal to give injections. Nevertheless, a significant number of patients arrange for a parent or partner to give their injections, a minor consequence being resulting lack of knowledge of the insulin doses taken.

A smaller literature suggests that some psychosocial aspects of injection therapy can be lessened in a proportion of patients by intensification of insulin therapy with insulin pumps (see below), or a multiple-injection regimen if a pen-injector is used [87, 88]. Studies have suggested reductions in depression and interpersonal sensitivity, and amelioration of aspects of anxiety [82].

CONTINUOUS SUBCUTANEOUS INSULIN INFUSION

Many ideas in science and medicine develop into useful tools only when the technology to support them becomes available. For clinical insulin administration it was the miniaturization of syringe pumps for delivery of hormones in laboratory animals that allowed the practice of pumped insulin delivery in humans to become a reality. Although conceived as a research tool, continuous subcutaneous insulin infusion (CSII) was born into a world where understanding of insulin pharmacokinetics was ill-developed, and measurement of blood glucose control yet to be revolutionized. As a consequence, initial results appeared little short of astounding when compared with the contemporary insulin regimens [89, 90], a promise not fulfilled when pump therapy later focused attention on the possibility of obtaining reasonable blood glucose control with insulin injections.

Nevertheless, CSII remains a useful therapeutic option where resources can justify the expense of infusion pumps, and in some patients who can make use of a flexibility of insulin administration unrivalled even by pen-injector regimens (see above). Furthermore, infused insulin provides overnight insulin delivery that is far closer to the physiological profile than that achieved by any extended-acting insulin preparation.

Concept and Implementation of CSII

It was part of the initial concept of CSII that pumping unmodified insulin into subcutaneous tissue would not be identical to delivering it directly into the circulation. Nevertheless, the pumps then available drove a syringe plunger forward at intervals of only seconds, providing more or less continuous subcutaneous insulin delivery throughout the day and night [91, 92]. With the recognition of the relatively slow absorption half-time of insulin from subcutaneous tissue (see below), and the inability of syringe systems to move in infinitesimal steps, later-generation pumps were activated as seldom as every 30 minutes, but still providing continual insulin delivery. This basal insulin delivery is supplemented by a boost at meal-times, in the early devices given as a fixed high-rate infusion, but soon substituted by bolus infusion of user-determined doses over a few seconds.

The early pumps were syringe drivers, but later devices were built around purpose-designed cartridges with fitted plungers, or even reservoir systems with peristaltic mechanisms [93]. Purpose-built devices allowed the development of user-friendly methods for changing basal insulin delivery rate and activating variable meal-time doses, and of electronic circuitry designed to medical safety standards. Development also led to a range of alarms to warn of pump failure, low insulin reservoir or obstruction of insulin delivery, and also, as the devices are battery powered, of impending battery exhaustion.

Insulin delivery was initially through fine infusion tubing implanted in the subcutaneous tissue of the anterior abdominal wall for up to 3 weeks. Recognition of the absence of pain sensation in subcutaneous tissue led to the use of standard butterfly (scalp vein) needles placed by the patients themselves, and changed every 1–3 days. Various purpose-designed cannulae have been introduced, including some with non-metallic (and therefore softer and less irritant) needles, and others with right-angled needles and self-adherent patches. Insulin compatibility with syringes and cannulae became the subject of considerable research [94], in respect of preservatives and cannula materials [95]. However, there has never been any real evidence that stability of insulin preparations was significantly affected over the short time intervals (1–3 days) typically used for any one syringe–cannula combination [96]. The insulin preparations used have, therefore, generally been identical or similar to standard unmodified formulations, but buffered preparations are usually preferred.

Provision must be made for the satisfactory and comfortable carriage of insulin pumps, the smallest of which approach the size of an old-fashioned pocket watch. Various forms of pocket, sling or pouch have been devised, worn on standard or purpose-designed belts or holsters, the profusion of ideas bearing witness to a problem never ideally solved.

Pharmacokinetics of Infused Insulin

The consequences of pharmacokinetics of infused insulin are easier to evaluate than those of depot injection therapy (see above), but not as simple as often believed. In the steady state, however, after infusion has been continuing at one rate for several (more than 5) hours, the absorption rate will simply equal the infusion rate, assuming negligible subcutaneous degradation. Nevertheless, even this assumes a steady state of capillary surface for absorption, and any change in this, due perhaps to warming of the skin or exercise, will have large and virtually immediate effects on insulin absorption rate, with plasma concentrations following more slowly to achieve a new steady state in 20–30 minutes. Thus even basal-rate infusions are unlikely to provide constant insulin delivery into the circulation.

In practice, most infusion pumps do not deliver insulin anything like continuously. However, if delivery is occurring at 30-minute intervals (which would not be unusual), in a patient with fast absorption half-times, plasma concentrations might oscillate by up to 30% in every half-hour [98]. Changes in the remote (effector) compartment would be much less than this, however (perhaps 10%), and probably acceptable clinically.

Insulin delivery rate into the circulation changes much more slowly than changes in subcutaneous infusion rate, including when starting and stopping infusions. In simple terms there is a need to build up a depot of insulin in the tissues to drive absorption by mass action. Because absorption increases as this depot is built up, the absorption rate rises with time in the form of a 'reverse' exponential (Figure 10) [99], the time to the new steady state absorption rate being determined by five times the half-time of subcutaneous absorption, namely 5 × 60–120 minutes, or 5–10 hours [98]. If, therefore, changes in basal rate infusion are to be made during the day for clinical reasons, they must be prospective by some hours, and allow additionally for insulin action occurring in a remote and delayed compartment. It should be noted, however, that where one infusion replaces another (when the cannula is changed), the rate of decline of insulin absorption from one site should parallel the rise from the new site.

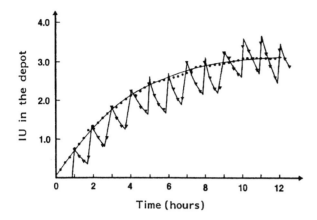

Figure 10 Accumulation of insulin in the subcutaneous depot from a 'continuous' insulin infusion pump delivering boluses of insulin every hour (from reference 98, with permission)

In principle, the absorption of the bolus meal-time dose of insulin given from a pump already *in situ* will be very similar to that of a subcutaneous injection of unmodified insulin. A small difference might be expected as a result of the effects on blood flow of the trauma of an injection, but any difference has not been formally investigated. The major practical difference, compared with multiple-injection therapy, might be expected to lie in the continuing basal infusion throughout the late postprandial period, which will add considerably to the hyperinsulinaemia resulting from the slow absorption of the bolus dose. Indeed, logically, basal infusion should cease just before a meal-time bolus dose is given, but this has not been tested in clinical practice.

Clinical Application of CSII

It is not intended here to give a complete guide to the practical clinical implementation of CSII, but only to draw together some of the features and problems of pumped subcutaneous insulin delivery, to allow it to be viewed in an appropriate perspective.

Achieved Metabolic Control on CSII

Early papers [89, 90] demonstrated improved blood glucose control in acute studies with pump therapy compared with insulin injection therapy, but the latter had not been optimized by education or by appropriate

choice of insulin regimen. It was soon shown that the improvements extended to other aspects of metabolism [100, 101], and that good blood glucose control could be maintained for some months. That such control could in fact be obtained for years has subsequently been demonstrated in the intervention trials of the effect of good control on complications, and it is clear that in such circumstances it remains better than non-optimized injection therapy [102, 103].

Studies performed under equivalent conditions of intensity have given less clear-cut messages. In very intensive studies, with doctor–patient interactions occurring virtually daily, multiple-injection therapy achieves almost identical blood glucose control to CSII [104]. In less intense studies, infusion pumps may have given better control [105, 106], but in these studies bovine ultralente insulin was used for basal insulin delivery by injection and may have adversely affected the achieved results. A hypothesis entertained at this time was that CSII might allow the achievement of better blood glucose control with less effort from the patients and their medical advisors [107]. However, long-term studies, performed in the regular diabetic clinic and under normal and similar intensities of management, failed to show any difference in overall blood glucose control when compared with conventional twice or three times daily isophane (NPH)-based injection regimens [77].

Given subsequent failure to demonstrate differences between overall control on multiple compared with twice-daily injections [79, 82], and the similarity of insulin delivery from multiple-injection regimens and pumps during the daytime, this might not now seem surprising. However, night-time insulin delivery in injection regimens is very different from that with CSII, the latter remaining the only satisfactory means of achieving anything like physiological pre-breakfast glucose concentrations in a significant number of patients [58, 108]. Thus, dramatic improvements in fasting blood glucose levels were demonstrated even in the studies in which overall control (judged by glycated haemoglobin concentrations) was no different from that achieved with injection therapy [77], and CSII additionally is the only means of obtaining fairly normal overnight profiles of ketone bodies [109]. The possibility that the lack of change in overall blood glucose levels might be explained by a lesser tendency of pump therapy to cause overnight asymptomatic hypoglycaemia has not been adequately addressed.

Indications for the Use of CSII

In the early days of pump therapy, CSII was presumed to be indicated for all patients with a special need for tight metabolic control [110], including such conditions as prepregnancy, symptomatic neuropathy, microalbuminuria, progressive retinopathy, growth retardation [111] and others. With the evidence that informed and thoughtful insulin injection therapy can achieve as good results in terms of glycated haemoglobin levels (see above), the rationale for these indications by themselves has disappeared. Similarly, the hope that patients with particularly unstable diabetes, typified by the young adolescent female with high insulin doses and intractable hyperglycaemia, might benefit from pump therapy, has not been fulfilled [112]. Nevertheless, there is some logic in using CSII in patients with recurrent overt or covert nocturnal hypoglycaemia on insulin injection therapy, given the more physiological insulin profile during the night. It is possible that such therapy might be most beneficial in those patients requiring higher doses of intermediate-acting insulin preparations to control blood glucose levels overnight, but this point has never been formally tested. There are reports of CSII being of value in patients with severe intractable hypoglycaemia at other times of day [110], but this needs to be confirmed with properly conducted studies.

One area where pumps did have a clear advantage over syringe injection therapy was in patients requiring a flexible life-style with varying meal-times. Such a life-style is difficult to accommodate successfully within the constraints of twice-daily injection therapy (see above), and syringe injections at lunch-time were not popular with patients [106]. Although this need was correctly identified by the use of CSII, a less expensive but still generally effective option has been provided by the pen-injector.

In short, the major clinical indication for CSII is patient preference over other intensive insulin regimens. Some patients simply feel in greater control of their diabetes when using a pump, a reassurance that may be very valuable to them [113]. CSII has been successfully used in young children [114] and in cooperative adolescents [115, 116], and good results do not appear to depend in general on educational level.

Insulin Dose Distribution

The insulin dose distribution for CSII closely parallels that found for multiple-injection therapy, and reflects physiological insulin delivery (see above). Thus, approximately half the dose is given at the basal insulin delivery rate, and the other half distributed between meals. Continuing absorption of the breakfast insulin dose through lunchtime may be significant if these meals are close together (4–5 hours), necessitating reduction of the second insulin bolus. For reasons that have not been determined, many well-controlled patients on CSII appear to need a disproportionate

amount of their meal-time insulin before the evening meal if good control is to be maintained during the evening.

Considerable efforts has been devoted to trying to understand the possible role of changes in basal infusion rate overnight in obtaining optimum control [117]. However, there is no good evidence of increased insulin requirement towards the end of the night in patients who are not insulin deficient, and simply using an adequate basal infusion rate will usually solve any problem of fasting hyperglycaemia [118, 119]. A particular problem can, however, occur in patients who use the flexibility of pump therapy to eat late in the evening (20.00–22.00 h). Any bolus of unmodified insulin given at this time will continue to be absorbed well into the night, and in conjunction with continuing basal rate insulin delivery can predispose to hypoglycaemia at 01.00–03.00 h. In these circumstances, programmed reduction of the basal delivery rate from the time of the evening meal may be useful.

It will be noted that it should be possible to combine pump therapy overnight with pen-injector therapy during the day. If this is done, then insulin pharmacokinetics would suggest initiating basal insulin infusion around 4 hours after the last main meal. The pre-breakfast insulin dose would need to be lower than that on conventional multiple-injection regimens.

Problems of Subcutaneous Insulin Infusion

System failure The most common forms of pump or cannula failure in early systems included displacement of the needle from subcutaneous tissue, disconnection of the cannula from the pump syringe/cartridge, and exhaustion of the insulin reservoir. The last problem should be detected by pressure sensors and alarms in any modern system, and disconnections can be avoided by appropriate locking devices. Pump failure or line blockage should also be detected by modern devices, and the user alerted. When failure of insulin delivery occurs in the basal state in an otherwise healthy patient, blood glucose concentration will rise to a plateau at 12–16 mmol/l (215–290 mg/dl) over about 8 hours [120], but ketone body concentrations go on increasing beyond this time, leading to acidosis in under 24 hours. Delivery of a meal-time insulin bolus before pump failure will delay decompensation, but consumption of carbohydrate as insulin concentrations fall will lead to more marked hyperglycaemia. Thus, advice to monitor blood glucose concentrations at least twice daily is a useful precaution against system failure. Patient education should ensure that the whole reservoir/cannula system is replaced in the event of unexpected hyperglycaemia or ketonuria. All patients on CSII should maintain supplies of syringes for emergencies.

Ketoacidosis   Ketoacidosis has been reported to be more common with CSII than with injection therapy, but when it occurs it is not usually associated with system failure. More common associations are with intercurrent illness [108], a probable explanation being that the absence of periods of gross hyperinsulinaemia overnight allows escape of ketone body levels in times of metabolic stress. There is a tendency for these episodes to be associated with hyperkalaemia, suggesting an acute onset. Nevertheless, every episode of ketoacidosis is clear evidence of failure of patient education, and the problem reinforces the need to provide recurrent advice on urinary ketone testing, regular self-monitoring of blood glucose, and action to increase insulin dosage during illness or for unexplained hyperglycaemia. A common error is for patients to increase preprandial insulin doses only, with resulting inadequacy of basal insulin delivery in the face of increased counter-regulatory hormone secretion.

Hypoglycaemia   Hypoglycaemia is not a greater problem with CSII than with insulin injection therapy for the same degree of overall blood glucose control [96]. Indeed, pump therapy may be helpful in some patients with hypoglycaemic problems. The most common error leading to hypoglycaemic coma is to ignore a series of low blood glucose concentrations (around 2.0 mmol/l, 36 mg/dl).

Infusion site problems   Some redness and soreness at the site of entry of the infusion needle through the skin is common, and usually suggests that the cannula is not being changed frequently enough. Frank infection is also much more common than with injection therapy, is generally staphylococcal, and again suggests poor hygiene. Chronic use of the same infusion site will result in lipohypertrophy and scarring, as with insulin injections (see above).

Poor blood glucose control   Poor blood glucose control on CSII may simply be a manifestation of the same problems that cause poor control on injection therapy. Some patients do, however, seem to have poor empathy with devices, and handle pumps to poor effect. More common is a less overt rejection of the pump, either as a constant reminder of diabetes, or through problems of depending on a machine for good health [96]. There is some evidence that many patients keen to start CSII are looking for an external solution to the management of their diabetes, but given the increased attention needed to use pumps effectively, these are just the patients who will fail to obtain benefit from them [121].

Patient acceptability   As well as poor control, covert psychological problems can lead to recurrent unexplained failure of the pump, or even in extreme cases

to inadequately explained damage to the device or cannula. However, portable pumps may also give rise to simple problems in terms of comfort while being worn, and cosmetic difficulties through their bulk. Careful attention therefore needs to be given to finding the most suitable method of carrying the pump in any individual. Proper advice is also necessary in respect of such activities as swimming or sexual intercourse, and for these and other purposes infusion may be discontinued for up to an hour if necessary [120]. Patients may also wish to discontinue pump usage for longer periods for activities such as dancing or sunbathing, when cover with an insulin injection may be helpful.

REFERENCES

1. Zuelzer GL. Uber Versuche einer specifischen Fermenttherapie des Diabetes. Z Exp Pathol Ther 1908; 5: 307–18.
2. Bliss M. The discovery of insulin. Edinburgh: Paul Harris, 1982.
3. Sanger F. Chemistry of insulin. Science 1959; 129: 1340–4.
4. Steiner DF, Kemmler W, Clark JL, Oyer PE, Rubenstein AH. The biosynthesis of insulin. In Steiner DF, Freinkel W (eds) Handbook of Physiology—Endocrinology I. Baltimore: Williams & Wilkins, 1972: pp 175–98.
5. Blundell T, Dodson G, Hodgkin D, Mercola D. Insulin: the structure in the crystal and its reflection in chemistry and biology. Adv Protein Chem 1972; 26: 279–402.
6. Romans RG, Scott DA, Fisher AM. Preparation of crystalline insulin. Indust Engineer Chem 1940; 32: 908–10.
7. Schlichtkrull J, Brange J, Christiansen AH, Hallund O, Heding LG, Jorgensen KH. Clinical aspects of insulin–antigenicity. Diabetes 1972; 21 (suppl. 2): 649–56.
8. Kung K, Do Y, Huang W et al. Total synthesis of crystalline insulin. Scientia Sinica 1966; 15: 544–61.
9. Teuscher A. Die biologische Wirkung von vollsynthetischem humanem Insulin bei Patienten mit Diabetes Mellitus. Schweiz Med Wschr 1979; 109: 743–7.
10. Ullrich A, Shine J, Chirgwin J, Pictet R, Tischer E, Rutter WJ, Goodman HM. Rat insulin genes: construction of plasmids containing the coding sequences. Science 1977; 496: 1313–19.
11. Villa-Komaroff L, Efstratiadis A, Broome S, Lomedico P, Tizard R, Naber SP, Chick WL, Gilbert W. A bacterial clone synthesizing pro-insulin. Proc Natl Acad Sci USA 1978; 75: 3727–31.
12. Jorpes JE. Recrystallized insulin for diabetic patients with insulin allergy. Arch Int Med 1949; 83: 363–71.
13. Berson SA, Yalow RS, Bauman A, Rothschild MA, Newerly K. Insulin-I^{131} metabolism in human subjects. Demonstration of insulin binding globulin in the circulation of insulin treated subjects. J Clin Invest 1956; 35: 170–90.
14. Mirsky IA, Kawamura K. Heterogeneity of crystalline insulin. Endocrinology 1966; 78: 1115–19.

15. Steiner DF, Hallund O, Rubenstein A, Cho S, Bayliss C. Isolation and properties of proinsulin, intermediate forms, and other minor components from crystalline bovine insulin. Diabetes 1968; 17: 725–36.

16. Welinder BS, Sørensen HH, Hansen B. Reversed-phase high-performance liquid chromatography of insulin. Resolution and recovery in relation to column geometry and buffer components. J Chromatog 1986; 361: 357–67.

17. Home PD, Mann NP, Hutchison AS, Park R, Walford S, Murphy M, Reeves WG. A fifteen-month double-blind cross-over study of the efficacy and antigenicity of human and pork insulins. Diabet Med 1984; 1: 93–8.

18. Alberti KGMM, Nattrass M. Highly purified insulins. Diabetologia 1978; 15: 77–80.

19. Home PD, Alberti KGMM. The new insulins. Drugs 1982; 24: 401–13.

20. Heding LG, Marshall MO, Persson B et al. Immunogenicity of monocomponent human and porcine insulin in newly diagnosed Type 1 (insulin-dependent) diabetic children. Diabetologia 1984; 27: 96–8.

21. Nakagawa S, Suda N, Kudo M, Kawasaki M. A new type of hypoglycaemia in a newborn infant. Diabetologia 1973; 9: 367–75.

22. Falholt K, Hoskam JAM, Karamanos BG, Süsstrunk K, Visvanathan N, Heding LG. Insulin specific IgE in serum of 67 diabetic patients against human insulin (Novo), porcine insulin, and bovine insulin. Four case reports. Diabetes Care 1983; 6: 61–5.

23. Koch M, Sodoyez JC, Sodoyez-Goffaux F, Dozio N, Di Silvio LS, Kurtz AB. Is quantitative assessment of insulin-autoantibodies and autoantibodies feasible? Diabetologia 1989; 32: 774–8.

24. Galloway JA, Bressler R. Insulin treatment in diabetics. Med Clin North Am 1978; 62: 663–80.

25. Heding LG, Persson B, Strongenberg M. B-cell function in newborn infants of diabetic mothers. Diabetologia 1980; 19: 427–32.

26. Reeves WG, Allen BR, Tattersall RB. Insulin-induced lipoatrophy: evidence for an immune pathogenesis. Br Med J 1980; 2: 1500–3.

27. Brange J. Galenics of insulin. Berlin: Springer, 1987.

28. von Dörzbach E, Müller R. Die Insulintherapie. Die Insulinpräparate. In Pfeiffer EF (ed.) Handbook of diabetes mellitus, pathophysiology and clinical considerations, vol. 2. Munich: Lehmann, 1971: pp 1087–111.

29. Hagedorn HC, Jensen DN, Krarup NB, Wodstrup I. Protamine insulinate. JAMA 1936; 106: 177–80.

30. Scott DA, Fisher AM. Studies on insulin with protamine. J Pharmacol Exp Ther 1936; 58: 78–92.

31. Krayenbühl C, Rosenberg T. Crystalline protamine insulin. Rep Steno Hosp 1946; 1: 60–73.

32. Hallas-Møller K, Petersen K, Schlichtkrull J. Crystalline and amorphous insulin–zinc compounds with prolonged action. Science 1952; 116: 394–9.

33. Nolte MS, Poon V, Grodsky GM, Forsham PH, Karam JH. Reduced solubility of short-acting insulins when mixed with longer-acting insulins. Diabetes 1983; 32: 1177–81.

34. Brange J, Ribel U, Hansen JF et al. Monomeric insulin obtained by protein engineering and their medical implications. Nature 1988; 333: 679–82.

35. Brange J, Owens DR, Kang S, Vølund A. Monomeric insulins and their experimental and clinical implications. Diabetes Care 1990; 13: 923–54.

36. Pingel M, Vølund A, Sørensen E, Sørensen AR. Assessment of insulin potency by chemical and biological methods. In Gueriguian JL, Bransome ED, Outschoorn AS (eds) Hormone drugs. Rockville: United States Pharmacopeial Convention, 1982; pp 200–7.

37. WHO Expert Committee on Biological Standardization. Thirty-seventh report. Geneva: WHO, 1987; pp 25–26.

38. Vølund Aa, Brange J, Drejer K, Jensen I, Markussen J, Ribel U, Sørensen AR, Schlichtkrull J. *In vitro* and *in vivo* potency of insulin analogues designed for clinical use. Diabet Med 1991; 8: 839–47.

39. Moses AC, Flier JS. Unconventional routes of insulin administration. In Alberti KGMM, Krall LP (eds) Diabetes annual 3. Amsterdam: Elsevier, 1987: pp 107–20.

40. Pontiroli AE, Pozza G. Intranasal administration of peptide hormones: factors affecting transmucosal absorption. Diabet Med 1990; 7: 770–4.

41. Bratusch-Marrain PR, Komjati M, Waldhäusl W. Pulsatile insulin delivery: physiology and clinical implications. Diabet Med 1987; 4: 197–200.

42. Binder C. A theoretical model for the absorption of soluble insulin. In Brunetti P, Alberti KGMM, Albisser AM, Hepp KD, Massi Benedetti M (eds) Artificial systems for insulin delivery. New York: Raven Press, 1983: pp 53–8.

43. Binder C. Absorption of injected insulin. Acta Pharmacol Toxicol 1969; 27 (suppl. 2): 1–87.

44. Turner RC, Grayburn JA, Newman GB, Nabarro JDN. Measurement of insulin delivery rate in man. J Clin Endocrinol Metab 1971; 33: 279–86.

45. Sherwin RS, Kramer KJ, Tobin JD et al. A model of the kinetics of insulin in man. J Clin Invest 1974; 53: 1481–92.

46. Heine R, Bilo HGJ, Sikkenck AC. Mixing short and intermediate acting insulins in the syringe: effect on postprandial blood glucose concentrations in type 1 diabetics. Br Med J 1985; 290: 204–5.

47. Brunfeldt K, Poulsen JE. Protamine-splitting enzyme from serum and subcutaneous tissue. Rep Steno Hosp 1953; 5: 51–61.

48. Thow JC, Johnston AB, Antiserov M, Home PD. Effect of raising injection site temperature on isophane insulin crystal dissociation. Diabetes Care 1989; 12: 432–4.

49. Hildebrandt P, Sejrsen P, Nielsen SL, Birch K, Sestoft L. Diffusion and polymerization determines the insulin absorption from subcutaneous tissue in diabetic patients. Scand J Clin Lab Invest 1985; 45: 685–90.

50. Koivisto VA, Fortney S, Hendler R, Felig P. A rise in ambient temperature augments insulin absorption in diabetic patients. Metabolism 1981; 30: 402–5.

51. Linde B. Dissociation of insulin absorption and blood flow during massage of a subcutaneous injection site. Diabetes Care 1986; 9: 570–4.

52. Binder C, Nielsen A, Jørgensen K. The absorption of an acid and neutral insulin solution after subcutaneous injection into different regions in diabetic patients. Scand J Clin Lab Invest 1967; 19: 156–63.

53. Larsen OA, Lassen NA, Quaade F. Blood flow through human adipose tissue determined with radioactive xenon. Acta Physiol Scand 1966; 66: 337–45.

54. Thow JC, Johnson AB, Marsden S, Taylor R, Home PD. Morphology of palpably abnormal injection sites

and effects on absorption of isophane (NPH) insulin. Diabet Med 1990; 7: 795-9.

55. Francis AJ, Hanning I, Alberti KGMM. The influence of insulin antibody levels on the plasma profiles and action of subcutaneously injected human and bovine short acting insulins. Diabetologia 1985; 28: 330-4.

56. Frid A, Linden B. Where do lean diabetics inject their insulin? A study using computed tomography. Br Med J 1986; 292: 1638.

57. Thow JC, Home PD. Insulin injection technique (editorial). Br Med J 1990; 301: 3-4.

58. Schiffrin A, Belmonte MM. Comparison between continuous subcutaneous insulin infusion and multiple injections of insulin. Diabetes 1982; 31: 255-64.

59. Kruszynska YT, Home PD, Hanning I, Alberti KGMM. Basal and 24-h C-peptide and insulin secretion in normal man. Diabetologia 1987; 30: 16-21.

60. Kruszynska YT, Home PD. Night-time metabolic changes in normal subjects in the absence of the dawn phenomenon. Diabète Métab 1988; 14: 437-42.

61. Campbell PJ, Bolli GB, Cryer PE, Gerich JE. Pathogenesis of the dawn phenomenon in patients with insulin-dependent diabetes mellitus. N Engl J Med 1985; 312: 1473-9.

62. Skor DA, White NH, Thomas L, Santiago JV. Influence of growth hormone on overnight insulin requirements in insulin dependent diabetics. Diabetes 1985: 34: 135-9.

63. Francis AJ, Hanning I, Alberti KGMM. The influence of insulin antibody levels on the plasma profiles and action of subcutaneously injected human and bovine short-acting insulins. Diabetologia 1985; 28: 330-4.

64. Pickup JC. Human insulin. Br Med J 1986; 292: 155-6.

65. Phillips M, Simpson RW, Holman RR, Turner RC. A simple and rational twice daily insulin regime. Quart J Med 1979; 191: 493-506.

66. Hildebrandt P, Berger A, Vølund AA, Kühl C. The subcutaneous absorption of human and bovine ultralente insulin formulations. Diabet Med 1985; 2: 355-9.

67. Home PD, Hanning I, Capaldo B, Alberti KGMM. Bioavailability of highly purified bovine ultralente insulin (letter). Diabetes Care 1983; 6: 210.

68. Owens DR. Human insulin. Clinical pharmacological studies in normal man. Lancaster: MTP, 1986.

69. Tunbridge FKE, Newens A, Home PD et al. A comparison of human ultralente- and lente-based twice daily injection regimens. Diabet Med 1989; 6: 496-501.

70. Tunbridge FKE, Newens A, Home PD et al. Double-blind cross-over trial of isophane (NPH)- and lente-based insulin regimens. Diabetes Care 1989; 12: 115-19.

71. Francis AJ, Hanning I, Alberti KGMM. The effect of mixing human soluble and human crystalline-zinc suspension insulin: plasma insulin and blood glucose profiles after subcutaneous injection. Diabet Med 1985; 2: 177-80.

72. Pedersen C, Høegholm A. A comparison of semisynthetic human NPH insulin and porcine NPH insulin in the treatment of insulin-dependent diabetes. Diabet Med 1985; 4: 304-6.

73. Clark AJL, Knight G, Wiles PG et al. Biosynthetic human insulin in the treatment of diabetes. Lancet 1982, ii: 354-7.

74. Lauritzen T, Pramming S, Gale E, Deckert T, Binder C. Absorption of isophane (NPH) insulin and its clinical implications. Br Med J 1982, 285: 159-62.

75. Holman RR, Steemson J, Turner RC. Sulphonylurea failure in type 2 diabetes: treatment with a basal insulin supplement. Diabet Med 1987; 4: 457-62.

76. Genuth S. Insulin use in NIDDM. Diabetes Care 1990; 13: 1240-64.

77. Marshall SM, Home PD, Taylor R, Alberti KGMM. A randomised crossover trial of continuous subcutaneous insulin infusion in the regular diabetic clinic. Diabet Med 1987; 5: 521-45.

78. Francis AJ, Home PD, Hanning I, Alberti KGMM, Tunbridge WMG. Intermediate acting insulin given at bedtime: effect on glucose concentrations before and after breakfast. Br Med J 1983; 286: 1173-6.

79. Small M, MacRury S, Boal A, Paterson KR, MacCuish AC. Comparison of conventional twice daily subcutaneous insulin administration and a multiple injection regimen (using the Novopen) in insulin-dependent diabetes mellitus. Diabetes Res 1988; 8: 85-9.

80. Paton JS, Wilson M, Ireland JT, Reith SB. Convenient pocket insulin syringe. Lancet 1981; i: 189-90.

81. Jefferson IG, Marteau TM, Smith MA, Baum JD. A multiple injection regimen using an insulin pen and pre-filled cartridged soluble human insulin in adolescents with diabetes. Diabet Med 1985; 2: 493-7.

82. Houtzagers CMGJ, Visser AP, Berntzen PA et al. Multiple daily injections improve self-confidence. Diabet Med 1989; 6: 512-19.

83. de Beaufort CE, Bruining GJ, Home PD, Houtzagers CMGJ, van Strik R. Overnight metabolic profiles in very young insulin-dependent diabetic children. Eur J Pediatr 1986; 145: 73-6.

84. Hardy KJ, Jones KE, Gill GV. Deterioration in blood glucose control in females with diabetes changed to a basal-bolus regimen using a pen-injector. Diabet Med 1991; 8: 69-71.

85. Steel JM, Home PD, Young RJ, Johnstone FD, Frier BM. Inter-relationships of insulin dose, plasma free insulin, and metabolic control in diabetic pregnancy. Diabetes Res Clin Pract 1987; 3: 1-7.

86. Schade DS, Santiago JV, Skyler JS, Rizza RA. Intensive insulin therapy. Amsterdam: Excerpta Medica. 1983.

87. Seigler DE, LaGreca A, Satin Citrin W, Reeves ML, Skyler JS. Psychological effects of intensification of diabetic control. Diabetes Care 1982; 5 (suppl. 1): 19-23.

88. Mazze RS, Lucido D, Shamoon H. Psychological and social correlates of glycemic control. Diabetes Care 1984; 7: 360-6.

89. Pickup JC, Keen H, Parsons JA, Alberti KGMM. Continuous subcutaneous insulin infusion: an approach to achieving normoglycaemia. Br Med J 1978; 1: 204-7.

90. Tamborlane WV, Sherwin RS, Genel M, Felig P. Reduction to normal of plasma glucose in juvenile diabetes by subcutaneous administration of insulin with a portable pump. New Engl J Med 1979; 300: 573-8.

91. Lauritzen T, Pramming S, Deckert T, Binder C. Pharmacokinetics of continuous subcutaneous insulin infusion. Diabetologia 1983; 24: 326-9.

92. Chisholm DJ, Kraegen EW, Hewett MJ, Furler S. Low subcutaneous degradation and slow absorption

of insulin in insulin-dependent diabetic patients during continuous subcutaneous insulin infusion at the basal rate. Diabetologia 1984; 27: 238–41.

93. Rothwell D. Technological aspects of CSII. Diabet Med 1984; 1: 32–4.

94. Lougheed WD, Woulfe-Flanagan H, Clement JR, Albisser AM. Insulin aggregation in artificial delivery systems. Diabetologia 1980; 19: 1–9.

95. Hansen B, Welinder BS, Johansen KB, Benned Hansen F, Balschmidt P. Insulin for delivery systems. In Brunetti P, Waldhäusl WK (eds) Advanced models for the therapy of insulin-dependent diabetes. New York: Raven Press 1987: pp 77–84.

96. Home PD, Marshall SM. Problems and safety of continuous subcutaneous insulin infusion. Diabet Med 1984; 1: 41–4.

97. Henriksen JE, Vaag A, Ramsgaard Hansen I, Lauritzen M, Djurhuus MS, Beck Nielsen H. Absorption of NPH (isophane) insulin in resting diabetic patients: evidence for subcutaneous injection in the thigh as the preferred site. Diabet Med 1991; 8: 453–7.

98. Hildebrandt P, Birch K, Jensen BM, Kühl C, Brange J. Absorption of subcutaneously infused insulin: influence of the basal rate pulse interval. Diabetes Care 1985; 8: 287–9.

99. Kraegen EW, Chisholm DJ. Insulin responses to varying profiles of subcutaneous insulin infusion. Diabetologia 1984; 26: 208–13.

100. Pickup JC, Keen H, Parsons JA, Alberti KGMM, Rowe AS. Continuous subcutaneous insulin infusion: improved blood glucose and intermediary metabolic control in diabetics. Lancet 1979; i: 1255–8.

101. Tamborlane WV, Sherwin RS, Genel M, Felig P. Restoration of normal lipid and amino acid metabolism in diabetic patients with a portable infusion pump. Lancet 1979; i: 1258–61.

102. Lauritzen T, Frost-Larsen K, Larsen H-W, Deckert T, Steno Study Group. Effect of 1 year of near-normal blood glucose levels on retinopathy in insulin dependent diabetics. Lancet 1983; i: 200–4.

103. Kroc Collaborative Study Group. Blood glucose control and the evolution of diabetic retinopathy and albuminuria. A preliminary multicenter trial. New Engl J Med 1984; 311: 365–72.

104. Reeves ML, Seigler DE, Ryan EA, Skyler JS. Glycemic control in insulin-dependent diabetes mellitus: comparison of out-patient intensified conventional therapy with continuous subcutaneous insulin infusion. Am J Med 1982; 72: 673–80.

105. Calabrese G, Bueti A, Santeusanio F et al. Continuous subcutaneous insulin infusion treatment in insulin-dependent diabetic patients: a comparison with conventional optimized treatment in a long term study. Diabetes Care 1982; 5: 457–65.

106. Home PD, Capaldo B, Burrin JM, Worth R, Alberti KGMM. A crossover comparison of continuous subcutaneous insulin infusion (CSII) against multiple insulin injections in insulin-dependent diabetic subjects: improved control with CSII. Diabetes Care 1982; 5: 466–71.

107. Skyler JS. Type 1 diabetes . . . regimens, targets, and caveats. Diabetes Care 1982; 5: 547–52.

108. Mecklenburg RS, Benson JW, Becker NM et al. Clinical use of the insulin infusion pump in 100 patients with type 1 diabetes. New Engl J Med 1982; 307: 513–18.

109. Home PD, Capaldo B, Alberti KGMM. The quality of metabolic control during open-loop insulin infusion in type 1 diabetes. In Mngola E (ed.) Diabetes 1982. Amsterdam: Excerpta Medica, 1982: pp 295–301.

110. Ward JD. Continuous subcutaneous insulin infusion (CSII): therapeutic options. Diabet Med 1984; 1: 47–50.

111. Tamborlane WV, Hintz RL, Bergman M, Genel M, Felig P, Sherwin RS. Insulin infusion-pump treatment of diabetes: influence of improved metabolic control on plasma somatomedin levels. New Engl J Med 1981; 305: 303–7.

112. Pickup JC, Home PD, Bilous RW, Alberti KGMM, Keen H. Management of severely brittle diabetes by continuous subcutaneous and intramuscular insulin infusion: evidence for a defect in subcutaneous insulin absorption. Br Med J 1981; 282: 347–50.

113. Shapiro J, Wigg D, Charles MA, Perley M. Personality and family profiles of chronic insulin-dependent diabetic patients using portable insulin infusion pump therapy: a preliminary investigation. Diabetes Care 1984; 7: 137–42.

114. de Beaufort CE, Houtzagers CMGJ, Bruining GJ et al. Continuous subcutaneous insulin infusion (CSII) versus conventional injection therapy in newly diagnosed diabetic children: two-year follow-up of a randomized prospective trial. Diabet Med 1989; 6: 766–71.

115. Schiffrin AD, Desrosiers M, Aleyassine H, Belmonte MM. Intensified insulin therapy in the type 1 diabetic adolescent: a controlled trial. Diabetes Care 1984; 7: 107–13.

116. de Beaufort CE, Bruining GJ. Continuous subcutaneous insulin infusion in children. Diabet Med 1987; 4: 103–8.

117. Renner RM, Piwernetz K, Hepp KD. Adequate insulin substitution at dawn with and without pump treatment. In Brunetti P, Waldhäusl WK (eds) Advanced models for the therapy of insulin-dependent diabetes. New York: Raven Press, 1987: pp 199–204.

118. Pickup JC. Pumps in practice: practical aspects of continuous subcutaneous insulin infusion (CSII). Diabet Med 1984; 1: 27–32.

119. Bending JJ, Pickup JC, Collins ACG, Keen H. Rarity of a marked dawn phenomenon in diabetic subjects treated by continuous subcutaneous insulin infusion. Diabetes Care 1985; 8: 28–33.

120. Pickup JC, Viberti GC, Bilous RW et al. Safety of continuous subcutaneous insulin infusion: metabolic deterioration and glycaemic auto regulation after deliberate cessation of infusion. Diabetologia 1982; 22: 175–9.

121. Bradley C, Gamsu DS, Moses JL et al. The use of diabetes specific perceived control and health belief measures to predict choice and efficacy in a feasibility study of continuous subcutaneous insulin infusion pumps. Psychol Health 1978; 1: 133–46.

122. Markussen J, Havelund S, Kurtzhals P, Andersen AS, Halstrøm J, Hasselager E et al. Soluble, fatty acid acylated insulins bind to albumin and show protracted action in pigs. Diabetologia 1996; 39; 281–8.

123. Myers S, Yakabu-Madus F, Johnson W, Baker J, Cusick V, Williams T et al. W99-S32: a soluble, basal insulin analogue (abstr). Diabetologia 1995; 38 (suppl. 1): A4.

124. Gliemann J, Gammeltoft S. The biological activity and the binding affinity of modified insulin determined

on isolated rat fat cells. Diabetologia 1974; 10: 105–13.

125. Spector AA. Fatty acid binding to plasma albumin. J Lipid Res 1975; 16: 165–79.

126. Jørgensen S, Vaag A, Langkjaer L, Hougaard P, Markussen J. NovoSol Basal: pharmacokinetics of a novel soluble long-acting soluble insulin analogue. Br Med J 1989; 299: 415–19.

127. Zeuzem S, Stahl E, Jungmann E, Zoltobrocki M, Schöffling K, Caspary WF. *In vitro* activity of biosynthetic human diarginylinsulin. Diabetologia 1990; 33: 65–71.

128. Vølund A, Brange J, Drejer K, Jensen I, Markussen J, Ribel U et al. *In vitro* and *in vivo* potency of insulin analogues designed for clinical use. Diabet Med 1991; 8: 839–47.

129. Fineberg SE, Fineberg NS, Anderson JH, Birkett M. Insulin immune response to LysPro human insulin therapy in insulin naïve type I and type II patients (abstr). Diabetologia 1995; 38 (suppl. 1): A4.

130. Ottesen JL, Nilsson P, Jami J, Weilguny D, Dührkop M, Bucchini D et al. The potential immunogenicity of human insulin and insulin analogues evaluated in a transgenic mouse model. Diabetologia 1994; 37: 1178–85.

131. Jørgensen LN, Dideriksen LH, Drejer K. Carcinogenic effect of human insulin analogue B10Asp in female rats (abstr). Diabetologia 1992; 35 (suppl. 1): A3.

132. Galloway JA, Chance RE. Approaches to insulin analogues. In Marshall SM, Home PD (eds) The diabetes annual 8. Amsterdam: Elsevier, 1994; pp 277–97.

133. Holman RR, Steemson J. OPID 174: a novel long-acting insulin preparation (abstr). Diabet Med 1989; 6 (suppl. 1): A41.

134. Talaulicar M, Willms B, Rosskamp R. Efficacy of HOE 901 following subcutaneous injection for four days in type 1 diabetic subjects (abstr). Diabetologia 1994; 37 (suppl. 1): A169.

135. Kang S, Brange J, Burch A, Vølund A, Owens DR. Subcutaneous insulin absorption explained by insulin's physicochemical properties. Evidence from absorption studies of soluble human insulin and insulin analogues in humans. Diabetes Care 1991; 14: 942–8.

136. Heinemann L, Starke AA, Heding L, Jensen I, Berger M. Action profiles of fast onset insulin analogues. Diabetologia 1990; 33: 384–6.

137. Kang S, Creagh FM, Peters JR, Brange J, Vølund A, Owens DR. Comparison of subcutaneous soluble human insulin and insulin analogues (AspB9; GluB27; AspB10; AspB28) on meal-related plasma glucose excursions in type 1 diabetic subjects. Diabetes Care 1991; 14: 571–7.

138. Anderson JH Jr, Brunelle RL, Vignati L. Insulin lispro improved postprandial glucose control and reduced hypoglycaemia rate in type 1 diabetes (abstr). Diabetologia 1995; 38 (suppl. 1): A3.

139. Brunelle RL, Anderson JH, Vignati L. Insulin lispro improves postprandial control in a large crossover study in patients with type II diabetes (abstr). Diabetologia 1995; 38 (suppl. 1): A3.

140. Nielsen FS, Jørgensen LN, Ipsen M, Voldsgaard AI, Parving H-H. Long-term comparison of human insulin analogue B10Asp and soluble human insulin in IDDM patients on a basal/bolus insulin regimen. Diabetologia 1995; 38: 592–8.

141. Binder C, Lauritzen T, Faber O, Pramming S. Insulin pharmacokinetics. Diabetes Care 1984; 7: 188–99.

142. Round PM, Olsen KJ, Home PD, for the B28-ASP UK Study Group. Improved blood glucose control with insulin analogue B28-ASP (abstr). Diabetologia 1996; 39 (suppl. 1): A24.

41

Alternative Routes for Insulin Delivery

Bernard Zinman and Elaine Y.L. Tsui

Department of Medicine, University of Toronto, Ontario, Canada

INTRODUCTION

The isolation and the first administration of insulin at the University of Toronto [1] revolutionized the management of insulin dependent diabetes mellitus (IDDM). Unfortunately, although we have made significant progress (in purifying this hormone; in making available large quantities of human insulin, both biosynthetic and semi-synthetic; in studying its physiologic actions, chemistry and kinetics), our ability to achieve physiologic insulin replacement remains elusive [2]. One of the major barriers to the latter is the lack of minute-to-minute feedback control of insulin secretion in response to the changing hormonal requirements of meals and exercise. Progress in the development of a glucose sensor has been disappointing and for the immediate future we will likely have to depend on 'open loop' insulin administration. The second most important barrier to physiologic insulin replacement relates to the route of administration. The subcutaneous route of insulin administration has served us well for more than 70 years but clearly, as will be illustrated, frustrates our attempts at achieving physiologic insulinemia.

These deficiencies in insulin therapy have long been recognized and several imaginative approaches at replacing insulin by alternative routes have been explored. This chapter will review the various routes of insulin administration and will examine critically their potential role in the clinical management of diabetes. The use of implantable pumps and artificial and bioartificial endocrine devices are dealt with in detail elsewhere (Chapters 42 and 43).

THE GOAL: PHYSIOLOGIC INSULIN REPLACEMENT

In the context of insulin replacement, it is useful to review briefly the physiology of insulin secretion and action. Insulin plays the pivotal role as the anabolic hormone responsible for metabolic fuel flux in relationship to carbohydrate, protein and fat metabolism. Insulin concentrations can vary severalfold over minutes, it is secreted into the portal circulation, is variably cleared by the liver [3] and has a short half-life (5 min). Insulin secretion by the B cell of the pancreas is acutely responsive to changes in nutrient intake and exercise. Insulin secretion is controlled by gut hormones, the composition of the absorbed nutrients and the autonomic nervous system. Ultimately, it is the interaction of these variables that determines the insulin secretory pattern. As an example, the response to exercise of moderate intensity in the fasted state is characterized by a 50% decrease in insulin secretion. By contrast, with strenuous exhaustive exercise insulin secretion has been shown to increase substantially, probably as a consequence of the hyperglycemia associated with this form of exercise. With exercise performed in the postprandial state (30-60 min after a meal), a more complex pattern of insulin secretion is required [4].

In addition, several investigators have suggested that the pulsatile nature of insulin secretion may be an important physiologic characteristic [5, 6]. Given these considerations, it is indeed not surprising that we have not easily achieved the challenge of physiologic insulin replacement with our current treatment regimens. Indeed, it is remarkable that we have been able to

International Textbook of Diabetes Mellitus, Second Edition. Edited by K.G.M.M. Alberti, P. Zimmet, R.A. DeFronzo, and H. Keen (Honorary)
© 1997 John Wiley & Sons Ltd

obtain the degree of metabolic regulation usually seen in IDDM with what are rather primitive techniques in comparison to normal B cell function.

The pursuit of alternative routes of insulin delivery in order to achieve glycemic normalization will undoubtedly be accelerated by the important findings of the Diabetes Control and Complications Trial (DCCT) [7]. It is evident from this large multicentred study involving 1441 patients with IDDM in the USA and Canada that improved diabetes control, as assessed by hemoglobin A_{1c}, translates into a substantial reduction in the risk of long-term microvascular complications. Interestingly, the relationship between elevated hemoglobin A_{1c} and microvascular complications is curvilinear and *any* improvement in hemoglobin A_{1c} results in an improved outcome for the microvascular complications. Unfortunately, there does not appear to be a threshold effect and thus glycemic normalization may well be required for complications to be entirely prevented. This extremely difficult challenge is currently not attainable for the vast majority of individuals with IDDM.

SUBCUTANEOUS ROUTE

The subcutaneous route of insulin delivery has undergone significant modifications over the years in order to improve metabolic control. Initially, only regular insulin (also referred to as soluble or crystalline zinc insulin) was available and most IDDM patients were treated with two injections daily. With the advent of modified insulins with longer durations of action (protamine zinc, lente, and NPH (neutral protamine Hagedorn)) there was a trend to use once-daily insulin injections. More recently, it was appreciated that insulin therapy should mimic physiologic secretion and that this cannot be obtained with one or two injections of modified insulins. Insulin replacement therapy is now being viewed in the context of providing insulin for meals and insulin for basal requirements. This concept has led to the development of continuous subcutaneous insulin infusion pumps (CSII) and multiple daily insulin (MDI) injection regimens.

However, despite our best efforts at duplicating physiologic insulin needs with the newer subcutaneous insulin treatment regimens (CSII and MDI), glycemic normalization remains an elusive goal. This is best illustrated by examining the metabolic outcomes in the intensively treated DCCT cohort. With highly selected IDDM volunteers, treated by multidisciplinary teams in diabetes centres, the attainment of the long-term goal of glycemic normalization was disappointingly infrequent. Indeed, although 40% of individuals achieved a normal hemoglobin A_{1c} at some time during their participation in the DCCT, less than 5% were able to maintain a normal hemoglobin A_{1c} for the entire duration

of the study. This result underscores the difficulties of achieving normoglycemia even with 'sophisticated' regimens of subcutaneous insulin administration, and continues to be a powerful stimulus to the search for alternative routes of insulin therapy.

One might ask, 'Why is the subcutaneous route of insulin delivery so inadequate?' As illustrated in Table 1, many variables determine insulinemia after a subcutaneous injection and as a consequence the resulting metabolic effect can also be quite variable. The demonstration that insulin action can vary considerably is illustrated by the observations that with repeat injections in the same subject using the same dose of insulin and a consistent anatomical site, the peak plasma insulin level may vary by 20–30% and the time between injection and peak plasma concentration can vary by 50% [8]. With glucose clamp studies, the amount of glucose needed to maintain euglycemia, a good measure of insulin action, can vary by as much as 35%. It is now well established that insulin kinetics are different when the arm, leg or abdomen is used as an injection site [9]. In addition, the dose of insulin being administered markedly affects the kinetics, and the larger the dose of insulin, the more delayed is the peak, as is the duration of action. It has been clearly shown that exercise involving an extremity in which insulin has been injected can lead to a rapid acceleration of insulin absorption, particularly if the exercise is performed shortly after the injection [10, 11]. Changes in ambient temperature as well as body temperature can also affect insulin kinetics. It has also been shown that different insulin species have different absorption characteristics; human insulin is absorbed more rapidly than animal insulins [12]. Thus, the interaction of these variables makes it difficult to predict precisely the metabolic consequence of a particular dose of insulin. (The kinetics of SC insulin is further discussed in Chapter 40.)

Table 1 Variables affecting the kinetics of subcutaneously administered insulin

- Site of injection
- Depth of injection
- Dose of insulin
- Exercise
- Ambient temperature
- Body temperature
- Insulin species

THE INTRAPERITONEAL ROUTE

Experience with the intraperitoneal route of insulin delivery has been obtained with implantable insulin pumps and in patients on continuous ambulatory peritoneal dialysis where the insulin is added to the dialysate [13-15]. In the latter circumstance, the dose of insulin is adjusted to the carbohydrate content of the dialysate and has resulted in remarkable glucose regulation without the need for subcutaneous injections in these patients. Naturally, our aim in using alternative routes of insulin delivery is to improve control and prevent complications and thus the use of insulin with CAPD is important therapeutically but not in the context of long-term physiologic replacement.

A substantial experience with implantable pumps which infuse insulin intraperitoneally has been accumulated [16-18]. Well over 100 patients have been studied using implantable pumps that deliver insulin intraperitoneally [19]. This topic will be reviewed extensively in Chapter 42. It is generally accepted that for implantable pumps the intraperitoneal route is the preferred site of insulin administration [20]. The major theoretical advantages of the peritoneal route of insulin delivery can be summarized as follows. The peritoneal cavity provides a large, easily accessible, well vascularized surface area for insulin absorption [21, 22]. In addition, insulin administered into the peritoneal cavity is absorbed into the portal circulation, mimicking the physiologic route of insulin secretion [22-25], and provides the opportunity for the liver to modulate peripheral insulinemia [26-29]. This may be particularly important if peripheral hyperinsulinemia is shown to be an important factor in the pathophysiology of macrovascular disease [30-32]. The kinetics of insulin administration via the peritoneal route are favourable and insulin profiles similar to that seen in non-diabetic individuals can be achieved [22-25]. Several studies have demonstrated that normalization of hepatic glucose production [33] and the concentrations of intermediary metabolites [27, 28, 34, 35] can be achieved with this route of insulin administration. Glycemic regulation similarly appears to be markedly improved as compared to subcutaneous insulin administration [36-38].

The major disadvantage of intraperitoneal insulin delivery is the need for an implantable pump, peritoneal catheter and the associated morbidity and costs of this treatment. The issues related to safety (i.e. the presence of a large reservoir of insulin in the implanted pump) and long-term catheter survival are continuing technological problems requiring further study. Based on these limitations, this route of insulin delivery continues to be experimental and appropriate for only a small select group of individuals with IDDM.

THE INTRAVENOUS ROUTE

The intravenous route of insulin delivery has been studied with external and implantable pumps, using both peripheral venous and large central venous access. The latter approach is essentially a modification of technology developed for long-term parenteral nutrition, chemotherapy and anticoagulant administration. A great deal of experience [39-42] has been achieved with this route of insulin administration since it has been used since the early 1970s [43]. When compared with CSII, the intravenous route was able to achieve similar levels of glycemic control as assessed by hemoglobin A_{1c}, with less glycemic variability and fewer episodes of hypoglycemia [44, 45]. Another important difference between the two routes of insulin administration was the impairment in counter-regulatory hormone responses to hypoglycemia seen with CSII while hypoglycemia counter-regulation was unaffected by the intravenous route [46]. This appeared to be related to the frequent mild hypoglycemia associated with CSII which leads to a blunting of the counter-regulatory hormone responses.

The major disadvantages of the intravenous route of delivery are similar to those described for intraperitoneal administration. Additional risks of this route are the development of phlebitis and thrombosis [42]. As with any peripheral route of insulin delivery, hyperinsulinemia will be a concomitant feature of glycemic normalization, and the impact of hyperinsulinemia particularly in relationship to macrovascular disease remains to be defined. Animal studies have demonstrated that the portal vein can be used effectively as a route of insulin administration [47-49]. Very few studies examining the portal route of insulin delivery have been performed in man. A recent small-scale short-term study in IDDM demonstrated the feasibility and efficacy of intraportal insulin infusion via the umbilical vein in controlling glucose metabolism [50]. Intermediary metabolites, counter-regulatory hormones and glycemia were all normalized without hyperinsulinemia.

THE NASAL ROUTE

The administration of drugs by nasal insufflation has been explored for many years. Indeed, for the treatment of diabetes insipidus, the use of intranasal desamino-D-arginine vasopressin (DDAVP) was an important therapeutic advance. This successful model of hormonal replacement has stimulated efforts to develop an intranasal route of insulin administration. Since insulin is much larger than DDAVP, efficient transmucosal diffusion requires the use of absorption-enhancing agents. Bile salts (sodium glucocholate, sodium deoxycholate), non-ionic polyethylene ether (Laureth-9) and fusidic acid derivatives (sodium tauridihydrofusidate) have been used with varying degrees of success in enhancing insulin absorption across the nasal mucosa in humans [51-56].

The metabolic and pharmacokinetic characteristics of insulin delivered by the intranasal route have been well documented. Serum insulin levels rise within 10–15 min, peak at approximately 60 min and are back to basal by 90–120 min. This pharmacokinetic pattern is very similar to that seen with intraperitoneal and intravenous administration. Insulin delivered by this route is biologically active and effectively controls postprandial hyperglycemia [57–61]. Unfortunately, despite the use of absorption enhancing agents, bioavailability is still low (approximately 10%) [53]. In addition, the major adverse effect of delivering insulin by this method is nasal congestion, rhinorrhea and discomfort. The effect of upper respiratory tract infections on absorption can also be a confounding problem which would undoubtedly change the pharmacokinetics. In addition, with current preparations, intranasal administration of insulin would provide appropriate insulin replacement for nutrient intake but would not be suitable for supplying the 24-hour basal requirements [62, 63].

Continued studies using novel approaches at improving absorption with phospholipid enhancers (didecanoylphosphatidylcholine) [64, 65], bioadhesive microspheres [66–68] and other bioadhesive systems [69] are being pursued. Of all the alternative routes of insulin delivery, intranasal insulin administration has shown the most promise and may become clinically useful if the problems of bioavailability and nasal irritation are successfully resolved.

THE PULMONARY ROUTE

Many drugs are administered by aerosol inhalation. This route of administration has not escaped investigation in the context of diabetes, and early animal studies have demonstrated that insulin delivered by this route maintains its biological activity [70–73]. The insulin appears to be absorbed primarily through the respiratory epithelium and recent studies have demonstrated that a dose of approximately 1 U insulin/kg body weight is well tolerated by humans and can improve fasting plasma glucose levels in individuals with non-insulin dependent diabetes mellitus [74]. The metering, absorption and bioavailability issues in relationship to the pulmonary administration of insulin remain to be resolved.

THE ORAL ROUTE

The administration of insulin orally when food is ingested is obviously an attractive approach to replacing meal-related insulin. However, it is also obvious that as a protein insulin will undergo rapid enzymatic digestion. To protect insulin from proteolytic digestion,

investigators have used various strategies, including positively charged liposomes [75–83] and coating the molecule with impermeable polymers [84]. In addition, oral delivery of insulin with water-in-oil microemulsions has been tried in IDDM [85]. The major problem with the oral route of insulin delivery is low bioavailability (1–4%) and variability in absorption [86]. Once again, in addition to meal-related insulin, investigators will have to develop slow-release insulin preparations to meet basal requirements.

THE RECTAL ROUTE

Studies have been performed using suppositories or micro-enemas combined with various absorption enhancers to determine whether insulin could be administered across the rectal mucosa [87–91]. Interestingly, it has been estimated that approximately 30% of the insulin absorbed from the rectum is delivered directly into the portal vein [88]. Peak plasma insulin levels occurred at 30–45 minutes, simulating physiologic insulin release for a meal [88]. Bioavailability is greater than with the oral route of insulin administration [92] and remarkably reasonable metabolic control has been achieved in some studies [88–91, 93]. Clearly, the side-effects of abdominal discomfort and rectal urgency and the unlikeliness that this route of administration would be acceptable to the vast majority of patients makes this a less promising alternative insulin delivery strategy.

OTHER ALTERNATIVE ROUTES

The administration of drugs by transdermal absorption has been successful, primarily in the context of slow continuous release. A newer innovative approach directed at facilitating the transfer of larger molecules across the skin involves the process of iontophoresis [62]. This technique involves the migration of ionic substances such as a highly ionized monomeric form of insulin by altering the lipophilic barriers to peptides with the application of a low level electrical current to the skin. This has been studied in animal models in which the biological effectiveness of insulin was maintained [94, 95]. Another innovative approach to insulin release involves the development of implantable materials containing insulin with predictable insulin release characteristics. These implants are composed of synthetic polymers and are generally most applicable for long-term basal replacement [96–99]. A further innovation involves introducing an oscillating magnetic field which can be externally controlled to regulate insulin delivery [100]. The safety and efficacy of these devices will require extensive testing.

Table 2 Alternative routes of insulin delivery

Route	Advantages	Disadvantages
Intraperitoneal	Portal absorption Good bioavailability Physiologic insulin profiles	Pump required Catheter blockage Infection risk Risk of large insulin reservoirs
Intravenous	Good bioavailability Physiologic insulin profiles	Pump required Catheter blockage Phlebitis Hyperinsulinemia
Intranasal	Physiologic insulin profiles Easy use No device required	Nasal irritation Low bioavailability Interference by respiratory infection
Pulmonary	Physiologic insulin profiles Simple device Easy use	Low bioavailability Variable absorption
Oral	Easy use Acceptable	Low bioavailability Variable absorption

To demonstrate that almost every approach has been tried, some investigators have used the conjunctiva as a means of delivering insulin in animal studies [101, 102]. This has not been attempted in humans and is unlikely to show much promise.

CONCLUSIONS

Many alternative routes of insulin delivery have been evaluated in order to achieve the goal of long-term glycemic normalization. These are summarized in Table 2. To date, none of these approaches appears to be clinically meaningful for the vast majority of individuals with IDDM. A significant breakthrough in technology will be required to make our current methods of delivering insulin obsolete. In the interim, intensive insulin treatment strategies involving MDI or CSII hold the most promise for improving glycemic regulation and thus preventing the long-term devastating complications of diabetes.

REFERENCES

1. Banting FG, Best CH, Collip JB, Campbell WR, Fletcher AA. Pancreatic extracts in the treatment of diabetes mellitus. Can Med Assoc J 1922; 12: 141-6.
2. Zinman B. The physiological replacement of insulin: an elusive goal. New Engl J Med 1989; 321: 363-70.
3. Polonsky KS, Rubenstein AH. C-peptide as a measure of the secretion and hepatic extraction of insulin: pitfalls and limitations. Diabetes 1984; 33: 486-94.
4. Nelson JD, Poussier P, Marliss EB, Albisser AM, Zinman B. Metabolic response of normal man and insulin-infused diabetics to postprandial exercise. Am J Physiol 1982; 242: E309-16.
5. Bratusch-Marrain PR, Komjati M, Waldhausl W. Pulsatile insulin delivery: physiology and clinical implications. Diabet Med 1987; 4: 197-200.
6. Paolisso G, Sgambato S, Torella R, Varricchio M, Scheen A et al. Pulsatile insulin delivery is more efficient than continuous infusion in modulating islet cell function in normal subjects and patients with type I diabetes. J Clin Endocrinol Metab 1988; 66: 1220-6.
7. The Diabetes Control and Complications Trial Research Group. The effect of intensive treatment of diabetes on the development and progression of long-term complications in insulin dependent diabetes mellitus. New Engl J Med 1993; 329: 977-86.
8. Galloway JA, Spradlin CT, Howey DC, Dupre J. Intrasubject differences in pharmacokinetic and pharmacodynamic responses: the immutable problem of present-day treatment? In Serrano-Rios M, Lefebvre PJ (eds) Diabetes 1985: proceedings of the 12th Congress of the International Diabetes Federation, Madrid, 23-28 September 1985. International congress series no. 700. Amsterdam: Excerpta Medica, 1986; 877-86.
9. Koivisto VA, Felig P. Alterations in insulin absorption and in blood glucose control associated with varying insulin injection sites in diabetic patients. Ann Intern Med 1980; 92: 59-61.
10. Berger M, Halban PA, Assal JP, Offord RE, Vranic M, Renold AE. Pharmacokinetics of subcutaneously injected tritiated insulin: effect of exercise. Diabetes 1979; 28: 53-7.
11. Zinman B, Vranic M, Albisser AM, Leibel BS, Marliss ED. The role of insulin in the metabolic response to exercise in diabetic man. Diabetes 1979; 28 (suppl): 76-81.
12. Gulan M, Gottesman IS, Zinman B. Biosynthetic human insulin improves postprandial glucose excursions in type I diabetes. Ann Intern Med 1987; 107: 506-9.
13. Gokal R. Continuous ambulatory peritoneal dialysis— 10 years on. Quart J Med 1987; 242: 464-72.
14. Crossley K, Kjell SI, Rand CM. Intraperitoneal insulin for control of blood sugar in diabetic patients during peritoneal dialysis. Br Med J 1971; 1: 269-70.
15. Balducci A, Slama G, Rottenbourg J, Baumelou A, Delage A. Intraperitoneal insulin in uraemic diabetics

undergoing continuous ambulatory peritoneal dialysis. Br Med J 1981; 283: 1021-3.

16. Point Study Group. One year trial of a remote controlled implantable insulin infusion system in type 1 diabetic patients. Lancet 1988; 2: 866-9.

17. Saudek C, Selam J-L et al. A preliminary trial of the programmable implantable medication system for insulin delivery. New Engl J Med 1989; 321: 574-9.

18. Pinget M, Tauber JP, Brunger J et al. Workshop of the AIDSPIT Study Group. Amsterdam, Jan 27-29, 1991.

19. Knatterud GL, Fisher M. International study group on implantable insulin delivery devices registry. Diabet Nutr Metab 1990; 3: 63-5.

20. Selam J-L. Implantable insulin pumps: long is the road. Diabet Med 1988; 5: 724-33.

21. Selam J-L, Charles MA. Devices for insulin administration. Diabetes Care 1990; 13: 955-79.

22. Schade DS, Eaton RP, Friedman NM, Spencer W. Prolonged peritoneal insulin infusion in diabetic man. Diabetes Care 1980; 3: 314-17.

23. Schade DS, Eaton RP, Davis T et al. The kinetics of peritoneal insulin absorption. Metabolism 1981; 30: 149-55.

24. Nelson JA, Stephen R, London ST et al. Intraperitoneal insulin administration produces a positive portal systemic blood insulin gradient in unanesthetized unrestrained swine. Metabolism 1982; 31: 969-72.

25. Selam J-L, Bergman RN, Raccah D et al. Determination of portal insulin absorption from the peritoneum using a novel nonisotopic method. Diabetes 1990; 39: 1361-5.

26. Giacca A, Caumo A, Galimberti G, Petrella G, Librenti MC, Scavini M et al. Peritoneal and subcutaneous absorption of insulin in type 1 diabetic subjects. J Clin Endocrinol Metab 1993; 77: 738-42.

27. Micossi P, Boxi E, Cristallo M et al. Chronic continuous intraperitoneal insulin infusion (CIPII) in type I diabetic patients non-satisfactorily responsive to continuous subcutaneous insulin infusion (CSII). Acta Diabetol Lat 1986; 23: 155-64.

28. Stevenson RW, Parsons JH, Alberti KGMM. Comparison of the metabolic responses to portal and peripheral infusion of insulin in diabetic dogs. Metabolism 1981; 30: 752-65.

29. Selam J-L, Raymond M, Jacquemimin J-L et al. Kinetics of insulin infused intraperitoneally via portable pumps. Diabète Métab 1985; 11: 170-3.

30. Alberti KGMM, Home PD, Capaldo B. Influence of delivery route of insulin in intermediary metabolism. In: Crepaldi G (ed.) Diabetes, obesity and hyperlipidemias. International Congress Series 681: Amsterdam: Elsevier, 1986; pp 471-6.

31. Stolar MW. Atherosclerosis in diabetes: the role of hyperinsulinemia. Metabolism 1988; 37: 1-9.

32. Ducimetiere P, Eschwege E, Papoz PK, Richard JL, Claude JR, Rosselen G. Relationship of plasma insulin levels to the incidence of myocardial infarction coronary artery disease mortality in a middle age population. Diabetologia 1980; 19: 205-10.

33. Monti LD, Piatti PM, Home PD, Tomson C, Alberti KGMM. The effect of intraperitoneal insulin delivery on carbohydrate metabolism in type 1 (insulin dependent) diabetic patients. Diabetes Res Clin Pract 1992; 15: 237-44.

34. Ruotolo G, Parlavecchia M, Taskinen M, Galimberti G, Zoppo A, Le N et al. Normalization of

35. Selam J, Kashyap M, Alberti KGMM, Lozano J, Hanna M, Turner D et al. Comparison of intraperitoneal and subcutaneous insulin administration on lipids, apolipoproteins, fuel metabolites, and hormones in type 1 diabetes mellitus. Metabolism 1989; 38: 908-12.

36. Irsigler R, Kritz H. Alternate routes of insulin delivery. Diabetes Care 1980; 3: 219-28.

37. Selam J-L, Slingeneyer A, Hedon B et al. Long-term ambulatory peritoneal insulin infusion of brittle diabetes with portable pumps. Comparison with intravenous and subcutaneous routes. Diabetes Care 1983; 6: 105-11.

38. Selam J, Raccah D, Jean-Didier N, Lozano JL, Waxman K, Charles MA. Randomized comparison of metabolic control achieved by intraperitoneal insulin infusion with implantable pumps versus intensive subcutaneous insulin therapy in type 1 diabetic patients. Diabetes Care 1992; 15: 53-8.

39. Albisser AM, Nomura M, Bahoric A. Pumped IV insulin in experimental diabetes. Diabetes Res 1986; 3: 255-61.

40. Rupp WM, Barbosa JJ, Blackshear PJ et al. The use of an implantable insulin pump in the treatment of type II diabetes. New Engl J Med 1982; 307: 265-70.

41. Irsigler K, Kritz H, Hagmuller G, Franetzki M, Prestele K, Thurow H, Geisen K. Long-term continuous intraperitoneal insulin infusion with an implanted remote controlled insulin infusion device. Diabetes 1981; 30: 1072-5.

42. Knatterud G, Fisher M. Reports from the International Study Group on Insulin Infusion Devices (ISGIID) 6th Meeting. Nice, June 22-23, 1990.

43. Slama G, Hautecouverture M, Assam R, Tchobroutsky G. One to five days continuous intravenous insulin infusion in seven diabetic patients. Diabetes 1974; 23: 733-8.

44. Gulan M, Perlamn K, Albisser M, Pyper J, Zinman B. Controlled crossover study of subcutaneous and intravenous insulin infusion in type 1 diabetes. Diabetes Care 1987; 10: 453-60.

45. Perlman K, Ehrlich RM, Filler RM, Albisser AM. Waveform requirements for metabolic normalization with continuous IV insulin delivery in man. Diabetes 1981; 30: 710-77.

46. Gulan M, Perlman K, Sole M, Albisser M, Zinman B. Counter-regulatory hormone responses preserved after long-term intravenous insulin infusion compared to continuous subcutaneous insulin infusion. Diabetes 1988; 37: 526-31.

47. Stevenson RW, Parsons JA, Alberti KGMM. Effect of intraportal and peripheral insulin on glucose turnover and recycling in diabetic dogs. Am J Physiol 1983; 244: E190-5.

48. Goriya Y, Bahoric A, Marliss EB, Zinman B, Albisser AM. The metabolic and hormonal responses to a mixed meal in unrestrained pancreatectomized dogs chronically treated by portal or peripheral insulin infusion. Diabetologia 1981; 21: 58-64.

49. Goriya Y, Bahoric A, Marliss EB, Zinman B, Albisser AM. Blood glucose control and insulin clearance in unrestrained diabetic dogs portal infused with a portable insulin delivery system. Diabetologia 1980; 19: 452-7.

50. Shisko PI, Kovalev PA, Goncharov VG, Zajarny IU. Comparison of peripheral and portal (via the umbilical vein) routes of insulin infusion in IDDM patients. Diabetes 1992; 41: 1042–9.

51. Moses AC, Gordon GS, Carey MC, Flier JS. Insulin administered intranasally as an insulin–bile salt aerosol: effectiveness and reproducibility in normal and diabetic subjects. Diabetes 1983; 32: 1040–7.

52. Moses AC. Nasal absorption of insulin. Pharm Weeklb [Sci] 1988; 10: 45–6.

53. Sinay IR, Schlimovich S, Damilano S, Cagide AL, Faingold MC et al. Intranasal insulin administration in insulin dependent diabetes: reproducibility of its absorption and effects. Horm Metab Res 1990; 22: 307–8.

54. Frauman AG, Jerums G, Louis WJ. Effects of intranasal insulin in non-obese type II diabetics. Diabetes Res Clin Pract 1987; 3: 197–202.

55. Nolte MS, Taboga C, Salamon E, Moses AC, Longenecker F et al. Biological activity of nasally administered insulin in normal subjects. Horm Metab Res 1990; 22: 170–4.

56. Bruce DG, Chisholm DJ, Storlien LH, Borkman M, Kraegen EW. Meal-time intranasal insulin delivery in type 2 diabetes. Diabetic Med 1991; 8: 366–70.

57. Salzman R, Manson JE, Griffing GT, Kimmerle R, Ruderman N et al. Intranasal aerosolized insulin: mixed meal studies and long-term use in type 1 diabetes. New Engl J Med 1985; 312: 1078–84.

58. El-Etr M, Slama G, Desplanque N. Preprandial intranasal insulin as adjuvant therapy in type II diabetics. Lancet 1987; ii: 1085.

59. Lassmann-Vague V, Thiers D, Vialettes B, Vague PH. Preprandial intranasal insulin. Lancet 1988; i: 367–8.

60. Kimmerle R, Griffing G, McCall A, Ruderman NB, Stoltz E, Melby JC. Could intranasal insulin be useful in the treatment of non-insulin dependent diabetes mellitus? Diabetes Res Clin Pract 1991; 13: 69–76.

61. Gizurarson S, Bechgaard E. Intranasal administration of insulin to humans. Diabetes Res Clin Pract 1991; 12: 71–84.

62. Kennedy FP. Recent developments in insulin delivery techniques. Current status and future potential. Drugs 1991; 42: 213–27.

63. Illum L, Davis SD. Intranasal insulin. Clin Pharmacokinet 1992; 23: 30–41.

64. Drejer K, Vaag A, Bech K, Hansen P, Sorensen AR, Mygind N. Intranasal administration of insulin with phospholipid as absorption enhancer: pharmacokinetics in normal subjects. Diabet Med 1992; 9: 335–40.

65. Hansen P, Drejer K, Engesgaard A, Guldhammer B, Hjortkjaer RK et al. Medium chain phospholipids enhance the transnasal absorption of insulin. Diabetes Res Clin Pract 1988; 5(suppl. 1): S164.

66. Illum L, Jorgensen H, Bisgaard H, Krogsgaard O, Rossing N. Bioadhesive microspheres as a potential nasal drug delivery system. Int J Pharmaceutics 1987; 39: 189–99.

67. Bjork E, Edman P. Degradable starch microspheres as a nasal delivery system for insulin. Int J Pharmaceutics 1988; 47: 233–8.

68. Bjork E, Bjurstrom S, Edman P. Morphologic examination of rabbit nasal mucosa after nasal administration of degradable starch microspheres. Int J Pharmaceutics 1991; 75: 73–80.

69. Illum L. Factors affecting nasal absorption of drugs. In Commelin, Midha (eds) Topics in pharmaceutical sciences, 1981. Stuttgart: Medpharm, 1992; pp 71–82.

70. Cresia DA, Saviolakis GA, Bostian HA. Efficacy of inhaled insulin: effect of adjuvant. FASEB J 1988; 2: A537.

71. Almer L-O, Truedsson A, Arboreluis MJ et al. Insulin inhalation—at last a breakthrough. Diabetes Res Clin Pract 1988; 5: S163.

72. Wigley FM, London JH, Wood SH, Shipp JC, Waldman RH. Insulin across respiratory mucosae by aerosol delivery. Diabetes 1971; 20: 552–6.

73. Elliott RB, Edgar BW, Pilcher CC, Quested C, McMaster J. Parenteral absorption of insulin from the lung in diabetic children. Aust Paediatr J 1987; 23: 293–7.

74. Laube BL, Georgopoulos A, Adams III GK. Preliminary study of the efficacy of insulin aerosol delivered by oral inhalation in diabetic patients. JAMA 1993; 269: 2106–9.

75. Shichiri M, Etani N, Kawamori R, Karasaki K, Okada A, Shigeta Y, Abe Y. Absorption of insulin from perfused rabbit small intestine *in vitro*. Diabetes 1973; 22: 459–65.

76. Shichiri M, Shimizu Y, Yoshida Y, Kawamori R, Fukuchi M, Shigeta Y, Abe H. Enteral absorption of water-in-oil insulin emulsions in rabbits. Diabetologia 1974; 10: 317–21.

77. Dapergolas G, Gregoriadis G. Hypoglycaemic effect of liposome-entrapped insulin administered intragastrically into rats. Lancet 1976; ii: 824–7.

78. Gregoriadis G. Liposomes in therapeutic and preventive medicine: the development of the drug-carrier concept. Ann NY Acad Sci 1978; 308: 343–70.

79. Hashimoto A, Kawada J. Effects of oral administration of positively charged insulin liposomes on alloxan diabetic rats: preliminary study. Endocrinol Jpn 1979; 26: 337–44.

80. Rowland RN, Woodley JF. The stability of liposomes *in vitro* to pH, bile salts and pancreatic lipase. Biochim Biophys Acta 1980; 620: 400–9.

81. Kawada J, Tanaka N, Nozaki Y. No reduction of blood glucose in diabetic rats after oral administration of insulin liposomes prepared under acidic conditions. Endocrinol Jpn 1981; 28: 235–8.

82. Weingarten C, Moufti A, Desjeux JF, Luong TT, Durand G, Devissaguet JP, Puisieux F. Oral ingestion of insulin liposomes: effects of the administration route. Life Sci 1981; 28(24): 2747–52.

83. Patel HM, Stevenson RW, Parsons JA. Use of liposomes to aid intestinal absorption of entrapped insulin in normal and diabetic dogs. Biochim Biophys Acta 1982; 716: 188–93.

84. Saffran M, Kumar GS, Savariar C, Burnham JC, Williams F, Neckers DC. A new approach to the oral administration of insulin and other peptide drugs. Science 1986; 233: 1081–4.

85. Cho YW, Flynn M. Oral delivery of insulin. Lancet 1989; 2: 1518–19.

86. Shenfield GM, Hill JC. Infrequent response by diabetic rats to insulin-liposomes. Clin Exp Pharmacol Physiol 1982; 9: 355–61.

87. Nishihata T, Okamura Y, Kamada A, Higuchi T, Yagi T, Kawamori R, Shichiri M. Enhanced bioavailability of insulin after rectal administration with enamine as adjuvant in depancreatized dogs. J Pharm Pharmacol 1985; 37: 22–6.

88. Yamasaki Y, Shichiri M, Kawamori R et al. The effectiveness of rectal administration of insulin suppository on normal and diabetic subjects. Diabetes Care 1981; 4: 454–8.

89. Hildebrandt R, Imus A, Lotz U, Schliack V. Effect of insulin suppositories in type 1 diabetic patients (preliminary communication). Exp Clin Endocrinol 1984; 83: 168–72.

90. Raz I, Kidron M, Bar-On H, Ziv E. Rectal administration of insulin. Israel J Med Sci 1984; 20: 173–5.

91. Ritschel WA, Ritschel GB. Rectal administration of insulin. Methods and findings. Exp Clin Pharmacol 1984; 6: 513–29.

92. Aungst BJ, Roger NJ, Shefter TS. Comparison of nasal, rectal, buccal, sublingual and intramuscular insulin efficacy and the effects of a bile salt absorption promoter. J Pharmacol Exp Ther 1988; 244: 23–7.

93. Nishihata T, Kamada A, Sakai K, Yagi T, Kawamori R et al. Effectiveness of insulin suppositories in diabetic patients. Pharm Pharmacol 1989; 4: 799–801.

94. Kari B. Control of blood glucose levels in alloxan diabetic rabbits by iontophorosis of insulin. Diabetes 1986; 35: 217–21.

95. Meyer BR, Katzeff HL, Eschbach JC, Trimmer J, Zacharias SH, Rosen S, Sibalis DT. Transdermal delivery of human insulin to albino rabbits using electrical current. Am J Med Sci 1989; 297: 321–5.

96. Brown L, Munoz C, Siemer L, Edelman E, Langer R. Controlled release of insulin from polymer matrices: control of diabetes in rats. Diabetes 1986; 35: 692–7.

97. Creque HM, Langer R, Folkman J. One month of sustained release of insulin from a polymer implant. Diabetes 1980; 29: 37–40.

98. Goosen MFA, Leung YF, O'Shea GM, Chou S, Sun AM. Long-acting insulin: slow release of insulin from a biodegradable matrix implanted in diabetic rats. Diabetes 1983; 32: 478–81.

99. Wang PY. Prolonged release of insulin by cholesterol-matrix implant. Diabetes 1987; 36: 1068–72.

100. Edelman ER, Kost J, Bobeck H, Langer R. Regulation of drug release from polymer matrices by oscillating magnetic fields. Biomed Mater Res 1985; 19: 67–85.

101. Chiou GCY, Chuang CY, Chang MS. Systemic delivery of insulin through eyes to lower the glucose concentration. J Ocul Pharmacol 1989; 5: 81–91.

102. Yamamoto A, Luo AM, Dodd-Kashi S, Lee VHL. The ocular route for systemic insulin delivery in albino rabbit. J Pharmacol Exp Ther 1989; 249: 249–55.

42

Implantable Pumps

Christopher D. Saudek

Johns Hopkins University School of Medicine, Baltimore, USA

INTRODUCTION

There is no doubt that clinical approaches to insulin delivery could be improved. Subcutaneous injection has been the rule since the first human use of insulin in Toronto in 1922. Many improvements have been made in insulin purification and adjustment of its absorption rate, but the vast majority of insulin-requiring diabetic patients continue to use a needle and a syringe to take conventional insulin injections one to four times daily, always aiming for the subcutaneous space.

Subcutaneous injection is imprecise, though, a fraction of the dose often being delivered intramuscularly [1], and even truly subcutaneous injection carries with it many uncontrollable variables [2]. The rate of delivery into the circulation, for example, differs depending on whether it is in a limb or the abdomen, the temperature of the skin, amount of exercise, and the degree of lipoatrophy that exists, to name just a few of the hard to control variables. Local exercise, temperature and vascularity are significant variables. Perhaps most important, subcutaneously injected insulin is delivered into the peripheral venous circulation, rather than via the physiologic route to the hepatic portal system.

Implantable insulin infusion pumps that deliver insulin into the peritoneal cavity offer the promise of being more acceptable to patients and more physiologically efficient—more acceptable because of the freedom from insulin injections, and more physiologically efficient because the insulin is delivered by basal–bolus patterns into the peritoneal space, where it is preferentially absorbed into the portal

system [3]. They also promise relief from the multiple daily injections that perhaps more than anything else are identified as the down side of diabetes self-care.

The development of implanted insulin pumps has been a laborious exercise in applied research. The necessary players were engineers who knew how to solve a variety of complex design issues and clinicians who knew the needs of people with diabetes. The technical challenges of designing a safe and effective delivery system were formidable. Insulin had to be modified to survive at body temperature for months at a time. Pumps had to be designed that would not harm the insulin or have excessive power requirements. Microelectronics had to assure reliable, durable transcutaneous communication. A series of safety features had to be incorporated that would eliminate the chance of unintended over-delivery of insulin. And even then, designs that appeared promising on the bench were foiled at an alarming rate when tried *in vivo*. Most troublesome of all is the still vexing problem of keeping the very tip of the insulin delivery catheter open and in contact with insulin-absorbing tissue. These have not been trivial exercises in biomedical engineering.

Brief consideration of the components that make up implanted insulin pumps will provide an overview of how the current systems operate, what developmental challenges have been overcome and what problems remain. The current status of implanted insulin pumps can then be better appreciated. By tracing this progress up to the present, we can begin to define the role that implanted insulin infusion pumps could play in regular diabetes management as well as what technical

International Textbook of Diabetes Mellitus, Second Edition. Edited by K.G.M.M. Alberti, P. Zimmet, R.A. DeFronzo, and H. Keen (Honorary)
© 1997 John Wiley & Sons Ltd

improvements can be expected in the short and long term.

THE ANATOMY OF IMPLANTED INSULIN INFUSION PUMPS (Figure 1)

The Casing

Each of the available pumps is housed in a titanium disk of 8–10 cm diameter, 1.8–3.0 cm thick, weighing 220–280 g with a full reservoir. The implant is not so much 'accepted' in the body as it is walled off. Encapsulation occurs over a period of months, a firm fibrous tissue capsule holding the pump firmly and painlessly in place under the skin, superficial to the abdominal rectus muscles. The main determinant of overall pump size is reservoir volume, which itself determines the interval patients can go between refills. The most significant advance in this respect is the use of highly concentrated (400 units/ml) insulin in the original Programmable Implantable Medication System (PIMS) and now the MiniMed Implantable Pump (MIP; MiniMed Technologies, Sylmar, CA). While other internal contents of pumps may eventually be miniaturized, unless even more concentrated insulin is used, it will be hard to further down-size the pumps by more than 25% or so, since more frequent refill would not be desirable.

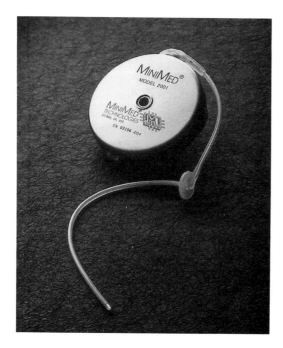

Figure 1   An implantable insulin infusion pump (MiniMed MMT-2001, version without side port)

The implanted pumps are clearly visible under the skin of thinner subjects but may be well hidden in people with some degree of adiposity. They are not uncomfortable or painful and not perceived as heavy. All degrees of physical activity and athletics are routinely permissible, although we do not recommend heavy contact sports.

It is most important that the capsule of the pump not become infected, since an established infection is virtually impossible to treat successfully without explantation. We therefore use aseptic techniques in refilling the devices. Post-operative infections have occurred rarely, and one case of apparent bacteremia-induced capsule infection has been reported [4]. Some centers have had repeated problems with skin breakdown over the site of implantation [5].

The Catheter

The catheter exits the pump, traverses the abdominal musculature, and delivers the insulin into the peritoneal space. It is surgically secured to the rectus muscles, with the tip floating freely in the abdominal cavity. In early trials, catheters often became grossly encapsulated within the peritoneum, blocking the exit of insulin and requiring laparoscopic surgery to clean the tissue off. With the development of more flexible, more biocompatible catheters, gross encapsulation is seen less often. The most frequent adverse event found in all the current implanted insulin pumps remains catheter blockage by small fibrin-containing plugs at the catheter tip, occurring at a rate of 10–20%/patient year. These catheter blocks, interestingly, usually present gradually and intermittently, with patients noticing less responsiveness to administered insulin or short periods of unresponsiveness. If complete blockage occurs, they resume subcutaneous insulin injections until the catheters can be surgically replaced (see below).

The Infusaid 1000 (Infusaid Co., Norwood, MA) took the lead in the development of a side port in the hub of the catheter where it meets the pump, allowing a needle to be passed transcutaneously into the proximal part of the catheter. This design permits detection of partial catheter blocks and the flushing of small intraluminal blocks within the catheter.

The Pump Module

The actual pumping mechanism that delivers insulin has required innovative engineering. The first approach, developed by Buchwald and colleagues at the University of Minnesota [6], was to take advantage of pressure exerted by a positive pressure Freon. However, the original Freon pressure-driven pump delivered at only one rate. To achieve variable rates, more sophisticated mechanisms were introduced. One suboptimal approach, for example, used a roller pump mechanism that was like a miniaturized tractor tread [7]. The problems were twofold: it required considerable electrical current to keep the pump going, causing a short battery life; and the mechanical pressure damaged the fragile insulin molecule.

The PIMS, invented by Fischell et al [8] at the Johns Hopkins University Applied Physics Laboratory and developed at the School of Medicine, took a different approach. A tiny positive displacement pump, developed originally by the National Aeronautics and Space Administration (NASA), provides an accurate pulse with minimal power requirement and minimal trauma to the insulin. Variations of this positive displacement pump are used in the MiniMed Implantable Pump.

The current Infusaid pump continues to rely on positive pressure Freon as the driving force, but incorporates a series of remotely controlled gates that regulate the flow of insulin out of the pump.

The Reservoir

Reservoirs in the current pumps are not static holding tanks. Rather, one surface is a moving diaphragm between the Freon chamber and the insulin reservoir. When the reservoir is full, the Freon chamber is collapsed; as the reservoir empties, the Freon chamber expands. Freon serves the purpose particularly well since its main physical property is to maintain essentially equal pressure regardless of volume. As the volume of the Freon chamber expands, more Freon vaporizes; as the volume contracts, Freon droplets develop; at all points, gas pressure exerted on the reservoir is constant. In the case of the Buchwald pump and its successors, positive pressure of Freon is the force that drives insulin delivery.

The most significant difference between the MIP and the Infusaid pump is the type of Freon used. Whereas the Infusaid reservoir is at positive pressure, in the MIP, Freon exerts a *less than atmospheric* pressure, i.e. a vacuum relative to atmosphere. This provides what is a significant safety feature in the MIP: insulin is *drawn into* the MIP during refills only when the refill needle is properly in place within the pump; and any leaks that occur in the MIP will draw tissue fluid back into the pump rather than causing an insulin leak.

The Electronics

Patient-driven communication from outside the body is the key to establishing variable-rate insulin delivery. Remotely controlled communication systems were not applied to insulin pumps until the 1980s. The issues raised primarily concern patient safety. It is immediately apparent, for example, that over-delivery is vastly more dangerous than under-delivery, since hyperglycemia and ketoacidosis develop gradually and are readily avoidable by conventional injections, whereas severe over-delivery could cause sudden, catastrophic hypoglycemia. It is also true that to control postprandial hyperglycemia, the rate of insulin delivery at mealtimes must be 10–100 times higher than that required as a basal rate. If a meal does not follow a mealtime dose of insulin, hypoglycemia will occur. Nevertheless, limits on insulin delivery can and are programmed in to prevent catastrophic insulin overdose.

Battery life is another significant factor in design of the electronics. No pumps have replaceable or rechargeable batteries, so the entire pump must be replaced surgically when the battery runs down. Current pumps have a life expectancy of about three years, and this battery life may improve in future pumps. Many of the subjects have had their original pumps electively replaced under local anesthesia, however, without significant problems.

The Insulin

Insulin is a highly unstable protein, subject to aggregation, precipitation and denaturation [9, 10]. Early approaches to preventing insulin aggregation included use of a viscous solution of glycerol [11]. A more practical solution was developed by Hoechst AG (Frankfurt, Germany), adding a surfactant material, polyethylene-polypropylene glycol (Genapol(R) [12]) that proved to be highly compatible in implanted pumps [13]. All pumps use this form of insulin at present.

The concentration of insulin determines the necessary reservoir volume and the refill interval. By using U-400 insulin, the MIP can plan reservoir refills only every three months. The Infusaid pump and other pumps use U-100 insulin.

CLINICAL USE OF IMPLANTED INSULIN PUMPS

Patient Selection

Patients implanted with insulin pumps thus far are carefully selected. The majority have documented type 1, insulin dependent diabetes, although about 50 patients with type 2 diabetes have been implanted. They are expected to monitor their own blood glucose three to four times daily, to come in regularly for research data collection as well as routine clinical management, and they are motivated to take part in a new form of treatment. Patients with serious co-morbidities, late stage diabetic complications, pregnancy and other factors which would interfere with completion of reliable studies have been excluded.

The restrictiveness of eligibility criteria, however, should not be over-emphasized. Over 100 patients have qualified at some centers. Subjects' ages range from 19 to 75, they have a range of body weights from thin to obese, and a variety of racial backgrounds and levels of formal education. While motivation to perform good self-care is a significant feature of the patient group, many have little formal education. It has not been our experience that management of the pump requires unusual intelligence.

Surgical Implantation

Dr Henry A. Pitt has developed the surgical techniques in use at Johns Hopkins. Pumps have been implanted under general anesthesia or with local anesthesia. About 45 min is required for preparation of the pump in the operating room, and the surgery itself takes a similar amount of time. The incision we prefer is midline, although some surgeons prefer a transverse incision cephalad to the pump. The abdominal location of the pump is determined by patient preference and topography of the abdomen, but it must be either above or below the beltline, not directly under the belt. After the initial incision, a subcutaneous pocket is formed, then a small incision is made through the abdominal musculature into the abdominal cavity. The catheter is placed freely in the abdomen, the proximal portion sutured to the fascia. The pump is then placed subcutaneously and also sutured in place. Closure is accomplished and the wound heals in the usual manner. Perioperative antibiotics (a second-generation cephalosporin) are given just before surgery.

Replacement of the pump and catheter or catheter alone is performed with local anesthetic. The original incision is re-opened, the pump and catheter removed. Any resistance in removing the catheter tip from the abdominal cavity is noted, since that suggests an adhesion. On a sterile side table, the pump is checked for stroke volume, rinsed if necessary, and a new catheter is attached. The pump is put in place, the catheter tip inserted through the same small incision through the abdominal muscles, and the pump pocket closed separately from cutaneous closure.

It is not uncommon to have a collection of serous fluid (seroma) for several weeks post-operatively. Some centers have used an abdominal wrap in the hope of reducing fluid accumulation; we have not found that useful. We do not drain the seroma unless it is so large as to threaten the integrity of the wound-healing, or unless we suspect infection. Antibiotics are re-started promptly if cellulitis, erythema or fever are noted.

Patients may remain hospitalized for 24 hours postoperatively in the absence of complications.

Complications of surgery are unusual. The most common would be some degree of inflammation surrounding the pump, particularly when replacing a pump into the same pump pocket. The most serious complication is undoubtedly infection of the pump pocket. Frank infection (positive cultures, pus in the pocket, inflammation) is rarely if ever curable. The usual course is explantation, followed several months later by re-implantation at a different site.

Routine Patient Use of Implanted Insulin Pumps

Insulin is delivered in a basal–bolus pattern, i.e. at a continuous low basal rate (usually about 0.5–1.0 units/hour) between meals and overnight, supplemented by boluses (e.g. 2–10 units) delivered before meals. Basal rates continue until changed by the patient, but at each mealtime the patient decides on the appropriate bolus dose, within limits established by the physician, places the external communicator over the pump and presses a button on the communicator, commanding the implant to deliver the intended bolus.

Pump refills are accomplished, as noted, every three months with the MIP and about every four weeks with the Infusaid pump. They are done at the physician's office, since the large amount of insulin put into the pump (2500–6000 units) would be exceedingly dangerous if self-administered erroneously. After aseptic preparation of the skin, and a drop of local anesthetic in the skin, a needle is passed into the pump reservoir. Old insulin is withdrawn and new insulin inserted, the whole procedure being painless and taking 10–15 minutes. The accuracy of insulin delivery by the pump can be estimated by comparing the amount of insulin actually withdrawn with what should be withdrawn based on the patient's insulin use. Under-delivery problems can be detected in this way.

Management of Complications

Patients are carefully instructed to keep conventional insulin supplies close at hand in case under-delivery occurs. If under-delivery is noted in the MIP, it is usually due to one of two problems; catheter block or back-flow through a slightly incompetent outlet valve due to micro-deposits of insulin. A rinse procedure with alkaline solution will correct the backflow condition, but if catheter blockage occurs, the catheter is surgically replaced under local anesthetic. The Infusaid pump experience has uncovered problems with insulin precipitation in the pump as well as a slow-down of insulin delivery for reasons that have not been specified.

A low battery condition (after 3.5 years' therapy, on average) is signaled in the MIP by an audible alarm, well before under-delivery would occur. As mentioned, this requires elective replacement of the battery.

In earlier experience with the pump developed by Siemens, skin erosion occurred at the corners of a rectangular pump. With the current pumps, skin erosion and other physical complications of pump placement are very unusual.

CLINICAL TRIALS OF IMPLANTED INSULIN PUMPS

Initial Trials

The first clinical use of implanted insulin pumps was by Buchwald et al in the 1970s, using the constant-rate Infusaid pump in a relatively large number of patients, primarily with non-insulin dependent diabetes mellitus (NIDDM) [14]. The first wave of variable rate pump trials took place in the early 1980s, with several relatively small experiences using pumps developed by the Sandia Corporation in collaboration with Schade, Eaton and colleagues [15], and Siemens, working with Irsigler et al [16]. While some success was achieved, the devices had short battery life, mechanical failures, and skin breakdown from the corners of the casing. Coincident with these experiences, PIMS was undergoing about four years of pre-clinical dog trial experience.

In 1986, PIMS entered clinical trials in 18 human subjects at the Johns Hopkins University and the University of California, Irvine [17]. For the first time, a variable rate pump was shown to treat IDDM in reliable fashion, free of a disabling rate of device failures for an average of three years continuously. Glycemic control was excellent, and there were no surgical or other safety hazards. Another generation of the Siemens pump was used in 20 subjects in Europe simultaneously, with less good results [18].

Current Trials

The two implanted insulin pumps currently in clinical trials, the MiniMed Implantable Pump Model 2000 (MIP) and the Infusaid Model 1000, are undergoing three major clinical trials at present:

The MiniMed Implantable Pump Trial in IDDM

The MIP in IDDM study is taking place in over 26 hospitals in the USA, France and elsewhere in Europe. Over 500 pumps have been implanted, starting in 1990. The trial is not randomized, but is designed to gain experience and collect data using the MIP in many practice-based as well as university centers. With the

exception of one interruption for a six-month FDA-imposed hold on new implantations in the USA while the cause and correction of the backflow anomaly was worked out, the trial has been continuous and successful. The rate of under-delivery is in the range of 15–30%/patient year, increasing with duration of implantation and with changes in manufacturing techniques for insulin. The alkaline rinse procedure was first used in 1992. By correcting backflow, it can clear about half the cases of under-delivery.

The Infusaid Trial in IDDM

The Infusaid clinical trial in IDDM began in 1989. Like the MiniMed trial, it is multicenter, carried out in Europe and the USA. Also like the MiniMed trial, it is not randomized, but is designed to expand experience with the Infusaid pump. There have been two long holds put on new implantations while problems with catheter breaks and septum leaks were addressed.

The Veterans' Affairs Trial in NIDDM

There are two crucial reasons to try implanted insulin pump therapy in type 2 diabetes [19]. First, as with IDDM, many people with NIDDM do not achieve good glycemic control despite multiple-dose insulin regimens; and second, there is concern that the peripheral hyperinsulinemia caused by subcutaneously delivered insulin may be particularly inadvisable in people already prone to accelerated atherosclerosis. Insulin delivered into the peritoneal space is not only more rapidly absorbed than insulin delivered subcutaneously, but produces less peripheral hyperinsulinemia [20], presumably due to the first-pass clearance of portally absorbed insulin by the liver.

The Veterans' Affairs (VA) Implanted Insulin Pump Study was therefore designed to test rigorously whether insulin delivered to people with NIDDM by implanted insulin pumps could control their diabetes as well as multiple-dose insulin delivered subcutaneously, and whether there are significant other advantages to the use of pumps in NIDDM. The MiniMed Implantable Pump was selected for use in the VA study, but the study was conceived and is being conducted entirely independent of corporate support, and this has made it possible to establish the first large-scale *randomized* trial comparing these modes of insulin delivery.

Preliminary results [21] presented in abstract form show that, consistent with the study objective, very good glycemic control was achieved with both the implanted pumps and multiple daily doses of insulin. There was, however, reduced glycemic variability in the patients treated with pumps, translating into a greatly reduced incidence of both severe and mild hypoglycemia in subjects assigned to implanted insulin pump therapy. The incidence of catheter block, however, seems to be higher in these overweight males.

FUTURE

The relatively near-term future of implanted insulin pump therapy can be relatively well visualized; the long-term future is, of course, less clear. Large clinical trials will allow application to regulatory agencies internationally, and there is a real prospect that implanted insulin pumps could become generally available therapy for diabetes within several years. This step would not only allow more people to benefit from a therapy that has had a high rate of patient satisfaction, but would allow further refinement of medical indications for its use, surgical and medical procedures for management of patients, and better definition of complication rates. It is fair to point out that no company has made a profit from implanted insulin pumps despite over 20 years of corporate investment in their development. At some point, the investment will have to provide some return which can then support further device improvements.

Scientifically, it will be of great interest to know the exact metabolic effects of insulin delivered into the peritoneal space and absorbed preferentially into the portal system. Some evidence suggests that, given equal concentrations, portally and peripherally delivered insulin have the same effect [22, 23]. This observation raises some interesting possibilities to explain the apparent decrease in the rate of hypoglycemia when insulin is delivered by implanted insulin pumps. Many questions remain to be answered with carefully controlled metabolic studies.

It is clear that certain device improvements will be made over the years, such as development of better catheters that allow the non-surgical correction of catheter tip blockage, smaller and more flexible external communication units, and somewhat smaller implanted devices (although reservoir volume will always limit the device miniaturization). Device and insulin changes are painfully slow in coming, not only because even the smallest change requires careful design, pre-clinical and clinical testing, but because new applications must be submitted to and approved by regulatory bodies.

The first question on everyone's mind when considering implanted insulin pumps, is whether, or when, they will become 'closed-loop', i.e. controlled automatically by an implanted sensor of blood glucose. To be sure, many laboratories have been and are working on glucose sensors, and continued progress is to be expected. The technical barriers are formidable, though, particularly to implanting a reliable, foolproof sensor

for years at a time. The first step may be to electronically interface a replaceable subcutaneous sensor with the permanently implanted delivery system. The holy grail of a fully automated, closed-loop implanted insulin pump may not be realized for decades. Were it to happen, though, it could rightly be put in the category of a technological 'cure' for diabetes, alongside another holy grail, islet cell transplantation without the need for immunosuppression.

SUMMARY

Implanted insulin pumps have developed from simple, single-rate devices through small and limited clinical trials to expanded clinical trials in which over 500 subjects now take part. They have been used to treat people with IDDM for over seven years continuously. The complications, especially blockage of the intraperitoneal catheter, are now well defined and clinically manageable, although they require a significant number of repeat surgical procedures. Implanted insulin pumps have a high degree of patient acceptance and enthusiasm. The therapy thus seems to be on the verge of becoming generally available. As advances are made to provide further ease of use and fewer interventions, the technology has the potential to improve the quality of life and the glycemic control of people with diabetes.

REFERENCES

1. Vaag A, Damgaard-Pedersen K, Lauritzen M, Hildebrandt P, Beck-Nielsen H. Intramuscular versus subcutaneous injection of unmodified insulin: consequences for blood glucose control in patients with Type 1 diabetes mellitus. Diabet Med 1990; 7: 335–42.
2. Zinman B. The physiologic replacement of insulin: an elusive goal. New Engl J Med 1989; 321: 363–70.
3. Duckworth WC, Saudek CD, Henry RR. Why intraperitoneal delivery of insulin with implantable pumps in NIDDM? Diabetes 1992; 41: 657–61.
4. Levy RP, Borchelt MD, Kremer RM, Francis SJ, O'Connor CA. *Haemophilus influenzae* infection of an implantable insulin-pump pocket. Diabetes Care 1992; 15: 1449–50.
5. Renard E, Bringer J, Jacques-Apostol D, Lauton D, Mestre C, Costalat G, Jaffiol C. Complications of the pump pocket may represent a significant cause of incidents with implanted systems for intraperitoneal insulin delivery. Diabetes Care 1994; 17: 1064–6.
6. Blackshear PJ, Rohde TD, Prosl F, Buchwald J. The implantable infusion pump: a new concept in drug delivery. Med Prog Technol 1979; 6: 149–61.
7. Irsigler K, Kritz H, Hagmuller G, Franetzki M, Prestele K, Thurow H, Geisen K. Long-term continuous intraperitoneal insulin infusion with an implantable remote-controlled insulin infusion device. Diabetes 1981; 30: 1072–5.
8. Saudek CD, Fischell RE, Swindle MM. The Programmable Implantable Medication System (PIMS):

design features and pre-clinical trials. Horm Metab Res 1990; 22: 201–6.

9. Grau U. Chemical stability of insulin in a delivery system environment. Diabetologia 1985; 28: 458–63.

10. Grau U. Insulin stability. In Hepp KD, Renner R (eds) Continuous insulin infusion therapy: experience from one decade. Stuttgart, FRG: Schattauer, 1985; pp 33–46.

11. Blackshear PJ, Rohde TD, Palmer JL, Wigness BD, Rupp WM, Buchwald H. Glycerol prevents insulin precipitation and interruption of flow in an implantable insulin infusion pump. Diabetes Care 1983; 6: 387–92.

12. Grau U, Seipke G, Obermeier R, Thurow H. Stabile Insulinlosungen fur authomatische Dosiergerate. In Petersen KG, Schluter KJ, Kerp L (eds) Neue Insuline. Freiburg: Freiburger Graphische Betriebe, 1982; pp 411–19.

13. Grau U, Saudek CD. Stable insulin preparation for implanted insulin pump: laboratory and animal trials. Diabetes 1987; 36: 1453–59.

14. Blackshear PJ, Shulman GI, Roussell AM, Nathan DM, Minaker KL, Rowe AM et al. Metabolic response to three years of continuous, basal rate intravenous insulin infusion in type II diabetic patients. J Clin Endocrin Metab 1985; 61: 753–60.

15. Schade DS, Eaton RP, Edwards WS et al. A remotely programmable insulin delivery system. Successful short-term implantation in man. J Am Med Assoc 1982; 247: 1848–53.

16. Irsigler K, Kritz H, Hagmuller G, Franetzki M, Prestele K, Thurow H, Geisen K. Long-term continuous intraperitoneal insulin infusion with an implantable remote-controlled insulin infusion device. Diabetes 1981; 30: 1072–5.

17. Saudek CD, Selam J-L, Pitt HA, Waxman K, Rubio M, Jeandidier N, Turner D, Fischell RE, Charles MA. A preliminary trial of the programmable implantable medication system for insulin delivery. New Engl J Med 1989; 321: 574–9.

18. Point Study Group. One year trial of a remote-controlled implantable insulin infusion system in type 1 diabetic patients. Lancet 1988; 2: 866–9.

19. Saudek CD, Duckworth WC. The Department of Veterans Affairs Implanted Insulin Pump Study. Diabetes Care 1992; 15: 567–70.

20. Micossi P, Cristallo M, Librenti MC, Petrella G, Galimberti G, Melandri M et al. Free-insulin profiles after intraperitoneal, intramuscular, and subcutaneous insulin administration. Diabetes Care 1986; 9: 575–8.

21. VA Study Group. Veterans' Affairs Implantable Insulin Pump Study: mean glycemia and hypoglycemia. Diabetes 1994; 43 (suppl. 1): 61A.

22. Ishida T, Chap Z, Chou J, Lewis RM, Hartley CJ, Entman ML, Field JB. Effects of portal and peripheral venous insulin infusion on glucose production and utilization in depancreatized, conscious dogs. Diabetes 1984; 33: 984–90.

23. Kryshak EJ, Butler PD, Marsh C, Miller A, Barr D, Polonsky K et al. Pattern of postprandial carbohydrate metabolism and effects of portal and peripheral insulin delivery. Diabetes 1990; 39: 142–9.

43

Artificial and Bio-artificial Pancreas Systems

Gérard Reach

Diabetes Department, Hôtel Dieu, Paris, France

INTRODUCTION: DIABETES THERAPY, A NAVIGATION BETWEEN TWO REEFS

Diabetes mellitus is a common disease afflicting 1–2% of the population, of whom 10% require the daily injection of insulin. Uncontrolled hyperglycaemia can lead to severe complications if the amount of injected insulin is too low and if blood glucose concentration remains in the high range [1]. By contrast, if too much insulin is injected, hypoglycaemia occurs [2]. Thus, the results of the Diabetes Control and Complications Trial (DCCT) indicate that if improving blood glucose control halves the rate of appearance and of progression of complications (retinopathy, nephropathy, neuropathy), it also trebles the risk of severe hypoglycaemia, despite intensive, but discontinuous, blood glucose monitoring [3].

The impact of hypoglycaemia, the most common side-effect of insulin treatment, and the one which diabetic patients fear most, cannot be overlooked. Severe hypoglycaemic attacks, leading to loss of consciousness, seem inevitable, since it is estimated that one patient in 10 has one coma a year, and that this risk increases when insulin therapy is intensified. Understandably, fear of hypoglycaemia is a major determinant of the reluctance of patients to adopt the techniques of intensified insulin therapy, which is one of the recommendations of the DCCT. This is one reason why normalization of HbA_{1c} is impossible in large groups of patients, even with intensified insulin therapy, and why pancreas transplantation is the only treatment currently capable of consistently *normalizing* glycated haemoglobin in type 1 diabetic patients.

Furthermore, to improve the quality of diabetes control, patients must continually adapt insulin dosage according to the results of self-monitoring of blood glucose levels and to the presence or absence of glucose in urine samples. Not only is this far from efficient, but it also represents a boring task, which only a machine can perform repeatedly without complaining. This is why the development of an artificial pancreas, a *machine* which can continuously administer insulin and be automatically controlled by concomitant blood glucose levels, has been considered as one of the ultimate objectives in diabetes research. It also corresponds, together with pancreatic tissue grafting, to one of the great expectations of diabetic patients.

ARTIFICIAL ORGANS

The European Society for Biomaterials defined an 'artificial organ' as 'a medical device that replaces, in part or in whole, the function of one of the organs of the body' [4]. It seems, therefore, that the first task in designing an artificial organ is to analyse the function of the natural organ. The function in need of replacement in the case of insulin dependent diabetes is the secretion of insulin by the pancreatic islet B cells, which has four characteristics: (a) it is continuous, even in the postabsorptive state, with rapid and transient peaks during meals: (b) it undergoes automatic regulation by blood glucose levels; (c) insulin is delivered into the portal blood system; (d) the endocrine pancreas is (of course) an internal organ placed within the body. None of these four characteristics can be applied to the

International Textbook of Diabetes Mellitus, Second Edition. Edited by K.G.M.M. Alberti, P. Zimmet, R.A. DeFronzo, and H. Keen (Honorary)
© 1997 John Wiley & Sons Ltd

current, discontinuous, administration of insulin via syringes, and only a different approach could lead to the development of an 'artificial pancreas'. It is also important to bear in mind two objectives in research towards improvement of the treatment of diabetes mellitus: (a) an improvement in the quality of diabetes control so as to prevent the late complications of the disease without increasing the risk of severe hypoglycaemia; and (b) an improvement in the patient's quality of life: it may be important that the artificial organ should be 'implantable' over a long term, as only this would permit the patient to consider himself cured. An external system might even be considered by a number of patients as useless, since it might not improve their quality of life: the challenge is therefore much more difficult than in the case of the artificial kidney [5, 6]. The new system must also be safe so that it adds no increased risk to a disease which can be relatively safely circumvented by syringe-injected insulin.

A major feature of insulin secretion, which is lacking in its restoration by current insulin therapy, is its continuous regulation by blood glucose level. The aim of this chapter is to describe two different approaches, one electromechanical, the other bio-artificial, to the concept of 'the artificial pancreas', by which insulin delivery would be automatically regulated, not just adapted by the diabetic patient, and to delineate the obstacles which have meant that such systems are not yet available.

ARTIFICIAL ELECTROMECHANICAL B CELLS

Methods were developed 25 years ago to monitor blood glucose continuously, either by modifying standard laboratory techniques adapted to continuous flow analysis, or by developing electrochemical biosensors. The results of the glucose concentration determinations could then be processed by a computer controlling the flow rate of a pump delivering insulin, creating the framework of an 'artificial B cell'. Interestingly, this application of the principle of the Clark oxygen electrode to the detection of glucose was proposed in the early 1970s, i.e. precisely when the first attempts at treating type 1 diabetic patients with *continuous* intravenous insulin infusion were made [7].

With these two technological advances it was possible to develop the bedside artificial system, referred to as the 'artificial pancreas'. The glucose sensor had the form of a flow-through chamber containing an enzymatic glucose electrode. A double lumen catheter indwelling in a vein was used to withdraw blood continuously in heparinized and diluted form. Blood was pumped to the glucose sensor chamber, and circulated inside it in contact with a membrane which served to protect the glucose oxidase responsible for the recognition of glucose which had crossed the membrane. The enzymatic layer was separated from the electrode by a secondary membrane aimed at screening off interferants such as ascorbate or urate. The hydrogen peroxide produced during glucose oxidation was able to cross this membrane and was oxidized on contact with the electrode, producing electrons. The current thus generated was analysed by a computer which, through a calibration procedure, transformed the result obtained electrically into an estimation of blood glucose concentration. A mathematical formula, or algorithm, was used to yield minute-by-minute from this estimation the necessary amount of insulin to be delivered by the system. This algorithm took into account not only the value of blood glucose concentration at a given time but also its derivative, the amount of insulin to be released being higher if blood glucose concentration was increasing than if it was stable or decreasing. This was necessary to avoid oscillations in blood glucose concentrations. Interestingly, this yielded an insulin delivery pattern during a glucose load which mimicked the biphasic insulin secretion profile of the natural B cell. Finally, the artificial system was also able to deliver either glucose or glucagon in case of overshoot hypoglycaemia, a feature which is shared not by the pancreatic B cell, but by its co-workers in the regulation of glucose homeostasis, the liver and the A cell of the islet of Langerhans, respectively.

These systems [8] were used early in such clinical situations as the treatment of diabetic ketoacidosis, haemodialysis, surgery, or the resection of insulinoma, and they were also used to achieve normoglycaemia for a short period of time after the onset of diabetes and to induce diabetes remission (review in [9]). However, the artificial pancreas has since become essentially a research tool. In the early 1980s it was recognized that it could be used to clamp blood glucose concentrations at a desired value, either in normal subjects or in diabetic patients. The importance of this new tool in diabetes research, i.e. determining the mechanisms of insulin sensitivity or the physiology of counter-regulation to hypoglycaemia, became such that an artificial pancreas is now present in many of the research departments interested in the physiology and pathophysiology of glucose homeostasis. However, concomitantly with the increasing investigational interest in the artificial pancreas, the devices progressively disappeared from the clinical departments and they never entered the homes of diabetic patients as routine therapy. Retrospectively, this is surprising.

Indeed, the artificial pancreas was developed exactly 20 years ago, a few years after the first walk of man on the moon, and it was believed at that time that the power of technology would make it possible to transform these bedside devices into miniaturized systems. Why did this not occur? Three possible explanations are considered here. The first, that miniaturization of the device was the problem, seems unlikely because progress in information technology has been such that the programs required to describe the rather simple algorithms used in artificial B cells could now be placed inside an almost invisible device. However, one should not forget that when the concept of an artificial B cell was under active development, microinformatics was in its prehistoric stage: microcomputers were non-existent at that time, and it may be that the concept was developed too soon. Similarly, the fact that no implantable programmable pump was available at that time suggests a second possible explanation. However, this is no longer an obstacle to the development of an implantable artificial pancreas, since in the mean time such pumps have been developed and their safety has been demonstrated (see Chapter 42). Coupling the pump to a glucose sensor should therefore now be possible, if a long-term glucose sensor were available. It is also interesting to speculate that the development of wearable pumps, making continuous insulin infusion possible, and of discontinuous blood glucose monitoring with test strips, have also contributed to the lack of success of bedside artificial pancreas systems in the management of acute metabolic situations (ketoacidosis, surgery, etc.). These complex and expensive devices were replaced by simple systems consisting of a wearable insulin pump, and of the cheap material required for capillary blood glucose monitoring, as well as by simple rules aimed at adapting insulin infusion in order to get the crude glucose regulation which is required in these acute situations.

A third explanation of the fact that artificial pancreas systems did not reach the stage at which they could be used in routine diabetes management therefore relates to the glucose sensor itself. Indeed, it was only possible to use these systems for perfect control of blood glucose levels in diabetic patients for short periods of time, since the patient needed to be connected to the device (which was the size of a television set); they required access to a blood vein, and pumped approximately 50 ml of blood per day. We can consider that these systems are at the same stage of development towards an artificial internal organ, as are the currently available artificial kidneys. The difference is that the treatment of end-stage renal failure is compatible with discontinuous dialysis sessions, whereas diabetes treatment requires the *continuous* control of blood glucose. Another difference is that clotting of a few fibres of an artificial kidney does not hinder the

function of the whole device. By contrast, even within a few hours of use, the membrane separating blood from glucose-oxidase rapidly becomes fouled with protein and blood cells, so that its exchange properties are altered, and frequent recalibration of the sensor is therefore required.

These obstacles have prompted some investigators such as Shichiri to propose another approach, in which a needle-type glucose sensor would be implanted in subcutaneous tissue [10]. Most of the studies, using the wick technique (cotton threads are implanted in the subcutaneous tissue over one hour, explanted, and glucose determined in the liquid collected from the wick), microdialysis, or ultrafiltration techniques, which have aimed to assay glucose directly in samples of subcutaneous interstitial fluid, have presented evidence [11–13] that the glucose concentration in the interstitial fluid is essentially identical to that in plasma under stationary conditions, as well as during changes in glucose concentration at rates comparable to those commonly observed during meals in diabetic patients. Thus, the control of diabetes in dogs with an artificial B cell sensing glucose in the subcutaneous tissue has also been demonstrated [14].

The sensor developed by Shichiri et al consisted of a platinum wire (the anode) placed inside a steel needle (the cathode). Glucose-oxidase was layered on the tip of the platinum wire melted to form a sphere, and the electrode was covered with polyurethane to make it biocompatible. This team next developed a wearable artificial pancreas system, which was able to normalize blood glucose concentration for a few days in diabetic patients [9]. Ten years after this first publication, however, one must admit that the reliability of glucose sensors has not been demonstrated sufficiently for it to be conceivable that a wearable, if not implantable, artificial pancreas will be commercially available in the near future. This failure has therefore led most investigators to consider that glucose sensors should be considered first as a way to replace the discontinuous monitoring of blood glucose currently achieved by diabetic patients with a continuous measurement, mainly with the aim of developing a hypoglycaemic alarm.

Indeed, this conceptual evolution of the topic, from an 'artificial pancreas', delivering insulin in a regulated way, to a simple *continuous* glucose monitoring system, is not surprising: it has coincided with the recognition of hypoglycaemia as one of the major problems faced by diabetic patients and diabetologists. Indeed, the development of self-monitoring of blood glucose (SMBG), which was made possible by the development of reagent strips, glucose meters and fingerprick systems, is now recognized as a milestone in the history of insulin therapy [15]. However, SMBG suffers from the fact that it is discontinuous, because the number of glucose determinations that the patient is willing to perform is limited by factors such as pain (limited but present), the time required for preparing the material and performing the test, and the simple fact that repeating a procedure is boring. People are sometimes willing to determine their blood glucose level 6 or 7 times a day when they are highly motivated (such as pregnant women), but this is certainly not true for the majority of the patients. A recent study in the USA indicated that only 40% of the patients monitored their blood glucose at least once a day [16]. If blood glucose concentration is determined only twice a day, SMBG will be unable to detect the occurrence of a hypoglycaemic attack, or to solve the problem of nocturnal hypoglycaemia.

The present and future of glucose sensors is described in Chapter 54.

BIO-ARTIFICIAL SYSTEMS

If insulin-dependent diabetes mellitus is due to the destruction of the cells which secrete insulin, the ultimate solution should be the graft of pancreatic tissue. Indeed, these cells have the property of responding rapidly to a glucose challenge, with a response proportional to the glucose concentration of the stimulating medium. There is a glucose sensor in B cells, and the machinery responsible for insulin exocytosis from the cell has a very prompt response time (within 1 min). Moreover, the cells have sensors for other nutrients which normally stimulate insulin secretion (amino acids, free fatty acids, hormones). In addition, unlike implantable pumps, pancreatic B cells have the potential for synthesizing insulin to restore reserves. Finally, the islet volume responsible for secretion of the daily insulin requirement (50 IU) is extremely small: 1 million islets of Langerhans represent a volume smaller than 1 ml. They could therefore be readily implantable.

So far, approximately 6000 insulin dependent diabetic patients have received a pancreatic, vascularized, graft, with a success rate of approximately 70%, and a patient survival rate of 90% at four years. Only a few patients (less than 10) have been successfully transplanted with isolated islets. These numbers are small when compared with those for kidney transplantation, even though insulin dependent diabetes is 10 times more frequent than end-stage renal failure. There are two explanations for the limited number of pancreas and islet transplantations. The first (shared with other organ transplantations) is the poor availability of transplantable tissue, especially for islet transplantation, since with the available techniques it is difficult

to obtain enough islets from one single donor. The second is more specific: as mentioned above, diabetes is not an immediately life-threatening disease, and unlike end-stage renal, cardiac or liver failure, does not justify the life-long use of immunosuppressive drugs. This explains why most of the grafts performed so far have been carried out in patients with diabetes-induced end-stage renal failure, justifying a combined kidney and pancreas transplantation. This strategy has meant that only patients who already have diabetic complications could be treated and has prevented the use of pancreas transplantation for the primary prevention of diabetic complications, which is still its main rationale.

This would only become feasible with islet xenografting (porcine islets, for instance, would represent an unlimited source of tissue), coupled with methods able to prevent islet rejection in the absence of immunosuppression: this is theoretically possible as islets can be rendered less immunogenic before they are transplanted. Three methods are being investigated. Two of these (islet immuno-alteration, and induction of tolerance) are described in Chapter 45. The present chapter describes the promise of a bio-artificial pancreas, in which islets are immuno-isolated in an artificial membrane, leading to the concept of cell immuno-isolation in a *bio-artificial organ*. Indeed, a bio-artificial pancreas represents a machine at the frontier between the two worlds of tissue transplantation and artificial organs, and its development is now considered as a major topic in these two different fields.

Several approaches are possible [17]: (a) vascular devices, in which blood of the host circulates in contact with a membrane (for instance through a semi-permeable hollow fibre) would be very similar to haemodialysers, the 'dialysate' compartment containing the islets being closed; (b) simpler systems, referred to as extravascular systems, include diffusion chambers, micro-encapsulated islets, and islets placed inside a hollow fibre, which may be implanted inside the peritoneal cavity or in the subcutaneous tissue. Whatever the geometry, however, it is important to understand what is really behind this attractive concept:

(1) The system works as a closed-loop insulin delivery system, not only 'correcting' diabetes, but preventing both hyper- and hypo-glycaemia.

(2) Islets of Langerhans can survive in an immuno-isolated state, although they are neither vascularized nor innervated.

(3) The membrane is biostable.

(4) The membrane is biocompatible. If a host reaction occurs, the function of the 'device' remains unaltered.

(5) The system is safe.

(6) It can be produced on an industrial basis, which means that all its parameters, including islets and membrane characteristics, can be defined.

(7) Finally, it can be prepared in a reproducible way and methods are developed for its storage until use.

Vascular Systems

Here the islets are placed outside a hollow fibre through which the recipient's blood circulates. This system would therefore be connected to a vascular shunt [18–22]. On the basis of the kinetic modelling of glucose and insulin transfer through the fibre [23], a system based on convective fluxes across the membrane was devised, and has yielded excellent kinetics *in vitro* [24] and *in vivo* in rats [25] and in dogs [26]. The correction of hyperglycaemia in diabetic rats with this system was demonstrated over a few hours [27]. However, the system awaits improvement in its haemocompatibility to avoid blood clotting inside the fibre.

A major effort in this field was made by the group working with Chick, who used a radically opposite approach. They focused on the haemocompatibility of the system, and reported the successful graft of a vascular device in dogs over several months in the absence of any heparinization of the animals, which only received aspirin [28, 29]. Hyperglycaemia was corrected, but the authors recognize that improvements in the kinetics of insulin release by this device are still required. This system was also used with xenogeneic, bovine islets, although the duration of diabetes correction was shorter [30].

A similar system was proposed by Calafiore et al, who implanted micro-encapsulated islets inside the wall of a dacron-based prosthesis connected to an arterial bypass. Plasma crossed the dacron meshes and perifused the islets, which were immunoprotected by the membrane of the microcapsules, and which released insulin into the bloodstream. This system was investigated in a small number of dogs [31] and in two diabetic patients [32].

It is obvious that the development of these systems is hindered by the need for vascular access and by its thrombotic risk: indefinite prevention of clotting represents a formidable challenge. This may be one reason why the subcutaneous site is the preferred site for glucose sensing (see Chapter 54) and why the intravenous route for insulin delivery by implantable pumps has now been abandoned: all the systems currently implanted infuse insulin into the peritoneal space (see Chapter 42).

Extravascular Systems

Diffusion Chambers

These are no longer investigated in their initial form (two disks of a piece of membrane separated by a ring), because of the severe fibrotic reaction elicited precisely by the disk form of the membranes [33]. More recently, however, a new design has been proposed, in which the membrane consists of a microporous membrane, covered with a second membrane capable of inducing neovascularization [34].

Micro-encapsulated Islets

Most of the studies are derived from the method initially published by Lim and Sun [35] using alginate, which is ionically cross-linked by polylysine to form the immunoprotective membrane. *In vitro* it was possible to demonstrate that, provided the capsule size is small, micro-encapsulated islets do respond to glucose by increasing their insulin release [36], and that the membrane provides immunoprotection to encapsulated insulin-secreting cells against the cytotoxic effect of antibodies present in the serum of newly diagnosed diabetic patients [37]. *In vivo* experiments with micro-encapsulated islets have indicated that they are able to provide long-term correction of hyperglycaemia in toxic, streptozotocin-induced models of diabetes in rats and mice, in BB rats and NOD mice [38–42]. Very recently, micro-encapsulated human islets were implanted in a type 1 diabetic patient, and diabetes was corrected for several months. However, the interest of this study is limited by the fact that this patient was under immunosuppressive therapy for a kidney graft [43]. It is essential to keep in mind that less optimistic results have also been published [44–47; review in 48]. It is universally accepted that fibrosis around implanted microcapsules is often observed, even though the phenomenon is not constant. The chemical nature of the membrane (in particular the respective percentages of mannuronic or glucuronic residues in the alginate used) might be a factor [49, 50], as might the fragile nature of the chemical bonding between alginate and polylysine, or simply the degree of purity of alginate used. The activation of complement [51] and of macrophages to elicit interleukin-1 [52] is a subject of concern, since interleukin-1 is known to induce fibrosis; furthermore it could cross the membrane and kill the islets [53]. This has led other groups to investigate other methods for micro-encapsulation, using non-soluble biomaterials known for their biocompatibility [54–56], or using islet coating with agarose [57] or barium alginate [58]. Globally, these novel methods are based on the use of a single material, which might prove to be more stable than the complex polyelectrolyte formed by alginate and polylysine.

Another point which deserves further investigation is the kinetics of insulin release by these systems *in vivo*. In all these studies, implantation of micro-encapsulated islets was considered to be successful when blood glucose (usually determined in a fasted state) was normalized. It should be pointed out that this can be achieved in rats by implanting a system releasing insulin without any regulation [59]. Such is not the case in diabetic humans, where a peak in insulin is necessary during or even before each meal. The only study which has tried to demonstrate the occurrence, during a glucose load, of an increase in plasma insulin in diabetic rats, in which chronic hyperglycaemia had been corrected by the peritoneal implantation of micro-encapsulated islets, was negative [60].

Finally, a major problem to consider is the size of the implant. It is clear that the volume of implanted material will be strongly dependent on the size of the microcapsules (since the volume of a sphere is proportional to the cube of the radius). It is therefore mandatory to set up methods for reducing the size of the microcapsules [61]. It is also necessary to design methods for recovering the micro-encapsulated islets if necessary from the cavity into which they have been implanted.

Macro-encapsulated Islets

First proposed by Archer [62], this method was successfully applied by Altman with fragments of human insulinoma seeded into pieces of semipermeable tubes, sealed and implanted in the peritoneal cavity of diabetic rats [63]. Less encouraging results were obtained when these fibres were implanted in pigs, where extensive fibrosis around the fibres was observed [64], and in experiments performed in rats by Zekorn [65]. More recently, two different American groups have published the successful effect of macro-encapsulated islets implanted either into the peritoneal cavity [66] or in the subcutaneous tissue of diabetic rats [67]. The implantation into the peritoneal cavity of 250 fibres containing dog islets was able to correct hyperglycaemia in diabetic dogs. Plasma glucose following a meal was not normal but returned to the normal range after two hours. Unfortunately no results concerning plasma insulin were shown [68]. Here also an important matter for consideration is the geometry of the system. What is the optimal geometry compatible with the length (several metres) necessary to accommodate the 500 000 islets required to correct diabetes in man?

Bio-artificial Pancreas: Unresolved Issues

As shown above, there is no doubt that islets can survive in an immuno-isolated state and that some of the systems proposed were able to correct diabetes in animals, although most of the studies only demonstrated the correction of fasting blood glucose with no data on the glycaemic and insulin profiles after a glucose load. Furthermore, most of them were performed in small laboratory animals. The scaling up of these systems remains a major issue, and it is not at all clear that this will not generate new, unexpected problems. For instance, it may be possible for an individual fibre containing islets to correct diabetes in a mouse, but the compact geometry required to form an implantable 10 metre long fibre would yield a device in which the supply of oxygen and nutrients to all the encapsulated islets would be problematic if the system were not richly neovascularized. This leads to the concept of a *bio-artificial organoid*. It will also be necessary to demonstrate the complete safety of the system, particularly its sterility: bacterial, viral and fungal hazards must be eliminated. Special attention will have to be paid to zoonoses in the case of porcine islet utilization. It may be that the bio-artificial concept will lead to an interest in the immuno-isolation of engineered cells, replacing the need for animal islets.

CONCLUSION: ARTIFICIAL PANCREAS, AN ELUSIVE GOAL?

Studies of both the artificial and the bio-artificial pancreas now have a 20-year history. There is no doubt that the recognition of the role of hyperglycaemia in the genesis of diabetic complications on the one hand, and of hypoglycaemia as a major obstacle to the implementation of intensive insulin therapy on the other, highlights the need to develop systems in which insulin would be delivered on a regulated basis. This would also alleviate the burden on patients of having to replace day after day, meal after meal, the complex regulation of insulin secretion normally achieved by pancreatic B cells. In the development of an artificial pancreas, it is clear that the difficulty in developing a biocompatible glucose sensor was largely underestimated, and that the present ambition (providing patients with a continuous glucose monitoring system without giving this system the responsibility of controlling an insulin pump) is much more modest. Nevertheless, a continuous glucose monitoring system may well play a major role in the next few years as a powerful tool for successful implementation of intensive insulin therapy, and its evaluation would pave the way for the development of an artificial B cell. Concerning

response to intravenous glucose infusion and test meal in rats with microencapsulated islets. Diabetologia 1991; 34: 542-54.

61. Lum ZP, Krestow M, Tai IT, Vacek I, Sun AM. Xenografts of rat islets into diabetic mice. An evaluation of new smaller capsules. Transplantation 1992; 53: 1180-83.

62. Archer J, Kaye R, Mutter G. Control of streptozotocin diabetes in Chinese hamsters by cultured mouse islet cells without immunosuppression: a preliminary report. J Surg Res 1980; 28: 77-85.

63. Altman JJ, Houlbert D, Callard P, McMillan P, Solomon BA, Rosen J et al. Long-term plasma glucose normalization in experimental diabetic rats with macroencapsulated implants of benign human insulinomas: Diabetes 1986; 35: 625-33.

64. Icard P, Penfornis F, Gotheil C, Boillot J, Cornec C, Barrat F et al. Tissue reaction to implanted bioartificial pancreas in pigs. Transpl Proc 1990; 22: 724-6.

65. Zekorn T, Siebers U, Filip L, Mauer K, Schmitt U, Bretzel RG et al. Bioartificial pancreas: the use of different hollow fibres as a diffusion chamber. Transpl Proc 1989; 21: 2748-50.

66. Lanza RP, Butler DH, Borland KM, Staruk JE, Faustman DL, Solomon BA et al. Xenotransplantation of canine, bovine, and porcine islets in diabetic rats without immunosuppression. Proc Natl Acad Sci USA 1991; 88: 11100-104.

67. Lacy PE, Hegre OD, Gerasimidi-Vazeou A, Gentile FT, Dionne KE. Maintenance of normoglycemia in diabetic mice by subcutaneous xenografts of encapsulated islets. Science 1991; 254: 1782-4.

68. Lanza RP, Borland KM, Lodge P, Caretta M, Sullivan S, Muller T et al. Treatment of severely diabetic pancreatectomized dogs using a diffusion-based hybrid pancreas. Diabetes 1992; 41: 886-9.

44

Complications of Insulin Therapy

S. Edwin Fineberg and James H. Anderson, Jr.

Department of Medicine, Indiana University School of Medicine, Indianapolis, USA

INTRODUCTION

Insulin Purification and Structure

Immunologic complications of insulin therapy have declined dramatically with the development of highly purified animal source and biosynthetic and semi-synthetic human insulins. Despite advances in purification techniques and biotechnology, insulin must still be administered as a pharmacologic agent, modified to extend activity, and delivered via a non-physiological route. Hypoglycemia and other complications due to the intrinsic activity of insulin as well as those attributable to faulty insulin injection techniques or delivery modes will continue to be seen until more physiologic therapies can be perfected.

Conventionally purified insulin preparations were produced by repeated recrystallization of pancreatic insulin extracts [1]. These insulins were substantially contaminated with non-insulin peptides [2]. Immunologic studies in patients treated with older insulins revealed antibodies to glucagon as well as other pancreatic peptides [3, 4]. With the application of gel and ion exchange chromatography, it became possible to reduce the proinsulin content of animal insulins from 3000 parts/million to less than 3 parts/million [5, 7]. Non-insulin pancreatic peptides are present in trace or undetectable concentrations in currently available highly purified porcine or bovine insulins [3, 6].

Semi-synthetic and biosynthetic human insulins are additionally purified using reversed-phase HPLC [7]. Semi-synthetic human insulin is chemically converted from purified porcine insulin by substitution of alanine

(B30) by threonine [8]. Biosynthetic human insulin is enzymatically derived from either an intact human proinsulin gene inserted in a non-pathogenic strain of *Escherichia coli* or alternatively from shortened synthetic proinsulin produced from genes inserted in yeast [9, 10]. Residual bacterial or yeast proteins from biosynthetic human insulins have not produced detectable antibody responses [11, 12].

This chapter will review immunological and non-immunological complications of insulin therapy (see Table 1). It should be noted that hypoglycemia unrelated to antibodies (see Chapter 60) remains the predominant complication of insulin therapy, followed by lipohypertrophy, and that problems resulting from immunologic reactions occur much less often.

IMMUNOLOGICAL COMPLICATIONS OF THERAPY

The Immunology of Pharmaceutical Insulins

Complications attributable to circulating antibodies and cellular immunity have not been totally averted, even with the *de novo* treatment of patients with human insulin [11]. Further, it is now known that insulin autoimmunity is common prior to the development of type 1 diabetes and very low levels of autoantibodies may be detected by ELISA in normal individuals [12, 13]. A list of potential immunogens found in insulin formulations can be found in Table 2, and factors affecting the immunogenicity of insulin are summarized in Table 3. Animal insulins are more

International Textbook of Diabetes Mellitus, Second Edition. Edited by K.G.M.M. Alberti, P. Zimmet, R.A. DeFronzo, and H. Keen (Honorary)
© 1997 John Wiley & Sons Ltd

Table 1 Complications of insulin therapy

Non-immunological	Immunological
Hypoglycemia	Insulin-related allergy—localized and systemic
Lipohypertrophy	Injection site lipoatrophy
Pseudoallergy (faulty injection technique)	Protamine allergy
Injection site infection	Antibody-related hypoglycemia
Insulin edema	Insulin resistance
DKA associated with CSII	Zinc allergy
	Immune complex-related disorders

DKA = diabetic ketoacidosis

Table 2 Possible immunogens in pharmaceutical insulins

Pancreas-derived	Biosynthetic
Insulin	Insulin
Animal proinsulin	Synthetic or human proinsulin
Non-insulin pancreatic peptide	Yeast or *Escherichia coli* peptides
Protamine	Protamine
Zinc	Zinc
Insulin covalent dimers	Insulin covalent dimers
Insulin degradation products	Insulin degradation products
Preservatives	Preservatives
Plasticizers	Plasticizers

immunogenic than human insulins [6, 11, 14, 15, 16]. Even the most highly purified beef insulin exceeds pork and human insulins in inciting circulating antibodies and in the incidence of insulin injection site lipoatrophy and local allergy [6]. Insulin antibody levels have been shown to be increased in individuals who are positive for HLA DR7, whereas lower levels were seen in those individuals positive for HLA B8, DR3 and C4 AQ0 [16]. There may be a link in immune responsiveness to genes for IgG heavy chains. There seems also to be an age relationship in the development of insulin antibodies, with younger type 1 diabetic patients being more prone to develop an immune response to porcine and human insulins than older patients with type 2 diabetes [17]. Patients previously treated with conventional insulin preparations not only had antibodies to insulin and non-insulin peptides, but also had high levels of antibodies directed against the animal proinsulins [18]. However, clinical trials with human biosynthetic proinsulin have demonstrated that human proinsulin is quite a weak immunogen [19].

It has been suggested that a substantial portion of the immunogenicity may be linked to insulin covalent dimers which form over time in therapeutic insulins [20]. Adverse storage conditions accelerate the formation of covalent insulin dimers [21]. Dimer-directed antibodies can be demonstrated in a high proportion of conventional insulin-treated individuals [22]. Formulations of insulin suspensions have been shown to be significantly more antigenic than soluble preparations

when injected subcutaneously, although lente and protamine insulins are equivalent [14]. There is also some evidence that if soluble insulin is delivered by continuous subcutaneous insulin infusion (CSII), this route may contribute to increased immunogenicity [23]. Intravenous insulin therapy with recrystallized human insulin has been shown to evoke antibody responses in the past [24]. Intraportal insulin delivery using highly concentrated human insulin delivered intraperitoneally also results in antibody formation [25].

Table 3 Factors affecting the development of insulin antibodies

Purity
Species of origin
HLA type
Patient age and/or type of diabetes
Formulation
Storage conditions

There is no question that a significant proportion of individuals treated with protamine insulins develop detectable antiprotamine antibodies [26]. However, such antibodies become a problem only rarely during the rapid reversal of heparin anticoagulation [27]. The presence of such antibodies does not predict protamine-related anaphylaxis [28]. Zinc present in various concentrations in insulin formulations may also precipitate local or systemic immune reactions [29].

Also, it is possible that insulin oxidation products as well as plasticizers in cap material, preservatives or diluents may contribute to insulin immunogenicity or to injection site reactions.

Altered Pharmacokinetics and Antibody-induced Hypoglycemia

There has been a continuing debate as to whether low or moderate anti-insulin antibody levels seen in clinical practice affect insulin pharmacokinetics and insulin dose requirements [30, 31]. When patients are transferred from conventional bovine to highly purified insulins, dose requirements may decrease by up to 14% [30]. Careful monitoring of glucose levels is advisable during the transfer of patients from conventional to highly purified porcine or human insulins [32]. In a study of the relationship of circulating antibodies to insulin dose, it has been shown that moderate doses of insulin (20–40 U/day) result in a predominant IgG1 and IgG2 response, whereas high doses (90–135 U/day) were associated with increased levels of IgG4 [33]. High levels of insulin antibodies result in inhibition of cellular binding of insulin (which may be demonstrated *in vitro*), and they may act as carrier proteins resulting in clearance by the reticuloendothelial system. In addition to causing insulin resistance, antibody binding of insulin may interfere with, or delay the onset of, insulin action following a pre-meal dosage [34, 84]. Such effects have been reported when radiotracer insulin binding in a liquid phase assay is $\geq 10\%$. The presence of insulin antibodies also interferes with the detection of insulin by immunoassay [35]. It is therefore advisable to measure free insulin levels in insulin-treated individuals after bedside precipitation of antibody-bound insulin by polyethylene glycol [36].

Anti-insulin antibodies may also serve as an insulin buffer, as first suggested by Dixon [37]. The reported benefits of such binding are a decrease in the incidence of diabetic ketoacidosis and prolonged insulin activity [37]. However, detrimental effects of such release of insulin are unpredicted hypoglycemia as well as delayed recovery from hypoglycemia and a disturbed time–action profile of insulin formulations and possibly metabolic instability [38]. Insulin antibody-mediated hypoglycemia has been reported in the insulin autoimmune syndrome, most commonly seen in women who are being treated with thioureas for hyperthyroidism [39]. Insulin antibody-related hypoglycemia has also been reported in insulin-treated patients and in patients whose antibodies arise spontaneously [40, 41].

Transplacental Transfer of Insulin Antibodies

Maternal insulin does not cross the placenta unless associated with anti-insulin antibodies. Heding and others have demonstrated that increased insulin levels seen in infants of diabetic mothers are associated with such transfer and that such insulin is present in immune complexes in the infant [42]. It has been proposed that transferred antibodies might increase the need for fetal insulin secretion and might lead to post-natal complications, such as post-partum hyperglycemia secondary to antibody binding or hypoglycemia secondary to islet B cell hypertrophy [42]. Macrosomia may be related to fetal serum insulin levels independent of glucose levels [43]. That other fetal complications of pregnancy in diabetes, such as an increased frequency of spontaneous abortions or perinatal deaths are related to insulin transfer has been suggested but not yet proven.

Insulin Hypersensitivity Reactions, Local Allergy, Pseudoallergic Reactions and Injection Site Infection

Allergic reactions to insulin therapy, which were once seen in up to 55% of patients, now occur in only 2–3% [44]. Most commonly, reactions are localized to insulin injection sites and occur within the first two weeks of therapy. Local injection site pseudoallergic reactions are due to intradermal injections of insulin. Such reactions are associated with marked pain at the site and occur rapidly after injection [45]. Injection sites become reddened within an hour and later become violet in color. Purulent reactions associated with intradermal injections have also been described. This is especially a problem for patients on CSII, in whom catheter-related infections have been reported regularly [46]. The risks of infection are small with ordinary subcutaneous injections [47]. Additionally, local reactions occasionally result from failure to permit isopropyl alcohol to dry properly, resulting in burning symptoms or rarely abscess formation at the injection site [48].

Local reactions due to hypersensitivity usually occur at least seven days after the initiation of therapy. Local reactions include immediate isolated wheal-and-flare reactions which are mediated by IgE antibodies to insulin and result in mast cell discharge [49]. Symptoms usually consist of itching and resolve rapidly within an hour. More commonly, IgG-mediated local reactions are biphasic and include wheal-and-flare reactions followed by a late-phase reaction which peaks at 4–6 hours and lasts for 24 hours. Symptoms of pain and erythema characterize this late phase. Induration at the site of such reaction may last several days. The late portion of a biphasic reaction may be secondary to an Arthus-like reaction in a highly sensitized patient associated with deposition of immune complexes in the affected sites. However, isolated Arthus reactions characterized by localized small vessel injury and neutrophilic infiltrates are rare [50]. Delayed tuberculin-like reactions, consisting of a deep 'hive' which develops after an 8–12 hour period and peaks within 24 hours, are mediated by cellular immunity. These reactions are often painful or pruritic and have well defined borders. Histologically, these reactions are characterized by perivascular cuffing with a mononuclear infiltrate [65]. Such reactions may take several days to resolve. In patients treated *de novo* with purified porcine, mixed beef/pork or human insulins, the incidence of local allergy was found to be 3.9, 12 and 2.4% respectively [44].

Localized skin reactions to insulin tend to remit spontaneously over a period of weeks as therapy is continued. Antihistamines, such as diphenhydramine, are useful in blocking wheal-and-flare reactions and may be used to ease patients' symptoms. Histamine blockers are ineffective in modifying late phase or tuberculin-like reactions. In some individuals, severe local reactions persist longer than 14–30 days. Proper injection technique should be emphasized and observed. Patients should then switch to human insulin if they are not already on this therapy.

If switching insulins is ineffective, then intradermal testing should be carried out to ascertain the least reactive insulin. During intradermal testing, reactivity to zinc sulfate should also be assessed together with a comparison of protamine and protamine-free insulins. Testing consists of the intradermal injection of 0.02 ml at 1:1 dilutions of U100 insulin, human, porcine and bovine insulins in phenol-saline diluent; 0.02 ml of a 700 µg/ml solution of zinc sulfate; 0.02 ml of histamine phosphate (0.1 mg/ml); and diluent alone. Histamine phosphate serves as a positive control and the saline serves as a negative control. Reactions should be observed at 20 minutes, 6 hours and 24 hours. Positive wheal-and-flare reactions should exceed the phenol saline control by 5 mm, 20 minutes after injection. Induration should exceed 1 cm. Patients should then be treated with the least reactive insulin. Zinc sulfate reactivity indicates the possible usefulness of protamine insulins which are low in zinc content. Zinc-free insulins may be available from the insulin manufacturers on a compassionate basis. If the above measures are not successful, then the following should be considered: (a) divide dosage and deliver into multiple sites; (b) use soluble insulin delivered by CSII; (c) add 1 µg of dexamethasone to each unit of insulin delivered (1 mg dexamethasone/1000 unit vial); and (d) add

systemic antihistamines [51, 52]. In addition, two relatively untested approaches have been suggested; cimetidine 300 mg three times a day, or oral insulin plus aspirin in individuals unresponsive to dermal desensitization [53, 54].

Systemic Allergy

Systemic allergy has been seen in less than 0.01% of patients treated with highly purified porcine and human insulins [52, 55]. Most commonly systemic allergy is characterized by cutaneous reactions such as urticaria, generalized rash, pruritus or paresthesias. Cardiorespiratory reactions include angioneurotic edema palpitations, pallor and circulatory collapse. Gastrointestinal manifestations have also been reported and include nausea, vomiting, cramps and diarrhea. Hematologic complications such as hemolytic anemia have also been reported [56].

Anaphylaxis due to insulin must be differentiated from anaphylaxis due to protamine hypersensitivity [57]. In only one case has anaphylaxis occurred in an individual who had interrupted treatment with protamine insulin. Reported mild protamine allergic reactions include flushing, urticaria and angioedema, often accompanied by transient hypotension. However, more prolonged hypotension, cardiac arrest or respiratory obstruction have also been reported. In addition, transient hematologic disorders have been seen. Anaphylaxis from either insulin or protamine is treated with life support measures, epinephrine by injection and possibly steroids in an intensive care setting [58].

Discontinuation of insulin is usually not advisable due to the possibility of future anamnestic reactions, but could be considered in individuals who might be responsive to diet or oral hypoglycemic agents. Desensitization with purified porcine and human insulins is successful in over 94% of individuals [51]. The mechanism of benefit from desensitization is unknown.

Skin Testing

Prior to desensitization, one should perform skin testing to determine the least reactive insulin. Begin with intradermal injections of 0.02 ml of neutral regular human insulin containing 0.001 units and proceeding to 0.01 and 0.1 units. If positive wheal-and-flare reactions are observed, test with porcine insulin in the same manner and then if positive, proceed to bovine insulin. A positive test results in a wheal-and-flare reaction 5 mm greater than negative control. If initial testing is negative, then proceed to test with 1 unit of insulin and if this is also negative, proceed to treat the patient with this insulin. If skin testing is positive, one should proceed to formal desensitization.

Desensitization

Desensitization should be carried out in a hospital setting with a syringe of 1:1000 epinephrine, life support equipment and an intravenous line in place. One should not mask reactions with prior administration of steroids or antihistamines. In medically stable patients in whom therapy ceased less than 24 hours prior to desensitization, administer one-third of the last dose of the same type of therapeutic insulin subcutaneously and increase the dosage by 5 units every 12 hours. If reactions occur, reduce to the previous dosage, otherwise begin therapy with intermediate-acting insulins when satisfactory metabolic control is achieved.

If reactions occur even with the reduction of dosage, if patients are medically unstable, or if the last insulin therapy was less than 24 hours prior to desensitization, proceed to a rapid desensitization protocol [59]. Using sterile saline, make a 1:1 dilution of U100 insulin and then serial 1:10 dilutions of the least reactive soluble U100 insulin down to 0.005 U/ml (50, 5, 0.5, 0.05 and 0.005 U/ml). Then every 20 minutes, beginning with 0.05 U/ml, administer increasing doses of insulin subcutaneously proceeding from 0.02 to 0.04 and 0.08 ml for each dilution. The absolute amounts of insulin injected would be from 0.001 to 4 units in 12 steps until a wheal-and-flare reaction is observed. If such a reaction or induration >1 cm is observed with 0.02 ml of the 0.05 U/ml solution, begin desensitization with 0.005 U/ml. Reduce the injectate by 2 dilution steps if higher concentrations produce a reaction. When patients tolerate the highest desensitization steps, double dose every 4 hours until metabolic stability is achieved. Patients should then be treated for 48–72 hours with injections of short-acting insulin at least every 6 hours, prior to switching to intermediate- or long-acting insulins. Rarely desensitization is not successful in a metabolically unstable individual. Then use of steroid therapy or delivery of soluble insulin by CSII may become necessary. An infrequent accompaniment of desensitization is the initiation of insulin resistance [60].

Insulin Antibody-mediated Resistance

Insulin antibody mediated insulin resistance has been previously estimated to occur in less than 1% of patients. Such resistance has been defined as an insulin requirement of ≥ 2.5 U/kg in adults and > 1.5 U/kg in children. The vast majority of individuals requiring high doses of insulin have insufficient antibody binding to account for increased insulin requirements [61]. Insulin antibody binding is determined in liquid phase

assays in which antibodies are assessed against fixed amounts of radiotracer insulin and varying amounts of non-labelled beef, pork and human insulins. Unlike the cross-reactivity which is usually seen with antibody levels in non-resistant patients, it is not uncommon to observe preferential binding of a heterologous population of antibodies for one species over all others. Predisposing factors for insulin resistance include a history of atopy, interrupted insulin therapy (especially with beef-containing insulins), and desensitization for systemic allergy [62]. In assessing patients for resistance, one should determine whether insulin therapy can be replaced with diet and/or oral hypoglycemic agents. Intercurrent illness, neoplasia, drugs, factitious insulin dosage and other known causes of insulin resistance should be actively sought. Patients on beef-containing insulins should be switched to highly purified porcine or human insulins, which are effective in the reduction of dose requirements in over 40% of individuals. If this measure proves to be ineffective, the institution of 40–80 mg of prednisone a day in a tapering manner over 4–6 weeks should be begun. Steroids have proven to be effective in about 50% of individuals. Steroid therapy must be approached with caution, since in responsive individuals it is not unusual to observe dramatic falls in insulin requirements with subsequent hypoglycemia. Sulfated beef insulin has also proved to be effective in the treatment of insulin resistance. If all of the above fail, the use of U500 porcine or human regular insulin (note, U500 human insulin is now available) administered 2–3 times per day, which in this concentrated form has delayed absorption characteristics and may prove effective in glycemic control and reduction of dose [63]. While antibody-mediated resistance in most patients spontaneously remits, patients have been seen whose resistance persisted for >5 years.

Injection Site Lipoatrophy

In contrast to reports of up to 55% incidence of insulin injection site lipoatrophy with older preparations of bovine insulins, *de novo* treatment with highly purified bovine insulin resulted in a 9% incidence [6]. There are only scattered reports of lipoatrophy with highly purified porcine or human insulins [64]. These hollowed-out areas are characterized by local loss of fat cells and are largely non-inflammatory in histologic appearance. Lipoatrophy occurs more often in individuals with dermal reactions to insulin and in young children. While lesions are usually limited to injection sites, they may also occur distally. In a study of 14 patients with lipoatrophy, Reeves demonstrated that lipoatrophic lesions occurred in individuals with high levels of circulating anti-insulin antibodies [65]. The edges of these lesions were characterized by deposition of immunologic proteins within dermal vessels, most commonly IgM and C3 or fibrin-fibrinogen. Reaccumulation of fat cells occurs over 90% of the time when highly purified porcine or human insulins are repeatedly injected into the affected areas [66, 67]. Once such areas are filled out, occasional injection of insulin is required to maintain normal appearance (see Figure 1). If reaccumulation of fat does not occur, injection of dexamethasone 4 μg/unit added to the insulin injection has been found to be effective in restoration of fat [68].

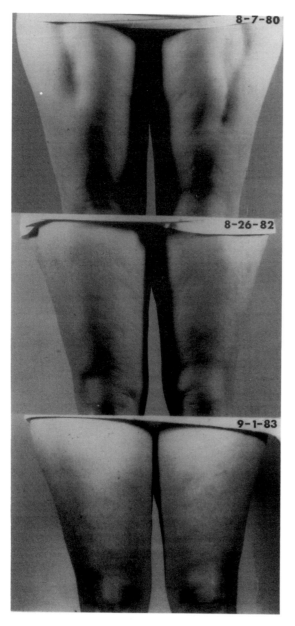

Figure 1 Injection site lipoatrophy (top panel) secondary to injection of beef-containing insulin. Repeated injections of highly purified soluble porcine insulin resulted in reaccumulation of lost fat (middle and lower panels). Photographs by courtesy of JA Galloway MD, Lilly Research Laboratories

Immune Complex-related Disorders in Diabetes—Possible Relationship Between Anti-insulin Antibodies and Diabetic Complications

Microangiopathy in diabetes has a similar histological appearance to lesions in immune complex disorders [69]. Elevated levels of immune complexes have been reported in individuals with advanced microvascular complications. However, there is little evidence to support the idea that insulin antibodies are contained in increased amounts within these complexes. Significant correlations have been found between soluble immune complexes, insulin dosage and evidence of small and large vessel damage [70]. *In vitro*, evidence has been presented that beef insulin–anti-insulin immune complexes are significantly more potent activators of procoagulant activity than pork or human insulin [71]. Thus it is possible, but not proven, that high levels of anti-insulin antibodies may indirectly relate to diabetic vasculopathy.

NON-IMMUNOLOGICAL COMPLICATIONS OF INSULIN THERAPY

Injection Site Lipohypertrophy

Hypertrophy of subcutaneous fat at sites of repeated insulin injections continues to be a common non-immunologic complication of therapy [72]. Hypertrophy of omental fat has also been reported to be a cause of catheter occlusion during the course of intraperitoneal delivery of concentrated insulin by implantable insulin pumps [73]. Such examples of fat cell hypertrophy are likely to result from the natural mitogenic activity of insulin. Pathologically, such fatty tumors are fibrous and have decreased vascularity. Patients often continue to select these injection sites due to their relative anesthesia. Avoidance of these areas is advisable due to their effects upon insulin absorption. Absorption from hypertrophic sites has been shown to be significantly impaired in studies by Young and co-workers utilizing clearance of ^{125}I insulin in 12 insulin-dependent patients [74]. If avoidance of affected sites does not result in regression and removal is desirable, liposuction is advised (see Figure 2) [75].

Insulin Edema

Edema associated with insulin therapy is an unusual and usually self-limited disorder. This is infrequently reported but should be suspected when the institution of insulin therapy is associated with a sudden weight gain over a short period. Although Leifer first reported insulin edema in 1928, the incidence of this condition

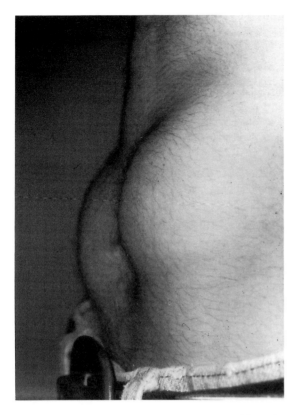

Figure 2 Injection site lipohypertrophy resulting from repeated injections into the same areas. Photograph by courtesy of JA Galloway MD, Lilly Research Laboratories

is unknown [76]. However, 3.5% of 491 patients in a series from Africa developed edema associated with malnutrition and insulin-induced hypoglycemia [77].

This complication of therapy has been most often reported after the initiation of insulin, following a large change in dosage, or following treatment for diabetic ketoacidosis. Perhaps the most dramatic reported results of sodium retention secondary to insulin therapy are congestive cardiac failure or ascites in individuals for whom a cardiac or renal etiology could not be demonstrated [78, 79]. Saudek and co-workers studied fluid retention in 5 individuals with poorly controlled diabetes and one with diabetic ketoacidosis during optimization of insulin therapy [80]. Sodium retention did not correlate with decreases in glycemia or ketonemia and was felt to be attributable in the past to a fall in glucagon levels. Others have proposed that persistent elevation of aldosterone or antidiuretic hormone during refeeding might play a role in the mechanisms of edema [81]. Wheatley and Edwards have demonstrated that there was an increased transcapillary albumin escape in three subjects whose edema followed the institution of excessive insulin [82]. Therapy consists of reduction in dosage. Diuretic therapy is usually not advisable. Recently, oral ephedrine has been used successfully in a patient with recurrent edema secondary to treatment

of poorly controlled diabetes. The mechanism may be correction of hyperaldosteronism [83].

REFERENCES

1. Galloway JA. Current trends in diabetes therapy. In Trends in pharmacological sciences vol 5, Amsterdam: Elsevier, 1984; pp 33-5.
2. Mirsky IA, Kawamura K. Heterogeneity of crystalline insulin. Endocrinology 1966; 78: 1115-19.
3. Fitz-Patrick D, Patel YC. Antibodies to insulin, pancreatic polypeptide, glucagon and somatostatin in insulin-treated diabetics. J Clin Endocrinol Metab 1981; 52: 948-52.
4. Bloom SR, Barnes AJ, Adiran TE, Polak JM. Autoimmunity in diabetes induced by hormonal contaminants of insulin. Lancet 1979: 1: 14-17.
5. Chance RE. Amino acid sequences of proinsulins and intermediates. Diabetes 1972; 21: 462-7.
6. Wilson RM, Douglas CA, Tattersall RB, Reeves WG. Immunogenicity of highly purified bovine insulin: a comparison with conventional bovine and highly purified human insulins. Diabetologia 1985; 28: 667-70.
7. Galloway JA, Chance RE. Human insulin rDNA: from rDNA through the FDA. In Lemberger L, Reidenberg MM (eds) Proceedings of the Second World Conference on Clinical Pharmacology and Therapeutics. Bethesda, MD: American Society for Pharmacology and Experimental Therapeutics 1984; pp 503-20.
8. Markussen J, Damgaard U, Pingel M, Snel L, Sorensen A, Sorensen E. Human insulin (NOVO): chemistry and characteristics. Diabetes Care 1983; 6 (suppl. 1): 4-8.
9. Frank BH, Pettee JM, Zimmerman RE, Burck PJ. The production of human proinsulin and its transformation to human insulin and C-peptide. In Rich DH, Gross R (eds) Peptides, synthesis-structure-function. Proceedings of the Seventh American Peptide Symposium. Rockford, IL: Pierce Cheurreal Co., 1981; pp 729-38.
10. Thim L, Hansen MT, Norris K, Hoegh I, Boel E, Forstom J et al. Secretion and processing of insulin precursors in yeast. Proc Natl Acad Sci USA, 1986; 83: 6766-70.
11. Fineberg SE, Galloway JA, Fineberg NS, Rathbun MJ, Hufferd S. Immunogenicity of recombinant DNA human insulin. Diabetologia 1983; 25: 465-9.
12. Palmer JP, Asplin CM, Clemons P, Lyen K, Tatpati O, Raghu PK, Paquette TL. Science 1983; 222: 1337-9.
13. Fineberg SE, Biegel AA, Durr KL, Hufferd S, Fineberg NS, Anderson JH. Presence of insulin autoantibodies as a regular feature of non-diabetic repertoire of immunity. Diabetes 1991; 40: 1187-93.
14. Fineberg SE, Galloway JA, Fineberg NS, Goldman J. Effects of species of origin, purification levels and formulation on insulin immunogenicity. Diabetes 1983; 32: 592-9.
15. Heding LG, Marshall MO, Persson B, Dahlquist G, Thalme B, Lindgren F et al. Immunogenicity of monocomponent human and porcine insulin in newly diagnosed type I (insulin-dependent) diabetic children. Diabetologia 1984; 27: 96-8.
16. Reeves WG, Barr D, Douglas CA, Gelsthorpe K, Hanning I, Skene A et al. Factors governing the human

immune response to injected insulin. Diabetologia 1984; 26: 266–71.

17. Fineberg NS, Fineberg SE, Galloway J. Does age at initiation of insulin therapy determine who will develop an immune response? Diabetes 1992; 41 (suppl. 1): 191A.

18. Klaff LJ, Vinik AI, Berelowitz M, Jackson WPU. Circulating antibodies in diabetes treated with conventional and purified insulins. S Afr Med J 1979; 54: 149–53.

19. Fineberg SE, Rathbun MJ, Hufferd S, Fineberg NS, Spradlin CT, Galloway JA, Frank BH. Immunologic aspects of human proinsulin therapy. Diabetes 1988; 37: 276–80.

20. Robbins DC, Mead PM. Free covalent aggregates of therapeutic insulins in the blood of insulin-dependent diabetics. Diabetes 1987; 36: 147–51.

21. Maislos M, Mead PM, Gaynor DH, Robbins DC. The source of circulating aggregates of insulin in type 1 diabetic patients is therapeutic insulin. J Clin Invest 1986; 77: 717–23.

22. Robbins DC, Cooper SM, Fineberg E, Mead PM. Antibodies to covalent aggregates of insulin in blood of insulin-using diabetic patients. Diabetes 1987; 36: 838–41.

23. Dahl-Jorgensen K, Torjensen P, Hanssen KF, Sandvik L, Aagenaes O. Increase in insulin antibodies during continuous subcutaneous insulin infusion and multiple-injection therapy in contrast to conventional treatment. Diabetes 1987; 36: 1–5.

24. Deckert T, Anderson OO, Grundahl E, Kerp L. Isoimmunization of man by recrystallized human insulin. Diabetologia 1972; 8: 358–61.

25. Georges LP, O'Brian JT, Davidson PC, Thornton KR, Fineberg SE, Fineberg NS and the MiniMed investigators. Intraperitoneal delivery of U400 insulin is immunogenic. Diabetes 1993; 42 (suppl.): 183A.

26. Kurtz AB, Gray RS, Markanday S, Nabarro JD. Circulating IgG antibody to protamine in patients treated with protamine insulins. Diabetologia 1983; 25: 322–4.

27. Kim R. Anaphylaxis masquerading as an insulin allergy. Delaware Med J 1993; 65: 17–23.

28. Weiler JM, Gellhaus MA, Carter JG, Meng RL, Benson PM, Hottel RA et al. A prospective study of the risk of an immediate adverse reaction to protamine sulfate during cardiopulmonary bypass surgery. J Allergy Clin Immunol 1990; 85: 713–19.

29. Bruni B, Campana M, Gamba S, Grassi G, Blatto A. A generalized allergic reaction to zinc in insulin preparation. Diabetes Care 1985; 8: 201.

30. Walford S, Allison SP, Reeves WG. The effect of insulin antibodies on insulin dose and diabetic control. Diabetologia 1982; 22: 106–10.

31. Haumont D, Dorchy H, Toussaint D, Despontin M. Exogenous insulin needs. Relationship with duration of diabetes, C-peptidemia, insulin antibodies and retinopathy. Helv Pediat Acta 1982; 37: 143–50.

32. Asplin CM, Hartog M, Goldie DJ. Change in insulin dosage, circulating free and bound insulin and insulin antibodies on transferring diabetics from conventional to highly purified porcine insulin. Diabetologia 1978; 14: 99–105.

33. Siddiqui MA, Wangnoo SK. Selective IgG subclass antibody response to insulin in diabetic patients receiving animal insulin replacement therapy. Int Arch Allergy Appl Immunol 1989; 89: 49–53.

34. Van Haeften TW, Bolli G, Dimitriadis GD, Gottesman IS, Horwitz DL, Gerich JE. Effect of insulin antibodies and their kinetic characteristics on plasma free insulin dynamics in patients with diabetes mellitus. Metabolism 1986; 35: 649–56.

35. Hayford JT, Thompson RG. Free and total insulin integrated concentrations in insulin dependent diabetes. Metabolism 1982; 31: 387–97.

36. Rudkowski R, Antony G. The effect of immediate polyethylene glycol precipitation on free insulin measurements in diabetic patients with insulin antibodies. Diabetes 1986; 35: 253–7.

37. Dixon K, Exon PD, Hughes HR. Insulin antibodies in the etiology of labile diabetes. Lancet 1972; 1: 343–7.

38. Bolli GB, Dimitriadis GD, Pehling GB, Baker BA, Haymond MW, Cryer PE, Gerich JE. Abnormal glucose counter-regulation after subcutaneous insulin in insulin-dependent diabetes mellitus. New Engl J Med 1984; 310: 1706–11.

39. Hirata Y, Tominaga M, Ito JI, Noguchi A. Spontaneous hypoglycemia with insulin autoimmunity in Graves' disease. Ann Intern Med 1974; 81: 214–18.

40. Anderson JH, Blackard WG, Goldman J, Rubenstein AH. Diabetes and hypoglycemia due to insulin antibodies. Am J Med 1978; 64: 868–73.

41. Albert SG, Popp DA. Hypoglycemia due to serum complexed insulin in a patient with insulin dependent diabetes mellitus. Diabetes Care 1984; 7: 285–90.

42. Heding LG, Persson B, Stangenberg M. β cell function in newborn infants of diabetic mothers. Diabetologia 1980; 19: 427–32.

43. Menon RK, Cohen RM, Sperling MA, Cutfield WS, Mimouni F, Khoury JC. Transplacental passage of insulin in pregnant women with insulin-dependent diabetes mellitus. Its role in fetal macrosomia. New Engl J Med 1990; 323: 309–15.

44. Galloway JA, Fireman P, Fineberg SE. Complications of insulin therapy: a brief review of four years experience with human insulin (rDNA). In Church J (ed.) Diabetes mellitus: achievements and skepticism. Royal Soc Med Int Congress and Symposium Series, vol 77. Oxford: Oxford University Press, 1984; pp 55–64.

45. Deckert T, Anderson OO, Poulsen JE. The clinical significance of highly purified pig insulin preparations. Diabetologia 1974; 10: 703–8.

46. Pietri A, Raskin P. Cutaneous complications of chronic continuous subcutaneous insulin infusion therapy. Diabetes Care 1981; 4: 624–6.

47. Koivisto VA, Felig P. Is skin preparation necessary before insulin injection? Lancet 1978; 1: 1072–3.

48. Leigh DA, Hough GW. Dangers of storing glass syringes in surgical spirit. Br Med J 1980; 281: 541–2.

49. deShazo RD, Mather P, Grant W, Carrington D, Frentz JM, Lueg M, Lauritano AA, Falholt K. Evaluation of patients with local reactions to insulin with skin tests and *in vitro* techniques. Diabetes Care 1987; 10: 330–6.

50. deShazo RD, Boehm TM, Kumar D, Galloway JA, Dvorak HF. Dermal hypersensitivity reactions to insulin: correlations of three patterns to their histopathology. J Allergy Clin Immunol 1982; 69: 229–37.

51. Galloway JA. Chemistry and clinical use of insulin in diabetes mellitus. In Galloway JA, Potvin JH, Shuman CR (eds) Diabetes mellitus. Indianapolis, IN: Eli Lilly Company, 1988; pp 105–37.

Complications of Insulin Therapy

52. Granic M, Renar IP, Metelko Z, Skrabalo Z. Insulin allergy. Diabetes Care 1986; 9: 99–100.

53. Chideckel EW, Mullin CJ, Michael BE. Cimetidine in insulin allergy. Diabetes Care 1981; 4: 503–4.

54. Holdaway IM, Wilson JD. Cutaneous allergy responsive to oral desensitization and aspirin. Br Med J Clin Res 1984; 289 (6458): 1565–6.

55. Hannauer L, Batson JM. Anaphylactic shock following insulin injection. Diabetes 1961; 10: 105–9.

56. Yamreudeewong W, Cavell RM, Hennan NE. Possible hemolytic anemia associated with human insulin therapy. Drug Intelligence Clin Pharm Ann Pharmacother 1990; 24: 887.

57. Weiler JM, Freiman P, Sharath MD, Metzger WJ, Smith JM, Richerson HB et al. Serious adverse reactions to protamine sulfate: are alternatives needed? Allergy Clin Immunol 1985; 75: 297–303.

58. Soto-Aguillar MC, deShazo RD, Waning NP. Anaphylaxis. Postgrad Med 1987; 82: 154–70.

59. Mattson JR, Patterson R, Roberts M. Insulin therapy in patients with systemic insulin allergy. Arch Intern Med 1975; 135: 818–21.

60. Witters LE, Ottman JL, Weir GC, Raymond LW, Lowell FC. Insulin antibodies in the pathogenesis of insulin allergy and resistance. Am J Med 1977; 63: 703–9.

61. Davidson JK, Fineberg SE, DeMeyts P, Fineberg NS, Galloway JA. Immunological and metabolic responses of patients with a history of antibody-induced beef insulin resistance to treatment with beef, pork, human and sulfated beef insulin. Diabetes Care 1992; 15: 702–4.

62. Davidson JK, DeBra DW. Immunological insulin resistance. Diabetes 1978; 27: 307–18.

63. Nathan DM, Axelrod L, Flier JS, Carr DB. U-500 insulin in the treatment of antibody-mediated insulin resistance. Ann Intern Med 1981; 94: 653–6.

64. Page MD, Bodansky JH. Human insulin and lipoatrophy. Diabetic Med 1992; 9: 779.

65. Reeves WG, Allen BR, Tattersall RB. Insulin-induced lipoatrophy: evidence for an immune pathogenesis. Br Med J 1980; 1: 1500–503.

66. Czyzyk A, Rogala H, Laweki J. Controlled study comparing treatment with monocomponent and conventional insulin in patients with lipoatrophy. Acta Diabetol Lat 1989; 26: 17–26.

67. Valenta LJ, Elias AN. Insulin induced lipodystrophy in diabetic patients resolved by treatment with human insulin. Ann Intern Med 1985; 102: 790–1.

68. Kumar D, Miller L, Mehtalia S. Use of dexamethasone in treatment of insulin lipodystrophy. Diabetes 1977; 26: 296–9.

69. Blumenthal HT, Hirata Y, Owens CT, Berns AW. A histo- and immunological analysis of the small vessel lesion of diabetes in the human and in the rabbit. In Siperstein MD, Wolwell AR, Meyer K (eds). Small blood vessel involvement in diabetes mellitus. Washington D.C.: American Institute of Biological Sciences, 1964: pp 279–87.

70. Iavicoli M, DiMario U, Pozzilli P, Canalese J, Ventriglia L, Galfo C, Andreani D. Impaired phagocytic function and increased immune complexes in diabetics with severe microangiopathy. Diabetes 1982; 31: 7–11.

71. Uchman B, Bang NU, Rathbun MJ, Fineberg NS, Davidson JK, Fineberg SE. Effect of insulin immune complexes in human blood monocyte and endothelial cell procoagulant activity. J Lab Clin Med 1988; 112: 652–9.

72. Galloway JA, Peck Jr FB, Fineberg SE, Spradlin CT, Marsden JH, Allemenos D, Ingulli-Fattic J. The US 'new patient' and 'transfer' studies. Diabetes Care 1982; 5 (suppl. 2): 135–9.

73. Pitt HA, Saudek CD, Zacur HA. Long-term intraperitoneal insulin delivery. Ann Surg 1992; 216: 483–91.

74. Young RJ, Hannan WT, Frier BM, Steel J, Duncan LJP. Diabetic lipohypertrophy delays insulin absorption. Diabetes Care 1984; 7: 479–80.

75. Bodansky HJ, Browning FS. Treatment of insulin lipohypertrophy with liposuction. Diabet Med 1992; 9: 395–6.

76. Leifer A. Case of insulin edema. JAMA 1928; 90: 610–11.

77. Shaper AG. The insulin-oedema syndrome in African diabetic subjects. Trans Roy Soc Trop Med Hyg 1966; 60: 519–25.

78. Sheehan JP, Sisam DA, Schumacher OP. Insulin-induced cardiac failure. Am J Med 1985; 79: 147–8.

79. Bronstein HD, Kantrowitz PA, Schaffner F. Marked enlargement of the liver and transient ascites with treatment of diabetic acidosis. New Engl J Med 1959; 261: 1314–18.

80. Saudek CD, Boulter PR, Knopp RH, Arky RA. Sodium retention accompanying insulin treatment of diabetes mellitus. Diabetes 1974; 23: 240–46.

81. Spark RF, Arky RA, Boulter PR, Saudek CD, O'Brian JT. Aldosterone and glucagon in the natriuresis of fasting. New Engl J Med 1975; 292: 1335–40.

82. Wheatley T, Edwards OM. Insulin oedema and its clinical significance: metabolic studies in three cases. Diabet Med 1985; 2: 400–4.

83. Hopkins DFC, Cotton SJ, Williams G. Effective treatment of insulin-induced edema using ephedrine. Diabetes Care 1993; 16: 1026–8.

84. Francis AJ, Hanning I, Alberti KGMM. The influence of antibody levels on the plasma profiles and action of subcutaneously injected human and bovine short acting insulins. Diabetologia 1985; 28: 330–34.

45

Islet Transplantation

Derek W.R. Gray and Peter J. Morris

John Radcliffe Hospital, Oxford, UK

There is now overwhelming evidence to implicate abnormal glucose control in the genesis of the angiopathic complications of diabetes mellitus [1, 2, 3, 4]. Normal or near-normal glucose homeostasis may slow or even halt the progression of diabetic angiopathy, both in experimental animals and in humans, although it is not known how early in the progression of the disease normal glucose homeostasis must be restored to have this effect.

In type 1 diabetes, insulin therapy, although controlling blood glucose levels to a greater or lesser extent, cannot replace the fine but complex physiological balance of normal islet hormone release which regulates glucose homeostasis. Even when insulin administration is intensive and carefully controlled, by either multiple daily injections or continuous subcutaneous infusion, blood glucose concentrations in patients with diabetes can swing widely outside the normal range [5, 6]. Combinations of hyperglycaemia, ketonaemia, hyperlipidaemia and other metabolic abnormalities occur, varying in intensity and duration, but with cumulative effects [7]. Although many trials of intensive insulin therapy have been undertaken, with largely inconclusive results, recent evidence suggests that even relatively modest improvements in glucose control have a detectable effect on diabetic complications [2]. Finally, the long-awaited results of the DCCT (Diabetes Control and Complications Trial) Research Group conclusively demonstrated that the better the glucose control the lower the incidence and progression of retinopathy, neuropathy and nephropathy [4].

Vascularized whole or segmental pancreas transplantation (see also Chapter 46) has been performed with increasing frequency over the past 25 years, mostly in diabetic patients with end-stage renal failure who require a kidney transplant and thus immunosuppression as well. The results have steadily improved and overall 1-year patient and graft survivals are at present better than 80% and 50% respectively [8] and may be as high as 90% and 80% respectively in some centres (H. Sollinger, personal communication); but there is still an appreciable morbidity [9] and patients given a pancreas transplant require more immunosuppression, have more complications and stay in hospital twice as long as patients given a kidney transplant alone [9]. Successful vascularized pancreas transplantation can restore normal metabolism [10–12]. However, the overall proportion of patients undergoing pancreas transplantation who maintain normal metabolic profiles is small, since many patients considered to have functioning pancreas allografts (in terms of not requiring insulin therapy) nevertheless demonstrate glucose intolerance, probably due in part to the effect of immunosuppressive drugs [13].

Vascularized pancreas transplantation is felt by most clinicians to be justifiable only in patients who have reached end-stage renal failure and require a renal transplant with appropriate immunosuppression. At this stage of the disease, most patients also have advanced retinopathy, neuropathy and vascular disease and it has scarcely been surprising that these changes have been found to be irreversible after pancreas transplantation. Rather more disappointing has been the lack of

International Textbook of Diabetes Mellitus, Second Edition. Edited by K.G.M.M. Alberti, P. Zimmet, R.A. DeFronzo, and H. Keen (Honorary)
© 1997 John Wiley & Sons Ltd

demonstrable effect on progression of complications such as retinopathy [14], although evidence is now accumulating that there is a beneficial effect on neuropathy, and possibly retinopathy, over a prolonged period [15, 16, 17].

Isolated pancreatic islet transplantation has a number of actual and theoretical advantages over vascularized pancreatic grafts: transplantation of a small volume of pure islet tissue is likely to be a relatively minor procedure with no exocrine complications: pretreatment might allow reduction of the immunogenicity of the islets; and storage by cryopreservation could permit optimal matching of donor and recipient, as well as transplantation of islets from more than one donor into single recipients. Fetal pancreas transplantation presents similar advantages, but also provides a graft in which B-cell replication can occur; however, the use of fetal tissue is associated with major ethical difficulties.

DEVELOPMENT OF ADULT ISLET ISOLATION AND TRANSPLANTATION TECHNIQUES

Early Techniques

Soon after the description of mouse pancreatic islet isolation by microdissection [18], Lacy and colleagues described a technique for rat islet isolation in which the pancreas was distended with a saline solution, minced, then exposed to collagenase and allowed to digest before separation of the islets from the dispersed tissue using a Ficoll density gradient [19, 20]. Transplantation of 600–800 islets from four to eight donors into the peritoneal cavity of syngeneic streptozotocin-induced diabetic recipients resulted in a reduction of urine glucose, and in a decrease of blood glucose levels to below 14 mmol/l (250 mg/dl) [20]. More uniform success was achieved by transplantation of islets into either the portal vein or splenic pulp than at other sites; there was also a suggestion that smaller numbers of islets could be transplanted successfully into sites with portal venous drainage than elsewhere, and still ameliorate the diabetic state [21, 22, 23, 24, 25].

Attempts were made to apply Lacy and Kostianovsky's technique to large animal pancreases such as those from the pig [26], monkey [27] and dog [28]. Despite claims of success, there was little convincing evidence of graft function [29]. These failures led to abandonment of any attempt at islet purification. Preparations of dispersed pancreas were used instead, not only in animal experiments, but also in clinical trials. Clinical trials of both autotransplantation and allotransplantation were attempted and success was claimed [30,

31, 32, 33], but there was little proof that these grafts functioned sufficiently to allow insulin independence. Additionally, the complications of portal venous hypertension and disseminated intravascular coagulation [34, 35] rendered dispersed pancreas transplantation unacceptable, despite the use of anticoagulation and enzyme inhibition (although one group has recently returned to this technique [36]).

Ductal Collagenase Injection Techniques

In 1981 Horaguchi and Merrell described a technique for the isolation of islets from the dog pancreas in which the excised pancreas was perfused retrogradely through the pancreatic duct with prewarmed collagenase at 37°C [37]. The gland was subsequently dispersed by chopping the attached portions of connective tissue and vasculature, then shaking the tissue in Hank's solution. Some purification of the tissue occurred during this process, apparently due to a proportion of the exocrine fragments undergoing disintegration. The volume of the preparation was small enough to be infused retrogradely into a branch of the splenic vein; normal or near-normal blood glucose levels were observed in dogs that underwent total pancreatectomy and subsequent intrasplenic transplantation of this partially purified islet preparation [37, 38]. Noel, Mintz and colleagues subsequently described the addition of a Ficoll density gradient to purify further the dispersed tissue obtained by a similar intraductal collagenase injection technique [39].

The improved results obtained by retrograde injection of collagenase solutions into the ducts of canine pancreases led to the development in our own laboratories of a method for isolation of human islets by intraductal collagenase injection [40]. In this technique a prewarmed collagenase solution was injected intraductally to distend the pancreas, then the gland was incubated for 25 min in a sterile beaker within a water bath at 39°C, after which the tissue was rapidly cooled and dispersed by teasing with forceps, in combination with rapid agitation. The islets were finally purified using a discontinuous density gradient technique (Figures 1 and 2). This technique was modified by Ricordi and colleagues [41], who placed the gland within a sealed chamber during the incubation phase, with a constant circulation of warm fluid to maintain temperature and constant agitation to encourage dispersion. Particles which separated from the digesting pancreas were kept in the chamber by a mesh screen of pore size 300 μm. Particles smaller than this could leave the chamber and were washed and salvaged. The advantage of this system was that the digestion time was controlled automatically, and the system has been widely adapted, with modifications [42], and used for isolation of islets from a number of species including the pig [43].

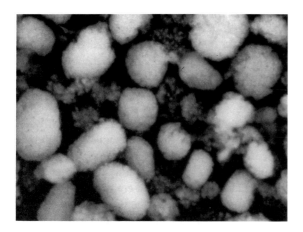

Figure 1 Isolated human islets obtained by ductal collagenase injection and subsequent purification on a Ficoll density gradient, stained with the supravital dye dithizone, which is islet specific (×40)

The dispersed pancreatic tissue produced from human pancreas by techniques such as intraductal digestion contains cleaved islets within a vast excess of exocrine particles, and the purification of the islet tissue presents a problem of considerable magnitude. The discontinuous Ficoll gradients originally introduced for purification of rodent islets have been applied successfully to human islet isolation [40], although the purification obtained was often very variable. Over the last 20 years many different approaches to islet purification have been investigated experimentally, including the use of a variety of alternative density media [44, 45, 46], separation by immunomagnetic beads [47], fluorescence-activated sorting [48], freezing [49] and culture techniques [50, 51]. The density gradient approach remains the most practical for dealing with the volume of tissue generated by digestion of human pancreas, and recent developments have concentrated on approaches for maximizing the differences in density between islet and exocrine tissue whilst maintaining islet viability using cold storage solutions originally designed for whole organ preservation [52, 53]. A commonly used density medium for human islet isolation combines Ficoll with EuroCollins organ perfusion solution to produce 'EuroFicoll' [54]. Other developments have concerned the practicalities of dealing with the large quantities of tissue generated by digestion of the human pancreas. Notable advances include the introduction of a centrifuge machine that allows large scale centrifugation of the digest from a whole pancreas as

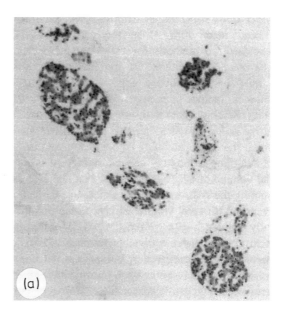

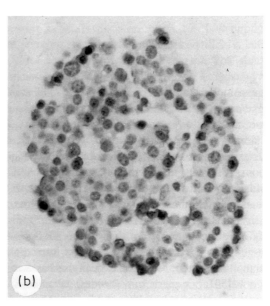

Figure 2 Isolated human islets obtained as in Figure 1: (a) stained with a two-layer immunoperoxidase technique for insulin (×50); (b) as (a), but stained for glucagon (×200)

a single manoeuvre [55], and also equipment for the production of continuous density gradients [53].

Techniques for Assessment of Islet Yield and Viability

The methods for islet isolation described above are in use, often with considerable modification, in a large number of laboratories throughout the world. Many centres are investigating ways to improve the yield of islets obtainable, with detailed research into the variables that affect collagenase digestion and density gradient separation. Comparison of the yield, purity and

year [72]. We have recently attempted to repeat these experiments in another rat isograft model using transplants of up to 3000 islets to both the kidney capsule and intraportal sites, and showed that normoglycaemia was maintained for over 18 months (indeed, for the lifespan of the particular breed of rat). Our findings were that normoglycaemia was maintained with transplants to both sites, IVGTT was almost normal and was maintained without graft failure (Leow et al, unpublished). The development of diabetic renal changes, notably glomerular basement membrane thickening, was prevented. The differing results may reflect a strain-specific phenomenon or possibly be related to the initial 'quality' of the islet transplants.

Metabolic Function of Canine Islet Transplants

Merrell and colleagues investigated the metabolic function of dogs given partially purified islet autografts transplanted by retrograde infusion into a branch of the splenic vein following total pancreatectomy [73, 74, 75]. These experiments showed that such islet grafts could maintain normal fasting glucose levels for over 2 years, but the K value during IVGTT was significantly lower than normal. Similar results have been obtained in dogs by both intrasplenic and intraportal autotransplantation of islets purified on Ficoll density gradients [76]. Of particular concern is the observation of Alejandro and colleagues that only three out of 15 dogs that received intraportal islet autografts sustained normal plasma glucose levels for more than 15 months after transplantation [76, 77]. Similar findings have been reported by other groups, although it is claimed that the graft failure is less common when the intrasplenic transplantation site is used.

Metabolic Function of Simian Islet Transplants

Following autotransplantation of islets in totally pancreatectomized cynomolgus monkeys we were able to show good early survival with normoglycaemia and islet tissue detectable on histological examination of the transplant site (Figure 4). In long-term metabolic studies of intraportal and intrasplenic islet autografts in cynomolgus macaques we also demonstrated a high rate of late autograft failure, with grafts failing between 3 months and 3 years after transplantation [78, 79]. Examination of a variety of parameters that might have influenced the survival of these autografts demonstrated that the only clear correlate with long-term function was B-cell function at 6 weeks (Figures 5 and 6) suggesting that the size of the functioning engrafted islet mass was important. The animals that maintained nearly normal glucose homeostasis for 3 years demonstrated

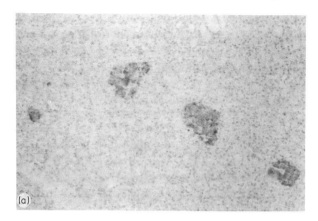

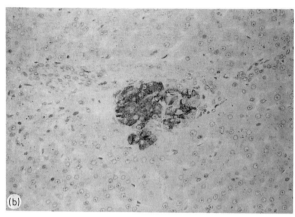

Figure 4 Paraffin sections of typical autografted cynomolgus islet tissue: (a) autografted into the spleen, stained for insulin (×95); (b) autografted into the liver via the portal vein, stained for insulin (×95)

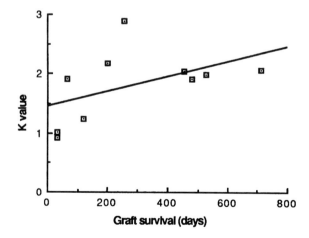

Figure 5 Correlation of graft survival and rate of fall in plasma glucose (K value, %/min) during 500 mg/kg intravenous glucose tolerance tests 6 weeks after intraportal islet autotransplantation ($n = 9$) in cynomolgus macaques

the greatest increase in insulin secretion following a glucose challenge at 6 weeks. The survival of islet grafts implanted in the spleen was no better than that of intraportal islet grafts, and subsequent studies of highly

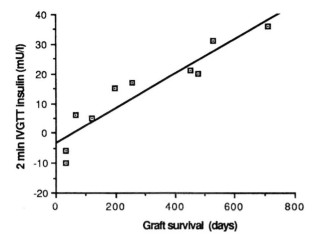

Figure 6 Correlation of graft survival and increase over basal fasting levels in plasma insulin 2 minutes after glucose injection during 500 mg/kg intravenous glucose tolerance tests 6 weeks after intraportal islet autotransplantation ($n = 9$) in cynomolgus macaques

purified islet transplants also showed graft failure after a few months, despite showing apparently better function than semi-purified grafts at 6 weeks. More recently it has been possible to achieve insulin independence with an islet autograft to the kidney capsule site in one animal [80], but this graft also failed after a few months, suggesting that the site probably plays little role in the failure of grafts in this model. Interestingly, histological examination of the graft revealed infiltration with chronic inflammatory cells, including lymphocytes, in this site.

Conclusions on the Long-term Metabolic Function of Islet Grafts

Our current knowledge on the long-term function of islet grafts remains unsatisfactory and incomplete. Models of islet autotransplantation in large animal models all point to graft failure after months or even 3 years, the cause of which is obscure. Whether it is related to inadequate graft mass and B-cell exhaustion, deleterious factors in particular transplant sites (for example the intraportal site) or an autoimmune response to islet autografts is uncertain. In rat models there are conflicting reports of short-term failure of islet autografts, with progression of diabetic renal changes, whilst we have found that long-term (life-long) maintenance of graft function is possible in at least one strain of rats and that glomerular basement membrane thickening is prevented if the blood glucose remains normal. In humans there are few long-term data, but one patient with an islet allograft that has functioned over 2 years, who achieved insulin independence at 2 months, with an acceptable but not normal IVGTT [81], is now showing signs of graft failure

(G. Warnock, personal communication). In contrast, there are claims of function of human islet autografts (performed after total pancreatectomy for pancreatitis) for up to 7 years [82].

REJECTION OF ALLOGENEIC ADULT ISLET TRANSPLANTS

The rejection of islet allografts has been most extensively studied in the rat and the mouse, and has been found to bear similarities to the rejection of vascularized organs and other tissue allografts in these species. Islet allograft rejection, in the absence of sensitization of the recipient, takes several days to develop, occurring less rapidly in sites such as the kidney capsule, perhaps due to reduced lymphatic drainage. Thus rat islets transplanted across a major histocompatibility barrier without treatment usually demonstrate function for 3–5 days after intraportal or intrasplenic grafting [25, 83] and for 7–8 days after renal subcapsular grafting [69, 83]. Other similarities between the rejection of islets and other tissues include second-set phenomena characteristic of immunological memory [84, 85] and T-cell dependency [86, 87].

The rejection of islets may be delayed by the use of immunosuppressive agents, but in general it has proved more difficult to suppress the rejection of islets than of vascularized organ allografts, including the pancreas [88]. Many different immunosuppressive agents, combinations and varied regimens have been investigated [29]. Some general conclusions can be drawn; most immunosuppressive agents require higher dosages to prevent islet rejection than rejection of vascularized organs, and tolerance to the islet allograft is rarely produced. This is especially true of cyclosporine use in rodents [89], and high plasma levels of cyclosporine must be achieved in dogs to prevent allograft rejection [90]. Recently introduced agents such as FK506 [91], mycophenolate [92] and deoxyspergualin [93] may be more effective for prevention of islet allograft rejection than previously available agents, but again the impression is that larger doses are required to prevent islet rejection than rejection of vascularized organs.

One of the fascinating aspects of islet transplantation research has been the way in which the technique lends itself to investigation of the rejection response. Thus islet transplantation experiments have been instrumental in the development of many of the central concepts in transplantation immunology. Early experiments showed that the rejection response was modified by culture of islets in a high oxygen environment [94], and since then a large number of experiments have been performed pretreating islets in various ways to reduce rejection by removal

Table 1 Effect of various islet pretreatments *in vitro* on islet allograft and xenograft survival in diabetic mice and rats. Diabetes was induced with at least 150 mg/kg (mouse) or 50 mg/kg (rat) streptozotocin; islets were transplanted across MHC or species barriers. Mean or median graft survival is indicated; rejection was taken to have occurred when serum glucose levels exceeded 14 mmol/l (250 mg/dl)

Authors	Donor	Recipient	Treatment	Survival (days)
		Mouse		
Yasunami et al, 1983 [95]	Rat	BALB/c	7 days culture at 37°C	46
Ricordi et al, 1987 [96]	Human	C57BL/6J	7 days culture at 24°C	40
Faustman et al, 1981 [97]	B10BR/6J	C57BL/6J	Anti-Ia + complement	>100
Morrow et al, 1983 [98]	B10.A	B10.G	Anti-Ia + complement	>100
Gores et al, 1986 [99]	B10BR	C57BL/6	Anti-Ia + complement	24
Faustman et al, 1984 [100]	B10BR/SJ	C57BL/6J	Anti dendritic cell + complement	>100
Hardy et al, 1984 [101]	Rat	B10BR	900 J/m^2 UV radiation	>100
O'Shea & Sun, 1986 [102]	Rat	BALB/c	Microencapsulation in poly-l-lysine membranes	80
		Rat		
Tucker et al, 1983 [103]	Wistar-Furth	Lewis	7–10 days culture in 95% O$_2$/5% CO$_2$ at 37°C	>100
Reece-Smith et al, 1983 [104]	Lewis	DA	Anti-Ia + complement	9
Tze & Tai, 1986 [105]	Lewis	ACI	Single islet cells in anti-Ia + complement	>100
Hardy et al, 1984 [101]	Lewis	ACI	900 J/m^2 UV radiation	>100
Sun et al, 1984 [106]	Outbred Wistar	Outbred Wistar	Microencapsulation in poly-l-lysine membranes	>100

of passenger leukocytes (Table 1) [95–106]. Some sites used for islet implantation have been found to provide protection against allograft rejection, and are compatible with the concept of privileged sites where the tissue appears to avoid detection by the immune system. Such sites include the anterior chamber of the eye [107], the cerebral ventricles [105] and the intra-abdominal testis [108]. Particularly interesting was the use of the intrathymic site, in conjunction with anti-lymphocyte serum (ALS) treatment, to produce tolerance to islet allografts [109], which has been shown to be based on clonal deletion of T cells [110]. A novel approach to prevention of rejection, first used for islets, is the concept of enclosing the tissue in a semi-permeable membrane with a pore size small enough to prevent ingress of immune cells and antibody but large enough to allow egress of nutrients and insulin. The potential for transplantation of allogeneic or even xenogeneic islets without immunosuppression is obvious. Early experiments along these lines experienced limited success, but recently two approaches, namely microencapsulation of the individual islets [106] and vascularized devices connected to the circulation [111] have been shown to function not only in rodent models but for prolonged periods in the dog model. There is intense commercial interest in the development of these devices, but it remains to be seen whether the problems of the fibrotic response to implanted tissue and poor long-term function of isolated islets can be overcome (see Chapter 43).

CLINICAL TRIALS OF ADULT HUMAN ISLET TRANSPLANTATION

Early Trials

By 30 June 1983, 159 islet tissue allografts had been reported to the International Pancreas Transplant Registry, but none of the patients had achieved insulin independence that could be attributed to the grafts [112]. The graft preparation techniques, transplantation sites and immunosuppressive protocols were highly varied, but did not include documented transplantation of purified adult islets. Techniques used in these early trials included one originally developed for the rat pancreas [30], which it is now generally agreed does not work for human pancreas, and dispersed pancreas transplantation without purification, which was definitely dangerous, resulting in portal hypertension and death [35].

Recent Trials

The application of intraductal collagenase digestion to the human pancreas [40] gave fresh impetus, and further attempts at human islet transplantation during the 1980s, although not successful in terms of achieving insulin independence, at least documented lack of toxicity and demonstrated for the first time unequivocal, repeatable C-peptide production [63].

The major advance came with the use of islet tissue combined from several donors. First short-term insulin independence [61], then long-term function were obtained [81]. The latter achievement was obtained using islets obtained from five donors (four of the islet preparations being cryopreserved), and one patient has remained free of insulin requirement for over 2 years [81], providing great encouragement to others working in the field and demonstrating the potential of islet transplantation. However, it is generally agreed that the use of islets from multiple human donors, whilst of great academic interest, is not of practical value for the routine treatment of type 1 diabetic patients. Admittedly, were it possible to obtain insulin independence using islets obtained from a single donor this would still not provide a practical solution for the routine treatment of the large numbers of diabetic patients needing it, particularly if the treatment were to be extended to those with type 2 diabetes. However, there would be enough donors to treat selected groups, such as those diabetic patients developing renal failure and requiring kidney transplantation. Since these patients already require immunosuppression for the kidney graft, all recent attempts at adult islet allotransplantation have been in this group. Several groups have been attempting single donor transplantation of purified islets, but have failed to obtain sufficient function to withdraw insulin. However, some progress has been made, with short-term insulin independence recently described following single-donor islet transplantation by the Milan group [113]. One of our own patients had a dramatic reduction in insulin requirements after transplantation of islets from a single donor, with maintenance of normal C-peptide levels for over 9 months, but did not become insulin independent.

Parallel to the attempts at human islet allotransplantation, a small number of patients undergoing total pancreatectomy for a variety of reasons have been given islet autografts, following digestion of the pancreas by the intraductal technique, often with very little purification. As mentioned above, in early trials it was autotransplantation of unpurified dispersed pancreas which produced cases of portal hypertension and death [35]. However, the difference in these more recent cases is probably the use of the intraductal digestion technique, which does result in smaller fragments of pancreas and probably a considerable degree of purification as well. It is interesting to note that documented histological and functional evidence of survival of these grafts has been obtained, and at least one graft has continued

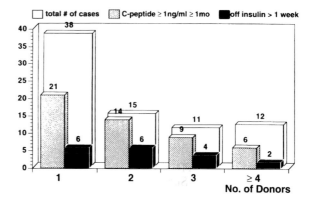

Figure 7 Results of human islet transplantation (1990–1992): Insulin independence and basal C-peptide according to number of donors. Data from the Islet Transplant Registry

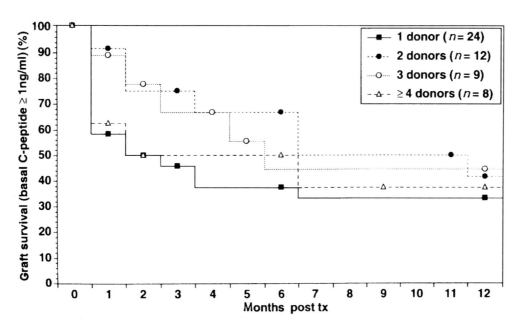

Figure 8 Results of human islet transplantation (1990–1992): One-year islet allograft survival according to the number of donors. Data from the Islet Transplant Registry

functioning for at least 7 years after total pancreatec-tomy, in contrast to the results of autotransplantation in monkeys [82]. These results have encouraged the same group to undertake a series of allografts of dispersed unpurified pancreatic tissue, again prepared using intra-ductal digestion, and so far insulin independence has been obtained in one case [36]. It remains to be seen if this technique can be performed safely; the prece-dent with this approach is not encouraging. The most recent results of islet transplantation are now collated by Drs Hering, Bretzel and Federlin as an Islet Trans-plant Registry run from Giessen, Germany. Figures 7 and 8 are drawn from data released by this registry.

ADULT ISLET XENOTRANSPLANTATION

The limited success of islet allotransplantation, usually requiring multiple donors, has been encouraging but has also highlighted the fact that this approach will not be practical for treating the large numbers of diabetic patients who could potentially benefit, because relatively few suitable human donor pancreases become available. The option of using non-human species as donors for pancreatic islet transplantation has the potential for solving the problem of obtaining sufficient tissue, but raises a further barrier, namely the xenograft rejection response. The barrier between species as regards xenotransplantation of vascularized grafts is described as either concordant or discordant. Concordant species are usually closely related and the graft is generally rejected by cellular mechanisms in a few days. Discordant species combinations are usually distantly related and vascularized xenografts are rejected within minutes, by antibody- and/or complement-mediated mechanisms which activate the clotting cascade and thrombose the organ. The use of concordant species such as non-human primates for human transplantation is likely to be both ethically and practically impossible. The most obvious practical species for human xenotransplantation is the pig, which is definitely discordant for vascularized xenografts into man. However, the situation regarding xenografts of islets is less certain. It is known that transplanted islets are not primarily vascularized and are therefore not susceptible to problems of thrombosis; indeed some models of islet transplantation have deliberately used a blood clot as a vehicle for transplantation [114]. A remarkable number of studies of islet xenotransplantation have been performed in rodent models, and have suggested that cellular rejection in these models is relatively easy to overcome [see 112 for review]. Unfortunately, rodents do not usually reject even vascularized xenografts in an immediate fashion, and are probably of limited value for prediction of the outcome of islet grafts in humans. A very

few studies have attempted xenotransplantation of islets into large animals, but the fate of xenogeneic islets transplanted into untreated recipients in a strain combination relevant to man, such as pig to non-human primate, has not been documented. Therefore, for some time it has remained an open question whether isolated islets of Langerhans, which are not primarily vascularized grafts, were susceptible to damage by hyperacute rejection. We showed that the targets for natural antibody in human serum were the same on both pig and rabbit tissue [115], and since rabbits are considerably easier to work with as laboratory animals, we chose to develop a technique for rabbit islet isolation [116] and subsequent xenotransplantation. As a substitute for human recipients we used cynomolgus monkeys, which are known to have natural antibodies against the same targets as the antibodies in human serum, including gal-a-1-3-gal. We showed that freshly isolated rabbit islets transplanted into untreated cynomolgus monkey recipients undergo extensive destruction within 6 hours with histological features typical of hyperacute rejection of vascularized organs, namely binding of natural antibody, infiltration by neutrophils and cell lysis [115]. We confirmed similar findings for a limited series of experiments transplanting pig islets instead of rabbit islets.

Further studies are now in progress, and it remains to be seen whether the antibody–complement barrier in man is likely to be as formidable for isolated islets as for vascularized organ xenografts.

RECURRENT AUTOIMMUNE DISEASE IN ISLET TRANSPLANTS

Recurrent Autoimmune Diabetes Mellitus in the Rodent

Two useful models of autoimmune diabetes have been developed by inbreeding in the rodent. The Bio-Breeding Laboratories (BB) rat and the non-obese dia-betic (NOD) mouse both develop diabetes mellitus with an autoimmune aetiology and with metabolic seque-lae similar to those of human type 1 diabetes mellitus. Both animals show features of B-cell destruction by autoimmune attack. Most of the studies of islet trans-plantation in spontaneously diabetic animals have been carried out in these two models. Islet transplantation carried out into these models results in temporary cure of diabetes, but then destruction of the graft results in hyperglycaemia. However, the problem is how to distinguish between graft rejection and recurrence of disease. The approach taken has generally been to make the recipients tolerant to the graft, either by inducing neonatal tolerance or by culturing the graft in such a way that rejection is inhibited by loss of passenger leukocytes. Using such models it should be possible to ascertain not only whether the disease recurs, but also whether there is MHC restriction of the disease process. The results show that disease recurrence does occur in both models, but unfortunately there are conflicting results suggesting that the disease recurrence either is [117, 118] or is not [119, 120, 121, 122] MHC-restricted. The differences may lie in the different protocols used and differing interpretation of the results. Possibly the latter view now prevails. The question is relevant to human transplantation, since if MHC restriction of the disease process were to be proved in humans, then MHC-mismatched grafts would be logical to prevent recurrence of disease (although the problem of rejection would remain).

Recurrent Autoimmune Diabetes Mellitus in Humans

Recurrent insulitis and B-cell destruction have been observed in segmental pancreas grafts from non-diabetic to type 1 diabetic identical twins [123]. This recurrent immune destruction, and subsequent return of diabetes mellitus, was prevented by the administration of an immunosuppressive protocol similar to that given to patients undergoing pancreas or kidney allografting [123]. The immunosuppressive protocols used after organ transplantation may well prevent the recurrence of significant B-cell autoimmunity, although recurrent autoimmune disease has been shown to damage both human kidney and liver allografts despite immunosuppression. However, if islet transplantation is attempted using reduced recipient immunosuppression, recurrent autoimmune disease may become a more significant problem, and strategies for overcoming both rejection and disease recurrence, such as intrathymic transplantation [109], may be necessary. It should be noted that these experiences do not shed any light on the question of MHC restriction of disease recurrence: it will be necessary to perform MHC-incompatible grafts into tolerant recipients before this can be settled, and this is not possible at present.

FETAL AND NEONATAL PANCREAS TRANSPLANTATION

The inherent capacity of fetal tissues to grow and develop may have applications in transplantation: in addition, the notion that fetal tissue might somehow be less prone to allograft rejection originally provided further impetus to this field of research [124, 125]. Although the first attempts at fetal pancreas transplantation in 1960 failed to reverse experimental diabetes consistently, exocrine atrophy was noted in sections taken from surviving fetal pancreas transplants [107].

Isografts of Fetal and Neonatal Pancreas

By 1973 amelioration of streptozotocin-induced diabetes had been obtained by transplantation of syngeneic fetal rat pancreas beneath the renal capsule [126]. Brown and colleagues went on to show that six syngeneic 17-day-old fetal rat pancreases transplanted beneath the renal capsule of streptozotocin-induced diabetic rats could restore both normal plasma glucose levels and normal plasma glucose profiles during IVGTT [127]. Subsequent experiments demonstrated that the fetal pancreas is not able to secrete insulin effectively in response to appropriate stimuli until it has undergone a period of maturation, and that this maturation is most likely to occur in an environment with normal or near-normal glucose concentrations [128, 129, 130, 131].

In initial experiments using neonatal pancreas to reverse diabetes, large numbers of collagenase-dispersed neonatal rat pancreases were transplanted into muscle or into the peritoneal cavity of rat recipients [132, 133]. Mauer and colleagues transplanted up to 25 syngeneic collagenase-dispersed neonatal rat pancreases into the peritoneal cavity to reverse the streptozotocin-induced diabetes, and even this did not entirely prevent the development of glomerular basement membrane thickening [132, 134]. Matas and colleagues subsequently dispersed the fetal pancreas with collagenase and used the portal vein site, reducing the number of pancreases needed to reverse diabetes to four [134]. Using this technique, fetal pancreas transplantation was subsequently shown to reverse mesangial thickening in streptozotocin-diabetic rats examined 7 months or more after transplantation [135].

Allografts of Fetal and Neonatal Pancreas

The notion that fetal pancreas allografts might be less prone to immunological rejection was refuted in a series of experiments carried out in our laboratories, where the complete destruction of fetal rat pancreas was demonstrated within 14 days of transplantation across a major histocompatibility barrier, despite insulin treatment of the recipients [136]. Lafferty described a beneficial effect of organ culture on the rejection of adult mouse thyroid allografts [137], an effect also observed on the rejection of isolated adult islets [138]. However, we could not find any significant effect of organ culture on the speed of fetal pancreas rejection [131]. Studies of immunosuppressive protocols previously shown to prevent the rejection of vascularized organ grafts in rodents proved relatively ineffective in preventing rejection of fetal pancreas. Protocols tested included passive enhancement [139] and active enhancement [140]. More complex approaches such as total lymphoid irradiation combined with bone marrow transplantation were more successful, but the radiation toxicity was considerable [141].

Another approach has been to disperse the fetal or neonatal tissue (usually with collagenase) and culture the tissue to form clusters of cells which are rich in islet tissue and have been termed fetal 'pro-islets' or 'islet-like cell clusters' (ICC). Culture in high oxygen concentration was reported to prevent rejection after allotransplantation in mice [142], although the effect was subsequently found to be strain dependent [143]. However, attempts to develop a large animal model in the mini-pig have not been consistently successful [144]. Further studies have recently examined the use of porcine ICC as xenografts in mice recipients, again with prolongation of graft survival using anti-CD4 antibody treatment [145].

Clinical Trials of Fetal and Neonatal Pancreas Transplantation

A surprisingly large number of trials of human fetal pancreatic tissue transplantation have been reported, mostly originating from countries of the former Soviet Union and from China. Despite claims of success, these reports are particularly difficult to evaluate as they have not been backed by sufficiently rigorous evidence. At present there remains a question mark as to whether any effect other than placebo has been obtained. Adequately documented studies have been reported from the USA and Australia, with no successful reversal of diabetes reported. More recently, intraportal transplants of neonatal porcine ICC xenografts have been undertaken in Sweden, again without demonstrable effect on insulin requirement, although production of porcine C-peptide was described in one case [146].

In conclusion, fetal and neonatal pancreatic tissue transplantation remains an interesting field with considerable potential, and current research is examining the growth factors concerned with the continued development of fetal and neonatal tissue after transplantation. Clinical trials have been greatly hindered by the lack of a successful large animal model, which has made the cause of the failure of clinical trials difficult to pinpoint.

FUTURE PROSPECTS

The past 10 years have seen great strides in islet transplantation, culminating in successful human islet transplantation with documented long-term function [81]. However, at the same time a number of important questions have been raised and barriers to the routine clinical application of islet transplantation have become clear. These include the potential of islet grafts for long-term function, the problems of providing sufficient quantities of human islets and the need to overcome xenograft rejection if non-human islets are used. The future of islet transplantation is likely to depend on the successful resolution of these problems, as well as many advances in the fields of islet isolation, preservation, physiology, transplantation technique and immunobiology.

REFERENCES

1. Brinchmann-Hansen O, Dahl-Jorgensen K, Sandvik L, Hanssen KF. Blood glucose concentrations and progression of diabetic retinopathy: the seven-year results of the Oslo study. Br Med J 1992; 304: 19–22.
2. Wang PH, Lau J, Chalmers TC. Meta-analysis of effects of intensive blood-glucose control on late complications of type 1 diabetes. Lancet 1993; 341: 1306–9.
3. Nathan DM. Long-term complications of diabetes mellitus. New Engl J Med 1993; 328: 1676–85.
4. DCCT Research Group. The effect of intensive treatment of diabetes on the development and progression of long-term complications in insulin-dependent diabetes mellitus. New Engl J Med 1993; 329: 977–86.
5. Mecklenburg RS, Benson EA, Benson JW et al. Acute complications associated with insulin infusion pump therapy: report of experience with 161 patients. JAMA 1984; 252: 3265–9.
6. Dahl-Jorgensen K, Brinchmann-Hansen O, Hanssen KF et al. Effect of near normoglycaemia for two years on progression of early diabetic retinopathy, nephropathy, and neuropathy: the Oslo study. Br Med J 1986; 293: 1195–9.
7. West KM, Ahuja MM, Bennett PH et al. Interretionships of microangiopathy, plasma glucose and other risk factors in 3583 diabetic patients: a multinational study. Diabetologia 1982; 22: 412–20.
8. Sutherland DER, Moudry KC, Fryd DS. Results of pancreas-transplant registry. Diabetes 1989; 38 (suppl 1): 46–54.
9. Rosen CB, Frohnert PP, Velosa JA, Engen DE, Sterioff S. Morbidity of pancreas transplantation during cadaveric renal transplantation. Transplantation 1991; 51: 123–7.
10. Ricordi C. (ed.) Pancreatic islet cell transplantation. Austin: R.G. Landes Company, 1992.
11. Sutherland DE, Najarian JS, Greenberg BZ, Senske BJ, Anderson GE, Francis RS, Goetz FC. Hormonal and metabolic effects of a pancreatic endocrine graft. Vascularized segmental transplantation in insulin dependent diabetic patients. Ann Intern Med 1981; 95: 537–41.
12. Pozza G, Bosi E, Secchi A et al. Metabolic control of type 1 (insulin dependent) diabetes after pancreas transplantation. Br Med J 1985; 291: 510–13.
13. Katz H, Homan M, Velosa J, Robertson P, Rizza R. Effects of pancreas transplantation on postprandial glucose metabolism. New Engl J Med 1991; 325: 1278–83.
14. Ramsay RC, Goetz FC, Sutherland DE et al. Progression of diabetic retinopathy after pancreas transplantation for insulin-dependent diabetes mellitus. New Engl J Med 1988; 318: 208–14.

15. Landgraf R, Nusser J, Muller W et al. Fate of late complications in type 1 diabetic patients after successful pancreas-kidney transplantation. Diabetes 1989; 38 (suppl 1): 33–7.

16. Ulbig M, Kampik A, Thurau S, Landgraf R, Land W. Long-term follow-up of diabetic retinopathy for up to 71 months after combined renal and pancreatic transplantation. Graefes Arch Clin Exp Ophthalmol 1991; 229: 242–5.

17. Scheider A, Meyer-Schwickerath E, Nusser J, Land W, Landgraf R. Diabetic retinopathy and pancreas transplantation: a 3-year follow-up. Diabetologia 1991; 34 (suppl 1): 95–9.

18. Hellerstrom C. A method for the microdissection of intact pancreatic islets of mammals. Acta Endocrinol 1964; 45: 122–32.

19. Lacy PE, Kostianovsky M. Method for the isolation of intact islets of Langerhans from the rat pancreas. Diabetes 1967; 16: 35–9.

20. Ballinger WF, Lacy PE. Transplantation of intact pancreatic islets in rats. Surgery 1972; 72: 175–86.

21. Kemp CB, Knight MJ, Scharp DW, Ballinger WF, Lacy PE. Effect of transplantation site on the results of pancreatic islet isografts in diabetic rats. Diabetologia 1973; 9: 486–91.

22. Gray BN, Watkins E. Prevention of vascular complications of diabetes by pancreatic islet transplantation. Arch Surg 1976; 111: 254–7.

23. Federlin K, Slijepcevic M, Helmke K. Islet transplantation in experimental diabetes of the rat. IV. The influence of transplantation site and of histocompatibility on islet function. Horm Metab Res 1976; 8: 97–101.

24. Feldman SD, Hirshberg GE, Dodi G, Raizman ME, Scharp DW, Ballinger WF, Lacy PE. Intrasplenic islet isografts. Surgery 1977; 82: 386–94.

25. Finch DR, Wise PH, Morris PJ. Successful intrasplenic transplantation of syngeneic and allogeneic isolated pancreatic islets. Diabetologia 1977; 13: 195–9.

26. Sutherland DE, Steffes MW, Bauer GE, McManus D, Noe BD, Najarian JS. Isolation of human and porcine islets of Langerhans and islet transplantation in pigs. J Surg Res 1974; 16: 102–11.

27. Scharp DW, Murphy JJ, Newton WT, Ballinger WF, Lacy PE. Transplantation of islets of Langerhans in diabetic rhesus monkeys. Surgery 1975; 77: 100–105.

28. Lorenz D, Lippert H, Tietz W et al. Transplantation of isolated islets of Langerhans in diabetic dogs. I. Results after allogeneic intraportal islet transplantation. J Surg Res 1979; 27: 181–92.

29. Sutherland DE. Pancreas and islet transplantation. I. Experimental studies. Diabetologia 1981; 20: 161–85.

30. Najarian JS, Sutherland DE, Matas AJ, Steffes MW, Simmons RL, Goetz FC. Human islet transplantation: a preliminary report. Transpl Proc 1977; 9: 233–6.

31. Valente U, Ferro M, Barocci S et al. Report of clinical cases of human fetal pancreas transplantation. Transpl Proc 1980; 12 (suppl 2): 213–17.

32. Cameron JL, Mehigan DG, Harrington DP, Zuidema GD. Metabolic studies following intrahepatic autotransplantation of pancreatic islet grafts. Surgery 1980; 87: 397–400.

33. Traverso LW, Abou-Zamzam AN, Longmire WP. Human pancreatic cell autotransplantation following total pancreatectomy. Ann Surg 1981; 193: 191–7.

34. Cameron JL, Mehigan DG, Broe PJ, Zuidema GD. Distal pancreatectomy and islet autotransplantation for chronic pancreatitis. Ann Surg 1981; 193: 312–17.

35. Mehigan DG, Bell WR, Zuidema GD, Eggleston JC, Cameron JL. Disseminated intravascular coagulation and portal hypertension following pancreatic islet autotransplantation. Ann Surg 1980; 191: 287–93.

36. Gores PF, Najarian JS, Stephanian E, Lloveras JJ, Kelley SL, Sutherland DER. Insulin independence in type 1 diabetes after transplantation of unpurified islets from single donor with 15-deoxyspergualin. Lancet 1993; 341: 19–21.

37. Horaguchi A, Merrell RC. Preparation of viable islet cells from dogs by a new method. Diabetes 1981; 30: 455–8.

38. Griffin SM, Alderson D, Farndon JR. Comparison of harvesting methods for islet transplantation. Br J Surg 1986; 73: 712–15.

39. Noel J, Rabinovitch A, Olson L, Kyriakides G, Miller J, Mintz DH. A method for large-scale high-yield isolation of canine pancreatic islets of Langerhans. Metabolism 1982; 31: 184–7.

40. Gray DWR, McShane P, Grant A, Morris PJ. A method for isolation of islets of Langerhans from the human pancreas. Diabetes 1984; 33: 1055–61.

41. Ricordi C, Lacy PE, Finke EH, Olack BJ, Scharp DW. Automated method for isolation of human pancreatic islets. Diabetes 1988; 37: 413–20.

42. Warnock GL, Kneteman NM, Evans MG, Dabbs KD, Rajotte RV. Comparison of automated and manual methods for islet isolation. Can J Surg 1990; 33: 368–71.

43. Ricordi C, Finke EH, Lacy PE. A method for the mass isolation of islets from the adult pig pancreas. Diabetes 1986; 35: 649–53.

44. Van Suylichem PTR, Wolters GHJ, Van Schilfgaarde R. The efficacy of density gradients for islet purification: a comparison of seven density gradients. Transpl Int 1990; 3: 156–61.

45. Buitrago A, Gylfe E, Henriksson C, Pertoft H. Rapid isolation of pancreatic islets from collagenase-digested pancreas by sedimentation through Percoll at unit gravity. Biochem Biophys Res Commun 1977; 79: 823–8.

46. James RFL, Lake SP, Chamberlain J, Bell PRF. Improved rat pancreatic islet isolation with intraductal collagenase digestion combined with BSA density-gradient centrifugation. Diabetes 1989; 38 (suppl 1): 273.

47. Muller-Ruchholtz W, Leyhausen G, Petersen P, Schubert G, Ulrichs K. A simple methodological principle for large-scale extraction and purification of collagenase-digested islets. Transpl Proc 1987; 19: 911–15.

48. Jiao L, Gray DW, Gohde DW, Flynn GJ, Morris PJ. *In vitro* staining of islets of Langerhans for fluorescence-activated cell sorting. Transplantation 1991; 52: 450–52.

49. Bank HL. A high yield method for isolation of rat islets of Langerhans using differential sensitivity to freezing. Cryobiology 1983; 20: 237–44.

50. Matas AJ, Sutherland DE, Kretschmer G, Steffes MW, Najarian JS. Pancreatic tissue culture: depletion of exocrine enzymes and purification of islets for transplantation. Transpl Proc 1977; 9: 337–9.

51. Hegre OD, Marshall S, Schulte BA, Hickey GE, Williams F, Sorenson RL, Serie JR. Non-enzymic *in*

vitro isolation of perinatal islets of Langerhans. In Vitro 1983; 19: 611–20.

52. Robertson GSM, Chadwick D, Contractor H et al. Storage of human pancreatic digest in University of Wisconsin solution significantly improves subsequent islet purification. Br J Surg 1992; 79: 899–902.

53. Chadwick DR, Robertson GSM, Rose S, Contractor H, James RFL, Bell PRF, London NJM. Storage of porcine pancreatic digest prior to islet purification: the benefits of UW solution and the roles of its individual components. Transplantation 1993; 56: 288–93.

54. Hering B. Islet xenotransplantation. In Ricordi C (ed.) Pancreatic islet cell transplantation. Austin: R.G. Landes Company, 1992; pp 313–35.

55. Lake SP, Bassett PD, Larkins A et al. Large-scale purification of human islets utilizing discontinuous albumin gradient on IBM 2991 cell separator. Diabetes 1989; 38 (suppl 1): 143–5.

56. Ricordi C, Gray DWR, Hering BJ et al. Islet isolation assessment in man and large animals. Acta Diabetol Lat 1990; 27: 185–95.

57. Gray DW, Morris PJ. The use of fluorescein diacetate and ethidium bromide as a viability stain for isolated islets of Langerhans. Stain Technol 1987; 62: 373–81.

58. Bank HL. Rapid assessment of islet viability with acridine orange and propidium iodide. In Vitro Cell Dev Biol 1988; 24: 266–73.

59. Lake SP, Chamberlain J, Bassett PD, London NJ, Walczac K, Bell PR, James RF. *In vivo* method for assessment of isolated human pancreatic islet function. Diabetes 1989; 38 (suppl 1): 296.

60. Warnock GL, Kneteman NM, Ryan E, Seelis REA, Rabinovitch A, Rajotte RV. Normoglycemia after transplantation of freshly isolated and cryopreserved pancreatic islets in type 1 (insulin-dependent) diabetes mellitus. Diabetologia 1991; 34: 55–8.

61. Scharp DW, Lacy PE, Santigo JV et al. Insulin independence after islet transplantation into type 1 diabetic patient. Diabetes 1990; 39: 515–18.

62. Tzakis AG, Ricordi C, Alejandro R et al. Pancreatic islet transplantation after upper abdominal exenteration and liver replacement. Lancet 1990; 336: 402–405.

63. Scharp DW, Lacy PE, Santiago JV et al. Results of our first nine intraportal islet allografts in type 1, insulin-dependent diabetic patients. Transplantation 1991; 51: 76–85.

64. Jindal RM, Soltys K, Yost F, Beer E, Tepper MA, Cho SI. Effect of deoxyspergualin on the endocrine function of the rat pancreas. Transplantation 1993; 56: 1275–8.

65. Osorio RW, Ascher NL, Jaenisch R, Freise CE, Roberts JP, Stock PG. Major histocompatibility complex class I deficiency prolongs islet allograft survival. Diabetes 1993; 42: 1520–27.

66. Qian T, Schachner R, Brendel M, Kong SS, Alejandro R. Induction of donor-specific tolerance to rat islet allografts by intrathymic inoculation of solubilized spleen cell membrane antigens. Diabetes 1993; 42: 1544–6.

67. Hellman B. Actual distribution of the number and volume of the islets of Langerhans in different size classes in non-diabetic humans of varying ages. Nature 1959; 184: 1498–9.

68. Kemp CB, Knight MJ, Scharp DW, Lacy PE, Ballinger WF. Transplantation of isolated pancreatic islets into the portal vein of diabetic rats. Nature 1973; 244: 447.

69. Reece-Smith H, DuToit DF, McShane P, Morris PJ. Prolonged survival of pancreatic islet allografts transplanted beneath the renal capsule. Transplantation 1981; 31: 305–6.

70. Reece-Smith H, McShane P, Morris PJ. Glucose and insulin changes following a renoportal shunt in streptozotocin diabetic rats with pancreatic islet isografts under the kidney capsule. Diabetologia 1982; 23: 243–6.

71. Orloff MJ, Macedo A, Greenleaf GE, Girard B. Comparison of the metabolic control of diabetes achieved by whole pancreas transplantation and pancreatic islet transplantation in rats. Transplantation 1988; 45: 307–12.

72. Hiller W, Klempnauer J. Long-term metabolic advantages of renal subcapsular over intraportal transplantation of isolated islets of Langerhans. Diabetes 1989; 38 (suppl 1): 301.

73. Cobb LF, Merrell RC. Intrasplenic islet autografts: insulin response to intravenous glucose challenge. Curr Surg 1983; 40: 36–9.

74. Merrell RC, Maeda M, Basadonna G, Marincola F, Cobb L. Suppression, stress, and accommodation of transplanted islets of Langerhans. Diabetes 1985; 34: 667–70.

75. Kakizaki K, Basadonna G, Merrell RC. Neural regulation of heterotopic islets of Langerhans. Surgery 1986; 100: 997–1002.

76. Alejandro R, Cutfield RG, Shienvold FL et al. Natural history of intrahepatic canine islet cell autografts. J Clin Invest 1986; 78: 1339–48.

77. Warnock GL, Rajotte RV. Critical mass of purified islets that induce normoglycemia after implantation into dogs. Diabetes 1988; 37: 467–70.

78. Sutton R, Gray DW, McShane P, Peters M, Morris PJ. Metabolic efficiency and long-term fate of intraportal islet grafts in the cynomolgus monkey. Transpl Proc 1987; 19: 3575–6.

79. Sutton R, Gray DW, Burnett M, McShane P, Turner RC, Morris PJ. Metabolic function of intraportal and intrasplenic islet autografts in cynomolgus monkeys. Diabetes 1989; 38 (suppl 1): 182–4.

80. Muller-Felber W, Landgraf R, Scheuer R et al. Diabetic neuropathy 3 years after successful pancreas and kidney transplantation. Diabetes 1993; 42: 1482–6.

81. Warnock GL, Kneteman NM, Ryan EA, Rabinovitch A, Rajotte RV. Long-term follow-up after transplantation of insulin-producing pancreatic islets into patients with type 1 (insulin-dependent) diabetes mellitus. Diabetologia 1992; 35: 89–95.

82. Farney AC, Najarian JS, Nakhleh RE, Lloveras G, Field MJ, Gores PF, Sutherland DER. Autotransplantation of dispersed pancreatic islet tissue combined with total or near-total pancreatectomy for treatment of chronic pancreatitis. Surgery 1991; 110: 427–39.

83. Gray DW, Reece-Smith H, Fairbrother B, McShane P, Morris PJ. Isolated pancreatic islet allografts in rats rendered immunologically unresponsive to renal allografts: the effect of the site of transplantation. Transplantation 1984; 37: 434–7.

84. Ziegler MM, Reckard CR, Barker CF. Long-term metabolic and immunological considerations in transplantation of pancreatic islets. J Surg Res 1974; 16: 575–81.

85. Scott J, Steffes MW, Lernmark A. Islet transplantation in mice differing in the I and S subregions of the H-2 complex. Effects of presensitization with skin allografts. Scand J Immunol 1982; 16: 9-15.

86. Naji A, Reckard CR, Ziegler MM, Barker CF. Vulnerability of pancreatic islets to immune cells and serum. Surg Forum 1975; 26: 459-61.

87. Shizuru JA, Gregory AK, Chao CT-B, Fathman CG. Islet allograft survival after a single course of treatment of recipient with antibody to L3T4. Science 1987; 237: 278-80.

88. Morris PJ, Finch DR, Garvey JF, Poole MD, Millard PR. Suppression of rejection of allogeneic islet tissue in the rat. Diabetes 1980; 29 (suppl 1): 107-112.

89. Dibelius A, Konigsberger H, Walter P, Permanetter W, Brendel W, Von Specht BU. Prolonged reversal of diabetes in the rat by transplantation of allogeneic islets from a single donor and cyclosporine treatment. Transplantation 1986; 41: 426-31.

90. Alejandro R, Cutfield R, Shienvold FL, Latif Z, Mintz DH. Successful long-term survival of pancreatic islet allografts in spontaneous or pancreatectomy-induced diabetes in dogs: cyclosporine-induced immune unresponsiveness. Diabetes 1985; 34: 825-8.

91. Yasunami Y, Ryu S, Kamei T. FK506 as the sole immunosuppressive agent for prolongation of islet allograft survival in the rat. Transplantation 1990; 49: 682-6.

92. Hao L, Calcinaro F, Gill RG, Eugui EM, Allison AC, Lafferty KJ. Facilitation of specific tolerance induction in adult mice by RS-61443. Transplantation 1992; 53: 590-95.

93. Stephanian E, Lloveras JJ, Sutherland DER et al. Prolongation of canine islet allograft survival by 15-deoxyspergualin. J Surg Res 1992; 52: 621-4.

94. Lafferty KJ, Woolnough J. The origin and mechanism of the allograft reaction. Immunol Rev 1977; 35: 231-62.

95. Yasunami Y, Lacy PE, Davie JM, Finke EH. Use of *in vitro* culture at 37°C to prolong islet xenograft survival (rat to mouse). Transpl Proc 1983; 15: 1371-2.

96. Ricordi C, Lacy PE, Sterbenz K, Davie JM. Low-temperature culture of human islets or *in vivo* treatment with L3T4 antibody produces a marked prolongation of islet human-to-mouse xenograft survival. Proc Natl Acad Sci USA 1987; 84: 8080-84.

97. Faustman D, Hauptfeld V, Lacy P, Davie J. Prolongation of murine islet allograft survival by pretreatment of islets with antibody directed to Ia determinants. Proc Natl Acad Sci USA 1981; 78: 5156-9.

98. Morrow CE, Sutherland DE, Steffes MW, Najarian JS, Bach FH. H-2 antigen class: effect on mouse islet allograft rejection. Science 1983; 219: 1337-9.

99. Gores PF, Mayoral J, Field MJ, Sutherland DE. Comparison of the immunogenicity of purified and unpurified murine islet allografts. Transplantation 1986; 41: 529-31.

100. Faustman DL, Steinman RM, Gebel HM, Hauptfeld V, Davie JM, Lacy PE. Prevention of rejection of murine islet allografts by pretreatment with anti-dendritic cell antibody. Proc Natl Acad Sci USA 1984; 81: 3864-8.

101. Hardy MA, Lau H, Weber C, Reemtsma K. Pancreatic islet transplantation. Induction of graft acceptance by ultraviolet irradiation of donor tissue. Ann Surg 1984; 200: 441-50.

102. O'Shea GM, Sun AM. Encapsulation of rat islets of Langerhans prolongs xenograft survival in diabetic mice. Diabetes 1986; 35: 943-6.

103. Tucker K, Suzuki M, Waldeck NJ, Jones G, Charles MA. Successful rat pancreatic islet allotransplantation without recipient immunosuppression. Cell Immunol 1983; 79: 403-6.

104. Reece-Smith H, McShane P, Morris PJ. Pretreatment of isolated adult islets with antibody. Effect on survival in allogeneic hosts. Transplantation 1983; 36: 228-30.

105. Tze WJ, Tai J. Intrathecal allotransplantation of pancreatic endocrine cells in diabetic rats. Transplantation 1986; 41: 531-4.

106. Sun AM, O'Shea GM, Goosen MF. Injectable microencapsulated islet cells as a bioartificial pancreas. Appl Biochem Biotechnol 1984; 10: 87-99.

107. Coupland RE. The survival and growth of pancreatic tissue in the anterior chamber of the eye of the albino rat. J Endocrinol 1960; 20: 69-77.

108. Selawry HP, Whittington K. Extended allograft survival of islets grafted into intra-abdominally placed testis. Diabetes 1984; 33: 405-6.

109. Posselt AM, Barker CF, Tomaszewski JE, Markmann JF, Choti MA, Naji A. Induction of donor-specific unresponsiveness by intrathymic islet transplantation. Science 1990; 249: 1293-5.

110. Posselt AM, Naji A, Roark JH, Markmann JF, Barker CF. Intrathymic islet transplantation in the spontaneously diabetic BB rat. Ann Surg 1991; 214: 363-73.

111. Sullivan SJ, Maki T, Borland KM et al. Biohybrid artificial pancreas: long-term implantation studies in diabetic, pancreatectomized dogs. Science 1991; 252: 718-21.

112. Sutherland DE. Pancreas and islet transplant registry statistics. Transpl Proc 1994; 16: 593-8.

113. Socci C, Falqui L, Davalli AM et al. Fresh human islet transplantation to replace pancreatic endocrine function in type 1 diabetic patients: report of six cases. Acta Diabetol 1991; 28: 151-7.

114. Gray DW, McShane P, Morris PJ. The effect of hyperglycemia on isolated rodent islets transplanted to the kidney capsule site. Transplantation 1986; 41: 699-703.

115. Hamelmann W, Gray DWR, Cairns TDJ et al. Immediate destruction of xenogeneic islets in a primate model. Transplantation 1994; 58: 1109-114.

116. Hamelmann W, Esmeraldo R, Gray DWR, Morris PJ. A simple method for isolation of islets from the rabbit pancreas. Transplantation 1994; 58: 390-92.

117. Tanada M, Salzler M, Lennartz K, Mullen Y. The effect of H-2 incompatibility on pancreatic beta cell survival in the non-obese diabetic mouse. Transplantation 1988; 45: 622-7.

118. Pipeleers D, Pipeleers-Marichal M, Markholst H, Hoorens A, Kloppel G. Transplantation of purified islet cells in diabetic BB rats. Diabetologia 1991; 34: 390-96.

119. Prowse SJ, Bellgrau D, Lafferty KJ. Islet allografts are destroyed by disease occurrence in the spontaneously diabetic BB rat. Diabetes 1986; 35: 110-14.

120. Weringer EJ, Like AA. Immune attack on pancreatic islet transplants in the spontaneously diabetic

biobreeding/Worcester (BB/W) rat is not MHC-restricted. J Immunol 1985; 134: 2383-6.

121. Woehrle M, Markmann JF, Silvers WK, Barker CF, Naji A. Transplantation of cultured pancreatic islets to BB rats. Surgery 1986; 100: 334-41.

122. Haskins K, Portas M, Bergman B, Lafferty K, Bradley B. Pancreatic islet-specific T-cell clones from non-obese diabetic mice. Proc Natl Acad Sci USA 1989; 86: 8000-8004.

123. Sibley RK, Sutherland DE, Goetz F, Michael AF. Recurrent diabetes mellitus in the pancreas iso- and allograft: a light and electron microscopic and immunohistochemical analysis of four cases. Lab Invest 1985; 53: 132-44.

124. Bretzel RG, Flesch BK, Brennenstuhl G, Greiner I, Hering BJ, Woehrle M, Federlin K. Rat pancreatic islet pretreatment with anti-MHC class II monoclonal antibodies and culture: *in vitro* MLIC test response does not predict islet allograft survival. Acta Diabetol 1993; 30: 49-56.

125. Tamsma JT, Schaapherder AFM, Van Bronswijk H et al. Islet cell hormone release immediately after human pancreatic transplantation: a marker of tissue damage associated with cold ischemia. Transplantation 1993; 56: 1119-23.

126. Brown J, Molnar IG, Clark W, Mullen Y. Control of experimental diabetes mellitus in rats by transplantation of fetal pancreases. Science 1974; 184: 1377-9.

127. Brown J, Clark WR, Molnar IG, Mullen YS. Fetal pancreas transplantation for reversal of streptozotocin-induced diabetes in rats. Diabetes 1976; 25: 56-64.

128. Mullen YS, Clark WR, Molnar IG, Brown J. Complete reversal of experimental diabetes mellitus in rats by a single fetal pancreas. Science 1977; 195: 68-70.

129. McEvoy RC, Hegre OD. Syngeneic transplantation of fetal rat pancreas. 3. Effect of insulin treatment on the growth and differentiation of the pancreatic implants after reversal of diabetes. Diabetes 1979; 28: 141-6.

130. Mandel TE, Georgiou H, Hoffman L, Carter WM, Koulmanda M, Dennington P. Proliferation of cultured and isografted fetal mouse pancreatic islets. Transpl Proc 1983; 15: 1362-5.

131. Garvey JF, Klein C, Millard PR, Morris PJ. Rejection of organ cultured allogeneic foetal rat pancreas. Surgery 1980; 87: 157-63.

132. Mauer SM, Steffes MW, Sutherland DE, Najarian JS, Michael AF, Brown DM. Studies of the rate of regression of the glomerular lesions in diabetic rats treated with pancreatic islet transplantation. Diabetes 1975; 24: 280-85.

133. Matas AJ, Sutherland DE, Payne WD, Eckhardt J, Najarian JS. A mouse model of islet transplantation using neonatal donors. Transplantation 1977; 24: 389-93.

134. Matas AJ, Payne WD, Grotting JC, Sutherland DE, Steffes MW, Hertel BF, Najarian JS. Portal versus systemic transplantation of dispersed neonatal pancreas. Transplantation 1977; 24: 333-7.

135. Steffes MW, Brown DM, Basgen JM, Mauer SM. Amelioration of mesangial volume and surface alterations following islet transplantation in diabetic rats. Diabetes 1980; 29: 509-15.

136. Garvey JF, Morris PJ, Millard PR. Early rejection of allogeneic foetal rat pancreas. Transplantation 1979; 27: 342-4.

137. Lafferty KJ, Bootes A, Dart G, Talmage DW. Effect of organ culture on the survival of thyroid allografts in mice. Transplantation 1976; 22: 138-49.

138. Lacy PE, Davie JM, Finke EH. Prolongation of islet allograft survival following *in vitro* culture (24°C) and a single injection of ALS. Science 1979; 204: 312-13.

139. Mullen Y. Specific immunosuppression for fetal pancreas allografts in rats. Diabetes 1980; 29 (suppl 1): 113-20.

140. Mullen Y, Shintaku IP. Fetal pancreas allografts for reversal of diabetes in rats. II. Induction of life-term-specific unresponsiveness to pancreas allografts across non-major histocompatibility complex barriers. Transplantation 1982; 33: 3-11.

141. Mullen Y, Gottlieb M, Shibukawa RL. Reversal of diabetes in rats by fetal pancreas allografts following TLI. Transpl Proc 1983; 15: 1355-8.

142. Simeonovic CJ, Lafferty KJ. The isolation and transplantation of foetal mouse proislets. Aust J Exp Biol Med Sci 1982; 60: 383-90.

143. Simeonovic CJ, Hodgkin PD, Donohoe JA, Bowen KM, Lafferty KJ. An analysis of tissue-specific transplantation phenomena in a minor histo-incompatibility system. Transplantation 1985; 39: 661-6.

144. Yoneda K, Mullen Y, Stein E, Clare-Salzler M, Ozawa A, Shevlin L, Danilovs J. Fetal pancreas transplantation in miniature swine. II. Survival of fetal pig pancreas allografts cultured at room temperature. Diabetes 1989; 38 (suppl 1): 213-16.

145. Koulmanda M, Mandel TE. Effect of anti-CD4 and anti-ICAM MAb on survival of fetal pig pancreas grafts in NOD mice. Transpl Proc 1994; 26: 3466.

146. Tibell A, Groth CG, Moller E, Korsgren O, Andersson A, Hellerstrom C. Pig-to-human islet transplantation in eight patients. Transpl Proc 1994; 26: 762-3.

46

Pancreas Transplantation

A. Tibell*, E. Christiansen†and C.G. Groth*

*Karolinska Institute, Huddinge, Sweden, and †Steno Diabetes Center, Gentofte, Denmark

INTRODUCTION

Pancreatic transplantation provides a surgical means of carrying out endocrine replacement therapy in diabetic patients. Following successful pancreatic transplantation, exogenous insulin injections can be discontinued and glucose metabolism becomes normal or near-normal. However, the benefits of pancreatic transplantation must be weighed against the operative risks and the hazards of the chronic immunosuppressive therapy required after transplantation.

CANDIDATES FOR PANCREATIC TRANSPLANTATION

The vast majority of diabetic patients undergoing pancreatic transplantation have received their pancreas graft in conjunction with a kidney transplantation. The question whether it is justifiable to expose the diabetic patient to a major surgical procedure followed by immunosuppressive treatment has thus been circumvented; these patients must undergo surgery and receive immunosuppression in any case.

Pancreatic transplantation has been performed either simultaneously with kidney transplantation, or after a successful kidney transplantation. The first attempt at such a combined transplantation was carried out by Kelly and Lillehei more than 25 years ago [1]. A number of transplant centers are now performing this procedure and worldwide some 6000 diabetic patients have undergone pancreatic transplantation, with the simultaneous procedure as the main approach.

In the simultaneous procedure, the patient undergoes only one surgical intervention, and the high-dose immunosuppressive treatment immediately after the transplantation is given only once. Since the kidney and the pancreas come from the same donor, the kidney can serve as a marker of rejection. A potential disadvantage of the simultaneous procedure is that surgical or other complications related to the pancreatic graft may cause some interference with the renal graft. The patients accepted for simultaneous transplantation constitute a subgroup of uremic diabetic patients who would otherwise have been accepted for renal transplantation alone. Difficulties with blood glucose control are an indication for pancreas transplantation. The general health of the patient should be reasonably well preserved and an upper age limit of approximately 50 years is usually applied.

The staged procedure involves two separate operations, and high doses of immunosuppressives must be given twice. Since the kidney comes from a different donor, it cannot serve as a marker of rejection of the pancreas. Most groups now prefer the simultaneous procedure, although the staged procedure may be suitable for diabetic patients who have a living related kidney donor. In such cases, common practice is to perform a kidney transplantation first, taking advantage of the related kidney graft, and to consider a cadaveric pancreatic transplantation later. Some patients who initially seem too sick to tolerate a simultaneous procedure make a marked recovery after receiving a kidney transplant, and may subsequently also be given a pancreas.

International Textbook of Diabetes Mellitus, Second Edition. Edited by K.G.M.M. Alberti, P. Zimmet, R.A. DeFronzo, and H. Keen (Honorary)
© 1997 John Wiley & Sons Ltd

Table 1 Preoperative evaluation

Obligatory	Exercise ECG
	Non-invasive evaluation of the peripheral vessels
	Upper GI series or gastroscopy
	Residual urine volume
	Electrophysiology of peripheral nerves, and cardiac beat-to-beat variation on provocation
	Fundus photography
	Fluorescein angiography
	Cr-EDTA-clearance
Optional	Coronary artery angiography
	Iliac artery angiography
	Cystoscopy
	Cystometry
	Renal biopsy

Over the years a small number of centers have explored the possibility of performing a pancreatic transplantation alone, in non-uremic diabetic patients. Earlier intervention might be expected to have a better effect on secondary complications. Most of the patients treated so far have had pre-uremic nephropathy or severe retinopathy. Others have had severe management problems such as hyperlabile diabetes, severe insulin resistance, and unawareness of hypoglycemia. Approximately 300 patients worldwide have undergone pancreas transplantation alone.

Pancreas transplantation is not a life-saving operation, and a number of potential complications are associated with the procedure. The benefits and risks should be discussed in detail with the patient. A written leaflet is useful in this context.

The following conditions constitute contraindications to transplantation in the diabetic patient: (a) current peripheral gangrene; (b) severe coronary insufficiency with angina; (c) cardiac decompensation; (d) severely incapacitating peripheral neuropathy, i.e. bedridden patients; and (e) severely incapacitating autonomic neuropathy, i.e. gastroparesis.

Diabetic patients who are candidates for pancreatic transplantation usually undergo a more extensive preoperative evaluation than do renal transplant candidates. The program used for the preoperative work-up at our hospital is outlined in Table 1. Pretransplant assessment of the retina is mandatory and, when indicated, photocoagulation should be performed before transplantation. Unless the retina is in a stable condition, the sudden improvement in glycemic control caused by pancreatic transplantation may cause a deterioration in the retinopathy [2].

RECIPIENT OPERATION AND THE POSTOPERATIVE COURSE

Most groups now use a pancreaticoduodenal graft which is placed intraperitoneally in the lower part of the recipient's abdomen. An arterial anastomosis is made to the iliac artery and a venous anastomosis is made to the recipient's common iliac vein or inferior vena cava (Figure 1). Some groups have performed the venous anastomosis to the portal vein or to one of its tributaries, thereby achieving splanchnic insulin delivery.

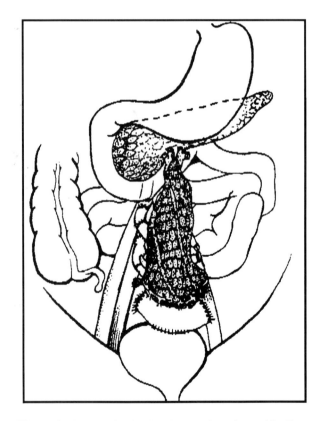

Figure 1 Pancreaticoduodenal transplantation with diversion of the pancreatic juice to the bladder of the recipient

Diversion of the graft exocrine secretion is usually performed to the recipient's bladder (Figure 1). Urinary diversion makes possible day-to-day monitoring of the graft by measurements of its exocrine excretion, as reflected by the urinary amylase levels [3]. There are, however, some disadvantages associated with this technique. The loss of alkaline pancreatic juice via the urine may result in metabolic acidosis, and oral supplementation with bicarbonate may be required [4]. Urinary tract infections and, in some instances, severe urinary tract symptoms probably caused by activation of the digestive pancreatic enzymes in the urine, have occurred in some patients [5]. In patients with more serious problems, a conversion to enteric drainage alleviates the symptoms [5]. At present, some 10–15% of patients with bladder-drained grafts require such a conversion [6].

Enteric exocrine diversion may also be applied as the primary procedure (Figure 2) [7]. However, this approach has not come into widespread use, partly because it seems to carry an increased risk of intra-abdominal infection. Moreover, the amylase excretion from the graft cannot be directly monitored. During the first weeks post-transplant, such monitoring can be accomplished by the use of an exteriorizing pancreatic duct catheter. However, intubation of the pancreatic duct increases the frequency of early and late graft pancreatitis. Therefore, we now rarely use pancreatic duct catheters [8].

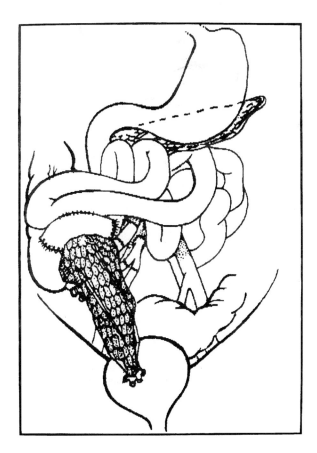

Figure 2 Pancreaticoduodenal transplantation with diversion of the pancreatic juice to the small bowel of the recipient

Duct-occluded segmental body and tail pancreatic grafts were commonly used in the early 1980s [9]. This procedure results in fibrosis and destruction of the exocrine part of the pancreas. The potential surgical advantages of 'eliminating' the exocrine part of the graft are offset by the loss of the various exocrine pancreatic markers that are important for diagnosing graft rejection. Today the duct occlusion technique is used rarely and only in recipients of combined renal and pancreatic grafts, in whom diagnosis of rejection is based on renal markers.

After pancreatic transplantation the blood glucose levels usually become normal or near-normal within hours and insulin administration can then be discontinued. Massive hyperamylasemia and inadequate blood glucose control in the early post-transplant period frequently indicate severe graft damage due to preservation injury, vascular thrombosis or severe rejection.

Surgical complications are more frequent after pancreatic transplantation than after renal transplantation. Graft thrombosis is the commonest technical cause of early graft loss. Consequently, many groups use anticoagulant protocols, such as low molecular weight dextran followed by aspirin. The increased frequency of local infectious complications may be due to contamination from the recipient's bowel or bladder or from the duodenal segment of the graft. Early severe graft pancreatitis, pancreatic fistulas and anastomotic leakages may also occur [10]. In many cases, symptoms and signs are surprisingly discrete in these diabetic and heavily immunosuppressed patients. The increased postoperative morbidity, when compared with renal grafting alone, is also accompanied by an increase in the mean hospitalization time.

PANCREATIC GRAFT MONITORING

Early after transplantation, the exocrine part of the pancreatic graft is monitored by daily measurements of serum amylase. In recipients of bladder-drained pancreatic grafts, the amylase level in the urine is also recorded daily. In patients with an exteriorizing pancreatic ductal catheter, measurements of the flow of juice and its amylase content provide hourly information concerning the condition of the graft.

The endocrine function of the graft is monitored by frequent measurements of blood glucose levels and of changes in the recipient's insulin requirement. Measurements of serum C-peptide levels indicate the insulin production of the graft. For long-term routine follow-up, glycated hemoglobin (HbA_{1c}) levels are regularly recorded. Intravenous and oral glucose tolerance tests are usually also included in the routine follow-up.

DIAGNOSIS OF REJECTION

For reasons not well understood, kidneys transplanted simultaneously with a pancreas seem more prone to rejection than kidneys transplanted alone [11, 12, 13]. Surprisingly, the pancreatic graft function usually remains unaffected while the kidney is being rejected. Sometimes symptoms and signs of rejection occur in both grafts, and in rare instances isolated pancreatic graft rejection has been encountered [13]. Paradoxically, a pancreas transplanted after a kidney often suffers rejection, and a similarly high incidence of rejection is seen when a pancreas is transplanted alone in non-uremic diabetic patients [14]. While the diagnosis of rejection in recipients of simultaneous grafts can generally be based on renal markers, the diagnosis of rejection in a pancreas transplanted after a kidney and in a pancreas transplanted alone must rely on pancreatic markers. Elevated blood glucose levels usually occur late in the rejection process, by which time the process in the exocrine pancreas may be difficult or even impossible to reverse by anti-rejection treatment [15]. Such differences in the timing of rejection have also been observed in animal experiments. Thus, in non-immunosuppressed dogs, rejection-type cellular infiltrates appear early in the exocrine tissue, at a time when the endocrine tissue is still unaffected [16].

An increase in plasma amylase levels may occur at the time of rejection, but it is also possible for levels to be unaffected [17]. Assays of more specific plasma markers, such as anionic trypsin, pancreas specific amylase or pancreas specific protein (PASP), have been found to correlate somewhat better with rejection but, even with these tests, the discrimination is rather poor [17, 18].

In recipients of bladder-drained pancreatic grafts, a drop in the urinary amylase excretion is commonly used as a marker of acute rejection [3]. The reliability of the test, however, has become a subject for debate. Apparently, urinary amylase excretion may vary for other reasons.

In grafts with an exteriorizing pancreatic duct catheter, a decrease in the amylase content of the pancreatic juice has been found to correlate closely with graft rejection [18]. Cytological examination of the juice has also proved helpful in this context [18, 19]. Indeed, lymphoblasts have been found in the juice 1 or 2 days prior to the decrease in amylase output. Biopsies have been used to verify rejection, but they carry a risk of complications, such as bleeding and fistulas, and should be used with caution.

In chronic rejection, a progressive deterioration in glycemic control is the most characteristic finding. In some cases bouts of hyperamylasemia have occurred weeks or months previously. These changes presumably reflect inflammation and perhaps outflow obstruction in the exocrine part of the graft.

PATIENT AND GRAFT SURVIVAL RATES

The International Pancreas Transplant Registry maintained at the University of Minnesota has for many years provided information on the patient and graft survival rates after pancreatic transplantation. Previously, the best patient survival figures were seen in the group of patients receiving a pancreas after kidney transplantation. This was not surprising, since these patients represented a selected population that had done well following a previous kidney transplant. However, recently this difference has disappeared and in the latest analysis the patient survival rates were similar, whether the procedure had been a simultaneous pancreas and kidney transplantation, a pancreas transplantation after a kidney transplantation, or a pancreas alone, the 1-year figures being 91%, 92% and 93%, respectively, with cardiovascular diseases the commonest cause of death. Thus, the patient survival figures are now similar to those seen after renal transplantation in diabetic patients.

With simultaneous pancreatic and renal transplantation and using the bladder diversion technique, the Registry figure for the 1-year pancreatic graft success rate is around 75%. The corresponding figures for grafts with enteric drainage and grafts with duct occlusion are 60% in both groups. Individual centers, however, have reported a 1-year graft success rate in the 70–80% range also with the latter two techniques [20, 21].

With pancreas transplantation after kidney transplantation, and pancreas transplantation alone, the pancreatic graft success rate has been lower. A possible explanation is the inadequacy of methods to diagnose rejection in these patients. Moreover, it seems that the rejection process may be more intense, at least in the recipients of pancreas transplants alone. However, the Minnesota group has recently reported improved results in these two groups. In their series, all grafts were performed with bladder diversion, which facilitated the diagnosis of rejection. Donor and recipient HLA-matching was performed and intensified rejection treatment was given as soon as the urinary amylase level declined. With this protocol, the 1-year pancreatic graft success rates were 70% and 61%, respectively [22].

It has been feared that the transplantation of a pancreas could, for immunological or other reasons, jeopardize the simultaneously transplanted kidney. However, a recent comparison of data from the Pancreas Transplant Registry and the UNOS Kidney Transplant Registry, has revealed a similar kidney survival, whether the kidney was transplanted in conjunction with a pancreas, or alone into the diabetic patients [22, 23].

Data concerning the long-term graft success rate are also now emerging. A recent analysis of the Stockholm series showed that of 65 pancreatic grafts that had been transplanted in combination with a kidney more than 5 years ago, 20 (31%) were functioning 5–9 years after the transplantation [24].

The question whether pancreatic transplantation has an impact on the life expectancy of the diabetic patient has not been finally settled. Data from Minneapolis, however, indicate that among diabetic patients with abnormal autonomic function those with a functioning pancreas transplant survive longer than those whose pancreas transplant failed. On long-term follow-up, survival in the former groups was also better than those not given a pancreas transplant [25].

BLOOD GLUCOSE CONTROL AFTER PANCREAS TRANSPLANTATION

Pancreas transplantation is the only therapeutic option by which normal fasting blood glucose concentrations can be obtained long-term in IDDM patients. Glycated hemoglobin (HbA$_{1c}$) also becomes normalized in a substantial proportion of pancreas transplant recipients (Figure 3) [26–28]. With an oral glucose tolerance test the 2-hour blood glucose level is normal in approximately two-thirds of the patients, and when an intravenous glucose tolerance test is performed, the k-value is normal in about half of the patients.

After pancreas transplantation glucose homeostasis depends on the insulin secretory capacity of the pancreatic B cells of the graft and the insulin sensitivity of the individual. The insulin secretory capacity depends on the number of B cells transplanted, the proportion of functioning B cells and the sensitivity of the B cells to nutrients. Insulin sensitivity is an important factor in determining hepatic glucose production and insulin-stimulated peripheral glucose uptake. A third factor is the blood glucose level, which itself influences glucose uptake in non-insulin dependent tissues. Glucose metabolism depends also on counter-regulatory hormones such as glucagon, epinephrine and norepinephrine, and on the incretin effect of the gastrointestinal hormones. Impairment in the function of any of these variables may affect glucose homeostasis and cause deterioration of the metabolic state or a recurrence of the diabetic state.

PANCREATIC B-CELL FUNCTION AND INSULIN SENSITIVITY

Several groups have conducted studies concerning the secretory capacity of the pancreatic graft B cells. The findings with direct measurements of insulin and C-peptide levels in the peripheral blood indicate that the B cells in the pancreatic graft may have a subnormal, normal or even enhanced insulin secretion. Detailed analysis of the data has made it clear, however, that several

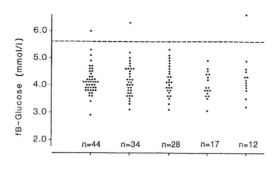
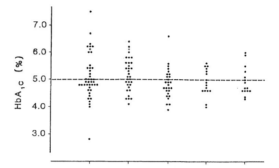
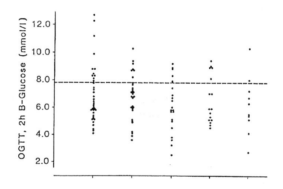
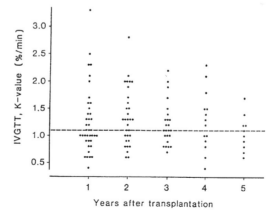

Figure 3 Long-term metabolic control in recipients of pancreatic grafts with enteric exocrine drainage, assessed by fasting blood glucose (fB-glucose), HbA$_{1c}$ and oral and intravenous glucose tolerance tests

confounding factors are involved. One such factor is a variation in the number of functioning B cells between pancreas transplant recipients. Most groups currently use pancreatic grafts consisting of the entire gland, but previously segmental grafts, consisting of the pancreatic body and tail only, were used by many groups, and some groups still use such grafts. Following transplantation, the islet mass may become reduced for a variety of reasons, including pancreatitis, graft rejection and graft fibrosis. B cells may also be lost because of drug toxicity. For example cyclosporine, which is given to all transplant patients, has been shown to have a toxic effect on B cells [29].

Furthermore, the vast majority of patients have received a graft with systemic venous drainage which eliminates the normal first-pass hepatic extraction of insulin [30, 31]. Consequently, insulin levels in the peripheral venous blood are 2–3 times higher than normal during fasting and after stimulation [30–34]. To avoid this unphysiological state, some groups have performed the venous anastomosis to the portal vein or to one of its tributaries, thereby achieving splanchnic insulin delivery [35]. By so doing they have indeed avoided peripheral hyperinsulinemia. However, whether this results in improved blood glucose control remains unclear. Furthermore, hyperinsulinemia may also be induced by increased insulin resistance, as discussed below. Finally, there are methodological problems concerning the analyses of insulin. Thus, cross-reactivity between insulin, proinsulin and 'proinsulin conversion intermediates' may affect the results of the insulin radioimmunoassay [31].

As with insulin, peripheral levels of C-peptide are often 2–3 times higher than normal, but the underlying reason is different. C-peptide is co-secreted by the B cells in equimolar amounts with insulin, but hepatic extraction of C-peptide is negligible and its metabolic clearance is constant over the physiological range of concentrations. Since C-peptide is degraded and excreted via the kidney, C-peptide turnover is highly dependent on renal function, and the elevated C-peptide levels may well be ascribed to the subnormal renal function that exists in many pancreas transplant recipients. Accordingly, the kinetics of C-peptide differ between transplant recipients and normal subjects and result in an increased half-life of C-peptide in pancreas recipients [30, 31].

Evaluated from insulin or C-peptide levels, the amount of insulin secreted in response to oral stimulation has been found to be either improved [30, 31, 34], similar [36], or slightly worse than in normal subjects [37]. However, only by using the 'deconvolution of peripheral C-peptide technique' [38] or mathematical modeling of concomitantly measured peripheral concentrations of insulin and C-peptide [39] can the actual secretion of insulin from the B cells be estimated. Thus, the calculated secretion of insulin in response to a meal stimulation has been found to be impaired

both in patients with a whole pancreas transplant [30] and in patients with a segmental transplant [31]. An impaired insulin secretion has also been found after oral glucose stimulation. The pancreas transplant recipients had a higher glycemic response [36, 40] and a lower postprandial stimulated insulin secretion when compared both to normal subjects and to non-diabetic kidney transplant patients on similar immunosuppression [36, 40]. In pancreas transplant recipients with abnormal glucose tolerance, insulin secretion was further reduced [40].

The effect of other B-cell secretagogues delivered intravenously, on glucose regulation and insulin secretion has also been studied. After stimulation with arginine during normoglycemia, insulin secretion has been found to be enhanced or similar to that in controls [27, 32, 41, 42]. Glucose potentiation of arginine-induced insulin secretion in whole organ graft recipients was found to be normal in some studies [42], but reduced in others [41]. When stimulation of the B cells was performed with glucagon, insulin secretion improved in a normal fashion [33]. Another important finding is that intravenous glucose stimulation resulted in a biphasic insulin response, even in transplant recipients with impaired glucose tolerance [27, 28, 32, 44]. Following combined stimulation with intravenous glucose and tolbutamide (the frequent sample intravenous glucose test, FSIGT), insulin secretion was found, somewhat surprisingly, to be higher in whole organ pancreatic transplant recipients than in normal controls [44, 45].

Glucose regulation and insulin secretion following B-cell stimulation with various intravenously administered secretagogues has also been compared between patients with whole organ pancreatic grafts, and those with segmental grafts. As expected, insulin secretion was reduced after arginine, after glucose potentiation of arginine-induced insulin secretion (Figure 4) [42], after glucagon [43] and after glucose alone during both first and second phase insulin secretion in the recipients of segmental grafts [44].

The various B-cell tests, oral as well as intravenous, are not equally sensitive for detecting minor alterations in B-cell function. As a result of enteric factors (the incretin effect) oral glucose stimuli induce a more pronounced B-cell stimulation than do intravenous glucose stimuli in normal subjects. In pancreas transplant recipients also, oral stimuli increase insulin secretion more than intravenous stimuli do [43] and the plasma levels of gastric inhibitory polypeptide (GIP), gastrin and glucagon-like peptide 1 (GLP-1) are elevated during oral glucose tolerance test (OGTT) and meal stimulation. This indicates that the enteroinsular axis and the incretin effect are indeed intact, although the transplanted pancreas is denervated [35, 37].

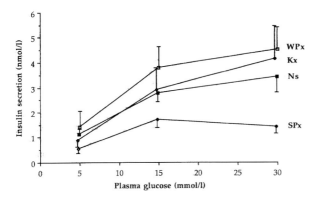

Figure 4 Glucose potentiation of arginine-induced insulin secretion in whole-organ pancreatic graft recipients (WPx), segmental pancreatic graft recipients (SPx), non-diabetic kidney graft recipients (Kx) and normal subjects (Ns)

Thus, the overall findings indicate that the number of functioning B cells in the graft is a major determinant of the quantity of insulin that can be secreted and of the B-cell adaptation to the insulin resistance present.

The other important factor that influences glucose metabolism after pancreatic transplantation is insulin sensitivity. Thus, insulin sensitivity has been found to be reduced by 60%, when assessed with the FSIGT [44, 45], and by 25%, when assessed with the conventional euglycemic hyperinsulinemic clamp technique [46]. This is not unexpected, since two of the immunosuppressive drugs given, prednisolone and cyclosporine, induce insulin resistance. Thus, hyperglycemia—and even 'steroid diabetes'—may occur in non-diabetic organ transplant recipients. In addition, hyperinsulinemia has been thought to cause insulin resistance by down-regulating the insulin receptor [47], but this mechanism is probably of minor importance. However, the insulin resistance encountered in transplanted diabetic patients does not seem to be caused by reduced muscle blood flow in the microvascular bed [48].

PANCREATIC A-CELL SECRETION AND COUNTER-REGULATION

In patients with long-standing diabetes, glucagon secretion is often deficient or even absent. Following pancreas transplantation, glucagon is secreted from the graft as well as from the patient's native pancreas. Indeed, several studies have shown that pancreas transplant recipients have basal hyperglucagonemia [34, 36, 37, 40]. A similar pattern of hyperglucagonemia has, however, also been found to exist in immuno-suppressed non-diabetic kidney transplant recipients [34, 36, 40, 42]. Further elevation of glucagon levels occurs following intravenous arginine stimulation [32, 42], whereas inappropriate suppression occurs during hyperglycemic clamping [34, 42]. Stimulation with

oral glucose or other nutrients causes a similar suppression of glucagon secretion in both patient groups [36, 37, 40]. These findings suggest that the hyperglucagonemia is related to immunosuppressive therapy. In pancreas transplant recipients with impaired glucose tolerance the inappropriate suppression of early glucagon secretion contributes indirectly to postprandial hyperglycemia [40].

Glucagon secretion plays an important role in glucose metabolism, especially as regards the counteraction of hypoglycemia by hepatic glycogenolysis. An improvement in recovery from insulin-induced hypoglycemia has, indeed, been reported in pancreas recipients as a result of an enhanced glucagon secretion [49]. In this context it was noted that normalization of epinephrine and growth hormone levels during hypoglycemia also occurred after pancreas transplantation [50]. As regards pancreatic polypeptide secretion, no increase was demonstrated in pancreas recipients during insulin-induced hypoglycemia. This indicates that no re-innervation of the pancreas graft takes place [49, 51].

Thus it is clear that fasting plasma glucose concentrations and HbA_{1c} can be restored to normal by pancreatic transplantation. The glycemic response to stimulation by meals or oral glucose becomes normal or near-normal. However, for a variety of reasons insulin secretion is not entirely normalized. The secretory demand on the B cells is increased due to insulin resistance caused by the treatment with prednisolone and cyclosporine. The improvement in glucagon secretion after pancreatic transplantation normalizes the counterregulation of hypoglycemia. The entero–insular axis and the incretin effect of the gastrointestinal hormones seem to be preserved, despite the denervated pancreas.

EFFECTS ON THE SECONDARY COMPLICATIONS

It was initially hoped that the secondary complications of diabetes would be halted or perhaps even reversed as a result of normoglycemia after successful pancreatic transplantation, but follow-up studies in a quite large series of patients show that the results are disappointing in this regard.

The progression of diabetic retinopathy was not affected during the first years after a successful pancreatic transplantation. In some patients, retinopathy actually worsened. However, 3–4 years after transplantation, stabilization or even an improvement has been observed by some groups [52]. Other groups have found no positive effect [53].

After combined renal and pancreatic transplantation, there is a definite improvement in neuropathy, but comparisons with the findings in recipients of renal grafts alone indicate that the improvement is mainly due to the reversal of uremia [54]. However, with longer follow-up, an additional advantage was found in patients who received a pancreas [55, 56, 57]. Recipients of pancreatic grafts alone also showed improvement or stabilization of sensory, motor and autonomic indices as compared to patients with failed grafts or no transplants [56].

Studies using vital microscopy and laser techniques indicate that pancreas transplantation may have a beneficial effect on microvascular reactivity in the skin. Thermoregulatory behavior and reoxygenation time also improved after transplantation [58, 59].

The finding that pancreatic transplantation has little or no effect on established diabetic neuropathy and retinopathy is presumably explained by the fact that the majority of the patients transplanted have had end-stage diabetic nephropathy. In most recipients of pancreas transplants alone, the secondary complications have also been relatively severe and the tissue destruction has probably been irreversible. Only if pancreatic transplantation is performed earlier can significant effects on the secondary complications be expected.

The hypothesis that the normalization of glycemic control may affect the secondary complications of diabetes if transplantation is performed earlier in the course of the disease derives strong support from experimental data and from observations concerning the development of nephropathy in renal grafts. Thus, in diabetic patients who have received a kidney transplant and a pancreas transplant, either simultaneously [60] or a few years later [61], the renal graft has been protected from developing the glomerular lesions characteristic of diabetes. However, when non-uremic patients with long-standing diabetes (15–29 years) were given a pancreas transplant alone, it was found that the glomerular lesions in their native kidneys had not improved even 5 years after the transplantation [62]. Thus, pancreatic transplantation prevented the development of diabetic lesions in a normal kidney but did not improve established diabetic lesions in native kidneys.

QUALITY OF LIFE

After successful pancreatic transplantation, insulin injections can be discontinued and all dietary restrictions abandoned. Such changes have considerable social and psychological implications for the patient. Several groups have now carefully analyzed the quality of life after pancreatic transplantation. In most of these studies, indicators of subjective health perception show an improvement [63, 64, 65]. The findings concerning physical well-being have, however, been conflicting [66]. Most diabetic patients certainly feel a strong relief following a successful pancreatic transplantation: a chronic disease has been cured.

SUMMARY

Approximately 6000 pancreatic transplantations have now been carried out worldwide and some 50 centers are actively pursuing pancreas transplant programs. The vast majority of the patients have received the pancreas graft in conjunction with a kidney transplantation, while a small group has been treated by pancreas transplantation alone. With few exceptions, the graft consists of the entire pancreas with a segment of its duodenum, and the pancreatic juice is usually diverted to the recipient's bladder. Pancreatic graft rejection is best monitored by using markers of exocrine function, since the endocrine function becomes impaired later in the rejection process. In recipients of simultaneous renal and pancreatic grafts the diagnosis of rejection is mainly based on renal markers. In many cases the relatively common surgical complications result in prolonged hospitalization after transplantation. Following pancreatic transplantation, the patient becomes insulin-independent and fasting blood glucose and glycated hemoglobin levels become normal or nearly normal. However, more sophisticated tests show that insulin secretion is subnormal in many patients. One important factor is that the transplanted islet mass may be insufficient. Furthermore, all patients suffer from insulin resistance which is due, among other things, to the immunosuppressive drugs currently used. Originally, it was hoped that the normoglycemia induced by pancreatic transplantation would alleviate the secondary complications of diabetes, but long-term follow-up in a considerable number of patients has made it clear that pancreatic transplantation has little or no effect on established secondary lesions. This is probably because the destructive changes in the tissues were already beyond the point of no return. There is evidence, however, that pancreatic transplantation can prevent secondary lesions. Thus kidney grafts in patients also given pancreatic grafts have been protected from the glomerular lesions characteristic of diabetes. The fact that the patients become insulin-independent and free of dietary restrictions has important social and psychological implications. Quality-of-life studies indicate that indicators of subjective well-being are significantly improved, but findings concerning physical state are less conclusive.

REFERENCES

1. Kelly WD, Lillehei RC, Merkel FK et al. Allotransplantation of the pancreas and duodenum along with the kidney in diabetic nephropathy. Surgery 1967; 61: 827–37.

2. The Kroc Collaborative Study Group. Diabetic retinopathy after two years of intensified insulin treatment. JAMA 1988; 260: 37-41.

3. Prieto M, Sutherland DER, Fernandez-Cruz L et al. Experimental and clinical experience with urinary amylase monitoring for early diagnosis of rejection in pancreas transplantation. Transplantation 1987; 43: 73-9.

4. Nghiem DD, Gonwa TA, Corry RJ. Metabolic effects of urinary diversion of exocrine secretions in pancreatic transplantation. Transplantation 1987; 43: 70-73.

5. Stephanian E, Gruessner RWG, Brayman KL et al. Conversion of exocrine secretions from bladder to enteric drainage in recipients of whole pancreaticoduodenal transplants. Ann Surg 1992; 216(6): 663-72.

6. Sollinger HW, Messing EM, Eckhoff DE et al. Urological complications in 210 consecutive simultaneous pancreas and kidney transplants with bladder drainage. Ann Surg 1993; 218: 561-70.

7. Tydén G, Tibell A, Groth CG. Pancreaticoduodenal transplantation with enteric exocrine drainage. Technical aspects. Clin Transplant 1991; 5: 36-9.

8. Tibell A, Brattström C, Kozlowski T et al. Management after clinical pancreas transplantation with enteric exocrine drainage. Transpl Proc 1994; 26: 1797-8.

9. Dubernard JM, Traeger J, Neyra P et al. A new method of preparation of segmental pancreatic grafts for transplantation: trials in dogs and man. Surgery 1978; 84: 633-40.

10. Hesse UJ, Sutherland DER, Simmons RL et al. Intra-abdominal infections in pancreas transplant recipients. Ann Surg 1986; 203: 153-62.

11. Nakache R, Mainetti L, Tydén G. Renal transplantation in diabetes mellitus: influence of combined pancreas-kidney transplantation on outcome. Transpl Proc 1990; 22: 624.

12. Hopt UT, Busing M, Schareck W, Muller GH. Differential immunostimulatory properties of combined pancreas-kidney and single-kidney allografts. Diabetes 1989; 38(suppl. 1): 251.

13. Gruessner RWG, Dunn DL, Tzardis PJ et al. Simultaneous pancreas and kidney transplantation versus single kidney transplantation and previous kidney transplants in uremic patients and single pancreatic transplants in non-uremic diabetic patients: comparison of rejection, morbidity and long-term outcome. Transpl Proc 1990; 22: 622-3.

14. Sutherland DER, Gruessner A, Moudry-Munns K. Report on results of pancreas transplantation in the United States, October 1987 to October 1991, from the United Network for Organ Sharing Registry. In Terasaki PI (ed) Clinical transplants 1991. Los Angeles: UCLA Tissue Typing Laboratory, 1991; pp 31-38.

15. Sutherland DER, Goetz FC, Najarian JS et al. One hundred pancreas transplants at a single institution. Ann Surg 1984; 200: 414-40.

16. Florack G, Sutherland DER, Sibley RK et al. Combined kidney and segmental pancreas allotransplantation in dogs. Transpl Proc 1985; 17: 374-7.

17. Brattström C, Tydén G, Reinholt F et al. Markers for pancreas graft rejection in humans. Diabetes 1989; 38(suppl. 1): 57-62.

18. Kubota K, Reinholt FR, Tydén G et al. Pancreas cytology for monitoring pancreatic grafts in the early postoperative period. Transpl Int 1992; 5: 133-8.

19. Steiner E, Klima G, Niederwisser D et al. Monitoring of the pancreatic allograft by analysis of exocrine secretion. Transpl Proc 1987; 19: 2336-8.

20. Tibell A, Brattström C, Wadström J et al. Improved results using whole-organ pancreaticoduodenal transplants with enteric drainage. Transpl Proc 1994; 26(2): 412-13.

21. Martin X, Lefrancois N, Marechal JM et al. Pancreas transplantation in Lyon: overall results. Diabetologia 1991; 34: 8-10.

22. Sutherland D. Pancreatic transplantation. An update. Diabet Rev 1993; 1(2): 152-65.

23. Cats S, Galton J. Effect of original disease in kidney transplant outcome. In Terasaki PI (ed) Clinical kidney transplantation. Los Angeles: UCLA Press, 1985; p III.

24. Brattström C, Tibell A, Tydén G et al. Outcome in 22 patients with pancreas transplants functioning beyond 5 years. Transpl Proc 1994; 26(2): 414-15.

25. Navarro X, Kennedy WR, Loewenson RB et al. Influence of pancreas transplantation on cardiorespiratory reflexes, nerve conduction and mortality in diabetes mellitus. Diabetes 1990; 39: 802-6.

26. Bolinder J, Tydén G, Tibell A, Groth CG, Östman J. Long-term metabolic control after pancreas transplantation with enteric diversion. Diabetologia 1991; 34(suppl. 1): S76-80.

27. Secchi A, Dubernard JM, La Rocca E, LeFrancois N, Melandri M, Martin X et al. Endocrinometabolic effects of whole versus segmental pancreas allotransplantation in diabetic patients—a two-year follow-up. Transplantation 1991; 51: 625-9.

28. Robertson RP, Diem P, Sutherland DER. Time related, cross-sectional and prospective follow-up of pancreatic endocrine function after pancreas allograft transplantation in type 1 diabetic patients. Diabetologia 1991; 34(suppl. 1): S57-60.

29. Nielsen JH, Mandrup-Poulsen T, Nerup J. Direct effect of cyclosporin A on human pancreatic cells. Diabetes 1986; 35: 1049-52.

30. Blackman JD, Polonsky KS, Jaspan JB, Sturis J, Cauter EV, Thistlewaite JR. Insulin secretory profiles and C-peptide clearance kinetics at 6 months and 2 years after kidney-pancreas transplantation. Diabetes 1992; 41: 1346-54.

31. Christiansen E, Andersen HB, Rasmussen K, Christensen NJ, Olgaard K, Kirkegaard P, et al. Pancreatic β-cell function and glucose metabolism in human pancreas and kidney transplantation. Am J Physiol 1993; 264 (Endocrinol Metab 27): E441-9.

32. Diem P, Abid M, Redmon JB, Sutherland DER, Robertson RP. Systemic venous drainage of pancreas allografts as independent cause of hyperinsulinemia in type 1 diabetic recipients. Diabetes 1990; 39: 534-40.

33. Osei K, Henry ML, O'Dorisio TM, Tesi RJ, Sommer BG, Ferguson RM. Physiological and pharmacological stimulation of pancreatic islet hormone secretion in type 1 diabetic pancreas allograft recipients. Diabetes 1990; 39: 1235-42.

34. Elahi D, Clark BA, McAloon-Dyke M, Wong G, Brown R, Shapiro M et al. Islet cell response to glucose in human transplanted pancreas. Am J Physiol 1991; 261(Endocrinol Metab 24): E800-808.

35. Clark JDA, Wheatley T, Brons IGM, Bloom SR, Calne RY. Studies of the entero-insular axis following pancreas transplantation: neural or hormonal control? Diabet Med 1989; 6: 813-17.

36. Katz H, Horman M, Velosa J, Robertson P, Rizza R. Effects of pancreas transplantation on postprandial glucose metabolism. New Engl J Med 1991; 325: 1278-83.

37. Nauck MA, Büsing M, Ørskov C, Siegel EG, Talartschik J, Baartz A et al. Basal and nutrient-stimulated pancreatic and gastrointestinal hormone concentrations in type 1 diabetic patients after successful combined pancreas and kidney transplantation. Clin Invest 1992; 70: 40-48.

38. Polonsky KS, Licinio-Paixao J, Given BD, Rue P, Falloway J, Karrison T, Frank B. Use of biosynthetic human C-peptide in measurement of insulin secretion rates in normal volunteers and type 1 diabetic patients. J Clin Invest 1986; 77: 98-105.

39. Vølund Aa, Polonsky KS, Bergman RN. Calculated pattern of intraportal insulin appearance without independent assessment of C-peptide kinetics. Diabetes 1987; 36: 1195-1202.

40. Christiansen E, Tibell A, Madsbad S, Vølund Aa, Rasmussen K, Schäffer L, Groth CG. Insulin release and glucose disposal in pancreas transplant recipients with impaired glucose tolerance. Diabetes 1992; 41(suppl. 1): 77A (abstr).

41. Teuscher AU, Seaquist ER. Insulin secretory reserve in human pancreas allograft recipients. Diabetes 1992; 41(suppl. 1): 78A (abstr).

42. Christiansen E, Tibell A, Groth CG, Rasmussen K, Pedersen O, Christensen NJ et al. β-cell secretory capacity in recipients of pancreas transplantation. Diabetes 1993; 42(suppl. 1): 53A (abstr).

43. Christiansen E, Tibell A, Rasmussen A, Tydén G, Madsbad S. Defects in quantitative and qualitative β-cell function following successful segmental pancreas transplantation. Transpl Proc 1993; 25(1): 1186-9.

44. Christiansen E, Tibell A, Vølund Aa, Rasmussen K, Tydén G, Pedersen O et al. Insulin secretion, insulin action and non-insulin-dependent glucose uptake in pancreas transplant recipients. J Clin Endocrinol Metab 1994; 79(6): 1561-9.

45. Osei K, Cottrel D, Henry ML, Tesi RJ, Ferguson RM, O'Dorisio TM. Minimal model analysis of insulin sensitivity and glucose-mediated glucose disposal in type 1 (insulin-dependent) diabetic pancreas allograft recipients. Diabetologia 1992; 35: 676-80.

46. Luzi L, Secchi A, Facchini F, Battezzatti A, Staudacher C, Spotti D, et al. Reduction of insulin resistance by combined kidney-pancreas transplantation in type 1 (insulin-dependent) diabetic patients. Diabetologia 1990; 33: 549-56.

47. Bar R, Gordon P, Roth J, Kahn C, DeMeyts P. Fluctuations in the affinity and concentrations of insulin receptors on circulating monocytes of obese patients. Effects of starvation, refeeding and dieting. J Clin Invest 1976; 58: 1123-35.

48. Boden G, DeSantis R, Chen X, Morris M, Badoza F. Glucose metabolism and leg blood flow after pancreas/kidney transplantation. J Clin Endocrinol Metab 1993; 76: 1229-33.

49. Diem P, Redmon JB, Munir A, Moran A, Sutherland DER, Halter JB, Robertson RP. Glucagon, catecholamine and pancreatic polypeptide secretion in type 1 diabetic recipients of pancreatic allografts. J Clin Invest 1990; 86: 2008-13.

50. Bolinder J, Wahrenberg H, Linde B, Tydén G, Groth CG, Östman J. Improved glucose counter-regulation after pancreas transplantation in diabetic patients with unawareness of hypoglycemia. Transpl Proc 1991; 23: 1667-9.

51. Luzi L, Battezzati A. Perseghin G, Bianchi E, Vergani S, Secchi A et al. Lack of feedback inhibition of insulin secretion in denervated human pancreas. Diabetes 1992; 41: 1632-9.

52. Ulbig N, Kampick A, Landgraf R et al. The influence of combined pancreatic and renal transplantation on advanced diabetic retinopathy. Transpl Proc 1987; 19: 3554-6.

53. Ramsey RC, Goetz FC, Sutherland DER et al. Progression of diabetic retinopathy after pancreas transplantation for insulin-dependent diabetes mellitus. New Engl J Med 1988; 318: 208-14.

54. Solders G, Wilczek H, Gunnarsson R et al. Effects of combined pancreatic and renal transplantation on diabetic neuropathy. Lancet 1987; 2: 1232-5.

55. Solders G, Tydén G, Persson A et al. Improvement in diabetic neuropathy four years after successful pancreatic and renal transplantation. Diabetologia 1991; 34: 125-7.

56. Kennedy WR, Navarro X, Goetz F et al. Effects of pancreatic transplantation on diabetic neuropathy. New Engl J Med 1990; 322: 1031-7.

57. Müller-Felber W, Landgraf R, Scheuer F et al. Diabetic neuropathy 3 years after successful pancreas and kidney transplantation. Diabetes 1993; 42: 1482-6.

58. Jörneskog G, Östergren J, Tydén G et al. Does combined kidney and pancreas transplantation reverse functional diabetic microangiopathy? Transpl Int 1990; 3: 167-70.

59. Abendroth P, Landgraf R, Milner WD et al. Course of diabetic microangiopathy after simultaneous pancreas and kidney transplantation. Transpl Proc 1988; 20: 874-5.

60. Wilczek H, Jaremko G, Tydén G et al. A pancreatic graft protects a simultaneously transplanted kidney from developing diabetic nephropathy; 1-6.5-year follow-up study. Transplantation (submitted).

61. Bilous RW, Mauer SM, Sutherland DER et al. The effects of pancreas transplantation on the glomerular structure of renal allografts in patients with insulin-dependent diabetes. New Engl J Med 1989; 321: 80-85.

62. Fioretto P, Mauer SM, Bilous RW et al. Effects of pancreas transplantation on glomerular structure in insulin-dependent diabetic patients with their own kidneys. Lancet 1993; 342: 1193-6.

63. Nakache R, Tydén G, Groth CG. Quality of life in diabetic patients undergoing combined pancreas-kidney transplantation and kidney transplantation only. Diabetes 1989; 38(suppl. 1): 40-42.

64. Piehlmeier W, Bullinger M, Nusser J, König A, Illner W-D, Abendroth D et al. Quality of life in type 1 (insulin-dependent) diabetic patients prior to and after pancreas and kidney transplantation in relation to organ function. Diabetologia 1991; 34(suppl. 1): S150-157.

65. Secchi A, DiCarlo V, Martinenghi S, La Rocca E, Caldara R, Spotti D et al. Effects of pancreas transplantation on life expectancy, kidney function and quality of life in uremic type 1 (insulin-dependent) diabetic patients. Diabetologia 1991; 34 (suppl. 1): S141-4.

66. Gross CR, Zehrer CL. Health-related quality of life outcomes of pancreas transplant recipients. Clin Transplant 1992; 6: 165-71.

Index

Index compiled by Campbell Purton